Brief Contents

Next-Generation NCLEX® (NGN)–Style Unfolding Case Studies appear at the end of every unit!

UNIT 1
Supporting the Patient Through the Health Care System
1. Clinical Judgment in Nursing Practice, 2
2. Communication and Collaboration, 17
3. Admitting, Transfer, and Discharge, 40
4. Documentation and Informatics, 52

UNIT 2
Vital Signs and Physical Assessment
5. Vital Signs, 70
6. Health Assessment, 110

UNIT 3
Special Procedures
7. Specimen Collection, 178
8. Diagnostic Procedures, 227

UNIT 4
Infection Control
9. Medical Asepsis, 260
10. Sterile Technique, 277

UNIT 5
Activity and Mobility
11. Safe Patient Handling and Mobility, 296
12. Exercise, Mobility, and Immobilization Devices, 324
13. Support Surfaces and Special Beds, 362

UNIT 6
Safety and Comfort
14. Patient Safety, 382
15. Disaster Preparedness, 417
16. Pain Management, 443
17. End-of-Life Care, 498

UNIT 7
Hygiene
18. Personal Hygiene and Bed Making, 520
19. Care of the Eye and Ear, 565

UNIT 8
Medications
20. Safe Medication Preparation, 586
21. Nonparenteral Medications, 608
22. Parenteral Medications, 659

UNIT 9
Oxygenation
23. Oxygen Therapy, 718
24. Airway Management, 753
25. Cardiac Care, 789
26. Closed Chest Drainage Systems, 799
27. Emergency Measures for Life Support, 821

UNIT 10
Fluid Balance
28. Intravenous and Vascular Access Therapy, 842
29. Blood Therapy, 895

UNIT 11
Nutrition
30. Oral Nutrition, 916
31. Enteral Nutrition, 940
32. Parenteral Nutrition, 966

UNIT 12
Elimination
33. Urinary Elimination, 984
34. Bowel Elimination and Gastric Intubation, 1018
35. Ostomy Care, 1038

UNIT 13
Care of the Surgical Patient
36. Preoperative and Postoperative Care, 1059
37. Intraoperative Care, 1095

UNIT 14
Dressings and Wound Care
38. Wound Care and Irrigation, 1110
39. Pressure Injury Prevention and Care, 1141
40. Dressings, Bandages, and Binders, 1162

UNIT 15
Home Care
41. Home Care Safety, 1198
42. Home Care Teaching, 1222

Appendix A: Terminology/Combining Forms: Prefixes and Suffixes, 1266

Answers to Clinical Judgment and Next-Generation NCLEX® Examination–Style Questions, 1269

Answers to Next-Generation NCLEX® (NGN)–Style Unfolding Case Studies, 1285

Index, 1299

T0294899

11TH EDITION

CLINICAL NURSING SKILLS & TECHNIQUES

Anne Griffin Perry, RN, MSN, EdD, FAAN
Professor Emerita
School of Nursing
Southern Illinois University—Edwardsville
Edwardsville, Illinois

Patricia A. Potter, RN, MSN, PhD, FAAN
Formerly, Director of Research
Patient Care Services
Barnes-Jewish Hospital
St. Louis, Missouri

Wendy R. Ostendorf, RN, MS, EdD, CNE
Contributing Faculty
Masters of Science in Nursing
Walden University
Minneapolis, Minnesota

Nancy Laplante, PhD, RN
Associate Professor of Nursing
Widener University
Chester, Pennsylvania

ELSEVIER

Elsevier
3251 Riverport Lane
St. Louis, Missouri 63043

Notice

Practitioners and researchers must always rely on their own experience and knowledge in evaluating and using any information, methods, compounds or experiments described herein. Because of rapid advances in the medical sciences, in particular, independent verification of diagnoses and drug dosages should be made. To the fullest extent of the law, no responsibility is assumed by Elsevier, authors, editors or contributors for any injury and/or damage to persons or property as a matter of products liability, negligence or otherwise, or from any use or operation of any methods, products, instructions, or ideas contained in the material herein.

Previous editions copyrighted 2022, 2018, 2014, 2010, 2006, 2002, 1998, 1994, 1990, 1986
International Standard Book Number 978-0-443-10718-4

Senior Content Strategist: Brandi Graham
Senior Content Development Manager: Lisa Newton
Content Development Specialist: Andrew Schubert
Publishing Services Manager: Julie Eddy
Senior Project Manager: Jodi Willard
Design Direction: Brian Salisbury

Printed in Canada

Last digit is the print number: 9 8 7 6 5 4 3 2 1

Working together
to grow libraries in
developing countries

www.elsevier.com • www.bookaid.org

As always, this book is dedicated to my children. To be their mother brings more joy, honor, and sense of pride than I could ever imagine. They and their loved ones are truly my shining stars. As they grow, things change, and I now dedicate this book to: My daughter Rebecca Lacey Perry Bryan; her husband Robert Donald Bryan; their three daughters Cora Elizabeth Bryan, Amalie Mary Bryan, and Noelle Anne Bryan; and their son Shepherd Charles Bryan. And to my son Mitch Perry-Cox and his husband Samuel Perry-Cox.
Anne Griffin Perry

For 44 years I have had the pleasure and honor to collaborate with Dr. Anne Perry on our many textbook projects. Anne has always offered her keen criticism, insight, and patient reflection when we have the ongoing challenges of creating a textbook. Her work is always contemplative and scholarly. Thanks, Anne, for a wonderful and rewarding journey.
Patricia A. Potter

For those who continue to support, inspire, and influence me daily, I thank you for this, as it is an essential part of my life and allows me to continue to be part of this great resource. And to my husband; I could not do this without your love and absolute support.
Wendy R. Ostendorf

For my husband Phil, who is my greatest support system and a wonderful partner to share this life with. For my children Chris and Charlotte and their growing families; I remain proud of you all and know I am blessed to have this family.
Nancy Laplante

About the Authors

ANNE GRIFFIN PERRY, RN, MSN, EdD, FAAN

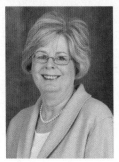

Dr. Anne Griffin Perry, Professor Emerita at Southern Illinois University—Edwardsville, was faculty at Saint Louis University and is a Fellow in the American Academy of Nursing. She received her BSN from the University of Michigan, her MSN from Saint Louis University, and her EdD from Southern Illinois University—Edwardsville. Dr. Perry is a prolific and influential author and speaker. An author for more than 40 years, her work includes four major textbooks (*Essentials for Nursing Practice, Fundamentals of Nursing, Nursing Interventions & Clinical Skills*, and *Clinical Nursing Skills & Techniques*) and numerous journal articles, abstracts, and nursing research and education grants. She has presented numerous papers at conferences across the United States and internationally. She was one of a few key consultants on *Mosby's Nursing Video Skills* and *Mosby's Nursing Skills Online*.

Dr. Perry is passionate about nursing education and has been involved in education since 1973, first as an instructor and then achieving the rank of Professor and assuming various leadership roles at Saint Louis University School of Nursing. She was a Professor and Associate Dean and Interim Dean at Southern Illinois University—Edwardsville. She has investigated and published findings regarding topics that include weaning from mechanical ventilation, use of the therapeutic intervention scoring system, critical care, and validation of nursing diagnoses.

PATRICIA A. POTTER, RN, MSN, PhD, FAAN

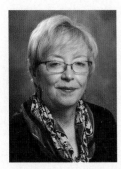

Dr. Patricia A. Potter received her diploma in nursing at Barnes Hospital School of Nursing, her BSN at the University of Washington in Seattle, and her MSN and PhD at Saint Louis University in St. Louis, Missouri. A groundbreaking author for more than 40 years, her work includes two major textbooks (*Fundamentals of Nursing* and *Clinical Nursing Skills & Techniques*) and publications in numerous professional journals. She has been an unceasing advocate of research, evidence-based practice and quality improvement in her roles as administrator, educator, and researcher.

Dr. Potter has devoted a lifetime to nursing education, practice, and research. She spent a decade teaching at Barnes Hospital School of Nursing and Saint Louis University. She entered into a variety of managerial and administrative roles, ultimately becoming Director of Nursing Practice at Barnes-Jewish Hospital. In that capacity she sharpened her interest in the development of nursing practice standards and in the measurement of patient outcomes in defining nursing practice. Her passion prior to retirement was in the area of nursing research, specifically cancer family caregiving, the cancer patient symptom experience, fall prevention, and the effects of compassion fatigue on nurses. One of her more significant projects involved development of an inpatient Innovation Unit, which was designed to incorporate current evidence into the selection and development of a unique work team and the creation of a care delivery model and innovative care practices. She currently is an active volunteer at a local hospice program. Dr. Potter was most recently the Director of Research for Patient Care Services at Barnes-Jewish Hospital in St. Louis, Missouri, before her retirement in 2017.

WENDY R. OSTENDORF, RN, MS, EdD, CNE

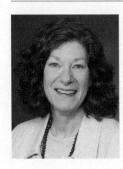

Dr. Wendy R. Ostendorf received her BSN from Villanova University, her MS from the University of Delaware, and her EdD from the University of Sarasota. She currently serves as a contributing faculty in the Master of Science in Nursing at Walden University. She has contributed more than 30 chapters to multiple nursing textbooks and has served as author for two major textbooks: *Nursing Interventions & Clinical Skills* and *Clinical Nursing Skills & Techniques*. She has presented more than 25 papers at conferences at the local, national, and international levels.

Professionally, Dr. Ostendorf has a diverse background in pediatric and adult critical care. She has taught at the undergraduate, master's, and doctoral levels for 35 years. With decades of practice as a clinician, her educational experiences have influenced her teaching philosophy and perceptions of the nursing profession.

NANCY LAPLANTE, PhD, RN

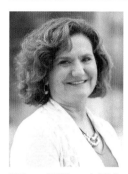

Dr. Nancy Laplante received her BSN from William Paterson University in Wayne, New Jersey; her MSN in Community Health from West Chester University in West Chester, Pennsylvania; and her PhD from Widener University in Chester, Pennsylvania. Dr. Laplante is also an advanced holistic nurse.

Dr. Laplante is an Associate Professor of Nursing at Widener University and also serves as the Director of the Accelerated RN to BSN to MSN program and Director of the RN to MSN bridge program. She teaches undergraduate courses in population health and teaches graduate courses in technology, health policy, assessment and evaluation, population health, and epidemiology. Dr. Laplante teaches primarily in online formats and enjoys being able to connect with a diverse group of students both nationally and internationally.

Dr. Laplante strives to engage all students in respectful dialogue. She believes teaching is a collaborative process between students and faculty and that there is a reciprocal relationship as we learn from one another. As an advanced holistic nurse, she incorporates self-care, self-responsibility, spirituality, and reflection in her teaching and seeks to be a role model for her students.

Dr. Laplante's research interests include creating a presence in online learning environments, health care applications of the Internet of Things (IoT), the image of nursing, and self-care practices for students and peers. Dr. Laplante has presented at local, national, and international conferences and has published recently in the areas of IoT and holistic nursing practice. In addition to her teaching and Director responsibilities, Dr. Laplante serves as a committee member and reader for doctoral nursing students. She believes this role is important to mentor and support the next generation of nursing scientists.

Contributors

Charlotte Biersmith, MSN, RN
Clinical Informatics Coordinator
Atrium Health
Charlotte, North Carolina

Eileen Costantinou, MSN, RN, NPD-BC
Senior Practice Specialist (retired)
Center for Practice Excellence
Barnes-Jewish Hospital
St. Louis, Missouri

Jane Fellows, MSN, COCN-AP
Wound/Ostomy Clinical Nurse Specialist
Advanced Clinical Practice
Duke University Health System
Durham, North Carolina

Nancy Laplante, PhD, RN, AHN-BC
Associate Professor
School of Nursing
Widener University
Chester, Pennsylvania

Nelda Kay Martin, RN, MSN, ANP-BC, CCNS
Clinical Nurse Specialist
Heart and Vascular
Barnes-Jewish Hospital
St. Louis, Missouri

Kathleen Michels, MBA, MSN, RN, CWOCN
Wound, Ostomy, Continence Clinical Nurse Educator
Clinical Professional Practice
The University of Chicago
Chicago, Illinois

Wendy R. Ostendorf, EdD, RN, CNE
Contributing Faculty
Masters in Nursing
Walden University
Minneapolis, Minnesota

Anne Griffin Perry, RN, MSN, EdD, FAAN
Professor Emerita
Nursing
Southern Illinois University—Edwardsville
Edwardsville, Illinois

Theresa Pietsch, PhD, RN, CRRN, CNE
Associate Professor
Dean of the School of Nursing and Health Sciences
School of Nursing and Health Sciences
Neumann University
Aston, Pennsylvania

Patricia A. Potter, RN, MSN, PhD, FAAN
Director of Research (retired)
Patient Care Services
Barnes-Jewish Hospital
St. Louis, Missouri

Amy E. Reed, RN, BSN, MSN, PhD
Assistant Professor
School of Nursing
Southern Illinois University—Edwardsville
Edwardsville, Illinois

Patti Stockert, BSN, MS, PhD
President, Retired
College of Nursing
Saint Francis Medical Center College of Nursing
Peoria, Illinois

Lauren Swanson, DNP, CRNA
Anesthesia
Society Hill Anesthesia Consultants
Philadelphia, Pennsylvania

CONTRIBUTORS TO PREVIOUS EDITIONS

We would like to acknowledge the following people who contributed to previous editions of *Clinical Nursing Skills & Techniques*.

Jeannette Adams, PhD, MSN, APRN, CRNI
Michelle Aebersold, PhD, RN, CHSE, FAAN
Della Aridge, RN, MSN
Elizabeth A. Ayello, PhD, MS, BSN, RN, CS, CWOCN
Sylvia K. Baird, BSN, MM

Marianne Banas, MSN, RN, CCTN, CWCN
Nicole Bartow, RN, MSN
Margaret Benz, RN, MSN, CSANP
Barbara J. Berger, MSN, RN
Lyndal Guenther Brand, RN, BSN, MSN
Peggy Breckinridge, RN, BSN, MSN, FNP
Victoria M. Brown, RN, BSN, MSN, PhD

Tim Buchanan, MSN
Gina Bufe, RN, BSN, MSN(R), PhD, CS
Hope Bussenius, DNP, APRN, FNP-BC, FAANP
Gale Carli, MSN, MHed, BSN, RN
Ellen Carson, PhD
Maureen Carty, MSN, OCN
Aurelie Chinn, RN, MSN

Mary F. Clarke, MA, RN

Janice C. Colwell, RN, MS, CWOCN

Charlene Compher, PhD, RD, CNSC, LDN, FADA

Kelly Jo Cone, RN, BSN, MS, PhD, CNE

Dorothy McDonnell Cooke, RN, PhD

Eileen Costantinou, RN, BSN, MSN

Sheila A. Cunningham, RN, BSN, MSN

Pamela A. Cupec, RN, MS, ONC, CRRN, ACM

Ruth Curchoe, RN, MSN, CIC

Rick Daniels, RN, BSN, MSN, PhD

Mardell Davis, RN, MSN, CETN

Carolyn Ruppel d'Avis, RN, BSN, MSN

Patricia A. Dettenmeier, RN, BSN, MSN(R), CCRN

Wanda Cleveland Dubuisson, BSN, MN

Christine Durbin, PhD, JD, RN

Sharon J. Edwards, RN, MSN, PhD

Martha E. Elkin, RN, MSN

Deborah Oldenburg Erickson, RN, BSN, MSN

Debra Farrell, BSN, CNOR

Linda Fasciani, RN, BSN, MSN

Susan Fetzer, BS, BSN, MSN, MBA, PHD

Cathy Flasar, MSN, APRN, BC, FNP

Marlene S. Foreman, BSN, MN, RNCS

Carol P. Fray, RN, MA

Leah W. Frederick, RN, MS, CIC

Kathleen Gerhart-Gibson, MSN, RN, CCRN

Paula Goldberg, RN, MS, MSN

Lorri A. Grahan, DNP-L, MSN, RN

Paula Gray, DNP, CRNP, NP-C

Thelma Halberstadt, EdD, MS, BS, RN

Amy Hall, PhD, MS, BSN, RN

Roberta L. Harrison, PhD, RN, CRRN

Linda C. Haynes, PhD, RN

Diane Hildwein, RN, BC, MA

Maureen B. Huhmann, MS, RD

Nancy C. Jackson, RN, BSN, MSN, CCRN

Stephanie Jeffers, PhD, RN

Ruth L. Jilka, RD, CDE

Teresa M. Johnson, RN, MSN, CCRN

Alaine Kamm, BSN, MSN

Judith Ann Kilpatrick, RN, DNSC

Carl Kirton, RN, BSN, MA, CCRN, ACRN, ANP

Lori Klingman, MSN, RN

Stephen D. Krau, PhD, CNE

Marilee Kuhrik, RN, MSN, PhD

Nancy S. Kuhrik, RN, MSN, PhD

Diane M. Kyle, RN, BSN, MS

Nancy Laplante, PhD, RN, AHN-BC

Louise K. Leitao, RN(c), BSN, MA

Gail B. Lewis, RN, MSN

Carol Ann Liebold, RN, BSN, CRNI

Ruth Ludwick, PhD, MSN, BSN, RNC, CNS

Mary Kay Macheca, MSN(R), RN, CS, ANP, CDE

Jill Feldman Malen, RN, MS, NS, ANP

Mary K. Mantese, RN, MSN

Elizabeth Mantych, RN, MSN

Tina Marrelli, MSN, MA, RN

Nelda K. Martin, APRN, BC, CCNS, ANP

Kristin L. Mauk, PhD, DNP, RN, CRRN, GCNS-BC, GNP-BC, FAAN

Karen A. May, PHD

Angela McConachie, FNP, DNP

Mary Mercer, RN, MSN

Rita Mertig, MS, BSN, RNC, CNS

Norma Metheny, PhD, MSN, BSN, FAAN

Mary Dee Miller, RN, BSN, MS, CIC

Theresa Miller, PhD, MSN, MHA, RN

Nancy Mirarchi, MSN, RN, CNOR

Sharon M.J. Muhs, MSN, RN

Kathleen Mulryan, RN, BSN, MSN

Lynne M. Murphy, RN, MSN

Elaine K. Neel, RN, BSN, MSN

Meghan G. Noble, PhD, RN

Marsha Evans Orr, RN, BS, MS, CS

Pamela L. Ostby, RN, MSN, OCN®

Dula F. Pacquiao, EdD, RN, CTN

Jennifer Painter, MSN, APRN, CNS, RN-BC, OCN, AOCNS

Jeanne Marie Papa, MBE, MSN, ACNP-BC, CCRN

Jill Parsons, PhD, RN

Ann Petlin, RN, MSN, CCNS, CCRN-CSC, ACNS-BC, PCCN

William Pezzotti, DNP, CRNP, AGACNP-BC

Theresa Pietsch, PHD, RN, CRRN, CNE

Sharon Phelps, RN, BSN, MS

Jacqueline Raybuck Saleeby, PhD, RN, CS

Catherine A. Robinson, BA, RN

Judith Roos, RN, MSN

Diane Rudolphi, MS, RN

Mary Jane Ruhland, MSN, RN, BC

Jan Rumfelt, RNC, MSN, EdD

Linette M. Sarti, RN, BSN, CNOR

Felicia Schaps, MSN-Ed, BSN, RN, CRNI, OCN, CNSC, lgCN

Phyllis Ann Schiavone, MSN, CRNP

Lois Schick, MN, MBA, CPAN, CAPA

Kelly M. Schwartz, RN, BSN

April Sieh, RN, BSN, MSN

Marlene Smith, RN, BSN, MEd

Julie S. Snyder, MSN, RNC

Laura Sofield, MSN, APRN, BC

Sharon Souter, MSN, BSN

Amy Spencer, MSN, RN-BC

Martha A. Spies, RN, MSN

Paula Ann Stangeland, PhD, RN, CRRN

Patricia A. Stockert, RN, BSN, MS, PhD

E. Bradley Strecker, RN, PhD

Virginia Strootman, RN MS CRNI

Sandra Ann Szekely, RN, BSN

Donna L. Thompson, MSN, CRNP, FNP-BC, CCCN

Lynn Tier, RN, MSN, LNC

Nancy Tomaselli, RN, MSN, CS, CRNP, CWOCN, CLNC

Riva Touger-Decker, PhD, RD, FADA

Anne Falsone Vaughan, MSN, BSN, CCRN

Cynthia Vishy, RN, BSN

Pamela Becker Weilitz, MSN(R), RN, CS, ANP

Rita Wunderlich, MSN, PhD

Carolyn C. Wright-Boon, MSN BSN

Joan Domigan Wentz, MSN, RN

Laurel Wiersema, RN, MSN

Pamela E. Windle, MS, RN, NE-BC, CPAN, CAPA, FAAN

Terry L. Wood, PhD, RN

Patricia H. Worthington, MSN, RN, CNSC

Rhonda Yancey, BSN, RN

Valerie Yancey, PhD, RN, HNC, CHPN

Reviewers

Dawn Anderson, RN
Staff RN
Evelyn's House
BJC Hospice
St. Louis, Missouri

Lisa Sharon Doget, DNP, MSN, RN
Director, ADN Program
Chaffey College
Rancho Cucamonga, California

Matthew Douglass, MSN, RN, AOS, CPN
Nursing Faculty
College of Eastern Idaho
Idaho Falls, Idaho

Candace Magan Evans, RN, MSN, DNP
Assistant Professor of Nursing
Mississippi University for Women
Columbus, Mississippi

Susan Pendergrass, MSN, MEd, FNP-BC
APRN—Florida Department of Health
Nassau County, Florida

Emily Rozek, EdD, RN-BC, CCRN-K
Program Director, Undergraduate Nursing Studies
Lourdes University
Toledo, Ohio

Lauren Swanson, DNP, CRNA
Anesthesia
Society Hill Anesthesia Consultants
Philadelphia, Pennsylvania

Preface

The evolution of technology and knowledge influences the way we teach clinical skills to nursing students and improves the quality of care possible for every patient. However, the foundation for success in performing nursing skills remains having a competent, well-informed nurse who thinks critically when making clinical judgments, asks the right questions at the right time, and makes timely decisions. That outcome is the driving factor behind this new edition.

In this eleventh edition of *Clinical Nursing Skills & Techniques*, we have maintained the same format from our tenth edition of the textbook. These features have proven popular among students and faculty. Each chapter opens by introducing students to key concepts: Practice Standards integrated within the skills, Principles for Practice, Person-Centered Care, Evidence-Based Practice, and Safety Guidelines. These are streamlined into a quick, easy-to-read bulleted format. Our approach emphasizes yet simplifies these important concepts.

Students will find that this edition of *Clinical Nursing Skills & Techniques* provides a comprehensive resource that will serve them well throughout their nursing education and into their clinical practice careers. This edition has a new chapter, "Clinical Judgment in Nursing Practice," which focuses on the very important need for students to develop clinical judgment skills, including critical thinking and use of the nursing process. The elements of clinical judgment are integrated within the skills of the text.

Recently the National Council of State Boards of Nursing (NCSBN) has emphasized the importance of sound nursing clinical judgment as the core of competent and safe patient care. In support of the NCSBN initiative, this edition of *Clinical Nursing Skills & Techniques* maintains another **feature from our previous edition:** unit openers. Each unit opener is designed to emphasize the importance of clinical judgment when applying specific knowledge and standards of care in order to safely and correctly perform the skills within the unit. In addition, each unit ends with a Next-Generation NCLEX® (NGN)–style Unfolding Case Study. Each case study challenges students to apply critical thinking when forming clinical judgments during use of the nursing process: recognizing and analyzing assessment cues, setting priorities, selecting interventions, and evaluating outcomes.

CLASSIC FEATURES

- A **Skills and Procedures** list and **Objectives** list open each chapter.
- **Comprehensive coverage** is given to basic, intermediate, and advanced nursing skills and procedures.
- **The nursing process format** provides a consistent presentation that helps students apply the process while learning each skill.
- An **extensive full-color art program** helps students master the material covered.
- **Practice Standards** highlight the evidence-based standards incorporated into skills content. **Supplemental Standards** include additional scientific resources pertaining to the chapter topic.

- **Evidence-Based Practice** sections present students with the newest scientific evidence for topics related to the procedures presented. Recent research findings are discussed, and their implications for patient care are explored. Newest evidence is also incorporated into the skills steps.
- **Patient-Centered Care** now has a new title, **Person-Centered Care**, to emphasize the importance of inclusivity in health care for all persons. These sections prepare students to recognize the importance of having patients partner in performing skills in a compassionate and coordinated way based on respect for a patient's autonomy, cultural and communication preferences, values, and needs.
- **Safety Guidelines** sections cover global recommendations on the safe execution of the particular skill sets covered in each chapter.
- **Rationales** are given for steps within skills so students learn the *why* as well as the *how* of each skill. Rationales include citations from the current literature.
- **Delegation** guidelines are now **Delegation and Collaboration** guidelines. These guidelines describe how to communicate with the patient care team and the nurse's responsibility when delegating to assistive personnel. In addition, interdisciplinary collaboration includes the disciplines commonly involved in support and performance of each procedure.
- **Clinical Judgment** alerts notify students of the key steps within a skill where clinical judgment is needed to consider patient safety and how to adapt skills to meet individual patient needs.
- **Evaluation** sections highlight the steps students must take to evaluate the outcomes of the skills performed.
- **Teach-Back** is included in each evaluation section to demonstrate to students how to phrase a Teach-Back question appropriately.
- **Unexpected Outcomes and Related Interventions** sections inform students to be alert for potential problems and help them determine appropriate nursing interventions.
- **Documentation** sections follow the evaluation discussion and alert students to what information should be documented in the health care record.
- **Hand-Off Reporting** follows the Documentation section and alerts students to what is reported during patient hand-off and emergent situations.
- **Special Considerations** sections include additional considerations when performing the skill for specific populations of patients or in specific settings and may include **Patient Education, Pediatrics, Older Adults, Populations With Disabilities, and Home Care.**
- **Quick Response codes** (scan with smartphone or tablet with camera to view video clips) in select Skills and Procedural Guidelines link video clips that allow students to view the video immediately after reading the implementation section of the skill.
- **Glossary** (on Evolve) defines key terms.
- **Additional Review Questions** (on Evolve) include a brand-new set of unique questions for every chapter.

- **TEACH for RN Instructor Manual** helps you capitalize on the new clinical material in the text, skills video series, and online course.
- As with the tenth edition, an **Image Collection** is available with *Clinical Nursing Skills & Techniques*.

ADDITIONAL FEATURES OF THIS EDITION

This eleventh edition includes the following elements to enhance student learning:

- **Clinical Judgment and Next-Generation NCLEX® Examination–Style Questions**
  - Each chapter ends with five chapter-specific, reflective clinical review questions. These questions are designed to have the student reflect on chapter-specific content. Some of these questions require the students to select the correct option(s). Other questions are open ended and require the student to apply chapter information to a recent clinical or laboratory experience. These questions also provide the instructor excellent discussion points for postclinical conference or self-study.
- **Unit Openers and End-of-Unit Next-Generation NCLEX® (NGN)–style questions reflecting the six new format questions for the Next-Generation NCLEX® Examination**
  - Unit openers describe to the student the importance of clinical judgment to perform the skills safely and correctly within the unit. This knowledge comes from the student's nursing and prerequisite courses in the biological, physical, and psychosocial sciences. These openers also demonstrate to the student the impact of environmental factors and interprofessional collaboration on safe patient care.
  - End-of-unit Next-Generation NCLEX® (NGN)–style unfolding case studies challenge the student to apply critical thinking and clinical judgment. These case studies include the six new format questions developed for the Next-Generation NCLEX® Examination.

Contents

UNIT 1

Supporting the Patient Through the Health Care System, 1

1 Clinical Judgment in Nursing Practice, 2
   Patricia A. Potter
   Clinical Judgment in Nursing Practice, 2
   Critical Thinking Evolving Case Study, 3
   Critical Thinking Competencies, 4
   Levels of Critical Thinking, 7
   Components of Critical Thinking in the Clinical Judgment Model, 8
   Evaluation of Clinical Judgments, 13

2 Communication and Collaboration, 17
   Nancy Laplante
   Purpose, 17
   Practice Standards, 17
   Supplemental Standards, 17
   Principles for Practice, 17
   Person-Centered Care, 18
   Evidence-Based Practice, 19
   Safety Guidelines, 19
   Skill 2.1 Establishing the Nurse-Patient Relationship, 20
   Skill 2.2 Communicating With Patients Who Have Difficulty Coping, 26
   Skill 2.3 Communicating With a Cognitively Impaired Patient, 31
   Skill 2.4 Communicating With Colleagues, 33
   Skill 2.5 Workplace Violence and Safety, 35

3 Admitting, Transfer, and Discharge, 40
   Nancy Laplante
   Purpose, 40
   Practice Standards, 40
   Supplemental Standards, 40
   Principles for Practice, 40
   Person-Centered Care, 41
   Evidence-Based Practice, 41
   Safety Guidelines, 41
   Admitting Process, 42
   Transfer Process, 45
   Discharge Process, 47

4 Documentation and Informatics, 52
   Charlotte Biersmith
   Purpose, 52
   Practice Standards, 52
   Supplemental Standards, 53
   Principles for Practice, 53
   Person-Centered Care, 54
   Evidence-Based Practice, 55
   Safety Guidelines, 55
   Confidentiality, 55
   Legal Guidelines in Documentation, 56
   Guidelines for High-Quality Documentation, 57
   Methods of Documentation, 58
   Common Electronic Health Record Data Screens, 58

Documentation Formats, 61
   Verbal Reporting, 62
   Procedural Guideline 4.1 Giving a Hand-off Report, 62
   Incident or Adverse Event Occurrence Reports, 63
   Procedural Guideline 4.2 Adverse Event Reporting, 64
   Home Care Documentation, 64
   Long-Term Health Care Documentation, 65
   UNIT 1: Supporting the Patient Through the Health Care System:
       Next-Generation NCLEX® (NGN)–Style Unfolding Case Study, 67

UNIT 2

Vital Signs and Physical Assessment, 69

5 Vital Signs, 70
   Anne Griffin Perry
   Purpose, 70
   Practice Standards, 70
   Supplemental Standards, 71
   Principles for Practice, 71
   Person-Centered Care, 71
   Evidence-Based Practice, 71
   Safety Guidelines, 71
   Skill 5.1 Measuring Body Temperature, 72
   Skill 5.2 Assessing Radial Pulse, 82
   Skill 5.3 Assessing Apical Pulse, 86
   Skill 5.4 Assessing Respirations, 91
   Skill 5.5 Assessing Arterial Blood Pressure, 95
   Procedural Guideline 5.1 Noninvasive Electronic Blood Pressure
       Measurement, 104
   Procedural Guideline 5.2 Measuring Oxygen Saturation
       (Pulse Oximetry), 105

6 Health Assessment, 110
   Patricia A. Potter
   Purpose, 110
   Practice Standards, 111
   Supplemental Standards, 111
   Principles for Practice, 111
   Person-Centered Care, 111
   Evidence-Based Practice, 111
   Safety Guidelines, 112
   Assessment Techniques, 113
   Preparation for Assessment, 115
   Physical Assessment of Various Age-Groups, 116
   Skill 6.1 General Survey, 117
   Skill 6.2 Head and Neck Assessment, 126
   Skill 6.3 Thorax and Lung Assessment, 132
   Skill 6.4 Cardiovascular Assessment, 140
   Skill 6.5 Abdominal Assessment, 151
   Skill 6.6 Genitalia and Rectum Assessment, 157
   Skill 6.7 Musculoskeletal and Neurological Assessment, 162
   Procedural Guideline 6.1 Monitoring Intake and Output, 170
   UNIT 2: Vital Signs and Physical Assessment: Next-Generation
       NCLEX® (NGN)–Style Unfolding Case Studies, 175

UNIT 3

Special Procedures, 177

7   Specimen Collection, 178
     Anne Griffin Perry
     Purpose, 178
     Practice Standards, 178
     Supplemental Standards, 179
     Principles for Practice, 179
     Person-Centered Care, 179
     Evidence-Based Practice, 179
     Safety Guidelines, 179
     Skill 7.1 Urine Specimen Collection: Midstream (Clean-Voided) Urine;
          Sterile Urinary Catheter, 179
     Procedural Guideline 7.1 Collecting a Timed Urine Specimen, 185
     Skill 7.2 Measuring Occult Blood in Stool, 187
     Skill 7.3 Measuring Occult Blood in Gastric Secretions (Gastroccult), 190
     Skill 7.4 Collecting Nose and Throat Specimens for Culture, 192
     Skill 7.5 Obtaining Vaginal or Urethral Discharge Specimens, 196
     Procedural Guideline 7.2 Collecting a Sputum Specimen by
          Expectoration, 199
     Skill 7.6 Collecting a Sputum Specimen by Suction, 200
     Skill 7.7 Obtaining Wound Drainage Specimens, 203
     Skill 7.8 Collecting Blood Specimens and Culture by Venipuncture
          (Syringe and Vacutainer Method), 206
     Skill 7.9 Blood Glucose Monitoring, 215
     Skill 7.10 Obtaining an Arterial Specimen for Blood Gas Measurement, 220

8   Diagnostic Procedures, 227
     Wendy R. Ostendorf
     Purpose, 227
     Practice Standards, 227
     Supplemental Standards, 227
     Principles for Practice, 227
     Person-Centered Care, 228
     Evidence-Based Practice, 228
     Safety Guidelines, 228
     Skill 8.1 Intravenous Moderate Sedation, 229
     Skill 8.2 Contrast Media Studies: Arteriogram (Angiogram), Cardiac
          Catheterization, and Intravenous Pyelogram, 234
     Skill 8.3 Care of Patients Undergoing Aspirations: Bone Marrow
          Aspiration/Biopsy, Lumbar Puncture, Paracentesis, and
          Thoracentesis, 240
     Skill 8.4 Care of a Patient Undergoing Bronchoscopy, 246
     Skill 8.5 Care of a Patient Undergoing Endoscopy, 250
     **UNIT 3: Special Procedures: Next-Generation NCLEX®
          (NGN)–Style Unfolding Case Study, 256**

UNIT 4

Infection Control, 259

9   Medical Asepsis, 260
     Patti Stockert
     Purpose, 260
     Practice Standards, 260
     Supplemental Standards, 260
     Principles for Practice, 260
     Person-Centered Care, 262
     Evidence-Based Practice, 262
     Safety Guidelines, 262
     Skill 9.1 Hand Hygiene, 263
     Skill 9.2 Caring for Patients Under Isolation Precautions, 267

10   Sterile Technique, 277
     Patti Stockert
     Purpose, 277
     Practice Standards, 277
     Principles for Practice, 277
     Person-Centered Care, 278
     Evidence-Based Practice, 278
     Safety Guidelines, 278
     Skill 10.1 Applying and Removing Cap, Mask, and Protective
          Eyewear, 279
     Skill 10.2 Preparing a Sterile Field, 282
     Skill 10.3 Sterile Gloving, 287
     **UNIT 4: Infection Control: Next-Generation NCLEX® (NGN)–Style
          Unfolding Case Study, 293**

UNIT 5

Activity and Mobility, 295

11   Safe Patient Handling and Mobility, 296
     Patricia A. Potter
     Purpose, 296
     Practice Standards, 296
     Supplemental Standards, 296
     Principles for Practice, 296
     Person-Centered Care, 297
     Evidence-Based Practice, 297
     Safety Guidelines, 298
     Skill 11.1 Using Safe and Effective Transfer Techniques, 298
     Procedural Guideline 11.1 Wheelchair Transfer Techniques, 311
     Skill 11.2 Moving and Positioning Patients in Bed, 313

12   Exercise, Mobility, and Immobilization Devices, 324
     Patricia A. Potter
     Purpose, 324
     Practice Standards, 325
     Principles for Practice, 325
     Person-Centered Care, 325
     Evidence-Based Practice, 325
     Safety Guidelines, 326
     Skill 12.1 Promoting Early Activity and Exercise, 326
     Procedural Guideline 12.1 Performing Range-of-Motion Exercises, 331
     Procedural Guideline 12.2 Applying Graduated Compression (Elastic)
          Stockings and Sequential Compression Device, 337
     Procedural Guideline 12.3 Assisting With Ambulation (Without Assist
          Devices), 342
     Skill 12.2 Assisting With Use of Canes, Walkers, and Crutches, 345
     Skill 12.3 Care of a Patient With an Immobilization Device, 355

13   Support Surfaces and Special Beds, 362
     Anne Griffin Perry
     Purpose, 362
     Practice Standards, 362
     Supplemental Standards, 362
     Principles for Practice, 362
     Person-Centered Care, 364
     Evidence-Based Practice, 365
     Safety Guidelines, 365
     Procedural Guideline 13.1 Selection of a Pressure-Redistribution
          Support Surface, 365
     Skill 13.1 Care of the Patient on a Support Surface, 368
     Skill 13.2 Care of the Patient on a Special Bed, 373
     **UNIT 5: Activity and Mobility: Next-Generation NCLEX®
          (NGN)–Style Unfolding Case Study, 379**

UNIT 6
Safety and Comfort, 381

14   Patient Safety, 382
      Eileen Costantinou
      Purpose, 382
      Practice Standards, 383
      Supplemental Standards, 383
      Principles for Practice, 383
      Person-Centered Care, 383
      Evidence-Based Practice, 383
      Safety Guidelines, 384
      Skill 14.1 Fall Prevention in Health Care Settings, 384
      Skill 14.2 Designing a Restraint-Free Environment, 394
      Skill 14.3 Applying Physical Restraints, 398
      Procedural Guideline 14.1 Fire, Electrical, and Chemical Safety, 405
      Skill 14.4 Seizure Precautions, 408

15   Disaster Preparedness, 417
      Nancy Laplante
      Purpose, 417
      Practice Standards, 417
      Supplemental Standards, 417
      Principles for Practice, 418
      Person-Centered Care, 421
      Evidence-Based Practice, 422
      Safety Guidelines, 422
      Skill 15.1 Care of a Patient After Biological Exposure, 424
      Skill 15.2 Care of a Patient After Chemical Exposure, 430
      Skill 15.3 Care of a Patient After Radiation Exposure, 434
      Skill 15.4 Care of a Patient After a Natural Disaster, 438

16   Pain Management, 443
      Patricia A. Potter
      Purpose, 443
      Practice Standards, 444
      Supplemental Standards, 444
      Principles for Practice, 444
      Person-Centered Care, 444
      Evidence-Based Practice, 445
      Safety Guidelines, 445
      Skill 16.1 Pain Assessment and Basic Comfort Measures, 446
      Skill 16.2 Nonpharmacological Pain Management, 453
      Skill 16.3 Pharmacological Pain Management, 460
      Skill 16.4 Patient-Controlled Analgesia, 466
      Skill 16.5 Epidural Analgesia, 472
      Skill 16.6 Local Anesthetic Infusion Pump for Analgesia, 479
      Skill 16.7 Moist and Dry Heat Applications, 482
      Skill 16.8 Cold Application, 489

17   End-of-Life Care, 498
      Nancy Laplante
      Purpose, 498
      Practice Standards, 498
      Principles for Practice, 498
      Person-Centered Care, 499
      Evidence-Based Practice, 500
      Safety Guidelines, 500
      Skill 17.1 Supporting Patients and Families in Grief, 500
      Skill 17.2 Symptom Management at the End of Life, 504
      Skill 17.3 Care of the Body After Death, 510
      **UNIT 6: Safety and Comfort: Next-Generation NCLEX®
      (NGN)–Style Unfolding Case Study, 516**

UNIT 7
Hygiene, 519

18   Personal Hygiene and Bed Making, 520
      Anne Griffin Perry
      Purpose, 520
      Practice Standards, 520
      Supplemental Standards, 521
      Principles for Practice, 521
      Person-Centered Care, 521
      Evidence-Based Practice, 521
      Safety Guidelines, 521
      The Skin, 522
      The Oral Cavity, 523
      The Hair, 524
      The Nails, 524
      Skill 18.1 Complete or Partial Bed Bath, 524
      Procedural Guideline 18.1 Perineal Care, 534
      Procedural Guideline 18.2 Bathing With Use of Chlorhexidine Chloride
          Gluconate (CHG) Disposable Washcloths, Tub, or Shower, 536
      Skill 18.2 Oral Hygiene, 538
      Procedural Guideline 18.3 Care of Dentures, 542
      Skill 18.3 Performing Mouth Care for an Unconscious or Debilitated
          Patient, 544
      Procedural Guideline 18.4 Hair Care—Combing and Shaving, 547
      Procedural Guideline 18.5 Hair Care—Shampooing Using Disposable
          Dry Shampoo Cap, 550
      Skill 18.4 Performing Nail and Foot Care, 551
      Procedural Guideline 18.6 Making an Occupied Bed, 557
      Procedural Guideline 18.7 Making an Unoccupied Bed, 561

19   Care of the Eye and Ear, 565
      Wendy R. Ostendorf
      Purpose, 565
      Practice Standards, 565
      Principles for Practice, 565
      Person-Centered Care, 565
      Evidence-Based Practice, 566
      Safety Guidelines, 566
      Procedural Guideline 19.1 Eye Care for Comatose Patients, 566
      Procedural Guideline 19.2 Taking Care of Contact Lenses, 567
      Skill 19.1 Eye Irrigation, 570
      Skill 19.2 Ear Irrigation, 573
      Skill 19.3 Care of Hearing Aids, 577
      **UNIT 7: Hygiene: Next-Generation NCLEX® (NGN)–Style Unfolding
      Case Study, 583**

UNIT 8
Medications, 585

20   Safe Medication Preparation, 586
      Wendy R. Ostendorf
      Practice Standards, 587
      Supplemental Standards, 587
      Principles for Practice, 587
      Person-Centered Care, 596
      Evidence-Based Practice, 603
      Safety Guidelines, 603
      Nursing Process, 603
      Reporting Medication Errors, 605
      Patient and Family Caregiver Teaching, 605

21 Nonparenteral Medications, 608
Anne Griffin Perry
Purpose, 608
Practice Standards, 608
Supplemental Standards, 609
Principles for Practice, 609
Person-Centered Care, 609
Evidence-Based Practice, 609
Safety Guidelines, 609
Skill 21.1 Administering Oral Medications, 610
Skill 21.2 Administering Medications Through a Feeding Tube, 618
Skill 21.3 Applying Topical Medications to the Skin, 623
Skill 21.4 Administering Ophthalmic Medications, 629
Skill 21.5 Administering Ear Medications, 635
Skill 21.6 Administering Nasal Instillations, 638
Skill 21.7 Using Metered-Dose Inhalers (MDIs), 642
Skill 21.8 Using Small-Volume Nebulizers, 649
Procedural Guideline 21.1 Administering Vaginal Medications, 653
Procedural Guideline 21.2 Administering Rectal Suppositories, 655

22 Parenteral Medications, 659
Amy E. Reed
Purpose, 659
Practice Standards, 659
Supplemental Standards, 660
Principles for Practice, 660
Person-Centered Care, 660
Evidence-Based Practice, 660
Safety Guidelines, 660
Skill 22.1 Preparing Injections: Ampules and Vials, 664
Procedural Guideline 22.1 Mixing Parenteral Medications in One Syringe, 670
Skill 22.2 Administering Intradermal Injections, 673
Skill 22.3 Administering Subcutaneous Injections, 677
Skill 22.4 Administering Intramuscular Injections, 685
Skill 22.5 Administering Medications by Intravenous Push, 692
Skill 22.6 Administering Intravenous Medications by Piggyback and Syringe Pumps, 699
Skill 22.7 Administering Medications by Continuous Subcutaneous Infusion, 705
UNIT 8: Medication Administration: Next-Generation NCLEX® (NGN)–Style Unfolding Case Study, 713

UNIT 9

Oxygenation, 717

23 Oxygen Therapy, 718
Anne Griffin Perry
Purpose, 718
Practice Standards, 718
Supplemental Standards, 718
Principles for Practice, 718
Person-Centered Care, 719
Evidence-Based Practice, 719
Safety Guidelines, 719
Skill 23.1 Applying an Oxygen-Delivery Device, 720
Skill 23.2 Administering Oxygen Therapy to a Patient With an Artificial Airway, 727
Skill 23.3 Using Incentive Spirometry, 730
Skill 23.4 Care of a Patient Receiving Noninvasive Positive Pressure Ventilation, 734
Procedural Guideline 23.1 Use of a Peak Flowmeter, 739
Skill 23.5 Care of a Patient on a Mechanical Ventilator, 742

24 Airway Management, 753
Lauren Swanson
Purpose, 753
Practice Standards, 753
Supplemental Standards, 753
Principles for Practice, 753
Person-Centered Care, 754
Evidence-Based Practice, 754
Safety Guidelines, 754
Skill 24.1 Performing Oropharyngeal Suctioning, 755
Skill 24.2 Suctioning: Open for Nasotracheal/Pharyngeal and Artificial Airways, 759
Procedural Guideline 24.1 Closed (In-Line) Suction, 769
Skill 24.3 Performing Endotracheal Tube Care, 770
Skill 24.4 Performing Tracheostomy Care, 778

25 Cardiac Care, 789
Wendy R. Ostendorf
Purpose, 789
Practice Standards, 789
Supplemental Standards, 789
Principles for Practice, 789
Person-Centered Care, 789
Evidence-Based Practice, 789
Safety Guidelines, 791
Skill 25.1 Obtaining a 12-Lead Electrocardiogram, 791
Skill 25.2 Applying a Cardiac Monitor, 794

26 Closed Chest Drainage Systems, 799
Anne Griffin Perry
Purpose, 799
Practice Standards, 799
Supplemental Standards, 799
Principles for Practice, 799
Person-Centered Care, 802
Evidence-Based Practice, 802
Safety Guidelines, 802
Skill 26.1 Managing Closed Chest Drainage Systems, 803
Skill 26.2 Assisting With Removal of Chest Tubes, 813
Skill 26.3 Autotransfusion of Chest Tube Drainage, 817

27 Emergency Measures for Life Support, 821
Nelda Kay Martin
Purpose, 821
Practice Standards, 821
Supplemental Standards, 821
Principles for Practice, 821
Person-Centered Care, 821
Evidence-Based Practice, 823
Safety Guidelines, 824
Skill 27.1 Inserting an Oropharyngeal Airway, 824
Skill 27.2 Using an Automated External Defibrillator, 827
Skill 27.3 Resuscitation Management, 830
UNIT 9: Oxygenation: Next-Generation NCLEX® (NGN)–Style Unfolding Case Study, 839

UNIT 10

Fluid Balance, 841

28 Intravenous and Vascular Access Therapy, 842
Wendy R. Ostendorf
Purpose, 842
Practice Standards, 842

Supplemental Standards, 842
Principles for Practice, 843
Person-Centered Care, 844
Evidence-Based Practice, 844
Safety Guidelines, 844
Skill 28.1 Insertion of a Peripheral Intravenous Device, 846
Skill 28.2 Regulating Intravenous Flow Rates, 861
Skill 28.3 Changing Intravenous Solutions, 867
Skill 28.4 Changing Infusion Tubing, 871
Skill 28.5 Changing a Peripheral Intravenous Dressing, 874
Procedural Guideline 28.1 Discontinuing a Peripheral Intravenous
    Device, 878
Skill 28.6 Managing Central Vascular Access Devices, 879

29   Blood Therapy, 895
     Patricia A. Potter
     Purpose, 895
     Practice Standards, 895
     Supplemental Standards, 895
     Principles for Practice, 896
     Person-Centered Care, 897
     Evidence-Based Practice, 897
     Safety Guidelines, 898
     Skill 29.1 Initiating Blood Therapy, 900
     Skill 29.2 Monitoring for Adverse Transfusion Reactions, 908
     **Unit 10: Fluid Balance: Next-Generation NCLEX® (NGN)–Style
     Unfolding Case Study, 913**

UNIT 11

Nutrition, 915

30   Oral Nutrition, 916
     Patti Stockert
     Purpose, 916
     Practice Standards, 916
     Supplemental Standards, 917
     Principles for Practice, 917
     Person-Centered Care, 917
     Evidence-Based Practice, 918
     Safety Guidelines, 919
     Skill 30.1 Performing a Nutrition Screening, 919
     Skill 30.2 Assisting an Adult Patient With Oral Nutrition, 925
     Skill 30.3 Aspiration Precautions, 931

31   Enteral Nutrition, 940
     Patti Stockert
     Purpose, 940
     Practice Standards, 940
     Supplemental Standard, 940
     Principles for Practice, 940
     Person-Centered Care, 941
     Evidence-Based Practice, 941
     Safety Guidelines, 941
     Skill 31.1 Insertion and Removal of a Small-Bore Feeding Tube, 942
     Skill 31.2 Verifying Placement of a Feeding Tube, 949
     Skill 31.3 Irrigating a Feeding Tube, 953
     Skill 31.4 Administering Enteral Nutrition: Nasogastric, Nasointestinal,
         Gastrostomy, or Jejunostomy Tube, 955
     Procedural Guideline 31.1 Care of a Gastrostomy or Jejunostomy
         Tube, 962

32   Parenteral Nutrition, 966
     Patricia A. Potter
     Purpose, 966
     Practice Standards, 966
     Supplemental Standards, 966
     Principles for Practice, 966
     Person-Centered Care, 968
     Evidence-Based Practice, 968
     Safety Guidelines, 968
     Skill 32.1 Administering Central Parenteral Nutrition, 970
     Skill 32.2 Administering Peripheral Parenteral Nutrition With Lipid (Fat)
         Emulsion, 975
     **UNIT 11: Nutrition: Next-Generation NCLEX® (NGN)–Style Unfolding
     Case Study, 981**

UNIT 12

Elimination, 983

33   Urinary Elimination, 984
     Wendy R. Ostendorf
     Purpose, 984
     Practice Standards, 984
     Supplemental Standards, 984
     Principles for Practice, 984
     Person-Centered Care, 985
     Evidence-Based Practice, 985
     Safety Guidelines, 985
     Procedural Guideline 33.1 Assisting With Use of a Urinal, 986
     Skill 33.1 Insertion of a Straight or an Indwelling Urinary Catheter, 987
     Skill 33.2 Care and Removal of an Indwelling Catheter, 998
     Procedural Guideline 33.2 Bladder Scan, 1003
     Skill 33.3 Performing Catheter Irrigation, 1004
     Skill 33.4 Applying an Incontinence Device, 1008
     Skill 33.5 Suprapubic Catheter Care, 1013

34   Bowel Elimination and Gastric Intubation, 1018
     Jane Fellows
     Purpose, 1018
     Practice Standards, 1018
     Principles of Practice, 1018
     Person-Centered Care, 1019
     Evidence-Based Practice, 1019
     Safety Guidelines, 1019
     Procedural Guideline 34.1 Providing and Positioning a Bedpan, 1020
     Procedural Guideline 34.2 Removing Fecal Impaction Digitally, 1022
     Skill 34.1 Administering an Enema, 1024
     Skill 34.2 Insertion, Maintenance, and Removal of a Nasogastric Tube for
         Gastric Decompression, 1029

35   Ostomy Care, 1038
     Jane Fellows
     Purpose, 1038
     Practice Standards, 1038
     Supplemental Standards, 1038
     Principles for Practice, 1038
     Person-Centered Care, 1039
     Evidence-Based Practice, 1040
     Safety Guidelines, 1040
     Skill 35.1 Pouching a Colostomy or an Ileostomy, 1040
     Skill 35.2 Pouching a Urostomy, 1046
     Skill 35.3 Catheterizing a Urinary Diversion, 1050
     **UNIT 12: Elimination: Next-Generation NCLEX® (NGN)–Style
     Unfolding Case Study, 1054**

UNIT 13

Care of the Surgical Patient, 1057

36 Preoperative and Postoperative Care, 1059
Wendy R. Ostendorf
Purpose, 1059
Practice Standards, 1059
Supplemental Standards, 1059
Principles for Practice, 1060
Person-Centered Care, 1060
Evidence-Based Practice, 1060
Safety Guidelines, 1060
Skill 36.1 Preoperative Assessment, 1061
Skill 36.2 Preoperative Teaching, 1065
Skill 36.3 Patient Preparation for Surgery, 1075
Skill 36.4 Providing Immediate Anesthesia Recovery in the Postanesthesia Care Unit, 1079
Skill 36.5 Providing Early Postoperative (Phase II) and Convalescent Phase (Phase III) Recovery, 1087

37 Intraoperative Care, 1095
Nancy Laplante
Purpose, 1095
Practice Standards, 1095
Supplemental Standards, 1095
Principles for Practice, 1095
Person-Centered Care, 1096
Evidence-Based Practice, 1097
Safety Guidelines, 1097
Skill 37.1 Surgical Hand Antisepsis, 1098
Skill 37.2 Donning a Sterile Gown and Closed Gloving, 1102
UNIT 13: Care of the Surgical Patient: Next-Generation NCLEX® (NGN)–Style Unfolding Case Study, 1106

UNIT 14

Dressings and Wound Care, 1109

38 Wound Care and Irrigation, 1110
Kathleen Michels
Purpose, 1110
Practice Standards, 1110
Supplemental Standards, 1110
Principles for Practice, 1110
Person-Centered Care, 1113
Evidence-Based Practice, 1113
Safety Guidelines, 1114
Procedural Guideline 38.1 Performing a Wound Assessment, 1114
Skill 38.1 Performing a Wound Irrigation, 1117
Skill 38.2 Removing Sutures and Staples, 1122
Skill 38.3 Managing Wound Drainage Evacuation, 1128
Skill 38.4 Negative-Pressure Wound Therapy, 1133

39 Pressure Injury Prevention and Care, 1141
Kathleen Michels
Purpose, 1141
Practice Standards, 1141
Supplemental Standards, 1141
Principles for Practice, 1141
Person-Centered Care, 1145
Evidence-Based Practice, 1145
Safety Guidelines, 1146
Skill 39.1 Risk Assessment, Skin Assessment, and Prevention Strategies, 1146
Skill 39.2 Treatment of Pressure Injuries, 1154

40 Dressings, Bandages, and Binders, 1162
Anne Griffin Perry
Purpose, 1162
Practice Standards, 1162
Supplemental Standards, 1162
Principles for Practice, 1162
Person-Centered Care, 1165
Evidence-Based Practice, 1165
Safety Guidelines, 1166
Skill 40.1 Applying a Dressing (Dry and Moist Dressings), 1166
Skill 40.2 Applying a Pressure Bandage, 1175
Skill 40.3 Applying a Transparent Dressing, 1178
Skill 40.4 Applying a Hydrocolloid, Hydrogel, Foam, or Alginate Dressing, 1181
Procedural Guideline 40.1 Applying Rolled Gauze and Elastic Bandages, 1187
Procedural Guideline 40.2 Applying an Abdominal Binder, 1191
UNIT 14: Dressings and Wound Care: Next-Generation NCLEX® (NGN)–Style Unfolding Case Study, 1194

UNIT 15

Home Care, 1197

41 Home Care Safety, 1198
Nancy Laplante
Purpose, 1198
Practice Standards, 1198
Principles for Practice, 1198
Person-Centered Care, 1199
Evidence-Based Practice, 1199
Safety Guidelines, 1199
Skill 41.1 Home Environment Assessment and Safety, 1200
Skill 41.2 Adapting the Home Setting for Clients With Cognitive Deficits, 1209
Skill 41.3 Medication and Medical Device Safety, 1216

42 Home Care Teaching, 1222
Theresa Pietsch
Purpose, 1222
Practice Standards, 1222
Supplemental Standards, 1222
Principles for Practice, 1222
Person-Centered Care, 1223
Evidence-Based Practice, 1223
Safety Guidelines, 1223
Skill 42.1 Teaching Clients to Measure Body Temperature, 1224
Skill 42.2 Teaching Blood Pressure and Pulse Measurement, 1227
Skill 42.3 Teaching Intermittent Self-Catheterization, 1232
Skill 42.4 Using Home Oxygen Equipment, 1236
Skill 42.5 Teaching Home Tracheostomy Care and Suctioning, 1243
Skill 42.6 Teaching Medication Self-Administration, 1248
Skill 42.7 Managing Feeding Tubes in the Home, 1253
Skill 42.8 Managing Parenteral Nutrition in the Home, 1257
UNIT 15: Home Care: Next-Generation NCLEX® (NGN)–Style Unfolding Case Study, 1264

Appendix A: Terminology/Combining Forms: Prefixes and Suffixes, 1266

Answers to Clinical Judgment and Next-Generation NCLEX® Examination–Style Questions, 1269

Answers to Next-Generation NCLEX® (NGN)–Style Unfolding Case Studies, 1285

Index, 1299

UNIT 1
Supporting the Patient Through the Health Care System

The skills in Unit 1 include chapters on Clinical Judgment and Communication and Collaboration. These are essential knowledge elements that enable you to think critically when caring for patients while selecting and performing skills. Patients enter the health care system through a variety of settings and in various levels of health. When nurses apply therapeutic communication principles, they are better able to perform the nursing process and make the clinical judgments needed to help patients transition through all phases of care and in all health care settings. Collaboration, likewise, is essential. You will collaborate with other health care professionals to gather data to gain a full picture of a patient's health care problems and associated needs when being admitted to a health care setting, during a transition period, and prior to discharge.

Scientific evidence informs us and provides a scope of knowledge that directs us in the type of assessment information we need to learn when communicating with patients and families. For example, the newest scientific evidence recommends the frequency of certain types of health screenings. In an outpatient center, during an initial admission, such evidence-based knowledge directs how a nurse interacts with patients to learn what they know about a particular screening and their own screening habits. The screening guidelines direct the type of questions a nurse poses (e.g., What does the patient know about the frequency of screening or its purpose?).

Sound clinical judgments cannot be made without applying evidence and using excellent communication skills. Therapeutic and collaborative communication enables us to become recipients of the type and depth of information we need to make informed clinical decisions. Effective communication is also a part of professional documentation—the conveying of relevant and accurate information that describes a patient's clinical course and response to nursing care.

The transition of patients through admission, transfer, and discharge, regardless of setting, requires an organized approach and emphasis on having accurate assessment information about patients. The methods we use to support patients in these phases of care depend in part on what we have learned from patients by using therapeutic communication. The same applies to our ability to collaborate effectively with colleagues. When a patient enters a hospital, the nurse becomes responsible for gathering as thorough a health history as possible to form a meaningful patient database. That database changes over time. During transfers within or between other health care settings, the information pertinent to a patient's clinical care must be communicated and documented for other health care providers to use. Discharge is a critical time, requiring nurses to fully understand a patient and family caregiver's willingness and ability to follow the health care guidelines and restrictions needed for successful recovery.

Entering a health care setting is stressful for a patient. Initially, there is uncertainty about a disease condition, procedures to be performed, and competence of health care staff, to name a few. Therapeutic communication can defuse some of that stress, enabling a nurse to form trust and then be able to obtain a thorough history database. Communication techniques are essential to help patients who have difficulty coping or understanding their health care experience. The exchange of information we learn about patients with other health care providers then becomes important for continuity of care and maintenance of quality care standards.

1 | Clinical Judgment in Nursing Practice

OUTLINE

Clinical Judgment in Nursing Practice, p. 2
Critical Thinking Evolving Case Study, p. 3
Critical Thinking Competencies, p. 4
Levels of Critical Thinking, p. 7
Evaluation of Clinical Judgments, p. 13

OBJECTIVES

Mastery of content in this chapter will enable you to:
- Explain the relationship between critical thinking and clinical judgment in nursing practice.
- Explain the value of applying a clinical judgment model in nursing practice.
- Examine the components of critical thinking in clinical decision making.
- Examine the factors influencing diagnostic reasoning when making clinical judgments.
- Analyze benefits of clinical experiences that contribute to critical thinking.
- Apply critical thinking attitudes during assessment of a patient condition.
- Explain how to apply intellectual standards during the nursing process.
- Evaluate the ability to make accurate clinical decisions when performing nursing skills.

MEDIA RESOURCES

- http://evolve.elsevier.com/Perry/skills
- Review Questions
- Audio Glossary
- Case Studies
- Answers to Clinical Judgment and Next-Generation NCLEX® Examination–Style Questions
- Printable Key Points

Pause for a moment. What do you think about before making a decision? Depending on the nature of the problem, you may think about past experiences, reflect on your knowledge about the problem, or consider the time you have and the desire to be accurate, or you might react to intuition. These factors and more involve the critical thinking needed to make a judgment and decision about how to solve the problem.

Every day you think critically without realizing it. When your computer flashes an error warning or your cell phone does not take you to a desired application, you think about the actions you took before the error, consider possible causes of the problem, and correct a keystroke or reboot the device. If you decide to walk your dogs, go to the door, and notice that it is raining, you decide to change into your raincoat. These simple examples show how you use basic critical thinking skills when you make daily decisions.

For a professional nurse, critical thinking is more complicated. You care for patients with unique, complex health care problems that can change within minutes. Critical thinking becomes embedded in your everyday practice, as it involves knowing as much as possible about each patient and sorting out the information into patterns to identify problems, recognize changes, and make appropriate clinical care decisions under pressure. This applies when performing nursing skills. You consider what you know about a patient, your knowledge base, and your experience in performing the skill, and then you make a clinical judgment in deciding how to adapt the skill for the patient's best outcomes.

Critical thinking and clinical judgment are essential processes for safe, efficient, and skillful nursing care. Sound critical thinking enables you to face each new experience and problem involving a patient's care with open-mindedness, confidence, and continual inquiry. It is a process mastered only through experience, commitment, and an active curiosity toward learning.

CLINICAL JUDGMENT IN NURSING PRACTICE

A patient's health care needs initiate the process of clinical judgment and clinical decision making (Dickison et al., 2019). Registered nurses (RNs) are responsible for making accurate and appropriate clinical decisions that ensure patients receive safe, appropriate, timely, and effective nursing interventions. A **clinical judgment** is defined by the National Council of State Boards of Nursing [NCSBN] (2019) as the observed outcome of critical thinking and decision making. Another definition for clinical judgment is a conclusion about a patient's needs or health problems that leads to taking or avoiding action, using or modifying standard approaches, or creating new approaches based on the patient's response (Tanner, 2006). It is a process that uses nursing knowledge, experience, and critical thinking to observe and assess presenting situations, identify a prioritized patient concern, and generate the best possible evidence-based solutions to make the decisions needed to deliver safe patient care (NCSBN, 2019).

Clinical decision making separates professional nurses from technicians or other assistive personnel (AP). For example, an RN observes for changes in a patient's condition, collects and analyzes data about the changes, recognizes and identifies new and potential problems, plans nursing interventions (including nursing skills), and takes immediate action when the patient's clinical condition worsens. Nurses direct AP to perform basic aspects of care based on patient need; AP do not have the knowledge or experience to analyze why or when patients' clinical conditions change and what strategies are required. Good clinical decision making requires you to use your clinical judgment in investigating and analyzing all aspects of a clinical problem and then applying scientific and nursing knowledge to choose the best course of action.

A Model for Clinical Judgment

Clinical judgments made by thinking critically and making sound decisions are at the core of professional nursing competence. Fig. 1.1

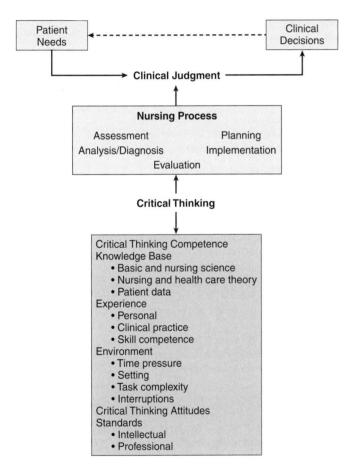

FIG. 1.1 Clinical judgment model for nursing. *(Adapted from Kataoka-Yahiro, M., & Saylor, C. [1994]. A critical thinking model for nursing judgment, Journal of Nursing Education, 33[8]:351; Glaser, E. [1941]. An experiment in the development of critical thinking. New York: Bureau of Publications, Teachers College, Columbia University; Miller, M., & Malcolm, N. [1990]. Critical thinking in the nursing curriculum, Nursing and Health Care, 11:67; Paul, R. W. [1993]. The art of redesigning instruction. In Willsen, J., & Blinker, A. J. A. [Eds.]. Critical thinking: How to prepare students for a rapidly changing world. Santa Rosa, CA: Foundation for Critical Thinking; Perry, W. [1979]. Forms of intellectual and ethical development in the college years: A scheme., New York: Holt, Rinehart, & Winston; and National Council State Boards of Nursing [NCSBN] [Winter 2019]. Next Generation NCLEX News: Clinical Judgment Measurement Model. https://www. ncsbn.org/NGN_Winter19.pdf.)*

offers a model for clinical judgment. The model explains the many variables involved as you make decisions and clinical judgments about your patients. The model for this textbook is research based and is the work of a number of nurse scholars, researchers, and the NCSBN (Kataoka-Yahiro & Saylor, 1994; Miller & Malcolm, 1990; Paul, 1993; NCSBN, 2019).

As you begin your professional nursing education, your knowledge and clinical experiences will build the competence you need to apply the clinical judgment model. The model is not offered for you to try to apply every element or component to each patient situation. But it does contain the elements that allow you to make the right clinical decisions in every type of patient situation. Each patient poses a unique situation for applying the model. For example, when you care for a patient who has respiratory problems because of pneumonia, you will apply knowledge about respiration and oxygenation and pneumonia, physically listen to lung sounds, reflect on criteria as to whether the patient requires airway suctioning, and consider data gathered after interviewing the patient to offer patient-centered care easing anxiety related to shortness of breath. In contrast, when you care for a patient who has respiratory problems because of fractured ribs, you will apply knowledge about ventilation and oxygenation and the pain associated with fractures, examine chest excursion, consider pain-relief approaches, and review data gathered after interviewing the patient to offer patient-centered care for promoting pain relief. The clinical judgment model offers a valuable conceptual approach to understanding the nature of nursing practice.

CRITICAL THINKING EVOLVING CASE STUDY

A 68-year-old patient had abdominal surgery for a colon resection and removal of a tumor yesterday. The nurse finds the patient lying supine in bed with arms held tightly over the abdomen. The facial expression is tense. The nurse checks the patient's surgical wound, observing the condition of the dressing. The patient winces when the nurse gently performs palpation around the surgical incision. The nurse assesses when the patient was last turned and repositioned laterally on the side. The patient responds, "Not since last night." The nurse also says, "Show me where you are having pain." The patient points to the incision and says, "It hurts too much to move." The nurse assesses the patient with a pain-rating scale and obtains a pain score of 7 on a scale of 0 to 10. The nurse refers to the electronic health record (EHR), noting that the patient last received an analgesic 5 hours ago. The nurse considers the information observed and gathered to determine that the patient's priority problem is pain, in addition to reduced mobility. The nurse decides to take action by administering an analgesic that is ordered to be given as needed every 4 hours and obtaining assistance from AP to position the patient more comfortably.

In this case example, the nurse begins by referring to knowledge about abdominal surgery and the effects on the colon when a tumor is removed. Recognition that a patient problem exists by gathering and assessing information (e.g., clinical data, observation of patient behavior, electronic health record [EHR]), analyzing information about the problem (e.g., is it anticipated or unexpected, what cues form patterns?), interpreting the information (reviewing assumptions and evidence, recognizing the patterns), and making conclusions specifically about the problem (diagnosis) involves clinical judgment. As a critical thinker, the nurse considers what is important in the clinical situation (based on knowledge and experience), contemplates and explores alternatives (what to assess further), considers ethical principles (patient choice about pain control), identifies the patient's problems (pain and mobility), and makes informed decisions about the care of the patient (types of skills to perform). The nurse forms a clinical judgment by applying **critical thinking**, the ability to think in a systematic and logical manner with the willingness to question and reflect on the reasoning process. This allows the nurse to make appropriate clinical decisions in the patient's care.

Critical thinking helps you to focus on the important issues in any clinical situation and make decisions that produce desired patient outcomes—in the case study example, reduced pain and improved mobility for the patient. The nurse in the case study first learned about the importance of early mobility after surgery when reading the nursing and scientific literature on the concept of mobility and deconditioning. Learning that pain reduces mobility was the result of caring for previous patients. When immobility is prolonged, patients become susceptible to complications such as deep vein thrombosis and pneumonia. Applying this knowledge, the nurse decides to implement pain-relief measures first so that the patient can become more mobile.

Critical thinkers question, are honest in facing personal biases, and reflect on information for answers and deeper meanings in order to understand their patients. Critical thinking is a way of thinking about clinical situations by asking questions such as:

- Why does the patient have this condition?
- How does the condition normally affect a patient physically and psychologically?
- Are the signs and symptoms shown by the patient what I would expect for the condition or situation?
- Are there signs and symptoms associated with worsening of the condition?
- What do I really know about this patient's situation?
- What other ways can I collect data to help me understand the problem more fully?
- Do I require more information?
- What care options (including nursing skills) do I have?
- Are there ways I need to adapt a skill based on the patient's clinical situation?

Nurses rely on a critical thinking process to look at each unique patient situation and determine which identified assumptions are true and relevant when making accurate clinical judgments. The nursing process is described by the American Nurses Association (ANA) as the framework nurses use to apply critical thinking in nursing practice for making clinical decisions (ANA, 2021). The ANA describes the process as including six steps: assessment, diagnosis, outcome identification, planning, implementation, and evaluation (ANA, 2021). Six cognitive skills interact, enabling nurses to apply the nursing process when making clinical judgments involving clinical decision making (Dickison et al., 2019). The six cognitive skills are recognize cues, analyze cues, prioritize problems/diagnoses, generate solutions, take actions, and evaluate outcomes (Fig. 1.2) (NCSBN, 2019).

The purpose of the nursing process is to diagnose and treat human responses (e.g., patient symptoms, need for knowledge) to patients' health problems. It encompasses significant actions taken by RNs and is the core of practice for the RN to deliver holistic, patient-centered care (ANA, 2021). The format for the nursing process is unique to the discipline of nursing and provides a common language and process for nurses to "think through" patients' clinical problems while applying critical thinking.

CRITICAL THINKING COMPETENCIES

Critical thinking competencies are the cognitive processes a nurse uses to make clinical judgments about the care of patients

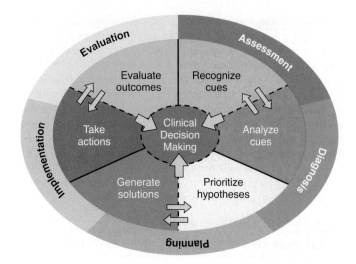

FIG. 1.2 Five-step nursing process. (*Copyright © NCSBN. All rights reserved.*)

(Kataoka-Yahiro & Saylor, 1994). These include general critical thinking, specific critical thinking in clinical situations, and specific critical thinking in nursing. General critical thinking processes include the scientific method, problem solving, and decision making. Specific critical thinking competencies include diagnostic reasoning and clinical decision making. The specific critical thinking competency in nursing is the nursing process.

General Critical Thinking
Scientific Method
The scientific method is a methodical way to solve problems by using reasoning. It is a systematic, ordered approach to gather data and solve problems. Health care researchers, including nurse scientists, use the scientific method when testing research questions. The scientific method has five steps:
1. Identify the problem.
2. Collect data.
3. Formulate a question or hypothesis.
4. Test the question or hypothesis.
5. Evaluate results of the test or study.

Table 1.1 offers an example of a nursing practice issue solved by applying the scientific method in a research study.

Problem Solving
Patients routinely present problems in nursing practice. For example, a home care nurse learns that a patient has difficulty taking medications regularly. The patient is unable to describe which medications have been taken for the past 3 days. The medication bottles are labeled and filled. The nurse must solve the problem of why the patient is not following the prescribed medication schedule. The nurse knows that when the patient was discharged from the hospital, five medications were ordered. The nurse learns that the patient also takes two over-the-counter medications regularly. When the nurse has the patient prepare the medications, the nurse notices that the patient has difficulty seeing the medication labels. The patient can describe the medications to take but is uncertain about the times of administration. The nurse recognizes a problem and recommends having the patient's pharmacy relabel the medications in larger lettering. In addition, the nurse shows the patient examples of pill organizers that will help in sorting the medications by time of day for a period of 7 days. During a follow-up visit, the nurse finds that the patient has organized the medications correctly

TABLE 1.1

Using the Scientific Method to Solve Nursing Practice Questions

Clinical Problem: The incidence of a health care–associated infection, *Clostridium difficile (C. diff)* infection, has increased on a hospital general medicine unit. The nursing staff on the unit practice committee, an infection control specialist, and a clinical nurse specialist in medicine meet to discuss factors that may be contributing to the problem. They note that visitors are inconsistent in the use of antiseptic hand rubs. A staff member questions whether the use of hand rubs is the best approach for this type of infection.

Identify the problem.	The incidence of *C. difficile* has increased among patients on a general medicine unit.
Collect data.	Staff members review the literature about the nature of *C. difficile* infection and the hand-hygiene antiseptic techniques recommended to prevent the infection. Staff members search the literature for studies that have investigated hand-hygiene practices of visitors of hospitalized patients. Staff members review performance improvement reports to monitor the occurrence of *C. difficile* on the unit. The infection control specialist is asked to discuss the trends within the hospital in the incidence of *C. difficile*.
Form a research question to study the problem.	Does visitor use of antiseptic hand rub with chlorhexidine versus handwashing with soap and water reduce incidence of *C. difficile* infection in medical patients?
Answer the question.	The nurse specialist and a small team of staff members create a 4-month study approved by the hospital research board. Patients' visitors are asked to use a chlorhexidine rub on their hands before entering and leaving patient rooms. Visitors switch to handwashing with soap and water for the next 2 months. The infection control specialist tracks the incidence of *C. difficile* infection over the 4 months.
Evaluate the results of the study. Does the study answer the research question?	Compare the incidence of *C. difficile* infection for the 2-month period when each hand-hygiene method was used.

and is able to read the labels without difficulty. The nurse obtained information that correctly clarified the cause of the patient's problem and tested a solution that proved successful.

Effective **problem solving** requires you to obtain information that clarifies the nature of a problem, suggest possible solutions, and try the solution over time to evaluate that it is effective. In the case of a nursing skill, a solution is an action that adapts a skill to minimize the effects of the problem. For example, when administering perineal care, if a patient has limited mobility due to painful arthritis of the hips, it will be difficult to access the perineal area and cleanse the patient effectively. Offering a pain medication prior to perineal care and positioning the patient onto the side, instead of the traditional dorsal recumbent position, are ways to address the patient's immobility problem and provide proper hygienic care.

Intuition is one problem-solving approach that relies on one's inner sense. It is the ability to understand something immediately, without the need for conscious reasoning. Intuitive thinking is commonly invoked for well-structured and familiar decision tasks, whereas analytic thinking is triggered for ill-structured and unfamiliar decision tasks (Dickison et al., 2019). For example, we think automatically when we carry out daily routines, but we must consciously think about new tasks or ones that are posing challenges to complete. Intuition is often perceived as being a form of guessing and therefore inappropriate in making nursing decisions. However, Tanner (2006) explained that less experienced nurses, including students, may rely more heavily on analytic reasoning, whereas experienced nurses are more likely to use intuitive reasoning based on their clinical experiences with numerous patients. Experienced nurses sense "red flags" when something goes wrong with a patient, when something just does not look right. Perhaps they have seen the problem before (such as a wound that is separating and forming yellow drainage), or they know to anticipate a problem because of their knowledge base. Responding intuitively enables quick action, but it must then be complemented with thoughtful reasoning and judgment to ensure that the proper response has occurred.

Decision Making

When you face a problem and choose a course of action from several options, you are making a decision. Basic decision making goes hand in hand with problem solving and problem resolution. Following a set of criteria helps you make a thorough and thoughtful decision. The criteria may be personal, based on an organizational policy or standard, or, in the case of nursing, based on a professional standard (e.g., ethical standard, standard for confidentiality).

For example, people make decisions when they choose a health care provider. An individual must first recognize and define the problem (the need for a health care provider) and assess all options (e.g., consider a recommended health care provider or choose one whose office is close to home). The person weighs each option against a set of personal criteria (experience, friendliness, reputation, location), tests possible options (talks directly with the different health care providers), considers the consequences of the decision (examines pros and cons of selecting one provider over another), and makes a final decision. Although the set of criteria follows a sequence of steps, decision making involves moving back and forth when considering all criteria. This process leads to informed conclusions that are supported by evidence and reason.

Specific Critical Thinking
Diagnostic Reasoning

In the earlier Critical Thinking case study in this chapter, once the nurse gathered information about the patient's discomfort and mobility limitation, **diagnostic reasoning** began.

Diagnostic reasoning is a cognitive process that involves applying cognitive skills, knowledge, and experience to diagnose and treat patients (Royce et al., 2019). It requires being able to understand

and think through clinical problems, gather information about the problem, analyze individual cues, understand the meaning of evidence, and know when you have enough information to decide on an accurate diagnosis. Caution is needed with this process. Often a nurse will oversimplify a patient's problem and, when the problem is viewed too narrowly, will not make the appropriate clinical decision. It is critical for accurate diagnostic reasoning to not only focus on a patient's primary problem but to consider relevant strengths and weaknesses of patients, their histories, and their environments. Diagnostic error occurs when one fails to consider the correct diagnosis, often by limiting the data used to make a decision or not being deliberative when reflecting on all problems a patient may present (Royce et al., 2019).

Once a diagnosis is made, one considers different factors associated with the problem and then decides on the interventions for those factors to best meet the needs of a patient. Accurate problem recognition (e.g., nursing diagnosis) is necessary before choosing solutions and implementing action. Diagnostic error is a common cause of medical error by health care providers and is often a result of faulty interpretation, synthesis, or judgment of available information (LaManna et al., 2019).

> Continuing the case study, the nurse enters the patient's room and finds the patient to be restless, short of breath, and stating, "I have this terrible pain in my chest." What might such a change indicate? Diagnostic reasoning begins when you interact with a patient or make physical or behavioral observations. An expert nurse sees the context of a patient situation (e.g., patient just had major surgery; has been inactive; and is at risk for blood pooling in the lower extremities, which can cause clots to form in the circulation and then break off and travel to the lung).

The nurse observes patterns and themes (e.g., symptoms that include shortness of breath, sharp chest pain, a cough that produces pink mucus, and irregular heart rate) and makes a clinical judgment quickly (e.g., a clot may have dislodged and traveled to the lung's circulation, requiring a quick medical response). The information that a nurse collects and analyzes leads to a diagnosis of a patient's condition (e.g., *impaired gas exchange*). Nurses do not make medical diagnoses, but they do assess and monitor each patient closely and compare a patient's signs and symptoms with those that are common to a medical diagnosis (e.g., in the case study, a pulmonary embolus). Nurses think critically during diagnostic reasoning, understanding the nature of problems and patients' responses through data assessment and analysis to enable selection of proper therapies.

Often you cannot make a precise diagnosis during your first meeting with a patient. Sometimes you sense that a problem exists but do not have enough data to make a specific diagnosis. Some patients' physical conditions limit their ability to tell you about symptoms. Others choose to not share sensitive and important information during your initial assessment. Some patients' behaviors and physical responses become observable only under conditions not present during your initial assessment. How you interpret this information is part of critical thinking and clinical judgment. When uncertain of a diagnosis, continue to collect data. Critically analyze changing clinical situations until you can determine a patient's unique situation. Diagnostic accuracy helps health care providers identify the nature of a problem more quickly and select appropriate medical therapies.

Clinical Decision Making

When you face a clinical problem involving a patient and need to choose an action from several options, you are making clinical decisions. Clinical decision making focuses on resolving a patient's problem such as how to best perform a nursing skill. For example, a home health nurse observes that a patient requires assistance with accessing and cooking food due to visual and mobility problems. The nurse applies judgment in making a clinical decision that identifies the problem (impaired ability to prepare food) and then chooses the best nursing interventions (e.g., large labels attached to food products, utensils with special handles). The ability to make clinical decisions develops over time and is affected by a number of factors. A nursing research study examining studies involving clinical decision making in nursing practice found these themes (Nibbelink & Brewer, 2018):

- Nursing experience and associated factors
- Organization and unit culture
- Understanding patient status
- Situation awareness

Experience. Nursing experience relates to time spent in clinical practice as well as personal experience (Nibbelink & Brewer, 2018). Experience can increase nurses' self-confidence, which promotes their ability to ask questions, consider options for patient care, and implement interventions. Experience also influences nurses' use of standard protocols in nursing practice. The use of protocols becomes second nature for experienced nurses but is particularly useful for unusual situations. Inexperienced nurses use protocols to regularly support decision making and enhance confidence in decisions. Part of experience is collaboration with other health care providers. Experienced nurse colleagues provide advice and confirmation of thinking to other nurses (Nibbelink & Brewer, 2018).

Organization and Unit Culture. Organization and unit culture influences decision making. Organizational decision-making factors such as use of informal rules, leadership on a nursing unit, and personalities of nurse colleagues provide informal influence over nurse decision making that could influence patient care both positively and negatively (Nibbelink & Brewer, 2018). Nurses must not permit organization and unit culture to be the sole factor in their decision making, especially if it discounts the importance of the nurse's scientific knowledge base.

Understanding the Patient Status. Understanding patient status is associated with knowledge, developed over a period of time. To better understand a patient's status, a nurse must invest time through physical presence with the patient to support decision making. This is part of knowing the patient. Knowing the patient is an in-depth knowledge of a patient's patterns of responses within a clinical situation and knowing the patient as a person (Tanner et al., 1993). Knowing a patient has two components: a nurse's understanding of a specific patient, and the nurse's subsequent selection of interventions. It relates to a nurse's experience with caring for patients with similar conditions, time spent in a specific clinical area, and having a sense of closeness with patients (Tanner et al., 1993). For example, an expert nurse who has worked on a general surgery unit for many years has cared for a patient for the past 2 days. The nurse is familiar with how the patient is progressing physically and mentally. When the patient begins to experience a change (e.g., a slight fall in blood pressure, becoming less responsive), the nurse knows that something is wrong, suspects that the patient may be bleeding internally, and takes action. Because of the nurse's clinical experience and knowing the patient, the expert nurse can make a clinical decision and act more quickly than a new nurse can be expected to act.

Foster your ability to know a patient and understand a patient's situation, using these guidelines:

- Spend enough time during initial and follow-up patient assessments to observe patient behavior and measure physical and psychosocial findings to improve knowledge of your patients. Determine what is important to them and make a positive emotional connection.

- Know trends and a patient's normal physical and psychological patterns for a clinical condition over time so that you can identify when patients require a change in their treatment plan.
- Know a patient's typical behaviors, schedules, and preferences at home to help guide you with their stay in a health care agency. This allows you to adjust and provide individualized patient-centered care.
- When talking with patients, listen to their accounts of their experiences with illness, watch them, and come to understand how they typically respond (Tanner, 2006).
- Consistently check on patients to assess and monitor problems to help you identify how clinical changes develop over time.
- Ask to have the same patient assigned to you over consecutive days.

Situation Awareness. Situation awareness, the ability to understand the present state of a clinical situation, affects clinical decision making. Types of patient information nurses use to help develop situation awareness include patient diagnoses, understanding of the importance of the information collected, prediction of potential patient outcomes to facilitate planning of care, and individual factors such as self-confidence and assertiveness (Nibbelink & Brewer, 2018). Situation awareness and knowing a patient are closely interrelated.

Knowing that multiple factors influence your decision making, you will learn to face a patient problem by critically analyzing available data to determine the most relevant information and ideas and then discard unnecessary data until a later time. Following a set of questions or criteria about the data helps you to make thorough and thoughtful decisions (Box 1.1). These types of questions are helpful when a nurse begins or completes a work shift or reviews a patient's history and progress.

Making accurate patient-centered clinical decisions requires you to prioritize your nursing interventions. Do not assume that certain health situations produce automatic priorities. For example, a patient who has surgery is anticipated to experience a certain level of postoperative pain, which often becomes a priority for care. However, if the same patient is having severe anxiety that increases pain perception, you focus on ways to relieve the anxiety before pain-relief measures will be effective.

BOX 1.1

Clinical Decision-Making Questions

Questions About a Problem
- Is the problem clear and understandable?
- Is the problem important or a priority in the patient's care?
- What does the problem mean to the patient?

Questions About Your Perspective
- Are you looking at the problem from the view of _____? Why?
- How might someone with an opposite view see the problem?
- How does your view compare with that of the patient?

Questions About Assumptions
- You are assuming _____. How does that affect your analysis of the problem? Does it bias you?
- What might you assume instead? Is there another option?

Questions About Evidence
- What evidence (data about patient, scientific evidence about the type of problem) supports your assumption?
- Is there a reason to doubt the evidence? Does it apply to this specific situation?
- What further evidence is needed?

BOX 1.2

Clinical Decision Making for Groups of Patients

- Identify the nursing diagnoses and collaborative problems of each patient.
- Analyze the diagnoses/problems and decide which are most urgent based on basic needs, the patients' changing or unstable status, and problem complexity.
- Consider the time it will take to care for patients whose problems are of high priority (e.g., do you have the time to restart a critical intravenous [IV] line when medication is due for a different patient?).
- Consider the resources you have to manage each problem, assistive personnel (AP) assigned with you, other health care providers, and patients' family members.
- Involve patients and/or their family as decision makers and participants in care.
- Decide how to combine activities to resolve more than one patient problem at a time.
- Decide which, if any, nursing care procedures to delegate to AP so that you can spend your time on activities requiring professional nursing knowledge.
- Discuss complex cases with other members of the health care team. This ensures a smooth transition in care throughout a patient's health care experience.

Clinical decision making is complicated, especially when nurses work in settings where they are assigned to multiple patients in fast-paced and unpredictable environments. To prioritize patient problems in such situations, use decision criteria that include factors such as the clinical condition of the patient, an examination of the advantages and disadvantages of each option, Maslow's hierarchy of needs, the risks involved in treatment delays, environmental factors (time and staff resources available for delegation), and patients' expectations of care to determine which patients have the highest priorities. For you to manage the wide variety of problems associated with groups of patients, skillful, prioritized clinical decision making is critical (Box 1.2).

Consider this: Think about a patient you have been assigned to recently. Based on that individual patient's needs and health problems, what evidence-based information might you seek to provide evidence-based nursing care?

LEVELS OF CRITICAL THINKING

Your ability as a nurse to develop and apply critical thinking when making clinical judgments evolves over time. The three levels of critical thinking describe how critical thinking develops (Box 1.3).

Basic Critical Thinking

Beginning nursing students are task oriented. They focus on performing skills and organizing nursing care activities rather than delivering skills within the context of their patients' specific clinical situations. At the basic level of critical thinking, a learner trusts that experts have the right answers for every problem. Thinking is concrete and based on a set of rules or principles. For example, as a nursing student you use a hospital procedure manual to confirm how to change an intravenous (IV) dressing. You will follow the procedure step-by-step without adjusting it to meet a patient's unique needs (e.g., positioning to minimize the patient's pain or mobility restrictions). Your inexperience does not allow you to anticipate how to individualize the procedure when problems arise. A basic critical thinker learns to accept the diverse opinions and values of experts (e.g., instructors and staff nurse preceptors).

BOX 1.3

Levels of Critical Thinking

Basic

- Answers to complex problems are perceived as either right or wrong (e.g., when an intravenous [IV] fluid is not infusing correctly, the rate must be regulated correctly).
- A single solution usually resolves each problem (e.g., adjusting the rate instead of trying to position the patient's arm to prevent catheter kinking).
- This is an early step in developing critical thinking.

Complex

- Make clinical decisions more independently.
- Creativity allows nurses to generate many ideas quickly, be able to change viewpoints, and create original solutions to problems.
- Thinking abilities and initiative to look beyond expert opinion begins to change.
- Learn that alternative and perhaps conflicting solutions exist.
- Consider different options from routine procedures.
- Gather additional information and take a variety of different approaches for the same therapy.

Commitment

- Able to consider a wider array of clinical alternatives for a patient's situation.
- Recognize that sometimes a proper action is the decision to not act or to delay an action until a later time based on experience and knowledge.
- Able to apply all elements of the clinical judgment model almost automatically.

Complex Critical Thinking

Complex critical thinkers begin to rely less on experts and trust their own decisions. For example, while teaching a patient how to use an inhaler, you recognize that your patient cannot deliver a dose correctly. Rather than refer to a procedure manual and repeat the same approach, you adapt by offering an inhaler the patient can activate and instruct the patient on how to better coordinate inhaling with delivery of a medication dose. You analyze the clinical situation (e.g., weakness in patient's hands) and examine choices more independently.

> Building on the previous case study, when the nurse enters the patient's room the patient is restless and short of breath and states, "I have this terrible pain in my chest." Thinking critically, the nurse wonders if something other than the abdominal incision is causing the discomfort. The nurse asks, "Is the pain you're feeling now different from before I gave you your medication?" The patient tells the nurse that the pain feels sharper, in the chest. The nurse quickly takes a set of vital signs; the heart rate, which was 88 beats/min and regular 1 hour ago is now 102 beats/min and irregular. The nurse calls the health care provider to report the change in the patient's condition.

The nurse thought outside the box. Rather than assume that the patient had incisional pain, more data were gathered and the nurse recognized that the patient possibly was experiencing a life-threatening condition, possibly a pulmonary embolus. In complex critical thinking, each solution has benefits and risks that you weigh before making a final decision. Thinking becomes more innovative.

Commitment

The third level of critical thinking is commitment (Kataoka-Yahiro & Saylor, 1994). At this level you anticipate when to make choices without assistance from others and accept accountability for decisions made. At the commitment level, you decide on an action or belief that is based on the available alternatives and support it. Because you take accountability for the decision, you consider the results of the decision and determine whether it was appropriate.

COMPONENTS OF CRITICAL THINKING IN THE CLINICAL JUDGMENT MODEL

The model for clinical judgment (see Fig 1.1) defines the outcome of critical thinking through the application of the nursing process as clinical judgment. Patient needs initiate the process of clinical judgment, and clinical decisions complete the process (Dickison et al., 2019). The model is relevant to patients' health care problems in a variety of health care settings. The model includes six components of critical thinking in nursing judgment:

- Critical thinking competence (e.g., diagnostic reasoning and clinical decision-making ability)
- Knowledge
- Experience
- Environment
- Attitudes
- Standards

The six components combined guide nurses in making sound clinical judgments necessary for relevant and appropriate clinical decisions.

Competence

The critical thinking competencies discussed earlier are essential for guiding you in applying the nursing process in making accurate clinical judgments. There is an additional competence—the ability to perform nursing skills (e.g., hands-on procedures, physical examination techniques) proficiently. When you are still a basic critical thinker you will perform skills carefully and cautiously, following policy and procedure. Skills can create a distraction, making it difficult for you as a new nurse to focus on applying the nursing process in an individualized and systematic way. When you become more adept at gathering patient-centered data, identifying patient problems, and planning appropriate nursing interventions, you evolve into a complex critical thinker. At that point nursing skills become more like second nature and are adapted to each patient's unique needs. You will develop competence as you continue to practice and perform nursing skills. Clinical judgment points incorporated into the skills chapters are designed to help you reflect and learn how to apply clinical judgment while performing a skill.

Knowledge Base

A nurse's knowledge base varies according to educational experience that includes basic nursing education, continuing education courses, and additional college degrees. A nurse also builds knowledge by reading the nursing literature (especially research-based literature) to maintain current knowledge of nursing science and theory. **Evidence-based knowledge**, or knowledge based on research or clinical expertise, makes nurses better-informed critical thinkers. Thinking critically and learning about scientific concepts prepares you to better anticipate and identify patient problems by understanding their origin and nature.

Evidence-based practice (EBP) guides you in making accurate, timely, and appropriate clinical decisions. It is an interprofessional process for applying the newest scientific knowledge available in health care sciences to the patient's bedside. For example, checking the pH of gastric content (see Chapter 32) prior to feeding a patient through an enteral tube and using the research-based Braden Scale to routinely assess a patient's risk for skin breakdown (see Chapter 39) are examples of using evidence at the bedside. This textbook includes evidence-based references throughout, demonstrates how to use evidence in nursing procedures or skills, and provides the scientific guidelines to perform skills more effectively and improve patient outcomes. See Table 1.2 for a review of the EBP process.

A nurse's knowledge base includes information and theory from the basic sciences, humanities, behavioral sciences, and nursing science. Nurses apply this knowledge by thinking holistically about patient problems. For example, a nurse's broad knowledge base offers a physical, psychological, social, moral, ethical, and cultural view of patients and their health care needs. The depth and extent of scientific knowledge influence a nurse's ability to think critically about nursing problems. The most critical source of knowledge a nurse applies in critical thinking is patient data. Patient data include:

- Observations of patient behavior and clinical signs
- Direct physical examination
- Interview with patient and family caregivers
- Electronic health record (EHR) resources
- Diagnostic data

A complex or committed clinical thinker gathers a thorough but also an appropriate **patient-centered** database. This means you do not simply gather patient data based on preselected categories found on an assessment recording form. Instead, you apply scientific knowledge to anticipate what assessment data are required for a specific patient. For example, if a patient is known to have diabetes mellitus, you will apply what the patient knows about the effects of this metabolic disorder and will attend more closely to the patient's actual or expected clinical signs and symptoms. A patient with diabetes mellitus is at risk for circulatory problems, so you assess peripheral pulses and the condition of any existing wound (e.g., Is it healing?). A patient with diabetes mellitus is also at risk for visual alterations, so a more extensive examination of vision is needed compared with a patient with no known visual risks. Patient data guide your assessment. Each data point raises questions about the nature of a patient's problem and what additional data are needed. It creates a picture of what makes the patient unique.

The nurse in the case study earned a bachelor's degree in education, taught high school for 1 year, and is now in the second year as an RN. Taking additional classes in health ethics and population health will add to a knowledge base preparing the nurse for a range of patient situations. The nurse's experience as a staff nurse has

---

TABLE 1.2	
The Evidence-Based Practice (EBP) Process	
Step 1: Cultivate a spirit of inquiry.	
Step 2: Ask a clinical question in the following format: Population, Intervention or Issue, Comparison population, Outcome, Time (PICOT) PICOT example: In medical patients (P) does the use of teach-back (I) compared with teach-back and a follow-up call-back system (C) improve patient medication adherence (O) during the first 60 days of discharge (T)?	Consistently question or challenge what you do as a nurse. Is this the best practice approach? Think about a patient care problem or area of interest that is time consuming, costly, or not logical. Work with mentors and clinical librarians to clarify your question. Be specific with key words.
Step 3: Search the most relevant scientific journals and standards.	Use concise key terms for your search (a librarian is a great resource). Use research journals and nonresearch resources, including government and professional websites, agency procedure manuals, performance improvement reports, and computerized bibliographical databases. Peer-reviewed articles are preferable because they have been evaluated by a panel of experts familiar with the subject matter of the article.
Step 4: Critically review the evidence.	The review of evidence determines if there is evidence that answers your question. Follow this checklist for each source of evidence (Centre for Evidence-Based Medicine, n.d.). • Does this study address a clearly focused question? • Did the study use valid methods to address this question? • Are the results of the study valid and important? • Will the results help you provide better care for your patients?
Step 5: Apply or integrate evidence along with clinical expertise, patient preferences, and values in making a practice decision or change.	As an individual you can recommend practice changes during staff meetings or policy and procedure review. An EBP team is ideal to apply evidence in a manner that integrates well with existing practice for all affected disciplines.
Step 6: Evaluate outcomes of change.	Know which outcomes to measure and how to collect the measures consistently. Gather baseline data of your outcome (e.g., fall rate, infection incidence, patient satisfaction score). Then gather data over time after practice change has been made. Do results show that change was effective?
Step 7: Communicate results.	Share results (regardless of outcome) by talking with colleagues, discussing in staff meetings, presenting in workshops or seminars, submitting an abstract for a poster presentation, and publishing an article.

EBP, Evidence-based practice.

allowed for development of knowledge about a variety of surgical procedures, the effects of different medications, and physical and psychological responses patients typically show to their treatment.

Experience

Nursing is a practice discipline. Clinical learning experiences are necessary to acquire decision-making skills and clinical judgment and gain competence in performing nursing skills. In clinical situations you learn from observing, sensing, talking with patients and families, providing hands-on care, and reflecting actively on all experiences. Clinical experience is the laboratory for developing and testing approaches that you safely adapt or revise to fit the setting, a patient's unique qualities, and the experiences you have from caring for previous patients. With experience you begin to understand clinical situations (including how to successfully complete a skill), anticipate and recognize cues from patients' health data, and interpret the patterns of data as relevant or irrelevant. As experience develops you will identify and build your personal set of cases with identifiable patterns and typical outcomes that can provide valuable background knowledge when dealing with a current situation (National Health Service [NHS], n.d.). Experience with nursing skills teaches you how to best organize and adapt a skill without sacrificing safe principles. Learn to value all patient experiences. Each experience is a stepping stone for building new knowledge, obtaining skills, and inspiring innovative thinking.

> The nurse in the case study was finishing the last year in nursing school while working as an assistive personnel (AP) in a nursing home. Spending time interacting with older-adult patients and giving basic nursing care as an AP provided the nurse valuable learning experiences, which have been applied in work with other patients as an RN. The nurse developed good interviewing skills, gained an understanding of the importance of the family in an individual's health, and learned to become a patient advocate. By learning that older adults need more time to perform activities such as eating and bathing, the nurse is able to adapt these skill techniques.

Environment

Environmental factors (e.g., task complexity, time pressure, family input, system factors, medical hierarchy, resource factors, and high workload) influence clinical decision making (Beldhuis et al., 2021). Critical thinking does not occur in a void. Nurses process patient data and knowledge applicable to patients' situations and then critically make judgments, all within the context of patients' conditions and environmental factors. Task complexity is an example. A patient with multiple health problems and/or one who requires numerous nursing procedures performed in a short period of time threatens clinical decision making. There are multiple data cues a nurse must sort and interpret, affecting the ability to make quick and clear decisions. If a nurse feels time pressure, either because another patient requires attention or because a procedure is due (e.g., medication), attention to making a clear decision is threatened. As patients' clinical conditions change, expert nurses are able to recognize the changes more quickly, consider knowledge pertaining to the situations, judge whether information is adequate, and attend to making clear decisions. An expert nurse will consider the risks and consequences if actions are not taken to improve a patient's clinical course.

Timeliness in making decisions affects patient outcomes. When making a clinical decision you must act in a timely manner when you see a pattern of data suggesting a problem that requires immediate action. You will learn in a health care setting how and when to communicate, who the leaders of your team are, and expectations the team has for managing problems. Whether a health care setting encourages autonomy is also a factor. Patient harm will occur if you hesitate and do not act on your diagnostic conclusions or judgment.

Tips for critical thinking within the health care environment context include (NHS, n.d.):

- Use the data you have gathered to enlist help, support, and advice from colleagues and the wider interprofessional team.
- Know your own limitations and when you need help.
- Collaborate with colleagues, listen, and be respectful of their ideas.
- Make judgments and prioritize these judgments based on the current patient and do not be distracted by other patients or tasks at the moment.
- Identify a role model whom you believe is a competent decision maker. Watch and question how your role model makes decisions.

Critical Thinking Attitudes

The fifth component of critical thinking is attitudes. Paul (1993) defined 11 attitudes of inquiry that define the central features of a critical thinker and how a successful critical thinker approaches a problem (Table 1.3).

> The case study patient is displaying anxiety. Shortness of breath continues, and the medical staff are on their way to confirm the nature of the breathing problem. The nurse will display curiosity by seeking further information. The nurse will also use discipline in forming questions and conducting a thorough assessment to find the source of the patient's anxiety.

Attitudes of inquiry involve an ability to recognize that problems exist, to consider the context of those problems, and to recognize that there is a need for evidence to support what you think is true. Critical thinking attitudes are guidelines for how to approach a problem and make the correct decision.

Confidence

Confidence is the belief in oneself, one's judgment and psychomotor skills, and one's possession of the knowledge and the ability to think critically. When you are confident, you feel certain about accomplishing a task or goal such as performing a procedure or making a nursing diagnosis. Confidence grows with experience in recognizing your strengths and limitations. You shift your focus from your own needs (e.g., remembering what assessment data mean or how to perform a procedure) to a patient's needs. When you lack confidence in knowing whether a patient's condition is clinically changing or in performing a nursing skill, you become anxious about not knowing what to do and may hesitate to make a necessary decision. Always be aware of the extent and limits of your knowledge. Never perform a procedure unless you have the knowledge base and feel confident. Patient safety is a priority. Confidence builds trust between you and your patients.

Thinking Independently

As you gain new knowledge, you learn to consider a wide range of ideas and concepts before making a judgment. You become open-minded to new concepts and interventions outside of what you learn in school. This does not mean that you ignore other people's ideas. Instead, you learn to consider all sides of a situation.

TABLE 1.3

Critical Thinking Attitudes and Applications in Nursing Practice

Critical Thinking Attitude	Application in Practice
Confidence	The nurse, gaining more experience in reasoning and decision making, does not hesitate to disagree and be troubled, thereby acting as a role model to colleagues. Speak with conviction to a patient when you begin an intervention. Do not lead a patient to think that you are unable to perform care safely. Always be well prepared before performing a nursing activity. Encourage a patient to ask questions.
Thinking independently	As you acquire new knowledge and experiences, examine your beliefs under new evidence. Be open-minded about different interventions. Read the scientific literature, especially when there are different views on the same subject. Talk with other nurses and share ideas about nursing interventions.
Fairness	Listen to both sides of a discussion. If a patient or family member complains about a co-worker, listen to the story, and speak with the co-worker as well. If a staff member labels a patient uncooperative, assume the care of that patient with openness and a desire to meet the patient's needs.
Responsibility and authority	Ask for help if you are uncertain about how to perform a nursing skill. Refer to a policy and procedure manual to review steps of a skill. Report any problems immediately. Follow standards of practice in your care.
Risk taking	If your knowledge causes you to question a health care provider's order, do so. Be willing to recommend alternative approaches to nursing care when colleagues are having little success with patients, especially if your ideas are supported by scientific evidence.
Discipline	Be thorough in whatever you do. Use known scientific and practice-based criteria for activities such as assessment and evaluation. Take time to be thorough and manage your time effectively.
Perseverance	Be cautious of an easy answer that avoids uncomfortable situations. If co-workers give you information about a patient and some fact seems to be missing, clarify the information or talk to the patient directly. If problems of the same type continue to occur on a nursing division, bring co-workers together, look for a pattern, and find a solution.
Creativity	Look for different approaches if interventions are not working for a patient. For example, a patient in pain may need a different positioning or distraction technique. When appropriate, involve the patient's family in adapting your approaches to care methods used at home.
Curiosity	Always ask why. Be willing to challenge tradition. A clinical sign or symptom often indicates a variety of problems. Explore and learn more about a patient so as to make appropriate clinical judgments.
Integrity	Recognize when your opinions conflict with those of a patient; review your position and decide how best to proceed to reach outcomes that will satisfy everyone. Do not compromise nursing standards or honesty in delivering nursing care.
Humility	Recognize when you need more information to make a decision. When you are new to a clinical division, ask for an orientation to the area. Ask registered nurses (RNs) regularly assigned to the area for assistance with approaches to care.

A critical thinker does not accept another person's ideas without question. When thinking independently, you challenge the ways that others think, and you look for rational and logical answers to problems. You raise important questions about your practice. For example, why do patients on your nursing unit fall? When nurses ask questions and look for the evidence behind clinical problems, they are thinking independently; this is an important aspect of EBP.

Fairness

A critical thinker deals with situations justly. This means that you do not let bias or prejudice affect your decisions. Look at a situation objectively and consider all viewpoints to understand the situation completely before making a decision. Having a sense of imagination helps you develop an attitude of fairness. Imagining what it is like to be in your patient's situation helps you see it with new eyes and appreciate its complexity.

Responsibility and Accountability

Responsibility is the knowledge that you are accountable for your decisions, actions, and critical thinking. When caring for patients,

you are responsible for correctly performing nursing care skills based on standards of practice. Standards of practice are the minimum level of performance accepted to ensure high-quality care. For example, you do not take shortcuts (work-arounds) when you give a patient a medication (e.g., skipping a step—failing to identify a patient, preparing medication doses for multiple patients at the same time). Professional nurses are responsible for competently performing nursing therapies and making clinical decisions about patients. As an RN, you are answerable or accountable for your decisions, the outcomes of your actions, and knowing the limits and scope of your practice.

Risk Taking

People often associate taking risks with danger. But risk taking does not always have negative outcomes. A critical thinker will take risks when trying different ways to solve problems. The willingness to take risks, without harming a patient, comes from experiences with similar clinical problems. Trying different approaches to motivating a patient to eat, involving dependent patients more in self-hygiene, or using nonpharmacological approaches to pain relief may pose risk but can be highly beneficial. When taking risks, follow safety guidelines, analyze any potential dangers to a patient, involve the patient in any decisions, and act in a reasoned, logical, and thoughtful manner.

Discipline

A disciplined thinker misses few details when assessing a patient, considering care options and resources, or making decisions about nursing interventions.

> For example, continuing the previous case study, the patient is experiencing incisional and chest pain. Instead of asking the patient only, "How severe is your pain on a scale of 0 to 10?" the nurse knows the need to ask more specific questions about the character of the pain (e.g., "What makes the pain worse?" "Show me exactly where it hurts." "How would you describe the pain?").

Being disciplined helps you identify problems more accurately and select the most appropriate interventions.

Perseverance

A critical thinker is determined to find effective solutions to patient care problems. This is especially important when problems remain unresolved or recur. Learn as much as possible about a problem before deciding on various approaches to care. Persevering means to keep looking for more resources until you find a successful approach. It often requires creativity, such as trying different communication approaches with a patient who has had throat surgery or does not speak your language.

Creativity

Critical thinking combined with creativity allows you to become more flexible and find original solutions to specific problems when traditional interventions are not effective. Creativity involves original thinking. This means that you find solutions outside the standard routines of care while still following standards of practice. Creativity motivates you to think of options and unique approaches. For example, a home care nurse must find a way to help an older patient with arthritis have greater mobility in the home. The patient has difficulty lowering and raising up in a chair because of pain and limited range of motion in the knees. The nurse uses wooden blocks to elevate the chair legs so that the patient can sit and stand with little discomfort while making sure that the chair is safe to use.

Curiosity

A critical thinker's favorite question is "Why?" As you gather and analyze patient information, data patterns appear that are not always clear. Having a sense of curiosity (asking yourself "What if?") motivates you to inquire further (e.g., question family or health care provider, review the scientific literature) and investigate a clinical situation so that you get all the information you need to make a decision.

Integrity

Critical thinkers question and test their own knowledge and beliefs. Your personal integrity as a nurse builds trust from your coworkers. Nurses face many dilemmas or problems in everyday clinical practice, and everyone makes mistakes at times. People of integrity are honest and willing to admit to mistakes or inconsistencies in their own behavior, ideas, and beliefs. A professional nurse always tries to follow the highest standards of practice.

Humility and Self-Awareness

It is important for you to admit to any limitations in your knowledge and skill. Critical thinkers admit what they do not know and try to find the knowledge needed to make proper decisions. It is common for a nurse to be an expert in one area of clinical practice but a novice in another because the knowledge in all areas of nursing is unlimited. A patient's safety and welfare are at risk if you do not admit your inability to deal with a practice problem. Always remain self-aware by internally clarifying your biases, inclinations, strengths, and limitations. Recognize when thinking is being affected by your emotions or self-interest. You must rethink a situation; learn more; and use the new information to form opinions, draw conclusions, and take action.

> The patient in the case study continues to have chest pain and shortness of breath. As the nurse waits for the medical team to arrive, the nurse assumes responsibility for the patient's welfare until treatment can be initiated. The nurse acts independently by keeping the patient comfortable in the chair (to avoid movement that could worsen the condition), explaining steps being taken by the health care team, and gathering additional assessment data. The nurse displays discipline in further assessing the patient's condition: rechecking vital signs, observing the abdominal wound and incision, and talking to allay anxiety and note if there is a change in consciousness. The nurse knows not to diagnose the patient medically. When the health care provider arrives, the nurse objectively reports what happened once the patient sat up in the chair, the symptoms displayed, and how those symptoms have changed.

Standards for Critical Thinking

The sixth component of critical thinking includes intellectual and professional standards (Kataoka-Yahiro & Saylor, 1994).

Intellectual Standards

Paul (1993) identified intellectual standards (Box 1.4) universal for critical thinking. An intellectual standard is a guideline or principle for rational thought. You apply these standards during all steps of the nursing process. For example, when you consider a

---

BOX 1.4

Intellectual Standards

- Clear—Plain and understandable (e.g., clarity in how one communicates)
- Precise—Exact and specific (e.g., focusing on one problem and possible solution)
- Specific—To mention, describe, or define in detail
- Accurate—True and free from error; getting to the facts (objective and subjective)
- Relevant—Essential and crucial to a situation (e.g., a patient's changing clinical status)
- Plausible—Reasonable or probable
- Consistent—Expressing consistent beliefs or values
- Logical—Engaging in correct reasoning from what one believes in a given instance to the conclusions that follow
- Deep—Containing complexities and multiple relationships
- Broad—Covering multiple viewpoints (e.g., patient and family)
- Complete—Thoroughly thinking and evaluating
- Significant—Focusing on what is important and not trivial
- Adequate (for purpose)—Satisfactory in quality or amount

patient problem, apply the intellectual standards of preciseness, accuracy, and consistency in measurement to make sure that you have all the data you need to make sound clinical decisions. During planning, apply standards such as logic and significance so that the plan of care is meaningful and relevant to a patient's needs. Routine use of intellectual standards in clinical practice prevents you from performing critical thinking haphazardly.

> In the case study, the health care provider orders a lung scan and chest x-ray and places the patient on bed rest. Blood tests are also ordered in anticipation of placing the patient on anticoagulation (to prevent further clot formation). The nurse asks the health care provider whether there are risks to be considered regarding the wound, and should the patient receive an anticoagulant (relevant question)? The nurse also asks if additional pain medication can be given at this time to manage the patient's surgical incision pain during the x-ray procedures (logical decision). By applying intellectual standards, the nurse is a competent partner in managing the patient's care, showing the ability to anticipate possible clinical problems.

Professional Standards

Professional standards for critical thinking refer to ethical criteria for nursing judgments, evidence-based criteria used for evaluation, and criteria for professional responsibility (Paul, 1993). Professional practice standards improve patient outcomes and maintain a high-quality level of nursing care. Using available scientific evidence and best practice guidelines found in professional standards is part of the decision-making process (NHS, n.d.).

Excellent nursing practice reflects ethical standards. Being able to focus on a patient's values and beliefs helps you make clinical decisions that are just, respectful of a patient's choices, and beneficial to a patient's well-being. Critical thinkers maintain a sense of self-awareness through conscious awareness of their own beliefs, values, and feelings and the multiple perspectives that patients, family members, and peers present in clinical situations. Critical thinking also requires the use of evidence-based criteria for making clinical judgments. These criteria are ideally scientifically based on research findings or practice based on standards developed by clinical experts. Examples are the clinical practice guidelines developed by individual clinical agencies and national organizations such as the American Association of Critical-Care Nurses (AACN) or the Oncology Nursing Society (ONS). A clinical practice guideline includes standards for the treatment of select clinical conditions such as stroke, deep vein thrombosis, and pressure injuries. Another example is clinical criteria used to categorize clinical conditions, such as the criteria for staging pressure injuries (see Chapter 39) and rating phlebitis (see Chapter 28). Evidence-based evaluation criteria set the minimum requirements for ensuring appropriate and high-quality care.

The standards of professional responsibility that a nurse tries to achieve are the standards cited in nurse practice acts, institutional practice guidelines, and professional organizations' standards of practice (e.g., the ANA Standards of Professional Performance). These standards "raise the bar" for the responsibilities and accountabilities that a nurse assumes in practice.

EVALUATION OF CLINICAL JUDGMENTS

When making clinical decisions about patients, nurses consciously consider if their judgments were accurate and whether the correct and appropriate decisions were made. This is a form of self-evaluation. Evaluation is also a step in the nursing process that methodically determines if nursing care approaches successfully led to desired or expected patient outcomes. Both evaluation processes go hand in hand in developing strong clinical judgment skills.

Reflection

Reflection is like instant replay. It is not intuitive. It involves a deliberate examination and review of one's own reasoning, purposefully visualizing a situation and taking the time to honestly review everything you remember about it (Royce et al., 2019). Reflection is a cognitive skill that demands conscious effort to look at a situation with an awareness of one's own beliefs, values, and practice, enabling you to learn from experiences and incorporate that learning in improving patient care outcomes (Patel & Metersky, 2021). It also leads to knowledge development in nursing. When you are engaged in caring for patients, reflective reasoning improves the accuracy of making diagnostic conclusions. Reflection complements clinical judgment because to be effective it involves description, critical analysis, synthesis, and evaluation (Galutira, 2018). Gathering information about a patient, reflecting on the meaning of your findings, and exploring the possible meaning of those findings improve your ability to problem solve. Reflection lessens the guesswork in decision making. Always be cautious in using reflection. Reliance on it can block thinking and not allow you to look at newer evidence or subtle aspects of situations that you have not encountered. Box 1.5 lists steps of a model for using reflection in your practice.

Reflective journaling is an approach for developing self-evaluation skills. It involves keeping a written record of your clinical experiences in a personal journal. It is a record of personal thoughts, daily events, and evolving insights, and it provides a foundation for creativity, guidance, self-awareness, understanding, and spiritual development (Dimitroff, 2018). Always keep journal entries confidential so that if someone else reads your journal, patients' identity is protected and they cannot be identified. Returning to the journal after each clinical experience gives you the chance to record the perceptions you had during patient care and better develop the ability to apply theory in practice. Often

---

BOX 1.5

Model for Reflection

REFLECT: This model can be used individually or as a process shared with others.

R—*R*ecall the events. Review the facts about a situation and describe what happened.

E—*E*xamine your responses. Think about or discuss your thoughts and actions at the time of the situation.

F—Acknowledge *f*eelings: Identify any feelings you had during the situation.

L—*L*earn from the experience: Review and highlight what you learned from the situation—for example, your patient's responses and your actions.

E—*E*xplore options: Think about or discuss your options for similar situations in the future.

C—*C*reate a plan of action: Create a plan for how to act in future similar situations.

T—Set a *t*ime: Set a time by which your plan of action will be completed.

Adapted from Barksby, J., et al. [2015]. A new model of reflection for clinical practice, *Nursing Times, 111*(34/35):21–23.

reflections are on things that go wrong; however, reflecting on things that went well can be just as rewarding and useful. Journaling improves your observational and descriptive skills. Writing skills improve as you learn to clearly describe concepts applied in practice (e.g., suffering, hope, powerlessness). Here are examples of questions to pose in a journal:

- What did I learn from the experience?
- Did I respond appropriately in this situation? If not, how should I have responded?
- What were the consequences of my actions? Whom did they affect and in what way?
- How might I act differently in the future?
- Was I working from tradition or evidence-based practices?

Meeting With Colleagues

A way to develop and evaluate critical thinking skills is to regularly meet with colleagues such as fellow students or nurses, faculty members, or preceptors to discuss and examine work experiences and validate decisions. Connecting with others helps you learn

that you do not need to know everything because support is available from other colleagues. Willingness to learn from practice and honesty to account for a clinical situation or experience are important. In addition, the persons with whom you share reflection must be trustworthy and approachable (Galutira, 2018). When nurses have a formal way to discuss their experiences, the dialogue allows for questions, differing viewpoints, and sharing of expertise. When they can discuss their practices, the process validates good practice and also offers challenges and constructive criticism.

Critical Thinking Synthesis

Critical thinking is a reasoning process by which you cognitively apply and analyze your thoughts, actions, and knowledge to make sound clinical judgments. As a beginning nurse, you will learn the steps of the nursing process and begin to incorporate the elements of critical thinking into your clinical experiences (Fig. 1.3). The two processes are interdependent in making the clinical judgments necessary for appropriate clinical decision making.

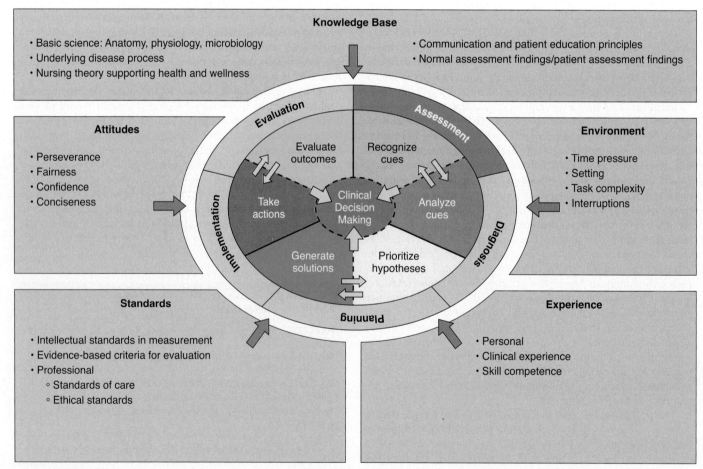

Fig. 1.3 Synthesis of critical thinking with the nursing process. (*Clinical judgment measurement model. Copyright © NCSBN. All rights reserved.*)

◆ **CLINICAL JUDGMENT AND NEXT-GENERATION NCLEX® EXAMINATION–STYLE QUESTIONS**

1. The nurse is preparing to care for a patient receiving hospice care who has been living at home with her spouse. She has ovarian cancer with metastasis to the brain, which was diagnosed 1 year ago. The patient has had "do not resuscitate" (DNR) directives in place for several years. Before providing care, the nurse reviews yesterday's nursing notes.

Highlight the findings that require the nurse to conduct further assessment.

Health History	Nurses' Notes	Vital Signs	Laboratory Results
1634: Patient in bed, reporting pain of 5 on a 0-to-10 scale, which she says is "about what it always is." Height: 163 cm (64 inches); weight: 45.8 kg (101 lb). VS: T 37.2°C (99.0°F); HR 62 beats/min; RR 14 breaths/min; BP 102/68 mm Hg. SpO$_2$ 98% on RA. Spouse reports patient did not eat anything for breakfast or lunch today, stating, "I'm just not hungry."			

2. The nurse performs an assessment and documents this information in the electronic health record (EHR).

Health History	Nurses' Notes	Vital Signs	Laboratory Results
1634: Patient in bed, reporting pain of 5 on a 0-to-10 scale, which she says is "about what it always is." Height: 163 cm (64 inches); weight: 45.8 kg (101 lb). VS: T 37.2°C (99.0°F); HR 62 beats/min; RR 14 breaths/min; BP 102/68 mm Hg. Spo$_2$ 98% on RA. Spouse reports patient did not eat anything for breakfast or lunch today, stating, "I'm just not hungry." Spouse confirms she drank about 4 ounces of water earlier in the day. **0902:** Patient sitting up in bed; appears to have eaten half of a scrambled egg. States, "I don't want any more; I'm starting to feel a little bit nauseated." Offered water; refused by patient. Pain rated at 6 on a 0-to-10 scale. Oxycodone, 5 mg PO administered. Assessment reveals T 37.2°C (99.0°F); HR 64 beats/min; RR 16 breaths/min; BP 108/68 mm Hg. SpO$_2$ 97% on RA. Skin thin and transparent. Weak but equal grip in upper and lower extremities.			

The nurse analyzes the findings to determine the patient's condition. Choose the *most likely* options for the information missing from the statement below by selecting from the lists of options provided.

The patient is at high risk for **1 [Select]** as evidenced by **2 [Select]**.

Options for 1	Options for 2
Dehydration	Pain of 6 on 0-to-10 scale
Lymphedema	Decreased fluid intake
Sepsis	Fatigue
Skin dryness	Hypotension

3. The nurse determines the priority for the plan of care.

Choose the *most likely* options for the information missing from the statement below by selecting from the list of options provided.

The **priority** for the patient at this time is to **[Word Choice]** and **[Word Choice]**.

Word Choices
Manage pain
Help the patient to walk
Moisturize skin
Prevent further metastasis
Facilitate fluid intake

4. Choose three interventions the nurse will plan to include in the plan of care to meet the patient's priority needs.

- o Continue to administer oxycodone as prescribed.
- o Require the patient to perform hygiene care for exercise.
- o Ask patient to identify favorite nonalcoholic beverages.
- o Encourage regular ambulation several times daily.
- o Monitor vital signs at every nursing visit.
- o Contact the health care provider to admit patient to hospital.
- o Teach spouse about the pathophysiology of ovarian cancer.

5. As the nurse administers morning medication followed by hygiene care, the patient says, "I've made peace with dying, but I'm very worried about my husband. He's been taking care of me full-time for a year, and I don't know what he's going to do when I'm gone. It seems like he's already slipping into a deep depression."

Which of the following nursing responses are appropriate? **Select all that apply.**

- o "Why do you think your spouse has depression?"
- o "It sounds like you care about your spouse very much."
- o "If I were you, I would tell him to get a job to get out of the house."
- o "I can understand why you are concerned about your spouse."
- o "Can you explain how you have made peace with dying?"
- o "I am sure he will grieve, but eventually he will be okay."
- o "We can talk about this after we finish your hygiene care."
- o "I think you should tell your spouse how concerned you are."

6. One week later, the nurse is assigned to visit the patient at home again and performs an assessment.

For each patient finding, indicate whether the interventions instituted last week by the nurse were effective or not effective.

Previous Patient Finding	Current Patient Finding	Effective	Not Effective
Pain rated at 5 on 0-to-10 scale	Pain rated at 5 on 0-to-10 scale		
Had consumed very few oral fluids	Spouse confirms patient is drinking several glasses of water daily		
Expressed concern about spouse	States, "I talked with my spouse about how I feel."		
Ate half of scrambled egg before becoming nauseated	Reports eating one scrambled egg daily		
Skin thin and transparent	Skin dry		

Visit the Evolve site for Answers to the Clinical Judgment and Next-Generation NCLEX® Examination–Style Questions.

REFERENCES

American Nurses Association (ANA), Nursing Scope and Standards of Practice, American Nurses Association: *Nursing: scope and standards of practice*, ed 4, Silver Spring MD, 2021, ANA.

Beldhuis IE, et al: Cognitive biases, environmental, patient and personal factors associated with critical care decision making: a scoping review, *J Crit Care* 64:144–153, 2021. https://www.sciencedirect.com/science/article/pii/S0883944121000733?via%3Dihubhttps://www.sciencedirect.com/science/article/pii/S0883944121000733?via%3Dihub. Accessed November 28, 2023.

Centre for Evidence-Based Medicine: *Critical appraisal tools*, n.d. https://www.cebm.net/2014/06/critical-appraisal/. Accessed November 28, 2023.

Dickison P, et al: Integrating the National Council of State Boards of Nursing Clinical Judgment Model Into Nursing Educational Frameworks, *J Nurs Educ* 58(2):72, 2019.

Dimitroff LJ: *Journaling: a valuable tool for registered nurses*, American Nurse, 2018. https://www.myamericannurse.com/journaling-valuable-registered-nurses/. Accessed November 28, 2023.

Galutira GD: Theory of reflective practice in nursing, *Int J Nurs Sci* 8(3):51–56, 2018.

Kataoka-Yahiro M, Saylor C: A critical thinking model for nursing judgment, *J Nurs Educ* 33(8):351, 1994.

LaManna JB, et al: Teaching diagnostic reasoning to advanced practice nurses: positives and negatives, *Clin Simul Nurs* 26:24–31, 2019.

Miller M, Malcolm N: Critical thinking in the nursing curriculum, *Nurs Health Care* 11:67, 1990.

National Council of State Boards of Nursing (NCSBN): *Next Generation NCLEX News: Clinical Judgment Measurement Model*, winter 2019. https://www.ncsbn.org/publications/NGN-News-Winter-2019. Accessed November 28, 2023.

National Health Service (NHS): *Effective practitioner: clinical decision making*, n.d, http://www.effectivepractitioner.nes.scot.nhs.uk/media/254840/clinical%20decision%20making.pdf. Accessed November 28, 2023.

Nibbelink CW, Brewer BB: Decision-making in nursing practice: an integrative literature review, *J Clin Nurs* 27(5-6):917–928, 2018.

Patel KM, Metersky K: Reflective practice in nursing: a concept analysis, *Int J Nurs Knowl* 33(3):180–187, 2022. doi:10.1111/2047-3095.12350.

Paul RW: The art of redesigning instruction. In Willsen J, Blinker AJA, editors: *Critical thinking: how to prepare students for a rapidly changing world*, Santa Rosa, CA, 1993, Foundation for Critical Thinking.

Royce CS, et al: Teaching critical thinking: a case for instruction in cognitive biases to reduce diagnostic errors and improve patient safety, *Acad Med* 94(2):187–194, 2019.

Tanner CA, et al: The phenomenology of knowing the patient, *J Nurs Scholarsh* 25:273, 1993.

Tanner CA: Thinking like a nurse: a research-based model of clinical judgment in nursing, *J Nurs Educ* 45(6):204, 2006.

2 | Communication and Collaboration

SKILLS AND PROCEDURES

Skill 2.1 **Establishing the Nurse-Patient Relationship, p. 20**

Skill 2.2 **Communicating With Patients Who Have Difficulty Coping, p. 26**

Skill 2.3 **Communicating With a Cognitively Impaired Patient, p. 31**

Skill 2.4 **Communicating With Colleagues, p. 33**

Skill 2.5 **Workplace Violence and Safety, p. 35**

OBJECTIVES

Mastery of content in this chapter will enable you to:
- Explain the communication process.
- Identify the purposes of therapeutic communication in various phases of the nurse-patient relationship.
- Develop skills for therapeutic communication in various phases of the nurse-patient relationship.
- Create a plan to communicate therapeutically with patients or family caregivers who have difficulty coping because of feelings such as anxiety, anger, and depression.
- Develop therapeutic communication skills for communication with cognitively impaired patients.
- Develop skills for effective communication with colleagues.
- Outline strategies to prevent workplace violence.

MEDIA RESOURCES
- http://evolve.elsevier.com/Perry/skills
- Clinical Review Questions
- Audio Glossary
- Answers to Clinical Judgment and Next-Generation NCLEX® Examination–Style Questions
- Case Studies
- Skills Performance Checklists
- Printable Key Points

PURPOSE

Communication is the interaction between two or more people. Effective communication positively influences how nursing care is delivered and how satisfied patients are with that care. Your responsibility to effectively communicate extends beyond the patient to include family caregivers and all members of the health care team. The purpose of this chapter is to provide a framework to develop effective communication skills that are essential to the delivery of patient-centered care and to creating a safe workplace environment for patients and the health care team.

PRACTICE STANDARDS
- The Joint Commission (TJC), 2023: National Patient Safety Goals—Patient identification
- U.S. Department of Health and Human Services (USDHHS) Office of Minority Health, 2021—Cultural and Linguistic Competency

SUPPLEMENTAL STANDARDS
- Trans Student Educational Resources (TSER), 2021: Definitions

PRINCIPLES FOR PRACTICE
- Communication is an interaction between two or more people that involves the exchange of information between a sender and a receiver, involving the expression of emotions, ideas, and thoughts through verbal (words or written language) and nonverbal (behaviors) exchanges (Fig. 2.1).
- Therapeutic communication is a process of information exchange between a nurse and patient based on mutual respect and engagement (Xue & Fellow, 2021).
- Communication skills provide information and comfort, promote understanding, clarify misinformation, help in developing plans of care, promote interprofessional collaboration, and facilitate wellness through patient and family caregiver teaching.
- Communication includes both spoken and written words. To send an accurate message, the sender of verbal communication needs to be aware of the tone, volume, and cadence (pace or rate) of their voice.
- Nonverbal communication is all behavior that conveys messages without the use of words. This type of communication includes body movement, physical appearance, personal space, and touch. Be aware of body language, which includes posture, body position, gestures, eye contact, facial expression, and

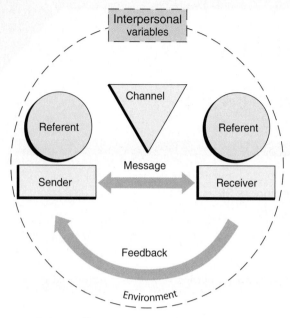

FIG. 2.1 Communication is a two-way process.

BOX 2.2	
Select LGBTQ+ Terms and Definitions	
Sex assigned at birth	Assignment and classification of people as male, female, intersex, or another sex assigned at birth.
Cisgender/cis	Someone who exclusively identifies as the sex assigned at birth.
Transgender/trans	Those who do not identify or exclusively identify with the sex assigned at birth.
Gender identity	One's internal sense of being male, female, neither of these, both, or other gender(s).
Transition	One's process of developing and assuming a gender expression to match their gender identity. Transition can include coming out to one's family, friends, and/or co-workers; changing one's name and/or sex on legal documents; hormone therapy; and possibly (although not always) some form of surgery.
Bigender	One who identifies as two genders. Can also identify as multigender.
Gender fluid	A changing ("fluid") gender identity and/or presentation.

Adapted from Trans Student Educational Resources (TSER). *Definitions*. (2021). <https://transstudent.org/about/definitions/>

movement. For clarity, make sure that nonverbal communication is consistent with the spoken word.

PERSON-CENTERED CARE

- Offer language assistance to individuals who have limited English proficiency (LEP) and/or other communication needs, at no cost to them, to facilitate timely access to all health care and services. Inform all patients of the availability of language assistance services clearly and in their preferred language, verbally and in writing (USDHHS, 2021) (Box 2.1).

BOX 2.1
Communicating With Patients Who Speak Different Languages
• Federal law requires linguistic services for patients with limited English proficiency (LEP).
• Health care agencies that receive federal funds are required to provide services in a language that a patient with LEP can understand.
• Professional interpreters improve communication, promote appropriate use of resources, and significantly increase patient and clinician satisfaction.
• Language interpretation requires bilingual fluency and the ability to switch fluidly between two languages while interpreting the meaning and tone of what has been said from one language to another.
• In choosing an in-person, a telephonic, or a video interpreter, consider resources available and the needs for your specific type of clinical situation.
• Talk in short units and pause frequently to promote accuracy of interpretation.

From AHRQ PSNet with permission from the Agency for Healthcare Research and Quality. The original WebM&M was written by Leah S. Karliner, MD, MAS: *When patients and providers speak different languages* (serial online: https://psnet.ahrq.gov/web-mm/when-patients-and-providers-speak-different-languages). Published April 1, 2018.

- Apply principles of inclusivity and respect to ensure that communication products and strategies adapt to the specific cultural, linguistic, environmental, and historical situation of each population or audience of focus (Centers for Disease Control and Prevention [CDC], 2022).
- Be mindful to address a person by the preferred pronouns (she/her, he/him, they/them) and that there are preferred terms for the LGBTQ+ community as to how one identifies; these are always changing (TSER, 2021) (Box 2.2).
- Communicate on the patient's level, considering the individual patient's vocabulary, educational background, and the effects of illness, without using a patronizing, condescending, or stigmatizing attitude (Steele, 2023).
- Therapeutic communication: Assess verbal and nonverbal patient communication needs, respect the patient's personal values and beliefs, allow time for communication, encourage the patient to verbalize feelings, and evaluate the effectiveness of communication (National Council of State Boards of Nursing [NCSBN], 2019).
- Acknowledge that many people with English as a secondary language are highly literate in a non-English language. Similarly, recognize that people may not be literate in their primary language, and avoid assuming that people with English as a secondary language will understand written information when it is translated into their primary language (CDC, 2022).
- Create a therapeutic environment: Identify external factors (e.g., stressors, family dynamics) that could interfere with the patient's recovery; make appropriate patient room assignments (NCSBN, 2019).
- Avoid dehumanizing language; for example, instead of using the terms *diabetics, the homeless,* and *disabled persons,* use *people with diabetes, people who are experiencing homelessness,* and *people who are experiencing [condition or disability type]* (CDC, 2022).

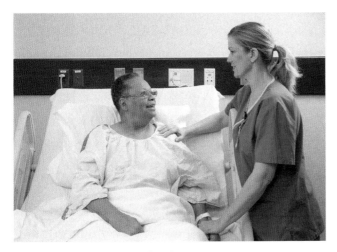

FIG. 2.2 An open, relaxed posture conveys interest.

- Be aware of cultural differences such as the use of touch and religious and ethnic practices because these influence methods of communication (Fig. 2.2).
- Adopt a flexible, respectful attitude that also communicates interest in a patient to bridge any communication barriers that exist because of cultural differences between a patient and caregiver.
- Provide easy-to-understand print and multimedia materials and signage in languages commonly used by populations in the health care agency service area (USDHHS, 2021).
- Listen to what and how a patient communicates, including content and verbal and nonverbal messages. Some patients express themselves clearly without difficulty. However, indirect and nonverbal cues communicate a patient's needs (e.g., pain, perceived stress).
- When teaching, try to have a family caregiver present with whom to reinforce the content of the instruction. Use language-appropriate print and multimedia materials. This is necessary for family caregivers to provide needed support when patients return home.

EVIDENCE-BASED PRACTICE

Nurses at Risk for Incivility and Bullying

Incivility and bullying comprise a wide range of disruptive, repetitive, and ineffective behaviors, including criticism and humiliation, and negative acts by an individual in a position of power with the intention to cause fear (Rutherford et al., 2019). Incidences of bullying between nurses, referred to as horizontal or lateral violence, and bullying of nurses by patients are underreported and sometimes difficult to recognize; however, some reports show that as many as 85% of nurses report experiencing bullying sometime in their career (Green, 2020). Research has begun to look closely at these acts, examining the reasons nurses feel they are at risk and the impact of bullying, to develop interventions aimed at prevention and supporting victims:
- Physical responses to bullying include somatic disturbances, fatigue, and risk for hypertension, heart disease, and maladaptive responses to stress. Psychological impacts include anxiety, depression, and posttraumatic stress disorder, which can occur even years after a bullying incident (Rutherford et al., 2019).

- Additional disorders and symptoms reported by victims include sleep disorders; reduced self-esteem; fear or lack of desire to go to work; excessive food consumption or reduced appetite; increased consumption of tobacco, alcohol, and/or drugs; and repeated sensations of irritability and anger (Bambi et al., 2019).
- Victims often choose to transfer units, leave their organization, or leave the nursing profession entirely (Bambi et al., 2019). There are financial implications for health care organizations for paid sick leave and the use of employee assistance programs. Hiring new nurses because victims have left their positions can cost an organization over $20,000 per person (Rutherford et al., 2019).
- Nurses feel they are targets for bullying because of their work environment, because they were new nurses, because there was an abuse of power, and because of the nature of the work they do.
- Organizations must support new nurses and manage relational attributes of the nursing work environment to reduce workplace bullying (Anusiewicz et al., 2020).
- Nursing students and professionals have used journaling to lessen the effects of bullying and create greater awareness to help them be part of creating a civil environment. Education to enhance awareness has also been highlighted as a means to prevent bullying (Bambi et al., 2019; Rutherford et al., 2019).
- Interventions to confront these problems include sensitizing nurses, managers, and administrators; organizing prevention education events; acquiring communication and conflict management skills; adopting zero tolerance strategies; and establishing codes of conduct that explicitly condemn unacceptable behaviors (Bambi et al., 2019).
- Formal and informal nursing leaders need education on fostering and sustaining favorable nursing work environments. Leaders need to set realistic expectations regarding the level of expertise for new nurses and ensure that new nurses are appropriately assigned patients based on acuity. New nurses need a gradual and fair increase in patient acuity workloads. (Anusiewicz et al., 2020).
- Form antibullying support groups in which victims feel safe to join and identify perpetrators. This allows nurses to seek help earlier and avoid prolonged trauma (Green, 2020).

SAFETY GUIDELINES

- Establish and understand the purpose of personal interaction. This is an essential quality of effective communication.
- Guide an interaction depending on the patient's condition and response. Patient needs remain the focus. For example, you establish that the purpose of the interaction is patient teaching. However, if the patient has just learned about the death of a loved one and expresses the need to talk about the death, you encourage this conversation and remain flexible and creative in the interaction. Or, if the patient complains of increased pain, provide an analgesic prior to implementing additional care plan needs.
- Control external factors in both the environmental setting (temperature of room, privacy issues) and the psychological setting (emotional state of the nurse and patient) that influence or hinder communication. When you are talking with a patient about a personal concern, privacy is important.

✦ SKILL 2.1 Establishing the Nurse-Patient Relationship

A therapeutic nurse-patient relationship is the foundation of nursing care and involves using a variety of patient-centered therapeutic communication skills (Box 2.3). The primary goal of therapeutic communication for a nurse is to promote patients' wellness and personal growth. Therapeutic communication empowers patients to make decisions but differs from social communication in that it is person centered, and goal directed with limited personal disclosure from the professional.

BOX 2.3

Therapeutic Communication Techniques

Technique: Active Listening
Definition: An active process of receiving information and examining one's reaction to messages received
Example: Consider the cultural practices of your patient, maintain appropriate eye contact, and be receptive to nonverbal communications.
Therapeutic Value: Nonverbally communicates your interest and acceptance to a patient
Nontherapeutic Threat: Failure to listen, interrupting patient

Technique: Broad Openings
Definition: Encouraging patient to select topics for discussion
Example: "Can you tell me what you're thinking about?"
Therapeutic Value: Indicates your acceptance and valuing of patient's initiative
Nontherapeutic Threat: Domination of interaction by nurse; rejecting responses

Technique: Restating
Definition: Repeating main thought that patient has expressed
Example: "You say that your mother left you when you were 5 years old."
Therapeutic Value: Indicates that you are listening and validates, reinforces, or calls attention to something important that has been said
Nontherapeutic Threat: Lack of validation of your interpretation of message; being judgmental; reassuring; defending

Technique: Clarification
Definition: Attempting to improve your understanding of words, vague ideas, or patient's unclear thoughts or asking patients to explain what they meant
Example: "I'm not sure what you mean. Could you tell me again?"
Therapeutic Value: Helps to clarify patient's feelings, ideas, and perceptions and provide an explicit correlation between them and patient's actions
Nontherapeutic Threat: Failure to probe; assumed understanding

Technique: Reflection
Definition: Directing back to patient ideas, feelings, questions, or content
Example: "You're feeling tense and anxious, and it's related to a conversation you had with your sister last night?"
Therapeutic Value: Validates your understanding of what patient is saying and signifies empathy, interest, and respect for patient
Nontherapeutic Threat: Stereotyping patient's responses; inappropriate timing of reflections; inappropriate depth of feeling of reflections; inappropriate to the cultural experience and educational level of the patient

Technique: Humor
Definition: Discharging energy through comic enjoyment of the imperfect
Example: "This gives a whole new meaning to 'Just relax'."
Therapeutic Value: Can promote insight by making conscious any repressed material, resolving paradoxes, tempering aggression, and revealing new options; is a socially acceptable form of sublimation
Nontherapeutic Threat: Indiscriminate use; belittling patient; screen to avoid therapeutic intimacy

Technique: Informing
Definition: Demonstrating skills or giving information
Example: "I think it would be helpful for you to know more about how your medication works."
Therapeutic Value: Helpful in patient education about relevant aspects of patient's well-being and self-care
Nontherapeutic Threat: Giving advice

Technique: Refocusing
Definition: Asking questions or making statements that help patient expand on a topic of importance
Example: "I think it would be helpful if we talk more about your relationship with your father."
Therapeutic Value: Allows patient to discuss central issues related to problem and keeps communication process goal directed
Nontherapeutic Threat: Allowing abstractions and generalizations; changing topics

Technique: Sharing Perceptions
Definition: Asking patient to verify your understanding of what patient is thinking or feeling
Example: "You're smiling, but I sense that you're really very angry with me."
Therapeutic Value: Conveys your understanding to patient and has potential for clearing up confusing communication
Nontherapeutic Threat: Challenging patient; accepting literal responses; reassuring; testing; defending

Technique: Theme Identification
Definition: Clarifying underlying issues or problems experienced by patient that emerge repeatedly during nurse-patient relationship
Example: "I've noticed that in all the relationships that you've described, you've been hurt or rejected by the man. Do you think this is an underlying issue?"
Therapeutic Value: Allows you to best promote patient's exploration and understanding of important problems
Nontherapeutic Threat: Giving advice; reassuring; disapproving

Technique: Silence
Definition: Using silence or nonverbal communication for a therapeutic reason
Example: Sitting with patient and nonverbally communicating interest and involvement
Therapeutic Value: Allows patient time to think and gain insights, slows the pace of the interaction, and encourages patient to initiate conversation while conveying your support, understanding, and acceptance
Nontherapeutic Threat: Questioning patient; asking for "why" responses; failing to break a nontherapeutic silence

Technique: Suggesting
Definition: Presenting alternative ideas for patient's consideration relative to problem solving
Example: "Have you thought about organizing your medications on a daily schedule? For example, you could use a pill organizer that allows you to sort out medicines to be taken each day or over a week."
Therapeutic Value: Increases patient's perceived options or choices
Nontherapeutic Threat: Giving advice; inappropriate timing; being judgmental

Adapted from Steele, D. (2023). *Keltner's psychiatric nursing* [9th ed]. St. Louis: Elsevier.

Social communication involves equal opportunity for personal disclosure, and both participants seek to have personal needs met (Steele, 2023). Nurses do not routinely share intimate details of their personal lives with patients. However, they use personal self-disclosure (e.g., outside interests, thoughts about local news, experience as a nurse) cautiously in selected situations. There are times when empathy is essential to establishing and maintaining the nurse-patient relationship. Empathy is being sensitive; it conveys an understanding of a patient's and/or family's feelings and communicating this understanding to them.

Barriers to therapeutic communication include giving an opinion, offering false reassurance, making disingenuous or insincere comments, being defensive, showing approval or disapproval, stereotyping, and asking, "Why?". The use of "why" questions causes increased defensiveness in patients and hinders communication. The therapeutic nurse-patient relationship is goal directed, with a patient moving toward productive modes of interpersonal functioning.

Delegation

All health care providers must practice effective communication. The skill of establishing therapeutic communication cannot be delegated to assistive personnel (AP). Direct the AP about:
- The proper way to interact verbally and nonverbally with select patients
- The need to keep all patient communication confidential
- Ways to arrange the environment to ensure privacy and confidentiality
- Special considerations pertaining to communication with patients who are cognitively or sensorially impaired, older adults, children, or those who are anxious and potentially violent

Interprofessional Collaboration

The nurse provides a role model for effective communication for members of the health care team.

STEP	RATIONALE

ASSESSMENT

1. Prepare for orientation phase of therapeutic communication. Formulate individualized goals for what you want to learn about the patient, consider time allocation (e.g., patient acuity and medical priorities), form initial questions, and mentally prepare to keep one's mind clear of other concerns or distractions. Select the assessment questions most relevant to the clinical situation.	Preparation is part of a planned communication process that facilitates interaction. Planning for the orientation phase helps to identify actual or potential problems, current health status, and experience. Without preparation, a risk exists for casual, non–goal-oriented communication.
2. Identify patient using at least two identifiers (e.g., name and birthday or name and medical record number) according to agency policy.	Ensures correct patient. Complies with The Joint Commission standards and improves patient safety (TJC, 2023).
3. Assess patient and family caregiver health literacy. What is the patient's primary language? *Option:* Use a standardized health literacy assessment tool such as the Short Assessment of Health Literacy—Spanish and English (SAHL-S&E); Rapid Estimate of Adult Literacy in Medicine—Short Form (REALM-SF); or Short Assessment of Health Literacy for Spanish Adults (SAHLSA-50) (CDC, 2023).	Determines degree to which individuals have the ability to find, understand, and use information and services to make informed health-related decisions and actions for themselves and others (CDC, 2023). Tools provide a direct comparison of health literacy in speakers of English and Spanish, the languages most frequently spoken in the United States (CDC, 2023).
4. Assess patient's ability to hear. Be sure that hearing aid is functional if worn (see Chapter 19). Be sure that patient hears and understands words.	Patients with hearing deficits require techniques to enhance hearing reception (e.g., speaking in normal tone, speaking so patient can see face).
5. Determine how the patient would like to be addressed. Address patient by name and introduce yourself and your role on the health care team ("Hello, my name is Jane Smith, and I am the registered nurse assigned to take care of you today.") Use clear, specific communication, including verbal and nonverbal techniques (e.g., good eye contact; relaxed, comfortable position) to provide information and clarify concerns (see Fig. 2.2). Create a climate of warmth and acceptance.	Congruent verbal and nonverbal communication expresses warmth and respect and helps to establish rapport. The quality of communication in interactions between nurse and patient has important influences on patient outcomes.
6. Assess the following during initial interaction: patient's perceived needs, coping strategies, defenses, and adaptation styles.	Recurrent themes in patient's responses help to identify problem areas related to health status (e.g., avoidance of questions, request for information, expression of a loss).
7. Determine patient's need to communicate (e.g., constant use of nurse call system, crying, patient who does not understand an illness or who has just been admitted).	Patients in need of support, comfort, knowledge, or encouragement benefit from individualized meaningful communication.
8. Observe patient's pattern of communication and verbal or nonverbal behavior (e.g., gestures, tone of voice, eye contact).	Observation determines type and manner of communication that you will use.

STEP	RATIONALE

Clinical Judgment *In times when you must wear a face mask (e.g., during the COVID-19 pandemic), keep in mind the impact on communication. An older adult may not feel comfortable discussing advance directives, those with hearing impairments may have more difficulty, and people with dementia usually interpret facial expressions correctly. Be mindful of gestures, tone, and body language; approach the patient from the front and make sure to respectfully speak at eye level (Schlög & Jones, 2020).*

    a. Observe for signs that patient has barriers in being allowed to communicate that may indicate abuse or human trafficking.

Avoiding eye contact and social interaction and not being allowed to be by themselves or speak for themselves are indications of abuse and human trafficking (State of Nevada, 2021).

9. Assess reason patient needs health care. Ask patient about health status, lifestyle, support systems, patterns of health and illness, and strengths and limitations.

Nature of illness affects patient's coping ability and effectiveness in communicating needs and concerns. For example, patients who are fearful of a cancer diagnosis and patients who are having joint replacement surgeries probably have differing needs and concerns.

10. Assess and reflect on variables about yourself and patient that normally influence communication. Examples of these variables include culture, experience, coping ability, and verbal/nonverbal behaviors (see illustration).

Communication is a dynamic process influenced by interpersonal and intrapersonal variables. By assessing factors that influence communication, you can more accurately assess a patient's perception of health status (Steele, 2023).

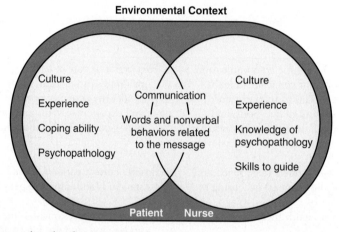

STEP 10 Essential and influencing variables of the therapeutic communication environment. (Adapted from Steele, D. [2023]. *Keltner's psychiatric nursing* [9th ed.]. St. Louis: Elsevier.)

11. Assess personal barriers to communicating with a patient (e.g., bias toward patient's condition, anxiety from inexperience).

Barriers prevent conveying empathy and caring and obtaining relevant assessment information.

12. Assess patient's use of language and ability to speak. Does patient have difficulty finding words or associating ideas with accurate word symbols? Does patient have difficulty with expression of language and/or reception of messages?

Assessment determines need for special techniques to address the communication needs of patients with limited English proficiency (LEP), hearing impairments, or literacy levels (USDHHS, 2021). Examples include picture boards, computers, sign language, or a medical interpreter (see illustration).

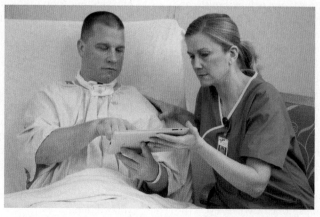

STEP 12 Communication tools for patient who cannot speak.

STEP	RATIONALE
13. Assess resources available in selecting communication methods:	
a. Review information in electronic health record (EHR) and reflect on your past patient communication experiences.	Relying totally on information from patient restricts the quality of interaction. Additional resources provide insight into best methods of communicating.
b. Consult with family, health care provider, and other health care team members concerning patient's condition, problems, and impressions.	Collaboration with health care team members facilitates your response to patient based on integration of knowledge. Seek information from family after patient approval. Patient privacy must be maintained.
14. Before initiating the working phase of nurse-patient relationship, assess patient's readiness to work toward goal attainment. "We want to work together with you to improve your health. I want to take some time together to learn what your expectations of care and goals are that you feel are important for you to recover."	Patient's goals are identified and agreed on by effective communication skills such as restating and clarifying.
15. Consider when patient is due to be discharged or transferred from health care agency. Share that information with patient and family caregiver.	This allows you to anticipate the amount of time available to work with patient and when termination of relationship is to occur.

PLANNING

1. Expected outcomes following completion of procedure:	
• Patient expresses ideas, fears, and concerns clearly, asks questions, and openly expresses relief of anxiety.	Once patients are able to talk directly about emotions, the focus is on coping more effectively with them (Steele, 2023). Asking questions shows an openness to communication.
• Patient's health care goals are identified and achieved.	Interaction remains patient focused.
• Patient verbalizes understanding of information communicated by nurse.	This provides a means to build trust and develop a knowledge base for patient to make decisions.
2. Before engaging in the working phase, prepare patient physically (e.g., provide comfort and pain-relief measures, provide for hygiene or elimination), provide a quiet environment, maintain privacy, and reduce distractions or interruptions before beginning discussion.	Taking care of basic needs promotes an environment for interaction and decreases patient distractions and interruptions.
3. Prepare necessary communication aids and initial communication approach.	
a. Use appropriate communication tools such as surface pads or other electronic devices for patients whose initial language is not English.	Electronic devices such as surface pads help with communication and provide translation resources.
b. Prepare open-ended questions to identify strategies for developing a realistic plan to meet identified health goals of patients (e.g., "Let's talk more about the goals you shared earlier for this hospitalization/visit to the health care agency").	Open-ended questions promote goal attainment and avoid risk of misinterpretation.

IMPLEMENTATION

1. Working phase:	
a. Observe patient's nonverbal behaviors, including body language.	Congruence between patient's verbal and nonverbal behaviors ensures that you receive the correct message.
b. If verbal behaviors do not match nonverbal behaviors, seek clarification from patient.	
2. Explain purpose of interaction when information is to be shared.	Information and explanation decrease anxiety about the unknown.
3. Use therapeutic communication skills throughout working phase (see Box 2.3).	Fosters open, interactive communication, with patient as a participant and the focus of the discussion.
4. Use questions carefully and appropriately. Ask one question at a time and allow sufficient time to answer. Use direct questions. Use open-ended statements as much as possible, such as, "Tell me about how you're feeling today."	This helps patients express themselves and allows you to obtain thorough information about needs and concerns.
5. Explore ways the health care team can meet patient's expectations in seeking health care.	Conducting interactions focused on patient's expectations conveys a level of interest in patient's needs.

STEP	RATIONALE
6. Encourage patient to ask for clarification at any time during the communication.	This gives patient a sense of control and keeps channels of communication open.
7. Set mutual goals.	
a. Use therapeutic communication skills such as restating, reflecting, and paraphrasing to identify and clarify strategies for attainment of mutually agreed-on goals (see Box 2.3).	For communication between nurse and patient to be effective, both need to possess the skills and knowledge required for participation within the communicative interaction.
b. Discuss and prioritize patient's perceived problem areas.	A patient, nonjudgmental, supportive approach minimizes patient anxiety.
c. Provide information to patients and help them to express needs and feelings.	Patient can respond to help, develop workable solutions based on goals, and fully participate in a realistic plan for well-being.

Clinical Judgment *Avoid asking questions about information that may not yet have been disclosed to the patient (e.g., human immunodeficiency virus [HIV] status, diagnostic test results). Avoid asking "why" questions; this causes increased defensiveness in the patient and prevents communication.*

STEP	RATIONALE
d. Avoid communication barriers (see Box 2.3).	Barriers result in a message not being received, being distorted, or not being understood.
8. Termination phase:	
a. Prepare by identifying methods of summarizing and synthesizing information pertinent for patient's aftercare (e.g., "What are your plans for follow-up once you return home to maintain your health status?").	Effective communication by summarizing and synthesizing information reinforces behavior change.
b. Use therapeutic communication skills to discuss discharge or termination issues and guide discussion related to specific patient changes in thoughts and behaviors.	Reinforces behaviors/skills learned during working phase of relationship.
c. Summarize with patient what you discussed during interaction, including goal setting and achievement.	Signals the close of interaction and allows you and patient to depart with the same idea. The termination phase consists of evaluation and summary of progress toward prescribed goals. Provides a sense of closure and mutual understanding.
9. For hospitalized patients, place nurse call system within patient's reach and raise side rails (as appropriate) and lower bed to lowest position, locking into position.	Ensures patient can call for assistance if needed. Ensures patient safety and prevents falls.

EVALUATION

1. Observe patient's verbal and nonverbal responses to your communication, noting willingness to share information and concerns during orientation phase.

    Verbal and nonverbal feedback reveals patient's interest and willingness to communicate and reflects patient's ability to form a therapeutic relationship.

2. Note your response to patient and patient's response to you. Reflect on effectiveness of therapeutic techniques used in establishing rapport with patient.

    Sensitivity to one's ability in using therapeutic communication skills improves ability to adjust techniques when necessary.

3. During working phase, evaluate patient's ability to identify and begin working toward identified goals. Elicit feedback (verbal and nonverbal) to determine success of goal attainment. During each therapeutic interaction, evaluate patient's health status in relation to identified goals. Reevaluate and identify barriers if patient goals are not met.

    Feedback is an essential step in evaluating new behaviors. Modifications are necessary if goals cannot be met.

4. During termination phase, summarize and restate. Reinforce patient's strengths, outline issues still requiring work, and develop an action plan.

    Evaluates patient progress in terms of attainment of mutually agreed-on goals.

5. **Use Teach-Back:** "I want to be sure that you understand the action plan following your discharge. We developed it together, taking into consideration your progress thus far and your strengths and limitations. Describe your action plan." Review the action plan or give patient/family caregiver the plan in a written/other format if patient/family caregiver is not able to teach back correctly.

    Teach-back is a technique for health care providers to ensure that they have explained medical information clearly so that patients and families understand what is communicated to them (Agency for Healthcare Research and Quality [AHRQ], 2023).

STEP	RATIONALE
Unexpected Outcomes	**Related Interventions**
1. Patient continues to verbally and nonverbally express feelings of anxiety, fear, anger, confusion, distrust, and helplessness. Patient often responds to internal and external factors and cues.	• Reassess patient's level of anxiety, fear, and distrust. Attempt to determine the cause of anxiety or fear. • Repeat message to patient at a later time. • Determine influence affecting clear communication (e.g., cultural issues, language issues, literacy issues, physical limitations).
2. Feedback between you and the patient reveals a lack of understanding and ineffective communication.	• Assess for and remove barriers to communication, such as literacy level, foreign language issues (USDHHS, 2021). • Repeat message using another approach if possible. • Consider cultural norms associated with eye contact, use of touch, personal space, and nonverbal behaviors. • Avoid using medical terms that patient does not understand.
3. You are unable to acquire information about patient's ideas, fears, and concerns. Communication techniques do not promote patient's willingness to communicate openly. Trust is not established. Goals are not identified and therefore cannot be achieved.	• Use alternative communication techniques to promote patient's willingness to communicate openly. • Offer another professional with whom patient can talk to obtain necessary information.
4. Family caregiver answers for patient even when patient can answer.	• Direct question to patient, using patient's name. • Acknowledge answer given by family caregiver, then state that you are interested in patient's response. • Resume interaction after family caregiver has left or encourage family caregiver to take a break for coffee or a meal.

Documentation

- Document communication pertinent to patient's health, response to illness or therapies, and responses that demonstrate understanding or lack of understanding (include verbal and nonverbal cues).
- Document teach-back and any changes to teaching plan.

Hand-Off Reporting

- Report any relevant information obtained through patient's verbal and nonverbal behaviors to members of health care team.

Special Considerations

Patient Education

- Use gestures, pictures, and role playing to help patient understand educational topic. Consider literacy status; determine if patient can access health information adequately. Be alert to words that patient seems to understand, and use them frequently.
- Individualize patient teaching to meet patient needs. Always conduct teaching with the purpose of meeting patient's learning needs with consideration for patient's preferred methods for learning.

Pediatrics

- Communicating with children requires an understanding of feelings and thought processes from the child's perspective (Hockenberry et al., 2024).
- Use vocabulary that is familiar to the child based on level of understanding (age and developmental level). Try to be on same eye level as patient.
- Understand the child's cognitive, developmental, and functional level to select most appropriate communication techniques.

Some age-appropriate communication techniques include storytelling and drawing (Hockenberry et al., 2024).

Older Adults

- Make sure that older-adult patients with visual or hearing impairment use assistive devices such as eyeglasses, large-print reading material, or hearing aids to assist in communication (Touhy & Jett, 2022).
- Be aware of any cognitive or sensory impairment. Assess each patient individually, and avoid stereotyping older adults who have cognitive or sensory impairments (Touhy & Jett, 2022).
- It is important to understand the value of effective communication skills, history, and personality among older adults in terms of providing both human and therapeutic responses. Regression to earlier defenses is normal and adaptive with this population, particularly when facing illness.

Populations With Disabilities

- Patients with intellectual and developmental disabilities (IDDs) may require you to take more time to get to know them as a person, their community, and their needs for additional support (Sullivan et al., 2018).
- Address the patient directly; use the patient's preferred communication method and tools; slow down communication; involve family caregivers, but be attentive to inappropriate taking over of decision making (Sullivan et al., 2018).

Home Care

- Identify primary family caregiver for patient, and adapt techniques to assess level of understanding regarding patient's condition.
- Incorporate communication into patient's daily activities (e.g., bathing and dressing).

✦ SKILL 2.2   Communicating With Patients Who Have Difficulty Coping

Patients in the health care setting may have difficulty coping with an illness or the health care environment itself for a variety of reasons and thus experience anxiety, anger, and/or depression. You can help the patient decrease or manage ineffective coping symptoms and behaviors through therapeutic communication. Examples of factors that cause anxiety are newly diagnosed illness, separation from loved ones, threat associated with diagnostic tests or surgical procedures, and expectations of life changes. How successfully a patient copes with anxiety depends in part on previous experiences, the presence of other stressors, the significance of the event causing anxiety, and the availability of supportive resources. There are four stages of anxiety with corresponding behavioral manifestations: mild, moderate, severe, and panic (Box 2.4).

Anger is the common underlying factor associated with potential for violence. Patients become angry for a variety of reasons. Anger is often directly related to a patient's experience with illness, or it is associated with previous problems. In the health care setting the nurse has frequent contact with patients and thus often becomes the target of their anger. Understanding how to use de-escalation skills is a useful technique to manage an angry or violent patient and help ensure a safe health care environment for other patients and health care personnel (Sharma & Gupta, 2022).

Depression is a state of feelings that is more than just sadness. It is a common psychiatric condition that affects a person's ability to function in day-to-day activities. There are many symptoms of depression, the most common being apathy, feelings of sadness, fatigue, guilt, poor concentration, sleep disturbances, and suicidal thoughts. Depression results in both subjective and objective behaviors and patient reports of increased physical complaints (Box 2.5). Some patients report feeling anxious when depressed.

Delegation

The skill of communicating therapeutically with a patient who has difficulty coping cannot be delegated to assistive personnel (AP). Direct the AP about:
- Basic communication skills needed to interact verbally and nonverbally with anxious, angry, or depressed patients
- When to contact the nurse if the patient's behavior or mood changes

---

BOX 2.4

Behavioral Manifestations of Anxiety: Stages of Anxiety

Mild Anxiety
- Increased auditory and visual perception
- Increased awareness of relationships
- Increased alertness
- Able to problem solve

Severe Anxiety
- Focus on fragmented details
- Headache, nausea, dizziness
- Unable to see connections between details
- Poor recall

Moderate Anxiety
- Selective inattention
- Decreased perceptual field
- Focus only on relevant information
- Muscle tension; diaphoresis

Panic State of Anxiety
- Does not notice surroundings
- Feeling of terror
- Unable to cope with any problem

BOX 2.5

Symptoms of Depression

Common Symptoms
- Apathy
- Decreased socialization
- Sadness
- Sleep disturbances
- Hopelessness
- Helplessness
- Worthlessness
- Guilt
- Anger

Other Symptoms
- Fatigue
- Decrease in performance of activities of daily living
- Thoughts of death
- Decreased libido
- Feeling inadequate
- Psychomotor agitation
- Verbal berating of self
- Spontaneous crying
- Dependency, passiveness

From Steele, D. (2023). *Keltner's psychiatric nursing* (9th ed.). St. Louis: Elsevier.

- Their role in the use of de-escalation techniques
- Appropriate safety measures for themselves and other patients

Interprofessional Collaboration

The nurse collaborates with the health care team to identify effective coping mechanisms unique to the patient.

STEP	RATIONALE

ASSESSMENT

1. Identify patient using at least two identifiers (e.g., name and birthday or name and medical record number) according to agency policy. Then provide a brief, simple introduction; introduce yourself and explain purpose of interaction.
2. Assess patient's/family caregiver's health literacy.

Ensures correct patient. Complies with The Joint Commission standards and improves patient safety (TJC, 2023).
Ineffective coping behaviors may limit amount of information patient can understand.
Determines degree to which individuals have the ability to find, understand, and use information and services to make informed health-related decisions and actions for themselves and others (CDC, 2023).

3. Assess factors influencing communication with patient (e.g., environment, timing, presence of others, values, experiences, need for personal space because of heightened anxiety).

Identifies effective communication strategies.

STEP	RATIONALE
4. Observe for physical, behavioral, and verbal cues that indicate that patient is anxious, such as dry mouth, sweaty palms, anxious tone of voice, frequent use of nurse call system, difficulty concentrating, wringing of hands, and statements such as "I'm scared."	Anxiety interferes with usual manner of communication and thus interferes with patient's care and treatment. Extreme anxiety interferes with comprehension, attention, and problem-solving abilities.
5. Assess for possible factors causing patient anxiety (e.g., hospitalization, unknown diagnosis, fatigue).	Understanding the source of anxiety helps in patient support and communication.
6. Discuss possible causes of patient's anxiety, anger, or depression with family members, including past history of the illness, if necessary.	Gathering information about patient from a family perspective is useful because family provides new information or understanding of the situation (Steele, 2023).
7. Assess for physical, behavioral, and verbal cues that indicate that patient is depressed, such as feelings of sadness, tearfulness, difficulty concentrating, increase in reports of physical complaints, and statements such as "I'm sad/depressed."	Depression interferes with usual manner of communication and thus with patient's care and treatment. If depression is severe, it interferes with comprehension, attention, and problem-solving abilities.
8. Assess for possible factors causing patient's depression (e.g., acute or chronic illness, personal vulnerability, recent loss).	Patient's depressive state is sometimes unknown. Understanding the possible cause of depression helps in patient support and communication.
9. Observe for behaviors that indicate that the patient is angry (e.g., pacing, clenched fist, loud voice, throwing objects) and/or expressions that indicate anger (e.g., repeated questioning of nurse, not following requests, aggressive outbursts, threats).	Anger is a normal expression of frustration or response to feeling threatened. However, its expression often interferes with or blocks communication and interactions.
10. Assess factors that influence the angry patient's communication, such as refusal to adhere to treatment goals, use of sarcasm or displaying hostile behavior, having a low frustration level, or being emotionally immature.	Allows you to accurately evaluate the situation or patient experiences that block or facilitate communication.
11. Assess for resources (e.g., social worker, pastoral care, or family) available to help in communicating with potentially violent patient.	This helps to clarify cause and intervention required to deal with patient's anger.
12. Assess for underlying medical conditions that may potentially lead to violent behavior.	Patients with medical conditions such as traumatic brain injury (TBI), dementia, or drug/alcohol withdrawal may exhibit hostile, aggressive behaviors (Steele, 2023).

Clinical Judgment *With some violent behaviors (e.g., physical aggression) you may not be able to de-escalate the situation. When this potential exists, know whom to call for assistance (e.g., trained psychology technicians, security staff). Personal safety is paramount (see agency policy).*

PLANNING

1. Expected outcomes following completion of procedure:	
• Patient discusses factors causing anxiety, anger, or depression.	Reflects success in making patient sense trust and ability to communicate openly.
• Patient can discuss methods to cope with anxiety, anger, or depression.	Reflects knowledge about resources made available (e.g., use of deep-breathing exercises, guided imagery) to cope with situations that cause anxiety, anger, or depression.
• Patient states that sensations of anxiety or depression are reduced.	Communication techniques ease symptoms associated with anxiety and depression and allow patient to focus on problem.

Clinical Judgment *First acknowledge and take care of anxious patient's physical and emotional discomfort, but avoid dwelling on physical complaints. Focus on understanding patient, providing feedback and helping to problem solve, and providing atmosphere of warmth and acceptance.*

• Patient no longer exhibits verbal and nonverbal expressions of anger.	De-escalation techniques successfully allow patient to express anger in a constructive way (Sharma & Gupta, 2022).
2. Prepare for therapeutic intervention by considering patient goals, time allocation, and resources.	Allows patient to establish rapport, achieve a sense of calm, and begin to analyze source of anxiety, depression, and anger.
3. Recognize personal level of anxiety and consciously try to remain calm (breathe slowly and deeply, relax pelvic floor muscles) when communicating with an anxious, angry, or depressed patient. Be aware of nonverbal cues that indicate own anxiety (e.g., body language, posture, cadence of speech). Remain nonjudgmental.	Your anxiety can increase a patient's anxiety. Your personal feelings and values may negatively affect interaction with patient.

STEP	RATIONALE
4. Prepare a quiet, calm area, allowing ample personal space.	Decreasing stimuli has a calming effect. Invasion of personal space increases anxiety, anger, or depression.
5. Prepare for de-escalation for an angry patient. a. Pause to collect own thoughts, feelings, and reactions.	Awareness and control of your reaction and responses facilitate more constructive interaction.
b. Listen carefully to determine what patient is saying.	Clarification of patient need or concern may help to de-escalate situation.
c. Prepare the environment to de-escalate a potentially violent patient:	Potentially violent patient needs to be in an environment with decreased stimuli and have protection from injury to self or others. Encourages patient's expression of anger rather than provoking it.
(1) Encourage other people, particularly those who provoke anger, to leave room or area.	Avoids pressuring patient; helps to prevent injury if anger becomes out of control.
(2) Maintain an adequate distance and open exit. Position yourself closest to door to facilitate escape from a potentially violent situation. Do not block exit so patient feels that escape is unattainable.	Prevents feeling of being trapped for both you and patient. Feeling trapped may cause a violent outburst. Safety of both parties is paramount.
(3) When anger begins to disturb others, close door. This is particularly important when patient becomes agitated.	Agitation and anxiety can spread to others. Some hospital rooms are equipped with security windows and cameras to allow for observation of patients.

Clinical Judgment *Some patients are disruptive to one another, especially those who are hyperactive, intrusive, or threatening or exhibit bizarre behaviors. For these patients, first try the least-restrictive measures before using more restrictive measures such as seclusion.*

(4) Reduce disturbing factors in room (e.g., noise, drafts, inadequate lighting).	Reduces irritants that may heighten anger.

IMPLEMENTATION

1. Use appropriate nonverbal behaviors and active listening skills such as staying with patient at bedside and having a relaxed posture. Focus on understanding the patient's issues.	Patients experiencing emotionally charged situation may not comprehend a verbally delivered message. Nonverbal messages to patient express interest and help alleviate anxiety.
2. Use appropriate verbal techniques that are clear and concise to respond to anxious patient. Use brief statements that acknowledge current state of feelings and provide direction to patient, such as, "It seems to me that you're anxious" or "I notice that you seem to want to be alone. Would you like to go to your room to rest?"	Promotes effective communication so patient can explore reasons for anxiety, anger, or depression. Appropriate techniques and statements provide reassurance.
3. Help patient acquire alternative coping strategies such as progressive relaxation, slow deep-breathing exercises, and visual imagery (see Chapter 16).	Coping strategies are nonpharmacological mechanisms to help the patient reduce anxiety and depression and, in some cases, reduce anger.
4. Provide necessary comfort measures such as analgesics, positioning, or hygiene.	Pain heightens patient's anxiety or depression and can contribute to anger.
5. Use open-ended questions, such as "Tell me about how you're feeling" or "You seem sad. Tell me about your sadness."	Encourages patient to continue talking, facilitating an in-depth discussion of symptoms.
6. Encourage and reward small decisions and independent actions. When necessary, make decisions that patients are not ready to make. Present situations that require no decision making.	Depressed patients are often overly dependent and indecisive.
7. Accept patients as they are and focus on their positive aspects. Provide positive feedback.	Depressed patients often have low self-esteem. This approach helps to focus on their strengths.
8. Be honest and empathic.	Honesty and empathy facilitate the development of trust.

Clinical Judgment *If your patient seems depressed, ask about suicidal ideation. Ask, "Have you had thoughts about hurting yourself? Have you felt like you don't want to live anymore?" If the patient endorses suicide, ask whether they have a plan. A patient with a well-developed plan is at increased risk for suicide. Risk factors include depression, previous suicide attempt, chronic mental disorders (especially those associated with chronic pain), serious illness, social isolation, and alcohol/drug use. Patients should be evaluated with a validated, age-appropriate screening tool and referred to appropriate mental health professional in agency (if available). Institute measures to ensure safety of patient (Steele, 2023).*

STEP	RATIONALE
9. De-escalation for an angry patient	
a. Maintain personal space. It may be necessary to have someone with you and to keep the room door open. Position yourself between patient and the exit.	Use of personal space may help to de-escalate patient's anger. Maintain a moderate distance without appearing guarded (Sharma & Gupta, 2022).
b. Maintain nonthreatening verbal and nonverbal approach using a calm, reassuring tone of voice. Use open body language with a concerned, nonthreatening facial expression, maintaining eye contact, open unfolded arms, relaxed posture, and a safe distance. Use gestures that are slow and deliberate rather than sudden and abrupt.	Decreases chance of misinterpretation of message and is less threatening. A relaxed atmosphere prevents further escalation. Creates climate of acceptance for patient.
c. Use therapeutic silence and allow patient to vent feelings. Use active listening for understanding. Do not argue with patient.	Often de-escalates anger. Anger expends emotional and physical energy; patient runs out of momentum and energy to maintain anger at high level. Arguing escalates anger.
d. Respond to anger therapeutically; avoid becoming defensive or angry and encourage verbal expression of anger.	Some depressed patients are angry; understand that anger is a symptom of their depression. Verbal expression often reduces tension.
e. Answer questions calmly and honestly as appropriate. If patient asks power-struggle–type question (challenging or confrontational type) (e.g., "Who said you were in charge?"), redirect and set limits by giving clear, concise expectations. Inform patient of potential consequences without sounding threatening and follow through with consequences if patient does not change behaviors.	A calm, clear communication style helps to set limits on power-struggle–type questions, provides structure for the interaction, and helps defuse anger (Steele, 2023).
f. If patient is making verbal threats to harm others, remain calm yet professional and continue to set limits on inappropriate behavior.	Angry patient loses ability to process information rationally and therefore may impulsively express anger through intimidation.

Clinical Judgment *If imminent harm to another person is present on discharge, notify proper authorities (e.g., nurse manager, security). A potentially violent patient can be impulsive and explosive; therefore you need to keep personal safety skills in mind. In this case, avoid touch.*

g. If patient appears to be calm and anger is defused, explore alternatives to situation or feelings of anger.	Processing with patient can prevent future explosive outbursts and teach patient effective ways of dealing with anger.

EVALUATION

1. Observe for continuing presence of physical signs and symptoms or behaviors reflecting anxiety, anger, or depression.	Observation determines extent to which planned interaction relieved patient's emotions.
2. Ask patient to describe ways to cope with anxiety, depression, or anger in the future and make decisions about own care.	This measures patient's ability to assume more health-promoting behavior.
3. Evaluate patient's ability to discuss factors causing anxiety, depression, or anger.	This measures patient's ability to attend to or focus on area of concern.
4. Note patient's ability to answer questions and problem solve.	Determines whether anger has lessened so patient is able to focus on alternative coping skills.
5. Use Teach-Back: "I want to be sure I explained options that will help you manage your anxiety in addition to medication. Describe a few of the exercises we discussed that will help you manage your anxiety." Revise your instruction now or develop a plan for revised patient/family caregiver teaching if patient/family caregiver is not able to teach back correctly.	Teach-back is a technique for health care providers to ensure that they have explained medical information clearly so that patients and families understand what is communicated to them (AHRQ, 2023).

Unexpected Outcomes

1. Physical signs and symptoms of anxiety/anger continue. Your interaction has increased patient's anxiety/anger; source of anxiety/anger is not resolved.

2. Patient displays difficulty making decisions by avoiding your efforts at focusing discussion or is unable to discuss real concerns. Anxiety/anger/depression continues to prevent problem solving.

Related Interventions

- Use refocusing or distraction skills such as relaxation or guided imagery to reduce anxiety (Steele, 2023).
- Reassess factors and remove or alter factors contributing to anxiety/anger.
- Take charge with calm, firm directions. Give as-needed (prn) medications as ordered for anxiety/agitation/escalating behaviors.
- Make sure that fellow staff members are available to help if necessary.
- Be clear and direct when communicating with patient to avoid misunderstanding.
- When used appropriately, touch helps control feelings of panic.

STEP	RATIONALE
3. Depressive behaviors continue; interaction has been ineffective at relieving depressive symptoms or patient reports suicidal ideation with or without plan.	• Continue to use therapeutic communication skills but try different techniques. • Refer patient to mental health professional for consultation regarding use of pharmacological agents and/or formal psychotherapy to treat depression. • Refer patient to mental health professional for evaluation and possible admission to an inpatient psychiatric treatment facility.

Documentation

- Document cause of patient's anxiety/anger/depression, any exhibited signs and symptoms of behaviors, and any methods used to enhance coping. Include direct quotes from patient demonstrating patient viewpoint.
- Document de-escalation technique used and patient's response to de-escalation efforts.
- Document your evaluation of patient and family caregiver learning.

Hand-Off Reporting

- Report methods used to relieve anxiety/anger/depression and patient's response to ensure continuity of care between nurses.
- Report technique used to de-escalate and patient's response to nurse in charge.

Special Considerations

Patient Education

- Teaching patient and family caregiver to identify possible sources of anxiety such as illness, hospitalization, knowledge deficits, or other known stressors gives patient knowledge of anxiety and increases patient's sense of control.
- Patients experiencing emotionally charged situations do not always comprehend instruction. Focus on understanding patient, making sure the patient correctly understands information, providing feedback, helping patient to problem solve, and providing an atmosphere of safety, warmth, and acceptance.
- Teaching patient and family caregiver to identify possible factors that contribute to angry outbursts may give patient a sense of control.
- Once anger has been de-escalated, teach patient new adaptive methods of coping with anger.
- Teach patient and family caregiver to identify possible sources and signs of depression. Knowledge of depression increases patient's sense of control over feelings of depression.

Pediatrics

- Children often demonstrate anxiety through physical and behavioral signs but are unable to express anxiety verbally. Some children express anxiety through restless behavior, physical complaints, or behavioral regression. Note any changes in child's behavior that occur during illness or hospitalization (Hockenberry et al., 2024).
- Set limits for inappropriate behaviors exhibited by child, such as a time-out. Apply such limits immediately because children tend to have less internal control over their own behaviors (Hockenberry et al., 2024).
- Children often demonstrate symptoms of depression that differ from those of adults. They manifest depression through physical (increased somatic complaints) and behavioral (poor school performance, social isolation) signs and are often unable to express it verbally. Some children express depression through restless behavior or behavioral regression. It is important to note any changes in a child's behavior that occur during illness or hospitalization (Hockenberry et al., 2024).

Older Adults

- Anxiety is common in older adults. Patients often become ritualistic and intent on performing activities a certain way. Anxiety develops as a result of a specific event or a general pattern of change (e.g., decline in health) (Touhy & Jett, 2022).
- Psychosocial factors such as anxiety and confusion, lack of mobility, and spatial organization of a long-term care facility are factors that decrease social contacts, thus hindering communication with peers and health care providers. This leads to further feelings of isolation, boredom, and increased anxiety.
- Older adults who are socially isolated have multiple medical problems and are more likely to have anxious and/or depressive symptoms. In addition, they are less likely to seek care for these symptoms.
- Depression among older adults is a major health concern. It is important to differentiate between depression and any underlying medical illness such as cognitive impairment (Touhy & Jett, 2022).
- Suicide risk is increased in older adults because of loss of life partner, health status, independence, and social support system or financial losses (Steele, 2023).

Populations With Disabilities

- Change in needs or a negative life event, such as loss of a support animal, loved one, or special caregiver, can lead to crisis. Assess and monitor family caregivers for stress, and advocate for respite care as needed (Sullivan et al., 2018).

Home Care

- Anticipation of a home care visit may increase a patient's anxiety and leads to exacerbation of symptoms.
- Personal safety for nurse against potentially violent patient or family caregiver extends to all health care settings, including patient's home. Assess patient's home and physical surroundings, including possible exits. You may be in a potentially dangerous situation while giving care to patient at home because you are without support from other staff members. Do not enter the home if you feel unsafe; call for help.
- Depression is often present among members who live together in home care settings. Educate family caregivers about how to identify symptoms. Manage depression based on patient's presenting behaviors, with consideration of any cognitive/physical impairment.

✦ SKILL 2.3 Communicating With a Cognitively Impaired Patient

The act of communicating and expressing oneself is affected by a person's cognitive ability. The need to receive, process, and integrate information from multiple sources is especially difficult for persons with a cognitive impairment (Hastings et al., 2021). Acute cognitive impairment or delirium is largely reversible and may be caused by conditions such as infection, polypharmacy, and metabolic changes. Once the cause is identified and treated, the patient's mental status returns to a baseline condition. Chronic types of cognitive impairments are irreversible and progressive. These include dementia (Alzheimer disease, vascular dementia, frontotemporal dementia), traumatic brain injury (TBI), and human immunodeficiency virus (HIV)–related cognitive dysfunction.

Cognitive impairments accompanied by communication deficits hinder a patient's ability to initiate conversation, communicate needs, and participate in self-care. Because it is time-consuming to interact with these patients, they may be deprived of human contact, which leads to depression, detachment, and isolation. Patients with cognitive impairments may also be at risk for physical status changes such as infection, falls and injury, and poor nutrition.

Delegation

The skill of communicating therapeutically with a cognitively impaired patient cannot be delegated to assistive personnel (AP). Direct the AP about:

- The proper communication skills needed to interact verbally and nonverbally with the cognitively impaired patient
- Notifying nurse if patient's ability to communicate worsens
- The possible causes and signs and symptoms of the patient's cognitive impairment and implications for communicating

Interprofessional Collaboration

- Lack of a high-quality relationship with the patient can negatively affect patient outcomes; collaborate with health care providers to communicate effectively.

STEP	RATIONALE
ASSESSMENT	
1. Identify patient using at least two identifiers (e.g., name and birthday or name and medical record number) according to agency policy.	Ensures correct patient. Complies with The Joint Commission standards and improves patient safety (TJC, 2023).
2. When you first meet a patient whom you expect to be cognitively impaired, approach from the front. Assess for the physical, behavioral, and verbal cues that indicate that a patient is cognitively impaired. Assess orientation status of patient (person, place, time) and perform a mini-mental examination (see Chapter 6).	You may startle and upset a patient if you touch them unexpectedly or approach from behind. If the patient is unable to think, speak, or understand, you need to adjust communication strategies to communicate effectively.
3. Assess patient's/family caregiver's health literacy with the simplest literacy screening tool.	Determines degree to which individuals have the ability to find, understand, and use information and services to make informed health-related decisions and take actions for themselves and others (CDC, 2023). Memory and verbal fluency are strongly associated with health literacy, even among those with subtle cognitive dysfunction. A lower level of literacy is associated with lower memory and verbal fluency.
4. Review electronic health record (EHR) and assess for possible factors causing patient's cognitive impairment (e.g., acute or chronic illness, fever, medications, fluid and electrolyte imbalance).	Understanding the possible cause of mental decline helps in conferring with medical team on appropriate therapy and has implications for short-term and long-term communication strategies.
5. Assess factors influencing communication with patient (e.g., environment, timing, presence of others, values, experiences, prior sensory loss, poor concentration).	Understanding factors that influence communication helps you to identify effective communication strategies (Steele, 2023).
6. Discuss possible causes of patient's cognitive impairment with family caregivers, including current illness, duration, treatment regimen, and past medical history.	Gathering information about patient from a family perspective is useful because family provides new information or understanding of the situation. It is important to establish patient's baseline mental status.
7. Discuss with family how patient typically communicates with them. Consider these questions: Does the patient lose train of thought, struggle to organize words logically, need more time to understand what you're saying, or curse or use offensive language? (Mayo Clinic, 2021).	Allows you to anticipate pattern of patient's communication so you can use effective communication strategies. Common types of conversation patterns include (Mayo Clinic, 2021): • Having trouble with finding the right word • Substituting words • Describing an object rather than naming it • Repeating words, stories, or questions • Mixing together unrelated ideas or phrases • Losing a train of thought • Speaking less often
8. Ascertain the most effective means of communication with patient (e.g., verbal or written communication, picture board).	Knowing how best to communicate and using alternative communication methods can help identify patient's needs.

STEP	RATIONALE

PLANNING

1. Expected outcome following completion of procedure:
   - Patient can communicate physical and emotional discomfort needs to nurse.

Use of relevant communication techniques enables patient to express needs (e.g., physical and emotional discomforts) effectively, given the limitations related to cognitive impairment.

2. Prepare for communication by considering type of cognitive impairment, communication impairments, time allocation, and resources.

Effective communication allows you to establish rapport with patient and have a high-quality nurse-patient interaction.

3. Be aware of your nonverbal cues that can affect communication with the cognitively impaired patient (e.g., body language, posture, cadence of speech). Remain nonjudgmental.

Frustration in communication with patients with cognitive impairment may negatively affect interaction with patient.

4. Prepare environment physically by providing a quiet, calm area. Reduce distractions such as external noises.

Decreasing stimuli has a calming effect. Ensuring that the environment is quiet and free from distractions enhances the communication experience.

IMPLEMENTATION

1. Approach patient from the front, and face patient when speaking.

This strategy avoids startling the patient and helps to ensure that patient both sees and hears you.

2. Provide brief, simple introduction. Introduce yourself, show respect, and explain purpose of interaction (Steele, 2023).

Symptoms associated with cognitive impairment limit amount of information that patient can understand.

3. Use appropriate nonverbal behaviors and active listening skills such as staying with patient at bedside or using touch appropriately.

Nonverbal messages to patient express your interest and convey empathy. Use of touch may help with concentration and reassurance.

4. Use clear and concise verbal techniques to respond to patient (Mayo Clinic, 2021). Be patient. Use simple language and speak slowly; use short and simple sentences, be connected, and offer comfort. Ask yes-or-no questions.

Appropriate techniques and statements provide reassurance to cognitively impaired patient.

5. Ask one question at a time and allow time for response. Avoid rushing patient. Do not interrupt patient (Steele, 2023).

This gives patient time to process the information and respond.

6. Repeat sentences using a steady voice and avoid raising your voice or being too quick to guess what patient is trying to express.

Repetition allows time for patient to respond. Attempting to guess what the patient is saying is frustrating for the patient if you misinterpret their message or pressure them to respond.

7. Use augmentative and assistive communication (AAC) devices such as pictogram grid, talking mats, objects, and surface pads to facilitate communication.

Talking mats are communication aids that use picture symbols; the patient can place relevant images below a visual scale to indicate feelings.

8. Make sure that patient is wearing eyeglasses or hearing aids to help with communication.

Some patients with cognitive impairments forget about eyeglasses or hearing aids and need to be reminded to use these to improve clarity of communication.

9. Do not argue with patient or correct patient if mistakes are made.

Arguing can lead to increased frustration and agitation.

10. Maintain meaningful interactions with patients and use creative modes of communication based on patient's comfort level and abilities.

Meaningful interactions help patient engage with family or community and surroundings and help reduce a sense of isolation and detachment.

11. Use individualized coping strategies such as progressive relaxation, slow deep-breathing exercises, or visual imagery.

Helps to reduce some anxiety associated with confusion and difficulties in communication.

EVALUATION

1. Observe patient's response for clarity and understanding of messages sent and received.

Observation determines extent to which cognitively impaired patients can express themselves.

2. Observe verbal and nonverbal behaviors.

Observation reveals if patient is comfortable and needs have been met.

3. **Use Teach-Back:** "I want to be sure I explained how this picture board will help you communicate with your family. Tell me how to use the picture board to show your wife that you want to take a shower or take a walk together." Revise your instruction now or develop a plan for revised patient/family caregiver teaching if patient/family caregiver is not able to teach back correctly.

Teach-back is a technique for health care providers to ensure that they have explained medical information clearly so that patients and families understand what is communicated to them (AHRQ, 2023).

STEP	RATIONALE

Unexpected Outcomes

1. Messages that are sent and received are not understood.

2. Patient becomes frustrated, and communication with nurse becomes more challenging.

Related Interventions

- Continue to use therapeutic communication skills when interacting with cognitively impaired patient. Be creative in using alternative strategies (e.g., involving family members).
- Speak to patient as an adult and give time to process information.
- Use verbal and nonverbal methods to convey empathy with patient's frustration.
- Allow for periods of adequate rest; make frequent attempts to interact to minimize social isolation.

Documentation

- Document objective and subjective behaviors (associated with cognitive impairment) that patient is displaying and objective behaviors (associated with cognitive impairment) observed.
- Document the methods used to communicate with the patient and patient's response.
- Document your evaluation of patient and family caregiver learning.

Hand-Off Reporting

- Report the methods used to communicate and patient's response.

Special Considerations
Patient Education

- Teach patient and family caregiver how to use various methods to communicate such as picture board or communication aids.
- Make teaching modifications with a consideration of impaired concentration and memory related to patient's cognitive status (e.g., present a small amount of material at a time; use simple and short phrases; repeat information as needed).

Pediatrics

- Children may exhibit cognitive impairments because of acute or chronic metabolic or neurological conditions. Know the child's developmental level when identifying communication strategies. Use pictures and drawings for patients who are unable to read.

Older Adults

- Many older adults have cognitive impairments that can pose serious barriers to the reliability of your assessment findings; therefore it is important to use effective verbal and nonverbal communication strategies. Poor communication can compromise care, leading to increased anxiety and frustration.
- Patients who have cognitive impairments may exhibit tantrum-like behaviors in response to real or perceived frustration. Use distraction techniques to remove a cognitively impaired older-adult patient from disturbing stimuli or redirect patient to activity that is pleasurable (Touhy & Jett, 2022).

Populations With Disabilities

- Assess patient's ability for decision making; many patients can participate to some extent if provided accommodations (Sullivan et al., 2018).

Home Care

- Include the family caregiver and friends in learning and using effective communication strategies.
- Address potential issues of driving, getting lost, and home safety each time you see the patient.
- Encourage regular physical activity, social activity, hobbies, and intellectual stimulation, as well as a healthy diet. Research links these approaches to the maintenance of cognitive function.

◆ SKILL 2.4 Communicating With Colleagues

In health care settings, communicating is a key part of everyday practice. You communicate with patients, family members, members of the interprofessional health care team, and external colleagues. This communication occurs face-to-face, over the phone, and in writing. The quality of these interactions is a key component of error prevention; clarity, comprehension, and adherence to treatment plans; and patient outcomes. TJC publishes National Patient Safety Goals, one of which is to "improve the effectiveness of communication among caregivers" (TJC, 2023). Collaboration among all health care professionals increases team members' awareness of one another's type of knowledge and skills, leading to continued improvement in clinical judgment, decision making, and patient outcomes.

SBAR (Situation, Background, Assessment, Recommendation) is one system that allows for structured communication among health care team members, allowing a way to set expectations for communication and provide a means to avoid omitting important information in hand-off reporting (see Chapters 3 and 4). SBAR has been shown to improve the quality of communication among health care providers,

enhance perspectives of patient safety, and reduce medical errors, resulting in improved quality of care and reduced cost for medical care (Dung, 2021). SBAR is an interprofessional, simple communication technique that can improve the overall culture of safety while increasing health care provider satisfaction.

Creating a civil work environment and enhancing communication are the responsibilities of all health care providers. Policies geared toward eliminating workplace incivility should be implemented, as uncivil acts can lead to poor quality of nursing care (Alshehry et al., 2019). All nurses should be proactive in recognizing, preventing, approaching, reporting, and intervening with uncivil acts to protect one another from these types of behaviors and avoid negative impacts on patient care (Alshehry et al., 2019). Conflicts among colleagues can indirectly influence the therapeutic nurse-patient relationship and negatively affect the delivery of care and patient and health care provider satisfaction. If conflicts are not resolved, they can escalate into workplace bullying, which is abusive conduct that is threatening, humiliating, or intimidating and interferes with a productive work environment (Clark, 2019).

Effective communication is necessary to resolve conflict among members of the health care team before situations escalate. Good communication in the form of conflict resolution skills can decrease the risk of conflict and its negative effects. Health care agencies need to be proactive to create healthy work environments with a shared philosophy of civility and respect (Clark, 2019).

Delegation

The skill of communicating effectively with colleagues can be delegated to assistive personnel (AP). Instruct the AP about:

- The proper communication skills needed to effectively interact verbally and nonverbally with colleagues to promote respectful communication

Interprofessional Collaboration

All members of the health care team should be expected to practice effective and respectful communication.

- Reflection on the way one wishes to live and perceptions of practice can help reduce incidences of uncivil behavior (Anusiewicz et al., 2020). This can be done individually and as a routine part of team meetings.
- Self-care workshops can be a means to enhance resilience and well-being and to create healing and healthy work environments (Barrett, 2019).

STEP	RATIONALE
ASSESSMENT	
1. Identify purpose of interaction with colleague.	This sets the stage for the interaction; all participants in the communication exchange are aware of purpose of conversation.
2. Assess factors influencing communication with others (e.g., environment, timing, workplace dynamics, presence of others' cultural beliefs and values, prior experiences).	Assessment allows you to accurately evaluate any barriers to communication or issues that may need to be considered to maintain open, clear channels of communication.
3. Consider level of stress in the situation; do you feel uncomfortable or threatened?	Feeling threatened results in a sympathetic stress response that can impair judgment, emotional control, and ability to communicate clearly.
PLANNING	
1. Prepare for communication with members of the health care team who may have differing needs or concerns. Example: If you feel stressed, try to relax, and perform deep breathing to consciously relax muscles of pelvic floor.	Effective communication allows members of the health care team to establish rapport and have a high-quality interaction. Adapt own style of communicating (e.g., relaxation) to meet the needs of the health care team.
2. Be aware of your nonverbal cues that affect communication with others. Remain nonjudgmental.	Frustration in communication may negatively affect interaction with others.
3. Prepare environment physically; go to a quiet, calm area. Reduce distractions such as external noises.	Factors to consider include privacy, noise control, seating space, and convenience to help ensure the space needed for effective teamwork.
4. Be aware of hierarchical differences among members of the health care team (e.g., nurse manager, charge nurse, staff nurse, physician, therapist) as a common barrier to effective communication and collaboration.	The hierarchical nature of health care can be a barrier to effective communication (Anusiewicz et al., 2020).
IMPLEMENTATION	
1. Approach colleagues from the front and face them when speaking. Maintain appropriate eye contact.	This strategy ensures that colleague both sees and hears you and conveys an attitude of respect.
2. Provide brief, simple introduction; introduce yourself and explain purpose of interaction.	This strategy ensures that colleague understands purpose of interaction.
3. Be aware of your own body language and tone. Assume an open stance; do not fold arms across your chest.	Nonverbal messages convey empathy. Be aware of how your nonverbal communication style may affect others.
4. Acknowledge and respond to a range of views. Allow for equal time for all parties to participate in expressing opinions.	Understand the perspectives of others, and support the value of collaboration and teamwork.
5. Use oral communication skills such as: ask open-ended questions; do not assume; do not interrupt; do not blame others. Provide feedback. Use active listening and recognize nonverbal triggers. Ask for clarification when necessary.	Effective communication skills are essential for communicating information and resolving conflict.
6. Use a range of workplace written communication methods (e.g., oral, written notes, memos, letters, charts, diagrams).	Standardized communication such as the SBAR method of communication can help streamline information exchanges and promote patient safety (Dung, 2021).
7. Encourage discussion of both positive and negative feelings to increase the chances of both parties expressing all of their concerns.	Discussion fosters active listening and understanding. All members of the exchange are valued, and their contributions are recognized.

STEP	RATIONALE
8. Summarize key themes in the discussion and help develop alternative solutions to the issue.	Conflict resolution involves examining alternative solutions to an issue. It values the influence of system solutions in achieving effective functioning among colleagues (Clark, 2019).

EVALUATION

STEP	RATIONALE
1. Confirm clarity and understanding of messages sent and received.	Determines extent to which members of the exchange understand.
2. Observe verbal and nonverbal behaviors.	Observation reveals if there are any negative emotions or further concerns that contradict a message.

Unexpected Outcomes	Related Interventions
1. Messages that are sent and received are not understood.	• Continue to use therapeutic communication skills when interacting with others. Be creative in using alternative strategies.
2. Frustration among colleagues persists, and communication becomes more challenging.	• Continue to have empathy, and use active listening to better understand colleagues. • Consult with manager or team leader to provide group meeting to address specific issues.
3. Bullying behaviors (verbal attacks, threats, spreading rumors and gossip, public ridicule, purposefully withholding vital information) occur (Clark, 2019).	• Follow agency protocol to report behaviors immediately, and seek assistance of agency security personnel.

✦ SKILL 2.5 Workplace Violence and Safety

Workplace violence targeting health care workers is a widely recognized problem. Examples of workplace violence include direct physical assaults (with or without weapons), written or verbal threats, physical or verbal harassment, bullying, and homicide (Occupational Safety and Health Administration [OSHA], 2016). The American Hospital Association (AHA) in collaboration with the International Association for Healthcare Security and Safety (IAHSS) recommends action steps for hospital leaders to build a safer workplace (AHA, 2021). This framework guides leaders in building a culture of safety, mitigating risk, violence intervention, and supporting trauma survivors. In order to mitigate violence, leaders can develop a threat management team to address violence and institute a zero-tolerance policy for all workplace violence. De-escalation is the ability to organize one's thinking and calmly respond to a threatening situation in a manner that helps one avoid a potential crisis (Crisis Prevention Institute [CPI], 2022). A workplace violence hazard assessment must be conducted to assess risk factors prior to implementing de-escalation techniques.

Services should be implemented to investigate any violent incident as well as to provide debriefing for health care staff involved in an incident to help minimize prolonged trauma effects.

Delegation

All health care providers must practice de-escalation techniques. The skill of intervening during a violent event cannot be delegated to assistive personnel (AP). Direct the AP to:
• Assess for potential hazards and risk factors for patient violence
• Notify the nurse of any hazards or risk factors
• Confirm understanding of de-escalation techniques

Interprofessional Collaboration

• Workplace safety is the responsibility and concern of all members of the health care team.
• The nurse will participate in prevention, identification, and interventions to promote safety and address workplace violence.

STEP	RATIONALE

ASSESSMENT

STEP	RATIONALE
1. Assess baseline knowledge of agency staff regarding workplace violence.	It is imperative that staff be aware of the agency's emergency management plan to maintain a safe environment for patients, family caregivers, and health care staff.
2. Identify organizational risk factors for workplace violence: • Lack of agency policies and staff training for recognizing and managing escalating hostile and assaultive behaviors from patients, clients, visitors, or staff • Working when understaffed—especially during mealtimes and visiting hours • High worker turnover • Inadequate security and mental health personnel (OSHA, 2016)	Identifies factors in a work setting that if not addressed make health care staff unequipped to manage violent situation.

STEP	RATIONALE
3. Identify patient- and setting-related risk factors for workplace violence: patients who are experiencing unrelieved pain, showing mood-altering behaviors, or are impaired due to ethyl alcohol (ETOH)/drugs. High-risk settings include the emergency department, psychiatric units, and geriatric long-term care facilities (OSHA, 2016).	Identifies factors within a work setting that increase risk of health care workers being exposed to violent behavior.
4. Assess patient for signs and symptoms of potentially violent behavior: recent stressors or losses (e.g., job loss, divorce); history of confirmed psychiatric disorder; history of drug or alcohol (ETOH) abuse or aggression; content of speech and tone of voice indicating agitated state (loud voice, angry tone); escalating verbal and nonverbal behaviors, including cursing or name-calling, pacing, and clenched fists.	All are risk factors for violence.

PLANNING

1. Expected outcomes following completion of procedure:	
• Potentially violent patient situations are avoided and/or minimized.	Participation in workplace violence prevention programs helps nurses to address potential problems before they arise and ultimately reduces the likelihood of workers being assaulted (AHA, 2021).
• Incident reporting and debriefing occur when indicated.	Established policies ensure the reporting, documentation, and monitoring of incidents and near misses helps identify root causes and helps prevent future incidents of violence (OSHA, 2016).

Clinical Judgment *Research has shown a link between nurses' experience of workplace bullying and poor patient care (Anusiewicz et al., 2020). All health care providers are responsible for maintaining a safe work environment and reporting risks/incidents.*

IMPLEMENTATION

1. Use notification system for identifying high-risk patients: label or color-code medical records; supply potentially violent patients with different colored socks.	Indicates to health care team patients most likely to commit a violent act. Acknowledges the value of a safe, healthful, violence-free workplace.
2. Remove opportunity for any type of weapon to be used by patients or visitors (bodily fluids, medical supplies, meal tray and utensils, personal items, furniture).	Managing threats of violence involves recognizing potential weapons and taking a proactive approach to minimizing use of those items (AHA, 2021).
Be aware of personal space with patient who may try to bite, hit with fists, or throw bodily fluids. Observe body stance (clenched fists, feces in hands).	Removing the potential risk and stimulus can eliminate and block the opportunity to act.
3. Do not work alone if feeling uncomfortable with a patient. Use measures to prevent or control workplace hazards.	Use of physical barriers (guards, door locks), metal detectors, panic buttons, better lighting, and accessible exits can reduce employee exposure.
4. Make sure all staff are trained to cope with physical and verbal abuse by using the following de-escalation techniques (CPI, 2022):	Victims of hospital violence are most often untrained or newly hired nurses, so prepare by training them with proven strategies for safely defusing anxious, hostile, or violent behavior at the earliest possible stage. This includes teaching them to look for warning signs, ask for help if they feel unsafe, and report any violent or suspicious behavior to a supervisor.
a. Be empathetic and nonjudgmental.	When someone says or does something you perceive as weird or irrational, try not to judge or discount their feelings. Whether you think those feelings are justified, they are real to the other person. Pay attention to them (CPI, 2022).
b. Respect personal space.	If possible, stand 1½ to 3 feet away from a person who is escalating. Allowing personal space tends to decrease a person's anxiety and can help you prevent acting-out behavior (CPI, 2022).
c. Use nonthreatening nonverbal behaviors.	The more a person loses control, the less they hear your words—and the more the person reacts to your nonverbal communication. Be mindful of your gestures, facial expressions, movements, and tone of voice (CPI, 2022).

STEP	RATIONALE
d. Avoid overreacting. Remain calm, rational, and professional.	Although you cannot control the person's behavior, how you respond to that behavior will have a direct effect on whether the situation escalates or defuses (CPI, 2022).
e. Focus on feelings.	Facts are important, but how a person feels is the heart of the matter. However, some people have trouble identifying how they feel about what is happening to them (CPI, 2022).
f. Ignore challenging questions.	Answering challenging questions often results in a power struggle. When a person challenges your authority, redirect their attention to the issue at hand (CPI, 2022).
g. Set limits.	If a person's behavior is belligerent, defensive, or disruptive, give them clear, simple, and enforceable limits. Offer concise and respectful choices and consequences (CPI, 2022).
h. Choose wisely what you insist on.	It is important to be thoughtful in deciding which rules are negotiable and which are not. For example, if a person does not want to shower in the morning, try to allow them to choose the time of day that feels best (CPI, 2022).
i. Allow silence for reflection.	Although it may seem counterintuitive to let moments of silence occur, sometimes it is the best choice. It can give people a chance to reflect on what is happening and how they need to proceed (CPI, 2022).
j. Allow time for decisions.	When people are upset, they may not be able to think clearly. Give them a few moments to think through what you have said (CPI, 2022).
k. Use concise, simple language.	Elaborate and technical terms are difficult for an impaired person to understand (Sharma & Gupta, 2022).
5. Notify security staff to intervene if patient begins unruly behavior or if additional information is needed to determine potential for violence. (See agency policy for how to notify security.)	If a patient begins to exhibit unruly behavior, you may request a security consultation to determine whether the patient poses a threat. If officers identify danger, a patient will undergo a safety assessment including a detailed search of personal effects for any weapons or dangerous items.
6. If an incident occurs, initial steps are first aid and emergency care for the injured workers and prevention of further injury.	Following a violent incident, first determine the extent of injuries and establish priorities of treatment.
7. Debrief using standard postincident procedures and services. The purpose of an investigation should be to identify the root cause of the incident.	Root causes refer to all possible causes associated with the incident of violence. If the root cause is not addressed and/or corrected, it will inevitably recreate the conditions for another incident to occur (OSHA, 2016).

Clinical Judgment *The nursing code of ethics and antibullying policies need to be strictly enforced. Nurses need a safe space to voice their concerns on bullying within the organization (Shorey & Wong, 2021).*

8. Refer colleague to any agency program for medical and psychological counseling and debriefing for staff who have experienced and witnessed assaults or violent incidents.	A strong follow-up program for these workers will not only help them address these problems but also help prepare them to confront or prevent future incidents of violence (OSHA, 2016).

EVALUATION

1. Evaluate staff comprehension of workplace violence program and de-escalation strategies.	Ensures staff preparation for any violent events. Require annual certification for all staff in safety training.
2. Monitor prevention impact. Evaluate prevalence of such incidents on a regular basis.	Data determine need to revise training or to assist select individuals with prevention techniques.
3. If there is a violent incident, evaluate safety of all persons involved. Provide prompt medical treatment for victims of workplace violence.	Worker well-being is critical to maintain safety and stability of work environment.
4. If there is an incident, immediately evaluate the effectiveness of the de-escalation techniques implemented. Victims of an assault, as well as their co-workers, need the opportunity to discuss their concerns and feelings about the event as a way to debrief.	A critical incident debriefing suggests ways to prevent similar incidents in the future. Critical incidents can cause emotional reactions that affect health care workers' ability to function.

STEP	RATIONALE
Unexpected Outcomes	**Related Interventions**
1. There is a violent incident between patient and nursing staff.	• Notify the agency's interprofessional response team. • Provide immediate treatment to persons injured. • Report the presence of a weapon immediately to a manager, a supervisor, or security (AHA, 2021). • Implement postincident procedures (root cause analysis and follow-up debriefing for staff).
2. De-escalation techniques are ineffective.	• Further workplace violence prevention training is necessary for staff.

Documentation

- Document hazard assessment and strategies used to promote a safe environment for incident involving patient.
- Document escalating behaviors exhibited by patient, any injuries, de-escalation techniques used by staff (effective and not effective), any treatment, and outcome of incident.

Hand-Off Reporting

- Provide detailed assessment of potentially hazardous situation.
- Report patients who are flagged as high risk for potentially violent behaviors.
- Report strategies implemented to prevent escalating behaviors.
- Report any violent incidents and outcomes associated with the incidents.

✦ CLINICAL JUDGMENT AND NEXT-GENERATION NCLEX® EXAMINATION–STYLE QUESTIONS

The nurse is caring for an 89-year-old patient with Alzheimer disease. The patient was admitted after becoming violent at home and attempting to hit the 50-year-old daughter, who is the primary family caregiver. During the altercation, the patient fell and now has a superficial laceration to the left side of the head and bruising around the left eye and is holding his left arm, which has a bruise at the elbow. Emergency services were called to assist; the daughter states the patient has never been physically violent in the past. She is tearful and states, "I can't believe my father attacked me." History reveals a progressive decline in mood and appetite over the past 3 months. Current body mass index (BMI) is 22. Currently the patient is exhibiting a heightened level of confusion and expressions of anger.

1. Choose four assessment findings the nurse will plan to communicate immediately with the primary health care provider.
   1. Daughter's grief
   2. Holding left arm
   3. Bruising of left eye
   4. Current heightened confusion
   5. Superficial laceration of the head
   6. Mood changes over the past 3 months
   7. New behavior involving physical altercation
2. Which of the following communication strategies will the nurse choose to use when talking directly with this patient? **Select all that apply.**
   1. Engage in active listening.
   2. Stand beside the patient to talk.
   3. Repeat sentences calmly as needed.
   4. Give the patient an electronic device to use when talking.
   5. Allow time for the patient to respond after asking a question.
3. The patient's daughter asks the nurse several questions about the patient's condition. Which of the following nursing statements is/are appropriate when responding to the daughter? **Select all that apply.**
   1. "I assume you understand your father's condition."
   2. "You're feeling tense and anxious."
   3. "I think you're being too hard on the patient."
   4. "I can empathize with how you're feeling."
   5. "Let's sit together so I can answer your questions."

4. Once the patient has been admitted to a medical unit for observation, which of the following communication techniques will the nurse use? **Select all that apply.**
   1. Respect the patient's personal space.
   2. Scold the patient for his behavior.
   3. Speak kindly even if the patient is verbally unkind.
   4. Suggest that the family caregiver intervene first if the patient acts out.
   5. Avoid overreacting to the patient's behavior.
5. Several months later, the patient is seeing the primary health care provider. The daughter tearfully reports that the patient has further cognitive impairment and rarely verbalizes. Which nursing response is appropriate?
   1. "He would likely respond if you would talk more to him."
   2. "This was expected since your father has Alzheimer disease."
   3. "Have you done something that makes him want to talk less?"
   4. "I am very sorry; this must be difficult for you to experience."

Visit the Evolve site for Answers to the Clinical Judgment and Next-Generation NCLEX® Examination–Style Questions.

REFERENCES

Agency for Healthcare Research and Quality (AHRQ): *Teach-back: intervention*, 2023. https://www.ahrq.gov/patient-safety/reports/engage/interventions/teachback.html.

Alshehry AS, et al: Influence of workplace incivility on the quality of nursing care, *J Clin Nurs* 28:4582, 2019.

American Hospital Association (AHA): *Creating safer workplaces: a guide to mitigating violence in health care settings*, 2021. https://www.aha.org/system/files/media/file/2021/10/creating-safer-workplaces-guide-to-mitigating-violence-in-health-care-settings-f.pdf. Accessed September 15, 2023.

Anusiewicz CV, et al: How does workplace bullying influence nurses' abilities to provide patient care? A nurse perspective, *J Clin Nurs* 29:4148, 2020.

Bambi S, et al: Negative interactions among nurses: an explorative study on lateral violence and bullying in nursing work settings, *J Nurs Manag* 27(4):749, 2019.

Barrett CA: Self-care: a holistic nurse imperative, *Beginnings* 39(3):14, 2019.

Centers for Disease Control and Prevention (CDC): *What is health literacy*, 2023. https://www.cdc.gov/healthliteracy/learn/index.html.

Centers for Disease Control and Prevention (CDC): *Preferred terms for select population groups & communities, gateway to health communication*, 2022. https://www.cdc.gov/healthcommunication/Preferred_Terms.html. Accessed September 15, 2023.

Clark CM: *Accused of workplace bullying: What happens next?* 2019. https://www.americannursetoday.com/accused-workplace-bullying/. Accessed September 15, 2023.

Crisis Prevention Institute (CPI): *CPI's top 10 de-escalation techniques revisited*, 2022. https://www.crisisprevention.com/Blog/CPI-s-Top-10-De-Escalation-Tips-Revisited. Accessed September 15, 2023.

Dung NT: Effectiveness of SBAR communication tool on patient safety: an integrative review, *J Nurs Sci* 4:147, 2021.

Green C: The hollow: a theory on workplace bullying in nursing practice, *Nurs Forum* 56:433, 2021.

Hastings SN, et al: Video-enhanced care management for medically complex older adults with cognitive impairment, *JAGS* 69:77, 2021.

Hockenberry MJ et al: *Wong's nursing care of infants and children*, ed 12, St. Louis, 2024, Elsevier.

Mayo Clinic: *Alzheimer's and dementia: Tips for effective communication*, 2021. https://www.mayoclinic.org/healthy-lifestyle/caregivers/in-depth/alzheimers/art-20047540. Accessed September 15, 2023.

National Council of State Boards of Nursing (NCSBN): *Test plan for the National Council Licensure Examination for Registered Nurses*, 2019. https://www.ncsbn.org/2019_RN_TestPlan-English.pdf. Accessed September 15, 2023.

Occupational Safety and Health Administration (OSHA): *Guidelines for preventing workplace violence for healthcare and social service workers*, 2016, U.S. Department of Labor Occupational Safety and Health Administration. https://www.osha.gov/Publications/osha3148.pdf . Accessed September 15, 2023.

Rutherford DE, et al: Interventions against bullying of prelicensure students and nursing professionals: an integrative review, *Nurs Forum* 54(1):84, 2019.

Schlög M, Jones CA: *Maintaining our humanity through the mask: mindful communication during COVID-19*, 2020. https://agsjournals.onlinelibrary.wiley.com/doi/10.1111/jgs.16488. Accessed September 15, 2023.

Sharma N, Gupta V: *Therapeutic communication*, 2022. https://www.ncbi.nlm.nih.gov/books/NBK567775/. Accessed September 15, 2023.

Shorey S, Wong PZE: A qualitative systematic review on nurses' experiences of workplace bullying and implications for nursing practice, *J Adv Nurs* 77:4306, 2021.

State of Nevada: *Warning signs of human trafficking*, 2021. https://ag.nv.gov/Human_Trafficking/HT_Signs/. Accessed September 15, 2023.

Steele D: *Keltner's Psychiatric nursing*, ed 9, St. Louis, 2023, Elsevier.

Sullivan WF, et al: Primary care of adults with intellectual and developmental disabilities: 2018 Canadian consensus guidelines, *Can Fam Physician* 64:254, 2018.

The Joint Commission (TJC): *2023 National Patient Safety Goals*, Oakbrook Terrace, IL, 2023, The Commission. https://www.jointcommission.org/standards/national-patient-safety-goals/.

Touhy T, Jett K: *Ebersole & Hess' gerontological nursing and healthy aging*, ed 6, St. Louis, 2022, Elsevier.

Trans Student Education Resources (TSER): *Definitions*, 2021. https://transstudent.org/about/definitions/. Accessed September 15, 2023.

U.S. Department of Health and Human Services (USDHHS), Office of Minority Health: *Cultural and linguistic competency*, 2021. https://www.minorityhealth.hhs.gov/omh/browse.aspx?lvl=1&lvlid=6. Accessed September 15, 2023.

Xue W, Fellow CHM: Therapeutic communication within the nurse–patient relationship: a concept analysis, *Int J Nurs Pract* 27:e12938, 2021.

3 | Admitting, Transfer, and Discharge

OUTLINE

Purpose, p. 40

Practice Standards, p. 40

Supplemental Standards, p. 40

Principles for Practice, p. 40

Person-Centered Care, p. 41

Evidence-Based Practice, p. 41

Safety Guidelines, p. 41

Admitting Process, p. 42

Transfer Process, p. 45

Discharge Process, p. 47

OBJECTIVES

Mastery of content in this chapter will enable you to:
- Explain the role communication plays in maintaining continuity of care through a patient's admission, transfer, and discharge from an acute care agency.
- Outline the purpose and importance of discharge planning.
- Examine the ongoing needs of patients in the discharge planning process.
- Explain the role of a patient's family caregiver in the admission, transfer, or discharge process.

MEDIA RESOURCES

- http://evolve.elsevier.com/Perry/skills
- Clinical Review Questions
- Audio Glossary
- Answers to Clinical Judgment and Next-Generation NCLEX® Examination–Style Questions
- Printable Key Points

PURPOSE

The coordination of resources and planning a patient's care from admission to discharge or from one level of care to the next is a key role of a nurse. Nurses identify patients' ongoing health care needs and anticipate physical, psychological, and social deficits that have implications for patients to resume normal activities after discharge. A nurse involves appropriate family caregivers in a plan of care; provides interventions, including health education; and assists in making health care resources available to patients. Clinical judgment is important in discharge planning when you apply knowledge of a patient's condition, anticipate the type of needs that might be required as the patient transitions to another agency or home, and then recommend or provide interventions.

PRACTICE STANDARDS

- Agency for Healthcare Research and Quality (AHRQ), 2019—Medication reconciliation
- The Joint Commission (TJC), 2023b—National Patient Safety Goals

- U.S. Department of Health and Human Services (DHHS), 2023—Health information privacy

SUPPLEMENTAL STANDARDS

- Trans Student Educational Resources (TSER), n.d.: Definitions

PRINCIPLES FOR PRACTICE

- Assist patients and family caregivers in becoming partners in care, sharing in the process of decision making.
- Integrate patient care across health care settings, services, health care providers, and care levels to maintain a continuum of care.
- Transitional care involves nursing actions implemented to ensure coordination and continuity of care for patients who transfer between different settings or levels of care.
- Transitions of care require careful communication among providers about necessary interventions to be continued or planned to ensure patient safety (CMS, 2019).
- Screen patients on admission to a health care agency for possible discharge needs to ensure that appropriate teaching is

completed to ensure a safe discharge (Toney-Butler and Unison-Pace, 2022).

PERSON-CENTERED CARE

- When caring for patients, assess for possible health disparities. Factors that contribute to a person's ability to attain good health include race or ethnicity, sex, sexual identity, age, disability, socioeconomic status, and geographical location. You will learn about these factors as you form relationships and care for patients. These factors may influence how you approach discharge planning.
- Be aware of how cultural variables will affect your patient and family caregiver assessment, approach to nursing care, and teaching during admission, transfer, or discharge. It is essential to involve the patient and family caregiver in making decisions about care activities.
- Providing patient-centered care from an intercultural nursing perspective allows you to view patients as unique individuals while considering their cultural needs. Communicating effectively with patients from various cultures allows for optimal delivery of patient care (Tuohy, 2019).
- Teaching occurs throughout the admission process with incorporation of a variety of patient-specific strategies and use of teach-back to confirm patient understanding (AHRQ, 2023a).
- In an emergency situation or if the patient is unable to perform aspects of their care, teach family caregivers about the rationale for any procedures and routines to be used in the patient's care.

EVIDENCE-BASED PRACTICE

Errors in Patient Transitions

Transitions in health care happen frequently, with patients being newly admitted, transferred to other units within or outside a health care agency, and discharged. Hand-offs are a leading cause for medical error, as they pose a major problem in communication for all providers to give and receive complete and accurate information (Burns et al., 2021). Transitions from one setting to another can be complicated and dangerous due to medication errors, lapses in communication, and the complexity of treatment plans (Gonzalez et al., 2021). Nurses take an active role in the coordination and implementation of patient transitions and therefore need to be aware of the following risks associated with transitions and develop nursing interventions to safely assist patients:

- Lack of communication among incoming and outgoing nurses in the intensive care unit (ICU) during a shift-to-shift handover was found to be the main cause of reduced safety, including delayed treatment, medical errors, and patient injury or death (Ahn et al., 2021).
- Lack of a standardized handover system was a major contributing factor to communication failure within the ICU. The actual information handed over was inconsistent, with insufficient and nonspecific details, resulting in inappropriate decision making (Ahn et al., 2021).
- In a study of nurses, communication failures were found to be a leading cause of patient harm; as patients transition from the emergency department (ED) to inpatient units, complete and accurate communication was needed for care planning but lacking (Cross et al., 2019).
- Four domains were identified in Ahn and colleagues' study to support an effective communication process, detailing some challenges for each domain and proposed interventions for

nurses: (1) sender, (2) receiver, (3) message, and (4) environment (Ahn et al., 2021):
- *Sender*—Oftentimes, nurses feel pressured to be perfect and reported lack of time for communication working in a high-pressure environment of the ICU. A culture of support is recommended to acknowledge and encourage each other for difficult shifts; encourage continuous conversations about difficulties of handovers to come to common ground among units.
- *Receiver*—Communication was one directional, not allowing nurses to ask questions; nurses were often fearful of being perceived incompetent if they asked questions. Nurses need to actively participate in the handover by asking appropriate questions and providing feedback. Having a checklist for hand-off can help prevent information omission.
- *Message*—Disorganized, repetitive reports and incomplete information were common communication barriers reported. Proper training on how to effectively conduct a hand-off report is necessary.
- *Environment*—Unstructured reports, distractions, and pressure to complete reports and transition the patient were barriers. Checklists to ensure complete information, allowing sufficient time and careful planning, limiting interruptions and distractions, and seeking help from others were strategies highlighted to facilitate communication and a safe transition for the patient.
- Hand-off improvement tools can allow for better communication and be adapted to meet the needs of a particular unit and patient transition (Burns et al., 2021).
- An interprofessional video conference between a hospital-based team and post–acute care providers to discuss patients discharged from inpatient services to post–acute care sites has been found to improve transitions. Communication and coordination errors, incorrect follow-up appointments, lack of review of the discharge summary, missing documentation of inpatient care, pharmacy issues, confusion about medical equipment, and postoperative needs were discovered; once identified, these issues were addressed by the interprofessional team to improve transitions and prevent patient harm (Gonzalez et al., 2021).

SAFETY GUIDELINES

- At all points of care, identify whether a patient has a sensory or communication need (e.g., hearing aid, glasses, need for an interpreter) and ensure that assistance is available.
- Identify if a patient uses any assistive devices and be sure that each is provided and deemed safe to use.
- Include the patient, family caregiver, and health care team early in planning care to promote successful transition through the health care system.
- Consider the patients' educational background, health literacy level, and ability to find, understand, and use information and services to make informed health-related decisions and actions for themselves (Centers for Disease Control and Prevention [CDC], 2023).
- Coordinate the health care providers who contribute to a patient's care needs to develop a plan of care for discharge to ensure a safe transition to home or an alternate care agency.
- Collaborate with other health care personnel (e.g., registered dietitian nutritionist, social worker, pharmacist, physical therapist) to assess appropriate resources needed as a patient transitions through the health care system.

ADMITTING PROCESS

Patients enter health care systems through a variety of locations (e.g., hospital, clinic, or physician's or health care provider's offices). The admission process is typically the first experience a patient has with a health care agency, and there are common procedures for admitting patients to these settings. A patient admitted through the emergency department (ED) will have a different experience and may not be a reliable resource for admission information because of acute conditions, pain, or level of consciousness. Family caregivers can provide pertinent information for the hospital records for the ED patient or for a patient who cannot provide this information (e.g., a patient with advanced dementia).

Role of the Admission Personnel

Admission officers, secretaries, and technicians are the personnel involved in the preliminary admission process such as interviewing patients and reviewing information about insurance coverage, demographic data, and agency procedures. The admission personnel initiate and maintain a courteous and professional relationship with patients while providing information about their safety, legal rights, and privacy. A private interview area gives patients and family caregivers a place to reveal important identifying information, including a patient's full legal name, age, birth date, address, next of kin, health care provider, religious or cultural preferences, occupation, and type of insurance.

The admission personnel secures an identification (ID) band legibly stating a patient's full legal name, hospital or agency number, health care provider, and birth date to the patient's wrist. If a patient has any known documented allergies, an allergy band will also be placed on the wrist. Health care providers use information from the ID band to identify a patient when performing treatments or procedures. In many agencies an ID band contains a patient's unique bar code that then makes it easy to identify a patient for all ordered procedures; bar code scanning is also used for medication administration and has been shown to help reduce medication errors (Mulac et al., 2021). If a patient is unconscious, identification must wait until family caregivers arrive. Hospital staff provide a patient who has been a victim of crime with an anonymous name on their ID band under the agency's "blackout" or "do not publish" procedure.

A patient's legal rights are met by instructing the patient or legal guardian to read the general consent form for treatment. The Centers for Medicare and Medicaid Services (CMS) (2023) requires that all patients receive information regarding their rights related to health care services at admission; otherwise, the hospital will not receive reimbursement for services (Box 3.1). The CMS requires that information be available in multiple languages and

---

BOX 3.1

Patients' Rights Provided for by the Centers for Medicare and Medicaid Services

Standard 1: Notice of Rights
- A hospital must protect and promote each patient's rights.
- A hospital must inform each patient whenever possible or, when appropriate, the patient's representative of the patient's rights in advance of furnishing or discontinuing patient care.
- The hospital must have a process for prompt resolution of patient grievances and must inform each patient whom to contact to file a grievance.

Standard 2: Exercise of Rights
- The patient has the right to participate in the development and implementation of a plan of care.
- The patient or their representative has the right to make informed decisions regarding care.
- The patient's rights include being informed of health status, involved in care planning and treatment, and able to request or refuse treatment. This right must not be construed as a mechanism to demand the provision of treatment or services deemed medically unnecessary or inappropriate.
- The patient has the right to formulate advance directives and have hospital staff and practitioners who provide care in the hospital comply with these directives.
- The patient has the right to have a family member or representative of their choice and a personal health care provider notified promptly of admission to the hospital.

Standard 3: Privacy and Safety
- The patient has the right to personal privacy.
- The patient has the right to receive care in a safe setting.
- The patient has the right to be free from all forms of abuse or harassment.

Standard 4: Confidentiality of Patient Record
- The patient has the right to confidentiality of clinical records.
- The patient has the right to access information contained in clinical records within a reasonable time frame.

Standard 5: Restraint or Seclusion
- The patient has the right to be free from physical or mental abuse and corporal punishment.
- The patient has the right to be free from restraints or seclusion of any form that is not medically necessary or is used as a means of coercion, discipline, convenience, or retaliation by staff. A restraint is any manual method, physical or mechanical device, material, or equipment that immobilizes or reduces the ability of a patient to move the arms, legs, body, or head freely. A drug used as a restraint is a medication used to manage the patient's behavior or to restrict the patient's freedom of movement and is not a standard treatment or dosage for the patient's medical or psychiatric condition. Seclusion is the involuntary confinement of a patient alone in a room or area from which the patient is physically prevented from leaving.
- A restraint does not include devices such as orthopedically prescribed devices, surgical dressings or bandages, protective helmets, or other methods that involve the physical holding of a patient for the purpose of conducting routine physical examinations or tests, to protect the patient from falling out of bed, or to permit the patient participation in activities without the risk of physical harm (this does not include a physical escort).
- A restraint or seclusion can be used only if needed to improve the patient's well-being and if less restrictive interventions have been determined to be ineffective.
- The use of a restraint or seclusion must be selected only when other less restrictive measures have been found to be ineffective to protect the patient or others from harm and in accordance with the order of a physician or other licensed independent practitioner.
- This order must never be written as a standing order or on an as-needed basis (i.e., prn). The order must be followed by consultation with the patient's treating physician as soon as possible if someone other than the patient's treating physician or health care provider ordered the restraint or seclusion.

Patients' Rights Provided for by the Centers for Medicare and Medicaid Services—cont'd

- The use of a restraint or seclusion must be:
  - In accordance with a written modification to the patient's plan of care and implemented in the least restrictive manner possible.
  - In accordance with safe and appropriate restraining techniques and ended at the earliest possible time.

- The condition of the restrained or secluded patient must be assessed, monitored, and reevaluated continually.
- All staff who have direct patient contact must have ongoing education and training in the proper and safe use of restraints and seclusion.

Adapted from Centers for Medicare and Medicaid Services. (2023). *State operations manual appendix A—survey protocol, regulations and interpretive guidelines for hospitals, discharge planning.* https://www.cms.gov/Regulations-and-Guidance/Guidance/Manuals/downloads/som107ap_a_hospitals.pdf Accessed August 8, 2023.

BOX 3.2

The Joint Commission Patients' Rights Standards

- Right to an appropriate level of care
- Right to receive safe care
- Respect for cultural values and religious beliefs
- Privacy
- Consent obtained for recording or filming for purposes other than the identification, diagnosis, or treatment of patients
- Confidentiality of information
- Recognition and prevention of potential abuse situation
- Notification of unanticipated outcomes
- Involvement in care decisions
- Information on risks and benefits of investigational studies
- End-of-life care
- Advance directives
- Organ procurement
- Right to have advance directives and to have them followed
- Freedom from unnecessary restraints
- Informed consent for various procedures
- Right to refuse care
- Right to have pain believed and relieved
- Communication with administration
- Education

From The Joint Commission (TJC): *Comprehensive accreditation manual for hospitals,* Oakbrook Terrace, IL, 2023, Author.

BOX 3.3

Advance Directives

- Advance care planning is a process that guarantees the respect of the patient's values and priorities about future care at the end of life.
- An advanced directive (AD) is a set of legal documents helpful to clinicians and family members for making critical decisions on behalf of the patient, whereas they might become incapable.
- The timely completion of AD is critical and requires that the person's values and preferences are discussed and documented per time.
- AD may include a living will, durable power of attorney for health care, or notarized handwritten document.
- Most ADs include information regarding the patient's preferences for interventions (e.g., antibiotics, hydration, feeding, use of ventilators, cardiopulmonary resuscitation, analgesia), life-sustaining treatments, resuscitation, and a surrogate decision maker.
- A copy of the document should be available in the patient's electronic health record (EHR). If not available, the substance of the advance directive should be documented in the EHR, and a family member should be asked to bring the advance directive to the hospital.
- All health care providers should be aware of the patient's AD.
- The SOP model (Shared decision making with Oncologists and Palliative care specialists) is an example for the implementation of Do-Not-Resuscitate preferences in patients, and the U.S. Advance Care Plan Registry is a database that contains all types of end-of-life documents and makes them available to all clinicians on the web.
- Witnesses for an advance directive document should not be medical personnel, nor should they be related to the patient or heirs to the patient's estate. A social worker often fulfills this requirement.

Adapted from National Institutes of Health. (2022). *Advance care planning and advance directives: an overview of the main critical issues.* https://www.ncbi.nlm.nih.gov/pmc/articles/PMC8847241/. Accessed August 8, 2023.

alternate formats (e.g., audio, visual, written). Other regulatory agencies such as The Joint Commission (TJC) also require agencies to provide for specific patient rights (Box 3.2).

Advance care planning (ACP) is a process that supports adults in understanding and sharing their personal values, life goals, and preferences regarding future care (National Institutes of Health [NIH], 2022). The Patient Self-Determination Act, effective December 1, 1991, requires all Medicare- and Medicaid-recipient hospitals to provide patients with information about their right to accept or reject medical treatment. At the time of registration, patients receive information about advance directives and are referred to appropriate resources if they want to discuss advance directives or receive help in completing an advance directive document (Box 3.3).

On admission, patients must also receive information about the Health Insurance Portability and Accountability Act (HIPAA), a federal law finalized in 2003 to protect the privacy of patient health information, referred to as *protected health information* (PHI) (U.S. Department of Health and Human Services [DHHS], 2022a). Health information refers to any information (oral or recorded) in any form that is created or received by a health care provider, health plan, public health authority, employer, life insurer, school or university, or health care clearinghouse and relates to the past, present, or future physical or mental

health or condition of any individual; the provision of health care to an individual; or the past, present, or future payment for the provision of health care to an individual (DHHS, 2022b). Individually identifiable health information is information that is a subset of health information, including demographic information (e.g., age, Social Security number, e-mail address) collected from an individual. Numerous resources are available for health care providers and individuals, including documents that summarize patient rights, how information is protected, and who can look at and receive someone's health information (DHHS, 2023). Review agency-specific policies and procedures related to HIPAA and stay informed on updates.

Role of the Nurse

When patients receive health care before admission (e.g., home health, long-term care), nurses from the sending agencies provide appropriate information regarding the patients' conditions and reasons for transfer to receiving nurses for continuity of care. Admitting personnel collaborate with receiving nursing staff to ensure that a patient's room assignment is based on the patient's condition, health care needs, developmental level, activity level, expected length of stay, and personal preferences. For example, the best room for an older adult patient who is acutely ill, at risk for falls, and receiving multiple treatments is one close to the nurses' workstation.

When a patient is admitted through the ED and stabilized, a nurse notifies the nursing unit of a transfer and reports on the patient's admission information. Typical information includes the patient's name; admitting health care provider; chief complaint; any treatments or testing completed (e.g., medications administered, intravenous [IV] fluids infusing); treatment outcomes; allergies; and pertinent information related to the patient's admitting diagnosis (e.g., initial vital signs, level of consciousness). The ED nurse also shares pertinent observations about the patient's behavior (e.g., anxiety, fear) and level of knowledge regarding need for health care with the nursing staff to foster continuity of care and help the patient and family caregivers cope with a new environment.

Patients may go to a health care agency several days in advance for necessary preoperative diagnostic testing or to attend preoperative education classes. Other patients have contact with health care providers for the first time when they arrive at a hospital or outpatient surgical center. Patients admitted to a health care agency on the morning of a surgical procedure or treatment are "same-day" admissions. A nurse provides basic instructions about the purpose of the surgery or treatment, preparatory procedures, and routine postsurgical or posttreatment care. Admission and consent forms, diagnostic tests, preoperative patient teaching (see Chapter 36), and instructions are usually completed before the actual day of surgery.

Nurses actively coordinate the initial admission process for all patients, being mindful of their clinical conditions. On receiving a patient, note the patient's level of fatigue and comfort. A critically ill patient who has undergone extensive examination and treatment procedures immediately may be fatigued, leaving little time available for you to orient the patient and family caregiver to the unit or learn of the patient's fears or concerns. When patients enter a health care agency for elective treatment, you have more time to prepare them psychologically for hospitalization.

Admission Assessment

Each agency sets a time frame for completion of an admission assessment (maximum time, 24 hours). The admission assessment cannot be delegated to assistive personnel (AP); however, AP can assist with preparing a patient's room with equipment needed before admission, gathering and securing the patient's personal care items, escorting and orienting the patient and family caregiver to the nursing unit, and collecting ordered specimens.

On admission of a patient to a patient care area, a registered nurse completes a thorough nursing assessment. You will assess the patient and family caregiver's health literacy level first to ensure that the patient and/or family caregiver has the capacity to find, understand, and use information and services to make informed health-related decisions and actions for themselves and others (CDC, 2023). You may ask family caregivers to leave the room during the assessment unless the patient requires or asks for assistance. Review any advance directives and ensure that necessary diagnostic testing is ordered or completed. Before gathering data from the patient, identify the patient using at least two identifiers (e.g., name and birthday or name and medical record number) according to agency policy to ensure you have the correct patient (TJC, 2023b). Check this information against the patient's ID wristband.

It is important to greet the patient and family caregivers in a cordial manner, and if available, write the names of the nurse and AP on a whiteboard in the patient's room. Address patients by their preferred names and determine if there is a need for a professional translator to assist you, either in person or through a remote translator service. Assess whether a patient has a hearing impairment that would prevent you from gathering necessary information. Assist the patient in storing personal items at the bedside. Complete clothing and valuables listing sheet (see agency policy). Valuables should be sent home with family caregiver when possible or stored in an agency safe.

Complete your admission assessment in accordance with agency policies (see Chapters 5 and 6); however, if the patient is having acute physical or psychological problems, perform a focused assessment and complete the remainder of the admission assessment later. It is important to document the patient's level of discomfort (see Chapter 16) and assess for fall risk. TJC requires accredited hospitals to conduct fall risk assessment using fall risk scales appropriate for the patients being served (see Chapter 14) (Joint Commission International [JCI], 2018). Your assessment for fall risk should include conditions that create fall risk. For example, you may ask the patient to walk so that you can observe gait and movement to determine if there is weakness or instability in the lower extremities. Review the patient's EHR for a history of neurological disorders, bone disease, coagulation disorders, or medications that could put the patient at a greater risk for falls and/or injuries (see Chapter 14).

Some health care agencies are now requiring assessment of risk for obstructive sleep apnea (OSA) in surgical patients (see Chapter 37). Consider using the STOP-Bang questionnaire—an easy-to-use screening tool that is reliable and concise, with eight yes-or-no questions (Olson et al., 2023). Other areas to assess include psychosocial needs (need for a sitter or video monitoring; any signs of agitation, restlessness, hallucinations, depression, suicidal ideations, or substance abuse) and nutritional needs (appetite, changes in body weight, need for nutritional consultation based on body mass index [BMI] calculated from measured height and weight on admission) (Toney-Butler & Unison-Pace, 2022).

Allow the patient to express a personal perception of illness and health needs, as well as reasons for admission including expectations for care. A holistic approach to assessment includes a review of health status based on standards such as elimination, respiration, nutrition and metabolism, activity and exercise, self-concept, values and beliefs, cultural factors, social support, and cognitive function. Your application of clinical judgment involves synthesizing all assessment information to begin forming decisions about the patient's health care needs. A priority is to assess a patient's skin integrity, providing baseline data, and any current skin breakdown at admission. Use a reliable and valid risk for pressure injury development scale, such as the Braden Scale, to assess risk for potential skin breakdown (Chapter 39). If the pressure injury is not present on admission but develops later, it is considered a hospital-acquired condition and has both financial and quality-of-care consequences that may be reported to various regulatory entities (Miller et al., 2019).

Medication reconciliation is another essential component of the admission assessment. You compare medications prescribed at time of admission with those the patient has been taking at home. Reconciliation allows for a complete understanding of what the patient was prescribed and what medications the patient is actually taking, reducing the risk of medication errors (Agency for Healthcare Research and Quality [AHRQ], 2019; TJC, 2023b). As patients are admitted or transferred to new units, new medications are often added or existing medications are changed (AHRQ, 2019). Obtain a detailed medication history, including prescribed, over-the-counter (OTC), and alternative therapies such as herbs and hormones. Instruct family caregivers to take all medications home because they should not be left at the bedside. Document history of allergies including type of substance and a description of the reaction that the patient has previously experienced. If not already on the patient, place an allergy armband listing allergies to foods, drugs, latex, or other substances, and document allergies according to agency policy. Make a good faith effort to obtain detailed information; as databases continue to evolve, there will be enhanced opportunity to share information across systems.

At the completion of the assessment, take some time to orient the patient and family caregiver to the room, the nurse call button, and the nursing unit and demonstrate any equipment use. Ensure that the patient knows to call for help if needed while in the bathroom by using the emergency call light and, if necessary, demonstrate its use. Raise side rails (as appropriate) and lower bed or stretcher to lowest position, locking into position. Implement Universal Fall Precautions immediately, and if a patient has been determined to be at risk for falling, implement measures specific to reduce those risk factors (see Chapter 14). Explain the visiting hours and their purpose (i.e., to provide time to administer needed procedures and give patient time to rest) and mealtimes in case a family caregiver plans to assist the patient. If the agency allows smoking in designated areas, discuss the smoking policy and identify the areas for the patient and family caregiver.

Ensure that the patient understands any procedures and tests that are ordered by the health care provider. Introduce staff members when possible, including the nurse manager in charge of the unit, and explain that person's role in overseeing the unit and solving problems. Complete learning readiness and learning needs assessment for the patient and family caregiver as per agency policy. Provide comfort care as needed and discuss the specific fall risks and measures taken to promote the patient's safety. Instruct the patient to ask for help before getting out of bed. Before leaving the patient's room, ensure that the bed is in the lowest position and the nurse call system is in reach.

Once your assessment is complete, you will document history and assessment findings in the electronic health record (EHR) or chart and begin to make the clinical decisions necessary to develop a nursing plan of care. Document your evaluation of patient and family caregiver learning using teach-back techniques (AHRQ, 2023a). If the patient has an advance directive, place a copy in the EHR (NIH, 2022) (see Box 3.2). Notify the health care provider of the patient's arrival and report any unusual findings. If not already provided, secure admission orders from the health care provider.

Special Considerations for Patient Admissions

Hospitalization is a major crisis for many patients, including children, who feel stress from separation from family caregivers, loss of control, bodily injury, and pain. Separation anxiety is most common from middle infancy throughout the toddler years, especially ages 16 to 30 months. Preschoolers are better able to tolerate brief periods of separation, but their protest behaviors are subtler than those in younger children (e.g., refusal to eat, difficulty sleeping, withdrawing from others). School-age children can cope with separation but have an increased need for parental security and guidance (Hockenberry et al., 2022).

To assist children with coping, explain the rooming-in and visiting policies of the agency and encourage family caregivers' involvement in the child's care. Allow them to help with routine care activities (e.g., bathing, eating) and, when possible, to remain with the child during procedures. Parental input during the admission assessment is essential because parents can provide input on the child's normal behavior and deviations caused by illness.

Hospitalized older adults are at risk for functional declines such as new-onset incontinence, malnutrition, deconditioning, pressure injuries, and falls due to the effects of treatments or the clinical progress of their conditions. Interventions that retain functional status (e.g., physical therapy, nutrition consultation) require providing coordinated interprofessional care (Touhy & Jett, 2022). Elderly patients at increased risk of falling are those who have been admitted recently and are unfamiliar with surroundings, have acute illness, take four or more medications, or have been relocated recently. Visual, auditory, and mobility changes that occur with aging also often lead to falls in hospitalized older-adult patients (Touhy & Jett, 2022).

TRANSFER PROCESS

Patients transfer to different patient care units and health care agencies to receive alternate forms and levels of therapy and services and to have essential care continued closer to home. The goal of a transfer of care is to continue health care to avoid therapeutic interruptions or omissions that may hinder progress toward recovery. Involve the patient and family caregiver in setting goals and expectations for care. Collaborate early with health care providers and members of the interprofessional team to ensure efficient patient transfer with optimal patient outcomes. Social workers and case managers play a key role in coordinating services at new receiving health care agencies.

When patients move between units or agencies for diagnosis, treatment, and ongoing care, there is a safety risk at each interval. Providing a hand-off report of a patient to another unit is essential to clearly communicate information about the patient's care, treatment, services, and current condition and any recent or anticipated changes in order to meet patient safety goals (TJC, 2023a). The TJC recommends the following actions to ensure high-quality hand-offs:

- Determine what information is critical to communicate to ensure a safe transition.
- Have a set of standardized tools and methods to communicate.
- Include some form of face-to-face or remote voice communication (telephone, video conference).
- Combine and communicate information from multiple sources at one time.
- There is a minimum set of information a receiver needs:
  - Sender contact information; illness assessment; patient summary, including events leading up to illness or admission; hospital course; ongoing assessment; and plan of care
  - To-do action list; contingency plans; allergy list; code status; medication list; dated laboratory tests; dated vital signs
- Communicate hand-off/transfer reports face-to-face in a location free from nonemergency interruptions.
- Include interprofessional team members and, if appropriate, the patient and family caregiver. Use this time to consult, discuss, and ask and answer questions.
- Use EHRs and other technologies (e.g., apps, patient portals, telehealth) to enhance hand-offs—do not rely on them as the sole means to communicate patient information.

Mnemonics incorporated into transfer forms such as SBAR (*Situation, Background, Assessment, Recommendation*); I PASS the BATON (*Introduction, Patient, Assessment, Situation, Safety concerns, Background, Actions, Timing, Ownership, Next*);

SHARQ (Situation, History, Assessment, Recommendations/Result, Questions); and ANTICipate (Administrative Data, New clinical information, Tasks to be performed, Illness severity, and Contingency plans for changes) are examples of formats to use to facilitate effective hand-offs that can be tailored for different clinical areas and/or purposes (AHRQ, 2023b).

In the ED, when a patient is transferred from one agency to another, a nurse completes the transfer in compliance with the Emergency Medical Treatment and Labor Act (EMTALA) (CMS, 2021a). EMTALA is a federal law intended to protect patients from being transferred against their wishes and thus defines how an appropriate agency-to-agency transfer is accomplished. Although this law primarily affects the ED, it is important to know EMTALA and the transfer policies for inpatient transfers within the agency itself. Many health care agencies follow the same policies for all patient transfers.

Role of the Nurse

The skill of assessment and decision making conducted during transfers cannot be delegated to AP. Ensure that you have the correct patient to transfer by identifying the patient using at least two identifiers (e.g., name and birthday or name and medical record number) according to agency policy (TJC, 2023b). Review the transfer order in collaboration with the health care provider and members of the interprofessional team, assessing the reason for the patient's transfer (e.g., change in condition, services available at the agency, patient or family caregiver preferences regarding patient's location) and statement of the patient's stability for transfer. Review the receiving agency (when applicable) and assess individuals at high risk for transitional care problems (e.g., older adults with multiple health issues, depression, non-English speakers, patients with sensory impairments, low-income patients) to allow for better continuity of care and improved patient outcomes (Touhy & Jett, 2022). Complete medication reconciliation as per agency policy, checking the patient's current orders for transfer against the most recent medication administration record and the original, prehospitalization medication list (AHRQ, 2019). When transferring to a new agency, contact the receiving agency and arrange for an appropriate patient bed. Confirm the willingness of the agency to accept the patient.

Explain the purpose of transfer thoroughly, and provide time to discuss the patient's and family caregiver's feelings and expectations about the change in care setting. The health care provider is legally responsible for releasing the patient from medical care. Keep in mind that the patient also has the legal right to refuse transfer against medical advice. As necessary, obtain the patient's written consent to transfer. If the patient is unable to consent, the family caregiver may provide this consent. Inform patients of transfer plans in a timely manner, and give adequate time for psychological preparation (TJC, 2023a). Confirm that the patient and family caregiver understand transfer and procedures; allow time to ask questions and provide feedback.

In the event of a clinical emergency in which the patient and family caregiver are unable to consent, this consent is waived, and the patient is transferred to a higher level of care based on the clinical judgment of the health care provider requesting the transfer. Be sure to perform a final assessment (including vital signs, airway, patency of IV lines and accuracy of infusion rate, and patient's level of consciousness), and document assessment findings along with a note about the patient's physical stability. Compare these data with previous findings to determine if there are changes in the patient's condition.

The method of transport will vary on the basis of the patient's current physical condition. Consult your agency policy and assess if the patient needs to be transferred by wheelchair or stretcher; you may also seek social worker involvement if necessary. If the patient's status and safety require life-support equipment, the staff assisting with the transfer need to have had appropriate training in life-support measures. Before transferring, determine if the patient needs pain relief or other medications for symptom management and ensure that family caregivers have been notified of the transfer if they are not with the patient. Your goal is to safely transfer the patient, maintaining the patient's vital signs and physiological status.

Direct the AP to help the patient to dress, gather, and secure personal belongings and any equipment (i.e., wheelchair, oxygen tank) that goes with the patient, and escort the patient to the nursing unit or transport area. Ensure that the patient has all necessary forms for transfer, including copies of medical records, radiology films, and laboratory tests.

Accurate information is necessary for the receiving agency to assume the patient's care; make sure that documentation in the patient's record is complete. Complete the nursing care transfer form according to the agency policy. Document the patient's status, including vital signs, relevant assessment findings specific to patient's condition, nursing plan of care, date and time of transfer, and method of transport on the appropriate transfer form. You will also document your evaluation of patient and family caregiver learning and code status when indicated (e.g., "do not resuscitate" [DNR] for patient being transferred by emergency medical transport).

If you are transferring a patient to a different nursing unit within the same agency, the entire health care record will accompany the patient whether it be an EHR or paper chart. Before transfer, make the patient as comfortable as possible, so you may need to perform therapies such as suctioning or dressing change prior to transfer. Help transfer the patient to a stretcher or wheelchair using safe patient handling techniques (see Chapter 11). Inspect the patient's alignment and positioning. Inspect and confirm that any necessary equipment to be used for transfer is functioning appropriately (e.g., oxygen tanks are full) and that other devices are secured properly (e.g., central lines, IV lines) if they are still needed.

If a patient is being transferred outside the agency, an appropriate person accompanies the patient to the transport vehicle. Call the receiving agency or unit to notify of the impending transfer and patient's status (check agency policy). Notify the nurse in charge or nurse assuming care of the patient so that the patient receives better continuity of care at the time of arrival.

Determine if the receiving agency/unit or nurse has questions about the patient's care, providing for clear communication during the hand-off report. The nurse receiving the patient documents the patient's arrival at the agency or unit by recording the date and time of arrival, reason for transfer, method of transport, patient's condition, and care provided at time of arrival.

Special Considerations for Patient Transfers

A transfer frequently creates anxiety for a patient and family caregivers. Carefully repeat instructions about the transfer when the patient and family caregiver are better able to understand your explanation. In this situation, be sure to have the patient restate any critical information using the teach-back method. Teach-back is a technique for health care providers to evaluate learning, ensuring that they have explained medical information clearly and that patients and their families understand what is communicated to them (AHRQ, 2023a).

Some patients are more vulnerable to transfer and transitions in health care and require extra attention. For example, you will need to collaborate with social workers to assist a homeless patient to secure a shelter placement prior to discharge (Canham et al., 2019). Children need their parents' comfort and security; thus, make sure that parents are well informed about the rationale for a planned or emergent transfer of a pediatric patient. Involve older children in any discussion regarding transfers (Hockenberry et al., 2022). Allow a parent to accompany the child in the transfer. When transferring an elderly patient to a new agency, keep in mind that relocation is stressful. Ensure that significant support people are still accessible and that the patient is thoroughly oriented to the new surroundings. Also make sure that the patient can take important memorabilia and has an opportunity to make decisions about care (Touhy & Jett, 2022).

It is important that all patients receive the level of services appropriate to their physical and mental health needs. Participation of a social worker or discharge planner in the transfer process ensures that transfer to a long-term care agency is appropriate. On a patient's arrival at the long-term care agency, you will complete a Resident Assessment Instrument (RAI). The RAI consists of the minimum data set (MDS), resident assessment protocols, and utilization guidelines specified in state operations guidelines (Touhy & Jett, 2022). Essential components of successful transfer to a long-term care agency are accurate communication of medication lists and advance directives. Possible use of a standardized transfer form can help in accurate communication.

DISCHARGE PROCESS

Early and comprehensive discharge planning facilitates the transition of a patient from a health care agency to the most independent level of care, whether that is home or another agency. The overall goal of discharge planning is to provide the most appropriate level and quality of care throughout all stages of a patient's illness.

The discharge planning process should be comprehensive and interprofessional, including all family caregivers who are involved in the care of the patient. From the time of admission, you will assess a patient's discharge needs using nursing history data, including assessments of a patient's physical health, functional status, psychosocial support system, financial resources, health values, cultural and ethnic background, level of education, and barriers to care that need to be addressed. Clinical judgment involves collecting data on an ongoing basis, anticipating what the patient's long-term needs will be, and making clinical decisions regarding specific care recommendations. Also review ongoing assessment data during your shift of care (e.g., physical examinations and discussions with patient and health care provider). All patients can be at risk for readmission; however, there are certain conditions that have higher readmission rates: septicemia, heart failure, diabetes mellitus with complications, chronic obstructive pulmonary disease, pneumonia, acute and unspecified renal failure, schizophrenia and other psychotic disorders, and cardiac arrythmia (Weiss & Jiang, 2021). Being mindful of these conditions and using better discharge planning with better care coordination can help patients avoid preventable readmissions.

Collaborate with the interprofessional team to assess what will be a patient's anticipated needs after discharge, their eligibility for home care reimbursement, and/or the need for discharge to a skilled care agency. Ask these questions: "Does the patient have an injury or illness that makes it difficult to leave home (e.g., requires the aid of supportive devices such as a wheelchair or walker; requires the use of special transportation; needs the assistance of a family caregiver)?" "Does the patient have a "skilled need" that requires skills from a specific health care provider?" "What is the capability of a family caregiver to provide a patient needed resources and hands-on care?"

Be sure that the discharge plan is culturally appropriate (e.g., learn the patient's preferences and values about continuing health care after discharge). In addition to including cultural preferences, assess for current barriers to learning (e.g., age, fatigue, pain, lack of motivation). Assess patient's and family caregiver health literacy to ensure the capacity to obtain, communicate, process, and understand basic health information (CDC, 2023). This will help you plan the appropriate way to provide information for the patient (e.g., printed material is written at proper reading level). Every hospitalized patient requires patient-centered discharge planning, and it is equally essential for any patient permanently moving to a different health care agency. The trend toward shorter lengths of stay in acute care settings makes discharge planning increasingly difficult but all the more essential.

TJC identifies the elements of a comprehensive discharge planning model (Box 3.4). In addition, CMS (2019) provides a guide in the form of a discharge checklist for patients and family caregivers. The checklist helps patients be proactive, with questions to ask

---

> **BOX 3.4**
>
> ### Joint Commission International Recommendations for Discharge Planning Process
>
> - Improve hand-off communications.
>   - Patient and family caregiver are included so that they can clarify information and ask and answer questions.
>   - Optimally done face-to-face between health care providers; verbal communication should supplement written records so that there is the opportunity to clarify information.
>   - The patient's EHR is kept current.
> - Discharge patients effectively: "5 *D*s of discharge" ensures successful continuity of care and care outcomes.
>   - Diagnosis—Does the patient understand the diagnosis and reason for being in a health care agency?
>   - Drugs—Does the patient know each medication, the reason for the medication, when to take the medication, and how to administer it? Also, does the patient have the resources to purchase or retrieve medications?
>   - Diet—Does the patient understand the dietary restrictions? Does the patient need a registered dietitian consult?
>   - Doctor follow-up—Does the patient know when to see the doctor next? Can the patient make the appointment and obtain transportation?
>   - Directions—Is there any education needed to increase the patient's ability to achieve optimal health? Does the patient understand this education?
> - Accommodate language and literacy needs.
> - Overcome cultural barriers.
> - Meet age-related needs.
> - Communicate accurate medical orders and test results.
>
> Adapted from Joint Commission International. (2018). *Communicating clearly and effectively to patients: how to overcome communication challenges in health care.* https://store.jointcommissioninternational.org/assets/3/7/jci-wp-communicating-clearly-final_(1).pdf Accessed August 8, 2023.

regarding their health needs after discharge, signs and symptoms to watch out for, creating and reviewing their medication list, and recovery and support needs after discharge.

Development of a discharge plan with outcomes mutually accepted by a patient and health care providers is essential. A discharge plan should result in a written document and is based on the following information (CMA, 2022):

- Where and how a patient will get care after discharge
- Support groups available (family caregivers, friends, hired help)
- Health care problems that might occur after discharge
- Medication reconciliation
- Arrangement of necessary equipment or supplies
- Resources available to help the patient to cope with and manage illness
- Resources available to assist the patient with costs associated with care

Avoidable hospital readmissions can be reduced with effective discharge planning and transition processes and by enhancing coaching, education, and support for patient self-management (Institute for Healthcare Improvement [IHI], 2023). The discharge process can be simple or complex and occurs in three phases: acute, transitional, and continuing care. In the acute phase, medical attention dominates discharge planning efforts (e.g., patient needing a cardiac procedure not available in current health care agency is transferred to one where this can be performed). During the transitional phase, the need for acute care is still present, but its urgency declines, and patients begin to address and plan for their future health care needs (e.g., a patient recovering from a hip replacement may need inpatient rehabilitation before going home). In the continuing care phase, patients are able to participate in planning and implementing continuing care activities needed after discharge (e.g., a patient needing more permanent placement is discharged to a skilled nursing facility [SNF]). In health care agencies these phases can occur very quickly, even within hours.

The greatest challenge in effective discharge planning is communication. Patients and families should be full partners in the discharge planning process and thus should be engaged in discussing what will be needed to make the transition in care safe and effective (CMA, 2022). When team members communicate during handoffs, consultations, or interprofessional discharge planning rounds, a patient's discharge readiness should be a central topic.

Communication is enhanced if an organization has a discharge coordinator or case manager. Staff members in these roles thoroughly assess what each patient's needs will be at discharge, identify available and needed resources, and link patients and families to these resources (e.g., community agencies, Meals on Wheels, rehabilitation sites). The staff also coordinate services (e.g., home health) as appropriate and may also follow up on patients' progress after discharge.

The Hospital Consumer Assessment of Healthcare Providers and Systems (HCAHPS) tool measures patients' perceptions of their hospital stay from admission through discharge. The HCAHPS tool is the first national standardized survey instrument (CMS, 2021b). Patients are asked to rate their hospital stay after discharge through the HCAHPS survey, which contains 29 questions asking patients about their recent hospital stay. There are 19 core questions about critical aspects of a patients' hospital experiences: communication with nurses and health care providers, the responsiveness of hospital staff, the cleanliness and quietness of the hospital environment, communication about medicines, discharge information, overall rating of the hospital, and would they recommend the hospital (CMS, 2021b).

Role of the Nurse

The skills of assessment, health problem identification, care planning, and patient education involved in discharging patients cannot be delegated to assistive personnel (AP). The AP assists nurses in gathering and securing personal items and any supplies that the patient will take with them. The AP may transport the patient to the discharge transport vehicle.

If a patient's destination at discharge will be the home, assess the patient's and family caregiver's learning needs as soon as possible (e.g., psychomotor skills, medication management, symptom recognition). Engaging the patient and family caregivers in the assessment supports person- and family-centered nursing. Consult with the interprofessional team regularly to know what the patient's likely discharge destination will be. Engage a patient and family caregiver as partners in the discharge teaching plan by having them identify their goals and concerns about discharge to help improve understanding of health care needs and ability to achieve self-care at home. A goal, for example, could be that the patient can perform activities of daily living independently once home. Determine if there is a need for any change to the physical arrangement of the home (see Chapter 41).

Prior to the day of discharge, provide information and, if appropriate, contact information about community health care resources (e.g., medical equipment companies, Meals on Wheels, adult day care) and determine the need for referrals. Conduct teaching sessions, including content related to the following topics as appropriate: description of what life at home will be like; review of medications and dosing schedules; warning signs of possible health problems; explanation of test results; explanation of how to provide therapies or use home medical equipment; review of restrictions resulting from health alterations; and when to make follow-up appointments. Give the patient and family caregiver an opportunity to practice new equipment, providing feedback to ensure the patient or family caregiver can use the equipment safely and correctly. A combination of written and verbal information is effective in improving patient satisfaction and knowledge (AHRQ, 2023b). In some settings electronic programs are available that allow you to tailor patient-specific media instructions. Use appropriate materials such as pamphlets, books, or multimedia resources, and refer the patient to reliable and current Internet resources. Document and communicate the patient's and family caregiver's response to teaching and proposed discharge plan to other health care team members for continuity of education.

Day of Discharge

On the day of discharge, encourage the patient and family caregiver to ask any remaining questions or discuss issues related to home care. You may also want to talk to them separately to ensure that all have a chance to speak freely of any lingering concerns. A final opportunity to demonstrate learned skills is helpful. You can use teach-back to ask patients and family caregivers questions related to specific discharge instructions; for example, ask the patient to tell you how and when they will take a new medication. The teach-back method allows you to check patients' understanding by stating in their own words what they need to know or do about their health (AHRQ, 2023a).

To ensure you are discharging the correct patient, identify the patient using at least two identifiers (e.g., name and birthday or name and medical record number) according to agency policy (TJC, 2023b). Check the health care provider's discharge orders for prescriptions, change in treatments, or need for special medical equipment. If orders are not complete, there can be delays in the discharge process. Confirm that delivery and setup of equipment is in place (e.g., hospital bed, oxygen) before patient arrives home; often, discharge planning and social work staff will assist with this coordination. Determine whether the patient or family caregiver has arranged for transportation. Obtain a copy of the list of valuables signed by the patient and have security or appropriate administrator deliver valuables to the patient. Complete medication reconciliation per agency policy and check discharge medication orders against the medication administration record and home medication list. Provide the patient with prescriptions or pharmacy-dispensed medications ordered by the health care provider. In some settings pharmacists or pharmacy technicians will deliver discharge medications to patients before they leave the hospital. Be sure to offer a final review of information needed to facilitate safe medication self-administration. Do not simply ask, "Do you understand your medications? Any questions?" Instead, take each medication and ask the patient to explain to you its purpose, when to take it, and what (if any) problems might develop. Also provide information on follow-up appointments to the patient's health care provider's office. Arrange for patient or family caregiver to visit the business office if they have any questions or concerns about financial payment.

Assistive personnel (AP) can provide privacy and assistance as the patient dresses and packs all personal belongings. The AP can check closets and drawers for belongings and acquire a utility cart to move patient's belongings. The AP can also obtain a wheelchair for the patient. The nurse will transport patients leaving by ambulance on stretchers.

Complete documentation of the patient's discharge on the discharge summary (Box 3.5). Give the patient a signed copy of the form and keep one copy in the patient's chart if using paper versions of this form. Document unresolved problems and description of arrangements made for resolution in nurses' notes in the EHR or chart; if the discharge form is not a paper copy, document the electronic version in the EHR. Document the patient's vital signs and status of health problems at time of discharge in nurses' notes in EHR or chart. Document your evaluation of patient and family caregiver learning.

Help the patient to a wheelchair or stretcher using safe patient handling and transfer techniques (see Chapter 11). The nurse, AP, or transport team member will escort the patient to the entrance of the agency where the source of transportation is waiting (see agency policy). Before helping the patient to move from the wheelchair, lock the wheelchair wheels. Help the patient to transfer into the transport vehicle and help place personal belongings in the vehicle. If transferring from a stretcher to an ambulance, work collaboratively with the ambulance team to transfer the patient to the vehicle. On return to the nursing unit, notify admitting or the appropriate department of the time of discharge. Notify housekeeping of the need to clean the patient's room.

Elements of a Written Discharge Summary Form

- Mode of discharge: ambulatory, wheelchair, stretcher
- Instructions for self-care activities: activity, diet, medications, and special treatments such as wound care, self-catheterization, and tracheostomy care
- Reconciled list of discharge medications with dose, frequency, route, reasons for change in medication or for newly prescribed medications
- Signs and symptoms of complications or drug reactions for which to be observant
- Signs and symptoms that patient should consider normal
- Correct settings for any equipment required
- Planned follow-up appointment at health care provider's office, clinic
- Name and contact information of health care provider and/or nursing unit
- Explanation of pertinent emergency procedures
- Patient's signature, showing understanding of instructions

Adapted from National Quality Forum. (2023). *Patient safety final technical report: spring 2022 cycle.* https://www.qualityforum.org/Publications/2023/01/Patient_Safety_Final_Report_-_Spring_2022_Cycle.aspx. Accessed August 8, 2023.

Special Considerations for Patient Discharges

Assess a patient's fatigue and pain levels before beginning any instruction. Keep focused on the important teaching topics to cover. Ensure that all patient education has been completed, and allow the patient and family caregivers enough time to ask questions. Collaborate with the health care providers who contribute to a patient's care needs to develop a plan of care for discharge to ensure a safe transition to home or an alternate care agency. Include and document the name and phone number of the pharmacy that the patient uses.

For pediatric patients, once the family caregivers have learned how to perform any necessary caregiver skills, have them assume care before the child returns home. Many hospitals incorporate a trial period requiring a family to manage care before the child's discharge home (Hockenberry et al., 2022). Older adults and their family caregivers often overestimate their ability to manage care after discharge. They also disagree about what postdischarge care includes. Make referrals to home care to address needs associated with functional decline and help prevent readmission to the hospital.

Assess the availability and skill of the primary family caregiver (e.g., spouse or friend): Assess time availability, ability, and willingness to give care; emotional and physical stamina; knowledge of caregiving requirements; and type of relationship held with patient. Assess additional resources, including friends or neighbors who are available to help. Inform the patient or family caregiver and patient's health care provider about decision to accept or not accept patient for admission to home care agency.

✦ CLINICAL JUDGMENT AND NEXT-GENERATION NCLEX® EXAMINATION–STYLE QUESTIONS

An 85-year-old patient has been admitted to an acute surgical unit after a fall at home, which resulted in a fracture of the right shoulder. The patient also has a headache and mild confusion. Surgery has been scheduled for the next day. History reveals Parkinson disease, hypertension, and uncontrolled type 2 diabetes mellitus. The 88-year-old spouse states the patient needs assistance with cutting food but self-feeds otherwise and can bathe and dress independently. The patient uses a walker to ambulate at home and a wheelchair during outings. Assessment reveals a stage 1 pressure injury on the left hip; a small bruise on the right side of the forehead; bilateral hand tremors; slight agitation; and an inability to remember how the injuries occurred and the trip to the hospital. The patient is oriented to person, recognizes spouse, and reports extreme shoulder pain. Vital signs: T 36.8°C (98.2°F); HR 90 beats/min; RR 18 beats/min; BP 142/96 mm Hg. Blood glucose 122. SpO₂ 98% on RA.

1. Complete the following sentence by selecting from the list of word choices below.

The nurse will first address the patient's **[Select 1]**, followed by the patient's **[Select 2]**.

Options for 1	Options for 2
Confusion	Nutrition status
Stage 1 pressure injury	Hand tremors
Blood glucose	Blood pressure
Mobility	Shoulder pain

2. When creating the plan of care, when would the nurse anticipate performing medication reconciliation? **Select all that apply.**
1. Each time medication is to be given
2. Prior to transfer to another level of care
3. At the change of every shift
4. During the discharge process
5. Once every 24 hours

3. The nurse is preparing the patient for surgery to repair the right shoulder injury. Which **priority** assessment finding would the nurse report to the surgeon?
1. Blood pressure 140/90
2. Ate cookies the spouse brought
3. Shoulder pain 6 out of 10
4. Limited range of motion in affected arm

4. The patient was returned to the surgical unit following surgery. Which of the following tasks would the nurse delegate to assistive personnel? **Select all that apply.**
1. Perform a neurological check.
2. Administer opioid medication.
3. Perform oral and denture hygiene.
4. Document intake and output.
5. Change dressing over pressure injury.

5. The nurse has completed discharge teaching. Which patient statement requires nursing intervention?
1. "I will take extra pain medication when my shoulder hurts more."
2. "I plan to use the wheelchair when I am out shopping so that my spouse can push me."
3. "I have asked my spouse to make a follow-up appointment for me with the surgeon."
4. "I called my insurance to see if they will cover the cost of my dressings."

Visit the Evolve site for Answers to Clinical Judgment and Next-Generation NCLEX® Examination–Style Questions.

REFERENCES

Agency for Healthcare Research and Quality (AHRQ): *Medication reconciliation*, 2019. https://psnet.ahrq.gov/primers/primer/1/medication-reconciliation. Accessed August 8, 2023.

Agency for Healthcare Research and Quality (AHRQ): *Teach-Back: intervention*, 2023a. https://www.ahrq.gov/patient-safety/reports/engage/interventions/teachback.html. Accessed August 8, 2023.

Agency for Healthcare Research and Quality (AHRQ): *TeamSTEPPS Fundamentals Course: module 3. Communication*, 2023b. https://www.ahrq.gov/teamstepps/instructor/fundamentals/module3/igcommunication.html. Accessed August 8, 2023.

Ahn JW, et al: Critical care nurses' communication challenges during handovers: a systematic review and qualitative meta-synthesis, *J Nurs Manag* 29:623, 2021.

Burns J, et al: Handoffs in radiology: minimizing communication errors and improving care transitions, *JACR* 18:1297, 2021.

Canham SL, et al: Health supports needed for homeless persons transitioning from hospitals, *Health Soc Care Community* 27(3):531, 2019.

Centers for Disease Control and Prevention (CDC): *What is health literacy?* 2023. https://www.cdc.gov/healthliteracy/learn/index.html. Accessed August 8, 2023.

Center for Medicare Advocacy (CMA): *Discharge planning: rights and procedures for Medicare beneficiaries in various care settings*, 2022. https://www.medicareadvocacy.org/medicare-info/discharge-planning/. Accessed August 8, 2023.

Centers for Medicare and Medicaid Services (CMS): *Your discharge planning checklist: for patients and their caregivers preparing to leave a hospital, nursing home, or other care setting*, 2019. https://www.medicare.gov/pubs/pdf/11376-discharge-planning-checklist.pdf. Accessed August 8, 2023.

Centers for Medicare and Medicaid Services (CMS): *Emergency Medical Treatment & Labor Act (EMTALA) Technical Advisory Group*, 2021a. https://www.cms.gov/Regulations-and-Guidance/Legislation/EMTALA/emtalatag. Accessed August 8, 2023.

Centers for Medicare and Medicaid Services (CMS): *HCAHPS: patients' perspectives of care survey*, 2021b. https://www.cms.gov/Medicare/Quality-Initiatives-Patient-Assessment-Instruments/HospitalQualityInits/HospitalHCAHPS. Accessed August 8, 2023.

Centers for Medicare and Medicaid Services (CMS): *State operations manual Appendix A—survey protocol, regulations and interpretive guidelines for hospitals, discharge planning*, 2023. https://www.cms.gov/Regulations-and-Guidance/Guidance/Manuals/downloads/som107ap_a_hospitals.pdf. Accessed August 8, 2023.

Cross R, et al: Nursing handover of vital signs at the transition of care from the emergency department to the inpatient ward: an integrative review, *J Clin Nurs* 28:1010, 2019.

Gonzalez MR, et al: ECHO-CT: an interdisciplinary videoconference model for identifying potential post-discharge transition-of-care events, *J Hosp Med* 16:93, 2021.

Hockenberry MJ, et al: *Wong's essentials of pediatric nursing*, ed 11, St. Louis, 2022, Elsevier.

Institute for Healthcare Improvement (IHI): Reduce avoidable readmissions, 2023. http://www.ihi.org/Topics/Readmissions/Pages/default.aspx. Accessed August 8, 2023.

Joint Commission International (JCI): *Communicating clearly and effectively to patients: how to overcome common communication challenges in health care*, 2018. https://store.jointcommissioninternational.org/assets/3/7/jci-wp-communicating-clearly-final_(1).pdf. Accessed August 8, 2023.

Miller MW, et al: *Reduction of hospital-acquired pressure injuries using a multidisciplinary team approach: a descriptive study*, 2019. https://www.medscape.com/viewarticle/913251. Accessed August 8, 2023.

Mulac A, et al: Barcode medication administration technology use in hospital practice: a mixed-methods observational study of policy deviations, *BMJ Qual Saf* 30:1021, 2021.

National Institutes of Health (NIH): *Advance care planning and advance directives: an overview of the main critical issues*, 2022. https://www.ncbi.nlm.nih.gov/pmc/articles/PMC8847241/. Accessed August 8, 2023.

Olson E, et al: *Surgical risk and the preoperative evaluation and management of adults with obstructive sleep apnea*, 2023, UpToDate. https://www.uptodate.com/contents/surgical-risk-and-the-preoperative-evaluation-and-management-of-adults-with-obstructive-sleep-apnea. Accessed May August 8, 2023.

The Joint Commission (TJC): *Comprehensive accreditation manual for hospitals*, Oakbrook Terrace, IL, 2023a, Author.

The Joint Commission (TJC): *2023 National patient safety goals*, Oakbrook Terrace, IL, 2023b, Author. https://www.jointcommission.org/standards/national-patient-safety-goals/. Accessed August 8, 2023.

Toney-Butler TJ, Unison-Pace WJ: *Nursing admission assessment and examination*, 2022. https://www.ncbi.nlm.nih.gov/books/NBK493211/. Accessed August 8, 2023.

Touhy T, Jett K: *Ebersole and Hess' Gerontological Nursing & Healthy Aging*, ed 16, St. Louis, 2022, Elsevier.

Tuohy D: Effective intercultural communication in nursing, *Nurs Stand* 34(2):35, 2019.

Trans Student Education Resources (TSER): *Definitions*, n.d. https://transstudent.org/about/definitions/. Accessed August 8, 2023.

U.S. Department of Health and Human Services (DHHS): *Summary of the HIPAA privacy rule*, Washington, DC, 2022a, Office for Civil Rights.

U.S. Department of Health and Human Services (DHHS): *Your rights under HIPAA*, 2022b. https://www.hhs.gov/hipaa/for-individuals/guidance-materials-for-consumers/index.html. Accessed August 8, 2023.

U.S. Department of Health and Human Services (DHHS): *Health information privacy*, 2023. https://www.hhs.gov/hipaa/index.html. Accessed August 8, 2023.

Weiss AJ, Jiang HJ: *Statistical brief 278*, 2021. https://www.hcup-us.ahrq.gov/reports/statbriefs/sb278-Conditions-Frequent-Readmissions-By-Payer-2018.jsp. Accessed August 8, 2023.

4 | Documentation and Informatics

SKILLS AND PROCEDURES

Procedural Guideline 4.1 **Giving a Hand-Off Report, p. 62**

Procedural Guideline 4.2 **Adverse Event Reporting, p. 64**

OBJECTIVES

Mastery of content in this chapter will enable you to:

- Discuss the features of electronic information systems available to health care providers.
- Compare measures to maintain confidentiality of patient information.
- Identify the purposes of a patient health care record.
- Discuss the elements of an SBAR (*S*ituation, *B*ackground, *A*ssessment, *R*ecommendation) hand-off report and when it would be used.
- Explain the features and benefits of an electronic documentation system.

- Compare the approaches used with charting by exception and problem-oriented documentation when a patient's condition unexpectedly changes.
- Explain how to complete a nursing flow sheet.
- Explain guidelines used in documentation of home care and long-term care.
- Discuss the accurate completion of adverse event reports and when they should be completed.

MEDIA RESOURCES

- http://evolve.elsevier.com/Perry/skills
- Review Questions
- Audio Glossary
- Answers to Clinical Judgment and Next-Generation NCLEX® Examination–Style Questions

- Case Studies
- Printable Key Points
- Skills Performance Checklists

PURPOSE

Health care documentation is anything entered in electronic or written format into a patient's health care record. Documentation of patient care includes a great deal of information. It is an essential component of health care delivery because when it is done correctly and appropriately, it is a form of communication that ensures better continuity of care to patients, increases interaction among health care providers, and improves patient safety (Sermersheim et al., 2020). It is important that you know how to document and report data and apply the information for patient care. The patient health care record is a legal document because it reflects the assessment findings of health care providers, the patient care provided, and an evaluation of outcomes achieved. Patient safety requires that the information included in the patient health care record be objective and timely.

Most health care agencies and systems maintain individual patient information using an electronic health record (EHR) (Box 4.1; Fig. 4.1). An EHR is a digital version of a patient's traditional paper chart. EHRs are real-time, patient-centered records that make information available instantly and securely to authorized users (HealthIT.gov, 2019). The EHR software stores patient information in a digital format. This digitized information or database can be communicated in real time to health care providers who

have access to that system (Harrington, 2019). Informatics refers to the property and structure of information or data. Nursing informatics is the nursing practice specialty that combines nursing science, computer science, and information science to record, organize, and communicate patient information (Healthcare Information and Management Systems Society [HIMSS], 2023).

PRACTICE STANDARDS

- Centers for Medicare and Medicaid Services (CMS), 2022: Final Rule—Principles for documentation practice, home care standards
- Office of the National Coordinator for Health Information Technology (ONC), 2022: Interoperability Standards—Documentation guidelines
- HealthIT.gov, 2018: Safer Guides—Electronic health record safety
- Institute for Safe Medication Practices (ISMP), 2021: List of Error-Prone Abbreviations—Standardized abbreviations
- The Joint Commission (TJC), 2023a: National Patient Safety Goals—Patient identification
- U.S. Department of Health and Human Services (DHHS), 2022: The HIPAA Privacy Rule—Health information privacy

BOX 4.1

Health Care Informatics

- Health information system (HIS)—a group of systems used within a health care organization to support and enhance health care. An HIS has two major types of information systems: a clinical information system (CIS) and an administrative information system. Together, the two systems operate to make the entry and communication of data and information more efficient.
- Clinical information system (CIS)—includes entry of clinical data by health care providers and monitoring systems; order entry systems; and laboratory, radiology, and pharmacy systems. A monitoring system includes devices that automatically monitor biometrics (e.g., vital signs, oxygen saturation). Some devices electronically send information to a nursing documentation system automatically to

reduce nursing workload. The primary purpose of clinical documentation should be to support patient care and improve clinical outcomes through enhanced communication.
- Computerized provider order entry (CPOE) is an example of an order entry system. It allows health care providers to directly enter orders for patient care into an EHR from any computer in the HIS.
- Nursing information system (NIS)—system used to record nursing care activities, most often organized according to the nursing process. The system will support all aspects of nursing practice. Data can also be used for administration, education, and research activities.

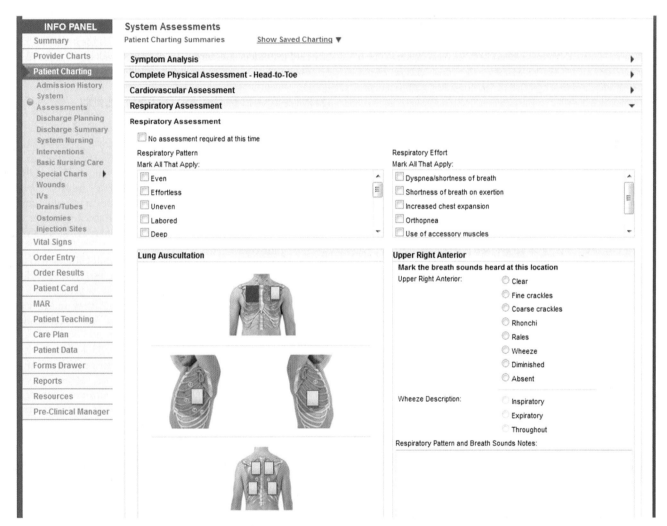

FIG. 4.1 Computerized documentation provides many benefits. (*From Williams PA: Fundamental concepts and skills for nursing, ed 3, St. Louis, 2022, Elsevier.*)

SUPPLEMENTAL STANDARDS

- American Nurses Association (ANA), 2022: Nursing Informatics Scope and Standards of Practice
- Petersen C, et al., 2018: American Medical Informatics Association Code of Professional and Ethical Conduct—Ethical principles for documentation practice

PRINCIPLES FOR PRACTICE

- All members of the health care team are legally and ethically obligated to keep patient information confidential.
- The Health Insurance Portability and Accountability Act of 1996 (HIPAA) protects patients' private health information. HIPAA governs all areas of health information management

---

BOX 4.2

Guidelines for Safe Use of Electronic Health Record

- Sign in to the electronic health record (EHR) using only your password.
- Never share passwords; keep your password private.
- Only open EHRs for patients for whom you are caring.
- Review assessment data, problems identified (nursing diagnoses), goals and expected outcomes, and interventions and patient responses during contact with each patient before data entry.
- Follow procedures for entering information in all appropriate program functions.
- Review previously documented entries with those that you enter, noting if there is significant change in patient's status. Report changes to patient's health care provider.
- The copy-and-paste features in EHRs should be avoided.
- Do not leave information about a patient displayed on a monitor where others can see it.
- Follow agency confidentiality procedures for documenting sensitive material such as diagnosis of human immunodeficiency virus (HIV) infection.
- Know and implement agency protocol for correcting documentation errors.
- Never create, change, or delete records unless your agency provides you with this authority.
- Software systems have a system for backup files. If you inadvertently delete part of the permanent record, follow agency policy.
- Save information as documentation is completed.
- Protect printouts from computerized records. Shredding printouts and logging in the number of copies generated by each health care provider minimizes duplicate records and protects the confidentiality of patient information.
- Sign off when you leave the computer.

---

including patient records, coding, security, and reimbursement (DHHS, 2022).
- The Security Rule and the Privacy Rule of HIPAA provide standards for the protection of EHR information (DHHS, 2022). Guidelines and strategies for safe computer charting are included in Box 4.2.
- Accreditation agencies such as TJC specify guidelines for documentation and require health care agencies to monitor and evaluate the appropriateness of patient care and patient outcomes (TJC, 2023b).
- The AMIA (Peterson et al., 2018) and ANIA (Matney & Settergren, 2018) have set standards for professional and ethical conduct in the use of EHRs and support for interprofessional terminology for documentation used in EHRs.
- Documentation occurs within the context of the nursing process, including documenting evidence of the frequency of patient assessments; problem identification; treatment interventions, including patient and family caregiver teaching; discharge planning; and meeting patient safety goals set by the CMS (2022). Reimbursement for patient health care encounters is dependent on how well patient safety measures are evident in the patient outcomes and documented in the EHR. It is essential to know the standards of your own health care agency.
- Although there are some health care agencies in which EHRs may not be fully implemented, CMS (2022) has incentivized the transition to EHRs by a set of reimbursement rates.
- Standardizing nursing terminology and classification of nursing interventions and patient outcomes results in clear communication of the health care provided (see Box 4.2). This standardization

is integral to yield EHR information required for measuring quality, demonstrating patient safety, meeting legal standards, and achieving reimbursement-related criteria (Matney & Settergren, 2018).
- Standardizing the classification of nursing interventions and nursing outcomes is designed to enhance the efficiency, accuracy, and quality of documentation. In addition, standardization enables data mining that supports the data analytics necessary to determine risks for patient groups. These analytics help incorporate clinical decision support systems that assist in decision making and care planning. Examples of clinical decision supports are safe medication procedures through scanning bar-coded medications and providing drug alerts for possible allergies or interactions.
- Integral to EHR documentation in a health care system is the interoperability of the system (ONC, 2022). Interoperability refers to the ability to de-silo the information documented by each health care provider, not only within a single health care agency, but also within all the partners and participants, including patients, within a health care system. This means all health care providers can access all data in the EHR to make clinical decisions.

PERSON-CENTERED CARE

- A patient's record or chart is a confidential, permanent legal document containing information relevant to a patient's health care. Health care providers document information about a patient's health care after each patient contact. The EHR is a real-time continuing account of a patient's health status and needs, interventions provided, diagnostic test results, and responses to therapy. The clinical record should include a patient's story in as much detail as is required to retell the story for clarity and accuracy.
- Patients' health records and reports communicate specific information about their health status and the interventions that all health care team members contribute toward improving their health. Clear interprofessional communication and documentation are necessary to provide efficient and effective health care and achieve targeted patient outcomes.
- Patient hand-off reports (see Procedural Guideline 4.1) are a standardized approach to communication of patient information among caregivers.
- Reports may be verbal, written, or electronic exchanges of information among caregivers (Fig. 4.2). Reports include

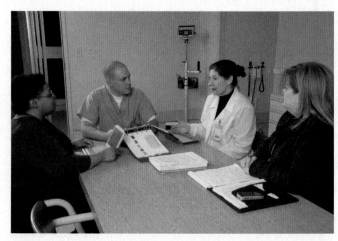

FIG. 4.2 Communication among members of the health care team.

individualized information about a patient's clinical status, observations made about their behavior, data pertaining to diagnostic tests, and directions for changes in therapy.

- Common reports given include end of shift hand-offs, telephone reports, transfer reports, and adverse event reports (see Procedural Guideline 4.2). Including a patient in a bedside shift report can also improve patient satisfaction.

EVIDENCE-BASED PRACTICE

Electronic patient health care records serve as databases of health care data and thus provide sources of information for promoting patient safety within health care agencies (Harrington, 2019). These databases require that the right data are input at the right time in the right place for interprofessional health care team members to take the right actions (Harrington, 2019). In 2014 the Office of the National Coordinator of Health Information Technology released the Safety Assurance Factors for EHR Resilience (SAFER), a series of toolkits that offer recommended best practices to align implementation of EHRs with strategies to ensure their safe use (Agency for Healthcare Research and Quality [AHRQ], 2014). One of the toolkits includes a clinical process guide for clinician communication (Box 4.3) (HealthIT.gov, 2018). Examples of how the information in these databases can be used to improve patient care, while also giving warnings as to current limitations with EHRs, are:

- Use of an EHR has proved to be helpful in management of heart failure patients. EHR data can be used for risk stratification for this patient population. Data entered on these patients can be quickly disseminated across the entire health care team (Kao, 2022).

BOX 4.3

Clinical Process Guide for High-Quality Clinician Communication

- Urgent clinical information is delivered to clinicians in a timely manner, and delivery is documented in the electronic health record (EHR).
- The EHR allows for multiple health care providers to view a patient chart simultaneously.
- The EHR includes the capability for clinicians to review the status of their electronic communications.
- Messages clearly display the individual who initiated the message and the time and date it was sent.
- The EHR facilitates provision of all necessary information for referral and consultation request orders before transmission.
- The EHR facilitates accurate routing of clinician-to-clinician messages and enables forwarding of messages to other clinicians.
- Clinicians are able to electronically access current patient and clinician contact information (e.g., e-mail address, telephone, and fax numbers) and identify clinicians currently involved in a patient's care.
- Electronic message systems include the capability to indicate the urgency of messages.
- The EHR displays time-sensitive and time-critical information more prominently than less urgent information.
- EHR design facilitates clear identification of clinicians who are responsible for action or follow-up in response to a message.
- Mechanisms exist to monitor the timeliness of acknowledgment and response to messages.

Adapted from *HealthIT.gov. Safer guides,* 2018. https://www.healthit.gov/topic/safety/safer-guides Accessed February 27, 2023.

- Research is being conducted into how an EHR can be used to predict central line–associated bloodstream infections (CLABSIs) in a patient, as CLABSIs are associated with increased morbidity, mortality, and health care costs. Data pulled from the EHR can be run through a predictive algorithm that targets risk of these infections (Rahmani et al., 2022).
- A review of several EHR systems in acute care hospital settings indicated improved efficiency and reduced rates of documentation errors, falls, and infections (McCarthy et al., 2019).
- Any error documented in the patient's EHR has capacity to cause harm. Downtime events, periods of time when the EHR is not available for use, can be especially dangerous and lead to errors (Kaipio, 2020).
- Small inefficiencies or design flaws seriously impact clinician workload and patient safety. The EHR for a given agency must be efficient, dynamic, and meet the needs of various users and patient populations. Not all EHR systems are created equal (Dunn Lopez, 2021).
- Confusing interfaces and security measures can disrupt workflow and communication and create incentives for clinicians to develop unsafe workarounds (AHRQ, 2019).

SAFETY GUIDELINES

A patient's EHR is a legal document that reflects all aspects of the patient's care while in a health care setting. As a result, there are standards that all health care agencies integrate into documentation systems to ensure that care delivered represents safe practices. Standards include the following:

- Standard documentation categories include allergy entries, fall risk information, intravenous (IV) fluid rates, and patient-identifying information.
- Information entered into an EHR must be accurate, thorough, and current because all health care providers rely on the information to deliver and coordinate patient care.
- Inaccurate or incomplete documentation or falsification of information can result in medical and nursing therapies that are unnecessary, inappropriate, or delayed, all potentially resulting in negative patient outcomes.
- The Institute for Safe Medication Practices (ISMP, 2021) requires health care agencies to standardize abbreviations, symbols, acronyms, and dose designations and establish a list of abbreviations that should **never** be used. It is essential to know the abbreviation list of the agency in which you work and to use only the accepted abbreviations, symbols, and measures (e.g., metric) so that all documentation is accurate and in compliance with standards. For example, the abbreviation for *every day (qd)* is no longer used (see Chapter 20). If a treatment or medication is needed daily, the written order or care plan should write out the word *"daily"* or *"every day."* The abbreviation *qd (every day)* can be misinterpreted to mean *O.D. (right eye)*.

CONFIDENTIALITY

You are legally and ethically obligated to keep information about patients confidential. Do not disclose information about a patient's status to other patients, family members (unless the patient grants permission), or health care staff not involved in the patient's care. HIPAA requires the DHHS to establish national standards for EHR transactions and national identifiers for providers, health plans, and employers. These standards are designed to improve the efficiency and effectiveness of the U.S. health care system through the widespread use of electronic data interchange. HIPAA addresses the security and privacy of personal health information that identifies the individual, such as demographic data (name, age, social security number, telephone); facts that relate to an individual's past, present, or future physical or mental health conditions; provision of care; and payment for provision of care.

Only health care providers directly involved in a specific patient's care have legitimate access to the EHR. Other professionals may use records for data gathering, research, or education only after gaining permission from appropriate agency, state, and federal institutions. Security mechanisms for information systems use a combination of passwords and physical restrictions such as firewalls and antivirus and antispyware programs to protect information. You must know your agency's policies for the proper use of passwords and ensure that a computer terminal is not left unattended when patient information is still displayed.

Security Mechanisms for Privacy and Confidentiality

There are legal implications associated with the use of electronic documentation. Anyone can access a computer within a health care agency and gain information about almost any patient unless proper security mechanisms are in place. Most clinical information system (CIS) security mechanisms use a combination of logical and physical restrictions to protect information. For example, an automatic sign-off is a safety mechanism that logs a user out of a computer system after a specific time period of inactivity. Other security measures include firewalls and the installation of antivirus

and spyware-detection software. Physical securing measures include placing computers or file servers in restricted areas or using privacy filters for computer screens so they are not visible to visitors or other people who have no computer access. This form of security has limited benefit, especially if an organization uses mobile wireless devices such as notebooks, personal computers (PCs), and smartphones. These devices are easily misplaced or lost and can fall into the wrong hands.

Access codes along with passwords are frequently used for authenticating authorized access to electronic records. A password is a collection of alphanumeric characters and symbols that a user types into a computer sign-on screen before accessing a program. *When using a health care agency computer system, do not share your computer password with anyone under any circumstances.* A good system requires frequent changes in personal passwords to prevent unauthorized persons from accessing and tampering with the system.

LEGAL GUIDELINES IN DOCUMENTATION

It is critical for you to be aware of the legal guidelines for documentation and reporting (Table 4.1). Five common issues in malpractice caused by inadequate or incorrect documentation include the following:
- Failing to document the correct time of events
- Failing to document verbal orders (VOs) or have them signed

---

TABLE 4.1

Legal Guidelines for Documentation and Reporting

Guidelines	Rationale	Correct Action
Use only your unique user identification and password to log into the EHR.	An electronic signature is associated with each user log-in identification and password.	Protect the security of your user identification and password. Once logged on to the computer, do not leave the computer screen unattended.
Do not document retaliatory or critical comments about patient or care by other health care professionals.	Statements can be used as evidence of nonprofessional behavior or poor quality of care.	Enter only objective descriptions of patient's behavior; use quotations for patient's comments.
Need to add patient information into record.	Forgot to chart during a shift.	Back-time to the appropriate time and date or document in real time with note that this is a late entry.
Correct all errors promptly.	Errors in documenting can lead to errors in treatment.	Avoid rushing to complete charting; be sure that information is accurate.
Document all facts.	Record must be accurate and reliable.	Be certain that entry is factual; do not speculate or guess.
If order is questioned, document that you sought clarification.	If you perform an order known to be incorrect, you are just as liable for prosecution as the health care provider.	Do not document "provider made error." Instead, chart that "provider was called to clarify order for analgesic."
Chart only for yourself.	You are accountable for information that you enter into chart.	Never chart for someone else. **Exception:** If caregiver has left unit for day and calls with information that needs to be documented, include the name of the source of information in the entry and that the information was provided via telephone.
Avoid using generalized, empty phrases such as "status unchanged" or "had good day."	Specific information about patient's condition or case can be deleted accidentally if information is too generalized.	Use complete, concise descriptions of care.
If your agency uses paper documentation, only use a black pen with legible handwriting. Do not erase, apply correction fluid, or scratch out errors made while documenting in a paper record.	Charting becomes illegible; it appears as if you were attempting to hide information or deface record.	Draw single line through error, write word *error* above it, and sign your name or initials. Then document note correctly. Check agency policy.

EHR, Electronic health record.

- Charting actions in advance to save time
- Documenting incorrect data
- Failing to give a report or giving an incomplete report to an oncoming shift of coworkers

GUIDELINES FOR HIGH-QUALITY DOCUMENTATION

High-quality documentation and reporting must have the following characteristics.

Factual

Factual data contain descriptive, objective information about what you see, hear, feel, and smell. This includes data from physical examinations and observations of patients' clinical changes. The only subjective data included in a record are what the patient actually verbalizes. Write subjective information with quotation marks, using the patient's exact words whenever possible. For example, document: "Patient states, 'My stomach hurts.'"

Accurate

The use of exact measurements in documentation establishes accuracy. Use standard measures or descriptors. For example, charting that an abdominal wound is "5 cm (2 inches) in length without redness, edema, or drainage" is more descriptive than "large wound healing well." It is essential to avoid unnecessary words, any assumptions, and irrelevant details.

Complete

The information within a recorded entry or a report must be complete, containing appropriate and essential information. A complete entry offers a thorough view of a patient situation. The criteria for reporting and documenting information for specific types of health problems or nursing activities can be found in Table 4.2.

Concise

Documentation of concise data is clear, to the point, and easy to understand. Avoid using unnecessary words and irrelevant detail. An example of a concise note follows:

> Patient ambulated with one person assistance 200 feet down hallway, gait slow but steady, heart rate 78 bpm before exercise, 82 bpm upon returning to room.

An example of a less concise note of the same event is as follows:

> Patient ambulated down nursing unit hallway approximately 200 feet. The patient's gait is slow but steady. Heart rate before exercise 78 beats/min, on returning to bed in room heart rate 82 beats/min. Patient seemed to enjoy walk.

The concise statement provides a more succinct description of the patient's ambulation and includes the most important information.

Current

Current documentation includes making timely entries in a patient's record, which avoids omissions and delay in patient care (ONC, 2022). To increase accuracy and decrease unnecessary duplication, many health care agencies locate EHRs near a patient's bedside, which facilitates immediate documentation of care activities. The use of a computer on wheels (COW) or workstation on wheels (WOW) can prove to be useful for real-time documentation. Document the following activities or findings at the time of occurrence:

- Vital signs
- Pain assessment and evaluation
- Administration of medications and treatments
- Preparation for diagnostic tests or surgery
- Change in patient's status and who was notified
- Treatment for a sudden change in patient's status
- Patient response to intervention
- Admission, transfer, discharge, or death of a patient

TABLE 4.2

Examples of Criteria for Reporting and Documenting

Topic	Criteria to Report or Document
Assessment	
Subjective data	Description of episode/event in patient's words in quotation marks. Clarify onset, location, description of condition (severity; duration; frequency; precipitating, aggravating, and relieving factors)
Patient behavior	Onset, behaviors exhibited (e.g., anxiety, confusion, hostility), precipitating factors
Objective data (e.g., rash, tenderness, breath sounds)	Onset, location, description of condition (severity; duration; frequency; precipitating, aggravating, and relieving factors)
Nursing Interventions and Evaluation	
Treatments (e.g., enema, bath, dressing change)	Time administered, equipment used (if appropriate), patient's response (objective and subjective changes) compared with previous treatment (e.g., "rated pain 2 on a scale of 0-10 during dressing change" or "patient reported no abdominal cramping during enema")
Medication administration	During administration, document: time medication given, dose, route, any preliminary assessment (e.g., pain level, vital signs), patient response or effect of medication. Example: 1200: "Pain reported at 7 (scale 0-10)." Acetaminophen 6500 mg given PO. 1230: Patient reports pain: "Pain at level 2 (scale 0-10) at 1330" or "Pruritus and hives developed over lower abdomen 1 hour after penicillin was given"
Patient teaching	Information presented using teach-back; method of instruction (e.g., discussion, demonstration, videotape, booklet); patient response, including questions and evidence of understanding such as return demonstration or change in behavior
Discharge planning	Measurable patient goals or expected outcomes, progress toward goals, need for referrals

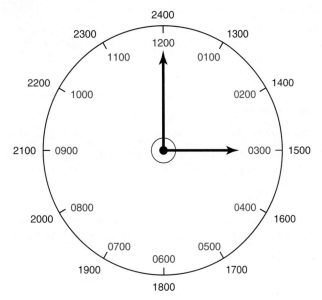

FIG. 4.3 Military Time Clock. Instead of two 12-hour cycles, the military clock is one 24-hour time cycle (e.g., 3 p.m. is 1500 military time).

Most health care agencies use military time, a 24-hour system that avoids misinterpretation of a.m. and p.m. times. Military time is recommended for documenting the time of events. The military clock ends with midnight at 2400 and begins 1 minute after midnight at 0001. For example, 1:00 p.m. is 1300 military time; 10:22 a.m. is 1022 military time. Fig. 4.3 compares military and civilian times. An EHR generates time of entry when you submit an entry. However, this time can be manually adjusted in the EHR as needed.

Organized

Information entered in a health care record facilitates communication when it is documented in a logical order. To document notes about complex situations in an organized fashion, first think about the situation and then make decisions about what information and words you need to include before beginning to enter data in the health care record. Application of your critical thinking skills and the nursing process will help you document clearly and comprehensively in a logical order. For example, an organized entry would describe a patient's pain, your assessment and resultant interventions, and the patient's response to treatment.

Recorded Signature

It is necessary to clearly know who enters information into the health care record. ONC standards (2022) require that "all entries in medical records be dated and a method established to identify the authors of entries," which is accomplished when you sign in with your unique log-on name and password. Thus each entry in a patient's record includes your full name and credentials because the EHR generates your name and credentials when the entry is submitted.

METHODS OF DOCUMENTATION

A nursing information system (NIS) method of documenting is often selected by a nursing administration to reflect the philosophy of the department. The type of forms and how they are formatted electronically or in a written format is dictated by the documentation system software chosen by a health care agency. For example,

many acute care agencies, outpatient and ambulatory settings, and rehabilitation and long-term care facilities use the terminology of Nursing Interventions Classification (NIC) and Nursing Outcomes Classification (NOC) (Aini et al., 2023). Another Classification system, the International Classification for Nursing Practice (ICNP), is a unified nursing language system that supports the standardization of nursing documentation at the point of care (ICNP, 2019). The ICNP, NIC, and NOC are included in electronic care planning and documentation systems across the globe.

A problem-oriented medical record (POMR) is a structured interprofessional method of documenting narratives that emphasizes a patient's nursing diagnoses or medical diagnoses or problems. When you use POMR, the method organizes data using the nursing process, which facilitates communication about patient needs. Data are organized by a problem or diagnosis. Ideally, all members of the health care team contribute to the list of identified patient problems. This approach helps to coordinate an individualized plan of care with the following sections: database, problem list, care plan, and progress notes.

In a source record, a patient's chart is organized so that each discipline (e.g., nursing, medicine, social work, respiratory therapy) has a separate section in which to document data. This traditional method of charting is seen less often today. The advantage of a source record is that it is easy for caregivers to locate the proper section of the record in which to make entries. A disadvantage of the source record is that information about a specific problem may be distributed throughout the record. The method makes it difficult to find chronological information about patient care or how the team is coordinating care to meet all the patient's needs. The patient's story is fragmented.

COMMON ELECTRONIC HEALTH RECORD DATA SCREENS

The patient EHR contains comprehensive evidence of a patient's health status. It includes a variety of screens within an NIS to facilitate quick and comprehensive documentation. Use of these screens helps avoid duplication of information within the record. The same screens can be found in the forms used in paper records.

Admission Nursing History

You complete a comprehensive nursing history to gather baseline assessment data when a patient is admitted to a health care setting. The type of health care setting influences the scope of assessment categories. Use the admission data to form a plan of care and compare it with any changes in a patient's condition (see Chapter 3). The nursing history guides you through a complete assessment and physical examination (see Chapter 6) to identify relevant nursing diagnoses or problems for the patient's care plan. Examples of information included in the nursing history are patient allergies, primary spoken and written language, advance directives, disabilities, mobility/fall risk assessment, and medication history and reconciliation (see Chapter 20).

Flow Sheets and Graphics

Flow sheets and graphic records permit concise documentation of nursing information and help to track trends of patient data over time. The screens are especially useful for the documentation of routine observations or repeated specific measurements for a patient such as vital signs (see Chapter 5), intake and output (see Chapter 28), hygiene measures, medication administration (see Chapter 20), and pain assessment (see Chapter 16). Flow sheets use a format or system for entry of information, usually every

Summary

Adult Overview

Adult Overview

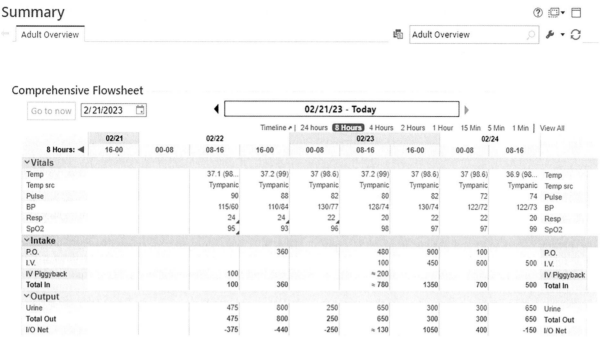

Comprehensive Flowsheet

Go to now 2/21/2023

02/21/23 - Today

Timeline ↗ | 24 hours **8 Hours** 4 Hours 2 Hours 1 Hour 15 Min 5 Min 1 Min | View All

8 Hours: ◀	02/21 16-00	00-08	02/22 08-16	16-00	00-08	02/23 08-16	16-00	02/24 00-08	08-16	
˅Vitals										
Temp			37.1 (98...	37.2 (99)	37 (98.6)	37.2 (99)	37 (98.6)	37 (98.6)	36.9 (98...	Temp
Temp src			Tympanic	Tympanic	Tympanic	Tympanic	Tympanic	Tympanic	Tympanic	Temp src
Pulse			90	88	82	80	82	72	74	Pulse
BP			115/60	110/84	130/77	128/74	130/74	122/72	122/73	BP
Resp			24	24	22	20	22	22	20	Resp
SpO2			95	93	96	98	97	97	99	SpO2
˅Intake										
P.O.				360		480	900	100		P.O.
I.V.						100	450	600	500	I.V.
IV Piggyback			100			≈ 200				IV Piggyback
Total In			100	360		≈ 780	1350	700	500	Total In
˅Output										
Urine			475	800	250	650	300	300	650	Urine
Total Out			475	800	250	650	300	300	650	Total Out
I/O Net			-375	-440	-250	≈ 130	1050	400	-150	I/O Net

FIG. 4.4 Graphic and intake-output record, electronic version. (© 2023 Epic Systems Corporation.)

24 hours (Fig. 4.4). When documenting a significant change that you recognize on a flow sheet, describe the change in the progress notes, including the patient's response to nursing interventions. For example, if a patient's blood pressure becomes dangerously low, document in the progress notes the blood pressure, relevant assessment data such as pallor or dizziness, and any interventions to raise the blood pressure (e.g., increase in IV fluid infusion per health care provider order). Also include an evaluation of the interventions such as repeated blood pressures and relief of dizziness. Licensed practical nurses and other health care providers such as assistive personnel (AP) may have the responsibility to document on nursing flow sheets or screens.

Patient Education Records

Many health care agencies have an education record that identifies patients' knowledge base about their diagnosis(es), treatments, and medications. The goal of patient and family caregiver education is to promote healthy behaviors and self-care by involving the patient and/or family caregiver in decisions, which improve health outcomes. Standards for patient education include assessment of health literacy level and teaching needs, functional abilities, learning styles, and readiness to learn. You will base patient education needs on the assessment and then teach patients about topics such as safe and effective use of medications, nutrition and dietary modifications, safe use of medical equipment, pain control, rehabilitative methods to promote and improve functional abilities, and self-care activities (ONC, 2022). When documenting in a patient education record, be specific about the information and/or skills taught, information given to the patient, and the results of the teach-back method of evaluating patient understanding of education topics.

Patient Care Summary

Many health care agencies have software systems that are designed with a concise set of information in the form of a patient care summary. This summary offers a broad overview of a patient's current

health care status and plan of care. Thus it gives you a valuable worksheet for a shift of care. A copy can be printed for each patient during each shift. Data are updated automatically as new orders and nursing decisions enter the system. The patient care summary generally includes the following:
- Basic demographic data (e.g., age, religion)
- Primary medical diagnosis
- Current health care provider's orders (e.g., diet, activity, dressing changes)
- Plan of care
- Nursing orders or interventions (e.g., skin care, comfort measures, teaching)
- Scheduled tests and procedures
- Safety precautions used in the patient's care
- Factors related to activities of daily living
- Nearest relative/guardian or person to contact in an emergency
- Emergency code status
- Allergies

Acuity Records

Many health care agencies use a patient acuity system as a method of determining what an equitable distribution of nurse staffing is based on the intensity of patient needs on the unit (Johnston & Strusowski, 2022). Patient acuity measurements serve as a guide for determining staffing needs on a nursing unit. An acuity documentation system determines the hours of nursing care and number of staff required for a nursing unit.

Oftentimes, you will enter acuity data into a computerized system in the morning, using the guidelines of the specific acuity system. The administrative staff collect the acuity data electronically and use them to make appropriate staffing decisions. Acuity levels allow the nursing staff to compare patients with one another. For example, an acuity system might rate bathing patients from 1 to 5 (1 is totally dependent, 5 is independent); a patient returning from surgery who requires frequent monitoring and extensive care has an acuity level of 1. On the same continuum another patient awaiting discharge after a successful recovery from surgery has an acuity level of 5. Accurate acuity ratings justify the number and qualifications of staff needed to safely care for patients on a particular unit.

Standardized Care Plans

In any health care setting, you are responsible for providing a nursing plan of care for each patient. The plan of care can take several forms (e.g., individual electronic care plan and standardized care plans). With the growth of EHRs within health care institutions, documentation systems typically include software programs for creating individualized and standard nursing care plans. These programs use standardized nursing language including nursing diagnostic language (e.g., International Classification for Nursing Practice [ICNP]) and NOC and NIC taxonomies. A standardized care plan is generated from the data compiled from patient assessment information. These plans incorporate several nursing diagnoses or problems in a single nursing or interprofessional plan. The systems improve documentation and facilitate high-quality care based on scientific evidence and proven experience (Ostensen et al., 2022).

After completing a nursing assessment, identify the patient's nursing diagnosis(es) or health problem(s) and select the appropriate standardized care plan(s) for the patient's EHR. Always individualize each plan for a patient. Most standardized care plans allow for the addition of patient-specific outcomes and target dates for achieving these outcomes.

One disadvantage of standardized care plans is an increased risk that the unique, individualized therapies needed by patients will go unrecognized. Standardized care plans do not replace clinical judgment and decision making. In addition, care plans need to be updated on a regular basis to ensure that content is current and appropriate.

Critical Pathways

Critical pathways are a system of care plan documentation that incorporates the goals and important treatment interventions for a specific health condition on the basis of best practices and the expected progress of a patient. A critical pathway system includes documenting, monitoring, and evaluating clinical variances from the expected standards. Key interventions and expected outcomes are established within an expected time frame for specific diseases (e.g., knee replacement surgery and stroke) (Fig. 4.5). Variances are unexpected occurrences, unmet goals, and interventions not specified within the critical pathway time frame and reflect a positive or negative change. A positive variance occurs when a patient progresses more rapidly than the pathway expected (e.g., use of a Foley catheter is discontinued a day early). A negative variance occurs when the activities on the critical pathway do not happen as predicted or outcomes are unmet (e.g., oxygen therapy is necessary for a new-onset breathing problem). Document the variance and include causative factors, actions taken, patient response, and outcomes. Over

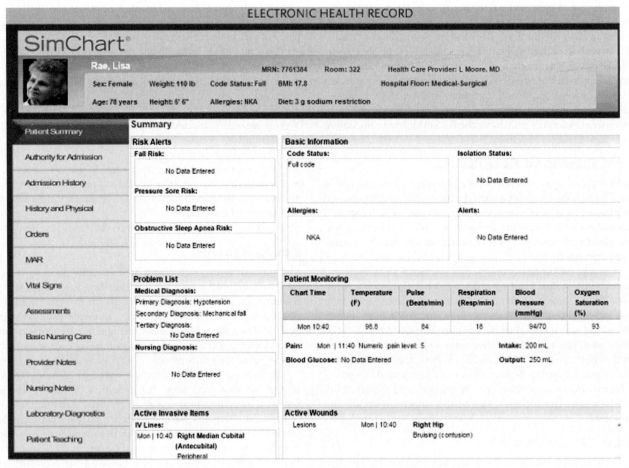

FIG. 4.5 Example of sections/information available in an electronic health record (EHR).
(Copyright © Elsevier 2019. SimChart www.evolve.elsevier.com.)

Discharge Summary Information

- Use clear, concise descriptions in patient's own language.
- Provide step-by-step description of how to perform a procedure (e.g., home medication administration). Reinforce explanation with printed instructions for the patient to take home.
- Provide a detailed list of all prescribed medications.
- Identify precautions to follow when performing self-care or procedures (e.g., dressing change) or taking medications.
- Review any restrictions that may relate to activities of daily living (e.g., bathing, ambulating, driving).
- Review signs and symptoms of complications to report to health care provider.
- List names and phone numbers of health care providers and community resources for the patient to contact.
- Identify any unresolved problem(s), including plans for follow-up and continuous treatment.
- List actual time of discharge, mode of transportation, and who accompanied patient.

time the recurrence of similar variances leads the health care team to revise a critical pathway, particularly if it affects quality of care or length of stay.

Discharge Summaries

A discharge summary includes essential information for a patient, family caregiver, and health care agency (Box 4.4) and is based on data obtained from the discharge planning process. Discharge planning is a comprehensive process, with emphasis placed on preparing a patient for discharge from a health care agency.

ONC (2022) has standards for patient and family education necessary for effective discharge planning. When a patient is discharged from a health care agency, the members of the health care team prepare a discharge summary. It provides important information relating to the patient's ongoing health problems and need for health care after discharge. Include in the discharge summary the reason for hospitalization; significant findings; current status of the patient (e.g., clinical condition, current treatments); all the medications the patient should take on discharge; and the teaching plan that is given to the patient, family caregiver, home care, rehabilitation, or long-term care facility (TJC, 2023a). Copies of the discharge summary should be given to the patient, family caregiver, and receiving health care agency and forwarded to the patient's health care provider. These summaries play a significant role in the continuity of care that is the basis of patient safety.

DOCUMENTATION FORMATS

A variety of documentation formats (organizational approaches for entering information) exist for documenting patient information and progress. The documentation system format selected usually reflects the philosophy of the health care agency. The same documentation format is used throughout a specific health care agency. There are several acceptable formats for documenting health care data.

Narrative Documentation

Narrative charting uses a storylike free-text format to document specific information about a patient's conditions and nursing care, usually presented in chronological order. It is useful in emergency situations when the time and order of events are important. Organize a narrative in a clear, concise way (e.g., by using the nursing process to order the data), for example:

> A 61-year-old patient was admitted through the emergency department with the chief complaint of shortness of breath. Patient presents with respirations 30, BP 110/68, heart rate 88 beats/min, temp 37.6°C (99.7°F). Chest x-ray obtained per order from provider. Radiological results show right and left pleural effusion. Patient states, "I have had a hard time getting my breath for the past week." Denies chest pain. Preparing patient for insertion of bilateral chest tubes.

Charting by Exception

Charting by exception (CBE) is a system of documentation that aims to eliminate redundancy, makes documentation of routine care more concise, emphasizes abnormal findings, and identifies trends in clinical care. CBE is a shorthand method for documenting on the basis of clearly defined standards of practice and predetermined criteria for nursing assessments and interventions. This system involves completing a flow sheet that incorporates standard assessment and intervention criteria by placing a check mark in the appropriate standard box on the flow sheet to indicate normal findings and routine interventions. These predefined standards used to document nursing assessments are called "within defined limits" (WDL) or "within normal limits" (WNL). Automated documentation in a computerized system allows you to select a WDL statement or to choose other statements from a drop-down menu that allows description of any unexpected findings. You write a narrative nurse's note only when there is an exception to the established standard criteria or when abnormal data are present. Assessments are standardized on forms, so all health care providers evaluate and document findings consistently.

The presumption with CBE is that you assessed the patient, and all standards are met unless otherwise documented. Changes in a patient's condition require thorough and precise descriptions of what happened, actions taken, and patient response to treatment. Legal risks in using CBE include difficulty in proving safe care if you are not disciplined in documenting exceptions.

Problem-Oriented Medical Records

A POMR is a structured method of documenting narratives that emphasizes a patient's problems or diagnoses. This method organizes data using the nursing process, which facilitates communication about patient needs to all members of the health care team. This approach helps to coordinate an individualized plan of care with the following sections: database, problem list, care plan, and progress notes.

Patient Database

A database contains all available information pertaining to a patient. This section is the foundation for identifying patient problems or diagnoses and planning care. The database remains active and current for each patient and is revised as new data become available.

Problem List

The problem list includes the patient's physiological, psychological, sociocultural, spiritual, developmental, and environmental needs identified as problems or diagnoses. The list is created after analyzing assessment data for a patient. Identify, list, and date priority problems in chronological order to serve as an organizing guide for the patient's care and progress. Add new problems as they are identified during the ongoing nursing assessment. When a problem is resolved, document the date and indicate that the problem is resolved.

Plan of Care

All disciplines involved in a patient's care contribute to the development of an interprofessional plan of care for a specific problem. For example, for a patient having a nutritional deficit, you may recommend feeding approaches, and a registered dietitian may recommend types of dietary supplements. Care plan standards require that a plan of care be developed for all patients on admission to a health care agency (TJC, 2023a). In general, these plans include nursing diagnoses, expected outcomes, interventions, and evaluations.

Progress Notes

Health care team members use progress notes to monitor and document the progress of a patient's problems and response to interventions. Narrative notes using problem-oriented formats, flow sheets, and discharge summaries collectively document patient progress.

VERBAL REPORTING

Structured verbal communication, with health care providers who report in the SBAR (Situation, Background, Assessment, Recommendation) format, is a concrete approach for framing conversations, especially critical ones that require immediate attention and action. SBAR originates from its use in the Navy. Health care organizations such as the Institute for Healthcare Improvement and the National Health Service recognize SBAR as an effective communication tool (Lo et al., 2021). The SBAR format is a reliable and validated communication tool that has shown a reduction in adverse events in a hospital setting, improvement in communication among health care providers, and promotion of patient safety (Lo et al., 2021). The SBAR format allows for an easy and focused way to set expectations for what the interprofessional team will communicate. SBAR promotes efficient, timely, and person-centered communication. This method is used primarily for verbal communication when a patient's condition changes, for a brief targeted report (e.g., as a preprocedure or postprocedure report), or as a change-of-shift hand-off report (see Procedural Guideline 4.1).

PROCEDURAL GUIDELINE 4.1 *Giving a Hand-off Report*

In addition to written documentation, you provide a verbal change-of-shift report to the next nurse assuming responsibility for patient care. In many clinical settings this hand-off report occurs at a patient's bedside. Bedside reporting is a process of exchanging vital patient information, responsibility, and accountability between the off-going and oncoming nurses in an effort to ensure safe continuity of care and the delivery of best clinical practices (Becker et al., 2021). The consequences of failed communication during hand-offs are medication errors, inaccurate patient plans, delay in transfer of patients to critical care, delay in hospital discharges, and repetitive diagnostic testing (Becker et al., 2021). Giving hand-off reports face to face can increase patient satisfaction and improve outcomes (Becker et al., 2021). The face-to-face hand-off allows you to ask questions and clarify any misinformation. It is also a way to more actively involve patients in decisions regarding their plan of care.

However, there can be patient dissatisfaction issues if hand-off reports are not done well. Research has shown dissatisfaction from difficulties understanding the report and medical jargon, tiredness as a result of information being repeated multiple times, lack of privacy, anxiety over incorrect information or too much information, and inconsistency with how the bedside shift report was conducted (Sermersheim et al., 2020). It is important for the patient to feel included and comfortable with the bedside report. Although the use of a mobile computer can aid in giving a thorough report to the oncoming nurse, do not let it distract you from the patient in front of you. During hand-offs, mnemonics in the form of SBAR may increase the memory of important steps and provide a structured and standardized process to follow.

Delegation

The skill of giving a hand-off report cannot be delegated to assistive personnel (AP). Direct the AP to:
- Report to a nurse any clinical change (e.g., increased pain, patient requests, changes in vital signs) so that any assessments, validation, or changes in the patient's condition can be included in the hand-off report.

Equipment

EHR worksheets, patient care summary, critical pathway or interprofessional treatment plan, EHR (if implemented by agency)

Steps

1. Plan to use an organized format for delivering the report that provides a description of patient needs and problems. SBAR (Situation, Background, Assessment, Recommendation) can be used to organize and streamline a report.
2. If giving a report at bedside, identify the patient using at least two identifiers (e.g., name and birthday or name and medical record number) according to agency policy (TJC, 2023a).
3. Gather information from documentation sources, AP report, or other relevant documents.

Clinical Judgment *Report only relevant and current information to next shift to ensure staff's timely responsiveness.*

4. Prioritize information on the basis of patient's problems and nursing diagnoses.
5. For each patient include the following:
   - Situation: Patient's name, gender, age, chief complaint on admission, and current situation.
   - Background information: Allergies, emergency code status (i.e., do not resuscitate [DNR]), medical and surgical histories, special needs as related to any physical challenges (e.g., blind, hearing deficit, amputee), and vaccinations.
   - Assessment data: Objective observations and measurements you made during the shift; emphasis on any recent changes. Include any relevant information reported by patient, family caregiver, or health care team members such as laboratory data and diagnostic test results. Include therapies or treatments administered during shift and expected outcomes (e.g., medication

PROCEDURAL GUIDELINE 4.1 *Giving a Hand-off Report—cont'd*

changes, use of oxygen, referral visits). Describe education given in the teaching plan and patient's/family caregiver's ability to demonstrate learning. Report on evaluation by explaining patient's response and whether outcomes are met. Review patient's progress toward discharge during each change-of-shift report.

- **R**ecommendation: Explanation of the priorities to which oncoming nurse/health care provider must

attend, including referrals, nursing orders, and core measures.

6. Ask staff from oncoming shift if they have any questions regarding information provided. Clarify any confusion or misinformation.

7. If report given at bedside, encourage patient to ask questions; are there any decisions the patient wishes to add to treatment plan?

Telephone and Verbal Orders

Telephone orders (TOs) occur when a health care provider gives therapeutic orders over the phone to a registered nurse (RN). Verbal orders (VOs) occur when a health care provider gives therapeutic orders to an RN while they are standing in proximity to each other. Use of VOs is discouraged except in urgent or emergent situations. TOs and VOs often occur at night or during emergencies; they should be used only when absolutely necessary and not for the sake of convenience. It is wise to have a second person listen to TOs, and some agency policies require it. Box 4.5 provides guidelines for accurate TOs and VOs.

When receiving a TO or VO, enter the complete order into the computer using the computerized provider order entry (CPOE) software, or write it out on a provider's order entry sheet so that it can be entered into the computer as soon as possible. After you receive an order, use the read-back process to ensure you are entering the correct order. Read back to the provider exactly what you were told. For example:

> I am going to read that back to you: Change IV fluid to lactated Ringer solution with potassium chloride 20 mEq/L to run at 125 mL/h STAT. Is that correct?

Do not enter an order for a health care provider without confirmation via read-back. Ensure all pieces necessary for entering the order are given to you, such as dose, rate, time, and frequency.

INCIDENT OR ADVERSE EVENT OCCURRENCE REPORTS

An adverse event is any event not consistent with the routine operation of a health care unit or routine care of a patient. Examples include patient falls, needlestick injuries, medication errors, or a visitor becoming ill. A standardized list of preventable, serious adverse events that may occur within a health care agency is depicted in Box 4.6. Completion of an adverse event occurrence report happens when there is actual or potential patient injury (near miss) that is not part of the patient record (Labrague, 2020). Document in the patient's record an objective description of what you observed and follow-up actions taken without reference to the incident report/occurrence report. A review of adverse events by an agency helps to identify high-risk trends in nursing care or daily unit operations that warrant correction. You complete a report even if an injury does not occur or is not apparent. The information from incident reports for a unit or hospital helps nursing staff explore causes and find solutions to prevent repeated incidents (Labrague, 2020). The reports are an important part of the quality improvement program of a unit and health care agency.

BOX 4.5

Guidelines for Telephone and Verbal Orders

- Only authorized staff (who are identified in a written policy by each agency) receive and document telephone orders (TOs) and verbal orders (VOs).
- Clearly identify the patient's name, room number, and diagnoses.
- Use clarification questions to avoid misunderstandings. Ask provider to repeat a word or phrase if needed.
- Enter TOs or VOs into the patient's EHR with date and time received, the complete order transcribed exactly as stated, and the name of health care provider giving order.
- Read back all TOs and VOs to health care provider.
- Follow agency policies. Some agencies require TOs and VOs to be reviewed and signed by two nurses.
- The health care provider cosigns each TO and VO within the time frame required by each agency (usually 24 hours).

BOX 4.6

Examples of Serious Reportable Events Occurring Within a Health Care Agency

- Surgery or other invasive procedure performed on the wrong patient
- Unintended retention of foreign object in a patient after surgery or invasive procedure
- Delay in treatment
- Patient death or serious injury associated with:
  - Use of restraints or bedrails
  - Use or function of a device in patient care in which device is used for or functions other than intended
  - A fall
  - Electrical shock
  - Elopement
  - Medication error
  - Unsafe administration of blood products
  - Suicide
- Stage 3 or 4 pressure injury acquired after admission to a health care agency

From the Joint Commission: *Most commonly reviewed sentinel event types*, Oakbrook Terrace, IL, 2021, The Joint Commission. https://www.jointcommission.org/-/media/tjc/documents/resources/patient-safety-topics/sentinel-event/most-frequently-reviewed-event-types-2020.pdf. Accessed August 10, 2023.

PROCEDURAL GUIDELINE 4.2 *Adverse Event Reporting*

Adverse event reports are important sources of data for enhancing understanding of underlying causes of events that, when analyzed, can improve patient safety (Labrague, 2020). You are an active participant in examining the cause of errors and redesigning systems to minimize the same type of errors in the future. By focusing on systems rather than individual failures, there is greater opportunity to improve patient safety (Labrague, 2020). For example, when a patient is administered the wrong medication by a nurse, a review of the event focuses primarily on the medication process as opposed to blaming the nurse for the error.

Delegation
The skill of adverse event reporting cannot be delegated to assistive personnel (AP). Instruct the AP to:
* Report to a nurse any event such as a fall, incorrect treatment, or adverse reaction observed or performed by the AP.
* Report to a nurse any pertinent information about the event so that a report can be completed.

Interprofessional Collaboration
* When more than one health care provider is in a patient room at the time of an incident and both witness the event, review the event together. Each witness should tell you what happened. Use direct quotations.

Equipment
Adverse occurrence event report system (likely this will be a separate application from your EHR)

Steps
1. When you witness an adverse event, assess the extent of any injury to patient or others, including patient's subjective report and objective physical examination findings.
2. If the adverse event involves an injury, take steps to restore individual's safety such as stabilizing patient's position after a fall and assessing for further injuries.
3. When patient sustains an injury, call the health care provider immediately.
4. Use clinical judgment skills to systematically and carefully assess what was involved in the event. Either report the event as witnessed or determine from AP specifically what occurred.
5. Notify the risk-management department per agency protocol.

Clinical Judgment *Prepare the report on any questionable event. Do not avoid reporting because of concerns that punitive actions will occur if reports are filed.*

6. Provide any treatment ordered or prepare patient for any diagnostic tests (e.g., x-ray).
7. When visitor or staff member sustains an injury, refer to emergency department or appropriate treatment setting.
8. Complete adverse occurrence event report form as follows:

Clinical Judgment *Document on report form as quickly as possible. The closer to the event, the more accurate the documentation.*

   a. Document time of event and describe in chronological order exactly what occurred or was observed, using objective findings and observations. Document nurse involved, condition of patient when discovered or observed, and observation of factors that possibly contributed to incident (e.g., in the case of a fall, presence of wet floor, extension cord). Use language that does not allow for subjective interpretation. Do not include personal opinions or feelings.
   b. Describe measures taken by any caregivers at time of event.
   c. Document victim's interpretation of event by using quotes. If there were witnesses, use quotation marks to frame their statements.
9. Submit completed report and notify your management team per agency policy.
10. When patient is involved, document events of incident in patient's chart.
   a. Enter only objective description of what happened.
   b. Document any assessment and intervention activities initiated as a result of event.
   c. Do not duplicate all information from report.
   d. Do not document in record that an occurrence report was completed.
11. Submit the report promptly with the risk-management department or designated people.
12. Conduct an adverse event huddle. For example, in the case of a fall, huddle with members of the interprofessional team to critique nature of the fall event and identify possible preventive strategies in the future. Postevent huddles may reduce the risk of repeat incidents. Staff who participate in postevent huddles have been found to have positive perceptions of teamwork support for risk reduction and a safety culture (Jones et al., 2019).

HOME CARE DOCUMENTATION

Home care for patients continues to grow with shorter hospitalizations and increasing numbers of older adults requiring home care services. Medicare has specific guidelines for establishing eligibility for home care reimbursement. For example, for home infusion therapy, there are parameters set for the type of intravenous medication administered (CMS, 2022). Documentation when caring for a patient in the home has different implications than in other areas of nursing. One primary difference is that the patient and family caregiver rather than the nurse witness the majority of care.

In addition, documentation systems need to provide the entire health care team with the necessary information to work together effectively (Box 4.7). The smooth transition from hospital to home is critical for patient safety. If, for example, medications are not clearly indicated and described in the hospital-to-home transition, this has a negative impact on home care and may result in a readmission to the hospital. Clear and complete documentation is both the quality control and the justification for reimbursement from Medicare, Medicaid, or private insurance companies. Computerized patient records are evolving in the home care setting (Sarzynski et al., 2019).

Forms for Home Care Documentation

The usual forms used to document home care include the following:
- Patient assessment
- Referral source information/intake form
- Discipline-specific care plans
- Health care provider's plan of treatment
- Medication sheet
- Clinical progress notes
- Miscellaneous (conference notes, verbal order forms, telephone calls)
- Discharge summary
- Reports to third-party payers

LONG-TERM HEALTH CARE DOCUMENTATION

Increasing numbers of older adults and disabled people in the United States require care in long-term health care facilities. Standardized protocols for assessment and care planning for long-term health care agencies are mandated by the Long-Term Care Facility Resident Assessment in the Omnibus Budget Reconciliation Act of 1989 (OBRA).

You are responsible for assessing the patient and coordinating the plan of care in the long-term health care agency. Clear documentation supports the care process for patients through communication among the interprofessional health care providers of nurses, social workers, recreational therapists, and dietitians. The fiscal support for long-term care residents depends on the justification of nursing care as demonstrated in sound and consistent documentation of the services rendered.

✦ CLINICAL JUDGMENT AND NEXT-GENERATION NCLEX® EXAMINATION-STYLE QUESTIONS

A 68-year-old patient is hospitalized following lithotripsy of renal calculi. Medications documented on admission include vitamin D 600 IU one tablet PO once daily and atorvastatin 10 mg one tablet PO once daily. There are no known drug allergies. As the nurse performs an assessment several hours after the procedure, the patient reports back pain at a level of 5 on a 0-to-10 scale that radiates to the lower abdomen, as well as mild nausea and cramping. The patient denies chest pain and breathing difficulty. The health care provider prescribed ondansetron 16 mg by dissolvable film and acetaminophen 650 mg PO every 4 to 6 hours.

1. The nurse prepares to administer ondansetron and acetaminophen when the patient states, "I don't want the acetaminophen. I want something stronger for the pain. However, I will take the other medication." How will the nurse document this patient response in the electronic health record?
   1. "Patient refuses acetaminophen and requests "something stronger." Provider notified. Ondansetron 16 mg by dissolvable film administered."
   2. "Patient appears to be drug seeking by refusing to take acetaminophen."
   3. "Patient only took ondansetron 16 mg dissolvable film for nausea."
   4. "Patient uncooperative with medication administration; refused acetaminophen and would only accept ondansetron."

2. The patient attempts to go to the bathroom without using the nurse call system and falls. The nurse finds the patient on the floor and assesses the right wrist to be tender, edematous, and reddened. Select three actions the nurse will take at this time.
   1. Assess extent of other potential injuries to the patient.
   2. Report the fall to the nurse manager of the unit.
   3. Contact the health care provider to report the situation.
   4. Request that the provider place an order for an x-ray of the right wrist.
   5. File an incident report in the patient's electronic health record.
   6. Scold the patient for getting up without using the nurse call system.
   7. Document the sequence of events that took place before and after the fall.

3. The patient's family arrives to see the patient and is concerned about the fall. Which nursing response is appropriate when the family requests to see the patient's electronic health record?
   1. "Because you are the patient's nearest relative, I can make the record available."
   2. "The health record can only be released to you after the patient is discharged."
   3. "Tell me why you are concerned about the fall, and I can answer your questions."
   4. "We cannot legally give you access to the health record unless the patient consents."

4. After performing an assessment before bedtime, the nurse documents more information in the health record. Which entry is reflective of appropriate documentation?
   1. Family caregiver is questioning whether staff were involved in causing patient's fall.
   2. Patient resting in bed, positioned on left side with right wrist elevated on pillow.
   3. Fall that took place earlier was likely precipitated by water left on floor by housekeeper.
   4. Filled out incident report after patient fell earlier in the evening.

5. The following morning, the nurse assesses the patient again after learning that the wrist x-ray was negative for fracture. Which of the following patient statements demonstrates that nursing actions from the prior evening and night were effective? **Select all that apply.**
   1. "My wrist pain is a 7 on a 0-to-10 scale."
   2. "I have been using my nurse call system when I need to go to the bathroom."
   3. "It looks like I have less swelling in my right hand and wrist this morning."
   4. "Is it time for my next pain medication yet?"
   5. "I am going to keep this soft brace on my wrist for comfort the next few days."

Visit the Evolve site for Answers to Clinical Judgment and Next-Generation NCLEX® Examination-Style Questions.

REFERENCES

Agency for Healthcare Research and Quality (AHRQ): *Safety assurance factors for her resilience: SAFER guides,* Office of the National Coordinator for Health Information Technology, 2014. https://psnet.ahrq.gov/issue/safety-assurance-factors-ehr-resilience-safer-guides. Accessed February 27, 2023.

Agency for Healthcare Research and Quality (AHRQ): *Patient safety network: electronic health records,* 2019. https://psnet.ahrq.gov/primer/electronic-health-records. Accessed February 27, 2023.

Aini N, et al. The effect of standardized nursing terminology education program on quality of nursing documentation: A systematic review. *Malaysian J Med Health Sci* 19:125-134, 2023.

American Nurses Association (ANA): *Nursing informatics: scope and standards for practice,* ed 3, Silver Spring, MD, 2022, ANA.

Becker S, et al: Implementing and sustaining bedside shift report for quality patient-centered care, *J Nurs Care Qual* 36(2):125–131, 2021.

Centers for Medicare and Medicaid Services (CMS): Final rule, 42 CFR, Part 412, 413, 424, 495, May 16, 2022.

Dunn Lopez K, Chin CL, Leitão Azevedo RF, et al: Electronic health record usability and workload changes over time for provider and nursing staff following transition to new her, *Appl Ergon* 93:103359, 2021.

Harrington L: *Future model for nursing documentation: extinction, Nurse Leader,* 17(2):113-116, 2019.

Healthcare Information and Management Systems Society (HIMSS): *What is nursing informatics?* 2023. https://www.himss.org/resources/what-nursing-informatics. Accessed February 27, 2023.

HealthIT.gov: *SAFER guides,* 2018. https://www.healthit.gov/topic/safety/safer-guides. Accessed February 28, 2023.

HealthIT.gov: *What is an electronic health record?* 2019. https://www.healthit.gov/faq/what-electronic-health-record-ehr. Accessed February 28, 2023.

Institute for Safe Medication Practices (ISMP): *List of error-prone abbreviations,* 2021. https://www.ismp.org/recommendations/error-prone-abbreviations-list. Accessed February 28, 2023.

International Classification for Nursing Practice: *Nursing diagnosis and outcome statements.* Updated 2019, Geneva, Switzerland, 2019, Author.

Johnston D, Strusowski T: Defining the complexity of patients through an acuity tool: a scoping review, *J Oncol Navig Survivor* 13(4):135–147, 2022.

Jones KJ, et al: The impact of post-fall huddles on repeat fall rates and perceptions of safety culture: a quasi-experimental evaluation of a patient safety demonstration project, *BMC Health Serv Res* 19:650, 2019.

Kao D: Electronic health records and heart failure, *Heart Fail Clin* 18(2):201–211, 2022.

Kaipio J: Physicians' and nurses' experiences on EHR usability: comparison between the professional groups by employment sector and system brand, *Int J Med Inform* 134:104018, 2020.

Labrague LJ, et al: The association of nurse caring behaviours on missed nursing care, adverse patient events and perceived quality of care: a cross-sectional study, *J Nurs Manag* 28(8):2257–2265, 2020.

Lo L, et al: Can SBAR be implemented with high fidelity and does it improve communication between healthcare workers? A systematic review, *BMJ Open* 11:1–9, 2021.

Matney S, Settergren R: *Inclusion of interprofessional terminology standards in electronic health records, position statement of the American Nursing Informatics Association Board of Directors,* 2018. https://www.ania.org/assets/documents/position/terminologyStandardsPosition.pdf. Accessed February 28, 2023.

McCarthy B, et al: Electronic nursing documentation interventions to promote or improve patient safety and quality care: a systematic review, *J Nurs Manag* 27:491–501, 2019.

Office of the National Coordinator for Health Information Technology (ONC): *2022 Interoperability Standards Advisory–reference edition.* https://www.healthit.gov/isa/sites/isa/files/inline-files/2022-ISA-Reference-Edition.pdf. Accessed February 28, 2023.

Østensen E, et al: Facilitating the implementation of standardized care plans in municipal healthcare, *Comput Inform Nurs* 40(2):104–112, 2022.

Petersen C, et al: American Medical Informatics Association (AMIA) code of professional and ethical conduct 2018, *J Am Med Inform Assoc* 25(11):1579–1582, 2018.

Rahmani K, et al: Early prediction of central line associated bloodstream infection using machine learning, *Am J Infect Control* 50(4):440–445, 2022.

Sarzynski E, et al: Eliciting nurses' perspectives to improve health information exchange between hospital and home health care, *Geriatr Nurs* 40:277–283, 2019.

Sermersheim E, et al: Improving patient throughput with an electronic nursing handoff process in an academic medical center: a rapid improvement event approach, *JONA* 50(3):174–181, 2020.

The Joint Commission: *Most commonly reviewed sentinel event types,* Oakbrook Terrace, IL, 2021, Author. https://www.jointcommission.org/-/media/tjc/documents/resources/patient-safety-topics/sentinel-event/most-frequently-reviewed-event-types 2020.pdf?db=web&hash=6739433300D8DA4CF9F69DEB79B3A2BE&hash=6739433300D8DA4CF9F69DEB79B3A2BE. Accessed February 27, 2023.

The Joint Commission: *2023 National Patient Safety Goals,* Oakbrook Terrace, IL, 2023a, Author. https://www.jointcommission.org/standards/national-patient-safety-goals/. Accessed February 28, 2023.

The Joint Commission: *Comprehensive accreditation manual,* Oakbrook Terrace, IL, 2023b, Author.

U.S. Department of Health and Human Services (DHHS): *The HIPPA privacy rule,* 2022. https://www.hhs.gov/hipaa/for-professionals/privacy/index.html. Accessed August 10, 2023.

Supporting the Patient Through the Health Care System: Next-Generation NCLEX® (NGN)–Style Unfolding Case Study

PHASE 1

QUESTION 1.

The nurse has documented an intake assessment for a client who has come to see the primary health care provider for an annual examination.

Highlight the findings that require **immediate** follow-up by the nurse.

History and Physical	Nurses' Notes	Vital Signs	Laboratory Results

1008: Client is here for an annual examination. States they are concerned about having some type of disorder and are afraid of what today's examination might reveal. About 8 months ago, client reports finding blood in their stool and occasional drops of blood in the toilet. No change in diet. Denies abdominal pain or tenderness but states, "Sometimes it burns when I urinate." States that passing stool is difficult at least 2 to 3 times weekly. Has been taking an opioid pain reliever for several weeks following a knee replacement. Has a family history of colon cancer. Alert and oriented × 4; lung sounds clear to auscultation; S_1S_2 present with no murmur heard; bowel sounds present × 4 quadrants; strength in all extremities equal. Vital signs: T 36.8°C (98.2°F); HR 102 beats/min; RR 22 breaths/min; BP 148/86 mm Hg; SpO$_2$ 99% on RA.

QUESTION 2.

For each asessment finding, indicate whether it is associated with colon cancer, constipation, or urinary tract infection. Any finding may be associated with more than 1 condition. Each finding will be associated with at least 1 condition.

Client Assessment Finding	Colon Cancer	Constipation	Hemorrhoids
Blood in stool			
Drops of blood in toilet			
Hard to pass stool			
Taking an opioid drug			

PHASE 2

QUESTION 3.

Choose the **most likely** options for the information missing from the statement below by selecting from the list of word choices provided.

The **priority** at this time is to address the [Word Choice] and the [Word Choice].

Word Choices
Increased heart rate
Elevated blood pressure
Blood in stool
Confusion
Fear of a potential diagnosis
Drops of blood in toilet

QUESTION 4.

The nurse is reviewing the vital signs and the documentation of the client's history. For each client concern, determine whether the nurse's plan to report the concern to the health care provider right away is indicated or not indicated.

Client Concern	Indicated	Not Indicated
Blood pressure 148/86 mm Hg		
Report of blood in stool		
Taking an opioid drug		
History of knee replacement		
Respiratory rate 22 breaths/min		
Difficulty passing stool		

PHASE 3

QUESTION 5.

The nurse is preparing to provide teaching to the client after the health care provider has performed an examination and ordered diagnostic testing.

Which teaching would the nurse provide? **Select all that apply.**

○ Confirm that blood in stool is a common finding.
○ Discourage the addition of whole grains to the diet.
○ Provide information about preparation for colonoscopy.
○ Increase intake of water to at least eight (8-ounce) glasses daily.
○ Explain that an antiinflammatory drug will be given for urinary burning.
○ Report an increase in blood in the stool or toilet to the health care provider immediately.
○ Be certain to take temperature at least twice daily to monitor for infection.
○ Reassure that there is no reason to be concerned about an unfavorable diagnosis.

QUESTION 6.

The client underwent all ordered diagnostic testing and was diagnosed with hemorrhoids and with constipation related to opioid use after knee replacement surgery. The opioid drug was discontinued. Two weeks later, the client follows up with the health care provider. Vital signs: T 36.8°C (98.2°F); HR 88 beats/min; RR 18 breaths/min; BP 118/70 mm Hg; SpO_2 99% on RA.

For each current client finding, indicate whether the nurse would document the client's condition as improved or unchanged.

Current Client Findings	Document as Improved	Document as Unchanged
Blood pressure 118/70 mm Hg		
Temperature 36.8°C (98.2°F)		
Notes drops of blood in toilet		
Reports relief from fear of an unfavorable diagnosis		
Easy stool passage most days of the week		

UNIT 2
Vital Signs and Physical Assessment

Any clinical decision about a patient is complex, requiring a nurse to gather sufficient assessment data that will reveal the cues indicating the patient's health-related problems. In order to recognize cues, a nurse identifies significant data from many sources. Whether a patient presents with common symptoms of a back sprain or symptoms of an upper respiratory infection, a clinical decision cannot be made without sufficient information. When assessment is thorough, common sets of cues reveal patterns, which, when analyzed critically, reveal patient problems and nursing diagnoses. A thorough assessment is comprehensive and patient centered.

Patient assessment includes a health assessment that incorporates the use of physical examination skills and direct patient questioning to uncover subjective and objective data about a patient's health status. Chapter 6 presents the comprehensive categories you may choose to include when performing a health assessment. However, the amount of data you gather in any clinical situation during a health assessment depends on the time you have with patients and the complexity and urgency of their problems. In addition, you make clinical judgments as to what you should further assess when certain signs are discovered. For example, if you notice swelling of a patient's ankle (edema), consider the meaning and what further assessments are necessary. You might question: The edema may be associated with a circulatory problem; therefore you should palpate peripheral pulses. If you observe a patient walking with an unsteady gait, that cue alone prompts you to examine if the source is neurological or musculoskeletal.

Patient assessment also includes obtaining vital signs. At times vital signs will be the primary reason you will assess a patient, as in the case of a routine check following a procedure. Vital signs reveal the stability of a patient's vital functions. When a vital sign is found to be abnormal or significantly different from a patient's baseline findings, you will then conduct appropriate health assessments to determine if other cues exist. For example, if a patient registers a fever on a thermometer, you will also palpate the skin for warmth, and note if the skin is diaphoretic.

When you analyze the various cues available from a health assessment and vital signs, there may be additional data available in the form of relevant laboratory and diagnostic test results. These data can help to confirm the findings from the health assessment. When a patient presents with pallor and a thready pulse, a low hematocrit offers a cue to the problem of poor oxygenation.

A nurse decides if assessment is complete for a specific clinical situation after connecting data gathered with a patient's presentation. Anticipating the type of data to be expected, based on a patient's self-reported problem or a health care provider's medical diagnosis, prompts a nurse to be thorough. In addition, anticipating what to assess aids in analyzing the meaning of assessment findings. When the data reveal unexpected findings, any potential problems need to be explored further. Patient assessment is central to providing the data needed for nurses to make sound clinical judgments regarding identification of patient problems and nursing diagnoses.

5 | Vital Signs

SKILLS AND PROCEDURES

Skill 5.1 **Measuring Body Temperature, p. 72**

Skill 5.2 **Assessing Radial Pulse, p. 82**

Skill 5.3 **Assessing Apical Pulse, p. 86**

Skill 5.4 **Assessing Respirations, p. 91**

Skill 5.5 **Assessing Arterial Blood Pressure, p. 95**

Procedural Guideline 5.1 **Noninvasive Electronic Blood Pressure Measurement, p. 104**

Procedural Guideline 5.2 **Measuring Oxygen Saturation (Pulse Oximetry), p. 105**

OBJECTIVES

Mastery of content in this chapter will enable you to:
- Identify when it is appropriate to assess each vital sign.
- Explain factors that cause variations in body temperature, pulse, respirations, blood pressure, and oxygen saturation.
- Evaluate patient's disease process, cognition, age, and other factors when selecting sites for temperature, pulse, and blood pressure assessments.
- Analyze a patient's oral, rectal, axillary, tympanic membrane, and temporal artery temperatures.
- Explain factors that cause variations in pulse rate.
- Analyze a patient's radial and apical pulses.
- Evaluate the significance of a pulse deficit.
- Explain factors that cause variations in respiratory rate.
- Analyze a patient's respirations.
- Explain factors that cause variations in blood pressure.

- Evaluate factors in selecting an extremity for blood pressure measurement.
- Explain the benefits and disadvantages of using an automatic blood pressure machine.
- Analyze a patient's blood pressure.
- Explain factors that cause variations in SpO_2 values.
- Analyze a patient's oxygenation status (SpO_2) using pulse oximetry.
- Discuss how clinical judgment is essential in determining when to measure vital signs.
- Determine when it is appropriate to delegate vital sign measurements to nursing assistive personnel.
- Evaluate the effectiveness of nursing interventions to promote or maintain normal vital signs.
- Demonstrate accurate documentation and reporting of vital sign measurement.

MEDIA RESOURCES

- http://evolve.elsevier.com/Perry/skills
- Clinical Review Questions
- Audio Glossary
- ▶ Video Clips
- Animations
- Case Studies

- NSO Nursing Skills Online
- Answers to Clinical Judgment and Next-Generation NCLEX® Examination-Style Questions
- Skills Performance Checklists
- Printable Key Points

PURPOSE

Vital signs, temperature, pulse, blood pressure, respirations, and oxygen saturation reflect the physiological status of the body and its response to physical, environmental, and psychological stressors. Pain, a subjective symptom, may often be referred to as a vital sign (see Chapter 16). Assess a patient's level of comfort and pain during vital sign measurements and according to agency policy (The Joint Commission [TJC], 2023).

Vital signs reveal sudden changes in a patient's condition, changes that occur progressively over time, and a patient's response to therapy. Any difference between a patient's normal baseline measurement and present vital signs may indicate the need for nursing therapies and medical interventions. Vital signs are also

important in evaluating a patient's response to therapy—for example, how a patient with a fever responds to antipyretics, how a patient in pain responds to opioids, or how a patient with hypertension responds to medication.

PRACTICE STANDARDS

- Muntner et al., 2019: American Heart Association Scientific Statement: Measurement of Blood Pressure in Humans—Auscultatory methods
- The Joint Commission (TJC), 2023: National Patient Safety Goals—Patient identification
- Whelton et al., 2018: Guideline For The Prevention, Detection, Evaluation, and Management of High Blood Pressure in

Adults: Report of the American College of Cardiology/American Heart Association Task Force on Clinical Practice Guidelines—Categories of hypertension

SUPPLEMENTAL STANDARDS

- American Association of Critical-Care Nurses (AACN), 2017: AACN Practice Alert: Obtaining Accurate Noninvasive Blood Pressure Measurement in Adults

PRINCIPLES FOR PRACTICE

- Vital signs are included in a routine physical assessment (see Chapter 6).
- Equipment must be clean, functional, properly calibrated, and appropriate for the patient's size, age, condition, and characteristics.
- Select equipment on the basis of the patient's condition and characteristics (e.g., do not use an adult-size blood pressure cuff for a child or a small cuff on an overweight adult).
- Control or minimize environmental factors that affect vital signs. For example, assessing a patient's temperature in a warm, humid room may yield a value that is not a true indicator of the patient's condition.
- Know the patient's usual range of vital signs. These values can differ from the acceptable range for a patient's age or health status. The patient's usual values serve as a baseline for comparison with later findings.
- Always obtain a baseline measurement of vital signs on first contact with a patient to provide a means for comparison with later vital sign measurements.
- Obtain a baseline measurement of vital signs before an invasive procedure (e.g., bronchoscopy, cardiac catheterization).
- Frequency of vital sign measurements depends on the specific patient's condition (Box 5.1). Apply sound clinical judgment to determine which vital sign to measure, when to obtain measurements, and the frequency of assessments.

PERSON-CENTERED CARE

- Vital sign measurements can require removing clothing or exposing areas considered inappropriate or offensive to patients from other cultures. You must be sensitive to each patient's need for privacy and observe cultural norms. Provide privacy or obtain a gender-congruent health care provider when taking a rectal temperature or performing apical pulse assessment.
- Always inform patients about their vital sign measurements. Many patients monitor their own vital signs at home and can be valuable partners in letting you know which values are normal for them.
- Be sensitive to the fact that procedures that are normally noninvasive may produce anxiety because of cultural variables of touch, privacy, and gender.
- Consult the health care provider and family decision maker regarding giving information to the patient about abnormal vital signs.
- Diversity practices are important when communicating with the patient and family. Language that is inclusive of the patient, family, and in some cases a cultural leader is critical to effective communication about the patient's health, needs for medications and diet to help regulate blood pressure and pulse, and so on (Stenhouse, 2021; Meyer et al., 2018).

EVIDENCE-BASED PRACTICE

Assessing Respirations

Respiratory rate has a strong relationship with mortality; some experts believe it is a better predictor than blood pressure or pulse of patient deterioration (Takayama et al., 2019). Often a patient's respiratory rate is the first sign of a declining physiological status. Assessment of respiratory rate is an accurate predictor of cardiac arrest and patient deterioration (Rolfe, 2019). Nurses are front line providers and often the first professionals to observe a change in respiratory rate (Lamberti, 2020; Harry et al., 2020). Evidence-based interventions include:

- Obtain a 60-second assessment when a patient has low, high, or irregular respirations (Harry et al., 2020).
- Obtain a respiratory assessment when the patient is not aware (Hill et al., 2018; Rolfe, 2019).
- Use of a consistent counting method when obtaining the respiratory rate increases accuracy (Harry et al., 2020).
- Obtaining a routine respiratory rate assessment helps to identify early respiratory compromise (Lamberti, 2020).
- Avoid counting respirations for 15 seconds and multiplying by 4 or counting for 30 seconds and multiplying by 2; these methods contribute to errors (Harry et al., 2020; Rolfe, 2019).
- Pulse oximetry values are a component of respiratory assessment, but not a standalone measure, and should not take the place of assessing respiratory rate (Elliott & Baird, 2019).

SAFETY GUIDELINES

- Use sound clinical judgment by communicating clearly with members of the health care team when assessing and analyzing patient's vital signs.
- Analyze vital signs to interpret their significance and use clinical judgment to make decisions about appropriate nursing interventions.
- Do not share devices for measuring vital signs among patients. Sharing these devices can increase the spread of COVID-19 and other communicable diseases within the agency.
- Blood pressure cuffs and pulse oximetry sensors can apply excessive pressure on fragile skin. Rotate sites during repeated measurements to decrease the risk for skin breakdown.
- Know a patient's medical history, therapies, and prescribed medications. Some illnesses or treatments cause predictable

---

BOX 5.1

When to Measure Vital Signs

- On admission to a health care agency
- When assessing a patient during home care visits
- In a health care agency on a routine schedule according to a health care provider's order or agency's standards of practice
- Before, during, and after a surgical or invasive diagnostic/treatment procedure
- Before, during, and after transfusion of any type of blood products
- Before, during, and after the administration of medications or therapies that affect cardiovascular, respiratory, or temperature-control functions
- Before, during, and after nursing interventions influencing a vital sign (e.g., before and after patient previously on bed rest ambulates, before and after patient performs range-of-motion exercises)
- When patient reports specific symptoms of physical distress (e.g., feeling "funny" or "different")
- When patient's general physical condition changes (e.g., loss of consciousness, increased intensity of pain)

vital sign changes. Most medications affect at least one of the vital signs.

- Provide latex-free equipment, including blood pressure cuffs and pulse oximeter probes, when a patient has or is suspected of having a latex allergy.
- Collaborate with the health care providers, as needed, to determine the frequency of vital sign assessment for each patient. Following surgery or treatment intervention, measure vital signs more frequently to detect complications. In a clinic or outpatient setting, take vital signs before the health care provider examines the patient and after any invasive procedures.
- When a patient's physical condition worsens, it is important to monitor the vital signs as often as every 5 to 15 minutes. Use

your clinical judgment to determine when more frequent assessments are necessary.

- Analyze the results of all vital sign measurements. Do not interpret vital signs results in isolation. You need to know related physical signs or symptoms and be aware of the patient's ongoing health status.
- Verify, communicate, and document significant changes in vital signs. Baseline measurements allow you to identify changes in vital signs. When vital signs appear abnormal, ask another nurse to repeat the measurement.
- Inform the health care provider when vital signs become abnormal and report any changes to the nurse in charge.

✦ SKILL 5.1   Measuring Body Temperature

 Video Clip

Body temperature is the difference between the amount of heat produced by body processes and the amount lost to the external environment. The core temperature, or temperature of the deep body tissues, is under control of the hypothalamus and remains within a narrow range. Skin or body surface temperature fluctuates dramatically as it rises and falls with the changing temperature of the surrounding environment.

The body tissues and cells function best within a relatively narrow temperature range, from 36°C to 38°C (96.8°F to 100.4°F), but no single temperature is normal for all people. Body temperature is lowest in the early morning and slowly trends upward with the normal range, peaking in late afternoon or early evening. For healthy young adults the average oral temperature is 37°C (98.6°F). In clinical practice, nurses learn the temperature range of individual patients. An acceptable temperature range for adults depends on age, gender, range of physical activity, hydration status, and state of health (Fig. 5.1).

Many factors affect body temperature, but physiological and behavioral control mechanisms act to maintain a constant core temperature. For example, the mechanism of peripheral vasodilation increases blood flow to the skin, which increases the amount of heat radiated to the environment. Control mechanisms have failed when heat produced by the body is not equal to heat lost to the environment. For example, patients without sweat gland function are unable to tolerate warm temperatures because they cannot adequately cool themselves. Fever occurs when heat-loss mechanisms are unable to keep pace with excess heat production, resulting in an abnormal rise in body temperature. When an individual has a febrile condition (i.e., pyrexia), use temperature-control measures such as controlling environmental temperatures, removing external coverings, and administering ordered antipyretics to achieve better temperature control.

The purpose of measuring body temperature is to obtain a representative average temperature of core body tissues. Average usual temperature varies, depending on the measurement site used. Research findings from numerous studies are contradictory; however, it is generally accepted that rectal temperatures are usually 0.5°C (0.9°F) higher than oral temperatures. Axillary and tympanic membrane temperatures are usually 0.5°C (0.9°F) lower than oral temperatures. Sites reflecting core temperature are more reliable indicators of body temperature than sites reflecting surface temperatures (Kiekkas et al., 2019) (Box 5.2).

To ensure accurate temperature readings you need to measure each site correctly. Use the same site when repeated measurements are necessary or when comparing temperature measurements over time. Each site has advantages and limitations (Box 5.3). You need to determine the safest and most accurate site for a patient.

A variety of thermometers are commonly available to measure body temperature (Box 5.4; Figs. 5.2, 5.3, 5.4, 5.5). The mercury-in-glass thermometer, once the standard device found in the clinical setting, is now prohibited because of the potential mercury hazards. However, mercury-in-glass thermometers can still be found in patients' homes. In addition, COVID-19 increased the use of tympanic and noncontact measurements from the skin as alternatives to mercury thermometers (Erdem et al., 2021). Current research notes greater accuracy in temperature assessment when the same device (e.g., noncontact skin, tympanic, electronic thermometer) is used to obtain serial body temperature assessments (Sweeting et al., 2022).

Delegation

The skill of temperature measurement can be delegated to assistive personnel (AP). Direct the AP by:

- Communicating the appropriate route, device, and frequency of temperature measurement

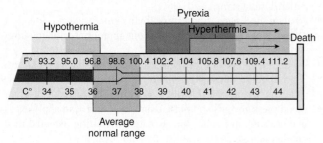

FIG. 5.1 Ranges of normal temperature values and abnormal body temperature alterations.

BOX 5.2

Core and Surface Temperature Measurement Sites

Core Site	Surface Site
• Rectum	• Skin
• Tympanic membrane	• Oral cavity
• Temporal artery	• Axilla
• Esophagus	
• Pulmonary artery	
• Urinary bladder	

BOX 5.3

BOX 5.3

Advantages and Limitations of Select Temperature Measurement Sites

Oral

Advantages
- Easily accessible, requires no position change
- Comfortable for patient
- Provides accurate surface temperature reading
- Reflects rapid change in core temperature
- Reliable route to measure temperature in intubated patients

Limitations
- Causes delay in measurement if patient recently ingested hot or cold fluids or foods, chewed gum, or smoked
- Do not use with patients who have had oral inflammatory process, oral surgery, or facial trauma; are unable to position thermometer in mouth; or have shaking chills or history of seizures
- Not recommended for children younger than 5 years or confused, unconscious, or uncooperative patients (Hockenberry et al., 2024; Sims et al., 2018)
- Do not use with patients who are hypothermic (Sims et al., 2018)
- Risk for body fluid exposure

Tympanic Membrane

Advantages
- Easily accessible site, without disturbing, waking, or repositioning patient
- Found to be most accurate method in critically ill patients when compared with oral, axillary, and rectal (Mogensen et al., 2018a; Mogensen et al., 2018b)
- Standard practice for measuring body temperature in children 2 years and older (Hockenberry et al., 2024)
- No body fluid exposure
- Used for patients with tachypnea without affecting breathing
- Sensitive to core temperature changes
- Very rapid measurement (2–5 seconds)
- Unaffected by oral intake of food or fluids or smoking
- Not influenced by environmental temperatures

Limitations
- More variability of measurement than with other core temperature devices
- Not recommended for children younger than 1 month because ear canal anatomy prohibits infrared sensor from seeing tympanic membrane (Hockenberry et al., 2024)
- Requires removal of hearing aids before measurement
- Requires disposable sensor cover with only one size available
- Otitis media and cerumen impaction distort readings
- Do not use in patients who have had surgery of the ear or tympanic membrane
- Does not accurately measure core temperature changes during and after exercise
- Affected by ambient temperature devices such as incubators, radiant warmers, and facial fans
- Does not obtain continuous measurements

Rectal

Advantages
- Argued to be reliable when oral temperature is difficult or impossible to obtain
- Not influenced by ambient temperature

Limitations
- Lags behind core temperature during rapid temperature changes
- Not used for patients with diarrhea or those who have had rectal surgery, rectal disorders, bleeding tendencies, or neutropenia
- Requires positioning and is often source of patient embarrassment and anxiety
- Risk for body fluid exposure and stool-borne pathogens (Kiekkas et al., 2019)
- Requires lubrication
- Not used for routine vital signs in newborns
- Readings influenced by impacted stool

Axilla

Advantages
- Safe and inexpensive
- Recommended for infants younger than 1 month (Hockenberry et al., 2024)

Limitations
- Long measurement time
- Measurement lags behind core temperature during rapid temperature changes
- Requires continuous positioning
- Not recommended for detecting fever in infants and young children; use rectal thermometer for correct assessment
- Requires exposure of thorax, which can result in temperature loss, especially in newborns
- Affected by exposure to the environment, including time it takes to place thermometer
- Underestimates core temperature in older adults and children (Fitzwater et al., 2019)

Skin

Advantages
- Inexpensive
- Provides continuous reading
- Safe and noninvasive
- Used for neonates

Limitations
- Measurement lags behind other sites during temperature changes, especially during hyperthermia
- Impaired adhesion from diaphoresis or sweat
- Affected by environmental temperature
- Cannot be used for patients with allergy to adhesives

Temporal Artery

Advantages
- Easy to access without position change
- Very rapid measurement
- Comfortable with no risk of injury to patient or nurse
- Eliminates need to disrobe or unbundle
- Can be used for children (Kiekkas et al., 2019)
- Reflects rapid change in core temperature
- Sensor cover not required

Limitations
- Inaccurate with head covering or hair on forehead
- Affected by skin moisture such as diaphoresis or sweating

- Explaining any precautions needed in positioning the patient (e.g., for rectal temperature measurement)
- Reporting the temperature values and any changes

Equipment

- Thermometer (selected on the basis of site used; see Box 5.3)
- Soft tissue or wipe
- Antiseptic swab
- Water-soluble lubricant (for rectal measurements only)
- Pen and vital sign flow sheet, record form, or electronic health record (EHR)
- Clean gloves (optional), plastic thermometer sleeve, disposable probe or sensor cover
- Towel

BOX 5.4

Types of Thermometers

Electronic Thermometer (see Fig. 5.2)

- Thermometer is a rechargeable battery-powered display unit with a thin wire cord and a temperature-processing probe covered by a disposable cover.
- Within 1 minute after placement, the thermometer displays a digital temperature reading.
- Separate probes are available for oral and axillary temperature measurement (blue tip) and rectal temperature measurement (red tip).

Tympanic Membrane Thermometer

- The probe consists of an otoscope-like speculum with an infrared sensor tip that detects heat radiated from the tympanic membrane of the ear (see Fig. 5.3).
- Within seconds after placing in the ear canal and depressing the scan button, a digital reading appears on the display unit. A sound signals when the peak temperature has been measured.

Temporal Artery Thermometer

- An infrared scanner is swept across the forehead, lifted, and then placed behind the ear where a woman would normally place perfume. If the patient is diaphoretic, a scan just behind the ear verifies the measurement accuracy (see Fig. 5.4).
- Within seconds after scanning, a digital reading appears on the display unit.

Chemical Dot Single-Use or Reusable Thermometer

- Thermometer consists of thin strips of plastic with a temperature sensor at one end and chemically impregnated dots formulated to change color at different temperatures (see Fig. 5.5).
- Chemical dots on thermometer change color to reflect temperature reading, usually within 60 seconds.
- It is useful for screening temperatures, especially in infants, during invasive procedures, for a patient in protective isolation, and in orally intubated critical care patients.
- It is not appropriate for monitoring fever in acutely ill patients or for temperature therapies.
- It can be used at axillary or rectal site if covered by a plastic sheath, with a placement time of 3 minutes.
- Home disposable thermometers are useful for temperature screening but are not as accurate as nondisposable electronic thermometers.

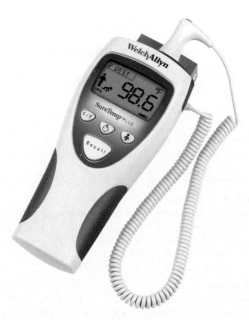

FIG. 5.2 Electronic thermometer with disposable plastic probe cover. (*Photo courtesy Welch Allyn.*)

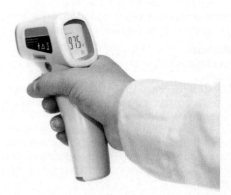

FIG. 5.4 A temporal artery thermometer measures the heat from blood flowing through the superficial temporal artery. (*From iStock. com/guvendemir.*)

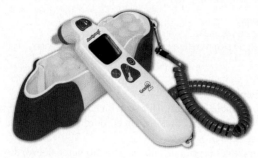

FIG. 5.3 Tympanic membrane thermometer with disposable plastic probe cover. (*Copyright © Covidien. All rights reserved.*)

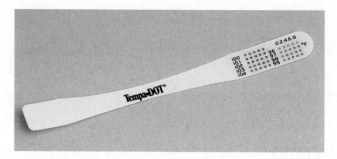

FIG. 5.5 Chemical dot, disposable, single-use thermometer.

STEP	RATIONALE

ASSESSMENT

1. Identify patient using at least two identifiers (e.g., name and birthday or name and medical record number) according to agency policy.	Ensures patient safety. Complies with The Joint Commission standards and improves patient safety (TJC, 2023).
2. Review patient's EHR to determine need to measure patient's body temperature.	

a. Note patient's risks for temperature alterations:
       • Expected or diagnosed infection
       • Open wounds or burns
       • White blood cell count below 5000/mm³ or above 12,000/mm³
       • Immunosuppressive drug therapy
       • Injury to hypothalamus
       • Exposure to temperature extremes
       • Blood product infusion
       • Hypothermia or hyperthermia therapy
	Certain conditions place patients at risk for temperature alterations and require more frequent temperature measurement and nursing assessment.

b. Determine previous baseline temperature and measurement site (if available) from patient's EHR.	Allows you to assess for change in condition. Provides comparison with future temperature measurements.
3. Assess patient's/family caregiver's health literacy.	Determines degree to which individuals have the ability to find, understand, and use information and services to make informed decisions and actions for themselves and others (Centers for Disease Control and Prevention [CDC], 2023).
4. Perform hand hygiene.	Reduces transmission of microorganisms.
5. Assess for factors that normally influence temperature:	Allows you to accurately assess for presence and significance of temperature alteration.
• Age	Older adults have narrower range of temperature than younger adults.

Clinical Judgment *No single temperature is normal for all people. A temperature within an acceptable range in an adult may reflect a fever in an older adult. Undeveloped temperature-control mechanisms in infants and children cause temperature to rise and fall rapidly.*

• Exercise	Muscle activity increases metabolism, which increases heat production and raises temperature.
• Hormones	Women have wider temperature fluctuations than men because of menstrual cycle hormonal changes, because body temperature varies during menopause, and because women have a thicker layer of subcutaneous fat.
• Stress	Stress elevates temperature.
• Environmental temperature	Infants and older adults are more sensitive to environmental temperature changes.
• Medications	Some drugs impair or promote sweating, vasoconstriction, or vasodilation or interfere with ability of hypothalamus to regulate temperature. Oxygen administered by nasal cannula at greater than 6 L can result in inaccurate temperature measurement using the oral and temporal route (Mason et al., 2017).
• Daily fluctuations	Body temperature normally changes 0.5°C to 1°C (0.9°F to 1.8°F) during a 24-h period. Temperature is lowest during early morning. Most patients have maximum temperature elevation around 4 p.m.; temperature falls gradually during night.
6. Determine appropriate measurement site and device for patient (see Box 5.3). Use disposable thermometer for patient on isolation precautions.	Identifies that patient's status contraindicates selection of a specific method or site.
7. Assess patient's knowledge of and prior experience with temperature measurement and feelings about procedure.	Reveals need for patient instruction and/or support.

STEP	RATIONALE

PLANNING

1. Expected outcomes following completion of procedure:
- Body temperature is within acceptable range for patient's age-group.
- Body temperature returns to baseline range following therapies for abnormal temperature.

2. Provide privacy and explain procedure and importance of maintaining proper position until temperature reading is complete.

3. Organize and set up any equipment needed to perform procedure.

4. If measuring oral temperature, verify that patient has not had anything to eat or drink and has not chewed gum or smoked within the past 20 minutes.

Thermoregulation is maintained.

Environmental factors that alter temperature are controlled.

Protects patient's privacy; reduces anxiety. Promotes cooperation.

Ensures more efficiency when completing an assessment.

Oral food and fluids, smoking, and gum can alter oral temperature (Mahabala et al., 2022; McClelland et al., 2021).

IMPLEMENTATION

1. Perform hand hygiene. Help patient to comfortable position that provides easy access to temperature measurement site.
  a. Sitting, or lying supine (oral, tympanic, temporal, axillary)
  b. Side lying with upper leg flexed (rectal)
2. Obtain temperature reading.
  a. Oral temperature (electronic):
   (1) *Optional:* Apply clean gloves when there is risk for exposure to respiratory secretions or facial or mouth wound drainage.
   (2) Remove thermometer pack from charging unit. Attach oral thermometer probe stem (blue tip) to thermometer unit. Grasp top of probe stem, being careful not to apply pressure on ejection button.
   (3) Slide disposable plastic probe cover over thermometer probe stem until cover locks in place (see illustration).

Ensures patient's comfort and accuracy of temperature reading.

An oral probe cover is removable without physical contact; thus this does not require gloves.

Charging provides battery power. Ejection button releases plastic cover from probe stem.

Soft plastic cover will not break in patient's mouth and prevents transmission of microorganisms between patients.

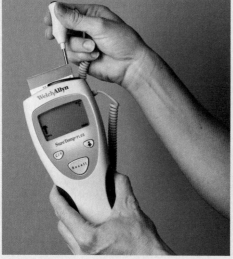 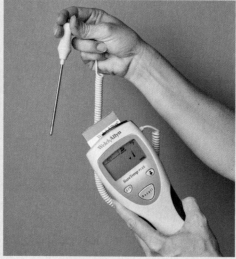

STEP 2a(3) Disposable plastic cover is placed over probe.

   (4) Ask patient to open mouth; observe for any inflammatory process such as mucositis. If present, consider an alternate route. Gently place thermometer probe under tongue in posterior sublingual pocket lateral to center of lower jaw (see illustration).

Oral inflammatory process can cause false elevations in temperature (Mahabala et al., 2022). Heat from superficial blood vessels in sublingual pocket produces temperature reading. With electronic thermometer, temperatures in right and left posterior sublingual pocket are significantly higher than in area under front of tongue.

STEP	RATIONALE

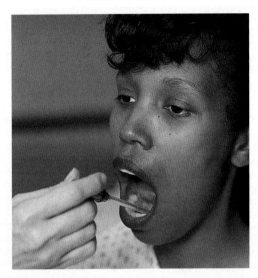

STEP 2a(4) Probe placed under tongue in posterior sublingual pocket.

(5) Ask patient to hold thermometer probe with lips closed and to refrain from talking while temperature is measured.	Maintains proper position of thermometer during recording.
(6) Leave thermometer probe in place until audible signal indicates completion and patient's temperature appears on digital display; remove thermometer probe from under patient's tongue. Note temperature reading.	Probe must stay in place until signal occurs to ensure accurate reading.
(7) Push ejection button on thermometer probe stem to discard plastic probe cover into appropriate receptacle. Return thermometer probe stem to storage position of thermometer unit.	Reduces transmission of microorganisms. Protects probe stem from damage. Returning thermometer probe stem automatically causes digital reading to disappear.
(8) If wearing gloves, remove, dispose in appropriate receptacle, and perform hand hygiene.	Reduces transmission of microorganisms.

b. Rectal temperature (electronic):

(1) With patient in side-lying or left lateral recumbent position with upper leg flexed, move aside bed linen to expose only anal area. Keep patient's upper body and lower extremities covered with sheet or blanket.	Maintains patient's privacy, minimizes embarrassment, and promotes comfort.
(2) Apply clean gloves. Cleanse anal region when feces and/or secretions are present. Remove soiled gloves, perform hand hygiene, and reapply clean gloves.	Maintains Standard Precautions when exposed to items soiled with body fluids (e.g., feces).
(3) Remove thermometer pack from charging unit. Attach rectal thermometer probe stem (red tip) to thermometer unit. Grasp top of probe stem, being careful not to apply pressure on ejection button.	Ejection button releases plastic cover from probe stem.
(4) Slide disposable plastic probe cover over thermometer probe stem until cover locks in place.	Soft plastic probe cover prevents transmission of infection between patients.
(5) Using a single-use package, squeeze a liberal amount of lubricant on tissue. Dip probe cover of thermometer, blunt end, into lubricant, covering 2.5 to 3.5 cm (1–1½ inches) for adult.	Lubrication minimizes trauma to rectal mucosa during insertion. Using a tissue allows adequate lubrication of probe.

Clinical Judgment *Rectal temperatures should not be routinely taken in infants younger than 1 month of age due to risk of rectal perforation (Hockenberry et al., 2024).*

(6) With nondominant hand, separate patient's buttocks to expose anus. Ask patient to breathe slowly and relax.	Fully exposes anus for thermometer insertion. Relaxes anal sphincter for easier thermometer insertion.
(7) Gently insert thermometer into anus in direction of umbilicus 3.5 cm (1½ inches) for adult (see illustration). Do not force thermometer.	Ensures adequate exposure against blood vessels in rectal wall.

STEP	RATIONALE

Clinical Judgment *If you cannot adequately insert thermometer into rectum or resistance is felt during insertion, remove thermometer, and consider alternative method for obtaining temperature. Never force thermometer.*

(8) Once positioned, hold thermometer probe in place until audible signal indicates completion and patient's temperature appears on digital display; remove thermometer probe from anus. Note temperature reading.

(9) Push ejection button on thermometer stem to discard plastic probe cover into appropriate receptacle. Wipe probe stem with antiseptic swab, paying particular attention to ridges where probe stem connects to probe. Allow probe stem to dry (10–20 seconds) and return probe stem to recording unit.

(10) Clean patient's anal area with soft tissue to remove lubricant or feces and discard tissue. Perform perineal hygiene as needed. Replace gown and linen.

(11) Remove and dispose of gloves in appropriate receptacle. Perform hand hygiene.

c. Axillary temperature (electronic):

(1) With curtain drawn around bed and/or room door closed, help patient to supine or sitting position. Move clothing or gown away from shoulder and arm.

(2) Remove thermometer pack from charging unit. Attach oral thermometer probe stem (blue tip) to thermometer unit. Grasp top of thermometer probe stem, being careful not to apply pressure on ejection button.

(3) Slide disposable plastic probe cover over thermometer stem until cover locks in place.

(4) Raise patient's arm away from torso. Inspect for skin lesions and excessive perspiration; if needed, dry axilla or select alternative site. Insert thermometer probe into center of axilla (see illustration), lower arm over probe, and place arm across patient's chest.

Probe must stay in place until signal occurs to ensure accurate reading.

Reduces transmission of microorganisms. Protects probe stem from damage. Returning thermometer probe stem automatically causes digital reading to disappear.

Reduces transmission of microorganisms. Provides for comfort and hygiene. Maintains patient's privacy and minimizes embarrassment.
Reduces transmission of microorganisms.

Maintains patient's privacy, minimizes embarrassment, and promotes comfort. Exposes axilla for correct thermometer probe placement.
Charging provides battery power. Ejection button releases plastic cover from probe stem.

Soft plastic probe cover prevents transmission of microorganisms between patients.
Maintains proper position of thermometer against blood vessels in axilla. Thermometer probe must be held close to the torso for accurate measurement (Ball et al., 2023).

Clinical Judgment *Do not use axilla if skin lesions are present, because local temperature is sometimes altered, and area may be painful to touch.*

(5) Once thermometer probe is positioned, hold it in place until audible signal indicates completion and patient's temperature appears on digital display; remove thermometer probe from axilla. Note temperature reading.

Thermometer probe must stay in place until signal occurs to ensure accurate reading.

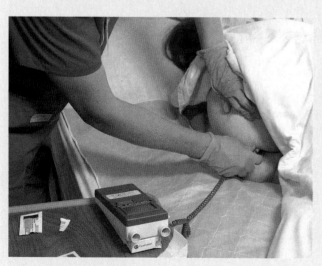

STEP 2b(7) Probe inserted into anus.

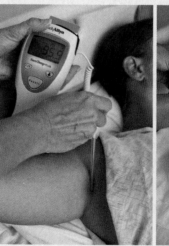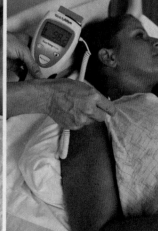

STEP 2c(4) Insert thermometer probe into center of axilla.

STEP	RATIONALE

(6) Push ejection button on thermometer stem to discard plastic probe cover into appropriate receptacle. Return thermometer stem to storage position of recording unit.

Thermometer probe must stay in place until signal occurs to ensure accurate reading. Returning thermometer stem to storage position automatically causes digital reading to disappear. Protects stem from damage.

(7) Replace linen or gown. Perform hand hygiene.

Restores comfort and a sense of well-being. Reduces transmission of infection.

d. Tympanic membrane temperature:

　(1) Help patient to assume comfortable position with head turned toward side, away from you. If patient has been lying on one side, use upper ear. Note if there is obvious presence of cerumen (earwax) in patient's ear canal.
　　NOTE: Obtain temperature from patient's right ear if you are right-handed, and from patient's left ear if you are left-handed.

Ensures comfort and facilitates exposure of auditory canal for accurate temperature measurement. Heat trapped in ear facing down causes falsely high temperature reading. Cerumen impedes lens cover of speculum. Switch to other ear or select alternative measurement site. The less acute the angle of approach, the better the probe seal.

　(2) Remove thermometer handheld unit from charging base, being careful not to apply pressure to ejection button.

Charging base provides battery power. Removal of handheld unit from base prepares it to measure temperature. Ejection button releases plastic probe cover from thermometer tip.

　(3) Slide disposable speculum cover over otoscope-like lens tip until it locks in place. Be careful not to touch lens cover.

Soft plastic probe cover prevents transmission of microorganisms between patients. Lens cover should not have dust, fingerprints, or cerumen obstructing optical pathway.

　(4) Insert speculum into ear canal following manufacturer instructions for tympanic probe positioning (see illustration).

Correct positioning of probe with respect to ear canal allows maximal exposure of tympanic membrane.

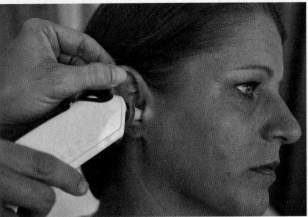

STEP 2d(4) Tympanic membrane thermometer with probe cover placed in patient's ear.

　(a) Pull ear pinna backward, up, and out for an adult. For children younger than 3 years, pull pinna down and back; point covered probe toward midpoint between eyebrow and sideburns. For children older than 3 years, pull pinna up and back (Hockenberry et al., 2024).

Ear tug straightens external auditory canal, allowing maximum exposure of tympanic membrane and therefore correctly positioning speculum (Hockenberry et al., 2024).

　(b) Fit speculum tip snugly in canal, pointing toward nose.
　Optional: Move thermometer in figure-eight pattern.

Gentle pressure seals ear canal from ambient air temperature, which alters readings by as much as 2.8°C (5°F).
Some manufacturers recommend movement of speculum tip in figure-eight pattern that allows sensor to detect maximum tympanic membrane heat radiation.

　(5) Once positioned, press scan button on handheld unit. Leave speculum in place until audible signal indicates completion and patient's temperature appears on digital display.

Pressing scan button causes detection of infrared energy. Speculum probe tip must stay in place until device has detected infrared energy noted by audible signal.

　(6) Carefully remove speculum from auditory meatus. Note temperature reading. Push ejection button on handheld unit to discard speculum cover into appropriate receptacle.

Reduces transmission of infection. Automatically causes digital reading to disappear.

STEP	RATIONALE

(7) If temperature is abnormal or second reading is necessary, replace probe cover and wait 2 minutes before repeating in same ear, or repeat measurement in other ear. Consider an alternative temperature site or instrument.

Lens cover must be free of cerumen to maintain optical path. Time allows ear canal to regain usual temperature.

(8) Return handheld unit to thermometer base.
(9) Perform hand hygiene

Protects sensor tip from damage.
Prevents transmission of infection.

e. Temporal artery temperature:
(1) Ensure that forehead is dry; dry with towel if needed.

Moisture and diaphoresis interfere with thermometer sensor (Wagner et al., 2021).

(2) Place sensor firmly on patient's forehead.
(3) Press red scan button with your thumb. Slowly slide thermometer straight across forehead while keeping sensor flat and firmly on skin (see illustration). Keeping scan button depressed, lift sensor after sweeping forehead and touch sensor on neck just behind earlobe. Read temperature when clicking sound during scanning stops. Release scan button.

Firm contact avoids measurement of ambient temperature.
Thermometer continuously scans for highest temperature when scan button is depressed. Area behind earlobe is less affected by diaphoresis and verifies temperature.

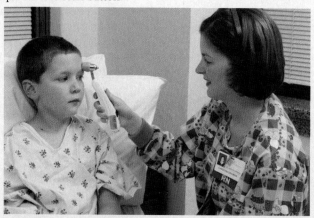

STEP 2e(3) Temporal thermometer sweeping across forehead.

(4) Gently clean sensor with alcohol swab; return to charging storage unit. Perform hand hygiene.

Maintains battery charge of thermometer unit. Prevents transmission of microorganisms.

3. Inform patient of temperature reading and document per agency policy.

Promotes participation in care and understanding of health status.

4. Help patient to a comfortable position.
5. Raise side rails (as appropriate) and lower bed to lowest position, locking into position.

Restores comfort and sense of well-being.
Ensures patient safety and prevents falls.

6. Place nurse call system in an accessible location within patient's reach.

Ensures patient can call for assistance if needed.

7. Perform hand hygiene.

Reduces transmission of microorganisms.

STEP	RATIONALE

EVALUATION

1. If you are assessing temperature for the first time, establish it as baseline if it is within acceptable range.

Used to compare future temperature measurements.

2. Compare temperature reading with patient's previous baseline and acceptable temperature range for patient's age-group.

Body temperature fluctuates within narrow range; comparison reveals presence of abnormality. Improper placement or movement of thermometer can cause inaccuracies. Second measurement with oral or rectal thermometer confirms initial findings of abnormal body temperature (Kiekkas et al., 2019).

3. If patient has fever, take temperature approximately 30 minutes after administering antipyretics and every 4 hours until temperature stabilizes.

Determines if temperature begins to fall in response to therapy.

4. Use Teach-Back: "I want to be sure I explained how to check your child's temperature at home. Show me how to swipe his forehead using the thermometer." Revise your instruction now or develop a plan for revised patient/family caregiver teaching if patient/family caregiver is not able to teach back correctly.

Teach-back is a technique for health care providers to ensure that they have explained medical information clearly so that patients and their families understand what is communicated to them (Agency for Healthcare Research and Quality [AHRQ], 2023).

Unexpected Outcomes

1. Patient has temperature 1°C (1.8°F) or more above usual range.

2. Patient has temperature 1°C (1.8°F) or more below usual range.

3. Unable to obtain temperature.

Related Interventions

- Initiate measures to lower body temperature, for example:
  - Cool room environment and reduce external coverings.
  - Keep clothing and bed linen dry.
  - Apply hypothermia blanket as ordered.
  - Administer antipyretics as ordered.
  - Increase fluid intake to at least 3 L daily (unless contraindicated).
- Initiate measures to raise body temperature, for example:
  - Apply warm blankets and, unless contraindicated, offer warm liquids.
  - Apply hyperthermia blankets if ordered.
  - Remove wet clothing or linen.
- Reassess correct placement of temperature probe or sensor.
- Choose alternative temperature measurement site.
- Obtain alternative temperature measurement device.

Documentation

- Document temperature and route as per agency policy.
- Document temperature after administration of specific therapies, such as blood or blood product transfusions.
- Document your evaluation of patient and family caregiver learning.

Hand-Off Reporting

- Report abnormal findings including route of assessment to nurse in charge or health care provider.
- Report measures taken to reduce or increase temperature and need for reassessment.

Special Considerations

Patient Education

- Identify patient's ability to initiate preventive health measures and recognize alteration in body temperature. Educate patient and family caregiver about measures to prevent body temperature alterations.
- Educate patients about risk factors for hypothermia and frostbite: fatigue; malnutrition; hypoxemia; cold, wet clothing; alcohol intoxication.
- Educate patients about risk factors for heatstroke: strenuous exercise in hot, humid weather; tight-fitting clothing in hot environments; exercising in poorly ventilated areas; sudden exposures to hot climates; poor fluid intake before, during, and after exercise.
- Educate patients that a fever is an expected response to an infection and the importance of taking and continuing antibiotics as directed until course of treatment for infection is completed.

Pediatrics

- Infants and young children may lose more heat to the environment because of their increased body surface area–to–volume ratios.
- Critically ill children sometimes have cool skin but a high core temperature because of poor perfusion to the skin.
- Newborns and neonates can develop hypothermia quickly owing to their immature ability to control internal temperature and exposure to heat loss (Hockenberry et al., 2024).
- Be consistent in use of measurement devices in the pediatric population to obtain accurate readings (Dante et al., 2020).
- Use axillary temperatures for screening purposes only for children up to 4 weeks of age (Dante et al., 2020; Franconi et al., 2018); axillary temperature cannot be relied on to detect a fever.
- Oral and rectal temperatures should be avoided in children up to 5 years old because of invasiveness (Franconi et al., 2018).
- Children may assume prone position for rectal temperature measurement.

- With children who cry or become restless, it is best to take temperature as the last vital sign.

Older Adults
- The temperature of older adults is at the lower end of the acceptable temperature range: 36°C (96.8°F).
- Temperatures reaching or exceeding 38.3°C (100.9°F) is serious in older adults and likely to be associated with serious bacterial or viral infections (Touhy & Jett, 2022).
- Oral temperature measurement is more reliable than tympanic membrane measurement because cerumen tends to be drier and cilia become stiff, contributing to buildup of cerumen impaction, which interferes with accurate tympanic temperature measurement.
- A decrease in sweat gland reactivity in the older adult results in a higher threshold for sweating at high temperatures, which can lead to hyperthermia (Touhy & Jett, 2022).

- Older adults are at high risk for hypothermia because of loss of subcutaneous fat that has insulating capacity, diminished sensation to cold, abnormal vasoconstrictor responses, and impaired shivering (Touhy & Jett, 2022).

Home Care
- Assess temperature and ventilation of patient's environment to determine existence of any environmental conditions that influence patient's temperature.
- In the home, some patients continue to use mercury-in-glass thermometers. Assess safe storage of these thermometers to protect from breakage and mercury spills. Educate patient and family caregiver on proper use of the thermometer, mercury hazards, and proper disposal of any mercury-containing devices. Suggest alternative temperature measurement devices for home use.

◆ SKILL 5.2   Assessing Radial Pulse

 Video Clip

The ejection of blood from the left ventricle of the heart distends the walls of the aorta. Because of the force of the blood exiting the heart, aortic distention creates a pulse wave that travels rapidly toward the extremities. When the pulse wave reaches a peripheral artery, you can feel it by palpating the artery lightly against underlying bone or muscle. The pulse is the palpable bounding of the blood flow. The number of pulsing sensations occurring in 1 minute is the pulse rate.

Assessing a patient's peripheral pulses determines the integrity of the cardiovascular system. An abnormally slow, rapid, or irregular pulse indicates the inability of the heart to deliver adequate blood to the body. In addition, a pulse deficit may be present. A pulse deficit is the difference between the apical heart rate (HR) and radial or pe-

ripheral pulse rate when obtained simultaneously over 1 minute. The strength or amplitude of a pulse reflects the volume of blood ejected against the arterial wall with each heart contraction. If the volume decreases, the pulse often becomes weak and difficult to palpate. In contrast, a full bounding pulse is an indication of increased volume.

The integrity of peripheral pulses indicates the status of blood perfusion to the area distributed by the pulse (Table 5.1). For example, assessment of the right femoral pulse determines whether blood flow to the right leg is adequate. If a peripheral pulse distal to an injured or treated area of an extremity feels weak on palpation, the volume of blood reaching tissues below the affected area may be inadequate, and an invasive intervention may be necessary.

TABLE 5.1

Pulse Sites

Site	Location	Rationale for Selection
Temporal	Over temporal bone of head, above and lateral to the eye	Easily accessible site to assess pulse in children
Carotid	Along medial edge of sternocleidomastoid muscle in neck	Easily accessible site used during physiological shock or cardiac arrest when other sites are not palpable
Apical	Fourth to fifth intercostal space at left midclavicular line	Site used to auscultate apical pulse
Brachial	Groove between biceps and triceps muscles at antecubital fossa	Site used to assess status of circulation to lower arm and auscultate blood pressure
Radial	Radial or thumb side of forearm at wrist	Common site to assess character of peripheral pulse and status of circulation to hand
Ulnar	Ulnar side of forearm at wrist	Site used to assess status of circulation to ulnar side of hand; also used to perform Allen test
Femoral	Below inguinal ligament, midway between symphysis pubis and anterior superior iliac spine	Site used to assess character of pulse during physiological shock or cardiac arrest when other pulses are not palpable; used to assess status of circulation to leg
Popliteal	Behind knee in popliteal fossa	Site used to assess status of circulation to lower leg
Posterior tibial	Inner side of each ankle, below medial malleolus	Site used to assess status of circulation to foot
Dorsalis pedis	Along top of foot between extension tendons of great and first toe	Site used to assess status of circulation to foot

You can assess any artery for pulse rate, but the radial and carotid arteries are commonly used because they are easy to palpate (Fig. 5.6). When a patient's condition suddenly worsens, the carotid site is recommended for finding a pulse quickly. Assessment of other peripheral pulse sites such as the brachial or femoral artery is unnecessary when routinely obtaining vital signs. Other peripheral pulses are assessed when a complete physical (see Chapter 6) is conducted or when the radial artery is not available for assessment because of surgery, trauma, or impaired blood flow.

Delegation

The skill of radial pulse measurement can be delegated to assistive personnel (AP) if a patient's condition is stable. The skill cannot be delegated when a patient's condition is unstable because the patient is at high risk for acute or serious cardiac problems, or when the nurse is evaluating a patient's response to a treatment or medication. Direct the AP by:

- Indicating the appropriate site for measuring pulse rate; frequency of measurement; and factors related to the patient's history such as risk for abnormally slow, rapid, or irregular pulse
- Reviewing the patient's usual pulse rate and significant changes to report to the nurse

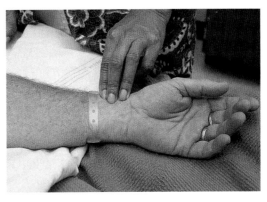
FIG. 5.6 Palpating radial pulse.

Interprofessional Collaboration

- If there is persistent tachycardia, bradycardia, or pulse irregularities, it often is necessary to collaborate with cardiac health care providers such as an advanced practice nurse or cardiologist.

Equipment

- Wristwatch with second hand or digital display
- Pen and vital sign flow sheet in electronic health record (EHR)

STEP	RATIONALE

ASSESSMENT

1. Identify patient using at least two identifiers (e.g., name and birthday or name and medical record number) according to agency policy.
2. Review patient's EHR to determine need to assess radial pulse:
   - History of heart disease
   - History of peripheral vascular disease
   - Cardiac dysrhythmia
   - Onset of sudden chest pain or acute pain from any site
   - Invasive cardiovascular diagnostic tests
   - Surgery
   - Large volume of intravenous (IV) fluid
   - Internal or external hemorrhage
   - Administration of medications that alter cardiac function
3. Determine previous pulse rate and measurement site (if available) from patient's record.
4. Assess patient's/family caregiver's health literacy.

5. Assess for factors that influence radial pulse rate and rhythm:

   - Age

   - Exercise

   - Position change

   - Medications

   - Temperature

Ensures patient safety. Complies with The Joint Commission standards and improves patient safety (TJC, 2023).
Certain conditions place patients at risk for pulse alterations. A history of peripheral vascular disease often alters pulse rate and quality.

Allows you to assess for change in condition. Provides comparison with future pulse measurements.
Determines degree to which individuals have the ability to find, understand, and use information and services to make informed health-related decisions and actions for themselves and others (CDC, 2023).
Allows you to anticipate factors that alter pulse, ensuring accurate interpretation.
Infant's HR at birth ranges from 80 to 160 beats/min at rest; by age 2, pulse rate slows to 65 to 100 beats/min; by adolescence, rate varies from 60 to 90 beats/min and remains so throughout adulthood (Hockenberry et al., 2024).
Physical activity increases HR: a well-conditioned patient may have a slower-than-usual resting HR that returns more quickly to resting rate after exercise.
HR increases temporarily when changing from lying to sitting or standing position.
Antidysrhythmics, sympathomimetics, and cardiotonics affect rate and rhythm of pulse; large doses of opioid analgesics can slow HR; general anesthetics slow HR; central nervous system stimulants such as caffeine can increase HR.
Fever or exposure to warm environments increases HR; HR declines with hypothermia.

STEP	RATIONALE
• Sympathetic stimulation	Emotional stress, anxiety, or fear stimulates sympathetic nervous system, which increases HR.
6. Perform hand hygiene.	Reduces transmission of microorganisms.
7. Assess for signs and symptoms of altered cardiac function such as presence of dyspnea, fatigue, chest pain, orthopnea, syncope, palpitations, edema of dependent body parts, cyanosis, or pallor of skin (see Chapter 6).	Physical signs and symptoms often indicate alteration in cardiac function, which affects radial pulse rate and rhythm.
8. Assess for signs and symptoms of peripheral vascular disease such as pale, cool extremities; thin, shiny skin with decreased hair growth; and thickened nails.	Physical signs and symptoms indicate alteration in local arterial blood flow.
9. Assess patient's knowledge of and prior experience with pulse measurement and feelings about procedure.	Reveals need for patient instruction and/or support.

PLANNING

1. Expected outcomes following completion of procedure:	
• Radial pulse is palpable, within usual range for patient's age.	Usual range for adults is 60 to 100 beats/min.
• Rhythm is regular.	Cardiac status is stable.
• Radial pulse is strong, firm, and elastic.	Radial artery is patent.
2. Provide privacy and explain procedure; encourage patient to relax as much as possible.	Protects patient's privacy, reduces anxiety, and promotes cooperation. Assessing radial pulse rate at rest allows for objective comparison of values.

Clinical Judgment *If patient has been active, wait 5 to 10 minutes before assessing pulse. If patient has been smoking or ingesting caffeine, wait 15 minutes before assessing pulse.*

3. Obtain and organize equipment needed to perform procedure.	Ensures more efficiency when completing procedure.

IMPLEMENTATION

1. Perform hand hygiene and help patient to assume a supine or sitting position.	Provides easy access to pulse sites.
2. If patient is supine, place patient's forearm straight alongside or across lower chest or upper abdomen (see illustration A). If sitting, bend patient's elbow 90 degrees and support lower arm on chair or on your arm. Place tips of first two or middle three fingers of hand over groove along radial or thumb side of patient's inner wrist (see illustration B). Slightly extend or flex wrist with palm down until you note strongest pulse.	Fingertips are most sensitive parts of hand to palpate arterial pulsation. Your thumb has pulsation that interferes with accuracy.

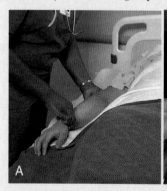 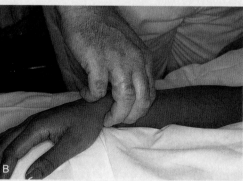

STEP 2 (A) Pulse check with patient's forearm at side with wrist extended. (B) Hand placement for pulse check. (From Yoost, B. L., & Crawford, L. R. [2016]. *Fundamentals of nursing: active learning for collaborative practice.* St. Louis: Elsevier.)

STEP	RATIONALE
3. Lightly compress pulse against radius, losing pulse initially; relax pressure so pulse becomes easily palpable.	Pulse assessment is more accurate when using moderate pressure. Too much pressure occludes pulse and impairs blood flow.
4. Determine strength of pulse. Note whether thrust of vessel against fingertips is bounding (4+); full increased, strong (3+); expected (2+); barely palpable, diminished (1+); or absent, not palpable (0).	Strength reflects volume of blood ejected against arterial wall with each heart contraction. Accurate description of strength improves communication among nurses and other health care providers.

STEP	RATIONALE
5. After palpating a regular pulse, look at watch second hand and begin to count rate. Count the first beat after the second hand hits the number on the dial; count as one, then two, and so on.	Rate is determined accurately only after pulse has been palpated. Timing begins with zero. Count of one is first beat palpated after timing begins.
6. If pulse is regular, count rate for 30 seconds and multiply total by 2.	A 30-second count is accurate for rapid, slow, or regular pulse rates.

Clinical Judgment *If pulse is irregular, count rate for a full 60 seconds. Assess frequency and pattern of irregularity, and compare radial pulses bilaterally. An inefficient contraction of heart fails to transmit pulse wave, resulting in an irregular pulse. A marked difference in pulse rate between radial sites may indicate that arterial flow is compromised to one extremity, and as a nurse you need to act.*

STEP	RATIONALE
7. Help patient to a comfortable position.	Restores comfort and sense of well-being.
8. Discuss findings with patient and document according to agency policy.	Promotes participation in care and understanding of health status.
9. Dispose of all contaminated supplies in appropriate receptacle; remove and dispose of gloves (if worn). Perform hand hygiene.	Prevents transmission of microorganisms.
10. Raise side rails (as appropriate) and lower bed to lowest position, locking into position.	Ensures patient safety and prevents falls.
11. Place nurse call system in an accessible location within patient's reach.	Ensures patient can call for assistance if needed.

EVALUATION

1. If assessing pulse for first time, establish radial pulse as baseline if it is within acceptable range. — Used to compare future pulse assessments.
2. Compare pulse rate and character with patient's previous baseline and acceptable range for patient's age. — Allows for assessment of change in patient's condition and presence of cardiac alteration.
3. **Use Teach-Back:** "I want to be sure I explained why it is important to check your pulse at home. Tell me which medication you are taking that would decrease your heart rate." Revise your instruction now or develop a plan for revised patient/family caregiver teaching if patient/family caregiver is not able to teach back correctly. — Teach-back is a technique for health care providers to ensure that they have explained medical information clearly so that patients and their families understand what is communicated to them (AHRQ, 2023).

Unexpected Outcomes

1. Patient has weak, thready, or difficult-to-palpate radial pulse.

2. An adult patient's pulse rate is less than 60 beats/min (bradycardia) or more than 100 beats/min (tachycardia).

Related Interventions

- Assess both radial pulses and compare findings.
- Observe for symptoms associated with ineffective tissue perfusion, including pallor and cool skin distal to weak pulse.
- Assess for swelling in surrounding tissues or any encumbrance (e.g., dressing or cast) that may impede blood flow.
- Obtain Doppler or ultrasound stethoscope to detect low-velocity blood flow (see Chapter 6).
- Auscultate apical pulse (see Skill 5.3).
- Assess for factors that decrease HR such as beta blockers and antiarrhythmic medications.
- Assess for factors that increase HR such as fever, acute pain, fear or anxiety, recent exercise, low blood pressure, blood loss, or inadequate oxygenation.
- Auscultate apical pulse (see Skill 5.3).
- Document pulse after administration of specific therapies, such as blood or blood product transfusions.
- Document your evaluation of patient and family caregiver learning.

Documentation

- Document pulse rate and site.

Hand-Off Reporting

- Report abnormal findings including route of assessment to nurse in charge or health care provider.

Special Considerations

Patient Education

- Patients taking certain prescribed cardiotonic or antidysrhythmic medications need to learn to assess their own pulse rates to detect side effects of medications.
- Patients undergoing cardiac rehabilitation need to learn to assess their own pulse rates to determine their response to exercise.
- Teach patients taking heart medications or starting a prescribed exercise regimen how to palpate one carotid artery and obtain carotid pulse rate.

Pediatrics

- Radial artery is difficult to assess in an infant. Apical, femoral, or brachial pulse is the best site for assessing pediatric HR and heart rhythm until 2 years of age (Hockenberry et al., 2024).

- Children often have a sinus dysrhythmia, which is an irregular heartbeat that speeds up with inspiration and slows down with expiration (Hockenberry et al., 2024).
- Breath holding in a child temporarily lowers pulse rate.

Older Adults

- Older adults have a reduced HR with exercise because of a decreased responsiveness to catecholamines.
- It takes longer for the HR to rise in the older adult to meet sudden increased demands that result from stress, illness, or excitement. Once elevated, the pulse rate of an older adult takes longer to return to normal resting rate.
- Peripheral vascular disease is more common among older adults, making radial pulse assessment difficult.

Populations With Disabilities

- Patients with a history of a stroke or peripheral extremity weakness may have differences in pulse strength.

✦ SKILL 5.3   Assessing Apical Pulse

 Video Clip

The apical pulse is the most reliable noninvasive way to assess cardiac function. The apical pulse rate is the assessment of the number and quality of apical heart sounds in 1 minute. A single apical pulse is the combination of two heart sounds: S_1 and S_2. S_1 is the sound of the tricuspid and mitral valves closing at the end of ventricular filling, just before systolic contraction begins. S_2 is the sound of the pulmonic and aortic valves closing at the end of the systolic contraction. As you listen for sound waves with a stethoscope, you will hear the characteristic "lub-dub" (S_1 and S_2) as a single pulsation.

A stethoscope (Fig. 5.7) is a closed cylinder that amplifies sound waves as they reach the surface of the body. The five major parts of the stethoscope are the earpieces, binaurals, tubing, bell, and diaphragm. The plastic or rubber earpieces should fit snugly and comfortably in your ears. Binaurals should be angled and strong enough that the earpieces stay firmly in place without causing discomfort. The earpieces follow the contour of the ear canal, pointing toward the face when the stethoscope is in place.

The polyvinyl tubing should be flexible and 30 to 45 cm (12–18 inches) in length; longer tubing decreases sound transmission. Stethoscopes can have one or two tubes. At the end of the tubing is the chest piece, consisting of a bell and diaphragm that you rotate into position depending on which part you choose to use.

The diaphragm is the larger, circular, flat-surfaced part of the chest piece. It transmits high-pitched sounds created by high-velocity movement of air and blood. Position the diaphragm to make a tight seal against a patient's skin. Exert enough pressure to complete the seal, leaving a temporary red ring on the patient's skin after you remove the diaphragm.

The bell is the cone-shaped part of the chest piece, usually surrounded by a rubber ring to avoid chilling the patient during placement. It transmits low-pitched sounds created by the low-velocity movement of blood. Hold the bell lightly against the skin for sound amplification.

Some stethoscopes have one chest piece that combines features of the bell and diaphragm. When you apply light pressure, the chest piece is a bell, whereas exerting more pressure converts the bell into a diaphragm. With the earpieces in your ears, tap lightly on the diaphragm and note which side you hear most clearly. This determines which side of the chest piece is functioning.

The stethoscope is a delicate instrument and requires proper care for optimal function. Remove the earpieces regularly and

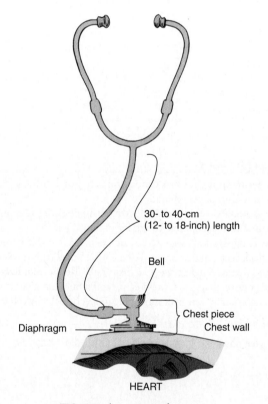

FIG. 5.7 Acoustic stethoscope.

clean them of cerumen (earwax). Health care–associated infections (HAIs), such as methicillin-resistant *Staphylococcus aureus* (MRSA), *Clostridium difficile*, and other multiple drug–resistant organisms (MDROs) can be transmitted by medical equipment such as a stethoscope, which can result in cross-contamination and HAI (Peacock et al., 2023; Marcos et al., 2019). Stethoscope hygiene is an important component of clinical care and can limit the contamination of stethoscopes with MDROs (Peacock et al., 2023). The Association of Operating Room Nurses (AORN, 2022) recommends that stethoscopes be cleaned before use with each patient according to the manufacturer's directions and agency policy.

Delegation

The skill of apical pulse measurement cannot be delegated to assistive personnel (AP). Often you measure the apical pulse when you suspect an irregularity in the radial pulse or when a patient's condition requires a more accurate assessment.

Interprofessional Collaboration

When apical radial pulse deficit is identified, collaborate with cardiac health care providers such as an advanced practice nurse or a cardiologist to determine if additional interventions such as medications are needed.

Equipment

- Stethoscope
- Wristwatch with second hand or digital display
- Pen and vital sign flow sheet in electronic health record (EHR)
- Antiseptic swab

STEP	RATIONALE

ASSESSMENT

1. Identify patient using at least two identifiers (e.g., name and birthday or name and medical record number) according to agency policy.	Ensures patient safety. Complies with The Joint Commission standards and improves patient safety (TJC, 2023).
2. Review patient's EHR to determine need to assess apical pulse: • History of heart disease • Cardiac dysrhythmia • Onset of sudden chest pain or acute pain from any site • Invasive cardiovascular diagnostic tests • Surgery • Large volume of intravenous (IV) fluid • Internal or external hemorrhage • Administration of medications that alter cardiac function	Certain conditions place patients at risk for heart rate (HR) alterations.
3. Determine previous pulse rate and measurement site (if available) from patient's record.	Allows you to assess for change in condition. Provides comparison with future pulse measurements.
4. Assess for factors that normally influence apical pulse rate and rhythm:	Allows you to anticipate factors that alter apical pulse, ensuring an accurate interpretation.
• Age	Infant's HR at birth ranges from 80 to 160 beats/min at rest; by age 2 pulse rate slows to 65 to 100 beats/min; by adolescence rate varies between 60 and 90 beats/min and remains so throughout adulthood (Hockenberry et al., 2024).
• Exercise	Physical activity increases HR. A well-conditioned patient may have a slower-than-usual resting HR that returns more quickly to resting rate after exercise.
• Position changes	HR increases temporarily when changing from lying to sitting or standing position.
• Medications	Antidysrhythmics, sympathomimetics, and cardiotonics affect rate and rhythm of pulse; large doses of narcotic analgesics can slow HR; general anesthetics slow HR; central nervous system stimulants such as caffeine can increase HR.
• Temperature of environment	Fever or exposure to warm environments increases HR; HR declines with hypothermia.
• Sympathetic stimulation	Emotional stress, anxiety, or fear stimulates sympathetic nervous system, which increases HR.
5. Assess patient's/family caregiver's health literacy.	Determines degree to which individuals have the ability to find, understand, and use information and services to make informed health-related decisions and actions for themselves and others (CDC, 2023).
6. Assess for presence of latex allergy. If patient has latex allergy, ensure that stethoscope is latex free.	Reduces risk of allergic reaction to stethoscope.
7. Perform hand hygiene.	Reduces transmission of microorganisms.
8. Assess for signs and symptoms of altered cardiac function such as presence of dyspnea, fatigue, chest pain, orthopnea, syncope, palpitations, edema of dependent body parts, cyanosis, or pallor of skin (see Chapter 6).	Physical signs and symptoms often indicate alteration in cardiac function, which affects radial pulse rate and rhythm.
9. Determine if patient measures apical HR at home. Assess patient's knowledge and skill level.	Determines level and type of instruction required by patient or family caregiver.
10. Assess patient's knowledge of and prior experience with apical pulse measurement and feelings about procedure.	Reveals need for patient instruction and/or support.

STEP	RATIONALE

PLANNING

1. Expected outcomes following completion of procedure:
   - Apical HR is within acceptable range.
   - Rhythm is regular.
2. Provide privacy and explain procedure.
3. Help patient to supine or sitting position. Move aside bed linen and gown to expose sternum and left side of chest.

4. Organize and set up any equipment needed and perform stethoscope hygiene according to agency policy prior to procedure.

5. Encourage patient to relax and not speak.

Adults average 60 to 100 beats/min.
Cardiovascular status is stable.
Protects patient's privacy; reduces anxiety. Promotes cooperation.
Exposes part of chest wall for selection of auscultatory site. Stethoscope diaphragm must touch skin for best sounds. Placing the stethoscope over a gown or clothing creates extraneous sounds and produces an inaccurate count.
Ensures more efficiency when completing an assessment. Reduces transmission of infection. Cleansing of stethoscope pieces before and after patient use has the potential to reduce HAIs (Peacock et al., 2023; AORN, 2022).
Patient's voice interferes with nurse's ability to hear sound when measuring apical pulse. Assessing apical pulse rate at rest allows for objective comparison of values.

Clinical Judgment *If patient has been active, wait 5 to 10 minutes before assessing pulse. If patient has been smoking or ingesting caffeine, wait 15 minutes before assessing pulse.*

IMPLEMENTATION

1. Perform hand hygiene. Locate anatomical landmarks to identify point of maximal impulse (PMI), also called *apical* impulse (see Chapter 6). The heart is located behind and to left of sternum with base at top and apex at bottom. Find angle of Louis just below suprasternal notch between sternal body and manubrium; it feels like a bony prominence (see illustration A). Slip fingers down each side of angle to find second intercostal space (ICS) (see illustration B). Carefully move fingers down left side of sternum to fifth ICS and laterally to left midclavicular line (MCL) (see illustration C). A light tap felt within area 1 to 2.5 cm (½–1 inch) of PMI is reflected from apex of heart (see illustration D).

Use of anatomical landmarks allows correct placement of stethoscope over apex of heart. This position enhances ability to hear heart sounds clearly. If unable to palpate PMI, reposition patient on left side. In presence of serious heart disease, you may locate PMI to left of MCL or at sixth ICS. PMI may not be palpated in obese adults or patients with severe pulmonary disease that has changed shape of thorax.

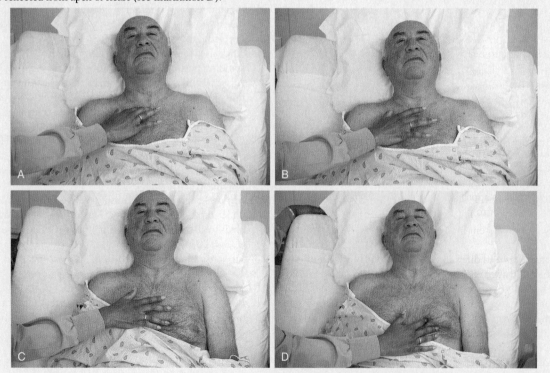

STEP 1 (A) Nurse locates sternal notch. (B) Nurse locates second intercostal space. (C) Nurse locates fifth intercostal space. (D) Nurse locates point of maximal impulse at fifth intercostal space at left midclavicular line.

STEP	RATIONALE

2. Place diaphragm of stethoscope in palm of hand for 5 to 10 seconds.

Warming of metal or plastic diaphragm prevents patient from being startled and promotes comfort.

3. Place diaphragm of stethoscope over PMI at fifth ICS, at left MCL, and auscultate for normal S1 and S2 heart sounds (heard as "lub-dub") (see illustrations).

Allow stethoscope tubing to extend straight without kinks that would distort sound transmission. Normal sounds S1 and S2 are high pitched and best heard with diaphragm.

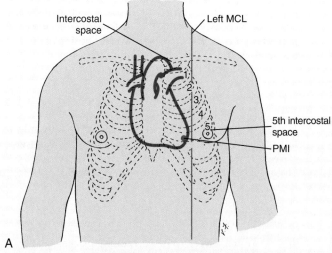
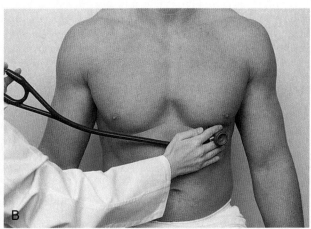

STEP 3 (A) Location of point of maximal impulse *(PMI)* in adult. (B) Listening to PMI in adult. *MCL,* Midclavicular line.

4. When you hear S1 and S2 with regularity, use second hand of watch and begin to count rate: when sweep hand hits number on dial, start counting with zero, then one, two, and so on.

Apical rate is determined accurately only after you are able to auscultate sounds clearly. Timing begins with zero. Count of one is first sound auscultated after timing begins.

5. If apical rate is regular, count for 30 seconds and multiply by 2.

You can assess regular apical rate within 30 seconds.

Clinical Judgment *When HR is irregular or patient is receiving cardiovascular medication, count for a full 1 minute (60 seconds). An irregular rate is more accurately assessed when measured over a longer interval.*

6. Note regularity of any dysrhythmia (S1 and S2 occurring early or late after previous sequence of sounds) (e.g., every third or every fourth beat is skipped).

Regular occurrence of dysrhythmia within 1 minute indicates inefficient contraction of heart and potential alteration in cardiac output.

Clinical Judgment *If apical rate is abnormal or irregular, repeat measurement or have another nurse conduct measurement. Original measurement may be incorrect. Second measurement confirms initial findings of an abnormal HR.*

7. Replace patient's gown and bed linen. Help patient to a comfortable position.

Restores comfort and sense of well-being.

8. Discuss findings with patient of pulse and document according to agency policy.

Promotes participation in care and understanding of health status.

9. Dispose of all contaminated supplies in appropriate receptacle; remove and dispose of gloves (if worn). Perform hand hygiene.

Reduces transmission of microorganisms.

10. Raise side rails (as appropriate) and lower bed to lowest position, locking into position.

Ensures patient safety and prevents falls.

11. Place nurse call system in an accessible location within patient's reach.

Ensures patient can call for assistance if needed.

12. Clean earpieces and diaphragm of stethoscope with alcohol swab routinely after each use. Perform hand hygiene.

Stethoscopes are frequently contaminated with microorganisms. Regular disinfection can control nosocomial infections. Reduces transmission of microorganisms.

STEP	RATIONALE

EVALUATION

1. If assessing pulse for first time, establish apical rate as baseline if it is within an acceptable range.

Used to compare future pulse assessments.

2. Compare apical rate and character with patient's previous baseline and acceptable range of HR for patient's age.

Allows you to assess for change in patient's condition and for presence of cardiac alteration.

3. **Use Teach-Back:** "I want to be sure I explained why it is important to check your heart rate at home. Tell me which medication you are taking that would decrease your heart rate." Revise your instruction now or develop a plan for revised patient/family caregiver teaching if patient/family caregiver is not able to teach back correctly.

Teach-back is a technique for health care providers to ensure that they have explained medical information clearly so that patients and their families understand what is communicated to them (AHRQ, 2023).

Unexpected Outcomes	Related Interventions
1. Adult patient's apical pulse is greater than 100 beats/min (tachycardia).	• Assess for factors that increase apical pulse such as fever, acute pain, fear or anxiety, recent exercise, low blood pressure, blood loss, or inadequate oxygenation. • Observe for signs and symptoms associated with abnormal cardiac function. • Notify charge nurse or health care provider of increased rate when abnormal for patient. Prepare for change in cardiac medication.
2. Patient's apical pulse is less than 60 beats/min (bradycardia).	• Assess for factors that decrease HR such as beta blockers and antiarrhythmic drugs. • Observe for signs and symptoms associated with abnormal cardiac function. • Have another nurse assess apical pulse. • Report findings to nurse in charge and/or health care provider. It may be necessary to withhold prescribed medications that alter HR until health care provider can evaluate need to alter dosage.
3. Patient's apical rhythm is irregular.	• Assess for pulse deficit: (a) nurse auscultates apical pulse while second provider palpates radial pulse (see Skill 5.2); (b) nurse begins 60-second pulse count by calling out loud when to begin counting pulses; (c) if pulse count differs, assess for other signs and symptoms of decreased cardiac output (see Chapter 6). • Report findings to nurse in charge and/or health care provider, who may order an electrocardiogram to detect cardiac conduction alteration.

Documentation

• Document apical pulse rate and rhythm according to agency policy. If apical pulse is not found at fifth ICS and left MCL, document location of PMI.
• Document measurement of apical pulse rate after administration of specific therapies per agency policy.
• Document your evaluation of patient and family caregiver learning.

Hand-Off Reporting

• Report abnormal findings including pulse deficit to nurse in charge or health care provider.

Special Considerations

Patient Education

• Teach family caregivers of patients taking prescribed cardiotonic or antidysrhythmic medications how to assess apical pulse rates to detect side effects of medications.

Pediatrics

• The PMI of an infant is usually located at the third to fourth ICS near the left sternal border.

• In infants and children younger than 2 years, an apical pulse is more reliable and is counted for 1 full minute because of possible irregularities in rhythm (Hockenberry et al., 2024).
• Breath holding in an infant or child temporarily lowers apical pulse rate.

Older Adults

• The PMI can be difficult to palpate in some older adults because the anterior-posterior diameter of the chest increases with age, and the heart becomes repositioned because of left ventricular enlargement (Touhy & Jett, 2022).
• When assessing older-adult women with sagging breast tissue, gently lift the breast tissue and place the stethoscope at the fifth ICS or the lower edge of the breast.
• Heart sounds are sometimes muffled or difficult to hear in older adults because of an increase in air space in the lungs.

Home Care

• Assess home environment to determine a quiet environment for auscultation of apical rate.

✦ SKILL 5.4   Assessing Respirations

▶ *Video Clip*

Respiration is the exchange of respiratory gases—oxygen (O_2) and carbon dioxide (CO_2)—between cells of the body and the atmosphere. Three processes of respiration are ventilation (i.e., mechanical movement of gases into and out of the lungs), diffusion (i.e., movement of oxygen and carbon dioxide between the alveoli and the red blood cells), and perfusion (i.e., distribution of red blood cells to and from the pulmonary capillaries).

Assess ventilation by observing the rate, depth, and rhythm of respiratory movements. Accurate assessment of respirations depends on recognizing normal thoracic and abdominal movements. Normal breathing is both active and passive. On inspiration the diaphragm contracts, and the abdominal organs move down to increase the size of the chest cavity. At the same time the ribs and sternum lift outward to promote lung expansion. On expiration the diaphragm relaxes upward, and the ribs and sternum return to their relaxed position (Fig. 5.8). During quiet breathing, the chest wall gently rises and falls. Expiration is an active process only during exercise, voluntary hyperventilation, and certain disease states. Altered breathing tends to be the first sign of clinical deterioration and is one of the most important indicators for predicting patient outcomes (Takayama et al., 2019).

Delegation

The skill of counting respirations can be delegated to assistive personnel (AP) unless the patient is considered unstable (i.e., complaints of dyspnea). Direct the AP by:
- Communicating the frequency of measurement and factors related to patient history or risk for increased or decreased respiratory rate or irregular respirations
- Reviewing any unusual respiratory values and significant changes to report to the nurse

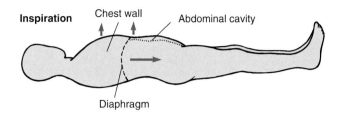
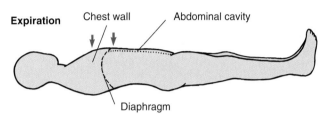

FIG. 5.8 Diaphragmatic and chest wall movement during inspiration and expiration.

Interprofessional Collaboration

- If patient has severe shortness of breath or persistent tachypnea, collaborate with a pulmonary health care provider, advanced practice nurse, or respiratory therapist for additional interventions such as medications or pulmonary chest physiotherapy.

Equipment

- Wristwatch with second hand or digital display
- Pen and vital sign flow sheet in electronic health record (EHR)

STEP	RATIONALE
ASSESSMENT	
1. Identify patient using at least two identifiers (e.g., name and birthday or name and medical record number) according to agency policy.	Ensures patient safety. Complies with The Joint Commission standards and improves patient safety (TJC, 2023).
2. Review patient's EHR to assess for factors that influence the patient's respirations.	Allows you to anticipate factors that influence respirations, ensuring a more accurate interpretation.
• Fever	Elevated body temperature increases oxygen demand and increases respiration rate and depth.
• Exercise	Respirations increase in rate and depth to meet need for additional oxygen and rid body of carbon dioxide.
• Diseases or trauma of chest wall or muscles	Certain conditions (e.g., fractured ribs, thoracic surgery, asthma, chronic lung disease) affect inspiration and/or expiration.
• Smoking	Chronic smoking changes pulmonary airways, resulting in increased respiratory rate at rest when not smoking.
• Medications	Opioid analgesics, general anesthetics, and sedative hypnotics depress rate and depth; amphetamines and cocaine increase rate and depth; bronchodilators cause dilation of airways, which ultimately slows respiratory rate.
• Neurological injury	Damage to brainstem impairs respiratory center and inhibits rate and rhythm.

STEP	RATIONALE

Clinical Judgment *Assess patients with difficulty breathing (dyspnea), such as those with heart failure or abdominal ascites or in late stages of pregnancy, in the position of greatest comfort. Repositioning may increase the work of breathing, which increases respiratory rate.*

4. Provide privacy and explain procedure to patient.	Protects patient's privacy; reduces anxiety, and promotes cooperation.
5. Organize and set up any equipment needed to perform procedure.	Ensures more efficiency when completing an assessment
6. Be sure that patient's chest is visible. If necessary, move bed linen or gown.	Ensures clear view of chest wall and abdominal movements.
7. Assess respirations after pulse measurement in an adult (see Skill 5.2).	Inconspicuous assessment of respirations immediately after pulse assessment prevents patient from consciously or unintentionally altering rate and depth of breathing.

IMPLEMENTATION

1. Perform hand hygiene and place patient's arm in relaxed position across abdomen or lower chest, leaving fingertips on the wrist, or place your hand directly over patient's upper abdomen.	A similar position used during pulse assessment allows respiratory rate assessment to be inconspicuous. Patient awareness of monitoring reduces respiratory rate by 2 breaths/min (Harry et al., 2020; Hill et al., 2018; Lamberti, 2020). Patient's or your hand rises and falls during respiratory cycle.
2. Observe complete respiratory cycle (one inspiration and one expiration).	Rate is accurately determined only after viewing a complete respiratory cycle. An inspiratory breath is half as long as an expiratory breath (Rolfe, 2019).
3. After observing a cycle, look at second hand of watch and begin to count rate: when sweep hand hits number on dial, begin time frame, counting one with first full respiratory cycle.	Timing begins with count of one. Respirations occur more slowly than pulse; therefore timing does not begin with zero.
4. If rhythm is regular, count number of respirations in 30 seconds and multiply by 2. If rhythm is irregular, less than 12, or greater than 20, count for 1 full minute (Lamberti, 2020; Harry et al., 2020).	Respiratory rate is equivalent to number of respirations per minute. Suspected irregularities require assessment for at least 1 minute (Box 5.5). Shorter count durations overestimate respiratory rate by 2–4 breaths (Takayama et al., 2019).
5. Note depth of respirations by observing degree of chest wall movement while counting rate. In addition, assess depth by palpating chest wall excursion or auscultating posterior thorax after you have counted rate (see Chapter 6). Describe depth as shallow, normal, or deep.	Character of ventilatory movement reveals specific disease states restricting volume of air from moving into and out of lungs.
6. Note rhythm of ventilatory cycle. Normal breathing is regular and uninterrupted. Do not confuse sighing with abnormal rhythm.	Character of ventilations reveals specific types of alterations. Periodically, people unconsciously take single deep breaths or sighs to expand small airways prone to collapse.

Clinical Judgment *Any irregular respiratory pattern or periods of apnea (cessation of respiration for several seconds) are symptoms of underlying disease in the adult; report this to the health care provider or nurse in charge. Further assessment and immediate intervention are often necessary.*

7. Replace bed linen and patient's gown. Help patient to a comfortable position.	Restores comfort and promotes sense of well-being.
8. Inform patient of respiratory rate and document according to agency policy.	Promotes participation in care and understanding of health status.
9. Dispose of all contaminated supplies in appropriate receptacle; remove and dispose of gloves (if worn). Perform hand hygiene.	Reduces transmission of microorganisms.
10. Raise side rails (as appropriate) and lower bed to lowest position, locking into position.	Ensures patient safety and prevents falls.
11. Place nurse call system in an accessible location within patient's reach.	Ensures patient can call for assistance if needed.

STEP	RATIONALE

EVALUATION

1. If assessing respirations for first time, establish rate, rhythm, and depth as baseline if within acceptable range.	Used to compare future respiratory assessment.
2. Compare respirations with patient's previous baseline and usual rate, rhythm, and depth.	Allows you to assess for changes in patient's condition and presence of respiratory alterations.
3. Correlate respiratory rate, depth, and rhythm with data obtained from pulse oximetry and ABG measurements if available.	Evaluations of ventilation, perfusion, and diffusion are interrelated.
4. **Use Teach-Back:** "I want to be sure I explained why you will be reminded to take deep breaths after surgery. Tell me why deep breathing is important." Revise your instruction now or develop a plan for revised patient/family caregiver teaching if patient/family caregiver is not able to teach back correctly.	Teach-back is a technique for health care providers to ensure that they have explained medical information clearly so that patients and their families understand what is communicated to them (AHRQ, 2023).

Unexpected Outcomes

1. Adult patient's respiratory rate is below 12 breaths/min (bradypnea) or above 20 breaths/min (tachypnea). Breathing pattern is sometimes irregular (see Box 5.5). Depth of respirations is increased or decreased. Patient complains of dyspnea.

2. Patient demonstrates Kussmaul, Cheyne-Stokes, or Biot respirations (see Box 5.5).

Related Interventions

- Assess for related factors, including obstructed airway, abnormal breath sounds, productive cough, restlessness, anxiety, and confusion (see Chapter 6).
- Help patient to supported sitting position (semi- or high-Fowler) unless contraindicated.
- Provide oxygen as ordered (see Chapter 23).
- Assess for environmental factors that influence patient's respiratory rate such as secondhand smoke, poor ventilation, or gas fumes.
- Notify health care provider or nurse in charge if alteration continues. Changes as little as 3 to 5 breaths/min can indicate a change in the patient's condition and are often the first sign of deterioration (Lamberti, 2020; Wheatley, 2019).
- Notify health care provider for additional evaluation and possible medical intervention.

Documentation

- Document respiratory rate, depth, and rhythm according to agency policy.
- Document measurement of respiratory rate after administration of specific therapies per agency policy.
- Document your evaluation of patient and family caregiver learning.
- Document the type and amount of oxygen therapy, if used, per agency policy.

Hand-Off Reporting

- Report abnormal findings to nurse in charge or health care provider.
- Report need for oxygen therapy.

Special Considerations

Patient Education

- Patients who demonstrate decreased ventilation (e.g., after surgery) often benefit from learning deep-breathing and coughing exercises (see Chapter 36).

BOX 5.5

Alterations in Breathing Pattern

Alteration	Description
Bradypnea	Rate of breathing is regular but abnormally slow (fewer than 12 breaths/min).
Tachypnea	Rate of breathing is regular but abnormally rapid (more than 20 breaths/min).
Hyperpnea	Respirations are labored, increased in depth, and increased in rate (greater than 20 breaths/min) (occurs normally during exercise).
Apnea	Respirations cease for several seconds. Persistent cessation results in respiratory arrest.
Hyperventilation	Rate and depth of respirations increase. Hypocarbia, an abnormally low level of carbon dioxide in the blood, may occur.
Hypoventilation	Respiratory rate is abnormally low; depth of ventilation may be depressed. Hypercarbia, an abnormally elevated level of carbon dioxide in the blood, may occur.
Cheyne-Stokes respiration	Respiratory rate and depth are irregular, characterized by alternating periods of apnea and hyperventilation. Respiratory cycle begins with slow, shallow breaths that gradually increase to abnormal rate and depth. The pattern reverses; breathing slows and becomes shallow, climaxing in apnea before respiration resumes.
Kussmaul respiration	Respirations are abnormally rapid and deep but regular; common in diabetic ketoacidosis.
Biot respiration	Respirations are abnormally shallow for two to three breaths, followed by irregular period of apnea.

- Instruct family caregiver to contact home care nurse or health care provider if unusual fluctuations in respiratory rate occur.

Pediatrics

- Assess respiratory rates before other vital signs or assessments if you are able to view movement of chest wall or abdomen. This allows assessment of rate and rhythm before child becomes anxious because of stranger anxiety or fear of other assessment procedures.
- Respiratory rate assessment on neonates and newborns may require auscultation with a stethoscope.
- Observe respiratory rate in infant or young child while chest and abdomen are exposed.
- Acceptable respiratory rate (breaths per minute) for newborns is 30 to 60; infant and toddlers (6 months to 2 years old) is 30; and children ages 3 to 12 years is 20 to 30 (Hockenberry et al., 2024).
- Neonates have shallow and irregular respirations; always count for a full minute.
- Children up to age 7 breathe abdominally; therefore respirations are observed by abdominal movement.

- An irregular respiratory rate and short apneic spells are normal for newborns.
- Use cardiorespiratory monitors for infants or newborns who are at risk for respiratory compromise or sustained apnea.

Older Adults

- Aging causes ossification of costal cartilage and downward slant of ribs, resulting in a more rigid rib cage, which reduces chest wall expansion. Kyphosis and scoliosis, frequent in older adults, may also restrict chest expansion.
- Depth of respirations tends to decrease with aging.
- Change in lung function with aging results in respiratory rates generally higher in older adults (Touhy & Jett, 2022).
- Some older adults depend more on accessory abdominal muscles than weakened thoracic muscles during respiration.

Home Care

- Assess for environmental factors in the home that influence patient's respiratory rate such as secondhand smoke, poor ventilation, gas or fireplace fumes, dust, and pets.

✦ SKILL 5.5   Assessing Arterial Blood Pressure

Blood pressure (BP) is measured in virtually all patients receiving health care. Accurate measurement of BP is essential to guide patient management, determine patient's response to interventions, and prevent adverse outcomes (AACN, 2017). BP is the force exerted by blood against the vessel walls. The peak pressure or systolic pressure occurs when the ventricles of the heart contract and force blood under high pressure into the aorta. When the ventricles relax, the blood remaining in the arteries exerts a minimal or diastolic pressure against the arterial walls at all times.

The standard unit for measuring BP is millimeters of mercury (mm Hg). The most common technique of measuring BP is auscultation with a sphygmomanometer and stethoscope. As the sphygmomanometer cuff is deflated, the five different sounds are heard over an artery. Each sound has unique characteristics (Fig. 5.9). BP is documented with the systolic reading (first sound) before the diastolic (beginning of the fifth sound). The difference between systolic and diastolic pressure is the pulse pressure. For a BP of 115/75 mm Hg, the pulse pressure is 40.

Recent validation and testing of automated oscillometric devices have demonstrated that these devices provide accurate BP measurement and are capable of accurately measuring serial BP to record patient responses to treatment. Both auscultatory methods are also considered acceptable for measuring BP in children and adolescents (Muntner et al., 2019).

Hypertension

Hypertension is a major factor underlying death from heart attack and stroke in the United States and Canada. Experts have determined criteria for the categories of hypertension (Whelton et al., 2018) (Table 5.2). Elevated BP, a designation for patients at high risk for developing hypertension, is between 120 and 129 mm Hg systolic blood pressure (SBP) and less than 80 mm Hg diastolic blood pressure (DBP). In these patients early intervention by adoption of healthy lifestyles reduces the risk of or prevents hypertension. Stage 1 hypertension is defined as SBP between 130 and 139 mm Hg or DBP between 80 and 89 mm Hg. Stage 2 hypertension is defined as SBP greater than 140 mm Hg or DBP greater than 90 mm Hg. The diagnosis of hypertension in adults requires the average of two or

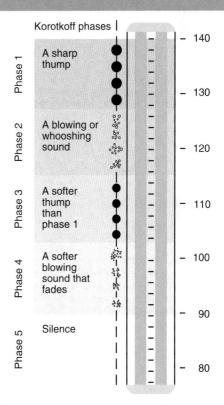

FIG. 5.9 The sounds auscultated during blood pressure measurement can be differentiated into five phases. In this example the blood pressure is 140/90 mm Hg.

more readings taken at each of two or more visits after an initial screening.

One BP measurement revealing a high SBP or DBP does not qualify as a diagnosis of hypertension. However, if you assess a high reading (e.g., 150/90 mm Hg), encourage the patient to practice healthy lifestyles, such as following a low-fat and low-sodium diet, getting exercise, and eating fresh fruits and vegetables; and

TABLE 5.2

Classification of Blood Pressure for Adults Ages 18 Years and Older[a]

BP Category[b]	Systolic (mm Hg)		Diastolic (mm Hg)
Normal	<120 mm Hg	And	<80 mm Hg
Elevated	120–129 mm Hg	And	<80 mm Hg
Hypertension			
Stage 1	130–139 mm Hg	Or	80–89 mm Hg
Stage 2	≥140 mm Hg	Or	≥90 mm Hg

[a]Based on the average of two or more readings taken at each of two or more visits after an initial screening. Patient is not taking antihypertensive drugs and is not acutely ill. When SBP and DBP fall into different categories, the higher category should be selected to classify the individual's blood pressure status. For example, 160/88 mm Hg should be classified as stage 2 hypertension.
[b]Individuals with SBP and DBP in two categories should be designated to the higher BP category. BP indicates blood pressure (based on an average of 22 careful readings obtained on 22 occasions).
DBP, Diastolic blood pressure; *SBP*, systolic blood pressure.
Data from Whelton, P. K., et al. (2018). Guideline for the prevention, detection, evaluation, and management of high blood pressure in adults: Report of the American College of Cardiology/American Heart Association Task Force on Clinical Practice Guidelines. Hypertension, *71*(6): e13.

TABLE 5.3

Recommendations for Blood Pressure Follow-Up

Initial Blood Pressure	Follow-up Recommended[a]
Normal	Recheck in 1 yr
Elevated	Recheck in 3–6 mo[b]
Stage 1 hypertension	Evaluate therapy within 3–6 mo[b]
Stage 2 hypertension	Evaluate therapy within 1 mo[b]
	For those with higher pressure (e.g., >180/110 mm Hg), evaluate and treat immediately or within 1 wk, depending on clinical situation and complications

[a]Modify the scheduling of follow-up according to reliable information about past blood pressure measurements, other cardiovascular risk factors, or target organ damage.
[b]Provide advice about lifestyle modifications.
Data from Whelton, P. K., et al. (2018). Guideline for the prevention, detection, evaluation, and management of high blood pressure in adults: Report of the American College of Cardiology/American Heart Association Task Force on Clinical Practice Guidelines. Hypertension *71*(6): e13, 2018.

encourage the patient to return for another checkup within 3 to 6 months (Table 5.3).

Hypotension

Hypotension occurs when the SBP falls to 90 mm Hg or below. Although some adults normally have a low BP, for most people a low BP is an abnormal finding associated with illness (e.g., hemorrhage or myocardial infarction). Orthostatic hypotension, also referred to as postural hypotension, occurs when a normotensive person develops symptoms (e.g., light-headedness or dizziness) and a significant drop in systolic pressure (greater than 20 mm Hg) or a drop by at least 10 mm Hg in diastolic pressure (Ball et al., 2023; Biswas et al., 2019). A loss of consciousness may occur in severe cases. Orthostatic changes in vital signs are effective indicators of blood volume depletion. Some medications cause orthostatic hypotension, especially in young patients and older adults. Orthostatic

hypotension is a risk factor for falls, especially among older adults with hypertension.

Blood Pressure Equipment

You measure arterial BP either directly (invasively) or indirectly (noninvasively). The direct method requires electronic monitoring equipment and the insertion of a thin catheter into an artery. The risks associated with invasive BP monitoring require a patient to be in an intensive care setting.

The more common, noninvasive method requires use of a sphygmomanometer and stethoscope. A sphygmomanometer includes a pressure manometer, an occlusive cloth or disposable vinyl cuff that encloses an inflatable rubber bladder, and a pressure bulb with a release valve that inflates the bladder. The aneroid pressure manometer has a glass-enclosed circular gauge containing a needle that registers millimeter calibrations. Before using the aneroid manometer, make sure that the needle is pointing to zero. The release valve of the sphygmomanometer that holds the pressure constant must be clean and freely movable in either direction.

Cloth or disposable vinyl compression cuffs contain an inflatable bladder and come in several different sizes. The size selected is proportional to the circumference of the limb that you are assessing. Ideally the width of the cuff should be 40% of the circumference (or 20% wider than the diameter) of the midpoint of the limb on which the cuff is to be used (Fig. 5.10). The bladder enclosed within the cuff should encircle at least 80% of the upper arm. Many adults require a large adult cuff. A regular-size cuff holds a bladder in the width of 12 to 13 cm (4.8–5.2 inches) and length of 22 to 23 cm (8½–9 inches). An improperly fitting cuff produces inaccurate BP measurements (Box 5.6).

Electronic or automatic BP machines consist of an electronic sensor positioned inside a BP cuff attached to an electronic processor (see Procedural Guideline 5.1). Electronic devices have limitations but are useful when frequent measurements are necessary (Box 5.7).

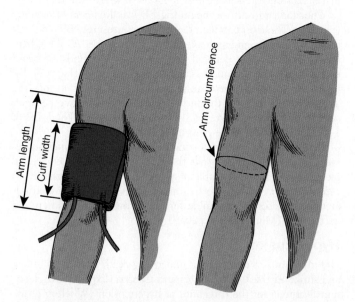

FIG. 5.10 Guidelines for proper blood pressure cuff size. Use correct cuff size, such that the bladder encircles 75% to 100% of the arm. Cuff width equals 20% more than upper arm diameter or 40% of circumference around upper arm and two-thirds of upper arm length. (Adapted from American Association of Critical-Care Nurses [AACN] [2016]: AACN Practice Alert: Obtaining accurate noninvasive blood pressure measurement in adults, *Critical Care Nurse* 36(3):212; and Muntner, P., et al. [2019]: American Heart Association Scientific Statement: Measurement of blood pressure in humans, *Hypertension* 73:e66.)

Common Mistakes in Blood Pressure Assessment

Error	Effect
Bladder or cuff too wide	False-low reading
Bladder or cuff too narrow or too short	False-high reading
Cuff wrapped too loosely or unevenly	False-high reading
Deflating cuff too slowly	False-high diastolic reading
Deflating cuff too quickly	False-low systolic and false-high diastolic reading
Arm below heart level	False-high reading
Arm above heart level	False-low reading
Arm not supported	False-high reading
Stethoscope that fits poorly or impairment of examiner's hearing, causing sounds to be muffled	False-low systolic and false-high diastolic reading
Stethoscope applied too firmly against antecubital fossa	False-low diastolic reading
Inflating too slowly	False-high diastolic reading
Repeating assessments too quickly	False-high systolic reading
Inaccurate inflation level	False-low systolic reading
Multiple examiners using different sounds for diastolic readings	False-high systolic and false-low diastolic reading

Delegation

The skill of BP measurement can be delegated to assistive personnel (AP) unless the patient is considered unstable. Direct the AP by:

- Explaining which limb for measurement, BP cuff size, and equipment (manual or electronic) to be used
- Communicating the frequency of measurement and factors related to the patient's history such as risk for orthostatic hypotension

Advantages and Limitations of Assessing Blood Pressure Electronically

Advantages
- Ease of use
- Efficient when frequent repeated measurements are indicated
- Stethoscope not required
- Allows blood pressure to be recorded more frequently, as often as every 15 seconds with accuracy

Limitations
- Expensive
- Requires source of electricity
- Requires space to position machine
- Sensitive to outside motion interference and cannot be used in patients with seizures, tremors, or shivers or patients unable to cooperate
- Not accurate in patients with irregular heart rate or hypotension or in conditions with reduced blood flow (e.g., hypothermia)
- Accuracy standards for electronic blood pressure machine manufacturers are voluntary
- Vulnerable to error among older adults and obese patients

- Reviewing the patient's usual BP values and significant changes or abnormalities to report to the nurse

Interprofessional Collaboration
- When a patient has an abnormal BP that does not respond to treatment, collaborate with cardiac health care providers.

Equipment
- Aneroid sphygmomanometer
- Cloth or disposable vinyl pressure cuff of appropriate size for patient's extremity (see Planning, Step 3)
- Stethoscope
- Antiseptic swab
- Pen and vital sign flow sheet or electronic health record (EHR)

STEP	RATIONALE

ASSESSMENT

1. Identify patient using at least two identifiers (e.g., name and birthday or name and medical record number) according to agency policy.

Ensures patient safety. Complies with The Joint Commission standards and improves patient safety (TJC, 2023).

2. Review patient's EHR to assess for risk factors for BP alterations:
- History of cardiovascular disease
- Renal disease
- Diabetes mellitus
- Circulatory shock (hypovolemic, septic, cardiogenic, or neurogenic)
- Acute or chronic pain
- Rapid intravenous (IV) infusion of fluids or blood products
- Increased intracranial pressure
- Postoperative status
- Gestational hypertension

Certain conditions place patients at risk for BP alteration.

3. Assess patient's/family caregiver's health literacy.

Determines degree to which individuals have the ability to find, understand, and use information and services to make informed health-related decisions and actions for themselves and others (CDC, 2023).

STEP	RATIONALE
4. Assess for factors that influence BP:	Allows you to anticipate factors that influence BP, ensuring a more accurate interpretation.
• Age	Acceptable values for BP vary throughout life (see Pediatric and Gerontological considerations).
• Gender	During and after menopause, women often have higher BPs than men of same age.
• Daily (diurnal) variation	BP varies throughout day; pressure is highest during the day between 10:00 a.m. and 6:00 p.m. and lowest in early morning.
• Weight	Obesity is an independent predictor of hypertension.
• Ethnicity	Incidence of hypertension is higher in certain racial/ethnic groups; people in these groups tend to develop more severe hypertension at an earlier age and have an increased risk for the complications of hypertension (Ogunniyi et al., 2021).
• Medications	Antihypertensives, diuretics, beta-adrenergic blockers, vasodilators, calcium channel blockers, angiotensin-converting enzyme (ACE) inhibitors, angiotensin receptor blockers (ARBs), and antidysrhythmics lower BP; opioids and general anesthetics also cause a drop in BP.
• Smoking	Causes vasoconstriction in the short term and atherosclerosis in the long term, increasing BP.
5. Determine previous baseline BP and site (if available) from patient's record. Determine any report of latex allergy.	Assesses for change in condition. Provides comparison with future BP measurements. If patient has latex allergy, verify that stethoscope and BP cuff are latex free.
6. Perform hand hygiene.	Reduces transmission of microorganisms.
7. Assess for factors that may influence BP measurement:	Allows you to anticipate for factors that may influence BP.
• Position	BP falls as person moves from lying to sitting or standing position; acceptable postural variations are less than 10 mm Hg (Ball et al., 2023; Hale et al., 2017).
• Exercise	Increase in oxygen demand by body during activity increases BP.
• Pain, anxiety, fear, or a full bladder	Sympathetic nervous system stimulation causes BP to rise. A full bladder increases SBP and DBP (Kallioinen et al., 2017).
• Smoking	Smoking results in vasoconstriction, a narrowing of blood vessels. SBP and DBP rise acutely and return to baseline approximately 20 to 30 minutes after stopping smoking, 30 minutes after chewing snuff, and 40 to 60 minutes after taking a nicotine tablet (Kallioinen et al., 2017).
8. Assess for signs and symptoms of BP alterations. In patient at risk for high BP, assess for headache (usually occipital), flushing of face, nosebleed, and fatigue in older adults. Hypotension is associated with dizziness; mental confusion; restlessness; pale, dusky, or cyanotic skin and mucous membranes; and cool, mottled skin over extremities.	Physical signs and symptoms indicate alterations in BP. Hypertension is often asymptomatic until pressure is very high. In hypotensive patients, BP measurement by palpation may be required.
9. Assess patient's knowledge of and prior experience with BP measurement and feelings about procedure.	Reveals need for patient instruction and/or support.

PLANNING

1. Expected outcome following completion of procedure: • BP is within acceptable range for patient's age.	Cardiovascular status is stable.
2. Provide privacy and explain procedure. Be sure that room is warm, quiet, and relaxing.	Protects patient's privacy; reduces anxiety. Promotes cooperation.
3. Determine best site for BP assessment. Avoid applying cuff to extremity when IV fluids are infusing, an arteriovenous shunt or fistula is present, patient has a peripherally inserted central catheter or midline catheter (AACN, 2017), or breast or axillary surgery has been performed on that side. In addition, avoid applying cuff to traumatized or diseased extremity or one that has a cast or bulky bandage. Use lower extremities when brachial arteries are inaccessible.	Inappropriate site selection may result in poor amplification of sounds, causing inaccurate readings. Application of pressure from inflated bladder temporarily impairs blood flow and can further compromise circulation in extremity that already has impaired blood flow.

Clinical Judgment For a patient who has had a mastectomy or lumpectomy, do not use the involved arm(s) for BP measurement if lymphedema is present (AACN, 2017).

STEP	RATIONALE
4. Select appropriate cuff size with a bladder of an adequate size capable of going around 75% to 100% of the arm (see Fig 5.10) (AACN, 2017; Muntner et al., 2019). Ensure that sphygmomanometer or electronic BP machine is in patient's room.	Use of improper cuff can cause measurement errors (Mickley et al., 2018; AANC, 2017) (see Box 5.6).
5. Organize and set up any equipment needed to perform procedure.	Ensures more efficiency when completing an assessment.
6. Ensure that patient has not exercised, ingested caffeine, or smoked for 30 minutes before assessing BP. Have patient rest at least 5 minutes before measuring lying or sitting BP and 1 minute before measuring standing BP.	Exercise causes false elevation in BP. Smoking increases BP immediately and for up to 15 minutes. Caffeine increases BP for up to 3 hours.
7. Explain to patient that you will measure BP. Have patient assume sitting or lying position. Allow the patient to rest 3 to 5 minutes before obtaining a BP (Mickley et al., 2018). Ask patient not to speak while you are measuring BP.	Reduces anxiety that falsely elevates readings. Deep breathing lowers BP. Talking to a patient during assessment increases BP. A higher BP measurement occurs if the patient has not rested or relaxed (Mickley et al., 2018). SBP and DBP of hypertensive and normotensive patients increase with talking (AACN, 2017).

IMPLEMENTATION

1. Perform hand hygiene. Perform stethoscope hygiene according to agency policy.	Reduces transmission of infection. Cleansing of stethoscope pieces before and after patient use have the potential to reduce health care–associated infection (HAIs) (Peacock et al., 2023; AORN, 2022)..
2. Prepare to obtain BP by auscultation.	
a. Upper extremity: With patient sitting or lying, position patient's forearm at heart level with palm turned up (AACN, 2017) (see illustration). Support arm on table or under your arm. If sitting, support back and instruct patient to keep feet flat on floor without legs crossed. If supine, patient should not have legs crossed.	If arm is extended and not supported, patient will perform isometric exercise that can increase diastolic pressure. Placement of arm above level of heart causes false-low reading; arm below the level of the heart creates false-high reading (AACN, 2017; Kallioinen et al., 2017). Not supporting the arm can falsely elevate SBP (AACN, 2017). BP measured with the back unsupported is higher than with the back supported (Ringrose et al., 2017). Legs crossed at the knees can significantly increase BP (Kallioinen et al., 2017).

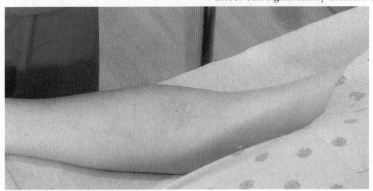

STEP 2a Patient's forearm supported on bed.

Clinical Judgment *There are special circumstances, such as bilateral arm trauma and bilateral arm lymphedema, in which the upper extremities cannot be used for BP measurement.*

b. Low er extremity: When upper extremities are inaccessible, lower extremity BP measures are obtained. **(1)** Calf BP measurements: Position the patient supine. **(2)** Thigh BP measurements: Place the patient prone. If the patient cannot be placed prone, position the patient supine with knee slightly bent (AACN, 2017; Ball et al., 2023).	Allows for application of BP cuff and placement of stethoscope over dorsalis pedis (calf measurement) and popliteal artery (thigh measurement).

Clinical Judgment *Patients with unstable vital signs, spinal surgeries, or orthopedic injuries cannot tolerate the prone position for thigh BP measurement; consult health care provider to determine if a calf BP measurement is acceptable.*

Clinical Judgment *Spinal cord–injured patients may be placed on rotational support surfaces. If thigh BP measurements are ordered, time obtaining the thigh BP measurement when the support surface rotates the patient to the prone position.*

STEP	RATIONALE

c. Expose extremity (arm or leg) fully by removing constricting clothing. Cuff may be placed over a sleeve as long as stethoscope rests on skin.

Ensures proper cuff application. Thin clothing <5 mm does not affect cuff inflation or BP measurements (Zhang et al., 2019).

3. Palpate brachial artery (arm, see illustration A) or popliteal artery (thigh) or dorsalis pedis artery or posterior tibial artery (calf).

Brachial artery measurement: With cuff fully deflated, position bladder of cuff 2 to 3 cm (1¼ inches) above antecubital fossa, at the level of the right atrium (midpoint of the sternum), above artery, by centering arrows marked on cuff over artery (AANC, 2017; Muntner et al., 2019) (see illustration B). If cuff does not have any center arrows, estimate center of bladder and place this center over artery. With cuff fully deflated, wrap it evenly and snugly around upper arm (see illustration C) or lower extremity.

Brachial artery is along groove between biceps and triceps muscles above elbow at antecubital fossa. Popliteal artery is just below patient's thigh, behind knee. Dorsalis pedis artery is on the top of the patient's foot, midpoint between the ankle and toes. The posterior tibial artery is behind the knee and above the Achilles tendon.

Placing bladder directly over artery ensures that you apply proper pressure during inflation. Loose-fitting cuff causes false-high readings.

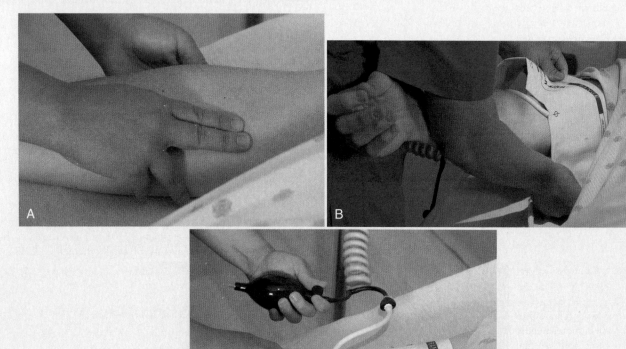

STEP 3 (A) Palpating brachial artery. (B) Aligning blood pressure cuff arrow with brachial artery. (C) Blood pressure cuff wrapped around upper arm.

Clinical Judgment *When a patient has a thigh BP measurement ordered, position cuff 2 to 3 cm (1¼ inches) above popliteal fossa (AACN, 2017).*

4. Position manometer gauge vertically at eye level. You should be no farther than 1 meter (approximately 1 yard) away.

Looking up or down at scale can result in distorted readings.

5. Auscultate BP.

  a. Two-step method:

    (1) Relocate brachial or popliteal pulse. Palpate artery distal to cuff with fingertips of nondominant hand while inflating cuff rapidly to pressure 30 mm Hg above point at which pulse disappears. Slowly deflate cuff and note point when pulse reappears. Deflate cuff fully and wait 30 seconds.

Estimating prevents false-low readings. Determine maximal inflation point for accurate reading by palpation. If unable to palpate artery because of weakened pulse, use ultrasonic stethoscope (see Chapter 6). Completely deflating cuff prevents venous congestion and false-high readings.

STEP	RATIONALE
(2) Place stethoscope earpieces in ears and be sure that sounds are clear, not muffled.	Ensure that each earpiece follows angle of ear canal to facilitate hearing.
(3) Relocate artery and place bell or diaphragm chest piece of stethoscope over it. Do not allow chest piece to touch cuff or clothing.	Proper stethoscope placement ensures best sound reception. Stethoscope improperly positioned causes muffled sounds that often result in false-low systolic and false-high diastolic readings. The stethoscope bell or diaphragm can be used for auscultatory readings (Muntner et al., 2019).
	The bell provides better sound reproduction, whereas the diaphragm is easier to secure with fingers and covers a larger area. Placing the stethoscope under the cuff increases the SBP and decreases the DBP measurement (Kallioinen et al., 2017).
(4) Close valve of pressure bulb clockwise until tight. Quickly inflate cuff to 30 mm Hg above patient's estimated systolic pressure.	Tightening valve prevents air leak during inflation. Rapid inflation ensures accurate measurement of systolic pressure.
(5) Slowly release pressure bulb valve and allow manometer needle to fall at rate of 2 to 3 mm Hg/s.	Too rapid a decline decreases SBP and increases DBP measurement (Kallioinen et al., 2017).
(6) Note point on manometer when you hear first clear sound. Sound will slowly increase in intensity.	First sound reflects SBP.
(7) Continue to deflate cuff gradually, noting point at which sound disappears in adults. Note pressure to nearest 2 mm Hg. Listen for 20 to 30 mm Hg after last sound and allow remaining air to escape quickly.	Beginning of last or fifth sound is indication of diastolic pressure in adults (Thomas & Pohl, 2022). In children, distinct muffling of sounds indicates diastolic pressure (Thomas & Pohl, 2022).
b. One-step method:	
(1) Place stethoscope earpieces in ears and be sure that sounds are clear, not muffled.	Earpieces should follow angle of ear canal to facilitate hearing.
(2) Relocate brachial or popliteal artery and place bell or diaphragm chest piece of stethoscope over it. Do not allow chest piece to touch cuff or clothing.	Proper stethoscope placement ensures optimal sound reception. Stethoscope improperly positioned causes muffled sounds that often result in false readings. Bell provides better sound reproduction, whereas diaphragm is easier to secure with fingers and covers larger area. Placing the stethoscope under the cuff increases the SBP and decreases the DBP measurement (Kallioinen et al., 2017).
(3) Close valve of pressure bulb clockwise until tight. Quickly inflate cuff to 30 mm Hg above patient's usual systolic pressure.	Tightening valve prevents air leak during inflation. Inflation above systolic level ensures accurate measurement of systolic pressure.
(4) Slowly release pressure bulb valve and allow manometer needle to fall at rate of 2 to 3 mm Hg/s. Note point on manometer when you hear first clear sound. Sound will slowly increase in intensity.	Too rapid a decline decreases SBP and increases DBP measurement (Kallioinen et al., 2017). First sound reflects systolic pressure.
(5) Continue to deflate cuff gradually, noting point at which sound disappears in adults. Note pressure to nearest 2 mm Hg. Listen for 10 to 20 mm Hg after last sound and allow remaining air to escape quickly.	Beginning of fifth sound is indication of diastolic pressure in adults. In children, distinct muffling of sounds indicates diastolic pressure (Thomas & Pohl, 2022).
6. Assess SBP by palpation:	
a. Locate and then continually palpate brachial, radial, or popliteal artery with fingertips of one hand. Inflate cuff to pressure 30 mm Hg above point at which you can no longer palpate pulse.	Ensures accurate detection of true systolic pressure once pressure valve is released.

Clinical Judgment *If unable to palpate artery because of weakened pulse, use a Doppler ultrasonic stethoscope (Fig. 5.11).*

STEP	RATIONALE
b. Slowly release valve and deflate cuff, allowing manometer needle to fall at rate of 2 mm Hg/s. Note point on manometer when pulse is again palpable.	Too rapid a decline decreases SBP and increases DBP measurement (Kallioinen et al., 2017). Palpation helps identify systolic pressure only.
c. Deflate cuff rapidly and completely. Remove cuff from patient's extremity unless patient condition requires repeated measurements.	Continuous cuff inflation or too slow deflation causes arterial occlusion, resulting in numbness and tingling of extremity.
7. The American Heart Association recommends average of two sets of BP measurement, 2 minutes apart. Use second set of BP measurements as baseline. If readings are different by more than 5 mm Hg, additional readings are necessary (Muntner et al., 2019; Whelton et al., 2018).	Two sets of BP measurements help to prevent false-positive readings based on patient's sympathetic response (alert reaction). Averaging minimizes effect of anxiety, which often causes first reading to be higher than subsequent measures (Kallioinen et al., 2017).

STEP	RATIONALE

Clinical Judgment *When upper extremities are inaccessible, use lower extremity; the ankle site is preferred. Ankle SBP measurement is slightly lower than arm measurement (Sheppard et al., 2020).*

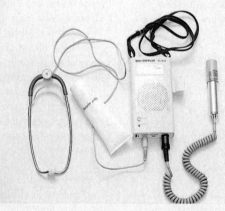

FIG. 5.11 Doppler. (From Ball, J. W., Dains, J. E., Flynn, J. A., Solomon, B. S., & Stewart, R. W. [2023]. Seidel's guide to physical examination: An interprofessional approach. St. Louis: Elsevier.)

STEP	RATIONALE
8. Remove cuff from patient's arm or leg unless you need to repeat measurement.	Continuous cuff inflation causes arterial occlusion, resulting in numbness and tingling of patient's arm/leg.
9. If this is first assessment of patient, repeat procedure on other arm or leg (Muntner et al., 2019).	Comparison of BP in both arms and legs detects circulatory problems. (Normal difference of 5–10 mm Hg exists between arms.) Use arm with higher pressure for repeated measurements.
10. Dispose of all contaminated supplies in appropriate receptacle; remove and dispose of gloves. Perform hand hygiene.	Reduces transmission of microorganisms.
11. Help patient return to comfortable position and cover upper arm or leg if previously clothed.	Restores comfort and provides sense of well-being.
12. Discuss findings with patient and document results per agency policy.	Promotes participation in care and understanding of health status.
13. Raise side rails (as appropriate) and lower bed to lowest position, locking into position.	Ensures patient safety and prevents falls.
14. Place nurse call system in an accessible location within patient's reach.	Ensures patient can call for assistance if needed.
15. Clean earpieces and diaphragm of stethoscope with alcohol swab as needed. Wipe cuff with agency-approved disinfectant if used between patients.	Controls transmission of microorganisms when nurses share stethoscope.
16. Perform hand hygiene.	Reduces transmission of microorganisms.

EVALUATION

1. If assessing BP for first time, establish baseline BP if it is within acceptable range.	Used to compare future BP measurements.
2. Compare BP reading with patient's previous baseline and usual BP for patient's age.	Allows you to assess for change in condition. Provides comparison with future BP measurements.
3. **Use Teach-Back:** "I want to be sure I explained why it is important to stand up slowly since you have high blood pressure. Tell me which of your medications might make you dizzy if you stand up too fast." Revise your instruction now or develop a plan for revised patient/family caregiver teaching if patient/family caregiver is not able to teach back correctly.	Teach-back is a technique for health care providers to ensure that they have explained medical information clearly so that patients and their families understand what is communicated to them (AHRQ, 2023).

Unexpected Outcomes	**Related Interventions**
1. Patient's BP is above acceptable range.	• Repeat measurement in other extremity and compare findings. • Verify correct size and placement of BP cuff. • Have another nurse repeat measurement in 1 to 2 minutes. • Report BP to nurse in charge or health care provider to initiate appropriate evaluation and treatment. • Administer antihypertensive medications as ordered.

STEP	RATIONALE
2. Patient's BP is not sufficient for adequate perfusion and oxygenation of tissues.	• Compare BP value to baseline. • Position patient in supine position to enhance circulation and restrict activity that decreases BP further. • Assess for signs and symptoms associated with hypotension, including tachycardia; weak, thready pulse; weakness; dizziness; confusion; and cool, pale, dusky, or cyanotic skin. • Assess for factors that contribute to low BP, including hemorrhage, dilation of blood vessels resulting from hyperthermia, anesthesia, or medication side effects. • Report BP to nurse in charge or health care provider to initiate appropriate evaluation and treatment. • Increase rate of IV infusion or administer vasoconstrictive drugs as ordered.
3. Unable to obtain BP reading.	• Determine that no immediate crisis is present by obtaining pulse and respiratory rate. • Assess for signs and symptoms of decreased cardiac output; if present, notify nurse in charge or health care provider immediately. • Use alternative sites or procedures to obtain BP: use Doppler ultrasonic instrument (see Chapter 6); palpate SBP.
4. Patient experiences orthostatic hypotension.	• Maintain patient safety. • Return patient to safe position in bed or chair.

Documentation

- Document BP and site(s) assessed.
- Document measurement of BP and any signs or symptoms of BP alterations after administration of specific therapies.
- Document your evaluation of patient and family caregiver learning.

Hand-Off Reporting

- Report abnormal findings to nurse in charge or health care provider.
- Report method of BP measurement.

Special Considerations

Patient Education

- Educate patient about risks for hypertension. People with family history of hypertension, premature heart disease, lipidemia, or renal disease are at significant risk. Obesity, cigarette smoking, heavy alcohol consumption, high blood cholesterol and triglyceride levels, and continued exposure to stress from psychosocial and environmental conditions are factors linked to hypertension.
- Primary prevention of hypertension includes lifestyle modifications (e.g., lose weight, exercise daily, reduce sodium and saturated fat intake, and maintain adequate intake of dietary potassium and calcium). Cigarette smoking is a significant risk factor; encourage patients to avoid tobacco in any form.
- Instruct primary caregiver to take BP at same time each day and after patient has had a brief rest. Take BP sitting or lying down; use same position and arm each time you take pressure.
- Instruct primary caregiver that if the BP is difficult to hear, it is probably caused by one of the following: cuff too loose, not large enough, or too narrow; stethoscope not over arterial pulse; cuff deflated too quickly or too slowly; or cuff not pumped high enough for systolic readings.

Pediatrics

- BP measurement is not a routine part of assessment in children younger than 3 years.
- For otherwise healthy children, BP need only be measured annually in healthy children 3 years of age through adolescence rather than during every health care encounter (Hockenberry et al., 2024).

- BP measurement can frighten children. Prepare child for squeezing feeling of inflated BP cuff by comparing sensation to elastic band on finger or a tight hug on the arm.
- Obtain BP in child before performing anxiety-producing tests or procedures.
- BP sounds are difficult to hear in children because of low frequency and amplitude. Using the bell of a pediatric stethoscope is often helpful.

Older Adults

- Older adults, especially frail older adults, have lost upper-arm mass, necessitating special attention to selection of BP cuff size.
- Skin of older adults is more fragile and susceptible to cuff pressure when measurements are frequent. More frequent assessment of skin under cuff or rotation of measurement sites is recommended (Touhy & Jett, 2022).
- Older adults have an increase in systolic pressure related to decreased vessel elasticity.
- Older adults often experience a fall in BP after eating, referred to as postprandial hypotension.
- Instruct older adults to change position slowly and wait after each change to avoid postural hypotension and prevent injuries.

Populations With Disabilities

- Obtain BP in the active arm in patients with unilateral muscle weakness or paralysis.

Home Care

- Assess home noise level to determine the room that provides the quietest environment for assessing BP.
- Instruct patient regarding the importance of an appropriate-size BP cuff for home use.
- Assess family's financial ability to afford a sphygmomanometer for performing BP evaluations on a regular basis. Recommend electronic devices or aneroid sphygmomanometers that have proven to be accurate according to standard testing and appropriate-size cuffs. Finger BP monitors are inaccurate.

PROCEDURAL GUIDELINE 5.1 *Noninvasive Electronic Blood Pressure Measurement*

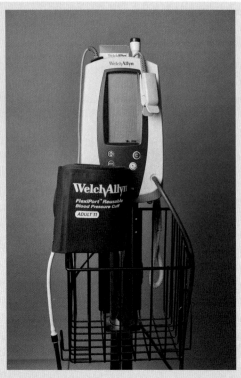

FIG. 5.12 Noninvasive electronic blood pressure machine. (*Photo courtesy of Welch Allyn.*)

Many different styles of electronic blood pressure machines are available to determine blood pressure automatically (Fig. 5.12). Electronic machines rely on an electronic sensor to detect the vibrations caused by the rush of blood through an artery. Although electronic blood pressure machines are fast, you must consider their advantages and limitations (see Box 5.7). The devices are used when frequent assessment is required, such as in critically ill or potentially unstable patients, during or after invasive procedures, or when therapies require frequent monitoring. However, automatic blood pressure measurements are often inaccurate when patients have an irregular heart rate (HR) or extremely low or high blood pressure. Always verify an assessment of an abnormal blood pressure by an electronic machine with a sphygmomanometer and stethoscope.

Delegation

The skill of blood pressure measurement using an electronic blood pressure machine can be delegated to assistive personnel (AP) unless the patient is considered unstable. Direct the AP by:
- Explaining the frequency and extremity to use for measurement
- Reviewing how to select appropriate-size blood pressure cuff for designated extremity and appropriate cuff for the machine
- Reviewing patient's usual blood pressure and reporting significant changes or abnormalities to the nurse

Equipment

Electronic blood pressure machine, blood pressure cuff of appropriate size as recommended by manufacturer, pen and vital sign flow sheet or electronic health record (EHR) per agency policy

Steps

1. Identify patient using at least two identifiers (e.g., name and birthday or name and medical record number) according to agency policy (TJC, 2023).
2. Assess risk factors for blood pressure alterations (see Skill 5.5, Assessment, Step 2) and determine patient's baseline blood pressure.
3. Determine appropriateness of using electronic blood pressure measurement. Patients with irregular HR, peripheral vascular disease, seizures, tremors, and shivering are not candidates for the device.
4. Assess patient's/family caregiver's health literacy.
5. Perform hand hygiene and explain procedure to patient. Determine best site for cuff placement; inspect condition of extremities.
6. Collect and bring appropriate equipment to patient's bedside. Select appropriate cuff size for patient extremity (Table 5.4) and appropriate cuff for machine. Electronic blood pressure cuff and machine must be matched by manufacturer and are not interchangeable.
7. Assist patient to a comfortable position, either lying or sitting. Plug device into electric outlet and place it near patient, ensuring that connector hose between cuff and machine reaches.
8. Locate on/off switch and turn on machine to enable device to self-test computer systems.
9. Remove constricting clothing to ensure proper cuff application.
10. Prepare blood pressure cuff by manually squeezing all the air out of the cuff and connecting it to connector hose.
11. Perform hand hygiene. Wrap flattened cuff snugly around extremity, verifying that only one finger can fit between cuff and patient's skin. Make sure that "artery" arrow marked on outside of cuff is placed correctly (see illustration).

TABLE 5.4

Correct Blood Pressure Cuff Size for Electronic Monitor[a]

Cuff Size	Limb Circumference (cm)
Small adult	17–25
Adult	23–33
Large adult	31–40
Thigh	38–50

[a]A 12- to 24-foot cord is required for adult blood pressure monitoring.

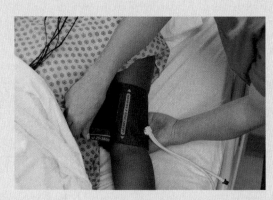

STEP 11 Aligning blood pressure cuff arrow with brachial artery.

PROCEDURAL GUIDELINE 5.1 *Noninvasive Electronic Blood Pressure Measurement—cont'd*

12. Verify that connector hose between cuff and machine is not kinked. Kinking prevents proper inflation and deflation of cuff.
13. Following manufacturer directions, set frequency control for automatic or manual and press the start button. The first blood pressure measurement pumps cuff to a peak pressure of approximately 180 mm Hg. After this pressure is reached, the machine begins a deflation sequence that determines the blood pressure. The first reading determines peak pressure inflation for additional measurements.
14. When deflation is complete, digital display provides most recent values and flash time in minutes that have elapsed since the measurement occurred (see illustration).

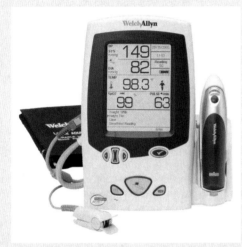

STEP 14 Digital electronic blood pressure display. *(Image courtesy of Hillrom.)*

Clinical Judgment *If unable to obtain blood pressure with electronic device, verify machine connections (e.g., plugged into working electrical outlet, hose-cuff connections tight, machine on, correct cuff). Repeat electronic blood pressure measurement; if unable to obtain, use auscultatory technique (see Skill 5.5).*

15. Set frequency of measurements and upper and lower alarm limits for systolic, diastolic, and mean blood pressure readings. Intervals between measurements can be set from 1 to 90 minutes. A nurse determines frequency and alarm limits on the basis of patient's acceptable range of blood pressure, nursing judgment, and health care provider order.

16. Obtain additional readings at any time by pressing the start button. Pressing the cancel button immediately deflates the cuff.
17. If frequent measurements are required, the cuff may be left in place. Remove it at least every 2 hours to assess underlying skin integrity and, if possible, alternate measurement sites.

Clinical Judgment *Frequent measurement by electronic blood pressure machines increases the risk of extremity pressure injuries, especially in vulnerable elders, patients with paralysis, and those with peripheral vascular diseases. Patients with abnormal bleeding tendencies are at risk for microvascular rupture from repeated inflations. Inspect the skin under the blood pressure cuff at regular intervals depending on the frequency of use.*

18. When patient no longer requires frequent blood pressure monitoring:
    a. Help patient return to a comfortable position, and cover upper arm or leg if previously clothed, to restore comfort and provide sense of well-being.
    b. Raise side rails (as appropriate) and lower bed to lowest position, locking into position, to ensure patient safety and prevent falls.
    c. Place nurse call system in an accessible location within patient's reach and instruct patient in use to ensure patient can call for assistance if needed.
    d. Wipe cuff with agency-approved disinfectant to reduce transmission of infection. Clean and store electronic blood pressure machine.
19. Perform hand hygiene.
20. Compare electronic blood pressure readings with auscultatory measurements to verify accuracy of electronic device.
21. Inform patient of blood pressure.
22. **Use Teach-Back:** "I want to be sure I explained why you need to keep your arm straight while the machine is taking your blood pressure. Tell me why it is important to remain still." Revise your instruction now or develop a plan for revised patient/family caregiver teaching if patient/family caregiver is not able to teach back correctly.
23. Document blood pressure and site assessed in EHR per agency policy; document any signs or symptoms of blood pressure alterations.
24. Report reason for electronic blood pressure and abnormal findings to nurse in charge or health care provider.

PROCEDURAL GUIDELINE 5.2 *Measuring Oxygen Saturation (Pulse Oximetry)*

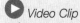 *Video Clip*

Pulse oximetry is the noninvasive measurement of arterial blood oxygen saturation, the percent to which hemoglobin is filled with oxygen. A pulse oximeter is a probe with a light-emitting diode (LED) connected by cable to an oximeter. The LED emits light wavelengths that are absorbed differently by the oxygenated and deoxygenated hemoglobin molecules. The more hemoglobin saturated by oxygen, the higher the oxygen saturation. Normally oxygen saturation (SpO_2) is greater than 95%. A saturation less than 90% is a clinical emergency in a patient without a chronic respiratory condition (Pagana et al., 2021).

Pulse oximetry measurement of SpO_2 is simple and painless and has few of the risks associated with more invasive measurements of oxygen saturation such as arterial blood gas sampling. A

Continued

PROCEDURAL GUIDELINE 5.2 *Measuring Oxygen Saturation (Pulse Oximetry)—cont'd*

vascular, pulsatile area is needed to detect the change in the transmitted light when making measurements with a finger probe. Conditions that decrease arterial blood flow such as peripheral vascular disease, hypothermia, pharmacological vasoconstrictors, hypotension, or peripheral edema affect accurate determination of oxygen saturation in these areas. For patients with decreased peripheral perfusion, you can apply an earlobe or forehead sensor (Seifi et al., 2018). Factors that affect light transmission such as outside light sources or patient motion also affect the measurement of oxygen saturation. Carbon monoxide in the blood, jaundice, and intravascular dyes can influence the light reflected from hemoglobin molecules.

In adults you can apply reusable and disposable oximeter probes to the earlobe, finger, toe, bridge of the nose, or forehead (Box 5.8). Pulse oximetry is indicated in patients who require ongoing monitoring during a procedure or who have an unstable oxygen status or are at risk for impaired gas exchange.

Delegation

The skill of SpO_2 measurement can be delegated to assistive personnel (AP). Direct the AP by:
- Communicating specific factors related to the patient that can falsely lower SpO_2
- Informing AP about appropriate sensor site and probe and to report any skin irritation from probe placement to nurse
- Notifying frequency of SpO_2 measurements for a specific patient
- Instructing to notify nurse immediately of any reading lower than SpO_2 of 95% or value for specific patient

---

BOX 5.8

Characteristics of Pulse Oximeter Sensor Probes and Sites

Finger Probe
- Easy to apply, conforms to various sizes

Earlobe Probe
- Clip-on smaller and lighter, although more positional than finger probe
- Yields strongest correlation with oxygen saturation
- Good when uncontrollable or rhythmic movements (e.g., hand tremors during exercise) are present
- Vascular bed least affected by decreased blood flow

Forehead Sensor
- Greater accuracy during decreased perfusion
- Reliable for patients on vasoactive medications
- Detects desaturation more quickly than other sites
- Does not require a pulsatile vascular bed
- Good when uncontrollable or rhythmic movements (e.g., hand tremors) are present
- Requires headband to secure sensor

Disposable Sensor Pad
- Can be applied to a variety of sites: earlobe of adult, nose bridge, palm or sole of infant
- Less restrictive for continuous oxygen saturation monitoring
- Expensive
- Contains latex
- Skin under adhesive may become moist and harbor pathogens
- Available in variety of sizes; pad can be matched to infant weight

---

- Instructing to refrain from using pulse oximetry to obtain heart rate (HR) because oximeter will not detect an irregular pulse

Interprofessional Collaboration
- The respiratory therapy and pulmonary health care providers may intervene for potential airway clearance measures, additional inhaled medications, or oxygen therapy when a patient has a persistent decrease in oxygen saturation.

Equipment
Oximeter, oximeter probe appropriate for patient and recommended by oximeter manufacturer, acetone or nail-polish remover if needed, pen and vital sign flow sheet or electronic health record (EHR) per agency policy

Steps
1. Identify patient using at least two identifiers (e.g., name and birthday or name and medical record number) according to agency policy (TJC, 2023).
2. Determine need to measure patient's oxygen saturation. Assess risk factors for decreased oxygen saturation (e.g., acute or chronic compromised respiratory problems, change in oxygen therapy, chest wall injury, recovery from anesthesia).
3. Assess patient's/family caregiver's health literacy.
4. Perform hand hygiene. Assess for signs and symptoms of alterations in oxygen saturation (e.g., altered respiratory rate, depth, or rhythm; adventitious breath sounds [see Chapter 6]; cyanotic appearance of nail beds, lips, mucous membranes, or skin; restlessness; difficulty breathing).
5. Determine if patient has a latex allergy; disposable adhesive sensors are made of latex.
6. Assess for factors that influence measurement of SpO_2 (e.g., oxygen therapy, respiratory therapy such as postural drainage and percussion, hemoglobin level, hypotension, temperature, nail polish, and medications such as bronchodilators).
7. Review patient's EHR for health care provider's order or consult agency procedure manual for standard of care for measurement of SpO_2.
8. Determine previous baseline SpO_2 (if available) from patient's record.
9. Perform hand hygiene.
10. Determine most appropriate patient-specific site (e.g., finger, earlobe, bridge of nose, forehead) for sensor probe placement by measuring capillary refill (see Chapter 6). If capillary refill time is greater than 2 seconds, select alternative site.
    - Site must have adequate local circulation and be free of moisture.
    - A finger free of black or brown nail polish is preferred.
    - If patient has tremors or is likely to move, use earlobe or forehead. Motion artifact is the most common cause of inaccurate readings.
    - If patient's finger is too large for the clip-on probe, as may be the case with obesity or edema, the clip-on probe may not fit properly; obtain a disposable (tape-on) probe.
11. Explain to patient the way you will measure oxygen saturation and the importance of breathing normally until reading is complete.

PROCEDURAL GUIDELINE 5.2 *Measuring Oxygen Saturation (Pulse Oximetry)—cont'd*

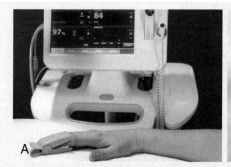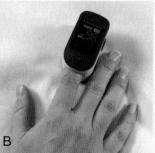

STEP 14 Oximeter sensor attached to finger.

12. Arrange equipment at the bedside.
13. Position patient comfortably.
14. Attach sensor to monitoring site (see illustration). If using finger, remove regular fingernail polish from digit with acetone or polish remover. If gel polish is in place, have it removed by patient or nail technician before monitoring, or choose alternate site. Gel-based manicures can result in overestimations of actual readings (Yek et al., 2019). Explain that clip-on probe will feel like a clothespin on the finger but will not hurt.

Clinical Judgment *Do not attach probe to finger, ear, or bridge of nose if area is edematous or skin integrity is compromised. Do not use earlobe and bridge of nose sensors for infants and toddlers because of skin fragility. Do not attach sensor to fingers that are hypothermic. Select ear or bridge of nose if adult patient has a history of peripheral vascular disease. Do not use disposable adhesive sensors if patient has a latex allergy. Do not place sensor on same extremity as electronic blood pressure cuff because blood flow to finger will be interrupted temporarily when cuff inflates and cause inaccurate reading that can trigger alarms.*

15. With sensor in place, turn on oximeter by activating power. Observe pulse waveform/intensity display and audible beep. Correlate oximeter pulse rate with patient's radial pulse.
16. Leave sensor in place 10 to 30 seconds or until oximeter readout reaches constant value and pulse display reaches full strength during each cardiac cycle. Inform patient that oximeter alarm will sound if sensor falls off or patient moves it. Read SpO_2 on digital display.
17. If you plan to monitor SpO_2 continuously, verify SpO_2 alarm limits preset by manufacturer at a low of 85% and a high of 100%. Determine limits for SpO_2 and pulse rate as indicated by patient's condition. Verify that alarms are on. Assess skin integrity under sensor probe every 2 hours; relocate sensor at least every 4 hours and more frequently if skin integrity is altered or tissue perfusion compromised.

18. If you plan intermittent or spot-checking of SpO_2, remove probe and turn oximeter power off.
19. **Use Teach-Back:** "I want to be sure I explained why you need to keep the probe on your finger. Tell me why this measurement is important and how moving your finger affects reading." Revise your instruction now or develop a plan for revised patient/family caregiver teaching if patient/family caregiver is not able to teach back correctly.
20. Discuss findings with patient.
21. Clean sensor and device per agency policy and store sensor in appropriate location. Perform hand hygiene.
22. Compare SpO_2 with patient's previous baseline, acceptable SpO_2. Correlate reading with data obtained from respiratory rate, depth, and rhythm assessment (see Skill 5.4).
23. Document SpO_2 on vital sign flow sheet; indicate type and amount of oxygen therapy used by patient during assessment; document any signs or symptoms of alterations in oxygen saturation in narrative nurses' notes.
24. Report abnormal findings to nurse in charge or health care provider.

◆ CLINICAL JUDGMENT AND NEXT-GENERATION NCLEX® EXAMINATION–STYLE QUESTIONS

A 30-year-old patient is admitted from the trauma unit following a motor-cycle-automobile accident. The patient has a fractured left femur and a fractured jaw, which has been wired closed during surgery. The nurse assesses that the patient has a cast on the left leg and an intravenous (IV) line in the right antecubital fossa through which the patient received IV opioids (morphine sulfate 10 mg) in the postanesthesia unit.

1. Which symptom would the nurse report immediately to the health care provider?
   1. Heart rate 64 beats/min
   2. Respirations 8 breaths/min
   3. Blood pressure 110/70 mm Hg
   4. Oxygen saturation 97%

2. Which finding that occurred over 2 hours alerts the nurse to a potential change in cardiac status?
   1. Oxygen saturation decrease from 98% to 96%
   2. Respiratory rate maintained at 14 breaths/min
   3. Heart rate increase from 88 beats/min to 98 beats/min
   4. Blood pressure decrease from 116/76 mm Hg to 98/50 mm Hg over 2 hours

3. The nurse has asked the assistive personnel to take a manual blood pressure to confirm the electronic reading. Which of the following actions by the AP can create a falsely elevated blood pressure? **Select all that apply.**
   1. Deflating the cuff too slowly
   2. Deflating the cuff too quickly
   3. Applying a loose-fitting cuff
   4. Positioning the patient's arm below the level of the heart
   5. Repeating the measurement too quickly

4. The patient later develops a fever. Which additional assessment finding does the nurse anticipate?
   1. Respirations 24 breaths/min
   2. Oxygenation 86%
   3. Heart rate 52 beats/min
   4. Blood pressure 90/60 mm Hg

5. Several days later, the patient is scheduled for discharge. The nurse has provided teaching to the patient and family caregiver.

   For each assessment finding, indicate whether nursing and collaborative interventions were effective or not effective.

Assessment Finding	Effective	Not Effective
Patient and family caregiver verbalize how to prepare nutritionally balanced liquids.		
The patient reports pain in jaw at 6 on a scale of 0 to 10.		
Patient and family caregiver state they will increase ambulation as per home physical therapy recommendations.		
Family caregiver verbalizes how to maintain oral hygiene measures.		

Visit the Evolve site for Answers to the Clinical Judgment and Next-Generation NCLEX® Examination-Style Questions.

REFERENCES

Agency for Healthcare Research and Quality (AHRQ): *Teach-back: intervention,* 2023. https://www.ahrq.gov/patient-safety/reports/engage/interventions/teach-back.html.

American Association of Critical-Care Nurses (AACN): *Obtaining accurate noninvasive blood pressure measurement in adults,* 2017. https://aacnjournals.org/ccnonline/article/36/3/e12/20666/Obtaining-Accurate-Noninvasive-Blood-Pressure. accessed November 5, 2023.

Association of Operating Room Nurses (AORN): Decreasing pathogen transmission from stethoscopes, *AORN J* 116(2):16, 2022.

Ball JW, et al: *Seidel's guide to physical examination,* ed 10 , St. Louis, 2023, Elsevier.

Biswas D, et al: Role of nurses and nurse practitioners in the recognition, diagnosis, and management of neurogenic orthostatic hypotension: a narrative review, *Int J Gen Med* 12:173–184, 2019.

Centers for Disease Control and Prevention (CDC): *What is health literacy,* 2023. https://www.cdc.gov/healthliteracy/learn/index.html.

Dante A, et al: Evaluating the interchangeability of forehead, tympanic, and axillary thermometers in Italian Paediatric Clinical Settings: results of a multicentre observational study, *J Pediatr Nurs* 52:e21, 2020.

Elliott M, Baird J: Pulse oximetry and the enduring neglect of respiratory rate assessment: a commentary on patient surveillance, *Br J Nurs* 28(19):1156.

Erdem N, et al: The comparison and diagnostic accuracy of different types of thermometers. *Turk J Pediatr* 63(3):434, 2021.

Fitzwater J, et al: A comparison of oral, axillary, and temporal artery temperature measuring devices in adult acute care, *Medsurg Nurs* 28(1):35–41, 2019.

Franconi I, et al: Digital axillary and non-contact infrared thermometers for children, *Clin Nurs Res* 27(2):180–190, 2018.

Hale G, et al: Treatment of primary orthostatic hypotension, *Ann Pharmacother* 51:417–428, 2017.

Harry ML, et al: Understanding respiratory rate assessment by emergency nurses: a health care improvement project, *J Emerg Nurs* 20(4):489, 2020.

Hill A, et al: The effects of awareness and count duration on adult respiratory rate measurements: an experimental study, *J Clin Nurs* 27:546–554, 2018.

Hockenberry MJ, et al: *Wong's nursing care of infants and children,* ed 12, St. Louis, 2024, Elsevier.

Kallioinen N, et al: Sources of inaccuracy in the measurement of adult patients' resting blood pressure in clinical settings: a systematic review, *J Hypertens* 35:421–441, 2017. https://www.uptodate.com/contents/mechanisms-causes-and-evaluation-of-orthostatic-hypotension.

Kiekkas P, et al: Temporal artery thermometry in pediatric patients: Systematic review and meta-analysis, *J Pediatr Nurs* 46:89–99, 2019.

Lamberti J: Respiratory monitoring in general care units, *Respir Care* 65(6):870, 2020.

Mahabala C, et al: A novel method for measuring sublingual temperature using conventional non-contact forehead thermometer, *F1000Res* 11:13, 2022.

Marcos PS, et al: Comparative assessment of the effectiveness of three disinfection protocols for reducing bacterial contamination of stethoscopes, *Infec Control Hosp Epidemiol* 41:120, 2019.

Mason T, et al: Equivalence study of two temperature-measurement methods in febrile adult patients with cancer, *Oncol Nurs Forum* 44(2):E82–E87, 2017.

McClelland M, et al: The immediate physiological effects of e-cigarette use and exposure to second-hand e-cigarette vapor. *Respir Care* 66(6):943–950, 2021.

Meyer C, et al: Research: 'One size does not fit all': Perspectives on diversity in community aged care, *Australas J Ageing* 37(4):268, 2018.

Mickley J, et al: Pilot application of varied equipment and procedural techniques to determine clinical blood pressure measurements, *J Diagn Med Sonogr* 34(6):446–457, 2018.

Mogensen CB, et al: Forehead or ear temperature measurement cannot replace rectal measurements, except for screening purposes, *BMC Pediatr* 18(1):15, 2018a. doi:10118/s12887-018-0994-1.

Mogensen CB, Vilhelmsen MB, Jepsen J, et al: Ear measurement of temperature is only useful for screening for fever in an adult emergency department, *BMC Emerg Med* 18(1):51, 2018b.

Muntner P, et al: American Heart Association Scientific Statement: Measurement of Blood Pressure in Humans, *Hypertension* 73:e66, 2019.

Ogunniyi M, et al: Race, ethnicity, hypertension, and heart disease. *J Am Coll Cardiol* 78(24):2460–2470, 2021.

Pagana KD, et al: *Mosby's Diagnostic and laboratory rest reference,* ed 15, St. Louis, 2021, Elsevier.

Peacock WF, et al: A new normal for clinician's third hand: stethoscope hygiene and infection prevention, *Am J Infec Control* 51:114, 2023.

Ringrose JS, et al: The effect of back and feet support on oscillometric blood pressure measurements, *Blood Press Monit* 22(4):213–216, 2017.

Rolfe S: The importance of respiratory rate monitoring, *Br J Nurs* 228(8):504–508, 2019. doi:10.12968/bjon.2019.28.8.504.

Seifi S, et al: Accuracy of pulse oximetry in detection of oxygen saturation in patients admitted to the intensive care unit of heart surgery: comparison of finger, toes, forehead and earlobe probes, *BMC Nurs* 17:15, 2018. doi:10.1186/s12912-018-0283-1.

Sheppard JP: Measurement of blood pressure in the leg: a statement on behalf of the British and Irish Hypertension Society, *J Human Hypertension* 34:418, 2020.

Sims M, et al: Selection of the most accurate thermometer devices for clinical practice, *Pediatr Nurs* 44(3):134-154, 2018.

Stenhouse R: Understanding equality and diversity in nursing practice, *Nurs Stand* 36(2):27, 2021.

Sweeting P, et al: Peripheral thermometry: Agreement between non-touch infrared versus not traditional modes in an adult population, *J Adv Nurs* 78(2):425, 2022.

Takayama A, et al: A comparison of methods to count breathing frequency, *Respir Care* 64(5):555–563, 2019.

The Joint Commission (TJC): *2023 National Patient Safety Goals*, Oakbrook Terrace, IL, 2023, The Joint Commission. https://www.jointcommission.org/standards/national-patient-safety-goals/.

Thomas G, Pohl MA: *Blood pressure measurement in the diagnosis and management of hypertension in adults*, 2022, UpToDate. https://www.uptodate.com/contents/blood-pressure-measurement-in-the-diagnosis-and-management-of-hypertension-in-adults. Accessed November 5, 2023.

Touhy TA, Jett, K: *Ebersole and Hess' Gerontological nursing and healthy aging*, ed 6, St. Louis, 2022, Elsevier.

Wagner M, et al: Comparison of a continuous noninvasive temperature to monitor core temperature measures during targeted temperature management. *Neurocrit Care* 34:449–455, 2021.

Wheatley I: Respiratory rate 3: how to take an accurate measurement, *Nurs Times* 114(7):11–12, 2019.

Whelton PK, et al: Guideline for the prevention, detection, evaluation, and management of high blood pressure in adults: Report of the American College of Cardiology/American Heart Association Task Force on Clinical Practice Guidelines, *Hypertension* 71(6):e13, 2018.

Yek JL, et al: The effects of gel-based manicure on pulse oximetry, *Singapore Med J* 60(8):432–435, 2019.

Zhang X, et al: Evidence-based nursing practice on the influences of different clothing thicknesses on blood pressure measurements of in patient, *Chinese Nurs Res* 33(13):2198–2204, 2019.

SKILLS AND PROCEDURES

Skill 6.1 **General Survey, p. 117**

Skill 6.2 **Head and Neck Assessment, p. 126**

Skill 6.3 **Thorax and Lung Assessment, p. 132**

Skill 6.4 **Cardiovascular Assessment, p. 140**

Skill 6.5 **Abdominal Assessment, p. 151**

Skill 6.6 **Genitalia and Rectum Assessment, p. 157**

Skill 6.7 **Musculoskeletal and Neurological Assessment, p. 162**

Procedural Guideline 6.1 **Monitoring Intake and Output, p. 170**

OBJECTIVES

Mastery of content in this chapter will enable you to:
- Explain the purposes of health assessment.
- Apply the techniques used with each physical assessment skill.
- Summarize the role physical assessment findings play in making clinical judgments about patient problems.
- Apply proper patient positioning during each phase of an examination.
- Discuss how to conduct a physical examination on patients from diverse cultures.
- Examine the approaches you can use to minimize the perception of discrimination that a transgender patient might have during a physical examination.
- Discuss techniques to promote a patient's physical and psychological comfort during an examination.
- Select necessary environmental preparations before an assessment.

- Identify pertinent data to collect from the nursing history before a physical examination.
- Evaluate normal physical findings for patients across the life span.
- Develop creative methods to incorporate health promotion and health teaching into an assessment.
- Explain the self-screening assessments commonly performed by patients.
- Evaluate preventive screenings and the appropriate age(s) for each screening.
- Plan how to perform physical assessment techniques and skills during routine nursing care.
- Explain the documentation of assessment findings on appropriate forms.
- Explain how to interpret abnormal findings when reporting to health care providers.

MEDIA RESOURCES

- http://evolve.elsevier.com/Perry/skills
- Review Questions
- Audio Glossary
- ▶ Video Clips
- Animations

- Case Studies
- Answers to Clinical Judgment and Next-Generation NCLEX® Examination–Style Questions
- Skills Performance Checklists
- Printable Key Points

PURPOSE

Health assessment is the cornerstone for nurses to gather information about patients and to make thoughtful and relevant clinical decisions about care. A health assessment includes a patient history, as well as physical assessment, the objective measurement of anatomical findings through the use of observation, palpation, percussion, and auscultation. Nurses gathering health assessment findings can reflect on scientific knowledge, the known condition of the patient, and the current therapies patients are receiving to make clinical judgments about the patient's health problems. This involves gathering data, recognizing cues, analyzing findings, and grouping significant findings into patterns of data (clusters) that reveal actual or potential nursing diagnoses (Table 6.1). Nurses perform systematic physical assessments regularly in every health care setting. Some are comprehensive, and others are focused and limited. For example, nurses perform a comprehensive assessment at the time a patient is admitted to an acute care unit or when home care services begin. In acute care settings, you perform a brief physical assessment at the beginning of each shift to identify changes in a patient's status for comparison with the previous assessment. In a clinic setting, an initial assessment is often lengthier, followed by shorter, more focused assessments during

TABLE 6.1

Development of an Individualized Nursing Diagnosis

Assessment Method	Findings	Patterns	Nursing Diagnosis
Inspection of skin	Skin along sacral area is intact. There is a 3-cm (1.2-inch) area of redness around coccyx; skin blanches on palpation. No blistering or skin lesions are observed.	There is tissue injury area around coccyx.	Risk for impaired skin integrity
Palpation of skin	Skin is moist from diaphoresis. There is tenderness to palpation at sacral area. Skin turgor is elastic.	Skin moisture promotes maceration.	
Historical data	Patient sustained fractured left leg. Patient is immobilized because of left leg traction.	Continued pressure is exerted over sacrum.	

subsequent visits. The length and depth of an assessment must be person centered, depending on a patient's presenting problem(s) and ongoing assessment findings. The information gathered is documented in the patient's database.

PRACTICE STANDARDS

- American Cancer Society (ACS), 2022: Cancer Facts & Figures
- The Joint Commission (TJC), 2023: National Patient Safety Goals—Patient identification

SUPPLEMENTAL STANDARDS

- Arnett DK et al., 2019: ACC/AHA Guideline on the Primary Prevention of Cardiovascular Disease: A Report of the American College of Cardiology/American Heart Association Task Force on Clinical Practice Guidelines

PRINCIPLES FOR PRACTICE

- An admission assessment involves a detailed review of a patient's condition and includes a nursing history, behavioral assessment, and physical examination.
- Use therapeutic communication techniques including open-ended questions to ensure that patients have exhausted descriptions before moving on in an assessment. For example, as a patient describes a symptom, you can say "Go on" to encourage more information sharing.
- Use critical thinking when applying clinical judgment to interpret and evaluate assessment findings.
- Initial assessment and examination provide a baseline for a patient's functional status and serve as a comparison for future assessment findings. Nurses use the information in making ongoing clinical decisions about the management of a patient's health problems.
- Demonstrate patient safety, comfort, and confidentiality during an examination.

PERSON-CENTERED CARE

- Conduct a patient-centered interview to learn about problems from the patient's perspective. Apply the RESPECT model during the assessment (Fig. 6.1).
- Show respect to patients and families in seeking involvement in planning care.
- The use of physical characteristics (e.g., skin color, shape of face) to distinguish a cultural group or subgroup is not appropriate (Ball et al., 2023). Do not confuse physical characteristics with cultural characteristics.

- When assessing a patient who identifies as transgender, consider throughout the assessment the potential prior negative experiences the patient had within the health care setting, including discrimination and physical or emotional abuse (Iwamato et al., 2021).
- Have patients explain symptoms by allowing details; meet patients on own terms.
- When cultural differences exist, attempt to fully understand what patients mean and know exactly what patients think you mean in words and actions (Ball et al., 2023).
- Be open to constant informing, communicating, and educating patients and family caregivers regarding patient care during an examination.
- Integrate health promotion and education into physical assessment activities. It is an ideal time to offer individualized patient teaching and to encourage promotion of health practices such as male genital self-examination, regular exercise (see Chapter 12), and a healthy diet (see Chapter 30).
- Patients should understand any risk factors and signs and symptoms that are being presented in detecting health problems (e.g., specific types of cancer [ACS, 2022]).
- Ensure that patients are comfortable and free from pain before beginning an examination and during an assessment.
- Communicate respect through proper use of distance, attention, eye contact, tone, and loudness of voice.
- When caring for gender-diverse patients, regularly practice gender-inclusive communication skills such as asking for pronouns and two-part gender identity (identity and sex assigned at birth) (Weingartner et al., 2022).
- Use a professional interpreter familiar with a patient's culture when English is not the patient's primary language.
- Consider only research-based information about health risks common to a cultural group when performing an assessment.
- Use gender-congruent health care providers to perform a physical assessment when possible.
- Ask permission before you touch a patient. Drape a patient thoroughly and use the bedside screen or curtains.

EVIDENCE-BASED PRACTICE

Health Assessment of Transgender and Gender-Diverse Patients

- Transgender and gender-diverse (TGD) patients experience health disparities and bias in health care settings (Weingartner et al., 2022). Research is growing with regard to understanding the health needs of the TGD population. A study conducted in Canada found that transgender individuals were more likely to live in lower-income neighborhoods, experience chronic physical and mental health conditions, and have higher health

The RESPECT Model

What is most important in considering the effectiveness of your cross-cultural communication, whether it is verbal, nonverbal, or written, is that you remain open and maintain a sense of respect for your patients. The RESPECT Model[1] can help you remain effective and patient-centered in all of your communication with patients.

Rapport
- Connect on a social level
- See the patient's point of view
- Consciously suspend judgment
- Recognize and avoid making assumptions

Empathy
- Remember the patient has come to you for help
- Seek out and understand the patient's rationale for his/her behaviors and illness
- Verbally acknowledge and legitimize the patient's feelings

Support
- Ask about and understand the barriers to care and compliance
- Help the patient overcome barriers; Involve family members if appropriate
- Reassure the patient you are and will be available to help

Partnership
- Be flexible
- Negotiate roles when necessary
- Stress that you are working together to address health problems

Explanations
- Check often for understanding
- Use verbal clarification techniques

Cultural competence
- Respect the patient's cultural beliefs
- Understand that the patient's views of you may be defined by ethnic and cultural stereotypes
- Be aware of your own cultural biases and preconceptions
- Know your limitations in addressing health issues across cultures
- Understand your personal style and recognize when it may not be working with a given patient

Trust
- Recognize that self-disclosure may be difficult for some patients; Consciously work to establish trust

Guide to Providing Effective Communication and Language Assistance Services
www.ThinkCulturalHealth.hhs.gov

OMH
U.S. Department of
Health and Human Services
Office of Minority Health

THINK
CULTURAL
HEALTH

FIG. 6.1 The RESPECT model.

service use compared with the general population (Abramovich et al., 2020). Specifically, the study found higher rates of asthma, chronic obstructive pulmonary disease (COPD), diabetes, and HIV and greater rates of mental health comorbidity (Abramovich et al., 2020).

- Assessment tools are being developed to measure a broad range of constructs that are important in understanding the psychological experience of individuals who identify as transgender or gender nonconforming (TGNC). In addition to gender dysphoria (the distress a person feels due to a mismatch between gender identity—the personal sense of gender and the sex assigned at birth), the constructs include impact of discrimination, minority stress, positive aspects of a TGNC identity, and psychosocial aspects of a medical transition (Shulman et al., 2017). Identification and use of nonstigmatizing language will be an ongoing challenge with all assessment tools for TGNC affirmative practice (Shulman et al., 2017).

- Always be culturally sensitive and thus aware that a patient may identify as TGNC.
- When caring for individuals who identify as TGNC, be aware of the high potential for mental health issues and self-harm (Abramovich et al., 2020).
- When conducting a physical examination, use a gender-affirming approach. Affirm gender identity by referring to the person's correct name and pronouns (Iwamato et al., 2021).
- Consider throughout an assessment the patient's prior negative experience with health care, including discrimination and mistreatment (Iwamato et al., 2021).

SAFETY GUIDELINES

- Prioritize an assessment on the basis of a patient's presenting signs and symptoms or health care needs. For example, when a patient develops sudden shortness of breath, first assess the lungs and thorax. If a patient is acutely ill, you may choose to assess only the involved body systems. Use clinical judgment to ensure that an examination is relevant and inclusive.

- Organize an examination. Compare both sides of the body for symmetry. If a patient becomes fatigued, offer rest periods. Perform painful or intrusive procedures near the end of an examination.
- In a comprehensive examination, use a head-to-toe approach following the sequence of inspection, palpation, percussion, and auscultation (except during abdominal assessment).
- Encourage a patient's active participation. Patients usually know about physical conditions and can let you know when certain findings are normal or when there have been changes.
- Follow Standard Precautions and infection control practices. Before assessment, know your patient's medical history to determine if there are specific concerns related to transmission of infectious agents to other patients and health care workers (Siegel et al., 2007, updated 2022). During an assessment you may have contact with body fluids and discharge. Always wear clean gloves when there are breaks in the skin, lesions, or wounds or when having contact with mucous membranes. In some circumstances you will need to wear a gown and face or eye protection.
- Maintain strict hand hygiene practices during examination, when your examination is interrupted, and especially after entry of data on mobile handheld devices (MHDs).
- Ask the patient about a latex allergy. The incidence of serious allergic reaction to latex has increased dramatically, and many supplies used during an assessment may contain latex (Ball et al., 2023).
- Document quick notes to facilitate accurate documentation. Inform a patient that you will be documenting the data.
- Document a summary of the assessment using appropriate medical terminology and in the order gathered. Use commonly accepted medical abbreviations to keep notes concise. Be thorough and descriptive, especially for abnormal findings.

ASSESSMENT TECHNIQUES

Use assessment techniques during each patient contact, including activities such as bathing, administering medications, and providing other therapies. Inspection, palpation, percussion, auscultation, and olfaction are the five basic assessment techniques. Each skill allows you to collect a broad range of physical data about patients. Incorporating assessment techniques into routine care is important. For example, you can use careful inspection while talking with a patient. This practice is an efficient use of time and will help you become more observant and better able to identify changes quickly. Nurses need experience to recognize normal variations among patients and ranges of normal for an individual. Remember, cultural diversity is one factor that influences both normal variations and potential alterations that you may find during an assessment. It is important to take the time needed to carefully assess each body part. Hurrying causes you to overlook significant signs and make incorrect conclusions about a patient's condition.

Inspection

Inspection is the visual examination of body parts or areas. An experienced nurse learns to make multiple observations almost simultaneously while becoming perceptive regarding any abnormalities. The secret is to always be observant. Think about normal findings and what to expect on the basis of a patient's reported condition, and then pay attention to the patient's actual data. For example, as you examine a patient with arthritis who is sitting, watch how the patient moves the lower extremities, consider the normal range of motion (ROM), and then compare with what to expect from arthritic changes. Analysis of your findings will lead to a clinical judgment as to whether there is an alteration. Watch all movements and look carefully at the body part that you are inspecting. It is important to know, recognize, and understand normal physical characteristics of patients of all ages before trying to distinguish abnormal findings.

Inspection requires good lighting and full exposure of body parts. Inspect each area for size, shape, color, symmetry, position, and the presence of abnormalities. If possible, inspect each area compared with the same area on the opposite side of the body. When necessary, use additional light such as a penlight to inspect body cavities such as the mouth and throat. *Do not hurry. Pay attention to detail.* Verify and clarify all abnormalities. If an abnormality is found, question the patient to gather subjective data to determine if this is a recent or long-term condition. Then decide if further information is needed. Let patient data and your knowledge of anatomy, physiology, and pathophysiology guide your inspection.

Palpation

Palpation uses the sense of touch. Through palpation the hands make delicate and sensitive measurements of specific physical signs. It detects resistance, resilience, roughness, texture, temperature, moisture, and mobility. You often use it with or after visual inspection. You will use different parts of the hand to detect specific characteristics. For example, the dorsum (back) of the hand is sensitive to temperature variations. The pads of the fingertips detect subtle changes in texture, shape, size, consistency, and pulsation of body parts. The palm of the hand is especially sensitive to vibration. You measure position, consistency, and turgor by lightly grasping a body part with the fingertips.

Help a patient relax and assume a comfortable position because muscle tension during palpation impairs the ability to detect abnormalities. Asking a patient to take slow, deep breaths enhances muscle relaxation. *Palpate tender areas last* because these could cause a patient to become tense and impede the assessment. Ask a patient to point out areas that are more sensitive and note any nonverbal signs of discomfort. Patients appreciate clean, warm hands; short fingernails; and a gentle approach. Palpation is either light or deep and is controlled by the amount of pressure applied with the fingers or hand. Light palpation precedes deep palpation. Consider a patient's condition, the area being palpated, and the reason for using palpation. For example, when a patient is admitted to the emergency department after an automobile accident, consider the factors surrounding the patient's injury and inspect the chest wall carefully before performing any palpation around the area of the ribs.

For light palpation, apply pressure slowly, gently, and deliberately, depressing approximately 1 cm (½ inch) (Fig. 6.2A). Check tender areas further, using light, intermittent pressure. After light palpation, you may use deeper palpation to examine the condition of organs (Fig. 6.2B). Depress the area that you are examining by approximately 2 cm (0.8 inch). Caution is the rule. Bimanual palpation involves one hand placed over the other while applying pressure. The upper hand exerts downward pressure as the other hand feels the subtle characteristics of underlying organs and masses. Seek the help of a qualified health care provider or nurse before attempting deep palpation.

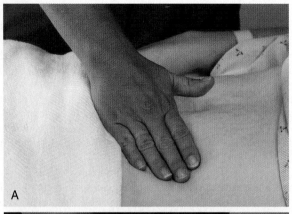

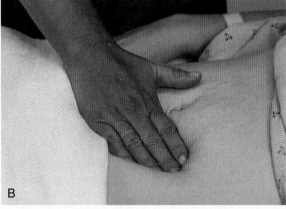

FIG. 6.2 (A) During light palpation, gentle pressure against underlying skin and tissues can be used to detect areas of irregularity and tenderness. (B) During deep palpation, depress tissue to assess condition of underlying organs. (*From Ball JW, et al: Seidel's guide to physical examination, ed 10, St Louis, 2023, Elsevier.*)

Percussion

Percussion involves tapping the body with the fingertips to vibrate underlying tissues and organs. The vibration travels through body tissues, and the character of the resulting sound reflects the density of underlying tissue. The denser the tissue, the quieter the sound. By knowing various densities of organs and body parts, you learn how to locate organs or masses, map their edges, and determine their size. An abnormal sound suggests a mass or substance such as air or fluid in a body cavity. The skill of percussion is used more often by advanced practice nurses (APNs) than by nurses in daily practice at the bedside.

Auscultation

Auscultation is listening with a stethoscope to sounds produced by the body. To auscultate correctly, listen in a quiet environment for both the presence of sound and its characteristics. To be successful in auscultation, you must first recognize normal sounds from each body structure, including the passage of blood through an artery, heart sounds, and movement of air through the lungs. These sounds vary according to the location in which they can be heard most easily. Likewise, you become familiar with areas that normally do not emit sounds. Practice listening to many normal sounds so that you can recognize abnormal sounds when they arise.

To auscultate, you need good hearing acuity, a good stethoscope, and knowledge of how to use the stethoscope properly (Box 6.1). A nurse cannot be successful at auscultation without knowing how to use a stethoscope correctly. Chapter 5 describes the parts of the acoustic stethoscope and use of the bell and diaphragm. Nurses with hearing disorders may purchase stethoscopes with greater sound amplification and may need to ask colleagues to verify some findings through auscultation. It is essential to place the stethoscope directly on a patient's skin because clothing

---

BOX 6.1

Using a Stethoscope

1. Place earpieces in both ears with tips of earpieces turned toward the face. *Lightly* blow against the diaphragm (flat side of chest piece). Now place the earpieces in both ears with the tips turned toward the back of the head and again blow against the diaphragm. Compare comfort in the ears and amplification of sounds with earpieces in both directions. After you have learned the right fit for the loudest amplification, wear the stethoscope the same way each time. Earpieces should fit snugly and comfortably.

2. If the stethoscope has both a diaphragm (flat side) and a bell (bowl shaped with a rubber ring), put earpieces in ears and lightly blow against the diaphragm. The chest piece can be turned to allow sound to be carried through either side (bell or diaphragm). If sound is faint, lightly blow into the bell. Then turn the chest piece and blow again against both the diaphragm and the bell. The diaphragm is used for higher-pitched heart sounds, bowel sounds, and lung sounds. The bell is used for lower-pitched heart sounds and vascular sounds.

3. When earpieces are in place and you are using the diaphragm, move the diaphragm lightly over the hair on your arm. The bristling sound mimics a sound heard in the lungs. When listening for significant sounds, hold the diaphragm still and firmly make a tight seal against the skin to eliminate extraneous sounds.

4. Place the diaphragm over the front of your chest directly on your skin and listen to your own breathing, comparing the bell and the diaphragm. Repeat the process while listening to your own heartbeat. Ask someone to speak in a conversational tone and note how the speech detracts from hearing clearly. When using a stethoscope, both you and the patient should remain quiet.

5. With the earpieces in your ears, gently tap the tubing. Note that it generates extraneous sounds. When listening to a patient, maintain a position that allows the tubing to extend straight and hang free. Movement may allow it to rub or bump objects, creating extraneous sounds. Kinked tubing muffles sounds.

6. *Care of a stethoscope:* Remove earpieces regularly and clean or remove cerumen (earwax). Keep the bell and diaphragm free of dust, lint, and body oils. Keep the tubing away from your body oils. Avoid draping the stethoscope around the neck next to the skin. To clean, wipe the entire stethoscope (e.g., diaphragm, tubing) with alcohol or soapy water. Be sure to dry all parts thoroughly. Follow manufacturer recommendations.

7. *Infection control:* Stethoscopes are the most common of all diagnostic tools used among nurses and are used on multiple patients. They are vectors for bacteria, including those that can cause heath care–associated infections (HAIs) (Knecht et al., 2019). A study by Venkatesan et al. 2019 examined 65 stethoscopes of practitioners and found 50.8% showed bacterial growth (gram-positive organisms). Further research is needed to determine whether stethoscope contamination actually results in infection in patients. However, strict adherence to disinfection practices can minimize cross-contamination and ensure patient safety in a hospital environment (Venkatesan et al., 2019). Follow agency infection control guidelines. Clean a stethoscope (diaphragm/bell) thoroughly with a disinfectant swab (e.g., isopropyl alcohol with or without chlorhexidine, benzalkonium, sodium hypochlorite) before reuse on another patient.

TABLE 6.2

Assessment of Characteristic Odors

Odor	Site or Source	Potential Causes
Alcohol	Oral cavity	Ingestion of alcohol; diabetes mellitus
Ammonia	Urine	Urinary tract infection, renal failure
Body odor	Skin, particularly in areas where body parts rub together (e.g., under arms, beneath breasts, perineal area)	Poor hygiene, excess perspiration (hyperhidrosis), foul-smelling perspiration (bromhidrosis)
	Wound site	Wound abscess; infection
	Vomitus	Abdominal irritation, contaminated food
Feces	Rectal area	Fecal incontinence; fistula
	Vomitus/oral cavity (fecal odor)	Bowel obstruction
Fetid, sweet odor	Tracheostomy or mucus secretions	Infection of bronchial tree (*Pseudomonas* bacteria)
Foul-smelling stools in infants	Stool	Malabsorption syndrome
Halitosis	Oral cavity	Poor dental or oral hygiene, gum disease; sinus infection
Musty odor	Casted body part	Infection inside cast
Stale urine	Skin	Uremic acidosis
Sweet, fruity ketones	Oral cavity	Diabetic acidosis
Sweet, heavy, thick odor	Draining wound	*Pseudomonas* (bacterial) infection

obscures and changes sound. Through auscultation there are four characteristics of sound:
- *Frequency:* Number of sound wave cycles generated per second by a vibrating object. The higher the frequency, the higher the pitch of a sound, and vice versa.
- *Loudness:* Amplitude of a sound wave. Auscultated sounds are described as loud or soft.
- *Quality:* Sounds of similar frequency and loudness from different sources. Terms such as *blowing* or *gurgling* describe quality of sound.
- *Duration:* Length of time that sound vibrations last. Duration of sound is short, medium, or long. Layers of soft tissue dampen the duration of sounds from deep internal organs.

Olfaction

Olfaction uses the sense of smell to detect abnormalities that go unrecognized by any other means. Some alterations in body function and certain bacteria create characteristic odors (Table 6.2).

PREPARATION FOR ASSESSMENT

Preparation of the environment, equipment, and patient facilitates a smooth assessment. Provide patients privacy to promote the comfort and efficiency of an examination. In a health care agency, close the door and pull privacy curtains. In the home, examine the patient in the bedroom. A comfortable environment includes a warm, comfortable temperature; a loose-fitting gown or pajamas for a patient; adequate direct lighting; control of outside noises; and precautions to prevent interruptions by visitors or other health care personnel. If possible, place the bed or examination table at waist level so that you can assess a patient easily. When using an examination table, be cautious and prevent patients from moving in a way that can precipitate falls. After an examination, return a bed to a safe height at the completion of the assessment or assist patient off the examination table and to a chair.

Preparing the Patient

Prepare patients both physically and psychologically for accurate assessments. A tense, anxious patient may have difficulty understanding questions, following directions, or cooperating with your instructions. To prepare a patient:
- Provide and maintain privacy.
- Implement comfort measures (e.g., positioning, hygiene) and provide the opportunity to empty the bowel or bladder (a good time to collect needed specimens).
- Minimize a patient's anxiety and fear by conveying an open, receptive, and professional approach. Using simple terms, thoroughly explain what will be done, what the patient should expect to feel, and how the patient can cooperate. Even if a patient appears unresponsive, it is still important to explain your actions.
- Establish an accepting rapport with transgender patients. When caring for individuals, one recommended approach to begin is to say, "Although I have limited experience caring for gender-diverse persons, it is important to me that you feel safe in my care" (Klein et al., 2018). Identify a patient's chosen gender identity and sex assigned at birth to help identify transgender patients. Use the patient's chosen name and pronoun (Klein et al., 2018).
- Provide access to body parts while draping areas that are not being examined.
- Reduce distractions. Turn down the volume on any music players or television.
- Eliminate drafts, control room temperature, and provide warm blankets.
- Help patients assume positions during assessments so that body parts are accessible and patients stay comfortable (Table 6.3). A patient's ability to assume positions depends on physical strength and limitations. Some positions are uncomfortable or embarrassing; keep a patient in position no longer than is necessary.

TABLE 6.3

Positions for Physical Assessment

Position	Areas Assessed	Rationale	Limitations
Sitting	Head and neck, back, posterior thorax and lungs, anterior thorax and lungs, breasts, axillae, heart, vital signs, upper extremities	Sitting upright provides full expansion of lungs and better visualization of symmetry of upper body parts.	Physically weakened or developmentally disabled patients are sometimes unable to sit. Use supine position with head of bed elevated instead.
Supine	Head and neck, anterior thorax and lungs, breasts, axillae, heart, abdomen, extremities, pulses	This is most normally relaxed position. It provides easy access to pulse sites.	If patient becomes short of breath easily, raise head of bed.
Dorsal recumbent	Head and neck, anterior thorax and lungs, breasts, axillae, heart, abdomen	Position is for abdominal assessment because it promotes relaxation of abdominal muscles.	Patients with painful disorders are more comfortable with knees flexed.
Lithotomy	Female genitalia and genital tract	This position provides maximal exposure of genitalia and facilitates insertion of vaginal speculum.	Lithotomy position is embarrassing and uncomfortable; thus examiner minimizes time that patient spends in it. Keep patient well draped. Patients with arthritis or other joint deformities may be unable to tolerate the position.
Left lateral	Rectum and vagina	Flexion of hip and knee improves exposure of rectal and genitourinary areas.	Joint deformities hinder patient's ability to bend hip and knee.
Prone	Musculoskeletal system	This position is for assessing extension of hip joint, skin, and buttocks.	Patients with cardiac and respiratory difficulties do not tolerate this position well.
Lateral recumbent	Heart	This position aids in detecting murmurs.	Patients with cardiac and respiratory difficulties do not tolerate this position well.
Knee-chest	Rectum	This position provides maximal exposure of rectal area.	This position is embarrassing and uncomfortable. Patients with arthritis or other joint deformities may be unable to assume this position.

- Pace assessment according to an individual's physical and emotional tolerance.
- Use a relaxed tone of voice and facial expressions to put a patient at ease.
- Encourage a patient to ask questions and report discomfort felt during the examination.
- Have a third person of patient's gender in the room during assessment of genitalia. This prevents a patient from accusing you of behaving in an unethical manner.

- At conclusion of an assessment, ask the patient if there are any concerns or questions.

PHYSICAL ASSESSMENT OF VARIOUS AGE-GROUPS

Children and Adolescents

- Routine assessments of children focus on health promotion and illness prevention, particularly for care of well children with

competent parenting and no serious health problems (Hockenberry et al., 2022). Focus on growth and development, sensory screening, dental examination, and behavioral assessment.
- Children who are chronically ill, disabled, in foster care, or foreign-born adopted may require additional assessments because of unique health needs or risks.
- When obtaining histories of infants and children, gather all or part of the information from parents or guardians.
- Parents may think that, as the examiner, you are testing or judging parental behavior. Offer support during examination and do not pass judgment.
- Call children by preferred names and address parents as "Mr. and Mrs. Brown" rather than by first names.
- Open-ended questions often allow parents to share more information and describe more of the child's problems.
- Older children and adolescents respond best when treated as adults and individuals and often can provide details about health history and severity of symptoms.
- The adolescent has a right to confidentiality. After talking with parents about historical information, arrange to be alone with the adolescent to speak privately and perform the examination.

Older Adults

- Do not assume that aging is always accompanied by illness or disability. Older adults can adapt to change and maintain functional independence (Touhy & Jett, 2022).
- A thorough assessment of an older adult provides critical information that can be used to maximize functional status and independence (Touhy & Jett, 2022).

- "Geriatric syndrome" is a term that refers to common health conditions in older adults who do not fit into distinct organ-based disease categories and often have multifactorial causes (Ward & Reuben, 2022). Examples of conditions include cognitive impairment, delirium, incontinence, malnutrition, falls, gait disorders, fatigue, and dizziness. There are formal assessment tools for gathering assessment data and at the same time reducing burden on the clinician; examples include (Ward & Reuben, 2022):
  - Ability to perform functional tasks and need for assistance
  - Fall history
  - Urinary and/or fecal incontinence
  - Pain
  - Sources of social support, particularly family or friends
  - Depressive symptoms
  - Vision or hearing difficulties
  - Whether the patient has specified a durable power of attorney for health care
- Provide adequate space for an examination, particularly if a patient uses a mobility aid.
- Plan the history and examination, considering an older adult's energy level, physical limitations, pace, and adaptability. You may need more than one session to complete the assessment (Touhy & Jett, 2022).
- Measure performance under the most favorable conditions. Take advantage of natural opportunities for assessment (e.g., during bathing, grooming, mealtime) (Touhy & Jett, 2022).
- Sequence an examination to keep position changes to a minimum. Be efficient throughout the examination to limit patient movement.

◆ SKILL 6.1 General Survey

The general survey begins a review of a patient's primary health problems, and it includes assessment of vital signs, height and weight, and consciousness and observation of general behavior and appearance. It provides information about characteristics of an illness and a patient's hygiene, skin condition, body image, emotional state, recent changes in weight, and developmental status. The survey reveals important information about a patient's behavior that influences how you communicate instructions and continue an assessment. Begin by establishing a positive therapeutic relationship built on courtesy, comfort, connection, and confirmation (Ball et al., 2023).

Delegation

The skill of completing the general survey cannot be delegated to assistive personnel (AP). Direct the AP to:
- Measure the patient's height and weight
- Obtain vital signs (VS) (not the initial set, but subsequent measurements if patient is stable)
- Monitor oral intake and urinary output
- Report a patient's subjective signs and symptoms to the nurse

Interprofessional Collaboration

- When assessment findings reveal abnormalities or changes in patient condition, communicate with the appropriate interprofessional team member (e.g., health care provider or physical therapist).

Equipment

- Stethoscope
- Sphygmomanometer and cuff
- Thermometer
- Digital watch or wristwatch with second hand
- Tape measure
- Clean gloves (use nonlatex if necessary)
- Tongue blade
- Appropriate electronic health record (EHR) or documentation form
- Penlight

STEP	RATIONALE
ASSESSMENT	
1. When beginning a physical examination, identify patient using at least two identifiers (e.g., name and birthday or name and medical record number) according to agency policy.	Ensures patient safety. Complies with The Joint Commission standards and improves patient safety (TJC, 2023).

STEP	RATIONALE
2. Check the electronic health record (EHR) for important information (e.g., previous assessment of lung sounds for a patient with a history of chronic obstructive pulmonary disease [COPD]; previous level of patient's abdominal pain) related to the assessment about to be performed. This includes previous vital signs and factors or conditions that may alter those values.	Establishes a baseline of expected information to be found during the physical examination, whether there is a change, and historical data related to the patient.
3. Note if patient has had any acute distress: difficulty breathing, pain, anxiety. If such signs are present, defer general survey until later and focus immediately on affected body system.	Signs establish priorities regarding which part of examination to conduct first.
4. Begin a conversation to assess patient's level of consciousness (LOC) and orientation. Observe the patient closely (Box 6.2).	Dementia and LOC influence ability to cooperate.
5. Connect with patient by using a gender-affirming approach. Identify yourself. Ask how patient would like to be addressed, then use correct name and pronouns. If patient is transgender, identify chosen gender identity and sex assigned at birth (Klein et al., 2018). Welcome others accompanying patient and ask about connections to patient (Ball et al., 2023).	Ensures a patient-centered approach. The introduction offers an opportunity to establish a partnership with patient and family.
6. Assess patient's/family caregiver's health literacy. If you identify need for an interpreter, determine availability of a professional interpreter. It is best to have an interpreter of the same gender who is older and mature. Have interpreter translate verbatim if possible.	Determines degree to which individuals have the ability to find, understand, and use information and services to make informed health-related decisions and actions (CDC, 2023b).
7. After reviewing medical history, confirm the primary reason for seeking health care with the patient (Ball et al., 2023): • "What would you like for us to do today?" • "What do you think is causing your symptoms?" Allow patient to tell personal story.	Keeps assessment focused on patient to ensure that perceived problems and expectations are addressed.
8. Identify patient's normal height, weight, and body mass index (BMI). If sudden gain or loss in weight has occurred, determine amount of weight change and period of time in which it occurred. Assess if patient is on a special diet or has recently been dieting for weight loss or following an exercise program. Use growth chart for children younger than 18 years.	The BMI is the most common method to assess nutritional status and total body fat (Ball et al., 2023). Healthy BMI is 18.5 to 24.9 (Ball et al, 2023). Most electronic health records (EHRs) calculate BMI automatically once height and weight are entered. Fluid retention is one factor that must be ruled out. A person's weight can fluctuate daily because of fluid loss or retention (1 L of water weighs 1 kg [2.2 pounds]).
9. Ask if patient has noticed any changes in condition of skin (e.g., dryness, changes in color or lack of pigment, changes in moles or new skin lesions).	Skin changes can indicate underlying illnesses (e.g., dry skin may be associated with hypothyroidism, changes in moles may indicate early signs of skin cancers) (Table 6.4).
10. Review patient's past fluid intake and output (I&O) records. Intake includes all liquids taken orally, by feeding tube, and parenterally. Liquid output includes urine, diarrhea stool, vomitus, drainage from fistulas and gastric suction, and drainage from postsurgical drainage tubes (see Chapter 38).	Fluid and electrolyte balance affects health and function in all body systems.

BOX 6.2

Characteristics of Dementia

Cognition
• Memory impaired: trouble recalling recent conversations, events, and appointments

Speech/Language
• Struggles to find words
• Conversation possibly incoherent

Activity
• Unchanged from usual behavior
• Difficulty performing tasks that require many steps

Mood and Affect
• Depressed
• Apathetic
• Uninterested

Delusions/Hallucinations
• Can be some delusions
• No hallucinations

Adapted from Ball JW, et al: *Seidel's guide to physical examination*, ed 10, St Louis, 2023, Elsevier.

STEP			RATIONALE

TABLE 6.4

Skin Color Variations

Color	Condition	Cause	Assessment Location
Bluish (cyanosis)	Increased amount of deoxygenated hemo-globin (associated with hypoxia and is a late sign of decreased oxygen levels)	Heart or lung disease, cold environment	Nail beds, lips, base of tongue, skin (severe cases)
Pallor (decrease in color)	Reduced amount of oxyhemoglobin	Anemia Shock	Face, conjunctivae, nail beds, palms of hands
	Reduced visibility of oxyhemoglobin resulting from decreased blood flow		Skin, nail beds, conjunctivae, lips
Loss of pigmentation	Vitiligo	Congenital autoimmune condition causing lack of pigment	Patchy areas on skin over face, hands, arms
Yellow-orange (jaundice)	Increased deposit of bilirubin in tissues	Liver disease, destruction of red blood cells	Sclerae, mucous membranes, skin
Red (erythema)	Increased visibility of oxyhemoglobin caused by dilation or increased blood flow	Fever, direct trauma, blushing, alcohol intake	Face; area of trauma; and areas at risk for pressure such as sacrum, shoulders, elbows, and heels
Tan-brown	Increased amount of melanin	Suntan, pregnancy	Areas exposed to sun: face, arms; areolae, nipples

11. Identify patient's general perceptions about personal health. Example: "How would you describe your general health compared with others your own age?" "What is your understanding of your diagnosis? The need for treatment?"

Patients may express strong emotions, setting the tone of the assessment interview and influencing the continued conversation and your plan for patient education later.

Clinical Judgment *During the assessment, look at the patient, not the computer screen of EHR. If you feel the need to use the device, do not let it distract you from assessment.*

12. Determine patient's history of any allergies or allergic reactions to latex, food, medications, or liquid topical preparations for the skin. Assess patient for risk factors for developing latex allergies (e.g., has high latex exposure [housekeeper, food handler, health care worker]; must avoid products containing latex [rubber bands, adhesive tape, certain paints or carpets]) and for food allergies such as nuts, shellfish, papaya, avocado, banana, peach, kiwi, or tomato.

Gloves are worn during certain aspects of the assessment. Repeated exposure to latex may result in the patient having more serious reactions, including asthma, itching, and anaphylaxis (Ball et al., 2023). Sensitivity to topical applications is common. Identification of food allergies ensures proper diet selection and avoidance of products containing food allergens, such as peanuts. Prior history of allergic reaction to medications usually leads to contraindication of medication.

13. Assess patient's knowledge, prior experience with physical assessment, and feelings about assessment and personal goals.

Reveals need for patient instruction and/or support. Transgender patients may experience discomfort during the physical examination because of negative past experiences (Klein et al., 2018).

PLANNING

1. Expected outcomes following completion of procedure:
   - Patient demonstrates alert, cooperative behavior without evidence of physical or emotional distress during assessment.
   - Patient provides appropriate subjective data related to physical condition.

Use calm and confident approach during assessment. Patient has no abnormal findings.

Patient is able to cooperate with assessment and communicate clearly.

2. Prepare patient by explaining that you will be doing a routine examination to check for areas of concern. Ask patient to tell you if any area that you examine hurts when touched.

Understanding promotes patient's cooperation. Pain is an important finding during assessment.

3. Anticipate topics that you can teach patient during this examination, including signs and symptoms of skin cancer and patient's identified fall risks.

Enables you to incorporate teaching during the examination.

4. Perform hand hygiene. Assemble necessary equipment and supplies at bedside.

Reduces transmission of infection. Promotes efficiency of examination.

5. Close room doors and/or bedside curtain.

Provides patient privacy.

6. Position patient initially, either sitting or lying supine with head of bed elevated.

Position makes it easy to examine patient.

7. Ensure patient that the assessment is routine and confidential.

Establishes trust with patient.

STEP	RATIONALE

IMPLEMENTATION

1. Perform hand hygiene. Throughout assessment, be observant and note patient's verbal and nonverbal behaviors.

2. Obtain temperature, pulse, respirations, and blood pressure unless taken within past 3 hours or if serious potential change is noted (e.g., change in LOC or difficulty breathing) (see Chapter 5). Inform patient of vital signs.

3. Ask to identify age.

4. If uncertain whether patient understands a question, rephrase or ask a similar question.

5. If patient's responses are inappropriate, ask short, to-the-point questions regarding information patient should know (e.g., "Tell me your name." "What is the name of this place?" "Tell me where you live." "What day is this?" "What month is this?" or "What season of the year is this?").

6. If patient is unable to respond to questions of orientation, offer simple commands (e.g., "Squeeze my fingers" or "Move your toes").

7. Assess affect and mood. Note if verbal expressions match nonverbal behavior and if appropriate to situation.

8. Watch patient interact with spouse or partner, older-adult, child, or family caregiver if possible. Be alert for indications of fear, hesitancy to report health status, or willingness to let someone else control assessment interview. Does partner or family caregiver have a history of violence, alcoholism, or drug abuse? Is person unemployed, ill, or frustrated with caring for a patient? Note if patient has any obvious physical injuries.

RATIONALE

Reduces transmission of infection. Behaviors may reflect specific physical abnormalities, allowing you to focus examination.

VS provide important information regarding physiological changes related to oxygenation and circulation.

Different physical characteristics and predisposition to certain illnesses are related to age.

Inappropriate response from a patient may be caused by language barriers or deterioration of mental status, preoccupation with illness, or decreased hearing acuity.

Measures patient's orientation to person, place, and time. Document exactly what the patient is oriented to. If disoriented in any way, include subjective and/or objective data rather than just documenting "disoriented."

LOC exists along a continuum ranging from full responsiveness to inability to consciously initiate meaningful behaviors to unresponsiveness to stimuli.

Reflects patient's mental and emotional status, consciousness, and feelings.

Suspect abuse in patients with obvious physical injury or neglect, who show signs of malnutrition, or who have ecchymosis (bruises) on extremities or trunk. Health care providers are often the first to identify evidence of abuse because patients may not be able to tell family or friends. Partners or caregivers may have history of abusive or addictive behaviors.

Clinical Judgment *Be discreet in how you conduct the interview. Ask direct questions about abuse in private. It is often necessary to delay this part of the assessment to a later time when the partner or caregiver is not present. Asking a partner or caregiver to leave during an assessment creates an awkward situation, but inquiring about possible abuse in front of an abuser puts a patient at risk for further abuse. Patients are more likely to reveal any problems when the suspected abuser is absent from the room.*

Clinical Judgment *In the case of transgender patients, consider routine screening for depression, anxiety, posttraumatic stress disorder, eating disorders, substance use, intimate partner violence, self-injury, bullying, truancy, homelessness, high-risk sexual behaviors, and suicidality (Klein et al., 2018). However, it is important to avoid assumptions that any concerns are secondary to being transgender.*

9. Observe for signs of abuse:
   a. *Child:* Unexplained burns, bites, bruises, broken bones, or black eyes. Also shows sudden changes in behavior or school performance; has not received help for physical or medical problems brought to the parents' attention; has learning problems not attributed to specific physical or psychological causes; physical injury inconsistent with parent's or caregiver's account of how injury occurred; lacks adult supervision.

   Blood on underclothing, pain in genital area, difficulty sitting or walking, pain on urination, vaginal or penile discharge, itching or unusual color in genital area.

Signals presence of child abuse or neglect (Johns Hopkins, 2022).

Indicates possible child sexual abuse (Ball et al., 2023; Hockenberry et al., 2022).

Clinical Judgment *If you suspect abuse, there is a validated brief Partner Violence Screen (PVS) for adults (Ball et al., 2023). Ask these questions: "Have you been hit, kicked, punched, or otherwise hurt by someone in the past year? Do you feel safe in your current relationship? Is there a partner from a previous relationship who is making you feel unsafe now? Assess safety: What are alternative living options? Who are alternative caregivers? What can be done to prevent future abuse? A pattern of findings indicating abuse usually mandates a report to a social service center (refer to state guidelines). Obtain immediate consultation with health care provider, social worker, and other support staff.*

   b. *Female, transgender woman:* Findings may reveal injury or trauma inconsistent with reported cause or obvious injuries to head, face, neck, breasts, abdomen, and genitalia (e.g., black eyes, abrasions, bruises/welts, broken nose, lacerations, broken teeth, strangulation marks, burns, human bites).

Suggests intimate partner violence (Ball et al., 2023). These signs also apply to male patient being abused by female partner.

STEP	RATIONALE

Clinical Judgment *Injuries from abuse are often located in areas under clothing and are not easily visible. Frequently a victim of abuse will wear clothing such as a turtleneck or long-sleeved shirt to hide bruises and other signs of abuse.*

    c. *Older adult:* Injury or trauma inconsistent with reported cause, injuries in unusual locations (e.g., neck or genitalia), pattern injuries (left when an object with which a person is struck leaves an imprint), parallel injuries (e.g., bilateral ecchymosis on upper arms, suggesting that patient was held and shaken), burns (shaped like cigarette, iron, rope), fractures, poor hygiene, and poor nutrition.

Indicates elder abuse/neglect (Ball et al., 2023; Touhy & Jett, 2022). Prolonged interval between injury and time patient sought medical care also indicates older-adult abuse or neglect. Risk of elder abuse is greater if the adult has had a history of mental illness, dementia, or living in a dependent situation (Ball et al., 2023).

10. Assess posture and position, noting alignment of shoulders and hips while patient stands and/or sits (bed or chair). Observe whether patient is slumped, is erect, or has bent posture (see illustration).

Reveals musculoskeletal problem, mood, or presence of pain.

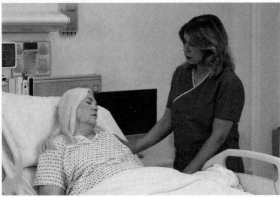

STEP 10 Observe patient's position and posture.

11. Assess body movements. Are they purposeful? Are there tremors of extremities? Are any body parts immobile? Are movements coordinated or uncoordinated?

May indicate neurological or muscular problem or emotional stress. See Skill 6.7 for more detailed musculoskeletal assessment.

12. Assess pattern of speech. Is it understandable and moderately paced? Is there association with patient's thoughts?

Alterations reflect neurological impairment, injury or impairment of mouth, improperly fitting dentures, differences in dialect or language, and some mental illnesses.

13. Observe hygiene and grooming for presence or absence of makeup, type of clothes (hospital or personal), and cleanliness. Hair, teeth, and nails are good places to assess for hygiene status.

Grooming may reflect activity level before examination, resources available to purchase grooming supplies, patient's mood, and self-care practices. It may also reflect culture, lifestyle, economic status, and personal preferences.

    a. Observe color, distribution, quantity, thickness, texture, and lubrication of hair.

Changes in hair may reflect hormonal changes, changes from aging, poor nutrition, or use of certain hair-care products.

    b. Inspect condition of nails (hands and feet). Note color, length, symmetry, cleanliness, and shape. Nails are normally transparent, smooth, and well rounded, with smooth, intact cuticle.

Changes indicate inadequate nutrition or grooming practices, nervous habits, or systemic diseases.

    c. Assess presence or absence of body odor.

Body odor may result from physical exercise, deficient hygiene, or physical or mental abnormalities. Inadequate oral hygiene or unhealthy teeth cause bad breath.

14. Inspect exposed areas of skin and ask if patient has noted any changes, including:

Patient is best source for skin changes. Determines presence of abnormalities and possible cancerous lesions.

Clinical Judgment *During inspection of the skin over body parts, note that transgender women may have breast development, feminine fat redistribution, reduced muscle mass, thin or absent body hair, softened and thinner skin, and testicles that have decreased in size or completely retract (Iwamato et al., 2021; Schneider & Chung, 2022). Transgender men may have facial and body hair growth, an enlarged clitoris, increased muscle mass, masculine fat redistribution, alopecia, and acne (Schneider & Chung, 2022).*

    a. Pruritus, oozing, bleeding

Itching could result from dry skin. Oozing could indicate infection, and bleeding may indicate a blood disorder.

STEP	RATIONALE

BOX 6.3

Malignant Melanoma Mnemonics: The ABCDE Rule of Melanoma

Here is a simple way to remember the characteristics that should alert you to the possibility of malignant melanoma.
A. *Asymmetry of lesion:* One half of spot does not match the other.
B. *Borders:* Irregular (ragged, notched, or blurred).
C. *Color:* The color is not the same all over, such as shades of brown or black, sometimes with patches of white, red, or blue.
D. *Diameter:* Usually greater than 6 mm, about the size of a pencil eraser. **NOTE:** These areas can be smaller at time of diagnosis.
E. *Evolving:* Changes noticed in existing lesions, especially if they are asymmetric.

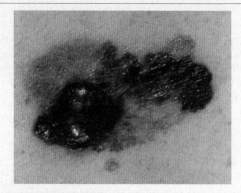

Data from American Academy of Dermatology Association, 2022. https://www.aad.org/public/diseases/skin-cancer/types/common/melanoma/symptoms. Accessed November 17, 2023.
Data and image from Ball JW, et al: *Seidel's guide to physical examination,* ed 10, St Louis, 2023, Elsevier.

---

b. Appearance of any spot, mole, bump, or nodule that does not look like others on the skin or has not healed. Look for: • A new, expanding, or changing growth • A sore that bleeds and/or does not heal after several weeks • A rough or scaly red patch, which might crust or bleed • Color that spreads from the border of a spot into surrounding skin • A mole (or other spot on the skin) that's new or changing in size/shape, oozing, scaly, or bleeding; redness extends beyond border of mole • A mole with an odd shape, irregular borders, or areas of different colors	These are key indicators that a lesion may be cancerous (ACS, 2020). Melanoma is an aggressive form of skin cancer; detection and prompt treatment are critical (Box 6.3).
c. Petechiae (pinpoint-size red or purple spots on skin caused by small hemorrhages in skin layers)	Petechiae may indicate serious blood clotting disorder, drug reaction, or liver disease.
15. Inspect skin surfaces. Compare color of symmetrical body parts, including areas unexposed to sun. Look for any patches or areas of skin color variation.	Changes in color can indicate pathological alterations (see Table 6.4). However, although color should assume an overall uniformity, there is often pigment variation that is sun related, trauma induced, or normal (Ball et al., 2023)

Clinical Judgment *Be alert for basal cell carcinomas: open sore that does not heal; flat, firm, pale or yellow areas, similar to a scar; raised reddish patches that might be itchy; small translucent, shiny, pearly bumps that are pink or red and which might have blue, brown, or black areas (ACS, 2020).*

16. Carefully inspect color of face, oral mucosa, lips, conjunctiva, sclera, palms of hands, and nail beds.	Abnormalities are easier to identify in areas of body where melanin production is lowest.

Clinical Judgment *When assessing the skin of a patient with bandages, cast, restraints, or other restrictive devices, note report of pain or tingling and areas of pallor, decreased temperature, decreased movement, and impaired sensation, which may indicate impaired circulation. Immediate release of pressure from the restrictive device may be necessary.*

Clinical Judgment *When assessing the skin of a patient who is exposed to medical adhesives (e.g., bandages, artificial airway stabilizers, catheter stabilization devices), observe for skin erythema, blistering, or tears. This is medical adhesive–related skin injury (MARSI) and can cause further skin injury and infection (Fumarola et al., 2020).*

17. Use ungloved fingertips to palpate skin surfaces to feel texture and moisture of intact skin. Make sure your hands are warm.	Changes in texture may be first indication of skin rashes in dark-skinned patients. Hydration, body temperature, and environment may affect skin. Older adults are prone to xerosis, presenting as dry, scaly skin (Touhy & Jett, 2022).
a. Stroke skin surfaces lightly with fingertips to detect texture of surface of skin. Note whether skin is smooth or rough, thick or thin, or tight or supple and if localized areas of hardness or lesions are present.	Localized texture changes result from trauma, surgical wounds, or lesions.

STEP	RATIONALE
b. Palpate any areas that appear irregular in texture.	Allows detection of localized areas of hardness and/or tenderness within subcutaneous skin layers.
c. Using dorsum (back) of hand, palpate for temperature of skin surfaces. Compare symmetrical body parts. Compare upper and lower body parts. Note distinct temperature difference and localized areas of warmth.	Skin on dorsum of hand is thin, which allows detection of subtle temperature changes. Cool skin temperature often indicates decreased blood flow. A stage 1 pressure injury may cause warmth and erythema (redness) of an area. Environmental temperature and anxiety may also affect skin temperature.

Clinical Judgment *In patients who receive routine injections (e.g., insulin, heparin), localized areas of hardness may be palpated over injection sites. Develop a plan to rotate injection sites systematically. Site rotation prevents local skin changes from repeated injections (Harding et al., 2021).*

18. Apply clean gloves. Inspect character of any body secretions; note color, odor, amount, and consistency (e.g., thin and watery, thick and oily). Remove gloves. Perform hand hygiene.	Description of secretions helps to indicate type of lesion, presence of infection, or if an existing wound is healing.
19. Assess skin turgor by grasping fold of skin on sternum, forearm, or abdomen with fingertips. Release skinfold and note ease and speed with which skin returns to place (see illustration).	With reduced turgor, skin remains suspended or "tented" for a few seconds before slowly returning to place, indicating decreased elasticity and possible dehydration. With altered turgor, provide measures for prevention of pressure injuries (see Chapter 39).

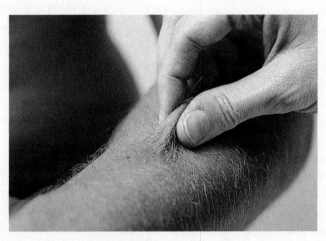

STEP 19 Checking skin turgor.

20. Assess condition of skin for pressure areas, paying particular attention to regions at risk for pressure (e.g., sacrum, greater trochanter, heels, occipital area, clavicles). If you see areas of redness, place fingertip over area, apply gentle pressure, and release. Look at skin color (EPUAP, NPIAP, PPPIA, 2019).	Normal reactive hyperemia (redness) is the visible effect of localized vasodilation, the normal response of the body to lack of blood flow to underlying tissue. Affected area of skin normally blanches with fingertip pressure. If area does not blanch, suspect tissue injury (EPUAP, NPIAP, PPPIA, 2019).

Clinical Judgment *When assessing darkly pigmented skin, visual inspection techniques to identify skin problems are ineffective. Skin inspection techniques for individuals with darkly pigmented skin must include assessment of temperature, edema, and changes in tissue consistency as compared with an adjacent or opposite area of the body (EPUAP, NPIAP, PPPIA, 2019).*

Clinical Judgment *With evidence of normal reactive hyperemia, reposition patient and develop a turning schedule if patient is dependent.*

21. When you detect a lesion, use adequate lighting to inspect color, location, texture, size, shape, and type (Box 6.4). Also note grouping (e.g., clustered or linear) and distribution (e.g., localized or generalized).	Observation of skin lesions allows for accurate description and identification.
a. Apply clean gloves if lesion is moist or draining. Gently palpate any lesion to determine mobility, contour (e.g., flat, raised, or depressed), and consistency (e.g., soft or hard).	Gentle palpation prevents rupture of underlying cysts. Gloves reduce transmission of microorganisms.
b. Note if patient reports tenderness with or without palpation.	Tenderness may indicate inflammation or pressure on body part.
c. Measure size of lesion (height, width, depth) with centimeter ruler.	Provides for baseline to assess changes in lesion over time.

STEP	RATIONALE

BOX 6.4

Types of Skin Lesions

Macule: Flat, nonpalpable change in skin color; smaller than 1 cm (0.4 inch) (e.g., freckle, petechia)

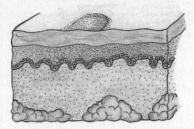

Vesicle: Circumscribed elevation of skin filled with serous fluid; smaller than 0.5 cm (0.2 inch) (e.g., herpes simplex, chickenpox)

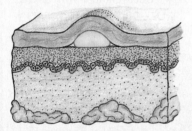

Papule: Palpable, circumscribed, solid elevation in skin; smaller than 0.5 cm (0.2 inch) (e.g., elevated nevus)

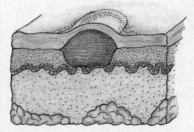

Pustule: Circumscribed elevation of skin similar to vesicle but filled with pus; varies in size (e.g., acne, staphylococcal infection)

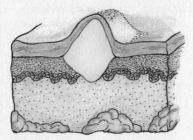

Nodule: Elevated solid mass, deeper and firmer than papule; 0.5–2 cm (0.2–0.8 inch) (e.g., wart)

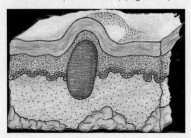

Ulcer: Deep loss of skin surface that may extend to dermis and frequently bleeds and scars; varies in size (e.g., venous stasis ulcer)

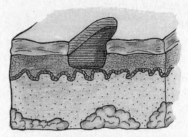

Tumor: Solid mass that may extend deep through subcutaneous tissue; larger than 1–2 cm (0.4–0.8 inch) (e.g., epithelioma)

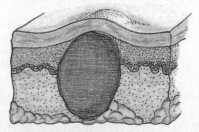

Atrophy: Thinning of skin with loss of normal skin furrow, with skin appearing shiny and translucent; varies in size (e.g., arterial insufficiency)

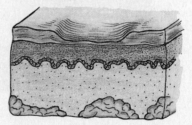

Wheal: Irregularly shaped, elevated area or superficial localized edema; varies in size (e.g., hive, mosquito bite)

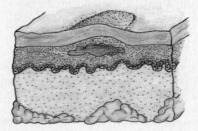

STEP	RATIONALE
22. If a patient has any type of medical device using adhesive, assess for patient's age, presence of dry skin, dehydration, malnutrition, certain medications (e.g., long-term use of corticosteroids, chemotherapeutic agents, antiinflammatory agents), dermatological conditions, radiation therapy, and medical conditions (e.g., diabetes, infection, immunosuppression, edema). Inspect skin around areas where adhesive was applied.	Risk factors for developing medical adhesive–related skin injury MARSI (Fumarola et al., 2020). There are three main categories of medical adhesive-related skin injury: mechanical (skin stripping, blistering, skin tears), dermatitis (irritation in response to the adhesive), and other (maceration and folliculitis) (Fumarola et al., 2020).
23. Remove gloves. Discard used supplies and gloves in proper receptacle. Proceed to next examination (Skill 6.2) or help patient to comfortable position. Perform hand hygiene.	Prevents transmission of infection.
24. Place nurse call system in an accessible location within patient's reach.	Ensures patient can call for assistance if needed.
25. Raise side rails (as appropriate) and lower bed to lowest position, locking into position.	Ensures patient safety and prevents falls.

EVALUATION

1. Observe throughout assessment for evidence of physical or emotional distress, which may alter assessment data.	Interaction during assessment reveals emotional problems. Maneuvers used during physical examination reveal presence of physical problems.
2. Compare assessment findings with normal characteristics.	Determines if problem is present or if change from general survey or any previous observations has occurred.
3. Ask patient if there is information about physical condition that you have not discussed.	Some patients think that it bothers you by asking questions unless an opportunity for questions is provided.
4. **Use Teach-Back:** State to patient, "I want to be sure I explained everything about the bleeding mole I found on your back. Tell me why it is important to see a dermatologist." Revise your instruction now or develop a plan for revised patient/family caregiver teaching if patient/ family caregiver is not able to teach back correctly.	Teach-back is a technique for health care providers to ensure that medical information has been explained clearly so that patients and their families understand what is communicated (AHRQ, 2023).

Unexpected Outcomes	Related Interventions
1. Patient demonstrates acute distress (e.g., shortness of breath, acute pain, severe anxiety)	• Respond immediately to identified need (e.g., repositioning, providing oxygen or medication as ordered). • Obtain vital signs. • Notify health care provider.
2. Patient has abnormal skin condition (e.g., change in color of a mole, dry texture, reduced turgor, lesions, or erythema).	• Identify contributing factors and prevent continued irritation or damage as appropriate. • Notify health care provider if cancerous lesion or healing problem is expected.
3. Patient is unwilling or unable to provide adequate information relating to identified concerns.	• Seek information from family caregivers if present. • Review patient's EHR for baseline data.

Documentation

- Document assessment findings and patient's VS.
- Describe alterations in patient's general appearance and patient's behaviors using objective terminology. Include patient's self-report of signs and symptoms.
- Document your evaluation of patient and family caregiver learning.

Hand-Off Reporting

- Report abnormalities and acute symptoms to nurse in charge or health care provider.

Special Considerations

Patient Education

- Explain to patient any findings that need further examination.

- During general survey, inform patient about normal range of VS for age and physical condition and normal weight for height and body frame.
- If patient is on a therapeutic diet, discuss any problems that involve preparing a diet or selecting food. The best form of weight reduction is to achieve gradual weight loss by increasing exercise and decreasing caloric intake. Refer to clinical dietitian for specific information.
- Teach patient how to do a skin self-examination (ACS, 2020):
  - The best time to do a skin self-examination is after a bath or shower. Check any moles, blemishes, or birthmarks from the top of your head to your toes. If you look at your skin regularly, you will know what's normal for you.
  - Face the mirror:
    - Check your face, ears, neck, chest, and belly. Women will need to lift their breasts to check the skin underneath.

- Check your underarm areas, both sides of your arms, the tops and palms of your hands, in between your fingers, and under your fingernails.
- Sit down:
  - Check the front of your thighs, shins, tops of your feet, in between your toes, and under your toenails.
  - Now use a hand mirror to look at the bottoms of your feet, your calves, and the backs of your thighs, first checking one leg and then the other.
- Stand up:
  - Use the hand mirror to check your buttocks, genital area, lower and upper back, and the back of your neck and ears. Or it may be easier to look at your back in the wall mirror using a hand mirror.
  - Use a comb or hair dryer to part your hair so that you can check your scalp.

Pediatrics

- Measurement of physical growth is a key element in evaluation of a child's health status. These physical growth parameters include height, length, weight, skinfold thickness, and arm and head circumference (Hockenberry et al., 2022). Use growth charts specific to child's age and condition.
- Weigh infants nude. Weigh children in light underclothes or gown.
- A child's interactions with parents offers valuable information regarding the child's behavior.

Older Adults

- An older adult's presenting signs and symptoms are often deceiving. An older adult has a diminished physiological reserve that sometimes masks the usual, or "classic," signs and symptoms of a disease. Signs and symptoms are often blunted or atypical (Touhy & Jett, 2022).

- Common skin changes with aging include generalized chronic itching, skin appears more transparent, flaking or scaling over extremities, skin appears to hang loosely on body frame, and tenting of skin when testing for turgor (Ball et al., 2023).
- Inspection of the feet is critically important in the presence of impaired circulation, impaired vision, and diabetes mellitus. Common foot conditions include ulceration, fungal infection, corns, calluses, bunions, plantar warts, and hammertoe.

Populations With Disabilities

- Determine if patient with a hearing, vision, or speech impairment needs a communication device to interact with you during an examination. Speak directly to a patient who has the capacity (Ball et al., 2023).
- An examination will take more time with patients who have intellectual or developmental disabilities (IDDs). Health checks require a proactive approach, including inviting adults with IDD for regular reviews and follow-up. This can reduce barriers to primary care appointments caused, for example, by lack of health literacy or by poverty. Scheduling extra time and planning to spread the tasks of a comprehensive review among other caregivers and over multiple appointments helps avoid the risk that encounters will deal only with current symptoms (Casson et al., 2018).
- Demonstrate a physical technique before using with patients who are nonverbal.

Home Care

- In the home the focus may be on the patient's ability to perform basic self-care tasks and whether complications have developed. The home assessment builds on all health concerns identified in health care settings.
- Use the same small portable scale provided by health agency to monitor weight changes.

◆ SKILL 6.2　Head and Neck Assessment

Examination of the head and neck includes assessment of the head, eyes, ears, nose, mouth, and sinuses. Assessment uses inspection, palpation, and auscultation, with inspection and palpation often used simultaneously. This assessment is especially important when a patient has had any form of head trauma. Common symptoms presented by patients with possible head and neck problems include headache and stiff neck (Ball et al., 2023).

Delegation

The skill of assessing the head and neck cannot be delegated to assistive personnel (AP). Direct the AP to:
- Observe/report any nasal discharge and nasal bleeding, headache or neck pain, and visual changes found during routine care (e.g., oral care, bathing) to the nurse for further assessment

Interprofessional Collaboration

- When assessment reveals abnormal findings or specific pathophysiological changes, communicate with the appropriate interprofessional team member available (e.g., health care provider or audiologist).

Equipment

- Stethoscope
- Clean gloves (use nonlatex if necessary)
- Tongue blade
- Penlight

STEP	RATIONALE

ASSESSMENT

1. When beginning an examination with the head and neck, identify patient and determine patient's level of consciousness (LOC), primary language, and literacy level as outlined in Skill 6.1, Assessment, Steps 1, 4, 5, and 6. Otherwise, these assessments need not be repeated.

Complies with The Joint Commission standards and improves patient safety (TJC, 2023).

STEP	RATIONALE
2. Check the EHR for history of any conditions (e.g., history of head trauma, radiation around head and neck, seizure disorder, blurred vision) that have implications for the assessment to be performed.	Establishes a baseline of expected findings to be found during the physical examination and the areas in which to focus the examination.
3. Review EHR for history of sexually transmitted disease, especially human papilloma virus (HPV).	History of HPV increases risk for mouth and oropharyngeal cancer (ACS, 2022).
4. Ask patient about history of headache, dizziness, neck pain, or stiffness in head or neck. Ask patient if there is history of difficulty moving neck.	Headaches and dizziness are signs of concussion and stress, symptoms of another underlying problem such as high blood pressure or a result of injury. Difficulty moving neck may indicate muscle strain, head injury, local nerve injury, or swollen lymph nodes.
5. Determine if patient has history of eye disease, diabetes mellitus, or hypertension.	Predispose patients to visual alterations requiring health care provider referral.
6. Ask if patient has had blurred vision, flashing lights, halos around lights, or reduced visual field.	These common symptoms indicate visual problems.
7. Ask if patient has had ear pain, itching, discharge, vertigo, tinnitus (ringing in the ears), or change in hearing. Does the patient use a personal audio device or system?	These signs and symptoms indicate infection or hearing loss. Personal audio systems are often listened to at unsafe volumes and for prolonged periods of time. Regular participation in such activities poses the serious threat of irreversible hearing loss (WHO, 2019a).
8. Review patient's occupational history.	Patient's occupation can create a risk of eye or ear injury—for example, computer work (potential for eye fatigue), working with chemicals (risk of splash injury to eye), or prolonged noise exposure (deafness).
9. Ask if patient has history of seasonal allergies, nasal discharge, epistaxis (nosebleeds), or postnasal drip.	History is useful in determining source of nasal and sinus drainage.
10. Assess if patient smokes or chews tobacco.	Risk factors for oropharyngeal cancer include any form of tobacco use and alcohol consumption, with a 30-fold increased risk for individuals who both smoke and drink heavily (ACS, 2022).
11. Assess patient's knowledge, prior experience with head and neck assessment, and feelings about procedure.	Reveals need for patient instruction and/or support.

PLANNING

1. Expected outcomes following completion of procedure:	
• Patient recognizes warning signs and symptoms of eye, ear, and sinus disease and head and neck cancer.	Awareness of warning signs improves adherence to reporting problems to health care provider.
• Patient identifies appropriate safety precautions to take for preventing occupational injury to head and neck.	Awareness of occupational safety precautions improves adherence to healthful behaviors.
• Patient exhibits good visual acuity, normal hearing, moist and intact oral mucosa, and head and neck without masses or lesions.	Patient has no abnormal findings.
2. Prepare patient by explaining that you will be completing routine examination of head and neck to check for areas of concern.	Understanding promotes patient's cooperation.
3. Anticipate topics that you can teach patient during examination (e.g., common symptoms of eye, ear, sinus, and mouth problems; occupational health safety).	Enables you to incorporate teaching during examination.
4. Perform hand hygiene. Assemble necessary supplies and equipment at bedside.	Reduces transmission of infection. Promotes efficiency of examination.
5. Close room doors or bed curtains.	Provides patient privacy.
6. Position patient sitting upright if possible.	Provides for more thorough examination of head and neck structures.

IMPLEMENTATION

1. Inspect head's position and facial features. Look for symmetry.	Head tilting to one side during a conversation may indicate hearing or visual loss. Neurological disorders such as paralysis often affect facial symmetry.
2. Assess eyes. (During examination, include discussion of signs and symptoms related to eye diseases and ways to prevent eye injury.)	

STEP	RATIONALE

a. Inspect position of eyes, color, condition of conjunctiva, and movement.

Asymmetrical positioning may reflect trauma or tumor growth. Differences in color are sometimes congenital; changes in color of conjunctiva (e.g., redness associated with infection) may be result of local infection or symptomatic of another abnormality (e.g., pale conjunctiva is associated with anemia).

b. Assess patient's near vision (ability to read newspaper or magazines) and far vision (ability to follow movement, read clock, watch television, or read signs at a distance).

Patient with visual acuity or visual field loss indicates need for support with self-care measures (e.g., feeding, bathing, hygiene, dressing) and teaching.

c. Inspect pupils for size, shape, and equality (see illustration).

Normal pupils are round, regular, and equal in size and shape and have consensual response to light and accommodation. Pinpoint pupils can indicate opioid use. Enlarged pupil unilaterally can indicate increased intracranial pressure.

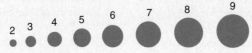

STEP 2c Pupil sizes in millimeters.

d. Test pupillary reflexes. To test reaction to light, dim room lights. If you cannot dim lights, cup hand over eye to temporarily shield light. As patient looks straight ahead, move penlight from side of patient's face and direct light on pupil. Observe pupillary response of both eyes, noting briskness and equality of reflex (see illustrations A and B).

Darkened room normally ensures brisk response of pupils to light. Pupil that is illuminated constricts. Pupil in other eye should constrict equally (consensual light reflex).

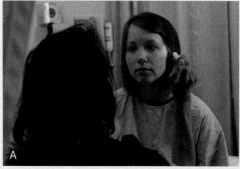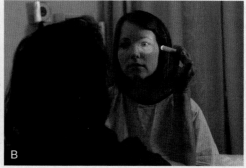

STEP 2d (A) Holding penlight to side of patient's face. (B) Illumination of pupil causes pupillary constriction.

(1) Test for accommodation by asking patient to look at you and then focus on distant object, which dilates the pupil. Then have patient shift back to looking at you (stay 7–8 cm [3–3.2 inches] from patient's nose) and observe for pupil constriction and convergence of eyes. **NOTE:** You can also ask patient to follow an object (e.g., finger, pen) with eyes from far to near point.

Absence of constriction, convergence, or an asymmetrical response requires further ophthalmological assessment (Ball et al., 2023).

Clinical Judgment *If visual abnormalities are suspected, have a health care provider perform ophthalmoscopic examination.*

3. Assess ears. During examination, discuss patient's risks for hearing loss and how to prevent.

a. Inspect outer ear and external auditory canal. Note any drainage, inflammation, or lesions (wear clean gloves if drainage present). Gently press against tragus and ask if patient notes discomfort.

Drainage, inflammation and pain on palpation may indicate external ear infection.

b. Note patient's response to questions and presence/use of hearing aid. Note if patient cups a hand behind the ear or tilts ear toward you while listening. If you suspect patient has hearing loss, check patient's response to your whispered voice one ear at a time. Stand behind and to side of patient, exhale and whisper into ear using a random combination of six letters and numbers (Ball et al., 2023). Repeat, gradually increasing voice intensity until patient correctly repeats the words.

Cupping and tilting suggest hearing loss.
Patients normally hear over 50% of words; fewer indicate hearing impairment (Ball et al., 2023).

STEP	RATIONALE

Clinical Judgment *For patient with obvious hearing impairment, speak clearly and concisely, stand so patient can see your face, stand toward patient's good ear, use low pitch, and avoid yelling. If hearing deficit is present, have a qualified nurse inspect patient's ears using an otoscope to check for impacted cerumen, external otitis, or allergic reactions to materials in hearing aids.*

4. Inspect nose.
   a. Inspect externally for shape, skin color, alignment, drainage, and presence of deformity or inflammation. Note color of mucosa and any lesions, discharge, swelling, or presence of bleeding. If drainage appears infectious, consult with health care provider about obtaining a specimen.

   Character of discharge and inflammation indicates allergy or infection. Perforation and erosion of septum and puffiness and/or increased vascularity of mucosa indicate habitual drug use.

   b. In patients with enteral tubes or nasotracheal (NT) tubes, inspect nares for pressure injury, excoriation, inflammation, or discharge. Use a penlight to look into each naris. Stabilize tube as needed (see Chapter 24). Also inspect skin around any adhesive stabilization device.

   Enteral tubes cause pressure on adjacent tissues and increase patient's risk for medical device–related pressure injuries (EPUAP, NPIAP, PPPIA, 2019). Adhesive device creates risk for MARSI (Fumarola et al., 2020).

   c. Inspect sinuses by palpating gently over frontal and maxillary areas. Use thumbs to apply pressure up and under eyebrows to assess frontal sinuses. Use thumbs to apply pressure over maxillary sinuses, about 0.4 cm (1 inch) below eyes (see illustration).

   Infection, allergy, or drug use sometimes causes tenderness.

5. Assess mouth. During examination, discuss signs and symptoms of oral cancer.
   a. Apply clean gloves. Inspect lips for color, texture, hydration, and lesions. Have patient remove lipstick.

   Normal lips are pink, moist, symmetrical, and smooth.

   b. Ask patient to open mouth wide. Inspect teeth and note position and alignment. Note color of teeth and presence of dental caries, tartar, and extraction sites.

   Reveals quality of hygiene and discoloring effects of cola, coffee, and tobacco. Teeth are normally smooth, white, and shiny.

   c. Inspect mucosa and gums. Determine if patient wears dentures or retainers and if they are comfortable. Remove dentures to visualize and palpate gums. Use tongue blade to lightly depress tongue and inspect oral cavity with penlight (see illustration). Inspect oral mucosa, tongue, teeth, and gums for color, hydration, texture, and obvious lesions.

   Dentures and retainers can cause chronic irritation. Normal mucosa is glistening, pink, smooth, and moist. Precancerous lesions can go unnoticed and progress rapidly.

   d. If oral lesions are present, palpate gently with gloved hand for tenderness, size, and consistency. Remove and dispose of gloves. Perform hand hygiene.

   Cancerous lesions tend to be hard and nontender.

6. Inspect and palpate the neck.

   Assesses function of neck muscles; lymph nodes; thyroid glands; and trachea.
   Detects muscle weakness, strain, and ROM.

   a. Neck muscles: Inspect neck for bilateral symmetry of muscles. Ask patient to slowly flex and hyperextend neck and turn head side to side.

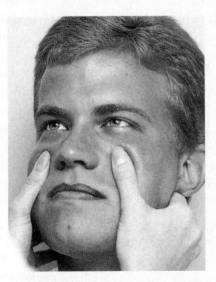

STEP 4c Palpation of maxillary sinus.

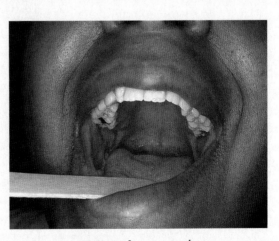

STEP 5c Inspect mouth.

b. Lymph nodes: With patient's chin raised and head tilted slightly, inspect area where lymph nodes are distributed and compare both sides (see illustration).

Lymph nodes are sometimes enlarged from infection or various diseases such as cancer.

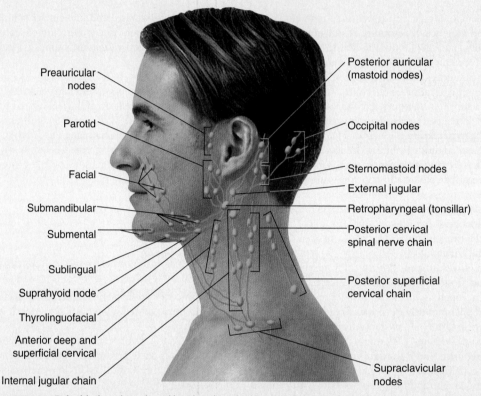

STEP 6b Palpable lymph nodes of head and neck. (*From Ball JW, et al: Seidel's guide to physical examination, ed 9, St Louis, 2019, Mosby.*)

(1) To examine lymph nodes more closely, have patient relax with neck flexed slightly forward. To palpate, face or stand to side of patient and use pads of middle three fingers of hand (see illustration). Palpate gently in rotary motion for superficial lymph nodes.

This position relaxes tissues and muscles.

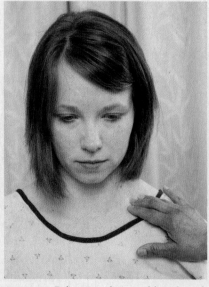

STEP 6b(1) Palpation of cervical lymph nodes.

STEP	RATIONALE
(2) Note if lymph nodes are large, fixed, inflamed, or tender.	Large, fixed, inflamed, or tender lymph nodes indicate local infection, systemic disease, or neoplasm.

Clinical Judgment *If you notice an enlarged lymph node, have a more experienced nurse or health care provider examine patient.*

STEP	RATIONALE
7. Discard used supplies and gloves in proper receptacle. Proceed to next examination (Skill 6.3) or help patient to comfortable position. Perform hand hygiene.	Prevents transmission of infection.
8. Place nurse call system in an accessible location within patient's reach.	Ensures patient can call for assistance if needed.
9. Raise side rails (as appropriate) and lower bed to lowest position, locking into position.	Ensures patient safety and prevents falls.

EVALUATION

1. Compare assessment findings with normal assessment characteristics or previous assessments.	Identifies abnormalities or changes in patient's condition.
2. Ask patient to describe common symptoms of eye, ear, sinus, or mouth disease.	Measures patient's ability to recognize abnormalities.
3. Ask patient to list occupational safety precautions for vision and hearing.	Knowledge allows patient to take safety precautions.
4. Use Teach-Back: "We talked about some of the signs and symptoms of injury to your ears due to your occupation. Tell me what you can do to reduce injury and potential hearing problems." Revise your instruction now or develop a plan for revised patient/family caregiver teaching if patient/family caregiver is not able to teach back correctly.	Teach-back is a technique for health care providers to ensure that medical information has been explained clearly so that patients and families understand what is communicated to them (AHRQ, 2023).

Unexpected Outcomes	Related Interventions
1. Patient has yellow nasal discharge, sneezing, and complaint of sinus pain.	• Reposition into semi-Fowler or other comfortable position to relieve sinus pain. • Monitor temperature for fever. • Notify health care provider if these are new findings.
2. Patient complains of severe headache and dizziness when standing.	• Respond immediately by obtaining heart rate and blood pressure. • Return patient to bed in position of comfort to minimize dizziness and relieve headache. • Identify contributing factors (e.g., stress, pain, or elevated blood pressure). • Notify health care provider.
3. Patient has mouth sore that bleeds easily, lump or thickening in cheek, white or red patch in mucosa, or lump involving lymph nodes.	• Notify health care provider.

Documentation

- Document all findings, including any abnormal findings such as hearing or visual loss, pain and its location, signs of infection, and characteristics of drainage.
- Document evaluation of patient and family caregiver learning.

Hand-Off Reporting

- Report any unexpected findings or changes to charge nurse or health care provider.

Special Considerations

Patient Education

- Explain the common visual changes associated with aging, including reduced acuity (presbyopia), loss of or a reduction in peripheral vision, reduced tearing, and sensitivity to glare or bright lights. Inform patients when to seek help from an eye-care professional.
- Teach the visually impaired patient and family caregivers how to make room adjustments at home to promote safer ambulation

(see Chapter 41). Self-help aids are available to help patient function independently with daily activities.
- Educate patients and family caregivers about strategies for preventing hearing loss (WHO, 2019b):
  - Immunize children against childhood diseases.
  - Immunize adolescent girls and women of reproductive age against rubella before pregnancy.
  - Do not insert any object into the ear and use earplugs/earmuffs in noisy situations.
  - Check if medicines you take affect hearing.
  - In case of ear problems, consult with your health care provider immediately.
  - Have your hearing tested regularly and wear a hearing device if advised to do so.

Pediatrics

- Some infants resist eye examination by closing eyes. Use distraction to encourage eye opening (Hockenberry et al., 2022).

- Headaches in children are usually caused by loss of sleep, poor nutrition, eye fatigue, and allergies. Children as young as 3 years of age can develop severe migraine headaches, but the symptoms are vague and difficult to diagnose (Hockenberry et al., 2022).
- Screen all babies for hearing loss by no later than 1 month of age, ideally before leaving a hospital after birth. If a baby does not pass a hearing screening, it is important to get a full hearing test as soon as possible, but no later than 3 months of age (CDC, 2022c).

Older Adults

- Older adults commonly have loss of peripheral vision caused by changes in the lens.
- Teach patients older than 65 years to have hearing checks when a change in hearing is noticed. Because of a lack of scientific evidence, the U.S. Preventive Services Task Force (USPSTF) concludes that the benefits and harms of screening for hearing loss in asymptomatic older adults are uncertain and that the balance of benefits and harms cannot be determined (Krist, 2021).

- Measuring visual acuity helps determine level of assistance that patient requires with daily living activities and ability of patient to safely ambulate and function independently within the home.

Populations With Disabilities

- Patients with limitations in cognitive function and adaptive behavior may be less likely to report visual symptoms or to have regular ophthalmic care. The method of screening may need to be individualized for patients with communication and perception limitations. Both vision and hearing limitations can have a disproportionate impact on adults who rely on sensory input to compensate for some of their disabilities (Sullivan et al., 2018).

Home Care

- Educate patients about proper techniques for maintaining glasses, contact lens, and hearing aids (see Chapter 19).
- Encourage use of helmets during bike riding, motorcycling, and contact sports to prevent head injuries.

◆ SKILL 6.3　Thorax and Lung Assessment

Assessment of the thorax and lungs detects alterations in ventilation and respiration. A patient's history will help you to anticipate physical changes that might be found. For example, a patient with a long history of smoking is likely to have abnormal lung sounds; a patient with recent chest trauma will have reduced chest excursion. When you confirm findings, you apply critical thinking in making clinical judgments about ways to improve the patient's ventilation or respiration. Assessment of the thorax and lungs is critical because alterations can be life threatening. Changes in respiration can occur quickly as a result of immobility (reduced lung sounds), infection (changed lung sounds), certain analgesic and sedative medications (reduced chest excursion and respirations), and fluid overload (changes in lung sounds). Use data from all body systems to determine the nature of pulmonary alterations.

You will use inspection, palpation, and auscultation during the examination.

Before assessing the thorax and lungs, know the landmarks of the chest (Fig. 6.3A–C). These landmarks help you identify findings and use assessment skills correctly. A patient's nipples, angle of Louis at the sternum, suprasternal notch, costal angle, clavicles, and vertebrae are key landmarks. Keep a mental image of the location of the lobes of the lung and the position of each rib (Fig. 6.4A–C). By knowing the position of each rib, you can better visualize the lobe of the lung being assessed. To begin, locate the angle of Louis on the anterior chest by palpating the "speed bump" at the manubriosternal junction where the second rib connects with the sternum. The angle is often visible and palpable. Count the ribs and intercostal spaces (ICSs; between the ribs) from this point. The

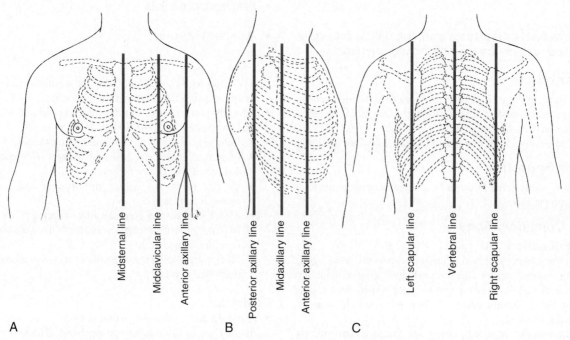

FIG. 6.3 Anatomical landmarks and order of progression for examination of thorax. (A) Anterior thorax. (B) Lateral thorax. (C) Posterior thorax.

number of each ICS corresponds with that of the rib just above it. The spinous processes of the third thoracic vertebra and the fourth, fifth, and sixth ribs help to locate the lung lobes laterally. The lower lobes project laterally and anteriorly (see Fig. 6.4B). Posteriorly, the tip or inferior margin of the scapula lies approximately at the level of the seventh rib (see Fig. 6.4C).

During the examination, use auscultation to listen to breath sounds with a stethoscope. You can hear these sounds best when a person breathes deeply through the mouth. Normal breath sounds include loud, high-pitched bronchial breath sounds over the trachea; medium-pitched bronchovesicular sounds over the mainstream bronchi, between the scapulae, and below the clavicles; and soft, breezy, low-pitched vesicular breath sounds over most of the peripheral lung fields. Adventitious sounds (abnormal breath sounds) result from air passing through fluid, mucus, or narrowed airways or from an inflammation between the pleural linings, indicating some form of pathology. The four types of adventitious sounds are crackles, rhonchi, wheezes, and pleural friction rubs (Table 6.5). First become familiar with normal breath sounds. Then learn to note the location and characteristics of the abnormal sounds, diminished breath sounds, or absence of breath sounds. One thing that assists in the classification of adventitious sounds is whether the sounds are continuous or intermittent. For example, rhonchi and wheezes are continuous sounds, whereas crackles are not. Crackles could be counted by the examiner as discrete acoustic events (Zimmerman & Williams, 2022). Also learn to note the pitch of adventitious sounds: wheezes and fine crackles are high pitched, whereas rhonchi and coarse crackles are low pitched (Zimmerman & Williams, 2022). Determine where in the respiratory cycle the abnormal sounds are heard.

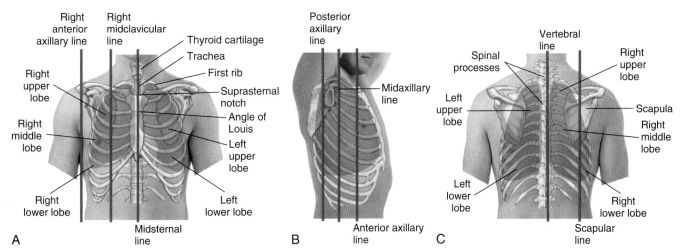

FIG. 6.4 Position of lung lobes in relation to anatomical landmarks. (A) Anterior position. (B) Lateral position. (C) Posterior position. (*From Ball JW, et al:* Seidel's guide to physical examination, *ed 9, St Louis, 2019, Mosby.*)

TABLE 6.5

Adventitious Breath Sounds

Sound	Site Auscultated	Cause	Character
Crackles	Most common in dependent lobes: right and left lung bases	The sound of airways snapping open, frequently occurring in interstitial lung disease, pulmonary edema from heart failure, and infection. Later, higher-pitched crackles often represent interstitial lung disease, whereas earlier and lower-pitched crackles tend more toward chronic obstructive lung disease.	Fine, short, interrupted crackling sounds heard during end of inspiration, expiration, or both; may or may not change with coughing; sound like crushing cellophane Medium crackles: lower, moister sounds heard during middle of inspiration; not cleared with coughing Coarse crackles: loud bubbly sounds heard during inspiration; not cleared with coughing
Rhonchi (sonorous wheeze)	Heard primarily over trachea and bronchi; if loud enough, can be heard over most lung fields	Fluid or mucus in larger airways causing turbulence; muscular spasm	Loud, low-pitched, continuous sounds heard more during expiration; sometimes cleared by coughing Sound like blowing air through fluid with a straw

TABLE 6.5

Adventitious Breath Sounds–cont'd

Sound	Site Auscultated	Cause	Character
Wheezes (sibilant wheeze)	Heard over all lung fields but more distinct over posterior lung fields	High-velocity airflow through severely narrowed or obstructed bronchus. Occurs in asthma, chronic obstructive lung disease, and focal masses.	High-pitched, musical sounds such as a squeak heard continuously during inspiration or expiration; usually louder on expiration. Not cleared with coughing. The duration, rather than pitch, of wheezing throughout the respiratory cycle is most predictive of the degree of pathology.
Pleural friction rub	Heard over anterior lateral lung field (if patient is sitting upright)	Inflamed pleura, parietal pleura rubbing against visceral pleura	Has grating quality heard best during inspiration; does not clear with coughing; heard loudest over lower lateral anterior surface

Data from Ball JW, et al: *Seidel's guide to physical examination,* ed 10, St. Louis, 2023, Mosby; Zimmerman, B. & William, D. Lung Sounds, National Library of Medicine StatPearls (Internet), 2022. https://www.ncbi.nlm.nih.gov/books/NBK537253/#article-36567.s2. Accessed March 17, 2023.

Delegation

The skill of assessing the lungs and thorax cannot be delegated to assistive personnel (AP). Direct the AP to:
- Measure the patient's respirations after the patient is confirmed stable.
- Report respiratory distress, chest pain, difficulty breathing, and changes in rate and depth.
- Keep head of bed elevated for a patient who has respiratory difficulties or is at risk for respiratory problems (e.g., aspiration).

Interprofessional Collaboration

- When assessment reveals changes in lung function or when assessments for specific pathophysiological changes reveal abnormal findings, communicate with the health care provider or respiratory therapist.

Equipment

- Stethoscope

STEP	RATIONALE

ASSESSMENT

1. When beginning a physical examination with an examination of the thorax and lungs, identify patient, determine patient's level of consciousness (LOC), primary language and health literacy as outlined in Skill 6.1, Assessment, Steps 1, 4, 5, and 6. Otherwise, these steps need not be repeated.

Complies with The Joint Commission standards and improves patient safety (TJC, 2023).

2. Check the electronic health record (EHR) for history of lung disease (e.g., asthma, bronchitis), chest trauma, and VS.

Establishes a baseline of expected information to be found during the physical examination and historical data that will help you focus the examination.

3. Assess history of tobacco (cigarette, cigar, pipe, or vaping with e-cigarette [electronic nicotine delivery system]) or marijuana use: type of tobacco, duration (number of years), and amount in pack-years (number of years smoking times number of packs smoked per day), age started, efforts to quit smoking with factors influencing success or failure, and extent of smoking by others at home or work (Ball et al., 2023). If patient has quit, determine length of time since smoking stopped. If patient vapes, determine device type and flavor preference and identify the mix of tobacco products used (Pearson et al., 2018).

Cigarette smoking is the most important risk factor for lung cancer, with risk increasing with both quantity and duration of smoking. Cigar and pipe smoking also increase risk. Another risk factor is exposure to secondhand smoke (ACS, 2022).

Even in small doses, inhaling the two primary ingredients found in e-cigarettes—propylene glycol and vegetable glycerin—is likely to expose users to a high level of toxins; the more ingredients inhaled, the greater the toxicity (Sassano et al., 2018; American Lung Association [ALA], 2022). The Food and Drug Administration has not found any e-cigarette to be safe and effective in helping smokers quit (ALA, 2022). Vaping can also cause chemical irritation and allergic or immune reactions to various chemicals or other substances in the inhaled vapors (Shmerling, 2022).

STEP	RATIONALE
4. Ask if patient has any of the following: *persistent cough* (productive or nonproductive), sputum production including color (yellow, green, *blood-streaked sputum*), *chest pain, worsening shortness of breath, a hoarse voice,* orthopnea, dyspnea during exertion, activity intolerance, or *recurrent bouts of pneumonia or bronchitis.*	Symptoms of respiratory alterations help to localize objective physical findings. Warning signals for lung cancer are in italics (ACS, 2022). Warning signals usually occur late.
5. Determine if patient lives or works in environment containing pollutants (e.g., radon, asbestos, arsenic, coal dust, or chemical irritants) or requiring exposure to radiation.	Exposure to radon gas, which is released from soil and can accumulate in indoor air, is the second-leading cause of lung cancer in the United States (ACS, 2022). Asbestos (particularly among people who smoke), radiation, air pollution, and diesel exhaust are also cancer risk factors. Patients with chronic respiratory disease (e.g., asthma) have symptoms aggravated by change in temperature and humidity, irritating fumes or smoke, emotional stress, and physical exertion.
6. Review history for known or suspected human immunodeficiency virus (HIV) infection; people who live or work in correctional facilities, long-term care facilities or nursing homes, and homeless shelters; health care workers who care for patients at increased risk for TB disease; immigration to the United States from a country where TB is prevalent (CDC, 2021b).	These are known risk factors for exposure to and/or development of TB.
7. Ask when patient last had a TB test.	Screens for presence of TB.
8. Ask if patient has history of persistent cough, hemoptysis (bloody sputum), unexplained weight loss, fatigue, night sweats, and/or fever.	Signs and symptoms of both TB and HIV infection.
9. Does patient have history of chronic hoarseness?	Hoarseness indicates laryngeal disorder or abuse of cocaine or opioids (sniffing).
10. Assess for history of allergies to pollen, dust, or other airborne irritants and to any foods, drugs, or chemical substances. Has patient had severe allergic reaction in past?	Allergic response is associated with wheezing on auscultation, dyspnea, cyanosis, and diaphoresis.
11. Review family history for cancer, TB, allergies, asthma, bronchitis, or emphysema (chronic obstructive pulmonary disease (COPD).	Familial history places patient at risk for lung disease.
12. Assess patient's knowledge, prior experience with chest examination and risk factors for lung problems, and feelings about procedure.	Reveals need for patient instruction and/or support.

PLANNING

1. Expected outcomes following completion of procedure:	
• Respirations are passive, diaphragmatic or costal, and regular (12–20 breaths/min in adult) with symmetrical expansion.	Characteristics of normal respirations.
• Breath sounds are clear to auscultation and equal bilaterally.	Air flows without interference or obstruction. Corresponding sides should sound the same.
• Patient is able to describe own risks and factors that predispose to lung disease.	Awareness of risks can improve patient adherence to healthy behavior.
2. Explain to patient the approach you will use to examine the chest and lungs to check for areas of concern.	Understanding promotes patient's cooperation.
3. Anticipate topics (e.g., tobacco use, occupational risks) that you can teach patient during examination.	Enables you to incorporate teaching during examination.
4. Perform hand hygiene. Prepare necessary supplies at bedside.	Reduces transmission of infection. Ensures efficient procedure.
5. Close room doors or bed curtains.	Provides patient privacy.
6. Position patient sitting upright. For bedridden patient, elevate head of bed 45 to 90 degrees. If unable to tolerate sitting, use supine and side-lying positions.	Promotes full lung expansion during examination. Patients with chronic respiratory disease may need to sit up throughout examination because of shortness of breath. May require help of another caregiver to position unresponsive patients.

IMPLEMENTATION

1. Remove patient's gown or drape from the posterior chest. Keep front of chest and legs covered. As examination progresses, remove gown from area being examined.	Avoids unnecessary exposure and provides full visibility of thorax. Allows direct placement of diaphragm or bell on patient's skin, which enhances clarity of sounds.

STEP	RATIONALE

2. As you proceed, explain all steps of procedure, encouraging patient to relax and breathe normally through mouth.

Anxiety alters respiratory function. Breathing through mouth decreases extraneous sounds from air passing through nose.

3. Posterior thorax:

   a. If possible, stand behind patient. Inspect thorax for shape and symmetry. Note any deformities, position of spine, slope of ribs, retraction of intercostal spaces (ICSs) during inspiration and bulging of ICSs during expiration, and symmetrical expansion during inspiration. Note anteroposterior diameter.

Allows for identification of impairment in chest expansion and any symptoms of respiratory distress. Normal chest contour is symmetrical. Child: shape of chest is almost circular, with anteroposterior diameter in 1:1 ratio. Adult: the anteroposterior diameter is ⅓ to ½ of side-to-side diameter. Chronic lung disease causes ribs to be more horizontal and increases anteroposterior diameter, resulting in "barrel chest." Patients with breathing problems assume postures that improve ventilation.

Clinical Judgment *When a patient holds the chest wall during breathing, it indicates localized chest pain. Assess the nature of pain, including specific location, onset, severity, precipitating factors, quality, region, and radiation.*

   b. Determine rate and rhythm of breathing (see Chapter 5). Examine thorax as a whole. Have patient relax.

   c. Systematically palpate posterior chest wall, costal spaces, and ICSs, noting any masses, pulsations, unusual movement, or areas of localized tenderness (see illustration). If patient voices pain or tenderness, avoid deep palpation. Palpate any suspicious mass lightly for shape, size, and qualities of lesion (see Skill 6.1). Do not palpate painful areas deeply.

Good time to count respirations, with patient relaxed and unaware of inspection. Awareness could alter respirations.

Palpation assesses further characteristics and confirms or supplements findings from inspection. Localized swelling or tenderness indicates trauma to ribs or underlying cartilage. A fractured rib fragment could be displaced.

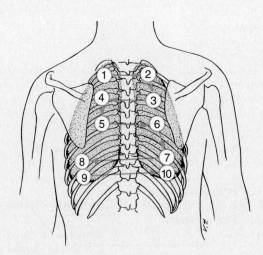

STEP 3c Pattern for assessment of posterior thorax.

   d. Assess chest expansion by standing behind patient and placing thumbs along spinal processes at tenth rib, with palms lightly contacting posterolateral surfaces (see illustration A). Keep thumbs about 5 cm (2 inches) apart, with thumbs pointing toward spine and fingers pointing laterally. Press hands toward patient's spine to form small skinfold between thumbs. After exhalation, patient takes deep breath. Note movement of thumbs (see illustration B) and symmetry of chest wall movement. Normally symmetrical separation of thumbs occurs during chest excursion 3 to 5 cm (1½–2 inches).

Palpation of chest expansion assesses depth of patient's breathing. This technique is a good measure to evaluate patient's ability to perform deep-breathing exercises. Limited movement on one side indicates that patient is voluntarily splinting during ventilation because of pain. Avoid allowing hands to slide over skin, which gives false measure of excursion.

STEP	RATIONALE

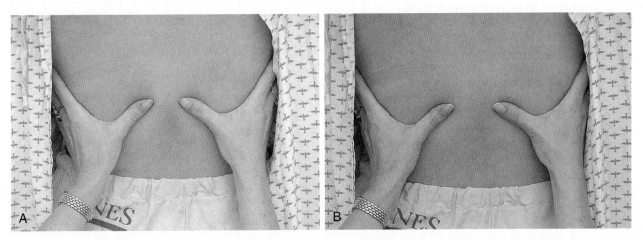

STEP 3d (A) Position of hands for palpation of posterior thorax excursion. (B) As patient inhales, movement of chest excursion separates nurse's thumbs.

e. Auscultate breath sounds. Instruct patient to take slow, deep breaths with mouth slightly open. For an adult, place diaphragm of stethoscope firmly on chest wall over ICSs (see illustration). Listen to an entire inspiration and expiration at each stethoscope position (see systematic pattern in Step 4c). If sounds are faint, as in obese patients, ask person to breathe harder and faster temporarily. Systematically compare breath sounds over right and left sides, listening for normal and adventitious sounds.

Assesses movement of air through tracheobronchial tree (Table 6.6). Recognition of normal airflow sounds allows detection of sounds caused by mucus or airway obstruction. Characterize sounds by length of inspiratory and expiratory phases.

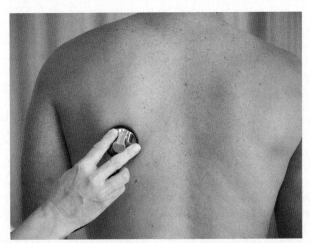

STEP 3e Auscultation with a stethoscope.

Clinical Judgment *Use caution when asking patients to breathe harder or faster, because inhaling and exhaling deeply or quickly can cause light-headedness.*

f. If you auscultate adventitious sounds, have patient cough. Listen again with stethoscope to determine if sound has cleared with coughing. See Table 6.5 for a description of adventitious breath sounds.

4. Lateral thorax:

a. Instruct patient to raise arms and inspect chest wall for same characteristics as reviewed for posterior chest.

b. Extend palpation and auscultation of posterior thorax to lateral sides of chest, except for excursion measurement (see illustration).

Coughing may clear adventitious sounds. Rhonchi are often eliminated or altered by coughing. Crackles and wheezes are not.

Improves access to lateral thoracic structures.

Locates abnormalities in lateral lung fields.

TABLE 6.6

Normal Breath Sounds

Type	Description	Location	Origin
Bronchial	Loud, harsh, and high-pitched sounds with hollow quality Heard best during expiration, lasting longer than inspiration (3:2 ratio)	Best heard over trachea or at the right apex	Created by air moving through trachea close to chest wall
Bronchovesicular	Midrange pitch and intensity Inspiratory phase equal to expiratory phase	Commonly heard over the upper third of the anterior chest, over the bronchioles lateral to sternum at first and second intercostal spaces; best heard posteriorly between scapulae	Created by air moving through large airways
Vesicular	Soft, breezy, and low-pitched sounds Inspiratory phase 3 times longer than expiratory phase	Best heard over posterior lung bases (Zimmerman & Williams, 2022)	Created by air moving through smaller airways.

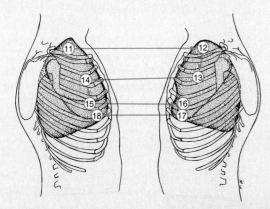

STEP 4b Pattern for assessment of lateral thorax.

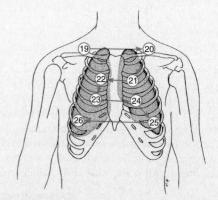

STEP 5d Pattern for assessment of anterior chest.

5. Anterior thorax:
   a. Inspect accessory muscles while patient is breathing: sternocleidomastoid, trapezius, and abdominal muscles. Note effort to breathe.

   b. Inspect width or spread of costal angle made by costal margins and tip of sternum. Angle is usually larger than 90 degrees between margins.
   c. Observe patient's breathing pattern, observing symmetry and degree of chest wall and abdominal movement. Respiratory rate and rhythm are more often assessed on anterior chest wall.
   d. Palpate anterior thoracic muscles and ribs for lumps, masses, tenderness, or unusual movement, following a systematic pattern across and down (see illustration).
   e. Palpate anterior chest excursion. Place hands over each lateral rib cage, with thumbs approximately 5 cm (2 inches) apart and angled along each costal margin. As patient inhales deeply, thumbs should symmetrically move apart 3 to 5 cm (1½–2 inches), with each side expanding equally.
   f. With patient sitting, auscultate anterior thorax following same pattern as in Step 5d. Begin above clavicles; move across and then down as during palpation. Compare right and left sides. Give special attention to lower lobes, where mucus commonly gathers.
6. Clean and store stethoscope. Proceed to next examination (Skill 6.4) or help patient to comfortable position. Perform hand hygiene.

Extent to which accessory muscles are used reveals degree of effort to breathe. Accessory muscles move little with normal passive breathing. Patients who require great effort and rely on these muscles may produce a grunting sound.
Indicates congenital, acquired, or traumatic alterations that may influence patient's chest expansion.

Assesses patient's effort to breathe: symmetrical, passive movement indicates no respiratory distress. A male patient's breathing is diaphragmatic, whereas a female's is more costal (Ball et al., 2023).
Localized swelling or tenderness indicates trauma to underlying ribs or cartilage.

Assesses depth of patient's breathing and ability to perform deep-breathing exercises. Certain abnormalities are evident if expansion is not symmetrical.

A systematic pattern of assessment comparing sides helps to identify abnormal sounds.

Reduces transmission of microorganisms.

STEP	RATIONALE
7. Place nurse call system in an accessible location within patient's reach.	Ensures patient can call for assistance if needed.
8. Raise side rails (as appropriate) and lower bed to lowest position, locking into position.	Ensures patient safety and prevents falls.

EVALUATION

1. Compare respiratory findings with normal assessment characteristics or previous assessments for thorax and lungs.	Determines presence of abnormalities or changes in patient's condition.
2. Have patient identify own risk factors and those factors leading to lung disease.	Demonstrates learning.
3. **Use Teach-Back:** "Let's review some of the risk factors your job poses for lung disease. Tell me what are the specific dangers to your lungs from what you use in your hair salon?" Revise your instruction now or develop a plan for revised patient/family caregiver teaching if patient/family caregiver is not able to teach back correctly.	Teach-back is a technique for health care providers to ensure that medical information has been explained clearly so that patients and their families understand what is communicated to them (AHRQ, 2023).

Unexpected Outcomes	Related Interventions
1. Patient has copious mucus production, audible inspiratory wheezing, or congested cough with thick mucus.	• Help patient cough by splinting chest; teach to inhale slowly through nose, exhale, and cough; encourage expectoration of mucus. • Auscultate breath sounds before and after cough to evaluate cough effectiveness. • Auscultate lungs for adventitious sounds. • Encourage increased oral intake (if permitted). • If unable to clear airway by coughing, suctioning may be indicated (see Chapter 24). • Monitor VS. • Notify health care provider.
2. Respirations are rapid or slow and irregular (see Chapter 5), and bulging of ICSs is present.	• Position patient more upright if appropriate. • Auscultate lungs for adventitious sounds. • Notify health care provider.
3. Patient presents with difficulty breathing; decreased breath sounds; rapid, shallow breathing; wheezing; cough (signs of atelectasis, collapse of portion of lung and alveoli).	• Reposition patient more comfortably with head of bed elevated. • Notify health care provider.

Documentation

- Document patient's respiratory rate and character; breath sounds, including type, location, and presence on inspiration, expiration, or both; changes noted after coughing; chest excursion; and other physical assessment findings.
- Document evaluation of patient and family caregiver learning.

Hand-Off Reporting

- Report abnormalities immediately to the charge nurse or health care provider.

Special Considerations

Patient Education

- Educate patients about risks of cigarette smoking and vaping. Individuals who stop smoking have the potential to live longer than those who continue to smoke. The probability of these individuals dying from lung cancer or other related causes continues to decline with further abstinence. Encourage patients who smoke to receive counseling to quit.
- The U.S. Preventive Services Task Force (USPSTF), the American Academy of Family Physicians (AAFP), and the American College of Chest Physicians recommend yearly lung cancer screening with low-dose computed tomography (LDCT) scans for people who are 50 to 80 years old and in fairly good health (ACS, 2023b) and currently smoke or have quit in the past 15 years.
- Have at least a 20 pack-year smoking history.
- Annual influenza vaccine reduces incidence of influenza. This is especially critical in high-risk patients. The Centers for Disease Control (CDC) recommends annual influenza vaccination for everyone age 6 months and older with any licensed influenza vaccine that is appropriate for the recipient's age and health status (CDC, 2022b).
- Explain to patients that exposure to radon, radiation, arsenic, and asbestos from occupational, medical, and environmental sources; air pollution; history of TB; and secondhand smoke contribute significantly to lung cancer (ACS, 2022).
- Discuss with patients the warning signs of lung cancer.

Pediatrics

- In children, observe for use of accessory muscles, which indicates respiratory distress. Retractions may involve intercostal, suprasternal, supraclavicular, or sternal muscles (Hockenberry et al., 2022).

- Use the bell of the stethoscope to auscultate lung sounds in children. Breath sounds are louder in children because of their thin chest walls.
- Children younger than 7 years normally exhibit noticeable abdominal or diaphragmatic movement. Older children and adults exhibit more costal or thoracic movement.
- Head bobbing and nasal flaring in infants are signs of significant respiratory distress (Hockenberry et al., 2022).
- The CDC (2023a) recommends routine administration of pneumococcal conjugate vaccine PCV13 for:
  - All infants as a series of 4 doses: 1 dose at 2 months, 4 months, 6 months, and 12 through 15 months.
  - Children who miss their shots or start the series later should still get the vaccine. The number of doses recommended and the intervals between doses will depend on the child's age when vaccination begins.

Older Adults

- Older adults have a costal angle (anteriorly) of slightly less than 90 degrees. The anteroposterior diameter sometimes increases from kyphosis.
- In older adults, chest expansion is reduced because of calcification of rib cartilage and partial contraction of inspiratory muscles.
- The CDC (2023a) recommends routine administration of pneumococcal conjugate vaccine (PCV15 or PCV20) for all adults 65 years or older who have never received any pneumococcal conjugate vaccine or whose previous vaccination history is unknown. If PCV15 was used, this should be followed by a dose of PPSV23 one year later. The minimum interval is 8 weeks and can be considered in adults with an immunocompromising condition, cochlear implant, or cerebrospinal fluid leak. If PCV20 is used, a dose of PPSV23 is NOT indicated.

◆ SKILL 6.4   Cardiovascular Assessment

Cardiovascular disease is the leading cause of death for men, women, and people of most racial and ethnic groups in the United States (CDC, 2022a); that's one in every four deaths. During a physical examination of the cardiovascular system, you want to identify any risks a patient may have for heart disease and any developing problems associated with existing disease. A patient who presents with signs or symptoms of heart (cardiac) problems such as chest pain may have a life-threatening condition that requires immediate attention. In this situation you act quickly and perform the parts of the examination that are absolutely necessary. This will reveal baseline heart function and any risks for heart disease. Patients tend to seek information about heart disease because it is so prevalent. You assess the heart, neck vessels, and peripheral circulation together because the systems work in unison. Then you can conduct a more thorough assessment when the patient is more stable.

Your assessment can determine the integrity of the circulatory system. Inadequate tissue perfusion results in an inadequate delivery of oxygen and nutrients to cells, a condition called *ischemia*. This is caused by constriction of vessels or occlusion (blockage) from clot formation. The effects of ischemia depend on the duration of the problem and metabolic needs of the tissues. Ischemia results in pain. If lack of oxygen to tissues is unrelieved, tissue necrosis (death) occurs. An *embolus* is a blood clot that breaks loose and travels through the circulation. If the clot obstructs circulation to the lungs or brain, it can be life threatening.

Begin assessment of the heart after examining the lungs because the patient is already in a suitable position with the chest exposed.

Assessment then proceeds to the neck vessels and ends with evaluating peripheral circulation. Use the skills of inspection, palpation, auscultation, and percussion during the examination.

Delegation

The skill of completing a comprehensive cardiovascular assessment cannot be delegated to assistive personnel (AP). Direct the AP to:
- Count peripheral pulses after vital signs (VS).
- Recognize skin temperature and color changes of affected extremities and report any changes to the nurse.
- Recognize changes in peripheral pulse rates and report any changes to the nurse.
- Report any occurrence of chest pain to the nurse immediately.

Interprofessional Collaboration

- When assessment reveals changes in cardiovascular function or when assessments for specific pathophysiological changes reveal abnormal findings, communicate with the appropriate interprofessional team member (e.g., health care provider or cardiac rehabilitation team).

Equipment

- Stethoscope
- Doppler stethoscope (optional)
- Penlight (optional)
- Conducting gel (if a Doppler stethoscope is used)
- Clean gloves (use nonlatex if appropriate)

STEP	RATIONALE

ASSESSMENT

1. When beginning a physical examination with the cardiovascular examination, identify patient and determine patient's level of consciousness (LOC), primary language, and health literacy as outlined in Skill 6.1, Assessment, Steps 1, 4, 5, and 6. Otherwise, these assessments need not be repeated.	Complies with The Joint Commission standards and improves patient safety (TJC, 2023).
2. Review EHR and confirm with patient any medications being taken for cardiovascular function (e.g., antiarrhythmics, antihypertensives, beta blockers, antianginals) and if patient knows their purpose, dosage, dosage schedule, and side effects.	Allows you to assess patient's adherence to and understanding of drug therapies. Medications for cardiovascular function cannot be taken intermittently.

STEP	RATIONALE
3. Ask if patient has experienced dyspnea, chest pain or discomfort, palpitations, excess fatigue, reduced ability to exercise, cough, leg pain or cramps, edema of the feet, rapid weight gain from fluid retention, cyanosis, fainting, and orthopnea. Ask if symptoms occur at rest or during exercise.	These are the cardinal symptoms of heart failure. Cardiovascular function is sometimes adequate during rest but not during exercise.
4. If patient reports chest pain, determine onset (sudden or gradual), precipitating factors, quality, region, and severity and if it radiates. Anginal pain is usually a deep pressure or ache that is substernal and diffuse, radiating to one or both arms, neck, or jaw.	Symptoms reveal acute coronary syndrome (heart attack) or coronary artery disease (CAD).

Clinical Judgment *The most common heart attack symptom in women is the same as in men—some type of chest pain or pressure that lasts more than a few minutes or comes and goes. However, women may experience neck pain or just dizziness and nausea with something that feels like heartburn. Jaw, back, and arm pain could be the only manifestation for women coming in, and chest discomfort could come later. The chest discomfort that many women report might not be crushing and thus might not seem as urgent. Being aware of the many combinations (e.g., nausea, jaw pain, heartburn, chest discomfort) and more subtle signs in women could be the key to quicker diagnoses and treatment (AHA, 2020).*

STEP	RATIONALE
5. Assess family history for heart disease, diabetes mellitus, high cholesterol and/or lipid levels, hypertension, stroke, or rheumatic heart disease.	Family history of these conditions increases risk for heart and vascular disease.
6. Ask patient about a personal history of any preexisting heart conditions (e.g., heart failure, congenital heart disease, CAD, dysrhythmias, murmurs), heart surgery, or vascular disease (e.g., hypertension, phlebitis, varicose veins).	Knowledge reveals patient's level of understanding of condition. Preexisting condition influences which examination techniques to use and expected findings.
7. Determine if patient experiences leg cramps; numbness or tingling in extremities; sensation of cold hands or feet; pain in legs; or swelling or cyanosis of feet, ankles, or hand. Ask about precipitating factors.	These are potential signs and symptoms of vascular disease.
8. If patient experiences leg pain or cramping in lower extremities, ask if it is relieved by walking or standing for long periods or if it occurs during sleep.	Relationship of symptoms to exercise clarifies if problem is vascular or musculoskeletal. Pain caused by vascular condition tends to increase with activity. Musculoskeletal pain is usually not relieved when exercise ends.
9. Ask patients about wearing tight-fitting underwear, hosiery, tight-fitting trouser socks, and sitting or lying in bed with legs crossed.	Tight hosiery around lower extremities and crossing legs can impair venous return, promoting clot formation.
10. Assess patient's knowledge, prior experience with cardiovascular examination and risks for heart problems, and feelings about procedure.	Reveals need for patient instruction and/or support.

PLANNING

1. Expected outcomes following completion of procedure:
   - Heart rate is 60–100 beats/min (adolescent through adult), without extra sounds or murmurs. BP within normal limits for patient.
   - Point of maximal impulse (PMI) is palpable at fifth intercostal space (ICS) at left midclavicular line in children older than 7 years of age and adults.
   - Patient describes risks for heart disease and changes in own behavior that could improve cardiovascular function.
   - Patient describes schedule, dosage, purpose, and benefits of medications being taken for cardiovascular function.
   - Carotid pulse is localized, strong, elastic, and equal bilaterally. No change occurs during inspiration or expiration; without carotid bruit.
   - Jugular veins distend when patient lies supine and flatten when patient is in sitting position.
   - Peripheral pulses are equal and strong (2+); extremities are warm and pink, with capillary refill less than 2 seconds. There is no dependent edema. Peripheral hair growth is symmetrical and evenly distributed, and the skin is free of lesions. Capillary refill is normal in fingers and toes.

Indicates normal rate and sinus rhythm.
Indicates patient's cardiovascular status is stable.

Indicates normal heart position.

Instruction about CVD risks may improve patient's health behavior habits.
Information related to health benefits may improve adherence to therapy.
This indicates a patent vessel.

Venous pressure is normal.

Peripheral circulation is intact.

STEP	RATIONALE
2. Explain to patient how you will proceed with routine examination of heart and vascular system to check for areas of concern.	Understanding promotes patient's cooperation.
3. Anticipate topics that you can teach patient during examination (e.g., risks for heart and vascular disease and disease prevention).	Enables you to incorporate teaching during examination.
4. Perform hand hygiene. Prepare necessary supplies at bedside. Close room curtains or door.	Reduces infection transmission. Promotes efficient examination. Provides privacy.
5. Help patient be as relaxed and comfortable as possible, using a calm tone of voice and purposeful actions.	An anxious or uncomfortable patient can have mild tachycardia, which alters findings.
6. Have patient assume semi-Fowler or supine position.	Provides adequate visibility and access to left thorax and mediastinum. Patient with heart disease often experiences shortness of breath while lying flat.

IMPLEMENTATION

1. As you proceed, explain procedure. Avoid facial gestures reflecting concern.	Patients with previously normal cardiac history may become anxious if you show concern, causing elevated heart rate.
2. Be sure that room is quiet.	Subtle, low-pitched heart sounds are difficult to hear.
3. Assess the heart:	
a. Form mental image of exact location of the heart (see illustration). Base of heart is the upper part, and apex is the bottom tip. Surface of right ventricle constitutes most of the anterior surface of the heart.	Visualization improves ability to assess findings accurately and determines possible source of abnormalities.
b. Find angle of Louis, felt as ridge in sternum approximately 5 cm (2 inches) below suprasternal notch (between sternal body and manubrium). Slip fingers down each side of angle to feel adjacent ribs. ICSs are just below each rib.	Provides you with landmarks to locate and assess heart sounds.
c. Find the following anatomical landmarks (see illustration):	Familiarity with landmarks allows you to describe findings more clearly and ultimately may improve assessment.
(1) Aortic area is at second ICS, right of patient's sternum, close to sternal border (1).	Listening to heart sounds too far away from sternal border decreases ability to hear them clearly.
(2) Pulmonic area is at second ICS, left of patient's sternum, close to sternal border (2).	
(3) Second pulmonic area is found by moving down to the left side of sternum to third ICS, at the left sternal border.	
(4) Tricuspid area (3) is located at fourth left ICS along sternum, close to sternal border.	
(5) Mitral area is found by moving fingers laterally to patient's left to locate fifth ICS at left midclavicular line (4). *This is typically the apex of the heart.*	
(6) Epigastric area (5) is at inferior tip of sternum.	

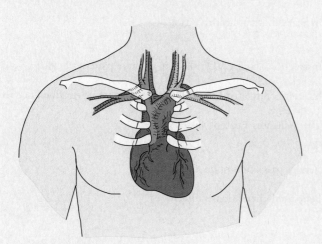

STEP 3a Anatomical position of heart.

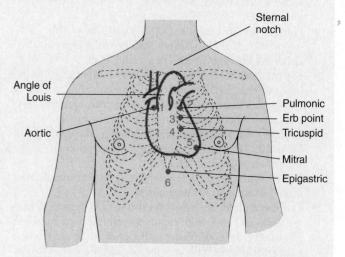

STEP 3c Anatomical sites for assessment of cardiac function.

STEP	RATIONALE

d. Stand to patient's right to inspect precordium with patient supine. Note any visible pulsations or exaggerated lifts. (Use a penlight to improve visualization.) Closely inspect area of apex.

Reveals size and symmetry of heart. Apical impulse may be visible at midclavicular line in fifth ICS. Apical impulse (PMI) may be visible only when patient sits up, bringing heart closer to anterior wall. Obesity obscures ability to visualize PMI.

e. Stay in same position. Palpate for pulsations (placing proximal half of four fingers together, lightly palpating, and then alternating with ball of hand) at all anatomical landmarks.

There should be no pulsations or vibrations. A thrill is a continuous palpable sensation, such as purring of a cat. A thrust is the upward lift felt when palpating the chest wall.

f. Locate PMI by palpating with fingertips along the fifth ICS in midclavicular line (see illustration). Note light, brief pulsation in area 1 to 2 cm (½–1 inch) in diameter at the apex.

In presence of serious heart disease, PMI is located to left of midclavicular line related to enlarged left ventricle. In chronic lung disease, PMI may be to right of midclavicular line as a result of right ventricular enlargement.

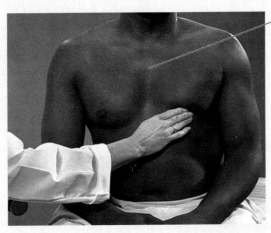

Angle of Louis

STEP 3f Palpation of point of maximal impulse. (*From Ball JW, et al: Seidel's guide to physical examination, ed 10, St Louis, 2023, Elsevier.*)

Clinical Judgment *Presence of a palpable thrill is not normal. Indicates a disruption of blood flow caused by a defect in heart valve or atrial septal defect. A stronger-than-expected impulse is a heave or lift, which indicates increased cardiac output or left ventricular hypertrophy. Report to health care provider.*

g. If palpating PMI is difficult, turn patient onto left side.

Maneuver moves heart closer to chest wall.

h. Inspect epigastric area and palpate abdominal aorta.
NOTE: You should feel a localized strong beat.

Rules out reduced blood flow or diffuse pulse, which indicates abnormality.

i. Auscultate heart sounds:

(1) Have patient sit up and lean slightly forward; then have patient lie supine; and end examination with patient in left lateral recumbent position (see illustrations A–C). In female patient it may be necessary to lift left breast to hear heart sounds more effectively.

Different positions help to clearly hear heart sounds. Sitting position is best to hear high-pitched murmurs (if present). Supine is common position to hear all sounds. Left lateral recumbent is best position to hear low-pitched sounds.

(2) While auscultating sounds at each anatomical landmark, ask patient not to speak but to breathe comfortably. Begin with diaphragm of stethoscope; alternate with bell. Use light pressure for bell. Inch stethoscope along; avoid jumping from one area to another. Do not try to hear all heart sounds at once.

Auscultation requires you to isolate each heart sound at all auscultation sites, especially in patients with soft heart sounds.

(3) Begin at apex or PMI; move systematically to aortic area, pulmonic area, Erb's point, tricuspid area, and mitral area (see illustration in Step 3c). (**NOTE:** Some examiners use reverse sequence.) S_1 is loudest at apex and is simultaneous with carotid pulse.

At normal slow rates S_1 is high pitched and dull in quality and sounds like a "lub." This sound precedes systolic phase of heart contraction.

(4) Listen for S_2 at each site. This sound is loudest at the aortic area. Heart sounds vary by pitch, loudness, and duration, depending on auscultatory site (Table 6.7).

Normal sounds S_1 and S_2 are high pitched and best heard with diaphragm. S_2 precedes diastolic phase and sounds like "dub."

STEP		RATIONALE

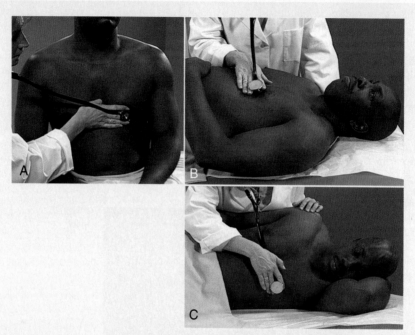

STEP 3i(1) Patient positions for auscultation of heart sounds. (A) Sitting. (B) Supine. (C) Left lateral. (*From Ball JW, et al: Seidel's guide to physical examination, ed 10, St Louis, 2023, Elsevier*).

TABLE 6.7

Heart Sounds According to Auscultatory Area

	Aortic	Pulmonic	Second Pulmonic	Mitral	Tricuspid
Pitch	$S_1 < S_2$	$S_1 < S_2$	$S_1 < S_2$	$S_1 > S_2$	$S_1 = S_2$
Loudness	$S_1 < S_2$	$S_1 < S_2$	$S_1 < S_2$[a]	$S_1 > S_2$[b]	$S_1 > S_2$
Duration	$S_1 > S_2$	$S_1 > S_2$	$S_1 > S_2$	$S_1 > S_2$	$S_1 > S_2$

[a]S_1 is relatively louder in second pulmonic area than in aortic area.
[b]S_1 may be louder in mitral area than in tricuspid area.
Adapted from Ball JW, et al: *Seidel's guide to physical examination*, ed 10, St Louis, 2023, Mosby.

(5) After both sounds are heard clearly as "lub-dub," count each combination of S_1 and S_2 as one heartbeat. Count number of beats for 1 minute.

Determines apical pulse rate.

(6) Assess heart rhythm by noting time between S_1 and S_2 (systole) and then time between S_2 and the next S_1 (diastole). Listen to full cycle at each auscultation area. Note regular intervals between each sequence of beats. There should be a distinct pause between S_1 and S_2.

Failure of heart to beat at regular intervals is a dysrhythmia (Table 6.8), which interferes with ability of heart to pump effectively.

(7) Assess for pulse deficit. When heart rate is irregular, compare apical and radial pulses. Auscultate apical pulse and then immediately palpate radial pulse. Also, you can ask a colleague to assess radial pulse while you simultaneously assess apical pulse. Difference in pulse rates is the pulse deficit.

Determines if pulse deficit (radial pulse is slower than apical) exists. Deficit indicates that ineffective contractions of heart fail to send pulse waves to periphery.

j. Auscultate for extra heart sounds at each site. Note pitch, loudness, duration, timing, location on chest wall, and where sound is heard in cardiac cycle.

Abnormal sounds include murmurs. Characteristics of murmurs help to identify contributing factors.

STEP		RATIONALE

TABLE 6.8

Abnormalities in Rates and Rhythms

Type	Findings	Description
Atrial fibrillation	Rapid, random contractions of atria cause irregular ventricular beats >100 beats/min and atrial beats at 200–350 beats/min.	Atria discharge rapidly, with some impulses not reaching ventricles. This condition occurs in rheumatic heart disease and mitral stenosis. It causes reduced cardiac output.
Sinus arrhythmia	Pulse rate changes during respiration, increasing at peak of inspiration and decreasing during expiration.	Blood is momentarily trapped in lungs during inspiration, causing a fall in stroke volume of heart.
Sinus bradycardia	Pulse rhythm is regular, but rate is <60 beats/min.	Sinoatrial node fires less frequently. This is common in well-conditioned athletes and with use of antiarrhythmic medications.
Sinus tachycardia	Pulse rhythm is regular, but rate is accelerated to >100 beats/min.	Exercise, emotional stress, and caffeine or alcohol ingestion are common factors that cause increased firing of sinoatrial node.
Premature ventricular contraction	Premature beat occurs before regularly expected heart contraction. Underlying rhythm can be any rate.	Ventricle contracts prematurely because of electrical impulse bypassing normal conduction pathway. It may occur so early that it is difficult to detect as second beat. It may be followed by a pause.

(1) Use stethoscope bell and listen for low-pitched extra heart sounds such as S_3 and S_4 gallops, clicks, and rubs. S_3, or a ventricular gallop, occurs just after S_2 at end of ventricular diastole. It sounds like "lub-dub-ee" or "Ken-tuc-ky." S_4, or an atrial gallop, occurs just before S_1 or ventricular systole. It sounds like "dee-lub-dub" or "Ten-nes-see."

4. Assess neck vessels:
   a. To assess carotid arteries, have patient remain in sitting position. Visualize position of artery (see illustration).
   b. Inspect neck on both sides for obvious arterial pulsations. Sometimes a pulse wave can be seen. *Option:* Use a penlight to improve visibility.
   c. Palpate each carotid artery separately with index and middle fingers around medial edge of sternocleidomastoid muscle. Ask patient to raise chin slightly, keeping head straight (see illustration) or slightly away from artery. Note rate and rhythm, strength, and elasticity of artery. Also note if pulse changes as patient inhales and exhales.

Premature rush of blood into a ventricle that is stiff or dilated or an atrial contraction pushing against a ventricle that is not accepting blood causes gallops.

Allows easier mobility of neck to expose artery for inspection and palpation.
Carotids are the only sites to assess quality of pulse wave. Experience is required to evaluate wave in relation to events of cardiac cycle.
If both arteries were occluded simultaneously, patient could lose consciousness from reduced circulation to brain. Turning head improves access to artery. A change indicates a sinus arrhythmia.

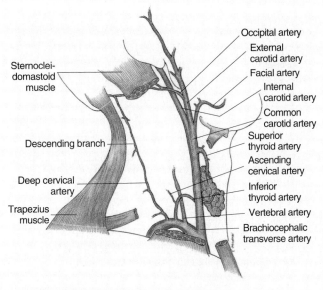

STEP 4a Anatomical position of carotid artery.

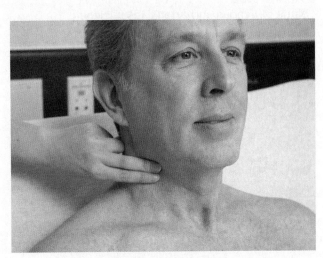

STEP 4c Palpate each carotid artery separately.

STEP	RATIONALE

Clinical Judgment *Do not palpate or massage the carotid artery vigorously. Stimulation of carotid sinus causes a reflex drop in heart rate and blood pressure. Never palpate both arteries simultaneously, as you could obstruct blood flow to the brain.*

d. Place bell of stethoscope over each carotid artery, auscultating for blowing sound (bruit) (see illustration). Ask patient to exhale and hold breath for a few heartbeats so that respiratory sounds do not interfere with auscultation (Ball et al., 2023).

Narrowing of lumen of carotid artery by arteriosclerotic plaques causes disturbance in blood flow. Blood passing through narrowed section creates turbulence and emits blowing or swishing sound. Normally you do not hear a bruit.

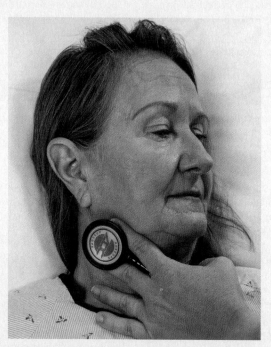

STEP 4d Auscultation for carotid artery bruit.

5. Peripheral vascular assessment:
a. Inspect lower extremities for changes in color and condition of skin (Table 6.9). Note skin and nail texture, hair distribution, venous patterns, edema, and scars or impaired skin integrity. Compare skin color with patient lying and standing.

Changes may reflect impaired peripheral circulation.

TABLE 6.9

Signs of Venous and Arterial Insufficiency

Assessment Criterion	Venous	Arterial
Pain	Aching; increases in evening and with dependent position	Burning, throbbing, cramping; increases with exercise
Paresthesia	None	Numbness, tingling, decreased sensation (most common in foot and toes)
Temperature	Normal to touch	Cool to touch
Color	Normal or cyanotic	Pale; worsened by elevation of extremity; dusky red when extremity is lowered
Capillary refill	Not applicable	>2 seconds (Ball et al., 2023)
Pulses	Present	Decreased or absent
Skin changes	Brown pigmentation around ankles	Thin, shiny skin; decreased hair growth; thickened nails
Ulcerations	Shallow ulcers around ankles (chronic venous stasis); edema apparent	Deep, well-defined at site of trauma or tips of toes

STEP	RATIONALE

b. Palpate edematous areas, noting mobility, consistency, and tenderness.

Helps to determine overall extent of edema.

c. Assess for pitting edema by pressing area firmly with one finger for 5 seconds and releasing. Depth of indentation determines severity (see illustration).
  2 mm: 1+ edema
  4 mm: 2+ edema
  6 mm: 3+ edema
  8 mm: 4+ edema

Limb edema is caused by right-sided heart failure (Ball et al., 2023). It is also classic sign of deep vein thrombosis (DVT), although this can be seen in other conditions; therefore, if DVT is suspected, diagnostic tests must be performed (Patel et al., 2019).

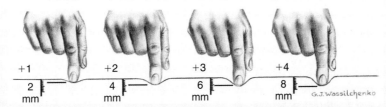

STEP 5c Assessing for pitting edema. (*From Ball JW, et al: Seidel's guide to physical examination, ed 9, St Louis, 2019, Mosby.*)

d. Use tape measure to measure circumference of leg.

Measuring circumference establishes baseline for future comparison. Development of edema, often a result of heart failure, will increase circumference.

e. Check capillary refill by grasping patient's fingernail or toenail and noting color of nail bed. Apply gentle, firm pressure to nail bed. Release quickly, watching for color change. Circulation is restored and normally returns to pink color in less than 2 seconds.

Capillary refill is measured in seconds; less than 2 seconds is brisk; greater than 4 seconds is sluggish.
Cold environmental temperature with vasoconstriction and vascular disease can delay refill. Local pressure from cast or bandage also slows refill.

f. Ask if patient experiences pain or tenderness and gently palpate for heat, firmness, or localized swelling of calf muscle, all of which are signs of phlebitis or DVT.

Three factors contribute to venous thrombus formation: (1) damage to a vessel wall, (2) alterations of blood flow, (3) alterations in blood constituents. The most frequent cause of a DVT is immobilization (e.g., following lengthy operative procedures, following an airplane flight lasting >8 hours).

Clinical Judgment *Homans sign (pain in calf on dorsiflexion of foot) is no longer considered a reliable indicator for the presence or absence of DVT (Ball et al., 2023) and is not a reliable test. If calf is swollen, tender, or red, notify patient's health care provider for further assessment and evaluation. If there is a strong suspicion of DVT, testing for Homans sign is contraindicated. If a clot is present, it may become dislodged from its original site during this test. This could result in a pulmonary embolism.*

g. Palpate peripheral arteries.
  (1) Start at most distal part of each extremity. Palpate each peripheral artery for equality, comparing side to side; elasticity of vessel wall (depress and release artery, noting ease with which it springs back to shape); and strength of pulse (force of blood against arterial wall), using the following rating scale (Ball et al., 2023):
  0   Absent, not palpable
  1+   Diminished, pulse barely palpable, weak and thready, and easy to obliterate
  2+   Normal pulse, easy to palpate
  3+   Full, easy to palpate, increases
  4+   Strong, bounding against fingertips; cannot be obliterated

Comparison of both arteries allows you to determine any localized obstruction or disturbance in blood flow. Pulses should be symmetrical side to side. If there is asymmetry, look for other factors related to impaired circulation.

  (2) Palpate radial pulse by lightly placing tips of first and second fingers in groove formed along radial side of forearm, lateral to flexor tendon of wrist (see illustration).

Pulse is relatively superficial and should not require deep palpation.

STEP	RATIONALE

(3) Palpate ulnar pulse by placing fingertips along ulnar side of forearm (see illustration).

Palpated when arterial insufficiency to hand is expected or when you assess for radial occlusion (e.g., during arterial blood gas sampling), which may affect circulation to hand.

(4) Palpate brachial pulse by locating groove between biceps and triceps muscles above elbow at antecubital fossa (see illustration). Place tips of first two fingers in muscle groove.

Artery runs along medial side of extended arm, requiring moderate palpation. If difficult to palpate, hyperextend arm to bring pulse site closer to the surface.

(5) Have patient lie supine with feet relaxed and palpate dorsalis pedis pulse. Gently place fingertips between great and first toe; slowly move fingers along groove between extensor tendons of great and first toe until pulse is palpable (see illustration).

Artery lies superficially and does not require deep palpation. Pulse may be congenitally absent.

(6) Palpate posterior tibial pulse by having patient relax and extend feet slightly. Place fingertips behind and below medial malleolus (ankle bone) (see illustration).

Artery is easily palpable with foot relaxed.

(7) Palpate popliteal pulse by having patient slightly flex knee with foot resting on table or bed. Instruct patient to keep leg muscles relaxed. Palpate deeply into popliteal fossa behind knee with fingers of both hands placed just lateral to midline. Patient may also lie prone to expose the artery (see illustration).

Flexion of knee and muscle relaxation improve accessibility of artery. Popliteal pulse is one of the more difficult pulses to palpate.

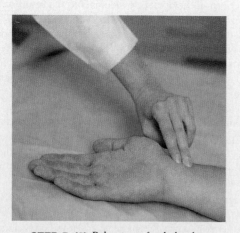

STEP 5g(2) Palpation of radial pulse.

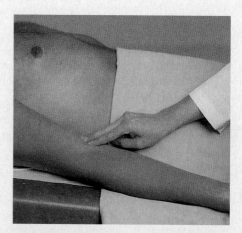

STEP 5g(4) Palpation of brachial pulse.

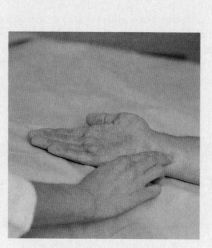

STEP 5g(3) Palpation of ulnar pulse.

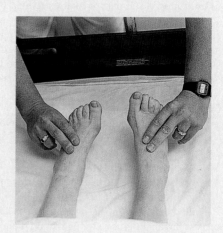

STEP 5g(5) Palpation of dorsalis pedis pulses.

STEP	RATIONALE

(8) Apply clean gloves. With patient supine, palpate femoral pulse by placing first two fingers over inguinal area below inguinal ligament, midway between pubic symphysis and anterosuperior iliac spine (see illustration).

Supine position prevents flexion in groin area, which interferes with artery access.

h. If pulses are difficult to palpate or are not palpable, use a Doppler instrument over pulse site:

(1) Apply conducting gel to patient's skin over pulse site or onto transducer tip of probe. Turn Doppler on.

Doppler amplifies sounds, allowing you to hear low-velocity blood flow through peripheral arteries.

(2) Gently apply ultrasound probe to skin, changing Doppler angle until pulsation is audible (see illustration). Adjust volume as needed. Wipe off gel from patient and Doppler.

Correct placement ensures good reception

6. Remove and discard gloves and used supplies in proper receptacle. Perform hand hygiene.

Reduces transmission of infection.

7. Proceed to next examination (Skill 6.5) or help patient to comfortable position.

Promotes patient comfort.

8. Place nurse call system in an accessible location within patient's reach.

Ensures patient can call for assistance if needed.

9. Raise side rails (as appropriate) and lower bed to lowest position, locking into position.

Ensures patient safety and prevents falls.

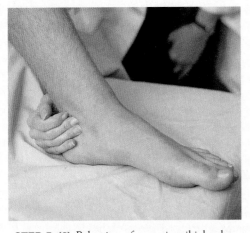

STEP 5g(6) Palpation of posterior tibial pulse.

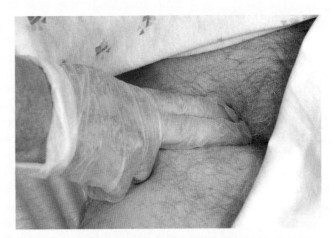

STEP 5g(8) Palpation of femoral pulse.

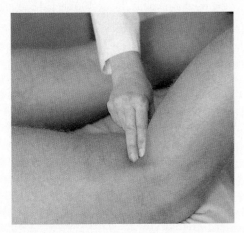

STEP 5g(7) Palpation of popliteal pulse with patient prone.

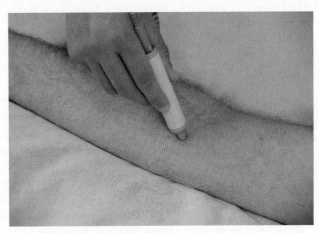

STEP 5h(2) Use of Doppler to assess brachial pulse.

STEP	RATIONALE

EVALUATION

1. Compare findings with normal assessment characteristics or previous assessments of heart and vascular system.

2. If heart sounds are not audible or pulses are not palpable, ask another nurse to confirm assessment.

3. Ask patient to describe own behaviors that increase risk for heart and vascular disease and how to adopt changes for better health.

4. Ask patient to describe schedule, dosage, purpose, and benefits of medications being taken for cardiovascular health.

5. **Use Teach-Back:** "I would like to make sure you understand some of the risks that can lead to heart disease and what can be done. Tell me how you think you can add exercise into your daily activities." Revise your instruction now or develop a plan for revised patient/family caregiver teaching if patient/family caregiver is not able to teach back correctly.

Determines presence of abnormalities or changes in patient's condition.
Validates assessment findings.

Demonstrates learning.

Demonstrates learning.

Teach-back is a technique for health care providers to ensure that medical information has been explained clearly so that patients and their families understand what is communicated to them (AHRQ, 2023).

Unexpected Outcomes	Related Interventions
1. Evaluation reveals: • Pulsations, vibrations, or both are palpable. These are the result of valvular problem, murmur, or both. • Extra heart sounds S_3 or S_4 are auscultated. Extra sounds indicate atrial or ventricular gallop.	• Prepare to obtain or assist with electrocardiogram (ECG). • Use communication techniques to keep patient calm. • Notify health care provider if this is a change in patient status.
2. Heart rate is irregular, with rate lower than 60 beats/min or higher than 100 beats/min.	• Check blood pressure. If low, dysrhythmia is contributing to inadequate cardiac output. • Observe for sensations or reports of dizziness or feeling "faint." • Notify health care provider. • Prepare to obtain ECG.
3. Decreased peripheral pulses noted. Potential sign of DVT.	• Recheck pulses using Doppler. • Notify health care provider. • Elevate extremity with decreased pulse.

Documentation

- Document quality (clear or muffled), intensity (weak or pounding), rate, and rhythm (regular, regularly irregular, or irregularly irregular) of heart sounds and quality and strength of peripheral pulses.
- Document additional cardiac findings, jugular vein distention, and condition of extremities.
- Document activity level and subjective data related to fatigue, shortness of breath, and chest pain.
- Document your evaluation of patient and family caregiver learning.

Hand-Off Reporting

- Report immediately to health care provider any irregularities in heart function and indications of impaired arterial blood flow.
- Report to health care provider changes in peripheral circulation, which may indicate circulatory compromise.

Special Considerations

Patient Education

- Explain risk factors for heart disease: high dietary intake of saturated fat or cholesterol, high blood cholesterol level, lack of regular exercise, smoking, obesity, excess alcohol intake, stressful lifestyle, hypertension, diabetes mellitus, and family history of heart disease (CDC, 2019).

- Refer patient (if appropriate) to resources available for controlling or reducing risks (e.g., nutrition counseling, exercise class, stress-reduction programs).
- Encourage patient to discuss with health care provider the need for periodic diagnostic testing (e.g., lipid panel, high-sensitivity C-reactive protein, natriuretic peptides) to assess CVD risk.
- Help patient find resources to help quit smoking because this lowers the risk for coronary heart disease and coronary vascular disease (ACS, 2023a). Nicotine in cigarette smoke causes vasoconstriction.
- Many health care providers continue to recommend a daily low dose of aspirin to prevent heart disease and DVT. However, the American Heart Association and American College of Cardiology have released guidelines, including that aspirin should be used infrequently in the routine primary prevention of atherosclerotic cardiovascular disease (ASCVD) because of lack of net benefit (Arnett et al., 2019). Patients should consult their health care provider about therapy.
- Atherosclerotic vascular changes can develop in childhood. Research has shown an accelerated burden of vascular changes and premature atherosclerosis among children and adolescents with well-established CVD risk factors (e.g., overweight/obesity, hypertension, dyslipidemia, smoke exposure) (Hartz & Ferranti, 2023). Parents should provide any child older than the age of 2 years with a heart healthy diet.

Pediatrics
- PMI is at fourth ICS at left midclavicular line in children younger than 7 years (Hockenberry et al., 2022).
- Capillary refill in infants is usually less than 1 second.
- It is not uncommon for children to have third heart sounds (S_3). Sinus arrhythmia occurs normally in many infants and children (Ball et al., 2023; Hockenberry et al., 2022). Continuous monitoring is recommended.
- Children have louder, higher-pitched heart sounds because of their thin chest walls.

Older Adults
- PMI may be difficult to find in an older adult because anteroposterior diameter of the chest deepens.
- Accidental massage of the carotid sinus during palpation of the carotid artery is a particular problem for older adults, causing a sudden drop in heart rate from vagal nerve stimulation.

- Older adults with hypertension benefit from regular monitoring of blood pressure (daily, weekly, or monthly). Home monitoring kits are available. Teach patient how to use them correctly.

Home Care
- The National Heart, Lung, and Blood Institute (2021) recommends the DASH eating plan to prevent CVD. Help patients in the home to adapt food preferences and meal preparation resources. The DASH eating plan (or DASH diet) requires no special foods and instead provides daily and weekly nutritional goals. This plan recommends:
  - Eating vegetables, fruits, and whole grains
  - Including fat-free or low-fat dairy products, fish, poultry, beans, nuts, and vegetable oils
  - Limiting foods that are high in saturated fat, such as fatty meats, full-fat dairy products, and tropical oils such as coconut, palm kernel, and palm oils
  - Limiting sugar-sweetened beverages and sweets

✦ SKILL 6.5 Abdominal Assessment

Abdominal assessment is complex because of the multiple organs located within and near the abdominal cavity. This area of the body is associated with many health complaints, but patients are also often reluctant to report problems because of being embarrassed by bowel or bladder dysfunction, reproductive problems, or urinary elimination problems. Abdominal pain is one of the most common symptoms that patients report when seeking medical care. It can be caused by alterations in organs, such as the stomach, gallbladder, kidneys, or intestines, or the pain may be the result of spinal or muscular injury. An accurate assessment requires matching the patient's history with a careful assessment of the location of physical symptoms (Table 6.10).

To perform an effective abdominal assessment, know the location and function of the underlying structures involved, including the lower pelvis, kidneys, rectum, genitalia, liver, gallbladder, stomach, spleen, appendix, pancreas, intestines, and reproductive organs (Fig. 6.5). An abdominal assessment is routine after abdominal surgery and for any patient who has undergone invasive diagnostic tests of the gastrointestinal (GI) tract to assess for the return of bowel function. It is also routine when patients present with abnormalities in GI function (e.g., diarrhea, constipation, cramping). The order of an abdominal assessment differs from that of other assessments. You begin with inspection and follow with auscultation. It is important to auscultate before percussion and then finally palpation because these maneuvers alter the frequency and character of bowel sounds (Mealie et al., 2022).

TABLE 6.10
Common Causes of Abdominal Pain

Condition	Physical Alteration	Physical Signs and Symptoms
Appendicitis	Obstruction of appendix associated with inflammation, perforation, and peritonitis. Patient often lies on back or side with knees flexed to decrease pain	Sharp pain directly over the irritated peritoneum 2–12 hours after onset. Often pain localizes in right lower quadrant between anterior iliac crest and umbilicus. Associated with rebound tenderness. Accompanied by anorexia, nausea, and vomiting.
Celiac disease	Damage to small intestine mucosa from ingestion of barley, rye, oats, and wheat	Foul-smelling diarrhea, abdominal distention, and symptoms of malnutrition may be present.
Cholecystitis	Obstruction of cystic duct causing inflammation or distention of gallbladder	*Murphy sign:* Apply gentle pressure below right subcostal arch and liver margin. Sharp pain and increased respiratory rate occur when patient takes a deep breath (Ball et al., 2023).
Constipation	Disruption in normal bowel pattern, which may occur with opioid use or inadequate fiber and fluid intake	Generalized discomfort accompanied by distention and palpation of a hard mass in the left lower quadrant. Nausea and vomiting may begin after several days.
Crohn disease	Chronic inflammatory disease of the ileum	Steady colicky pain in the right lower quadrant, with cramping, tenderness, flatulence, nausea, fever, and diarrhea. Often associated with bloody stools, weight loss, weakness, and fatigue. A tender mass of thickened intestine may be palpated in right lower quadrant.
Gastroenteritis	Inflammation of the stomach and intestinal tract	Generalized abdominal discomfort accompanied by anorexia, nausea, vomiting, diarrhea, abdominal cramping.

Continued

TABLE 6.10

Common Causes of Abdominal Pain–cont'd

Condition	Physical Alteration	Physical Signs and Symptoms
Pancreatitis	Inflammation of the pancreas associated with alcoholism, drug reaction, and gallbladder disease	Steady severe epigastric pain close to umbilicus radiates to back. Associated with abdominal rigidity and vomiting. Pain is unrelieved by vomiting, worsens by lying supine.
Paralytic ileus	Obstruction of the small bowel that occurs after abdominal surgery, from abdominal radiation, or from use of anticholinergic medications	Generalized severe abdominal distention, nausea, and vomiting; decreased/absent bowel sounds.
Peptic ulcers (gastric and duodenal)	Damage of gastrointestinal (GI) mucosa at any area of the GI tract May be caused by bacterial infection (*Helicobacter pylori*) or nonsteroidal antiinflammatory drugs (NSAIDs) Thought to be unrelated to stress Aggravated by smoking and excessive alcohol use Both caffeinated and decaffeinated coffee can increase acid production and worsen symptoms in individuals with ulcer disease (GI Society, 2022)	*Gastric ulcer:* Dull epigastric pain, localized midline. Early satiety; not usually relieved by food or antacids. *Duodenal ulcer:* Pain is episodic, lasting 30 minutes to 2 hours. It is located midline in epigastric region, may radiate around costal border to back; described as aching, burning, or gnawing. Typically occurs 1–3 hours after meals and at night (12 midnight to 3 a.m.). Often relieved by food/antacid. *Both (dyspepsia syndrome):* Complaints of fullness, epigastric discomfort, vague feeling of nausea, abdominal distention, and bloating; anorexia; weight loss.

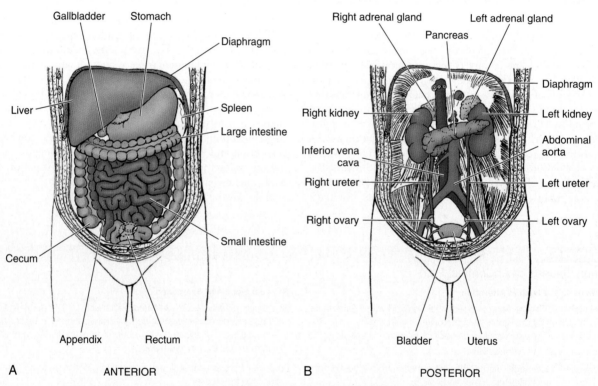

FIG. 6.5 Location of organs in abdomen. (A) Anterior. (B) Posterior. (*Adapted from* Mosby's expert 10-minute physical examinations, *ed 2, St. Louis, 2005, Mosby.*)

Delegation

The skill of abdominal assessment cannot be delegated to assistive personnel (AP). Direct the AP to:

• Report the development of abdominal pain and changes in the patient's bowel habits or dietary intake to the nurse.

Interprofessional Collaboration

• When assessment reveals changes in abdominal function or when assessments for specific pathophysiological changes reveal abnormal findings, communicate with the appropriate interprofessional team member, such as the health care provider, registered dietitian, urologist, ostomy nurse, or pain management team.

Equipment

• Stethoscope
• Tape measure
• Examination light
• Water-based marking pen

STEP	RATIONALE

ASSESSMENT

1. When beginning a physical examination with the abdominal examination, identify patient and determine patient's level of consciousness (LOC), health literacy, and primary language as outlined in Skill 6.1, Assessment, Steps 1, 4, 5, and 6. Otherwise, these assessments need not be repeated.

   Complies with The Joint Commission standards and improves patient safety (TJC, 2023).

2. Review EHR for family history of cancer, kidney disease, alcoholism, liver disease, hypertension, or heart disease.

   Information may reveal risk for significant abdominal alterations. For example, chronic alcohol ingestion causes GI and liver problems; heart failure can lead to abdominal bloating if severe.

3. Review patient's history for these risk factors: health care occupation, history of hemodialysis or intravenous (IV) drug use, household or sexual contact with hepatitis B virus (HBV) carrier, sexually active heterosexual person (more than one sex partner in previous 6 months), sexually active homosexual or bisexual man, international traveler in area of high HBV prevalence.

   These are risk factors for HBV exposure. Abdominal findings for hepatitis include jaundice, hepatomegaly, anorexia, abdominal and gastric discomfort, tea-colored urine, and clay-colored stools (Harding et al., 2021).

4. If patient has abdominal or low back pain, assess the character of pain in detail (see Chapter 16) (location, onset, frequency, precipitating factors, aggravating factors, type of pain, severity, course).

   Knowing pattern of characteristics of pain helps determine its source.

5. During the examination, carefully observe patient's movement and position such as lying still with knees drawn up, moving restlessly to find a comfortable position, or lying on one side or sitting with knees drawn up to chest.

   Positions assumed by patient reveal nature and source of pain (e.g., peritonitis, kidney stone, appendicitis). Patients with peritonitis lie still because movement aggravates pain. Supine position worsens acute pancreatitis pain; flexed knee, curved-back position brings relief. Patients with appendicitis lie on side or back with knees flexed in attempt to decrease muscle strain on abdominal wall.

6. Assess patient's normal bowel habits: frequency of stools; character of stools; recent changes in character of stools; measures used to promote elimination such as laxatives (including frequency), enemas, and dietary intake; and eating and drinking habits.

   Data compared with information from physical assessment may help identify cause and nature of elimination problems, allowing you to select appropriate nursing interventions. Overreliance on laxatives can cause GI problems.

7. Assess if patient has had recent weight changes or intolerance to diet (nausea, vomiting, cramping, especially in past week).

   Changes may indicate alterations in upper GI tract (e.g., stomach or gallbladder) or lower colon.

8. Assess for difficulty in swallowing, belching, flatulence, bloody emesis (hematemesis), black or tarry stools (melena), heartburn, diarrhea, or constipation.

   Indicative of GI alterations.

9. Ask if patient takes antiinflammatory medications (e.g., aspirin, steroids, nonsteroidal antiinflammatory drugs [NSAIDs]), iron supplements, or antibiotics.

   These medications may cause GI upset or bleeding. Iron can cause black-colored stools.

10. Assess patient's knowledge, prior experience with abdominal examination, and feelings about procedure.

    Reveals need for patient instruction and/or support.

PLANNING

1. Expected outcomes following completion of procedure:
   - Abdomen is soft and symmetrical, with smooth and even contour. No mass, distention, or tenderness is palpable. There are no forceful visible pulsations.

     These are normal abdominal assessment findings.

   - Bowel sounds are active and audible in all four quadrants.

     Indicates normal peristaltic activity.

   - Patient denies discomfort or worsening of existing discomfort following examination.

     Proper examination procedures have been implemented.

   - Patient describes personal risks and signs and symptoms of colorectal cancer.

     Instruction about colorectal cancer risks, signs, and symptoms may improve patient's health behavior habits.

2. Prepare patient by explaining how you will be completing routine examination of abdomen to check for areas of concern.

   Understanding promotes patient's cooperation.

STEP	RATIONALE
3. Anticipate topics during the examination that you can teach patient (e.g., warning signs of colorectal cancer, practices for promoting normal elimination, such as a high-fiber diet).	Allows you to incorporate instruction during physical assessment.
4. Ask if patient needs to empty bladder or defecate.	Palpation of full bladder causes discomfort and feeling of urgency and makes it difficult for patient to relax.
5. Perform hand hygiene. Prepare necessary supplies at bedside.	Reduces transmission of infection. Promotes efficient examination.
6. Close room curtains or door.	Provides patient privacy.
7. Help patient be as relaxed and comfortable as possible, using a calm tone of voice and purposeful actions. Be sure that room is warm.	Relaxation of abdomen allows you to conduct examination more successfully.
8. Position patient supine or in dorsal recumbent position with arms down at sides and knees slightly bent. *Option:* Place small pillow under patient's knees. Keep upper chest and legs draped.	Placing arms under head or keeping knees fully extended causes abdominal muscles to tighten. Tightening of muscles prevents adequate palpation. Draping maintains patient comfort and promotes relaxation.

IMPLEMENTATION

1. Move sheet or blanket to expose area from just above xiphoid process down to symphysis pubis.	Provides full visualization of abdomen.
2. Maintain conversation during assessment except during auscultation. Explain steps calmly and slowly.	Patient's ability to relax during assessment improves accuracy of findings. Talking interferes with hearing bowel sounds.
3. First ask patient to point to any tender areas of the abdomen.	*Assess painful areas last.* Manipulation of body part increases patient's pain and anxiety and makes remainder of assessment difficult to complete.
4. Begin with inspection and identify landmarks that divide abdominal region into quadrants. Boundary begins at tip of xiphoid process to symphysis pubis with line crossing and intersecting umbilicus, dividing abdomen into four equal sections (see illustration).	Location of findings by common reference point helps successive examiners confirm findings and locate abnormalities.
5. Inspect skin of surface of abdomen for color, scars, venous patterns, rashes, lesions, silvery white striae (stretch marks), and artificial openings (stomas). Observe skin lesions for characteristics described in Skill 6.1.	Scars reveal evidence that patient has had past trauma or surgery (especially if pigmented) (Mealie et al., 2022).). Striae indicate stretching of tissue from growth, obesity, pregnancy, ascites, or edema. Venous patterns reflect liver disease (portal hypertension). Artificial openings indicate bowel or urinary diversion (see Chapters 34 and 35).
6. If you note bruising of skin, ask if patient self-administers injections (e.g., heparin or insulin).	Frequent injections may cause bruising and hardening of underlying tissues.

Clinical Judgment *Bruising may also be a physical sign of abuse, accidental injury, or a bleeding disorder. When bruising is noted, additional information may be needed from the patient (see Skill 6.1).*

7. Inspect contour, symmetry, and surface motion of abdomen. Note any masses, bulging, or distention. (Flat abdomen forms a horizontal plane from xiphoid process to symphysis pubis. Round abdomen protrudes in convex sphere from horizontal plane. Concave abdomen sinks into muscular wall. All are normal.)	Changes in symmetry or contour reveal underlying masses, fluid collection, or gaseous distention. Everted umbilicus (protruding outward) indicates distention. Hernia also causes umbilicus to protrude upward.
8. If abdomen appears distended, note if distention is generalized. Look at flanks on each side.	Distention may be caused by the nine F's (*fat, flatus, feces, fluids, fibroid, full bladder, false pregnancy, fatal tumor, and fetus*) (Ball et al., 2023). If gas causes distention, flanks do not bulge. If fluid causes distention, flanks bulge. Tumors may cause more unilateral bulging or distention. Pregnancy causes symmetrical bulge in lower abdomen.
9. If you suspect distention, measure size of abdominal girth by placing tape measure under patient and around abdomen at level of umbilicus (see illustration). Use marking pen to indicate where tape measure was applied.	Consecutive measurements show any increase or decrease in abdominal distention. Make all subsequent measurements at same level of umbilicus to provide objective means to evaluate changes. Use water-based pen to make mark on abdomen for subsequent measurements.
10. If patient has an enteral tube connected to suction, turn off momentarily to check bowel sounds.	Sound of suction obscures bowel sounds.

STEP	RATIONALE

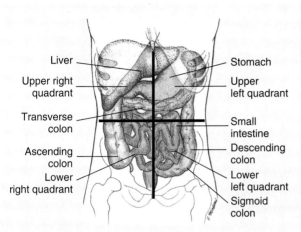

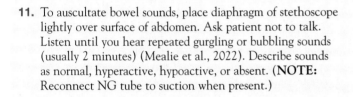

STEP 4 Division of abdomen into quadrants.

Labels: Liver; Upper right quadrant; Transverse colon; Ascending colon; Lower right quadrant; Stomach; Upper left quadrant; Small intestine; Descending colon; Lower left quadrant; Sigmoid colon

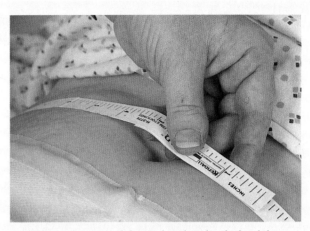

STEP 9 Measuring abdominal girth at level of umbilicus.

11. To auscultate bowel sounds, place diaphragm of stethoscope lightly over surface of abdomen. Ask patient not to talk. Listen until you hear repeated gurgling or bubbling sounds (usually 2 minutes) (Mealie et al., 2022). Describe sounds as normal, hyperactive, hypoactive, or absent. (**NOTE:** Reconnect NG tube to suction when present.)

Auscultation in all four quadrants is traditional but may be excessive because bowel sounds are readily transmitted throughout the abdomen (Mealie et al., 2022).

Normal bowel sounds occur irregularly every 5 to 15 seconds. Hypoactive bowel sounds are normal during sleep. However, hypoactive or absent sounds indicate slowing or cessation of gastric motility. Hyperactive bowel sounds mean there is an increase in intestinal activity, often due to diarrhea or after eating. Hyperactive bowel sounds may also indicate early intestinal obstruction or ileus. Always assess abdominal sounds together with symptoms such as gas, nausea, presence or absence of bowel movements and vomiting (MedLine Plus, 2020).

It is common for bowel sounds to be hypoactive after surgery for 24 hours or more, especially following abdominal surgery.

Clinical Judgment *Nausea and vomiting, increasing distention, and inability to pass flatus may accompany severe paralytic ileus.*

12. Place bell of stethoscope over epigastric region of abdomen and each quadrant. Auscultate for vascular (whooshing) sounds.

Determines presence of turbulent blood flow (bruit) through thoracic or abdominal aorta, which may indicate an aneurysm.

Clinical Judgment *If aortic bruit is auscultated, suggesting presence of an aneurysm, stop assessment and notify health care provider immediately. Percussion or palpation over abdominal bruit could rupture an already weakened vessel wall in the presence of an abdominal aneurysm.*

14. The next step of an abdominal examination is routinely percussion. Advanced practice nurses learn to percuss the four quadrants for presence of masses or fluid.

Technique helps reveal nature of abdominal distention (e.g., ascites, bloating). Tightness, for example, is not felt with obesity.

15. Lightly palpate over each abdominal quadrant, laying palm of hand with fingers extended and approximated lightly on abdomen. Keep palm and forearm horizontal. Pads of fingertips depress skin no more than 1 cm (½ inch) in gentle dipping motion. Palpate painful areas last. If you sense presence of an obvious mass, gently apply deep palpation.

Detects areas of localized tenderness, degree of tenderness, and presence and character of underlying masses or fluid. Palpation of sensitive area causes guarding (voluntary tightening of underlying abdominal muscles).

   a. Note muscular resistance, distention, tenderness, and superficial masses or organs while observing patient's face for signs of discomfort.

Patient's verbal and nonverbal cues may indicate discomfort from tenderness. Firm abdomen indicates active obstruction with buildup of fluid or gas.

   b. Note if abdomen is firm or soft to touch.

Soft abdomen is normal or reveals that obstruction is resolving.

16. Just below umbilicus and above symphysis pubis, palpate for smooth, rounded mass. While applying light pressure, ask if patient has sensation of need to void.

Detects presence of dome of distended bladder.

Clinical Judgment *Routinely check for distended bladder if patient has been unable to void, patient has been incontinent, or an indwelling Foley catheter is not draining well or has been removed recently.*

STEP	RATIONALE

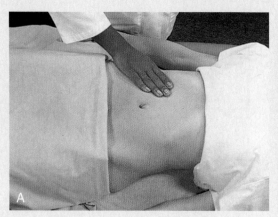 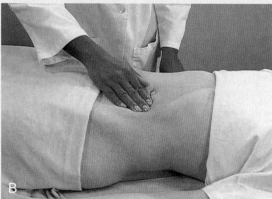

STEP 15 (A) Light palpation of abdomen. (B) Deep palpation of abdomen. (*From Ball JW, et al: Seidel's guide to physical examination, ed 10, St Louis, 2023, Elsevier.*)

17. If masses are palpated, note size, location, shape, consistency, tenderness, mobility, and texture.	Descriptive characteristics help to reveal type of mass.
18. Discard used supplies in proper receptacle. Perform hand hygiene.	Reduces transmission of infection.
19. Proceed to next examination (Skill 6.6) or help patient to comfortable position.	Promotes patient comfort.
20. Place nurse call system in an accessible location within patient's reach.	Ensures patient can call for assistance if needed.
21. Raise side rails (as appropriate) and lower bed to lowest position, locking into position.	Ensures patient safety and prevents falls.

EVALUATION

1. Compare assessment findings with previous assessment characteristics or normal findings to identify changes.	Determines presence of abnormalities or change in patient's condition.
2. Ask patient to describe own risks and signs and symptoms of colorectal cancer.	Demonstrates learning.
3. **Use Teach-Back:** "I would like to make sure that you understand the signs and symptoms of colorectal cancer. Tell me three changes in your bowel habits that might be signs of colorectal cancer." Revise your instruction now or develop a plan for revised patient/family caregiver teaching if patient/family caregiver is not able to teach back correctly.	Teach-back is a technique for health care providers to ensure that medical information has been explained clearly so that patients and their families understand what is communicated to them (AHRQ, 2023).

Unexpected Outcomes	Related Interventions
1. Abdomen protrudes symmetrically with skin taut; patient complains of tightness, and/or bowel sounds are hypoactive or absent. GI motility has ceased. Patient is vomiting. Signs suggest an obstruction.	• Keep patient on nothing by mouth (NPO) status. • Notify health care provider. • Encourage ambulation/activity as ordered. • Gastric decompression following insertion of NG tube sometimes may be necessary (see Chapter 34).
2. Hyperactive bowel sounds are evident with GI motility, often due to anxiety, diarrhea, overuse of laxatives, bowel inflammation, or reaction of intestines to certain foods.	• Patient may need to be NPO. • Contact health care provider. • Consult with registered dietitian if problem is dietary
3. Bladder is palpable over symphysis pubis and distended.	• Facilitate voiding by placing patient in sitting position or encourage to bear down (if not contraindicated); run water within hearing distance or have patient place hand in basin of warm water. • Use bladder scan to determine extent of bladder fullness (see Chapter 33). • If unable to void, urinary catheterization may be necessary (see Chapter 33). Contact health care provider for order.

Documentation

- Document appearance of abdomen, quality and location of bowel sounds, presence of distention, abdominal circumference, and presence and location of tenderness.
- Document patient's ability to void and defecate, including description of output.
- Document evaluation of patient and family caregiver learning.

Hand-Off Reporting

- Report serious abnormalities such as absent bowel sounds, presence of a mass, or acute pain to nurse in charge and health care provider.

Special Considerations

Patient Education

- Explain that factors such as diet, regular exercise, establishment of regular elimination schedule, and adequate fluid intake promote normal bowel elimination.
- If patient is a health care worker or has contact with blood or body fluids of affected people, encourage patient to receive series of three HBV vaccine doses.

Pediatrics

- The most common palpable abdominal mass in a child is feces, usually palpated in right lower quadrant (Hockenberry et al., 2022).
- Have a child stand erect and then lie supine during inspection of abdominal surface. Normal abdomen of infants and young children is cylindrical in erect position and flat in supine position. School-age children may have a rounded abdomen until 13 years of age when standing.
- In infants and children, skin of abdomen is usually taut and without wrinkles or creases.
- Infants and children until the age of 7 years are abdominal breathers.
- Some children perceive superficial palpation as tickling. Drawing attention to their laughter only causes it to increase. Have the children help by placing a hand on top of yours or on the abdomen with fingers separated and then palpate between fingers.

Older Adults

- Older adults often lack abdominal tone; underlying organs are more easily palpable.
- Constipation along with nausea, flatulence, and heartburn is common.
- Stress to older adults the importance of adequate fluid intake; regular exercise (see Chapter 12); and a diet with at least four servings daily of fresh fruit, vegetables, and high-fiber food to promote normal defecation.

Populations With Disabilities

- A patient with an intellectual or developmental disability (IDD) might have difficulty relaxing the abdomen.

✦ SKILL 6.6   Genitalia and Rectum Assessment

The best time to examine a patient's external genitalia is while performing routine hygiene measures or preparing to insert or care for a urinary catheter. An examination of female and male external genitalia is part of preventive health screenings. Male patients need to learn how to perform self-examinations of the genitalia to detect testicular cancer (ACS, 2018) (Box 6.5). You examine adolescents and young adults because of the growing incidence of sexually transmitted infections (STIs). The average age of menarche among girls has declined, and most male and female teenagers are sexually active by age 19 (Hockenberry et al., 2022). You can easily combine rectal and anal assessments with this examination because the patient assumes a lithotomy or dorsal recumbent position.

Delegation

The skill of assessing the genitalia and rectum cannot be delegated to assistive personnel (AP). Direct the AP to:
- Report presence of drainage in the perineal area or anus.
- Report if patient complains of difficulty voiding or pain in urethral or genital area.

BOX 6.5

Testicular Self-Examination

A testicular self-examination helps patients learn how their testicles normally look and feel so that an individual is more likely to notice subtle changes (Mayo Clinic, 2022). Although rare, testicular cancer appears as a lump on the testicle (first common symptom), or the testicle might be swollen or larger than normal (ACS, 2018). Most physicians recommend monthly testicular exams after puberty begins (ACS, 2018). Have patients call their health care providers if a lump or any other abnormality is found.

Genital Examination

1. Have patient perform the examination after a warm bath or shower when the scrotal sac is relaxed.
2. Have patient stand naked in front of a mirror: hold the penis in your hand out of the way and look for swelling of the scrotum. Then examine the head of the penis. Pull back the foreskin if uncircumcised to expose the glans.
3. Examine each testicle by using both hands, placing your index and middle fingers under the testicle and your thumbs on top. Gently roll each testicle between thumbs and fingers (see illustration).

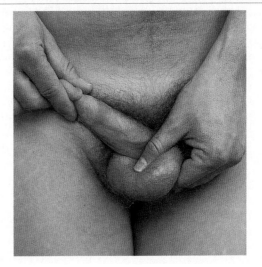

Continued

BOX 6.5

Testicular Self-Examination—cont'd

4. Observe and palpate the entire head of the penis in a clockwise motion, looking carefully for any bumps, sores, blisters or genital warts.
5. Feel for small, pea-size lumps on the front and side of the testicle. The lumps are usually painless and are abnormal.
6. Look at the opening (urethral meatus) at the end of the penis for discharge (see illustration).

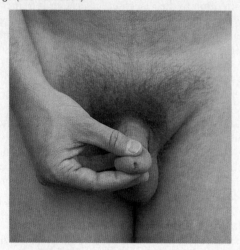

7. Look along the entire shaft of the penis for the same signs.
8. Separate pubic hair at the base of the penis and carefully examine the skin underneath.
9. Instruct patient to call the health care provider if abnormalities are noted.
10. **Use Teach-Back:** "I want to be sure I explained to you how to do a genital and testicular self-examination. Describe for me the steps you will follow to do a testicular self-exam." Document your evaluation of patient learning. Revise your instruction now or develop a plan for revised patient teaching if patient is not able to teach back correctly.

Data from American Cancer Society (ACS). Can testicular cancer be found early? Atlanta, 2018. https://www.cancer.org/cancer/testicular-cancer/detection-diagnosis-staging/detection.html. Accessed November 17, 2023; Mayo Clinic, Testicular Exam, 2022. https://www.mayoclinic.org/tests-procedures/testicular-exam/about/pac-20385252. Accessed November 17, 2023.
Illustrations from Ball JW, et al: *Seidel's guide to physical examination*, ed 10, St. Louis, 2023, Mosby.

Interprofessional Collaboration

- When assessment reveals changes in genitourinary (GU) function or when assessments for specific pathophysiological changes reveal abnormal findings, communicate with the appropriate interprofessional team member, such as the health care provider.

Equipment

- Examination light
- Clean gloves (use nonlatex if necessary)

STEP	RATIONALE

ASSESSMENT

1. When beginning a physical examination with a genital and rectal examination, identify patient and determine patient's level of consciousness (LOC), primary language, and health literacy as outlined in Skill 6.1, Assessment, Steps 1, 4, 5, and 6. Otherwise, these assessments need not be repeated.

Complies with The Joint Commission standards and improves patient safety (TJC, 2023).

2. Assessment of female patients:
   a. Review EHR or ask if patient has signs and symptoms of vaginal discharge, painful or swollen perianal tissues, or genital lesions.

   These signs and symptoms are consistent with an STI or other pathological condition.

   b. Review electronic health record (EHR) for symptoms or history of GU problems, including burning during urination (dysuria), frequency, urgency, nocturia, hematuria, or incontinence.

   Urinary problems are associated with gynecological disorders, including STIs.

   c. Ask if the patient has had signs of bleeding outside of normal menstrual cycle or after menopause or unusual vaginal discharge.

   These are warning signs for cervical and endometrial cancer or vaginal infection.

STEP	RATIONALE
d. Determine if patient has history of HPV; suspect persons who begin having sex at an early age or have had many sexual partners, although infection can occur with only one sexual partner. Several factors known to increase the risk of both persistent HPV infection and progression to cancer include a suppressed immune system, a high number of childbirths, and cigarette smoking.	These are risk factors for cervical cancer and can affect screening recommendations (ACS, 2022).
e. Review electronic health record (EHR) to determine if patient is older than 63; has a family history of breast or ovarian cancer; is obese; has personal history of breast cancer, endometriosis, or pelvic inflammatory disease; and is of tall adult height. Modifiable factors associated with increased risk include menopausal hormone therapy (previously referred to as hormone replacement therapy or HRT).	These are risk factors for ovarian cancer (ACS, 2022).
f. Determine if patient has excess body weight and insufficient physical activity. Other factors that increase estrogen exposure include the use of postmenopausal estrogen alone (continuous estrogen plus progestin does not appear to increase risk), late menopause, type 2 diabetes, and a history of polycystic ovary syndrome.	These are risk factors for endometrial cancer (ACS, 2022). Most (70%) endometrial cancers are attributed to excess body weight and insufficient physical activity and are thus preventable (ACS, 2022). Obesity and abdominal fatness each substantially increase the risk of uterine cancer, partly by increasing the amount of circulating estrogen, which is a strong risk factor.
g. Assess patient's knowledge, prior experience with risk factors and signs of cervical and other gynecological cancers, and feelings about procedure.	Reveals need for patient instruction and/or support.
3. Assessment of male patients:	
a. Review normal elimination pattern, including frequency of voiding; history of nocturia; character and volume of urine; daily fluid intake; symptoms of burning, urgency, and frequency; difficulty starting stream; and hematuria.	Urinary problems are directly associated with genital problems because of anatomical structure of men's reproductive and urinary systems.
b. Ask if patient has noted penile pain or swelling, genital lesions, or urethral discharge.	These are signs and symptoms of STIs.
c. Ask if patient has noted heaviness, painless enlargement, or irregular lumps of testis, and if testicular self-examination is performed regularly.	These signs and symptoms are early warning signs for testicular cancer. Determines need for education.
d. Ask if patient has noticed an enlargement in inguinal area and assess if intermittent or constant, associated with straining or lifting, and painful. Does coughing, lifting, or straining at stool cause pain?	Signs and symptoms indicate potential inguinal hernia.
e. Review electronic health record (EHR) to assess patient's age (risk increases with age), racial ancestry, and family history of prostatic cancer.	Risk factors for prostatic cancer (ACS, 2022). Black men in the United States and Caribbean have the highest documented prostate cancer incidence rates in the world (ACS, 2022).
f. Ask if patient has experienced weak or interrupted urine flow; difficulty starting or stopping urination; frequent urination, especially at night; blood in the urine; or pain or burning with urination. Assess if patient has continuing pain in lower back, pelvis, or upper thighs.	These are warning signs of advanced prostate cancer (ACS, 2022) and benign prostatic hypertrophy (BPH). Early-stage prostate cancer usually causes no symptoms.
g. Assess patient's knowledge of examination, risk factors, signs of BPH, and prostate and testicular cancer, as well as feelings about procedure.	Reveals need for patient instruction and/or support.
4. Assessment of all patients:	
a. Determine if patient has received human papillomavirus (HPV) vaccine.	The CDC (2021a) recommends routine HPV vaccination at 11 or 12 years of age for all children. Also recommends vaccination for everyone through age 26 years if not adequately vaccinated when younger. HPV vaccination is given as a series of either 2 or 3 doses, depending on age at initial vaccination. HPV vaccine not recommended for everyone older than age 26 years, as vaccine found to be less effective and most individuals already exposed to virus.

STEP	RATIONALE
b. Does patient have a history of rectal bleeding, black or tarry stools (melena), rectal pain, changes in bowel habits (constipation or diarrhea) or stool shape, abdominal cramping, decreased appetite and weight loss (unplanned)?	These are warning signs of colorectal cancer (ACS, 2022) and other gastrointestinal (GI) alterations.
c. Determine whether patient has strong family history of colorectal cancer, polyps, or chronic inflammatory bowel disease. Is patient's age older than 50? Is patient overweight, physically inactive, a long-term smoker, or high consumer of red or processed meat and alcohol? Does patient have a low calcium intake?	These are risk factors for colorectal cancer (ACS, 2022). More than half (55%) of colorectal cancers in the United States are attributable to potentially modifiable risk factors and thus preventable (ACS, 2022).
d. Inquire about dietary habits, including high fat intake, diet high in processed meats, or deficient fiber content (inadequate fruits and vegetables).	Colon cancer is often linked to diet high in fats and processed meats and low in fiber (ACS, 2022).
e. Assess medication history for use of laxatives or cathartic medications. Does patient have bloating, cramping, diarrhea or constipation (following use of laxative), thirst, or nausea?	Repeated use causes diarrhea and eventual loss of intestinal muscle tone (Frothingham, 2019).
f. Does patient routinely take codeine or iron preparations?	Codeine causes constipation. Iron turns stool black and tarry.
g. Assess patient's knowledge of risks and signs of colorectal cancer.	Provides baseline for patient education.
5. Assess patient's knowledge, prior experience with genital/ rectal examination, and feelings about procedure.	Reveals need for patient instruction and/or support.

PLANNING

1. Expected outcomes following completion of procedure:	
• Patient denies discomfort or worsening of existing discomfort following examination.	Proper examination procedures have been implemented.
• Patient is able to list warning signs of colorectal cancer: female patient—cervical, endometrial, and ovarian cancer; male patient—testicular and prostate cancer.	Demonstrates learning.
• Patient is able to discuss guidelines for HPV immunization.	Demonstrates learning.
• Male patient is able to perform genital self-examination.	Demonstrates learning.
2. Anticipate topics you can teach patient during examination (e.g., warning signs of rectal cancer or genital cancer).	Prepares you for incorporating teaching into assessment activities.
3. Ask if patient needs to empty bladder or defecate.	Promotes comfort during examination.
4. Perform hand hygiene. Prepare necessary supplies at bedside.	Reduces transmission of infection. Promotes efficient examination.
5. Close room curtains or door.	Provides patient privacy.
6. Keep upper chest and legs draped and keep room warm.	Maintains patient's comfort during examination, promoting relaxation.
7. Position patient:	
a. Female should lie in dorsal recumbent position with arms down at sides and knees slightly bent. Place small pillow under the knees.	Placing arms under head or keeping knees fully extended causes tightening of abdominal muscles.
b. Male should lie supine with chest, abdomen, and lower legs draped; or have him stand during examination.	

IMPLEMENTATION

1. Perform hand hygiene and apply clean gloves.	Prevents transmission of microorganisms.
2. Female genitalia examination. (Use this time to discuss woman's risk for STIs and signs and symptoms of cervical, ovarian, and endometrial cancers.)	

Clinical Judgment *The examination of genitalia can be a traumatic and anxiety-inducing procedure for transgender men and other transmasculine persons. Allow patient to have a support person in the room (Schneider & Chung, 2022).*

a. Expose perineal area, repositioning sheet as needed.	
b. Inspect surface characteristics of perineum and retract labia majora; observe for inflammation, edema, lesions, or lacerations. Note if there is any vaginal discharge. Presence of discharge may indicate need for a culture specimen (see Chapter 7).	Skin of perineum is smooth, clean, and slightly darker than other skin. Mucous membranes are dark pink and moist. Labia majora are symmetrical; may be dry or moist. Normally there is no vaginal discharge.

STEP	RATIONALE
3. Male genitalia examination. (Use this time to discuss man's risk for STIs and signs and symptoms of testicular cancer.)	
a. Expose perineal area. Observe genitalia for rashes, excoriations, or lesions.	Normally skin is clear without lesions.
b. Inspect and palpate penile surfaces (see also Box 6.5).	
(1) Inspect corona, prepuce (foreskin), glans, urethral meatus, and shaft. Retract foreskin in uncircumcised males. Observe for discharge, lesions, edema, and inflammation. Return foreskin to normal position.	Glans should be smooth and pink along all surfaces. Urethral meatus is slitlike and normally positioned at tip of glans. Foreskin should retract easily. Area between foreskin and glans is common site for venereal lesions.
c. Inspect and palpate testicular surfaces.	
(1) Inspect size, color, shape, and symmetry; note any lesions or swelling.	Left testicle is normally lower than right. Scrotal skin is usually loose, surface is coarse, and skin color is more deeply pigmented than body skin.
d. Palpate testes (see also Box 6.5). Use pads of fingers and thumbs to gently palpate tissue.	
(1) Note size, shape, and consistency of tissue. Most common symptom of testicular cancer is irregular, nontender fixed mass.	Testes are normally ovoid and approximately 2 to 4 cm (0.8–1.6 inches) in size, feel smooth and rubbery, and are free from nodules.
(2) Ask if patient experiences tenderness with palpation.	Testes are normally sensitive but not tender.
4. Assess rectum.	
a. Female patient remains in dorsal recumbent position or assumes side-lying (left lateral) position.	These positions allow for optimum visualization of the rectum.
b. Male patient stands and bends forward with hips flexed and upper body resting across examination table; examine nonambulatory patient lying in bed in left lateral position with hips and knees flexed (Ball et al., 2023).	

Clinical Judgment *Examine a patient in the position congruent with their identified gender, considering comfort and anatomy (Ball et al., 2023).*

STEP	RATIONALE
c. View perianal and sacrococcygeal areas by gently retracting buttocks with your nondominant hand.	Perianal skin is smooth, more pigmented, and coarser than skin covering buttocks.
d. Inspect anal tissue for skin characteristics, lesions, external hemorrhoids (dilated veins that appear as reddened skin protrusion), inflammation, rashes, and excoriation.	Anal tissues are moist and hairless; voluntary sphincter holds anus closed.
4. Remove and discard gloves and used supplies in proper receptacle. Perform hand hygiene.	Reduces transmission of infection.
5. Proceed to next examination (Skill 6.7) or help patient to comfortable position.	Promotes patient comfort.
6. Place nurse call system in an accessible location within patient's reach.	Ensures patient can call for assistance if needed.
7. Raise side rails (as appropriate) and lower bed to lowest position, locking into position.	Ensures patient safety and prevents falls.

EVALUATION

1. Compare assessment findings with previous assessment characteristics or normal findings to identify changes.	Determines presence of abnormalities or changes in patient's condition.
2. Ask patient to list warning signs of colorectal cancer: female patient: cervical, endometrial, and ovarian cancer; male patient: testicular and prostate cancer.	Demonstrates learning.
3. Ask male patient to explain how to perform self-examination of genitalia.	Demonstrates learning.
4. Ask patient to identify guidelines for HPV vaccination.	Demonstrates learning.
5. **Use Teach-Back:** "I would like to make sure that you understand the warning signs of (colorectal/ovarian/testicular/prostate) cancer. First, tell me some of the signs and symptoms of _____ cancer." Revise your instruction now or develop a plan for revised patient/family caregiver teaching if patient/family caregiver is not able to teach back correctly.	Teach-back is a technique for health care providers to ensure that medical information has been explained clearly so that patients and their families understand what is communicated to them (AHRQ, 2023).

STEP	RATIONALE
Unexpected Outcomes 1. Patient has vaginal/penile drainage and burning sensation during voiding. Women may have vaginal bleeding between menstrual periods. Symptoms may suggest STI.	**Related Interventions** • Notify health care provider. • Prepare to collect a culture specimen of the discharge. • Provide additional education.

Documentation

• Document appearance of genitalia, presence and description of any discharge, and any abnormal findings.
• Document patient's ability to void, including description of output.
• Document evaluation of patient learning.

Hand-Off Reporting

• Report any abnormalities such as presence of a mass or acute pain to nurse in charge and health care provider.

Special Considerations

Patient Education

• Tell patients with an STI to inform their sexual partners of the need to have an examination. Instruct patient to seek treatment as soon as possible if partner becomes infected with an STI.
• Discuss early detection of colorectal cancer. The USPSTF (2021) and ACS recommend screening for colorectal cancer for patients at average risk beginning at age 45 and up to 75 years of age. Evidence is strong to support screening in these age groups. Screening may include stool-based tests or visual examination of colon/rectum (e.g., colonoscopy). The USPSTF recommends for adults aged 76 to 85 years that clinicians selectively offer screening. Evidence indicates that the net benefit of screening all persons in this age group is small. It is important to consider the patient's overall health, prior screening history, and preferences (USPSTF, 2021). Patients at higher risk for colorectal cancer: personal history of colorectal cancer or certain types of polyps, family history of colorectal cancer, personal history of inflammatory bowel disease, confirmed or suspected hereditary colorectal cancer syndrome, personal history of getting radiation to the abdomen or pelvic area to treat a prior cancer (USPSTF, 2021).

Male Health Teaching

• The ACS recommends that beginning at age 50, men who are at average risk of prostate cancer and have a life expectancy of at least 10 years discuss with their health care provider the benefits and limitations of PSA testing and make an informed decision about whether to be tested. Black men and those with a close relative diagnosed with prostate cancer before the age of

65 should have this discussion beginning at age 45 (ACS, 2022).
• Explain warning signs of STIs: pain on urination and during sex, abnormal penile discharge, swollen lymph nodes, or rash or ulcer on skin or genitalia.
• Teach measures to prevent STIs: use of condoms, avoiding sex with infected partner, avoiding sex with people who have multiple partners, and using regular perineal hygiene.
• Teach patient how to perform genital self-examination (see Box 6.5).
• Discuss dietary planning and healthy lifestyle choices to maintain or improve colon health.

Female Health Teaching

• Teach patient about purpose and recommended frequency of Papanicolaou (Pap) smears and gynecological examinations. ACS recommends cervical cancer screening with an HPV test alone every 5 years for everyone with a cervix from age 25 until age 65 (NCI, 2020). If HPV testing alone is not available, people can get screened with an HPV/Pap cotest every 5 years or a Pap test every 3 years (NCI, 2020). For women older than 65, no screening is required if previous tests were normal (NCI, 2020).
• Explain warning signs of STIs: pain or burning on urination, pain during sex, pain in pelvic area, bleeding between menstruation, itchy rash around vagina, and abnormal vaginal discharge.
• Teach measures to prevent STIs (e.g., male partner's use of condoms, restricting number of sexual partners, avoiding sex with people who have several other partners, perineal hygiene measures).
• Reinforce the importance of performing perineal hygiene (as appropriate).

Pediatrics

• When examining the testes in a male infant, avoid stimulating the cremasteric reflex, which causes the testes to pull higher into the pelvic cavity.

Older Adults

• The decision to screen for colorectal cancer in adults aged 76 to 85 years should be an individual one.

✦ SKILL 6.7   Musculoskeletal and Neurological Assessment

A person's musculoskeletal and neurological status have a significant influence on the ability to perform daily activities, remain active, and be cognitively alert and involved. Much of this examination is performed when assessing other body systems and you suspect problems. During the general survey, you inspect gait, posture, and body position. The head and neck assessment may reveal possible neurological alterations. For example, while assessing head

and neck structures, assess neck ROM and examine select cranial nerves (CNs). A more thorough assessment of major bone, joint, and muscle groups and sensory, motor, and CN function is indicated in the presence of abnormalities. Use the skills of inspection and palpation during the musculoskeletal and neurological assessment. Integrate assessment into routine activities of care (e.g., while bathing or positioning the patient). Assessment of the musculoskeletal and neurological systems is important when a patient reports pain, loss of sensation, impairment of muscle function, or change in cognitive status (neurological). Prolonged illness or immobility may result in muscle weakness and atrophy. Neurological assessment is often conducted simultaneously because muscles may be weakened as a result of nerve involvement.

Delegation

The skill of assessing musculoskeletal and neurological function cannot be delegated to assistive personnel (AP). Direct the AP to:

- Report patients' problems with gait, balance, ROM, and muscle strength.
- Be informed of patients who are at risk for falls (e.g., unsteady gait, foot dragging).
- Help patients with muscular weakness with transfer and ambulation.

- Report any cognitive changes (e.g., loss of recent memory, inappropriate response to questions).

Interprofessional Collaboration

- When assessment reveals changes in musculoskeletal and neurological function or when assessments for specific pathophysiological changes reveal abnormal findings, communicate with the appropriate interprofessional team member such as the health care provider or physical therapist.

Equipment

- Cotton balls or cotton-tipped applicators
- Penlight
- Tape measure
- Tongue blade
- Tuning fork
- Reflex hammer

STEP	RATIONALE

ASSESSMENT

1. When beginning a physical examination with a musculoskeletal or neurological examination, identify patient and determine patient's level of consciousness (LOC), health literacy, and primary language as outlined in Skill 6.1, Assessment, Steps 1, 4, 5, and 6. Otherwise, these assessments need not be repeated.

Complies with The Joint Commission standards and improves patient safety (TJC, 2023).

2. Assess EHR for history of inadequate intake of calcium and vitamin D and not eating enough fruits and vegetables; excess intake of protein, sodium, and caffeine; inactive lifestyle; smoking; excess alcohol intake; losing weight.

These are modifiable risk factors for osteoporosis (Bone Health and Osteoporosis Foundation, 2023).

Also review EHR for age older than 50, female, menopause, family history of osteoporosis, low body weight/being small and thin, broken bones, or height loss.

These are nonmodifiable risk factors for osteoporosis (Bone Health and Osteoporosis Foundation, 2023).

3. Determine if patient has been screened (e.g., bone density) for osteoporosis.

The USPSTF (2018) recommends screening for osteoporosis with bone measurement testing in women 65 years and older and postmenopausal women younger than 65 years at increased risk of osteoporosis.

Current evidence is insufficient to assess the balance of benefits and harms of screening men for osteoporosis (USPSTF, 2018).

4. Ask patient to describe history of changes or problems related to bone, muscle, or joint function (e.g., recent fall, trauma, lifting heavy objects, bone or joint disease with sudden or gradual onset) and location of alteration.

History helps in assessing nature of musculoskeletal problem.

5. Assess height and weight (see Skill 6.1). Note if there is a height decrease in women older than 50 by subtracting current height from recall of maximum adult height.

Body mass index (BMI) less than 22 is a risk factor, and loss of height more than 7.5 cm (3 inches) is one of the first clinical signs of osteoporosis (Touhy & Jett, 2022).

6. Ask patient to describe nature and extent of musculoskeletal pain: location, duration, severity, predisposing and aggravating factors, relieving factors, and type of pain. If patient reports pain or cramping in lower extremities, ask if walking or stretching relieves or aggravates it. Assess distance walked and characteristics of pain before, during, and after activity.

Pain frequently accompanies alterations in bone, joints, or muscle. It has implications for comfort and also ability to perform activities of daily living (ADLs). Pain caused by certain vascular conditions tends to increase with activity.

7. Determine if patient uses analgesics, antipsychotics, antidepressants, nervous system stimulants, or recreational drugs.

These medications alter LOC or cause behavioral changes. Abuse of any drugs sometimes causes tremors, ataxia, and changes in peripheral nerve function.

8. Determine if patient has recent history of seizures or convulsions. Clarify sequence of events (aura, loss of muscle tone, falling, motor activity, loss of consciousness); character of any symptoms; and relationship to time of day, fatigue, or emotional stress (see Chapter 14).

Seizure activity often originates from central nervous system (CNS) alteration. Characteristics of seizure help determine its origin.

STEP	RATIONALE
9. Screen patient for headache, tremors, dizziness, vertigo, numbness or tingling of body part, visual changes, weakness, pain, or changes in speech.	These symptoms commonly result from CNS dysfunction. Identifying patterns aids in diagnosis.
10. Discuss with spouse, family member, or friends (as appropriate) any recent changes in patient's behavior (e.g., increased irritability, mood swings, memory loss, change in energy level).	Behavioral changes may result from intracranial pathology.
11. Determine if patient has noticed change in vision (cranial nerve [CN] I), hearing (CN VIII), smell, taste (CN VII), or touch.	Major sensory nerves originate from brainstem. These symptoms help to localize nature of problem during CN examination.
12. If patient displays sudden acute confusion (delirium), review history for drug toxicity (e.g., anticholinergics, digoxin, antihistamines, antipsychotics, benzodiazepines, opioid analgesics, sedative-hypnotics, steroids), serious infections, metabolic disturbances (e.g., diabetes mellitus), heart failure, and severe anemia.	Delirium is one of most common mental disorders in older people (Touhy & Jett, 2022), but it also occurs in children.
13. Review history for head or spinal cord injury, meningitis, congenital anomalies, neurological disease, or psychiatric counseling.	These neurological symptoms or behavioral changes help to focus assessment on possible cause.
14. Assess patient's knowledge, prior experience with neuromuscular assessment and knowledge of osteoporosis, and feelings about procedure.	Reveals need for patient instruction and/or support.

PLANNING

1. Expected outcomes following completion of procedure:	
• Patient demonstrates erect posture; strong grasp; steady gait, with arms swinging freely at side.	Indicates normal alignment, gait, and muscle strength.
• There is bilateral symmetry of extremities in length, alignment, position, and skinfolds.	Indicates normal alignment and structure.
• Full active ROM is present in all joints, with good muscle tone and absence of contractures, spasticity, or muscular weakness.	Indicates normal ROM of joints.
• Patient is alert and oriented to person, place, and time. Behavior and appearance appropriate for condition and situation.	Indicates normal cerebral function.
• Patient demonstrates normal pupil reaction to light and accommodation (see Skill 6.2), normal external ocular movement (EOM), facial sensation intact, symmetrical facial expressions, soft palate and uvula midline and rise on phonation, gag reflex intact, speech clear without hoarseness, no difficulty swallowing.	Indicates normal functioning of CNs III, IV, V, VI, VII, IX, and X.
• Patient distinguishes between sharp and dull sensations and light touch on symmetrical areas of extremities. Position sense intact to lower extremities.	Indicates normal function of sensory nerves.
• Gait is coordinated, steady, with appropriate stance and swing phases. Romberg test negative.	Indicates normal cerebellar and motor system functioning.
• Patient able to explain risks for osteoporosis and falls.	Demonstrates learning.
2. Perform hand hygiene. Prepare necessary supplies at bedside.	Reduces transmission of infection.
3. Close room curtains or doors.	Provides for patient privacy.
4. Prepare patient:	
a. Integrate musculoskeletal and neurological assessments during other parts of physical assessment or during nursing care (e.g., when patient moves in bed, rises from chair, or walks).	You can conduct assessment as patient performs activities or goes through movements required during complete physical examination. Conserves patient's energy and allows observation of patient performing more naturally.
b. Plan time for short rest periods during a comprehensive assessment.	Movement of body parts and various maneuvers may tire patient. Always plan rest periods with older adults and very ill patients.

IMPLEMENTATION

1. Assess musculoskeletal system. (During examination, discuss any risks patient may have for falls or other injuries.)	Educates patient for fall prevention.
a. Make a general observation of extremities. Look at overall size, alignment, and symmetry. Note any gross deformity or bony enlargement.	General review pinpoints areas requiring in-depth assessment.

STEP	RATIONALE

b. Observe ability to use arms and hands for grasping objects (e.g., pen, utensils) and dressing self.

Assesses coordination and muscle strength.

c. To assess hand grasp strength, cross your hands and have patient grasp index and middle fingers of both of your hands and squeeze them as hard as possible (see illustration).

It is common for patient's dominant hand to be slightly stronger than nondominant hand. By crossing your hands, patient's right hand grasps your right hand. This helps with recall of which is patient's right/left hand.

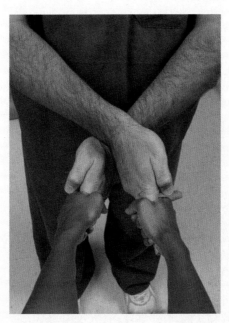

STEP 1c Assessing strength of hand grasps, comparing sides.

d. To assess strength of lower arms or legs, ask patient to extend or flex the joint being tested. Then have patient resist as you apply force against that muscle contraction. Have patient maintain pressure until told to stop. Compare symmetrical muscle groups. Note weakness and compare right with left.

Compares strength of symmetrical muscle groups. Upper and lower extremities on dominant side are usually stronger. Rate muscle strength on scale of 0 to 5 as follows:
- 0   No voluntary contraction
- 1   Slight contractility, no movement
- 2   Full ROM, passive
- 3   Full ROM, active
- 4   Full ROM against gravity, some resistance
- 5   Full ROM against gravity, full resistance

Each joint or muscle group requires different position for measurement.

e. Observe body alignment for sitting, supine, prone, or standing positions. Muscles and joints should be exposed and free to move to allow for accurate measurement.

f. Inspect gait as patient walks. Have patient use their assistive device (e.g., cane, walker) if appropriate. Observe for foot dragging, shuffling or limping, balance, presence of obvious deformity in lower extremities, and position of trunk in relation to legs.

Gait is more natural if patient is unaware of your observation. Assesses for neuro-musculoskeletal disorder. Foot dragging, limping, shuffling, and poor balance are risk factors for falls (see Chapter 14).

g. Perform the Banner Mobility Assessment Tool (BMAT) (Boynton et al., 2020) (see Chapter 12) or the Timed Up and Go (TUG) test (CDC, 2017) if patient is able to ambulate.

The BMAT assesses four functional tasks to identify the level of mobility a patient can achieve, revealing if assistance is needed (Boynton et al., 2020).

STEP	RATIONALE

Timed Up and Go test: Have adult wear regular footwear, sit back in comfortable chair, and use normal assistive devices, if needed. Have watch with a second hand. On the word "Go," begin timing as you have the patient stand from a sitting position without using chair arms for support, stand still momentarily, walk 10 feet (3 meters) in a line, turn around and return to chair, and sit back in chair without using chair arms for support. Observe gait and ability to stand.

The TUG test measures the progress of balance, sit to stand, and walking (CDC, 2017). It should be conducted as part of routine evaluation of older adults. The test helps to detect a person's risk for falls. Normally a person completes the task in less than 10 seconds; over 20 seconds is abnormal. The Timed Up and Go has shown excellent reliability in typical adults; in individuals with cerebral palsy, multiple sclerosis, Huntington's disease, or stroke; and in individuals with a spinal cord injury (Christopher et al., 2021). In the same study, predictive validity (e.g., predicting falls) was limited.

h. Stand behind patient and observe postural alignment (position of hips relative to shoulders). Look sideways at cervical, thoracic, and lumbar curves (see illustration).

Abnormal curves of posture include kyphosis (hunchback, exaggerated posterior curvature of thoracic spine), lordosis (swayback, increased lumbar curvature), and scoliosis (lateral spinal curvature). Postural changes indicate muscular, bone, or joint deformity; pain; or muscular fatigue. Head should be held erect.

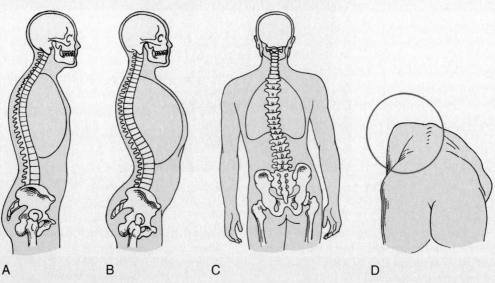

A   B   C   D

STEP 1h Observe spinal deformities. **(A)** Kyphosis. **(B)** Lordosis. **(C)** Scoliosis. **(D)** Scoliosis with patient bending forward.

i. Gently palpate bones, joints, and surrounding tissue in involved areas. Note any heat, tenderness, edema, stiffness, or resistance to pressure. Do not move joint when fracture is suspected or joint is apparently "frozen" by lack of movement over a long period of time.

Reveals changes resulting from trauma or chronic disease. Heat and tenderness indicate acute or chronic inflammation. ROM causes pain or injury.

j. Ask patient to put major joint through its full ROM (Table 6.11). Patients with deformities, reduced mobility, joint fixation, or weakness require passive ROM assessment (see Chapter 12). Observe equality of motion in same body parts:

Assessment of patient's normal ROM provides baseline for assessing later changes after surgery or inactivity.

(1) *Active motion:* (Patient needs no support or help, able to move joint independently.) Teach patient to move each joint through its normal range. Sometimes it is necessary to demonstrate and ask patient to mimic your movements.

Identifies muscle strength and detects limited ROM.

(2) Active assisted or *Passive motion:* Begin by assisting patient in moving joint. Joint may have full ROM, but patient does not have strength to move it independently. Then have patient relax and let you move the same joints passively until end of range is felt. Support extremity at joint. Do not force joint if there is pain or muscle spasm.

Determines ability to perform joint motion in presence of muscle weakness. Forcing joint causes injury and pain.

STEP	RATIONALE

TABLE 6.11

Assessing Range of Motion (ROM)[a]

Body Part	Assessment Procedure	ROM
Upper Extremities		
Neck	Bend head forward and then backward. Bend neck side to side. Turn head to look over each shoulder.	Flexion, lateral flexion, rotation
Shoulders	Raise both arms to vertical position level at sides of head.	Flexion
	Bring arm across upper chest to touch opposite shoulder.	Adduction
	Place both hands behind neck, with elbows out to sides.	External rotation and abduction
	Place both hands behind small of back.	Internal rotation
	Have patient make small circles with hands, with arms extended at shoulder level.	Circumduction
Elbows	Bend and straighten elbows.	Flexion and extension
	Place hands at waist with elbows flexed.	Internal rotation
Wrists	Flex and extend wrist (bend and straighten).	Flexion and extension
	Bend wrist to radial and then ulnar side.	Radial and ulnar deviation
	Turn palm upward and then downward.	Supination and pronation
Hands	Make a fist with both hands; open hand.	Flexion and extension
	Extend and spread fingers and thumb outward; bring back together.	Adduction and abduction
Lower Extremities		
Hips (with patient supine)	With knees extended, raise one leg upward.	Flexion and extension: Expect 90 degrees flexion
	Cross leg over other leg.	Abduction: Expect 45 degrees
	Swing legs laterally.	Adduction: Expect 30 degrees
	With knee flexed, hold ankle and rotate leg inward and outward.	Internal and external rotation: Expect 40–45 degrees
Knees (with patient sitting)	Raise foot, keeping knee in place.	Extension: Expect full extension and up to 15 degrees hyperextension
Ankles	With foot held off floor, point toes downward and bring them back toward knee.	Plantar flexion: Expect 45 degrees
		Dorsiflexion: Expect 20 degrees
Toes	Turn foot (sole) inward and sole outward.	Inversion and eversion: Expect to reach 5 degrees
	Bend toes down and back.	Flexion and hyperextension: Expect to reach 40 degrees

[a]This may be done actively by the patient (active range of motion [AROM]) or passively by the nurse (passive range of motion [PROM]).

   k. Assess muscle tone in major muscle groups. Normal tone causes mild, even resistance to movement through entire ROM.

2. Neurological assessment
   a. Assess LOC and orientation by asking patient to identify name, location, day of week, and year; note behavior and appearance. This can be completed during general survey.

   b. Assess CNs. (**NOTE:** CNs I [olfactory], II [optic], and VII [auditory] are assessed during head and neck examination).

If muscle has increased tone (hypertonicity), any sudden movement of joint is met with considerable resistance. Hypotonic muscle moves without resistance. Muscle feels flabby.

A fully conscious patient responds to questions spontaneously. As LOC declines, patient may show irritability, shortened attention span, or unwillingness to cooperate. As LOC continues to deteriorate, patient becomes disoriented to name, time, and place. Behavior and appearance reveal information about patient's mental status.

STEP	RATIONALE
(1) For CNs III (oculomotor), IV (trochlear), and VI (abducens), assess extraocular muscles (EOMs). Ask patient to look straight ahead without moving head and follow movement of your finger through six cardinal positions of gaze; measure pupillary reaction to light reflex and accommodation (see Skill 6.2) using penlight.	These CNs are those most likely to be affected by increasing intracranial pressure (ICP), which causes change in response or size of pupil; pupils may change shape (more oval) or react sluggishly. ICP impairs movements of EOMs. Accommodation is ability of eye to adjust vision from near to far distance.
(2) For CN V (trigeminal), apply light sensation with cotton ball to symmetrical areas of face. Also have patient tightly clench teeth and then palpate muscles over the jaw for tone (see illustration).	Sensations should be symmetrical; unilateral decrease or loss of sensation may be caused by CN V lesion.

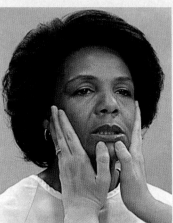

STEP 2b(2) Examination of the trigeminal cranial nerve. (*From Stewart RW, Dains JE, Ball JW, Solomon BS, Flynn JA. Seidel's guide to physical examination: interprofessional approach, ed 10, St Louis, 2023, Elsevier.*)

STEP	RATIONALE
(3) For CN VII (facial), note facial symmetry. Have patient frown, smile, puff out cheeks, and raise eyebrows.	Expressions should be symmetrical; Bell palsy causes drooping of upper and lower face; cerebral vascular accident (CVA) causes asymmetry.
(4) For CNs IX (glossopharyngeal) and X (vagus), have patient speak and swallow. Ask patient to say "ah" while you use tongue blade and penlight. Check for midline uvula and symmetrical rise of uvula and soft palate. Use tongue blade and place on posterior tongue to elicit gag reflex. For CN XII (hypoglossal), inspect tongue for symmetry, tremors, and movement toward nose and chin.	Damage to CN IX causes impaired swallowing; damage to CN X causes loss of gag reflex, hoarseness, and nasal voice. When palate fails to rise and uvula pulls toward normal side, this indicates a unilateral paralysis. Tongue should be symmetrical without tremors, atrophy, or abnormal deviation.
(5) For CNs XI (spinal accessory), have patient shrug shoulders against resistance.	Tests strength of sternocleidomastoid muscle.
Then have patient turn head toward each side against resistance.	Tests strength of trapezius muscle.
c. Assess extremities for sensation. Perform all sensory testing with patient's eyes closed so that patient is unable to see when or where a stimulus strikes skin. Use minimal stimulation initially, increasing gradually until patient is aware of it.	For all sensory stimulus testing, patient should note minimal differences side to side, correctly describe the sensation (sharp or dull, hot or cold), and recognize side of the body tested and location.
(1) *Pain:* Ask patient to indicate when sharp or dull sensation is felt as you alternately apply sharp and dull ends of a broken tongue blade to skin surface. Apply in symmetrical areas of extremities.	Patient should be able to distinguish sharp or dull sensations. Impaired sensations indicate disorders of spinal cord or peripheral nerve roots.

Clinical Judgment *Loss of sensation in feet is sign of peripheral neuropathy, common in those with long-term diabetes, whereas localized loss of sensation in toes is commonly a result of a neuroma (thickening of tissue around nerve).*

STEP	RATIONALE
(2) *Light touch:* Apply light wisp of cotton to different points along surface of skin in symmetrical areas of extremities.	Patient should be able to distinguish when touched.

STEP	RATIONALE

(3) *Position:* Grasp finger or toe, holding it by its sides with your thumb and index finger. Alternate moving finger or toe up and down. Ask patient to state when finger is up or down. Repeat with toes.

Patient should be able to distinguish movements of a few millimeters. Decreased/absent position sense may occur in spinal anesthesia, paralysis, or other neurological disorders.

d. Assess motor and cerebellar function:
(1) *Gait:* Have patient walk across room, turn, and come back. Similarly, note use of assistive devices. This is a good time to instruct on proper use of assistive devices.

Neurological and musculoskeletal disorders impair gait and balance.

(2) *Romberg test:* Have patient stand with feet together, arms at sides, both with eyes open and eyes closed (for 20–30 seconds). Protect patient's safety by standing at side; observe for swaying.

Romberg test should be negative; slight swaying is considered normal.

e. Assess deep tendon reflexes (DTRs):
0   No response
1+   Sluggish or diminished response
2+   Normal, active or expected response
3+   More brisk than expected; slightly hyperactive
4+   Very brisk; hyperactive, with clonus

This examination is usually performed by advanced practice nurses. Muscle spasticity and hyperactive reflexes may result from disorders such as stroke and paralysis. Diminished DTRs and muscle weakness may suggest electrolyte abnormalities or lower motor neuron disorders (e.g., amyotrophic lateral sclerosis [ALS] or Guillain-Barré syndrome).

3. Remove and discard gloves and used supplies in proper receptacle. Perform hand hygiene.

Reduces transmission of infection.

4. This is the end of the neurological and/or comprehensive examination. Ask patients if there are any questions about examination findings.

Promotes trust and partnership with patients.

5. Help patient to a comfortable position.

Restores comfort and sense of well-being.

6. Place nurse call system in an accessible location within patient's reach.

Ensures patient can call for assistance if needed.

7. Raise side rails (as appropriate) and lower bed to lowest position, locking into position.

Ensures patient safety and prevents falls.

EVALUATION

1. Compare muscle strength, posture and alignment, and ROM with previous physical assessment.

Determines presence of abnormalities or change in condition.

2. Compare neurological status with previous physical assessment.

Determines presence of abnormalities or change in condition.

3. Ask patient to explain personal risks for osteoporosis and falls.

Demonstrates learning.

4. **Use Teach-Back:** "It is important to know the reasons why you are at risk for falling. Let's review what we discussed during your examination. Tell me two reasons why you are at risk for falling." Revise your instruction now or develop a plan for revised patient/family caregiver teaching if patient/family caregiver is not able to teach back correctly.

Teach-back is a technique for health care providers to ensure that medical information has been explained clearly so that patients and families understand what is communicated to them (AHRQ, 2023).

Unexpected Outcomes	Related Interventions
1. Joints are prominent, swollen, and tender with nodules or overgrowth of bone in distal joints, indicating signs of arthritis.	• Consult with physical therapist to implement proper ROM exercises. • Determine patient's knowledge regarding use of antiinflammatory medications and nonpharmacological measures (see Chapter 16).
2. ROM is reduced in one or more major joints: shoulder, elbow, wrist, fingers, knee, hip.	• Notify health care provider if this is a change • Position patient comfortably and reduce mobility in extremity until cause of abnormal joint motion is clarified or determined.
3. Patient demonstrates weakness in one or more major muscle groups or has difficulty with gait or ability to walk and sit during Timed Up and Go test, indicating a fall risk.	• Place patient on fall precautions. • Provide patient safety when ambulating (see Chapter 12). • Notify health care provider.
4. Patient has changes in mental status and pupillary response or other neurological deficits.	• Notify health care provider immediately. • Continue to assess patient's vital signs and LOC closely. • Place on fall precautions.

Documentation

- Document posture, gait, muscle strength, ROM, LOC, cognition and orientation, pupillary and other CN responses, and sensation.
- Document evaluation of patient and family caregiver learning.

Hand-Off Reporting

- Report to nurse in charge or health care provider acute pain or sudden muscle weakness, change in LOC, or change in size or pupillary reaction, which require immediate treatment.

Special Considerations

Patient Education

- Teach patient about correct postural alignment. Consult with physical therapist to provide patient with exercises for improving posture.
- Encourage intake of calcium to meet the recommended daily allowance. Recommendation for daily dietary allowance for calcium in adults 19 to 50 years of age: 1000 mg/day; in female adults over age 50: 1200 mg/day; in male adults: 1000 mg/day (National Institutes of Health, 2022). Milk, yogurt, and cheese are rich natural sources of calcium.
- Explain to patients with low back pain that there are benefits from modification of work-related risk factors (e.g., lifting heavy weights, use of protective equipment), regular aerobic exercise, exercises that strengthen the back and increase trunk flexibility, and learning how to lift properly.
- Explain measures to ensure safety (e.g., use of ambulation aids or safety bars in bathrooms or stairways) for patients with sensory or motor impairments.

Pediatrics

- Examine infants carefully for musculoskeletal anomalies resulting from genetic or fetal insults. An examination includes review of posture, generalized movement, symmetry and skin creases of the extremities, muscle strength, and hip alignment.
- Normally the back of a newborn is rounded or C-shaped from the thoracic and pelvic curves.

- Scoliosis, lateral curvature of the spine, is an important childhood problem, especially in females, usually identified at puberty. (For closer examination, have child stand erect wearing only underclothes. Observe from behind, looking for asymmetry of shoulders and hips. Then observe from the back as child bends forward.) Uneven dress hems or trouser hems or uneven fit of clothing at the waist is an indication of scoliosis.
- Watching a child during play reveals information about musculoskeletal function.
- Children ages 13 to 19 years need 1300 mg of calcium daily with 400 International Units of vitamin D (Hockenberry et al., 2022).

Older Adults

- Older adults tend to assume a stooped, forward-bent posture with hips and knees somewhat flexed, arms bent at the elbows, and level of arms raised.
- Short, uncertain steps are characteristic of gait disturbance in older adults (Ball et al., 2023).
- Teach older adults about fall prevention. Make suggestions for modifications in the home environment to reduce the risk of falls (see Chapter 41).
- To reduce bone demineralization, teach older-adult patients about a proper weight-bearing exercise program (e.g., walking, low-impact aerobics, swimming) to be followed three or more times a week. Also teach about proper body mechanics and ROM exercises (see Chapter 12).
- Functional assessment is a measurement of an older person's ability to perform ADLs (Ball et al., 2023). When a patient is unable to perform self-care easily, determine need for assistive devices (e.g., zippers on clothing instead of buttons, elevation of chairs to minimize bending of knees and hips).

Populations With Disabilities

- Research has shown high rates of osteoporosis documented among adults with intellectual and developmental disabilities (IDDs); earlier screening is recommended beginning at younger ages (40 if living in an institution, 45 if community dwelling). Risk factors among women with IDs include inactivity, long-term anticonvulsant use, and possible Down syndrome (Sullivan et al., 2018).

PROCEDURAL GUIDELINE 6.1 *Monitoring Intake and Output*

 Video Clip

Measuring and documenting intake and output (I&O) during a 24-hour period is part of the assessment database for fluid and electrolyte balance (Table 6.12). You are responsible for accurate documentation of all intake (liquids taken orally, by enteral feedings, and parenterally) and output (urine, diarrhea, vomitus, gastric suction, and drainage from surgical tubes). Monitoring a patient on I&O requires cooperation and help from the patient and family caregivers. Accuracy is critical because health care providers will use this information when prescribing medications and intravenous (IV) fluids.

Monitor I&O for patients with a fever or edema, receiving diuretic therapy, or on restricted IV fluids. It is also important when a patient has electrolyte losses associated with vomiting, diarrhea, gastrointestinal (GI) drainage, or extensive open wounds such as burns. Total and evaluate a patient's I&O at the end of each shift or at specified times such as every 8 hours.

Significant alterations are apparent by comparing 24-hour totals over several days. Because fluid imbalance occurs at any time, be aware of I&O for all patients, even when documentation is not required.

Delegation

The skills of assessing I&O totals at the end of each shift; comparing 24-hour totals over several days; and monitoring and documenting IV therapy, wound or chest tube drainage, and tube feedings cannot be delegated to assistive personnel (AP). Direct the AP to:

- Use Standard Precautions related to body fluids, accurately measuring and documenting I&O for oral intake, urinary output, liquid diarrheal stools, vomitus and wound drainage, and using the metric system with standard containers.
- Report changes in patient's condition such as alteration in intake or changes in color, amount, or odor of output.

PROCEDURAL GUIDELINE 6.1 *Monitoring Intake and Output—cont'd*

TABLE 6.12

Adult Average Fluid Gains and Losses

Fluid Intake and Output	Volume (mL)	Fluid Intake and Output	Volume (mL)
Fluid Intake		**Fluid Output**	
Oral fluids	1100–1400	Kidneys	1200–1500
Solid foods	800–1000	Skin	500–600
Oxidative metabolism	300	Lungs	400
		Gastrointestinal	100
Total Gains	2200–2700	**Total Losses**	2200–2700

From Hall, J. E., & Hall, M. *Guyton and Hall textbook of medical physiology,* ed 14, Philadelphia, 2020, Elsevier.

Interprofessional Collaboration

- Accuracy in I&O collection may require the assistance of dietary assistants or a dietitian.
- When assessment reveals changes in fluid balance or when assessments for specific pathophysiological conditions reveal abnormal findings, communicate with the appropriate interprofessional team member (e.g., health care provider, dietitian).

Equipment

Sign to alert personnel of I&O measurement; daily I&O; electronic health record (EHR); graduated measuring container; bedpan, urinal, bedside commode, or urine "hat" (a receptacle that fits under the toilet seat); clean gloves; mask, eye protection, and gown (optional).

Steps

1. Identify patients with conditions that increase fluid loss (e.g., fever, diarrhea, vomiting, surgical wound drainage, chest tube drainage, gastric suction, major burns, or severe trauma).
2. Identify patients with impaired swallowing, unconscious patients, and those with impaired mobility.
3. Identify patients on medications that influence fluid balance (e.g., diuretics, steroids).
4. Assess signs and symptoms of dehydration and fluid overload (e.g., bradycardia versus tachycardia, hypotension versus hypertension, reduced skin turgor versus edema).
5. Weigh patients daily using the same scale, the same time of day, and with comparable clothing.
6. Monitor laboratory reports:
   - Urine specific gravity (normal is 1.010–1.030)
   - Hematocrit (Hct) (normal range is 38%–47% for females and 40%–54% for males)
7. Assess patient's/family caregiver's literacy level and knowledge of purpose and process of I&O measurement.
8. Explain to patient and family caregiver the reasons that I&O measurement is important.
9. Perform hand hygiene.
10. Measure and document all fluid intake:
    a. Liquids with meals, gelatin, custards, ice cream, popsicles, sherbets, ice chips (documented as 50% of measured volume [e.g., 100 mL of ice chips equals 50 mL of water]). Convert household measures to the metric system: 1 ounce equals 30 mL; therefore 12 ounces (soda can) equals 360 mL.
    b. Count liquid medicines such as antacids and fluids with medications as fluid intake.
    c. Calculate fluid intake from tube feedings (see Chapter 31).
    d. Calculate fluid intake from parenteral fluids, blood components, and total parenteral nutrition solutions (see Chapters 28, 29, and 31).

Clinical Judgment *To maintain accuracy, document intake as soon as you measure it. If more than one patient is in the same room, each must have urine receptacles labeled with name and bed location.*

11. Instruct patient and family caregiver to call you or the AP to empty contents of urinal, urine hat, or commode each time patient uses it. Have patient and family monitor incontinence, vomiting, and excessive perspiration and report these things to a nurse.
12. Inform patient and family caregiver that Foley catheter drainage bag and wound, gastric, or chest tube drainage are closely monitored, measured, and documented and who is responsible for this. Each patient must have a graduated container clearly marked with name and bed location and used only for the patient indicated.
13. Apply clean gloves. Measure drainage at the end of the shift or as indicated using appropriate containers and noting color and characteristics. If splashing is anticipated, wear mask, eye protection, and/or gown.
    a. Measure urine drainage using a "hat" that fits over toilet seat. Patient voids into hat and can then be accurately measured using a graduated container (see illustration).

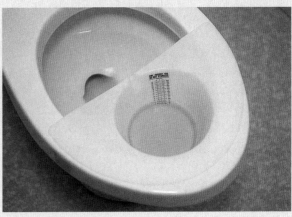

STEP 13a Urine "hat."

Continued

PROCEDURAL GUIDELINE 6.1 *Monitoring Intake and Output—cont'd*

b. Observe color and characteristics of urine in Foley tubing and drainage bag. Sometimes a measuring device is part of the drainage bag (see Chapter 33). Otherwise, measure with a graduated container.

c. Measure chest tube drainage by marking and documenting the time on the collection chamber at specified intervals (see illustration) (see Chapter 26). Chest tube collection devices are changed when they become full.

d. Measure Jackson-Pratt/Hemovac drainage with a medicine cup (see illustration) (see Chapter 38).

e. Measure gastric drainage or larger drainage pouches by opening clamp and pouring into graduated cup with a 240-mL capacity (see illustration).

14. Remove gloves and dispose of them in appropriate receptacle. Perform hand hygiene.

15. Note I&O balance or imbalance and report to health care provider any urine output less than 30 mL/h or significant changes in daily weight.

16. Document intake and output.

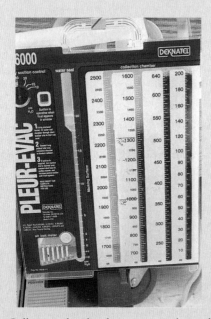

STEP 13c Collection chamber for measuring chest tube drainage.

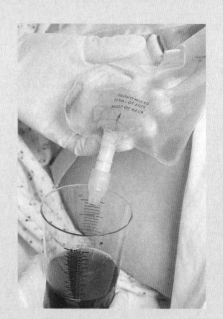

STEP 13e Measuring drainage from large drainage pouch.

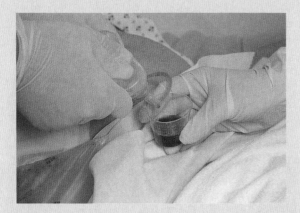

STEP 13d Measuring wound drainage through Jackson-Pratt drain.

✦ CLINICAL JUDGMENT AND NEXT GENERATION NCLEX® EXAMINATION-STYLE QUESTIONS

The nurse is admitting a new patient to the hospital from a long-term care agency. Vital signs include blood pressure 180/100 mm Hg, pulse 94 beats/min, respirations 24 breaths/min, temperature 36.9°C (98.4°F), and oxygen saturation 96% on room air. The electronic health record (EHR) shows:

- Demographics: Age 84, male, African American
- Social history: Used to consume alcohol regularly; quit drinking 20 years prior; smoked cigarettes between ages of 20 and 40; spouse deceased 1 year prior; lived alone before referral to long-term care agency
- Medical history: Hypertension, osteoarthritis, renal failure, Type 2 diabetes mellitus, congestive heart failure
- Current medication: Bisoprolol, metformin, potassium supplement, polyethylene glycol as needed for constipation
- Ambulates with a walker as needed
- Consumes renal diet

1. After completing a full assessment, which of the following information will the nurse report to the health care provider? **Select all that apply.**
   1. Respirations 24 breaths/min
   2. Expresses sadness over loss of spouse
   3. Reports consuming diet rich in fiber
   4. Crackles in lung bilaterally
   5. Pitting edema in lower extremities
   6. States, "I try to drink water instead of juices."
   7. Weight gain of 0.9 kg (2 pounds) overnight
   8. Capillary refill 4 seconds

2. Which type of assessment **best** indicates to the nurse that the patient is experiencing heart failure?
   1. Drinks water instead of juice
   2. Self-reported shortness of breath
   3. History of renal failure
   4. Rapid increase of weight overnight

3. When planning care for this patient, which task will the nurse assign to assistive personnel (AP)?
   1. Measuring intake and output during the shift
   2. Teaching how to reduce sodium in the diet
   3. Evaluating if pitting edema is increasing
   4. Assessing for ongoing crackles in the lungs

4. Which of the following assessment findings indicates to the nurse that the patient should use a walker for ambulation? **Select all that apply.**
   1. Pedal edema
   2. Shuffling gait
   3. Mild cognitive changes
   4. Report of peripheral neuropathy
   5. Oxygen saturation 96% on room air

5. Following administration of furosemide, the nurse reassesses the patient. When compared with the nurse's initial assessment, which current finding indicates that treatment was effective?
   1. Oxygen saturation 95% on room air
   2. Decreased crackles in lungs
   3. Temperature 37°C (98.6°F)
   4. Pulse rate 88 beats/min

Visit the Evolve site for Answers to Clinical Judgment and Next Generation NCLEX® Examination-Style Questions.

REFERENCES

Abramovich A, et al: *Assessment of health conditions and health service use among transgender patients in Canada*, 2020. https://jamanetwork.com/journals/jamanetworkopen/fullarticle/2769915. Accessed March 17, 2023.

Agency for Healthcare Research and Quality (AHRQ): *Teach-back: intervention*, 2023. https://www.ahrq.gov/patient-safety/reports/engage/interventions/teachback.html.

American Cancer Society: *Can testicular cancer be found early?* Atlanta, 2018, The Society. https://www.cancer.org/cancer/types/testicular-cancer/detection-diagnosis-staging/detection.html. Accessed November 7, 2023.

American Cancer Society: *How to spot skin cancer*, 2020. https://www.cancer.org/latest-news/how-to-spot-skin-cancer.html. Accessed March 17, 2023.

American Cancer Society: *Cancer facts & figures 2022*, Atlanta, 2022, The Society. https://www.cancer.org/research/cancer-facts-statistics/all-cancer-facts-figures/cancer-facts-figures-2022.html. Accessed November 7, 2023.

American Cancer Society: *How to quit using tobacco*, Atlanta, 2023a, The Society. https://www.cancer.org/healthy/stay-away-from-tobacco/guide-quitting-smoking.html. Accessed March 17, 2023.

American Cancer Society: *Lung cancer screening guidelines*. 2023b. https://www.cancer.org/health-care-professionals/american-cancer-society-prevention-early-detection-guidelines/lung-cancer-screening-guidelines.html. Accessed November 7, 2023.

American Heart Association: *Changing the way we view women's heart attack symptoms*, 2020. https://www.heart.org/en/news/2020/03/06/changing-the-way-we-view-womens-heart-attack-symptoms. Accessed November 7, 2023.

American Lung Association: *The impact of e-cigarettes on the lung*, 2022. https://www.lung.org/getmedia/e5325d10-11fa-4b17-aaed-312e135b4100/impact-of-ecigarettes-on-lung.pdf.pdf. Accessed November 7, 2023.

Arnett, DK, et al: 2019 ACC/AHA Guideline on the Primary Prevention of Cardiovascular Disease: A Report of the American College of Cardiology/American Heart Association Task Force on Clinical Practice Guidelines, *Circulation* 140(11):e596–e646, 2019.

Ball JW, et al: *Seidel's guide to physical examination*, ed 10, St. Louis, 2023, Mosby.

Bone Health and Osteoporosis Foundation: *Are you at risk?* 2023. https://www.bonehealthandosteoporosis.org/preventing-fractures/general-facts/bone-basics/are-you-at-risk/. Accessed March 17, 2023.

Boynton T, et al: The bedside mobility assessment tool, 2.0, *Am Nurse J* 15(7): 18–29, 2020.

Casson I, et al: Health checks for adults with intellectual and developmental disabilities in a family practice, *Can Fam Physician* 64(Suppl 2):S44–S50, 2018.

Centers for Disease Control and Prevention (CDC): *Timed up & go (TUG)*, 2017. https://www.cdc.gov/steadi/pdf/TUG_Test-print.pdf. Accessed March 17, 2023.

Centers for Disease Control and Prevention (CDC): *Know your risk for heart disease*, 2019. https://www.cdc.gov/heartdisease/risk_factors.htm. Accessed March 17, 2023.

Centers for Disease Control and Prevention (CDC): *HPV vaccination recommendations*, 2021a. https://www.cdc.gov/vaccines/vpd/hpv/hcp/recommendations.html. Accessed March 17, 2023.

Centers for Disease Control and Prevention (CDC): *Tuberculosis (TB) Disease and Latent TB infection: symptoms, risk factors & treatment*, 2021b, CDC. https://www.cdc.gov/tb/features/riskfactors/RF_Feature.html. Accessed March 17, 2023.

Centers for Disease Control and Prevention (CDC): *Heart disease facts*, 2022a. https://www.cdc.gov/heartdisease/facts.htm. Accessed March 17, 2023.

Centers for Disease Control and Prevention (CDC): *Prevent seasonal flu: vaccination information*, 2022b. https://www.cdc.gov/flu/prevent/index.html. Accessed March 17, 2023.

Centers for Disease Control and Prevention (CDC): *Screening and diagnosis of hearing loss*, 2022c. https://www.cdc.gov/ncbddd/hearingloss/screening.html. Accessed March 17, 2023.

Centers for Disease Control and Prevention (CDC): *Pneumococcal vaccine recommendations*, 2023a. https://www.cdc.gov/vaccines/vpd/pneumo/hcp/recommendations.html. Accessed March 17, 2023.

Centers for Disease Control and Prevention (CDC): *What is health literacy?* 2023b. https://www.cdc.gov/healthliteracy/learn/index.html.

Christopher A, et al: The reliability and validity of the Timed Up and Go as a clinical tool in individuals with and without disabilities across a lifespan: a systematic review, *Disabil Rehabil* 43(13):1799–1813, 2021.

European Pressure Ulcer Advisory Panel (EPUAP) and National Pressure Injury Advisory Panel (NPIAP) and Pan Pacific Pressure Injury Alliance (PPPIA): *Prevention and treatment of pressure ulcers/injuries: Clinical Practice Guidelines; The International Guideline*. 2019, EPUAP/NPIAP/PPPIA.

Frothingham S: *Common side effects of laxatives*, Healthline, 2019. https://www.healthline.com/health/laxatives-side-effects. Accessed March 17, 2023.

Fumarola S, et al: Overlooked and underestimated: medical adhesive-related skin injuries. Best practice consensus document on prevention. *J Wound Care* 29(Suppl 3c):S1–S24, 2020.

GI Society, Canadian Society of Intestinal Research: *Stomach ulcer diet*, 2022. https://badgut.org/information-centre/health-nutrition/diet-for-ulcer-disease/. Accessed March 17, 2023.

Harding MM, et al: *Lewis's medical-surgical nursing*, ed 11, St. Louis, 2021, Elsevier.

Hartz J, de Ferranti S: *Overview of risk factors for development of atherosclerosis and early cardiovascular disease in childhood*, UpToDate, 2023. https://www.uptodate.com/contents/overview-of-risk-factors-for-development-of-atherosclerosis-and-early-cardiovascular-disease-in-childhood. Accessed November 7, 2023.

Hockenberry MJ, et al: *Wong's essentials of pediatric nursing*, ed 11, 2022, Elsevier.

Iwamoto SJ, et al: Routine screening for transgender and gender diverse adults taking gender-affirming hormone therapy: a narrative review, *J Gen Intern Med* 36(5):1380–1389, 2021.

Johns Hopkins: *Child abuse and neglect: what is child abuse and neglect*, 2022. https://www.hopkinsmedicine.org/health/conditions-and-diseases/child-abuse-and-neglect. Accessed November 7, 2023.

Klein DA, et al: Caring for transgender and gender-diverse persons: what clinicians should know, *Am Fam Physician* 98(11):645–653, 2018.

Knecht VR, et al: Molecular analysis of bacterial contamination on stethoscopes in an intensive care unit, *Infect Control Hosp Epidemiol* 40:171–177, 2019.

Krist AH, et al: Screening for hearing loss in older adults: US Preventative Services Task Force recommendation statement, *JAMA* 325(12):1196–1201, 2021.

Mayo Clinic: *Testicular exam*, 2022. https://www.mayoclinic.org/tests-procedures/testicular-exam/about/pac-20385252. Accessed March 17, 2023.

MedLine Plus: *Abdominal sounds*, 2020, National Library of Medicine. https://medlineplus.gov/ency/article/003137.htm. Accessed August 11, 2023.

Mealie C, et al: *Abdominal exam*. National Library of Medicine StatPearls, 2022.

National Cancer Institute: *ACS's updated cervical cancer screening guidelines explained*, 2020. https://www.ncbi.nlm.nih.gov/books/NBK459220/. Accessed November 7, 2023.

National Heart, Lung, and Blood Institute (NHLBI): *DASH eating plan*, 2021. https://www.nhlbi.nih.gov/health-topics/dash-eating-plan. Accessed March 17, 2023.

National Institutes of Health (NIH): *Calcium: fact sheet for health professionals*, 2022. https://ods.od.nih.gov/factsheets/Calcium-HealthProfessional/. Accessed March 17, 2023.

Patel K: *Deep venous thrombosis*, 2019. http://emedicine.medscape.com/article/1911303-overview. Accessed March 17, 2023.

Pearson JL, et al: Recommended core items to assess e-cigarette use in population-based surveys, *Tob Control* 27:341–346, 2018.

Sassano MF, et al: Evaluation of e-liquid toxicity using an open-source high-throughput screening assay, *PLoS Biol* 16(3):e2003904, 2018.

Schneider A, Chung, P: *Transgender and gender diverse patient urologic care*. American Urological Association (AUA), 2022. https://www.auanet.org/meetings-and-education/for-medical-students/medical-students-curriculum/transgender-and-gender-diverse-patient-care. Accessed August 11, 2023.

Shulman GP, et al: A Review of contemporary assessment tools for use with transgender and gender nonconforming adults, *Psychol Sex Orientat Gend Divers* 4(3):304–313, 2017.

Siegel JD, et al and the Healthcare Infection Control Practices Advisory Committee: *2007 Guideline for isolation precautions: preventing transmission of infectious agents in healthcare settings*, 2007, last update May 2022. https://www.cdc.gov/infectioncontrol/pdf/guidelines/isolation-guidelines-H.pdf. Accessed March 17, 2023.

Shmerling RH: *Can vaping damage your lungs? What we do (and don't) know*, Harvard Health Publishing, Harvard Health blog, posted March 24, 2022. https://www.health.harvard.edu/blog/can-vaping-damage-your-lungs-what-we-do-and-dont-know-2019090417734. Accessed March 17, 2023.

Sullivan W, et al: Primary care of adults with intellectual and developmental disabilities: clinical practice guidelines, *Can Fam Physician* 64:254, 2018.

The Joint Commission (TJC): *2023 National patient safety goals*, Oakbrook Terrace, IL, 2023, The Joint Commission. https://www.jointcommission.org/standards/national-patient-safety-goals/. Accessed March 17, 2023.

Touhy T, Jett K: *Ebersole and Hess' Gerontological nursing & healthy aging*, ed 6, St. Louis, 2022, Elsevier.

U.S. Preventive Services Task Force (USPSTF): *Final recommendation statement: osteoporosis to prevent fractures: screening*, 2018. https://www.uspreventiveservicestaskforce.org/uspstf/recommendation/osteoporosis-screening. Accessed March 17, 2023.

U.S. Preventive Services Task Force (USPSTF): *Colorectal cancer screening*, 2021. https://www.uspreventiveservicestaskforce.org/uspstf/recommendation/colorectal-cancer-screening#:~:text=Recommendation%20Summary%20%20%20%20Population%20%20,that%20clinicians%20se%20...%20%20%20C%20. Accessed March 17, 2023.

Venkatesan KD, et al: Stethoscopes: a potential source of hospital acquired infection, *Int J Adv Med* 6(4):1322, 2019.

Ward KT, Reuben DB: *Comprehensive geriatric assessment*, UpToDate, 2022. https://www.uptodate.com/contents/comprehensive-geriatric-assessment. Accessed March 17, 2023.

Weingartner L, et al: *Gender-affirming care with transgender and genderqueer patients: a standardized patient case*, Association of American Medical Colleges, 2022, https://www.mededportal.org/doi/10.15766/mep_2374-8265.11249. Accessed March 17, 2023.

World Health Organization (WHO): *Safe listening devices and systems, a WHO-ITU standard*, 2019a. https://apps.who.int/iris/bitstream/handle/10665/280085/9789241515276-eng.pdf. Accessed March 17, 2023.

World Health Organization (WHO): *Hearing Loss: How to reduce it and prevent its impact*, 2019b. https://cdn.who.int/media/docs/default-source/documents/health-topics/deafness-and-hearing-loss/whd-2019-flyer.pdf. Accessed November 7, 2023.

Zimmerman B, Williams D: *Lung sounds*, National Library of Medicine Stat Pearls, 2022. https://www.ncbi.nlm.nih.gov/books/NBK537253/#article-36567.s2. Accessed March 17, 2023.

Vital Signs and Physical Assessment: Next-Generation NCLEX® (NGN)–Style Unfolding Case Study

PHASE 1

QUESTION 1.

The nurse has seen a client in the outpatient setting for the first time. Following the initial encounter, the nurse provides the documentation below.

Highlight the findings that require **immediate** follow-up by the nurse.

History and Physical	Nurses' Notes	Vital Signs	Laboratory Results
1204: Client is here to report "heartburn" that is increasing in frequency. Client states, "The older I get, the more I have this burning in my chest after I eat." Reports no recent changes in diet and no traveling in or out of the country. Works as a long distance truck driver, smokes 2 packs of cigarettes a day, and often eats at fast-food restaurants. The client is 52 years old and weighs 200 pounds (90.7 kg). Denies other symptoms, including abdominal discomfort or bloating, changes in bowel or bladder habits, chest pain, and respiratory difficulty or shortness of breath. Alert and oriented × 4; lung sounds clear to auscultation; S_1S_2 present without murmur; bowel sounds present × 4 quadrants; strength in all extremities equal. Vital signs: T 36.9°C (98.4°F); HR 72 beats/min; RR 14 breaths/min; BP 190/90 mm Hg; SpO_2 98% on RA.			

QUESTION 2.

The nurse considers information provided by the client.

Complete the following sentence by selecting from the list of options below.

The client is at highest risk for health complications based on the findings of **1 [Select]** and **2 [Select]**.

Options for 1	Options for 2
RR 14 breaths/min	SpO_2 98% on RA
Denial of bowel or bladder changes	Burning in chest after eating
BP 190/90 mm Hg	Heart rate 72 beats/min
S_1S_2 present without murmur	Aging

PHASE 2

QUESTION 3.

The client is seen by the health care provider, undergoes diagnostic testing, and returns to the office 2 weeks later. The nurse collects today's vital signs: T 37.9°C (100.2°F); HR 98 beats/min; RR 18 breaths/min; BP 210/100 mm Hg; SpO_2 95% on RA.

Choose the **most likely** options for the information missing from the statement below by selecting from the list of word choices below.

The nurse is concerned about the client's [**Word Choice**] and [**Word Choice**].

Word Choices
Temperature
Blood pressure
Heart rate
Respiratory rate
Oxygen saturation

QUESTION 4.

The health care provider has seen the client and assigned a diagnosis of gastrointestinal reflux disease (GERD) and hypertension. The nurse is planning care based upon the client's diagnoses and decides to offer instruction about hypertension and elimination of risk factors. Select 3 risk factors for hypertension that the nurse has identified in the patient's history

- Abnormal heart rate
- Overweight
- Burning sensation in chest
- Smokes cigarettes
- Limited opportunity to exercise
- Eats a low-fat diet

PHASE 3

QUESTION 5.

Several weeks later, the client presents to the emergency department with urticaria, a swollen tongue, and shortness of breath. Wheals are noted on the chest. Between breaths, the client tells the nurse, "I was trying to eat healthier; I decided to try some grilled shrimp, and now it is hard to breathe. I'm really scared." The nurse quickly reviews the client's history in the electronic health record and notes that the client has a history of smoking. Vital signs at this time include T 37.3°C (99.2°F); HR 114 beats/min; RR 28 breaths/min; BP 202/98 mm Hg; SpO$_2$ 89% on RA.

For each body system below, click to select the intervention the nurse will take at this time. Each body system may support more than 1 potential intervention.

System	Potential Interventions
Cardiovascular	o Document blood pressure. o Apply cardiac monitor. o Discuss cardiac rehabilitation with the client.
Respiratory	o Auscultate lungs. o Monitor oxygen saturation. o Teach cough and deep breathing exercises.
General	o Prepare to administer antibiotic for fever. o Stay with the client. o Document temperature.

QUESTION 6.

The client was intubated and then moved to intensive care. Current vital signs: T 37.3°C (99.2°F); HR 88 beats/min; RR 18 breaths/min; BP 118/70 mm Hg; SpO$_2$ 99% on RA. The nurse auscultates the lungs, which currently have no wheezes, rales, or rhonchi. Wheals are noted on the chest. For each current client finding, indicate whether the nurse will document the client's condition as an improvement or unchanged since the emergency department interventions.

Current Client Findings	Document as Improvement	Document as Unchanged
Temperature 37.3°C (99.2°F);		
Blood pressure 118/70 mm Hg		
SpO$_2$ 99%		
Lungs clear to auscultation		
RR 18 breaths/min		

UNIT 3
Special Procedures

Making clinical judgments about any patient is a complex process, and in many cases, you need to collect additional data from laboratory studies and diagnostic procedures. This information must be included in a patient's electronic health record (EHR) and physical assessment database. It is important to analyze cues from laboratory and/or diagnostic findings to determine if there are ongoing problems affecting the patient's health. It does not matter if the patient has a routine physical examination and needs a blood specimen, has a urinary tract infection and needs a clean-voided urinary specimen, or requires a cardiac catheterization; data from these studies provide valuable assessment data and cues, which are important to correctly identify a patient's health problems.

Collecting specimens from patients and preparing them for diagnostic tests are more than having knowledge about the procedure and necessary skills to correctly obtain a specimen. For many of the skills in this unit, you will need to use clinical judgment to assess a patient's ability to assist in specimen collection, identify any cultural considerations when obtaining specimens, and provide patient and family caregiver education to ensure successful specimen collection or prediagnostic procedure preparation and postprocedure care.

Most diagnostic procedures are done in an outpatient setting, and thus the time you spend with a patient before a procedure is limited. Patients receive information about scheduled tests when in a referring health care provider's office, in the mail, or online before a procedure. Your role may include validating what the patient knows about the procedure and clarifying questions. For example, does the patient understand the procedure, preprocedure requirements (e.g., nothing to eat or drink after midnight on the day of the procedure), any positioning requirements for the procedure, any local or moderate sedation involved, and postprocedure care? To make a sound clinical judgment, you need to assess the patient's educational needs and what is known, analyze this information, and determine an individualized patient and family caregiver education plan for preprocedure and postprocedure care.

The data you collect about a patient for a specific specimen collection or diagnostic test depends on more than the standard assessments for the skill. Environmental factors such as the complexity and urgency of the test influence your assessment. In some situations, your patient may have a lot of uncertainty and stress related to specimen collection and, more often, with diagnostic procedures. Your patient might be fearful of the outcome. In these situations, use therapeutic communication skills to holistically and fully assess and understand your patient's problems and concerns and implement nursing interventions related to your patient's fears and anxieties.

As you prepare for any of the skills in this unit, use your clinical judgment. Consider a patient's presenting condition and any risks for problems to determine if more assessment data are needed or if adjustments are necessary for how you prepare the patient for the test or procedure. Analyze the specimen or diagnostic procedure findings, and, as appropriate, communicate the findings to other members of the health care team. Plan and implement individualized nursing interventions to address postprocedure care or abnormal results. Use objective evaluation criteria to determine the patient's response to any postprocedure interventions or follow-up care.

7 | Specimen Collection

SKILLS AND PROCEDURES

Skill 7.1 **Urine Specimen Collection: Midstream (Clean-Voided) Urine; Sterile Urinary Catheter, p. 179**

Procedural Guideline 7.1 **Collecting a Timed Urine Specimen, p. 185**

Skill 7.2 **Measuring Occult Blood in Stool, p. 187**

Skill 7.3 **Measuring Occult Blood in Gastric Secretions (Gastroccult), p. 190**

Skill 7.4 **Collecting Nose and Throat Specimens for Culture, p. 192**

Skill 7.5 **Obtaining Vaginal or Urethral Discharge Specimens, p. 196**

Procedural Guideline 7.2 **Collecting a Sputum Specimen by Expectoration, p. 199**

Skill 7.6 **Collecting a Sputum Specimen by Suction, p. 200**

Skill 7.7 **Obtaining Wound Drainage Specimens, p. 203**

Skill 7.8 **Collecting Blood Specimens and Culture by Venipuncture (Syringe and Vacutainer Method), p. 206**

Skill 7.9 **Blood Glucose Monitoring, p. 215**

Skill 7.10 **Obtaining an Arterial Specimen for Blood Gas Measurement, p. 220**

OBJECTIVES

Mastery of content in this chapter will enable you to:
- Explain the rationale for the collection of each specimen.
- Identify special conditions necessary for collection of each specimen.
- Use patient education to promote patient cooperation during specimen collection.
- Identify measures to minimize anxiety and promote safety during specimen collection.
- Identify nursing responsibilities for processing a specimen after collection.
- Apply correct technique for collecting clean-voided, timed, and catheterized urine specimens.
- Apply correct technique for collecting specimens and cultures for blood and other body fluids.
- Apply correct technique to perform venipuncture.
- Apply infection control practices during specimen collection techniques.
- Apply correct technique to perform arterial puncture for blood gas measurement.
- Identify nursing responsibility for reporting laboratory results to the health care provider.

MEDIA RESOURCES

- http://evolve.elsevier.com/Perry/skills
- Clinical Review Questions
- Audio Glossary
- ▶ Video Clips

- **NSO** Nursing Skills Online
- Answers to Clinical Judgment and Next-Generation NCLEX® Examination–Style Questions
- Skills Performance Checklists
- Printable Key Points

PURPOSE

Laboratory test results aid in the diagnosis of health care problems, provide information about the stage and activity of a disease process, and measure a patient's response to therapy. Nurses are accountable for correctly collecting specimens, monitoring patient outcomes, and ensuring that these laboratory tests are performed and that results are shared with the interprofessional team in a timely manner.

PRACTICE STANDARDS

- Occupational Safety and Health Administration (OSHA), n.d.: Worker Protections Against Occupational Exposure To Infectious Diseases
- The Joint Commission (TJC), 2023: National Patient Safety Goals—Patient identification

SUPPLEMENTAL STANDARDS

- Centers for Disease Control and Prevention (CDC), 2022: CDCs Core Infection Prevention and Control Practices for Safe Healthcare Delivery in All Settings

PRINCIPLES FOR PRACTICE

- Proficiency and sound clinical judgment in obtaining specimens minimize patient discomfort, promote patient safety, and ensure accuracy and quality of diagnostic procedures.
- Everyone who handles body fluids is at risk for exposure. The use of hand hygiene and clean gloves or personal protective equipment is necessary to protect yourself and patients. Proper labeling on a container marked as a biohazard protects laboratory personnel and others who may come in contact with the specimen (OSHA, n.d.).
- Each health care agency may establish its own values for each test based on specific testing methods and standards, which are printed on the agency's laboratory forms. The value ranges are for normal, high, and low results. In addition, the agencies establish a critical value range. When questions arise, consult the health care agency procedure manual, or call the laboratory.

PERSON-CENTERED CARE

- Patients often experience embarrassment and/or discomfort when giving a sample of body excretions or secretions, especially urine, urogenital, or stool samples. It is important to provide patient privacy and handle excretions or secretions discreetly. When provided clear instructions, patients or a family caregiver are able to obtain specimens of urine, stool, and sputum without unnecessary exposure (Pagana et al., 2021).
- Consider both cultural and language barriers when delegating specimen collection to patients and family caregivers. Language barriers make it difficult to explain the purpose of tests and collection techniques. Providing repeated return demonstrations helps patient and/or family caregiver understand how to prepare for a test or how to perform a procedure (CDC, 2023; Miteva et al., 2022).

EVIDENCE-BASED PRACTICE

Prevention of Hemolysis in Blood Samples

Hemolysis is the breakdown of red blood cells (RBCs) resulting in the leakage of intracellular contents into the plasma, and it affects the accuracy of blood test results. Hemolysis of blood sampling is a leading cause of preanalytical laboratory errors and can result in inaccurate diagnoses, delays in treatment and in monitoring

disease progression, and increased cost of care (Krasowski, 2019; Burchill et al., 2021). When access to IV sites must be used, observed rates of hemolysis may be substantially reduced by placing the IV device at the antecubital site. Best practices that assist in reducing hemolysis rates include:

- For venipuncture, a large-bore needle is recommended over obtaining a blood sample from an IV site (Burchill et al., 2021; Emergency Nurses Association [ENA], 2018), because small needles increase pressure, leading to hemolysis.
- Use the antecubital region for optimal blood collection site (ENA, 2018).
- Avoid vigorous shaking of a blood sample because hemolysis may occur and invalidate test results (Pagana et al., 2021).
- Collect a blood specimen from the arm without an IV device if possible because IV fluids can influence test results (Ersoy et al., 2023; Pagana et al., 2021).
- Do not fasten the tourniquet for longer than 1 minute. Prolonged tourniquet application can cause stasis, localized acidemia, and hemoconcentration.
- Because the blood cells continue to live in the collection tubes, they will metabolize some of the components in the blood, which can result in alterations in the concentration of some blood components before analysis in the laboratory. Blood specimens should be promptly delivered to the laboratory for processing within 1 hour, depending on the test (Pagana et al., 2021).

SAFETY GUIDELINES

- Adapt to patient's need and physical and cognitive abilities to safely perform and/or participate in specimen collection procedures.
- Verify the type of procedure scheduled and the procedure site with the patient.
- Follow procedures for special conditions (e.g., iced specimens, special containers with preservatives) required for transport of specimens. Specific required prerequisite conditions include fasting and nothing by mouth (NPO) and may need to be completed before the collection of a specimen (Pagana et al., 2021).
- Follow agency policy regarding infection control practices and Standard Precautions (see Chapter 9) when collecting specimens of blood or body fluids (OSHA, n.d.; CDC, 2022).
- Properly label all specimens with patient's identification, date and time the specimen is obtained, name of the test, and source of the specimen/culture for each container (TJC, 2023). Label containers in the presence of the patient.
- Follow infection control practices for transporting and delivering specimens to the laboratory within the recommended time or ensure that they are stored properly for later transport.
- Follow precautions for collecting specimens from patients who are in protective isolation.

✦ SKILL 7.1   Urine Specimen Collection: Midstream (Clean-Voided) Urine; Sterile Urinary Catheter

 Video Clip

A urinalysis provides information about kidney or metabolic function, nutrition, and systemic diseases. Urine collection uses a variety of methods, depending on the purpose of the urinalysis and the presence or absence of a urinary catheter. Routine urinalysis includes measurement of nine or more elements, including urine pH, protein and glucose levels, ketones, specific gravity, white blood cell (WBC) count, and presence of bacteria and/or blood (Pagana et al., 2021).

Types of Urine Tests and Specimens

- A *random urine specimen for routine urinalysis* is collected using a specimen "hat" (Fig. 7.1), which you place under a toilet seat to collect voided urine. Then place approximately 120 mL of urine in a specimen container, properly labeled, and send to the laboratory. **NOTE:** Urine collected from a specimen "hat" is never used to determine the presence of bacteria and should never be

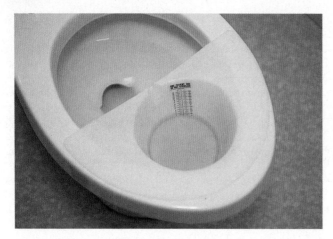

FIG. 7.1 Specimen hat.

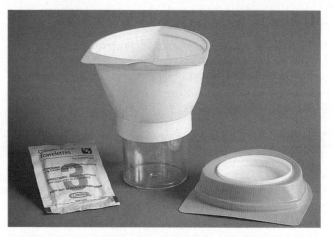

FIG. 7.2 Clean-voided specimen collection kit.

cultured. It is contaminated with surface bacteria from the patient's perineal area.

- A *culture and sensitivity (C&S) of urine* is performed to identify whether bacteria are present (culture) and to determine the most effective antibiotic for treatment (sensitivity). You collect specimens for C&S either as a clean-voided midstream specimen or under sterile technique from a urinary catheter. Urine collected by this method may also be analyzed for the same components as a routine urinalysis.
- A *timed urine specimen for quantitative analysis* requires urine to be collected over 2 to 72 hours. The 24-hour timed collection (see Procedural Guideline 7.1) is most common and allows for measurement and quantitative analysis of elements such as amino acids, creatinine, hormones, glucose, and adrenocorticosteroid excretion.
- *Chemical properties of urine* are tested by immersing a specially prepared test strip of paper (Chemostrip) into a clean urine specimen. The test detects the presence of glucose, ketones, protein, or blood not normally present in the urine. When the screening test for the presence of substances in the urine is positive, additional laboratory tests are used to determine a patient's diagnosis or measure the effectiveness of treatment.

Delegation

The skill of collecting urine specimens can be delegated to assistive personnel (AP). Direct the AP to:
- Obtain the specimens at a specified time as ordered or per protocol (identify type of urine specimen ordered and technique to use [e.g., clean catch])
- Position patient as necessary when mobility restrictions are present
- Report to the nurse if the urine is not clear (e.g., contains blood, cloudiness, or excess sediment)
- Report to the nurse when a patient is unable to initiate a stream or has pain or burning on urination

Interprofessional Collaboration
- Place signs and verbally communicate to other members of the health care team to save all urine when a patient is undergoing a timed urine specimen collection.

Equipment
- Completed identification labels with appropriate patient identifiers
- Completed laboratory requisition, including patient identification, date, time, name of test, and source of culture specimen
- Biohazard bag or container for delivery of specimen to laboratory (or container specified by agency)

Clean-Voided Urine Specimen
- Commercial kit for clean-voided urine (Fig. 7.2), containing:
  - Sterile cotton balls or antiseptic towelettes
  - Antiseptic solution (chlorhexidine or povidone-iodine solution)
  - Sterile water or normal saline
  - Sterile specimen container
  - Urine cup
- Clean gloves
- Soap, water, washcloth, and towel
- Bedpan (for nonambulatory patient), specimen hat (see Fig. 7.1) (for ambulatory patient)

Sterile Urine Specimen from Urinary Catheter
- 20-mL Luer-Lok for routine urinalysis or 3-mL safety Luer-Lok syringe for culture
- Chlorhexidine, or other disinfectant swab
- Clamp or rubber band
- Specimen container (nonsterile for routine urinalysis; sterile for culture)
- Clean gloves

STEP	RATIONALE

ASSESSMENT

1. Identify patient using at least two identifiers (e.g., name and birthday or name and medical record number) according to agency policy.

Ensures correct patient. Complies with The Joint Commission standards and improves patient safety (TJC, 2023).

STEP	RATIONALE
2. Review patient's electronic health record (EHR), including health care provider's order and nurses' notes.	Identifies purpose and ensures proper collection technique of urine sample.
3. Review EHR for any pathological conditions that may impair collection of urine specimen (e.g., enlarged prostate gland in men, urethral strictures) or have an impact on results (e.g., hematuria from menses; patient has undergone transurethral resection of the prostate [TURP]).	Identifies conditions that may hinder the ability to obtain a voided specimen, and identifies conditions when blood is expected in urine specimen.
4. Refer to agency procedures for specimen collection methods.	Agency policies may vary regarding collection and/or handling of specimens.
5. Assess patient's/family caregiver's health literacy.	Determines degree to which individuals have the ability to find, understand, and use information and services to make informed health-related decisions and actions for themselves and others (CDC, 2023).
6. Ask patient and check EHR for history of allergies. Check allergy bracelet.	Identifies if patient is allergic to antiseptic solution.
7. Perform hand hygiene. Assess patient's weight, level of consciousness, developmental level, ability to cooperate, and mobility.	Reduces transmission of microorganisms. This determines degree of help patient requires to position self and hold container.
8. Assess for signs and symptoms of urinary tract infection (UTI) (frequency, urgency, dysuria, hematuria, flank pain, fever; cloudy, malodorous urine).	These are indicators of UTI.
9. Assess patient's knowledge, prior experience with urine specimen collection, and feelings about procedure.	Reveals need for patient instruction and/or support.

PLANNING

1. Expected outcomes following completion of procedure:	
• Specimen free of contaminants, such as stool or toilet paper, is collected.	Proper collection technique prevents substances from changing normal characteristics of urine.
• Patient discusses purpose and benefits of specimen collection.	Evaluates patient's learning.
2. Provide privacy. Allow mobile patients to collect specimen in bathroom.	Privacy allows patient to relax and produce specimen more easily.
3. Explain the procedure and what is required of the patient.	Patients often prefer to obtain their own clean voided specimen but need appropriate education to correctly collect the sample.
4. Obtain and organize equipment labels, and requisition for urine specimen collection at bedside.	Ensures more efficient procedure.
5. Arrange for extra personnel to help if necessary.	Some patients are unable to assume positioning on bedpan if needed.

IMPLEMENTATION

1. Collect clean-voided urine specimen.	
a. Perform hand hygiene and apply clean gloves. Give patient cleaning towelette or towel, washcloth, and soap to clean perineum or help with cleaning perineum. Help bedridden patient onto bedpan to facilitate access to perineum. Remove and dispose of gloves. Perform hand hygiene.	Reduces transmission of microorganisms. Patients prefer to wash their own perineal areas when possible. Cleaning prevents contamination of specimen after urine passes from urethra.
b. Using aseptic technique, open outer package of commercial specimen kit.	Maintains sterility of equipment.
c. Apply clean gloves.	Prevents contact of microorganisms on your hands.
d. Pour antiseptic solution over cotton balls (unless kit contains prepared antiseptic towelettes).	Cotton ball or towelette is used to clean perineum.
e. Open specimen container, maintaining sterility of inside of specimen container, and place cap with sterile inside up. Do not touch inside of cap or container.	Contaminated specimen is most frequent reason for inaccurate reporting of urine C&S.

STEP	RATIONALE
f. Use aseptic technique to help patient or allow patient to independently clean perineum and collect specimen. Amount of help needed varies with each patient. Inform patient that antiseptic solution will feel cold.	Maintains patient's dignity and comfort.
(1) Male:	
(a) Hold penis with one hand; using circular motion and antiseptic towelette, clean meatus, moving from center to outside 3 times with different towelettes (see illustration). Have uncircumcised male patient retract foreskin for effective cleaning of urinary meatus and keep retracted during voiding. Return foreskin when done.	Reduces number of microorganisms at urethral meatus and moves from areas of least to most contamination. Return of foreskin prevents stricture of penis.
(b) If agency procedure indicates, rinse area with sterile water and dry with cotton balls or gauze pad.	Prevents contamination of specimen with antiseptic solution.
(c) After patient initiates urine stream into toilet or bedpan, have him pass urine specimen container into stream and collect 90 to 120 mL of urine (Pagana et al., 2021) (see illustration).	Initial urine flushes out microorganisms that normally accumulate at urinary meatus and prevents transfer into specimen.
(2) Female:	
(a) Either nurse or patient spreads labia minora with fingers of nondominant hand.	Provides access to urethral meatus.
(b) With dominant hand, clean urethral area with antiseptic swab (cotton ball or gauze). Move from front (above urethral orifice) to back (toward anus). Use fresh swab each time; clean 3 times; begin with labial fold farthest from you, then labial fold closest, and then down center (see illustration).	Prevents contamination of urinary meatus with fecal material. Cleaning down center last decreases contamination from labia.
(c) If agency procedure indicates, rinse area with sterile water and dry with cotton ball.	Prevents contamination of specimen with antiseptic solution.
(d) While continuing to hold labia apart, patient initiates urine stream into toilet or bedpan; after stream is achieved, pass specimen container into stream and collect 90 to 120 mL of urine (Pagana et al., 2021) (see illustration).	Initial stream flushes out resident microorganisms that accumulate at urethral meatus and prevents transfer into specimen.
g. Remove specimen container before flow of urine stops and before releasing labia or penis. Patient finishes voiding into bedpan or toilet. Offer to help with personal hygiene as appropriate.	Prevents contamination of specimen with skin flora. Prevents sediment from bladder from getting into specimen.

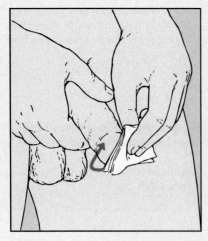

STEP 1f(1)(a) Cleaning technique (male).

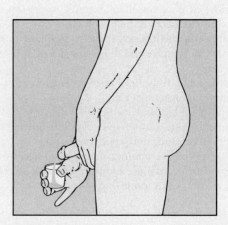

STEP 1f(1)(c) Collecting midstream urine specimen (male).

STEP	RATIONALE
h. Replace cap securely on specimen container, touching only outside.	Retains sterility of inside of container and prevents spillage of urine.
i. Clean urine from exterior surface of container.	Prevents transfer of microorganisms to others.
2. Collect urine from indwelling urinary catheter.	
a. Explain that you will use syringe without need to remove urine through catheter port and that patient will not experience any discomfort.	Minimizes anxiety when you manipulate catheter and aspirate urine with syringe from catheter port.
b. Explain that you will need to clamp catheter for 10 to 15 minutes before obtaining urine specimen and that urine cannot be obtained from drainage bag.	Allows urine to accumulate in catheter. Urine in drainage bag is not considered sterile.
c. Perform hand hygiene and apply clean gloves. Clamp drainage tubing with clamp or rubber band for as long as 15 minutes below site chosen for withdrawal (see illustration).	Permits collection of fresh sterile urine in catheter tubing rather than draining into bag.
d. After 15 minutes, position patient so catheter sampling port is easily accessible. Location of port is where catheter attaches to drainage bag tube (see illustration). Clean port for 15 seconds with disinfectant swab and allow to dry.	Prevents entry of microorganisms into catheter.
e. Attach needleless Luer-Lok syringe to built-in catheter sampling port (see illustration). Some needleless ports use blunt plastic valve or slip-tip syringe inserted into port diaphragm.	Guideline recommends use of Luer-Lok needleless system. Needleless system prevents injury by needlestick.
f. Withdraw 3 mL for culture or 20 mL for routine urinalysis.	Allows collection of urine without contamination. Proper volume is needed to perform test.

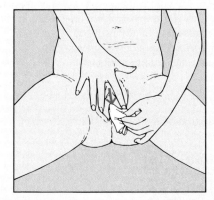

STEP 1f(2)(b) Clean from front to back, holding labia apart.

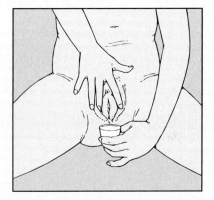

STEP 1f(2)(d) Collecting midstream urine specimen (female).

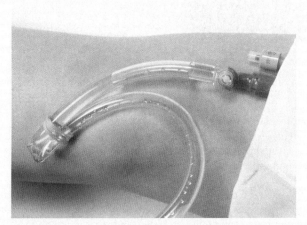

STEP 2c Rubber band used to clamp drainage tube.

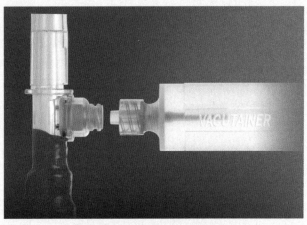

STEP 2d Port with syringe attached.

STEP	RATIONALE

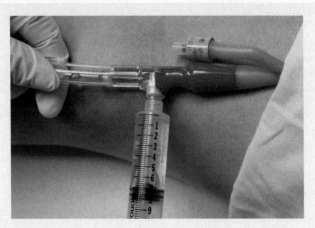

STEP 2e Access urinary catheter port with Luer-Lok syringe or syringe with blunt plastic valve.

g. Transfer urine from syringe into clean urine container for routine urinalysis or into sterile urine container for culture.	Prevents contamination of urine during transfer procedure.
h. Place lid tightly on container.	Prevents contamination of specimen by air and loss by spillage.
i. Unclamp catheter and allow urine to flow into drainage bag. Ensure that urine flows freely.	Allows urine to drain by gravity and prevents stasis of urine in bladder.
3. Check label, then securely attach label to container (not lid). In patient's presence, confirm label identifiers (two identifiers, specimen source, and collection date and time). If patient is female, indicate if she is menstruating.	Ensures that specimen is identified correctly for proper diagnosis (TJC, 2023).
4. Dispose of soiled supplies. Remove and dispose of gloves and perform hand hygiene.	Prevents transmission of microorganisms. Use appropriate disposal receptacle if patient is on hazardous drugs (Gorski et al., 2021).
5. Offer patient hand hygiene or provide time to wash hands.	Reduces transmission of microorganisms.
6. Help patient to a comfortable position.	Restores comfort and sense of well-being.
7. Raise side rails (as appropriate) and lower bed to lowest position, locking into position.	Ensures patient safety and prevents falls.
8. Place nurse call system in an accessible location within patient's reach.	Ensures patient can call for assistance if needed.
9. Send specimen and completed requisition to laboratory within 20 minutes. Refrigerate specimen if delay cannot be avoided.	Delay of analysis may significantly alter test results (Pagana et al., 2021).

EVALUATION

1. Inspect clean-voided specimen for contamination with toilet paper or stool.	Contaminants prevent specimen from being used.
2. Evaluate patient's urine C&S report for bacterial growth.	Routine cultures identify organism(s), and sensitivity study identifies antimicrobial medications that may be effective against pathogen.
3. Observe urinary drainage system in catheterized patient to ensure that it is intact and patent.	System must remain closed to remain sterile.
4. **Use Teach-Back:** "I want to be sure I explained the way to obtain a clean-voided specimen. Please repeat the steps back to me." Revise your instruction now or develop a plan for revised patient/family caregiver teaching if patient/family caregiver is not able to teach back correctly.	Teach-back is a technique for health care providers to ensure that they have explained medical information clearly so that patients and their families understand what is communicated to them (Agency for Healthcare Research and Quality [AHRQ], 2023).

STEP	RATIONALE

Unexpected Outcomes

1. Urine specimen is contaminated with stool or toilet paper.

2. Urine culture reveals bacterial growth (determined by colony count of more than 10,000 organisms per milliliter).

3. Lumen leading to balloon that holds catheter in place is punctured.

Related Interventions

- Repeat patient instruction and specimen collection. If unable to obtain specimen through clean voiding, patient may need catheterization.
- Report findings to health care provider.
- Administer medications as ordered.
- Monitor patient for fever and dysuria.
- Notify health care provider.
- Prepare for removal of existing catheter and insertion of new catheter.

Documentation

- Document method used to obtain specimen, date and time collected, type of test ordered, laboratory receiving specimen, characteristics of specimen, patient's tolerance to procedure of specimen collection, and time specimen sent to the lab.
- Document your evaluation of patient and family caregiver learning.

Hand-Off Reporting

- Report the type of urinalysis and date and time specimen was sent to laboratory.
- Report any abnormal findings to health care provider.

Special Considerations

Patient Education

- Discuss signs and symptoms of UTI with patient and family caregiver if appropriate.
- Explain significance of cleaning genital area before collecting specimen.

Pediatrics

- Use clean technique and apply a sterile plastic urine-collecting bag (Fig. 7.3) that adheres to the perineum of an infant or a non–toilet-trained child (Hockenberry et al., 2022).

Older Adults

- Older adults may need help in positioning to obtain specimen. In confused patients it may be necessary for the AP to help the patient collect a specimen (Touhy & Jett, 2022).

Populations With Disabilities

- Insertion of a urinary catheter to collect a urine sample may elicit different reactions for a person with a cognitive or

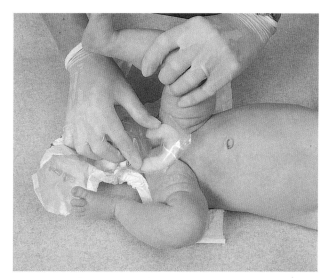

FIG. 7.3 Application of urine collection bag. (*From Warekois, R. S., & Robinson, R. [2012]. Phlebotomy worktext and procedures manual [3rd ed.]. St. Louis: Mosby.*)

learning disability. It is important to consider the needs of the individual and provide care in a sensitive and respectful manner (Tremayne et al., 2019).

Home Care

- Instruct a patient collecting a sample at home to keep it on ice until it reaches the laboratory to minimize bacterial growth before it is applied to a culture medium in the laboratory setting.

PROCEDURAL GUIDELINE 7.1 *Collecting a Timed Urine Specimen*

Some tests of renal function and urine composition require urine to be collected over 2 to 72 hours. The 24-hour timed collection is used most often and measures elements such as amino acids, creatinine, hormones, glucose, and adrenocorticosteroids. A timed urine collection provides a means to measure the concentration or dilution of urine.

To ensure the accuracy of a 24-hour timed urine specimen, the patient and staff must work together to collect all voided urine in a 24-hour period. Obtain an appropriate container with or without preservative from the laboratory; check agency or laboratory policy. The type of analysis for the 24-hour timed specimen determines the need for any preservative or the need to place the

Continued

PROCEDURAL GUIDELINE 7.1 *Collecting a Timed Urine Specimen—cont'd*

specimen container on ice during the 24 hours of collection time. If there is any question, consult with the lab for instructions. You may place the specimen container in the patient's bathroom or the "soiled" utility room. Post a sign to remind the patient and staff that a test is in progress.

Label the specimen container with all appropriate identification information and the number of containers sequentially if more than one container is needed. Confirm identifiers on labels with patient. Documentation and collection of all urine is necessary for an accurate test result.

Delegation

The skill of collecting a timed urine specimen can be delegated to assistive personnel (AP). Direct AP about:

- When timed collection begins, proper method to store the collected urine, where to place signs that a timed urine collection is in progress, and saving all urine

Interprofessional Collaboration

- Communicate with the interprofessional health care team the need to save all urine; include start date and time and stop date and time.

Equipment

Large collection bottle with cap, which usually contains a chemical preservative; bedpan, urinal, specimen hat, bedside commode, or pediatric potty-chair; graduated measuring container for intake and output (I&O) measurement; large basin to hold collection bottle surrounded by ice if immediate refrigeration is required; specimen identification label and completed laboratory requisition (with appropriate patient identifiers and specimen information); instructional signs that remind patient and staff of timed urine collection; clean gloves; biohazard plastic bag or container (see agency policy)

Steps

1. Identify patient using two identifiers (e.g., name and birthday or name and medical record number) according to agency policy (TJC, 2023).
2. Review health provider's order to determine specific test.
3. Assess patient's/family caregiver's health literacy.
4. Explain the reason for specimen collection, how patient can help, and that urine must be free of feces and toilet tissue.
5. Assess patient's knowledge, prior experience with timed urine collection, and feelings about procedure.
6. Place specimen collection container in the bathroom and, if indicated, in a pan of ice.
   a. Post signs to remind staff, family and visitors, and patient of timed urine collection on patient's door and toileting area.
   b. If patient leaves unit, be sure that personnel in receiving area collect and save all urine.

7. If possible, have patient drink two to four glasses of water about 30 minutes before times of collection to facilitate ability to void at the appropriate time for test to begin.
8. Perform hand hygiene and apply clean gloves. Discard the first voided specimen as the test begins. Indicate time test began on laboratory requisition. For accurate results the patient must begin the test with an empty bladder. Begin collecting all urine for designated time. Remove and dispose of gloves and perform hand hygiene.
9. Measure volume of each voiding if I&O is to be documented. Place all voided urine in labeled specimen bottle with appropriate additives.

Clinical Judgment *If a void is missed during the collection period, the timed urine collection procedure must start over, and previously collected urine must be discarded.*

10. Unless instructed otherwise, keep specimen bottle in specimen refrigerator or container of ice in bathroom to prevent decomposition of urine.
11. Encourage patient to drink two glasses of water 1 hour before timed urine collection ends. Encourage patient to empty bladder during last 15 minutes of urine collection period.
12. Perform hand hygiene and apply clean gloves. Collect final specimen at end of collection period. Label specimen (two identifiers, specimen source, collection date and time, number of bottle) in patient's presence, attach appropriate requisition, and send to laboratory. Dispose of all contaminated supplies in appropriate receptacle.
    NOTE: Use appropriate disposal receptacle if patient is on hazardous drugs (Gorski et al., 2021). Remove and dispose of gloves and perform hand hygiene.
13. Remove signs. Tell patient that specimen collection period is completed.
14. Raise side rails (as appropriate) and lower bed to lowest position, locking into position.
15. Place nurse call system in an accessible location within patient's reach.
16. **Use Teach-Back:** "I want to be sure I explained how you can help us collect a 24-hour urine specimen. Tell me what you need to do when you have to pass urine." Revise your instruction now or develop a plan for revised patient/family caregiver teaching if patient/family caregiver is not able to teach back correctly (AHRQ, 2023).
17. Place specimen in biohazard bag or container as per agency policy and deliver to appropriate laboratory.
18. Document time 24-hour specimen collection was completed and the time it was sent to lab.
19. Provide hand-off report to health care provider of any changes or abnormal findings.

✦ SKILL 7.2   Measuring Occult Blood in Stool

 Video Clip

Hemoccult testing is useful for screening for the presence of occult (not visible) blood in the stool for some urgent conditions such as bleeding gastrointestinal (GI) ulcers and localized gastric or intestinal irritation. Use caution; a false-positive result may occur if a patient has ingested red meat within 3 days of testing or is taking certain medications (e.g., iron). A false-negative result may occur if the patient is taking vitamin C (Pagana et al., 2021). The test measures microscopic amounts of blood in the stool. Normally a person loses small amounts of blood daily in the feces as a result of minor abrasions of the nasopharyngeal or oral mucosa. If more than 50 mL of blood enters the feces from the upper GI tract, the blood causes melena (darkening of feces). When blood is present, further testing is indicated to determine the source of the bleeding.

There are newer, more sensitive tests for colorectal cancer screening. The multitarget stool DNA test with fecal immunochemical test (sDNA-FIT) is recommend as an option for colorectal cancer screening (Anand & Liang, 2022). Another multitarget stool DNA test (MT-sDNA) or Cologuard is used in adults 45 to 75 years of age who are at average risk. This detects not only hemoglobin but also DNA mutations and methylation that may indicate the presence of colorectal cancer or precancerous advanced adenomas (Clebak et al., 2022).

Delegation

The skill of testing stool for occult blood can be delegated to assistive personnel (AP). Direct the AP to:
- Report immediately if any blood is detected and not discard stool from a positive test so the nurse may repeat the testing

Equipment
- Soap, water, washcloth, and towel
- Paper towel
- Clean gloves
- Wooden applicators

Hemoccult Test
- Cardboard Hemoccult slide (Fig. 7.4)
- Hemoccult developing solution

Hematest
- Hematest tablets (must be protected from moisture, heat, and light)
- Guaiac paper
- Clean container of tap water

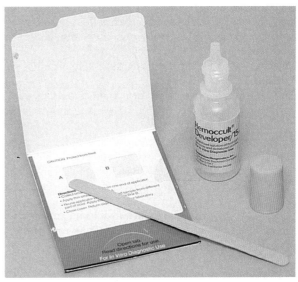

FIG. 7.4 Hemoccult testing kit for measuring occult blood.

STEP	RATIONALE

ASSESSMENT

1. Identify patient using at least two identifiers (e.g., name and birthday or name and medical record number) according to agency policy.

    Ensures correct patient. Complies with The Joint Commission standards and improves patient safety (TJC, 2023).

2. Review patient's electronic health record (EHR), including health care provider's order and nurses' notes. Note any health care provider's orders for medication or dietary modifications or restrictions before test.

    Specimens will be positive if contaminated by menstrual blood, hemorrhoid blood, or povidone-iodine. Diets rich in meats, green leafy vegetables, poultry, and fish may produce false-positive results.

3. Review patient's EHR for GI disorders (e.g., history of bleeding, colitis, or hemorrhoids).

    You can institute routine screening. Hemorrhoids can cause bleeding that may be misinterpreted as upper GI bleeding.

4. Review patient's EHR for any patient medications that contribute to bleeding.

    Anticoagulants increase risk for bleeding in GI tract, even from minor trauma to mucosa. Long-term use of steroids, nonsteroidal antiinflammatory drugs (NSAIDs), and acetylsalicylic acid (aspirin) can irritate mucosa and result in bleeding (Pagana et al., 2021).

5. Assess patient's/family caregiver's health literacy.

    Determines degree to which individuals have the ability to find, understand, and use information and services to make informed health-related decisions and actions for themselves and others (CDC, 2023).

STEP	RATIONALE
6. Perform hand hygiene. Assess patient's weight, level of consciousness, developmental level, ability to cooperate, and mobility.	Reduces transmission of microorganisms. Determines how much help is needed to properly position patient if a bedpan is used, ability of patient to cooperate during procedure, and level of explanation needed. To avoid embarrassment, patients often prefer to collect own stool specimen.
7. Assess patient's knowledge, prior experience with stool specimen collection, and feelings about procedure.	Reveals need for patient instruction and/or support.

PLANNING

1. Expected outcomes following completion of procedure:	
• Test for occult blood is negative.	Patient has only small amount or no blood in feces. Test specimen obtained correctly.
• Patient discusses purpose and benefits of testing stool for blood.	Validates learning.
2. Arrange for any needed dietary or medication restrictions.	Ensures accuracy of test results.
3. Provide privacy and explain procedure to patient and/or family caregiver. Discuss reason for specimen collection and how patient can help. Explain that feces must be free of urine and toilet tissue.	Protects patient's privacy; reduces anxiety. Promotes cooperation. Patient who understands procedure is more likely to cooperate and may be able to obtain specimen independently. Also prevents accidental disposal of specimen.
4. Organize and set up any equipment needed to perform procedure.	Ensures more efficiency when completing an assessment.
5. Arrange for extra personnel to help as necessary. Organize supplies at bedside.	Some patients are unable to assume positioning on a bedpan if needed to collect the stool specimen.

IMPLEMENTATION

1. Perform hand hygiene and apply clean gloves. Obtain uncontaminated stool specimen and place in clean, dry container not contaminated with urine, water, or toilet tissue.	Prevents transmission of microorganisms. Allows for accurate testing when specimen is not contaminated with other products.
2. Obtain two pieces of stool from two different areas of the specimen using a new wooden applicator for each of the two pieces.	Small specimen is sufficient for measuring blood content (Pagana et al., 2021).
3. Measure for occult blood.	
a. Perform Hemoccult slide test:	
(1) Open flap of Hemoccult slide. Apply thin smear of stool on paper in first box.	Guaiac paper inside box is sensitive to fecal blood content.
(2) Obtain second fecal specimen from different part of stool with a new applicator and apply thinly to second box of slide (see illustration).	Occult blood from upper GI tract is not always dispersed equally throughout stool. Findings of occult blood are more conclusive for GI bleeding when entire specimen is found to contain blood (Pagana et al., 2021).
(3) Close slide cover and turn slide over to reverse side. Open cardboard flap and apply 2 drops of Hemoccult developing solution on each box of guaiac paper (see illustration).	Developing solution penetrates underlying fecal specimen. Change in color of guaiac paper indicates blood.
(4) Read results of test after 30 to 60 seconds. Note color changes.	Ensures correct results. Bluish discoloration indicates occult blood (guaiac positive). No change in color of guaiac paper indicates negative results.
(5) Dispose of test slide in proper receptacle.	Reduces transfer of microorganisms.
b. Perform test using Hematest tablets:	Tablet contains solid form of developing solution.
(1) Place stool on guaiac paper. Then place Hematest tablet on top of stool specimen. Apply 2 to 3 drops of tap water to tablet, allowing water to flow onto guaiac paper.	Tap water dissolves Hematest tablet and thus dispenses developing solution over specimen and guaiac paper.
(2) Observe color of guaiac paper within 2 minutes.	Bluish discoloration is guaiac positive. Do not read color after 2 minutes. False findings may occur.
(3) Dispose of tablet and paper in proper receptacle.	Reduces transfer of microorganisms.
4. Wrap wooden applicator in paper towel, grasp in nondominant hand, remove gloves over wrapped applicator, discard soiled supplies, and perform hand hygiene.	Reduces transfer of microorganisms.

STEP	RATIONALE

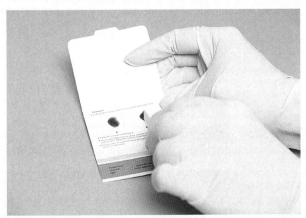

STEP 3a(2) Applying stool specimen to both spots on Hemoccult slide.

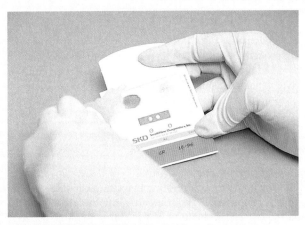

STEP 3a(3) Applying developing solution.

5. Raise side rails (as appropriate) and lower bed to lowest position, locking into position.

Ensures patient safety and prevents falls.

6. Place nurse call system in an accessible location within patient's reach.

Ensures patient can call for assistance if needed.

EVALUATION

1. Note color changes in guaiac paper.

Reveals blood in feces.

2. **Use Teach-Back:** "You may need to check your stool two more times for blood when you go home. I want to be sure I explained the procedure correctly. Tell me the steps you will use to collect this specimen." Revise your instruction now or develop a plan for revised patient/family caregiver teaching if patient/family caregiver is not able to teach back correctly.

Teach-back is a technique for health care providers to ensure that they have explained medical information clearly so that patients and their families understand what is communicated to them (AHRQ, 2023).

3. Note character of stool specimen.

Certain abnormal constituents of stool may be visible.

Unexpected Outcomes

1. Test for occult blood is positive.

Related Interventions

- Continue to monitor patient.
- Notify health care provider.

Documentation

- Document results of test and stool characteristics.
- Document your evaluation of patient and family caregiver learning.

Hand-Off Reporting

- Report positive test results to health care provider.

Special Considerations

Patient Education

- Teach patient and family caregiver how to apply stool to the Hemoccult slide from two different locations of the stool

specimen, close the flap, and return to the clinic or health care provider's office if appropriate.

- Teach patient and family caregiver to wrap wooden applicator in paper towel, grasp in nondominant hand, and remove gloves over wrapped applicator. Discard in proper receptacle. Perform hand hygiene.

Pediatrics

- Children of school age and older are concrete thinkers and often very curious. They may ask many questions about the test. Answer questions honestly and at child's level of understanding.

Allow child to watch, if desired, while performing test (Hockenberry et al., 2022).

- Testing reagent is often poisonous; therefore, keep it out of reach of the small child.

Older Adults

- Older adults may need help in positioning to obtain specimen. In confused patients it may be necessary for the AP or family caregiver to help the patient collect a specimen (Touhy & Jett, 2022).

Populations With Disabilities

- Collecting a stool specimen may elicit different reactions for a person with a cognitive disability. The family caregiver may be a valuable resource in obtaining this specimen (Mendes, 2018).

Home Care

- Many patients or family caregivers are instructed to collect specimens at home and return them to the clinic or health care provider's office. Be sure they know infection control principles.

✦ SKILL 7.3   Measuring Occult Blood in Gastric Secretions (Gastroccult)

Analysis of gastric secretions or emesis can detect blood that is not always visible. Gastroccult testing helps to reveal bleeding in the esophagus or stomach. The test can verify the presence of blood when red or black coloration of the gastric contents is noted or when the gastric contents or emesis has the appearance of coffee grounds. The test measures microscopic amounts of blood in the gastric secretions. It is a useful diagnostic tool for conditions such as upper gastrointestinal (GI) ulcers or bleeding. Because the test is easy to perform, patients are often taught how to test emesis in the home.

Delegation

The skill of Gastroccult testing can be delegated to assistive personnel (AP) for testing emesis (see agency policy). You cannot delegate the skill of Gastroccult testing to AP if the specimen is collected from a nasogastric (NG) or nasoenteral (NE) tube. Direct the AP to:

- Report immediately if blood or coffee-ground emesis is visible in NG or NE tube secretions
- Save specimen for repeat testing

Equipment

- Facial tissues
- Emesis basin
- Wooden applicator or 3-mL syringe
- Bulb or catheter tip syringe
- Cardboard Gastroccult test slide
- Gastroccult developing solution
- Clean gloves

STEP	RATIONALE
ASSESSMENT	
1. Identify patient using at least two identifiers (e.g., name and birthday or name and medical record number) according to agency policy.	Ensures correct patient. Complies with The Joint Commission standards and improves patient safety (TJC, 2023).
2. Review patient's electronic health record (EHR), including health care provider's order and nurses' notes. Note if occult blood was found previously in gastric secretions.	Identifies purpose of screening for occult blood in gastric secretions.
3. Review patient's EHR for patient's medical history for bleeding or GI disorders (e.g., history of bleeding, colitis) and drugs that predispose the patient to increased risk of bleeding.	You can institute routine screening. Anticoagulants increase risk for bleeding in GI tract, even from minor trauma to mucosa. Long-term use of steroids, nonsteroidal antiinflammatory drugs (NSAIDs), and acetylsalicylic acid (aspirin) can irritate mucosa.
4. Assess patient's/family caregiver's health literacy.	Determines degree to which individuals have the ability to find, understand, and use information and services to make informed health-related decisions and actions for themselves and others (CDC, 2023).
5. Assess patient's knowledge, prior experience with screening for occult blood in gastric secretions, and feelings about procedure.	Reveals need for patient instruction and/or support.
PLANNING	
1. Expected outcomes following completion of procedure:	
• Test for occult blood is negative.	Patient has only small or no amount of blood in gastric secretions.
• Patient discusses purpose and benefits of testing gastric contents for blood.	Validates learning.
2. Explain procedure to patient and/or family caregiver. Discuss why specimen collection is necessary.	Patient who understands procedure is more likely to be less anxious and more cooperative.

STEP	RATIONALE
3. Provide privacy and explain procedure.	Protects patient's privacy; reduces anxiety. Promotes cooperation.
4. Organize and set up any equipment needed to perform procedure.	Ensures more efficiency when completing an assessment.

IMPLEMENTATION

1. Perform hand hygiene. Apply clean gloves.	Reduces transmission of microorganisms.
2. Verify NG tube placement (see Chapter 31).	Ensures aspiration of gastric contents.
3. Obtain specimen.	
a. Disconnect suction or gravity drainage tube from NG or NE tube. Using a bulb or catheter tip syringe, aspirate 5 to 10 mL of fluid from NG or NE tube.	Only small amount of specimen is needed for testing.
b. To obtain sample of emesis, use 3-mL syringe or wooden applicator to obtain sample from emesis basin.	Small specimen is sufficient for measuring blood content.

Clinical Judgment *Observe specimen. If you find red blood or coffee-ground material, report these findings immediately to health care provider.*

4. Perform Gastroccult test:	
a. Using wooden applicator or syringe, apply 1 drop of gastric sample to Gastroccult blood test slide.	Sample must cover test paper for test reaction to occur.
b. Apply 2 drops of commercial developer solution over sample and 1 drop between positive and negative performance monitors (see illustration).	
c. Verify that performance monitor turns blue in 30 seconds.	Indicates proper function of testing paper.
d. After 60 seconds, compare color of gastric sample with that of performance monitor.	If sample turns blue, test is positive for occult blood. If sample turns green, it is negative for occult blood.
5. Dispose of test slide, wooden applicator, and syringe in proper receptacle. If needed, reconnect enteral tube to drainage system or suction. Remove and dispose of gloves. Perform hand hygiene.	Reduces transmission of microorganisms. Use appropriate disposal receptacle if patient is on hazardous drugs (Gorski et al., 2021).
6. Raise side rails (as appropriate) and lower bed to lowest position, locking into position.	Ensures patient safety and prevents falls.
7. Place nurse call system in an accessible location within patient's reach.	Ensures patient can call for assistance if needed.

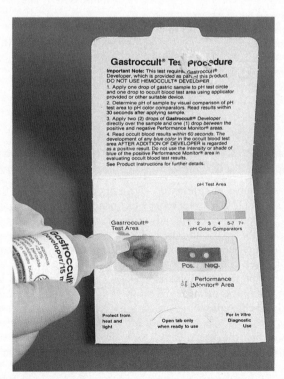

STEP 4b Applying developing solution to Gastroccult test area.

STEP	RATIONALE

EVALUATION

1. Note character of gastric secretions.

2. Note color changes in guaiac paper.
3. **Use Teach-Back:** "I want to be sure I explained the purpose and procedure for obtaining a specimen of your gastric secretions. Tell me why we are performing this test." Revise your instruction now or develop a plan for revised patient/family caregiver teaching if patient/family caregiver is not able to teach back correctly.

Blood may be visible, or coffee-ground material denoting blood may be observed.
Reveals blood in gastric secretions.
Teach-back is a technique for health care providers to ensure that they have explained medical information clearly so that patients and their families understand what is communicated to them (AHRQ, 2023).

Unexpected Outcomes

1. Test for occult blood is positive.

2. Bright red blood or coffee-ground secretions appear in nasogastric or nasoenteral tube or patient vomitus.

Related Interventions

- Continue to monitor patient.
- Notify health care provider.
- Notify health care provider immediately.

Documentation

- Document results of test and presence of any unusual characteristics of gastric contents.
- Document your evaluation of patient and family caregiver learning.

Hand-Off Reporting

- Report positive test results to health care provider.

Special Considerations

Patient Education

- Teach patient and family caregiver to contact the health care provider if specimen is positive for blood.
- Teach patient and family caregiver how to apply gastric emesis to the Gastroccult slide, close the flap, and return to the clinic or health care provider's office if appropriate.
- Teach patient and family caregiver to dispose of test slide, wooden applicator, and syringe in proper receptacle. Remove and dispose of gloves. Perform hand hygiene.

Pediatrics

- Children of school age and older are concrete thinkers and often very curious. They may ask many questions about the test. Answer questions honestly and at child's level of understanding. Allow child to watch, if desired, while performing test (Hockenberry et al., 2022).
- Testing reagent is often poisonous; therefore, keep it out of reach of the small child.

Older Adults

- In confused patients, the family caregiver may be necessary to help the patient collect and test the specimen for blood at home (Touhy & Jett, 2022).

Home Care

- Many patients or family caregivers can perform the Gastroccult test on emesis. Be sure they know infection control principles.

◆ SKILL 7.4 Collecting Nose and Throat Specimens for Culture

When patients have signs and symptoms of upper respiratory or sinus infection, a nose or throat culture is a simple diagnostic tool to identify the presence and type of microorganisms. You should obtain culture specimens before antibiotic therapy is initiated because antibiotics may interrupt the growth of the organisms in the laboratory. In addition, an antibiotic-free culture helps to ensure proper therapy so that the proper antibiotic or antiviral is prescribed. If a patient is receiving an antibiotic or antiviral, notify the laboratory and identify which specific antibiotics are being taken (Pagana et al., 2021).

Collection of a specimen from the nose and throat can cause discomfort and gagging because of sensitive mucosal membranes. It is important to collect a throat culture before mealtime or at least 1 hour after eating or drinking to decrease the chance of inducing vomiting.

Delegation

The skill of obtaining specimens from the nose and throat cannot be delegated to assistive personnel (AP).

Equipment

- Two sterile swabs in sterile culture tubes (flexible wire swab with cotton tip may be used for nose cultures)

- Nasal speculum (optional)
- Emesis basin or clean container (optional)
- Tongue blades and penlight
- Facial tissues/gauze
- Clean gloves

- Completed identification labels with proper patient identifiers
- Completed laboratory requisition (date, time, name of test, patient identification, source of culture)
- Biohazard plastic bag for delivery of specimen to laboratory (or container specified by agency)

STEP	RATIONALE

ASSESSMENT

1. Identify patient using at least two identifiers (e.g., name and birthday or name and medical record number) according to agency policy.

Ensures correct patient. Complies with The Joint Commission standards and improves patient safety (TJC, 2023).

2. Review patient's electronic health record (EHR), including health care provider's order and nurses' notes. Note if nose, throat, or both cultures are needed.

Identifies purpose of collecting nose or throat cultures and prevents exposing patient to unnecessary discomfort of repeated cultures.

3. Review patient's EHR to determine if patient has had a fever, chills, or other signs of infection.

Symptoms help reveal nature of problem.

4. Assess patient's/family caregiver's health literacy.

Determines degree to which individuals have the ability to find, understand, and use information and services to make informed health-related decisions and actions for themselves and others (CDC, 2023).

5. Ask if patient is experiencing postnasal drip, sinus headache or tenderness, nasal congestion, or sore throat, or has had exposure to others with similar symptoms.

Possible indicators for testing of nasal secretions.

6. Perform hand hygiene and apply clean gloves. Assess condition of posterior pharynx (see Chapter 6).

Reveals local inflammation or lesions of pharynx.

7. Inspect condition of nares and drainage from nasal mucosa and sinuses.

Reveals physical signs that indicate infection or allergic irritation. Clear drainage usually indicates allergy. Yellow, green, or brown drainage usually indicates infection.

8. Assess patient's knowledge, prior experience with nose or throat cultures, and feelings about procedure.

Reveals need for patient instruction and/or support.

PLANNING

1. Expected outcomes following completion of procedure:
   - There is no bacterial growth in specimens.
   - Patient does not experience bleeding of nasal mucosa.
   - Specimen is not contaminated.
   - Patient discusses purpose of nose and throat cultures.

Absence of bacterial infection.
Procedure is atraumatic.
Evidenced by results of laboratory analysis.
Validates learning.

2. Plan to do culture before mealtime or at least 1 hour after eating.

Procedure often induces gagging; timing decreases patient's chances of vomiting.

3. Provide privacy and explain procedure to patient and/or family caregiver. Discuss reason for specimen collection and how patient can help.

Protects patient's privacy; reduces anxiety. Promotes cooperation.

4. Explain that patient may have tickling sensation or gagging during swabbing of throat. Nasal swab may create urge to sneeze. Each procedure takes only a few seconds to complete.

Knowing that this is a normal response to the procedure may help patient relax.

5. Organize and set up any equipment needed to perform procedure.

Ensures more efficiency when completing an assessment.

6. Arrange for extra personnel to help, as necessary.

Some patients are unable to assume positioning independently for procedure.

IMPLEMENTATION

1. Have swab in tube ready for use. Loosen top so swab can be removed easily.

Allows you to grasp swab easily without danger of contamination. Most commercial tubes have tops that fit securely over end of swab. Allows touching outer tops without contaminating swab stick.

2. Ask patient to sit erect in bed or chair facing you. Acutely ill patient or young child may lie back against bed with head of bed raised to 45-degree angle in semi-Fowler position.

Provides easy access to nasal or oral structures.

STEP	RATIONALE

3. Collect throat culture.

    a. Perform hand hygiene and apply clean gloves.

    b. Instruct patient to tilt head backward. For patients in bed, place pillow behind shoulders.

    c. Ask patient to open mouth and say "ah." To visualize pharynx, depress tongue with tongue blade and note inflamed areas of pharynx or tonsils. Depress anterior third of tongue only and illuminate with penlight as needed.

Reduces transmission of microorganisms.
Facilitates visualization of pharynx.

Permits exposure of pharynx, relaxes throat muscles, and minimizes gag reflex.
Area to be swabbed should be visualized clearly.

Clinical Judgment *Do not attempt throat culture in a pediatric patient if you suspect acute epiglottitis because trauma from swab might cause increase in edema, resulting in occlusion of airway (Hockenberry et al., 2022).*

    d. Insert swab without touching lips, teeth, tongue, cheeks, or uvula.

    e. Gently but quickly swab tonsillar area side to side, making contact with inflamed or purulent sites (see illustration).

Prevents contamination with organisms from oral cavity (Pagana et al., 2021).
These areas contain most microorganisms.

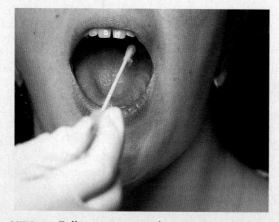

STEP 3e Collecting specimen from posterior pharynx.

    f. Carefully withdraw swab without touching oral structures.

Collects microorganisms from throat tissues without contamination from mouth and tongue.

4. Collect nasal culture:

    a. Perform hand hygiene and apply clean gloves.

    b. Encourage patient to blow nose, and then check nostrils for patency with penlight. Select nostril with greatest patency.

    c. In sitting position, have patient tilt head backward. Patients in bed should have small pillow behind shoulders.

    d. Gently insert nasal speculum in one nostril *(optional)*.

    e. Carefully pass swab into nostril until it reaches that part of mucosa that is inflamed or contains exudate. Rotate swab quickly. **NOTE:** If you need to obtain nasopharyngeal culture, use special swab on flexible wire that can be flexed downward to reach nasopharynx.

    f. Remove swab without touching sides of speculum or nasal canal.

    g. Carefully remove nasal speculum (if used) and place in basin. Offer patient facial tissue.

5. Insert swab into culture tube. Use gauze to protect your fingers while crushing ampule at bottom of tube to release culture medium (see illustrations).

Reduces transmission of microorganisms.
Clears nasal passages of mucus containing resident bacteria.

Provides access to nasal passages and facilitates visualization of nasal septum and sinuses.

Allows retraction of mucosa for easier swab insertion.
Swab should remain sterile until it reaches area to be cultured. Rotating swab covers all surfaces where exudate is present.

Prevents contamination of swab by resident bacteria.

Minimizes period of time that patient experiences discomfort.

Placing tip within culture medium maintains life of bacteria for testing.

STEP	RATIONALE

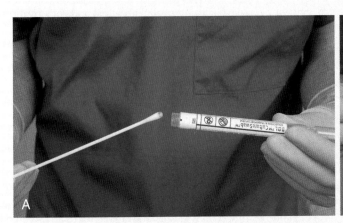 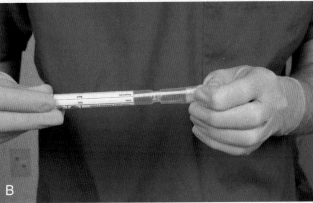

STEP 5 Activating culture tube. (A) Place swab into tube. (B) Crush end of tube to release liquid medium.

6. Place tip of swab into liquid medium and place top securely on top of tube. — Preserves specimen for testing.

7. Securely attach completed identification label and laboratory requisition to culture tube and confirm identifiers, specimen source, and collection date and time in front of patient (check agency policy). Note on laboratory requisition if patient is taking antibiotic or if specific organism is suspected (e.g., *Bordetella pertussis*). — Incorrect identification of specimen could result in diagnostic or therapeutic errors (TJC, 2023).

8. Enclose specimen in a biohazard bag (according to agency policy) and send immediately to laboratory. — Specimen not sent to laboratory immediately or refrigerated allows growth of organisms and inaccurate results.

9. Return patient to position of comfort. Remove and dispose of gloves and perform hand hygiene. — Provides for patient comfort. Reduces transmission of microorganisms.

10. Raise side rails (as appropriate) and lower bed to lowest position, locking into position. — Ensures patient safety and prevents falls.

11. Place nurse call system in an accessible location within patient's reach. — Ensures patient can call for assistance if needed.

EVALUATION

1. Check laboratory record for results of culture test. — Results reveal type of organisms in nose or pharynx and antibiotics most likely to be effective.

2. **Use Teach-Back:** "I want to be sure I explained the purpose and procedure for obtaining a throat culture. Please tell me why we are obtaining this culture." Revise your instruction now or develop a plan for revised patient/family caregiver teaching if patient/family caregiver is not able to teach back correctly. — Teach-back is a technique for health care providers to ensure that they have explained medical information clearly so that patients and their families understand what is communicated to them (AHRQ, 2023).

Unexpected Outcomes

1. Nose and throat cultures reveal bacterial growth.

2. Patient experiences minor nasal bleeding.

3. Specimen is contaminated.

Related Interventions

- Notify health care provider of findings.
- Administer medications as ordered.
- Apply mild pressure and ice pack over bridge of nose.
- Notify health care provider of patient's condition if bleeding continues.
- Repeat specimen collection.

Documentation

- Document appearance of nasal and oral mucosal structure; document specimen collection date and time, and document time and time sent to laboratory.
- Document your evaluation of patient and family caregiver learning.

Hand-Off Reporting

- Report unusual test results to health care provider.

Special Considerations

Patient Education

- Teach patient that procedure may cause slight discomfort and that gagging is common.
- Discuss reason for time delay in receiving culture results.

Pediatrics

- Allowing young children to visualize and examine speculum decreases their fear.
- Immobilization of child's head and arms is important when obtaining specimen. You should do this in a firm, gentle, kind manner. Ask another nurse to help if necessary.

- Ask parents to act as coach and suggest that they hold their child on their lap. Do not ask parents to restrain child (Hockenberry et al., 2022).
- Showing tongue blade and penlight to child and demonstrating how to say "ah" helps to decrease anxiety.
- School-age child will be more cooperative if given opportunity to ask questions about procedure and results.

Older Adults

- Some older adults need help in keeping mouth open to obtain specimen.
- Some older adults have poor dentition. Take care not to break a tooth, and consider removal of dentures (Touhy & Jett, 2022).

Populations With Disabilities

- Obtaining a nose or throat culture specimen in a patient with intellectual or cognitive disability may be perceived as a threat. Explain the procedure in short and simple sentences. Observe patient for warning signs of increased agitation or combativeness. If these occur, stop the procedure and give the patient time to calm down (Mendes, 2018).

✦ SKILL 7.5   Obtaining Vaginal or Urethral Discharge Specimens

Normally drainage from the vagina or urethra is thin, nonpurulent, whitish or clear, and small in amount. Factors such as poor hygiene practices can cause an accumulation of discharge. If a patient develops an increased amount of discharge or if there is a change in the character of discharge from the vagina or urethra, medical follow-up is necessary.

Patients most commonly requiring cultures of vaginal or urethral discharge have signs and symptoms of sexually transmitted infection (STI) or urinary tract infection (UTI). Patients suspected of having an STI may be embarrassed about their condition. Show respect and understanding toward a patient. When collecting vaginal or urethral specimens, work quickly and calmly, maintaining the patient's privacy at all times.

Delegation

The skill of obtaining vaginal or urethral discharge specimens cannot be delegated to assistive personnel (AP).

Interprofessional Collaboration

- Discuss any abnormal findings such as vaginal or urethral discharge or if signs and symptoms of STI or UTI are present with the health care team.

Equipment

- Sterile swab in sterile culture tube (commercially available culture tubes have swab and tube with ampule containing special transport medium)
- Sheet, blanket, or paper drape
- Clean gloves
- Penlight or gooseneck lamp
- Completed identification labels with proper patient identifiers
- Completed laboratory requisition (date, time, name of test, patient identification, source of culture)
- Biohazard plastic bag for delivery of specimen to laboratory (or container specified by agency)

STEP	RATIONALE

ASSESSMENT

STEP	RATIONALE
1. Identify patient using at least two identifiers (e.g., name and birthday or name and medical record number) according to agency policy.	Ensures correct patient. Complies with The Joint Commission standards and improves patient safety (TJC, 2023).
2. Review patient's electronic health record (EHR), including health care provider's order to determine if culture is to be vaginal or urethral.	Identifies purpose of culture. Patient may require one or both types of cultures.
3. Review patient's EHR to determine if patient has had a fever, chills, or other signs of infection.	Symptoms help reveal nature of problem.
4. Assess patient's/family caregiver's health literacy.	Determines degree to which individuals have the ability to find, understand, and use information and services to make informed health-related decisions and actions for themselves and others (CDC, 2023).

STEP	RATIONALE
5. Ask patient about dysuria, localized pruritus of genitalia, or lower abdominal pain.	Symptoms of urinary tract or vaginal infection.
6. If symptoms suggest STI, gather and document patient's sexual history.	Determines sexual activity and if there has been sexual contact with a person known to have an STI.
7. Perform hand hygiene and apply clean gloves. Position patient and assess condition of external genitalia and urethra, meatus, and vaginal orifice. Observe for redness; swelling; complaint of tenderness; and discharge that is whitish, mucoid, or purulent or a whitish discharge such as cottage cheese. Remove and dispose of gloves and perform hand hygiene. **NOTE:** This step may be done during collection.	Reduces transmission of microorganisms. Assessment findings and specimen test results reveal nature of problem.
8. Assess patient's knowledge, prior experience with vaginal or urethral swab, and feelings about procedure.	Reveals need for patient instruction and/or support.

PLANNING

1. Expected outcomes following completion of procedure: • Specimen is not contaminated. • Vaginal or urethral cultures do not reveal growth of microorganisms.	Results of laboratory test will reveal whether skin cells or mucosal cells have contaminated specimen. Evidence of absence of infection.
2. Provide privacy and explain procedure to patient and/or family caregiver. Discuss reason for specimen collection and how patient can help. Instruct female patient not to douche for 24 hours before culture is obtained. Male patient is not to urinate for 1 hour before urethral culture is obtained.	Protects patient's privacy; reduces anxiety. Patient who understands procedure is less anxious and more likely to cooperate. Douching of vaginal canal would remove discharge containing pathogens. Urinating by male washes secretions out of urethra (Pagana et al., 2021).
3. Organize and set up equipment needed to perform procedure.	Ensures more efficiency when completing an assessment.
4. Arrange for extra personnel, usually of the same gender as the patient, to assist in specimen collection. Organize supplies at bedside.	Some patients need gender-congruent caregivers to assist with positioning and obtaining the culture.

IMPLEMENTATION

1. Draw bedside curtains or close room door. Place "Do Not Enter" sign on door (if available).	Provides privacy for patient and demonstrates respect for patient's well-being.
2. Perform hand hygiene and apply clean gloves.	Reduces transmission of microorganisms.
3. Help patient to proper position, raise gown, and drape body parts to be exposed: a. *Female:* Dorsal recumbent position with sheet draped over each leg and genitalia. b. *Male:* Sitting on chair or bed or lying supine with sheet draped across lower trunk and genitalia.	Provides easy access to perineal area. Draping minimizes exposure of body parts, minimizing anxiety.
4. Direct light source onto perineum (may not be needed for male patient).	Allows better visualization of external urethral or vaginal structures.
5. Open culture tube and hold swab in dominant hand.	Provides for easier manipulation of swab during culture collection.
6. Instruct patient to deep breathe slowly.	Helps patient relax. Tensing of muscles around pelvic floor may cause discomfort during swabbing.
7. Obtain specimens. a. Female: (1) With nondominant hand, fully separate labia to expose vaginal orifice.	Exposes perineum and ensures that specimen is of vaginal discharge.
(2) Touch tip of swab into discharge pool, being careful not to touch skin or mucosa along perineum or vaginal canal. If no discharge is visible, gently insert swab 1 to 2.5 cm (⅓–1 inch) into vaginal orifice and rotate before removal.	Discharge contains greatest concentration of microorganisms.
(3) To expose urethral meatus, use nondominant hand to pull gently on labia minora upward and back to separate.	Allows better visualization of urethral orifice.

STEP	RATIONALE
(4) Use clean swab; gently apply to tip of meatus where discharge is visible. Avoid touching labia.	Discharge contains greatest concentration of microorganisms.

Clinical Judgment *If discharge near vagina appears different from discharge along perineum, collect separate specimens from each area because if two organisms are present, they could be cross-contaminated on a single swab. Label specimen with area of patient's body that you swabbed.*

STEP	RATIONALE
b. Male:	
(1) Grasp patient's penis proximal to glans with nondominant hand; if male is uncircumcised, gently retract foreskin.	Provides clear exposure of urethral meatus.
(2) Use dominant hand to hold swab. Apply gently to area of discharge at urinary meatus.	Discharge contains greatest number of microorganisms.
(3) If no discharge is apparent, health care provider may order swab to be introduced into urinary meatus. Hold male genitalia firmly but gently.	Excess manipulation can cause erection.
(4) Return foreskin to natural position.	Tightening of foreskin around shaft of penis can cause localized discomfort, edema, and potential necrosis.
8. Return each swab to culture tube and secure top.	Retains microorganisms within tube.
9. If using commercial culture tube, wrap ampule with gauze to prevent injury to your fingers while crushing. Immediately squeeze end of tube to crush ampule (see Skill 7.4). Push tip of swab into fluid medium.	Medium supports life of microorganisms until culture is analyzed.
10. Remove and dispose of gloves. Perform hand hygiene.	Reduces transmission of microorganisms. Use appropriate disposal receptacle if patient is on hazardous drugs (Gorski et al., 2021).
11. Label each culture tube with identification label, affix completed requisition, and confirm identifiers in front of patient.	Incorrect specimen identification could lead to diagnostic or therapeutic error (TJC, 2023).
12. Send specimen to laboratory immediately or refrigerate.	Bacteria multiply quickly. Prompt analysis ensures accurate results.
13. Help patient to a comfortable position, help with personal hygiene, and remove and discard drape. Perform hand hygiene.	Reinforces patient's sense of self-esteem.
14. Raise side rails (as appropriate) and lower bed to lowest position, locking into position.	Ensures patient safety and prevents falls. Reduces transmission of microorganisms.
15. Place nurse call system in an accessible location within patient's reach.	Ensures patient can call for assistance if needed.

EVALUATION

1. Review laboratory results for evidence of pathogens.	Results will reveal type of organisms present. Certain organisms are common to vaginal tract. Urethra should be free of microorganisms.
2. Continue to monitor whether discharge is present; if so, observe color and amount.	Characteristics of discharge indicate specific type of infection.
3. **Use Teach-Back:** "I want to be sure I explained the purpose and procedure for obtaining a vaginal culture. Please tell me the steps of this procedure." Revise your instruction now or develop a plan for revised patient/family caregiver teaching if patient/family caregiver is not able to teach back correctly.	Teach-back is a technique for health care providers to ensure that they have explained medical information clearly so that patients and their families understand what is communicated to them (AHRQ, 2023).

Unexpected Outcomes	Related Interventions
1. Vaginal or urethral cultures reveal growth of pathogenic microorganisms.	• Tell patient to receive treatment and to have sexual partners evaluated (Pagana et al., 2021). • Notify health care provider of findings and follow new orders. • Continue to monitor patient.
2. Specimen is contaminated with feces or epidermal cells.	• Repeat specimen collection.

Documentation

- Document the types of cultures obtained and date and time sent to laboratory.
- Document your evaluation of patient and family caregiver learning.

Hand-Off Reporting

- Report laboratory results to health care provider.
- Report abnormal findings such as redness or swelling; complaint of tenderness; and discharge that is whitish, mucoid, or purulent or a whitish cottage cheese–like discharge.

Special Considerations

Patient Education

- Discuss sexuality and safe sex practices with patient if appropriate.
- Patients with urethral or vaginal discharge often require instruction about perineal hygiene measures.
- If topical treatments (e.g., suppositories) are ordered, teach patient proper administration of medication (see Chapter 21).

Pediatrics

- A second nurse can help with specimen collection from an infant or young child by gently holding child's legs apart in froglike position. Have parent present to encourage cooperation.
- Parents should understand that obtaining vaginal specimen will not affect virginity of child.

Older Adults

- Older adults may need help in positioning to obtain specimen. In confused patients it may be necessary for the AP or family caregiver to help with the collection of the specimen (Touhy & Jett, 2022).

Populations With Disabilities

- Collecting vaginal or urethral culture may elicit different reactions for a person with an intellectual disability. It may be helpful to have family caregiver assist. Explain procedure in short clear sentences, carefully consider the needs of the individual, and provide care in a sensitive and respectful manner. Verify that all members of the health care team are aware of the patient's intellectual disability and appropriate interventions (Bobbette et al., 2020; Sullivan et al., 2018).
- When patients have physical disabilities, an assistant is often needed to position patient to obtain a culture.

PROCEDURAL GUIDELINE 7.2 *Collecting a Sputum Specimen by Expectoration*

Sputum is mucus produced by cells of the lungs, bronchi, and trachea. You collect a specimen either by having a patient cough and expectorate into a sterile specimen container or by suctioning into a sterile sputum trap (see Skill 7.6). In a healthy patient sputum production is minimal; a disease state can increase the amount and character of sputum. Sputum specimens are collected to identify cancer cells, for culture and sensitivity (C&S) testing, and for acid-fast bacillus testing to diagnose pulmonary tuberculosis.

Delegation

The skill of collecting a sputum specimen by expectoration can be delegated to assistive personnel (AP). Direct the AP to:

- Immediately report the presence of blood in the sputum or changes in patient's vital signs

Interprofessional Collaboration

- Discuss with the health care provider and a respiratory therapist to determine if patient needs a prescribed respiratory treatment to assist with obtaining sputum sample.

Equipment

Completed identification labels with appropriate patient identifiers; completed laboratory requisition, including appropriate patient identification, date, time, name of test, and source of specimen; small biohazard plastic bag for delivery of specimen to laboratory (or container as specified by agency); sterile specimen container with cover; clean gloves; facial tissues; emesis basin *(optional)*; toothbrush *(optional)*; disinfectant swab *(optional)*

Steps

1. Identify patient using at least two identifiers (e.g., name and birthday or name and medical record number) according to agency policy (TJC, 2023).
2. Provide opportunity to clean or rinse mouth with water. Patient should not use mouthwash or toothpaste because the products may alter test results.
3. Assess patient's/family caregiver's health literacy.
4. Assess patient's knowledge, prior experience with sputum collection, and feelings about procedure.
5. Provide privacy and explain procedure to patient.
6. Perform hand hygiene and apply clean gloves. Provide sputum cup and instruct patient not to touch the inside of the container.
7. Have the patient take three or four deep, slow breaths with full exhalation. Then take full inhalation followed immediately by a forceful cough, expectorating sputum directly into specimen container.
8. Repeat until 5 to 10 mL of sputum (not saliva) has been collected.
9. Secure lid on container tightly. If any sputum is present on outside of container, wipe it off with disinfectant.
10. Offer patient tissues after patient expectorates, dispose of tissues, and offer mouth care.
11. Securely attach properly completed identification label and laboratory requisition to side of specimen container (not lid). Confirm identifiers in patient's presence (TJC, 2023).
12. Enclose specimen in a biohazard bag.
13. Remove and dispose of gloves. Perform hand hygiene.
14. Help patient to a comfortable position.
15. Raise side rails (as appropriate) and lower bed to lowest position, locking into position.
16. Place nurse call system in an accessible location within patient's reach.
17. Send specimen to laboratory immediately.
18. **Use Teach-Back:** "I want to be sure I explained the way to obtain a sputum specimen. Please repeat the steps back to me." Revise your instruction now or develop a plan for revised patient/family caregiver teaching if patient/family caregiver is not able to teach back correctly (AHRQ, 2023).
19. Document time sputum specimen collection was completed and sent to lab.
20. Provide hand-off report to health care provider of any changes, abnormal findings, or respiratory distress.

✦ SKILL 7.6   Collecting a Sputum Specimen by Suction

 Video Clip

Although sputum production is minimal in a healthy state, disease states can increase the amount or change the character of sputum. Examination of sputum aids in the diagnosis and treatment of several conditions, ranging from simple bronchitis to lung cancer.

Suctioning is indicated to collect a sterile sputum sample or sputum from patients who are unable to spontaneously expectorate a sample for laboratory analysis. Sometimes suctioning provokes violent coughing, which can induce vomiting and constriction of pharyngeal, laryngeal, and bronchial muscles. In addition, it may cause hypoxemia or vagal overload, causing cardiopulmonary compromise and increased intracranial pressure.

Delegation

The skill of collecting sputum specimens by suction cannot be delegated to assistive personnel (AP).

Interprofessional Collaboration

- Discuss with the health care provider and a respiratory therapist to determine if patient needs prescribed respiratory treatment to assist with obtaining sputum sample.

Equipment

- Completed identification labels with proper patient identifiers
- Completed laboratory requisition, including patient identification, date, time, name of test, and source of culture specimen
- Suction device (wall or portable)
- Sterile suction catheter (size 14, 16, or 18 Fr [not large enough to cause trauma to nasal mucosa]) or suction catheter with sleeve (see Chapter 24)
- Sterile gloves and clean gloves
- Sterile water in container
- In-line specimen container or sputum trap
- Biohazard bag for delivery of specimen to laboratory (or a container as specified by agency)
- Oxygen therapy equipment if indicated
- Protective eyewear
- Disinfectant wipe
- Vital signs equipment and pulse oximeter

STEP	RATIONALE

ASSESSMENT

1. Identify patient using at least two identifiers (e.g., name and birthday or name and medical record number) according to agency policy.	Ensures correct patient. Complies with The Joint Commission standards and improves patient safety (TJC, 2023).
2. Review electronic health record (EHR) for health care provider's orders for type of sputum analysis and specifications (e.g., amount of sputum, number of specimens, time of collection, method to obtain). Acid-fast bacillus (AFB) testing requires three consecutive morning samples.	Specific test dictates when or how frequently specimens are collected. Ideal time to collect sputum is early morning because bronchial secretions tend to accumulate during the night. Bacteria also accumulate as secretions pool.
3. Assess patient's/family caregiver's health literacy.	Determines degree to which individuals have the ability to find, understand, and use information and services to make informed health-related decisions and actions for themselves and others (CDC, 2023).
4. Assess EHR for contraindication to airway suctioning: • Head injury/facial fractures • Croup • Epiglottitis • Laryngospasm	It is important to follow current clinical practice guidelines to prevent inadvertent injury to patient. These conditions pose risks with suctioning.
5. Assess when patient last ate meal (or had tube feeding).	It is best to obtain specimen 1 to 2 hours after or 1 hour before meal to minimize gagging, which can cause vomiting and aspiration.
6. Determine type of help needed by patient to obtain specimen.	Positioning, postural drainage, and deep-breathing and coughing exercises may improve ability to cough productively. Suctioning is indicated when patient is unable to cough and expectorate.
7. Perform hand hygiene and perform a respiratory assessment, including respiratory rate, depth, and pattern and color of mucous membranes. Measure BP and attach pulse oximeter and measure oxygen saturation	Respiratory status can depend on amount of sputum in tracheobronchial tree. Findings serve as presuction baseline.
8. Assess patient's knowledge, prior experience with collecting a sputum specimen by suctioning, and feelings about procedure.	Reveals need for patient instruction and/or support.

STEP	RATIONALE

PLANNING

1. Expected outcomes following completion of procedure:
   - Patient's respirations and oxygen saturation are same rate and character before and after procedure.
   - Patient maintains comfort level and experiences minimal anxiety.
   - Sputum is not contaminated by saliva or oropharyngeal flora.
   - Patient discusses purpose and benefit of sputum collection.
2. Provide privacy and explain steps of procedure and purpose. Instruct patient to breathe normally during suctioning to prevent hyperventilation.
3. Gather and organize supplies at bedside.
4. Prepare suction machine or device and determine whether it functions properly.
5. Position patient in high- or semi-Fowler position.

Specimen collection did not alter respiratory status.

Suctioning tends to cause anxiety.

Sputum must originate from tracheobronchial tree for accurate results.
Validates learning.
Reduces anxiety and promotes understanding and cooperation.

Ensures greater efficiency when completing procedure.
Verifies that equipment is working properly before suctioning procedure.
Promotes full lung expansion and facilitates ability to cough.

IMPLEMENTATION

1. Perform hand hygiene and apply clean glove to nondominant hand. Prepare suction machine or device and determine if it functions properly.

Reduces transmission of microorganisms. Adequate amount of suction is necessary to aspirate sputum.

Clinical Judgment *If patient has surgical incision or localized area of discomfort, have patient place pillow or hands firmly over affected area. Splinting of painful area minimizes muscular stretching and discomfort during coughing and thus makes cough more productive.*

2. Connect suction tube to adapter on sputum trap. Open sterile water (see Chapter 24).
3. Using sterile technique, apply sterile glove to dominant hand or use a clean glove if suction catheter has plastic sleeve.
4. With gloved hand, connect sterile suction catheter to rubber tubing on sputum trap.
5. Lubricate suction catheter tip with sterile water (*with suction off*).
6. Gently insert tip of suction catheter through nasopharynx, endotracheal tube, or tracheostomy tube without applying suction (see Chapter 24).
7. Gently and quickly advance catheter into trachea. Warn patient to expect to cough.
8. As patient coughs, apply suction for 5 to 10 seconds, collecting 2 to 10 mL of sputum.

Establishes suction that passes through sputum trap to aspirate specimen.
Tracheobronchial tree is sterile body cavity. Allows you to manipulate suction catheter without contamination.

Aspirated sputum will go directly to trap instead of to suction tubing.
Lubrication allows for easier insertion of catheter.

Minimizes trauma to airway as catheter is inserted.

Entrance of catheter into larynx and trachea triggers cough reflex.
Ensures collection of sputum from deep within tracheobronchial tree. Suctioning longer than 10 seconds can cause hypoxia and mucosal damage.

Clinical Judgment *Observe for changes in patient's pulse oximetry and cardiac rhythm throughout procedure to determine if there are significant changes, such as decreased oxygenation or increased/decreased heart rate during procedure, which may indicate the patient's need for supplemental oxygen during procedure.*

9. Release suction and remove catheter; turn off suction.
10. Detach catheter from specimen trap and dispose of catheter in appropriate receptacle.
11. Secure top on specimen container tightly. For sputum trap, detach suction tubing and connect rubber tubing on sputum trap to plastic adapter (see illustration).
12. If any sputum is present on outside of container, wipe it off with disinfectant.
13. Offer patient tissues after suctioning. Dispose of tissues in emesis basin or appropriate container.
14. Label specimen with identification label on side of specimen container (not lid). Confirm identifiers in front of patient (TJC, 2023). Place specimen in biohazard bag (or container specified by agency) and attach requisition.

Suction can damage mucosa if applied during withdrawal.
Decreases risk for spreading microorganisms.

Contains microorganisms within container, preventing exposure to personnel handling specimen.

Prevents spread of infection to people handling specimen.

Maintains cleanliness and comfort.

Incorrect identification could lead to diagnostic or therapeutic error. Plastic bag or container reduces risk for health care worker's exposure to sputum.

STEP	RATIONALE

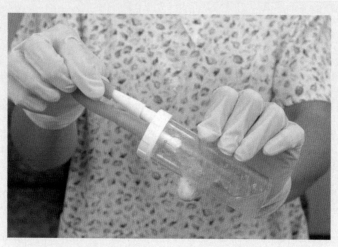

STEP 11 Closing sputum specimen trap.

15. Remove and dispose of gloves. Perform hand hygiene.
16. Offer patient mouth care if desired. Help patient to a comfortable position.
17. Raise side rails (as appropriate) and lower bed to lowest position, locking into position.
18. Place nurse call system in an accessible location within patient's reach.
19. Send specimen immediately to laboratory or refrigerate.

Reduces transmission of microorganisms.
Restores comfort and sense of well-being.

Ensures patient safety and prevents falls.

Ensures patient can call for assistance if needed.

Bacteria multiply quickly. Prompt analysis ensures accurate results.

EVALUATION

1. Observe patient's respiratory status throughout procedure, especially during suctioning. If in distress, measure oxygen saturation with pulse oximeter.
2. Note anxiety or discomfort in patient.

3. Observe character of sputum: color, consistency, odor, volume, viscosity, and/or presence of blood.
4. Refer to laboratory reports for test results.

5. **Use Teach-Back:** "I want to be sure I explained the purpose and procedure for obtaining a sputum specimen. Please tell me how I will obtain this sputum specimen." Revise your instruction now or develop a plan for revised patient/family caregiver teaching if patient/family caregiver is not able to teach back correctly.

Excessive coughing or prolonged suctioning can alter respiratory pattern and cause hypoxia. Determines oxygenation status.

Procedure can be uncomfortable. If patient becomes short of breath, anxiety will develop.
Characteristics may indicate disease type.

Indicates if abnormal cells or microorganisms are present in sputum.
Teach-back is a technique for health care providers to ensure that they have explained medical information clearly so that patients and their families understand what is communicated to them (AHRQ, 2023).

STEP	RATIONALE

Unexpected Outcomes

1. Patient becomes hypoxic with increased respiratory rate, effort, shortness of breath, and reduced oxygen saturation.

2. Patient remains anxious or reports discomfort from suction catheter.

3. Patient reports pain when coughing to produce sputum.

Related Interventions

- Discontinue suctioning immediately.
- Administer oxygen (if ordered).
- Notify health care provider of patient's condition.
- Continue to monitor patient's vital signs and pulse oximetry.

- Discontinue procedure until stable.
- Administer oxygen (if ordered).
- Notify health care provider of patient's change in condition.
- Continue to monitor patient's vital signs and pulse oximetry.

- Encourage patient who is recovering from surgical procedure to splint incision before coughing.
- Obtain order for pain medication as needed (prn).
- Inform health care provider of changes in patient's condition.

Documentation

- Document the method used to obtain specimen, type of test ordered, and date and time collected and transported to laboratory. Describe characteristics of sputum specimen. Describe patient's tolerance of procedure.
- Document your evaluation of patient and family caregiver learning.
- Document on specimen requisition if patient is receiving antibiotics and the name of the antibiotic.

Hand-Off Reporting

- Report any change in respiratory status and/or unusual sputum characteristics to nurse in charge or health care provider.
- Report abnormal findings to health care provider. If acid fast bacillus (AFB) sputum culture is positive, initiate appropriate isolation techniques.

Special Considerations

Patient Education

- Demonstrate proper splinting technique for postoperative patients.
- If aerosol treatment is indicated, teach patient purpose of procedure, explaining that it will stimulate coughing and sputum expectoration.

Pediatrics

- Children need very clear instructions or demonstration for deep breathing. Infants and young children will be unable to cooperate; aerosol treatment may be indicated.
- Use smaller catheter size for young children. It may be possible to elicit a cough by tickling the back of the throat with the suction catheter.

✦ SKILL 7.7   Obtaining Wound Drainage Specimens

When caring for a patient with a wound, assess the condition of the wound and observe for the development of infection. Localized inflammation, tenderness, and warmth at the wound site and purulent drainage are signs and symptoms of wound infection. A specimen of wound drainage is analyzed to determine the type and number of pathogenic microorganisms. Identification of the causative organism confirms an infection and provides guidelines for accurate treatment.

Always collect a wound culture sample from fresh exudate from the center of a wound, not the skin edge, after removing old drainage. Remove any antibiotic ointment or solution with water before obtaining the specimen. Collect the specimen before irrigating the wound (Pagana et al., 2021).

Resident colonies of bacteria on the skin grow in wound exudate and may not be the true causative organisms of infection. Use separate techniques to collect specimens for measuring aerobic versus anaerobic microorganisms. Aerobic organisms grow in superficial wounds exposed to the air. Anaerobic organisms grow deep within body cavities, where oxygen is not normally present.

Delegation

The skill of obtaining wound drainage specimens cannot be delegated to assistive personnel (AP).

Interprofessional Collaboration

- An interprofessional wound care team is a valuable resource if the wound has a foul odor or increase in drainage, or if the patient has an increase in temperature or reports discomfort.
- Consult infection control health care team members if wound is positive for organisms such as methicillin-resistant *Staphylococcus aureus* (MRSA) that require contact isolation (see Chapter 9). Communicate type of isolation precautions by posting a sign at the patient's bedside and documenting in the electronic health record (EHR).

Equipment

- Culture tube with swab and transport medium for aerobic culture
- For anaerobic cultures, obtain anaerobic culture tube from laboratory (Pagana et al., 2021)

- 5- to 10-mL safety syringe and 19-gauge needle
- Two pairs of clean gloves
- Two pairs of sterile gloves
- Protective eyewear
- Antiseptic swab
- Sterile dressing materials (determined by type of dressing)

- Paper or plastic disposable bag
- Completed specimen identification label with proper patient identifiers
- Completed laboratory requisition (date, time, name of test, patient identification, and source of culture specimen)
- Biohazard bag for delivery of specimen to laboratory (or container specified by agency)

STEP	RATIONALE

ASSESSMENT

1. Identify patient using at least two identifiers (e.g., name and birthday or name and medical record number) according to agency policy.

   Ensures correct patient. Complies with The Joint Commission standards and improves patient safety (TJC, 2023).

2. Review patient's electronic health record (EHR), including health care provider's order. Note if specimen is for aerobic or anaerobic culture.

   Specimens are taken from different sites and placed in different containers, depending on type of culture.

3. Review patient's EHR for fever and whether laboratory results report that white blood cell (WBC) count is elevated.

   Signs and symptoms indicate systemic infection.

4. Assess patient's/family caregiver's health literacy.

   Determines degree to which individuals have the ability to find, understand, and use information and services to make informed health-related decisions and actions for themselves and others (CDC, 2023).

5. Ask patient about extent and type of pain at wound site and use a scale of 0 to 10 to assess severity. If patient requires analgesic before dressing changes, give medication 30 minutes before beginning procedure to reach peak effect.

   Pain at wound site often increases with infection.

6. Determine when dressing change is scheduled (see Chapters 38 and 40). Perform wound assessment as part of actual procedure.

   Coordinating obtaining a wound culture with dressing change organizes care and assists with patient's comfort.

7. Perform hand hygiene and apply clean gloves. Remove old dressings covering wound. Fold soiled sides of dressing together and dispose of properly. Remove and dispose of gloves and perform hand hygiene. Apply sterile gloves to palpate wound. Observe for swelling, separation of wound edges, inflammation, and drainage. Palpate gently along wound edges and note tenderness or drainage. Remove and dispose of gloves and perform hand hygiene.

   Gloves minimize exposure to microorganisms. Signs indicate wound infection.

8. Assess patient's knowledge, prior experience with wound specimen collection, and feelings about procedure.

   Reveals need for patient instruction and/or support.

PLANNING

1. Expected outcomes following completion of procedure:
   - Wound culture does not reveal bacterial growth.
   - Culture swab is free of contamination from skin bacteria.
   - Patient discusses purpose and procedure for specimen collection.

   Wound remains free of pathogenic microorganisms.
   Test results indicate type of cells present.
   Validates learning.

2. Determine if analgesia is necessary. Administer analgesic 30 minutes before dressing change and/or specimen collection.

   Minimizes discomfort during procedure.

3. Provide privacy and explain reason for wound culture and how it will be collected.

   Protects patient's privacy; reduces anxiety. Promotes cooperation.

4. Explain that patient may feel tickling sensation when wound is swabbed.

   Anticipation of expected sensations minimizes anxiety.

5. Organize and set up equipment needed to perform procedure.

   Ensures greater efficiency when completing procedure.

6. Arrange for extra personnel to help, as necessary. Organize supplies at bedside.

   Some patients are unable to assume positioning independently for procedure.

STEP	RATIONALE

IMPLEMENTATION

1. Perform hand hygiene and apply clean gloves.

Reduces transmission of microorganisms.

2. Clean area around wound edges with antiseptic swab or sterile saline as ordered. Wipe from edges outward. Remove old exudate.

Removes skin flora, preventing possible contamination of specimen.

3. Discard antiseptic swab and remove and dispose of soiled gloves in appropriate receptacle. Perform hand hygiene.

Reduces spread of infection.

4. Open packages containing sterile culture tube and dressing supplies. *Apply sterile gloves.*

Provides sterile field for picking up and handling sterile supplies.

5. Obtain cultures.

Clinical Judgment *Handle all wound culture specimens as though they are capable of transmitting disease (Pagana et al., 2021).*

a. Aerobic culture
   (1) Take swab from culture tube, insert tip into wound in area of drainage, and rotate swab gently. Remove swab and return to culture tube (wrap outside of ampule with gauze to prevent injury to your fingers). Crush ampule of medium and push swab into fluid.

Swab should be coated with fresh secretions from within wound. Medium keeps bacteria alive until analysis is complete.

b. Anaerobic culture
   (1) Take swab from special anaerobic culture tube (obtained from the lab), swab deeply into draining body cavity of viable tissue, and rotate gently. Remove swab and return to culture tube.

Viable tissue means the tissues should be pink or red. Do not culture necrotic tissues. Specimen is taken from deep cavity where oxygen is not present. Carbon dioxide or nitrogen gas keeps organisms alive until analysis is complete.

   Or
   (2) Insert tip of syringe (without needle) into wound and aspirate 5 to 10 mL of exudate. Attach 19-gauge needle, expel all air, and inject drainage into special culture tube.

Sterile large-bore needle (19-gauge) allows exudate to be transferred from sterile syringe into special culture tube without contamination. Air injected into tube would cause organisms to die.

6. Remove and dispose of gloves. Perform hand hygiene.

Reduces transfer of microorganisms.

7. Place correct specimen label on each culture tube. Verify identifiers in front of patient (TJC, 2023). **NOTE:** Indicate on specimen if patient is receiving antibiotics.

Ensures correct results for correct patient.

8. Be sure that specimens are sent to laboratory within 30 minutes (Pagana et al., 2021).

Prompt analysis ensures accurate results.

9. Clean wound per health care provider's order. Apply new sterile dressing (see Chapters 38 and 40) using aseptic technique. Secure dressing with tape or ties.

Protects wound from further contamination; aids in absorbing drainage and debridement of wound.

10. Remove and dispose of gloves and soiled supplies in appropriate receptacle according to agency policy. Perform hand hygiene.

Reduces transmission of microorganisms.

11. Help patient to a comfortable position.

Promotes patient's ability to relax.

12. Raise side rails (as appropriate) and lower bed to lowest position, locking into position.

Ensures patient safety and prevents falls.

13. Place nurse call system in an accessible location within patient's reach.

Ensures patient can call for assistance if needed.

EVALUATION

1. Obtain laboratory report for results of cultures.

Report indicates if pathogenic organisms are identified.

2. Observe character of wound drainage.

Characteristics can reveal abnormal status and infection.

3. Observe edges of wound for redness and bleeding.

Indicates trauma to healing tissue.

4. **Use Teach-Back:** "I want to be sure I explained the purpose and procedure for obtaining a wound specimen. Please tell me in your own words how we will collect the specimen." Revise your instruction now or develop a plan for revised patient/family caregiver teaching if patient/family caregiver is not able to teach back correctly.

Teach-back is a technique for health care providers to ensure that they have explained medical information clearly so that patients and their families understand what is communicated to them (AHRQ, 2023).

STEP	RATIONALE
Unexpected Outcomes	**Related Interventions**
1. Wound cultures reveal bacterial growth.	• Monitor patient for fever, chills, or excessive thirst, which indicate systemic infection. • Inform health care provider of findings.
2. Wound culture is contaminated from superficial skin cells.	• Monitor patient for fever and pain. • Inform health care provider of findings. • Repeat collection of specimens as ordered.
3. Patient reports increased pain.	• Provide analgesia. • Notify health care provider.

Documentation

- Document types of specimens obtained, source, and time and date sent to laboratory, and describe appearance of wound and characteristics of any drainage.
- Document your evaluation of patient and family caregiver learning.
- Document patient's tolerance to procedure, dressing change, and response to analgesics.

Hand-Off Reporting

- Report any evidence of infection to the health care provider.

Special Considerations

Patient Education

- Instruct patient to inform you if procedure causes pain or if you need to stop because patient is unable to tolerate pain.
- Teach patient to assess status of wound for changes and signs and symptoms of infection.

Pediatrics

- If procedure is to be performed on a child and is anticipated to be painful, some agencies prefer performing it in area other than child's room to maintain feeling that child's room is safe place (Hockenberry et al., 2022).
- It is often helpful to have an additional nurse or other adult available to help with specimen collection in a young child or infant.

Older Adults

- Older adults may need help in positioning to change the dressing and obtain a wound culture. In confused patients it may be necessary for the AP or family caregiver to help with the collection of the specimen (Touhy & Jett, 2022).

Populations With Disabilities

- Changing a dressing and collecting wound culture may elicit different reactions in a person with an intellectual and developmental disability (IDD), particularly if it causes pain. If possible, give the patient an analgesic and time to process the procedure (Mendes, 2018).

◆ SKILL 7.8 | **Collecting Blood Specimens and Culture by Venipuncture (Syringe and Vacutainer Method)**

Blood tests are one of the most common diagnostic aids in the care and evaluation of patients. Tests allow health care providers to screen patients for early signs of physical illness, monitor changes in acute or chronic diseases, and evaluate responses to therapies.

In some health care agencies, you are responsible for collecting blood specimens; however, many agencies have specially trained phlebotomists who are responsible for drawing venous blood. Be familiar with your agency policies and procedures and your state nurse practice act regarding guidelines for drawing blood samples.

The three methods of obtaining blood specimens are (1) venipuncture, (2) skin puncture, and (3) arterial puncture. All procedures require sterile technique. Venipuncture is the most common method of obtaining blood specimens. This method involves inserting a hollow-bore needle into the lumen of a large vein to obtain a specimen using either a needle and syringe or a Vacutainer device that allows the drawing of multiple samples. Because veins are major sources of blood for laboratory testing and routes for intravenous (IV) fluid or blood replacement, maintaining their integrity is essential. You need to be skilled in venipuncture to avoid unnecessary injury to veins.

Skin puncture, also called *capillary puncture,* is the least traumatic method of obtaining a blood specimen. A sterile lancet or needle is used to puncture a vascular area on a finger or earlobe in

an adult or a child. You place a drop of blood on a test slide, wick a drop of blood to a test slide, or collect it within a thin glass capillary tube for laboratory analysis. Changes in health care economics and delivery result in the increased use of skin puncture. Point-of-care (POC) clinical laboratory tests at the bedside most frequently use skin puncture (Pagana et al., 2021).

Blood cultures aid in detection of bacteria in the blood. It is important that at least two culture specimens be drawn from two different sites. Because bacteremia may be accompanied by fever and chills, blood culture specimens should be drawn when these symptoms are present (Pagana et al., 2021). Bacteremia exists when both cultures grow the infectious agent. Only one culture growing bacteria is considered contamination. Draw all culture specimens before antibiotic therapy begins because the antibiotic may interrupt the growth of an organism in the laboratory. If the patient is receiving antibiotics, notify the laboratory and inform them of specific antibiotics the patient is receiving (Pagana et al., 2021).

Delegation

The skill of collecting blood specimens by venipuncture can be delegated to specially trained assistive personnel (AP). In some health care agencies, phlebotomists obtain the venipuncture samples. Agency and government regulations and policies differ regarding personnel who may draw blood specimens. Direct the AP to:

- Report any patient discomfort or signs of excessive bleeding from the puncture site to the nurse

Equipment

All Procedures

- 2% chlorhexidine in 70% alcohol, antiseptic swab, or check agency policy for use of other antiseptic solutions
- Clean gloves
- Small pillow or folded towel
- Sterile 2 × 2–inch gauze pads
- Tourniquet
- Adhesive bandage or adhesive tape
- Completed identification labels with proper patient identifiers
- Completed laboratory requisition (appropriate patient identification, date, time, name of test, and source of culture specimen)
- A biohazard bag for delivery of specimen to laboratory (or container specified by agency)
- Sharps container

Venipuncture With Syringe

- Sterile safety needles (20- to 21-gauge for adults; 23- to 25-gauge for children)

- Sterile 10- to 20-mL Luer-Lok safety syringes
- Needle-free blood transfer device
- Appropriate blood specimen tubes

Venipuncture With Vacutainer

- Vacutainer and safety access device with Luer-Lok adapter
- Sterile double needles (20- to 21-gauge for adults; 23- to 25-gauge for children)
- Appropriate blood specimen tubes

Blood Cultures

- Vacutainer holder
- Blood culture collection set (e.g., Safety-Lok with Luer connector)
- Two sets of anaerobic and aerobic culture bottles (check agency policy) that fit into Vacutainer holder

Central Venous Catheter (CVC) Collection

- Two empty 10-mL sterile syringes
- Sterile 10-mL normal saline (NS) flushes
- Vacutainer and safety access device Luer-Lok adapter
- Appropriate blood specimen tubes
- *Option:* Barrier isolation gown and/or sterile drape

STEP	RATIONALE

ASSESSMENT

1. Identify patient using at least two identifiers (e.g., name and birthday or name and medical record number) according to agency policy.

2. Review patient's electronic health record (EHR) for health care provider's orders for type of tests.

3. Review patient's EHR for possible risks associated with venipuncture: anticoagulant therapy, low platelet count, bleeding disorders (history of hemophilia).

4. Assess patient's/family caregiver's health literacy.

5. Determine if special conditions need to be met before specimen collection (e.g., patient allowed nothing by mouth [NPO], specific time for collection in relation to medication given, need to ice specimen).

6. Perform hand hygiene and assess patient for contraindicated sites for venipuncture: presence of IV infusion, hematoma at potential site, arm on side of mastectomy, or hemodialysis shunt.

7. Identify patient's risk for medical adhesive sensitivities. Review EHR to determine patient's age and history of dehydration, malnutrition, exposure to radiation therapy, underlying chronic conditions (e.g., diabetes mellitus, immunosuppression), and edema of the skin.

8. Identify if patient is allergic to latex or povidone-iodine (Betadine) or other antiseptic.

Ensures correct patient. Complies with The Joint Commission standards and improves patient safety (TJC, 2023).

Multiple samples are often needed. Health care provider's order is required.

Patient history may include abnormal clotting abilities caused by low platelet count, hemophilia, or medications that increase risk for bleeding and hematoma formation.

Determines degree to which individuals have the ability to find, understand, and use information and services to make informed health-related decisions and actions for themselves and others (CDC, 2023).

Some tests require meeting specific conditions to obtain accurate measurement of blood elements (e.g., fasting blood sugar, drug peak and trough level, timed endocrine hormone levels).

Reduces transmission of microorganisms. Drawing specimens from such sites can result in false test results or may injure patient. Samples taken from vein near IV infusion may be diluted or contain concentrations of IV fluids. Postmastectomy patient may have reduced lymphatic drainage in arm on operative side, increasing risk for infection from needlesticks. Never use arteriovenous shunt to obtain specimens because of risks for clotting and bleeding. Hematoma indicates existing injury to vessel wall.

Common risk factors for medical adhesive–related skin injury (MARSI) (Fumarola et al., 2020). Requires avoiding exposure to adhesives.

Exposure to topical agents can cause serious allergic reaction.

STEP	RATIONALE
9. Before drawing blood cultures, assess for systemic signs and symptoms of bacteremia, including fever and chills. 10. Assess patient's knowledge, prior experience with blood collection, and feelings about procedure.	Three blood culture samples should be drawn at least 1 hour apart beginning at the earliest signs of sepsis (Pagana et al., 2021). Reveals need for patient instruction and/or support.

Clinical Judgment *Some specimens have special collection requirements before or after specimen collection; examples follow:*
- *Cryoglobulin levels: Use prewarmed test tubes.*
- *Ammonia and ionized calcium levels: Place tube in ice for delivery to laboratory.*
- *Lactic acid levels: Do not use tourniquet.*
- *Vitamin levels: Avoid exposure of test tube to light.*

PLANNING

1. Expected outcomes following completion of procedure:	
• Venipuncture site shows no evidence of continued bleeding or hematoma after specimen collection.	Indicates that hemostasis has been achieved.
• Patient denies anxiety or discomfort.	Explanation relieves anxiety; procedure is performed quickly. Removal of painful stimulus lessens anxiety.
• An adequate sample is collected for testing (see agency policy or laboratory manual).	Appropriate laboratory analysis can be conducted.
• Patient discusses purpose, procedure, and benefits of venipuncture.	Validates learning.
2. Provide privacy and explain procedure to patient: describe purpose of tests; explain how sensation of tourniquet, antiseptic swab, and needlestick will feel.	Protects patient's privacy; reduces anxiety. Promotes cooperation.
3. Gather and organize equipment for blood specimen collection at bedside.	Ensures more efficiency when completing an assessment.

Clinical Judgment *Arrange for extra personnel for confused or pediatric patients who may not be able to remain still during venipuncture.*

IMPLEMENTATION

1. Raise or lower bed to comfortable working height.	Reduces strain on your back muscles and improves access to venipuncture site.
2. Perform hand hygiene and apply gloves. Help patient to supine or semi-Fowler position with arms extended to form straight line from shoulders to wrists. Place small pillow or towel under upper arm. (*Option:* Lower arm briefly so it fills veins in hand and lower arm with blood.)	Reduces transmission of microorganisms. Helps to stabilize extremity because arms are most common sites of venipuncture. Supported position in bed reduces chance of injury to patient if fainting occurs.
3. Apply tourniquet so it can be removed by pulling an end with single motion.	Tourniquet blocks venous return to heart from extremity, causing veins to dilate for easier visibility.
a. Position tourniquet 5 to 10 cm (2–4 inches) above venipuncture site selected (antecubital fossa site is most often used).	
b. Cross tourniquet over patient's arm (see illustration). May place it over gown sleeve to protect skin.	Older adult's skin is very fragile.
c. Hold tourniquet between your fingers close to arm. Tuck loop between patient's arm and tourniquet so you can grasp free end easily (see illustration).	Pull free end to release tourniquet after venipuncture.

Clinical Judgment *Palpate distal pulse (e.g., radial) below tourniquet. If pulse is not palpable, remove tourniquet, wait 60 seconds, and reapply it more loosely. If tourniquet is too tight, pressure will impede arterial blood flow.*

4. Do not keep tourniquet on patient longer than 1 minute (Pagana et al., 2021; ENA, 2018).	Prolonged tourniquet application causes stasis (Gorski et al., 2021).
5. Quickly inspect extremity for best venipuncture site, looking for straight, prominent vein without swelling or hematoma. Of three veins located in antecubital area, median cubital vein is preferred (see illustration).	Straight and intact veins are easiest to puncture.
6. Palpate selected vein with finger (see illustration). Note if vein is firm and rebounds when palpated or if it feels rigid or cordlike and rolls when palpated. *Avoid vigorously slapping vein, which can cause vasospasm.*	Patent, healthy vein is elastic and rebounds on palpation. Thrombosed vein is rigid, rolls easily, and is difficult to puncture.

| STEP | RATIONALE |

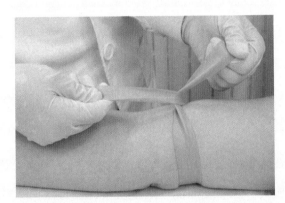

STEP 3b Cross tourniquet over arm.

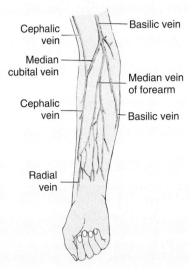

STEP 5 Location of antecubital veins.

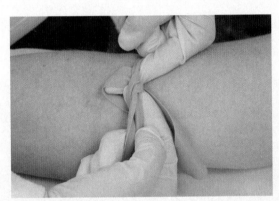

STEP 3c Tuck loop between patient's arm and tourniquet.

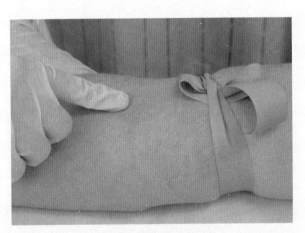

STEP 6 Palpate vein.

7. Obtain blood specimen.
   a. Syringe method
      (1) Have syringe with appropriate needle securely attached.
      (2) Clean venipuncture site with antiseptic swab, with first swab moving back and forth on horizontal plane, another swab on vertical plane, and last in circular motion from site outward for about 5 cm (2 inches) for 30 seconds. Allow to dry.
         (a) If drawing sample for blood alcohol level (BAL) or blood cultures, use only antiseptic swab rather than alcohol swab.
      (3) Remove needle cover and check needle for burrs.
      (4) Place thumb or forefinger of nondominant hand 2.5 cm (1 inch) below site and gently pull skin taut. Stretch skin steadily until vein is stabilized.
      (5) Hold syringe and needle at 15- to 30-degree angle from patient's arm with bevel up.

      (6) Slowly insert needle into vein, stopping when "pop" is felt as needle enters vein (see illustration).

Needle must not dislodge from syringe during venipuncture.
Antimicrobial agent cleans skin surface of resident bacteria so organisms do not enter puncture site. Allowing antiseptic to dry completes its antimicrobial task and reduces "sting" of venipuncture. Alcohol left on skin can cause hemolysis of sample and retraction of tissue away from puncture site.
Ensures accurate test results.

Burrs can cause damage to patient's veins.
Stabilizes vein and prevents rolling during needle insertion.

Reduces chance of penetrating both sides of vein during insertion. Bevel up decreases chance of contamination by not dragging bevel opening over skin and allows point of needle to first puncture skin, reducing trauma.
Prevents puncture through vein to opposite side.

STEP	RATIONALE
(7) Hold syringe securely and pull back gently on plunger.	Syringe held securely prevents needle from advancing. Pulling on plunger creates vacuum needed to draw blood into syringe. If plunger is pulled back too quickly, pressure may collapse vein.
(8) Observe for blood return (see illustration).	If blood flow fails to appear, needle may not be in vein.
(9) Obtain desired amount of blood, keeping needle stabilized.	Test results are more accurate when required amount of blood is obtained. You cannot perform some tests without minimal blood requirement. Movement of needle increases discomfort.
(10) After obtaining specimen, release tourniquet.	Reduces bleeding at site when needle is withdrawn.
(11) Apply 2 × 2–inch gauze pad without applying pressure. Quickly but carefully withdraw needle from vein.	Pressure over needle can cause discomfort. Careful removal of needle minimizes discomfort and vein trauma. Hematoma may cause compression injury (Gorski et al., 2021).
(12) Immediately apply pressure over venipuncture site with gauze or antiseptic pad for 2 to 3 minutes or until bleeding stops (see illustration). Observe for hematoma. Tape gauze dressing securely.	Direct pressure minimizes bleeding and prevents hematoma formation. Pressure dressing controls bleeding.
(13) Activate safety cover and immediately discard needle in appropriate container.	Prevents needlestick injury.
(14) Attach blood-filled syringe to needle-free blood transfer device. Attach tube and allow vacuum to fill tube to specified level. Remove and fill other tubes as appropriate (see illustration). Gently rotate each tube back and forth 8 to 10 times.	Additives prevent clotting. Shaking can cause hemolysis of red blood cells (RBCs) (Pagana et al., 2021; Krasowski, 2019).
b. Vacutainer system method	
(1) Attach double-ended needle to Vacutainer tube holder (see illustration).	Long end of needle is used to puncture vein. Short end fits into blood tubes.
(2) Have proper blood specimen tube resting inside Vacutainer holder but do not puncture rubber stopper.	Puncturing causes loss of tube vacuum.

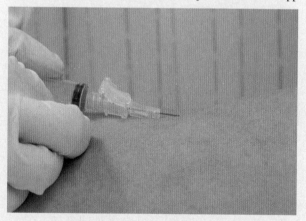

STEP 7a(6) Insert needle into vein.

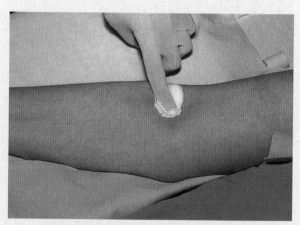

STEP 7a(12) Apply gauze to puncture site.

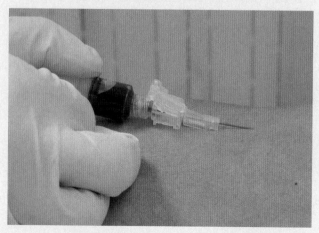

STEP 7a(8) Observe for blood return.

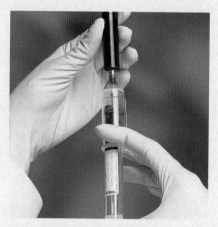

STEP 7a(14) Attach blood-filled syringe to needle-free blood transfer device.

STEP	RATIONALE
(3) Clean venipuncture site by following Step 7a(2) for antiseptic swab. Allow to dry.	Cleans skin surface of resident bacteria so organisms do not enter puncture site. Drying maximizes effect of antiseptic.
(4) Remove needle cover and inform patient that "stick" will occur, lasting only a few seconds.	Patient has better control over anxiety when prepared about what to expect.
(5) Place thumb or forefinger of nondominant hand 2.5 cm (1 inch) *below* site and gently pull skin taut. Stretch skin down until vein stabilizes.	Helps to stabilize vein and prevent rolling during needle insertion.
(6) Hold Vacutainer needle at 15- to 30-degree angle from arm with bevel up.	Smallest and sharpest point of needle will puncture skin first. Reduces chance of penetrating sides of vein during insertion. Keeping bevel up causes less trauma to vein.
(7) Slowly insert needle into vein (see illustration).	Prevents puncture on opposite side.
(8) Grasp Vacutainer securely and advance specimen tube into needle of holder (do not advance needle in vein).	Pushing needle through stopper breaks vacuum and causes flow of blood into tube. If needle in vein advances, vein may become punctured on other side.
(9) Note flow of blood into tube, which should be fairly rapid (see illustration).	Failure of blood to appear indicates that vacuum in tube is lost or needle is not in vein.
(10) After filling specimen tube, grasp Vacutainer firmly and remove tube. Insert additional specimen tubes as needed. Gently rotate each tube back and forth 8 to 10 times.	Vacuum in tube stops flow at amount to be collected. Grasping prevents needle from advancing or dislodging. Tube should fill completely because additives in certain tubes are measured in proportion to filled tube. Ensures proper mixing with additive to prevent clotting.
(11) After last tube is filled and removed from Vacutainer, release tourniquet.	Reduces bleeding at site when needle is withdrawn.
(12) Apply 2 × 2–inch gauze pad over puncture site without applying pressure and quickly but carefully withdraw needle with Vacutainer from vein.	Pressure over needle can cause discomfort. Careful removal of needle minimizes discomfort and vein trauma.

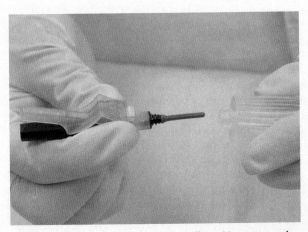

STEP 7b(1) Attach double-ended needle to Vacutainer tube.

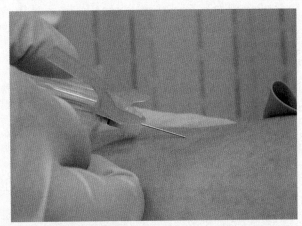

STEP 7b(7) Insert Vacutainer needle into vein.

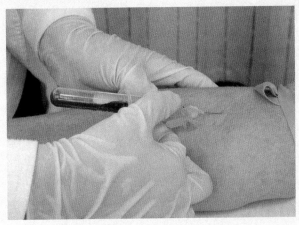

STEP 7b(9) Blood flowing into tube.

STEP	RATIONALE
(13) Immediately apply pressure over venipuncture site with gauze or antiseptic pad for 2 to 3 minutes or until bleeding stops. Observe for hematoma. Tape gauze dressing securely.	Direct pressure minimizes bleeding and prevents hematoma formation. Hematoma may cause compression and nerve injury. Pressure dressing controls bleeding.
c. Blood culture	
(1) Loosen tourniquet to prepare site and culture bottles. Clean venipuncture site with chlorhexidine antiseptic swab for 30 seconds or follow agency policy. Allow to dry.	Antimicrobial agent cleans skin surface so organisms do not enter puncture site or contaminate culture. Drying ensures complete antimicrobial action and decreases stinging.

Clinical Judgment *Culture specimens obtained through an IV catheter are often contaminated, and tests using specimens obtained in this manner are only done when catheter sepsis is suspected (Pagana et al., 2021).*

STEP	RATIONALE
(2) Remove protective flip-top overcap and prep the rubber septum of the blood culture bottles with alcohol swab; allow to dry for 1 minute.	Removes microorganisms from bottle septum.
(3) Reapply tourniquet and locate vein.	Dilates vein for easy visibility.
(4) Connect the Vacutainer holder to the Luer connector of the blood culture collection set.	Allows for needleless filling of culture bottles.
(5) Remove and dispose of gloves. Apply clean pair of gloves. Apply tourniquet.	Reduces risk of contaminating specimen.
(6) Perform venipuncture. When the needle is in the vein, secure it with tape or hold in place.	Ensures needle position is stabilized.
(7) Insert the aerobic bottle first into the Vacutainer holder and press down to penetrate the septum. Allow bottle to fill (approximately 10 mL). Repeat with anaerobic bottle.	Most bacteremias are caused by aerobic organisms. Aerobic bottles are more resistant to air and less likely to be contaminated.
(8) Gently rotate (do not shake) the bottles to mix the blood and broth.	Contributes to accuracy of test results.
(9) Place gauze pad over needle and remove gently. Apply pressure.	Controls hemostasis.
(10) Repeat venipuncture at another site (usually other arm).	Sampling paired blood cultures from venipunctures at separate sites improves detection of contamination of the blood cultures by skin bacteria.
d. Central venous catheter (CVC) collection	
(1) Apply a barrier gown or prepare a sterile drape work surface (see agency policy). Select appropriate port on IV catheter (see illustration). Turn off all IV pumps and clamp lumens (see Chapter 28).	Reduces transfer of microorganisms. If more than one lumen, select distal lumen if possible. Prevents dilution of sample with medication or total parenteral nutrition (TPN).
(2) Wipe all Luer-Lok caps with alcohol-wipe antiseptic solution or remove Luer-Lok alcohol-impregnated cap (DualCap system) (see illustration). Attach 10-mL saline prefilled syringe to selected port. Release clamp. Aspirate gently for blood return. Flush with 5 to 10 mL NS (check agency policy). Do not use syringe smaller than 10 mL. Remove syringe.	Use of 70% isopropyl alcohol–impregnated Luer-Lok cap (DualCap system) eliminates issue of wiping CVC ports adequately. Aspirating and flushing ensures patency of selected lumen and catheter in vein. Pressure from small syringe may damage catheter.

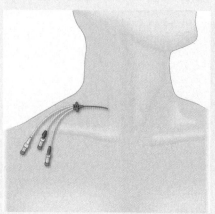

STEP 7d(1) Triple-lumen central venous catheter; select appropriate distal lumen port.

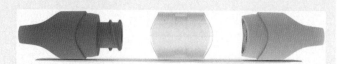

STEP 7d(2) DualCap system. Disinfects and protects both IV catheter needleless Luer access and end of IV tubing.

STEP	RATIONALE
(3) Wipe port with alcohol wipe. For **syringe method,** attach syringe to selected port, aspirate 5 mL of blood, and discard. Reclamp catheter. Wipe port, attach 10- to 20-mL Luer-Lok syringe, unclamp catheter, and aspirate desired amount of blood. Reclamp catheter and remove syringe. Clean catheter port with alcohol. To transfer blood from syringe to specimen tube, use Vacutainer holder with Luer-Lok attachment. Insert appropriate specimen tube into Vacutainer holder. Attach syringe to Luer-Lok attachment and fill desired tubes.	Discard ensures that blood sample is not contaminated with IV fluids, medication, or other products. Tubes have vacuum and automatically fill to necessary amount.
(4) For **Vacutainer method,** clamp catheter and attach needleless connecter to Vacutainer holder. Place blood tube into Vacutainer holder. Disinfect injection or access cap with alcohol. Insert Vacutainer needleless connector into injection or access cap, unclamp catheter, and advance blood tube into holder to activate blood flow. Allow blood to fill tube, clamp catheter, and discard first tube in appropriate biohazard container. Attach specimen tubes to Vacutainer with Luer-Lok adapter, unclamp catheter, and obtain blood specimens (see illustration).	Tubes have vacuum and automatically fill to necessary amount.
(5) After all specimens are collected, clamp catheter. Remove Vacutainer holder and needleless connector from injection or access cap and disinfect cap with alcohol.	Reduces risk for contamination by bloodborne pathogens.
(6) Attach 10-mL prefilled NS syringe and flush with 5 to 10 mL NS using push-pause method (see Chapter 28). Ensure positive pressure for lumen. Cap with spring automatically has positive pressure; therefore, syringe can be removed and lumen locked (see illustration). For caps without positive pressure, hold syringe plunger steady at completion of flush, lock off lumen with slide clamp, and remove syringe. Reattach alcohol-impregnated cap.	Push, pause creates turbulence that helps to clear lumen. Positive pressure prevents blood from flowing into tip of catheter and forming clot.
(7) Blood tubes contain additives; gently rotate back and forth 8 to 10 times. Remove gown or drape and dispose in receptacle.	Additives mix with blood to prevent clotting. Shaking can cause hemolysis of RBCs, producing inaccurate test results.
8. Check all tubes for any sign of external contamination with blood. Decontaminate with 70% alcohol if necessary.	Prevents cross-contamination. Reduces risk for exposure to pathogens present in blood.

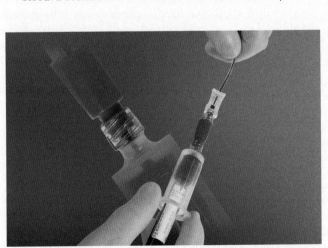

STEP 7d(4) Male Luer-Lok Vacutainer adapter attaches to port; blood draws directly into specimen tubes. (*Courtesy and copyright © Becton Dickinson.*)

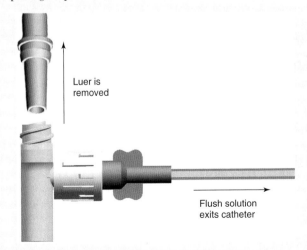

Luer is removed

Flush solution exits catheter

STEP 7d(6) Positive-pressure cap helps maintain patency of vascular access device. (*With permission, courtesy ICU Medical, San Clemente, CA.*)

STEP	RATIONALE
9. Securely attach properly completed identification label to each tube and affix proper requisition. Verify identifiers in front of patient (TJC, 2023).	Incorrect identification of specimen could result in diagnostic or therapeutic errors.
10. Place specimens in plastic biohazard bag and send to laboratory. Cultures must be sent to laboratory within 30 minutes (Pagana et al., 2021).	Minimizes spread of microorganisms. Prompt analysis ensures accurate results.
11. Dispose of syringe, needle, gauze, and other supplies in appropriate containers.	Safe disposal of supplies exposed to body fluids prevents transfer of microorganisms.
12. Remove and dispose of gloves and perform hand hygiene after specimen is obtained and any spillage is cleaned.	Reduces transmission of microorganisms. Use appropriate disposal if patient is on hazardous drugs (Gorski et al., 2021).
13. Help patient to a comfortable position.	Restores comfort and sense of well-being.
14. Raise side rails (as appropriate) and lower bed to lowest position, locking into position.	Ensures patient safety and prevents falls.
15. Place nurse call system in an accessible location within patient's reach.	Ensures patient can call for assistance if needed.

EVALUATION

1. Inspect venipuncture site for hemostasis.
2. Determine if patient remains anxious or fearful.
3. Check laboratory report for test results.
4. **Use Teach-Back:** "I want to be sure I explained the purpose and procedure for obtaining a blood specimen. Tell me why we are collecting this blood specimen." Revise your instruction now or develop a plan for revised patient/family caregiver teaching if patient/family caregiver is not able to teach back correctly.

Determines if bleeding has stopped or hematoma has formed.
Some patients require more blood tests in future. Address concerns and let patient express anxiety.
Reveals constituents of blood specimen.
Teach-back is a technique for health care providers to ensure that they have explained medical information clearly so that patients and their families understand what is communicated to them (AHRQ, 2023).

Unexpected Outcomes	Related Interventions
1. Hematoma forms at venipuncture site.	• Apply pressure using 2 × 2–inch gauze dressing. • Continue to monitor patient for pain and discomfort.
2. Bleeding at site continues.	• Apply pressure to site; patient may also apply pressure. • Monitor patient. • Notify health care provider.
3. Signs and symptoms of infection at venipuncture site occur.	• Notify health care provider.

Documentation
• Document method used to obtain blood specimen, date and time collected, type of test ordered, time specimen was sent to the laboratory, and description of venipuncture site.
• Document your evaluation of patient and family caregiver learning.

Hand-Off Reporting
• Report any STAT or abnormal test results to health care provider.

Special Considerations
Patient Education
• Instruct patient to briefly apply pressure (if able) to venipuncture site. Patients with bleeding disorders or those undergoing anticoagulant therapy should apply pressure for at least 5 minutes.
• Instruct patient to notify nurse or health care provider if persistent or recurrent bleeding or expanding hematoma develops at venipuncture site.

Pediatrics
• Explain procedure to child at developmentally appropriate age level and provide atraumatic care (Hockenberry et al., 2022).

• Because children often fear that loss of their blood is a threat to their lives, explain to them that their blood is continually being produced. An adhesive bandage gives them assurance that their blood will not leak out through puncture site (Hockenberry et al., 2022).
• Children's blood specimens are often obtained in a treatment room instead of in bed or room to maintain feeling that their room is a safe place (Hockenberry et al., 2022).
• When performing venipuncture on children, explore sources for vein access: scalp, antecubital fossa, saphenous, and hand veins.
• Application of eutectic mixture of local anesthetics (EMLA) cream to the venipuncture site may be ordered before the stick to reduce pain in infants and young children (Hockenberry et al., 2022).
• Vacutainers are not recommended in children under 2 years of age because of possible vein collapse with their use.

Older Adults
• Older adults have fragile veins that are easily traumatized during venipuncture (Touhy & Jett, 2022). Sometimes application of warm compresses may help in obtaining samples. Using small-bore catheter may be beneficial.

✦ SKILL 7.9   Blood Glucose Monitoring

Blood glucose monitoring (BGM) is an essential component of any diabetes self-management program (American Diabetes Association [ADA], 2023). The procedure is less painful than venipuncture, and the ease of the skin puncture method makes it possible for patients to perform this procedure at home. The development of reagent strips, home glucose monitors, and the skin puncture method has revolutionized home management care of patients with diabetes mellitus.

Blood glucose reflectance meters are lightweight and run on batteries (e.g., AccuChek III, OneTouch) (Fig. 7.5). After a drop of blood from the skin puncture is dropped or wicked onto a reagent strip, the meter provides an accurate measurement of blood glucose level in 5 to 50 seconds. Point-of-care (POC) blood glucose testing meters must be cleaned and disinfected after each patient use.

The meters differ in several ways, including amount of blood needed for each test, testing speed, overall size, ability to store test results in memory, cost of the meter, and cost of test strips (U.S. Food and Drug Administration [FDA], n.d.a). Some larger meters are voice activated, which provides support for the older adult or patient with visual impairments. Most meters now allow for the use of alternative site or forearm capillary testing. Improved technology introduced a method for glucose measurement that is now available on the market.

There are continuous glucose monitoring (CGM) systems, such as Dexcom G6 Continuous Monitoring (Dexcom G6 CGM). These systems have an implantable glucose sensor and compatible mobile app for adults with diabetes (FDA, n.d.b). The device uses a small sensor that is implanted just under the skin by a qualified health care provider during an outpatient procedure. CGM devices provide real-time blood glucose data, and the patient can access this information from a smartphone (Fig. 7.6). In addition, there are alerts for high and low blood glucose levels. Patients are also able to share glucose data with their family and health care providers.

Testing of glycosylated hemoglobin (HbA$_{1c}$) evaluates the amount of glucose available in the bloodstream over the 120-day life span of a red blood cell (RBC). HbA$_{1c}$ provides an accurate long-term index of a patient's average blood glucose level drawn by venous puncture (Pagana et al., 2021).

Delegation

Assessment of a patient's condition cannot be delegated to assistive personnel (AP). When the patient's condition is stable, the skill of obtaining and testing a sample of blood for blood glucose level can be delegated to AP. Direct the AP by:

- Explaining appropriate sites to use for puncture and when to obtain glucose levels
- Reviewing expected blood glucose levels and when to report unexpected glucose levels to the nurse so the nurse can retake blood glucose level as per agency policy

Interprofessional Collaboration

- Request the diabetes nurse educator for patients who need diabetic counseling and education.

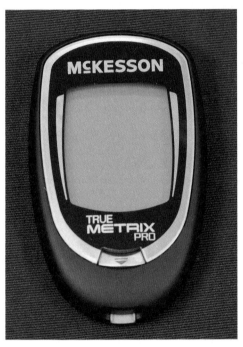

FIG. 7.5 Blood glucose monitor.

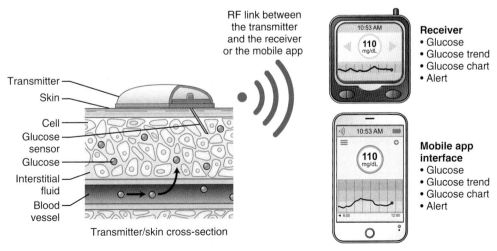

FIG. 7.6 Continuous glucose monitoring system with a fully implantable glucose sensor. (*From Melmed S, et al: Williams textbook of endocrinology, ed 14, St. Louis, 2020, Elsevier.*)

Equipment

- Antiseptic swab
- Cotton ball
- Lancet device, either self-activating or button activated
- Blood glucose meter (e.g., Accucheck III, OneTouch)
- Blood glucose test strips appropriate for meter brand used
- Clean gloves
- Paper towel

STEP	RATIONALE

ASSESSMENT

1. Identify patient using at least two identifiers (e.g., name and birthday or name and medical record number) according to agency policy.	Ensures correct patient. Complies with The Joint Commission standards and improves patient safety (TJC, 2023).
2. Review patient's electronic health record (EHR) for health care provider's order for time or frequency of measurement.	Health care provider determines test schedule on basis of patient's physiological status and risk for glucose imbalance.
3. Review patient's EHR to determine if risks exist for performing skin puncture (e.g., low platelet count, anticoagulant therapy, bleeding disorders).	Abnormal clotting mechanisms increase risk for local ecchymosis and bleeding.
4. Determine if specific conditions need to be met before or after sample collection (e.g., fasting, postprandial, after certain medications, before insulin doses).	Dietary intake of carbohydrates and ingestion of concentrated glucose preparations alter blood glucose levels.
5. Assess patient's/family caregiver's health literacy.	Determines degree to which individuals have the ability to find, understand, and use information and services to make informed health-related decisions and actions for themselves and others (CDC, 2023).
6. Assess area of skin to be used as puncture site. Inspect fingers or forearms for edema, inflammation, cuts, or sores. Avoid areas of bruising and open lesions.	Sides of fingers are commonly selected because they have fewer nerve endings.
	Measurements from alternative sites are meter specific and may be different from those at traditional sites. Puncture site should not be edematous, inflamed, or recently punctured because these factors cause increased interstitial fluid and blood to mix and also increase risk for infection.
7. For patient with diabetes who performs test at home, assess ability to handle skin-puncturing device. Patient may choose to continue self-testing while in hospital.	Patient's physical health may change (e.g., vision disturbance, fatigue, pain, disease process), preventing patient from performing test.
8. Assess patient's knowledge, prior experience with BGM, and feelings about procedure.	Reveals need for patient instruction and/or support.

PLANNING

1. Expected outcomes following completion of procedure:	
• Puncture site shows no evidence of bleeding or tissue damage.	Hemostasis is achieved. Lancet or needle did not puncture skin too deeply.
• Blood glucose measurements are accurate.	Normal fasting glucose is 70 to 110 mg/dL, indicating good metabolic control (Pagana et al., 2021). Values may vary slightly; check agency policy.
• Patient can verbalize procedure for self-monitoring blood glucose.	Demonstrates psychomotor learning.
• Patient explains test results.	Validates knowledge.
2. Provide privacy and explain procedure and purpose to patient and/or family caregiver. Offer patient and family caregiver opportunity to practice testing procedures. Provide resources/teaching aids for patient and family caregiver.	Protects patient's privacy; reduces anxiety. Promotes cooperation.
3. Organize and set up any equipment needed to perform procedure.	Ensures greater efficiency when completing procedure.

IMPLEMENTATION

1. Perform hand hygiene. Instruct adult to perform hand hygiene, including forearm (if applicable) with soap and water. Rinse and dry.	Promotes skin cleansing and vasodilation at selected puncture site. Reduces transmission of microorganisms.
2. Position patient comfortably in chair or in semi-Fowler position in bed.	Ensures easy accessibility to puncture site. Patient assumes position when self-testing.

STEP	RATIONALE
3. Apply clean gloves. Remove reagent strip from vial and tightly seal cap. Check code on test strip vial. Use only test strips recommended for glucose meter. Some newer meters do not require code and/or have disk or drum with 10 or more test strips.	Reduces transmission of microorganisms. Protects strips from accidental discoloration caused by exposure to air or light. Code on test strip vial must match code entered into glucose meter.
4. Insert strip into meter (refer to manufacturer directions) (see illustration). Do not bend strip, and do not touch the sensor where the specimen of blood is to be obtained. Meter turns on automatically.	Some machines must be calibrated; others require zeroing of timer. Each meter is adjusted differently.
5. Remove unused reagent strip from meter and place on paper towel or clean, dry surface with test pad facing up (see manufacturer directions).	Moisture on strip can alter accuracy of final test results.
6. Meter displays code on screen that must match code from test strip vial. Press proper button on meter to confirm matching codes. Meter is ready for use.	Codes must match for meter to operate. Meters have different messages that confirm that meter is ready for testing and blood can be applied.
7. Prepare single-use lancet or multiple-use lancet device. **NOTE:** Some meters recommend that this step be completed before preparing test strip. Remove cap from lancet device; insert new lancet. Some lancet devices have disk or cylinder that rotates to new lancet.	Never reuse a lancet because of risk of infection.
a. Twist off protective cover on tip of lancet. Replace cap of lancet device.	
b. Cock lancet device, adjusting for proper puncture depth.	Each patient varies as to depth of insertion needed for lancet to produce blood drop.
8. Obtain blood sample.	
a. Wipe patient's finger or forearm lightly with antiseptic swab and allow to dry. Choose vascular area for puncture site. In stable adults, select lateral side of finger. Avoid central tip of finger, which has denser nerve supply (Pagana et al., 2021).	Removes microorganisms from skin surface. Side of finger is less sensitive to pain.
b. Hold area to be punctured in dependent position. Do not milk or massage finger site.	Increases blood flow to area before puncture. Milking may hemolyze specimen and introduce excess tissue fluid (Pagana et al., 2021).
c. Hold tip of lancet device against area of skin chosen for test site (see illustration). Press release button on device. Some devices allow you to see blood sample forming. Remove device.	Placement ensures that lancet enters skin properly.
d. With some devices a blood sample begins to appear. Otherwise gently squeeze or massage fingertip until round drop of blood forms (see illustration).	Adequate-size blood sample is needed to test glucose.

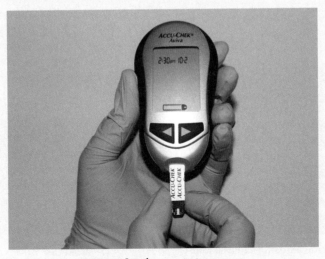

STEP 4 Load test strip into meter.

STEP	RATIONALE

9. Obtain test results.

   a. Be sure that meter is still on. Bring test strip in meter to drop of blood. Blood will be wicked onto test strip (see illustration). Follow specific meter instructions to be sure that you obtain adequate sample.

Exposure of blood to test strip for prescribed time ensures proper results.

Blood enters strip, and glucose device shows message on screen to signal that enough blood has been obtained.

Clinical Judgment *Do not scrape blood onto the test strips or apply it to wrong side of test strip. This prevents accurate glucose measurement.*

   b. Blood glucose test result will appear on screen (see illustration). Some devices "beep" when completed.

10. Turn meter off. Some meters turn off automatically. Dispose of test strip, lancet, and gloves in proper receptacles.

Meter is battery powered. Proper disposal reduces risk for needlestick injury and spread of infection.

11. Perform hand hygiene.

Reduces transmission of microorganisms.

12. Discuss test results with patient and encourage questions and eventual participation in care if this is a new diabetes mellitus diagnosis.

Promotes participation and adherence to therapy.

13. Help patient to a comfortable position.

Restores comfort and sense of well-being.

14. Raise side rails (as appropriate) and lower bed to lowest position, locking into position.

Ensures patient safety and prevents falls.

15. Place nurse call system in an accessible location within patient's reach.

Ensures patient can call for assistance if needed.

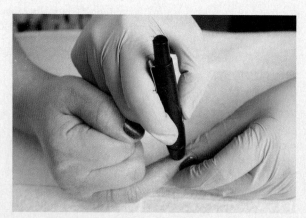

STEP 8c Prick side of finger with lancet. (*From Sorrentino SA, Remmert LN:* Mosby's textbook for nursing assistants, *ed 10, St. Louis, 2021, Elsevier.*)

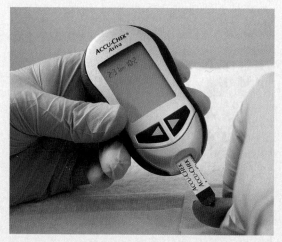

STEP 9a Touch test strip to blood drop. Blood wicks into test strip.

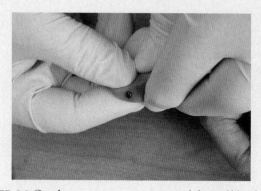

STEP 8d Gently squeeze puncture site until drop of blood forms.

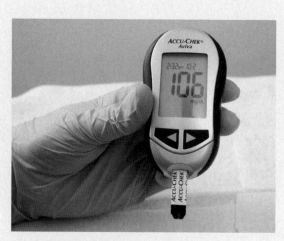

STEP 9b Results appear on meter screen.

STEP	RATIONALE

EVALUATION

1. Inspect puncture site for bleeding or tissue injury.
2. Compare glucose meter reading with normal blood glucose levels and previous test results.
3. **Use Teach-Back:** "I want to be sure I explained how to obtain a blood glucose reading. Show me the steps to obtain your blood glucose measurement." Revise your instruction now or develop a plan for revised patient/family caregiver teaching if patient/family caregiver is not able to teach back correctly.

Site can be source of discomfort and infection.
Determines if glucose level is normal.

Teach-back is a technique for health care providers to ensure that they have explained medical information clearly so that patients and their families understand what is communicated to them (AHRQ, 2023).

Unexpected Outcomes

1. Puncture site is bruised or continues to bleed.

2. Blood glucose level is above or below target range.

3. Glucose meter malfunctions.

Related Interventions

- Apply pressure.
- Notify health care provider if bleeding continues.
- Continue to monitor patient.
- Check if there are medication orders for deviations in glucose level.
- Notify health care provider.
- Administer insulin or carbohydrate source as ordered, depending on glucose level.
- Review instructions for troubleshooting glucose meter.
- Repeat test.

Documentation

- Document procedure and glucose level according to agency policy. Patient's glucose level may be automatically downloaded to EHR from the glucometer (check agency policy).
- Document action taken for an abnormal range for the patient's blood glucose.
- Describe patient response, including appearance of puncture site.
- Describe any patient education provided.
- Document your evaluation of patient and family caregiver learning.

Hand-Off Reporting

- Report abnormal blood glucose levels.
- Report interventions implemented to correct high or low blood glucose levels.

Special Considerations

Patient Education

- Provide information on where patient with diabetes mellitus can obtain testing supplies. When possible, teach with the same meter that patient will use at home.
- Provide patient with information on where to obtain help if glucose meter has malfunctioned.
- Stress importance of the timing of blood glucose levels, particularly in patients with diabetes mellitus.

Pediatrics

- Allow young children to choose puncture site; heel and great toe are common puncture sites in infants.

- Heel warming helps to obtain specimen from a neonate.
- Infection or abscess of the heel and necrotizing osteochondritis are the most serious complications of heelstick puncture in infants. To avoid osteochondritis, make sure that puncture is not deeper than 2 mm and is made at the outer aspect of the heel (Hockenberry et al., 2022).
- Allow young child with parent to demonstrate technique; incorporate a play activity for further understanding.

Older Adults

- Warming fingertips with warm water may facilitate obtaining specimen.
- Some older adults have vision or dexterity problems that interfere with performing self-fingersticks.

Home Care

- Provide information on correct disposal of sharps in nonpermeable and puncture-resistant container.
- Suggest that patient attend diabetic support group if needed.
- Be sure that patient's family caregiver can perform test when patient is ill or is unable to manipulate devices.
- Teach patient and family caregiver about the frequency of BGM and that it can be performed more frequently than prescribed if necessary.
- Teach patient and family how to document findings and how to retrieve results from the memory of the glucose meters.

✦ SKILL 7.10   Obtaining an Arterial Specimen for Blood Gas Measurement

You assess effectiveness of oxygenation and ventilation by measuring arterial blood gases (ABGs). Measurement of ABGs provides valuable information in assessing and managing a patient's respiratory and metabolic disturbances (Pagana et al., 2021). The parameters measured in an ABG assessment include arterial blood pH, partial pressure of oxygen (PaO_2), partial pressure of carbon dioxide ($PaCO_2$), and arterial oxygen saturation (SaO_2).

Each agency has a policy regarding who is allowed to obtain ABG samples. Many agencies allow nurses in specialty areas (e.g., critical care) to obtain them, others specify a certified respiratory therapist, and some require institutional certification of this skill.

Delegation

The skill of obtaining an ABG sample cannot be delegated to assistive personnel (AP).

Interprofessional Collaboration

- Inform the health care provider if bleeding from arterial puncture site occurs and about any changes in patient vital signs, level of consciousness, or restlessness.

- Communicate with the health care provider and respiratory therapist to determine if patient needs prescribed respiratory treatment or oxygen therapy for signs of respiratory distress.

Equipment

- Commercial blood gas kit or individual supplies, including:
- 3-mL heparinized syringe
  - 23- or 25-gauge needle with safety guard
  - Filter cap (allows expelling of air and retains blood)
  - Alcohol swabs (2)
  - 2 × 2–inch gauze pad
  - Tape
  - Heparin (1:1000 solution)
- Cup or plastic bag with crushed ice
- Clean gloves
- Protective eyewear
- Completed identification labels with proper patient identifiers
- Completed laboratory requisition with date, time, name of test, patient identification, and source of specimen
- Biohazard bag for delivery of specimen to laboratory (or container specified by agency)

STEP	RATIONALE
ASSESSMENT	
1. Identify patient using at least two identifiers (e.g., name and birthday or name and medical record number) according to agency policy.	Ensures correct patient. Complies with The Joint Commission standards and improves patient safety (TJC, 2023).
2. Review patient's electronic health record (EHR) for health care provider's order for time or frequency of measurement.	Health care provider determines test schedule on basis of patient's physiological status and risk for impaired oxygenation.
3. Review patient's EHR to identify medications that may influence ABG measurement (e.g., supplemental oxygen, anticoagulants, diuretics).	Certain medications increase risk for bleeding at puncture site or may cause hemoconcentration. Important to note and document if patient is prescribed supplemental oxygen.
4. Assess patient's/family caregiver's health literacy.	Determines degree to which individuals have the ability to find, understand, and use information and services to make informed health-related decisions and actions for themselves and others (CDC, 2023).
5. Assess for factors that influence ABG measurements:	Allows you to eliminate factors that interfere with accurate measurement.
a. Assess respiratory status, including rate, depth, rhythm, adventitious sounds, lung excursion (hypoventilation or hyperventilation), and use of accessory muscles.	Physical signs and symptoms may indicate need for ABG sample. Hypoventilation can cause retention of CO_2, and hyperventilation can cause decreased CO_2 levels.
b. Body temperature	Change in body temperature as little as 0.56°C (1°F) can alter ABG values (Hockenberry et al., 2022).
6. Review criteria for choosing site for ABG sample.	Prevents causing compromised circulation from puncture.

Clinical Judgment *Factors that contraindicate use of arterial site include amputation, contractures, localized infection, dressing or cast, mastectomy, and arteriovenous shunts.*

a. Assess collateral blood flow. *Perform Allen test.*	Allen test assesses collateral circulation before performing arterial puncture on radial artery. Positive Allen test result ensures that there is collateral circulation to hand in case thrombosis of radial artery occurs following puncture (Pagana et al., 2021).
(1) Perform hand hygiene and apply gloves. Have patient make tight fist and raise hand above heart.	Removes as much blood from hand as possible.
(2) Apply direct pressure to both radial and ulnar arteries (see illustration).	Obstructs arterial blood flow to hand.

STEP	RATIONALE
(3) Have patient lower and open hand (see illustration).	Fingers and hand should be pale and blanched, indicating lack of arterial blood flow.
(4) Release pressure over ulnar artery; observe color of fingers, thumbs, and hand (see illustration).	Flushing identifies that circulation through ulnar artery is good and that ulnar artery alone is capable of providing blood supply to entire hand. Therefore you can use radial artery for puncture.

Clinical Judgment *If there is no flushing in 15 seconds, Allen test result is negative, and you should repeat it on the other arm or choose another artery for puncture (Pagana et al., 2021).*

b. Assess accessibility of vessel.	Palpating, stabilizing, and performing venipuncture of superficial artery is easier. Superficial arteries are located at distal ends of extremities.
c. Assess tissue surrounding artery.	Muscle, tendon, and fat have decreased sensation to pain. Bony periosteum and nerves are highly sensitive to pain.
d. Assess that arteries are not directly adjacent to veins.	Helps reduce chance of venous puncture and possibility of inaccurate samples.
7. Assess arterial sites for use in obtaining specimen.	Arterial blood may be obtained from areas where strong pulses are palpable (i.e., radial, brachial, or femoral artery) (Pagana et al., 2021).

Clinical Judgment *Previous puncture sites or preexisting conditions may eliminate potential sites (see agency policy). Artery should be easily accessible.*

a. Radial artery	Safest, most accessible site for puncture. Is superficial, is not adjacent to large veins, usually has adequate collateral circulation by ulnar artery, and is relatively painless if periosteum is avoided. Used when Allen test result is positive.

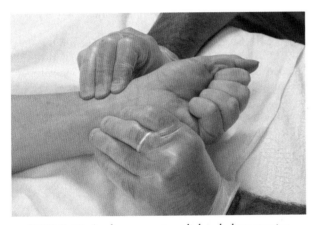

STEP 6a(2) Apply pressure to radial and ulnar arteries.

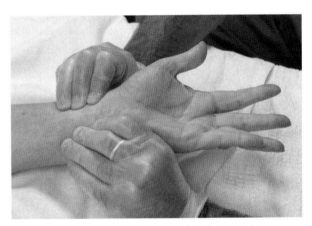

STEP 6a(3) Patient opening hand; note color.

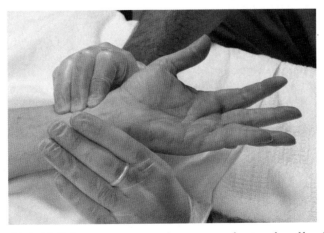

STEP 6a(4) Release pressure over ulnar artery and note color of hand.

STEP	RATIONALE
b. Brachial artery	Has reasonable collateral blood flow, is less superficial, is more difficult to palpate and stabilize, carries increased risk for venous puncture, and results in increased discomfort for patient if brachial nerve is punctured. Used when radial artery is inaccessible or Allen test result is negative.
c. Femoral artery	Nurses without specialized training should not use this artery. Has no adequate collateral flow if obstructed below inguinal ligament, is difficult to stabilize, is deep, and is directly adjacent to femoral vein. Is best artery to use in emergency (e.g., cardiac arrest or hypovolemic shock when pulses are difficult to palpate).
8. Remove and dispose of gloves. Perform hand hygiene.	Reduces transmission of infection.
9. Review the EHR for baseline ABG values for patient.	Provides baseline for comparison and evaluation of therapies.
10. Assess patient's knowledge, prior experience with obtaining ABGs, and feelings about procedure.	Obtaining blood specimen is painful. Patient who is knowledgeable will be more cooperative. Reveals need for patient instruction and/or support.

PLANNING

1. Expected outcomes following completion of procedure:	
• Patient's ABG values are within normal range.	Indicates adequate oxygenation.
• Patient's extremity distal to puncture remains warm and pink, has adequate capillary refill, and is free of pain.	Indicates adequate arterial circulation to extremity.
• Patient denies anxiety, and respiratory rate remains within baseline.	Anxiety increases respiratory rate, which can alter ABG results.
• Patient correctly discusses ABG procedure.	Indicates learning.
2. Prepare heparinized syringe (if not in commercial kit).	Heparin mixes with specimen to prevent clotting.
a. Aspirate 0.5 mL sodium heparin (1000 units/mL) into syringe from vial or ampule.	Prevents blood sample from clotting before reaching laboratory. Excessive heparin can affect pH of arterial sample.
b. Withdraw plunger entire length of syringe. Maintain asepsis.	Coats inside of barrel of syringe with heparin.
c. Eject all heparin in barrel out of syringe.	In hub of syringe, 0.15 to 0.25 mL of sodium heparin remains; 0.05 mL of sodium heparin adequately anticoagulates 1 mL of blood; 0.15 mL adequately anticoagulates 3 mL without affecting pH level.
3. Provide privacy and explain procedure.	Protects patient's privacy; reduces anxiety. Promotes cooperation.
4. Organize and set up any additional equipment needed to perform procedure at bedside.	Ensures more efficiency when completing an assessment.
5. Arrange for extra personnel to help if necessary.	Confused or pediatric patients may not be able to remain still during the collection of ABGs.

IMPLEMENTATION

1. Perform hand hygiene.	Reduces transmission of infection.
2. Palpate selected radial, femoral, or brachial site with fingertips.	Determines area of maximal impulse for puncture site.
3. Using radial artery, elevate patient's wrist with small pillow and ask patient to extend fingers downward. Stabilize artery by slight hyperextension of wrist.	Flexes wrist and positions radial artery closer to surface. Reduces mobility of artery and makes insertion of needle easier.
4. Apply clean gloves. Clean area of maximal impulse with alcohol swab or antiseptic swab (check agency or manufacturer recommendation). Wipe in circular motion away from site or use back-and-forth strokes. Allow to dry.	Reduces number of resident bacteria on surface of skin. Drying maximizes antibacterial effects.
5. Hold 2 × 2 inch–gauze pad with same fingers used to palpate artery.	Keeps gauze pad accessible for covering puncture site when necessary.
6. Use corner of sterile gauze pad or alcohol wipe to point to chosen site.	Maintaining location of artery improves likelihood of successful puncture.
7. Hold needle bevel up and insert at 45-degree angle into artery. Prepare patient for needlestick because radial sticks are painful.	Angle allows for better arterial flow into needle. Prepared patient will be less likely to withdraw arm.
8. Stop advancing needle when blood is noted returning into hub of needle or syringe.	Quick return of blood indicates that arterial flow is obtained. Prevents puncturing through both sides of artery.

STEP	RATIONALE
9. Allow arterial pulsations to pump 2 to 3 mL of blood into heparinized syringe slowly (see illustration).	Allowing pulsations to help fill syringe reduces presence of air bubbles in sample. Bubbles alter ABG results.
10. When sampling is complete, hold 2 × 2–inch gauze pad over puncture site, withdraw syringe and needle, and activate safety guard over needle.	Pad minimizes pulling of skin as needle is withdrawn. Decreases contamination from blood and accidental needlestick.
11. Apply pressure over and just proximal to puncture site with pad (see illustration).	Insertion of needle into artery is just proximal to insertion site through skin. Gauze absorbs any blood that might ooze from site.
12. Maintain continuous pressure on and proximal to site for 3 to 5 minutes (**NOTE:** extend continuous pressure to approximately 15 minutes if patient is undergoing anticoagulant therapy or has bleeding disorder) (Pagana et al., 2021). Have another nurse remove safety needle and attach filter cap to syringe (see Step 15) if prolonged pressure is needed.	To avoid hematoma formation, apply and hold pressure or apply a pressure dressing to arterial puncture site for 3 to 5 minutes (Pagana et al., 2021). Prevents delay in preparing syringe in ice.
13. Visually inspect site for signs of bleeding or hematoma formation.	Determines if continued need exists to exert pressure. Because artery rather than vein has been accessed, monitor puncture site for bleeding.
14. Palpate artery below or distal to puncture site.	Determines if pulse quality has changed, indicating alteration in arterial flow.
15. Take syringe, if not done by another nurse, remove safety needle, and discard needle in appropriate biohazard container. Attach filter cap to syringe (available in kit) to expel air or cover tip of syringe with 2 × 2–inch sterile gauze to expel air (see agency procedure). Some kits may have all supplies, including syringe with heparin, needle with safety needle cap, and filter cap that allows air to vent and not blood (see illustration).	Decreases chance of contamination from room air. Air bubbles in specimen can falsely elevate or decrease results, depending on patient's blood gas concentration.
16. Prepare syringe for laboratory analysis (according to agency policy).	
a. Place patient identification label on syringe in front of patient; confirm identifiers (TJC, 2023).	Ensures proper identification of sample.
b. Place syringe in cup of crushed ice (check agency policy).	Failure to place ABG sample can affect results of pH, PaO_2, and $PaCO_2$ (Pagana et al., 2021).
c. Attach properly labeled laboratory requisition to blood gas sample. Add appropriate patient data (e.g., hemoglobin, mode and flow of supplemental oxygen, and patient's body temperature) (check agency policy).	Prevents mislabeled specimens. Hemoglobin level, supplemental oxygen, and hypothermia or hyperthermia affects PaO_2 or $PaCO_2$ values.

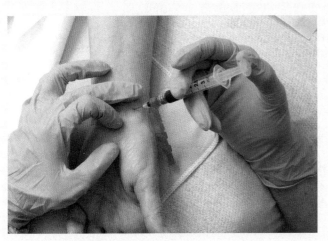

STEP 9 Blood flowing into syringe.

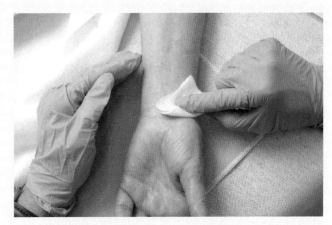

STEP 11 Apply firm pressure to arterial puncture site.

STEP	RATIONALE

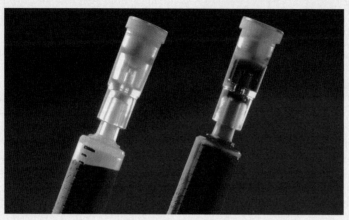

STEP 15 Filter-Pro Air Bubble Removal Device expels air safely from syringe without accidentally expelling blood and aerosolizing sample. *(With permission from Smiths Medical, Carlsbad, CA.)*

STEP	RATIONALE
17. Place sample in biohazard bag. Send sample to laboratory immediately.	Prevents alteration in gas tensions resulting from metabolic processes that continue after blood is drawn.
18. Remove and dispose of gloves and perform hand hygiene.	Reduces transmission of microorganisms. Use appropriate disposal if patient is on hazardous drugs (Gorski et al., 2021).
19. Assist patient to a comfortable position.	Restores comfort and sense of well-being.
20. Raise side rails (as appropriate) and lower bed to lowest position, locking into position.	Ensures patient safety and prevents falls.
21. Place nurse call system in an accessible location within patient's reach.	Ensures patient can call for assistance if needed.

EVALUATION

1. Inspect puncture site and area distal to puncture site for complications.	An artery can be obstructed, or important structures anatomically juxtaposed to an artery can be penetrated (Pagana et al., 2021).
2. Review results of sample as soon as possible.	Identifies any abnormality and expedites initiation of treatment.
3. **Use Teach-Back:** "I want to be sure I explained the way I will obtain your arterial blood gas specimen. Tell me the steps I will use to obtain this specimen." Revise your instruction now or develop a plan for revised patient/family caregiver teaching if patient/family caregiver is not able to teach back correctly.	Teach-back is a technique for health care providers to ensure that they have explained medical information clearly so that patients and their families understand what is communicated to them (AHRQ, 2023).

Unexpected Outcomes	Related Interventions
1. Patient has abnormal ABG values.	• Continue to monitor patient. • Notify health care provider of findings and obtain further orders.
2. Patient has hematoma formation at puncture site.	• Continue to monitor patient. • Notify health care provider.
3. Patient reports numbness, burning, or tingling at puncture site, indicating possible nerve injury.	• Monitor for hematoma formation. • Notify health care provider.

Documentation

- Document results of Allen test, location and condition of puncture site, patient's tolerance of procedure, use of supplemental oxygen, and time specimen was sent to the laboratory.
- Document your evaluation of patient and family caregiver learning.
- Document results of ABG.

Hand-Off Reporting

- Report ABG results to health care provider as soon as available.
- Report patient's fraction of inspired oxygen concentration (FiO_2) and any ventilator settings (e.g., tidal volume [V_t], respiratory frequency [RF], mode of ventilation).

Special Considerations

Patient Education

- Teach patient to report numbness, burning, and/or tingling in hand during and after radial artery puncture.

Pediatrics

- In neonatal and pediatric patients, you can use capillary blood gas. Procedures are similar to those for obtaining heelsticks.
- When dealing with neonatal patients, especially premature infants, normal values for ABGs often differ from those of adults.
- Arterial blood samples from punctures are painful and cause crying and breath holding that affect the accuracy of ABG values (decreases PaO_2) (Hockenberry et al., 2022).

Older Adults

- Pay special attention during interpretation of ABGs for patients with chronic pulmonary conditions. In these patients, compensatory mechanisms may allow normal pH in face of markedly elevated $PaCO_2$.

Populations With Disabilities

- This is a painful procedure, and patients with cognitive or intellectual disabilities may not be able to understand the procedure. Some patients may need some medication to reduce any procedure-related anxiety (Mendes, 2018).

◆ CLINICAL JUDGMENT AND NEXT-GENERATION NCLEX® EXAMINATION–STYLE QUESTIONS

1. An 84-year-old patient with a history of type 2 diabetes mellitus is admitted from the long-term care agency to the emergency department after developing mild confusion. Patient has an indwelling Foley catheter and is pulling it. The urine is dark, cloudy, and foul smelling. Vital signs include blood pressure 80/50 mm Hg, pulse 108 beats/minute, respirations 22 breaths/minute, temperature 38.4°C (101.2°F) and oxygen saturation 93% on room air. Which of the following laboratory specimens does the nurse anticipate will be ordered **initially** by the health care provider? Select 4 correct answers.
   1. Urine culture and sensitivity
   2. Stool specimen
   3. Blood cultures
   4. White blood cell count
   5. Electrolytes
   6. Urethral culture
   7. Throat culture

2. The experienced nurse is supervising a new nurse who is collecting the ordered urine specimen from a Luer-Lok catheter port. Which action by the new nurse requires the experienced nurse to intervene?
   1. Dons clean gloves prior to specimen collection.
   2. Clamps drainage tube with clamp for 15 minutes.
   3. Cleans catheter entry port and waits for disinfectant to dry.
   4. Aspirates 3 mL of urine into syringe attached to Luer-Lok.

3. Later in the day, the patient reports having a sore throat. Which action will the nurse take when obtaining a throat specimen that is ordered by the health care provider?
   1. Collect the specimen from the uvula.
   2. Elevate the head of the bed to 30 degrees.
   3. Pass the swab onto the tongue and then the throat.
   4. Insert the collection device while avoiding the lips and cheeks.

4. When collecting a blood glucose sample, the nurse notices the patient has multiple puncture sites on each fingertip that are reddened and painful. When two puncture sites are noted to be oozing with pus, which nursing action is appropriate?
   1. Clean fingertips by soaking in alcohol.
   2. Place adhesive bandages over all fingertips.
   3. Culture each fingertip separately.
   4. Notify the health care provider of the fingertip findings.

5. The nurse is preparing to measure a patient's blood glucose level. Which action is essential to accurately collecting the sample?
   1. Connect the glucometer to a corded power source.
   2. Use only lancets made by the glucometer's manufacturer.
   3. Match code on test strip to code on the glucometer.
   4. Sterilize the glucometer in an autoclave prior to use.

Visit the Evolve site for Answers to Clinical Judgment and Next-Generation NCLEX® Examination-Style Questions.

REFERENCES

Agency for Healthcare Research and Quality (AHRQ): *Teach-back: intervention,* 2023. https://www.ahrq.gov/patient-safety/reports/engage/interventions/teachback.html.

American Diabetes Association (ADA): *The big picture: checking your blood glucose,* 2023. https://www.diabetes.org/healthy-living/medication-treatments/blood-glucose-testing-and-control/checking-your-blood-sugar. Accessed March 18, 2023.

Anand S, Liang PS: A practical overview of the stool DNA test for colorectal cancer screening, *Clin Transl Gastroenterol* 13(4):e00464, 2022.

Bobbette N, et al: Adults with intellectual and developmental disabilities and interprofessional, team-based primary health care: a scoping review, *JBI Evid Synth* 18(7):1470, 2020.

Burchill CN, et al: Emergency nurses' knowledge, attitudes, and practices related to blood sample hemolysis prevention: an exploratory descriptive study, *J Emerg Nurs* 47(4):580, 2021.

Centers for Disease Control and Prevention (CDC): *CDC's Core infection prevention and control practices for safe healthcare delivery in all settings,* 2022. https://www.cdc.gov/infectioncontrol/guidelines/core-practices/index.html. Accessed March 18, 2023.

Centers for Disease Control and Prevention (CDC): *What is health literacy?,* 2023. https://www.cdc.gov/healthliteracy/learn/index.html.

Clebak KT, et al: Multitargeted stool DNA testing (Cologuard) for colorectal cancer screening, *Am Fam Physician* 105(2):198, 2022.

Emergency Nurses Association (ENA): Clinical practice guideline: Prevention of blood specimen hemolysis in peripherally-collected venous specimens, *J Emerg Nurs* 44(4):402, 2018.

Ersoy S, et al: A single-center prospective study of the effects of different methods of phlebotomy in the emergency department on blood sample hemolysis rates. *J Emerg Nurs* 49(1):134–139, 2023.

Fumarola S, et al: Overlooked and underestimated: Medical adhesive-related skin injuries. Best practice consensus document on prevention, *J Wound Care* 29(Suppl 3c):S1–S24, 2020.

Gorski L, et al: *Infusion therapy standards of practice,* ed 8, Norwood: Mass, 2021, Infusion Nurses Society (INS).

Hockenberry MJ, et al: *Wong's essentials of pediatric nursing*, ed 11, St. Louis, 2022, Elsevier.

Krasowski M: Hemolysis and lipemia interference with laboratory testing, *J Infus Nurs* 42(5):237–247, 2019.

Mendes A: Meeting the care needs of a person with dementia who is distressed, *Br J Nurs* 27(4):219, 2018.

Miteva D, et al: Impact of language proficiency on mental health service, use, treatment, and outcomes: "Lost in Translation", *Compr Psychiatry* 114:152299, 2022.

Occupational Safety and Health Administration (OSHA): *Worker protections against occupational exposure to infectious diseases*, n.d. https://www.osha.gov/bloodborne-pathogens/worker-protections. Accessed March 18, 2023.

Pagana KD, et al: *Mosby's diagnostic and laboratory tests reference*, ed 15, St. Louis, 2021, Mosby.

Sullivan WF, et al: Primary care of adults with intellectual and developmental disabilities: 2018 Canadian consensus guidelines, *Can Fam Physician* 64(4):254, 2018.

The Joint Commission (TJC): *2023 National Patient Safety Goals*, Oakbrook Terrace, IL, 2023, The Joint Commission. https://www.jointcommission.org/standards/national-patient-safety-goals/.

Touhy T, Jett K: *Ebersole and Hess' gerontological nursing and healthy aging*, ed 6, St. Louis, 2022, Mosby.

Tremayne P, et al. Care and management of indwelling urinary catheters for people with learning disabilities, *Learn Disabil Pract* 22(4): 2019.

U.S. Food and Drug Administration (FDA): *Blood glucose monitoring devices*, n.d.a. http://www.fda.gov/medicaldevices/productsandmedicalprocedures/invitrodiagnostics/glucosetestingdevices/default.htm. Accessed March 18, 2023.

U.S. Food and Drug Administration (FDA): *FDA approves first continuous glucose monitoring system with a fully implantable glucose sensor and compatible mobile app for adults with diabetes*, n.d.b. https://www.fda.gov/news-events/press-announcements/fda-approves-first-continuous-glucose-monitoring-system-fully-implantable-glucose-sensor-and. Accessed March 18, 2023.

Diagnostic Procedures

SKILLS AND PROCEDURES

Skill 8.1 **Intravenous Moderate Sedation, p. 229**

Skill 8.2 **Contrast Media Studies: Arteriogram (Angiogram), Cardiac Catheterization, and Intravenous Pyelogram, p. 234**

Skill 8.3 **Care of Patients Undergoing Aspirations: Bone Marrow Aspiration/Biopsy, Lumbar Puncture, Paracentesis, and Thoracentesis, p. 240**

Skill 8.4 **Care of a Patient Undergoing Bronchoscopy, p. 246**

Skill 8.5 **Care of a Patient Undergoing Endoscopy, p. 250**

OBJECTIVES

Mastery of content in this chapter will enable you to:

- Outline the physiological indications for diagnostic procedures.
- Explain the health care team collaboration and teamwork required before, during, and after procedures, including delegation to assistive personnel (AP).
- Summarize the appropriate physical and psychosocial assessments before, during, and after diagnostic procedures.
- Explain basic nursing responsibilities related to care of patients undergoing angiogram, cardiac catheterization, intravenous (IV) pyelogram, bone marrow aspiration/biopsy, lumbar puncture (LP), paracentesis, thoracentesis, bronchoscopy, and endoscopy.
- Explain nursing responsibilities related to the care of the patient undergoing IV sedation during diagnostic/surgical procedures.
- Examine the risks and complications associated with IV sedation, media studies, aspirations, bronchoscopy, and endoscopy.

MEDIA RESOURCES

- http://evolve.elsevier.com/Perry/skills
- Clinical Review Questions
- Audio Glossary
- Answers to Clinical Judgment and Next-Generation NCLEX® Examination–Style Questions
- Skills Performance Checklists
- Printable Key Points

PURPOSE

Diagnostic procedures are performed at patients' bedsides or in specially equipped rooms within a health care agency or outpatient care setting. Before preparing patients, check the agency protocol specific to the procedure you will be performing or with which you are assisting. Depending on the area in which you work, as a nurse you may be responsible for assessing a patient's knowledge of a procedure; preparing the patient physically and emotionally; providing a safe environment and emotional support throughout the procedure; providing preprocedure and postprocedure assessment, care, and documentation; and providing discharge teaching. The health care provider is responsible for providing the patient with an explanation of the test/procedure, risks, benefits, treatment options, and outcomes before the procedure as part of the *informed consent* process.

PRACTICE STANDARDS

- American Society of Anesthesiologists (ASA), 2018—Practice Guidelines for Moderate Procedural Sedation and Analgesia
- The Joint Commission (TJC), 2023: National Patient Safety Goals—Patient identification

SUPPLEMENTAL STANDARDS

- United States Department of Labor, n.d.: Occupational Safety and Health Administration, Workers' Protection Against Occupational Exposure to Infectious Diseases—Standard Precautions

PRINCIPLES FOR PRACTICE

- Nurses take steps to ensure that patients who require diagnostic testing understand their testing and postprocedural care requirements.
- Some tests require intravenous (IV) sedation along with the diagnostic procedure such as a gastrointestinal (GI) endoscopy; others require contrast media or aspirations.
- Diagnostic procedures pose some risk for patients. Understand the diagnostic procedure, including why it is needed, which preprocedure assessments are needed, expected outcomes, your role during the procedure, potential risks, actions appropriate in the event of unexpected outcomes, and appropriate postprocedural nursing care, to help ensure patient safety.
- IV sedation is used for diagnostic or surgical procedures that do not require complete or general anesthesia. Sedation classifications include "minimal," "moderate," or "deep" sedation/analgesia, depending on the depth of sedation (Lingappan, 2021).

American Society of Anesthesiologists (ASA) Physical Status Classification System

- ASA I = Normal healthy patient
- ASA II = Patient with mild systemic disease
- ASA III = Patient with severe systemic disease
- ASA IV = Patient with severe systemic disease that is a constant threat to life
- ASA V = Moribund patient who is not expected to survive without the operation
- ASA VI = Declared brain-dead patient whose organs are being removed for donor purposes

"E" is added if the procedure is performed as an emergency.

From American Society of Anesthesiologists (ASA). *ASA physical status classification system,* 2020, https://www.asahq.org/standards-and-guidelines/asa-physical-status-classification-system. Accessed March 9, 2023.

- The use of objective scales such as the American Society of Anesthesiologists (ASA) physical status classification system determines whether patients are at risk for undesirable outcomes (Box 8.1). Use of an objective scale can reduce the risk for complications by determining when it is wise to involve an anesthesiologist to help manage the care of a complicated patient condition.
- These scales also incorporate evidence-based guidelines to reduce the risk for sedation-induced complications such as cardiac arrhythmias, respiratory failure, renal failure, neurological disorders related to the use of paralytic agents, or bleeding disorders resulting from hepatic failure.

PERSON-CENTERED CARE

- Any diagnostic procedure can create a sense of powerlessness for patients. The unknown (e.g., not knowing what a test may reveal or not completely understanding what a test involves or feels like) can also create fear and anxiety.
- It is important to involve patients in discussions of what their procedures involve and give them an opportunity to ask questions. Learn what their concerns are because you may be able to alleviate them. For example, if a patient worries about being physically exposed during a procedure, communicate with procedure staff to see if there is a way to minimize exposure and use more draping.
- When a patient is chronically ill, is fatigued, or has decreased functional status, plan the diagnostic testing schedule to provide rest periods between multiple procedures performed on the same day. Ensure that the patient is stable before the next diagnostic procedure.
- Provide reassurance to a patient throughout a procedure. Most of these procedures cause moderate discomfort, and the patient is likely anxious. The patient often tolerates a procedure better if you remain close and explain each step.

EVIDENCE-BASED PRACTICE

Noninvasive Approaches to Pain Control

Patients undergoing bone marrow biopsies can experience a significant amount of pain. Recent research has examined alternative, complementary, and integrative approaches to caring for these patients to reduce pain, promote comfort, and lessen anxiety and stress. Noninvasive nursing approaches to pain control can be based on the following findings:

- Procedures such as a bone marrow biopsy cause anxiety in patients. Inhalation of lavender has demonstrated reduction in anxiety for this population (Abbaszadeh et al., 2020).
- Nonpharmacological interventions that have been used successfully as adjuvants to medication to reduce pain include music therapy and hypnosis (Gendron et al., 2019).
- Use of music resulted in a reduction in patient anxiety, reduction in procedure length, and decreased medication use during the procedure (Schandert et al., 2021).
- The use of music therapy in children with cancer has demonstrated a reduction in preoperative anxiety before invasive procedures (Giordano et al., 2020).

SAFETY GUIDELINES

Before a Procedure

- It is essential to be sure that the correct patient undergoes the correct procedure. Identify a patient by using a minimum of two identifiers, verifying the correct procedure (and site, when applicable). This includes verbal verification and written/computerized documentation of the preceding information on patient arrival, again in the procedure room, and just before starting a procedure (The Joint Commission [TJC], 2023).
- Assess for completion of relevant documentation (e.g., history and physical [H&P], signed procedure consent form, nursing assessment, and preanesthesia assessment) necessary for performing a safe procedure (ASA, 2018).
- Identify any medications for which uninterrupted dosing is required (e.g., anticonvulsants, antibiotics, certain cardiac medications). If the procedure requires a patient to have nothing by mouth (NPO), discuss medications with the health care provider to decide if the patient should take any medications before the procedure. When insulin or oral hypoglycemic medications are given to patients before procedures, arrange to have either the patients' meals or other nutritional support available on completion of the procedure.
- Verify that informed consent was obtained before administering any sedatives. The health care provider performing the procedure is responsible for obtaining informed consent from a patient (TJC, 2022). In some agencies after the health care provider discusses the procedure and obtains verbal consent, the registered nurse obtains the patient's signature on the consent form. (Check agency policy to determine if a consent form is required and the expectations of the nurse in this process.) *When there is no evidence of informed consent in the patient's electronic health record (EHR), hold any preprocedure medications that may alter the patient's level of consciousness and notify the health care provider performing the procedure and staff in any receiving area.*
- If English is not the patient's primary language, ensure that an official interpreter is used when obtaining consent, and document in the consent form.
- Make sure that emergency equipment (e.g., oxygen, suction, defibrillator) is available in the procedure area and has been checked to ensure function.
- Confirm presence and date of expiration for sedation reversal agents.

During a Procedure

- Procedure involving the use of radiation:
  - Minimize the amount of radiation exposure by using protective shielding devices such as a lead apron and goggles, radioprotective gloves, and/or thyroid shield.

- Monitor staff radiation exposure with the use of a dosimeter if necessary.
- Remain positioned as far away from the radiographic equipment as possible while performing required patient care.
- All procedures:
  - Monitor physiological parameters indicated by the procedure.
  - Position patients carefully to avoid musculoskeletal or neurological injury.
  - Label any specimens obtained during a procedure properly.

After the Procedure

- Assess for possible procedural complications and conduct appropriate assessments for early detection.

- Monitor oxygen saturation and vital signs (VS) to detect sedation failure and adverse effects (e.g., vomiting, hypoxic events). The use of continuous pulse oximetry (CPOX) has been shown to improve detection of desaturation (Harper et al., 2021).
- Know the use, side effects, and complications of the sedative and reversal agents to be administered.
- Be able to recognize cardiac dysrhythmias (see Chapter 25).
- Institute fall precautions until a patient has recovered from the effects of sedatives (see Chapter 14).
- Timely and complete neurovascular checks are critical to identify postprocedure limb ischemia or other arterial complications.

◆ SKILL 8.1   Intravenous Moderate Sedation

Certain diagnostic or therapeutic procedures require patients to receive intravenous (IV) moderate sedation. Moderate sedation/analgesia (also referred to as *conscious sedation*) produces a minimally depressed level of consciousness induced by the administration of pharmacological agents. The patient can respond to external stimuli (verbal or tactile), and the airway reflexes, spontaneous ventilation, and cardiovascular function are maintained (Lingappan, 2021). Moderate sedation improves a patient's cooperation with a procedure, allows a rapid return to preprocedure status, and minimizes the risk for injury. It often raises a patient's pain threshold and provides amnesia concerning the actual procedural events. In addition, no interventions are required during a procedure to maintain a patent airway, and spontaneous ventilation is adequate.

Deep sedation is one risk associated with moderate sedation when a patient's level of consciousness depresses past the point at which the patient can maintain a patent airway. Typically, certified registered nurse anesthetists (CRNAs), anesthesiologists, physicians, dentists, and oral surgeons are qualified providers of moderate sedation, and specifically trained registered nurses may assist in the administration (American Association of Moderate Sedation Nurses [AAMSN], 2022). Know the agency policy for recommended and maximum doses of medications and monitoring and documentation requirements when using IV sedation.

The most common types of medications used to achieve moderate sedation include benzodiazepines and opiates. Benzodiazepines include midazolam, lorazepam, and diazepam; they reduce anxiety and promote muscle relaxation (Lingappan, 2021). Midazolam also produces an amnesic effect. Opiates such as morphine sulfate or fentanyl help control pain while achieving sedation. Nonbarbiturate sedatives, such as propofol, provide a safe, rapid-acting hypnotic and may offer a faster recovery time than the combination of benzodiazepines and opiates.

Patient risks during IV sedation include hypoventilation, airway compromise, hemodynamic instability, and/or altered levels of consciousness that include an overly depressed level of consciousness or agitation and combativeness. Emergency equipment appropriate for the patient's age and size (see Chapter 27) and a staff competent in airway management, oxygen delivery, and use of resuscitation equipment are essential. During a procedure, patients need continuous monitoring. Monitor a patient's response to verbal commands during moderate sedation, except in patients who are unable to respond appropriately (e.g., those in whom age or development may impair bidirectional communication) or during procedures in which movement could be detrimental (ASA,

2018). During procedures in which a verbal response is not possible (e.g., oral surgery, restorative dentistry, upper endoscopy), check the patient's ability to give a "thumbs up" or other indication of consciousness in response to verbal or tactile (light tap) stimulation; this suggests that the patient will be able to control the airway and take deep breaths if necessary (ASA, 2018). Continuously monitor all patients by pulse oximetry. Measure blood pressure before sedation/analgesia is initiated; once moderate sedation/analgesia is established, continually monitor blood pressure (e.g., at 5-minute intervals) and heart rate during the procedure (ASA, 2018). Monitoring continues after the procedure.

Delegation

The skill of assisting with IV moderate sedation, including the preprocedure assessment, cannot be delegated to assistive personnel (AP).

Interprofessional Collaboration

- In most agencies a specially trained registered nurse or health care provider assesses and monitors a patient's level of sedation, airway patency, and level of consciousness. Roles in monitoring depend on scope-of-practice guidelines as determined by state regulations (see agency policy).

Equipment

- Personal protective equipment (PPE): gloves, mask, head cover, gown, eye protection
- Sedation as prescribed: benzodiazepines, opiates, propofol, and fentanyl
- Emergency equipment: crash cart, cardiac monitor/defibrillator, and endotracheal intubation/airway management equipment in various sizes and appropriate for patient's age
- Equipment for insertion of a peripheral IV catheter and IV fluids (see Chapter 28)
- Oxygen and airway supplies: bag and mask device, oral/nasopharyngeal airways
- Suction equipment (see Chapter 24)
- Blood pressure monitor
- Pulse oximeter or end-tidal carbon dioxide (CO_2) monitor
- Electrocardiogram (ECG) monitor
- Appropriate reversal drugs (e.g., flumazenil for reversal of benzodiazepines, naloxone for reversal of opiates) and labels for each
- Pain medication (opioids) for procedures anticipated to cause discomfort such as dizziness, disorientation, nausea, vomiting

STEP	RATIONALE

ASSESSMENT

1. Identify patient using at least two identifiers (e.g., name and birthday or name and medical record number) according to agency policy. Compare identifiers with information in patient's medication administration record (MAR) or electronic health record (EHR).	Ensures correct patient. Complies with The Joint Commission standards and improves patient safety (TJC, 2023).
2. Assess patient's/family caregiver's health literacy.	Determines degree to which individuals have the ability to find, understand, and use information and services to make informed health-related decisions and actions (CDC, 2023).
3. Refer to health care provider order and verify type of procedure scheduled and procedure site with patient.	Ensures correct procedure for correct patient.
4. Verify that a preprocedure medication reconciliation and history and physical (H&P) examination were completed.	Accrediting agencies such as the TJC (2023) require a documented preprocedure medication history and H&P before administration of procedural IV sedation.
5. Verify that informed consent was obtained before administering any sedatives.	Federal regulations, many state laws, and accreditation agencies such as The Joint Commission require informed consent for procedure. Patients should provide informed consent before any procedure (TJC, 2022).
6. Assess patient's history of adverse reaction to IV sedation (e.g., hemodynamic instability, nausea or vomiting, airway compromise, altered level of consciousness).	Patients with history of these reactions are at higher risk for procedural complications if IV sedation is used.
7. Verify patient's ASA physical status classification (see Box 8.1).	Patients with significant underlying conditions require consultation with a medical specialist (e.g., physician anesthesiologist, cardiologist, endocrinologist, pulmonologist, nephrologist, pediatrician, obstetrician, or otolaryngologist) before procedure (ASA, 2018).

Clinical Judgment *Consultation with an anesthesiologist is required if a patient has an ASA classification of 3 to 6 or history of or evidence for difficult intubation, sleep apnea, or complications related to sedation/anesthesia.*

8. Review EHR for history of airway abnormalities, liver failure, lung disease, heart failure, hypotonia, sleep apnea, and history of adverse reaction to sedatives (American College of Radiology [ACR], 2020).	These risk factors increase likelihood of adverse event (ACR, 2020).

Clinical Judgment *A Mallampati score can be used to predict a difficult intubation in patients with obstructive sleep apnea (OSA). This assessment is performed while the patient sits with the head in a neutral position and mouth open. Patients who receive a Mallampati score of 3 or 4 are often considered to be at increased risk of OSA (Sleep Foundation, 2023).*

9. Assess patient's current status or history for substance abuse or liver/kidney disease.	A history of substance abuse and/or liver/kidney disease usually requires dose adjustment of sedative agents.
10. Verify that patient has not ingested food or fluids, except for oral medications, for at least 4 h.	Because risk of moderate sedation is loss of airway protection, an empty stomach reduces risk for aspiration.
11. Determine if patient is allergic to latex, antiseptic, tape, medications used for induction, or anesthetic solutions.	Allergic reactions to latex or tape range from mild skin reaction to anaphylaxis. Common allergic reactions to local anesthetic agents include central nervous system (CNS) depression, respiratory difficulty, and hypotension.
12. Perform hand hygiene. Assess baseline heart rate, breath sounds, respiratory rate, blood pressure, level of consciousness, pain level, and oxygen saturation (SpO$_2$).	Establishes baseline for comparison during and after procedure.
13. Determine patient's height and weight.	Needed to calculate drug dosages.
14. Assess patient's baseline status via designated scoring system of agency. A variety of tools are available for scoring, including the Postanesthetic Discharge Scoring System (PADSS) (Table 8.1).	Establishes baseline for comparison after procedure.
15. Assess patient's knowledge, prior experience with IV sedation, and feelings about procedure.	Reveals need for patient instruction and/or support.

STEP	RATIONALE

TABLE 8.1

Postanesthetic Discharge Scoring System (PADSS)

		Score
Vital signs	±20% of preprocedure value	2
	±20–40% of preprocedure value	1
	±40% of preprocedure value	0
Activity	Steady gait, no dizziness, or meets preoperative level	2
	Requires assistance	1
	Unable to ambulate	0
Nausea and vomiting	No or minimal/treated with PO medication	2
	Moderate/treated with parenteral medication	1
	Severe/continues despite treatment	0
Pain	Minimal or no pain (0–3 numerical value)	2
	Moderate (4–6 numerical value)	1
	Severe (7–10 numerical value)	0
Surgical bleeding	None or minimal (no intervention required)	2
	Moderate/up to 2 dressing changes required	1
	Severe/more than 3 dressing changes required	0

BP, Blood pressure; *PO,* by mouth.
From American Society of PeriAnesthesia Nurses (ASPAN): 2021–2022 perianesthesia nursing standards, practice recommendations and interpretive statements. Cherry Hill, NJ, 2020, ASPAN; and Walke S, et al.: When to discharge a patient after endoscopy: a narrative review, *Clin Endosc* 55(1):8-14, 2022.

BOX 8.2

The Joint Commission Universal Protocol

- Verification of correct person, correct site, and correct procedure occurs.
- Procedure site is marked before moving to procedure area.
- A time-out is performed immediately before starting procedures.
- When patient is in preprocedure area (immediately before moving the patient to procedure room), a standardized list (e.g., paper, electronic, or other medium such as a wall-mounted white board) is used to review and verify that required items are available and accurately matched to the patient.

From The Joint Commission (TJC): *2023 National Patient Safety Goals,* Oakbrook Terrace, IL, 2023, The Joint Commission. https://www.jointcommission.org/standards/national-patient-safety-goals/.

PLANNING

1. Expected outcomes following completion of procedures:
   - Adhere to Universal Protocol (Box 8.2). — Maintains patient safety (TJC, 2023).
   - Patient's airway remains patent. — Moderate sedation is monitored successfully without progression to deep sedation.
   - Patient's pain acuity is equivalent to score of 4 or less on pain scale of 0 to 10. — Procedure managed to minimize patient's pain acuity.
2. Provide privacy and explain to patient that IV sedation will cause relaxation and amnesia but maintain wakefulness during procedure. If patient will not be able to verbalize because of nature of procedure, teach agreed-on nonverbal signals such as "yes," "no," and "pain." — Protects patient's privacy; reduces anxiety. Promotes cooperation.
3. Explain that close monitoring of vital signs (VS) and frequent checks to determine that patient is awake are normal and do not mean that there are problems. — Reduces patient anxiety during procedure.
4. Explain to patient major steps of procedure. — Reduces patient anxiety during procedure.
5. Organize and set up any equipment needed to perform procedure. — Ensures more efficiency when completing a procedure.
6. Position patient as needed for procedure.

IMPLEMENTATION

1. Perform hand hygiene. Apply clean gloves, mask, and other PPE as needed. Establish peripheral IV access (see also Chapter 28). — Reduces transmission of microorganisms. Provides access for administration of sedation and any emergency medications (as needed).

STEP	RATIONALE

TABLE 8.2

Modified Ramsay Sedation Scale

Minimal sedation (anxiolysis)	1	Anxious and agitated or restless or both
	2	Cooperative, oriented, and tranquil
Moderate sedation/analgesia (conscious sedation)	3	Responds to commands spoken in a normal voice
Deep sedation/analgesia	4	Brisk response to a light forehead tap or loud auditory stimulus
	5	Sluggish response to a light forehead tap or loud auditory stimulus
	6	No response to a light forehead tap or loud auditory stimulus

Data from Rasheed AM, et al.: Ramsay sedation scale and Richmond agitation sedation scale: a cross sectional study, *Dimens Crit Care Nurs* 38(2):90, 2019.

STEP	RATIONALE
2. Implement Universal Protocol for second time in presence of appropriate health care team members (as applicable) and in accordance with agency policy (see Box 8.2).	Ensures patient safety by correctly identifying correct patient with correct procedure.
3. During diagnostic procedure, monitor heart rate and SpO$_2$ continuously via pulse oximetry equipment. Some agencies also use end-tidal CO$_2$ monitoring (capnography) (ASA, 2018). Monitor patient's airway patency, respiratory rate and depth, blood pressure, and level of consciousness and responsiveness every 5 min (ACR, 2020). Keep oxygen and suction equipment nearby.	VS, oximetry, and capnography provide comparison with patient's baseline status. Oxygen and suction equipment may be required if there is any respiratory or CNS depression or in an emergent situation.
4. Observe for verbal or nonverbal evidence of pain, facial grimacing, and eye opening.	Physical responses indicate level of sedation.
5. Assess level of sedation using Modified Ramsay Sedation Scale (Table 8.2) or other criteria adopted by agency.	Determines patient's level of sedation. Numeric rating scale offers consistent assessment and accurate judgment of patient's changing status and verbal/physical stimulation (Rasheed, 2019).

Clinical Judgment *Report a Ramsay sedation score higher than 3 (responsive to commands only) to the health care provider (see Table 8.2).*

STEP	RATIONALE
6. Reposition patient as needed without interrupting diagnostic procedure.	Prevents pressure- and position-related injuries (ACR, 2020).
7. Dispose of all contaminated supplies in appropriate receptacle, remove and dispose of gloves, mask, and other PPE.	Reduces transmission of microorganisms. Use appropriate disposal receptacle if patient is receiving hazardous drugs (Blake, 2019; Oncology Nursing Society [ONS], 2018).
8. Help patient to a comfortable position.	Restores comfort and sense of well-being.
9. Raise side rails (as appropriate) and lower bed or stretcher to lowest position, locking into position.	Ensures patient safety and prevents falls.
10. Place nurse call system in an accessible location within patient's reach.	Ensures patient can call for assistance if needed.
11. Perform hand hygiene.	Reduces transmission of microorganisms.

EVALUATION

STEP	RATIONALE
1. Monitor patient throughout procedure using the Modified Ramsay Sedation Scale (or other criteria adopted by the agency).	Provides data to verify patient's expected return to baseline status.
2. After procedure: Use PADSS (see Table 8.1) and monitor level of consciousness, respiratory rate, SpO$_2$, blood pressure, heart rate and rhythm, and pain score according to agency policy (ACR, 2020) (e.g., every 5 minutes for at least 30 minutes, then every 15 minutes for an hour, and then every 30 minutes until patient meets discharge criteria).	Enables prompt detection of any airway compromise or protective reflexes caused by delayed action of medications.
3. Have patient's "designated driver" explain any postprocedure education and sign appropriate documents if patient is unable to sign.	Patients who receive conscious sedation are restricted from driving for 24 to 48 h, depending on procedure, type of sedation, and postprocedure restrictions.

STEP	RATIONALE
4. **Use Teach-Back:** "I want to be sure I explained what to do when you return home and your medications . Tell me what you know about the restrictions to follow and the medications you will be taking once you're home." Revise your instruction now or develop a plan for revised patient/family caregiver teaching if patient/family caregiver is not able to teach back correctly.	Teach-back is a technique for health care providers to ensure that they have explained medical information clearly so that patients and families understand what is communicated to them (Agency for Healthcare Research and Quality [AHRQ], 2023).

Unexpected Outcomes	Related Interventions
1. Oversedation, evidenced by decreasing SpO_2 (cyanosis, slow shallow respirations with periods of apnea), tachycardia, sedation score of 4 (exhibiting brisk response to light glabellar tap or loud auditory stimulus) or higher on Modified Ramsay Sedation Scale.	• Support patient's breathing with positioning and manual airway bagging. • Immediately notify health care provider. • Be prepared to administer reversal agents. Naloxone is for reversal of opioids, and flumazenil is for reversal of benzodiazepines.
2. Patient develops cardiac instability evidenced by irregular heart rate, change in pulse rate, or change in blood pressure.	• Initiate oxygen therapy, ensure IV access, and obtain ECG as ordered. • Immediately notify health care provider.

Documentation

- Document VS, SpO_2, end-tidal CO_2, and sedation level at baseline, then every 5 minutes during the procedure and every 15 minutes for at least 30 minutes after the procedure according to agency policy.
- Document dosage, route, and time of administration for drugs given during and after the procedure, including reversal agents.
- Document significant patient reactions during the procedure. Include IV fluids and blood products if administered.
- Document discharge teaching, medication reconciliation, discontinuation of IV access, final/discharge assessment, and to whom/how discharged (e.g., designated driver, ambulance/transporter, nursing home).
- Document your evaluation of patient and family caregiver learning.

Hand-Off Reporting

- Immediately report to patient's health care provider any respiratory distress, cardiac compromise, or unexpected altered mental status.

Special Considerations

Patient Education

- Explain that it is unlikely for patients to remember the procedure because of the amnesic effect of the sedative(s).
- Before the procedure, instruct patient to arrange for transportation home after the procedure because (at most agencies) patient will not be permitted to drive for 24 hours after receiving sedation.
- Provide patients and family caregivers with discharge instructions that include complications that may occur; how to manage complications; and physical signs and symptoms to report to the health care provider, including contact information and postprocedure medication reconciliation and instructions.

Pediatrics

- As compared with adults, differences exist in cognitive abilities and developmental status, respiratory mechanics, airway anatomy, drug metabolism, and toxic dosages (Lingappan, 2021).
- A preprocedure medical evaluation is required. The presedation assessment must take into consideration the limited speech and expressive capabilities of children. A child's behavioral state must be assessed before picking an agent, as this state may affect the choice of drug and the dose (Lingappan, 2021).
- During the preprocedure assessment, answer the parent's questions in a relaxed and confident manner. When communicating with children, consider the child's developmental stage.

Older Adults

- Closely monitor the effects of medications on patient's respiratory status and pulse. These drugs interfere with breathing or increase or decrease heart rate as a result of reduced drug clearance through the kidneys or liver (Touhy & Jett, 2022).
- Physical limitations of the patient, including hearing and vision loss, contribute to frustration and confusion, compounding the sense of loss of control.
- As a result of an aging liver, some medications are not metabolized as rapidly as they might be in younger patients.
- Chronic illness may complicate a patient's recovery.

Populations With Disabilities

- Provide enough time that patients can make specific health care needs clear (Sullivan, 2018).

Home Care

- Instruct patient to avoid making any legally binding decisions until at least 24 hours after the procedure.

Contrast media studies involve visualization of blood vessels and internal organs by intravascular injection of a radiopaque medium. An arteriogram (angiogram) permits visualization of the vasculature and arterial system of an organ (Fig. 8.1). Arteriography is usually performed by an interventional radiologist to diagnose arterial or venous occlusions; stenosis; emboli; thromboses; aneurysms; tumors; congenital malformations; or trauma to the brain, heart, lung, kidneys, or lower extremities.

Cardiac catheterization is a specialized form of angiography performed by an interventional cardiologist. An IV or intraarterial catheter introducer (Fig. 8.2) is inserted into the left or right side of the heart via a major peripheral vessel, usually the femoral artery and/or vein. Newer interventions are using the radial artery for these procedures as it reduces the risk of postprocedure complications such as bleeding (Kim et al., 2021). The test studies pressures within the heart, cardiac volumes, valvular function, and patency of coronary arteries. Cardiac catheterizations are performed in specially equipped laboratories (Fig. 8.3). A contrast medium is injected to allow for visualization of the structures and functions of the heart and lungs.

There are no definitive contraindications for a cardiac catheterization, but many of the contraindications are relative. They depend on the need for the procedure and related comorbidities of the patient. Most of these can be corrected before the procedure (Manda & Baradhi, 2022).

IV pyelography (IVP) is a venographic examination of the flow of radiopaque contrast medium through the kidneys, ureters, and bladder to identify obstruction, hematuria, stones, bladder injury, or renal artery occlusion. Dye is injected into a peripheral vein, and serial radiographs are taken over the subsequent 30 minutes.

Delegation

The skill of assisting with angiography and IVP can be delegated to AP if the patient is stable, and no IV sedation is used. Direct the AP about:

- When to obtain and report vital signs (VS), urinary output, and weight
- Which signs and symptoms to report to the nurse
- Accompanying the patient to the procedure room and helping specially trained and licensed radiology personnel with the specific angiography procedure

The skill of assisting with cardiac catheterization can be delegated to specially trained AP with a registered nurse continuously

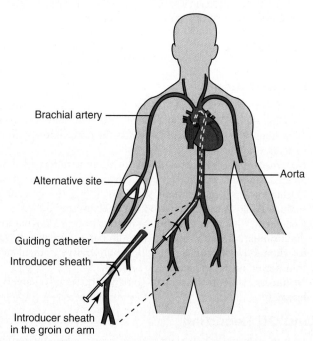

FIG. 8.2 A catheter introducer placed into a femoral artery or vein allows for threading the tip of a long, thin catheter into the right or left side of the heart during cardiac catheterization.

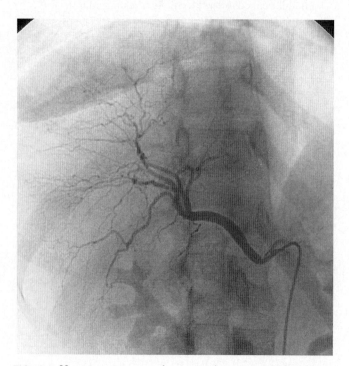

FIG. 8.1 Hepatic arteriogram shows a catheter passing through the common hepatic artery. (*From Long BW, et al.: Merrill's atlas of radiographic positioning & procedures, ed 15,. St. Louis, 2023, Elsevier.*)

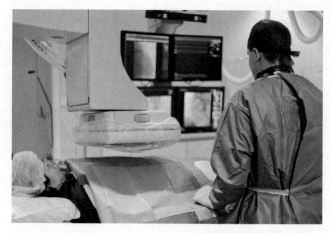

FIG. 8.3 Cardiac catheterization laboratory. (*From iStock.com/Image Supply.*)

present. The nurse provides continuous patient assessment and monitoring for serious complications. The AP helps with patient transport, positioning, and obtaining supplies.

Interprofessional Collaboration

- Contrast media studies require the collaboration of a specially trained health care team. The nurse works with the team, ensuring patient safety and advocating on the patient's behalf.

Equipment

- PPE: mask, sterile gown, head cover, eye protection, and clean and sterile gloves

- Sterile packs containing catheters/equipment for performing procedures
- Equipment for peripheral IV access and IV fluids
- Medications such as sedatives (e.g., diazepam, midazolam, propofol) for IV sedation or analgesics for relaxation and pain control
- Emergency equipment: oxygen, endotracheal intubation/airway management equipment, emergency cart, cardiac monitor/defibrillator, sedative reversal agents
- Pulse oximeter, end-tidal carbon dioxide (CO_2) monitor, blood pressure (BP) equipment, stethoscope

STEP	RATIONALE

ASSESSMENT

1. Identify patient using at least two identifiers (e.g., name and birthday or name and medical record number) according to agency policy. Compare identifiers with information in patient's medication administration record (MAR) or electronic health record (EHR). | Ensures correct patient. Complies with The Joint Commission standards and improves patient safety (TJC, 2023).

2. Assess patient's/family caregiver's health literacy. | Determines degree to which individuals have the ability to find, understand, and use information and services to make informed health-related decisions and actions (CDC, 2023).

3. Refer to health care provider order and verify type of procedure scheduled and procedure site with patient. | Ensures correct procedure and patient (TJC, 2023).

4. Verify that informed consent was obtained before administering any sedatives. | Federal regulations, many state laws, and accreditation agencies such as The Joint Commission require informed consent for procedure. Patients should provide informed consent before any procedure (TJC, 2022).

5. Determine if patient is taking anticoagulants, aspirin, or any nonsteroidal medication. | Some medications increase risk for bleeding and are often stopped before procedure (Bangalore et al., 2021).

6. Assess patient for history of any allergies to iodine dye or shellfish and whether patient has had previous reaction to contrast agent (Bangalore et al., 2021). If so, notify cardiologist or radiologist. | Allergic individuals may be at a mildly increased risk for developing adverse reactions to radiocontrast media. Hypoallergenic contrast medium is sometimes used.

7. Review EHR for contraindications:

   a. *All contrast media:* Pregnancy unless benefits of test outweigh risks to fetus. | Radioactive iodinated contrast media crosses blood-placental barrier.

   b. *Angiography:* Anticoagulant therapy, bleeding disorders, thrombocytopenia, dehydration, uncontrolled hypertension, renal insufficiency, and pregnancy. | Anticoagulants and bleeding disorders interfere with patient's blood-clotting abilities and may cause blood loss. However, a temporary hold on anticoagulant dosing is often preferred preprocedure over contraindication of procedure. Dehydration and renal insufficiency are contraindications to use of ionic radiographic contrast media because patient has impaired ability to excrete contrast media via kidneys.

   c. *Cardiac catheterization:* History of severe cardiomyopathy, severe dysrhythmias, uncontrolled heart failure (HF). | Introduction of catheter into myocardium increases risk for dysrhythmias (Pagana et al., 2021).

   d. *IVP:* History of dehydration, known renal insufficiency (with blood urea nitrogen [BUN] level >40 mg/100 mL) (Pagana et al., 2021). | Iodinated dye is sometimes nephrotoxic and worsens existing renal disease.

   e. Determine whether patient took metformin hydrochloride within previous 48 hours. If so, notify health care provider immediately. | Metformin hydrochloride may be continued unless the patient has severe renal dysfunction (Bangalore et al., 2021). Some continue the older practice of the medication being discontinued 1 day before procedure and 2 days after catheterization because of the possibility of causing lactic acidosis and acute nephropathy (Yale School of Medicine, 2022).

STEP	RATIONALE
8. Assess patient's bleeding and coagulation status (e.g., complete blood count [CBC], platelets, prothrombin time [PT], activated partial thromboplastin time [aPTT]/ international normalized ratio [INR]) and patient's renal function (e.g., BUN, creatinine levels) before procedure. Assess electrolytes (sodium and potassium).	Abnormal laboratory findings may contraindicate procedure because of potential complications of hemorrhage and/or renal failure. Report elevated BUN or creatinine levels because such patients are at risk for renal failure induced by contrast media (Pagana et al., 2021). Abnormal electrolytes may reveal possible electromechanical problems.
9. Perform hand hygiene. Obtain VS and peripheral pulses. For arterial procedures, mark patient's peripheral pulses before procedure. For cardiac catheterization, also auscultate heart and lungs and obtain weight.	Provides baseline data and locations for comparison with findings during and after procedure.
10. Assess patient's hydration status, including condition of mucous membranes, skin turgor, and recent 24-hour intake.	Severe dehydration can lead to renal failure (Pagana et al., 2019)
11. Determine type of arteriogram scheduled (e.g., carotid, femoral, brachial, radial). If cardiac catheterization, verify if test is for right or left side of heart or both. For IVP, ask if study is for one or both kidneys.	Enables you to anticipate patient teaching needs and postprocedure interventions.
12. Determine and document last time of ingested food, drink, or medications.	Prevents possible aspiration because patient is sedated. Excessive hydration causes dilution of contrast medium, making structures more difficult to visualize. Some agencies require patients should be on nothing by mouth (NPO) 8 h before procedure and others allow a clear liquid breakfast (Pagana et al., 2021).

Clinical Judgment *Exceptions occur for patients at risk for contrast media–induced renal impairment who are specifically instructed to drink increased fluids in the hours before the procedure or those instructed by the health care provider to take medications before the procedure. Good preprocedure hydration reduces the risk for renal impairment caused by contrast media (Pagana et al., 2021).*

STEP	RATIONALE
13. Review health care provider's orders for preprocedure medications, hydration, antihistamines, and IV sedation:	Increased sedation is necessary in anxious or confused patients. Increased hydration is often required for renal insufficiency and antihistamines for possible allergic reaction.
a. Atropine	Decreases salivary secretions and increases heart rate when bradycardia is present.
b. Diphenhydramine	Used prophylactically to block histamine and decrease allergic response.
c. Prednisone	Used with or without an antihistamine to decrease allergic response.
d. Preprocedural sedative	Decreases anxiety and promotes relaxation.
14. Assess patient's knowledge, prior experience with contrast media studies, and feelings about procedure.	Reveals need for patient instruction and/or support.

PLANNING

1. Expected outcomes following completion of procedure:	
• Patient does not experience any procedure or postprocedure complications such as significant changes in VS, bleeding, diminished or absent peripheral pulses, allergic response, or decreased or absent urine output.	Procedure performed without complication.
• Patient's pain acuity is equal to score of 4 or less on pain scale of 0 to 10. Expected site of discomfort includes soreness at catheter insertion site and possible backache.	Patient tolerates procedure.
• Patient tolerates increased fluid intake and urinates sufficiently (at least 30 mL/h or 0.5 mL/kg/h) to excrete radiographic dye.	Adequate renal function.
• Patient recovers from IV sedation without respiratory complications or change in level of consciousness.	Appropriate level of sedation.
2. Provide privacy and explain to patient purpose of and what will happen during procedure.	Protects patient's privacy; reduces anxiety. Promotes cooperation.
3. Have patient empty bladder before procedure.	Ensures that patient will not need to void during procedure.
4. Remove all of patient's jewelry, metal objects, and body piercings.	Eliminates objects that interfere with radiography visualization of vessels and could be conductive material during electrocautery.
5. Preprocedure preparation:	
a. *For IVP:* Verify that patient has completed necessary bowel preparation of orally administered evacuation preparation 24 hours before test and evacuation enema 8 hours before test (check agency policy).	Evacuated lower intestine and bowel improve visualization of urinary structures.

STEP	RATIONALE
b. *For cardiac catheterization:* Determine whether hair at site of catheter insertion needs clipping or preparation with antiseptic just before procedure. Allow antiseptic to dry. Do not shave site.	Reduces risk for site-related infection. Drying promotes maximal antibacterial activity. Shaving results in increased chance for infection.
6. For cardiac catheterization, it is common to verify availability of emergent cardiac surgery because of risk for complete coronary artery occlusion from dislodged plaque or inadvertent perforation of vasculature. Also verify patient's ASA classification before procedure (see Box 8.1).	Prepares backup plan for possible procedural outcomes that would necessitate emergency surgery.
7. Organize and set up any equipment needed to perform procedure.	Ensures more efficiency when completing a procedure.

IMPLEMENTATION

STEP	RATIONALE
1. Open and prepare supplies in procedure room using sterile technique (see Chapter 10).	Prevents transmission of microorganisms during needle insertion.
2. Prepare cardiac monitor, pulse oximeter, and/or end-tidal CO_2 monitor.	Provides easy access to equipment for monitoring patient status during and after procedure.
3. Perform hand hygiene and apply clean gloves and appropriate protective equipment.	Reduces transmission of microorganisms.
4. Provide IV access using large-bore cannula. Remove and dispose of gloves and perform hand hygiene.	Provides access for delivery of IV fluids and/or drugs.
5. Help patient assume a comfortable supine position on x-ray table. Some patients undergoing IVP may be in supine or in a slight Trendelenburg position. Immobilize extremity that will be injected. Pad any bony prominences.	For arterial procedures, patient may need to maintain position for 1 to 3 hours. Padding the bony prominences reduces the risk for impaired skin integrity.
6. Take time-out to verify patient's name, type of procedure to be performed, and procedure site with patient.	Time-out verification just before starting procedure includes health care provider and all involved personnel and is a safety precaution to prevent wrong patient, wrong site, and wrong procedure errors (TJC, 2023).
7. Begin monitoring VS, pulse oximetry (SpO_2), end-tidal CO_2; and, for arterial procedures, palpate peripheral pulses.	Data provide comparison with baseline to determine patient's response to procedure.
8. Inform patient that during injection of dye, it is common to experience some chest pain and a severe hot flash that is quite uncomfortable but lasts only a few seconds.	Dye causes feeling of warmth, flushing, or metallic taste shortly after injection.
9. All health care team members apply appropriate PPE (e.g., mask and goggles, sterile gown, head cover, sterile gloves).	Reduces transmission of microorganisms.
10. Physician cleanses arterial puncture site for catheter insertion (femoral, radial, carotid, or brachial) with antiseptic.	Reduces transmission of microorganisms.
11. Drape patient with sterile drapes, leaving puncture site exposed. Physician anesthetizes skin overlying arterial puncture site.	Maintains surgical asepsis. Provides local anesthetic to area of incision or puncture.
12. For arterial procedures, physician does the following:	
a. Punctures artery, inserts introducer (see Fig. 8.2) into artery, inserts guidewire through introducer and advances, and inserts flexible catheter over guidewire and advances into heart. Introducers allow for use of various procedure catheters depending on need (e.g., balloon angioplasty, stent placement, ablation).	Permits access to artery and coiling of catheter in artery.
b. Advances catheter to desired artery or cardiac chamber, removes guidewire, and injects contrast medium through catheter.	Permits radiographic visualization of structures, aneurysms, occlusions, or anomalies.
13. During dye injection, specialized machinery takes rapid sequence of x-ray films.	Permits radiographic records of visualization of dye through artery and any abnormalities present.
14. If iodinated dye is used, observe patient for signs of anaphylaxis, including respiratory distress, palpitation, itching, and diaphoresis.	Allergic reactions can be life threatening.
15. During cardiac catheterization, assist with measuring cardiac volumes and pressure.	Provides data related to cardiac output, central venous pressure (CVP), ventricular pressures, and pulmonary artery pressure.
16. Nurse administering IV sedation monitors levels of sedation, level of consciousness, and VS (see Skill 8.1).	Proper IV sedation does not cause loss of consciousness.

STEP	RATIONALE
17. Physician withdraws catheter and applies manual pressure to puncture site until homeostasis occurs (5 to 15 minutes or longer). Vascular closure device may be used.	Manual pressure for 5 to 15 minutes is often enough to stop active site bleeding. However, a certain amount of bed rest is needed to achieve reliable hemostasis. Check agency policy for postprocedure bed rest requirements. This may vary from 2 to 6 hours when no vascular closure device is used. Check agency policy for length of time a vascular closure device stays in place.

Clinical Judgment *Before removing catheter sheath, check health care provider's orders for instructions for treating a vasovagal reaction. Manual pressure applied to the groin/femoral area can stimulate the baroreceptors and cause a vasovagal reaction in which the patient becomes bradycardic and hypotensive. Vasovagal reactions are usually brief and self-limiting. When applying pressure to the groin after sheath removal, be alert for a vasovagal reaction and be prepared to treat it by lowering the head of the bed to the flat position and giving a bolus of IV fluids.*

STEP	RATIONALE
18. If a percutaneous coronary intervention (PCI) such as a percutaneous transluminal coronary angioplasty (PTCA) or directional coronary atherectomy (DCA) was performed during cardiac catheterization, a femoral introducer/sheath is often left in place and removed in several hours.	Postinterventional sheaths provide emergency access to vasculature in the event that coronary artery becomes occluded, allowing time for anticoagulants to wear off.
19. Dispose of all contaminated supplies in appropriate receptacle; remove and dispose of gloves and other PPE.	Reduces transmission of microorganisms. Use appropriate disposal receptacle if patient on hazardous drugs (Blake, 2019; ONS, 2018).
20. Raise side rails (as appropriate) and lower bed or stretcher to lowest position, locking into position.	Ensures patient safety and prevents falls.
21. Place nurse call system in an accessible location within patient's reach.	Ensures patient can call for assistance if needed.
22. Perform hand hygiene.	Reduces transmission of microorganisms.

23. Postprocedure
    a. For arterial procedures:
      (1) Keep affected extremity extended and immobilized after removal of sheath (see agency policy). Use orthopedic bedpan for female patient as needed for bowel or bladder evacuation while on bed rest.
      (2) Emphasize need to lie flat for 4 to 8 hours (and possibly overnight if sheath is left in groin).
      (3) Encourage patient to drink fluids after procedure.
	Helps prevent bleeding and formation of hematoma.
	
	Allows complete sealing of puncture site (Pagana et al., 2021).
	
	Facilitates elimination of contrast material and prevents renal damage (Pagana et al., 2021).

EVALUATION

1. Evaluate patient's body position and comfort during procedure.	Position can cause stress on insertion site and patient's musculoskeletal structures.
2. Monitor VS and SpO$_2$ and assess for signs of cardiac complications every 15 minutes for 1 hour, every 30 minutes for 2 hours, or until patient is stable.	Verifies patient's physiological status and evaluates effect of procedure. Signs of cardiac complications include chest pain or pressure, new dysrhythmias, and/or shortness of breath.

3. Monitor for complications:
    a. Perform neurovascular checks by palpating peripheral pulses on affected extremity and comparing right and left extremities for skin color, temperature, and sensation. Use Doppler ultrasonic stethoscope to locate pulses that are not palpable (see Chapter 6).
    b. Assess vascular access site for bleeding and hematoma.
    c. Auscultate heart and lungs and compare with preprocedure findings.
    d. Observe patient for possible delayed reaction to iodine dye (if used)—dyspnea, hives, tachycardia, and rash (Pagana et al., 2019).
	Enables prompt detection of circulatory impairment caused by intravascular clotting or bleeding at procedure site. Signs of reduced circulation include diminishing distal pulses and/or coolness, mottling, pallor, pain, numbness, and tingling in affected extremity.
	Verifies expected sealing of puncture.
	Evaluates patient response to procedure.
	
	Reaction may occur up to 6 hours after injection of dye.

4. Evaluate level of sedation, level of consciousness, and SpO$_2$. Use PADSS scale (see Table 8.1).	Determines patient's response to IV sedation.
5. Assess postprocedure laboratory values—CBC, prothrombin time, aPTT, INR, electrolytes, BUN/creatinine.	Detects changes in laboratory values that indicate onset of complications such as bleeding.
6. Have patient rate pain acuity on pain scale of 0 to 10.	Pain is an early sign of complications.

STEP	RATIONALE
7. Use Teach-Back: "I want to be sure I explained what to watch for if you start to have an allergic reaction after this procedure. Tell me what feelings would make you think you might be having an allergic reaction." Revise your instruction now or develop a plan for revised patient/family caregiver teaching if patient/family caregiver is not able to teach back correctly.	Teach-back is a technique for health care providers to ensure that they have explained medical information clearly so that patients and families understand what is communicated to them (AHRQ, 2023).

Unexpected Outcomes

1. Vasovagal response occurs (at time of femoral puncture or after procedure with femoral pressure). Symptoms include feeling faint, dizzy, and light-headed and possible momentary loss of consciousness. Bradycardia is caused by stimulation of vagus nerve via baroreceptors.

2. Evidence of oversedation:
   - Prolonged reduced level of consciousness.

3. Pedal pulses are nonpalpable bilaterally 2 hours after arteriogram with change in skin color and temperature.

4. Hematoma or hemorrhage is present at catheter insertion site.

5. Patient has allergic reaction to contrast medium with symptoms of flushing, itching, and urticaria.

6. Renal toxicity from contrast medium occurs: urine output less than 30 mL/h or 0.5 mL/kg/h.

7. Patient experiences retroperitoneal bleeding (when femoral access site is used):
   - Low back pain radiating to both sides of body (hallmark sign)
   - Tachycardia

Related Interventions

- Support airway (through positioning).
- Lower table or head of bed to flat position or Trendelenburg position if ordered.
- Be prepared to administer bolus of IV fluid (normal saline).
- See Skill 8.1.

- Assess pulse with Doppler.
- Immediately notify health care provider.

- Apply pressure over insertion site.
- Monitor catheter site every 15 to 30 minutes for 2 to 3 hours; follow agency protocol.
- Notify health care provider if interventions do not stop bleeding or if patient has symptoms of acute blood loss (hypotension, tachycardia, decreased level of consciousness).

- Monitor VS and observe for symptoms of anaphylaxis.
- Notify health care provider.
- Follow specific postprocedure orders related to findings.
- Prepare to administer antihistamine or epinephrine if ordered.

- Place on strict intake and output (I&O) monitoring.
- Monitor closely for signs of fluid overload.
- Review electrolyte, urea nitrogen, and creatinine levels.

- Prepare patient for emergency surgery.
- Monitor VS every 5 to 15 minutes.
- Monitor distal pulses hourly.

Documentation

- Document patient's status: VS, SpO_2/end-tidal CO_2, status of peripheral pulses for equality and symmetry, BP for hypotension, temperature and color of catheterized extremity, condition of IV site, and level of patient responsiveness.
- Document any drainage from puncture site, appearance of dressing, and condition of puncture site.
- Document your evaluation of patient and family caregiver learning.

Hand-Off Reporting

- Report to health care provider any VS change, excessive bleeding or increasing hematoma at puncture site, decreased or absent peripheral pulses, persistent pain, altered neurological status, dysrhythmias, decreased SpO_2 or increased end-tidal CO_2, or decreased responsiveness after sedation.

Special Considerations

Patient Education

- See Skill 8.1, Patient Education.
- Prepare patient to stay in the hospital if complications occur or if an intervention necessitates prolonged postprocedure vascular checks and cardiac monitoring.

Pediatrics

- Infants and children are particularly susceptible to the diuretic effects of radiocontrast dyes because of their small body size and immature renal/hepatic systems. In addition, those with congenital cardiac anomalies develop compensatory erythrocytosis and thus experience complications from dehydration quickly. Emphasize to the parent(s) or caregiver the importance of fluid intake with the child after the procedure. Urinary output should exceed 1 mL/kg/h (Hockenberry et al., 2022).

Older Adults

- Physical exposure and low room temperature contribute to hypothermia in frail older adults who are unable to communicate discomfort. Use heated blankets or forced-air heat to maintain core temperature at comfortable, safe levels (Harding et al., 2020).
- In older adults, slight alterations in VS or behavior are signs of impending problems; therefore, close monitoring is important.

Populations With Disabilities

- Cardiovascular disease is prevalent for people with intellectual and developmental disabilities (IDDs); screening may need to be done earlier than in general population and to promote prevention (Sullivan et al., 2018).

Home Care

- On discharge provide patient with written instructions to contact the health care provider (or affiliated emergency department) if any of the following occur after arteriogram or cardiac catheterization:
  - Bleeding from the catheterization puncture site; apply gentle pressure with a clean gauze or cloth
  - Formation of a knot or lump under the skin that increases in size
  - Worsening of a bruise or its movement down the extremity rather than disappearing
  - Pain at puncture site or in the extremity used for the catheterization
  - Extremity is pale and cool to the touch where arterial puncture is made
  - Appearance of redness, swelling, or warmth of the affected extremity
- It is helpful to have patient repeat (teach-back) the instructions back to you and to acknowledge clear understanding.
- After arteriogram or cardiac catheterization, instruct patient not to drive or climb stairs for 24 hours; to avoid sports, strenuous activity/housework, and lifting (e.g., groceries, children) for 3 days; and to avoid taking baths until wound is healed.
- On discharge after an IVP, instruct patient to:
  - Drink at least 1 to 2 L (64 ounces) of water to help flush the contrast medium through the kidneys.
  - Watch for signs of a delayed reaction to the contrast medium for 24 hours after the procedure and call the health care provider or go to the nearest emergency department.

♦ SKILL 8.3   Care of Patients Undergoing Aspirations: Bone Marrow Aspiration/Biopsy, Lumbar Puncture, Paracentesis, and Thoracentesis

Aspirations are sterile invasive procedures involving the removal of body fluids or tissue for diagnostic procedures (Table 8.3). Many are performed at the bedside or in a procedural unit with a nurse assisting. Informed consent is required for these invasive procedures.

Bone marrow aspiration is the removal of a small amount of the liquid organic material in the medullary canals of selected bones. The sternum and the posterior superior iliac crests are the most common in adults. The anterior or posterior iliac crests and the proximal tibia are the most common in infants (Hockenberry et al., 2022; Pagana et al., 2021). A biopsy is the removal of a core of marrow cells for laboratory analysis. Both aspiration and biopsy are used to diagnose and differentiate leukemia, certain malignancies, anemia, and thrombocytopenia. The marrow is examined in a laboratory to reveal the number, size, shape, and development of red blood cells (RBCs) and megakaryocytes (platelet precursors). Bone marrow cultures help differentiate infectious diseases such as tuberculosis (TB) or histoplasmosis. This procedure takes approximately 20 minutes to perform. Potential complications of bone marrow aspiration or biopsy include bleeding, especially if coagulopathy is present; infection; and, less commonly, organ puncture.

A lumbar puncture (LP), called a *spinal puncture* or *tap*, involves the introduction of a needle into the subarachnoid space of the spinal column. The purpose of the test is to measure pressure in the subarachnoid space; obtain cerebrospinal fluid (CSF) for visualization and laboratory examination; and inject anesthetic, diagnostic, or therapeutic agents. CSF is examined in a laboratory to help diagnose spinal cord tumors, CNS infections, hemorrhage, and degenerative brain disease. The procedure takes approximately 30 minutes to perform.

The major contraindication for LP is evidence of increased intracranial pressure (ICP). The LP causes a sudden release of pressure and possible herniation of the brain structures through the foramen magnum. This herniation compresses the brainstem, which contains the vital cardiac, respiratory, and vasomotor centers, causing sudden death. In elective LP, preprocedure computed tomography results are reviewed for evidence of brain shift to rule out increased ICP. In such cases, spinal punctures are contraindicated.

Abdominal paracentesis involves aspiration of peritoneal fluid from the abdomen. Cytological analysis of the aspirate determines presence of bacteria, blood, glucose, and protein to help diagnose the causes of an abdominal effusion. Paracentesis may also be a palliative measure to provide temporary relief of abdominal and respiratory discomfort caused by severe ascites. Lavage paracentesis, in which a lavage of solution is instilled and then withdrawn, is done to detect the presence of bleeding, as in cases of blunt abdominal trauma or tumor cells when cancer is suspected. Although not contraindicated, paracentesis is performed with caution in patients with coagulopathies, with portal hypertension accompanied by abdominal collateral circulation, and in those who are pregnant. The procedure takes approximately 30 minutes to perform.

Thoracentesis is performed to analyze or remove pleural fluid or instill medications intrapleurally. Cytological studies of specimens reveal presence of blood, white blood cells, glucose, amylase, lactate dehydrogenase (LDH), and cellular composition. Cytological specimens are also examined for malignancy, differentiated between transudative and exudative characteristics, and cultured for pathogens. The following cause transudate in the pleural space: ascites, cirrhosis (hepatic), heart failure, hypertension (pulmonary, systemic), nephritis, and nephrosis. Therapeutic thoracentesis relieves pain, dyspnea, and signs of pleural pressure. The test takes approximately 30 minutes to perform.

Delegation

The skill of assisting with aspirations can be delegated to AP if the patient is stable (check agency policy). However, assessment of the patient's condition must be completed by the nurse and cannot be delegated. Direct the AP about:

- Proper positioning of the patient during the procedure
- When to take and report VS
- Which signs and symptoms experienced by the patient should be reported immediately

TABLE 8.3

Summary of Aspiration Procedures

Aspiration Procedure	Preparation/Assessment Specific to Test	Position and Site	Special Considerations
Bone marrow aspiration	Assess complete blood count for abnormalities.	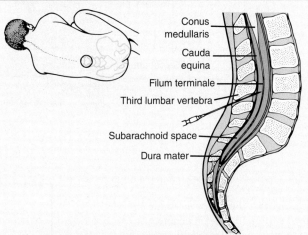Bone marrow aspiration from the iliac crest. *(From Ignatavicius, D. D., et al. [2020]. Medical-surgical nursing: concepts for interprofessional collaborative care [10th ed.]. St. Louis: Elsevier.)*	Patients with arthritis or orthopnea may have difficulty assuming the positions. Pressure is applied to the site following procedure.
Lumbar puncture	Assess neurological status, including movement, sensation, and muscle strength of legs to provide a baseline for comparison. Assess bladder for distention and determine last voiding; have patient empty bladder before procedure.	Conus medullaris Cauda equina Filum terminale Third lumbar vertebra Subarachnoid space Dura mater *(From Pagana, K. D., et al. [2021]. Mosby's diagnostic and laboratory test reference (15th ed.) St. Louis: Mosby.)*	*Risk for spinal headache:* Instruct patient to remain flat and logroll according to health care provider's orders. Observe for excessive drainage at site. Fluid loss at site can predispose patient to headache and infection.
Paracentesis	Assess bladder for distention and determine last voiding; have patient empty bladder before procedure. Weigh patient, inspect and palpate abdomen, and measure abdominal girth at largest point. Mark location.	*(From Pagana, K. D., et al. [2021]. Mosby's diagnostic and laboratory test reference (15th ed.). St. Louis: Mosby.)*	After fluid is removed, pressure on diaphragm is released, and breathing becomes much easier. *Risk for trauma:* Have patient empty urinary bladder before procedure.

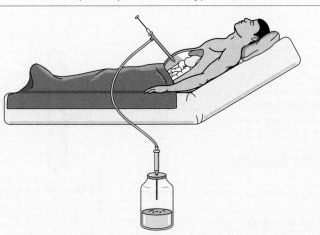

Continued

TABLE 8.3			
Summary of Aspiration Procedures–cont'd			
Aspiration Procedure	**Preparation/Assessment Specific to Test**	**Position and Site**	**Special Considerations**
Thoracentesis	Assess respiratory rate and depth, symmetry of chest on inspiration and expiration, cough, and sputum. Help patient remain still during procedure to prevent trauma to visceral pleura. Patient needs to hold breath and avoid coughing during procedure.	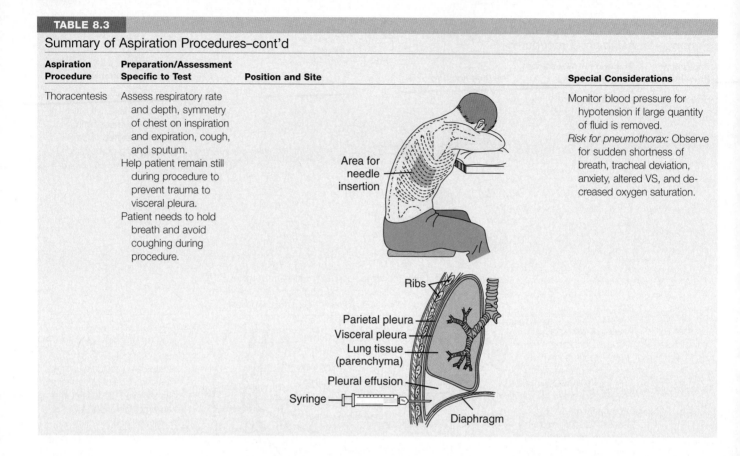 Area for needle insertion	Monitor blood pressure for hypotension if large quantity of fluid is removed. *Risk for pneumothorax:* Observe for sudden shortness of breath, tracheal deviation, anxiety, altered VS, and decreased oxygen saturation.

Ribs
Parietal pleura
Visceral pleura
Lung tissue (parenchyma)
Pleural effusion
Syringe
Diaphragm

Equipment

- PPE: masks, clean gloves, goggles, gowns, head cover, sterile gloves for all health care personnel performing the procedure
- Test tubes, sterile specimen containers, laboratory requisitions, and labels
- Analgesia (if ordered)
- Antiseptic solution
- 4 × 4–inch sterile gauze pads, tape, Band-Aid
- Sphygmomanometer, pulse oximeter/end-tidal CO_2 monitor
- Aspiration tray: Most agencies provide trays specific to the aspiration procedure. Standard tray includes antiseptic solution (e.g., povidone-iodine; chlorhexidine); gauze sponges (4 × 4–inch); sterile towels; local anesthetic solution (e.g., lidocaine 1%); two 3-mL sterile syringes with 16- to 27-gauge needles.

Additional Equipment for Specific Aspirations

- Bone marrow aspiration: two bone marrow needles with inner stylet (Fig. 8.4)
- LP: manometer to measure spinal pressure and at least four test tubes
- Paracentesis: IV fluids as ordered, vacuum bottles to collect fluid, stopcock with extension tubing, sterile collection containers, measuring tape
- Thoracentesis: vacuum bottles to collect fluid, stopcock with extension tubing

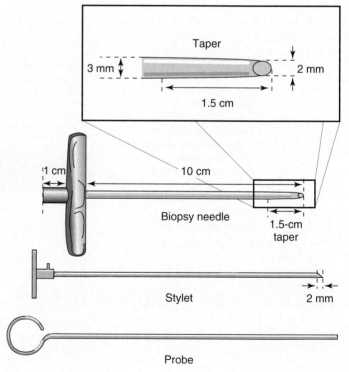

Taper
3 mm
2 mm
1.5 cm
1 cm
10 cm
Biopsy needle
1.5-cm taper
Stylet
2 mm
Probe

FIG. 8.4 Bone marrow biopsy needle showing shape and size. *(Courtesy and © Becton, Dickinson and Company.)*

STEP	RATIONALE

ASSESSMENT

1. Identify patient using at least two identifiers (e.g., name and birthday or name and medical record number) according to agency policy. Compare identifiers with information in patient's medication administration record (MAR) or electronic health record (EHR). — Ensures correct patient. Complies with The Joint Commission standards and improves patient safety (TJC, 2023).

2. Verify type of procedure scheduled, purpose, and procedure site with patient and EHR. — Ensures correct patient and procedure (TJC, 2023).

3. Verify that informed consent was obtained before administering any analgesia or antianxiety agents. — Federal regulations, many state laws, and accreditation agencies such as The Joint Commission require informed consent for procedure. Patients should provide informed consent before any procedure (TJC, 2022).

4. Review EHR for contraindications.
   a. *Lumbar puncture (LP):* Increased intracranial pressure (ICP), spinal deformities, and clotting disorders. Patient cannot maintain position during LP. — Factors can cause hemorrhage, and increased ICP may cause brainstem herniation.
   b. *Paracentesis:* Clotting or bleeding disorders, intestinal obstructions, and pregnancy. — Paracentesis in pregnant woman may injure fetus.
   c. *Bone marrow biopsy:* Patient cannot maintain position during procedure.
   d. *Thoracentesis:* Patient cannot maintain position during procedure.

5. If patient is unable to assume position for procedure (see Table 8.3), discuss with health care provider need for premedication for anxious patients. — Movement during procedure can cause complications such as bleeding and injury to nerves or tissue. Required position depends on site used for aspiration.

6. Assess patient's/family caregiver's health literacy. — Determines degree to which individuals have the ability to find, understand, and use information and services to make informed health-related decisions and actions for themselves and others (CDC, 2023).

7. Perform hand hygiene. Obtain VS, oxygen saturation (SpO_2)/end-tidal carbon dioxide (CO_2) value, and weight. For paracentesis, obtain abdominal girth measurement. (Use ink pen to mark measurement location for abdominal girth measurement.) For LP, assess lower extremity movement, sensation, and muscle strength. — Prevents transmission of microorganisms. Provides baseline for comparison with VS during and after procedure. Patients will have decreased abdominal girth and lose weight after paracentesis.

8. Instruct patient to empty bladder. — Reduces risk for bladder trauma during paracentesis. Promotes patient comfort.

9. Assess patient's coagulation status: use of anticoagulants, CBC, platelet count, clotting factors, aPTT/INR, and prothrombin time (PT). — Invasive procedures may be contraindicated in patients with coagulation disorders because of risk for bleeding (Pagana et al., 2021).

10. Determine whether patient is allergic to antiseptic, latex, or anesthetic solutions. — Precautions can be taken to decrease chance of allergic reactions.

11. Assess patient's character of pain and rate acuity on pain scale of 0 to 10. — Determines need for preprocedure analgesia. Pain control helps patients maintain proper position and tolerate aspiration procedure.

12. Assess patient's knowledge, prior experience with aspiration, and feelings about procedure. — Reveals need for patient instruction and/or support.

PLANNING

1. Expected outcomes following completion of procedure:
   - Patient describes purpose of procedure. — Demonstrates understanding and improves likelihood of cooperation.
   - Patient assumes and maintains required position and remains still throughout procedure. — Achieving level of patient comfort allows for correct position, which facilitates safe and timely completion of procedure.
   - There is no bleeding at needle insertion site. — Precautions during procedure prevent bleeding.
   - Amount of aspirate is sufficient to perform laboratory testing.
   - Patient's pain acuity score is 4 or less on pain scale of 0 to 10. — Procedure performed with minimal discomfort to patient.

STEP	RATIONALE
• VS, SpO_2, and end-tidal CO_2 remain within normal limits during and after aspiration procedure.	Removal of abdominal (ascites) or pleural fluid increases lung expansion and improves gas exchange.
• Patient undergoing paracentesis has reduced abdominal girth and improved respirations.	Fluid successfully removed from peritoneal space.
2. Provide privacy and explain procedure. Explain steps of skin preparation, anesthetic injection, needle insertion, and position required.	Protects patient's privacy; reduces anxiety. Promotes cooperation.
3. Organize and set up any equipment needed to perform procedure at the bedside.	Ensures more efficiency when completing a procedure.
4. If ordered, premedicate for pain 30 min before procedure. *Option:* In some cases, patients will receive antianxiety medications.	Pain and anxiety control helps patient to remain in position, minimizes discomfort from needle insertion, and decreases anxiety.
5. Before thoracentesis verify recent chest x-ray film examination.	Provides preprocedure baseline to determine location of pleural fluid.

IMPLEMENTATION

STEP	RATIONALE
1. Perform hand hygiene. Apply clean gloves. Don additional PPE if there is risk of splashing.	Reduces transmission of microorganisms.
2. Set up sterile tray or open supplies to make accessible for health care provider.	Maintains integrity of sterile field and promotes prompt completion of procedure.
3. Take time-out to verify patient's name, type of procedure to be performed, and procedure site with patient and health care team.	Time-out verification just before starting procedure includes health care provider and all personnel and is a safety precaution to prevent wrong patient, wrong site, and wrong procedure errors (TJC, 2023).
4. Help patient maintain correct position. Reassure patient while explaining procedure.	Decreases chance of complications occurring during procedure. Explanations increase patient comfort and relaxation.
a. Bone marrow	
• *Adults:* For sternal biopsy, place in supine position. For iliac crest biopsy, place patient in prone or lateral recumbent position.	Provides best access to bone containing marrow.
• *Children:* For iliac crest biopsy, place patient in prone or lateral recumbent position.	
b. LP	
• Position in lateral recumbent (fetal) position with head and neck flexed (see Table 8.3).	Provides full curvature and flexion of spinal column to allow maximal space between vertebrae.
c. Paracentesis	
• Position patient in bed in semi-Fowler position or sitting upright on side of bed or in chair with feet supported (see Table 8.3).	Position uses gravity to cause fluid to accumulate in lower abdominal cavity, where it is drained more easily.
d. Thoracentesis	
• Place patient in orthopneic position (upright position with arms and shoulders raised and supported on padded over-bed table) (see Table 8.3). If patient is unable to tolerate, assist to side-lying position with affected lung positioned upward.	Expands intercostal space for needle insertion.

Clinical Judgment *Emphasize to the patient the importance of remaining immobile during procedure to prevent trauma, especially with LP. Sudden movement is a risk for spinal cord nerve root damage. Sudden movement during paracentesis or thoracentesis risks damage of the abdominal or pulmonary structures. Also instruct patient not to cough, sneeze, or breathe deeply during the procedures because these actions increase the risk for needle displacement and damage of other structures.*

STEP	RATIONALE
5. Explain to patient that pain may occur when lidocaine (local anesthetic) is injected into tissues around site of needle or trocar insertion. Pressure may also occur when tissue or fluid is aspirated.	Aspiration is painful but lasts for only a few moments. If patient is having bone marrow aspiration, deep pressure feeling is frequently experienced as bone marrow is withdrawn (Pagana et al., 2019).
6. Physician and members of health care team in procedure apply sterile gloves, mask, gown, and goggles; physician cleans patient's skin with antiseptic solution and drapes site with sterile drape.	Removes surface bacteria from skin at area of puncture site. Creates sterile field.
7. Physician injects local anesthetic at insertion site and allows time for anesthesia to occur.	Provides optimal effect of local anesthesia.

STEP	RATIONALE
8. Physician inserts needle or trocar into spinal space or body cavity involved (see Table 8.3). To aspirate tissue or body fluids for specimen analysis, syringe is attached to trocar or needle, and aspirate is placed into specimen container.	Success depends on positioning, accurate insertion site, and patient remaining still.
9. Nurse assesses patient's condition during procedure, including respiratory status, VS if patient's condition indicates, and any complaints of pain or feelings of anxiety. Maintain conversation to provide distraction.	Identifies any changes that indicate complication.

Clinical Judgment *Increased or worsening abdominal or thoracic pain is significant in paracentesis and thoracentesis. Severe abdominal pain indicates a possible bowel perforation after paracentesis. Following thoracentesis, abdominal pain results from possible diaphragmatic, liver, or spleen perforation. Inspiratory chest pain results from perforation of the lung.*

STEP	RATIONALE
10. Note characteristics of aspirate:	
a. *Bone marrow aspirate:* Marrow may appear red or yellow.	Normal marrow.
b. *LP:* Document opening pressure; observe fluid for color, cloudiness, or blood.	Normal CSF is clear and colorless. Cloudiness is result of protein, which indicates an infection.
c. *Paracentesis:* Fluid may appear yellow, cloudy, bile-stained green, or blood tinged. Peritoneal lavage fluid may appear bright red.	Blood-tinged fluid is caused by traumatic tap. In patient with abdominal trauma, bloody lavage indicates active bleeding.
d. *Thoracentesis:* Pleural fluid may appear clear yellow, puslike, or cloudy.	Clear yellow is normal. Transudate and exudates are typically a yellow, straw color. Blood-tinged fluid indicates malignancy, pulmonary infarction, or severe inflammation. Puslike fluid indicates infection (empyema); milky fluid indicates chylothorax (i.e., leak from thoracic duct resulting in lymphatic drainage in pleural cavity).
11. Properly label specimens in presence of patient and transport to laboratory in proper containers. Label specimens in order of collection.	Ensures that correct laboratory results are assigned to right patient. Test tubes are numbered in sequence of collection (e.g., 1 through 4).
12. Physician removes needle/trocar and applies pressure over insertion site until drainage ceases. If necessary, help with direct pressure and application of a small gauze dressing.	Helps in hemostasis and secures insertion site.
13. All health care team members in procedure remove and dispose of protective equipment and discard in appropriate receptacle.	Reduces transmission of microorganisms.
14. Help patient to a comfortable postprocedure position.	Restores comfort and sense of well-being.
15. Raise side rails (as appropriate) and lower bed to lowest position, locking into position.	Ensures patient safety and prevents falls.
16. Place nurse call system in an accessible location within patient's reach.	Ensures patient can call for assistance if needed.
17. Perform hand hygiene.	Reduces transmission of microorganisms.

EVALUATION

1. Monitor level of consciousness, VS, lung sounds, and SpO$_2$/end-tidal CO$_2$. Check agency policy: sometimes physiological measures are obtained every 15 minutes for 2 hours.	Verifies patient's physiological status in response to procedure or any potential complications.
2. Inspect dressing over puncture site for bleeding, swelling, tenderness, and erythema. Inspect area under patient for bleeding. Avoid disrupting healing clot at site if pressure dressing is present.	Determines further blood loss from puncture site. Infection is potential complication (Pagana et al., 2021).
3. Evaluate character of patient's pain and whether pain acuity is a score of 4 or less on pain scale of 0 to 10.	Determines if patient is having increased pain to warrant postprocedure analgesia.
4. Following paracentesis, measure abdominal girth and respirations and compare with preprocedure measurements.	Determines amount of change in abdominal size and ability to ventilate.
5. **Use Teach-Back:** "I want to be sure that I explained what to expect or how you may feel after this procedure. Tell me what you know about what to expect." Revise your instruction now or develop a plan for revised patient/family caregiver teaching if patient/family caregiver is not able to teach back correctly.	Teach-back is a technique for health care providers to ensure that they have explained medical information clearly so that patients and families understand what is communicated to them (AHRQ, 2023).

STEP	RATIONALE
Unexpected Outcomes	**Related Interventions**
1. Oversedation occurs.	• See Skill 8.1.
2. Site complications occur:	• Notify health care provider and obtain further orders.
a. *Bone marrow:* Tenderness or erythema at site.	• Administer analgesic as ordered. • Continue to monitor site.
b. *LP:* (1) Postprocedure headache (PPH) is evidenced by headache, blurred vision, and tinnitus.	• Monitor fluid loss. • Physician may inject blood patch into epidural space. • Medicate for pain as ordered.
(2) Excess loss of CSF is indicated by decreased level of consciousness, hearing loss, dilated pupils, and decreased ICP.	• Maintain airway and monitor VS. • Transfer to intensive care unit (ICU) per physician order.
c. *Paracentesis:* Leakage of fluid from site and acute abdominal pain occur.	• Reinforce dressing; may also be instructed to place sterile collection bag over site. • Monitor VS and SpO$_2$/end-tidal CO$_2$. • Assess abdomen for bowel sounds.
d. *Thoracentesis:* Pneumothorax is evidenced by sudden dyspnea, tachypnea, and asymmetrical chest excursion.	• Administer oxygen. • Monitor VS, lung sounds, and SpO$_2$/end-tidal CO$_2$. • Anticipate chest x-ray film examination and possible chest tube insertion.

Documentation

• Document name of procedure; preprocedure preparation; location of puncture site; amount, consistency, and color of fluid drained or specimen obtained; duration of procedure; patient's tolerance (e.g., vital signs, SpO$_2$) and comfort level; laboratory tests ordered and specimen sent; type of dressing; postprocedure activities (e.g., chest x-ray film examination); and other procedure-specific assessments (e.g., extremity assessment, abdominal girth, level of consciousness).
• Document your evaluation of patient and family caregiver learning.

Hand-Off Reporting

• Immediately report to health care provider any change in vital signs and SpO$_2$, unexpected pain/discomfort, and any excessive drainage from dressing over puncture site.

Special Considerations

Patient Education

• Instruct patient that some people experience tenderness at the puncture site for several days after the study and that mild analgesia often helps to relieve some of the discomfort.

Pediatrics

• Conscious or unconscious sedation is commonly used. If using unconscious sedation, an anesthesiologist or nurse anesthetist is needed for the procedure.

• Prepare preschool children before the procedure; make a game out of having child recall the next procedural step, which can serve as a distraction (Hockenberry et al., 2022).

Older Adults

• Older adults with arthritis need help to stay in the required position.
• Older adults have reduced elastic lung recoil, weaker cough efficiency, and decreased chest expansion. Restlessness may indicate hypoxia following thoracentesis (Touhy & Jett, 2022).
• Be aware that older adults may have specific fears and anxiety related to postprocedural falling and fatigue.

Populations With Disabilities

• Involve family caregivers as needed in decision making; take extra time as needed to ensure the patient has expressed concerns (Sullivan et al., 2018).

Home Care

• Teach patients and family caregivers about specific postprocedure complications and when to report them to the health care provider.
• If patient is transferred to long-term care facility, ensure thorough communication between agencies regarding results of procedure and patient condition.

♦ **SKILL 8.4   Care of a Patient Undergoing Bronchoscopy**

Bronchoscopy is the examination of the tracheobronchial tree through a lighted tube containing mirrors. A flexible fiberoptic bronchoscope has lumens that allow both visualization and simultaneous administration of oxygen (Fig. 8.5). The fiberoptic bronchoscope is used for obtaining sputum, foreign bodies, and biopsy specimens. Laser ablation of endotracheal lesions may also be performed through a bronchoscope.

Bronchoscopy may be an emergency or elective procedure and is performed for diagnostic or therapeutic reasons. The main purposes of this procedure include aspirating excessive sputum or mucus plugs that airway suctioning cannot remove; visualizing the tracheobronchial tree for assessment of abnormalities of the mucosa, abscesses, aspiration pneumonia, strictures, and tumors; obtaining deep tissue biopsy and sputum specimens; and/or

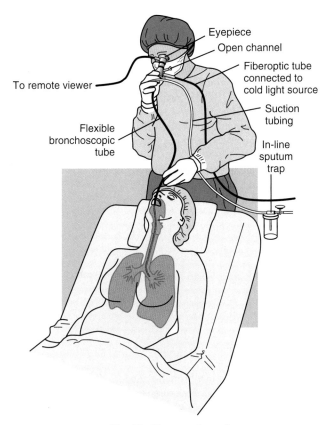

FIG. 8.5 Flexible fiberoptic bronchoscopy.

removing foreign bodies. This procedure is contraindicated in patients who cannot tolerate interruption of high-flow oxygen unless intubated. Potential complications of bronchoscopy include fever, hypoxemia, bronchospasm and/or laryngospasm, pneumothorax, aspiration, and hemorrhage (after biopsy) (Pagana et al., 2021).

The procedure is performed at the bedside or in a specially equipped endoscopy room. Usually, a pulmonary specialist or surgeon performs it in approximately 30 to 45 minutes.

Delegation

The skill of assisting with a bronchoscopy cannot be delegated to assistive personnel (AP). Direct the AP about:

- When to take and report VS (after initial assessment by registered nurse [RN])
- Helping position the patient appropriately (based on procedure and patient limitations)
- Immediately reporting to the nurse if patient has possible respiratory distress or is coughing up blood after the procedure

Interprofessional Collaboration

- In most agencies a registered nurse or health care provider assesses and monitors a patient's level of sedation, airway patency, and level of consciousness.

Equipment

- PPE: mask, gown, clean and sterile gloves, head cover, and goggles for all health care providers
- Bronchoscopy tray, if available from central supply, which includes flexible fiberoptic bronchoscope (see Fig. 8.5); 4 × 4–inch gauze sponges; local anesthetic spray (lidocaine); sterile tracheal suction catheters; diazepam, midazolam, or other sedative for IV sedation
- Oxygen, resuscitative equipment
- Pulse oximeter/end-tidal carbon dioxide (CO_2) monitor, cardiac monitor
- Sterile water-soluble lubricating jelly (**NOTE**: Petroleum-based lubricants are not used because of the hazard of aspiration and subsequent pneumonia.)
- Emesis basin
- Suction machine and connecting tube
- Blood pressure equipment

STEP	RATIONALE

ASSESSMENT

1. Identify patient using at least two identifiers (e.g., name and birthday or name and medical record number) according to agency policy. Compare identifiers with information in patient's medication administration record (MAR) or electronic health record (EHR).

Ensures correct patient. Complies with The Joint Commission standards and improves patient safety (TJC, 2023).

2. Verify type of procedure scheduled and procedure site with patient and EHR.

Ensures correct procedure for correct patient. Complies with The Joint Commission standards and improves patient safety (TJC, 2023).

3. Verify that informed consent was obtained before administration of any sedatives.

Federal regulations, many state laws, and accreditation agencies such as The Joint Commission require informed consent for procedure. Patients should provide informed consent before any procedure (TJC, 2022).

4. Determine purpose of procedure: for sputum aspiration, assessment, tissue biopsy, or removal of foreign body.

Anticipates equipment needs of physician and type of information to convey to patient during teaching.

5. Review health care orders for preprocedure medication (usually atropine and opioid or sedative).

Atropine decreases secretions and inhibits vagally stimulated bradycardia; opioids or sedatives relieve anxiety and decrease discomfort.

6. Assess patient's medical history for inability to tolerate interruption of high-flow oxygen unless intubated.

Determines need for oxygen administration during procedure.

STEP	RATIONALE
7. Assess patient's/family caregiver's health literacy.	Determines degree to which individuals have the ability to find, understand, and use information and services to make informed health-related decisions and actions for themselves and others (CDC, 2023).
8. Perform hand hygiene. Obtain baseline VS, pulse oximetry (SpO_2), and end-tidal CO_2 values.	Reduces transmission of microorganisms. Baseline data provide for comparison with findings during and after procedure.
9. Assess type of cough, sputum produced, and heart and lung sounds.	Provides for comparison with respiratory status during and after procedure.
10. Ask whether patient is allergic to local anesthetic used for spraying throat (usually lidocaine).	Allergy causes laryngeal edema or laryngospasm.
11. Assess time patient last ingested food/fluids or medications. Patient must be on nothing-by-mouth (NPO) status for at least 8 hours before a bronchoscopy; however, some medications may be taken before procedure by physician order.	Reduces risk for aspiration.
12. Assess patient's knowledge, prior experience with bronchoscopy, and feelings about procedure.	Reveals need for patient instruction and/or support.

PLANNING

1. Expected outcomes following completion of procedure:	
• Patient recovers from sedation without respiratory complications or change in level of consciousness.	Sedation adequate and patient tolerates procedure.
• Patient's pain acuity is 4 or less on pain scale of 0 to 10.	Minimal trauma caused by bronchoscope.
• Physician can observe, suction, and obtain specimens from tracheobronchial tree.	Indicates that purpose of procedure was achieved.
• Patient explains procedure and assumes appropriate position for procedure.	Demonstrates patient's understanding.
2. Provide privacy and explain procedure to patient.	Protects patient's privacy; reduces anxiety. Promotes cooperation.
3. Organize and set up any equipment needed to perform procedure.	Ensures more efficiency when completing a procedure.
4. In procedure room, drape patient to maintain privacy. In patient room, close room door or drapes.	Protects patient's privacy; reduces anxiety.
5. Administer atropine, opioid, or antianxiety agent 30 minutes before procedure.	Ensures that medication takes effect before procedure.
6. Remove and safely store patient's dentures and/or eyeglasses.	Minimizes chance of airway obstruction.

IMPLEMENTATION

1. Perform hand hygiene. Assess current IV access or establish a new IV access with large-bore cannula (see Chapter 28).	Reduces transmission of microorganisms. Provides immediate access for IV fluids or medications if emergency occurs.
2. Organize and open any equipment needed using sterile technique.	Ensures efficiency of procedure. Reduces microorganism transmission.
3. Help patient assume position desired by physician: usually semi-Fowler.	Provides maximal visualization of lower airway and adequate lung expansion.
4. Take time-out to verify patient's name, type of procedure, and procedure site with patient and health care team.	Time-out verification just before starting procedure includes health care provider and all personnel and is safety precaution to prevent wrong patient, wrong site, and wrong procedure errors (TJC, 2023).
5. Health team members assisting with procedure perform hand hygiene and apply PPE. Nurse prepares by positioning tip of suction catheter for easy access to patient's mouth.	Reduces transmission of microorganisms. Removes secretions to reduce risk for aspiration.
6. Physician usually sprays nasopharynx and oropharynx with topical anesthetic. Lidocaine is commonly used 10 to 15 minutes before procedure. When a patient is intubated or has tracheostomy, anesthetic spray is usually not needed.	Provides swift topical anesthesia of oropharynx. Topical anesthetic decreases gag reflex caused by passage of bronchoscope, thus improving safety and comfort.
7. Instruct patient not to swallow local anesthetic; provide emesis basin for expectorating it.	Reduces unintended anesthesia of esophagus.
8. Another physician or staff member attaches bronchoscope to machine light source.	Enhances visualization during procedure.

STEP	RATIONALE
9. Physician applies goggles, mask, and sterile gloves; introduces bronchoscope into mouth to pharynx; and passes it through glottis and into trachea and bronchi (see Fig. 8.5). More anesthetic spray may be used at glottis to prevent cough reflex. For intubated patients, flexible bronchoscope is introduced through their endotracheal tube.	Bronchoscope must be passed through upper airway structures to promote visualization of lower airways. Trachea and bronchi are observed for lesions and obstructions. Adaptor accompanies bronchoscope and is used for bag-valve mask or ventilator use.
10. Physician suctions mucus and performs bronchial washing with cytological specimens taken with wire brush or curette. Biopsy specimens may also be obtained.	Cytological specimens are obtained to diagnose carcinoma.
11. Help patient through procedure by providing explanations, verbal reassurance, and support.	Although premedicated and drowsy, remind patient not to change position and to cooperate. Reinforce that patient will be able to breathe during procedure.
12. Assess patient's VS, SpO$_2$, end-tidal CO$_2$, and breathing capacity during procedure; observe degree of restlessness, capillary refill, and color of nail beds.	Bronchoscope can cause feelings of suffocation and vasovagal response and laryngospasm. Because airway is partially occluded, patient can develop hypoxia during procedure.
13. Note characteristics of suctioned material. Expect small amount of blood mixed with aspirate because of tissue trauma.	Information used to document and report and make further patient observations.
14. Using gloved hand, wipe patient's mouth and nose to remove lubricant after bronchoscope is removed.	Promotes hygiene and comfort.
15. Instruct patient not to eat or drink until tracheobronchial anesthesia has worn off and gag reflex has returned, usually in 2 hours. Use tongue depressor to touch pharynx to test for presence of gag reflex.	Prevents aspiration.
16. Dispose of all contaminated supplies in appropriate receptacle; remove and dispose of gloves and other PPE.	Reduces transmission of microorganisms. Use appropriate disposal receptacle if patient is receiving hazardous drugs (Blake, 2019; ONS, 2018).
17. Help patient to a comfortable postprocedure position.	Restores comfort and sense of well-being.
18. Raise side rails (as appropriate) and lower bed to lowest position, locking into position.	Ensures patient safety and prevents falls.
19. Place nurse call system in an accessible location within patient's reach.	Ensures patient can call for assistance if needed.
20. Perform hand hygiene.	Reduces transmission of microorganisms.

EVALUATION

1. Monitor vital signs, SpO$_2$, and end-tidal CO$_2$.	Verifies physiological response to procedure.
2. Observe character and amount of sputum. Physician may order serial sputum collection for 24 hours for cytological examination.	Evaluates for complication of bronchial perforation, indicated by severe hemoptysis. Slight blood-tinged sputum is normal after this procedure.
3. Observe respiratory status closely; palpate for facial or neck crepitus (skin when palpated feels like crispy rice cereal).	Detects early sign of bronchial or esophageal perforation.
4. Assess for return of gag reflex. It usually returns in approximately 2 hours.	Helps prevent aspiration pneumonia, which is a risk until gag reflex returns.
5. **Use Teach-Back:** "I want to be sure I explained what are considered postprocedure normal and abnormal symptoms. Tell me what you know about these symptoms." Revise your instruction now or develop a plan for revised patient/family caregiver teaching if patient/family caregiver is not able to teach back correctly.	Teach-back is a technique for health care providers to ensure that they have explained medical information clearly so that patients and families understand what is communicated to them (AHRQ, 2023).

Unexpected Outcomes	Related Interventions
1. Vasovagal response caused by stimulation of baroreceptors during bronchoscope insertion, causing symptoms of: • Feeling nauseous, faint, dizzy, and/or light-headed • Diaphoresis with slow, steady pulse • Unconsciousness for a few seconds	• Lower head of table. • Support airway (positioning/suctioning). • Continue vital signs monitoring.
2. Laryngospasm and bronchospasm as evidenced by: • Sudden, severe shortness of breath	• Call physician immediately. • Support airway (positioning). • Prepare to administer oxygen. • Prepare emergency resuscitation equipment. • Anticipate possible cricothyrotomy.

STEP	RATIONALE
3. Hypoxemia as evidenced by: • Gradual shortness of breath • Decreasing level of consciousness	• Monitor SpO_2/end-tidal CO_2 values. • Maintain airway and breathing. Administer oxygen. • Notify physician immediately.
4. Hemorrhage as evidenced by: • Acute blood loss • Hypotension and tachycardia • Decreasing level of consciousness	• Notify physician immediately. • Monitor vital signs. • Be prepared to administer IV fluids.
5. Oversedation	• See Skill 8.1.

Documentation

- Document procedure(s) performed (e.g., biopsy); character of sputum; duration of procedure, patient's tolerance and, if any, complications; and the collection and disposition of specimen(s). Document time of gag reflex return.
- Document your evaluation of patient and family caregiver learning.

Hand-Off Reporting

- Report bleeding or respiratory distress following the procedure or any changes in VS beyond patient's normal limits to physician immediately. Report results of procedure to appropriate health care personnel.

Special Considerations

Patient Education

- Before the procedure, instruct patient to perform good mouth care to decrease risk for introducing bacteria into lungs during the procedure.
- In some cases, patients may receive IV sedation (see Skill 8.1, Patient Education).
- If ordered, teach patient how to perform controlled coughing techniques (Chapter 24) for obtaining serial sputum samples (see Chapter 7).

Pediatrics

- In children, the procedure is most frequently performed under general anesthesia to remove foreign bodies from the larynx or trachea. Follow-up care after the foreign body is removed includes chest physiotherapy, monitoring for respiratory distress, and education of parents.
- Children are at higher risk for hypoxemia than adults because of smaller bronchi, and the bronchoscope decreases the available breathing space.

Older Adults

- Physical exposure and room temperature contribute to hypothermia in frail older adults who are unable to communicate discomfort. Use warmed blankets or forced-air heat to maintain core temperature at comfortable, safe levels (Harding et al., 2020).
- Postprocedure restlessness often indicates hypoxemia or pain. Thoroughly assess pulmonary capacity before administering opioids, which may depress the respiratory centers.

Populations With Disabilities

- Assess the patient's capacity for decision making, and involve family caregivers as needed (Sullivan et al., 2018).

Home Care

- Instruct ambulatory care patients to notify the physician if the following symptoms develop: fever, chest pain or discomfort, dyspnea, wheezing, or hemoptysis.
- Throat discomfort is managed with throat lozenges or warm saline gargles.

◆ SKILL 8.5   Care of a Patient Undergoing Endoscopy

Endoscopy allows direct visualization of an internal organ or structure by means of a long, flexible fiberoptic scope. The tip of the scope has a light source and camera lens that allows visualization of the lining of structures such as the gastrointestinal (GI) tract, shoulder or knee joint, or intraperitoneal structures on a large display screen (Fig. 8.6). This skill focuses on GI endoscopic procedures. For visualization of the upper GI tract, esophagoscopy, gastroscopy, gastroduodenojejunoscopy (GDJ) or duodenoscopy, or, more frequently, esophagogastroduodenoscopy (EGD) is performed. This permits visualization of the esophagus, stomach, and duodenum in one examination. Besides direct observation, endoscopy enables biopsy of suspicious tissue, polyp removal, and performance of many other procedures such as direct visual guidance for fine-needle aspiration biopsies and dilation and stenting of strictures. For visualization of the hepatobiliary tree and pancreatic ducts, endoscopic retrograde cholangiopancreatography (ERCP) is performed. For visual examination of the lower GI tract, proctoscopy, sigmoidoscopy, or colonoscopy is performed. Typically, these patients receive IV moderate sedation.

Risks of endoscopic procedures include intestinal perforation, hemorrhage, peritonitis, aspiration, respiratory depression, and/or myocardial infarction secondary to vasovagal response. Endoscopic procedures are typically performed in procedure rooms.

Delegation

The skill of assisting with endoscopy cannot be delegated to assistive personnel (AP). Direct the AP about:

- When to take and report VS (after initial assessment by registered nurse [RN])
- Helping position the patient appropriately (based on procedure and patient limitations)
- Immediately reporting to the nurse if patient has possible abdominal or respiratory distress or is vomiting or coughing up blood after the procedure

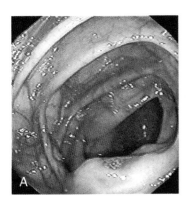 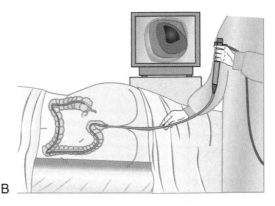 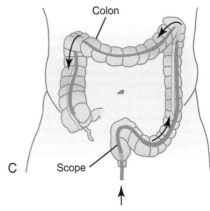

FIG. 8.6 (A) Scope view of healthy colon. (B) Overview of colonoscopy process. (C) Path of scope through colon.

Interprofessional Collaboration

- In most agencies a registered nurse or health care provider assesses and monitors a patient's level of sedation, airway patency, and level of consciousness. Roles in monitoring depend on scope-of-practice guidelines as determined by state regulations (see agency policy).

Equipment

- PPE: mask, gown, gloves, head cover, goggles for all health care personnel
- Endoscopy tray
- Fiberoptic endoscope and camera
- Solutions for biopsy specimens
- Local anesthetic spray
- Tracheal suction equipment (see Chapter 24)
- Blood pressure equipment
- Sterile water-soluble jelly
- Sterile gloves for physician
- Emesis basin
- IV fluid and equipment for IV start (optional)
- Diazepam, midazolam, or other sedative for IV sedation
- Sedative reversal agents
- Carbon dioxide source to inflate colon (for lower GI procedures)
- Oxygen, resuscitative equipment, SpO_2/end-tidal carbon dioxide (CO_2) monitor

STEP	RATIONALE

ASSESSMENT

1. Identify patient using at least two identifiers (e.g., name and birthday or name and medical record number) according to agency policy. Compare identifiers with information in patient's medication administration record (MAR) or electronic health record (EHR).

Ensures correct patient. Complies with The Joint Commission standards and improves patient safety (TJC, 2023).

2. Verify type of procedure scheduled and procedure site with patient and EHR.

Ensures correct procedure and patient. Complies with The Joint Commission standards and improves patient safety (TJC, 2023).

3. Verify that informed consent was obtained before administering sedation.

Federal regulations, many state laws, and accreditation agencies such as The Joint Commission require informed consent for procedure. Patients should provide informed consent before any procedure (TJC, 2022).

4. Determine purpose of procedure: biopsy, examination, or coagulation of bleeding sites.

Anticipates appropriate equipment needs.

5. Assess patient's/family caregiver's health literacy.

Determines degree to which individuals have the ability to find, understand, and use information and services to make informed health-related decisions and actions (CDC, 2023).

6. Perform hand hygiene. Determine if GI bleeding is present. Apply gloves if at risk for body fluid exposure. Observe character of emesis, stool, and nasogastric (NG) tube drainage for frank blood or material that looks like coffee grounds.

Reduces transmission of infection. Test is contraindicated in patients where the ampulla of Vater is not accessible, if there are esophageal diverticula, or if there is known pancreatitis (Pagana et al., 2021).

7. Obtain VS and SpO_2/end-tidal CO_2 values.

Baseline data provide for comparison with findings during and after procedure.

STEP	RATIONALE

Clinical Judgment *If patient is bleeding actively, physician may order lavage of the stomach and aspiration to clear clots before procedure is attempted.*

8. Verify that patient was on nothing-by-mouth (NPO) status for at least 8 h for endoscopy of upper GI tract.	Introduction of endoscope increases risk for vomiting resulting from stimulation of gag reflex (Pagana et al., 2021).
9. For lower GI studies (proctoscopy, sigmoidoscopy, or colonoscopy), verify that patient followed clear liquid diet for 2 days and has completed any ordered bowel-cleansing regimen.	An empty intestinal tract promotes endoscopic insertion and clear visualization of interior wall.
10. Assess patient's knowledge, prior experience with GI endoscopy, and feelings about procedure.	Reveals need for patient instruction and/or support.

PLANNING

1. Expected outcomes following completion of procedure:	
• Patient does not aspirate and has no postprocedure bleeding.	Indicates absence of complications and tolerance of procedure.
• Patient's pain acuity is 4 or less on pain scale of 0 to 10.	Indicates preprocedure analgesia effective in managing pain.
• Patient is without respiratory complications or change in level of consciousness.	Indicates patient recovers from sedation.
• Patient describes purposes and steps of procedure.	Documents patient understanding.
2. Prepare patient:	
a. Provide privacy and explain steps of procedure, including sensations to expect.	Protects patient's privacy; reduces anxiety. Promotes cooperation.
b. Organize and set up any equipment needed to perform procedure.	Ensures more efficiency when performing procedure.
c. Administer pain medication or preprocedure medication.	Promotes relaxation and reduces anxiety.

IMPLEMENTATION

1. Perform hand hygiene and apply PPE.	Reduces transmission of microorganisms.
2. Remove patient's eyeglasses, dentures, or other dental appliances.	Prevents damage to eyeglasses or damage/dislodgement of dental structures during intubation phase.
3. Organize and open equipment using sterile technique.	Ensures efficient procedure. Reduces transmission of infection.
4. Take time-out to verify patient's name, type of procedure, and procedure site with patient and health care team.	Time-out verification just before starting procedure includes health care provider and all personnel and is safety precaution to prevent wrong patient, wrong site, and wrong procedure errors (TJC, 2023).
5. Ensure that IV line is patent and administer IV sedation as ordered (see Skill 8.1) if certified.	Provides route for emergency medications and creates immediate conscious sedation.

Clinical Judgment *Nurse must be certified to administer IV sedation.*

6. Help patient assume proper position for procedure and apply appropriate drape.	Improves efficiency of procedure and ability of physician to visualize site. Drape provides comfort and minimizes exposure.
a. *Upper GI procedures:* Help patient maintain left lateral position.	Left lateral position allows easy passage of upper or lower endoscope. Provides airway clearance if patient gags and vomits gastric contents.
Lower GI procedures: Help patient maintain left lateral decubitus position. Drape patient for privacy.	Left lateral decubitus position provides access to lower GI tract.
7. Physician performs hand hygiene and puts on PPE.	Reduces transmission of microorganisms.
8. Upper GI procedures:	
a. Help physician spray nasopharynx and oropharynx with local anesthetic.	Topical anesthetic decreases gag reflex caused by passage of endoscope, thus improving safety and comfort.
b. Administer atropine if ordered.	Reduces quantity of secretions, therefore reducing risk for aspiration.
c. Position tip of suction catheter for easy access in patient's mouth.	Removes oral secretions to reduce risk for aspiration.
9. Lower GI procedures:	
a. Prepare lubricant for fiberoptic endoscope.	Facilitates passage of tubing.
10. Physician lubricates endoscope and slowly passes it into mouth or through anus to view esophagus, stomach, colon, or rectum and advances to desired depth while visualizing lining of structures.	Provides visualization of all structures to detect polyps, cancerous lesions, or areas of inflammation and stricture.

STEP	RATIONALE
11. Physician insufflates air through endoscope into upper GI tract or carbon dioxide into lower GI tract in case of colonoscopy.	Distends GI structures for better visualization. Carbon dioxide insufflation produces less postprocedure abdominal cramping than air insufflation because it is more readily absorbed.
12. Assist patient throughout procedure.	
a. Anticipate needs and promote comfort.	Patient is unable to speak after tube is passed into throat.
b. Tell patient what is happening as each part of procedure is carried out (e.g., abdominal cramping).	Reassures patient about procedure and how long it will last.
c. For upper GI procedures, suction if there are excessive oral secretions or vomitus.	Prevents aspiration of oral secretions or gastric contents.
13. Place tissue specimens in proper laboratory containers or on proper slides. Seal as needed. Mark date, time, and initials on all specimen containers before sending to laboratory.	Ensures proper specimen preservation and labeling and preparation of specimens for microscopic examination.
14. Help patient return to comfortable position.	Promotes relaxation.
15. Dispose of all contaminated supplies in appropriate receptacle; remove and dispose of gloves and other PPE.	Reduces transmission of microorganisms. Use appropriate disposal receptacle if patient is on hazardous drugs (Blake, 2019; ONS, 2018).
16. In recovery, after sedation resolves, inform patient not to eat or drink until gag reflex returns.	Reduces risk for aspiration.
17. Help patient to a comfortable postprocedure position.	Restores comfort and sense of well-being.
18. Raise side rails (as appropriate) and lower bed to lowest position, locking into position.	Ensures patient safety and prevents falls.
19. Place nurse call system in an accessible location within patient's reach.	Ensures patient can call for assistance if needed.
20. Perform hand hygiene.	Reduces transmission of microorganisms.

EVALUATION

1. Monitor VS and oxygen saturation according to agency policy, which can be every 15 minutes for 2 hours.	Patient monitoring during sedated GI endoscopy may detect changes in pulse, blood pressure, and level of sedation before clinically significant events occur (Dossa et al., 2021).
2. Assess for levels of sedation and consciousness (see Skill 8.1).	Determines patient's response to IV sedation.
3. Ask patient to describe pain acuity using pain scale of 0 to 10. Observe for pain.	Monitors for sudden abdominal pain, which can indicate rupture of abdominal organs.
4. Evaluate emesis or aspirate for frank or occult blood (see Chapter 7).	Monitors for GI bleeding.
If a lower endoscopy was completed, you should monitor the abdomen for increased size.	The size of the abdomen and bowel sounds are important to assess for perforation.
5. Assess for return of gag reflex, usually in 2 to 4 hours. Provide oral hygiene when gag reflex returns.	Determines when effects of anesthetic have disappeared. Gag reflex prevents aspiration.
6. **Use Teach-Back:** "I want to be sure I explained what you can eat and any activity limitations on returning home. Tell me what you know about what you can eat and type of activity to limit." Revise your instruction now or develop a plan for revised patient/family caregiver teaching if patient/family caregiver is not able to teach back correctly.	Teach-back is a technique for health care providers to ensure that they have explained medical information clearly so that patients and families understand what is communicated to them (AHRQ, 2023).

Unexpected Outcomes	Related Interventions
1. Vasovagal response caused by stimulation of baroreceptors during endoscope insertion as evidenced by:	• Lower head of table.
• Feeling nauseous, faint, dizzy, and/or light-headed	• Support airway.
• Diaphoresis with slow, steady pulse	
• Few seconds of unconsciousness	
2. For upper GI procedures:	
A. Laryngospasm and bronchospasm as evidenced by:	• Call physician immediately.
• Sudden, severe shortness of breath	• Support airway (positioning).
	• Prepare emergency resuscitation equipment.
	• Anticipate possible cricothyrotomy.
B. Hypoxemia as evidenced by:	• Monitor SpO_2/end-tidal CO_2 values.
• Gradual shortness of breath	• Maintain airway and breathing.
• Decreasing level of consciousness	• Notify physician immediately.

STEP	RATIONALE
C. Pulmonary aspiration as evidenced by: • Dyspnea, tachypnea, decreasing levels of oxygen saturation	• Support airway. • Follow specific postprocedural orders related to findings. • Monitor SpO_2/end-tidal CO_2 values.
3. For lower GI procedures: abdominal pain, fever, or bleeding, indicating damage to intestinal wall	• Continue to monitor VS. • Notify physician of findings.
4. Oversedation with decreasing level of consciousness	• See Skill 8.1.

Documentation

- Document the procedure, duration, VS and pulse oximetry, patient's tolerance, complications and interventions, and collection and disposition of specimen.
- Document your evaluation of patient and family caregiver learning.

Hand-Off Reporting

- Report onset of bleeding, abdominal pain, dyspnea, and VS changes to physician.

Special Considerations

Patient Education

- Upper GI endoscopy:
  - Explain method for endoscope insertion. Prepare patient for a slight feeling of not being able to breathe. Assure the patient that this feeling is common, but that air is delivered through the endoscope and suffocation will not occur.
  - Teach patient simple hand signals for pain or discomfort because it will be impossible to speak after the endoscope is positioned in the esophagus.
- Lower GI procedures (colonoscopy, sigmoidoscopy, proctoscopy):
  - Explain that it is normal to experience increased flatus and abdominal cramping.
  - Small amounts of blood in the stool are common if a biopsy specimen was taken.

Pediatrics

- Introduction of the endoscope in infants and small children who have a narrow and collapsible airway may result in respiratory distress.

Older Adults

- Older adults frequently have reduced drug clearance from decreased glomerular filtration rate (GFR) and nephron activity or decreased hepatic function. It is important to monitor the effects of medications given to older adults (Touhy & Jett, 2022).
- Because of age-related changes in older adults, the gastric mucosa is thinner, which increases the incidence of irritation, ulceration, and perforation (Touhy & Jett, 2022).
- Physical exposure and room temperature contribute to hypothermia in frail older adults who are unable to communicate discomfort. Use warmed blankets or forced-air heat to maintain core temperature at comfortable, safe levels (Harding et al., 2020).
- Some older adults experience dehydration, electrolyte imbalance, and exhaustion from pretest preparation. If the procedure is done on an ambulatory care basis, it is helpful to have someone stay with the patient for at least 24 hours.

Populations With Disabilities

- Gastrointestinal problems are common among people with intellectual and developmental disabilities (IDDs) and may be displayed as food aversions, behavior changes, or weight loss. Careful screening is needed (Sullivan et al., 2018).

Home Care

- Explain that patient might have hoarseness or a sore throat after an upper GI procedure. Patient can have ice chips or anesthetic lozenges after gag reflex returns.
- Instruct patient or family caregiver to notify physician if patient has a fever, abdominal pain, a rigid abdomen, and rectal bleeding or blood in stool.

✦ CLINICAL JUDGMENT AND NEXT GENERATION NCLEX® EXAMINATION–STYLE QUESTIONS

The nurse is caring for a 58-year-old patient who needs a lumbar puncture performed. The patient has a history of hypertension and began experiencing headaches with a fever 2 days ago. It is difficult for the patient to touch the chin to chest when the head is flexed by the health care provider. Currently the patient is taking ami___pine, 5 mg, twice daily. Vital signs include BP 102/62 mm ___g, pulse 64 beats/min, RR 12 breaths/min, T 39.1°C (102.4°F), and SPO₂ 97% on room air (RA). The patient's partner reports that the patient has been anxious and forgetful lately.

1. You are concerned this patient could experience increased intracranial pressure during the lumbar puncture. Which of the following symptoms are indicative of increased intracranial pressure? **Select all that apply**.
   1. Increased alertness
   2. Decreased headache
   3. Decreased respirations
   4. Sudden death
   5. Increased heart rate
2. Which equipment will the nurse gather before the lumbar puncture procedure?
   1. Otoscope
   2. Manometer
   3. Tuning fork
   4. Ophthalmoscope
3. Into which position will the nurse place the patient for the lumbar puncture?
   1. Semi-Fowler
   2. Lateral recumbent
   3. Lithotomy
   4. Supine
4. Following the lumbar puncture procedure, which of the following nursing interventions will be provided? **Select all that apply.**
   1. Assess for fluid loss.
   2. Withhold pain medication for 1 hour.
   3. Anticipate chest x-ray examination.
   4. Ambulate patient as soon as procedure ends.
   5. Monitor for cerebrospinal fluid leakage at the puncture site.
5. Which patient finding, after the procedure, requires the nurse to alert the health care provider?
   1. Pulse rate 90 beats/min
   2. Tenderness at the puncture site
   3. Headache rated at 8 on a 0-to-10 scale
   4. Continued temperature 39.1°C (102.4°F)

Visit the Evolve site for Answers to the Clinical Judgment and Next Generation NCLEX® Examination-Style Questions.

REFERENCES

Abbaszadeh R, et al: The effect of lavender aroma on anxiety of patients having bone marrow biopsy, *Asian Pac J Cancer Prev* 21(3):771–775, 2020.
Agency for Healthcare Research and Quality (AHRQ): *Teach-back: intervention*, 2023. https://www.ahrq.gov/patient-safety/reports/engage/interventions/teachback.html.
American Association of Moderate Sedation Nurses (AAMSN): *Scope of practice*, 2022. https://aamsn.org/resources/pdfs/sedation-related-pdfs/registered-nurse-csrn-scope-of-practice.
American College of Radiology (ACR): *ACR-SIR practice parameter for sedation/analgesia*, 2020, The American College of Radiology. https://www.acr.org/-/media/acr/files/practice-parameters/sed-analgesia.pdf. Accessed August 11, 2023.
American Society of Anesthesiologists (ASA): Practice guidelines for moderate procedural sedation and analgesia 2018: a report by the American Society of Anesthesiologists Task Force on Moderate Procedural Sedation and Analgesia, the American Association of Oral and Maxillofacial Surgeons, American College of Radiology, American Dental Association, American Society of Dentist Anesthesiologists, and Society of Interventional Radiology, *Anesthesiology* 128:437, 2018.
Bangalore S, et al: Evidence-based practices in the cardiac Catheterization laboratory: a scientific statement from the American Heart Association. *Circulation* 144:e107–e119, 2021.
Blake K: USP <800>: Gaining compliance through implementation of a hazardous drug control program. *CJON* 23:324–326, 2019.
Centers for Disease Control and Prevention (CDC): *What is health literacy*, 2023. https://www.cdc.gov/healthliteracy/learn/index.html.
Dossa F, et al: Sedation practices for routine gastrointestinal endoscopy: a systematic review of recommendations. *BMC Gastroenterol* 21:22, 2021.
Gendron N, et al: Pain assessment and factors influencing pain during bone marrow aspiration: a prospective study. *PLoS One* 14(8):e0221534, 2019.
Giordano F, et al: The influence of music therapy on preoperative anxiety in pediatric oncology patients undergoing invasive procedures. *Arts Psychol* 68:101649, 2020.
Harding MM, et al: *Lewis's medical-surgical nursing: assessment and management of clinical problems*, ed 11, St. Louis, 2020, Elsevier.
Harper J, et al: Determination of oxygen saturation compared to a prescribed target range using continuous pulse oximetry in acutely unwell medical patients. *BMC Pulm Med* 21:332, 2021.
Hockenberry MJ, et al: *Wong's essentials of pediatric nursing*, ed 11, St. Louis, 2022, Mosby.
Kim Y, et al: Assessment of the conventional radial artery with optical coherent tomography after the snuffbox approach. *CARDIOL J* 28(6):849–854, 2021.
Lingappan AM: *Sedation*, 2021. https://emedicine.medscape.com/article/809993-overview. Accessed August 11, 2023.
Manda Y, Baradhi K: *Cardiac catheterization risks and complications*. Treasure Island, FL, 2022, StatPearls Publishing.
Oncology Nursing Society (ONS): *Toolkit for safe handling of hazardous drugs for nurses in oncology*, 2018. https://www.ons.org/clinical-practice-resources/toolkit-safe-handling-hazardous-drugs-nurses-oncology.
Pagana KD, et al: *Mosby's diagnostic and laboratory test reference*, ed 15, St. Louis, 2021, Elsevier.
Rasheed AM, et al: Ramsay sedation scale and Richmond agitation sedation scale: a cross-sectional study, *Dimens Crit Care Nurs* 38(2):90, 2019.
Schandert L, et al: Music Intervention: nonpharmacologic method to reduce pain and anxiety in adult patients undergoing bone marrow procedures. *Clin J Oncol Nurs* 25(3):314–320, 2021.
Sleep Foundation: *Mallampati score and predicting sleep apnea*, 2023. https://www.sleepfoundation.org/sleep-apnea/mallampati-score. Accessed August 11, 2023.
Sullivan WF, et al: Primary care of adults with intellectual and developmental disabilities: 2018 Canadian consensus guidelines, *Can Fam Physician* 64:254, 2018.
The Joint Commission (TJC): *Informed consent: more than getting a signature*, 2022. https://www.jointcommission.org/-/media/tjc/newsletters/quick-safety-21-update-4-4-22.pdf. Accessed August 11, 2023.
The Joint Commission (TJC): *2023 National Patient Safety Goals*, Oakbrook Terrace, IL, 2023, The Joint Commission. https://www.jointcommission.org/standards/national-patient-safety-goals/.
Touhy TA, Jett KF: *Ebersole and Hess' gerontological nursing and healthy aging*, ed 6, St. Louis, 2022, Elsevier.
Yale School of Medicine: *Metformin and iodinated contrast*, 2022. https://medicine.yale.edu/diagnosticradiology/patientcare/policies/glucophage/. Accessed August 11, 2023.

PHASE 1

QUESTION 1.

A client comes to urgent care reporting lower pelvic discomfort.

Highlight the findings that require **immediate** follow-up by the nurse.

History and Physical	Nurses' Notes	Vital Signs	Laboratory Results

1228: Client reports to urgent care reporting 3 days of worsening pain upon urination, abdominal discomfort, and fatigue. The urinary pain is described as "burning" in nature and occurring with each urination. The patient states, "I constantly feel as if I have to urinate, but when I go to the bathroom, very little urine will come out." The patient also states she has experienced a thick vaginal discharge for the past 2 days that "smells awful" and is yellowish-green in color. Sexual history reveals unprotected intercourse with partner and one other individual recently. Alert and oriented × 4; lung sounds clear to auscultation; S_1S_2 present without murmur; bowel sounds present × 4 quadrants; strength in all extremities equal. Lower abdominal tenderness in the LLQ and RLQ upon gentle palpation. Vital signs: T 38.4°C (101.2°F); HR 78 beats/min; RR 20 breaths/min; BP 124/78 mm Hg; SpO_2 98% on RA.

QUESTION 2.

The nurse considers information provided by the client.

Complete the following sentence by selecting from the lists of word choices below.

The nurse determines the patient's priorities and prepares to perform the following: [**Word Choice**] and [**Word Choice**].

Word Choices
Assessment of nature of fatigue
Neurologic exam
Collection of clean voided urine specimen
Breast examination
Vaginal discharge specimen

PHASE 2

QUESTION 3.

The nurse prepares to talk with the health care provider.

Complete the following sentence by selecting from the list of word choices below.

The client needs that the nurse will **prioritize** communicating to the health care provider include [**Word Choice**] and [**Word Choice**].

Word Choices
Reduced urinary output
Qualities of vaginal discharge
Burning on urination
Blood pressure
Temperature
Urinary frequency

QUESTION 4.

The client is seen by the health care provider, who then enters diagnostic testing orders in the electronic health record (EHR).

Complete the following sentence by selecting the *most likely* options from the list of word choices below.

The nurse anticipates that the health care provider will order diagnostic testing of [**Word Choice**] and [**Word Choice**].

Word Choices
Blood glucose
Urinalysis
Cardiac enzymes
Vaginal discharge culture
Stool sample
Lactic acid

PHASE 3

QUESTION 5.

The nurse assists the health care provider with collections of samples during a pelvic examination of the client. Select 2 conditions the samples will be tested for when sent to the laboratory.

- Mpox
- Syphilis
- Hepatitis
- Gonorrhea
- Chlamydia
- Genital herpes
- Human immunodeficiency virus

QUESTION 6.

The patient's condition continues to deteriorate over the next 24 hours. The patient drives to the emergency department and is admitted to a general medical floor for intravenous antibiotics and monitoring. When the client develops new symptoms, including an increasing fever, headache, and inability to lower the chin to the neck, the health care provider orders a lumbar puncture. The nurse provides teaching to the client before the diagnostic test.

Select the patient statements that the nurse evaluates as demonstrating an understanding of the test.

- "Prior to the test, you will check my neurologic status."
- "I will lie on my side during the test."
- "My lower leg strength will be evaluated before the test."
- "Before the test, I must go to the bathroom to empty my bladder."
- "It is important that you help me sit up and get in a chair after the puncture is done."
- "I can expect that my headache may get worse after this lumbar puncture is done."
- "A needle is going to be placed in an area around the spinal cord space during the lumbar puncture."

Health care–associated infection (HAI) is a growing problem as new virulent organisms evolve and patients present with not only infection but also serious comorbidities. Clinical judgment in selecting the appropriate skills for infection control requires the application of knowledge about the nature of infection, the pathology of different types of infection, and a patient's susceptibility and risks for infection. Knowing a patient's susceptibility and risks requires a thorough and focused assessment of the patient's clinical condition and common risk factors. Basic infection control techniques, called Standard Precautions, are the evidence-based approaches that apply in the care of all patients. These techniques reduce the spread of infection being transmitted from nurses to patients and reduce the transfer of infection to nurses directly by patients. It is important to follow medically aseptic Standard Precautions because health care environments have sources of infection everywhere, including from work surfaces in patient rooms and common work areas, from patients' bodily fluids, and from visitors' and health care workers' hands. It is critical that you form an **infection control conscience**, the highest form of patient advocacy. It means anticipating sources of infection, understanding the risks to you and to patients, and providing the procedures necessary to reduce infection transmission.

Hand hygiene and clean gloving are two of the most common medically aseptic skills you will perform. However, clinical judgment is necessary to perform these skills correctly and at the appropriate times during patient care. You must always anticipate what the gloves have touched and what your next care activity involves. For example, you will perform hand hygiene and then apply clean gloves before bathing patients. During the bath, you clean the patient's perineal area. Gloves should immediately be removed, followed by handwashing and reapplication of clean gloves to complete the bath. The body fluids that adhere to the gloves during perineal care cannot then touch clean areas of the patient's body.

When you work in environments where invasive procedures occur, sterile aseptic techniques are necessary. This is the norm in areas such as the operating room, interventional procedure areas, and special treatment rooms. Using skills such as sterile gloving or creating a sterile field reduces infection transmission when foreign sterile objects such as a urinary catheter, intravenous catheter, or nasotracheal suction catheter are introduced into the body. Sterile objects must remain sterile, and proper aseptic technique achieves this goal. When you do not work in special procedure areas but a procedure is planned to be performed at a patient's bedside, anticipate how to use sterile aseptic technique in that situation. The risks for accidental contamination of a sterile work field at the bedside are higher than when you work in a more controlled procedure room.

Clinical judgment plays a role in deciding when to use medical versus sterile aseptic techniques. Consider caring for a patient with leukemia, a form of cancer. Your scientific knowledge informs you of the patient's increased risk for reduced immune function by nature of the disease. In addition, you know that the chemotherapy the patient receives can further lower immunity. The combination of reduced immunity and chemotherapy makes the patient highly susceptible to infection. The use of Standard Precautions limits transmission of organisms that are normally transmitted through routine patient contact. However, when your assessment reveals patient risks, such as a skin tear or pressure injury, you will decide if more aggressive infection control techniques are needed, such as use of sterile gloves during a dressing change. Depending on the degree to which the patient's immune system is depressed, consultation with infection control professionals could be necessary to implement Contact Precautions in this case to protect the patient from microorganism exposure.

9 | Medical Asepsis

SKILLS AND PROCEDURES

Skill 9.1 **Hand Hygiene, p. 263**

Skill 9.2 **Caring for Patients Under Isolation Precautions, p. 267**

OBJECTIVES

Mastery of content in this chapter will enable you to:

- Apply critical thinking in the prevention of the transmission of infection.
- Explain medical asepsis principles for patient care.
- Identify nursing care measures intended to break the chain of infection.
- Determine how each element of the infection chain contributes to infection.
- Identify the factors that influence nursing staff adherence with hand hygiene.
- Demonstrate proper procedures for hand hygiene.
- Demonstrate correct isolation precautions.
- Explain differences in special tuberculosis precautions compared with Airborne Precautions.

MEDIA RESOURCES

- http://evolve.elsevier.com/Perry/skills
- Clinical Review Questions
- Audio Glossary
- ▶ Video Clips
- NSO Nursing Skills Online
- Answers to Clinical Judgment and Next-Generation NCLEX® Examination–Style Questions
- Skills Performance Checklists
- Printable Key Points

PURPOSE

Infection prevention and control practices reduce or eliminate sources and transmission of infection. This is done by breaking links in the chain of infection. Infection prevention and control practices are designed to protect patients and health care providers from disease. Medical asepsis, or clean technique, includes procedures used for reducing the number of organisms and preventing their transfer. Surgical asepsis, or sterile technique (see Chapter 10), refers to procedures used to eliminate all organisms from an area.

Health care–associated infections (HAIs) are infections that patients develop while being treated in medical facilities. The Centers for Disease Control and Prevention (CDC) (2023a) explain that it is difficult to determine with certainty where a pathogen is acquired since patients may be colonized with or exposed to potential pathogens outside of the health care setting before receiving health care. In addition, patients may develop infections caused by those pathogens when exposed to the conditions associated with delivery of health care. Patients also move about within hospitals (CDC, 2023a).

A hospital is one of the most likely settings for patients to acquire infections. Staff, patients, and environmental factors support a high population of pathogens that are resistant to antibiotics. Health care workers transmit many HAIs by direct contact during the delivery of care, and HAIs are also related to procedures or equipment used during procedures (Monegro et al., 2023). Nurses play a critical role in prevention of infection in all health care settings. Evidence shows that combining evidence-based practice, a culture of safety, teamwork, and communication can decrease HAIs (Agency for Healthcare Research and Quality [AHRQ], 2023a).

PRACTICE STANDARDS

- Association of periOperative Registered Nurses (AORN), 2021: Guidelines for Perioperative Practice
- Centers for Disease Control and Prevention (CDC), 2021a: Hand Hygiene in Healthcare Settings: Healthcare Providers
- Centers for Disease Control and Prevention (CDC), Siegel JD et al., and the Healthcare Infection Control Practices Advisory Committee, 2023a: 2007 Guideline for Isolation Precautions: Preventing Transmission of Infectious Agents in Healthcare Settings
- The Joint Commission (TJC), 2023: National Patient Safety Goals—Patient identification

SUPPLEMENTAL STANDARDS

- World Health Organization (WHO), 2021: SAVE LIVES—Clean Your Hands: Annual Global Campaign
- World Health Organization (WHO), 2020: Hand Hygiene for All Initiatives: Improving Access and Behaviour in Health Care Facilities

PRINCIPLES FOR PRACTICE

- Hand hygiene practices comprise a major principle of infection control and are essential to safe patient care.
- Patients in all health care settings are at risk of becoming colonized or infected as a result of an impaired immune response, exposure to an increased number of pathogenic organisms, and the performance of invasive procedures (Tejiram & Sava, 2019).

- Determine a patient's susceptibility to infection. Age, nutritional status, stress, disease processes, and forms of medical therapy place patients at risk (Casadevall & Pirofski, 2018; Virology Research Services, 2019).
- Recognize elements of the chain of infection and initiate measures to prevent the onset and spread of infections. The presence of a pathogen does not mean that an infection will occur. Infection occurs in a cycle, often referred to as the *chain of infection*. An infection develops if this chain remains intact (Fig. 9.1). In patient care it is important to use infection control practices to break an element of the chain so as not to transmit infection (Table 9.1). The six elements in the chain are:
  - An infectious agent or pathogen
  - A reservoir or source for pathogen growth
  - A portal of exit from the reservoir
  - A mode of transmission
  - A portal of entry to the host
  - A susceptible host

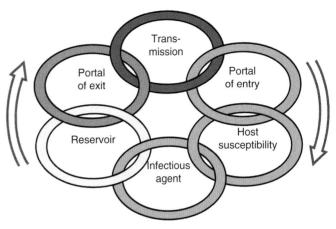

FIG. 9.1 Chain of infection.

TABLE 9.1

Breaking the Chain of Infection

Element of Infection Chain	Medical Asepsis Practices
Infectious agent (pathogenic organism capable of causing disease)	Clean contaminated objects. Clean, disinfect, and sterilize.
Reservoir (site or source of microorganism growth)	Perform hand hygiene before and after patient contact with appropriate antiseptic (e.g., chlorhexidine) or soap and water. Control and contain sources of body fluids and drainage. Bathe patient with soap and water, chlorhexidine, or disposable bath. Change soiled dressings. Dispose of soiled tissues, dressings, or linen in moisture-resistant bags. Place syringes, uncapped hypodermic needles, and intravenous needles in designated puncture-proof containers. Keep table surfaces clean and dry. Do not leave bottled solutions open for prolonged periods. Keep reusable solutions tightly capped. Keep surgical wound drainage tubes and collection bags patent. Empty and dispose of drainage suction bottles according to agency policy, and keep wounds covered.
Portal of exit (means by which microorganisms leave a site)	Respiratory • Avoid talking, sneezing, or coughing directly over wound or sterile dressing field. • Cover nose and mouth when sneezing or coughing. • Wear mask if experiencing respiratory tract infection. Urine, feces, emesis, and blood • Wear clean gloves when handling blood and body fluids. • Wear gowns and eyewear if there is a chance of splashing fluids. • Handle all laboratory specimens as if infectious.
Transmission (means of spread)	Reduce microorganism spread: • Perform hand hygiene. • Use personal set of care items for each patient. • Avoid shaking bed linen or clothes; dust with damp cloth. • Avoid contact of soiled item with uniform. • Discard any item that touches the floor. • Follow Standard Precautions or select transmission-based isolation precautions.
Portal of entry (site through which microorganism enters a host)	Skin and mucosa • Maintain skin and mucous membrane integrity; lubricate skin, offer frequent hygiene, turn and position. • Cover wounds as needed. • Clean wound sites thoroughly. • Dispose of used needles in puncture-proof container. Urinary • Keep all drainage systems closed and intact, maintaining downward flow.
Host (patient)	Reduce susceptibility to infection. Provide adequate nutrition. Ensure adequate rest. Promote body defenses against infection. Provide immunizations.

- Principles of hand hygiene, use of barrier (personal protective equipment) techniques, and routine environmental cleaning are examples of medical asepsis. These principles are common in the health care and home environment (e.g., washing hands before preparing food). Consistently incorporate the basic principles of medical asepsis into all patient care activities.
- Teach principles of hand hygiene to patients and family caregivers to decrease illnesses and prevent spreading of germs while in the hospital, at home, or in the community (CDC, 2023c; Yoon et al., 2020). Good hand hygiene is particularly important in helping prevent the spread of COVID-19 and other respiratory illnesses.

PERSON-CENTERED CARE

- Nurses are responsible for educating patients and their families about infection control, including information concerning signs and symptoms of infection, disease transmission, methods of prevention, knowledge of the infectious process, and appropriate use of aseptic techniques and barrier protection.
- Infection can require isolation. This may lead to anxiety, loneliness, depression, or changes in self-concept or body image (Purssell et al., 2020).
- Know the cultural views and preferences of your patients. Some may rely on alternative health care practices that require education on medical asepsis.
- When a patient from another culture requires isolation, carefully assess the meaning of isolation and use that knowledge in how you explain to the patient and family caregiver the therapeutic purpose of isolation (Giger & Haddad, 2021).

EVIDENCE-BASED PRACTICE

Hand Hygiene

The most important recommendation in evidence-based guidelines on how to prevent HAIs is for health care workers to correctly perform hand hygiene before and after every patient encounter (CDC, 2022; Sands & Aunger, 2020). Patients' practice of hand hygiene can also help reduce HAIs (Manresa et al., 2020). Evidence-based guidelines for proper hand hygiene include:
- Alcohol-based products are more effective for standard handwashing or hand antisepsis than soap or antiseptic soaps (CDC, 2023b, 2023e; Gupta & Lipner, 2020). Moreover, brisk alcohol-based rinses or gels containing emollients cause substantially less skin irritation and dryness than plain or antimicrobial soaps (CDC, 2023f; Gupta & Lipner, 2020).
- Handwashing with plain soap sometimes results in paradoxical increases in bacterial counts on the skin (Health Protection Surveillance Centre, 2022).
- Following the WHO's Five Moments for Hand Hygiene guidelines and adhering to hand hygiene practices among health care providers is increased through goal setting, incentives, and accountability (WHO, 2021) (Fig. 9.2).
- Soap and water are still necessary for hand hygiene if hands are visibly soiled or when caring for patients infected with *Clostridium difficile* (CDC, 2019a, 2022; Kiersnowska et al., 2021).
- Use soap and water or alcohol-based hand sanitizers for hand hygiene with COVID-19 and respiratory syncytial virus (RSV). Higher levels of hand hygiene have been associated with lower COVID-19 morbidity and mortality (Szczuka et al., 2021).

SAFETY GUIDELINES

- Hand hygiene with an appropriate alcohol-based hand antiseptic or soap and water is an essential part of patient care and

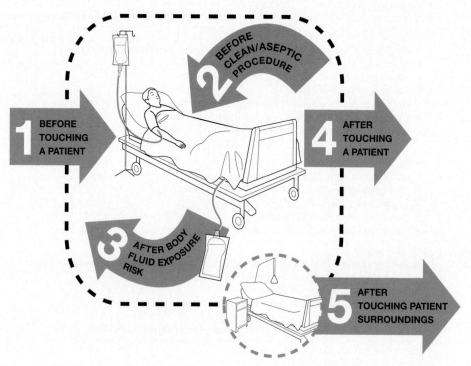

FIG. 9.2 My Five Moments for Hand Hygiene. (*From World Health Organization: About SAVE lives: clean your hands: 5 moments for hand hygiene, 2021. https://www.who.int/campaigns/world-hand-hygiene-day.*)

infection prevention and is a priority for patient safety (CDC, 2023f; Sands & Aunger, 2020).

- Do not wear artificial nails and extenders because of bacterial buildup.
- Fingernails should not be longer than 0.625 cm (¼ inch) in length, and nail polish should not be chipped. Evidence supports decreased effectiveness of hand hygiene with longer nails and gel-based polishes. There are no recommendations regarding nail polish color (Wałaszek et al., 2018).

- Consistently incorporate the basic principles of medical asepsis into patient care.
- Ensure that patients, family caregivers, and health care workers follow "cough hygiene practices" (see Table 9.2).
- Protect fellow health care workers from exposure to infectious agents through proper use and disposal of equipment.
- Be aware of body sites where HAIs are most likely to develop (e.g., urinary or respiratory tract). This enables you to direct preventive measures.

✦ SKILL 9.1 Hand Hygiene

 Video Clip

Hand hygiene is the most important and basic technique in preventing and controlling transmission of infection (CDC, 2023a). Hand hygiene is a general term that applies to handwashing, antiseptic hand wash, antiseptic hand rub, or surgical hand antisepsis. Handwashing is washing hands with plain soap and water. An antiseptic hand wash is washing hands with water and soap or other detergents containing an antiseptic agent. An antiseptic hand rub is the application of an antiseptic hand rub product to all surfaces of dry hands to reduce the number of microorganisms present. Surgical hand antisepsis is the use of an antiseptic hand wash or antiseptic hand rub before surgery by surgical personnel to eliminate transient and reduce resident hand flora (see Chapter 37).

The decision to perform a specific hand hygiene technique depends on four factors: (1) the intensity or degree of contact with patients or contaminated objects, (2) the amount of contamination that may occur with the contact, (3) the patient or health care worker's susceptibility to infection, and (4) the procedure or activity to be performed (Denton & Hallam, 2020; Hillier, 2020). It is a critical responsibility for all health care workers to follow these guidelines for appropriate hand hygiene (CDC, 2023a; WHO, 2022) (see Fig. 9.2).

- Wash hands with either a nonantibacterial soap and water or an antibacterial soap and water when they are visibly dirty or soiled with blood or other body fluids, before eating, and after using the toilet.
- Wash hands with soap and water, rather than using an alcohol-based hand rub, if exposed to spore-forming organisms such as *Clostridium difficile*. Handwashing mechanically removes spores from hands.
- If hands are not visibly soiled, use an alcohol-based hand rub for routinely decontaminating hands in the following clinical situations:
  - Before and after having direct contact with patients

- Before and after direct contact with a patient's intact skin (e.g., when taking a pulse or blood pressure or lifting a patient)
- Before clean/aseptic procedure
- Before applying sterile gloves and inserting an invasive device such as indwelling urinary catheters and intravenous peripheral vascular catheters
- After contact with blood, body fluids or excretions, mucous membranes, nonintact skin, or wound dressings
- After contact with inanimate objects (including medical equipment and patient surroundings) in the immediate vicinity of the patient
- When moving from a contaminated body site to a clean body site during patient care
- After removing gloves

Delegation

The skill of hand hygiene is performed by all caregivers. Hand hygiene is not optional.

Interprofessional Collaboration

- Members of the health care team should serve as role models for one another and provide reminders when hand hygiene is missed or incomplete.

Equipment

Antiseptic Hand Rub

- Alcohol-based waterless antiseptic containing emollients

Handwashing

- Easy-to-reach sink with warm running water
- Antimicrobial or regular soap
- Paper towels
- Disposable nail cleaner (optional)

STEP	RATIONALE

ASSESSMENT

1. Inspect surface of hands for breaks or cuts in skin or cuticles. Cover any skin lesions with a dressing before providing care. If lesions are too large to cover, you may be restricted from direct patient care.

Open cuts or wounds can harbor high concentrations of microorganisms. Agency policy may prevent nurses from caring for high-risk patients if open lesions are present on hands (Broussard & Kahwaji, 2023; WHO, 2021).

STEP	RATIONALE
2. Inspect hands for visible soiling.	Visible soiling requires handwashing with soap and water.
3. Inspect condition of nails. Natural tips should be no longer than 0.625 cm (¼ inch) long. Be sure that fingernails are short, filed, and smooth.	Subungual areas of hands harbor high concentrations of bacteria. Long nails and chipped or old polish increase the number of bacteria residing on hands (CDC, 2021a).

Clinical Judgment *The CDC (2023a) recommends artificial fingernails and extenders not be worn by health care personnel who have contact with high-risk patients. Artificial nail applications increase microbial load on hands (Wałaszek et al., 2018).*

PLANNING

1. Expected outcomes following completion of procedure:	
• Hands and areas under fingernails are clean and free of debris.	Transient bacteria have been removed.
• Skin of hands is without irritation or breakdown.	Proper hand hygiene technique used.
• Patient and/or family caregiver perform hand hygiene appropriately in health care or home setting.	Reduces infection transmission. Family caregivers often have primary responsibility for adherence to recommended infection control practices (CDC, 2023a).

IMPLEMENTATION

STEP	RATIONALE
1. Push wristwatch and long uniform sleeves above wrists. Avoid wearing rings. If worn, remove during hand hygiene.	Provides complete access to fingers, hands, and wrists. The skin underneath rings carries higher bacterial count; bacteria include gram-negative bacilli, enterobacteria, and *Staphylococcus aureus* (AORN, 2021).
2. Antiseptic hand rub:	In the absence of visible soiling of hands, approved alcohol-based products for hand disinfection are preferred over antimicrobial or plain soap and water because of their superior microbiocidal activity, reduced drying of the skin, and convenience (CDC, 2023a).
a. According to manufacturer directions, dispense ample amount of product into palm of one dry hand (see illustration).	Use enough product to cover hands thoroughly.
b. Rub hands together, covering all surfaces of hands and fingers with antiseptic (see illustration).	Ensures complete antimicrobial action.
c. Rub hands together until alcohol is dry. Allow hands to dry completely before applying gloves.	Provides enough time for product to work.
3. Handwashing using regular or antimicrobial soap:	
a. Stand in front of sink, keeping hands and uniform away from sink surface. (If hands touch sink during handwashing, repeat sequence.)	Inside of sink is contaminated area. Reaching over sink increases risk of touching edge, which is contaminated.

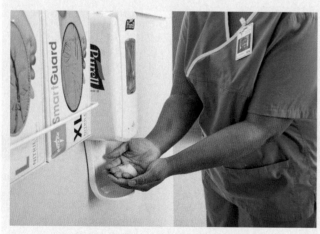

STEP 2a Apply waterless antiseptic to hands.

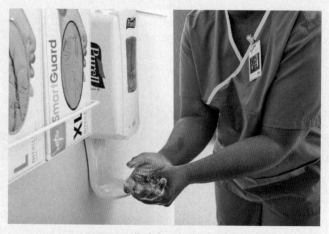

STEP 2b Rub hands thoroughly.

STEP	RATIONALE
b. Turn on water (see illustration), push knee pedals laterally, or press pedals with foot to regulate flow and temperature.	Knee pads within operating room and treatment areas are preferred to prevent hand contact with faucet. Faucet handles are likely to be contaminated with organic debris and microorganisms (AORN, 2021).
c. Avoid splashing water against uniform.	Microorganisms travel and grow in moisture.
d. Regulate flow of water so that temperature is warm.	Warm water removes less of protective oils on hands than hot water.
e. Wet hands and wrists thoroughly under running water. Keep hands and forearms lower than elbows during washing.	Hands are the most contaminated parts to wash. Water flows from least to most contaminated area, rinsing microorganisms into sink. Ensure that all surfaces of hands and fingers are cleaned.
f. Apply the amount of antiseptic soap recommended by the manufacturer and rub hands together to thoroughly lather hands (see illustration).	Ensure that all surfaces of hands and fingers are cleaned. Soap cleans by emulsifying fat and oil and lowering surface tension. Friction and rubbing mechanically loosen and remove dirt and transient bacteria. Interlacing fingers and thumbs ensures that all surfaces are cleaned. Adequate time is needed to expose skin surfaces to antimicrobial agent.

Clinical Judgment *The decision whether to use an antiseptic soap or an alcohol-based hand rub depends on whether the hands are visibly soiled, the type of infectious microorganism, the procedure you will perform, and the patient's immune status.*

STEP	RATIONALE
g. Perform hand hygiene using plenty of lather and friction for at least 20 seconds. Interlace fingers and rub palms and back of hands with circular motion at least five times each. Keep fingertips down to facilitate removal of microorganisms.	Hands should be washed with soap and water for at least 20 seconds when visibly soiled, before eating, and after using the restroom (Hillier, 2020).
h. Areas underlying fingernails are often soiled. Clean them with fingernails of other hand and additional soap or with disposable nail cleaner.	Area under nails can be highly contaminated, which increases risk for transmission of infection from nurse to patient.
i. Rinse hands and wrists thoroughly, keeping hands down and elbows up (see illustration).	Rinsing mechanically washes away dirt and microorganisms.
j. Dry hands thoroughly from fingers to wrists with paper towel or single-use cloth.	Drying from cleanest (fingertips) to least clean (wrist) avoids contamination (Toney-Butler et al., 2023). Drying hands prevents chapping and roughened skin. Do not tear or cut skin under or around nail.
k. If used, discard paper towel in proper receptacle.	Wet towel and hands allow transfer of pathogens from faucet by capillary action.
l. To turn off hand faucet, use clean, dry paper towel; avoid touching handles with hands (see illustration). Turn off water with foot or knee pedals (if applicable).	

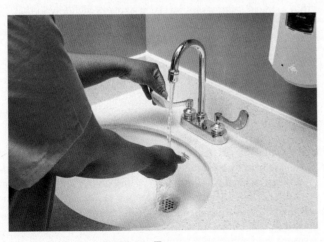

STEP 3b Turn on water.

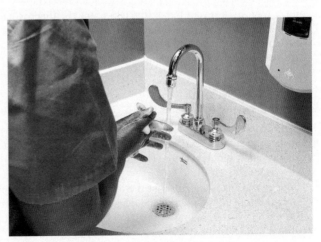

STEP 3f Lather hands thoroughly.

STEP	RATIONALE

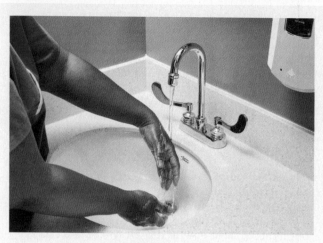

STEP 3i Rinse hands.

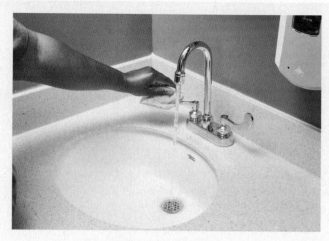

STEP 3l Turn off faucet.

m. If hands are dry or chapped, use small amount of lotion or barrier cream dispensed from individual-use container.

Helps to minimize skin dryness. There is risk of organism growth in lotion; therefore, only apply after patient care activities are complete. Only use lotions or creams approved by your health care agency because they have been selected to not interact with hand sanitizing products (CDC, 2021a).

EVALUATION

1. Inspect surface of hands for obvious signs of dirt or other contaminants.

2. Inspect hands for dermatitis or cracked skin.

3. **Use Teach-Back:** "I want to be sure you understand the proper way to wash your hands. Explain to me the times when you should wash your hands thoroughly." Revise your instruction now or develop a plan for revised patient/family caregiver teaching if patient/family caregiver is not able to teach back correctly.

Determines if hand hygiene is adequate.

Breaks in skin integrity increase risk for transmission of microorganisms.

Teach-back is a technique for health care providers to ensure that medical information has been explained clearly so that patients, families, and/or health care providers understand what is communicated to them (AHRQ, 2023b).

Special Considerations

Patient Education

• Instruct patient and family caregiver in proper techniques and situations for hand hygiene (including visiting health care agencies) (CDC, 2023c).

• Patients who are educated about the risks for infections play an important role in improving hand hygiene adherence in health care settings by reminding visitors and health care workers to perform hand hygiene (Chadwick, 2019; Lastinger et al., 2017).

Older Adults

• The impact of infections is greater in older adults. Hand hygiene by staff attending older adults is of utmost

importance and must be an ongoing continuing education requirement.

Home Care

• Evaluate patient and family caregiver to determine understanding of the transmission of infection and ability and motivation to perform hand hygiene correctly.

• Evaluate hand hygiene facilities in the home to determine the possibility of contamination, proximity of the facilities to the patient, and ability to maintain supplies and equipment.

✦ SKILL 9.2 Caring for Patients Under Isolation Precautions

 Video Clip

When a patient has a known or suspected source of colonization or infection, health care workers follow specific infection prevention and control practices to reduce the risk of cross-contamination to other patients (CDC, 2016b, 2023a; Marra, 2019). Standard Precautions include a group of infection prevention practices that apply to all patients, regardless of suspected or confirmed infection status, in any setting in which health care is delivered (CDC, 2016b, 2023a). These include hand hygiene, use of personal protective equipment (PPE, including gloves, gown, mask, eye protection, or face shield, depending on the anticipated exposure), and safe injection practices (CDC, 2023a) (see Table 9.2, Tier One). Standard Precautions require you to wear clean gloves before coming in contact with mucous membranes, nonintact skin, blood, body fluids, or other infectious material. It is not necessary to wear gloves when simply entering and then leaving a patient room. However, you wear clean gloves routinely when performing a variety of procedures. Wear a mask and protective eyewear when there is the risk of splash of blood or other body fluids to the eyes or mouth. Masks are worn during a procedure (e.g., suctioning) or when certain sterile procedures such as changing a central line dressing are performed.

Assess the need for PPE for each task you plan and for all patients, regardless of their diagnoses. Because of increased attention to the prevention of bloodborne pathogens and tuberculosis (TB) (Box 9.1), the CDC (2019c) and Occupational Safety and Health Administration (OHSA) (2011) have stressed the importance of barrier protection. The CDC (2019b) published revised guidelines for the routine practices for occupational infection prevention and control. The updated recommendations in this document are aimed at the leaders and staff of Occupational Health Services and the administrators and leaders of health care organizations and are intended to facilitate the provision of occupational infection prevention and control services to health care personnel. The CDC (2023a) also published revised guidelines for *Isolation Precautions: Preventing Transmission of Infectious Agents in Healthcare Settings*, important standards that are incorporated into this skill.

In many cases the application of Standard Precautions may be insufficient to reduce microorganism transmission. For that reason, the CDC has a Tier Two level (Table 9.2) of precautions, described as transmission-based precautions, or isolation. The transmission-based precautions are for patients who are known or suspected to be infected or colonized with infectious agents, including certain epidemiologically important pathogens, which requires additional control measures to effectively prevent transmission (CDC, 2023a). Tier Two (see Table 9.2) includes precautions designed for care of patients who are known or suspected to be infected, or colonized, with microorganisms transmitted by the contact, droplet, or airborne route (CDC, 2019b) or by contact with contaminated surfaces. The three types of transmission-based precautions—Airborne, Droplet, and Contact Precautions—may be combined for diseases that have multiple routes of transmission (e.g., chickenpox). Whether used singly or in combination, you use them in addition to Standard Precautions.

Multidrug-resistant organisms (MDROs) such as methicillin-resistant *Staphylococcus aureus* (MRSA) and vancomycin-resistant enterococci (VRE) have become increasingly common as a cause of colonization and HAIs. MRSA is a frequently identified pathogen associated with increased mortality. Data collected from hospitals over the past 6 years show a decrease in the incidence of bacteremia caused by MRSA (CDC, 2021b). VRE, another MDRO, poses a greater risk to immune-compromised and debilitated patients and is associated with antibiotic and device use (Davis et al., 2020). *C. difficile* infection is one of the most common and costly HAIs (CDC, 2019a). In most instances, patient susceptibility to *C. difficile* infection requires prior treatment with antibiotics. Unlike MRSA and VRE, *C. difficile* is more difficult to eliminate from the environment because it is a spore-forming organism, meaning that it can remain on surfaces in its dormant state for long periods of time. No matter which MDRO is involved, the most common means of transmission is by way of a health care worker's hands. To reduce the risk of cross-contamination among patients, use Contact Precautions (see Table 9.2) in addition to Standard Precautions when caring for these patients.

BOX 9.1

Special Tuberculosis Precautions

The Centers for Disease Control and Prevention (CDC) published guidelines for preventing tuberculosis (TB) transmission in health care agencies in response to a resurgence of TB in the United States associated with the increasing incidence of human immunodeficiency virus (HIV) infection, TB infection transmission in health care settings, and increasing immigration from countries with a high incidence of TB (CDC, 2023f; Cole et al., 2020).

- Current CDC guidelines for preventing and controlling TB focus on early detection of infection, preventing close contact with patients with active TB disease, and applying effective infection control measures in health care settings. Suspect TB in any patient with respiratory symptoms lasting longer than 3 weeks accompanied by other suspicious symptoms, such as unexplained weight loss, night sweats, fever, and a productive cough often streaked with blood.
- Consider the potential for infectious pulmonary or laryngeal TB from documented positive acid-fast bacillus (AFB) smear

or culture, cavitation on chest x-ray film, or history of recent TB exposure.
- Isolation for patients with suspected or confirmed TB includes placing the patient on Airborne Precautions in a single-patient negative-pressure room.
- Health care workers who care for patients with suspected or confirmed TB must wear special respirators (e.g., N95 or P100) (CDC, 2023d). These respirators are high-efficiency particulate masks that can filter particles at a 95% or better efficiency (CDC, 2023g; OSHA, 2011).
- The CDC now recommends the use of the QuantiFERON-TB Gold test (QFT-GIT) or the T-SPOT in place of the traditional TB skin test (CDC, 2016a). Both are interferon-gamma release assay (IGRA) blood tests. The advantages of an IGRA test are that it does not boost responses measured by subsequent tests and the results, results are available in 24 hours, and tests are not subject to reader bias.

TABLE 9.2

Centers for Disease Control and Prevention Isolation Guidelines

Standard Precautions (Tier One) for Use With All Patients

- Standard Precautions apply to blood, blood products, all body fluids, secretions, excretions (except sweat), nonintact skin, and mucous membranes.
- Perform hand hygiene before direct contact with patients; between patient contacts; after touching blood, body fluids, secretions, excretions, or contaminated items; and immediately after removing gloves.
- Hand hygiene: Wash hands with either a nonantimicrobial sop or antimicrobial soap and water when hands are visibly soiled or contaminated with blood or body fluids. When hands are not visibly soiled or contaminated with blood or body fluids, use an alcohol-based hand rub to perform hand hygiene.
- Personal protective equipment (PPE): Wear gloves for touching blood, body fluids, secretions, excretions, and contaminated items; and for touching mucous membranes and nonintact skin.
- PPE: Wear a gown during procedures and patient-care activities when contact of clothing/exposed skin with blood/body fluids, secretions, and excretions is anticipated.
- PPE: Wear a mask, eye protection (goggles), and face shield during procedures and patient-care activities likely to generate splashes or sprays of blood, body fluids, and secretions, especially suctioning and endotracheal intubation. During aerosol-generating procedures on patients with suspected or proven infections transmitted by respiratory aerosols (e.g., tuberculosis, COVID-19), wear a fit-tested N95 or higher respirator in addition to gloves, gown, and face/eye protection.
- Soiled patient care environment: Handle in a manner that prevents transfer of microorganisms to others and to the environment, wear gloves if visibly contaminated, and perform hand hygiene.
- Environmental control: Develop procedures for routine care, cleaning, and disinfection of environmental surfaces, especially frequently touched surfaces in patient-care areas.
- Bedclothes/Linen: Handle in a manner that prevents transfer of microorganisms to others and to the environment (e.g., hold dirty linen away from uniform/gown).
- Handling of needles and other sharps: Do not recap, bend, break, or hand-manipulate used needles; if recapping is required, use a one-handed scoop technique only; use safety features when available; place all used sharps in puncture-resistant container.
- Patient resuscitation: Use disposable (when possible) mouthpiece, resuscitation bag, or other ventilation devices to prevent contact with mouth and oral secretions.
- Patient placement: Prioritize for single-patient room if patient is at increased risk of transmission, is likely to contaminate the environment, does not maintain appropriate hygiene, or is at increased risk of acquiring infection or developing adverse outcome following infection.
- Respiratory hygiene and cough etiquette: Have patients cover the nose or mouth when sneezing or coughing; use tissues to contain respiratory secretions and dispose in nearest waste container; perform hand hygiene after contact with respiratory secretions and contaminated objects or materials; contain respiratory secretions with procedure or surgical mask; sit at least 3 feet away from others if coughing.
- Safe injection practices: Use a sterile, single-use, disposable needle and syringe for each injection given, and prevent contamination of injection equipment and medication. Whenever possible, use of single-dose vials is preferred over multiple-dose vials, especially when medications will be administered to multiple patients.

Transmission-Based Precautions (Tier Two) for Use With Specific Types of Patients

Category	Infection/Condition	Barrier Protection
Airborne Precautions (droplet nuclei smaller than 5 microns)	Measles, chickenpox (varicella), disseminated varicella zoster, COVID-19, RSV, pulmonary or laryngeal tuberculosis	Private-room, negative-pressure airflow of at least 6–12 exchanges per hour via HEPA filtration; mask or respiratory protection device, N95 respirator (depending on condition)
Droplet Precautions (droplets larger than 5 microns; being within 3 feet of patient)	Diphtheria (pharyngeal), rubella, streptococcal pharyngitis, pneumonia or scarlet fever in infants and young children, pertussis, mumps, *Mycoplasma* pneumonia, meningococcal pneumonia or sepsis, pneumonic plague	Private-room or cohort patients; mask or respirator (refer to agency policy)
Contact Precautions (direct patient or environmental contact)	Colonization or infection with multidrug-resistant organisms such as VRE and MRSA, *C. difficile*, *Shigella*, and other enteric pathogens; major wound infections; herpes simplex; scabies; varicella zoster (disseminated); respiratory syncytial virus in infants, young children, or immunocompromised adults	Private-room or cohort patients (see agency policy), gloves, gowns; patients may leave the room for procedures or therapy if infectious material is contained or covered and placed in a clean gown and hands cleaned
Protective environment	Allogeneic hematopoietic stem cell transplants	Private room; positive airflow with ≥12 air exchanges per hour; HEPA filtration for incoming air; mask to be worn by patient when out of room during times of construction in area

HEPA, High-efficiency particulate air; *MRSA*, methicillin-resistant *Staphylococcus aureus*; *VRE*, vancomycin-resistant enterococci.
Adapted from Centers for Disease Control and Prevention (CDC), et al: *2007 Guideline for Isolation Precautions: Preventing Transmission of Infectious Agents in Health Care Settings, 2019.* https://www.cdc.gov/infectioncontrol/pdf/guidelines/isolation-guidelines-H.pdf.

Other types of isolation precautions have been initiated for patients who are neutropenic, are receiving chemotherapy, or have contracted infectious diseases outside the scope of the second tier of precautions. In these types of situations, follow organizational policy.

Delegation

The skill of caring for patients on isolation precautions can be delegated to assistive personnel (AP). However, the nurse must assess the patient's status and isolation indications. Instruct the AP about:

- Reason patient is on isolation precautions
- Precautions for bringing equipment into the patient's room
- Special precautions regarding individual patient needs such as transportation to diagnostic tests

Interprofessional Collaboration

- When a patient develops an infection and the causative organism is unclear, collaborate with the infection control specialist to determine proper transmission control procedures.

- Communication of isolation precautions is key between all health care workers who come in contact with the isolated patient so that there is no breach in precautions.

Equipment

- PPE determined by type of isolation required: clean gloves, mask, eyewear or goggles, face shield, and gown (gowns may be disposable or reusable, depending on agency policy)
- Other patient care equipment (as appropriate) (e.g., hygiene items, medications, dressing supplies, sharps container, disposable blood pressure [BP] cuff)
- Soiled linen bag and trash receptacle
- Sign for door indicating type of isolation and/or for visitors to come to the nurses' station before entering room
- TB isolation
  - Room with negative airflow
  - N95 or P100 respirator

STEP	RATIONALE

ASSESSMENT

1. Identify patient using at least two identifiers (e.g., name and birthday or name and medical record number) according to agency policy.

Ensures correct patient. Complies with The Joint Commission standards and improves patient safety (TJC, 2023).

2. Assess patient's medical history for possible indications for isolation (e.g., risk factors for TB or other communicable disease, major draining wound, or purulent productive cough).

Mode of transmission for infectious microorganism determines type and degree of precautions followed.

3. Review laboratory test results (e.g., body fluid/tissue culture, acid-fast bacillus [AFB] smears, changes in white blood cell [WBC] count).

Reveals type of microorganism for which patient is being isolated, body fluid in which it was identified, and whether patient is immunosuppressed.

4. Review precautions for specific isolation system, including appropriate barriers to apply (see Table 9.2). Consider types of care measures that you will perform while in patient's room (e.g., medication administration or dressing change).

Ensures adequate protection. Allows you to organize care items for procedures and time spent in patient's room.

5. Assess patient's/family caregiver's knowledge, experience, and health literacy.

Determines degree to which individuals have the ability to find, understand, and use information and services to make informed health-related decisions and actions for themselves and others (CDC, 2023h).

6. Assess whether patient has known latex allergy. If allergy is present, refer to agency policy and resources available to provide full latex-free care. Apply allergy arm band.

Identifies patient risk and protects patient from serious allergic response.

7. Assess patient's knowledge, prior experience with isolation, and feelings about isolation. Review nursing care plan notes or confer with colleagues regarding patient's emotional state and reaction/adjustment to isolation.

Provides opportunity to plan for patient's need for emotional support and teaching.

8. Assess patient's goals or preferences for how isolation will be performed or what patient expects.

Allows care to be individualized to patient.

PLANNING

1. Expected outcomes following completion of procedure:
   - Patient asks for information about disease transmission.

Active interaction reveals patient's willingness and/or ability to communicate and be taught and understand information.

   - Patient explains purpose of isolation.

Instruction about precautions improves patient's ability to cooperate in care.

2. Explain purpose of isolation and precautions for patient and family caregiver to take. Offer opportunity to ask questions.

Improves patient's and family caregiver's ability to participate in care and minimizes anxiety. Identifies opportunity for planning social interaction and diversional activities.

3. Close room door.

Provides privacy and is often required as part of isolation procedure.

STEP	RATIONALE

IMPLEMENTATION

1. Perform hand hygiene (see Skill 9.1).

Reduces transmission of microorganisms.

2. Prepare all equipment to be taken into patient's room. In many cases dedicated equipment such as stethoscopes, BP equipment, and thermometers should remain in room until patient is discharged. If patient is infected or colonized with resistant organism (e.g., vancomycin-resistant enterococcus, methicillin-resistant *Staphylococcus aureus*), equipment remains in room and is thoroughly disinfected before removal (see agency policy).

Prevents you from making more than one trip into room. The CDC recommends use of dedicated noncritical patient care equipment (CDC, 2019b, 2023d). Use EPA-registered disinfectants that have microbiocidal (i.e., killing) activity against the pathogens most likely to contaminate the patient care environment (CDC, 2023a).

3. Prepare for entrance into isolation room. Ideally, before applying PPE, step into patient's room and stay by door. Introduce yourself and explain care that you are providing. If this is not possible, or patient is on Airborne Precautions, apply PPE outside of the room.

Proper preparation ensures protection from microorganism exposure. Allows patient to see you without PPE and without exposing yourself to risk of infection transmission.

a. Apply gown, being sure that it fully covers torso from neck to knees and from arms to end of wrist and wraps around the back, covering all outer garments (CDC, 2023a). Pull sleeves down to wrist. Tie securely at neck and waist (see illustration).

Prevents transmission of infection; protects you when patient has excessive drainage or discharges.

b. Apply either surgical mask or fitted respirator. Secure ties or elastic band at middle of head and neck. Next fit flexible band to nose bridge. Be sure mask or respirator fits snugly to face and below chin. Fit-check of respirator mask is required (see Box 9.2) (CDC, 2023d; NIOSH, 2021).

Prevents exposure to airborne microorganisms or microorganisms from splashing of fluids.
A respirator mask is a specialized filtering mask that provides a high level of protection against droplet and airborne transmitted diseases.

c. If needed, apply eyewear or goggles snugly around face and eyes. If you wear prescription glasses, side shields may be used.

Protects you from exposure to microorganisms that may occur during splashing of fluids.

d. Apply clean gloves (select according to hand size). (**NOTE:** Wear unpowdered, latex-free gloves if you, the patient, or another health care worker has latex allergy.) Bring glove cuffs over edge of gown sleeves (see illustration).

Reduces transmission of microorganisms.

Clinical Judgment *As you work in patient room, keep hands away from face. Work from clean to dirty surfaces (CDC, 2023a). If gloves become heavily soiled, remove and change to continue care activities.*

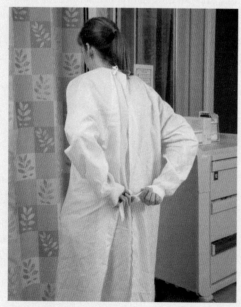

STEP 3a Tie isolation gown at waist.

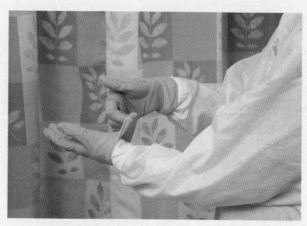

STEP 3d Apply gloves over edge of gown sleeves.

STEP	RATIONALE

BOX 9.2

Fit Testing for Respirator Masks

- The Occupational Safety and Health Administration (OSHA) (29 CFR 1910.134) requires a medical evaluation and a respirator fit test before the employee uses the respirator in the workplace (NIOSH, 2018; NIOSH, 2021).
- The test evaluates whether the respirator forms a tight seal on the employee's face to provide protection. The fit test benefits the employee by ensuring that the employee has the correct model and size of respirator (NIOSH, 2018; NIOSH, 2021).
- Fit testing is done with any tight-fitting respirator such as a filtering face piece respirator, elastomeric half and full face piece respirators, a self-contained breathing apparatus, and tight-fitting powered-air purifiers (NIOSH, 2021).
- A fit test is required annually and as needed if the health care employee experiences a change that could impact the seal (i.e., facial surgery, dental work)

- Fit testing is specific to the brand/model/size of a respirator. If a different respirator is to be used, the employee is required to have fit testing for the new model (NIOSH, 2021).
- Facial hair such as beards, sideburns, or moustaches, which grow along the face where the mask seals, interfere with the facepiece seal. This prevents the employee from achieving maximum protection with the respirator (NIOSH, 2018).
- Two types of fit testing exist (NIOSH, 2021):
  - Qualitative testing: This is a pass/fail test. The employee's sensory system must respond appropriately to a test agent while wearing the respirator. In this test, the test agent triggers a taste, smell, or involuntary cough in the employee.
  - Quantitative testing: Specific numeric value must be achieved. Test is done using an instrument to measure effectiveness of respirator mask.

---

4. Enter patient's room. Arrange supplies and equipment. (**NOTE:** If equipment will be reused, place on clean paper towel.)	Prevents extra trips entering and leaving room. Minimizes contamination of care items.
5. If patient is on TB precautions, instruct to cover mouth with tissue when coughing and to wear disposable surgical mask when leaving room.	Reduces TB microorganism transmission (CDC, 2023f).
6. Assess vital signs (see Chapter 5).	
a. If patient is infected or colonized with resistant organism (e.g., vancomycin-resistant enterococci [VRE], MRSA), equipment remains in room, including stethoscope and BP cuff (CDC, 2019b).	Decreases risk of infection being transmitted to another patient.
b. If stethoscope is to be reused, clean earpieces and diaphragm or bell with 70% alcohol or agency-approved germicide. Set aside on clean surface.	Systematic disinfection of stethoscopes with 70% alcohol or approved germicide minimizes chance of spreading infectious agents between patients (Boulée et al., 2019).
c. Use individual or disposable thermometers and BP cuffs when available.	Prevents cross-contamination.

Clinical Judgment *If disposable thermometer indicates a fever, assess for other signs/symptoms. Confirm fever using an alternative thermometer. Do not use electronic thermometer if patient is suspected or confirmed to have C. difficile infection (McDonald et al., 2018).*

7. Administer medications (see Chapters 20, 21, and 22).	
a. Give oral medication in wrapper or cup.	Handle and discard supplies to minimize transfer of microorganisms.
b. Dispose of wrapper or cup in plastic-lined receptacle.	
c. Continue wearing gloves when administering an injection.	Reduces risk of exposure to blood.
d. Discard needleless syringe or safety sheathed needle into designated sharps container.	Needleless devices should be used to reduce risk of needlesticks and sharps injuries to health care workers.
8. Administer hygiene. Encourage patient to ask any questions or express concerns about isolation. Provide informal teaching at this time.	Hygiene practices further minimize transfer of microorganisms. Quality time should be spent with patient when in room.
a. Avoid allowing isolation gown to become wet; carry wash basin outward away from gown; avoid leaning against wet tabletop.	Moisture allows organisms to travel through gown to uniform.

Clinical Judgment *When there is a risk for excess soiling, wear a gown impervious to moisture.*

b. Help patient remove own gown; discard in leak-proof linen bag.	Reduces transfer of microorganisms.
c. Remove linen from bed; avoid contact with isolation gown. Place in leak-proof linen bag.	Handle linen soiled by patient's body fluids to prevent contact with clean items.
d. Provide clean bed linen.	
e. Change gloves and perform hand hygiene if gloves become excessively soiled and further care is necessary. Re-glove.	Reduces transmission of microorganisms.

STEP	RATIONALE
9. Collect specimens (see Chapter 7).	
a. Place specimen container on clean paper towel in patient's bathroom and follow procedure for collecting specimen of body fluids.	Container will be taken out of patient's room; prevents contamination of outer surface.
b. Follow agency procedure for collecting specimen of body fluids (see Chapter 7).	
c. Transfer specimen to container without soiling outside of container. Place container in plastic bag and place label on outside of bag or per agency policy. Label specimen in front of patient (TJC, 2023). Perform hand hygiene and re-glove if additional procedures are needed.	Specimens of blood and body fluids are placed in well-constructed containers with secure lids to prevent leaks during transport. Proper labeling prevents diagnostic error.
d. Check label on specimen for accuracy. Send to laboratory (warning labels are often used, depending on agency policy). Label containers of blood or body fluids with biohazard sticker (see illustration).	Ensures that health care providers who transport or handle containers are aware of infectious contents.
10. Dispose of linen, trash, and disposable items.	
a. Use sturdy moisture-impervious bags to contain soiled articles. Use double bag, if necessary, for heavily soiled linen or heavy wet trash.	Linen or refuse should be contained totally to prevent exposure of personnel to infectious material.
b. Tie bags securely at top in knot (see illustration).	
11. Remove all reusable pieces of equipment. Clean any contaminated surfaces with hospital-approved disinfectant (Marra, 2019) (see agency policy).	All items must be properly cleaned, disinfected, or sterilized for reuse.
12. Resupply room as needed. Have staff colleague hand new supplies to you. Help patient to a comfortable position.	Limiting trips of personnel into and out of room reduces exposure to microorganisms. Restores comfort and sense of well-being.

Clinical Judgment *Before leaving the room, assess if the patient is experiencing negative effects of isolation, such as anxiety or depression. Spend time listening to the concerns expressed by the patient. Make sure the patient has access to a telephone, television, reading material, computer, and Internet as appropriate. These activities can help decrease the social isolation that may occur (Purssell et al., 2020).*

13. Leave isolation room. Order of removal of PPE depends on what you wear in room. This sequence describes steps to take if all barriers were worn. PPE worn in room must be removed before leaving room.	Order of removal minimizes exposure to any infectious material on barriers.
a. Remove gloves. Remember: outside of gloves is contaminated. Remove one glove by grasping cuff and pulling glove inside out over hand. Hold removed glove in gloved hand (see illustration) while sliding fingers of ungloved hand under remaining glove at wrist. Peel glove off over first glove. Discard gloves in proper waste container.	Technique prevents contact with contaminated outer surface of glove. Change gloves between exposures to body sites and patient equipment. Inadequate glove changes and hand hygiene can lead to contamination, increasing the risk of health care–associated infections (HAIs) (CDC, 2019b).

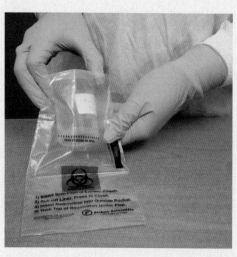

STEP 9d Place specimen container in biohazard bag.

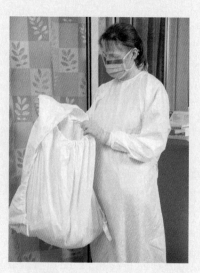

STEP 10b Tie bag securely.

STEP	RATIONALE

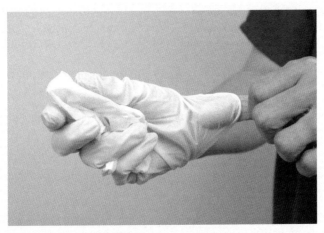

STEP 13a Remove gloves.

b. Remove eyewear, face shield, or goggles. Handle by headband or earpieces. Discard in proper waste container.

Outside of goggles/eyewear is contaminated. Hands have not been soiled.

c. Remove gown. Untie neck strings and then untie back strings of gown. Allow gown to fall from shoulders (see illustration); touch inside of gown only. Remove hands from sleeves without touching outside of gown. Hold gown inside at shoulder seams and fold inside out into bundle; discard in proper waste container.

Hands do not come in contact with soiled front of gown.

d. Remove mask. If mask secures over ears, remove elastic from ears and pull mask away from face. For tie-on mask, untie *bottom* mask string and then top strings, pull mask away from face (see illustration A), and drop into proper waste container (see illustration B). (Do not touch outer surface of mask.)

Ungloved hands are not contaminated by touching only elastic or mask strings. Prevents top part of mask from falling down over uniform.

Clinical Judgment *If patient is on TB precautions, place reusable mask in labeled paper bag for storage, being careful not to crush mask (check agency policy for number of times reusable masks can be used).*

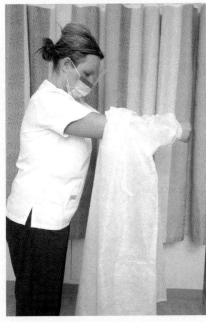

STEP 13c Remove gown by allowing it to fall from shoulders.

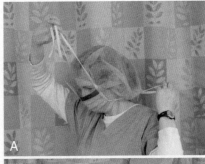
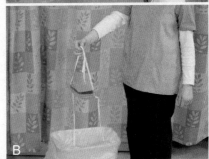

STEP 13d (A) Pull mask away from face. (B) Drop into trash receptacle.

STEP	RATIONALE
e. Perform hand hygiene. If patient is being treated for *C. difficile* infection, clean hands with soap and water.	Reduces transmission of microorganisms. Alcohol-based hand rubs are not effective against the spores of *C. difficile*.
f. Retrieve wristwatch and stethoscope (unless items must remain in room).	
g. Explain to patient when you plan to return to room. Ask whether patient requires any personal care items. Offer books, magazines, and audiotapes.	Diversions can help to minimize boredom and feeling of social isolation.
h. Raise side rails (as appropriate) and lower bed to lowest position, locking into position.	Ensures patient safety and prevents falls.
i. Place nurse call system in an accessible location within patient's reach.	Ensures patient can call for assistance if needed.
j. Dispose of all contaminated supplies and equipment in proper manner (see agency policy). Perform hand hygiene.	Prevents transmission of microorganisms.
k. Leave room and close door if necessary. Close door if patient is on Airborne Precautions or in negative-airflow room.	Maintains negative-airflow environment and reduces transmission of microorganisms.

EVALUATION

1. Observe patient's and family caregiver's use of isolation precautions when visiting.	Promptly identifies any improper use of a precaution.
2. While in room, ask if patient has had sufficient chance to discuss health problems, course of treatment, or other topics important to the patient.	Measures patient's perception of adequacy of discussions with caregivers.
3. **Use Teach-Back:** "I want to be sure I explained when these precautions for reducing infection are needed. Tell me what you will do to reduce the spread of infection while in your room." Revise your instruction now or develop a plan for revised patient/family caregiver teaching if patient/family caregiver is not able to teach back correctly.	Teach-back is a technique for health care providers to ensure that they have explained medical information clearly so that patients and their families understand what is communicated to them (AHRQ, 2023b).

Unexpected Outcomes

1. Patient avoids social and therapeutic discussions.

2. Patient or health care worker displays symptoms of latex allergy.

Related Interventions

- Confer with family caregiver and/or significant other and determine best approach to reduce patient's sense of loneliness and depression.
- Notify health care provider/employee health and treat sensitivity or allergic reaction appropriately.
- Use latex-free gloves for future care activities.

Documentation

- Document procedures performed and patient's response to social isolation. Also document any patient or family caregiver education performed and reinforced.
- Document type of isolation in use and the microorganisms (if known).

Hand-Off Reporting

- Share type of isolation precautions and how patient has been responding to social isolation.
- Share any related infectious disease testing results.

Special Considerations

Patient Education

- Teach visitors and family caregivers how to follow the recommended isolation precautions when visiting a patient.

Pediatrics

- Isolation creates a sense of separation from family and loss of control. A strange environment adds to the confusion that a child feels during isolation. Preschoolers are unable to understand the cause-effect relationship for isolation. Older children may be able to understand cause but still fantasize. Initiate age-appropriate activities that can be done in the isolation room for the child.

- Children require simple explanations (e.g., "You need to be in this room to help you get better.") Show all barriers to a child. Actively involve parents in any explanations. Let the child see your face before applying a mask so that the child does not become frightened.

Older Adults

- Isolation can be a particular concern for older adults, especially those who have signs and symptoms of anxiety, confusion, or depression. Many times, patients become more confused when confronted with a nurse using barrier precautions or when left in a room with the door closed (Purssell et al., 2020). Nurses must assess need for closing a door (negative-airflow room) along with safety of patient and additional safety measures that may need to be taken.
- Assess older adults for signs of depression such as loss of appetite or decrease in verbal communications. If necessary, report to the health care team for appropriate interventions.

Home Care

- Although isolation precautions followed in the hospital are not directly applicable to home care, caregivers should be aware of potential sources of contamination in the home.

✦ CLINICAL JUDGMENT AND NEXT GENERATION NCLEX® EXAMINATION–STYLE QUESTIONS

An 86-year-old patient is admitted to an acute care hospital from home. The patient reports pain all over the body after falling earlier in the day after a period of sudden dizziness. The nurse reviews the electronic health record (EHR), which documents a history of hypertension and heart failure. The medication record includes lisinopril 10 mg once daily, metoprolol 25 mg once daily, furosemide 20 mg once daily, and digoxin 0.125 mg once daily. VS: BP 118/82 mm Hg, pulse 58 beats/min, RR 20 breaths/min, T 37.2°C (99.2°F) and SpO$_2$ 98% on room air. Physical assessment reveals numerous new and faded bruises on the patient's face, left arm, and legs. There is a 1-cm (0.4-inch) open wound on the left elbow. The nurse assists the patient with removing pants and notes dampness and two soaked incontinence pads. The patient acknowledges ongoing incontinence issues. There is a 2 × 2–cm (0.78 x 0.78–inch) open wound on the coccyx, which is draining a moderate amount of thin yellow fluid.

1. Complete the following sentence by selecting from the list of word choices below.

The assessment findings that require immediate follow-up include **[Word Choice]**, **[Word Choice]**, and **[Word Choice]**.

Word Choices
Dizziness
Elbow wound
BP 118/82
Pulse 58 beats/min
SPO$_2$ 98%
Open wound on coccyx
Urinary incontinence
T 37.2°C (99.2°F)

2. The nurse is preparing to clean and dress the patient's wounds. Which action will the nurse take before performing these tasks?
   1. Clean hands with betadine
   2. Rub alcohol wipes over hands
   3. Wash hands with soap and water
   4. Perform a surgical scrub on the hands

3. The patient is diagnosed with MRSA. Which type of precaution will the nurse institute by the nature of MRSA's transmission?
   1. Contact
   2. Droplet
   3. Airborne
   4. Standard only

4. After providing hygiene care, which action will the nurse take **first** before exiting the patient's room?
   1. Remove gloves one at a time
   2. Untie neck string of gown
   3. Take off face mask
   4. Perform hand hygiene

5. While hospitalized, the patient's fever increases, and a diagnosis of tuberculosis is made. Which type of precaution will the nurse institute at this time?
   1. Contact
   2. Droplet
   3. Airborne
   4. Standard only

Visit the Evolve site for Answers to Clinical Judgment and Next Generation NCLEX® Examination–Style Questions.

REFERENCES

Agency for Healthcare Research and Quality (AHRQ): *AHRQ's healthcare-associated infections program*, 2023. https://www.ahrq.gov/hai/index.html. Accessed November 26, 2023.

Agency for Healthcare Research and Quality (AHRQ): *Teach-back: intervention*, 2023. https://www.ahrq.gov/patient-safety/reports/engage/interventions/teachback.html.

Association of periOperative Registered Nurses (AORN): *Guidelines for perioperative practice*, Denver, 2021, AORN.

Boulée D, et al: Contemporary stethoscope cleaning practices: What we haven't learned in 150 years, *Am J Infect Control* 47(3):238–242, 2019. doi:10.1016/j.ajic.2018.08.005.

Broussard I, Kahwaji I: Universal precautions. In: *StatPearls* [Internet]. Treasure Island, FL, 2023, StatPearls Publishing. https://www.ncbi.nlm.nih.gov/books/NBK470223/. Accessed November 26, 2023.

Casadevall A, Pirofski L: What is a host? Attributes of individual susceptibility, *Infect Immun* 86(2):e00636-17, 2018. doi:10.1128/IAI.00636-17. https://iai.asm.org/content/86/2/e00636-17. Accessed November 26, 2023.

Centers for Disease Control and Prevention (CDC): *Interferon-Gamma Release Assays (IGRAs) – blood tests for TB infection*, 2016a. https://www.cdc.gov/tb/publications/factsheets/testing/igra.htm. Accessed November 26, 2023.

Centers for Disease Control and Prevention (CDC): *Transmission-based precautions*, 2016b. https://www.cdc.gov/infectioncontrol/basics/transmission-based-precautions.html. Accessed November 26, 2023.

Centers for Disease Control and Prevention (CDC): *Antibiotic resistant infections in the United States*, 2019a. https://www.cdc.gov/drugresistance/pdf/threats-report/2019-ar-threats-report-508.pdf. Accessed November 26, 2023.

Centers for Disease Control and Prevention (CDC): *Infection control in healthcare personnel: infrastructure and routine practices for occupational infection prevention and control services*, 2019b. https://www.cdc.gov/infectioncontrol/pdf/guidelines/infection-control-HCP-H.pdf. Accessed November 26, 2023.

Centers for Disease Control and Prevention (CDC): *TB infection control in healthcare settings*, 2019c. https://www.cdc.gov/tb/topic/infectioncontrol/TBhealthCareSettings.htm. Accessed November 26, 2023.

Centers for Disease Control and Prevention (CDC): *Hand hygiene in healthcare settings: healthcare providers*, 2021a. https://www.cdc.gov/handhygiene/providers/index.html. Accessed November 28, 2023.

Centers for Disease Control and Prevention (CDC): *Methicillin-resistant Staphylococcus aureus*, Atlanta, 2021b, Centers for Disease Control and Prevention.

Centers for Disease Control and Prevention (CDC): *When and how to wash your hands*, 2022. http://www.cdc.gov/features/handwashing. Accessed November 26, 2023.

Centers for Disease Control and Prevention (CDC), Siegel JD, Healthcare Infection Control Practices Advisory Committee: *2007 Guideline for isolation precautions: preventing transmission of infectious agents in healthcare settings—recommendations to the Healthcare Infection Control Practices Advisory Committee (HICPAC), Updated 2019*, Washington, DC, 2023a, CDC. http://www.cdc.gov/hicpac/2007IP/2007isolationPrecautions.html. Accessed November 28, 2023.

Centers for Disease Control and Prevention (CDC): *Hand hygiene in healthcare settings: show me the science*, 2023b. https://www.cdc.gov/handhygiene/science/index.html. Accessed November 28, 2023.

Centers for Disease Control and Prevention (CDC): *Handwashing in communities: clean hands save lives*, 2023c. https://www.cdc.gov/handwashing/index.html. Accessed November 28, 2023.

Centers for Disease Control and Prevention (CDC): *Isolation precautions*, 2023d. https://www.cdc.gov/infectioncontrol/guidelines/isolation/index.html. Accessed November 28, 2023.

Centers for Disease Control and Prevention (CDC): *Show me the science: when to use hand sanitizers in community settings*, 2023e. Accessed November 28, 2023.

Centers for Disease Control and Prevention (CDC): *Tuberculosis*, 2023f. https://www.cdc.gov/tb/default.htm. Accessed November 28, 2023.

Centers for Disease Control and Prevention (CDC): *Types of masks and respirators*, 2023g. https://www.cdc.gov/coronavirus/2019-ncov/prevent-getting-sick/types-of-masks.html#:~:text=CDC%20recommends%20that%20specially%20labeled,for%20use%20by%20healthcare%20personnel. Accessed November 28, 2023.

Centers for Disease Control and Prevention (CDC): *What is health literacy*, 2023h. https://www.cdc.gov/healthliteracy/learn/index.html.

Chadwick C: Infection control 4: good hand-hygiene practice for hospital patients. *Nursing Times* 115(9):27–29, 2019.

Cole B, et al: Essential Components of a Public Health Tuberculosis Prevention, Control, and Elimination Program: Recommendations of the Advisory Council for the Elimination of Tuberculosis and the National Tuberculosis Controllers Association, *MMWR* 69(7):1–27, 2020. https://www.cdc.gov/mmwr/volumes/69/rr/rr6907a1.htm. Accessed November 26, 2023.

Davis E, et al: Epidemiology of Vancomycin-Resistant *Enterococcus faecium* and *Enterococcus faecalis* colonization in nursing facilities, *Open Forum Inf Dis* 7(1):ofz553, 2020.

Denton A, Hallam C: Principles of asepsis 1: the rationale for using aseptic technique. *Nursing Times* 116:38–41, 2020. https://www.nursingtimes.net/clinical-archive/infection-control/principles-of-asepsis-1-the-rationale-for-using-aseptic-technique-14-04-2020/. Accessed November 26, 2023.

Giger J, Haddad L: *Transcultural nursing: assessment and intervention*, ed 8, St. Louis, 2021, Elsevier.

Gupta MK, Lipner SR: Hand hygiene in preventing COVID-19 transmission, *Cutis* 105(5):233–234, 2020.

Health Protection Surveillance Centre: *A strategy for the control of antimicrobial resistance in Ireland*, 2022. https://www.lenus.ie/bitstream/handle/10147/43701/3916.pdf;jsessionid=E006F3B509E08FF4737221A5870F4184!sequence=1. Accessed November 26, 2023.

Hillier MD: Using effective hand hygiene practice to prevent and control infection, *Nurs Stand* 35(5):45–50, 2020. doi:10.7748/ns.2020.e11552.

Kiersnowska ZM, et al: Hand hygiene as the basic method of reducing *Clostridium difficile* infections (CDI) in a hospital environment, *Ann Agric Environ Med* 28(4):535–540, 2021.

Lastinger A, et al: Use of a patient empowerment tool for hand hygiene, *Am J Infect Control* 45(8):824–829, 2017. doi:10.1016/j.ajic.2017.02.010.

Manresa Y, et al: Improving patients' hand hygiene in the acute care setting: Is staff education enough? *Am J Infect Control* 48(9):1100–1101, 2020.

Marra A: *Hospital infection control: proper isolation procedures*, 2019. https://www.infectiousdiseaseadvisor.com/home/decision-support-in-medicine/hospital-infection-control/proper-isolation-procedures/. Accessed November 26, 2023.

McDonald E: *Clinical practice guidelines for clostridium difficile infection in adults and children: 2017 update by the Infectious Diseases Society of America (IDSA) and Society for Healthcare Epidemiology of America (SHEA)*, 2018. https://www.idsociety.org/practice-guideline/clostridium-difficile/. Accessed November 26, 2023.

Monegro AF, et al: Hospital-acquired infections. In: *StatPearls* [Internet]. Treasure Island, FL, 2023, StatPearls Publishing. https://www.ncbi.nlm.nih.gov/books/NBK441857/. Accessed November 28, 2023.

National Institute for Occupational Safety and Health (NIOSH): *Filtering out confusion: frequently asked questions about respiratory protection, fit testing.* By Krah J., Shamblin M., and Shaffer R. Pittsburgh, PA: U.S. Department of Health and Human Services, Centers for Disease Control and Prevention, National Institute for Occupational Safety and Health, DHHS (NIOSH) Publication 2018–129, 2018. https://doi.org/10.26616/NIOSHPUB2018129. Accessed November 26, 2023.

National Institute for Occupational Safety and Health (NIOSH): *The respiratory protection information trusted source: Fit test FAQs*, 2021. https://www.cdc.gov/niosh/npptl/topics/respirators/disp_part/respsource3fittest.html. Accessed November 26, 2023.

Occupational Safety and Health Administration (OSHA): *Infectious disease: final rule*, 29 CFR Part 1910, *Fed Reg* 75:87, 2011.

Purssell E, et al: Impact of isolation on hospitalised patients who are infectious: systematic review with meta-analysis, *BMJ Open* 10:e030371, 2020. doi:10.1136/bmjopen-2019-030371.

Sands M, Aunger R: Determinants of hand hygiene compliance among nurses in US hospitals: a formative research study, *PLoS One* 15(4):e0230573, 2020. https://doi.org/10.1371/journal.pone.0230573. Accessed November 26, 2023.

Szczuka Z, et al: The trajectory of COVID-19 pandemic and handwashing adherence: findings from 14 countries, *BMC Public Health* 21(1):1791, 2021.

Tejiram S, Sava J: Emergency general surgery in the immunocompromised surgical patient. In Brown C, Inaba K, Martin M, et al., editors: *Emergency general surgery*, Cham, 2019, Springer.

The Joint Commission (TJC): *2023 National patient safety goals*, Oakbrook Terrace, IL, 2023, The Joint Commission. https://www.jointcommission.org/standards/national-patient-safety-goals/.

Toney-Butler TJ, et al: Hand hygiene. [Updated 2023 July]. In: *StatPearls* [Internet]. Treasure Island (FL): StatPearls Publishing; 2023 July. https://www.ncbi.nlm.nih.gov/books/NBK470254/. Accessed November 26, 2023.

Virology Research Services: *What determines susceptibility to virus infection?* 2019. https://virologyresearchservices.com/2019/07/29/susceptibility-to-virus/#:~:text=Multiple%20innate%20factors%20(e.g.%2C%20age,person%20exposed%20to%20a%20virus. Accessed November 26, 2023.

Wałaszek MZ, et al: Nail microbial colonization following hand disinfection: a qualitative pilot study, *J Hosp Infect* 100(2):207–210, 2018.

World Health Organization (WHO): *Hand hygiene for all initiative: improving access and behaviour in health care facilities*, 2020. https://www.who.int/publications/i/item/9789240011618. Accessed November 26, 2023.

World Health Organization (WHO): *SAVE LIVES—clean your hands: annual global campaign*, 2021. https://www.who.int/campaigns/world-hand-hygiene-day. Accessed November 26, 2023.

World Health Organization (WHO): *The evidence for clean hands*, 2022. https://www.who.int/teams/integrated-health-services/infection-prevention-control/hand-hygiene/guidelines-and-evidence. Accessed November 26, 2023.

Yoon S, et al: *Importance of patient hand hygiene education and accessibility of hand sanitizers*, 2020. https://infectioncontrol.tips/2020/10/22/importance-of-patient-hand-hygiene-education-and-accessibility-of-hand-sanitizers/. Accessed November 26, 2023.

10 | Sterile Technique

SKILLS AND PROCEDURES

Skill 10.1 **Applying and Removing Cap, Mask, and Protective Eyewear, p. 279**

Skill 10.2 **Preparing a Sterile Field, p. 282**

Skill 10.3 **Sterile Gloving, p. 287**

OBJECTIVES

Mastery of content in this chapter will enable you to:
- Discuss settings where surgical aseptic techniques are necessary.
- Explain conditions when surgical asepsis is necessary.
- Identify the principles of surgical asepsis.
- Explain the importance of organization and caution when using surgical aseptic techniques.

- Apply and remove a cap, mask, and protective eyewear correctly.
- Identify individuals at risk for a latex allergy.
- Demonstrate the following skills: preparing a sterile field, applying sterile gloves using open-glove method, and applying a sterile drape correctly.
- Utilize principles of surgical asepsis to maintain a sterile field.

MEDIA RESOURCES

- http://evolve.elsevier.com/Perry/skills
- Clinical Review Questions
- Audio Glossary
- ▶ Video Clips

- **NSO** Nursing Skills Online
- Answers to Clinical Judgment and Next-Generation NCLEX® Examination–Style Questions
- Skills Performance Checklists
- Printable Key Points

PURPOSE

Sterile technique and aseptic practices maintain an area that is free from pathogenic organisms, serve to isolate an operative area from the unsterile environment, and maintain a sterile field for surgery and invasive procedures. Proper sterile asepsis minimizes patient exposure to infection-causing agents, thus reducing the patient's risk for infection. These techniques are common in the operating room (OR), labor and delivery area, and major diagnostic areas, but they are also used at the bedside (e.g., when inserting an intravenous [IV] line or urinary catheter).

PRACTICE STANDARDS

- Association of periOperative Registered Nurses (AORN), 2023: Guidelines for Perioperative Practice
- Centers for Disease Control and Prevention (CDC): 2022: CDCs Core Infection Prevention and Control Practices for Safe Healthcare Delivery in All Settings
- The Joint Commission (TJC), 2023: National Patient Safety Goals—Patient identification

PRINCIPLES FOR PRACTICE

- The majority of sterile technique practices are used in the OR or in diagnostic procedure areas, including applying a mask, protective eyewear, and a cap; performing a surgical hand scrub; applying a sterile gown; and applying sterile gloves.

- Medical asepsis is the use of procedures to decrease the number of microorganisms and prevent spread of infection. As with medical asepsis, proper hand hygiene with an appropriate cleaner or antiseptic is required before initiating any sterile procedure.
- Surgical aseptic technique is also used at the bedside in the following situations: during procedures that require intentional puncture of the skin or insertion of devices into an area of the body that is normally sterile (e.g., sterile dressing change) or in a situation in which skin integrity is compromised because of incision or burn (Box 10.1).
- When sterile procedures are carried out in the OR or procedure area, health care providers must follow a series of steps to maintain sterile asepsis: applying a mask, protective eyewear, and cap; performing a surgical hand scrub; and applying a sterile gown and gloves.
- When sterile procedures such as a sterile dressing change are carried out at the bedside, the health care provider must perform hand hygiene and apply sterile gloves. When the risk of splash is present, other personal protective equipment (PPE) is required.
- When completing a sterile procedure at the bedside, communicate with the patient about which steps are being taken to prevent infection, including which actions the patient should avoid to keep the field sterile. These actions include avoiding sudden body movements, refraining from touching sterile supplies, and avoiding coughing or talking over the sterile area.

Principles of Surgical Asepsis

1. All items used within a sterile field must be sterile.
2. A sterile barrier that has been permeated by punctures, tears, or moisture must be considered contaminated.
3. Once a sterile package is opened, a 2.5-cm (1-inch) border around the edges is considered unsterile.
4. Tables draped as part of a sterile field are considered sterile only at table level.
5. If there is any question or doubt about the sterility of an item, the item is considered to be unsterile.
6. Sterile people or items contact only sterile areas; unsterile people or items contact only unsterile areas.
7. Movement around and in the sterile field must not compromise or contaminate the field.
8. A sterile object or field out of the range of vision or an object held below a person's waist is contaminated.
9. A sterile object or field becomes contaminated by prolonged exposure to air; stay organized and complete any procedure as soon as possible.

PERSON-CENTERED CARE

- Whether performed in a hospital, ambulatory care setting, the patient's home, or health care provider's office, invasive procedures such as starting an intravenous (IV) line or inserting a urinary catheter pose a risk for infection. It is your responsibility to protect patients from infection by adhering strictly to the principles of surgical asepsis when performing invasive procedures or when helping with such a procedure and to intervene to stop it when a break in sterile technique occurs. TJC encourages nurses to "speak up" in these instances (TJC, 2023).
- Perioperative nurses practice "surgical conscience," a moral obligation to guard surgical asepsis and protect patients by reducing preventable adverse events that often lead to poor patient outcomes (Duff et al., 2022). The nurse knows correct surgical asepsis practices and patient safety principles and recognizes when the principles are not followed. The nurse feels bad (conscience) about patient safety and takes action to correct the problem and prevent adverse patient outcomes (Duff et al., 2022).
- Take into consideration the patient's cultural background or beliefs when sterile asepsis is required. Individualized patient-centered education for patients and family caregivers before any aseptic procedure reduces fears and misconceptions about sterile asepsis attire. This also provides an opportunity for patients and family caregivers to ask questions and express their concerns regarding surgical attire.

EVIDENCE-BASED PRACTICE

Preventing Surgical Site Infections

Recommendations for prevention of surgical site infections (SSIs), such as performing patient-centered education, inserting devices only when necessary, using sterile technique, and removing devices that are no longer needed, have decreased the number of health care–associated SSIs. SSIs are associated with a twofold to elevenfold increase in mortality; are the costliest health care–associated

infection (HAI), with an estimated annual cost of $3.3 billion; and are associated with an average extended hospital stay of 9.7 days and additional cost of $20,000 per patient experiencing an SSI (CDC, 2023a). Prevention of SSI is a complex process that requires nursing intervention before, during, and after surgery (Boga, 2019). Prevention is supported by the following nursing interventions:

- Prevention of contamination of a sterile work area can be done by minimizing traffic; comprehensive cleaning and disinfecting; changing skin preparation; administering antibiotics; and removing watches, jewelry, and artificial nails (CDC, 2021; Tennat & Rivers, 2021; Wałaszek et al., 2018).
- Covering a sterile field with a sterile cover protects the field from bacterial contamination and maintains the sterility of the field for up to 24 hours (Wistrand et al., 2021).
- Use of additional antiseptics such as chlorhexidine reduces bacterial count on the patient's skin (AORN, 2023; Christian et al., 2020; Seidelman et al., 2023). Avoid removing hair at the surgical site unless necessary. If hair removal is necessary, use clippers rather than a razor before the patient enters the operating room (Institute for Healthcare Improvement [IHI], 2023; Seidelman et al., 2023).
- Collaborate with health care provider to maintain patient glucose less than 150 mg/dL during and after surgery (IHI, 2023; Seidelman et al., 2023).
- Most health care agencies have policies against artificial nails, gels, and acrylic overlays (Aluise et al., 2020; Blackburn et al., 2020). The subungual area (under a fingernail) of the hand contains a high concentration of bacteria, more specifically coagulase-negative staphylococci and gram-negative rods, and fungal growth. These organisms are not removed effectively after hand hygiene.
- Preoperative prevention measures support using a dual agent (e.g., alcohol plus iodine or chlorhexidine) skin preparation. Intraoperative measures include using wound edge protectors for abdominal procedures and using triclosan-coated antibacterial sutures (Andersen, 2019). Evidence supports use of postoperative prevention measures including negative pressure wound therapy for high-risk procedures such as abdominal and vascular cases (Shiroky et al., 2020).

SAFETY GUIDELINES

- Follow Standard Precautions with all patients (CDC, 2022; TJC, 2023).
- Review agency policies and procedures before performing a sterile procedure.
- Assess the potential for splash and/or transmission of infection before choosing the barrier to be used, such as masks or protective eyewear.
- Nurses use barrier techniques to decrease the transmission of microorganisms from health care personnel and the environment to a patient.
- Remain organized while performing any sterile procedure; keep bedside surfaces free of clutter.
- Remember that hand hygiene is essential before and after initiating any sterile procedure to reduce HAIs (Singhal et al., 2023; Toney-Butler et al., 2022).
- Apply the principles of surgical asepsis when conducting any sterile procedure.

♦ SKILL 10.1 Applying and Removing Cap, Mask, and Protective Eyewear

Although masks and caps are usually worn in surgical procedure areas (e.g., the operating room [OR]), certain aseptic procedures performed at a patient's bedside also require the application of additional personal protective equipment (PPE), such as eyewear, gown, and gloves. For example, it may be agency policy for a nurse to wear a mask during the changing of a central line dressing or insertion of a peripherally inserted central catheter (PICC). Other policies might require that a nurse wear a mask and a cap to secure hair during dressing changes on a patient with extensive burns or a central line (Gorski et al., 2021). During the COVID-19 pandemic, health care agency policies required employees to wear masks indoors, when in close contact with others, and if there was a possibility the employee would be exposed to or in contact with someone with the COVID-19 virus; many health care agencies continue to enforce these policies post pandemic (OSHA, 2021). When there is a risk of splattering blood or body fluid, there is also the need to apply protective eyewear (Association of Surgical Technologists [AST], 2017). This skill summarizes how to apply a mask, cap, and protective eyewear, which are not considered sterile. The additional application of clean or sterile gloves depends on the type of procedure being performed.

Assess a patient's potential for acquiring an infection and the splash risk before deciding whether to apply a mask (e.g., Does the patient have a large open wound? Is the patient immunosuppressed? Is there a splash risk from the wound?). If you wear a mask, change it when it becomes moist or soiled (e.g., splattered with blood). Wear eyewear when there is a risk of body fluids splashing into your eyes.

Delegation

The skill of applying and removing cap, mask, and protective eyewear is required of all health care providers when working in areas in which sterile procedures are performed. However, the procedures performed at a patient's bedside that require a cap, mask, or eyewear generally cannot be delegated to assistive personnel (AP). The skill of applying PPE can be delegated to the AP. Instruct the AP:

- To be available to hand off equipment or help with patient positioning during a sterile procedure; the AP is not trained to hand off items to a sterile field
- Regarding the importance of not contaminating the sterile field

Interprofessional Collaboration

- Members of the health care team should serve as role models for one another and provide reminders when sterile technique is missed or incomplete.

Equipment

- Surgical mask (different types are available for people with different skin sensitivities)
- Surgical cap (**NOTE:** Use in OR, outpatient surgery, and labor and delivery suites, or if agency policy requires in specific departments or during sterile procedures at the bedside. Use to secure hair if there is a possibility of contamination of a sterile field.)
- Hairpins, rubber bands, or both
- Protective eyewear (e.g., goggles or glasses with appropriate side shields). *Option:* Clean or sterile gloves (applied after cap, mask, or eyewear are applied). See Chapter 9 and Skill 10.3.

STEP	RATIONALE

ASSESSMENT

1. Review type of sterile procedure to be performed and consult agency policy for use of mask/caps/protective eyewear.

Not all sterile procedures require a mask, cap, or protective eyewear. Ensures that nurse and patient are properly protected.

2. If you or other health care providers have symptoms of a respiratory infection, either avoid participating in procedure or apply a mask.

A greater number of pathogenic microorganisms reside within the respiratory tract when infection is present.

3. Assess patient's risk for infection (e.g., older adult, neonate, or immunocompromised patient).

Some patients are at a greater risk for acquiring an infection; thus, use additional protective barriers.

Clinical Judgment *Related factors and risk factors are individualized based on patient's condition or needs.*

PLANNING

1. Expected outcome following completion of procedure:
   - Patient does not develop signs of localized infection (e.g., redness, tenderness, edema, drainage) or systemic infection (e.g., fever, change in white blood cell [WBC] count) 24 hours after procedure.

Indicates lack of microorganism transfer to patient and sterile field.

2. Prepare equipment and inspect packaging for integrity and exposure to sterilization.

Ensures availability of equipment and sterility of supplies before procedure begins.

IMPLEMENTATION

1. Perform hand hygiene (see Chapter 9).

Reduces transient microorganisms on skin.

2. *Option:* In cases in which you are performing or assisting with a procedure at a patient's bedside, apply a clean gown if there is a risk of splatter or soiling. Apply the gown with opening to the back. Be sure that it covers all outer garments. Pull sleeves down to wrist. Tie securely at neck and wrist.

Proper gowning prevents transmission of infections when patient has excessive drainage or discharges.

STEP	RATIONALE

3. Prepare to apply a cap.

   a. If hair is long, comb back behind ears and secure.

   b. Secure hair in place with pins.

   c. Apply cap over head as you would apply hairnet. Be sure that all hair fits under edges of cap (see illustration).

4. Apply a mask.

   a. Find top edge of mask, which usually has thin metal strip along edge.

   b. Hold mask by top two strings or loops, keeping top edge above bridge of nose.

   c. Tie two top strings at top of back of head, over cap (if worn), with strings above ears (see illustration). Alternatively, place loops over ears.

   d. Tie two lower ties snugly around neck with mask well under chin (see illustration).

   e. Gently pinch upper metal band around bridge of nose.

5. Apply protective eyewear.

   a. Apply protective glasses, goggles, or face shield comfortably over eyes and check that vision is clear (see illustration).

   b. Be sure that face shield fits snugly around forehead and face.

Rationale column:

Cap must cover all hair entirely.

Long hair should not fall down or cause cap to slip and expose hair.

Loose hair hanging over sterile field or falling dander contaminates objects on sterile field.

Pliable metal fits snugly against bridge of nose.

Position prevents contact of hands with clean facial part of mask. Mask covers all of nose.

Position of ties at top of head provides tight fit. Strings over ears may cause irritation.

Tying prevents escape of microorganisms through sides of mask as you talk and breathe.

Pinching prevents microorganisms from escaping around nose and eyeglasses from steaming up.

Positioning affects clarity of vision.

Snug fitting ensures that eyes are fully protected.

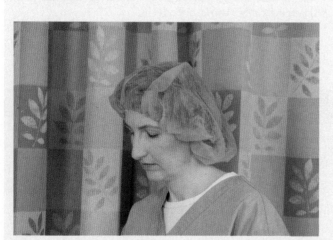

STEP 3c Apply cap over head, covering all hair.

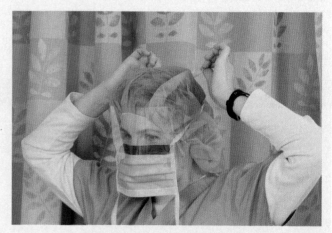

STEP 4c Tie top strings of mask.

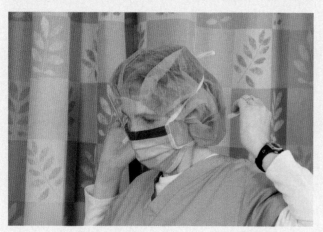

STEP 4d Tie bottom strings of mask.

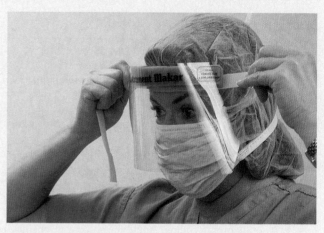

STEP 5a Apply face shield over cap.

STEP	RATIONALE

6. If performing a sterile procedure, apply sterile gown (see Skill 37.2) at this time. After applying cap, mask, and eyewear, you will apply clean gloves for nonsterile procedures and sterile gloves (see Skill 10.3) for sterile procedures. Pull up clean gloves to cover each wrist (see illustration). **NOTE:** Provide a latex-free environment if patient or health care worker has a latex allergy.

7. Remove protective barriers.
   a. Remove gloves first if worn (see Chapter 9 or Skill 10.3). Remove gloves by grasping cuff and pulling glove inside out over hand. Hold removed glove in hand. Slide fingers of ungloved hand under remaining glove at wrist (see illustration). Peel glove off over first glove. Discard gloves in proper container.

   Proper removal prevents contamination of hair, neck, and facial area.

   b. Remove eyewear. Avoid placing hands over soiled lens. **NOTE:** If wearing a face shield, remove it before removing mask.

   Proper removal prevents transmission of microorganisms.

   c. Remove gown by unfastening neck ties and pulling away from neck and shoulders. Touching only inside of gown, turn gown inside out, roll or fold into a bundle, and discard.

   Front and sleeves of gown are contaminated. This method of disposal prevents transmission of infection.

   d. Untie bottom strings of mask. First hold strings, untie top strings, and pull mask away from face while holding strings. Remove mask from face and discard in proper receptacle (see illustrations).

   Proper removal prevents top part of mask from falling down over uniform. If mask falls and touches uniform, uniform will be contaminated.

   e. Grasp outer surface of cap and lift from hair.
   f. Discard cap in proper receptacle and perform hand hygiene.

   Proper removal minimizes contact of hands with hair. Routine reduces transmission of infection.

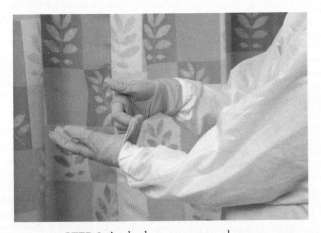

STEP 6 Apply gloves over gown sleeves.

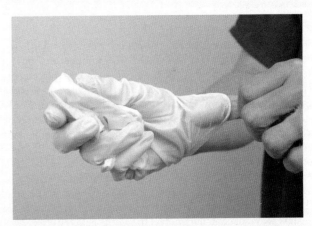

STEP 7a Remove second glove while holding soiled glove.

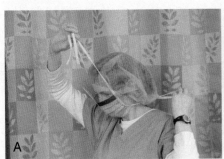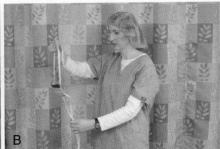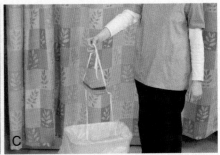

STEP 7d (A) Untie top mask strings. (B) Remove mask from face. (C) Discard mask.

STEP	RATIONALE

EVALUATION

1. Following the procedure, assess patient for signs of systemic infections or local area of body treated for drainage, tenderness, edema, or redness.

2. **Use Teach-Back:** "I want to be sure I explained why personal protective equipment is used. Please explain to me why you and your family caregiver need to wear personal protective equipment and show me how you will put it on." Revise your instruction now or develop a plan for revised patient/family caregiver teaching if patient/family caregiver is not able to teach back correctly.

Assessment rules out presence of localized infection.

Teach-back is a technique for health care providers to ensure that medical information has been explained clearly so that patients and families understand what is communicated to them (Agency for Healthcare Research and Quality [AHRQ], 2023).

Unexpected Outcomes

1. Redness, heat, edema, pain, or purulent drainage develops at wound or treatment site 2 or more days following the surgical procedure, indicating possible infection.

Related Interventions

- Notify health care provider of change in condition of affected area and initiate appropriate treatments as ordered.

Documentation

- No documentation is required for using PPE.

Hand-Off Reporting

- No reporting required for using PPE.

Special Considerations
Home Care

- Instruct family caregiver about specifics of when to use PPE and how to dispose of it properly.
- Determine ability of family caregiver to use equipment safely.
- Observe for signs and symptoms of infection.

✦ SKILL 10.2 Preparing a Sterile Field

 Video Clip

When performing sterile aseptic procedures, you need a sterile work area in which objects can be handled with minimal risk for contamination. A sterile field provides a sterile surface for placement of sterile equipment. Sterile drapes establish a sterile field around a treatment site such as a surgical incision, venipuncture site, or site for introduction of an indwelling urinary catheter. Sterile drapes also provide a work surface for placing sterile supplies and manipulating items with sterile gloves. After a sterile kit is opened, the inside surface of the cover can be used as a sterile field. Once you create a sterile field, you are responsible for performing the procedure and making sure that the field is not contaminated. Cover the sterile field with a sterile cover if not using sterile materials right away. This prevents bacterial contamination of the sterile field (AORN, 2022).

Delegation

Surgical technicians may prepare a sterile field (see agency policy); however, assistive personnel (AP) cannot. Direct the AP to:
- Help with patient positioning and obtaining any necessary supplies

Interprofessional Collaboration

- All members of the surgical team are mindful to ensure that all maintain a sterile field.

Equipment

- Sterile pack (commercial or institution wrapped)
- Sterile drape or kit that is to be used as a sterile field
- Sterile gloves (optional)
- Sterile solution and equipment specific to a procedure
- Waist-high table/countertop surface
- Appropriate personal protective equipment (PPE): gown, mask, cap, protective eyewear (see agency policy)

STEP	RATIONALE

ASSESSMENT

1. Identify patient using at least two identifiers (e.g., name and birthday or name and medical record number) according to agency policy.
2. Assess for latex allergies.

Ensures correct patient. Complies with The Joint Commission standards and improves patient safety (TJC, 2023).

A review may reveal latex allergies and determine the need to use latex-free supplies.

STEP	RATIONALE
3. Verify in agency policy and procedure manual that procedure requires surgical aseptic technique.	Some procedures require medical rather than surgical aseptic technique.
4. Assess patient's/family caregiver's health literacy.	Determines degree to which individuals have the ability to find, understand, and use information and services to make informed health-related decisions and actions for themselves and others (CDC, 2023b).
5. Assess patient's comfort, positioning, oxygen requirements, and elimination needs before preparing for procedure.	Certain procedures that require a sterile field may last a long time. Anticipates patient's needs so that patient can relax and avoid any unnecessary movement that might disrupt procedure.
6. Instruct patient and family caregiver not to touch work surface or equipment during procedure.	Instruction prevents contamination of sterile field.
7. Check sterile package integrity for punctures, tears, discoloration, moisture, or any other signs of contamination. Check expiration date if applicable. If using commercially packaged supplies or those prepared by agency, check for sterilization indicator (marker that changes color when exposed to heat or steam).	Inspection of packaging ensures that only sterile items are presented to sterile field (AORN, 2023).
8. Anticipate number and variety of supplies needed for procedure.	Not all sterile kits contain sufficient amounts or types of supplies. Failure to have necessary supplies causes you to leave sterile field, increasing risk for contamination.
9. Assess patient's knowledge, prior experience with a sterile field, and feelings about procedure.	Reveals need for patient instruction and/or support.

PLANNING

STEP	RATIONALE
1. Ask visitors to step out briefly during procedure. Instruct staff helping with procedure not to move.	Traffic or movement can increase potential for contamination through spread of microorganisms by air currents.
2. Expected outcomes after completion of procedure:	
• Sterile field is not contaminated.	Correct surgical aseptic practice is performed.
• Patient is not exposed to microorganisms.	Lack of exposure prevents likelihood of infection transmission.
3. Complete all other nursing interventions (e.g., medication administration, suctioning patient) before beginning procedure.	Prepare sterile fields as close as possible to time of use to reduce potential for contamination (AORN, 2023).
4. Arrange equipment at bedside.	Ensures availability before procedure and prevents break in sterile technique. (**NOTE:** Povidone-iodine and chlorhexidine are not considered sterile solutions and require separate work surfaces for preparation.)
5. Provide privacy. Position patient comfortably for specific procedure to be performed. If a body part is to be examined or treated, position patient so that area is accessible. Have AP help with positioning as needed.	Patient should be able to lie still in one position comfortably during procedure. Movement can contaminate sterile field.
6. Explain to patient purpose of procedure and importance of sterile technique.	Explanation ensures patient's ability to cooperate with procedure. Performing patient teaching before procedure reduces need to talk during procedure, which can cause air-droplet contamination of sterile area.

IMPLEMENTATION

STEP	RATIONALE
1. Perform hand hygiene (see Chapter 9).	Hand hygiene reduces number of microorganisms on hands, thus reducing transmission to patient. Do not allow rinse water to run down arms onto clean hands (i.e., arms are considered dirty).
2. Apply PPE as needed (consult agency policy) (see Skills 10.1 and 10.3).	PPE controls spread of airborne microorganisms.
3. Select a clean, flat, dry work surface above waist level.	A dry work surface is needed for a sterile field. A sterile object placed below a person's waist is considered contaminated.
4. Prepare sterile work surface.	
a. Use sterile commercial kit or pack containing sterile items.	
(1) Place sterile kit or pack on the dry and clean work surface.	Sterile object placed above waist is considered sterile.

STEP	RATIONALE
(2) Open outside cover (see illustration) and remove package from dust cover. Place on work surface.	Inner kit remains sterile.
(3) Grasp outer surface of tip of outermost flap.	Outer surface of package is not sterile. There is a 2.5-cm (1-inch) border around any sterile drape or wrap that is considered not sterile and can be touched with clean fingers.
(4) Open outermost flap away from body, keeping arm outstretched and away from sterile field (see illustration).	Reaching over sterile field contaminates it.
(5) Grasp outside surface of edge of first side flap.	Outer border is considered unsterile.
(6) Open side flap, pulling to side, allowing it to lie flat on table surface. Keep arm to side and not over sterile surface (see illustration).	Drape or wrapper should lie flat so that it does not accidentally rise up and contaminate inner surface or sterile contents.
(7) Repeat Step 4a(6) for second side flap (see illustration).	
(8) Grasp outside border of last and innermost flap (see illustration). Stand away from sterile package and pull flap back, allowing it to fall flat on table. Kit is ready to be used.	Outer border is considered unsterile. Never reach over a sterile field.
b. Open sterile linen-wrapped package.	
(1) Place package on clean, dry, flat work surface above waist level.	Sterile items placed below waist level are considered contaminated.
(2) Remove sterilization tape seal and unwrap both layers following same steps (see Steps 4a[2] through 4a[8]) as for sterile kit (see illustration).	Linen-wrapped items have two layers. The first is a dust cover. The second layer must be opened to view chemical indicator.
(3) Use opened package wrapper as sterile field.	Inner surface of wrapper is considered sterile.

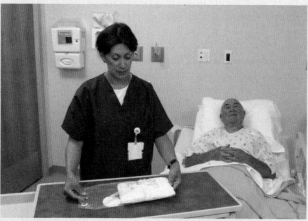

STEP 4a(2) Open outside cover of sterile kit.

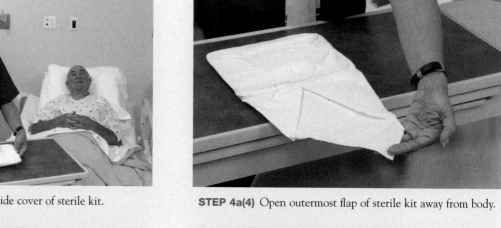

STEP 4a(4) Open outermost flap of sterile kit away from body.

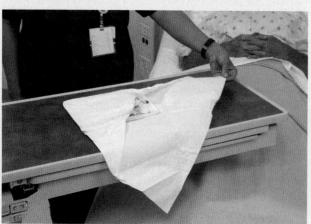

STEP 4a(6) Open first side flap, pulling to side.

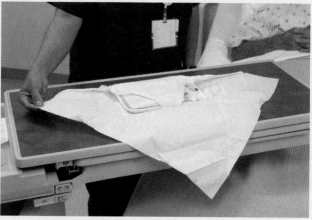

STEP 4a(7) Open second side flap, pulling to side.

STEP	RATIONALE

c. Prepare sterile drape.

(1) Place pack containing sterile drape on flat, dry surface and open as described (see Steps 4a[2] through 4a[8]) for sterile package.

Packaged drape remains sterile.

(2) Apply sterile gloves (*optional*, see agency policy). You may touch outer 2.5-cm (1-inch) border of drape without wearing gloves.

Sterile object remains sterile only when touched by another sterile object. Gloves are not necessary as long as fingers grasp the 2.5-cm (1-inch) unsterile border of the drape.

(3) Using fingertips of one hand, pick up folded top edge of drape along 2.5-cm (1-inch) border. Gently lift drape up from its wrapper without touching any object. Discard wrapper with other hand.

If sterile object touches any nonsterile object, it becomes contaminated.

(4) With other hand, grasp an adjacent corner of drape and hold it straight up and away from body. Allow drape to unfold, keeping it above waist and work surface and away from body (see illustration). (Carefully discard wrapper with other hand.)

An object held below a person's waist or above chest is contaminated.
Drape can now be placed properly with two hands.

(5) Holding drape, position bottom half over top half of intended work surface (see illustration).

Proper positioning prevents nurse from reaching over sterile field.

(6) Allow top half of drape to be placed over bottom half of work surface (see illustration).

Proper positioning creates flat, sterile work surface for placement of sterile supplies.

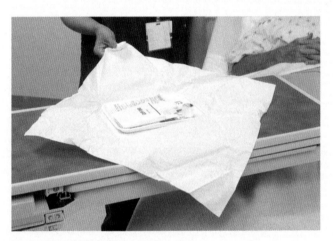

STEP 4a(8) Open last and innermost flap.

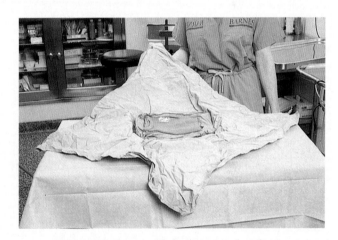

STEP 4b(2) Open sterile linen-wrapped package.

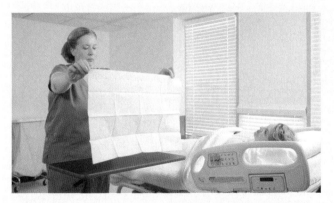

STEP 4c(4) Grasp corners of sterile drape, and then hold up and away from body. (*From Elsevier: Clinical skills: essentials collection, St. Louis, 2021, Elsevier.*)

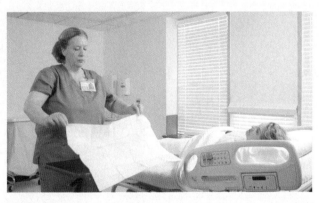

STEP 4c(5) Position bottom half of sterile drape over top half of work space. (*From Elsevier: Clinical skills: essentials collection, St. Louis, 2021, Elsevier.*)

STEP	RATIONALE
5. Add sterile items to sterile field.	
a. Open sterile item (following package directions) while holding outside wrapper in nondominant hand.	Use of nondominant hand frees dominant hand for unwrapping outer wrapper.
b. Carefully peel wrapper over nondominant hand.	Item remains sterile. Inner surface of wrapper covers hand, making it sterile.
c. Be sure that the wrapper does not fall down onto the sterile field. Place the item onto the field at an angle (see illustration). Do not hold arms over sterile field.	Secured wrapper edges prevent flipping wrapper and contaminating contents of sterile field (AORN, 2023).

Clinical Judgment *Do not flip or toss objects onto sterile field.*

STEP	RATIONALE
d. Dispose of outer wrapper.	Disposal prevents accidental contamination of sterile field.
6. Pour sterile solutions.	
a. Verify contents and expiration date of solution.	Verification ensures proper solution and sterility of contents.
b. Place receptacle for solution near table/work surface edge. Sterile kits have cups or plastic molded sections into which fluids can be poured.	Proper placement prevents reaching over sterile field during pouring of solution.
c. Remove sterile seal and cap from bottle in upward motion.	Upward movement prevents contamination of bottle lip.
d. With solution bottle held away from field and bottle lip 2.5 to 5 cm (1 to 2 inches) above inside of sterile receiving container, slowly pour needed amount of solution into container. Hold bottle with label facing palm of hand (see illustration).	Edge and outside of bottle are considered contaminated. Slow pouring prevents splashing. Sterility of contents cannot be ensured if cap is replaced.
	Prevents label from becoming wet and illegible.

Clinical Judgment *When liquids permeate sterile field or barrier, it is called strikethrough and results in contamination of the sterile field.*

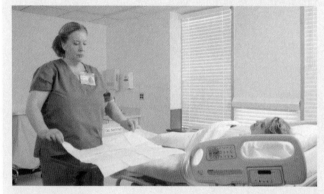

STEP 4c(6) Allow top half of drape to be placed over bottom half of work surface. *(From Elsevier: Clinical skills: essentials collection, St. Louis, 2021, Elsevier.)*

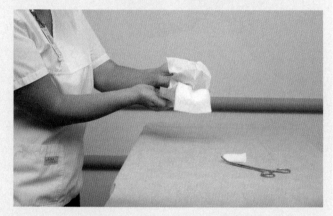

STEP 5c Add items to sterile field.

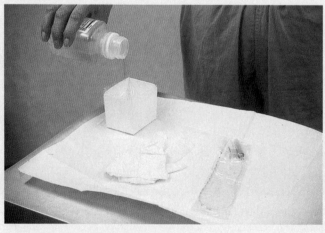

STEP 6d Pour solution into receiving container on sterile field.

STEP	RATIONALE
7. Help patient to a comfortable position.	Restores comfort and sense of well-being.
8. Place nurse call system in an accessible location within patient's reach.	Ensures patient can call for assistance if needed.
9. Raise side rails (as appropriate) and lower bed to lowest position, locking into position.	Ensures patient safety and prevents falls.
10. Remove and dispose of supplies and gloves and perform hand hygiene.	Prevents transmission of microorganisms.

EVALUATION

1. Observe for breaks in sterile field.
2. **Use Teach-Back:** "I want to be sure I explained the procedure that was performed and the steps used to prevent infection. Please tell me some of the things that can be done to prevent infection." Revise your instruction now or develop a plan for revised patient/family caregiver teaching if patient/family caregiver is not able to teach back correctly.

A break in sterile field requires you to set up new sterile field.
Teach-back is a technique for health care providers to ensure that they have explained medical information clearly so that patients and their families understand what is communicated to them (AHRQ, 2023).

Unexpected Outcomes

1. Sterile field comes in contact with contaminated object, or liquid splatters onto drape, causing strikethrough.

2. Sterile item falls off sterile field.

Related Interventions

• Discontinue field preparation and start over with new equipment.

• Open another package containing new sterile item and add to field unless field becomes contaminated, in which case a new sterile field would need to be established.

Documentation

• No documentation is required for this set of skills.

Hand-Off Reporting

• No reporting is required for this set of skills.

Special Considerations

Home Care

• Most care procedures in the home setting involve clean technique. If a sterile environment is ordered, the patient and family caregiver need to be aware of the principles that apply to the sterile environment. For example, teach the family caregiver how to correctly use package wrapper as a sterile drape/barrier when applying a sterile dressing or the correct procedure for removing sterile item from package.

 SKILL 10.3 **Sterile Gloving**

▶ *Video Clip*

Sterile gloves help prevent the transmission of pathogens by direct and indirect contact. Nurses apply sterile gloves before performing sterile procedures such as inserting urinary catheters, assisting with surgical procedures, or applying sterile dressings. Sterile gloves do not replace hand hygiene.

It is important to verify whether the patient or health care providers have a latex allergy. When allergies are present, select latex-free gloves. Repeated exposure to latex can lead to a latex allergy, in which case latex-free gloves would need to be used. Box 10.2 lists risk factors for a latex allergy. Latex proteins enter the body through skin or mucous membranes, intravascularly, or via inhalation. Reactions to latex range from mild to severe (Box 10.3).

Gloves must be the proper size. The gloves should not stretch so tightly over the fingers that they can tear easily, yet they need to be tight enough that objects can be picked up easily. Sterile

Risk Factors for Latex Allergy

- Spina bifida
- Multiple surgeries or medical procedures
- High latex exposure (e.g., health care workers, housekeepers, food handlers, tire manufacturers, workers in industries that use gloves routinely)
- Rubber industry workers
- Personal or family history of allergies
- There is a connection between an allergy to latex and an allergy to avocados, bananas, chestnuts, kiwis, and passion fruits. These foods have some of the identical allergens that are found in latex.

Adapted from Mayo Clinic: *Diseases and conditions: latex allergy*, 2022. https://www.mayoclinic.org/diseases-conditions/latex-allergy/symptoms-causes/syc-20374287. Accessed March 31, 2023.

Levels of Latex Reactions

The three types of common latex reactions (in order of severity) are as follows:

1. *Irritant contact dermatitis:* skin reaction isolated to the area of contact.
   a. Symptoms: red, dry, itchy, and irritated skin
2. *Type IV allergic contact:* allergic reaction to chemicals used in latex processing. Symptoms may take 24 to 48 hours to appear.
   a. Symptoms: dry, red skin; rash; itchy rash; small blisters (papules)
3. *IgE-mediated allergic reaction (Type I):* could be life threatening, and reactions can start as soon as 2 to 3 minutes after contact, up to several hours.
   a. Symptoms: hives, swelling, runny nose, nausea, abdominal cramps, dizziness, low blood pressure, bronchospasm, anaphylaxis (shock)

Adapted from Centers for Disease Control and Prevention (CDC): *Contact dermatitis and latex allergy*, 2016. https://www.cdc.gov/oralhealth/infectioncontrol/faqs/latex.html. Accessed September 25, 2023.

gloves are available in various sizes (e.g., 6, 6½, 7). They are also available in "one size fits all" or "small," "medium," and "large."

Delegation

Assisting with skills that include the application and removal of sterile gloves may be delegated to assistive personnel (AP). However, most procedures that require the use of sterile gloves cannot be delegated to AP. Instruct the AP about:
- The reason for using sterile gloves for a specific procedure

Equipment

- Package of proper-size sterile gloves, latex or synthetic non-latex. If patient has a latex allergy, ensure that gloves are latex free and powder free.

STEP	RATIONALE

ASSESSMENT

1. Consider the type of procedure to be performed and consult agency policy on use of sterile gloves. In some institutions, double gloving has been recommended for the operating room (OR) (Zhang et al., 2021).

2. Consider patient's risk for infection (e.g., preexisting condition and size or extent of area being treated).

3. Select correct size and type of gloves, and examine glove package to determine if it is dry and intact with no water stains.

4. Use nonpowdered gloves.

5. Inspect condition of hands for cuts, hangnails, open lesions, or abrasions. In some settings, you are allowed to cover any open lesion with a sterile, impervious transparent dressing (check agency policy). In some cases, presence of such lesions may prevent you from participating in a procedure.

6. Assess patient for the following risk factors before applying latex gloves:
   a. Previous reaction to the following items within hours of exposure: adhesive tape, dental or face mask, golf club grip, ostomy bag, rubber band, balloon, bandage, elastic underwear, intravenous (IV) tubing, rubber gloves, condom (Allergy & Asthma Network, 2023)
   b. Personal history of asthma, contact dermatitis, eczema, urticaria, rhinitis
   c. History of food allergies, especially avocado, banana, peach, chestnut, raw potato, kiwi, tomato, papaya

Ensures proper use of sterile gloves when needed. Evidence supports the use of double gloving and double gloving with an indicator glove system to decrease the risk of percutaneous injury; this provides an effective barrier to bloodborne pathogen exposure (AORN, 2023; Zhang et al., 2021).

Knowledge of risk directs you to follow added precautions (e.g., use of additional protective barriers) if necessary.

Torn or wet package is considered contaminated. Signs of water stains on package indicate previous contamination by water.

The U.S. Food and Drug Administration (FDA) passed a ruling that powdered gloves may no longer be used owing to increased risk of hypersensitivity and allergic reactions (FDA, 2020).

Cuts, abrasions, and hangnails tend to ooze serum, which possibly contains pathogens. Breaks in skin integrity permit microorganisms to enter, increasing the risk for infection for both patient and nurse (AORN, 2023).

Risk factors determine level of patient's risk for latex allergy.

Items are known to lead to latex allergy.

Patients with a history of these conditions are at higher risk of having a reaction (Allergy & Asthma Network, 2023).

Patients with a history of food allergies are at higher risk of developing a reaction.

STEP	RATIONALE
d. Previous history of adverse reactions during surgery or dental procedure	Previous history suggests allergic response.
e. Previous reaction to latex product	Previous reaction suggests allergic response.
7. Assess patient's/family caregiver's health literacy.	Determines degree to which individuals have the ability to find, understand, and use information and services to make informed health-related decisions and actions for themselves and others (CDC, 2023b).
8. Assess patient's knowledge, prior experience with sterile gloving, and feelings about procedure.	Reveals need for patient instruction and/or support.

Clinical Judgment *Related factors and risk factors are individualized on the basis of the patient's condition or needs.*

PLANNING

1. Expected outcomes after completion of procedure:	
• Patient does not develop signs or symptoms of infection after procedure.	Lack of signs of infection indicates that microorganisms are not introduced into sterile body cavities or sites (such as skin or urinary tract).
• Patient does not develop latex sensitivity or latex allergy reaction.	Patient at risk for latex allergy is not exposed to latex proteins.

Clinical Judgment *Synthetic nonlatex gloves (latex free/powder free) must be used when patients are at risk for or if nurse has sensitivity or allergy to latex.*

IMPLEMENTATION

STEP	RATIONALE
1. Apply sterile gloves.	
a. Perform thorough hand hygiene (see Skill 9.1). Place glove package near work area.	Hand hygiene reduces number of bacteria on skin surfaces and transmission of infection. Proximity to work area ensures availability before procedure.
b. Remove outer glove package wrapper by carefully separating and peeling apart sides (see illustration).	Proper removal prevents inner glove package from accidentally opening and touching contaminated objects.
c. Grasp inner package and lay on clean, dry, flat surface at waist level. Open package, keeping gloves on inside surface of wrapper (see illustration).	Sterile object held below waist is contaminated. Inner surface of glove package is sterile.
d. Identify right and left glove. Each glove has a cuff approximately 5 cm (2 inches) wide. Glove dominant hand first.	Proper identification of gloves prevents contamination by improper fit. Gloving of dominant hand first improves dexterity.
e. With thumb and first two fingers of nondominant hand, grasp glove for dominant hand by touching only inside surface of cuff.	Inner edge of cuff will lie against skin and thus is not sterile.
f. Carefully pull glove over dominant hand, leaving a cuff and being sure that cuff does not roll up wrist. Be sure that thumb and fingers are in proper spaces (see illustration).	If outer surface of glove touches hand or wrist, it is contaminated.

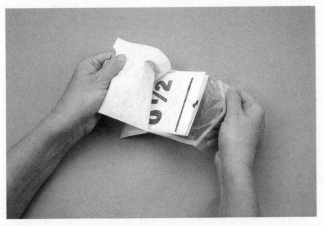

STEP 1b Open outer glove package wrapper.

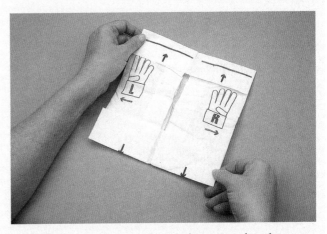

STEP 1c Open inner glove package on work surface.

STEP	RATIONALE
g. With gloved dominant hand, slip fingers underneath cuff of second glove (see illustration).	Cuff protects gloved fingers. Sterile touching prevents glove contamination.
h. Carefully pull second glove over fingers of nondominant hand (see illustration).	Contact of gloved hand with exposed hand results in contamination.

Clinical Judgment *Do not allow fingers and thumb of gloved dominant hand to touch any part of exposed nondominant hand. Keep thumb of dominant hand abducted back.*

i. After second glove is on, interlock hands together and hold away from body above waist level until beginning procedure (see illustration).	Ensures smooth fit over fingers and prevents contamination.
2. Perform procedure.	
3. Remove gloves.	
a. Grasp outside of one cuff with other gloved hand; avoid touching wrist.	Procedure minimizes contamination of underlying skin.
b. Pull glove off, turning it inside out, and place it in gloved hand.	Outside of glove does not touch skin surface.
c. Take fingers of bare hand and tuck inside remaining glove cuff (see illustration). Peel glove off inside out and over previously removed glove. Discard both gloves in receptacle.	Fingers do not touch contaminated glove surface.
d. Perform thorough hand hygiene.	Hand hygiene protects health care worker from contamination resulting from any unseen tears or pinholes in gloves; also removes powder from hands to prevent skin irritation.

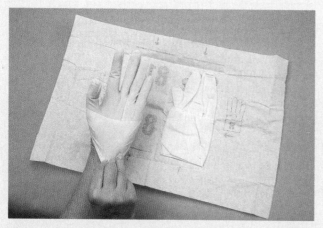

STEP 1f Pick up glove at cuff of dominant hand and insert fingers. Pull glove completely over dominant hand (example is for left-handed person).

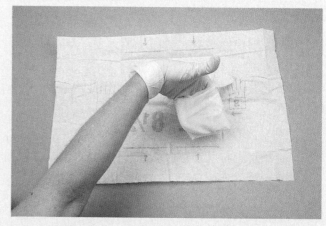

STEP 1g Pick up glove for nondominant hand.

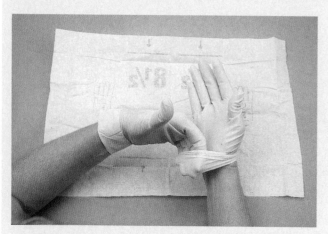

STEP 1h Pull second glove over nondominant hand.

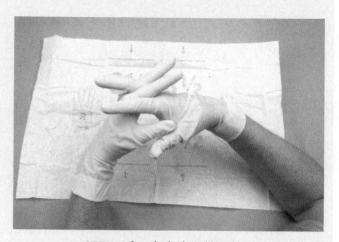

STEP 1i Interlock gloved hands.

STEP	RATIONALE
4. Help patient to a comfortable position.	Restores comfort and sense of well-being.
5. Place nurse call system in an accessible location within patient's reach.	Ensures patient can call for assistance if needed and promotes safety and prevents falls.
6. Raise side rails (as appropriate) and lower bed to lowest position, locking into position.	Ensures patient safety and prevents falls.

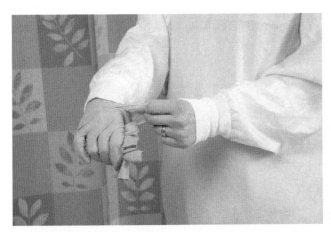

STEP 3c Remove second glove by turning it inside out.

EVALUATION

1. Assess patient for signs of infection, focusing on area treated.
2. Assess patient for signs of latex allergy.
3. **Use Teach-Back:** "I want to be sure I explained why I used sterile gloves for this procedure. Please explain to me why I needed to use sterile gloves." Revise your instruction now or develop a plan for revised patient/family caregiver teaching if patient/family caregiver is not able to teach back correctly.

Improper technique contributes to development of an infection.
Assessment establishes baseline for patient's reaction to latex.
Teach-back is a technique for health care providers to ensure that they have explained medical information clearly so that patients and their families understand what is communicated to them (AHRQ, 2023).

Unexpected Outcomes

1. Patient develops localized signs of infection (e.g., urine becomes cloudy or odorous; wound becomes painful, edematous, or reddened with purulent drainage).

2. Patient develops systemic signs of infection (e.g., fever, malaise, increased white blood cell count).

3. Patient develops allergic reaction to latex (see Box 10.3).

Related Interventions

- Contact health care provider and implement appropriate treatments as ordered.

- Contact health care provider and implement appropriate treatments as ordered.
- Immediately remove source of latex.
- Bring emergency equipment to bedside. Have epinephrine injection ready for administration and be prepared to initiate IV fluids and oxygen.

Documentation

- It is not necessary to document application of gloves. Document specific procedure performed and patient's response and status.
- In the event of a latex allergy reaction, document patient's response. Note type of response and patient's reaction to emergency treatment.

Hand-Off Reporting

- Report specific reason for procedure, patient's response to procedure, and response to education.

- In the event of a patient latex allergy, report the patient response and reaction to emergency treatment.

Special Considerations

Patient Education

- Patient with a known latex allergy should wear a medical alert bracelet or tag and carry a wallet card stating, "latex allergy."
- Individuals with known latex allergies should always carry a quick-acting oral antihistamine and an epinephrine auto-injector.

✦ CLINICAL JUDGMENT AND NEXT GENERATION NCLEX® EXAMINATION–STYLE QUESTIONS

A 68-year-old patient is admitted to the hospital for lung surgery related to a tumor in the lower lobe of the left lung. The patient has a 40 pack-year history of smoking and a history of hypertension, history of angina, and myocardial infarction. The patient has an indwelling Foley catheter with dark, foul-smelling urine. The patient confides in the nurse about anxiety over the upcoming surgery and possible diagnosis of cancer. VS: BP 106/74 mm Hg, HR 110 beats/min, RR 22 breaths/min, T 38.2°C (100.8°F), and SPO₂ 98% on room air. The nurse notices that the patient seems restless during the assessment, which reveals crackles in the lungs bilaterally. A chest x-ray shows bilateral infiltrates in the bases of both lungs.

1. Highlight the assessment findings in the paragraph above that require immediate follow-up by the nurse.
2. The patient is cared for as an inpatient over the following days and surgery is rescheduled. When returning to the hospital for surgery, the patient states, "I always get a rash when I wash dishes and wear rubber gloves." Which of the following actions will the nurse take? **Select all that apply**.
   1. Notify the surgeon immediately.
   2. Reassure that this is a normal reaction.
   3. Ask if other symptoms occur such as shortness of breath.
   4. Document the statement in the electronic health record.
   5. Tell the patient they will not be washing dishes at the hospital.
3. The nurse receives the patient into the operating room to begin a series of procedures and surgery. Which of the following actions will the nurse take at this time? **Select all that apply**.
   1. Perform hand hygiene.
   2. Confirm the patient's latex allergy.
   3. Verify the patient with one identifier.
   4. Make sure all equipment needed is present.
   5. Place sterile kit at level of the hip.
4. When working in a sterile field, an instrument accidentally touched the edge of the drape. Which nursing action is appropriate?
   1. Obtain a new sterile instrument.
   2. Wipe the instrument off with alcohol.
   3. Use the instrument, as the field is sterile.
   4. Ask the surgeon what to do with the instrument.
5. During the procedure, the assisting nurse notices that there is a small hole in a glove. Which action will the nurse take?
   1. Apply a new sterile glove over the one with a hole.
   2. Continue the procedure because a small hole is not significant.
   3. Use the hand with the glove that does not have a hole for the remainder of the surgery.
   4. Remove the damaged gloves, perform hand hygiene, and put on new sterile gloves.

Visit the Evolve site for Answers to Clinical Judgment and Next Generation NCLEX® Examination–Style Questions.

REFERENCES

Agency for Healthcare Research and Quality (AHRQ): *Teach-Back: intervention*, Rockville, MD, 2023, AHRQ. https://www.ahrq.gov/health-literacy/quality-resources/tools/literacy-toolkit/healthlittoolkit2-tool5.html.

Allergy & Asthma Network: *Latex allergy*, 2023. https://allergyasthmanetwork.org/allergies/latex-allergy/. Accessed September 25, 2023.

Aluise M, et al: The effects of nail products including polish, gel, and acrylic nails on infection rates in the healthcare setting, *North Dakota Nurse* 89(2):10, 2020.

Andersen BM: Prevention of postoperative wound infections. In Andersen BM, editor: *Prevention and control of infections in hospitals*, Cham, Switzerland, 2019, Springer. https://link.springer.com/chapter/10.1007/978-3-319-99921-0_33.

Association of periOperative Registered Nurses (AORN): *Key takeaways: guidelines for sterile field*, 2022. https://www.aorn.org/article/2022-10-10-Sterile-Technique-Questions-Answered. Accessed March 31, 2023.

Association of periOperative Registered Nurses (AORN): *Guidelines for perioperative practice*, Denver, 2023, AORN.

Association of Surgical Technologists (AST): *AST guidelines for best practices in use of eye protection during surgical procedures*, 2017, Association of Surgical Technologists. http://www.ast.org/uploadedFiles/Main_Site/Content/About_Us/ASTGuidelinesEyeProtection.pdf. Accessed September 25, 2023.

Blackburn L, et al: Microbial growth on the nails of direct patient care nurses wearing nail polish, *Onc Nurs Forum* 47(2):1–10, 2020.

Boga SM: Nursing practices in the prevention of post-operative wound infection in accordance with evidence-based approach, *Int J of Caring Sci* 12(2):1229–1235, 2019.

Centers for Disease Control and Prevention (CDC): *Clean hands count for healthcare providers*, 2021. https://www.cdc.gov/handhygiene/providers/index.html. Accessed March 31, 2023.

Centers for Disease Control and Prevention (CDC): *CDC's core infection prevention and control practices for safe healthcare delivery in all settings*, 2022. https://www.cdc.gov/infectioncontrol/guidelines/core-practices/index.html. Accessed March 31, 2023.

Centers for Disease Control and Prevention (CDC): *Surgical site infection event*, 2023a. https://www.cdc.gov/nhsn/pdfs/pscmanual/9pscssicurrent.pdf. Accessed March 31, 2023.

Centers for Disease Control and Prevention (CDC): *What is health literacy?* 2023b. https://www.cdc.gov/healthliteracy/learn/index.html.

Christian HJ, et al: Chlorhexidine bathing for infection prevention, *North Dakota Nurse* 89(2):9, 2020.

Duff J, et al: What does surgical conscience mean to perioperative nurses? An interpretive description, *Collegian* 29:147–153, 2022.

Gorski LA, et al: Infusion therapy standards of practice, 8th edition, *J Inf Nurs* 44(5):S1–S224, 2021.

Institute for Healthcare Improvement (IHI): *Changes to prevent surgical site infection*, 2023. http://www.ihi.org/resources/Pages/Changes/ChangestoPreventSurgicalSiteInfection.aspx. Accessed March 31, 2023.

Occupational Safety and Health Administration (OSHA): *Protecting workers: guidance on mitigating and preventing the spread of COVID-19 in the workplace*, 2021. https://www.osha.gov/coronavirus/safework. Accessed March 31, 2023.

Seidelman JL, et al: Surgical site infection prevention: a review, *JAMA* 329(3):244–252, 2023.

Shiroky J, et al: The impact of negative pressure wound therapy for closed surgical incisions on surgical site infection: a systematic review and meta-analysis, *Surgery* 167(6):1001–1009, 2020.

Singhal H, et al: *Wound infection treatment and management*, 2023. https://emedicine.medscape.com/article/188988-treatment#d11. Accessed March 31, 2023.

Tennat K, Rivers CL: *Sterile technique*, 2021, National Library of Medicine Stat Pearls. https://www.ncbi.nlm.nih.gov/books/NBK459175/. Accessed March 31, 2023.

The Joint Commission (TJC): *2023 National patient safety goals*, Oakbrook Terrace, IL, 2023, The Commission. https://www.jointcommission.org/en/standards/national-patient-safety-goals/. Accessed March 31, 2023.

Toney-Butler TJ, et al: *Hand hygiene*, Treasure Island (FL), 2023, StatPearls.

U.S. Food & Drug Administration (FDA): *Medical device bans*, 2020. https://www.fda.gov/medical-devices/medical-device-safety/medical-device-bans. Accessed March 31, 2023.

Wałaszek MZ, et al: Nail microbial colonization following hand disinfection: a qualitative pilot study, *J Hosp Infect* 100(2):207–210, 2018.

Wistrand C, et al: T Time-dependent bacterial air contamination of sterile fields in a controlled operating room environment: an experimental intervention study, *J Hosp Inf* 110:97–102, 2021.

Zhang Z, et al: Effectiveness of double-gloving method on prevention of surgical glove perforations and blood contamination: a systematic review and meta-analysis, *J Adv Nurs* 77(9):3630–3643, 2021.

PHASE 1

QUESTION 1.
A client comes to the emergency room for evaluation. The triage nurse conducts an initial assessment.

Highlight the findings that could indicate an infectious process and require **immediate** follow-up by the nurse.

History and Physical	Nurses' Notes	Vital Signs	Laboratory Results
0248: Client in the emergency department after returning from a vacation. States, "I started to feel unwell while flying home yesterday." This morning, the client awoke with a productive cough, chills, fever, diarrhea, weakness, and vomiting. Alert and oriented × 4; lung sounds with rhonchi; S_1S_2 present without murmur; bowel sounds present × 4 quadrants; tenderness noted near the umbilicus; strength diminished yet equal in all extremities. Vital signs: T 39.6°C (103.2°F); HR 86 beats/min; RR 18 breaths/min; BP 134/98 mm Hg; SpO_2 93% on RA.			

QUESTION 2.
The client is moved into an examination room in the emergency department. The emergency nurse reviews the triage nurse's notes.

Complete the following sentence by selecting from the list of word choices below.

Before entering the client's room, the triage nurse dons **[Word Choice]** and **[Word Choice]**.

Word Choices
Clean gloves
A mask
A cap
A pair of goggles
Sterile gloves

PHASE 2

QUESTION 3.
The health care provider evaluates the client and orders diagnostic testing. It is determined that the client has a C. *difficile* infection and a urinary tract infection. The client's testing was negative for COVID-19 and influenza.

Complete the following sentence by selecting from the list of options below.

The client needs that the nurse will address include following **1 [Select]** Precautions and **2 [Select]**.

Options for 1	Options for 2
Standard	Washing hands regularly
Airborne	Explaining how to avoid *C. difficile*
Droplet	Encouraging fluids
Contact	Collecting repeat vital signs

QUESTION 4.
The client is admitted for observation to a medical unit. Later in the shift, the medical unit nurse assesses the client.

For each client concern the nurse observes, determine whether reporting the concern to the health care provider is indicated or not indicated.

Client Concern	Indicated	Not Indicated
Blood pressure 90/60 mm Hg		
Urinary output <30 mL/hr		
Family at the bedside		
Several episodes of watery diarrhea		
Respiratory rate 12 breaths/min		

PHASE 3

QUESTION 5.

The health care provider orders an indwelling urinary catheter to be placed. Which of the following actions would the nurse take when donning sterile gloves? **Select all that apply.**

○ Perform hand hygiene.
○ Apply glove to dominant hand first.
○ Roll cuff of applied glove over the wrist.
○ Hold gloved hands close to body after application.
○ Slip hand underneath cuff of second glove after first glove is applied.
○ Lay unopened package of sterile gloves on chest-high flat surface.
○ Grab glove for dominant hand by touching the glove's inside surface or cuff.

QUESTION 6.

The client remained hospitalized for several days, receiving treatment. Today's nursing evaluation includes this documentation.

History and Physical	Nurses' Notes'	Vital Signs	Laboratory Results

1644: Client sitting up in bed watching television. Alert and oriented × 4; lung sounds clear to auscultation. Productive cough noted; mucus with tinges of blood seen. S_1S_2 present without murmur; bowel sounds present × 4 quadrants, no tenderness upon gentle palpation; strength diminished yet equal in all extremities. Vital signs: T 37.7°C (99.9°F); HR 80 beats/min; RR 16 breaths/min; BP 120/82 mm Hg; Spo_2 98% on RA. No episodes of watery diarrhea for 24 hours.

For each current client finding, indicate if the client's condition has improved or declined.

Current Client Findings	Improved	Declined
Blood pressure 120/82 mm Hg		
Temperature 37.7°C (99.9°F)		
No watery diarrhea in 24 hours		
No abdominal tenderness		
Mucus with tinges of blood		

UNIT 5
Activity and Mobility

Safe activity and mobility practices are important for preventing injury to both health care providers and patients. Health care agencies are responsible for providing you with safety information, training, and resources to use when transferring, positioning, and lifting patients, but it is your responsibility to use these correctly. Safe patient handling and mobility skills must be used in any activity that involves moving patients. These skills incorporate knowledge regarding patient size and weight, the nature of the skill, and the body movements required to move or position an individual safely. Your knowledge and skill in using safe patient handling and mobility, along with use of assistive equipment, ensure safe patient transfer, ambulation, and positioning without injury to your patient or yourself.

To maintain your safety prior to positioning or transferring patients, use your clinical judgment to assess a patient's condition and any risks that might be created during movement, your knowledge and skill level for safe patient handling, and presence of environmental factors that pose risk for injury. For example, assess your patients and determine if they understand the procedure or present risks for being unable to assist with movement. Consider factors in your patient's condition, such as balance, weight, weight-bearing ability, and cognitive status, which can either facilitate or impede safe patient positioning. Assess if your patient can understand directions about positioning. Determine what resources, such as a lift team or hydraulic lift devices, are available. Assess for obstacles in the environment that make positioning difficult. Critically think about your prior experience in safely transferring and positioning patients. What worked? What did not work? What resources did you use? What resources were missing? Determine the number of people needed to safely transfer your patient, and plan and

discuss the steps of the procedure before initiating the transfer. Using clinical judgment in the assessment and analysis of data assists in planning and implementing safe patient transfer and positioning.

Safe mobility practices include early progressive activity and exercise. Early activity decreases length of hospital stays and improves posthospital rehabilitation. Use your clinical judgment to correctly assess and analyze data to support a patient's mobility plan. For example, data collected in an outpatient setting for stable or recovering patients will include access to exercise areas, routine activity, and frequency of the activity. However, patients recovering from a myocardial infarction will require assessment of activity tolerance because they will need a prescribed, graduated activity plan. Your knowledge about your patients and their disease processes will assist you in assessing and planning appropriate activity. The skills in this unit outline specific mobility exercises and use of assistive devices. Your clinical judgment guides you in individualizing activity interventions for your patient's level of health and evaluating your patient's response to activity.

There are, however, situations in which immobile patients require support surfaces and special beds to prevent complications of immobility. In these situations, patients have conditions such as paralysis, bilateral leg amputations, and obesity that place them at risk for pressure injuries. To provide safe patient care, use your clinical judgment to continually assess and analyze your patient to determine if a support surface is necessary to prevent pressure injuries. Use the health care agency's skin care/wound care resource nurse to determine the best surface for your specific patient. When caring for patients on a support surface, recognize and analyze cues to determine the patient's response to and tolerance of the support surface.

11 | Safe Patient Handling and Mobility

SKILLS AND PROCEDURES

Skill 11.1 **Using Safe and Effective Transfer Techniques, p. 298**

Procedural Guideline 11.1 **Wheelchair Transfer Techniques, p. 311**

Skill 11.2 **Moving and Positioning Patients in Bed, p. 313**

OBJECTIVES

Mastery of content in this chapter will enable you to:

- Discuss principles of safe patient handling and mobility (SPHM) as they apply to patient situations.
- Explain the importance of using SPHM devices when moving, positioning, transferring, and mobilizing patients.
- Take part in a functional mobility assessment for determining the type of approach to use and amount of help needed to move, position, transfer, and mobilize patients safely.

- Demonstrate positioning, transfer, and mobilization procedures to follow to ensure patient and nurse safety.
- Explain positioning techniques for the supported Fowler, semi-Fowler, supine, and 30-degree lateral side-lying positions.
- Discuss the procedures for helping a patient move up in bed, helping a patient to a sitting position, logrolling a patient, and transferring a patient from a bed to a chair and transferring from a chair to a bed.

MEDIA RESOURCES

- http://evolve.elsevier.com/Perry/skills
- Clinical Review Questions
- Audio Glossary
- ▶ Video Clips

- **NSO** Nursing Skills Online
- Answers to Clinical Judgment and Next-Generation NCLEX® Examination–Style Questions

PURPOSE

Overexertion and bodily reaction is the second leading nonfatal injury or illness event occurring in workplaces in the United States (National Safety Council, 2023). Nurses experience overexertion injuries from nonimpact injuries or illnesses resulting from excessive physical effort during manual lifting, moving, repositioning patients, and working in awkward positions (Fig. 11.1). Common worker activities include lifting, pulling, pushing, holding, and carrying (National Safety Council, 2023). Health care agencies are required to provide employees with safety information and training to use when transferring, positioning, lifting, and mobilizing patients. Safe patient handling and mobility (SPHM) involves the use of assistive devices to ensure that patients can be mobilized safely and that care providers avoid performing high-risk manual patient-handling tasks (U.S. Department of Veterans Affairs, 2021). The correct use of assistive devices reduces the work effort and a care provider's risk of injury and improves the safety and quality of patient care.

It also is important for health care workers to use good body mechanics when performing patient-handling activities (Box 11.1). Refer to the SPHM policies and procedures of the agency in which you work. In acute care facilities the proper use of SPHM techniques mobilizes patients easily, gently, earlier, and progressively without risking injury. In early and progressive mobility programs, SPHM promotes preservation of patient functional status and

improves clinical outcomes (U.S. Department of Veterans Affairs, 2021). When performing the skills in this chapter, it is essential to use SPHM techniques and principles.

PRACTICE STANDARDS

- Occupational Safety and Health Administration (OSHA), 2014: Safe Patient Handling: Preventing Musculoskeletal Disorders in Nursing Homes—Guidelines for transfer and positioning of patients
- Occupational Safety and Health Administration (OSHA), n.d.a: Worker Safety in Hospitals—Safe patient handling
- Veterans Health Administration (VHA), 2014: VHA Safe Patient Handling and Mobility Algorithms (2014 revision)—Safe patient handling
- The Joint Commission (TJC), 2023: National Patient Safety Goals—Patient identification

SUPPLEMENTAL STANDARDS

- Association of Perioperative Nurses, 2018: Guideline for safe patient handling and movement

PRINCIPLES FOR PRACTICE

- Key principles in determining the SPHM techniques and technology used for patients are knowing if a patient is weight

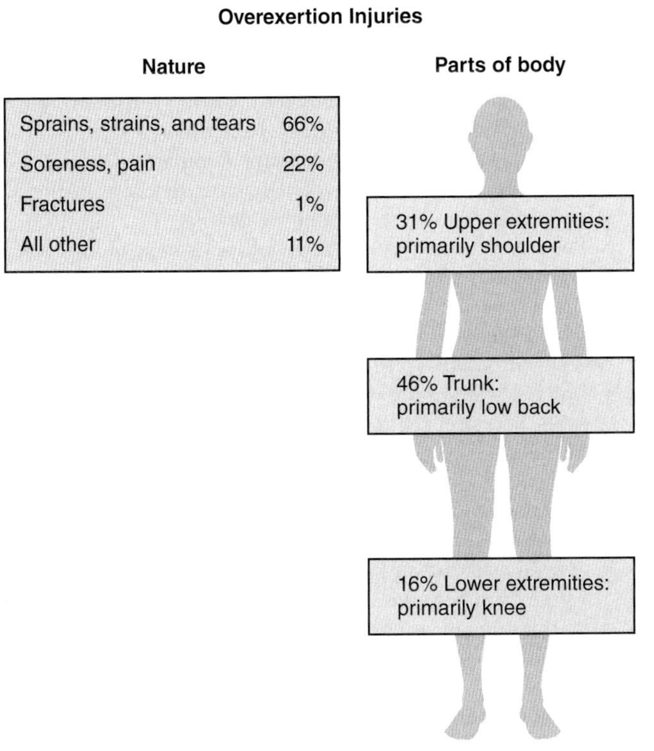

Overexertion Injuries

Nature		Parts of body
Sprains, strains, and tears	66%	
Soreness, pain	22%	
Fractures	1%	
All other	11%	

31% Upper extremities: primarily shoulder

46% Trunk: primarily low back

16% Lower extremities: primarily knee

FIG. 11.1 Overexertion injuries. (*Adapted from National Safety Council [NSC]: NSC Injury Facts: Overexertion and bodily reaction [website], 2023. https://injuryfacts.nsc.org/work/safety-topics/overexertion-and-bodily-reaction/. Accessed August 23, 2023.*)

BOX 11.1

Principles of Safe Body Mechanics When Transferring and Positioning Patients

Mechanical lifts and lift teams are essential when patient is unable to help move. When a patient is able to help, remember these principles:
- The lower the center of gravity, the greater the stability of the nurse.
- The equilibrium of an object is maintained as long as the line of gravity passes through its base of support.
- Facing the direction of movement prevents abnormal twisting of the spine.
- Dividing balanced activity between arms and legs reduces the risk for back injury.
- Leverage, rolling, turning, or pivoting requires less work than lifting.
- When friction is reduced between the object to be moved and the surface on which it is moved, less force is required to move it.

---

bearing and the patient's weight and height, strength, and ability to cooperate and provide help (Matz, 2019).
- Have the proper training to assist patients to move or position while using safe patient-handling equipment.
- Patients who are at high risk for complications from improper positioning and injury during transfer include those with poor nutrition, poor circulation, loss of sensation, alterations in bone formation or joint mobility, and impaired muscle development.
- During a patient transfer, avoid using your weight to lift patients. Instead, have patients use their strength during transfers and repositionings when possible (Bergman & De Jesus, 2022).
- Be careful not to let patients wrap their arms around your head during a transfer (Bergman & De Jesus, 2022).
- A comprehensive SPHM program includes integrating use of safe patient-handling and mobilization equipment, practices for

improving patient mobility, use of patient risk assessments, a hospital infrastructure for maintaining and servicing equipment, patient hand-off procedures, and staff training (Dennerlein et al., 2017).

PERSON-CENTERED CARE

- Ultimately if patients are alert and oriented, it is their choice to increase mobility and activity level. Consider a patient's knowledge, cultural beliefs, and attitudes about the loss of independent activity and the willingness to participate in activity when developing a plan of care.
- A study involving patients who survived cerebrovascular accidents revealed that patients described their bodies as uncontrollable, unresponsive, and untrustworthy (Stott, 2021). Many felt disembodied as they tried to assert control over their "object" body. Patients had altered perceptions such as limb heaviness, absence, pain, or unresponsiveness when they attempted to mobilize (Stott, 2021). Assessment of and consideration of patient perceptions of mobility should be a part of your approach to improving patient mobility.
- Use simple language when you provide patients with information about the complications of immobility and their unique risks.
- Consider the circumstances surrounding a patient's loss of independent activity and mobility to ensure that a plan of care is realistic and attainable.
- Understand to what extent a patient chooses to have a family caregiver involved to learn transfer and positioning techniques for home care.

EVIDENCE-BASED PRACTICE

Efficacy of Safe Patient-Handling and Mobility Programs

Health care organizations have SPHM programs to reduce patient and health care worker injuries. A literature review of the evaluation of SPHM programs revealed substantial injury reductions after program implementation (Teeple et al., 2017). The interventions used in these programs had greater injury reduction the longer the duration of patient follow-up. The greatest effects were found in intensive care unit interventions (Teeple et al., 2017). SPHM programs can reduce injuries by using several strategies:
- Use of SPHM practices improved significantly when SPHM programs were in place.
- Staff had more positive attitudes toward patient-handling equipment and increased use of specific patient-handling equipment (Risør et al., 2017).
- Research has revealed factors that affect staff's use of safe patient-handling devices: patient unable to help with lift/transfer, size/weight where staff member needed assistance to help lift/transfer, availability of others who could assist with manual lift, devices functioning properly and having supplies available, and devices being easy to retrieve from storage (Schoenfisch et al., 2019). Consider these factors to better prepare and plan for a patient's safe transfer.
- Research has shown that a comprehensive safe patient-handling program that combines management commitment, patient risk assessments, employee involvement, policies, SPHM equipment and maintenance, staff training, and maintenance is needed (OSHA, n.d.b).
- A multicomponent SPHM program has been found to be effective in reducing patient-handling injuries among nurses (Choi & Cramer, 2016).

- Research involving nurses who experienced chronic low back pain showed a reduction in back pain and an increase in the number of properly executed horizontal and vertical patient transfers after nurses participated in spine strengthening exercise and formal education about SPHM (Járomi et al., 2018).

SAFETY GUIDELINES

Professional standards and guidelines, such as those from the American Nurses Association (ANA, 2021), the American Association for Safe Patient Handling and Movement (AASPHM, 2016), and the Centers for Disease Control and Prevention (CDC, 2023a) concerning the use of assistive equipment and devices to transfer and position patients safely are invaluable for the safety of you and your patients. Follow these guidelines in the performance of skills in this chapter:

- Routine servicing and maintenance of safe patient-handling equipment and wheelchair is needed (OSHA, n.d.b).
- It can actually take much longer to gather a team of colleagues to manually lift a patient than to find and use lifting equipment. Using SPHM devices to transfer patients takes fewer personnel and about 5 minutes less, overall, than manual transfers (OSHA, n.d.b).
- Communicate clearly with members of the health care team. During hand-off communication, share information about the patient's level of mobility, any restrictions, type of assistive devices used, and methods being used to transfer, reposition, or ambulate.
- Clear the immediate environment where a patient will stand and walk of any obstacles or clutter.
- During any patient task, a caregiver may lift no more than 15.9 kg (35 lb) of a patient's weight (body, head, limbs) (VHA, 2014).
- Mentally review the steps of a transfer before beginning to ensure safety of both you and the patient.

- Monitor a patient's activity tolerance throughout any extended ambulation or period of time sitting in a chair or wheelchair.
- Stand on patient's weak side when assisting a patient able to stand (Fairchild & O'Shea, 2022). Exceptions:
  - Patient who has weakness from a unilateral stroke. You may stand on the strong side if you are the only one present (depending on degree of limb weakness).
  - Patients who are postoperative following knee or hip surgery. If patients are toe-touch weight bearing, stand on the strong side if you are the only one assisting. That is the side on which the knee would buckle.
- Wheelchair safety—pushing a wheelchair:
  - Precheck your route where possible, identify likely hazardous spots, and alter the route if necessary.
  - Stand close to the wheelchair, keeping your spine upright with your elbows slightly bent; avoid stooping and overreaching.
  - Keep your elbows "soft" to absorb stresses.
  - As you walk forward, use the power in your legs to produce forward momentum.
- Raise the side rail on the side of the bed opposite of where you are standing to prevent the patient from falling out of bed on that side.
- Make sure all personnel have been trained in how lift and friction-reducing devices (FRDs) function before they are used.
- Educate patients and/or family caregivers about how equipment functions to reduce their anxiety and enlist their cooperation.
- Arrange equipment (e.g., intravenous [IV] lines, feeding tube, Foley catheter) so that it will not interfere with the transfer process.
- Evaluate patient for correct body alignment and pressure injury (PI) risks after a transfer.

◆ SKILL 11.1   Using Safe and Effective Transfer Techniques

 Video Clip

Patient transfer involves moving a patient from one flat surface to another, from a bed to a stretcher, and from a bed to a wheelchair (Bergman & De Jesus, 2022). Safe transfer involves use of safe patient handling and mobility (SPHM) techniques (including use of lift devices) for assisting dependent patients or helping patients with restricted mobility to attain positions to regain or maintain optimal independence. It also benefits patients psychologically by increasing their social activity and mental stimulation and providing a change in environment (Huether & McCance, 2020).

Safe transfer involves the use of friction-reducing devices (FRDs), which fall into three categories: air-assisted transfer devices, friction-reducing slide sheets and tubes, and transfer and roller-type boards (Baptiste-McKinney & Halvorson, 2018). Such devices provide patients comfort during transfer and repositioning processes. The use of FRDs also promotes in-bed mobility, potentially reduces risk of pressure injuries, provides ease of movement for patients and caregivers, and reduces the spinal load during a transfer (Baptiste-McKinney & Halvorson, 2018). Research has shown that slide board and air-assisted devices significantly reduce hand force, shoulder flexion, muscle activities of caregivers, and patients' head acceleration compared with a drawsheet (Hwang et al., 2019). It is critical that the correct techniques be applied when using FRDs. Patient lift equipment is also important for safe lifting.

Properly designed lift equipment (e.g., ceiling lifts and power lifts) reduces the biomechanical load and physical stress associated with patient lifting and transferring tasks (Kucera et al., 2019).

Before transferring patients, use clinical judgment by considering the type of problems a patient can develop. For example, a patient who has been immobile for several days or longer is often weak or dizzy or sometimes develops initial orthostatic hypotension (OH); consider the pathology causing the patient's immobility, the patient's risks for not tolerating standing or possibly falling during a transfer, and the options you have for a safe transfer. Always use a transfer belt, and if there is any doubt about a safe transfer, obtain assistance when transferring patients. Follow the principles of proper body mechanics (see Box 11.1) when you are required (within safe patient-handling guidelines) to lift a patient or any patient care equipment. The guidelines will reduce lumbar injury. Remember that injuries are related not only to lifting. Activities that involve bending and twisting (e.g., carrying supplies and equipment and pushing and pulling equipment) can also cause injury.

Delegation

The skill of safe and effective transfer techniques can be delegated to trained assistive personnel (AP). A nurse is responsible for initially assessing a patient's readiness and functional ability to transfer. Direct the AP by:

- Assisting and supervising; moving patients who are transferred for the first time after prolonged bed rest, extensive surgery, critical illness, or spinal cord trauma
- Explaining the patient's mobility restrictions, changes in blood pressure (BP) to look for, or sensory alterations that may affect safe transfer (e.g., medicated or confused)
- Explaining what to observe and report back to the nurse, such as dizziness or the patient's ability/inability to assist

Interprofessional Collaboration

- Consult with physical therapist (PT) on best transfer method for patient. PTs use their knowledge of proper body mechanics, ergonomic safety, and injury and fall prevention to train members of the multidisciplinary health care team in SPHM (Wren & Burlis, 2020).

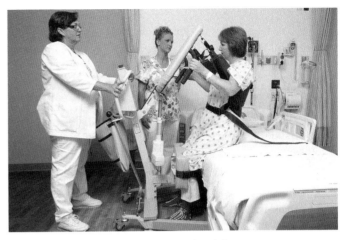

FIG. 11.2 Standing lift.

Equipment

- Gait belt, sling, or lap board (as needed)
- Nonskid shoes, bath blankets, and pillows
- Chair with arms, or wheelchair (position chair at 45- to 60-degree angle to bed, lock brakes, remove footrests, and lock bed brakes)
- Stretcher (position next to bed, lock brakes on stretcher, lock brakes on bed)

- Lateral transfer device: sliding board or inflatable air-assisted transfer device
- Mechanical/hydraulic lift (use frame, canvas strips or chains, and hammock or canvas strips)
- *Option:* Stand-assist lift device (Fig. 11.2)
- *Option:* Clean gloves (If there is risk of touching soiled linen)

STEP	RATIONALE

ASSESSMENT

STEP	RATIONALE
1. Identify patient using at least two identifiers (e.g., name and birthday or name and medical record number) according to agency policy.	Ensures correct patient. Complies with The Joint Commission standards and improves patient safety (TJC, 2023).
2. Refer to patient's electronic health record (EHR) for most recently documented weight and height for patient.	Data determine if mechanical transfer device or FRD is needed for transfer.
3. Review history for previous fall and if patient has a fear of falling (applicable for patient transferring from bed to chair).	Previous fall history and fear of falling are individual fall risk factors. Fear of falling is related to a patient's physical performance, such as balance and gait (Schoene et al., 2019). Having a fear of falling can alter one's gait and willingness and security in being mobile (Liu et al., 2021).
4. Review EHR for previous mode of transferring to bed or chair (if applicable) that was used.	Ensures consistency in how to assist with transfer.
5. Review patient's EHR for presence of neuromuscular deficits, motor weakness or incoordination, calcium loss from bone, cognitive and visual dysfunction, and altered balance.	Certain conditions increase risk of tripping, falling, or sustaining potential injury during fall.
6. Assess patient's/family caregiver's health literacy.	Determines degree to which individuals have the ability to find, understand, and use information and services to make informed health-related decisions and actions for themselves and others (CDC, 2023b).
7. Assess patient's cognitive status including ability to follow verbal instructions, short-term memory, and recognition of physical deficits and limitations to movement.	Patient transfers are best facilitated when patient is able to cooperate and follow instructions. More assistance may be needed from colleagues to transfer patients who are cognitively impaired.

Clinical Judgment *Patients with conditions such as dementia, head trauma, or degenerative neurological disorders may have perceptual cognitive defects that create safety risks. If the patient has difficulty comprehending, simplify instructions. Explain one step at a time and be consistent.*

STEP	RATIONALE
8. Perform hand hygiene.	Reduces transmission of microorganisms.
9. Assess the patient's mobility: administer the Banner Mobility Assessment Tool (BMAT 2.0) (Matz, 2019; Boynton et al., 2020):	The BMAT 2.0 is an updated tool that assesses four functional tasks to identify the level of mobility a patient can achieve (Matz, 2019). The assessment aids in determining a patient's level of mobility and recommends assistive devices needed to safely lift, transfer, and mobilize a patient.

STEP	RATIONALE

Level 1: Sit and Shake: Have patient pivot from a semireclined position (head of bed ≥30 degrees) to the edge of the bed and maintain an unsupported seated balance for up to 1 minute (to allow for blood pressure compensation). Then ask patient to reach across the midline with one hand and shake your hand; have the patient repeat with the other hand.

If patient fails to sit and shake: Use total lift with sling and/or positioning sheet and/or straps, and/or use lateral transfer devices such as rollboard, friction-reducing (slide sheets/tube) or air-assisted device.

Level 2: Stretch and Point: Have the patient sit upright and unsupported on the side of the bed or in a chair. Then instruct patient to extend one leg, straighten the knee (knee remains below hip level), pump the ankle (dorsiflexion/plantar flexion) at least three times, and repeat with the other leg and ankle.

If patient fails to stretch and point: Requires same SPHM equipment as Level 1. When working to progress Level 2 patients, a powered sit-to-stand lift, which allows the patient to safely assume an upright position and bear weight through one or both legs, may be appropriate.

Level 3: Stand: Have the patient sit upright unsupported on the side of the bed or in a chair, with feet positioned about shoulder-width apart. Then instruct the patient to move from a seated position to standing upright. Patients should shift their weight forward while raising the buttocks from the surface and rising. Patient should hold for a count of five. Note patient's proprioception (awareness of position of body) and balance.

If patient fails to stand: Use same type of SPHM equipment as Level 2 patients for tasks such as quick transfers from bed to toilet. Use assistive device (cane, walker, crutches, prosthetic leg[s]) to complete stand.

Level 4: Walk (march in place and advance step): Ask patient to march in place at bedside, then ask patient to step forward and back with each foot. Patient should display stability while performing tasks. Assess for stability and safety awareness.

If patient cannot walk: May require Level 3 SPHM equipment (e.g., a stand aid) for quick transfers from bed to toilet. Following good practice guidelines, initially use walking/ambulation belt, vest, or pants and a lift; consistent with best practice, use the patient's walker, cane, crutches, or prosthetic leg(s) to complete the maneuver. Use nonpowered raising/stand aid (default to powered sit-to-stand lift if no stand aid available), or use total lift with ambulation accessories, or use assistive device (cane, walker, crutches).

Clinical Judgment *Do not rely on self-report from patient or family caregiver as to patient's ability to sit, stand, or ambulate. You need an objective assessment to accurately determine a patient's capabilities.*

10. While assessing mobility, note any weakness, dizziness, or risk for OH (e.g., previously on bed rest, first time arising from supine position after surgical procedure, history of dizziness when arising).	Determines risk of fainting or falling during transfer. Immobilized patients have decreased ability of autonomic nervous system to equalize blood supply; specifically, after 3 minutes of standing (or 3 minutes of sitting upright), a decrease of ≥20 mm Hg in systolic BP or a decrease of ≥10 mm Hg in diastolic BP indicates that a patient has OH (Biswas et al., 2019).
	Neurogenic orthostatic hypotension (nOH) is a sustained reduction in BP on standing that is caused by autonomic dysfunction and is common among patients with neurodegenerative disorders (e.g., Parkinson disease). In this situation a systolic BP drop of ≥20 mm Hg (or ≥10 mm Hg diastolic) on standing with little or no compensatory increase in heart rate is consistent with nOH (Biswas et al., 2019).
11. Assess previous activity tolerance, noting patient fatigue during sitting and standing (previous transfer).	Determines ability of patient to help with transfer.
12. Assess sensory status including central and peripheral vision, adequacy of hearing, and presence of peripheral sensation loss.	Visual field loss decreases patients' ability to see in direction of transfer and may affect balance. Peripheral sensation loss decreases proprioception. Patients with visual and hearing losses need transfer techniques and communication methods adapted to their deficits.

Clinical Judgment *Patients with hemiplegia may "neglect" one side of the body (inattention to or unawareness of one side of body or environment), which distorts perception of the visual field. If patient experiences neglect of one side, instruct to scan all visual fields when transferring.*

13. Assess level of comfort (e.g., joint discomfort, muscle spasm), and if pain is present measure character of pain and pain severity using scale of 0 to 10. Offer prescribed analgesic 30 minutes before transfer. (**NOTE:** Patient will require assistance when analgesic has been given.)	Pain reduces patient's motivation and ability to be mobile. Pain relief before a transfer enhances patient's ability to participate.
14. Assess patient's level of motivation such as eagerness versus unwillingness to be mobile and perception of value of exercise.	Will affect patient's desire to engage in activity.
15. Assess previous mode of transfer in home setting (if applicable).	Providing appropriate aids greatly enhances transfer ability at home.
16. Assess patient's vital signs (VS) just before transfer.	Baseline measures will determine if VS changes that occur during activity indicate activity intolerance (see Chapter 5).
17. Analyze assessment data and refer to mobility status and safe-handling algorithms (e.g., Veterans Affairs Safe Patient Handling App), available in most agencies, to determine if a lift device or mechanical transfer device is needed and the number of people needed to help with transfer (see illustrations A and B). **Do not start procedure until all required caregivers are available.**	Algorithms provide guidelines to ensure safe patient handling, reducing risk of injury to patient and caregivers (VHA, 2014).

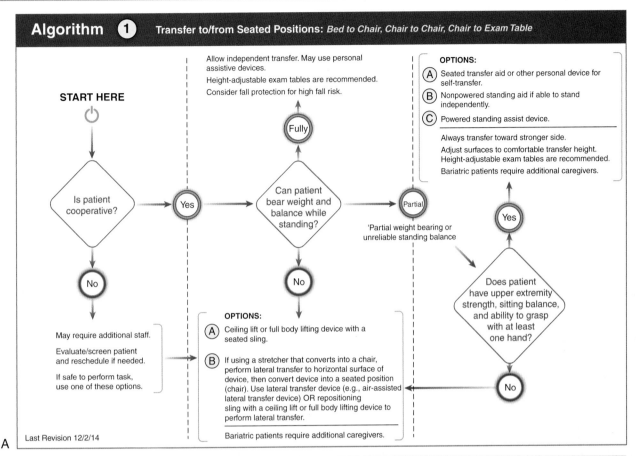

Algorithm ① Transfer to/from Seated Positions: *Bed to Chair, Chair to Chair, Chair to Exam Table*

START HERE

Is patient cooperative?

No → May require additional staff.

Evaluate/screen patient and reschedule if needed.

If safe to perform task, use one of these options.

Yes → Can patient bear weight and balance while standing?

Fully → Allow independent transfer. May use personal assistive devices.
Height-adjustable exam tables are recommended.
Consider fall protection for high fall risk.

No → OPTIONS:
(A) Ceiling lift or full body lifting device with a seated sling.
(B) If using a stretcher that converts into a chair, perform lateral transfer to horizontal surface of device, then convert device into a seated position (chair). Use lateral transfer device (e.g., air-assisted lateral transfer device) OR repositioning sling with a ceiling lift or full body lifting device to perform lateral transfer.
Bariatric patients require additional caregivers.

Partial → 'Partial weight bearing or unreliable standing balance

Does patient have upper extremity strength, sitting balance, and ability to grasp with at least one hand?

Yes → OPTIONS:
(A) Seated transfer aid or other personal device for self-transfer.
(B) Nonpowered standing aid if able to stand independently.
(C) Powered standing assist device.

Always transfer toward stronger side.
Adjust surfaces to comfortable transfer height.
Height-adjustable exam tables are recommended.
Bariatric patients require additional caregivers.

No →

Last Revision 12/2/14

A

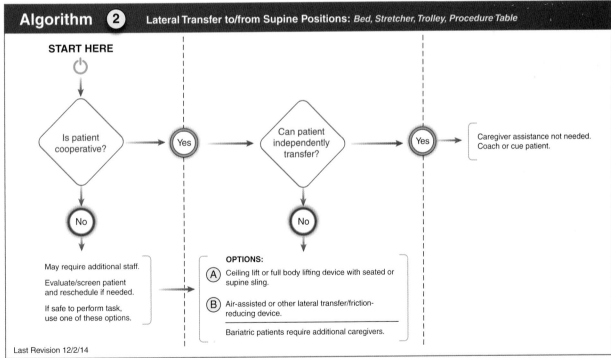

Algorithm ② Lateral Transfer to/from Supine Positions: *Bed, Stretcher, Trolley, Procedure Table*

START HERE

Is patient cooperative?

No → May require additional staff.

Evaluate/screen patient and reschedule if needed.

If safe to perform task, use one of these options.

Yes → Can patient independently transfer?

Yes → Caregiver assistance not needed. Coach or cue patient.

No → OPTIONS:
(A) Ceiling lift or full body lifting device with seated or supine sling.
(B) Air-assisted or other lateral transfer/friction-reducing device.
Bariatric patients require additional caregivers.

Last Revision 12/2/14

B

STEP 17 (A) Veterans Health Administration (VHA) Safe Patient Handling and Mobility Algorithm 1. (B) VHA Safe Patient Handling and Mobility Algorithm 2. (*From VHA Safe Patient Handling and Mobility Algorithms, 2014 revision [website]. https://behealthyswhrcin.org/wp-content/uploads/2017/11/VHA-Safe-Patient-Handling-algorithms.pdf.*)

STEP	RATIONALE
18. Assess patient's knowledge, prior experience with transfer, and feelings about procedure.	Reveals need for patient instruction and/or support.

PLANNING

STEP	RATIONALE
1. Expected outcomes following completion of procedure: • Patient sits on side of bed without dizziness, weakness, or OH. • Patient tolerates increased activity in chair. • Patient can bear more weight on the lower extremities. • Patient transfers without injury. • Patient transfers with minimal discomfort.	Precautions during transferring prevent vascular compromise. Gradual increase in number of transfers and period of time out of bed increases tolerance and endurance. Repeated transfers usually result in improved strength/endurance and greater patient independence. Proper techniques avoid injury to patient and caregivers. Transfer procedures performed correctly.
2. Close room door and bedside curtain. Prepare environment; remove any obstacles impeding transfer.	Provides for patient privacy and safety.
3. Obtain and organize equipment/lift device for transfer at bedside. Perform hand hygiene.	Ensures more efficient procedure. Reduces transmission of microorganisms.
4. Explain to patient how you are going to prepare for transfer technique and safety precautions to be used. Explain benefits and reasons for getting up in a chair.	Provides for clearer understanding by patient. Motivates patient to be involved in transfer.

IMPLEMENTATION

STEP	RATIONALE
1. Assist patient from lying to sitting position on edge of bed. **a.** With patient in supine position in bed, raise head of bed 30 to 45 degrees and lower bed, level with your hips. Raise upper side rail on side where patient will exit bed. Apply nonskid shoes or socks. **b.** If patient is fully mobile, allow to sit up on side of bed independently, using side rail to raise up. **c.** If patient needs assistance to sit on side of bed, turn patient onto side facing you while standing on side of bed where patient will sit. **(1)** Stand opposite patient's hips. Turn diagonally to face patient and far corner of foot of bed. **(2)** Place your feet apart in wide base of support with foot closer to head of bed in front of other foot. **(3)** Place your arm nearer to head of bed under patient's lower shoulder, supporting the head and neck. Place your other arm over and around patient's thighs (see illustration). **(4)** Move patient's lower legs and feet over side of bed as patient uses side rail to push and raise the upper body. Pivot weight onto your rear leg as you allow patient's upper legs to swing downward (see illustration). **Do not lift legs.** At same time, continue to shift weight to your rear leg and guide patient in elevating trunk into upright position	Minimizes strain on your back during patient transfer. Patient can use side rails for lifting upward into sitting position. Technique incorporates body mechanics into transfer move to sitting position.
2. Lower bed so that patient can sit on the side of the bed with feet on floor for 2 to 3 minutes. Have patient alternately flex and extend feet and move lower legs up and down without touching floor. Ask if patient feels dizzy; if so, check BP. Have patient relax and take a few deep breaths until any dizziness subsides or balance is gained. If dizziness lasts more than 60 seconds or if systolic BP has dropped at least 20 mm Hg within 3 minutes of sitting upright, return patient to bed. Recheck BP.	Foot placement allows patient to achieve balance while sitting. Exercise promotes circulation and provides range of motion. Allows patient's circulation to equilibrate to reduce chance of OH. After 3 minutes of standing (or 3 minutes of sitting upright), a decrease of ≥20 mm Hg in systolic BP or a decrease of ≥10 mm Hg in diastolic BP indicates OH (Biswas et al., 2019).

Clinical Judgment *Anticipate risk for fall. Remain in front of patient until patient regains balance and continue to provide physical support to weak or cognitively impaired patient.*

STEP	RATIONALE

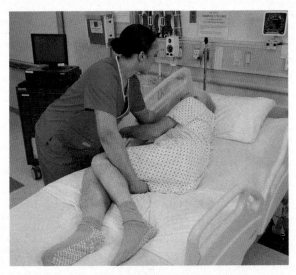

STEP 1c(3) With one arm under patient's shoulders and other under thighs, nurse prepares to assist patient to sitting position.

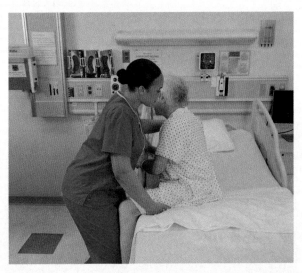

STEP 1c(4) Nurse moves patient's lower legs and feet over side of bed.

3. **Transfer patient from bed to chair** (*Options:* Use seated transfer aid [see Procedural Guideline 11.1] or powered stand-assist device):

   a. Apply clean gloves if bed linen is soiled. Have chair in position at 45-degree angle with one side against bed, facing foot of bed.

   b. Be sure patient's feet are comfortably flat on the floor with the hip and knees at a 90-degree angle. Help patient apply stable, nonskid shoes/socks.

   c. **Patient can bear weight and balance** while standing during transfer.

      (1) Stand by bedside and allow patient to transfer independently.

   d. **Patient has partial weight bearing or unreliable standing balance** but is cooperative and has upper extremity strength and sitting balance (VHA, 2014).

      (1) Apply gait belt (see illustration). Be sure that it completely encircles patient's waist. Belt buckle is in front of patient. Belt should fit snugly, being sure two fingers fit between the belt and patient's body. Do not place belt over any intravenous lines, wounds, drains, or tubes. You may need to adjust belt once patient stands.

      (2) Place patient's weight-bearing or strong leg on floor under the patient and the weak or non–weight-bearing foot forward on floor.

      (3) Hold the gait belt with both hands and fingers pointing up along patient's sides. Caregivers should never plan to push, pull, lift, or catch patients with use of gait belt

      (4) Spread your feet apart. Flex hips and knees, aligning knees with patient's knees (see illustration).

Rationale column:

Positions chair with easy access for transfer.

Provides patient stability when transferring. Shoes/socks prevent slipping on floor.

Key criteria for determining transfer method (Matz, 2019).

Caregiver assistance not needed; stand by for safety as needed.

Use stand-and-pivot technique with one caregiver (*Option:* powered stand-assist device).

NOTE: If a caregiver is required to lift more than 15.9 kg (35 lb) of a patient's weight, then the patient should be considered to be fully dependent, and assistive devices should be used for transfer (Matz, 2019).

Transfer belt allows you to maintain stability and balance of patient during transfer and reduces risk for falling (Matz, 2019).

Patient will stand on stronger or weight-bearing leg initially, raising torso.

Provides patient stability and allows you to direct patient's movement.

Ensures balance with wide base of support. Flexing knees and hips lowers your center of gravity to object to be raised; aligning knees with those of patient stabilizes knees when patient stands.

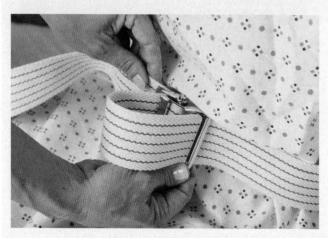

STEP 3d(1) Placement of gait belt.

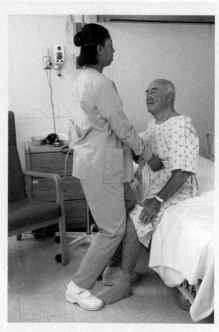

STEP 3d(4) Nurse flexes hips and knees, aligns knees with patient's knees, and grasps gait belt with palms up.

STEP	RATIONALE
(5) Rock patient up to standing position on count of three while straightening hips and legs and keeping knees slightly flexed (see illustration). While rocking patient in back-and-forth motion, make sure that your body weight is moving in the same direction as patient's to ensure that you and patient are moving in same direction simultaneously. Unless contraindicated, patient may be instructed to use hands to push up if applicable.	Rocking motion gives patient's body momentum and requires less muscular effort to lift.
(6) Maintain stability of patient's weaker leg with your knee (if needed).	Ability to stand can often be maintained in weak limb with support of knee to stabilize.
(7) Pivot on stronger foot near chair while bearing weight.	Maintains support of patient while allowing adequate space for patient to move. Always transfer toward stronger side (VHA, 2014).
(8) Instruct patient to use armrests on chair for support and ease into chair (see illustration).	Increases patient stability.
(9) Flex hips and knees while lowering patient into chair.	Prevents injury from poor body mechanics.
(10) Assist patient to assume proper alignment in sitting position. Provide support for weakened extremity (as needed). You can use a sling or lap board to support an injured or flaccid arm.	Prevents injury to patient from poor body alignment.
(11) Proper alignment for sitting position: head erect, vertebrae in straight alignment. Body weight is evenly distributed on buttocks and thighs. Thighs are parallel and in horizontal plane. Both feet are supported flat on floor, and ankles are comfortably flexed. A 2.5- to 5-cm (1- to 2-inch) space is maintained between edge of seat and popliteal space on posterior surface of knee.	Prevents stress on intravertebral joints. Prevents increased pressure over bony prominences and reduces damage to underlying musculoskeletal system.
(12) To return patient to bed from wheelchair, follow steps in Procedural Guideline 11.1 Step 7.	

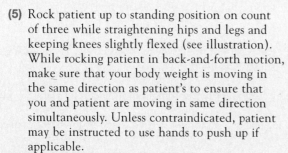

STEP	RATIONALE

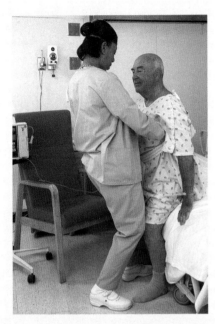

STEP 3d(5) Nurse rocks patient (who is able to bear weight on strong leg) to standing position.

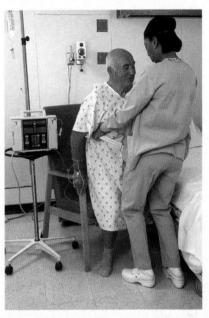

STEP 3d(8) Patient uses armrests and is pivoted to sit in chair.

e. Transfer patient from bed to chair. If patient is limited cognitively, is uncooperative, or has weight-bearing precautions with upper body strength or caregiver must lift more than 15.9 kg (35 lb), use a full body sling lift with minimum of two or three caregivers (Matz, 2019). Follow manufacturer lift guidelines to apply correctly.

Research supports use of mechanical lifts to prevent musculoskeletal injuries (OSHA, 2014; OSHA, n.d.a). Use of ceiling-mounted lifts is a popular choice (when available) because of location in each patient's room and ease of application.

Clinical Judgment *Patient who requires a lift will not initially be assisted to sit on side of bed. Lift will be applied with patient lying supine in bed, and then patient will be moved directly to chair.*

Clinical Judgment *Patients with new hip replacements who have hip precautions should not use a Hoyer lift because it may promote hip flex >90 degrees, which is contraindicated for patients with posterior hip precautions.*

(1) Bring mechanical floor lift to bedside or lower ceiling lift and position properly.

Ensures safe elevation of patient off bed.

(2) Be sure chair is available along one side of bed, facing foot of bed. Allow adequate space to maneuver the lift.

Prepares environment for safe use of lift and subsequent transfer of patient into chair.

Clinical Judgment *If patient demonstrates weakness or paralysis of one side of the body, place chair on patient's strong side.*

(3) Raise bed to safe working height with mattress flat. Lower side rail on side near chair.

Allows you to use proper body mechanics.

(4) Have second nurse positioned at opposite side of bed.

Maintains patient safety, preventing fall from bed.

(5) Roll patient on side away from you.

Positions patient for placement of lift sling.

(6) Place hammock or canvas strips under patient to form sling. With two canvas pieces, lower edge fits under patient's knees (wide piece), and upper edge fits under patient's shoulders (narrow piece). Place sling under patient's center of gravity and greatest part of body weight.

Two types of seats are supplied with mechanical/hydraulic lift: Hammock style is better for patients who are flaccid, weak, and need support; canvas strips can be used for patients with normal muscle tone. Be sure hooks face away from patient's skin.

(7) Roll patient back toward you as second nurse gently pulls hammock (straps) through.

Ensures that sling is in proper position before lift.

(8) Return patient to supine position. Be sure that hammock or straps are smooth over bed surface. Sling should extend from shoulders to knees (hammock) to support patient's body weight equally.

Completes positioning of patient on mechanical/hydraulic sling.

(9) Remove patient's glasses if worn.

Swivel bar is close to patient's head and could break eyeglasses.

(10) Roll the horseshoe base of floor lift under patient's bed (on side with chair).

Positions lift efficiently and promotes smooth transfer.

STEP	RATIONALE
(11) Lower horizontal bar to sling level by following manufacturer's directions. Lock valve if required.	Positions hydraulic lift close to patient. Locking valve prevents injury to patient.
(12) Attach hooks on strap (chain) to holes in sling. Short chains or straps hook to top holes of sling; longer chains hook to bottom of sling (see manufacturer's directions).	Secures hydraulic lift to sling.
(13) Elevate head of bed to Fowler position and have patient fold arms over chest.	Positions patient in sitting position. Prevents patient injury.
(14) If the lift is electric, push the button to raise the patient off the bed. If the lift is nonelectric, pump the hydraulic handle by using long, slow, even strokes until patient is raised off bed (see illustration A). For ceiling lift, turn on control device to move lift (see illustration B).	Ensures safe support of patient during elevation.
(15) Use lift to raise patient off bed and use steering handle to pull lift from bed as you and another nurse maneuver patient to chair. Have second nurse alongside patient.	Lifts patient off the bed safely; nurse's position reduces any risk of patient falling from sling.
(16) Roll base of lift around chair with one nurse guiding patient's legs. Release check valve slowly or push the button down and lower patient into chair (see manufacturer's directions) (see illustration).	Positions lift in front of chair into which patient is to be transferred. Safely guides patient into back of chair as seat descends.

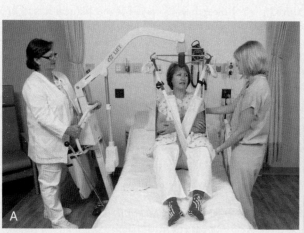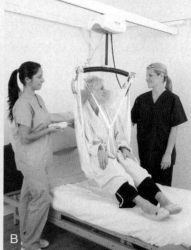

STEP 3e(14) (A) Hydraulic lift raises patient off bed mattress. (B) Electric control raises patient in ceiling lift. (*Courtesy Handicare USA, Inc*).

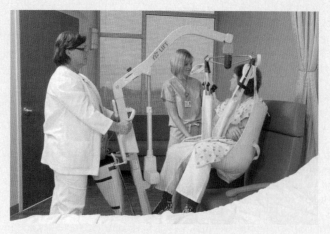

STEP 3e(16) Use of hydraulic lift lowers patient into chair.

STEP	RATIONALE
(17) Close check valve, if needed, as soon as patient is down in chair and straps can be released. Newer lifts may not need this step (see manufacturer's directions).	If valve is left open, boom may continue to lower and injure patient.
(18) Remove straps and roll mechanical/hydraulic lift out of patient's path.	Prevents damage to skin and underlying tissues.
(19) Check patient's sitting alignment and correct if necessary. Keep lift straps in place.	Prevents injury from poor posture.
4. Perform lateral transfer from bed to stretcher. (A number of FRDs are available to assist with lateral transfers both in and out of beds or stretchers. This skill summarizes the use of slide boards and sheets, mechanical lifts, and air-assisted FRDs.)	The three-person lift (using only a drawsheet) for horizontal transfer from bed to stretcher is no longer recommended and is discouraged as it is used inappropriately (Matz, 2019). Physical stress can be decreased significantly by using a slide board or friction-reducing board positioned under drawsheet beneath patient. In addition, patient is more comfortable when this method is used.
a. *Patient can assist* (refer to patient's weight last documented).	Patient's level of strength and weight determine level of help required for safe transfer.
(1) A caregiver is only needed to stand by for safety, with stretcher and bed locked in flat position, as patient moves to stretcher (VHA, 2014). Surface of stretcher should be ½ inch lower for lateral move.	Promotes patient's independent mobility.
b. If patient is not able to independently transfer and is <91 kg (200 lb), use an FRD and/or lateral transfer board.	Prevents the need for nurse to lift patient. If any caregiver is required to lift more than 15.9 kg (35 lb) of a patient's weight, then the patient should be considered to be fully dependent and an assistive device should be used for transfer (Matz, 2019; OSHA, n.d.a).

Clinical Judgment *Air-assisted devices float patients from an air-layered surface directly across to another surface (bed, stretcher). They can also be used for repositioning. Indicated for patients with compromised skin integrity, pressure injuries, multiple trauma, or burns; oncology patients experiencing severe pain; and bariatric patients (Baptiste-McKinney & Halvorson, 2018).*

(1) Lateral transfer FRD (e.g., friction-reducing sheet, slide board) or air-assisted device (see illustrations):	Maintains alignment of spinal column. Ensures that bed does not move inadvertently.
i. Apply clean gloves if there is risk of soiling. Lower head of bed as much as patient can tolerate, then raise bed to comfortable working height. Be sure to lock bed brakes.	Reduces transmission of microorganisms. Eases positioning on an FRD. Prevents accidental patient fall during transfer.
ii. Cross patient's arms on chest.	Prevents injury to arms during transfer.
iii. Lower side rails. To place transfer device (slide board) or deflated air-assisted mattress under patient, position two nurses on side of bed toward which patient will be turned. Position third nurse on other side of bed.	Distributes weight equally between nurses.
iv. Fanfold drawsheet on both sides.	Provides strong handles to grip drawsheet without slipping.
v. On count of three, logroll patient onto side toward the two nurses. Turn patient as one unit with smooth, continuous motion.	Maintains body in alignment, preventing stress on any body part.
vi. Place slide board or *option: deflated mattress of air-assisted device* under drawsheet (see illustrations). Spread out deflated mattress on bed under patient as you would a new sheet.	Positions patient for board or mattress placement. Prevents friction from contact of skin with board or mattress.
vii. Warn that patient will be rolling over hard or irregular surface. Ask patient to roll toward the one nurse on other side of bed staying aligned (see illustration). Roll out deflated air mattress to cover bed mattress. Gently turn patient onto supine position to center over FRD.	Positions patient onto board or mattress surface.
viii. Be sure board or mattress is centered under patient. Secure patient to air-assisted mattress (see illustration).	Centering patient ensures transfer of torso and lower extremities.

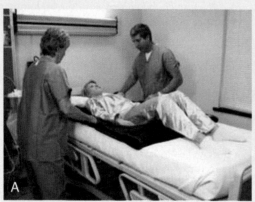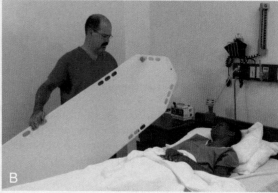

STEP 4b(1) (A) Friction-reducing sheet. (B) Slide board friction-reducing device. (A *from EZ way, Inc.,* *Clarinda, IA.*)

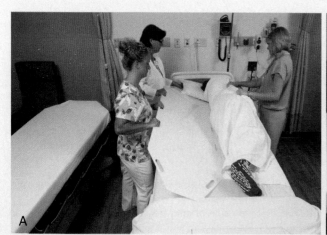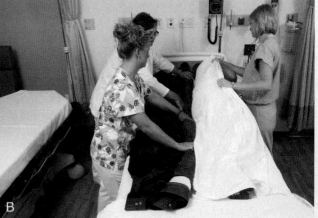

STEP 4b(1)vi (A) Two caregivers placing slide board under drawsheet with third caregiver assisting. (B) Two caregivers placing deflated air-assisted transfer device under patient with third caregiver assisting.

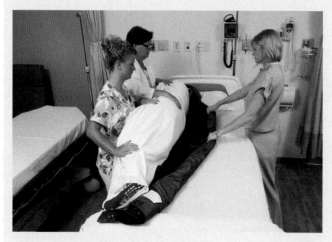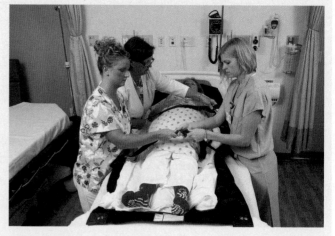

STEP 4b(1)vii Patient rolls over mattress to opposite side, while other caregiver unrolls air-assisted device.

STEP 4b(1)viii Secure safety straps over patient on air-assisted device.

STEP	RATIONALE
ix. Line up stretcher so that surface is ½ inch lower than bed mattress. Lock brakes on stretcher. Instruct patient not to move	Ensures that stretcher does not move inadvertently during transfer.
x. *Option:* At this time inflate the mattress. Then secure safety straps over patient (if air-assisted mattress used).	Provides for smooth transfer with no shear force. Protects from accidental fall during transfer.
xi. Two nurses position themselves on side of stretcher while third nurse positions self on side of bed without stretcher. All three nurses place feet widely apart with one foot slightly in front of the other and grasp FRD.	Promotes easy transfer.

Clinical Judgment *For patients with stage 3 or 4 pressure injuries, take care to avoid shearing force against skin.*

Clinical Judgment *Option: Position a nurse at the head of patient's bed to protect and support the head if patient is weak or unable to help.*

xii. Holding the edges of slide board or air-inflated mattress, one nurse counts to three, and the two nurses slide board or mattress to stretcher, positioning patient onto stretcher (see illustrations). The third nurse pushes and guides slide board or mattress in place.	Slide board provides slippery surface to reduce friction against sheets and allows patient to transfer easily to stretcher.

Clinical Judgment *Air-assisted devices have a limitation. Once a transfer begins, the friction-reduction capability contributes to an increase in momentum, making it more difficult to stop the transfer. Use caution to be sure the patient does not slide beyond or even off the stretcher or bed to which the patient is being transferred (Baptiste-McKinney & Halvorson, 2018).*

xiii. Position patient in center of stretcher. Turn patient to side to remove slide board. Air mattress can remain in place deflated. Raise head of stretcher if not contraindicated. Raise stretcher side rails. Cover patient with blanket.	Provides for patient comfort.

Clinical Judgment *An air-assisted device can be left under a patient when deflated. A device is waterproof, antibacterial, and made of antistain nylon.*

c. *If patient is not able to independently transfer and is >91 kg (200 lb), use a ceiling lift or full body-lifting device with seated or supine sling (VHA, 2014) (see illustration) with a minimum of three caregivers (Baptiste-McKinney and Halvorson, 2018; VHA 2014).*	Use of mechanical devices ensures patient and caregiver safety.

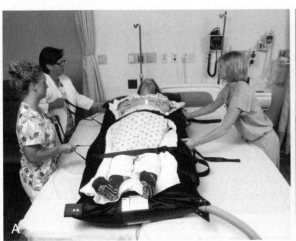 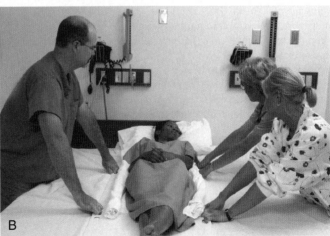

STEP 4b(1)xii (A) Transfer of patient to stretcher using air-assisted transfer device. (B) Transfer of patient to stretcher using slide board.

STEP	RATIONALE

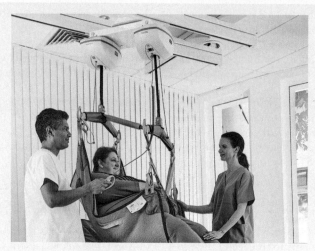

STEP 4c Bariatric lift. *(Photo courtesy of Arjo, Inc.)*

5. After transferring patient to bed, chair, or stretcher, be sure patient is positioned comfortably.	Ensures patient safety.
6. Place nurse call system in an accessible location within patient's reach.	Ensures patient can call for assistance if needed.
7. Raise side rails (as appropriate) and lower bed to lowest position, locking into position.	Ensures patient safety and prevents falls.
8. Remove and dispose of gloves (if used) and perform hand hygiene.	Reduces transmission of microorganisms.

EVALUATION

1. Monitor VS. Ask if patient feels dizzy or tired. Evaluate character of pain and severity of pain as reported by patient on a pain scale of 0 to 10.	Evaluates patient's response to postural changes and activity.
2. Note patient's behavioral response to transfer.	Reveals level of motivation and self-care potential.
3. Be sure to check condition of patient's skin (dependent areas) after each transfer.	Determines if injury to skin has occurred.
4. Use Teach-Back: "I want to be sure I explained the steps we are going to use to transfer you to the chair. Tell me the steps we are going to take to transfer you safely." Revise your instruction now or develop a plan for revised patient/family caregiver teaching if patient/family caregiver is not able to teach back correctly.	Teach-back is a technique for health care providers to ensure that they have explained medical information clearly so that patients and their families understand what is communicated to them (Agency for Healthcare Research and Quality [AHRQ], 2023).

Unexpected Outcomes	Related Interventions
1. Patient is unable to comprehend or is unwilling to follow directions for transfer.	• Reassess continuity and simplicity of your instruction. • Determine if patient is tired or in pain; allow for rest period before transferring. • Consider medicating for pain (if indicated). • Consider using hydraulic lift.
2. Patient sustains injury on transfer.	• Evaluate incident that led to injury (e.g., inadequate assessment, change in patient status, improper use of equipment). • Complete adverse event (see Chapter 4) according to agency policy.
3. Patient is unable to stand for time required to transfer to chair.	• Consider use of lateral transfer slide board or hydraulic lift.

Documentation

- Document procedure, including pertinent observations: weakness, level of pain, ability to follow directions, weight-bearing ability, balance, strength, ability to pivot, length of time to perform activity, number of personnel needed to help, assistive device used, and patient's response.
- Document your evaluation of patient and family caregiver learning.

Hand-Off Reporting

- Report transfer ability, patient response, and help needed to next shift or other caregivers.
- Report progress or remission to rehabilitation staff (PT, occupational therapist).

Special Considerations

Patient Education

- Teach patient and family caregiver the importance of increasing activity out of bed.
- Instruct family caregiver on how to assess a patient's tolerance to increased activity.
- Inform patients that mechanical transfer devices are used for comfort and safety. Studies have shown that patients feel more comfortable and secure when a mechanical transfer device is used (OSHA, n.d.b).

Pediatrics

- Whenever possible, transporting a child (who is bed bound) by stretcher outside confines of room increases environmental stimuli and provides social contact with others (Hockenberry et al., 2022).

Older Adults

- A health concern that threatens the function of an older adult, particularly during a transfer from bed to chair, is the risk for falls (see Chapter 14). Assess the patient for the risk for falls on admission, and implement a protocol to prevent falls (Harding et al., 2020).

Populations With Disabilities

- Follow SPHM algorithms for patients with cognitive impairment.

Home Care

- Have family caregiver practice and demonstrate transfer to chair skill in hospital to achieve success before taking patient home. Alternatively, have patient (if living alone) practice transfer skills in bed that will be used at home. Teach patient to transfer to a chair with arms for ease of rising and sitting.
- Home should be free of hazards (e.g., throw rugs, electric cords in walkways, slippery floors).
- If wheelchair is used as chair, access must be possible through all doors, and space for transfer must be available in bedroom and bathroom.

PROCEDURAL GUIDELINE 11.1 *Wheelchair Transfer Techniques*

Purpose

Wheelchair safety is very important. Patients who use wheelchairs can sustain falls, pressure injuries, and even choking if seat belts used on wheelchairs are applied too loosely (enabling a patient's torso to slide down so that the belt becomes a choking hazard). Transporting patients without proper application or use of safety features such as antitip bars, brakes, or side rails may lead to patient ejection, collisions, or entrapped limbs. Wheelchair prescription, posture, training, and maintenance are also critical components of safety for patients who use wheelchairs routinely. Transferring a patient from a bed to a wheelchair encompasses the same steps and principles discussed in Skill 11.1. This procedural guideline focuses on the safety precautions to follow when a weight-bearing patient is being transferred to a wheelchair.

Delegation

The skill of transferring a patient to or from a wheelchair can be delegated to assistive personnel (AP). Direct the AP by:

- Assessing and supervising when moving patients who are transferring for the first time after prolonged bed rest, extensive surgery, critical illness, or spinal cord trauma
- Explaining the patient's mobility restrictions, changes in blood pressure, or sensory alterations that may affect safe transfer

Interprofessional Collaboration

- Consult with physical therapist and/or occupational therapist about proper type of wheelchair for a patient and best transfer technique.

Equipment

Transfer belt, nonskid shoes, wheelchair, transfer board

Steps

1. Identify patient using at least two identifiers (e.g., name and birthday or name and medical record number) according to agency policy (TJC, 2023).
2. Review electronic health record (EHR) to assess patient's weight, height, and strength; cognition; level of pain; and balance during previous transfer.
3. Assess patient's health literacy level, knowledge, and experience with wheelchair transfers (CDC, 2023b).
4. Perform hand hygiene. Complete a full assessment, including the Banner Mobility Assessment Tool (BMAT) for functional ability (see Skill 11.1) to determine patient's ability to tolerate and help with transfer.
5. Check wheelchair locks, wheels, and footplates for proper functioning before use.
6. Explain to patient the steps you will be taking to help in transfer.
7. **Transferring patient from a wheelchair to bed** (patient is cooperative and partially weight bearing) **using pivot technique:**
   a. Adjust the height of the bed to the level of the seat of the wheelchair (when possible).
   b. Position wheelchair with one wheel against the side of the bed midway between the head and foot of the bed, with the wheelchair facing toward the foot of the bed. Remove the armrest nearest the side of the bed.
   c. Lock both wheels of the wheelchair. Locks are located above the rims of the wheels. Push handle forward to lock.
   d. Raise the footplates.
   e. Place a gait belt on patient (see Skill 11.1). Be sure that it completely circles patient's waist. Be sure that it is snug. Do not place the belt over intravenous lines, incisions, drains, or tubes.
   f. Have patient place hands on armrests and stand by as you have patient move to the front of the wheelchair.

Continued

PROCEDURAL GUIDELINE 11.1 *Wheelchair Transfer Techniques—cont'd*

g. Stand slightly in front of patient to guard and protect throughout the transfer.

h. Instruct patient to stand at a count of three as you place both hands (palms up) under gait belt while bending your knees.

i. Allow patient to stand a few seconds. Be sure patient is not dizzy and has good balance. Pivot with patient while turning to face away from the side of the bed. Then have patient sit on the edge of the mattress. Be sure patient is firmly sitting and not slipping off edge of bed.

j. Raise head of bed to 45 degrees. With patient sitting on the edge of the bed, place your arm nearest the head of the bed under patient's shoulder while supporting the head and neck. Place your other arm under patient's knees. Bend your knees and keep your back straight.

k. Tell patient to help lift the legs when you begin to move. On a count of three, standing with a wide base of support, raise patient's legs as you pivot the body and lower the shoulders onto the bed. Remember to keep your back straight.

l. Help patient return to bed and lower head of bed so patient may assume a comfortable position.

8. Transferring patient from a wheelchair to bed (patient is non–weight bearing and unable to stand but is cooperative and has upper body strength) **using transfer board:**

a. Follow Steps 7a through 7f.

b. Be sure seat of the wheelchair is level with the top of the bed mattress. Position a transfer board by placing it across the bed to the chair so patient can slide across it. Be sure the board overlaps the chair and mattress so that it will not slip out of place. Then have patient use hands on wheelchair arms to raise hips up and place the other part of the board under the patient's buttock that is closest to the bed (see illustration).

c. Stand in front of patient. Have patient lift and move to the front of the wheelchair.

d. Place your legs on the outside of patient's legs. Be sure that patient's feet are on the floor. Grasp the gait belt (palms up) along both of patient's sides. Have patient place one hand on the slide board and the other on the mattress surface.

e. Bend your knees, and on a count of three have patient use the arms to slide across the board from the chair to the bed.

Clinical Judgment *If the patient is struggling, attempt to assist the patient or a lift device will need to be used.*

f. Have patient sit on edge of bed, slightly above where the bed bends when elevated. This prevents having to move patient up in the bed.

g. Assist patient by raising the legs as you pivot the patient's body, moving legs back onto mattress, and position in comfortable position.

9. Place nurse call system in an accessible location within patient's reach; instruct patient in use.

10. Raise side rails (as appropriate) and lower bed to lowest position, locking into position. Perform hand hygiene.

11. Monitor vital signs after patient has been transferred. Ask if patient feels dizzy, fatigued, or in pain.

12. Note patient's behavioral response to transfer.

13. Use Teach-Back: "I want to be sure I explained what to do as I move you from the chair to the bed. Tell me how you can help move to the bed." Revise your instruction now or develop a plan for revised patient/family caregiver teaching if patient/family caregiver is not able to teach back correctly.

14. Document patient's ability to tolerate transfer (fatigue, level of pain) and level of assistance required.

15. Hand-off reporting: Report any intolerance to transfer to next nurse caring for patient.

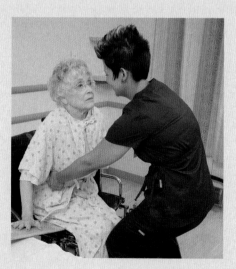

STEP 8b Patient transferring from wheelchair to bed using a lateral transfer board.

Video Clip

Patients with impaired nervous or musculoskeletal system functioning or increased weakness and patients restricted to bed rest benefit from therapeutic positioning. Correct positioning maintains patients' body alignment and comfort. Immobilized patients require frequent repositioning to reduce the risk of pressure injuries (PIs), reduced ventilation, muscle contractures, and deep vein thrombosis. Traditionally, health care agencies have recommended turning and repositioning patients at least every 2 hours if they are in bed; however, the frequency of turning is based on dated research (Chew et al., 2018). In addition, the 2-hour turning recommendation was made when foam and air mattresses where not yet used. Turning frequency should be based on patient condition. However, at a minimum, follow agency policy for the frequency of repositioning and turning patients. With the use of pressure-relieving mattresses (see Chapter 39), the turning frequencies for patients at risk of developing a PI can be longer compared with patients who are not on pressure-relieving devices (Chew et al., 2018). The type of positioning also affects development of PIs. A 30-degree lateral side-lying position has been found to be more effective than supine and 90-degree lateral positioning because a 30-degree lateral side-lying position minimizes tissue interface pressure, especially to the sacrum, enhancing blood flow and transcutaneous oxygen levels to the tissues (Chew et al., 2018).

Patients often move about in bed, assuming positions that increase their risk for PIs. Patients routinely slip down in bed, so routine monitoring is needed. Caregivers are at risk for injuring during positioning of patients unless safe patient handling and mobility (SPHM) principles are followed.

Delegation

The skills of moving and positioning patients in bed and maintaining correct body alignment can be delegated to assistive personnel (AP). Direct the AP by:

- Explaining any moving and positioning restrictions and type of safe patient-handling devices needed
- Designating specific times throughout the shift that AP must reposition the patient
- Providing information regarding patient's individual needs for body alignment (e.g., patient with spinal cord injury or severe contractures), ability to help, and number of other caregivers needed to help

Interprofessional Collaboration

- Patients who require assistance with repositioning often have musculoskeletal disorders that affect how their limbs can be positioned. Consult with physical therapist (PT) or occupational therapist (OT) for the best positioning and whether there is a need for limb braces.

Equipment

- Pillows, friction-reducing device (FRD)/slide sheet/tube
- Appropriate safe patient-handling assistive device (e.g., FRD such as slide board or slide sheet, ceiling lift, or mechanical floor lift)
- Therapeutic boots/splints (optional)
- Trochanter roll
- Hand rolls
- Clean gloves

STEP	RATIONALE

ASSESSMENT

1. Identify patient using at least two identifiers (e.g., name and birthday or name and medical record number) according to agency policy).

   Ensures correct patient. Complies with The Joint Commission standards and improves patient safety (TJC, 2023).

2. Refer to patient's electronic health record (EHR) for most recent documented weight and height for patient.

   Factors help to determine type of safe patient-handling device or FRD that is needed for moving patient up in bed.

3. Check health care provider's orders for any restrictions in movement before positioning patient, such as spinal cord injury; hip fracture; respiratory difficulties; neurological conditions; or presence of incisions, drains, or tubing.

   Some positions may be contraindicated to prevent patient injury.

4. Assess patient's/family caregiver's health literacy.

   Determines degree to which individuals have the ability to find, understand, and use information and services to make informed health-related decisions and actions for themselves and others (CDC, 2023b).

5. Perform hand hygiene.

   Reduces transmission of microorganisms.

6. Assess patient's range of motion (ROM) (see Chapter 6) and current body alignment while patient is lying down.

   Provides baseline data for later comparisons. Determines ways to improve position and alignment.

7. Examine patient to assess for risk factors that contribute to complications of immobility.

   Risk factors require patient to be repositioned more frequently.

   a. *Reduced sensation:* Cerebrovascular accident (CVA), spinal cord injury, or neuropathy

   Reduces patient awareness of pressure on involved body part. Patient is unable to position body part and protect it from pressure.

   b. *Impaired mobility:* Traction, arthritis, CVA, spinal cord injury, bone fractures, joint surgery, or other contributing disease processes

   These diseases and conditions have potential for decreased ROM. Loss of function caused by CVA or spinal injury can lead to contractures.

   c. *Impaired circulation:* Arterial insufficiency

   Predisposes patient to PI due to poor tissue perfusion.

STEP	RATIONALE
d. *Age:* Very young, older adult	Premature and young infants require frequent turning because their skin is fragile. Normal physiological changes of aging predispose to greater risks for developing complications of immobility.
8. Assess patient's level of consciousness (see Chapter 6).	Determines need for special aids or devices. Patients may not understand instructions and may be unable to help with positioning.
9. Assess patient for presence of pain; assess character of pain and rate severity on a scale of 0 to 10 (see Chapter 16).	Pain reduces patient's motivation and ability to be mobile. Pain relief before transfer enhances patient participation.
10. Perform a thorough assessment of condition of patient's skin, especially over bony prominences (see Chapter 39). Know patient's Braden score and level of risk for developing a PI.	Skin condition and risks for breakdown provide baseline to determine effects of positioning and frequency required. Routine positioning reduces occurrence of PIs.

Clinical Judgment *A Braden Scale score of 18 indicates that patient is at risk for pressure injury (PI) development. The results of a study showed that of the six subscales, the activity subscale was the most sensitive and specific in predicting PI (Lim et al., 2019). However, the overall results showed that the Braden Scale remained the most predictive of PI development (Lim et al., 2019). Apply clinical judgment. Even if the Braden Scale score shows low risk, if a patient has any area of risk on a subscale, a corresponding plan of care is needed.*

STEP	RATIONALE
11. Assess patient's vision and hearing (see Chapter 6).	Sensory deficits affect patient's ability to cooperate during repositioning.
12. Apply clean gloves (as needed) to assess for presence of incisions, drainage tubes, and equipment (e.g., traction). Empty drainage bags before positioning. Remove and dispose of gloves. Perform hand hygiene.	Alters positioning procedure and type of position in which to place patient. Eliminates barriers to moving patient. Reduces transmission of microorganisms.
13. Assess motivation of patient and ability of family caregivers to participate in moving and positioning if patient is to be discharged home.	Indicates level of instruction needed before discharge.

PLANNING

1. Expected outcomes following completion of procedure: • Patient retains ROM.	Correct positioning allows patient to achieve optimal joint mobility and alignment.
• Patient's skin shows no evidence of breakdown.	Frequent position changes may decrease occurrence of PI.
• Patient's comfort level increases.	Proper positioning reduces stress on joints.
• Patient's level of independence in completing bathing and grooming activities (ADLs) increases.	Maintaining good body alignment and joint mobility increases patient's overall mobility.
2. If patient perceives level of pain to be enough to avoid movement, offer an analgesic 30 minutes (if ordered) before repositioning.	Will lessen discomfort when positioning extremities. **NOTE:** An analgesic may not be available as frequently as a patient will require turning.
3. Obtain additional caregivers and/or necessary lift or transfer devices to perform positioning.	Safe-handling algorithms (see agency policy) determine number of caregivers and type of devices needed to position a patient if lifting is required (VHA, 2014). Ensures more efficiency when completing the procedure.
4. Close room door or bedside curtains. Explain procedure and what is expected of the patient.	Provides for patient's privacy; reduces anxiety. Promotes cooperation.

IMPLEMENTATION

1. Perform hand hygiene.	Reduces transmission of microorganisms.
2. Raise level of bed to comfortable working height, level with your elbows. Remove all pillows and any devices used in previous position.	Raises level of work toward your center of gravity and reduces risk for back injuries. Reduces interference from bedding during positioning procedure.
3. Assist patient to move up in bed:	This is not a one-person task unless patient can reposition independently (VHA, 2014). Pulling patients who have migrated in bed with a pull sheet carries an extremely high risk of caregiver injury (Matz, 2019).
a. Patient can fully assist.	Technique promotes patient independence.
(1) Stand at bedside to help with positioning of tubing and equipment as patient moves.	Prevents accidental tube dislodgement.
(2) Have patient place feet flat on mattress, grasp either side rails or overhead trapeze and, on a count of three, have patient lift hips up and push legs so body moves up in bed.	Technique prevents shear and friction against skin.
(3) Position for comfort.	

STEP	RATIONALE
b. Patient cannot independently assist:	
(1) Use a repositioning aid such as an FRD (slide board or slide sheet) or air-assisted lateral transfer device or a lifting device (VHA, 2014).	Repositioning device reduces friction as patient is moved up in bed.
(2) Patient weighs <91 kg (200 lb): Use FRD and two to three caregivers (Nelson, 2015).	Reduces musculoskeletal stress on caregivers.
(3) Patient weighs >91 kg (200 lb): Use FRD (e.g., slide board or slide sheet) and at least three caregivers (Nelson, 2015).	Reduces musculoskeletal stress on caregivers
i. Using an FRD with three nurses, position patient supine with head of bed flat. A nurse stands on each side of bed.	Prevents friction from contact of skin with board.
ii. Remove pillow from under head and shoulders and place it at head of bed.	Allows you to move patient freely up to head of bed.
iii. Turn patient side to side to place FRD under drawsheet on bed, with device extending from shoulders to thighs or ankles.	Centering device ensures repositioning of entire trunk and extremities.
iv. Return patient to supine position.	
v. Have two caregivers grasp drawsheet (one on each side of bed) firmly and have third nurse hold FRD at end of bed.	Drawsheet slides easily upward, reducing friction and shear, allowing patient to move up in bed easily.
vi. Place feet apart with forward-backward stance. Flex knees and hips. On count of three, shift weight from back to front leg and move patient and drawsheet to desired position up in bed (see illustration). **(Do not lift patient.)**	Sheet slides easily across FRD. Positions patient smoothly without exerting shear against skin and without risk of injury to nurses.
c. Patient unable to assist:	
(1) Use ceiling lift with supine sling or floor-based lift and two or more nurses to move and position patient up in bed (see Skill 11.1).	Repositioning patients manually is associated with high risk of musculoskeletal injury (Matz, 2019).

Clinical Judgment *Protect patient's heels from shearing force by having another caregiver lift heels while moving patient up in bed.*

4. Position patient in bed in one of the following positions while ensuring correct body alignment. In all cases protect pressure areas.	Prevents injury to patient's musculoskeletal system and integument. Even positioning patient side to side requires use of SPHM techniques.
a. Determine if patient can assist.	Determines degree of risk in repositioning patient and the technique required to safely help patient. **NOTE:** If a caregiver is required to lift more than 15.9 kg (35 pounds) of a patient's weight, then the patient should be considered to be fully dependent, and assistive devices should be used for positioning (Matz, 2019).

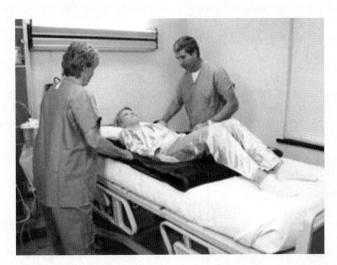

STEP 3b(3)vi Moving patient up in bed using friction-reducing device. (*From EZ Way, Inc., Clarinda, IA.*)

STEP	RATIONALE
b. For a patient who can assist fully, begin by having patient lie supine and move up in bed following Steps 3a(1)–(3). For a patient unable to assist independently, follow Step 3b.	Proper technique based on patient's level of mobility reduces risk of patient and caregiver injury.
c. Supported semi-Fowler position or Fowler position (two nurses):	
(1) With patient lying supine, position pillows using two caregivers.	Increases comfort.
(2) Rest head against mattress or on small pillow.	Prevents flexion contractures of cervical vertebrae.
(3) Place pillows under and along patient's left and right hip and back. Logroll patient slightly to position pillow on each side.	"Floating" of hip on pillow reduces PI risk.
(4) Use pillows to support arms and hands if patient does not have voluntary control or use of hands and arms.	Prevents shoulder dislocation from effect of downward pull of unsupported arms, promotes circulation by preventing venous pooling, and prevents flexion contractures of arms and wrists.
(5) Place pillows lengthwise under each leg (midthigh to ankle) to support the knee in slight flexion (avoids hyperextension) and to allow the heels to float.	Prevents hyperextension of knee and occlusion of popliteal artery from pressure from body weight. Heels should not be in contact with bed. Floating heels prevents prolonged pressure of mattress on heels.
(6) Raise head of bed 45 to 60 degrees if not contraindicated (see illustration).	Improves ventilation and increases patient's ability to socialize and relax.
d. Hemiplegic patient positioned in supported semi-Fowler or Fowler position (two nurses):	

Clinical Judgment   *A patient who has had a cerebrovascular accident (CVA) may have problems with muscle tone that could affect your ability to position appropriately. Consider consulting with physical therapist (PT) or occupational therapist (OT) for special limb braces.*

STEP	RATIONALE
(1) With patient lying supine, position pillows using two caregivers.	Increases comfort. Patient will have very limited mobility.
(2) Position head on small pillow with chin slightly forward. If patient is totally unable to control head movement, avoid hyperextension of neck.	Prevents hyperextension of neck. Too many pillows under head may cause or worsen neck flexion contracture.
(3) Place pillows under and along patient's left and right hip and back, being sure patient is as anatomically straight as possible. Logroll patient slightly to position pillow on each side.	"Floating" of hip on pillow reduces PI risk. Aligning patient counteracts tendency to slump toward affected side.
(4) Provide support for involved arm and hand by placing arm away from patient's side and supporting elbow with pillow.	Paralyzed muscles do not automatically resist pull of gravity as they do normally. As a result, shoulder subluxation, pain, and edema may occur.
(5) Place rolled blanket (trochanter roll) or pillows firmly alongside patient's legs to further help prevent the patient from leaning toward the affected side.	Ensures proper alignment. Prevents external rotation of hips, which contributes to muscle contractures.
(6) Support feet in dorsiflexion with therapeutic boots or splints (see illustration).	Prevents plantar flexion contractures or footdrop by positioning patient's ankle in neutral dorsiflexion. Positions foot so heel is aligned in opening of splint to prevent pressure. There are boots or splints made with thick padding to cushion heel and prevent a PI.

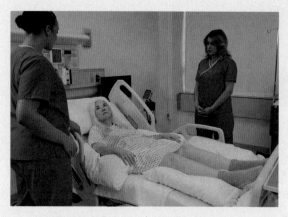

STEP 4c(6) Supported semi-Fowler position.

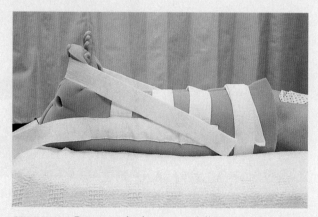

STEP 4d(6) Patient with placement of therapeutic foot boots.

STEP	RATIONALE
(7) Elevate head 30 to 60 degrees according to patient's tolerance. For example, those with increased risk for PI remain at a 30-degree lateral angle (see Chapter 39).	Improves ventilation and cardiac output; decreases intracranial pressure. Improves patient's ability to swallow and helps prevent aspiration of food, liquids, and gastric secretions.
e. Patient placed in supported supine position (two nurses):	
(1) With patient lying supine and head of bed flat, use two caregivers to position pillows.	Necessary for properly aligning patient.
(2) Place pillow under upper shoulders, neck, and head.	Maintains correct alignment and prevents flexion contractures of cervical vertebrae.
(3) Place pillows under and along patient's left and right hip and back. Logroll patient slightly to position pillow on each side.	"Floating" of hip on pillow reduces PI risk.
(4) Place pillows lengthwise under each leg (midthigh to ankle) to support the knee in slight flexion (avoids hyperextension) and to allow the heels to float.	Prevents hyperextension of knee and occlusion of popliteal artery from pressure from body weight. Heels should not be in contact with bed. Floating heels prevents prolonged pressure of mattress on heels.
(5) *Option:* Place patient's feet in therapeutic boots or splints.	Maintains feet in dorsiflexion. Prevents plantar flexion contractures or footdrop.
(6) Place pillows under pronated forearms, keeping upper arms parallel to patient's body (see illustration).	Reduces internal rotation of shoulder and prevents extension of elbows. Maintains correct body alignment.

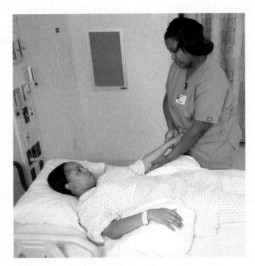

STEP 4e(6) Supported supine position with pillows in place.

STEP	RATIONALE
(7) *Option:* Place hand rolls in patient's hands. Consider PT referral for use of hand splints.	Reduces extension of fingers and abduction of thumb. Maintains thumb slightly adducted and in opposition to fingers.
f. Position hemiplegic patient in supine position (two nurses):	
(1) With patient lying supine and head of bed flat, use two caregivers to position.	Necessary for properly aligning patient.
(2) Place folded towel or small pillow under shoulder of affected side.	Decreases possibility of pain, joint contracture, and subluxation. Maintains mobility in muscles around shoulder to permit normal movement patterns.
(3) Keep affected arm away from body with elbow extended and palm up. Position affected hand in one of recommended positions for flaccid or spastic hand. (Alternative is to place arm out to side, with elbow bent and hand toward head of bed.)	Maintains mobility in arm, joints, and shoulder to permit normal movement patterns. (Alternative position counteracts limitation of ability of arm to rotate outward at shoulder [external rotation]. External rotation must be present to raise arm overhead without pain.)
(4) Place folded towel under hip of involved side.	Diminishes effect of spasticity in entire leg by controlling hip position.
(5) Flex affected knee 30 degrees by supporting it on elongated pillow or folded blanket.	Slight flexion breaks up abnormal extension pattern of leg. Extensor spasticity is most severe when patient is supine.

STEP	RATIONALE
(6) Support feet with soft pillows placed against sole of feet at right angle to leg. (*Option:* Use soft foot boot.)	Maintains foot in dorsiflexion and prevents footdrop. Pillows prevent stimulation to ball of foot by hard surface, which has tendency to increase muscle tone in patient with extensor spasticity of lower extremity.
g. Position patient in 30-degree lateral (side-lying) position (two nurses).	Position is recommended to prevent development of PIs, reducing direct contact of trochanter with support surface (see Chapter 39).
(1) With patient lying supine, lower head of bed completely or as low as patient can tolerate. One nurse on each side of bed.	Provides position of comfort for patient and removes pressure from bony prominences on back.
(2) Lower side rails. Alternately turn patient side to side to place an FRD (slide board or sheet) underneath patient's drawsheet. Then position patient by having one nurse pull drawsheet toward side of bed in opposite direction toward which patient is to be turned. Align patient straight, then roll side to side to remove FRD.	Provides room for patient to turn to side. If a caregiver is required to lift more than 15.9 kg (35 lb) of a patient's weight, then the patient should be considered to be fully dependent and an assistive device should be used (Matz, 2019).
(3) Keep patient's leg straight on side on which patient will lie when turned. Flex patient's knee of other leg with foot staying on mattress. Nurse on side to which patient is to be turned places one hand on patient's upper bent knee and other hand on patient's shoulder (see illustration).	Use of leverage makes turning to side easy.
(4) Using knee and shoulder for leverage, nurse rolls patient onto side (see illustration).	Rolling decreases trauma to tissues. In addition, patient is positioned so leverage makes turning easy.
(5) Place pillow under patient's head and neck.	Maintains alignment. Reduces lateral neck flexion. Decreases strain on sternocleidomastoid muscle.
(6) Nurse facing patient places hands under patient's dependent shoulder and brings shoulder blade slightly forward (see illustration).	Prevents patient's weight from resting directly on shoulder joint.
(7) Position both of patient's arms in slightly flexed position. Support upper arm with pillow level with shoulder. Support other arm against mattress or small pillow (for comfort).	Decreases internal rotation and adduction of shoulder. Supporting both arms in slightly flexed position protects joint. Ventilation improves because chest is able to expand more easily.
(8) Nurse facing patient's back places hands under dependent hip and realigns hip so angle from upper hip to mattress is approximately 30 degrees (see illustration).	The 30-degree lateral position reduces pressure on trochanter; designed to prevent PI.

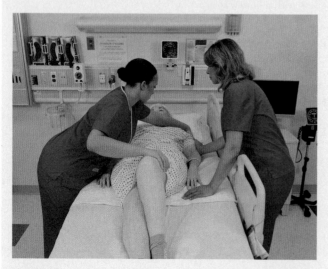

STEP 4g(3) Nurse facing patient, holding hands on shoulder and bent knee.

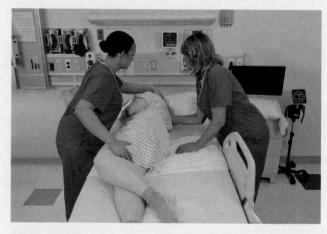

STEP 4g(4) Nurse using knee and shoulder for leverage, turning patient onto side.

STEP	RATIONALE
(9) Place tuck-back pillow behind patient's back. (Make by folding pillow lengthwise. Smooth area is slightly tucked under patient's back.)	Provides support to maintain patient on side.
(10) Place pillow under semiflexed upper leg level at hip from groin to foot (see illustration).	Flexion prevents hyperextension of leg. Maintains leg in correct alignment. Prevents pressure on bony prominences.
(11) *Option:* Place pillows or sandbags (if available) parallel against plantar surface of dependent foot. May also use ankle-foot orthotic on feet if available.	Maintains dorsiflexion of foot.

h. Logroll patient (three nurses):

Clinical Judgment *A registered nurse supervises and helps assistive personnel (AP) when there is a health care provider's order to logroll a patient. Patients with spinal cord injuries or who are recovering from neck, back, or spinal surgery need to keep the spinal column in straight alignment to prevent further injury.*

(1) With patient lying supine, place small pillow between patient's knees.	Prevents tension on spinal column and adduction of hip.

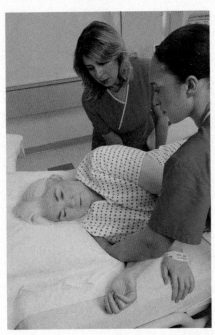

STEP 4g(6) Nurse facing patient's back realigns shoulder.

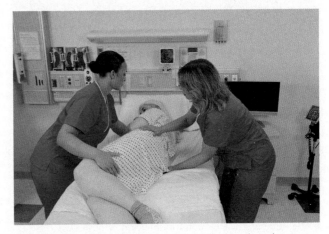

STEP 4g(8) Nurse facing patient's back realigns hip.

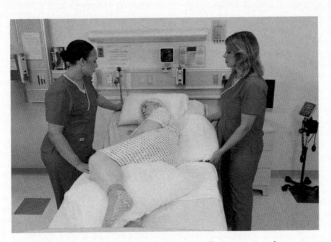

STEP 4g(10) Final placement of pillow, groin to foot.

STEP	RATIONALE

(2) Cross patient's arms on chest.

Prevents injury to arms.

(3) Position two nurses on side toward which patient is to be turned and one nurse on side where pillows are to be placed behind patient's back (see illustration). This nurse also supports patient's neck as needed.

Distributes weight equally between nurses during turning. Prevents lateral flexion of patient's neck if muscles are weakened.

(4) Fanfold drawsheet along backside of patient.

Provides strong handles for nurses to grip drawsheet without slipping.

(5) With one nurse grasping drawsheet at lower hips and thighs and the second nurse grasping drawsheet at patient's shoulders and lower back, roll patient as one unit in a smooth, continuous motion on count of three (see illustration). **Do not lift patient.**

Maintains proper alignment by moving all body parts at the same time, preventing tension or twisting of spinal column.

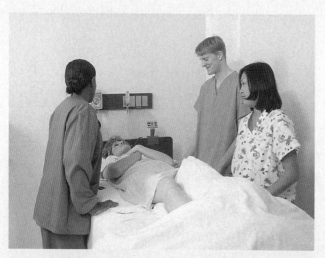

STEP 4h(3) Preparing patient for logrolling.

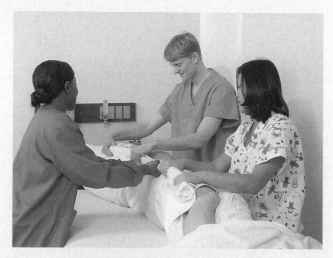

STEP 4h(5) Logrolling patient onto side.

(6) Nurse on opposite side of bed places pillows firmly along length of patient for support.

Maintains patient in side-lying position.

(7) Gently lean patient as a unit back toward pillows for support. Place patient's feet in therapeutic boots or splints.

Ensures continued straight alignment of spinal column, preventing injury. Prevents foot drop.

5. Be sure patient feels comfortable in new position.

Gives patient sense of well-being.

6. Raise side rails (as appropriate) and lower bed to lowest position, locking into position.

Ensures patient safety and prevents falls.

7. Place nurse call system in an accessible location within patient's reach.

Ensures patient can call for assistance if needed.

8. Perform hand hygiene.

Reduces transmission of microorganisms.

STEP	RATIONALE

EVALUATION

1. Assess patient's respiratory status, body alignment, position, and level of comfort on an ongoing basis. Patient's body should be supported by adequate mattress, and vertebral column should be without observable curves.

Determines effectiveness of positioning and patient's tolerance. Additional supports (e.g., pillows, bath blankets) may be added or removed for comfort and correct body alignment.

Clinical Judgment *Ongoing evaluation is critical, as patient is in best position to indicate when developing symptoms require repositioning.*

2. Observe for changes in joint ROM.
3. Observe for areas of erythema or breakdown involving skin, especially in dependent areas (see Chapter 39).
4. **Use Teach-Back:** "I want to be sure I explained the steps we are going to use to move and position you in bed. Please repeat the steps you can follow to help us move you up in bed." Revise your instruction now or develop a plan for revised patient/family caregiver teaching if patient/family caregiver is not able to teach back correctly.

Early identification of muscle contracture development is critical.
Provides ongoing observation regarding patient's skin. Indicates early PI formation or improper positioning of body part.
Teach-back is a technique for health care providers to ensure that they have explained medical information clearly so that patients and their families understand what is communicated to them (AHRQ, 2023).

Unexpected Outcomes

1. Joint contractures develop or worsen.

2. Skin shows localized areas of erythema and breakdown.

3. Patient avoids moving.

Related Interventions

- Increase frequency of ROM exercises to affected and immobilized areas (see Chapter 12).
- Consider PT consultation for different positioning.
- Increase frequency of repositioning.
- Use a different FRD.
- Place a turning schedule above patient's bed.
- Provide appropriate skin care (see Skill 39.1).
- Medicate with analgesia as ordered by health care provider to ensure patient's comfort before moving.
- Allow pain medication to take effect before repositioning.

Documentation

- Document positioning change, time of change, FRD used, and observations (e.g., condition of skin, joint movement, ventilation).
- Document evaluation of patient learning.

Hand-Off Reporting

- Report observations of patient's tolerance of position changes to nurse at change of shift.
- Report skin or joint complications to health care provider.

Special Considerations
Patient Education

- Teach patient ways to help with positioning and provide opportunity for return demonstration.
- A patient's values and beliefs about the nature of pain and pain management might affect willingness to accept pain control measures needed for frequent repositioning.
- For patients who are in any way sensitive to personal contact, be patient and explain in depth why it is necessary to take the steps required for proper positioning.
- Explain to patients the added comfort provided in using FRD devices during positioning.

Pediatrics

- Due to the generally smaller size and frame of young children, it is common for nurses and family members to use the basic

drawsheet when repositioning these patients. Nurses will manually lift children. These lifting efforts may have the potential to cause serious injury (Baptiste-McKinney & Halvorson, 2018).
- As the prevalence of obesity continues to increase in the United States, children can weigh up to 136 kg (300 lb). The use of FRDs can make care tasks much more comfortable (Baptiste-McKinney & Halvorson, 2018).

Older Adults

- Most long-term care facilities have mechanical lifts for vertical and sit-to-stand transfers, but little attention has been given to FRDs for repositioning residents. Most facilities do not have equipment available (Baptiste-McKinney & Halvorson, 2018).

Home Care

- Teach patient and family caregiver signs and symptoms of PI and contractures to observe for in the home.
- Teach family caregiver how to position patient, especially when caring for infant, young child, or confused or unconscious patient. Be sure family caregiver has assistance from another individual if patient's weight dictates.

✦ CLINICAL JUDGMENT AND NEXT-GENERATION NCLEX® EXAMINATION–STYLE QUESTIONS

A 62-year-old patient is 1 week post–cerebrovascular accident (CVA; stroke) that resulted in paralysis of the left arm and leg. Current vital signs include blood pressure 146/84 mm Hg, pulse 88 beats/min, respirations 14 breaths/min, temperature 37.1°C (98.8°F), and oxygen saturation 99% on room air. The nurses assesses that the patient has a facial droop on the left side yet can speak clearly. The electronic health record (EHR) shows the patient has been having difficulty eating due to impaired swallowing. There is some return in function of the left leg, as the patient can move the toes and foot but cannot bend the left knee. During a physical therapy consultation, the patient showed normal strength in the right arm and leg.

1. A nurse is planning to transfer the patient to a chair at the bedside. Which of the following assessments will the nurse perform before the transfer? **Select all that apply**.
   1. Dietary history
   2. Orientation
   3. Current weight
   4. Blood pressure
   5. BMAT score
   6. Activity tolerance prior to CVA
2. Which of the following factors does the nurse identify that place the patient at risk for injury during transfer? **Select all that apply**.
   1. Impaired nutrition
   2. Reduced circulation
   3. Loss of sensation
   4. Blood pressure 146/84 mm Hg
   5. Reduced joint mobility
3. Immediately before transferring the patient, which action will the nurse take?
   1. Be sure the patient is wearing soft slippers.
   2. Place wheelchair at a 90-degree angle to the bed.
   3. Ensure that gait belt will fit appropriately around patient.
   4. Allow family members to perform the initial transfer to chair.
4. The patient has regained most strength in the left side after several days. Which task will the nurse delegate to assistive personnel (AP)?
   1. Transfer patient to wheelchair for discharge.
   2. Assess range of motion of left knee.
   3. Teach about home safety when ambulating.
   4. Evaluate the best transfer method for the patient at home.
5. When providing hand-off communication to the oncoming nurse, which information will the current nurse provide as the **priority**?
   1. "The patient sat in a chair for 30 minutes today."
   2. "Blood pressure before transfer was 146/84 mm Hg; after transfer, it was 98/68 mm Hg."
   3. "The physical therapist came to work on the patient's range of motion this afternoon."
   4. "The walker the patient was using became wobbly, so we got another one to use."

Visit the Evolve site for Answer to Clinical Judgment and Next-Generation NCLEX® Examination–Style Questions.

REFERENCES

Agency for Healthcare Research and Quality (AHRQ): *Teach-Back: intervention*, Rockville, MD, 2023, AHRQ. https://www.ahrq.gov/health-literacy/quality-resources/tools/literacy-toolkit/healthlittoolkit2-tool5.html.

American Association for Safe Patient Handling and Movement (AASPHM): *Healthcare recipient sling and lift hanger bar compatibility guidelines*, 2016. https://www.hcergo.org/wp-content/uploads/2015/10/AASPHM-Sling-Hanger-Bar-Guidelines-2016.pdf. Accessed August 25, 2023.

American Nurses Association (ANA): *Safe patient handling and mobility interprofessional standards*, ed 2, Silver Spring, MD, 2021, American Nurses Association.

Baptiste-McKinney A, Halvorson B: The use of friction-reducing devices in a safe patient handling and mobility program, *Int J SPHM* 8(3):132–141, 2018.

Bergman R, De Jesus O: *Patient care transfer techniques*, National library of medicine: Stat Pearls, October 2022. https://www.ncbi.nlm.nih.gov/books/NBK564305/. Accessed August 25, 2023.

Biswas D, et al: Role of nurses and nurse practitioners in the recognition, diagnosis, and management of neurogenic orthostatic hypotension: a narrative review, *Int J Gen Med* 12:173–184, 2019.

Boynton T, et al: The Bedside Mobility Assessment Tool 2.0, *American Nurse*, 2020. https://www.myamericannurse.com/the-bedside-mobility-assessment-tool-2-0/.

Centers for Disease Control and Prevention (CDC): *Safe Patient Handling and Mobility (SPHM)*, The National Institute for Occupational Safety and Health (NIOSH), 2023a, https://www.cdc.gov/niosh/topics/safepatient/default.html.

Centers for Disease Control and Prevention (CDC): *What is health literacy?* 2023b. https://www.cdc.gov/healthliteracy/learn/index.html.

Chew HSJ, et al: Turning frequency in adult bedridden patients to prevent hospital-acquired pressure ulcer: a scoping review, *Intl Wound J* 15(2):225–236, 2018.

Choi J, Cramer E: Reports from RNs on safe patient handling and mobility programs in acute care hospital units, *J Nurs Adm* 46(11):566–573, 2016.

Dennerlein JT, et al: Lifting and exertion injuries decrease after implementation of an integrated hospital-wide safe patient handling and mobilisation programme, *Occup Environ Med* 74:336–343, 2017.

Fairchild SL, O'Shea R: *Pierson and fairchild's principles and techniques of patient care*, ed 7, St. Louis, 2022, Saunders.

Harding M, et al: *Lewis's Medical-surgical nursing: assessment and management of clinical problems*, ed 11, St Louis, 2020, Elsevier.

Hockenberry MJ, et al: *Wong's essentials of pediatric nursing*, ed 11, St Louis, 2022, Elsevier.

Huether SE, McCance KL: *Understanding pathophysiology*, ed 7, St Louis, 2020, Mosby.

Hwang J, et al: Commercially available friction-reducing patient-transfer devices reduce biomechanical stresses on caregivers' upper extremities and low back, *Hum Factors* 61(7):1125–1140, 2019.

Járomi M, et al: Back School programme for nurses has reduced low back pain levels: a randomised controlled trial, *J Clin Nurs* 27(5–6):e895–e902, 2018.

Kucera K, et al: Factors associated with lift equipment use during patient lifts and transfers by hospital nurses and nursing care assistants: a prospective observational cohort study, *Int J Nurs Stud* 91:35–46, 2019.

Lim E, et al: Using the Braden subscales to assess risk of pressure injuries in adult patients: a retrospective case-control study, *Int Wound J* 16(3):665–673, 2019.

Liu M, et al: Fear of falling is as important as multiple previous falls in terms of limiting daily activities: a longitudinal study, *BMC Geriatr* 21(1):350, 2021. https://bmcgeriatr.biomedcentral.com/articles/10.1186/s12877-021-02305-8. Accessed August 25, 2023.

Matz M: *Patient handling and mobility assessments*, ed 2, The Facility Guidelines Institute, 2019. https://www.fgiguidelines.org/wp-content/uploads/2019/10/FGI-Patient-Handling-and-Mobility-Assessments_191008.pdf. Accessed August 25, 2023.

National Safety Council (NSC): *NSC injury facts: overexertion and bodily reaction*, 2023. https://injuryfacts.nsc.org/work/safety-topics/overexertion-and-bodily-reaction/. Accessed August 25, 2023.

Nelson A: Assessment *criteria and care plan for safe patient handling and movement*, 2015, VISN 8 Patient Safety Center Tampa, Fl https://www.medline.com/media/mkt/clinical-solutions/safe-patient-handling-program/tools/tools-pdf/OTH_Safe-Patient-Handling-Movement-Instructions.pdf. Accessed August 25, 2023.

Occupational Safety and Health Administration (OSHA): *Worker safety in hospitals*, n.d.a. OSHA. https://www.osha.gov/dsg/hospitals/. Accessed August 25, 2023.

Occupational Safety and Health Administration (OSHA): *Safe patient handling; busting the myths*, n.d.b. https://www.osha.gov/sites/default/files/3.1_Mythbusters_508.pdf. Accessed August 25, 2023.

Occupational Safety and Health Association (OSHA): *Safe patient handling—preventing musculoskeletal disorders in nursing homes*, 2014, OSHA Publication

3108. https://www.osha.gov/Publications/OSHA3708.pdf. Accessed August 25, 2023.

Risør B, et al: A multi-component patient-handling intervention improves attitudes and behaviors for safe patient handling and reduces aggression experienced by nursing staff: a controlled before-after study, *Appl Ergon* 60:74–82, 2017.

Schoene D, et al: A systematic review on the influence of fear of falling on quality of life in older people: is there a role for falls? *Clin Interv Aging* 14:701–719, 2019.

Schoenfisch AL, et al: Use of assistive devices to lift, transfer, and reposition hospital patients, *Nurs Res* 68(1):3–12, 2019.

Stott H: Embodied perceptions of immobility after stroke. In Vindrola-Padros C, Vindrola-Padros B, Lee-Crossett K, editors: *Immobility and medicine*, Singapore, 2021, Palgrave Macmillan. https://link.springer.com/chapter/10.1007/978-981-15-4976-2_8#citeas. Accessed August 25, 2023.

Teeple E, et al: Outcomes of safe patient handling and mobilization programs: a meta-analysis, *Work* 58(2):173–184, 2017.

The Joint Commission (TJC): *2023 National patient safety goals*, Oakbrook Terrace, IL, 2023, The Commission. https://www.jointcommission.org/standards_information/npsgs.aspx.

U.S. Department of Veterans Affairs: *Public health: Safe Patient Handling and Mobility (SPHM)*, 2021. https://www.publichealth.va.gov/employeehealth/patient-handling/. Accessed August 25, 2023.

Veterans Health Administration (VHA): *VHA safe patient handling and mobility algorithms*, 2014 revision. https://behealthyswhrcin.org/wp-content/uploads/2017/11/VHA-Safe-Patient-Handling-algorithms.pdf.

Wren ME, Burlis TL: An innovative experiential interprofessional education activity using physical therapy students to teach medical students how to safely handle patients, *J Interprofessional Educ Prac* 19:100309, 2020. https://profiles.wustl.edu/en/publications/an-innovative-experiential-interprofessional-education-activity-u. Accessed August 25, 2023.

12 | Exercise, Mobility, and Immobilization Devices

SKILLS AND PROCEDURES

Skill 12.1 **Promoting Early Activity and Exercise, p. 326**

Procedural Guideline 12.1 **Performing Range-of-Motion Exercises, p. 331**

Procedural Guideline 12.2 **Applying Graduated Compression (Elastic) Stockings and Sequential Compression Device, p. 337**

Procedural Guideline 12.3 **Assisting With Ambulation (Without Assist Devices), p. 342**

Skill 12.2 **Assisting With Use of Canes, Walkers, and Crutches, p. 345**

Skill 12.3 **Care of a Patient With an Immobilization Device, p. 355**

OBJECTIVES

Mastery of content in this chapter will enable you to:

- Identify significant assessment data to be collected before assisting a patient with exercise and ambulation.
- Discuss implications for preventing deconditioning and deep vein thrombosis (DVT) in hospitalized inpatients.
- Identify the evidence that supports early activity and exercise in patient care.
- Explain how to plan a safe exercise program for a patient.
- Discuss indications for performing range-of-motion (ROM) exercises.
- Identify the risks for patients to develop DVT.

- Explain safety measures to use when ambulating patients with assist devices.
- Interpret evaluation findings to determine a patient's response to wearing compression stockings or sequential compression devices.
- Create plans to assist patients with ambulation, ambulation with the use of an assist device, ROM exercises, and applying elastic stockings and a sequential compression device.
- Create teaching plans for safety in the home while using an assist device.

MEDIA RESOURCES

- http://evolve.elsevier.com/Perry/skills
- Review Questions
- Audio Glossary
- ▶ Video Clips
- Case Studies

- Answers to Clinical Judgment and Next-Generation NCLEX® Examination–Style Questions
- Skills Performance Checklists
- Printable Key Points

PURPOSE

Regular physical activity and exercise contribute to individuals' physical and emotional well-being. The American Heart Association (AHA, 2023a; 2023b) has described the benefits of physical activity: elevates mood and attitude, promotes physical fitness, boosts energy, helps in stress management, promotes better sleep, and improves self-image. Promoting activity and exercise is a principle that you apply in the care of patients in all phases of illness and in all health care settings. When promoting activity, it is important to do so in a safe manner, especially for patients who are functionally impaired and in need of your physical assistance.

Functional decline (e.g., the loss of the ability to perform self-care or activities of daily living [ADLs]) may result from not only illness or adverse treatment effects but also physical deconditioning. Prolonged inactivity (e.g., during ill health; after injury, surgery, or hospitalization; or due to an inactive lifestyle) subjects the human body to negative physiological processes, particularly in older adults. As a result, there is a loss of function sometimes termed *disuse syndrome* (Santy-Tomlinson, 2021). Inactivity and reduced activity impact all body systems, including the musculoskeletal, cardiovascular, and respiratory systems; cognition; and the skin. The musculoskeletal effects of prolonged immobility include muscle myopathy and atrophy, resulting in musculoskeletal deconditioning (Santy-Tomlinson, 2021). When cardiac deconditioning develops, the stroke volume is reduced, with an associated increase in resting heart rate and signs of orthostatic intolerance (e.g., dizziness upon standing).

Inactivity has become a problem as a result of the COVID-19 pandemic. The older population experienced two main negative effects: (1) Individuals no longer felt safe leaving their homes and moving around in their communities, and (2) those who usually visited and supported them at home could no longer do so in a way that was meaningful (Santy-Tomlinson, 2021). As a result, many individuals entering health care agencies are already physically deconditioned due to their prior social isolation. There is an urgent and growing need to shift focus from just avoiding deconditioning to promoting reconditioning (Arora, 2022). Encouraging activity and exercise to promote rehabilitation and reablement in hospitals, long-term care, and community programs serves to improve long-term health outcomes and prevent loneliness (Arora, 2022).

Because deconditioning results in numerous physical changes, it is a particular risk for hospitalized patients, who can spend most of their time in bed even when able to walk. Recently, hospitals have made efforts to increase inpatients' activity and mobility levels as soon as possible to prevent hospital-acquired deconditioning. This includes even those patients hospitalized in critical care units. Interprofessional early mobility protocols, such as that developed by the American Association of Critical Care Nurses, have shown success through the application of evidenced-based guidelines for assessing patient eligibility, mobility progression, tolerance assessment, and reevaluation (Bach & Hetland, 2022; Linke et al., 2020; Schallom et al., 2020). Well-designed protocols include the input and implementation by physicians, nurses, respiratory therapists, physical therapists, and occupational therapists. The early mobility protocols use patient outcomes such as time from admission (to nursing unit) to first occurrence of formal activity (e.g., sitting on side of bed) and frequency of ambulation (Linke et al., 2020). When patients are transferred out of intensive care to general nursing units, early mobility protocols should continue. Early mobility guidelines involving physical therapy are part of rapid recovery protocols in orthopedic patients (Taylor et al., 2022).

Nurses play an important role in increasing the overall activity of all patients, including those in the community, hospitalized patients, and patients in rehabilitation and long-term care settings. The Physical Activity objectives for *Healthy People 2030* reflect the strong state of the science supporting the health benefits of regular physical activity among youth and adults (Office of Disease Prevention and Health Promotion [ODPHP], n.d.). The promotion of early exercise and mobility as a daily therapy for patients in all health care settings is basic to competent nursing practice. In patients at risk for being immobile, preventive actions minimize the effects of deconditioning and help prevent complications such as thromboembolic disease and deep vein thrombosis (DVT).

PRACTICE STANDARDS

- Bach & Hetland, 2022: A Step Forward for Intensive Care Unit Patients: Early Mobility Interventions and Associated Outcome Measures
- Badireddy & Mudipalli, 2023: Deep Vein Thrombosis Prophylaxis
- The Joint Commission (TJC), 2023: National Patient Safety Goals—Patient identification
- U.S. Department of Health and Human Services, 2018: Physical Activity Guidelines for Americans, 2nd edition

PRINCIPLES FOR PRACTICE

- Regular physical activity includes participation in moderate- and vigorous-intensity physical activities and muscle-strengthening activities (USDHHS, 2018).
- Changes in a patient's mobility and activity can result from a variety of health problems (e.g., musculoskeletal, cardiovascular, neurological) and therapeutic measures (e.g., prescribed bed rest or reduced activity from sedation). Direct nursing measures to maintain and/or restore optimal mobility and decrease the hazards associated with immobility.
- It is important to act aggressively and implement early activity and mobility once hospitalized patients are physiologically stable and able to respond to verbal stimulation.

- Research has shown that both aerobic (endurance) and muscle-strengthening (resistance) physical activity are beneficial (USDHHS, 2018).
- When caring for patients with reduced mobility, consider that immobilization often leads to emotional, intellectual, sensory, and sociocultural alterations. For young and older adults, immobility may alter employment, family role functions, and social interactions. Such changes can lead to altered self-concept, lowered self-esteem, and depression.
- Bed rest or limited walking (only sitting up in a chair) during hospitalization causes deconditioning, a primary factor for loss of walking independence in hospitalized older adults (American Academy of Nursing [AAN], 2021). Loss of walking independence increases the length of hospital stay, the need for rehabilitation services, new nursing home placement, and risk for falls both during and after discharge from the hospital.

PERSON-CENTERED CARE

- Respect patient preferences for degree of active engagement in the care process (e.g., activity and exercise).
- Assess each patient's expectations concerning activity and exercise and determine the patient's perception of what is normal or acceptable.
- Always assess a patient's level of physical and emotional comfort before implementing activity or exercise therapies. Patients with pain, nausea, or fatigue are less motivated to engage in physical activity. Patients who are anxious or afraid of injury often resist participation.
- Perceived self-efficacy is a judgment of capability and applies to a person's willingness to engage in an activity such as exercise. Ask patients to what extent exercise is enjoyable. Find out what patients believe about the ability to exercise. This factor is positively associated with adult physical activity (ODPHP, n.d.).
- When helping with exercises or ambulation, keep in mind that these activities may place patients in positions that can be embarrassing. Provide a garment that protects a patient's privacy. Many cultures emphasize modesty, and patients from these cultures may not participate in treatment measures for fear of being exposed.

EVIDENCE-BASED PRACTICE

Physical Activity Guidelines for Americans

The Physical Activity Guidelines for Americans are evidence-based guidelines for helping Americans maintain or improve personal health through physical activity (AHA, 2023a; AHA, 2023b; USDHHS, 2018). The guidelines were developed after an extensive review of the scientific literature on physical activity and health. Research shows that everyone benefits from regular physical activity: men and women of all races and ethnicities, young children to older adults, women who are pregnant or postpartum (first year after delivery), people living with a chronic condition or a disability, and people who want to reduce their risk of chronic disease (USDHHS, 2018). These guidelines offer a tool for nurses to use whenever educating patients and families about exercise and health promotion. The following are key activity guidelines for adults (USDHHS, 2018):

- Adults should move more and sit less throughout the day. Some physical activity is better than none. Adults who sit less and do any amount of moderate-intensity to vigorous physical activity gain some health benefits.

- For substantial health benefits, adults should do at least 150 minutes (2 hours and 30 minutes) to 300 minutes (5 hours) a week of moderate-intensity or 75 minutes (1 hour and 15 minutes) to 150 minutes (2 hours and 30 minutes) a week of vigorous-intensity aerobic physical activity, or an equivalent combination of moderate-intensity and vigorous aerobic activity. Preferably, aerobic activity should be spread throughout the week.
- Additional health benefits are gained by engaging in physical activity beyond the equivalent of 300 minutes (5 hours) of moderate-intensity physical activity a week.
- Adults should also do muscle-strengthening activities of moderate or greater intensity and that involve all major muscle groups on 2 or more days a week, as these activities provide additional health benefits.

SAFETY GUIDELINES

- When assisting patients with any form of ambulation, apply safe patient-handling (SPH) techniques (see Chapter 11). Have extra personnel help as needed.

- During any form of ambulation, use SPH devices and nonskid footwear that is well fitted, secure on your feet, and supportive as you walk.
- Be sure a patient's assist device is in good condition. Know how to properly prepare and use a device so that you can teach patients or family caregivers how to use it safely and correctly.
- Prepare patients for activity. Make sure that vital signs are stable, patients are rested and not overly tired, and pain is under control.
- Address a patient's fear of falling, if present. Ask patients: "How do you feel about walking? Have you have fallen recently? How do you intend to remove risks for falling?"
- Use appropriate clinical guidelines (see agency protocols) for advancing a patient's activity level. Consult with a physical therapist.
- When using canes, walkers, or crutches:
  - No loose rugs, trailing cables, and clutter on the floor. Keep entrance to all rooms clear.
  - NEVER allow patient to use a walking aid on stairs.

✦ SKILL 12.1 Promoting Early Activity and Exercise

In primary care a patient-centered approach ensures that individuals set goals for activity and exercise that are physically and mentally beneficial and readily achievable. A patient-centered exercise program must be relevant and suited to patient preferences and resources. In setting activity goals, people can consider doing a variety of activities both indoors and outdoors with proper social distancing—for example, a brisk walk in the neighborhood with friends for 45 minutes 3 days a week and walking to lunch twice a week may be appropriate for someone who wants to increase both physical activity, socialization, and engagement (AHA 2023a; AHA, 2023b; USDHHS, 2018). A patient who loves gardening might plan regular yard work as part of aerobic activity. Develop and implement a holistic plan of care that enhances a patient's overall physical fitness.

Before starting any exercise program, be sure the patient's health care provider has cleared the patient for regular activity and has recommended the preferred target heart rate zone. Then teach patients how to calculate a safe target heart rate to use for monitoring their response to exercise. Begin by teaching patients how to measure their own resting heart rate; typically it is easier to learn how to measure a carotid pulse. Once patients are comfortable measuring their own pulse, calculate target rates that are desirable during exercise. The AHA (2023a) recommends that a target heart rate during moderate intensity activities is about 50%–70% of maximum heart rate, while during vigorous physical activity it's about 70%–85% of maximum.

Calculation of target rate zone:

Maximum heart rate = 220 beats/min − Person's age (for adults)

Example:

Start with a patient's maximum heart rate: 220 − Patient's age

For a 50-year-old patient: 220 − 50 = 170 beats/min

Multiply 170 by 50%, then multiply 170 by 85% to calculate zones based on activity level

Safe target heart rate zone = 85 to 144 beats/min

As a nurse, you may work in outpatient settings with the opportunity to plan health promotion activities. It is crucial to educate patients and family caregivers about the importance of regular physical activity and exercise and how these activities can be done safely during daily routines.

In acute and tertiary care, a nurse focuses on increasing or maintaining a patient's level of activity for functional health. Recently, hospitals have been developing clinical protocols to increase inpatients' activity and mobility levels as soon as possible to prevent deconditioning and other complications of immobilization (Schallom et al., 2020). Many health care agencies are adopting programs of early mobility in which there is no provider order necessary to initiate mobility. It is automatic unless there is a specific order to not initiate mobility. When patients are transferred out to general nursing units, early mobility protocols should continue. This is often a challenge because staff nurses on general units often have difficulty routinely ambulating patients because of overall patient care demands, access to equipment, or unfamiliarity with transfer skills (see Chapter 11). Some health care agencies have special mobility teams or mobility assistants to engage patients in early ambulation and activity. Your role is to anticipate and engage patients in activity and exercise (e.g., sitting on side of bed, progressing to chair, walking) as soon as physical stability occurs and as often as possible. Monitoring patients' conditions is critical because clinical change is common. You will make clinical decisions as to whether it is appropriate for a patient to participate or continue in a mobility protocol based on ongoing evaluation.

Delegation

The skill of promoting early activity and exercise for patients can be delegated to assistive personnel (AP) trained in transfer and assisted ambulation skills. In the outpatient setting, education regarding activity and exercise cannot be delegated. Direct the AP by:

- Explaining the level of progressive mobility a patient has achieved

- Explaining if there are any weight-bearing precautions or if patient needs to use an assist device
- Explaining criteria for stopping assisted ambulation or sitting if patient cannot tolerate activity

- PT can develop a complete exercise program to fit the needs of a patient.
- Collaborate with the health care provider on how to adapt exercise routine to a patient's chronic illness.

Interprofessional Collaboration

- An interprofessional team will provide support for an inpatient early mobility protocol.
- Physical Therapy (PT) can recommend the type of assist device a patient may require to ambulate safely (see Skill 12.2).

Equipment

- Inpatient—pulse oximeter, gait belt, appropriate assist devices (see Skill 12.2)
- Outpatient—depends on type of exercise recommended (e.g., 2.2-kg [5-lb] weights, resistance bands, walking shoes)

STEP	RATIONALE

ASSESSMENT

1. Identify patient using at least two identifiers (e.g., name and birthday or name and medical record number) according to agency policy.	Ensures correct patient. Complies with The Joint Commission standards and improves patient safety (TJC, 2023).
2. Review patient's electronic health record (EHR) for conditions that could influence or contraindicate mobility/exercise (e.g., dysrhythmias, recent myocardial infarction, stroke, paralyzed extremity, neuromuscular disease, peripheral neuropathy, current pregnancy). *Inpatient:* Review health care provider's order for early mobility or exercise program. *Outpatient:* Obtain health care provider clearance for outpatient exercise.	Examples of conditions that may contraindicate or require adjustments to activity. Patients should have medical clearance to begin activity/exercise program.
3. Assess patient's/family caregiver's health literacy.	Determines degree to which individuals have the ability to find, understand, and use information and services to make informed health-related decisions and actions for themselves and others (CDC, 2023).
4. Perform hand hygiene. Gather baseline assessment of vital signs (VS) and oxygen saturation (if available).	Reduces transmission of microorganisms. Allows you to later evaluate patient's response to activity/exercise.
5. Assess character of patient's pain and ask patient to rate pain on scale of 0 to 10.	Determines if there is need for an analgesic before mobilizing or ambulating inpatient. In outpatient settings, data will allow you to counsel patient as to best time to try more strenuous exercise.
6. Determine patient's age and then calculate target heart rate range. Confirm with health care provider desired target range (as appropriate).	Provides a heart rate target for safe exercise tolerance. Heart rate during moderately intense activities is about 50% to 70% of your maximum heart rate, whereas heart rate during hard physical activity is about 70% to 85% of the maximum heart rate (AHA, 2023a).
7. Assess patient's knowledge and beliefs regarding current health status and confidence in being capable of performing exercise (including fear of falling).	Perceived self-efficacy is a judgment of capability. The outcomes that people anticipate depend largely on their judgments of how well they will be able to perform in given situations. Fear of falling has been shown to be associated with the occurrence of falls in community-dwelling older adults (Asai et al., 2022).
8. Inpatient Early Progressive Mobility Interventions—to begin in intensive care unit (ICU) (Bach & Hetland, 2022).	Protocol established for ICU patients; however, protocols have been adapted for different levels of mobility for patients not in ICUs.

Clinical Judgment *Each patient care unit may have different screening criteria based on the patient population that it commonly sees. For example, some ICUs or clinical units may use a MOVEN acronym, with N indicating neurological assessment. The following is an example developed for ICU patients (Schallom et al., 2020).*

PERFORM SAFETY SCREENING (MOVE)

M: Assess patient's myocardial stability. • No evidence of active myocardial ischemia has occurred over past 24 hours. • No dysrhythmia requiring new antidysrhythmic drug has occurred over past 24 hours.	Ensures cardiac stability. Exercise can initiate ischemic attack or worsen dysrhythmias.

STEP	RATIONALE
O: Assess oxygenation status; must be adequate on: • FiO_2 ≤0.6 • Positive end-expiratory pressure PEEP (on ventilator) <10 cm H_2O • *Option:* Heart rate <120 beats/min at rest, respiratory rate <28 breaths/min **V:** Patient on minimal vasopressors • No increase of any vasopressor has occurred for past 2 hours. **E:** Patient engages to voice of caregiver. • Patient responds appropriately to verbal stimulation/commands.	Use of activity assessment criteria allows for safe early ambulation (Linke et al., 2020; Schallom et al., 2020). Change in vasopressor dose could lead to side effects such as tachycardia, dysrhythmias, and blood pressure (BP) changes such as orthostatic hypotension (Burchum & Rosenthal, 2022). Patient must be alert and responsive, able to follow directions.

9. Outpatient assessment.
    a. Identify patient's activity/exercise history:
        • Describe the type of regular daily exercise you perform at home.
        • How many minutes a week do you participate in moderately intensive exercise (vigorous walking, cycling, dancing)?
        • On a scale of 0 to 5 with 0 being no daily exercise and 5 strenuous regular exercise daily, how would you rate yourself?
        • How long have you been regularly exercising daily?
    b. Determine if patient has social support from peers, family, or spouse.
    c. Assess if patient has access to facility or area to exercise. Is neighborhood considered safe (i.e., physically safe, as in having sidewalks and being in good repair, versus threats)?
    d. Consider patient's age, income level, time available to exercise, rural resident, overweight or obesity, being disabled.
    e. Have patient rate level of quality of life based on current activity level.

Provides information on patient's motivation or willingness to exercise regularly.
Allows you to plan exercise that complements and advances patient's activity level.

Factors positively associated with adult physical activity (ODPHP, n.d.).
Absence of facility or sense of safety discourages activity/exercise.

Factors negatively associated with adult participation in activity (ODPHP, n.d.).
Serves as baseline to measure long-term benefits of exercise.

PLANNING

1. Expected outcomes following completion of procedure:
    • **Inpatient:** Patient will progress from sitting on edge of bed to sitting in chair 20 minutes 3 times a day (TID).
    • **Inpatient:** Patient will progressively increase ambulation distance during hospital stay.
    • **Outpatient:** Patient will identify and develop an exercise and activity program to perform.
    • **Outpatient:** Patient will adhere to exercise plan that includes 150 minutes of weekly moderate-intensity activity.
    • **Outpatient:** Patient will report a perceived improvement in overall mobility and quality of life (**NOTE:** Some institutions may use a scale for measurement).

Early progressive mobility protocol is designed with progressive levels of exercise to promote improved patient function, reduce length of hospital stay, and improve patients' perceived quality of life.
Relevant and appropriate exercise plan increases adherence.

Meets objective of ODPHP (n.d.) guidelines for physical activity.

Exercise promotes positive mood, attitude, and self-image.

2. **Inpatient:** Consult with PT regarding role in protocol to provide planned active resistance exercise for patients. If PT is available in home health, consult regarding types of exercises suited for outpatient's mobility restrictions.
3. **Inpatient:** Explain precautions that will be taken to prevent falls during ambulation (gait belt, assisted walking, monitoring for dizziness).
4. **Inpatient:** As patient progresses to ambulating, try to schedule ambulation around patient's other activities.
5. **Inpatient:** If patient reporting pain, consider administering ordered analgesic 30 minutes before exercise.
6. **All patients:** Explain benefits and reasons for activity/exercise. Do so in a way that matches patient's beliefs and values regarding recovery or maintaining health.

Progressive resistance exercise (PRE) is method of increasing ability of muscles to generate force.

Patients may have a fear of falling. Explanation may relieve anxiety.

Avoids overexertion of patient. Organizes nursing care activities.

Pain control enhances patient's ability to ambulate.

Measures patient's sense of self-efficacy and ability to perform a given activity successfully.

STEP	RATIONALE

IMPLEMENTATION

1. **Inpatient Early Progressive Mobility Interventions** (Bach & Hetland, 2022): Each patient's medical status and ability to participate in mobility dictate the start level. Work closely with interprofessional team to coordinate a plan. The following levels are an example to use:

Clinical Judgment *The following levels are designed for critically ill patients. General nursing units may advance patients more quickly (e.g., active instead of passive exercise).*

Level 1
- Initiate passive ROM exercises TID (see Procedural Guideline 12.1).
- Turn patient at least every 2 hours or more frequently on the basis of the assessment for risk of pressure injury.
- Help patient to sitting position in bed (e.g., stretcher chair or elevating head of bed to 45 degrees) and maintain for 20 minutes TID.
- Obtain a PT consultation for active resistance exercise.

This level is designed for patients who are medically unstable to tolerate activity and/or have bed rest orders because of a medical condition.

Level 2
- Continue passive ROM exercises TID.
- Turn patient at least every 2 hours.
- Help patient to sitting position in bed and maintain for 20 minutes TID.
- Initiate sitting patient on edge of bed or lift patient to chair.
- Active resistance exercise by PT.

Patient begins to progress and is starting to be able to sit independently on edge of bed or tolerate sitting up in a chair.

Principles of active resistance exercise: (1) to perform small number of repetitions until fatigue, (2) to allow sufficient rest between exercises for recovery, and (3) to increase resistance as ability to generate force increases.

Level 3
- Continue passive ROM exercises TID.
- Turn at least every 2 hours.
- Help patient to sitting position in bed and maintain for 20 minutes TID; sitting on edge of bed unsupported (but supervised).
- Active transfer to chair with the goal of the patient sitting up in chair 20 minutes TID.
- Active resistance exercise by PT.

Patient progresses to transfer training, prewalking activities. Patient can still be in ICU during this phase or on nursing unit.

Level 4
- Continue passive ROM TID.
- Turn at least every 2 hours.
- Active transfer to chair with patient sitting up in chair 20 minutes TID sitting on edge of bed unsupported (but supervised).
- PT to continue with active resistance strengthening program.
- Initiate ambulation. Apply gait belt (if needed). Have patient ambulate (marching in place, walking in halls) (see Procedural Guideline 12.3 and Skill 12.2). **NOTE:** Ambulation time/distance should increase daily during hospitalization.

Patients can still be in ICU during this phase or out on a general nursing unit. Progression of mobility (amount of help required and distance walked) should occur until hospital discharge.

2. Outpatient exercise and activity promotion
   a. Initiate an exercise program that contains any of the following components:
      - Warm-up (5 to 10 minutes)
      For a brisk walk: walk slowly for 5 to 10 minutes.
      For a run: walk briskly for 5 to 10 minutes.
      Balance exercises
      - Flexibility/stretching exercises
      Endurance exercises
      - Cool-down (5 minutes)

   b. Recommend strength training for adults.

Warm-up directs needed blood flow to muscles and prepares body for exercise. Begin by doing an activity and movement pattern of individual's chosen exercise, but at a low, slow pace that gradually increases in speed and intensity (Mayo Clinic, 2021).
Flexibility exercises prevent tightness of muscles and improve joint ROM, both of which can impede a person's function. Do after warm-up (Mayo Clinic, 2021).
Cool-downs allow for a gradual recovery of preexercise heart rate and BP (Mayo Clinic, 2021). Continue a workout session for 5 minutes or so, but at a slower pace and reduced intensity.
Strength training has been shown to improve strength and bone density and can be beneficial for older adults.

STEP	RATIONALE
c. USDHHS (2018) and AHA (2023a; 2023b) recommend aerobic exercise: at least 150 minutes per week of moderate exercise or 75 minutes per week of vigorous exercise (or combination of moderate and vigorous activity). This includes activities such as climbing stairs; playing sports; or aerobic activities such as walking, jogging, swimming, or biking.	Designed to improve overall cardiovascular health.
d. Recommend balance exercises for older adults to decrease risk of falls. Have patient be sure to have something sturdy nearby on which to hold (wall or chair) if unsteady. Follow this link for safe balance exercises (Johns Hopkins, 2023): https://www.hopkinsmedicine.org/health/wellness-and-prevention/fall-prevention-exercises.	Helps to improve person's balance while standing or sitting and may decrease risk of falls.
e. As a person progresses, add strengthening exercises such as use of weights or resistance bands (that come in varying strengths). Start by using light weights at first, then gradually add more. Perform at least 2 days per week, but don't exercise the same muscle group on any 2 days in a row (National Institute on Aging, 2021).	Improves balance and helps an individual stay independent and make everyday activities feel easier, like getting up from a chair, climbing stairs, and carrying groceries (National Institute on Aging, 2021).
f. Recommend patient perform cool-down (5 minutes) after exercising (Mayo Clinic, 2021): • To cool down after a brisk walk, walk slowly for 5–10 minutes. • To cool down after a run, walk briskly for 5–10 minutes. • To cool down after swimming, swim laps leisurely for 5–10 minutes.	Exercises help muscles relax and become more flexible.

EVALUATION

1. Measure VS and oxygen saturation during activity/exercise and compare findings with baseline and target heart rate range.	Determines patient's exercise tolerance.

Clinical Judgment *During exercise in the acute care setting, ongoing monitoring is critical. Assess for onset of dizziness, vertigo, shortness of breath, fatigue, nausea, and pain, and consider use of scales (e.g., Borg Rating of Perceived Exertion). Measure heart rate, respiratory rate, oxygen saturation, and, if dizziness does develop, BP (with patient sitting) (Dean et al., n.d.).*

Clinical Judgment *Terminate exercise if dizziness lasts 60 seconds or fainting or diaphoresis occurs; change in breathing pattern occurs with increase in accessory muscle use, extreme fatigue, or severe dyspnea with respiratory rate greater than baseline by >20 breaths/min (Myszenski, 2017).*

2. Evaluate character of patient's pain and rate severity using 0-to-10 pain scale.	Exercises can increase muscle discomfort.
3. Monitor number of steps or estimated distance during walking.	Provides objective measure of ambulation progression.
4. After patient has reached Level 4 of inpatient mobility protocol or after outpatient has been exercising over 2–3 months, evaluate level of confidence in performing exercises.	Determines self-efficacy and likelihood of continued participation in exercise.
5. **Use Teach-Back:** "We've talked about doing a warm-up and cool-down as part of your exercise plan. Tell me why each is important." Revise your instruction now or develop a plan for revised patient/family caregiver teaching if patient/family caregiver is not able to teach back correctly.	Teach-back is a technique for health care providers to ensure that they have explained medical information clearly so that patients and their families understand what is communicated to them (Agency for Healthcare Research and Quality [AHRQ], 2023).

Unexpected Outcomes	Related Interventions
1. Patient has abnormal VS response or decrease in oxygen saturation requiring termination of exercise. (In home setting be sure that patient or family caregiver knows patient's normal pulse range and when to terminate exercise.)	• Return patient to chair or bed immediately using SPH principles. • Notify health care provider. • Continue to monitor VS until patient's condition stabilizes.
2. Patient develops chest pain/discomfort during exercise.	• Return patient to chair or bed immediately using SPH principles. • Notify health care provider. • Prepare for possible electrocardiogram. • Continue to monitor VS until patient's condition stabilizes. • In home setting have caregiver call 9-1-1.

Documentation

- Document results of patient screening, type of exercise implemented, preexercise and postexercise assessments, and patient's tolerance.
- Document your evaluation of patient and family caregiver learning.

Hand-Off Reporting

- Report to health care provider any signs or symptoms indicative of exercise intolerance.

Special Considerations

Patient Education

- Teach patients that physically active occupations can count toward meeting the key guidelines for physical activity, as can active transportation choices (walking or bicycling). All types of aerobic activities can count, as long as they are of sufficient intensity (e.g., mowing the lawn, vacuuming). For health benefits, the total amount of moderate intensity to vigorous physical activity is more important than the length of each physical activity episode (AHA 2023a; AHA, 2023b; USDHHS, 2018).
- In the inpatient setting, teach a family caregiver how to be a coach for encouraging and safely assisting patients with ambulation (see agency protocol).
- Inform patients of the benefits of early mobilization and how it specifically relates to their recovery (e.g., reduced length of stay in an ICU, fewer days in hospital).

Pediatrics

- The USDHHS (2018) guidelines for active children and adolescents include:
  - Preschool-age children (ages 3 through 5 years) should be physically active throughout the day to enhance growth and development.
  - Children and adolescents ages 6 through 17 years should do 60 minutes (1 hour) or more of moderate-intensity to vigorous physical activity daily. Most of the 60 minutes or more per day should be either moderate-intensity or vigorous aerobic physical exercise. As part of the 60 minutes, children and adolescents should include muscle-strengthening physical activity at least 3 days a week and bone-strengthening physical activity at least 3 days a week.

Older Adults

- The USDHHS (2018) guidelines for older adults include:
  - As part of weekly physical activity, older adults should do multicomponent physical activity that includes balance training as well as aerobic and muscle-strengthening activities.
  - Older adults should determine the appropriate level of effort for physical activity relative to level of fitness.
  - Older adults with chronic conditions should understand whether and how these conditions affect one's ability to do regular physical activity safely.
  - Older adults who cannot do 150 minutes of moderate-intensity aerobic activity a week because of chronic conditions should be as physically active as abilities and conditions allow.

Populations With Disabilities

- The USDHHS (2018) guidelines for adults with chronic disease or disabilities include:
  - Perform at least 150 minutes (2 hours and 30 minutes) to 300 minutes (5 hours) a week of moderate-intensity or 75 minutes (1 hour and 15 minutes) to 150 minutes (2 hours and 30 minutes) a week of vigorous aerobic physical activity, or an equivalent combination of moderate-intensity and vigorous aerobic activity.
  - Perform muscle-strengthening activities of moderate or greater intensity that involve all major muscle groups on 2 or more days a week, as these activities provide additional health benefits.
  - Adults with chronic conditions or disabilities who are not able to meet these key guidelines should engage in regular physical activity according to personal abilities and should avoid inactivity.

Home Care

- Teach outpatient or family caregiver how to measure carotid or radial pulse, the normal range for the patient, how to monitor exercise tolerance based on target heart range, and when to notify health care provider about problems.
- Have patient or family caregiver keep diary to document exercise activities, progression, and patient response.

PROCEDURAL GUIDELINE 12.1 *Performing Range-of-Motion Exercises*

Patients are at risk to sustain a reduction in joint range of motion (ROM) as a result of injury to an extremity, disuse as a result of pain or neuromuscular disease (e.g., stroke), or after prolonged bed rest. The easiest intervention to maintain joint mobility for patients and one that can be coordinated with a variety of care activities is the use of ROM exercises. *Range of motion* refers to the distance a joint can be moved in a certain direction (e.g., rotating, flexing, abduction) or the amount of freedom during joint movement. ROM helps maintain movement and flexibility of muscles within joints, preventing development of contractures. In the example of patients who have experienced cerebrovascular accidents (strokes), a study has shown that the use of passive ROM exercises prevents local joint complications and also improves motor function after stroke (Hosseini et al., 2019). Performing ROM exercises early

and regularly during the acute phase of illness can enhance return of motor function, particularly when patients continue a rehabilitation program after hospitalization. Frequency is important. The study by Hosseini et al. (2019) found ROM exercises to be helpful when performed 6 times daily. ROM exercises are active, passive, or active assisted:

Active: Patient independently moves a limb against gravity
Active Assisted: Caregiver is needed to help a patient move a limb against gravity
Passive: Caregiver performs the exercise, moving joint through ROM

Always encourage patients to be as active and independent as possible in every aspect of activities of daily living (ADLs) (Table 12.1). Teach family caregivers how to assist. Incorporate passive ROM in bathing and feeding activities. Collaborate with

Continued

PROCEDURAL GUIDELINE 12.1 *Performing Range-of-Motion Exercises—cont'd*

TABLE 12.1

Incorporating Active Range-of-Motion Exercises Into Activities of Daily Living

Joint Exercised	Activity of Daily Living	Movement
Neck	Nodding head "yes"	Flexion
	Shaking head "no"	Rotation
	Moving right ear to right shoulder	Lateral flexion
	Moving left ear to left shoulder	Lateral flexion
Shoulder	Reaching to turn on overhead light	Flexion, extension
	Reaching to bedside stand for book	Hyperextension
	Rotating shoulders toward chest	Internal rotation
	Rotating shoulders toward back	External rotation
Elbow	Eating, bathing, shaving, grooming	Flexion, extension
Wrist	Eating, bathing, shaving, grooming	Flexion, extension, ulnar/radial deviation
Fingers and thumb	All activities requiring fine-motor coordination (e.g., writing, eating, painting)	Flexion, extension, abduction, adduction, opposition
Hip	Walking	Flexion, extension, hyperextension
	Moving to side-lying position	Flexion, extension, abduction
	Moving from side-lying position	Extension, adduction
	Rolling feet inward	Internal rotation
	Rolling feet outward	External rotation
Knee	Walking	Flexion, extension
	Moving to and from side-lying position	Flexion, extension
Ankle	Walking	Dorsiflexion, plantar flexion
	Moving toe toward head of bed	Dorsiflexion
	Moving toe toward foot of bed	Plantar flexion
Toes	Walking	Extension, hyperextension
	Wiggling toes	Abduction, adduction

patients to develop schedules for ROM activities. Passive ROM exercises begin as soon as a patient's ability to move an extremity or joint is lost. Carry out movements slowly and smoothly, through a prescribed range, just to the point of resistance. ROM exercises should not cause pain.

Delegation

The skill of performing ROM exercises can be delegated to trained assistive personnel (AP). Patients with spinal cord injuries, burns, or orthopedic trauma usually require ROM exercises by professional nurses or physical therapists (PT). Direct the AP to:
- Perform exercises slowly and provide adequate support to each joint being exercised
- Not exercise joints beyond the point of resistance or to the point of fatigue or pain
- Be aware of a patient's individual limitations or preexisting conditions such as arthritis that affect ROM

Interprofessional Collaboration
- PT recommends specific types of strengthening, ROM, and active resistance exercises.

Equipment
- No mechanical or physical equipment needed; clean gloves (*option*)

Steps

1. Identify patient using at least two identifiers (e.g., name and birthday or name and medical record number) according to agency policy (TJC, 2023).
2. Review patient's EHR for physical assessment findings that could affect exercise performance (e.g., pain in joint, reduced skin integrity or presence of wound near joint, presence of deformity, level of consciousness and ability to attend), health care provider's orders (e.g., any ROM restrictions for medical reasons), medical diagnosis, medical history, and progress.
3. Assess patient's/family caregiver's health literacy.
4. Assess patient's current level of fatigue and ability to cooperate with exercises.
5. Perform hand hygiene. Assess patient's baseline joint function. Observe for obvious limitations in joint mobility, redness over joints; palpate for warmth over joint, joint tenderness, and presence of deformities or edema. Note baseline ROM for affected joints.
6. Assess character of patient's pain or discomfort including rating pain severity (on a scale of 0 to 10) before exercises. Determine if patient would benefit from pain medication before beginning ROM exercises; then administer analgesic 30 minutes before exercise.
7. Assess patient's/family caregiver's knowledge, experience, and readiness to learn (e.g., perceived ability to perform exercise, perceived benefit of exercise). Explain in plain language reason for the ROM exercises and describe and demonstrate exercises to be performed.
8. Perform hand hygiene and apply clean gloves if wound drainage or skin lesions are present.
9. Help patient to a comfortable position, preferably sitting or lying down.
10. When performing passive and active assisted ROM exercises (Table 12.2), support joint by holding or cradling distal part of extremity or using cupped hand to support joint (see illustrations).

PROCEDURAL GUIDELINE 12.1 *Performing Range-of-Motion Exercises—cont'd*

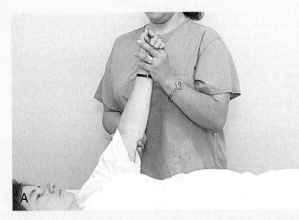 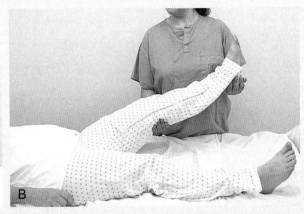

STEP 10 (A) Support joint by cradling distal part of extremity. (B) Use cupped hand to support joint.

TABLE 12.2

Range-of-Motion Exercises

Body Part	Type of Joint	Type of Movement	Range (Degrees)	Primary Muscles
Neck, cervical spine	Pivotal	*Flexion:* Bring chin to rest on chest.	45	Sternocleidomastoid
		Extension: Return head to erect position.	45	Trapezius
		Hyperextension: Bend head back as far as possible.	10	Trapezius
		Lateral flexion: Tilt head as far as possible toward each shoulder.	40–45	Scalenes
		Rotation: Turn head as far as possible in circular movement.	180	Sternocleidomastoid, upper trapezius
Shoulder	Ball and socket	*Flexion:* Raise arm from side position forward to position above head.	45–180	Coracobrachialis, biceps brachii, deltoid, pectoralis major
		Extension: Return arm to position at side of body.	180	Latissimus dorsi, teres major, triceps brachii
		Shoulder extension: Move arm behind body, keeping elbow straight.	0–60	Latissimus dorsi, teres major, deltoid
		Internal rotation: With elbow flexed and shoulder abducted, rotate shoulder by moving arm until thumb is turned inward and toward back.	70–90	Pectoralis major, latissimus dorsi, teres major, subscapularis
		External rotation: With elbow flexed and shoulder abducted, move arm until thumb is upward and lateral to head.	90	Infraspinatus, teres major, deltoid

Continued

PROCEDURAL GUIDELINE 12.1 *Performing Range-of-Motion Exercises—cont'd*

TABLE 12.2

Range-of-Motion Exercises–cont'd

Body Part	Type of Joint	Type of Movement	Range (Degrees)	Primary Muscles
		Circumduction: Move arm in full circle (circumduction is combination of all movements of ball-and-socket joint).	360	Deltoid, coracobrachialis, latissimus dorsi, teres major
Elbow	Hinge	*Flexion:* Bend elbow so that lower arm moves toward its shoulder joint and hand is level with shoulder.	150	Biceps brachii, brachialis, brachioradialis
		Extension: Straighten elbow by lowering hand.	150	Triceps brachii
Forearm	Pivotal	*Supination:* Turn lower arm and hand so that palm is up.	70–90	Supinator, biceps brachii
		Pronation: Turn lower arm so that palm is down.	70–90	Pronator teres, pronator quadratus
Wrist	Condyloid	*Flexion:* Move palm toward inner aspect of forearm.	80–90	Flexor carpi ulnaris, flexor carpi radialis
		Extension: Move fingers and hand posterior to midline.	70–80	Extensor carpi radialis brevis, extensor carpi radialis longus, extensor carpi ulnaris
		Hyperextension: Bring dorsal surface of hand back as far as possible.		Extensor carpi radialis brevis, extensor carpi radialis longus, extensor carpi ulnaris
		Radial deviation: Bend wrist medially toward thumb.	Up to 30	Flexor carpi radialis brevis, extensor carpi radialis brevis, extensor carpi radialis longus
		Ulnar deviation: Bend wrist laterally toward fifth finger.	30	Flexor carpi ulnaris, extensor carpi ulnaris
Fingers	Condyloid hinge	*Flexion:* Make fist.	90	Lumbricales, interosseus volaris, interosseus dorsalis
		Extension: Straighten fingers.	90	Extensor digiti quinti proprius, extensor digitorum communis, extensor indicis proprius
		Hyperextension: Bend fingers back as far as possible.	30–60	Extensor digitorum

PROCEDURAL GUIDELINE 12.1 *Performing Range-of-Motion Exercises—cont'd*

TABLE 12.2

Range-of-Motion Exercises–cont'd

Body Part	Type of Joint	Type of Movement	Range (Degrees)	Primary Muscles
		Abduction: Spread fingers apart.	30	Interosseus dorsalis
		Adduction: Bring fingers together.	30	Interosseus volaris
Thumb	Saddle	*Flexion:* Move thumb across palmar surface of hand.	90	Flexor pollicis brevis
		Extension: Move thumb straight away from hand.	90	Extensor pollicis longus, extensor pollicis brevis
		Abduction: Extend thumb laterally (usually done when placing fingers in abduction and adduction).	30	Abductor pollicis brevis and longus
		Adduction: Move thumb back toward hand.	30	Adductor pollicis obliquus, adductor pollicis transversus
		Opposition: Touch thumb to each finger of same hand.		Opponens pollicis, opponens digiti minimi
Hip	Ball and socket	*Flexion:* Move leg forward and up.	110–120	Psoas major, iliacus, sartorius
		Extension: Move leg back beside other leg.	90–120	Gluteus maximus, semitendinosus, semimembranosus
		Abduction: Move leg laterally away from body.	30–50	Gluteus medius, gluteus minimus
		Adduction: Move leg back toward midline position and beyond if possible.	20–30	Adductor longus, adductor brevis, adductor magnus
		Internal rotation: Turn foot and leg toward other leg.	45	Gluteus medius, gluteus minimus, tensor fasciae latae
		External rotation: Turn foot and leg away from other leg.	45	Obturatorius internus, obturatorius externus, quadratus femoris, piriformis, gemellus superior and inferior, gluteus maximus

Continued

PROCEDURAL GUIDELINE 12.1 *Performing Range-of-Motion Exercises—cont'd*

TABLE 12.2

Range-of-Motion Exercises–cont'd

Body Part	Type of Joint	Type of Movement	Range (Degrees)	Primary Muscles
		Circumduction: Move leg in circle.	120–130	Psoas major, gluteus maximum, gluteus medius, adductor magnus
Knee	Hinge	*Flexion:* Bring heel back toward back of thigh.	120–130	Biceps femoris, semitendinosus, semimembranosus, sartorius
		Extension: Return leg to floor.	120–130	Rectus femoris, vastus lateralis, vastus medialis, vastus intermedius
Ankle	Hinge	*Dorsal flexion:* Move foot so that toes are pointed upward.	20–30	Tibialis anterior
		Plantar flexion: Move foot so that toes are pointed downward.	45–50	Gastrocnemius, soleus
Foot	Gliding	*Inversion:* Turn sole of foot medially.	35 or less	Tibialis anterior, tibialis posterior
		Eversion: Turn sole of foot laterally.	10 or less	Peroneus longus, peroneus brevis
Toes	Condyloid	*Flexion:* Curl toes downward.	30–60	Flexor digitorum, lumbricalis pedis, flexor hallucis brevis
		Extension: Straighten toes.	30–60	Extensor digitorum longus, extensor digitorum brevis, extensor hallucis longus
		Abduction: Spread toes apart. *Adduction:* Bring toes together.	15 or less 15 or less	Abductor hallucis, interosseus dorsalis Adductor hallucis, interosseus plantaris

PROCEDURAL GUIDELINE 12.1 *Performing Range-of-Motion Exercises—cont'd*

11. Complete exercises in head-to-toe sequence. Repeat each movement 5 times during an exercise session with sessions performed up to 6 times a day (do not perform during sleep hours). Inform patient how these exercises can be incorporated into ADLs (see Table 12.1).

Clinical Judgment *When resistance is noted within a joint, do not force joint motion. Consult with health care provider or physical therapist.*

12. Once exercises are completed, help patient to comfortable position.
13. Place nurse call system in an accessible location within patient's reach, raise side rails (as appropriate), and lower bed to lowest position, locking into position.

14. Perform hand hygiene.
15. For active ROM, observe patient performing each exercise. *Option:* Measure joint motion using a goniometer to determine level of improvement.
16. Ask patient while exercising to describe any discomfort and rate pain on a pain scale.
17. **Use Teach-Back:** "Let's review what I discussed about ways to practice ROM at home. Tell me some exercises you can do at home." Revise your instruction now or develop a plan for revised patient/family caregiver teaching if patient/family caregiver is not able to teach back correctly.
18. Document exercises performed and patient's tolerance in a chart.
19. Report any new onset of pain in a joint or reduction in ROM to health care provider.

PROCEDURAL GUIDELINE 12.2 *Applying Graduated Compression (Elastic) Stockings and Sequential Compression Device*

▶ *Video Clip*

Patients who are immobile are at risk for thrombus formation. A thrombus is an accumulation of platelets, fibrin, clotting factors, and the cellular elements of the blood attached to the interior wall of a vein or artery, which sometimes occludes the lumen of a blood vessel. Three factors contribute to venous thrombus formation: (1) damage to a vessel wall (e.g., injury during surgical procedures), (2) alterations of blood flow (e.g., slow blood flow in calf veins associated with bed rest), and (3) alterations in blood constituents (e.g., a change in clotting factors or increased platelet activity). These three factors are referred to as the Virchow triad (Huether et al., 2020). One of the dangers of a deep vein thrombosis (DVT) is the development of a pulmonary embolus (PE). A PE occurs when a part of the thrombus or clot (located in the deep veins) breaks off and travels to the lungs and then blocks the pulmonary artery, altering the blood supply to lung tissue. PE has a variety of presenting features, ranging from no symptoms to shock or sudden death. The most common presenting symptom is dyspnea followed by pleuritic chest pain and cough (Thompson et al., 2022). However, many patients, including those with large PE, have mild or nonspecific symptoms or are asymptomatic (Thompson et al., 2022). You will practice in numerous situations in which deep vein thrombosis (DVT) must be prevented, especially during perioperative care (see Chapter 36).

Numerous risk factors for DVT influence the Virchow triad (see Box 12.1) (Cleveland Clinic, 2019; Harding et al., 2020). Signs of a DVT usually occur on one side of the body at a time, including swelling in the affected leg or arm; warm, cyanotic skin; and pain or tenderness in the affected extremity. A patient may report cramping or soreness. If a DVT is suspected, keep patient calm and quiet in bed and notify the health care provider.

There are well-established clinical standards for the prevention of VTE, published by the American Society of Hematology (ASH) (Anderson et al., 2019; ASH, 2022; Badireddy & Mudipalli, 2023):
• Provide pharmacological VTE prophylaxis (anticoagulant therapy) in acutely or critically ill inpatients at acceptable bleeding risk.

BOX 12.1

Risk Factors for Deep Vein Thrombosis

- Injury to a vein, often caused by:
  - Fractures
  - Severe muscle injury
  - Major surgery (e.g., involving the abdomen, pelvis, hip, or legs)
- Slow blood flow, often caused by:
  - Confinement to bed (e.g., caused by a medical condition or after surgery)
  - Limited movement (e.g., a cast on a leg to help heal an injured bone)
  - Sitting for a long time, especially with crossed legs
  - Paralysis
- Increased estrogen, often caused by:
  - Use of birth-control methods that contain estrogen or hormone therapy for menopause symptoms
  - Pregnancy, for up to 3 months after giving birth
- Certain chronic medical illnesses such as:
  - Heart disease, lung disease, cancer and its treatment, inflammatory bowel disease, and some kidney disorders
- Other factors include:
  - Previous DVT or PE
  - Family history of DVT or PE
  - Age (risk increases as age increases)
  - Obesity
  - A catheter located in a central vein

DVT, Deep vein thrombosis; *PE,* pulmonary embolism.
From Centers for Disease Control and Prevention (CDC): *Venous thromboembolism (blood clots)* (website). 2022. https://www.cdc.gov/ncbddd/dvt/index.html, Accessed April 4, 2023.

• Use mechanical prophylaxis (compression stockings, intermittent sequential compression devices [SCDs], intermittent mobile compression devices (MCDs) when bleeding risk is unacceptable.
• Conditional recommendations include:
  • Not to use VTE prophylaxis routinely in long-term care patients or outpatients with minor VTE risk factors

Continued

PROCEDURAL GUIDELINE 12.2 *Applying Graduated Compression (Elastic) Stockings and Sequential Compression Device—cont'd*

- Use graduated compression stockings or low-molecular-weight heparin in long-distance travelers only if there is a high risk for VTE

Nurses promote mechanical prophylaxis in at-risk patients by initiating early ambulation; applying intermittent sequential compression devices (SCDs), intermittent mobile compression devices (MCDs), or compression stockings; and applying foot pumps. Elastic compression stockings offer compression of 15–18 mm Hg and are indicated for use for bedridden or partly ambulatory patients. By reducing the resting vein diameter, the stockings increase venous flow and prevent venous stasis and thrombosis (Berszakiewicz, 2020). Elastic compression stockings, SCDs, and MCDs improve the calf muscle pump function and reduce the amount of both venous reflux and venous volume, in turn normalizing ambulatory venous pressure in limbs with venous insufficiency (Berszakiewicz, 2020). Beyond simply overcoming stasis, some forms of mechanical VTE prophylaxis also have fibrinolytic properties to combat the hypercoagulable component of the Virchow triad (Shatri & Ipinge, 2023). MCDs have added benefits of increasing femoral vein flow and reducing leg swelling with continuous use while mobilizing (Ramakrishna et al., 2021).

All SCDs pump blood into deep veins, thus removing pooled blood and preventing stasis. When a compression cuff deflates, the veins refill and, because of the intermittent nature of the system, will ensure periodic flow of blood through the deep veins as long as there is a supply. Compression stockings in contrast function more by preventing venous distention. An SCD increases the hydrostatic pressure on the extracellular interstitial spaces, which may increase blood flow and decrease edema. The effects of compression stockings are aided by muscular activity of the limb and may be less effective in immobile patients. SCDs are preferred due to their improved efficacy and better patient adherence (Insin et al., 2021). Using an additional device, such as a SCD plus graduated compression stockings, offers no additive benefit regarding VTE outcomes.

Venous plexus foot pumps promote venous return by pumping blood through compression, mimicking the natural action of walking (Fig. 12.1). The muscles in the foot, however, are much less compressible, and the overall blood volume in the plantar venous plexus is much smaller in comparison to the calf, which therefore requires larger compressive forces to obtain similar effects seen with stockings. This increased pressure requirement is often the cause of increased pain and discomfort during application of venous foot pumps and poorer patient adherence.

Delegation

The skill of applying and maintaining graduated stockings, intermittent SCDs, or mobile compression devices (MCDs) may be delegated to assistive personnel (AP). The nurse initially determines the size of elastic stockings/sleeves and assesses the patient's lower extremities for any signs and symptoms of a DVT or impaired circulation. Direct the AP to:

- Remove the SCD sleeves (exception: MCDs may remain on) before allowing a patient to get out of bed
- Report nurse if a patient's calf appears larger than the other or is red or hot, if the patient complains of calf pain, or if there are signs of allergic reactions to elastic (redness, itching, or irritation)
- Report if there is redness, itching, or irritation on the legs (signs of allergic reactions to elastic)
- Report if the patient is routinely removing the compression device from the legs

Equipment

Tape measure; powder or cornstarch (optional); graduated compression stockings or Velcro compression device sleeves; SCD/MCD insufflator with air hoses attached; compression device pump (*option*: cotton stockinette with MCD); hygiene supplies

Steps

1. Identify patient using at least two identifiers (e.g., name and birthday or name and medical record number) according to agency policy (TJC, 2023).
2. Review EHR for order for SCDs/MCDs or graduated compression stocking.
3. Review EHR to assess patient for risk factors for developing DVT (Box 12.2). One option is to use the Wells score, an objective measure for screening outpatients' and inpatients' risk for a DVT (The Constans score is used for assessing upper extremity risk for DVT) (American Academy of Family Physicians, 2019).
4. Assess patient's/family caregiver's health literacy.
5. Perform hand hygiene. Assess for contraindications for use of elastic stockings or compression devices:
   a. Dermatitis or open skin lesions on area to be covered by stockings/sleeves
   b. Recent skin graft to lower leg
   c. Decreased arterial circulation in lower extremities as evidenced by cyanotic, cool extremities and/or gangrenous conditions affecting the lower limb(s)
   d. Presence of signs or symptoms of a DVT (Manipulation could cause a clot in a vein within the leg to dislodge.)

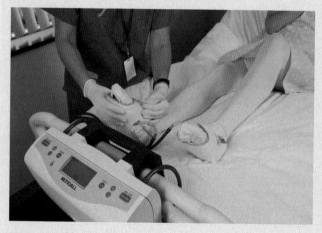

FIG. 12.1 Venous plexus foot pump with bedside controls. (*Courtesy Tyco Healthcare Group LP.*)

PROCEDURAL GUIDELINE 12.2 *Applying Graduated Compression (Elastic) Stockings and Sequential Compression Device—cont'd*

BOX 12.2

Wells Score

Parameter	Score
Active cancer (patient receiving treatment for cancer within previous 6 months or currently receiving palliative treatment)	1
Paralysis, paresis, or recent plaster immobilization of lower extremities	1
Recently bedridden for 3 days or more, or major surgery within previous 12 weeks requiring general or regional anesthesia	1
Localized tenderness along distribution of the deep vein system	1
Entire leg swollen	1
Calf swelling at least 3 cm (1.2 inches) more when compared with asymptomatic leg	1
Pitting edema localized to symptomatic leg	1
Collateral superficial veins	1
Previously documented DVT	1
Alternative diagnosis as likely or greater than that of DVT	−2

Wells scoring system for DVT: −2 to 0, low probability; 1 to 2, moderate probability; 3 to 8, high probability.

DVT, Deep vein thrombosis.
From Bruce, B and Brenner, B.: Deep vein thrombosis risk stratification, Medscape. https://emedicine.medscape.com/article/1918446-overview. Accessed April 5, 2023.

6. Assess condition of patient's skin and circulation to the legs. Palpate pedal pulses, note any palpable veins, and inspect skin over lower extremities for edema, skin discoloration, blistering, warmth, or presence of lesions.
7. Assess patient's or family caregiver's knowledge or experience regarding previous use of elastic compression stockings or compression devices.
8. Explain procedure and reason for applying elastic stockings/SCD/MCD to prevent DVT.
9. Close room curtains or door to provide privacy. Position patient in supine position.
10. Perform hand hygiene. Bathe patient's legs as needed. Dry thoroughly. Perform hand hygiene.
11. **Apply graduated compression stocking:**
    a. Use tape measure to measure patient's leg to determine proper elastic stocking size (follow package directions).
    b. *Option:* Apply a small amount of powder or cornstarch to legs, provided patient does not have sensitivity.
    c. Turn elastic stocking inside out: Place one hand into stocking, holding heel of stocking. Take other hand and pull stocking inside out until reaching the heel (see illustration).

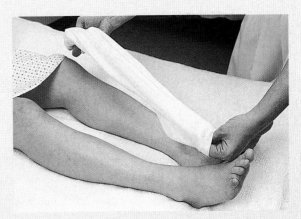

STEP 11c Turn stocking inside out; hold heel and pull through.

d. Place patient's toes into foot of elastic stocking up to the heel, making sure that stocking is smooth (see illustration).

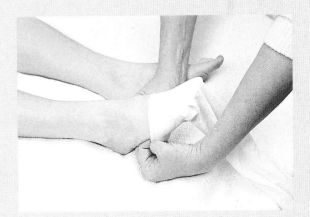

STEP 11d Place toes into foot of stocking.

e. Slide remaining portion of stocking over patient's foot, making sure that toes are covered. Make sure that foot fits into toe and heel position of stocking. Stocking will now be right side out (see illustration).

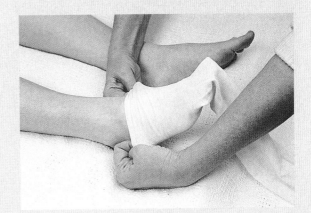

STEP 11e Slide remaining part of stocking over foot.

Continued

PROCEDURAL GUIDELINE 12.2 *Applying Graduated Compression (Elastic) Stockings and Sequential Compression Device—cont'd*

f. Slide stocking up over patient's calf until sock is completely extended. Be sure that stocking is smooth and that no ridges or wrinkles are present (see illustration).

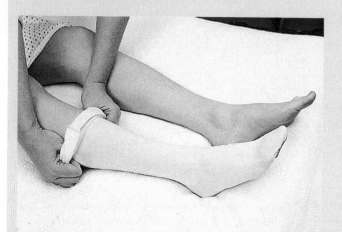

STEP 11f Slide sock up leg until completely extended.

g. Instruct patient to not roll stockings partially down, to avoid wrinkles, to avoid crossing legs, and to elevate legs while sitting.
12. **Apply SCD sleeve(s):**
   a. Remove SCD sleeves from plastic cover; unfold and flatten onto bed.
   b. Arrange SCD sleeve under patient's leg according to leg position indicated on inner lining of sleeve.
   c. Place patient's leg on SCD sleeve. Back of ankle should line up with ankle marking on inner lining of sleeve.
   d. Position back of knee with popliteal opening on inner sleeve (see illustration).

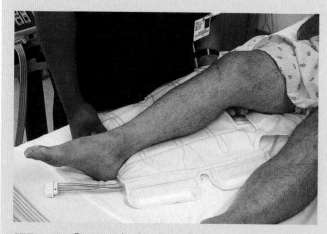

STEP 12d Position back of patient's knee with popliteal opening.

e. Wrap SCD sleeve securely around patient's leg. Check fit of SCD sleeve by placing two fingers between patient's leg and sleeve (see illustration).

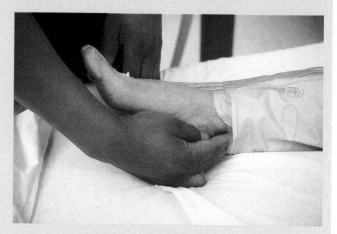

STEP 12e Check fit of sequential compression device sleeve.

f. Attach SCD sleeve connector to plug on mechanical unit. Arrows on connector line up with arrows on plug from mechanical unit (see illustration).

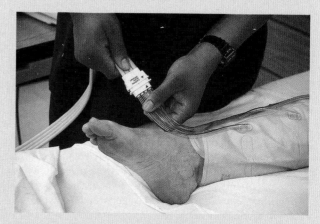

STEP 12f Align arrows when connecting plug to mechanical unit.

g. Turn mechanical unit on. Green light indicates that unit is functioning. Monitor functioning SCD through one full cycle of inflation and deflation.
13. **Apply MCD sleeve (one example of a product is shown):**
   a. A cotton stockinette may be provided along with the calf sleeves. Apply over patient's calves (*option*).
   b. Wrap the sleeve smoothly around the patient's calf and fasten it beginning at the top, moving toward the bottom.

PROCEDURAL GUIDELINE 12.2 *Applying Graduated Compression (Elastic) Stockings and Sequential Compression Device—cont'd*

c. Place two fingers between patient's calf and sleeve to be sure it is snug but not too tight (see illustrations).

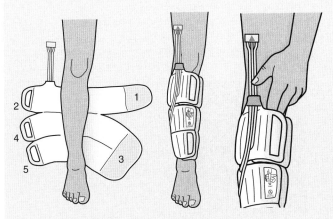

STEP 13c Application of sleeve to calves.

d. The device has two identical extension tubes (see illustrations). Use either end of the extension tube to connect to the sleeve or device pump.

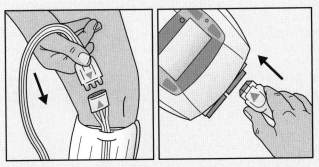

STEP 13d Application of mobile compression device connector hose to pump.

(1) Connect one end of the extension tube to the sleeve connector. The white arrows should be pointed toward each other.

(2) Connect the other end of the extension tube to the device pump. The white arrow should be facing upward.

e. Press the power switch located at the back of the device to ON position (see illustration). After turning the device on, the Configuration Setup Screen is shown on the LCD screen, and the sleeves should immediately start to inflate from the bottom to the top.

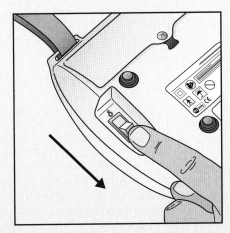

STEP 13e Powering on mobile compression device.

f. Wait 60 seconds for the automatic operation of the device. The device automatically identifies which sleeves are connected, selects the suitable treatment mode, and will display information on the main LCD screen.

14. Position patient comfortably, then place nurse call system in an accessible location within the patient's reach. When wearing MCD sleeves, a patient may walk with device in place (see illustration).

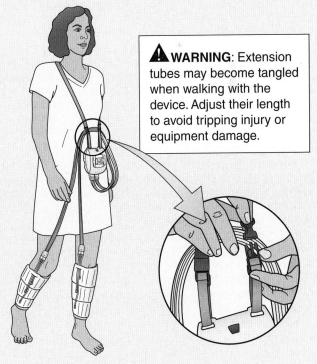

⚠ WARNING: Extension tubes may become tangled when walking with the device. Adjust their length to avoid tripping injury or equipment damage.

STEP 14 Walking with mobile compression device.

Continued

PROCEDURAL GUIDELINE 12.2 *Applying Graduated Compression (Elastic) Stockings and Sequential Compression Device—cont'd*

Clinical Judgment *Caution patient to not exit bed and walk with SCDs in place. Have patient call for assistance. However, the patient may walk with MCD in place.*

15. Raise side rails (as appropriate) and lower bed to lowest position, locking into position. Perform hand hygiene.
16. All compression stockings and devices should be worn only during daytime activities and removed for resting and at night due to poor tolerance and the risk of increased edema of distal, less compressed leg segments. Remove compression stockings or SCD/MCD sleeves at least once per shift (e.g., long enough to inspect skin for irritation or breakdown and to determine patient's comfort level).
17. Evaluate skin integrity and circulation to patient's lower extremities as ordered (see agency policy).
18. **Use Teach-Back:** "We have reviewed the signs and symptoms you might have if a clot forms in your leg. Tell me what those symptoms are and what you should do." Revise

your instruction now or develop a plan for revised patient/family caregiver teaching if patient/family caregiver is not able to teach back correctly.
19. Document condition of lower extremities, application of stockings/SCDs/MCDs, and patient response to education.
20. Hand-off reporting: Report to health care provider or nurse in charge any signs that may indicate formation of DVT.

PROCEDURAL GUIDELINE 12.3 *Assisting With Ambulation (Without Assist Devices)*

▶ *Video Clip*

Early ambulation for hospitalized patients is important in preventing deconditioning. The benefits of ambulation include maintenance of muscle tone, strength, and joint flexibility and function of the respiratory, circulatory, and gastrointestinal systems. Use a gait belt when you help a patient ambulate to increase patient safety and decrease a patient's fall risk. Measure distances a patient walks in estimated feet or yards instead of charting "ambulated to nurses' station and back." Some health care organizations will have markers along floorboards designating distances, or a pedometer may be used and the patient can take it home as an incentive to continue walking.

Illness or trauma usually reduces activity tolerance, and some conditions cause disabilities, resulting in the need for help with walking or the use of assist devices such as crutches, canes, or walkers/rollators (see Skill 12.2). Patients who increase their walking distance before discharge improve their ability to independently perform basic activities of daily living (ADLs), increase activity tolerance, and have a faster recovery after surgery (Walia et al., 2018). A recent study has shown that early ambulation (within 4 hours following surgery) improved functional status, decreased the incidence of complications, and shortened postoperative hospital stays in older patients undergoing spinal surgery (Huang, 2021).

When helping a patient up and out of bed or a chair, there is a risk for orthostatic hypotension. Orthostatic hypotension or postural hypotension is a drop in blood pressure (BP) that occurs when a patient changes from a horizontal to a vertical position. A drop in BP greater than 20 mm Hg in systolic pressure or 10 mm Hg in diastolic pressure with symptoms of dizziness, light-headedness, nausea, tachycardia, pallor, and fainting indicates orthostatic hypotension (Harding et al., 2020). When a

patient moves from a lying to a sitting position, dangling on the side of the bed (sitting on the edge of the bed with patient moving legs back and forth) and making sure the legs can touch the floor can minimize the onset of orthostatic hypotension by allowing the circulatory system to equilibrate. After dangling, have the patient stand; if able to stand without dizziness, proceed with ambulation. Use safety precautions before and during ambulation to control for orthostatic hypotension and subsequent falling.

Delegation
The skill of assisting patients with ambulation can be delegated to assistive personnel (AP). Direct the AP to:
- Apply safe patient handling principles when assisting patient out of bed or chair.
- Review steps to ensure the patient is not having orthostatic hypotension when rising from a lying position in bed to sitting. Check patient's BP before ambulation.
- Immediately return a patient to the bed or chair if nausea, dizziness, pale complexion, or diaphoresis occur (Biswas et al., 2019). Report these signs and symptoms to the nurse immediately.
- Apply safe, nonskid shoes/socks and ensure that the environment is free of clutter and there is no moisture on the floor before ambulating patient.

Equipment
Gait/transfer belt; nonskid shoes/socks; stethoscope, sphygmomanometer, pulse oximeter (as needed); *option:* pedometer

Steps
1. Identify patient using at least two identifiers (e.g., name and birthday or name and medical record number) according to agency policy (TJC, 2023).

PROCEDURAL GUIDELINE 12.3 *Assisting With Ambulation (Without Assist Devices)—cont'd*

2. Review EHR for patient's most recent activity history, including distance ambulated, use of assist device, activity tolerance, balance, and gait. Note history of orthostatic hypotension and any medications, chronic illnesses, gait alterations, or a history of falling.
3. Review most recently documented weight for patient and any report describing patient's ability to stand and bear weight.
4. Review health care provider's order for ambulation; note any mobility, range-of-motion (ROM), or weight-bearing restrictions.
5. Assess patient's/family caregiver's health literacy.
6. Perform hand hygiene. Assess patient's physical readiness to ambulate:
   a. Assess baseline resting heart rate, BP, oxygen saturation (when available), and respirations (see Chapter 5).
   b. If patient's strength and endurance have been affected by illness or deconditioning, assess ROM and muscle strength (see Chapter 6) of lower extremities while patient is in bed.
   c. Ask if patient feels excessively tired or is currently having any pain. Assess character of pain and rate severity pain scale of 0 to 10. Discomfort may delay ambulation. Offer an analgesic 30 minutes before ambulation to improve patient's tolerance to exercise.

Clinical Judgment *Do not administer an analgesic that could make the patient feel dizzy.*

   d. Assess the patient's mobility (ability to sit up, stand) by using the Banner Mobility Assessment Tool (BMAT) (see Chapter 11) (Matz et al., 2019).
7. Assess patient's response to commands and ability to cooperate during ambulation.
8. Apply patient's BMAT score to a safe-handling algorithm (available in most agencies) to determine if patient needs to walk with assist of a movable lift. Do not start procedure until all required caregivers are available.
9. Assess patient for any hearing or visual deficits (see Chapter 6) to ensure patient can see walking path and hear your instructions.
10. Check patient's environment for any barriers or safety risks. When walking, it is helpful within a hospital or rehabilitation center to walk in an area where handrails are on the walls and chairs are near.
11. Assess patient's or family caregiver's knowledge and experience regarding ambulation with assistance and patient's goals for ambulating.
12. Determine the best time to ambulate, considering all scheduled activities.
13. If this is the first time ambulating or if patient has been unsteady in the past, have a chair or wheelchair positioned close to the path you choose for ambulation. *Option:* The patient can push a wheelchair, using it for stability, or can use a rollator. Move patient quickly into a safe sitting position if patient becomes unstable.
14. Provide privacy. Organize equipment.
15. Remove sequential compression devices (SCDs) from patient's legs, if present (Exception: may wear mobile

compression devices [MCDs] while walking) (see Procedural Guideline 12.2).
16. Explain to patient in simple language how you are going to prepare for ambulation (e.g., gait belt application, use of wheelchair or rollator, distance planned to walk). Discuss benefits of walking and risks that you are adapting for to reduce chance of falling.
17. If hands became soiled during assessment, perform hand hygiene.
18. Assist patient from supine position to sitting position on edge of bed:
   a. With patient in supine position in bed, raise head of bed 30 to 45 degrees and place bed in low position, level with your hips. Raise upper side rail on side where patient will exit bed. Apply nonskid shoes or socks. If patient is fully mobile, allow sitting up on side of bed independently, using a side rail to raise up.
   b. If patient needs assistance to sit on side of bed, turn patient sideways facing you while standing on side of bed where patient will sit.
   c. Stand opposite patient's hips. Turn diagonally to face patient and far corner of foot of bed.
   d. Place your feet apart in wide base of support with foot closer to head of bed in front of other foot.
   e. Place your arm nearer to head of bed under patient's lower shoulder, supporting the head and neck. Place your other arm over and around patient's thighs (see illustration).

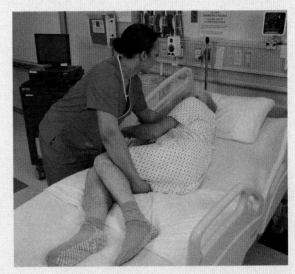

STEP 18e Nurse places arm over patient's thighs and other arm under patient's shoulder.

   f. Move patient's lower legs and feet over side of bed as patient uses side rail to push and raise the upper body. Pivot weight onto your rear leg as you allow patient's upper legs to swing downward (see illustration). **Do not lift legs.** At same time, continue to shift weight to your rear leg and guide patient in elevating the trunk into upright position.

Continued

PROCEDURAL GUIDELINE 12.3 *Assisting With Ambulation (Without Assist Devices)—cont'd*

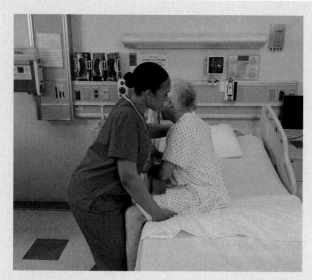

STEP 18f Nurse shifts weight to rear leg and elevates patient to sitting position.

19. Allow patient to sit on the side of the bed with feet on floor for 2 to 3 minutes (see illustration). Have patient alternately flex and extend feet and move lower legs up and down without touching floor. Ask if patient feels dizzy; if so, check BP. Have patient relax and take a few deep breaths until dizziness subsides and balance is gained. If dizziness lasts more than 60 seconds or if systolic BP has dropped at least 10 mm Hg within 3 minutes of sitting upright, return patient to bed (Biswas et al., 2019). Recheck BP.

20. Apply gait belt. Be sure that it completely encircles a patient's waist below the belly button. Belt should fit snugly; be sure two fingers fit between the belt and patient's body. Avoid placing belt over any intravenous (IV) lines, incisions, or drainage tubes. You may need to adjust belt once patient stands.

21. If patient is alert and can bear weight and balance while standing, allow to stand independently. Assist by holding gait belt to offer balance assistance.

22. If patient cannot bear weight or balance to stand independently but is stable to attempt ambulation, use an ambulation lift or ceiling lift with gait harness if available (see Chapter 11). Patient can walk with support of this mechanical device.

23. Confirm with patient distance to ambulate.

24. If patient has an intravenous (IV) line, place the IV pole on the same side as the site of infusion and instruct patient where to hold and push the pole while ambulating. It is best if another caregiver can push the IV pole.

25. If a Foley catheter is present, carry the bag below the level of the bladder and prevent tension on the tubing.

26. For orthopedic patients, stand on patient's unaffected side. For patients with neurological deficits (e.g., stroke), stand on the affected side. *For all other patients requiring assistance to maintain balance while weight bearing, stand on involved side.*

27. Grasp belt firmly with one hand, palm facing down (see illustration). Take a few steps, guiding patient with one hand grasping the gait belt and the other hand placed under the elbow of the patient's flexed arm.

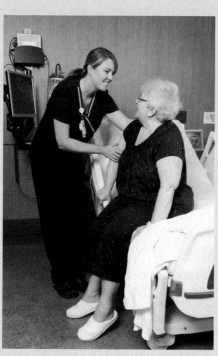

STEP 19 Patient sits on side of bed.

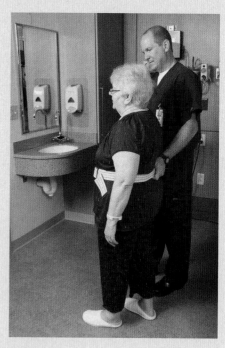

STEP 27 Nurse grasps gait belt firmly palm down.

PROCEDURAL GUIDELINE 12.3 *Assisting With Ambulation (Without Assist Devices)—cont'd*

28. When ambulating in a hallway, position patient between yourself and the wall. Encourage patient to use handrails if available (see illustration).

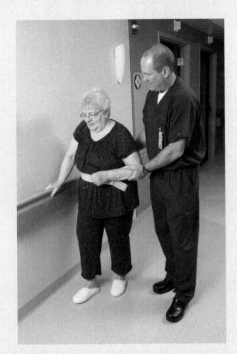

STEP 28 Help patient by providing balance support under patient's flexed arm.

29. Observe how patient walks (posture, gait, balance) and determine distance patient can safely continue walking. Measure pulse and respirations as needed.

30. Return patient to bed or chair (independent transfer or use of mechanical lift) and help patient to assume a comfortable position. Place the nurse call system in an accessible location within patient's reach.

31. Raise side rails (as appropriate) and lower bed to lowest position, locking into position. Perform hand hygiene.

32. **Teach-Back:** "Let's review what we discussed about taking steps in your home to have a safe path for safe walking. Tell me how you can prepare the rooms in your home." Revise your instruction now or develop a plan for revised patient/family caregiver teaching if patient/family caregiver is not able to teach back correctly.

33. Document time or distance ambulated, any changes in VS, and patient's tolerance (symptoms such as pain and fatigue).

34. Report to health care provider any incident of orthostatic hypotension or patient's unexpected intolerance to exercise.

✦ SKILL 12.2   Assisting With Use of Canes, Walkers, and Crutches

Patients with impaired mobility may require an ambulatory assist device to provide stability and balance to safely walk. An assist device is any device (e.g., cane, walker) that is designed, made, or adapted to help a person perform a particular task or function. A device increases stability during ambulation; supports weak extremities; or reduces the load on weight-bearing structures such as hips, knees, or ankles. Although the use of an assist device is to promote safety, falls often occur as a result of improper use or fit of a device (American Academy of Orthopedic Surgeons, 2020; Bateni et al., 2018).

When choosing the proper mobility assist device, several factors need to be considered. The first factor is the main reason the patient needs the assist device. For example, a cane is an option for patients with arthritis, pain, or injury on one lower extremity or only mildly impaired balance. Canes are considered the least stable of assist devices for mobility, and therefore patients who use them safely must have adequate balance, upper body strength, and dexterity (Sehgal et al., 2021). Another factor to consider is the amount of weight a patient needs the device to support. In the case of crutches, a patient's full weight can be exerted against crutch tips. Older adults rarely use crutches because they require a tremendous amount of upper body strength. Walkers provide a larger base of support for patients with impaired balance or lower body weakness (Sehgal et al., 2021) (Fig. 12.2). They are also helpful for patients who cannot bear weight through one lower extremity (e.g., after knee or hip surgery). Two-wheeled rolling walkers are more functional and easier to maneuver than standard walkers without wheels. A four-wheeled rolling walker, also called a

rollator, is helpful for higher-functioning patients with good balance (Sehgal et al., 2021).

One of the most important aspects of using an assist device is to ensure a proper fit. Some studies suggest that assist devices may interfere with the legs' lateral movement, which impacts the user's ability to have compensatory stepping reactions in the case of a lateral loss of balance (Bateni et al., 2018). Research suggests that walkers can limit the success of compensatory reactions more than canes, thus increasing the risk of falls more than canes (Bateni et al., 2018). Research suggests that a high percentage of assist devices may be inappropriate, of incorrect height, or used incorrectly.

There are a variety of ambulatory assist devices. For example, there are three types of canes: straight canes, quad canes (Fig. 12.3), and tripod canes. Always consult with a licensed physical therapist (PT) to choose the proper assist device, fit the device, and instruct the patient on the correct gait technique. Selection of an appropriate device depends on a patient's age, diagnosis, muscular coordination, weight-bearing status, and ease of maneuverability. Use of assist devices may be temporary (e.g., during recovery from a fractured extremity or orthopedic surgery) or permanent (e.g., a patient with paralysis or permanent weakness of the lower extremities). As a nurse, you help patients use their devices correctly during ambulation. Always have a gait belt on the patient and stand slightly behind and off to the side of the patient (on the weak/affected side or on the strong/unaffected side if the patient has an orthopedic condition). Table 12.3 reviews the features of each type of assist device and the procedure for proper measurement.

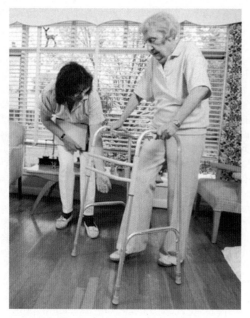

FIG. 12.2 Patient using walker.

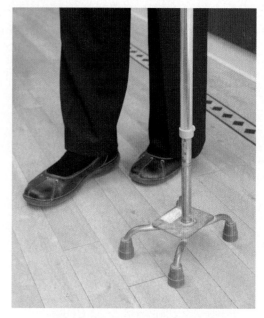

FIG. 12.3 Bottom of quad cane.

TABLE 12.3

Types of Assist Devices

Type of Device	Features	Measurement
Canes: lightweight, easily movable devices, extend approximately waist high, made of wood or metal. Three types: straight, quad (see Fig. 12.3)., and tripod.	Straight canes provide support and balance for patients with mild balance or strength impairments. Quad canes often used for patients who have unilateral weakness (i.e., stroke); have a larger base of support than straight canes. Tripods have smaller base than quad but provide better stability than a straight cane. Patient keeps cane on the strong side, opposite of the injury, pain, or weakness (unless instructed otherwise by a health care provider) (Health in Aging Foundation, 2019). Nurse stands on the patient's weak side for support.	Correct length of a cane or walker is measured from the wrist to the floor (Health in Aging Foundation, 2019): • Have patient wear normal shoes. • Let patient's arm hang loosely at the side. • Nurse measures distance from wrist to floor (should be about the same as the distance from the floor to the point of greater trochanter). • Adjust cane or walker so that the top of it is that same distance from the floor. • Have patient place hand on the cane or walker handle. If the length is correct, there is a 20- to 30-degree bend in the elbow.
Walkers: extremely light, movable devices, made of metal tubing (see Fig. 12.2). They have four widely placed, sturdy legs. They can also have two to four wheels.	Has a wide base of support, providing stability and security when walking. Beneficial for patients with arthritis or pain (especially of the knees and hips) on both sides. Medium to bad balance and gait problems. General weakness or weakness of both legs (Health in Aging Foundation, 2019).	Have patient step inside walker (see steps above for fitting).
Crutches: wooden or metal staff. Two types of crutches: double-adjustable Lofstrand (Fig. 12.4) or forearm crutch, and the axillary wooden or metal crutch.	Use of crutches is usually temporary (e.g., after ligament damage to knee). Some patients such as those with paralysis of the lower extremities need crutches permanently. Crutches remove weight from one leg; used by patients who must transfer more weight to their arms than is possible with canes.	Measurements include the patient's height, angle of elbow flexion, and distance between crutch pad and axilla. Measure standing: Position crutches with crutch tips at 15 cm (6 inches) laterally to side and 15 cm in front of patient's feet (tripod position). Crutch pads should be 3.75 to 5 cm (1½ to 2 inches) or 2 to 3 finger widths under axilla (Fig. 12.5) with the elbows slightly flexed (American College of Foot and Ankle Surgeons, 2022). Adjust height of handgrips so that patient's elbow is slightly flexed or grip sits at approximate height of wrist crease. Both height of crutch and handgrip dimensions are adjustable on a well-made crutch.

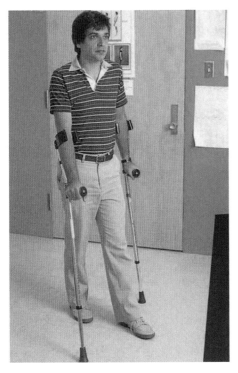

FIG. 12.4 Double adjustable Lofstrand or forearm crutch.

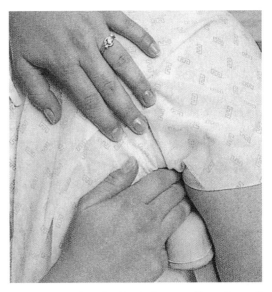

FIG. 12.5 Crutch pad is 2 to 3 finger widths under axilla.

- Apply safe, well-fitted nonskid shoes on patient and ensure that the environment is free of clutter and there is no moisture on the floor before ambulating patient

Interprofessional Collaboration

- PT will determine appropriate assist device and type of gait to be used for patient.

Equipment

- Ambulation device (crutch, walker, cane)
- Safety device (gait belt)
- Well-fitting, flat, nonskid shoes for patient
- *Option:* pedometer
- *Option:* Goniometer for measurement of the degree of joint range of motion (ROM)

Delegation

The skill of assisting patients with ambulation using assist devices can be delegated to assistive personnel (AP). The nurse conducts the initial assessment when a patient is ambulating for the first time. Direct the AP to:
- Have a patient dangle after lying in bed, before ambulation
- Immediately return a patient to the bed or chair if nausea, dizziness, pale complexion, or diaphoresis occurs and report these signs and symptoms to the nurse immediately

STEP	RATIONALE

ASSESSMENT

1. Identify patient using at least two identifiers (e.g., name and birthday or name and medical record number) according to agency policy.

Ensures correct patient. Complies with The Joint Commission standards and improves patient safety (TJC, 2023).

2. Complete assessment steps in Procedural Guideline 12.3, Steps 2 to 12.

Determines patient's ability to ambulate with a device and readiness for learning necessary gaits and precautions.

3. Determine patient's or family caregiver's prior experience and knowledge of type of device to be used in ambulating.

Allows patient to verbalize concerns. Patients who have been immobile may be hesitant to ambulate. Family caregiver may be hesitant to learn how to help with ambulation.

4. Assess degree of physical assistance that patient needs. PT will likely make this recommendation.

For safety, another person may be needed initially to help with patient ambulation. Allow patient as much independence as possible.

PLANNING

1. Expected outcomes following completion of procedure:
   - Patient ambulates using assist device without injury.
   - Patient is able to ambulate without excessive fatigue or dizziness and with return of VS to baseline 3 to 5 minutes after rest.

Appropriate level of assistance with device ensures patient's safety.
Assist device chosen requires minimal exertion. Patient tolerates exercise.

   - Patient demonstrates correct use of assist device, gait pattern, and weight-bearing status.

Demonstrates learning and physical ability to use device.

STEP	RATIONALE
2. Explain to patient how you are going to prepare for ambulation (e.g., transfer technique out of bed and safety precautions to be used while walking). Explain benefits and reasons for activity/exercise. Do so in a way that matches patient's educational level and beliefs and values regarding recovery or maintaining health.	Exercise self-efficacy is an important predictor of the adoption and maintenance of exercise behaviors.
3. Explain and demonstrate specific gait technique to patient or family caregiver.	Teaching and demonstration enhance learning, reduce anxiety, and encourage cooperation.
4. Check for appropriate height and fit of assist device. If PT has seen patient, the device should be at appropriate height. **NOTE:** *This is usually done when patient is standing at side of bed and is stable. See Table 12.3.*	Ensures that patient is able to ambulate successfully without injury using device.
5. Make sure that ambulation device has rubber tips. In the case of a walker, check tips or function of brakes.	Prevents device from slipping.

Clinical Judgment *Remove obstacles such as throw rugs (in the home) and electrical cords from walking path. Wipe up any spills immediately. Avoid crowds. Crowds increase the risk of the crutch, cane, or walker being kicked or jarred and patient losing balance.*

IMPLEMENTATION

1. Perform hand hygiene.	Reduces transmission of microorganisms.
2. If using crutches, have patient report any tingling or numbness in upper torso while ambulating.	Helps to indicate that crutches are being used incorrectly or that they are wrong size.
3. Help patient from lying position to side of bed (see Procedural Guideline 12.3) or up from chair.	Ensures that patient is stable and ready to ambulate.
4. Allow patient to sit on edge of bed for a few minutes. Have patient alternately flex and extend feet and move lower legs. Ask if patient feels dizzy. Have patient relax and take a few deep breaths until dizziness subsides and balance is gained.	Determines ability to tolerate standing. Immediately return a patient to the bed or chair if nausea, dizziness, paleness, or diaphoresis occurs or if systolic blood pressure dropped at least 10 mm Hg within 3 minutes of sitting upright (Biswas et al., 2019). Recheck blood pressure.
5. Apply gait belt around patient's waist (see Procedural Guideline 12.3). Be sure that it completely encircles a patient's waist below the belly button. Belt should fit snugly; be sure two fingers fit between the belt and patient's body. Avoid placing belt over any intravenous lines, incisions, or drainage tubes. You may need to adjust belt once patient stands.	Belt controls patient's center of mass during mobility, assisting with balance. Controls descent if a fall occurs, and reduces chance of grabbing patient's upper extremities.
6. Help patient stand at bedside. Hold gait belt along patient's back, under gait belt with your palms facing up. Reassess height of assist device to make sure that it is correct size. Have patient stand fully erect with shoulders back and looking ahead (not at floor). At this time, assess patient's ability to bear weight (e.g., does patient have discomfort, unsteady stance?) and balance.	Ensures that patient begins ambulation with correct posture and position.
7. If patient is unsteady, position in chair or return to bed immediately.	Patient may require strengthening exercises or evaluation of balance by PT.
8. Confirm with patient distance planned for ambulation.	Determines mutual goal.
9. Implement ambulation around patient's other activities.	Taking scheduled rest periods between activities reduces patient fatigue.
10. **Walk with cane** (steps are the same with standard, tripod, or quad cane).	

Clinical Judgment *Patients with quad cane may walk more slowly. Gait will vary on the basis of the nature of a patient's weakness or limited mobility.*

a. Have patient hold cane on strong/unaffected side. Direct patient to place cane forward 10 to 15 cm (4 to 6 inches) and slightly to the side of the foot, keeping most of body weight on good foot (Health in Aging Foundation, 2019). Allow approximately 15- to 30-degree elbow flexion.	Offers most support when on stronger side of body. Cane and weaker leg work together with each step.

STEP	RATIONALE
b. To begin, have patient move the cane and weak/affected leg forward together about 15 to 25 cm (6 to 10 inches) (American Academy Orthopedic Surgeons, 2020). The cane and weak/affected leg swing and strike the ground at the same time.	Distributes body weight equally. Body weight is supported by cane and strong leg.
c. With patient's weight supported on both the cane and weak leg, finish step by advancing strong/unaffected leg even with the cane. When first walking with the cane, this provides better balance.	Aligns patient's center of gravity. Returns patient body weight to equal distribution.
d. Repeat sequences as patient tolerates. Once comfortable, have patient advance cane and weak/affected leg together and then the stronger/unaffected leg can advance 15 to 25 cm (6 to 10 inches) past the cane.	Mimics a more normal gait once patient has balance.
11. Crutch walking (Use appropriate crutch gait determined by PT):	To use crutches, patient supports self with hands and arms; therefore ability to balance body in upright position and stamina are necessary. Type of crutch gait depends on patient's weight-bearing status.
a. Four-point gait:	This is most stable crutch gait. It provides at least three points of support at all times. Patient must be able to bear weight on both legs. Patient moves each leg alternately with each opposing crutch so three points of support are on floor all the time. Often used when patient has some form of paralysis (e.g., children with spastic cerebral palsy) (Hockenberry et al., 2022). May also be used for arthritic patients.
(1) Begin in tripod position (see illustration). Have patient lean slightly forward, placing the crutch tips about 15 cm (6 inches) to the side and in front of each foot (Warees et al., 2022). Have patient place weight on good foot and handgrips, not under arms.	Improves balance by providing wide base of support. Patient should have posture of erect head and neck, straight vertebrae, and extended hips and knees.
(2) Move right crutch tip forward 10 to 15 cm (4 to 6 inches) (see illustration A).	Crutch and foot position is similar to arm and foot position during normal walking.
(3) Begin step as if patient were going to use the weaker foot or leg but, instead, shifts weight to the crutch (American Academy of Orthopedic Surgeons, 2020). Have patient move left foot forward to level of left crutch (see illustration B).	
(4) Move left crutch tip forward 10 to 15 cm (4 to 6 inches) (see illustration C).	
(5) Move right foot forward to level of right crutch (see illustration D).	
(6) Repeat above sequence. (As patient becomes stronger, distance to advance crutches can increase to 30 cm [12 inches].	
b. Three-point gait:	Requires patient to bear all weight on the one strong foot. Weight is borne on strong/unaffected leg and then on both crutches. Weak/affected leg does not touch ground during three-point gait. May be useful for patient with broken leg or sprained ankle.
(1) Begin in tripod position (see illustration A) with patient standing on strong weight-bearing foot.	Improves patient's balance by providing wide base of support.
(2) Advance both crutches 15 cm (6 inches) and weak/affected leg, keeping foot of weak leg off floor (see illustration B).	
(3) Move weight-bearing strong leg forward, stepping on floor (see illustration C).	
(4) Repeat sequence.	

STEP	RATIONALE

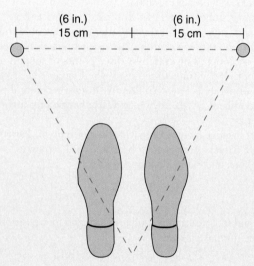

STEP 11a(1) Tripod position.

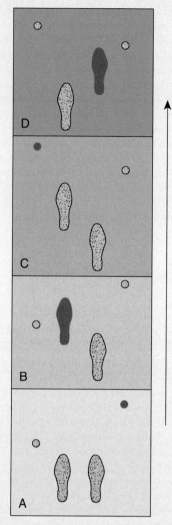

STEP 11a(2-5) Four-point gait. Solid feet and crutch tips show foot and crutch tip movement in each of four phases. (Read from bottom to top.) (A) Right tip moves forward. (B) Left foot moves toward left crutch. (C) Left crutch tip moves forward. (D) Right foot moves toward right crutch.

  c. Two-point gait:

    Requires at least partial weight bearing on each foot. Is faster than four-point gait. Requires more balance because only two points support body at one time.

  (1) Begin in tripod position (see illustration A).
  (2) Move left crutch and right foot forward (see illustration B).
  (3) Move right crutch and left foot forward (see illustration C).
  (4) Repeat sequence.

    Improves patient's balance by providing wide base of support.
    Crutch movements are similar to arm movement during normal walking; patient moves crutch at same time as opposing leg.

  d. Swing-through gait:

    Used by patients whose lower extremities are weakened or who wear weight-supporting braces on their legs.

  (1) Begin in tripod position.

    This is the easier of two swinging gaits. It requires the ability to partially bear body weight on both legs.

  (2) Move both crutches forward.
  (3) Lift and swing both legs to crutches, letting crutches support body weight.
  (4) Repeat two previous steps.

STEP	**RATIONALE**

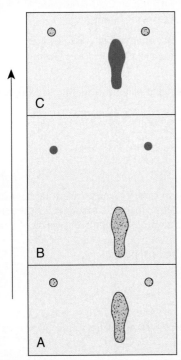

STEP 11b(1-3) Three-point gait with weight borne on unaffected right leg. Solid foot and crutch tips show weight bearing in each phase (A–C). (Read from bottom to top.)

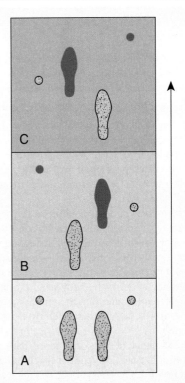

STEP 11c(1-3) Two-point gait. Solid areas indicate weight-bearing leg and crutch tips (A–C). (Read from bottom to top.)

e. Swing-to gait (see illustration):

   (1) Begin in tripod position. Support on strongest leg.
   (2) Advance the left and right crutch, then the left and right legs are advanced.

   (3) Lift and swing legs up to crutches.
   (4) Repeat previous steps.

Requires that patient have the ability to bear partial weight on both feet.
Improves patient's balance by providing wide base of support.
Initial placement of crutches increases patient's base of support so that when body swings forward, patient is moving center of gravity toward additional support provided by crutches.

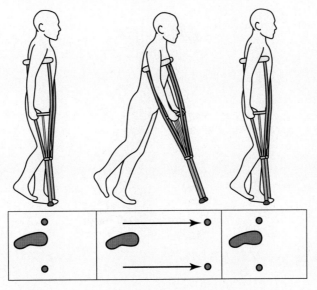

STEP 11e Swing-to gait.

STEP	RATIONALE
12. Ascending stairs with railing and crutches (partial weight bearing, one leg):	Climbing stairs with use of a railing is safest way for patient with crutches to ascend stairs.

Clinical Judgment *This skill will most likely be done in the home. Patients should not climb stairs until crutches can be handled well (UW Medicine, 2019). There is a risk for falling using this technique. Monitor patient's balance carefully. If patient cannot ascend or descend stairs easily with crutches, PT typically recommend patients scoot their bottoms up and down stairs (UW Medicine, 2019).*

STEP	RATIONALE
a. Have patient begin in tripod position while standing on strong weight-bearing leg and bearing weight on crutch.	Improves patient's balance by providing wide base of support.
b. Have the patient hold the handrail for support with one hand (strong leg next to railing if possible). You will carry the crutch positioned next to the handrail as the patient places the other crutch under the axilla of the weak/affected side.	Ensures patient safety.
c. Stay behind the patient, holding on to the gait belt. Then have the patient place weight on the crutches and step up with the strong weight-bearing foot, holding handrail (UW Medicine, 2019) (see illustration A).	Prepares patient to transfer weight to strong leg when ascending first stair. Achieves balance. Stronger leg provides base of support. Maintaining balance reduces risk of a fall.
d. The patient straightens the strong knee, pushes down on crutches, and lifts the body weight, bringing the weak/affected leg and then the crutch up the stair (see illustration B). Be sure the crutch tip is completely on the stair.	Prevents accidental tripping.
e. Repeat sequence of steps, instructing patient to climb one stair at a time until patient reaches top of stairs (see illustration C). Observe patient's balance and level of fatigue.	Patient's tolerance determines frequency of practice.
f. *Option: Going up stairs without crutches, using patient's seat.* Have patient sit on the lower stair. Have patient (or caregiver) place crutches as far up the stairs as possible. Then patient will move them to the top while progressing up the stairs (UW Medicine, 2019).	Safest way to ascend stairs (UW Medicine, 2019). Reaching for inaccessible crutches could lead to a fall.
(1) In the seated position, have patient reach behind with both arms, then use arms and strong weight-bearing foot/leg to lift up one step.	Weight remains off affected leg.
(2) Repeat this process one step at a time (move crutches farther up if there are additional stairs) until patient reaches top of stairs.	

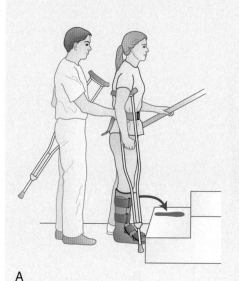
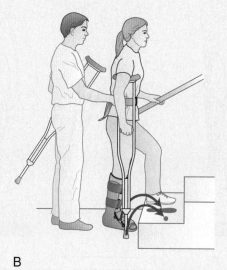
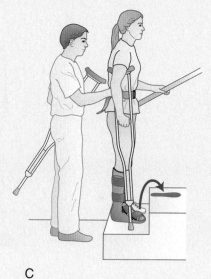

A   B   C

STEP 12(c-e) Ascending stairs with crutches.

STEP	RATIONALE

13. Descending stairs with a railing and crutch (partial weight bearing, one leg):

Clinical Judgment *There is a risk for falling using this technique. Monitor patient's balance carefully.*

a. Have patient begin in tripod position while bearing weight on strong/unaffected leg and crutch.

Improves patient's balance by providing wide base of support. Prepares patient to release support of body weight maintained by crutches.

b. Have the patient stand close to the edge of the top step. Then have the patient hold the handrail with one hand (strong leg next to railing if possible). You will carry the crutch positioned next to the handrail as the patient places the other crutch under the axilla of the weak/affected side. Stand in front of the patient to be able to guide during a possible fall (see illustration A). Do not hold patient's hand (UW Medicine, 2019).

Promotes patient's balance.

c. Have the patient bend the strong knee while lowering the crutch down to the step below and then moving the weak/affected leg down a step (see illustration B).

Maintains weight-bearing support.

d. Patient then supports body weight evenly between handrail, strong leg, and crutch. Be sure that patient has good balance (see illustration C).

Maintains balance.

e. Caution patient not to hop while descending stairs.

Hopping could injure leg and create risk for fall.

f. *Option:* **Going down stairs without crutches using patient's seat.** Have patient sit on the top step. Place crutches down the stairs by sliding them to the lowest possible point on the stairway. Then continue to move them down as patient progresses down the stairs (UW Medicine, 2019).

Safest way to descend stairs (UW Medicine, 2019). Reaching for inaccessible crutches could lead to a fall. Moving down by seat avoids risk of losing balance and falling down the stairs.

(1) In the seated position, have patient reach behind with both arms, and then use arms and strong weight-bearing foot/leg to lift bottom down step.

Weight remains off affected leg

(2) Repeat this process one step at a time (moving crutches down if there are additional stairs) until patient reaches bottom of stairs.

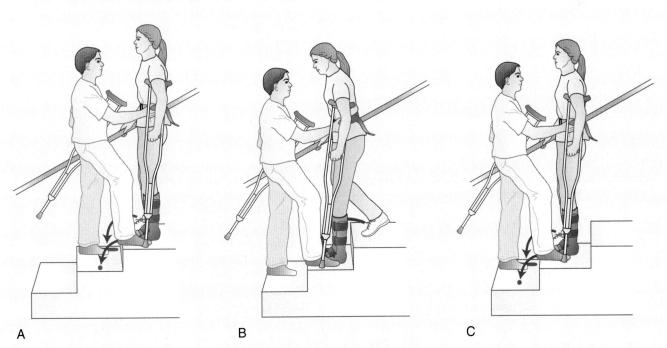

A   B   C

STEP 13(b-d) Descending stairs with crutches.

STEP	RATIONALE
14. Ambulating with walker:	Patients who are able to bear partial weight use walkers or rollators.
a. Have patient stand straight in center of walker and grasp handgrips on upper bars. **Do not allow patient to lean over walker.**	Patient balances self before attempting to walk.
b. Have patient move walker comfortable distance forward, about 15 to 20 cm (6 to 8 inches). Patient then takes step forward with weak/affected leg first and follows through with strong/unaffected leg into walker (Mayo Clinic, 2022). Instruct patient not to advance leg past the front bar of walker. If patient has equal strength in both legs, it makes no difference which leg advances first.	Provides broad base of support between walker and patient. Patient then moves center of gravity toward walker. Keeping all four feet of walker on floor is necessary to prevent tipping walker.
c. If patient has difficulty bearing weight on weak leg, have patient slowly hop to center of walker using strong leg, supporting weight on hands. *Caution: Do not hop using a rollator.*	Hopping creates a fall risk
d. Instruct patient not to try to climb stairs with walker unless patient has specific walker for steps.	Patient should use handrails as alternative. Using walker could cause a fall.
15. After ambulation, help patient back to bed or chair and help assume comfortable position.	Promotes patient comfort.
16. Place nurse call system in an accessible location within patient's reach.	Ensures patient can call for assistance if needed.
17. Raise side rails (as appropriate) and lower bed to lowest position, locking into position.	Ensures patient safety and prevents falls.
18. Perform hand hygiene.	Prevents transmission of infection.

EVALUATION

1. After ambulation, obtain patient's VS, observe skin color, and evaluate comfort and energy levels.	Evaluates how patient tolerated ambulation and whether there was progress. Assesses stage of patient's illness and degree of convalescence when evaluating process.
2. Evaluate patient's subjective statements regarding experience.	Evaluates activity tolerance.
3. Evaluate patient's gait pattern: observe body alignment in standing position and balance during gait.	Determines if patient is using supportive aids for ambulation correctly. Keep in mind patient's previous manner of ambulating when assessing gait.
4. **Use Teach-Back:** "You have done well walking with your walker. We reviewed with your wife how to place a gait belt and why it is important to use. Show me how to place the gait belt correctly." Revise your instruction now or develop a plan for revised patient/family caregiver teaching if patient/family caregiver is not able to teach back correctly.	Teach-back is a technique for health care providers to ensure that they have explained medical information clearly so that patients and their families understand what is communicated to them (AHRQ, 2023).

Unexpected Outcomes	Related Interventions
1. Patient is unable to ambulate because of fear of falling, physical discomfort, upper body muscles that are too weak to use assist device, or lower extremities that are too weak to support body.	• Consult with PT about possible exercise program to strengthen muscles or other alternative methods for ambulation. • Provide analgesic for discomfort. • Discuss with patient fears or concerns about walking using assist device.
2. Patient sustains an injury.	• Notify health care provider. • Return patient to bed if injury is stable. Otherwise, have lift team transfer patient to bed. • Document per institution/agency policy.
3. When using a cane or walker, patient bends over and does not stand straight.	• Reinforce correct posture.

Documentation

- Document assessment findings, type of assist device and gait patient used, amount of help required, distance walked, and activity tolerance.
- Document your evaluation of patient and family caregiver learning.

Hand-Off Reporting

- Immediately report any injury sustained during attempts to ambulate, alteration in VS, or inability to ambulate to nurse in charge or health care provider.

Special Considerations

Patient Education

- Teach patients who use a walker to examine the frame daily. Patient should observe for signs of bending or deformation of the frame, protruding screws that can scratch, and loose or missing screws that weaken the frame joints. Assess handgrips for cracks or signs of being loose.
- Teach patients to use the arms of a chair rather than the assist device to get leverage when getting up from a chair; the device is likely to tip if used for this purpose.
- Blistering or soreness of the hands can result from continual pressure between the hand and the handle of a crutch. Advise patient to release pressure intermittently and wear gloves or pad the handle to reduce friction.
- Instruct patient that, if wearing shoes with varying heel sizes, the crutches, canes, and walkers may need to be adjusted to maintain the proper height.
- Caution patients when using an assist device: **Don't** look down. Look straight ahead as you normally do when you walk. **Don't** walk on slippery surfaces. **Avoid** snowy, icy, or rainy conditions. **Don't** put *any* weight on the affected foot if your doctor has so advised.

Pediatrics

- Forearm crutches are usually the best choice for children. The crutches do not put pressure on nerves and blood vessels under the arm. Forearm crutches have a flexible cuff that surrounds the forearm just below the elbow. This helps to reduce arm strain and gives the user more independence (St. Jude's Children's Research Hospital, 2022).
- An option for children who are just learning to walk would be front- or rear-rolling walkers.

Older Adults

- Patients using walkers and who wish to carry items should attach a basket and put the items inside.
- Emphasize to an older adult the importance of using a cane and/ or walker routinely when one is recommended by a health care provider. In a study, 75% of participants who reported falling were not using their device at the time of fall despite stating that canes help prevent falls. Reasons for nonuse included the belief that it was not needed, forgetfulness, that the device made the person feel old, and inaccessibility (Luz et al., 2017).

Populations With Disabilities

- If an individual regularly uses a prescribed walker to perform activities of daily living (ADLs), and if the person uses the walker to travel from room to room in the home, the individual would likely be found disabled under current Social Security Administration (SSA) regulations (Viner Disability Law, 2023).
- There are mobile frame walkers for one-handed use available to patients with disabilities. The frame has a central handgrip that enables the frame to be held and moved using one hand. Caution: a one-handed frame does not offer as much support as gripping the frame with both hands. Patients should use this type of walker only if recommended by a health care provider.

Home Care

- Teach patient how to use the ambulation aid on various terrains (e.g., carpet, stairs, rough ground, inclines) in the home. Teach patient how to maneuver around obstacles such as doors and how to use the aid when transferring to and from a chair, toilet, and tub.
- Teach family caregivers how to help and what to observe to ensure that an assist device is used correctly.
- Tennis balls cut and placed on the rubber tips of a walker can be helpful for ease of movement on carpeted surfaces (Health in Aging Foundation, 2019).
- Tell patient to not hold onto assist device to get in and out of a chair. The device is not stable enough. Patient should push up with the hands on the arms of the chair and only take hold of the device once standing. Have patient practice this with a health care professional.
- Do not use assist devices to enter a shower. If patient needs to access a wet room or shower, ask the advice of an occupational therapist. It is safer to install grab rails in the bathroom.

✦ SKILL 12.3 Care of a Patient With an Immobilization Device

Immobilization devices increase stability of bones and joints, support extremities, or reduce the load on weight-bearing structures such as hips, knees, or ankles (Table 12.4). A splint immobilizes and protects a body part. Slings provide support, immobilization, and elevation of the arm or shoulder after injury or surgery. An abduction splint or pillow is used after hip replacement surgery to maintain a patient's legs in an abducted position so that the new joint remains stable. Cloth and foam splints, known as immobilizers, provide long-term immobilization (Fig. 12.6). Orthotic devices or orthoses maintain joint(s) in a position that enables patients to maximize the movement they can produce (facilitation); prevent, correct, or compensate

for deformity or contracture; and reduce weight or forces being taken through a limb.

Medical device–related pressure injuries (MDRPI) can result from the use of devices designed and applied for diagnostic or therapeutic purposes. In the case of immobilization devices or orthotics, the resultant injury generally mirrors the pattern or shape of the device (Pittman & Gillespie, 2020). It is a nursing responsibility to carefully assess the skin before device placement, be sure the device supports an extremity as intended, and be hypervigilant, evaluating the condition of the skin on an ongoing basis. In addition, if a device is applied too tightly or incorrectly, there can be compression causing reduction in circulation to the extremity.

TABLE 12.4

Immobilization Devices

Device	Uses and Benefits	Features
Soft splints	• Temporary splints reduce pain and prevent tissue damage from further motion immediately after an injury (e.g., fracture or sprain). • Air splints, Thomas splints, and improvised splints from material on hand are examples of temporary splints applied in emergency situations.	• Available commercially or can be made for almost any body part. • Velcro or buckle closures permit these devices to be adjusted to fit a body part of almost any size and shape.
Molded splints	• Provide support to patients with chronic injuries or diseases such as arthritis. • Maintain the body part in a functional position to prevent contractures and muscle atrophy during the period of disuse.	• Made of plastic, which can be cleaned with a washcloth and warm soap and water. • Can be removed quickly for assessment of the skin or a wound.
Abduction pillow	• Permits a patient to be turned without changing the position of the healing limb. • Prevents dislocation of the hip prosthesis.	• The pillow is easily removed for nursing care (e.g., skin care, dressing changes, neurovascular assessments).
Immobilizers	• Immobilizers treat sprains and dislocations that do not require complete and continuous immobilization in a cast or traction.	• Common types of immobilizers include cervical collars (soft or hard), belt-type shoulder immobilizers, and knee immobilizers.
Braces	• Support weakened structures during weight bearing. • Chest and abdominal braces (Boston brace) immobilize the thoracic and lumbar vertebral column to treat scoliosis (curvature of the spine). • Lumbar braces support lumbar and sacral tissues after spinal surgery. • Leg and foot braces hold the thigh, leg, and foot in functional positions for weight bearing and ambulation.	• Made of sturdy materials such as leather, metal, and molded plastic.

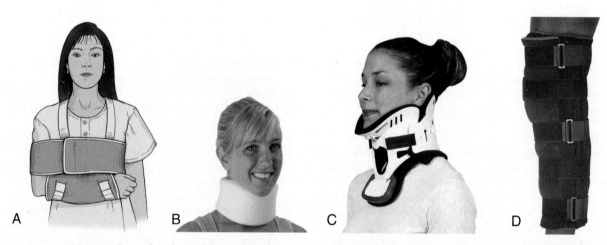

FIG. 12.6 Examples of immobilizers. (A) Shoulder/arm immobilizer. (B) Soft cervical collar. (C) Hard cervical collar. (D) Knee immobilizer. (*A from Chudnofsky CR, Chudnofsky AS: Roberts and Hedges' clinical procedures in emergency medicine and acute care, St. Louis, 2020, Elsevier; B–D used with permission from Ossur Americas. All rights reserved.*)

Delegation

The skill of caring for a patient wearing a brace, splint, or sling can be delegated to assistive personnel (AP). Direct the AP by:
• Reviewing prescribed schedule of wear and activities allowed wearing device
• Reviewing special observations that might be required based on device
• Instructing to inform the nurse if the patient complains of pain, rubbing, or pressure from the brace, splint, or sling or if a change occurs in condition of patient's skin under device

Interprofessional Collaboration

• Physical therapy (PT) and occupational therapy (OT) will fit patients for certain devices (e.g., brace and sling).
• A professional orthotist is skilled in making and fitting orthopedic appliances (e.g., splints).

Equipment

• Brace, splint, or commercially prepared sling
• Cotton shirt or gown
• Clean gloves
• Cotton webbing or bandage (optional)
• Towel, washcloth, soap, and basin with water

STEP	RATIONALE

ASSESSMENT

1. Identify patient using at least two identifiers (e.g., name and birthday or name and medical record number) according to agency policy.

    Ensures correct patient. Complies with The Joint Commission standards and improves patient safety (TJC, 2023).

2. Review patient's EHR for medical history, previous and current activity level, description of the condition requiring immobilization, and medical order for device.

    Reveals patient's current and previous health status and purpose for immobilization. Medical order required for use of devices.

3. Perform hand hygiene. Inspect area of skin in contact with immobilization device or area that will be covered by a newly applied device (apply clean gloves if risk of contacting body fluids).

    Reduces transmission of microorganisms. Provides baseline to monitor for skin breakdown. Immobile and older patients are particularly vulnerable.

Clinical Judgment *When assessing for medical device–related pressure injuries (MDRPI), remove only those devices that can be safely removed. "Nonremovable" includes devices that are not normally removed during patient care (e.g., casts) and situations in which the patient has a health care provider order to "not remove." Skin under the edges of nonremovable devices can be assessed if it can be done without displacing the device.*

4. Palpate temperature, pulse, and sensation of extremity distal to where device is to be applied. Perform hand hygiene.

    Provides baseline to measure circulation and neurosensory status. Reduces transmission of microorganisms.

5. Assess patient's/family caregiver's health literacy.

    Determines degree to which individuals have the ability to find, understand, and use information and services to make informed health-related decisions and actions (CDC, 2023).

6. Assess patient's/family caregiver's knowledge and experience with immobilization devices.

    Reveals need for patient instruction and/or support.

7. Assess patient for discomfort. If pain is present, assess character and rate severity on a scale of 0 to 10.

    Provides baseline to determine if immobilization device affects comfort.

8. Refer to PT or OT to determine type of device to be used, desired position, and amount of activity and movement permitted.

    Provides direction in proper fit and use of device.

PLANNING

1. Expected outcomes following completion of procedure:
    - Patient's skin remains intact, warm, without signs of injury, blistering, or pressure, and with normal sensation.

        Device applied correctly without skin irritation.

    - Patient and family caregiver verbalize purpose, correct application, and care of the device.

        Demonstrates learning.

    - Patient reports a temporary increase in pain during device application.

        Normal response to device application.

    - Patient uses the device correctly, including schedule of wear, activity limitations, and positioning.

        Able to perform self-care wearing device.

2. Provide privacy by closing room curtains or doors and prepare environment.

    Ensures comfortable, organized environment.

3. Explain to patient and family caregiver purpose of device and how it will be applied.

    Promotes understanding needed for self-care of device.

IMPLEMENTATION

1. Perform hand hygiene. Assist patient to a comfortable position: apply upper extremity brace/splint/sling with patient sitting upright; apply lower extremity brace with patient lying down.

    Reduces transmission of microorganisms. Facilitates correct, aligned placement of brace/splint/sling.

2. Apply clean gloves if risk of contacting body fluids. Prepare skin that will be enclosed in brace/splint/sling by cleaning skin with soap and water; rinse, pat dry, and change any dressings (if present). If applying a back brace, put a thin cotton shirt or gown on patient. Ensure that there are no wrinkles to cause pressure.

    This protects skin and keeps brace clean. Smooth cotton clothing between the brace and skin protects skin from irritation and absorbs moisture.

3. Inspect device for wear, damage, or rough edges.

    Decreases potential for skin breakdown and maintains correct alignment.

4. Apply brace/splint/sling as directed by health care provider, orthotist, PT, or OT. Be sure application provides for the alignment and support indicated in the order.

    Proper application of the brace/splint/sling is important to avoid skin breakdown, pressure injuries, neurovascular compromise, calluses, or worsening of deformity.

    a. Apply even tension on any bandage or gauze padding that is ordered to be applied against skin; wrap distal to proximal.

    Prevents trapping of blood and fluid distal to immobilization device.

STEP	RATIONALE
b. Prevent padding from gathering or bunching.	Prevents irritation to underlying tissues.
c. Support joints when you position and apply the device.	Reduces risk of musculoskeletal injury during movement.
5. Apply commercial sling:	
a. Be sure correct size is chosen. Place elbow into close side of sling, aligning arm into sling and slipping wrist and hand through open side of sling or through separate Velcro enclosure (see Fig. 12.6A).	Commercially available slings secure arm to chest for added support and have padding on strap for comfort.
b. Enclose Velcro strap around arm, place strap around patient's neck, and tighten buckle until it fits snugly.	
c. Position arm so that the hand and forearm are higher than elbow.	
6. Remove and dispose of gloves. Perform hand hygiene.	Reduces transmission of microorganisms.
7. Teach patient and family caregiver prescribed schedule of wear and activities while in device as directed by health care provider, PT, or OT.	Proper use of brace/splint/sling facilitates healing and mobility and reduces pain and stress.
8. Reinforce instruction regarding signs to report to health care provider: skin breakdown, painful pressure, or rubbing.	Device may need to be adjusted. Changes may also be required because of growth or atrophy, when muscles regain or lose strength, or after reconstructive surgery.
9. Teach patient/family caregiver how to care for brace/splint/sling:	Maintains integrity of device.
a. When not in use, store metal braces upright in a safe but easily accessible location.	Prevents deformity or bending of brace.
b. Store splints of molded materials away from heat.	Prevents melting and deformation of splint.
c. Treat any leather material with leather preservative.	Prevents drying or cracking.
d. Keep brace clean, dry, and in good working order. Clean plastic parts with a damp cloth and thoroughly dry. Clean metal brace joints with a pipe cleaner, and oil weekly. Remove rust with steel wool, and clean metal parts with a solvent.	Maintains function and integrity of devices.
10. Assist patient in ambulating with brace/splint/sling in place.	Determines if patient is able to ambulate safely.
11. Observe while patient or family caregiver applies and removes brace/splint/sling.	Promotes patient independence; demonstration confirms level of learning skill.
12. Help patient to a comfortable position.	Gives patient a sense of well-being.
13. Place nurse call system in an accessible location within patient's reach.	Ensures patient can call for assistance if needed.
14. Raise side rails (as appropriate) and lower bed to lowest position, locking into position.	Ensures patient safety and prevents falls.
15. Dispose of supplies or dirty linen. Perform hand hygiene.	Reduces transmission of microorganisms.

EVALUATION

1. Inspect area of skin underneath device for redness or skin breakdown. If allowed, remove device briefly to thoroughly assess skin integrity.	Monitors for development of MDRPI.
2. Palpate temperature, pulse, and sensation of extremity distal to device. Check capillary refill by pressing on toe or finger (see illustration).	Screens for changes in circulation due to compression of device against skin.
3. Inspect alignment of the limb after application of device.	Device is designed to support limb in a stable position.
4. Ask patient to describe any discomfort, then evaluate character of pain and have patient rate severity on a pain scale after device application.	Application of device may cause temporary discomfort, but eventually the support it offers reduces pain.
5. Use Teach-Back: State to the patient, "I want to be sure I explained clearly the need for the brace/splint/sling, how to maintain the device, and the limitations related to the device. Please tell me ways you will use this brace/splint/sling safely." Revise your instruction now or develop a plan for revised patient/family caregiver teaching if patient/family caregiver is not able to teach back correctly.	Teach-back is a technique for health care providers to ensure that they have explained medical information clearly so that patients and their families understand what is communicated to them (AHRQ, 2023).

STEP	RATIONALE

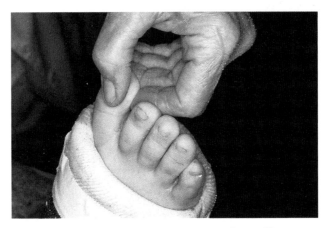

STEP 2 Inspecting toe to assess capillary refill.

Unexpected Outcomes

1. Patient reports increased severity in pain after application of the device.

2. Patient develops area of pressure with redness, skin breakdown.

Related Interventions

- Reposition extremity.
- Administer analgesics as ordered to maintain patient's comfort level.
- Increase frequency of neurovascular checks.
- Inform health care provider.
- Inspect device for proper fit and positioning and for areas of damage, wear, or rough edges.
- Provide appropriate skin care (see Chapter 39).
- Inform health care provider.
- Inform orthoptist, PT, or OT so that adjustments to device can be made.

Documentation

- Document assessments of skin integrity, neurovascular status, application of and type of device, schedule of wear, activity level, movement permitted, patient's tolerance of procedure, and instructions given to patient and family caregiver.
- Document observations about patient's or family caregiver's ability to apply device, ambulate, and remove device.
- Document your evaluation of patient/family caregiver learning.

Hand-Off Reporting

- Report to health care provider any unexpected outcomes.

Special Considerations

Patient Education

- When a patient has an immobilization device, instruct to inspect skin daily for pressure or areas of breakdown. Involve family caregiver as appropriate.
- Give patients a list of medical suppliers in the community to obtain new sling or elastic wrap for splints.

Pediatrics

- If a child's extremity has been immobilized for a long time, perform upper body strengthening exercises to condition and strengthen arms and shoulders (Hockenberry et al., 2022).
- Monitor children closely to ensure that they do not remove an immobilization device.
- Recognize that bracing in adolescents affects body image and self-esteem.

Older Adults

- Lightweight immobilization devices are less restrictive for older adults.
- Older adults may have decreased sensation, so carefully assess fit of immobilization device (Touhy & Jett, 2022).

Home Care

- Remind patient to inspect and clean immobilization device weekly.

✦ CLINICAL JUDGMENT AND NEXT GENERATION NCLEX® EXAMINATION–STYLE QUESTIONS

The nurse is caring for a patient who is 70 years old and newly postoperative for a total left knee replacement 18 hours ago. The patient lives alone at home. The patient's medical history includes hypertension and osteoarthritis. Average blood pressure readings are approximately 150–160/84–90 mm Hg. Surgeon orders include early mobility protocol and bearing weight on the left leg. Last night after surgery, the patient was able to sit in a chair for 30 minutes and rated the pain level then as 4 on a scale of 0 to 10.

1. The patient received an analgesic 30 minutes ago before planned ambulation. Which of the following signs would indicate to the nurse that the patient should not be ambulated at this time? **Select all that apply**.
   1. Dyspnea
   2. Pain at Level 4 in left knee
   3. Dizziness
   4. Reduced ROM, left knee
   5. Fear of increased pain

2. The physical therapist has fitted the patient for a walker. The patient is to be monitored for a target heart rate of 75% of maximum heart rate. The nurse will discontinue ambulation if the patient's heart rate raises higher than which amount?
   1. 150 beats/min
   2. 220 beats/min
   3. 115 beats/min
   4. 112 beats/min

3. The patient is prepared to ambulate. Which action will the nurse tell the patient to accomplish **first**?
   1. "Step forward with your weaker leg."
   2. "Move your center of gravity toward the walker."
   3. "Balance yourself in the center of the walker."
   4. "Move the walker about 6 to 8 inches forward."

4. The nurse has provided the patient's family with teaching about safe walker use at home. Which family member statement demonstrates that teaching was effective?
   1. "We can cut golf balls to put on the rubber tips of the walker."
   2. "It is important to take the walker into the shower to stay stable."
   3. "The walker can be used to balance when getting up from a chair."
   4. "Walkers can be used inside and outside the house, as well as on inclines."

5. The nurse has provided the patient with teaching about safe walker use at home. Indicate whether the patient's statement demonstrates an understanding of this teaching or requires further nursing intervention.

Patient Statement	Demonstrates Understanding	Requires Nursing Intervention
"I will use my walker only if I feel weak."		
"All four feet of the walker need to stay on the floor."		
"I can use my walker when I need to go upstairs."		
"The first step I take needs to be with my affected leg."		
"I should never lean over my walker."		

Visit the Evolve site for Answers to Clinical Judgment and Next Generation NCLEX® Examination–Style Questions.

REFERENCES

Agency for Healthcare Research and Quality (AHRQ): *Teach-Back: intervention,* 2023. https://www.ahrq.gov/patient-safety/reports/engage/interventions/teachback.html.

American Academy of Orthopedic Surgeons: *Ortho info: how to use crutches, canes, and walkers,* 2020. https://orthoinfo.aaos.org/en/recovery/how-to-use-crutches-canes-and-walkers/. Accessed April 5, 2023.

American Academy of Family Physicians: Diagnosing VTE: Guidelines from the American Society of Hematology, *Am Fam Physician* 100(11):716–717, 2019.

American Academy of Nursing: *Choosing wisely,* 2021. https://www.aannet.org/initiatives/previous-initiatives/choosing-wisely. Accessed April 5, 2023.

American Heart Association (AHA): *American Heart Association recommendations for physical activity in adults and kids,* 2018, AHA. http://www.heart.org/HEARTORG/GettingHealthy/PhysicalActivity/FitnessBasics/American-Heart-Association-Recommendations-for-Physical-Activity-in-Adults_UCM_307976_Article.jsp#.VkjC8aSFOpo. Accessed April 4, 2023.

American Heart Association (AHA): *Target heart rates chart,* 2021, AHA. https://www.heart.org/en/healthy-living/fitness/fitness-basics/target-heart-rates. Accessed April 4, 2023.

American Heart Association (AHA): *How much physical activity do you need?* 2023a. https://www.heart.org/en/healthy-living/fitness/fitness-basics/aha-recs-for-physical-activity-infographic. Accessed April 4, 2023.

American Heart Association (AHA): *American Heart Association recommendations for physical activity in kids infographic,* 2023b. https://www.heart.org/en/healthy-living/fitness/fitness-basics/aha-recs-for-physical-activity-in-kids-infographic. Accessed April 4, 2023.

American Society of Hematology (ASH): *Clinicians: ASH clinical practice guidelines on venous thromboembolism,* 2023. https://www.hematology.org/education/clinicians/guidelines-and-quality-care/clinical-practice-guidelines/venous-thromboembolism-guidelines. Accessed April 4, 2023.

Anderson D, et al: American Society of Hematology 2019 guidelines for management of venous thromboembolism: prevention of venous thromboembolism in surgical hospitalized patients, *Blood Adv* 3(23):3898–3944, 2019.

Arora A: Time to move again: from deconditioning to reconditioning, *Age Ageing* 51(2):afab227, 2022. https://academic.oup.com/ageing/article/51/2/afab227/6520503. Accessed April 5, 2023.

Asai T, et al: The association between fear of falling and occurrence of falls: a one-year cohort study, *BMC Geriatr* 22(1):393, 2022.

Bach C, Hetland B: A step forward for intensive care unit patients: early mobility interventions and associated outcome measures, *Crit Care Nurse* 42(6):13–24, 2022.

Badireddy M, Mudipalli V: *Deep venous thrombosis prophylaxis,* Treasure Island, FL, 2023, Stat Pearls.

Berszakiewicz A, et al: Compression therapy in venous diseases: current forms of compression materials and techniques, *Postepy Dermatol Alergol* 37(6):836–841, 2020.

Biswas D, et al: Role of nurses and nurse practitioners in the recognition, diagnosis, and management of neurogenic orthostatic hypotension: a narrative review, *Int J Gen Med* 12:173–184, 2019.

Burchum JR, Rosenthal LD: *Lehne's pharmacology for nursing care,* ed 10, St. Louis, 2022, Elsevier.

Centers for Disease Control and Prevention (CDC): *What is health literacy?* 2023. https://www.cdc.gov/healthliteracy/learn/index.html.

Cleveland Clinic: *Deep Vein Thrombosis (DVT),* 2022. https://my.clevelandclinic.org/health/diseases/16911-deep-vein-thrombosis-dvt. Accessed April 4, 2023.

Dean E, et al: *Safe prescription of mobilizing patients in acute care settings: what to assess, what to monitor, when not to mobilize and how to mobilize and progress,* SAFEMOB task force, n.d. https://physicaltherapy.med.ubc.ca/files/2012/05/SAFEMOB_Final18673.pdf. Accessed April 4, 2023.

Harding M, et al: *Lewis's medical-surgical nursing: assessment and management of clinical problems,* ed 11, St. Louis, 2020, Elsevier.

Health in Aging Foundation: *Tip sheet: choosing the right cane or walker,* 2019. https://www.healthinaging.org/tools-and-tips/tip-sheet-choosing-right-cane-or-walker. Accessed April 5, 2023.

Hockenberry MJ, et al: *Essentials of pediatric nursing,* ed 11, St. Louis, 2022, Elsevier.

Hosseini Z, et al: The effect of early passive range of motion exercise on motor function of people with stroke: a randomized controlled trial, *J Caring Sci* 8(1):39–44, 2019. https://www.ncbi.nlm.nih.gov/pmc/articles/PMC6428159/?msclkid=124f5ac5cf9911ecb72cfde1f2420bfc. Accessed April 5, 2023.

Huang J, et al: Benefits of early ambulation in elderly patients undergoing lumbar decompression and fusion surgery: a prospective cohort study, *Orthop Surg* 13(4):1319–1326, 2021.

Huether SE, et al: *Understanding pathophysiology,* ed 7, St. Louis, 2020, Mosby.

Insin P, et al: Prevention of venous thromboembolism in gynecological cancer patients undergoing major abdominopelvic surgery: a systematic review and network meta-analysis, *Gynecol Oncol* 161(1):304–313, 2021.

Johns Hopkins: *Fall prevention: balance and strength exercises for older adults*, 2023. https://www.hopkinsmedicine.org/health/wellness-and-prevention/fall-prevention-exercises. Accessed April 4, 2023.

Linke CA, et al: Early mobilization in the ICU: a collaborative, integrated approach, *Crit Care Explor* 2(4):e0090, 2020. https://www.ncbi.nlm.nih.gov/pmc/articles/PMC7188418/. Accessed April 5, 2023.

Luz C, et al: Do canes or walkers make any difference? Nonuse and fall injuries, *Gerontologist* 57(2):211–218, 2017.

Matz M, et al: *Patient handling and mobility assessments*, ed 2, 2019, *The Facility Guidelines Institute*. http://www.fgiguidelines.org/wp-content/uploads/2019/10/FGI-Patient-Handling-and-Mobility-Assessments_191008.pdf. Accessed April 5, 2023.

Mayo Clinic: *Aerobic exercise: how to warm up and cool down*, 2021. https://www.mayoclinic.org/healthy-lifestyle/fitness/in-depth/exercise/art-20045517. Accessed April 4, 2023.

Mayo Clinic: *Healthy lifestyle: tips for choosing and using walkers*, 2022. https://www.mayoclinic.org/health-lifestyle/healthy-aging/multimedia/walker/sls-20076469. Accessed April 4, 2023.

Myszenski A: *The essential role of lab values and vital signs in clinical decision making and patient safety for the acutely ill patient*, 2017, Physical Therapy.com. https://www.physicaltherapy.com/articles/essential-role-lab-values-and-3637?msclkid=5c382b0ccf9511ec93f331742db5b40c. Accessed April 4, 2023.

National Institute on Aging (NIA): *Four types of exercise can improve your health and mobility*, 2021. https://www.nia.nih.gov/health/four-types-exercise-can-improve-your-health-and-physical-ability#strength. Accessed April 4, 2023.

Office of Disease Prevention and Health Promotion (ODPHP): *Physical activity*, Healthy people 2030, n.d., US Department of Health and Human Services. https://health.gov/healthypeople/objectives-and-data/browse-objectives/physical-activity. Accessed April 5, 2023.

Pittman J, Gillespie C: Medical device–related pressure injuries, *Crit Care Nurs Clin North Am* 32(4):533–542, 2020.

Ramakrishna R, et al: Use of a mobile intermittent pneumatic compression device (vekroosan) in mobile patients with chronic venous disease, *J Hematol* 10(1):8–13, 2021.

Santy-Tomlinson: The musculoskeletal implications of deconditioning in older adults during and following COVID-19, *Int J Orthop Trauma Nurs* 42:100882, 2021. https://www.ncbi.nlm.nih.gov/pmc/articles/PMC8223128/. Accessed April 5, 2023.

Sehgal M, et al: Mobility assistive device use in older adults, *Am Fam Physician* 103(12):737–744, 2021.

Schallom M, et al: One-year outcomes after implementation of an ICU early mobility protocol, *Crit Care Nurse* 40(4):e7–e17, 2020.

Shatri A, Ipinge TK: Recent incidence of deep-vein thrombosis in surgical departments, 2015-2022: a systematic review. *Undergraduate Res Health J* 1(1):11–15, 2023.

Taylor AJ, et al: Outcomes of an institutional rapid recovery protocol for total joint arthroplasty at a safety net hospital, *J Am Acad Orthop Surg Glob Res Rev* 6(3):e21.00173, 2022.

The Joint Commission (TJC): *2023 National patient safety goals*, Oakbrook Terrace, IL, 2022, The Joint Commission. https://www.jointcommission.org/standards/national-patient-safety-goals/hospital-national-patient-safety-goals/. Accessed April 5, 2023.

Thompson BT, et al: *Clinical presentation, evaluation, and diagnosis of the nonpregnant adult with suspected acute pulmonary embolism*, UpToDate, 2022. https://www.uptodate.com/contents/clinical-presentation-evaluation-and-diagnosis-of-the-nonpregant-adult-with-suspected-acute-pulmonary-embolism?topicRef=8253&source=see_link. Accessed April 4, 2023.

Touhy T, Jett K: *Gerontological nursing & healthy aging*, ed 6, St. Louis, 2022, Elsevier.

U.S. Department of Health and Human Services (USDHHS): *Physical activity guidelines for Americans*, ed 2, Washington, DC, 2018, U.S. Department of Health and Human Services. https://health.gov/sites/default/files/2019-09/Physical_Activity_Guidelines_2nd_edition.pdf. Accessed April 4, 2023.

UW Medicine: *How to use crutches: step-by-step instructions and safety tips*, 2019. https://healthonline.washington.edu/sites/default/files/record_pdfs/How-Use-Crutches.pdf. Accessed April 5, 2023.

Viner Disability Law: *How using a walker may impact your disability claim*, 2023. https://denversocialsecuritydisability.com/how-using-a-walker-may-impact-your-disability-claim/#:~:text=If%20you%20make%20regular%20use%20of%20a%20prescribed,under%20the%20Social%20Security%20Administration%E2%80%99s%20%28SSA%29%20current%20regulations. Accessed April 5, 2023.

Walia S, et al: Early mobilization in the ICU: Assessing a standardized early mobility protocol on neurological patients, *Neurology* 90(Suppl 15), 2018.

Warees M, et al: *Crutches*, Treasure Island (FL), *Stat Pearls*, 90(15): Supplement P4.323, 2022.

U.S. Department of Veterans Affairs: *Safe patient handling for everyone around the world*, n.d. https://www.publichealth.va.gov/docs/employeehealth/SPHM-Solutions-Everywhere-for-Everyone.pdf#. Accessed April 5, 2023.

13 | Support Surfaces and Special Beds

SKILLS AND PROCEDURES

Procedural Guideline 13.1 **Selection of a Pressure-Redistribution Support Surface, p. 365**

Skill 13.1 **Care of the Patient on a Support Surface, p. 368**

Skill 13.2 **Care of the Patient on a Special Bed, p. 373**

OBJECTIVES

Mastery of content in this chapter will enable you to:
- List the different types of support surfaces and specialty beds used for pressure redistribution.
- Explain why preventive nursing care remains essential when using support surfaces and specialty beds.
- Discuss how prone-positioning specialty beds improve oxygenation in selected patients.
- Explain guidelines for placing patients on support surfaces and specialty beds.

- Compare and contrast differences between mattress support surfaces and specialty beds.
- Discuss the mechanisms by which skin breakdown can occur on a support surface, specialty bed, or wheelchair seat cushion.
- Choose the steps for correct placement of a patient on a support surface or specialty bed.

MEDIA RESOURCES

- http://evolve.elsevier.com/Perry/skills
- Review Questions
- Audio Glossary

- Answers to Clinical Judgment and Next-Generation NCLEX® Examination–Style Questions
- Skills Performance Checklists
- Printable Key Points

PURPOSE

Pressure injuries (PIs) are a major problem that affects patient comfort, length of stay in health care agencies, and health care costs (European Pressure Ulcer Advisory Panel, National Pressure injury Advisory Panel, Pan Pacific Pressure Injury Alliance [EPUAP/NPIAP/PPPIA], 2019). Nursing assessment for PIs is key to prevention and timely interprofessional interventions, especially in critical care areas (Cox et al., 2022).

A support surface is one type of intervention designed to prevent PI. A device provides pressure redistribution and an environment more conducive to PI healing. Support surfaces redistribute interface pressure by conforming to the contours of the body so that pressure is redistributed over a larger surface area rather than concentrated on a more circumscribed location (Nix & Milne, 2024). Nursing assessment identifies those patients at risk for PI development or those with PIs who should be placed on a support or specialty bed.

PRACTICE STANDARDS

- Wound, Ostomy, and Continence Nurses Society (WOCN), 2016: Guidelines for prevention and management of pressure ulcers (injuries)
- National Pressure Injury Advisory Panel (NPIAP), 2019: Clinical Practice Guideline
- The Joint Commission (TJC), 2023: National Patient Safety Goals—Patient identification

SUPPLEMENTAL STANDARDS

- European Pressure Ulcer Advisory Panel, National Pressure Injury Advisory Panel, and Pan Pacific Pressure Injury Alliance (EPUAP/NPIAP/PPPIA), 2019: Treatment of Pressure Ulcers/Injuries: Quick Reference Guide
- McNichol LL et al., 2022: Wound, Ostomy, and Continence Nurses Society Core Curriculum: Wound Management

PRINCIPLES FOR PRACTICE

- Factors contributing to PI formation are both extrinsic (e.g., pressure, moisture, friction and shear, medical devices) and intrinsic (e.g., malnutrition, loss of sensation, impaired mobility, aging skin, impaired mental status, infection, incontinence, and low arteriolar pressure) (Bambi et al., 2022; Serraes et al., 2018).
- PIs are localized injuries to the skin and/or underlying tissue, usually over a bony prominence such as the heel or sacrum. These injuries are a result of unrelieved pressure or pressure in combination with shear and/or friction and result in chronic wounds (McNichol et al., 2020; Tomova-Simitchieva et al., 2018; WOCN, 2016).
- The major cause of pressure injuries is unrelieved pressure. The greater the pressure and the longer it is applied, the greater the likelihood for PI development. When external pressure on the tissues exceeds 32 mm Hg (the capillary closing pressure), the network of capillaries collapses. Pressure interrupts the delivery

of oxygen and nutrients to the cells and the removal of metabolic waste products, resulting in tissue ischemia and tissue necrosis.

- Frequent repositioning, which temporarily relieves pressure, is the backbone of prevention protocols. No support surface or mattress totally eliminates the need for competent nursing care. It is your responsibility to use appropriate turning schedules for patients in bed or in a chair. Use lift teams and lifting devices to transfer patients from a regular bed to a special support surface (see Chapter 11).
- Support surfaces are specialized devices (e.g., mattress overlays, mattress replacements, integrated bed systems, seat cushions, or seat cushion overlays) that redistribute pressure and are designed for management of tissue loads, microclimate, shear, and/ or other therapeutic functions (Edsberg, 2022; NPUAP, 2019).
- Support surfaces reduce pressure by redistributing it over a larger surface area. The extent to which a support surface reduces pressure is characterized in two ways. The first is preventive, in which pressure is not consistently reduced below 32 mm Hg (e.g., foam, air, or gel overlay). The second is therapeutic, in

which pressure is consistently reduced below 32 mm Hg (e.g., powered overlay air mattress or low-air-loss mattress).

- Therapeutic surfaces are for patients at high risk for PI development or for those with existing PIs (Nix & Milne, 2024; EPUAP/NPIAP/PPPIA, 2019). Support surfaces are one intervention for redistributing pressure; they are used in conjunction with other PI risk-reduction strategies (see Chapter 39) (Rae et al., 2018).
- Support surfaces also reduce friction and shear and provide temperature and moisture control. A support surface reduces shear and friction by strategic placement of surfaces and covers that allow for low-friction patient positioning without excessive sliding (Nix & Milne, 2024).
- Support surfaces may provide a microclimate control function. Excess moisture of the skin is a well-known factor associated with PI development. Control of temperature at the interface surface (patient–bed boundary) helps to maintain normal skin temperature, which in turn inhibits sweating and lowers skin hydration (Nix & Milne, 2024). Table 13.1 provides a comparison of support surfaces.

TABLE 13.1

Support Surfaces

Category and Mechanism of Action	Indications for Use	Advantages	Disadvantages
Support Surfaces and Overlays			
Foam Overlay (Available as an Overlay or in a Full Mattress)			
Reduces pressure; the cover (top) can reduce friction and shear. Foam overlays and cushions are single use and designed for a specific weight limit and life span.	Use for moderate- to high-risk patients. Specific products (e.g., elastic foam and memory foam) are useful with certain patients. Assess patient to determine the best foam overlay.	One-time charge. No setup fee. Cannot be punctured. Available in various sizes (e.g., bed, chair, operating room table). Little maintenance. Does not need electricity.	Elevates body temperature. Increases risk for patient dehydration. Hot and may trap moisture. Limited life span. Plastic protective sheet needed for incontinent patients or patients with draining wounds. **NOTE:** Not indicated for those with existing stage 3 or 4 PIs.
Water Overlay (Available as an Overlay or in a Full Mattress)			
Redistributes pressure and pressure points because surface provides lower interface pressure than standard mattresses. Flotation assists by redistributing patient's weight evenly over entire support surface.	Use for high-risk patients.	Readily available. Some control over motion sensations. Easy to clean.	Easily punctured. Fluid motion may make procedures (e.g., positioning, transfer, CPR) difficult. Maintenance is needed to prevent microorganism growth. Needs a heater to control temperature. Difficult to raise and lower head of bed.
Gel Overlay			
Redistributes pressure because of surface; provides flotation by redistributing patient's weight evenly over entire support surface.	Use for moderate- to high-risk patients. Use for patients who are wheelchair dependent.	Low maintenance. Easy to clean. Multiple-patient use. Effective in reducing shear. Impermeable to needle punctures.	Heavy. Difficult to repair. Expensive. Lacks airflow, which can result in increased skin moisture and skin temperature. Variable friction control.
Nonpowered Air-Filled Overlay			
Redistributes pressure by lowering mean interface pressure between patient's tissue and overlay.	Use for moderate- to high-risk patients. Use for patients who can reposition themselves.	Easy to clean. Multiple-patient use. Low maintenance. Lightweight. Durable.	Damaged by punctures from needles and sharps. Requires routine monitoring to determine adequate inflation pressure. Patient transfers out of bed can be difficult.

Continued

TABLE 13.1

Support Surfaces—cont'd

Category and Mechanism of Action	Indications for Use	Advantages	Disadvantages
Low-Air-Loss Overlay (Available as an Overlay or in a Full Mattress)			
Maintains constant and slight air movement against patient's skin; redistributes pressure; assists in managing the heat and humidity (microclimate) of the skin.	Use for moderate- to high-risk patients. May be used alone or in combination with alternating pressure, lateral rotation, and air-fluidized technology (Mackey & Watts, 2022).	Easy to clean. Maintains constant inflation. Deflates to facilitate transfer and CPR. Manages heat and humidity (microclimate) and moisture control. Fabric covering overlay is air permeable, bacteria impermeable, and waterproof. Reduces shear and friction. Setup provided by manufacturer.	Damaged by needles and sharps. Can be noisy. Requires electricity; some are available with short backup battery. In home, may need to purchase backup generator in case of loss of electrical power.
Specialty Beds			
Air-Fluidized Bed			
Bedframe contains silicone-coated beads and provides pressure redistribution by means of the fluidlike medium that is created by forcing air through beads, resulting in immersion and envelopment of the patient.	Use for high-risk patients. Use for patients with stage 3 or 4 PIs or burns.	Less frequent turning or repositioning. Improved patient comfort. Becomes firm for CPR or other treatments when device is turned off. Reduces shear, friction, and edema to site. May facilitate management of copious wound drainage or incontinence. Setup provided by manufacturer.	Continuous circulation of warm, dry air may increase patient risk for dehydration. Possible increase in room temperature. Patient may experience disorientation. Patient transfer is difficult. Heavy. Expensive. May not be wide enough for use with obese patients or patients with contractures. Patient cannot lie prone because of risk of suffocation.
Low-Air-Loss Bed			
Bedframe with series of connected air-filled pillows. The flow of air controls the amount of pressure in each pillow and assists in managing the heat and humidity (microclimate) of the patient's skin. Redistributes pressure.	Use for patients who need pressure redistribution, those who cannot be repositioned frequently, or those who have skin breakdown on more than one surface. Contraindicated in patients with unstable spinal column.	Can raise and lower head and foot of bed. Easy transfer into and out of bed. Setup provided by manufacturer.	Portable motor can be noisy. Bed surface material slippery; patients can easily slide down mattress or out of bed when being transferred.
Rotation Therapy			
Provides continuous passive motion to promote mobilization of pulmonary secretions and low air loss and provides pressure redistribution.	Used primarily to facilitate pulmonary hygiene in patients with acute respiratory conditions. Should not be used when the patient is hemodynamically unstable.	Reduces pulmonary complications associated with restricted mobility.	Does not reduce shear or moisture. Cannot be used with cervical or skeletal traction. Possible motion sickness initially.

CPR, Cardiopulmonary resuscitation.
Data from Mackey D, Watts C: Therapeutic surfaces for bed and chair. In McNichol LL et al, editors: *WOCN core curriculum wound management,* ed 2, Mt. Laurel, NJ, 2022, Wound, Ostomy, and Continence Nurses Society (WOCN).

PERSON-CENTERED CARE

- Complete a thorough patient assessment, including determining individual needs, health care provider needs, and location of the patient.
- Features of a support surface must match a patient's unique pressure-reduction needs (McNichol et al., 2022; McNichol et al., 2020; McNichol et al., 2015).

- Be aware of patient and family's financial considerations. These are expensive beds, and a patient may not be able to afford this in a home care environment. Ensure that the family caregivers understand and are able to use other pressure-relieving and skin-care interventions (e.g., frequent position change, individualized skin care).
- Educate patient/family caregivers about the advantages, disadvantages, and methods of operation of all support devices to ensure their proper use in all settings.

- Be sensitive and aware of patient's cultural and religious preferences. Some patients and family caregivers may have limited English communication. When this is the situation, provide for an interpreter early.
- Be sensitive to a patient's need for gender congruent caregivers and privacy.

EVIDENCE-BASED PRACTICE

Support Surfaces and Prevention of Pressure Injuries

Pressure injuries can be partially controlled by an appropriate support surface (Nix & Milne, 2024). Evidence suggests that pressure-redistribution devices can reduce the incidence of pressure injuries when the correct surface is matched to patient needs (Bambi et al., 2022). Pressure reduction and relief are major nursing interventions for the prevention of PIs (NPIAP, 2019; Borchert, 2022).

- Alternating pressure mattresses are superior to a standard hospital mattress (Bambi et al., 2022; Haesler, 2018).
- Active support surfaces (e.g., alternating air pressure mattresses, air-fluidized support surfaces, and low-air-loss support surfaces) are more effective than foam overlays (Mackey & Watts, 2022; Haesler, 2018; Serraes et al., 2018).
- There is insufficient evidence to support one support surface for pressure redistribution over another for the prevention of PIs (Bambi et al., 2022).
- Although support surfaces are effective in the treatment of PIs, they are not a substitute for routine positioning and thorough skin assessment (Bambi et al., 2022; McInnes et al., 2018; Rae et al., 2018).
- Pressure distribution surfaces should be used in the operating room for individuals assessed to be at high risk for PI development, especially older adults and bariatric patients. Pressure redistribution has been associated with a decreased incidence of postoperative PIs.

SAFETY GUIDELINES

- Perform complete and routine skin assessments, as per agency protocol, to determine patient's risk for PIs.
- A complete patient assessment includes use of appropriate validated pressure injury risk scales, such as the Braden Scale, which include factors such as presence of shear and friction and a patient's mobility and continence status (see Chapter 39).
- Perform complete and routine assessments to determine patient's risk for medical device–related pressure injuries (MDRPIs). Inspect skin under device at point where device exits the patient's

body region (e.g., nasogastric tube, endotracheal/tracheal tubes, indwelling catheters, wound drainage systems) (Haesler, 2017; Padula et al., 2017).

- Perform complete and routine assessments to determine patient's risk for medical adhesive–related skin injury (MARSI). Know impact of patient's age and history of dehydration, malnutrition, exposure to radiation therapy, underlying chronic conditions (e.g., diabetes mellitus, immunosuppression), and edema, all of which increase patients' risk for MARSI. Inspect under any adhesive material used to secure dressings, medical equipment, sterile barriers, and so on (Fumarola et al., 2020).
- Select a support surface based on patient's risk for developing PIs, such as prior PIs, impaired mobility, need for microclimate control (control of heat and humidity of patient's skin), reduction of shear, and size and weight of patient (Rae et al., 2018).
- Know the reason for and extent of a patient's reduced mobility. A patient who is not easy to reposition or who has PIs involving multiple surfaces benefits from pressure-redistribution support devices (Rae et al., 2018; Serraes et al., 2018).
- Use special underpads designed for the support surface to control moisture exposure from incontinence (Nix & Milne, 2024). Do not use plastic-backed incontinence pads, which increase the number of layers between the patient and the support surface and as a result decrease the effectiveness of pressure redistribution (Mackey & Watts, 2022). Have an incontinence-management plan in place.
- Do not place a patient in the prone position while using these support surfaces. During the COVID-19 pandemic, critically ill patients had life-threatening declines in oxygenation status. Recent findings regarding the use of proning—moving a patient to a lying face down (prone) position—showed improved patient oxygenation status and clinical outcomes in patients with respiratory failure associated with COVID-19 (Shelhamer et al., 2021; Wiggerman et al., 2020). Placing critically ill patients in the prone position requires manual positioning and disconnecting and reconnecting equipment. To date, specialty support surfaces are not designed for proning a patient. Because of the soft air/fluid-filled mattresses and hard surfaces, there is a risk for patient suffocation.
- Continue to provide basic prevention care measures against the hazards of immobility (e.g., regular skin assessment, turning, correct positioning, range-of-motion exercises).
- Use safe patient-handling techniques and proper body mechanics when positioning or working with patients (see Chapter 11).
- Educate family caregivers about the advantages, disadvantages, and methods of operation of all support devices to ensure their proper use in all settings.

PROCEDURAL GUIDELINE 13.1 *Selection of a Pressure-Redistribution Support Surface*

Delegation

The selection of a pressure-redistribution support device cannot be delegated to assistive personnel (AP).

Interprofessional Collaboration

- Communicate with the interprofessional team, including the health care provider, skin-care specialist, and physical therapy provider to determine optimal support surface.
- Coordinate with agency discharge planning and social work services to ensure patient is provided with correct support surface in skilled nursing facility or at home as needed.

Equipment

Pressure injury risk assessment tool, such as the Braden Scale (see agency policy) (see Chapter 39); body chart, tape measure, and/or camera to document existing areas of impaired skin integrity; clean gloves; electronic health record (EHR); skin-care products

Steps

1. Identify patient using at least two identifiers (e.g., name and birthday or name and medical record number) according to agency policy (TJC, 2023).

Continued

PROCEDURAL GUIDELINE 13.1 *Selection of a Pressure-Redistribution Support Surface—cont'd*

2. Check agency policy regarding implementing a support surface.
   a. Obtain a health care provider's order. This is usually required for a patient to obtain third-party reimbursement.
   b. Consult with health care agency case manager or social worker to help with patient's financial eligibility and terms and length of third-party reimbursement for the surface.
   c. Consult with agency home care or discharge planning services if the device is anticipated for long-term use. Specific procedures and evaluations are needed for continuity of surface when patient is transferred to extended care or discharged home.
3. Review EHR for patient weight and weight distribution and the following risk factors/comorbidities: advanced age, fever, poor dietary intake of protein, diastolic pressure <60 mm Hg, hemodynamic instability, generalized edema, and anemia (Mackey & Watts, 2022; WOCN, 2016).
4. Assess patient's/family caregiver's health literacy.
5. Perform hand hygiene. Apply clean gloves if drainage or open wound present.
6. Assess patient's risk for skin breakdown by using a risk assessment tool. Include mobility and ability to reposition.
7. Assess patient for risks for medical adhesive–related skin injury (MARSI): history of dehydration, malnutrition, exposure to radiation therapy, underlying chronic conditions (e.g., diabetes mellitus, immunosuppression), and edema of the skin. Inspect skin under any adhesive or securing devices for items such as nasogastric tubes, urinary catheters, and wound dressings (Fumarola et al., 2020).
8. Assess patient's existing and past PIs, including location, condition of skin and stage, areas of blistering, abnormal reactive hyperemia, and abrasion.
9. Assess the presence of medical devices (e.g., catheters, feeding tubes, and so on) and determine patient's risk for medical device–related pressure injuries (MDRPIs) (Haesler, 2017; Rae et al., 2018). Remove and dispose of gloves. Perform hand hygiene.
10. Assess character of patient's pain, and rate acuity on a pain scale of 0 to 10.
11. Determine the need for a pressure-reduction surface from assessment data.
12. Identify patient factors when selecting an appropriate surface (Fig. 13.1):
    a. Braden Scale score ≤18
    b. Does patient need pressure redistribution (e.g., you cannot reposition the patient, or there is an existing PI)?
    c. Is the surface needed for short- or long-term care? A short-term surface is usually needed for an acute illness and hospitalization. A long-term surface is usually needed for extended or home care.
    d. What is the potential comfort level achieved by the surface? If patient is sensitive to noise, a device with a loud motor will increase discomfort.
    e. Are patient and family caregivers cooperative and adherent to repositioning? In addition, are they aware that a support surface should never replace repositioning? Is adequate help available for repositioning? In a home setting a support surface is often necessary when the

family caregiver or patient is unable to reposition independently or help with repositioning.
    f. Does the support surface have a potential to interfere with patient's independent functioning? The height of the overlay and its soft edge may affect patient's ability to transfer, and a high-air-loss bed is not appropriate for a patient who needs to get into and out of bed frequently.
    g. What are patient's financial limitations?
    h. If patient is using the device in the home, what are the environmental limitations? Will the home and existing electrical service accommodate the surface selected? Can the family caregivers in the home manage the surface?
    i. How durable is the product? Is the surface easily subjected to puncture? How easily can the surface be cleaned?
    j. Does patient need pressure-relief surfaces in a chair/wheelchair?
13. Choose the appropriate surface (see Table 13.1). Place at-risk patients on a pressure-reduction surface or high-specification foam mattress and not on a standard hospital mattress (Mackey & Watts, 2022; WOCN, 2016; NPUAP, 2019).
    a. Pressure-redistribution devices redistribute the pressure/load over the control area of the patient's body to reduce the overall pressure and avoid areas of localized pressure (WOCN, 2016). Surfaces providing pressure redistribution include therapeutic mattress replacements, nonpowered and powered (e.g., moving) surfaces, low-air-loss beds and mattresses, and air-fluidized beds (Mackey & Watts, 2022; McNichol et al., 2020). Pressure-redistribution surfaces are also used in the operating room for individuals who are at high risk or for lengthy procedures (Bambi et al., 2022).
    b. Use a nonpowered support surface if patient can assume a variety of positions without bearing weight on a PI without "bottoming out." Bottoming out makes the support surface ineffective because it is inadequate for patient's weight and the body sinks too deeply into the surface.

Clinical Judgment *The hand check method to assess for "bottoming out" of static or overlay mattresses, integrated bed mattresses, or certain support surfaces is not reliable and is no longer recommended (Nix & Milne, 2024; Mackey & Watts, 2022; EPUAP/NPIAP/PPIA, 2019).*

    c. Select a powered support surface when patient cannot assume a variety of positions without bearing weight on a PI, if patient fully compresses the nonpowered support surface, or if the PI does not show evidence of healing. Alternating or powered mattresses are associated with a lower incidence of PIs compared with standard mattresses (Mackey & Watts, 2022).
    d. High-specification foam is effective in decreasing the incidence of PIs in fairly high-risk patients, including older adults and patients with fractures of the neck and femur (WOCN, 2016).

PROCEDURAL GUIDELINE 13.1 *Selection of a Pressure-Redistribution Support Surface—cont'd*

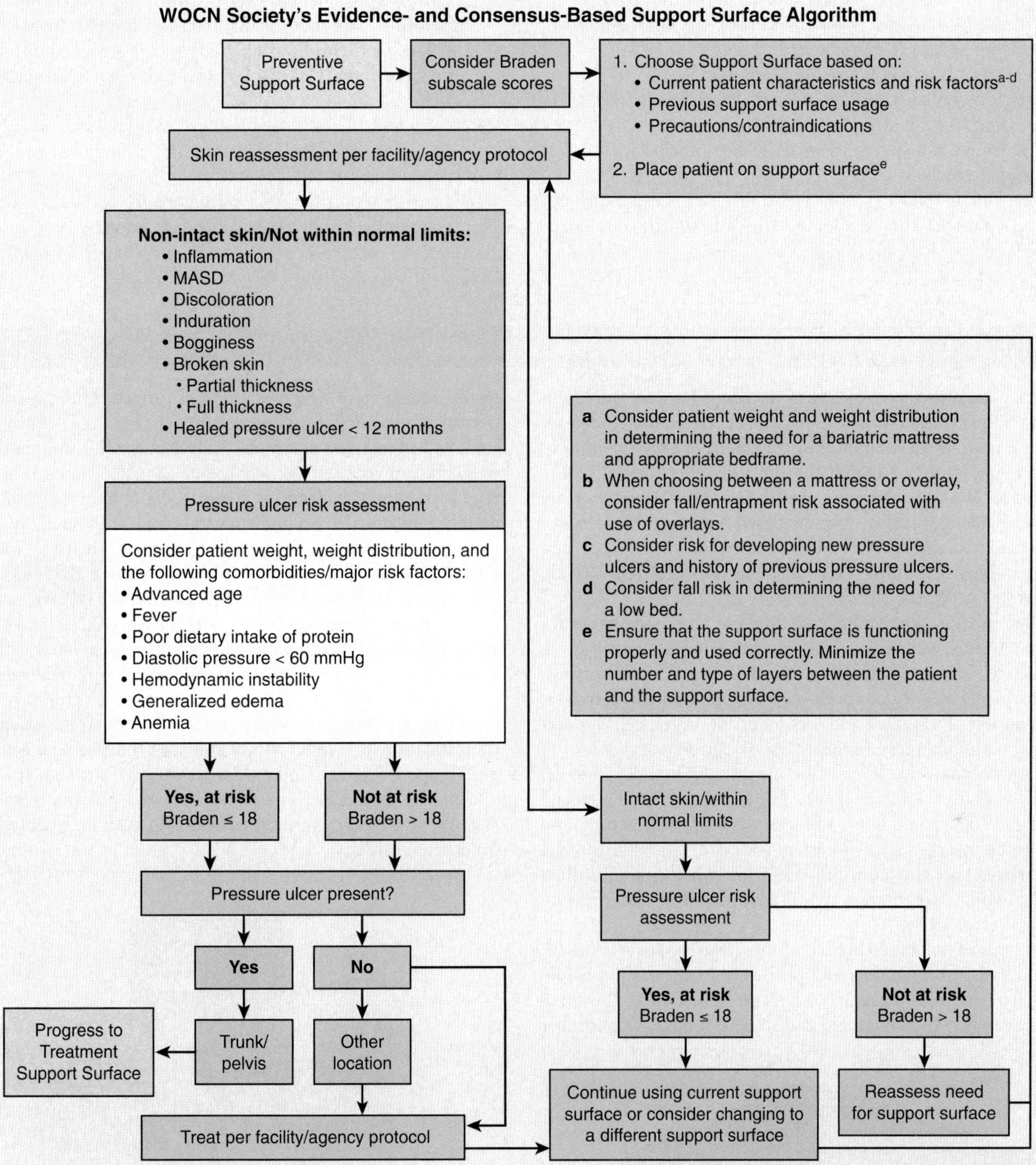

WOCN Society's Evidence- and Consensus-Based Support Surface Algorithm

FIG. 13.1 Flow diagram for ordering specialty beds.

e. Patients with burns or stage 3 or 4 PIs (Chapter 39) often benefit from an air-fluidized bed (Mackey & Watts, 2022).

f. When excess moisture is a potential risk, a support surface that controls the microclimate is important to control skin moisture and temperature (Nix & Milne, 2024; NPUAP, 2019).

14. Provide privacy and explain procedure to patient or family caregiver.

15. Assess patient's/family caregiver's knowledge, prior experience with PI or support surfaces, and expectations if support surface is to be used at home.

16. Apply appropriate support surface to patient's bed. Follow manufacturer's directions.

17. Perform hand hygiene. Apply clean gloves. Regularly inspect condition of skin and existing PIs for evidence of healing according to agency policy to evaluate changes in skin and effectiveness of therapy.

Continued

PROCEDURAL GUIDELINE 13.1 *Selection of a Pressure-Redistribution Support Surface—cont'd*

18. Remove and dispose of gloves. Perform hand hygiene.
19. Observe for side effects associated with specific pressure-reducing surface (e.g., nausea, dizziness).
20. Help patient to a comfortable position.
21. Raise side rails (as appropriate) and lower bed to lowest position, locking into position.
22. Place nurse call system in an accessible location within patient's reach.
23. **Use Teach-Back:** "I want to be sure I explained clearly why you need this special mattress to protect your skin. Tell me why this mattress is necessary to protect your skin." Revise your instruction now or develop a plan for revised patient/family caregiver teaching if patient/family caregiver is not able to teach back correctly.
24. Document PI risk assessment and skin assessment, type of support surface selected, and patient response to the specific support surface.
25. Hand-off report: Notify health care provider of any changes to patient's skin or existing pressure injuries.

✦ SKILL 13.1   Care of the Patient on a Support Surface

There are numerous support surfaces to reduce pressure on tissues overlying bony prominences. These devices are recommended for prevention and, in some situations, treatment of pressure injuries (PIs). It is important to match the pressure-relief surface to the patient. The Wound, Ostomy, and Continence Nurses Society (WOCN) Evidence- and Consensus-Based Support Surface Algorithm, located on the WOCN website, is a valuable resource that a wound ostomy care nurse (WOCN) can use (McNichol et al., 2015; Mackey & Watts, 2022).

Support surfaces are available in different sizes and shapes for chairs, mattresses, stretchers, and procedure and operating room tables (Nix & Milne, 2024). They can be categorized as mattress, chair, or wheelchair overlays or as mattress replacements. An overlay rests on top of a surface and uses foam, air, water, gel, or combinations to provide pressure relief (Fig. 13.2).

A flotation pad is made of a silicone or polyvinyl chloride gel enclosed in a vinyl-covered square. The pad serves as an artificial layer of fat to protect bony surfaces such as the sacrum and greater trochanters. These flotation pads are available for the bed or wheelchair. In addition, there are wheelchair air-filled cushions, which are battery powered and allow for pressure adjustment (Fig. 13.3).

Foam is also available in chair cushions, overlays, mattresses for beds, and pads for stretchers and operating room and procedure tables. There are two types of foam mattresses. One is the foam mattress overlay, which has a flat and smooth surface, foam rubber peaks, an egg-crate structure, or a cut surface. The egg-crate foam overlay is used only for patient comfort (Fig. 13.4). Place one on top of a bed mattress and place a sheet over the foam mattress pad overlay to prevent soiling and provide ease of cleaning. The second type is the high-specification foam specialty mattress, which completely replaces the hospital mattress and is covered by a loose-fitting cover intended to protect the specialty mattress and minimize friction and shear. There is no evidence that one type of high-specification foam is better than another (NPIAP, n.d.).

Air mattress overlays are either nonpowered or powered and consist of interconnected air cells or cushions inflated with a motorized blower. More complex air mattresses contain several layers of tubes or support cells. These mattresses use a pressure-cycling device to intermittently inflate and deflate or to maintain a constant inflation and slight air movement in the mattress. A nonpowered support surface is inflated with a simple air blower after the mattress has been placed on a bed. In addition to mattress and bed systems, air support overlays are available as chair, wheelchair, and toilet seat cushions.

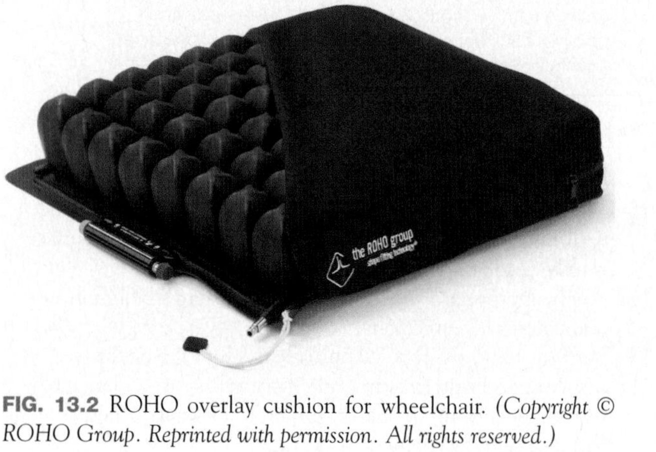

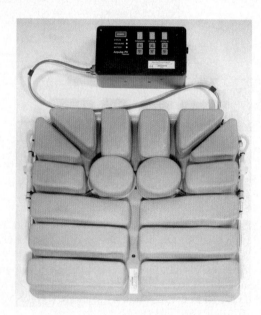

FIG. 13.2 ROHO overlay cushion for wheelchair. (*Copyright © ROHO Group. Reprinted with permission. All rights reserved.*)

FIG. 13.3 Air-filled cushion for wheelchair. (*Copyright © Aquila Corporation. Reprinted with permission. All rights reserved.*)

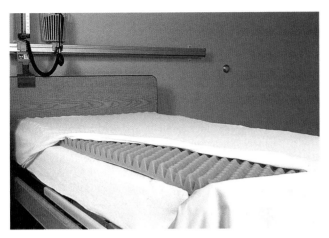

FIG. 13.4 Egg-crate foam overlay.

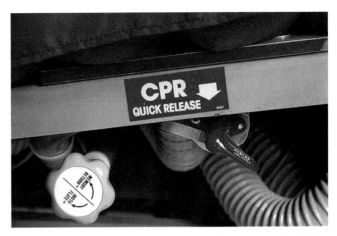

FIG. 13.5 Cardiopulmonary resuscitation (CPR) switch deflates low-air-loss bed to provide hard surface.

An integrated bed system is a bedframe and support surface combined into a single unit. With these integrated beds system, the features of both the frame and support surface must be evaluated for support needed and patient safety (Nix & Milne, 2024). An integrated air mattress connects with a pressure-cycling device that intermittently inflates and deflates sections of the mattress, creating a cycling effect that minimizes pressure on bony prominences.

Another available option is an air-integrated replacement mattress instead of the conventional mattress. These mattresses may also be fully integrated into the bed. Air mattresses are usually for patients with moderate to high risk for skin breakdown. You must deflate air mattresses before initiating cardiopulmonary resuscitation (CPR) (Fig. 13.5). Many agencies have purchased air-integrated replacement mattresses to replace their standard hospital mattresses because of improved skin and wound outcomes.

Another preventive intervention is a low-pressure seat cushion overlaid on a wheelchair or a dry, nonpowered flotation mattress system that you overlay on a bed (Fig. 13.6). Through a system of controlled dynamics, a cushion maintains low pressures by distributing pressure across a patient's body surface, reducing friction and shear.

Support surfaces aid in reducing pressure on a patient's skin but do not replace regular repositioning, meticulous skin assessment and skin care, or range-of-motion exercises. The appropriate assessment of a patient and selection of a pressure-redistribution surface is a nursing and health care team responsibility (see Procedural Guideline 13.1).

Delegation

The skill of placing a patient on a support surface can be delegated to assistive personnel (AP). However, the nurse must first complete the assessment, determine the need for a support surface, and select the specific surface. Some types of support surfaces require that a manufacturer's representative set up and maintain the support system. Direct the AP to:
- Report any changes in a patient's skin; the nurse then evaluates condition of the skin
- Continue to regularly turn and reposition a patient and seek help for patient position changes as necessary in bed or wheelchair
- Monitor the normal functioning of the support device such as inflation and deflation cycles and report to the nurse any changes in these cycles or leakage of air, water, or gel

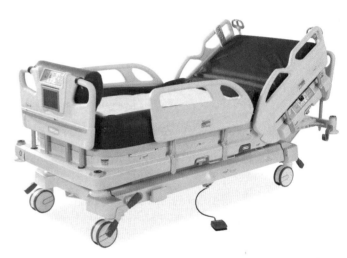

FIG. 13.6 Combination air-fluidized, low-air-loss bed. (*Copyright © 2023 Baxter International Inc. Reprinted with permission. All rights reserved.*)

Interprofessional Collaboration

- Coordinate care activities with health care provider, wound ostomy care nurse (WOCN), physical therapist, and manufacturer's representative from the specific support surface provider to ensure that patient receives correct support surface and that surface is used correctly.

Equipment

- Pressure injury risk-assessment tool (see agency policy) (see Chapter 39)
- Mattress and/or chair overlay support surface of choice: foam overlays, air mattress overlay, bed with integrated surface, air-integrated replacement mattress (**NOTE:** Some patients may require both mattress and chair overlay support surface.)
- Sheet(s)
- Clean gloves (if soiled linen is being handled)
- Standard bedframe (with mattress) if overlay is to be used (optional)

STEP	RATIONALE

ASSESSMENT

1. Identify patient using at least two identifiers (e.g., name and birthday or name and medical record number) according to agency policy.

Ensures correct patient. Complies with The Joint Commission standards and improves patient safety (TJC, 2023).

2. Review patient's electronic health record (EHR) for health care provider's order.

Health care provider's order is usually required to ensure third-party payment of support surface.

3. Assess patient's/family caregiver's health literacy.

Determines degree to which individuals have the ability to find, understand, and use information and services to make informed health-related decisions and actions for themselves and others (Centers for Disease Control and Prevention [CDC], 2023).

Clinical Judgment *Prepare to have these assessments completed before representative from specialty bed provider comes to assist with bed setup. In some cases, the manufacturer's representative may need to observe this assessment.*

4. Perform hand hygiene. Apply clean gloves if open wound present. Determine patient's risk for PI formation or progression of an existing injury using a valid assessment tool (e.g., Braden Scale) and assess for risk factors for pressure injuries (e.g., nutritional deficits, shear stress, friction, alterations in mobility and sensory perception, moisture, and abnormal serum albumin and hemoglobin levels) (see Chapter 39).

Reduces transmission of microorganisms.

Risk assessment tools provide an objective measure of risk that is consistent over time (NPUAP, 2019; Borchert, 2022).

Clinical Judgment *Patients with unstable conditions do not always tolerate turning or positioning required for thorough assessment or the application of a support surface mattress. Frequently assess patient and, if necessary, reposition patient or apply support surface in two steps.*

5. Perform skin assessment (see Chapters 6 and 38). Inspect condition of skin, especially over dependent sites, at bony prominences, and under and near medical devices. Remove and dispose of gloves (if worn). Perform hand hygiene.

Provides baseline to determine change in skin integrity or in existing pressure injury. Medical devices apply pressure directly or indirectly to underlying skin and tissues and increase risk for pressure injury (Borchert, 2022; Black & Kalowes, 2016).

6. Assess for dehydration, malnutrition, exposure to radiation, and underlying chronic conditions. Observe skin for edema and under existing dressings, securement devices, and anywhere adhesive is used to secure device, dressing, and so on. Determine risk for and presence of medical adhesive–related skin injury (MARSI).

Common risk factors for MARSI. Pressure injuries can begin with skin injury from medical adhesives and progress to worsening stages (Fumarola et al., 2020).

7. Assess character of patient's pain and rate acuity on a pain scale of 0 to 10.

Provides baseline to determine patient's response to therapy and comfort needs.

Clinical Judgment *Some patients experiencing pain need pain medication before application of support surface of choice or transfer to another bed (WOCN, 2016; EPUAP, 2019).*

8. Assess patient's knowledge, prior experience with support surfaces, and feelings about procedure.

Reveals need for patient instruction and/or support.

PLANNING

1. Expected outcomes following completion of procedure:
   - Patient's skin is without new areas of erythema or mottling.

   Mottling represents hypoxia, which is an abnormal physiological response in tissues under pressure.

   - Existing PI shows signs of healing.

   Skin remains free of new PIs. Support surface does not interfere with circulation to dependent areas.

   - Patient expresses improved level of comfort with reduced acuity.

   Equalized pressures have eliminated localized areas of discomfort.

2. Provide privacy and explain purpose of mattress and method of application to patient and family caregiver.

Protects patient's privacy, reduces anxiety, and promotes cooperation.

3. Organize and set up any specific equipment for support surface.

Ensures more efficiency when transferring patient from hospital bed to support surface bed/mattress.

4. Arrange for extra personnel to help as necessary.

Some patients are unable to assume positioning or transfer independently for procedure. Assistance from other caregivers reduces risk for friction and shear in transfer to new surface.

STEP	RATIONALE

IMPLEMENTATION

1. Perform hand hygiene. Apply clean gloves (if linens are soiled or wet). Transfer patient to a chair or stretcher, depending on mobility and type of device being applied.

Prevents transmission of microorganisms.

2. Apply support surface to bed or prepare alternative bed (bed may be occupied or unoccupied). Keep sharp objects away from air mattress or air-surface bed.

   a. Replacing mattress:

      (1) Apply mattress to bedframe after removing standard hospital mattress.

The mattress will be stored by supply or housekeeping personnel. In some instances, mattress replacements are standard procedure.

      (2) Apply one sheet over mattress. Keep linens between surfaces to a minimum.

Sheet reduces soiling. Multiple layers decrease surface effectiveness of the pressure-relieving mattress (Mackey & Watts, 2022).

   b. Preparing an air mattress/overlay:

      (1) Apply deflated mattress flat over surface of bed mattress. (There may be directions on pad indicating which side to place up.)

Provides smooth, even surface.

      (2) Bring any plastic strips or flaps around corners of bed mattress.

Secures air mattress in place.

      (3) Attach connector on air mattress to inflation device. Inflate mattress to proper air pressure using a manual air pump or electric blower.

Mattresses vary as to requiring one-time or continuous inflation cycle. Check inflation daily. Manufacturer's directions indicate desired air pressure designed to distribute patient's body weight evenly. Directions are included with each mattress.

      (4) Place one sheet over air mattress, being sure to eliminate all wrinkles.

Prevents soiling of mattress; reduces direct contact of skin with plastic surface. Wrinkles can cause pressure.

Clinical Judgment *Avoid placing excessive linens and incontinence pads on top of support surface. This can interfere with functioning of support surface (Nix & Milne, 2024; Mackey & Watts, 2022).*

      (5) Check air pumps to be sure that pressure cycle alternates.

Alternating airflow mattress produces intermittent cycling, inflating only parts of mattress at any one time. Intermittent cycle continually alternates pressure against skin and soft tissue.

   c. Install an air-surface bed:

      (1) Obtain and place linen on bed.

In some instances, an air-surface bed is available in patient rooms. If not, an ordering system exists to obtain the specialty bed and specific linen as needed (see agency policy).

      (2) Place switch in "prevention" mode.

In "prevention" mode, surface pressures change automatically with patient position to equalize pressure and eliminate points of pressure.

Clinical Judgment *Most pressure-relieving beds in the hospital and home care setting are equipped with a cardiopulmonary resuscitation (CPR) switch to instantly lower head section from an elevated position and deflate the mattress to provide a firm surface for chest compressions (see Fig. 13.5).*

3. Use available personnel and help patient transfer into bed.

Safe transfer reduces risk of shear or friction to skin when placed on new support surface (Edsberg, 2022).

4. Position patient comfortably as desired over support surface. Reposition routinely.

Location of existing PI might influence type of positioning (Edsberg, 2022; Mackey & Watts, 2022).

5. Remove and dispose of gloves and perform hand hygiene.

Reduces transmission of microorganisms.

6. Raise side rails (as appropriate) and lower bed to lowest position, locking into position.

Ensures patient safety and prevents falls.

7. Place nurse call system in an accessible location within patient's reach.

Ensures patient can call for assistance if needed.

8. Perform hand hygiene.

Reduces transmission of microorganisms.

EVALUATION

1. Reassess patient's risk for PI formation at routine intervals; follow agency policy.

Documents change in status, which is critical for evaluating continued need for therapeutic surface.

STEP	RATIONALE
2. Assess "bottoming out" of support surface. Observe for at least 2.5 cm (1 inch) of space between the support surface and the patient's skin surface. Less than 2.5 cm (1 inch) indicates bottoming out (Mackey & Watts, 2022).	Bottoming out means there is inadequate support for the patient's weight and the body may sink so deeply into the surface that the bony prominences are resting on the underlying bedframe or chair. When this occurs, the support surface is ineffective and a change in support surface is necessary (Mackey & Watts, 2022).

Clinical Judgment *The prior method of assessing for "bottoming out" by placing your hand between the patient and the support surface is a subjective method. This was the hand-check method and is no longer recommended (Nix & Milne, 2024; NPIAP, 2019; Mackey & Watts, 2022; NPUAP, 2015).*

STEP	RATIONALE
3. Inspect and compare condition of patient's skin according to agency policy to determine changes in skin integrity, PI status, and effectiveness of support surface.	Determines if PIs develop or if condition of existing sores changes.
4. Ask patient to describe character of pain and rate acuity on a scale of 0 to 10.	If pressure-relief mattress is effective, patient generally experiences less discomfort.
5. Evaluate functioning of support surface periodically.	Regular inspection of mechanical components of mattress ensures proper functioning (Mackey & Watts, 2022).
6. **Use Teach-Back:** "I want to be sure I explained why you are using this special bed surface. Tell me how this bed will protect your skin." Revise your instruction now or develop a plan for revised patient/family caregiver teaching if patient/family caregiver is not able to teach back correctly.	Teach-back is a technique for health care providers to ensure that they have explained medical information clearly so that patients and their families understand what is communicated to them (Agency for Healthcare Research and Quality [AHRQ], 2023).

Unexpected Outcomes / **Related Interventions**

1. Patient develops localized areas of abnormal reactive hyperemia for longer than 30 minutes, mottling, swelling, and tenderness with evidence of breakdown.
   - Modify skin-care regimen.
   - Increase frequency of skin assessment.
   - Increase types of pressure-relief interventions.
   - Check for proper inflation of support surface.
   - Revise turning schedule.
   - Consult with skin-care expert.
   - Notify health care provider.
   - Notify manufacturer's representative if surface is not functioning properly.

2. Existing PIs or areas of pressure fail to heal or increase in size or depth.
   - Modify skin-care regimen.
   - Revise turning schedule.
   - Consult with skin-care expert.
   - Notify health care provider.

3. Patient expresses discomfort while on support surface.
   - Evaluate need for analgesia or mild sedation.
   - Evaluate need to modify or change support surface.
   - Reposition patient more frequently.
   - Unless contraindicated, provide back massage. Do not massage reddened areas or bony prominences because massage to these areas causes breaks in surface capillaries and contributes to skin and tissue injury (Borchert, 2022).

Documentation

- Document type of support surface applied, extent to which patient tolerated procedure, and condition of patient's skin.
- Document your evaluation of patient and family caregiver learning.

Hand-Off Reporting

- Report evidence of new PI formation or worsening of existing PIs to nurse in charge, health care provider, or WOCN.

Special Considerations
Patient Education

- Explain patient's specific risks of immobility and PI formation to patient and family caregivers (see Chapter 38).

- Instruct in proper use of positioning and pressure-relief methods. Caution family against rubbing reddened areas of skin.
- Explain purpose and function of the pressure-redistribution support surface. Include reminder that the surface augments care and does not replace the need for turning and pressure-relief maneuvers.
- Explain precautions regarding sharp objects and fire hazards.

Pediatrics

- Various pain assessment tools have been developed specifically for use in children (see Chapter 16).
- When caring for a child who is on a support surface, pediatric evidence-based skin protection and wound care are priorities of care. Care practices include selecting products that promote skin integrity and wound healing and prevention of skin injuries

(including medical device–related pressure injuries [MDRPIs] and MARSIs) (Lund & Singh, 2022).

- Parents can support older school-age children by reinforcing why a specialty bed is needed (Hockenberry et al., 2022).

Older Adults

- Implement preventive measures because aging skin is drier, thinner, and less pressure sensitive, increasing the risk for skin breakdown (Touhy & Jett, 2022).
- Adding mattress overlays changes the bed height. Use care when transferring and teaching family caregiver to transfer a patient from bed to chair.

Populations With Disabilities

- Patients who are confused or cognitively impaired may have difficulty understanding the need for and application of

the support surface (Bobbette et al., 2020; Sullivan et al., 2018).

Home Care

- Most of the devices can be adapted for home use on a standard twin bed or hospital bed.
- Base selection on patient needs and environmental assessment. For example, a patient on total bed rest who smokes is not an ideal candidate for a foam mattress because of the potential for fire; a patient with pets that sleep in the bed is not suited for an air-filled mattress because of the risk for puncture.
- Address concerns in the home setting related to need for a backup generator or other plan to maintain the support surface during power outages.

◆ **SKILL 13.2** **Care of the Patient on a Special Bed**

Air-suspension beds support a patient's weight on air-filled cushions. There are two types of systems: low air loss and high air loss. A low-air-loss system minimizes pressure and reduces shear. In this type of system, air flow assists in managing the heat and humidity (microclimate) of the patient's skin (Mackey & Watts, 2022; WOCN, 2016). If a patient has large stage 3 or 4 pressure injuries (PIs) on multiple turning surfaces of the skin, a low-air-loss bed or air-fluidized bed may be indicated (Tomova-Simitchieva et al., 2018). If wounds are not healing, a change in support surface is indicated and should be matched to patient's needs (Mackey & Watts, 2022).

Air-fluidized, high-air-loss beds provide for selective drying and do not increase insensible fluid losses. For patients requiring high air loss under a body part (e.g., under the buttocks), you can substitute high-air-loss cushions. It is also possible to adapt the air-suspension beds to individual patient needs with specialty cushions for positioning, foot support, and lateral arm supports.

Another adaptation of the air-suspension bed is the low-air-loss bed. Low air loss provides airflow to assist in managing the heat and humidity (microclimate) of the skin. Low air loss may be used alone or in combination with alternating pressure, lateral rotation, and air-fluidized technology and may be incorporated into overlays, mattresses, bed systems, and chair cushions (Mackey & Watts, 2022).

An air-fluidized therapy bed distributes a patient's weight evenly over its support surface. In this type of system, pressure redistribution occurs by means of a fluidlike medium that is created by forcing temperature-controlled air through fine ceramic microspheres (WOCN, 2016; Nix & Milne, 2024). The bed minimizes pressure and reduces shearing force and friction through the principle of fluidization (Fig. 13.7). These beds are the most expensive support surfaces and are commonly used for patients with burns, skin flaps, and multiple stage 3 and 4 PIs (Mackey & Watts, 2022).

Air-fluidized beds are useful in the care of patients who require minimal movement to prevent skin damage by shearing force and for patients who experience significant pain when being turned or positioned (e.g., burn patients, those who have undergone extensive skin grafts or have existing pressure injuries, and victims of multiple trauma). Patients tend to perspire and lose body fluids while on the bed because the surface of the filter sheet warms. As patients perspire, moisture is quickly absorbed into the circulating microspheres. Diaphoresis often goes undetected; therefore, insensible fluid loss is not always evident until a patient develops fluid

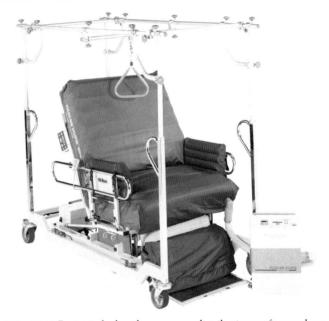

FIG. 13.7 Bariatric bed with pressure-redistribution surface and programmable continuous lateral rotation therapy. Low-air-loss mattress replacement. (*Copyright © 2023 Baxter International Inc. Reprinted with permission. All rights reserved.*)

and electrolyte imbalances. You need to monitor the patient's fluid balance status carefully.

A valuable resource in the care of a morbidly obese patient (a person who weighs more than 45.45 kg [100 lb] above ideal weight) is the bariatric bed (see Fig. 13.7). The newer bariatric beds provide pressure redistribution and have programmable continuous lateral rotation. The bariatric bed is capable of allowing upright or sitting positions, patient transport, and in-bed scale use. The full-function hand controls also allow you to change the bed position and thus facilitate care while reducing risk for staff injury when moving a patient. The bed is slightly wider than a standard hospital bed, but it is within the guidelines for standard door width, which allows movement into and out of a room without difficulty. Most bariatric beds are capable of supporting weights up to 454 kg (1000 lb).

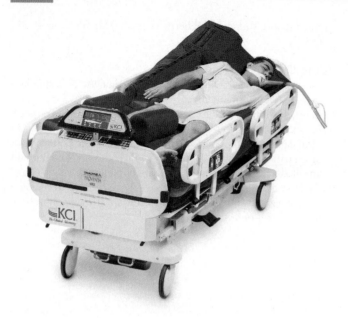

FIG. 13.8 Lateral rotation bed. (*Tria Dyne™ Therapy System. Courtesy KCI Licensing, Inc., 2013.*)

A continuous lateral rotation bed is used for the prevention and treatment of certain cardiopulmonary conditions and helps maintain skeletal alignment while providing constant rotation (Fig. 13.8). The bed rotates a patient in a continual side-to-side pattern of 40 degrees or less (Mackey & Watts, 2022). The patient is never placed in a prone position on this bed. A rotation bed does not eliminate the need for meticulous ongoing skin assessment and routine manual repositioning (Nix & Milne, 2024). It is used in the care of patients with spinal cord injuries or multiple traumas (Mackey & Watts, 2022). There is an emergency lever that can quickly interrupt rotation when needed. To initiate cardiopulmonary resuscitation (CPR), return the bed to the horizontal position and lock in place. The constant motion often leads to sensory distress for patients, especially older adults. This is associated with the constant kinetic stimulation, the limited visual field, and inner ear disequilibrium. Be aware of these complications and provide necessary emotional support.

Delegation

The skill of placing a patient on a specialty bed can be delegated to assistive personnel (AP). However, first the nurse completes the assessment, determines the need for a support surface, and selects the specific bed. Some types of support surfaces require that the manufacturer's representative set up and maintain the support system. Direct the AP to:

- Notify the nurse of any changes in the patient's skin.
- Continue to turn and reposition the patient regularly and seek help for patient position changes, as necessary. This is not always necessary for patients who are on beds that have continuous lateral rotation.
- Monitor the normal functioning of the air-suspension bed such as inflation and deflation cycles and report to the nurse any changes in these cycles.
- Notify the nurse if the patient becomes disoriented or restless or complains of nausea.

Interprofessional Collaboration

- The health care provider, WOCN, physical therapist, and manufacturer's representative from the specialty bed provider are involved in patient care to ensure that the bed is set up correctly and that the patient receives correct pressure redistribution.

Equipment

- Disposable bed pads, if indicated
- Clean gloves (optional)
- Foam positioning wedges if indicated
- Special sheet (if appropriate, supplied by manufacturer)
- Mechanical lift (if indicated)

STEP	RATIONALE
ASSESSMENT	
1. Identify patient using at least two identifiers (e.g., name and birthday or name and medical record number) according to agency policy.	Ensures correct patient. Complies with The Joint Commission standards and improves patient safety (TJC, 2023).
2. Review patient's electronic health record (EHR) for health care provider's order.	Health care provider's order is usually required to ensure third-party payment of support surface.
3. Review patient's serum electrolyte levels if available.	Movement of air through mattress causes water loss through the skin and increases patient's risk for dehydration (Mackey & Watts, 2022).
4. Assess patient's/family caregiver's health literacy.	Determines degree to which individuals have the ability to find, understand, and use information and services to make informed health-related decisions and actions for themselves and others (CDC, 2023).
5. Determine if patient needs frequent weights.	Scales are available in some air-suspension beds and as underbed units for patients who need to be weighed frequently or those who cannot be moved for weighing.
6. Perform hand hygiene. Apply clean gloves. Determine patient's risk for PI formation using a valid assessment tool (e.g., Braden Scale) and assess for risk factors for pressure injuries (e.g., nutritional deficits, shear stress, friction, alterations in mobility and sensory perception, moisture, and abnormal serum albumin and hemoglobin levels) (see Chapter 39).	Reduces transmission of microorganisms. Risk assessment tools provide an objective measure of risk that is consistent over time (WOCN, 2016).

STEP	RATIONALE
7. Inspect condition of skin, especially over dependent sites and bony prominences and areas exposed to medical adhesives (e.g., IV sites, nasogastric tubes), which increases risk for medical adhesive–related skin injury (MARSI). Note appearance of existing PI and determine stage of injury (see Chapter 39). Remove and dispose of gloves. Perform hand hygiene.	Provides baseline to determine patient's response to therapy and comfort needs. Reduces transmission of microorganisms. MARSI increases patient's risk for progression to pressure injuries (Fumarola et al., 2020).

Clinical Judgment *Patients with unstable conditions do not always tolerate turning or positioning required for thorough assessment or the application of a support surface mattress.*

STEP	RATIONALE
8. Assess character of patient's pain and rate acuity on a pain scale of 0 to 10.	Provides baseline to determine patient's response to therapy and comfort needs.

Clinical Judgment *Some patients experiencing pain need pain medication before transfer to support surface or another bed (WOCN, 2016; NPUAP, 2019).*

STEP	RATIONALE
9. Assess risk of complications from air-fluidized beds.	
a. Dehydration	Patients may become dehydrated with use of this bed because of insensible fluid loss.
b. Aspiration	Inability to elevate head of bed is limited to placing foam wedges under patient's head and shoulders.
c. Difficulty with patient positioning	Repositioning is limited to use of foam wedges.
d. Level of orientation	Patients may be at risk for developing delirium from dehydration and floating sensation with air-fluidized bed.
10. Assess patient's knowledge, prior experience with support surfaces, and feelings about procedure.	Reveals need for patient instruction and/or support.

PLANNING

STEP	RATIONALE
1. Expected outcomes following completion of procedure:	
• Patient's skin is without erythema or mottling.	Mottling represents hypoxia, which is an abnormal physiological response in tissues under pressure.
• Existing PI shows signs of healing.	Skin remains free of new PIs. Support surface or specialty bed does not interfere with circulation to dependent areas.
• Patient expresses improved level of comfort with reduced pain acuity.	Equalized pressures have eliminated localized areas of discomfort.
2. Provide privacy and explain purpose of bed and method of application to patient and family caregiver.	Protects patient's privacy, reduces anxiety, and promotes cooperation.
3. Organize and set up any specific equipment for bed.	Ensures more efficiency when completing procedure.
4. Review instructions provided by manufacturer.	Promotes safe and correct use of bed.
5. Obtain additional personnel needed to transfer patient to bed.	Ensures safety by having sufficient personnel for transfer. Assistance from other caregivers reduces risk for friction and shear in transfer to new surface.
6. For patients with moderate to severe pain, premedicate approximately 30 minutes before transfer to bed.	Promotes patient's comfort and ability to cooperate during transfer to bed. Decreases patient's energy expenditure.

IMPLEMENTATION

STEP	RATIONALE
1. Perform hand hygiene. Apply clean gloves (if linens are soiled or wet).	Prevents transmission of microorganisms.
2. Transfer patient to bed using appropriate transfer techniques (see Chapter 11). Bed surface is sometimes slippery; therefore do not attempt transfers without help.	Appropriate safe patient-handling techniques maintain alignment and reduce risk of injury during procedure. Manufacturer's representative adjusts bed to patient's height and weight.
3. Once patient has been transferred, turn bed on by depressing switch; regulate temperature.	Turning on bed allows pressure cushions to adjust automatically to preset levels to minimize pressure, friction, and shear.
4. Position patient and perform range-of-motion exercises as appropriate.	Promotes comfort and reduces contracture formation.
5. To turn patient, position bedpans, or perform other therapies, turn on appropriate bed setting. Once you have completed the procedure, return bed to previous setting.	The appropriate bed settings create a firm bed surface, which facilitates turning and positioning the patient or performing procedures such as urinary catheterization. **NOTE:** Patient does not receive pressure relief while bed is in this mode.
6. Use special features of bed as needed.	
a. Scales	Facilitates ability to obtain routine weights.
b. Portable transport units to maintain inflation when primary power is interrupted	Provides for continuous pressure reduction.

STEP	RATIONALE
c. Specialty cushions or wedges for positioning, providing pressure relief, reducing moisture, preventing patient from sliding down in bed, or relieving weight from orthopedic devices	Reduces pressure, friction, and shearing forces.
d. Lateral rotation, which allows approximately 40 degrees or less of turning (Mackey & Watts, 2022)	Reduces pressure and assists in control of pulmonary secretions.

Clinical Judgment *Never place a patient in prone position on an air-fluidized bed or on a continuous lateral rotation bed because of the chance of suffocation.*

Clinical Judgment *Verify settings, following all nursing procedures. Underinflation or improper functioning of certain air mattresses, low air loss bed, or air-fluidized bed may result in tissue damage. Overinflation can result in too firm a surface and create pressure damage.*

STEP	RATIONALE
7. Remove and dispose of gloves and perform hand hygiene.	Reduces transmission of microorganisms.
8. Help patient to a comfortable position.	Restores comfort and sense of well-being.
9. Raise side rails (as appropriate) and lower bed to lowest position, locking into position.	Ensures patient safety and prevents falls.
10. Place nurse call system is in an accessible location within patient's reach.	Ensures patient can call for assistance if needed.
11. Perform hand hygiene.	Reduces transmission of microorganisms.

EVALUATION

1. Reassess patient's risk for PI formation at routine intervals.	Documents change in status, which is critical for evaluating continued need for therapeutic bed.
2. Assess "bottoming out" of pressure-relief mattress or seat cushion. Observe for at least 2.5 cm (1 inch) of space between the support surface and the patient's skin surface. Less than 2.5 cm (1 inch) indicates bottoming out (Mackey & Watts, 2022).	Bottoming out means there is insufficient support and the patient's bony prominences are resting on the underlying bedframe or chair. When this occurs, there must be a change in support surface (Mackey & Watts, 2022).

Clinical Judgment *The prior method of assessing for "bottoming out" by placing your hand between the patient and the support surface is a subjective method. This was the hand-check method and is no longer recommended (Nix & Milne, 2024; NPIAP, 2019; Mackey & Watts, 2022; NPUAP, 2015).*

3. Inspect and compare condition of patient's skin every 8 hours or according to agency policy to determine changes in skin integrity, PI status, and effectiveness of support surface.	Determines if PIs develop or if condition of existing injuries changes.
4. Ask patient to describe pain and rate any discomfort on a scale of 0 to 10.	If specialty bed surface is effective, patient generally experiences less discomfort.
5. Review fluid and electrolyte status.	Fluidized and air-loss beds can cause fluid and electrolyte disturbances in some patients, especially in patients with fever and those with hemodynamic instability.
6. Evaluate functioning of support surface periodically.	Regular inspection of mechanical components of support surface/mattress ensures proper functioning.
7. **Use Teach-Back:** "I want to be sure I explained the purpose of this bed and why it turns side to side. Tell me why we placed you on this type of bed and how you might feel." Revise your instruction now or develop a plan for revised patient/family caregiver teaching if patient/family caregiver is not able to teach back correctly.	Teach-back is a technique for health care providers to ensure that they have explained medical information clearly so that patients and their families understand what is communicated to them (AHRQ, 2023).

Unexpected Outcomes	Related Interventions
1. Existing areas of skin breakdown or PIs fail to heal, or they increase in size and depth.	• Modify skin-care regimen. • Increase frequency of skin assessment. • Change types of pressure-relief interventions. • Check for proper function of bed • Revise turning schedule. • Consult with skin-care expert. • Notify health care provider. • Notify bed supplier if bed malfunctions.
2. Patient becomes nauseated.	• Provide short-term antiemetic such as prochlorperazine. If using lateral rotation, obtain antiemetic order around the clock. • If using lateral rotation, decrease cycle frequency. • Notify health care provider.

Documentation

- Document transfer of patient to bed, amount of help needed for transfer, tolerance of procedure, and condition of skin.
- Document your evaluation of patient and family caregiver learning.

Hand-Off Reporting

- Report changes in condition of skin, level of orientation, nausea, and electrolyte levels to health care provider.

Special Considerations

Patient Education

- Explain function and purpose of specialty bed.
- Explain the need to continue to change position at intervals to diminish the effects of immobility.
- Explain the need for adequate fluid intake because bed surface sometimes causes dehydration.

Pediatrics

- The air-suspension bed is used commonly with older children and for children with significant burns. Make sure that instructions are age appropriate and include any restrictions such as raising the head of the bed.
- Parents need to know that the child may have some dizziness and/or nausea when first placed on the air-fluidized or other specialty bed. This is because of the flotation sensation and will disappear as the child becomes adjusted to the bed.

Older Adults

- Some hospitalized older adults experience misperceptions of their environment that are intensified by the constant flotation of these types of beds. The specialty bed in combination with medications can increase the older adult's risk for confusion and agitation (Richbourg, 2022; Touhy & Jett, 2022).

Populations With Disabilities

- Patients with intellectual disabilities or who are confused may have difficulty adjusting to specialty beds, especially those beds that give the patient a sensation of movement and/or increase noise in the environment (Bobbette et al., 2020: Sullivan et al., 2018). Observe these patients for increased confusion, which may result in the need to review other specialty bed options.

Home Care

- The air-fluidized bed weighs between 772 and 954 kg (1700 and 2100 lb); therefore the company leasing the bed needs to inspect the home for accessibility and structural support.
- Consult with social worker or case manager to determine third-party reimbursement. Thorough documentation of skin condition is essential in obtaining reimbursement.
- A version of the air-fluidized bed is available for home use for renting or purchase; the bed rental company is responsible for proper cleaning.
- Instruct family caregiver in importance of maintaining patient hydration and skin care.
- Instruct family caregiver regarding steps to take in the event of a power failure. This may include purchasing a backup generator for the home.

✦ CLINICAL JUDGMENT AND NEXT-GENERATION NCLEX® EXAMINATION–STYLE QUESTIONS

1. The nurse is caring for a 48-year-old patient who was involved in a motor vehicle accident that resulted in quadriplegia (causing loss of sensation and movement below the neck). The patient is on an air-suspension bed with lateral rotation due to blistering over bony prominences. The AP contacts the nurse to report skin changes over the patient's buttocks and left hip.

   Select whether the following potential nursing actions are indicated or not indicated for the patient at this time.

Nursing Action	Indicated	Not Indicated
Perform a full skin assessment		
Modify existing repositioning schedule		
Verify that the bed is working properly		
Request a consultation with a WOCN specialist		
Avoid cleansing the skin around the injury to minimize tissue trauma		

2. During a full assessment, the nurse gathers the data listed below. Which of the following findings alert the nurse that the patient may need a pressure-reduction support surface? **Select all that apply**.
   1. Braden Scale score of 12
   2. Blood pressure 96/68 mm Hg
   3. Healed pressure injury from 12 months ago
   4. Anemia
   5. Urine and bowel incontinence

3. The patient has been provided with a support surface. Which of the following activities can the nurse delegate to the AP for the care of the patient at this time? **Select all that apply.**
   1. Assessing redness over a bony prominence
   2. Regular turning and repositioning
   3. Selecting a wheelchair support surface
   4. Determining support surface function
   5. Reporting changes in patient orientation or behavior

4. The patient has been changed to an air-fluidized bed. The nurse anticipates potential problems with the bed and assesses for which of the following issues? **Select all that apply.**
   1. Back pain from lack of firm support
   2. Dehydration from the amount of warm circulating air
   3. Problems moving the patient out of bed because of body submersion
   4. Ability to successfully manage ongoing episodes of incontinence
   5. Difficulty moving the bed to another location because of its weight

5. The nurse is performing a final assessment before the patient is transferred to a long-term care agency. Which assessment finding demonstrates that nursing care to reduce skin injury has been effective?
   1. Redness on buttocks and left hip
   2. Reduction in Braden Scale score
   3. Blood pressure 110/78 mm Hg
   4. Respirations 18 breaths/min

Visit the Evolve site for Answers to Clinical Judgment and Next-Generation NCLEX® Examination–Style Questions.

REFERENCES

Agency for Healthcare Research and Quality (AHRQ): *Teach-Back: intervention,* 2023. https://www.ahrq.gov/patient-safety/reports/engage/interventions/teachback.html.

Bambi AA, et al: Reducing the incidence and prevalence of pressure injury in adult ICU patients with support surfaces use: a systematic review, *Adv Skin Wound Care* 35(5):263, 2022.

Black J, Kalowes P: Medical device-related pressure ulcers, *Chronic Wound Care Manag Res* 3:9, 2016.

Bobbette N, et al: Adults with intellectual and developmental disabilities and interprofessional, team-based primary health care: a scoping review, *JBI Evid Synth* 18(7):1470, 2020.

Borchert K: Pressure injury prevention: Implementing and maintaining a successful plan and program. In McNichol LL, et al., editors: *WOCN core curriculum wound management,* ed 2, Philadelphia, 2022, Wolters Kluwer.

Centers for Disease Control and Prevention (CDC): *What is health literacy?* 2023. https://www.cdc.gov/healthliteracy/learn/index.html.

Cox J, et al: Pressure injuries in critical care patients in US Hospitals, *J Wound Ostomy Continence Nurs* 49(1); 21, 2022.

Edsberg L: Pressure and shear injuries. In McNichol LL, et al., editors: *WOCN core curriculum wound management,* ed 2, Philadelphia, 2022, Wolters Kluwer.

European Pressure Ulcer Advisory Panel, National Pressure Injury Advisory Panel, and Pan Pacific Pressure Injury Alliance (EPUAP/NPIAP/PPPIA): *Treatment of pressure ulcers/injuries: quick reference guide,* Emily Haesler (ED), 2019, EPUAP/NPIAP/PPPIA.

Fumarola S, et al: Overlooked and underestimated: medical adhesive-related skin injuries. Best practice consensus document on prevention, *J Wound Care* 29(Suppl 3c):S1–S24, 2020.

Haesler E: Evidence summary: pressure injuries: preventing medical device related pressure injuries, *Wound Pract Res* 25(4):214, 2017.

Haesler E: Evidence summary: Pressure injuries: active support surfaces for prevention and treating pressure injuries, *Wound Pract Res* 26(1):50, 2018.

Hockenberry MJ, et al: *Wong's essentials of pediatric nursing,* ed 11, St. Louis, 2022, Elsevier.

Lund C, Singh C: Skin and wound care for neonatal and pediatric populations, In McNichol LL, et al., editors: *WOCN core curriculum wound management,* ed 2, Philadelphia, 2022, Wolters Kluwer.

Mackey D, Watts C: Therapeutic surfaces for bed and chair. In McNichol LL, et al., editors: *WOCN core curriculum wound management,* ed 2, Philadelphia, 2022, Wolters Kluwer.

McInnes E, et al: Support surfaces for treating pressure ulcers, *Cochrane Database Syst Rev* 10(10):CD009490, 2018. https://www.cochrane.org/CD009490/WOUNDS_support-surfaces-treating-pressure-ulcers. Accessed November 5, 2023.

McNichol LL, Ratliff C, Yates S: *Wound, Ostomy, and Continence Nurses Society core curriculum: wound management,* ed 2, Philadelphia, 2022, Wolters Kluwer.

McNichol L, et al: Choosing a support surface for pressure injury prevention and treatment, *Nursing* 50(2):41–44, 2020.

McNichol L, et al: Identifying the right surface for the right patient at the right time: generation and content validation of an algorithm for support surface selection, *J Wound Ostomy Continence Nurs* 42(1):19, 2015.

National Pressure Injury Advisory Panel (NPIAP): *Hand-check method: Is it an effective method to monitor for bottoming out? National Pressure Ulcer Advisory Position Statement,* 2015. https://cdn.ymaws.com/npuap.site-ym.com/resource/resmgr/position_statements/hand-check-position-statemen.pdf. Accessed November 5, 2023.

National Pressure Injury Advisory Panel (NPIAP): *Clinical practice guideline—2019,* Westport, MA, 2019, The Association.

National Pressure Injury Advisory Panel (NPIAP): *Support surface standards initiative (S31): Terms and definitions related to support surface,* n.d. https://npiap.com/page/S3I?&hhsearchterms=%22support+and+surfaces%22. Accessed March 2023.

National Pressure Ulcer Advisory Panel (NPUAP) Support Surfaces Standard Initiative: *Pressure ulcer treatment recommendations: clinical practice guidelines,* Washington, DC, 2019, National Pressure Ulcer Advisory Panel.

Nix DP, Milne CT: Pressure redistribution support surfaces. In Bryant RA, Nix DP, editors: *Acute & chronic wounds: intraprofessionals from novice to expert,* ed 6, St. Louis, 2024, Elsevier.

Padula CA, et al: Prevention of medical device-related pressure injuries associated with respiratory equipment use in a critical care unit, *J Wound Ostomy Continence Nurs* 44(2):138, 2017.

Rae KE, et al: Support surfaces for the treatment and prevention of pressure ulcers: a systematic literature review, *J Wound Care* 27(8):467, 2018.

Richbourg L: Skin and wound care for the geriatric population. In McNichol LL, Ratliff CR, editors: *WOCN core curriculum wound management,* ed 2, Philadelphia, 2022, Wolters Kluwer.

Serraes B, et al: Prevention of pressure ulcers with a static air support surface: systemic review, *Int Wound J* 15(3):333, 2018.

Shelhamer MC, et al: Prone positioning in moderate to severe acute respiratory distress syndrome due to COVID-19: a cohort study and analysis of physiology, *J Intensive Care Med* 36(2):241, 2021.

Sullivan WF, et al: Primary care of adults with intellectual and developmental disabilities: 2018 Canadian consensus guidelines, *Can Fam Physician* 64:254, 2018.

The Joint Commission (TJC): *2023 National patient safety goals,* Oakbrook Terrace, IL, 2023, The Joint Commission. https://www.jointcommission.org/standards/national-patient-safety-goals/.

Tomova-Simitchieva T, et al: Comparing the effects of 3 different pressure ulcer prevention support surfaces on the structure and function of heel and sacral skin: an exploratory cross-over trial, *Int Wound J* 15(3):429, 2018.

Touhy T, Jett K: *Ebersole and Hess' Gerontological nursing & healthy aging,* ed 6, St. Louis, 2022, Mosby.

Wiggerman N, et al: Proning patients with COVID-19: a review of equipment and methods, *Hum Factors* 62(7):1069, 2020.

Wound, Ostomy, and Continence Nurses Society (WOCN): *Guideline for prevention and management of pressure ulcers (injuries): WOCN clinical practice guideline series,* ed 2, Mt. Laurel, NJ, 2016, Author.

UNIT 5

Activity and Mobility: Next-Generation NCLEX® (NGN)–Style Unfolding Case Study

PHASE 1

QUESTION 1.

A client has been brought to the emergency room for evaluation by their spouse. The triage nurse conducts an initial assessment.

Highlight the findings that require **immediate** follow-up by the nurse.

History and Physical	Nurses' Notes	Vital Signs	Laboratory Results

1341: 50-year-old client brought to the emergency department by spouse, who reports client has experienced progressive weakness over the past few days. History positive for multiple sclerosis. Over the past few months, client has experienced an increase in peripheral neuropathy and has been sitting in a wheelchair more often. Client appears sleepy yet is able to be awakened upon command; lung sounds clear; S_1S_2 present without murmur; bowel sounds present × 4 quadrants; strength weak yet equal in all extremities. 5-cm (2-inch) reddened and nonblanchable area on sacrum; no breakdown noted. Vital signs: T 39.0°C (102.2°F); HR 62 beats/min; RR 12 breaths/min; BP 110/70 mm Hg; SpO_2 98% on RA.

QUESTION 2.

The client is taken by wheelchair into an examination room in the emergency department.

Complete the following sentence by selecting from the lists of options below.

The nurse anticipates that the client is at high risk for **1 [Select]** due to **2 [Select]**.

Options for 1	Options for 2
Muscle weakness	Respiratory rate 12 breaths/min
Falls	Reddened area on sacrum
Pressure injury	Peripheral neuropathy
Respiratory distress	Increased time in wheelchair

PHASE 2

QUESTION 3.

Because of the client's weakness and neuropathy, the client is at risk for injury due to falls.

Complete the following sentence by selecting from the lists of options below.

The nurse will obtain a **1 [Select]** and **2 [Select]** to increase client safety.

Options for 1	Options for 2
Cervical collar	Gait belt
Lumbar brace support	Drug allergy arm band
Fall risk arm band	Splints for the feet

QUESTION 4.

The health care provider examined the client and diagnosed the client with an exacerbation of multiple sclerosis and a urinary tract infection. The client is admitted to a medical unit for monitoring and antibiotic therapy. The nurse on the medical unit is planning care for the client.

Determine whether the following potential nursing actions are indicated or not indicated for the plan of care.

Potential Nursing Action	Indicated	Not Indicated
Delegate teaching of range-of-motion (ROM) exercises to assistive personnel (AP).		
Monitor oxygen saturation during any activity.		
Perform an assessment using the Braden Scale.		
Obtain foam overlay for bed.		
Massage nonblanchable area on sacrum.		

PHASE 3

QUESTION 5.

The client has been sitting in a wheelchair for 45 minutes. Which of the following actions would the nurse take when transferring the client back to bed? **Select all that apply**.

- ○ Perform hand hygiene.
- ○ Use a gait belt during the transfer process.
- ○ Assess range of motion before transferring.
- ○ Determine client's level of consciousness before moving.
- ○ Instruct client to avoid using wheelchair armrests to rise.
- ○ Move client as quickly as possible to bed after standing from chair.
- ○ Adjust bed height 5 cm (2 inches) below the wheelchair seat height prior to transfer.

QUESTION 6.

The nurse has transferred the client from the wheelchair to the bed.

For each body system, select the client assessment findings that would indicate a successful outcome of the transfer. Each body system may support more than 1 client assessment finding that would indicate a successful outcome of the transfer.

Body System	Client Assessment Findings
Cardiovascular	○ Blood pressure 80/50 mm Hg ○ Pulse 74 beats/min ○ Heart regular rate and rhythm
Respiratory	○ Oxygen saturation 96% on RA ○ Respiratory rate 24 breaths/min ○ Lungs clear bilaterally
General	○ Reports feeling weak ○ States, "I am dizzy" ○ Temperature 37.1°C (98.8°F)

UNIT 6
Safety and Comfort

Patient safety and comfort are two important basic human needs. Managing a patient's health care environment, reducing risks for patient injury, and knowing how to respond in hazardous emergency situations require good clinical judgment and decision making. Critical thinking applied during patient assessment identifies patient safety risks such as falls so that you can identify problems accurately and take appropriate precautions based on your scientific knowledge and evidence-based safety standards. For example, assessment of a patient's risk factors compared with the common risk factors associated with falls offers direction for specific steps to take to prevent the patient from falling. If you assess that a patient has visual problems and an unsteady gait, you apply knowledge of the types of interventions that best match the patient's risks. You assist with suggesting ways to modify the patient's home environment. Having night lights in bathrooms and marking edges of stairs in bright yellow are appropriate for patients with visual alterations. Use of handrails on stairs and elimination of throw rugs are interventions suited to patients with gait problems. Safety procedures must be patient centered to be effective.

Comfort is one of the most common patient needs that nurses manage. When you care for a patient experiencing pain or other uncomfortable symptoms, direct the patient's assessment based on knowledge of the physiology of pain and the patient's condition, the mechanisms by which pain therapies relieve pain, and the patient's unique presentation of the pain experience. Your own experience in assisting patients with pain management is also valuable in making clinical judgments for subsequent patients. A patient-centered approach to assessment allows patients to make decisions about methods for pain relief and thus assists you in selecting appropriate nonpharmacological versus pharmacological comfort measures. Critical thinking applied to pain management requires anticipation of symptoms and physical changes patients may experience based on their clinical conditions. For example, when a patient has pain related to an arthritic knee, pharmacological measures for pain relief in addition to safe support for ambulation are required. If the patient's pain is from a surgical incision, pharmacological measures and physical support of the incision to minimize stress are necessary.

Procedures such as patient-controlled analgesia (PCA), epidural analgesia, and local anesthesia pumps pose special risks and therefore require your critical thinking to ensure patient safety. Because PCA is self-managed by a patient, you know that a priority is providing the patient the information necessary to ensure safe medication administration. Critical thinking applies assessment data about a patient's ability and readiness to manipulate the PCA device to judge the appropriateness of the therapy for the patient. Epidural analgesia is an invasive procedure; therefore a part of skill competency is implementing strict infection control principles to reduce patient risk.

Therapeutic nurse-patient relationships are important with regard to effectively delivering any skill. Such relationships are crucial when supporting patients in need of end-of-life or palliative care. Good clinical judgments are based on understanding the patient and family as a unit. A thorough assessment of the impact of a terminal or long-term chronic condition on the patient's emotional, social, and physical well-being and the application of knowledge about the grief response allow you to choose appropriate palliative support measures.

14 | Patient Safety

SKILLS AND PROCEDURES

Skill 14.1 **Fall Prevention in Health Care Settings, p. 384**

Skill 14.2 **Designing a Restraint-Free Environment, p. 394**

Skill 14.3 **Applying Physical Restraints, p. 398**

Procedural Guideline 14.1 **Fire, Electrical, and Chemical Safety, p. 405**

Skill 14.4 **Seizure Precautions, p. 408**

OBJECTIVES

Mastery of content in this chapter will enable you to:

- Identify the features of a culture of safety.
- Discuss the importance of national standards for patient safety.
- Discuss current evidence regarding fall prevention.
- Describe the components of a nursing assessment focused on patient safety.
- Examine how clinical judgment is involved in identifying nursing interventions specific for reducing patients' risks for falls.

- Explain the rationale for approaches used to create a restraint-free environment.
- Identify nursing interventions taken in the event of a fire, electrical shock, or chemical spill.
- Discuss precautions used to prevent injury in patients who are restrained.
- Identify nursing interventions for a patient who experiences generalized seizures.
- Evaluate the efficacy of safety interventions.

MEDIA RESOURCES

- http://evolve.elsevier.com/Perry/skills
- Clinical Review Questions
- Audio Glossary
- ▶ Video Clips

- **NSO** Nursing Skills Online
- Answers to Clinical Judgment and Next-Generation NCLEX® Examination–Style Questions
- Skills Performance Checklists
- Printable Key Points

PURPOSE

Reducing the risk of harm associated with the delivery of health care is a national health care policy priority. Making patients safe is a responsibility of every professional nurse. The World Health Organization (WHO) offers a simple definition of patient safety: a health care discipline that aims to prevent and reduce risks, errors, and harm that occur to patients during provision of health care (WHO, 2023). Patient safety requires effective communication, teamwork, critical thinking, and timely clinical decisions. As part of the health care team, you will engage in all activities that support a patient-centered safety culture. Key features of a culture of safety are the determination to achieve consistently safe operations in health care agencies, blame-free environments in which individuals are free to report errors or near misses without fear of reprimand or punishment, collaboration across ranks and disciplines to seek solutions to patient safety problems, and organizational commitment of resources to address safety concerns (Agency for Healthcare Research and Quality [AHRQ], 2019a). You are accountable as a member of a health care team to support a culture of safety.

Patient safety requires the recognition that each patient is the source of control and full partner in providing compassionate and coordinated care based on respect for each patient's preferences, values, and needs (QSEN, 2020). The QSEN safety competency is stated as "Minimizes risk of harm to patients and providers through both system effectiveness and individual performance." The QSEN skills for safety competency include the following:

- Demonstrate effective use of technology and standardized practices that support quality and safety.
- Demonstrate effective use of strategies to reduce risk of harm to self or others.
- Use appropriate strategies to reduce reliance on memory.
- Communicate observations or concerns related to hazards and errors to patients, families, and the health care team.
- Use organizational error reporting systems for near miss and error reporting.
- Participate appropriately in analyzing errors and designing improvements.
- Use national patient safety resources for professional development and to focus attention on safety in care settings.

Patient safety is not optional. You will apply clinical judgment when following the principles of safety relevant to all nursing activities. Following national safety standards in practice improves the likelihood you will achieve favorable patient outcomes.

PRACTICE STANDARDS

- Centers for Medicare and Medicaid Services (CMS), 2020: Survey Protocol, Regulations, and Interpretive Guidelines for Hospitals—Standards for use of physical restraints
- Health Research and Educational Trust (HRET), 2016: Preventing Patient Falls—Fall risk factor assessment and solutions
- The Joint Commission (TJC), 2023: National Patient Safety Goals—Patient identification
- Quality and Safety Education for Nurses (QSEN) Institute, 2020: QSEN Competencies—Patient-centered care, patient safety, and quality improvement

SUPPLEMENTAL STANDARDS

- Stevens JA, Burns ER, 2015: A CDC Compendium of Effective Fall Interventions: What Works for Community-Dwelling Older Adults
- Rogers S, et al., 2021: CDC STEADI: Best Practices for Developing an Inpatient Program to Prevent Older Adult Falls After Discharge
- Centers for Disease Control and Prevention (CDC), 2021: STEADI—Older Adult Fall Prevention

PRINCIPLES FOR PRACTICE

- The integration of evidence-based practice (EBP) into nursing skills and procedures promotes a safer health care environment and improves patient outcomes.
- You are responsible for applying clinical judgment and critical thinking skills when using the nursing process; assessing each patient for inherent safety risks, any environmental hazards that threaten safety, and potential risks associated with procedures; and planning and intervening appropriately to maintain a safe environment.
- The Joint Commission's Speak Up campaign was developed to help patients and their advocates become active in their care (TJC, 2019). Encourage patients and family caregivers to report any questionable safety events to you as soon as possible.
- It is essential that health care providers share information about any patient injury, learn from errors, and participate in the trending and evaluation of those errors.

PERSON-CENTERED CARE

- Person-centered care is defined by the International Council of Nurses (ICN) as "valuing and respecting the characteristics, attributes, and preferences of the patient, such as cultural and religious beliefs, and incorporating them into the planning and implementation of nursing care, services or programs design" (ICN, 2021).
- Partnering with patients and their caregivers in the care process through sharing information, inviting their opinion, and collaborating with them facilitates patient-centered care and communication (Kwame & Petrucka, 2021).
- Patients and family caregivers should be treated with dignity and respect, be active partners in all aspects of their care, contribute to the development and improvement of health care facilities and systems, and be partners in research and the education of health care professionals (Institute for Patient- and Family-Centered Care [IPFCC], 2022). Begin by learning about a patient's background and expressing concern for the patient's physical and emotional health.
- Research has shown that areas in which patient-centered hospital care can be improved include improving responsiveness to patient needs, the discharge experience, and patient-clinician interactions. To improve responsiveness, use proactive nursing rounds; for the discharge experience, participate in interprofessional rounds and postdischarge calls; and to improve clinician-patient interactions, be accountable for specific desired behaviors set according to hospital standards (Aboumatar et al., 2015).
- Being hospitalized or living in an assisted-living facility places patients at risk for injury in an unfamiliar and confusing environment. Normal life cues such as a bed without side rails and the direction one usually takes to the bathroom are absent. Thought processes and coping mechanisms are affected by physical and psychological illness and the accompanying emotions. Therefore patients are more vulnerable to injury.
- For patients of diverse cultural backgrounds, vulnerability to injury may be intensified. Health care providers are responsible for protecting all patients, regardless of their cultural background. Most adverse events are related to failures of communication; therefore it is important to be particularly attentive to communication during assessment. For example, use approaches that recognize a patient's cultural background (e.g., an interpreter or simple language) so appropriate questions can be raised to clearly reveal health behaviors and risks.
- Enhance a patient's safety by considering the whole person and seeing each care situation through "the patient's eyes" and not just from your perspective. The following include some specific patient-centered safety guidelines:
  - Support patients emotionally and empower them to express their values and preferences and ask questions without being inhibited (Betancourt et al., 2021).
  - When restraints are needed, clarify their meaning to the patient and family. Some patients may view restraining an older adult to be disrespectful. Similarly, some survivors of war or persecution view restraints as imprisonment or punishment.
  - Collaborate with family caregivers in accommodating a patient's cultural perspectives regarding restraints. Removing restraints when family is present shows respect and caring for a patient.
  - Be familiar with agency restraint protocol. Identify potential areas for negotiation with a patient's and family's preferences such as using a mitten versus arm restraints.
  - Inform patients and family caregivers of the reasons a patient is at risk for falls. It is important for patients to know their risks, the options that exist to promote safety, and the potential consequences of not following precautions.

EVIDENCE-BASED PRACTICE

Fall Prevention

Falls are the most common adverse events reported in hospitalized older adults (LeLaurin & Shorr, 2019). Falls in hospitals are associated with longer length of stay and poorer patient outcomes. Falls that occur in hospitals typically result in physical injury such as bruises, hip fractures, and head injuries. Research has shown that falls and fall injuries can be prevented by completing an individualized patient assessment, developing a patient-centered fall prevention plan, and executing the plan consistently (Dykes et al., 2020). Key elements of fall prevention involve developing and implementing

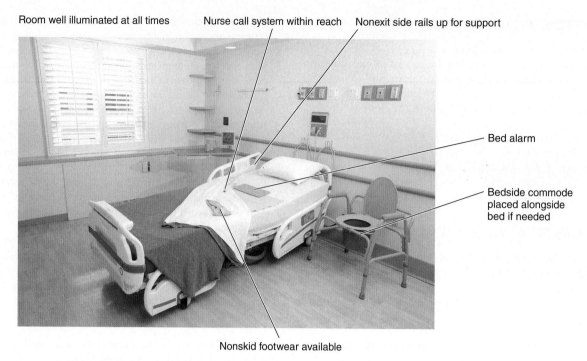

Room well illuminated at all times   Nurse call system within reach   Nonexit side rails up for support

Bed alarm

Bedside commode placed alongside bed if needed

Nonskid footwear available

FIG. 14.1 Patient room environment with bed positioned low, floor mat in place, and side rails positioned up.

multifactorial strategies that address modifiable risk factors such as medication management, exercise interventions, and environmental modifications (Montero-Odasso et al., 2021). In the community setting, falls are also a frequent occurrence. Research has shown that exercise interventions are associated with fall-related benefit, but adherence levels vary. Integrating strength and balance exercises tailored to the capacity of the person into daily activities, such as bending from the knees when opening a drawer or standing on toes to reach a cabinet, has shown promise (Szanton et al., 2021).

- Promote early mobility in hospitalized patients (see Chapter 11) and collaborate with physical therapy providers to ensure that appropriate gait training (if needed) and assistive devices are used.
- Implement Universal Fall Precautions for all acute care patients and then tailor multiple interventions specific to the patient's own fall risk factors (see Skill 14.1).
- Implement the use of checklists that incorporate hospital-approved fall prevention interventions. The checklist has shown promise for improving adherence to each intervention and reducing the incidence of falls. Checklists can be used during change-of-shift hand-offs to determine whether all prevention interventions are in place before accepting care of a patient (Johnston & Magnan, 2019).
- In the community setting, the National Institute on Aging (NIA, 2020) recommends four types of exercise to improve health and physical ability. These include endurance, strength, balance, and flexibility.

- The CDC makes an evidence-based toolkit available through the Stopping Elderly Accidents, Deaths, and Injuries (STEADI) initiative (CDC, 2021).

SAFETY GUIDELINES

- Accurate patient identification before any procedures is crucial to patient safety. Use at least two patient identifiers (TJC, 2023).
- Safety begins with a patient's immediate environment (Fig. 14.1). Always keep a bed in the low position with the nurse call system easily accessible. The nurse call/bed-control system allows patients to adjust bed positions and signal caregivers for help. Explain to patients and visiting family caregivers how to operate a call system correctly, and then use teach-back to confirm understanding and have them demonstrate use of device.
- Always be alert to conditions within a patient's environment that pose risks for patient injury (e.g., personal care items out of reach, hazards along walking paths, liquid spilled on the floor, poorly functioning equipment).
- Follow agency policy and procedure in the agency where you work. Do not use work-arounds when performing skills or procedures. A work-around occurs when a person improvises, takes shortcuts, or works around intended work practices.
- Communicate clearly to other health care providers the plan of care, including procedures to be performed, procedures completed, and patient response. Communicate all important test results to the right staff person in a timely manner (TJC, 2023).

◆ SKILL 14.1   **Fall Prevention in Health Care Settings**

A report from the Health Research and Educational Trust (HRET, 2016) commissioned by The Joint Commission (TJC) noted that an estimated 700,000 to 1,000,000 people fall in U.S. hospitals each year and that 30% to 35% of those patients sustain a fall-related

injury, and approximately 11,000 falls are fatal. Patient falls resulting in injury have remained one of the most frequently reviewed sentinel events by The Joint Commission (TJC, 2021). A fall may result in fractures, bruises, lacerations, or internal bleeding, leading to increased diagnostic tests and treatments, extended hospital stays, and discharge to rehabilitation or long-term care instead of home. Falls have been identified by the Centers for Medicare and Medicaid Services (CMS, 2020) as a preventable or "never" event that should never occur. Therefore in October 2008 CMS stopped reimbursing hospitals for costs related to patient falls (Fehlberg et al., 2017). Fall prevention is a priority in all health care settings. It requires a culture of safety in which all health care providers are mindful of the fall risks existing within health care settings combined with the fall risks created by patients' health conditions and are thus proactive in providing fall prevention strategies.

Falls are clearly multifactorial. Many different conditions can contribute to a single patient fall (Berry & Kiel, 2022; TJC, 2015). The risk factors for falls include two categories: patient related (intrinsic) and hospital environment and working process related (extrinsic). In international and national studies examining risk factors for falls, common risks are found for all patients (Berry & Kiel, 2022; HRET, 2016) (Table 14.1). In an effort to anticipate a patient's fall risk, health care settings use validated fall risk assessment tools that include risk factors that have been identified from the scientific literature. The number of risks identified for a specific patient is computed into a fall risk score (e.g., high, medium, and low). The most common risk assessment tools used in hospitals are the Morse Fall Scale, the STRATIFY scale, and the Hendrich II Fall Risk Model (Berry & Kiel, 2022; Callis, 2016). Once a patient's fall risks have been identified, partner with the patient to affirm those risks and select evidence-based interventions (usually multiple strategies) that appropriately target the patient's risks (Berry & Kiel, 2022).

Universal Fall Precautions are called "universal" because they apply to all patients regardless of fall risk. Universal Fall Precautions revolve around keeping a patient's environment safe and comfortable. Although the choice regarding which precautions to emphasize may vary by agency, a good starting list was recommended by the Agency for Healthcare Research and Quality (AHRQ, 2013). This list is current today:

- Familiarize the patient with the environment.
- Have the patient demonstrate use of the nurse call system.
- Maintain nurse call system within reach.
- Keep the patient's personal possessions within patient safe reach.
- Have sturdy handrails in patient bathrooms, room, and hallway.
- Place the hospital bed in low position when a patient is resting in bed; raise bed to a comfortable height when the patient is transferring out of bed.

TABLE 14.1	
Risk Factors for Falls in Hospitalized Patients	
Intrinsic Factors	**Extrinsic Factors**
History of previous fall	Communication issues
Behavioral	• Frequency of rounding
• Patient does not seek assistance for toileting	• Inconsistent or incomplete communication of patient risk for falls between caregivers
• Patient did not know, forgot, or chose not to use nurse call system	Fall prevention education for patient and family is not used or is inconsistently used
Altered cognition	Physical hazards
• Dementia, sedation, delirium	• Liquids on floor
• Patient awareness and acknowledgment of own risk for falls	• Electrical cords near walking path
Altered mobility	• Uses IV pole to walk
• Lower extremity weakness	• Wears compression stocking with cords
• Abnormal gait	Increased use of restraints (Miake-Lye et al., 2013)
• Shuffling and stumbling	Decreased efforts by hospital staff to mobilize patients (Miake-Lye et al., 2013)
• Requires assistance with mobility and/or assistive device	Inappropriate or no footwear
Sensory deficit	
• Needs corrective lenses	
• Wears hearing aids	
• Hard of hearing and does not wear hearing aids	
Medications	
• Benzodiazepines	
• Antipsychotics	
• Antidepressants	
• Opiates	
• Barbiturates	
• Antihistamines	
• Anticonvulsants	
• Sedatives	
• Antihypertensives	
• Diuretics	
Toileting problems	
• Takes diuretics	
• Has urgency or frequency	
Disease conditions causing:	
• Dizziness	
• Peripheral neuropathy	
• Pain (especially in lower extremities)	
• Hypotension	

IV, Intravenous.

- Keep hospital bed brakes locked.
- Keep wheelchair wheel locks in "locked" position when stationary.
- Keep nonslip, comfortable, well-fitting footwear on the patient.
- Use night lights or supplemental lighting.
- Keep floor surfaces clean and dry. Clean up all spills promptly.
- Keep patient care areas uncluttered.
- Follow safe patient-handling practices.

Fall prevention is not simple. Even after adopting Universal Fall Precautions, it is recommended that additional individualized interventions be used based on patients' fall risks. However, there is still no conclusive evidence for any particular set of interventions that will consistently prevent falls, even though numerous individual nursing fall prevention interventions have been tested (Fehlberg et al., 2017). AHRQ (2013) recommends these tips:

- **Fall prevention must be balanced with other priorities for the patient.** The patient is usually not in the hospital because of falls, so attention is naturally directed elsewhere. Yet a fall in a sick patient can be disastrous and prolong recovery.
- **Fall prevention must be balanced with the need to mobilize patients.** It may be tempting to leave patients in bed to prevent falls, but patients need to transfer and ambulate to maintain their strength and to avoid complications of bed rest.
- **Fall prevention is one of many activities needed to protect patients from harm during their hospital stay.** How should fall prevention be reinforced while maintaining enthusiasm for other priorities, such as infection control?
- **Fall prevention is interprofessional.** All health care providers need to cooperate to prevent falls. How should the right information about a patient's fall risks get to the right member of the team at the right time?
- **Fall prevention needs to be individualized.** Each patient has a different set of fall risk factors, so care must thoughtfully address each patient's unique needs. For example, patients with urinary urgency will benefit from diuretics given in the early morning and bedside toilets.

The Joint Commission (TJC) Center for Transforming Healthcare aims to prevent inpatient falls with injury (HRET, 2016).

Seven hospitals in the United States worked with the Center and successfully reduced the total number of falls and falls with injury by creating awareness among staff, empowering patients to take an active role in their own safety, using validated fall risk assessment tools, engaging patients and their families in fall safety programs, providing hourly rounding that included proactive toileting, and engaging all hospital staff to ensure that no patient walked unaccompanied (HRET, 2016).

Delegation

The skill of assessing and communicating a patient's risks for falling cannot be delegated to assistive personnel (AP). Skills used to prevent falls can be delegated. Direct the AP by:

- Explaining a patient's specific fall risks and associated prevention measures needed to minimize risks
- Explaining environmental safety precautions to use (e.g., bed locked in low position, nurse call system within easy reach)
- Explaining specific patient behaviors (e.g., disorientation, wandering) that are precursors to falls and that should be reported to the registered nurse (RN) immediately

Interprofessional Collaboration

- Physical therapists (PTs) assess and develop individualized treatment plans including exercises to improve strength, mobility, and balance.
- Occupational therapists (OTs) assess influences from the person, the person's normal activity roles and routines, and the environment to maximize independence while reducing fall risk.

Equipment

- Standardized and valid fall risk assessment tool (HRET, 2016)
- Hospital bed with side rails; *Option:* low bed
- Nurse call system
- Gait belt for assisting with ambulation
- Wheelchair and seat belt (as needed)
- Optional safety devices: bed alarm pad, no-slip floor mat, wedge cushion, head protective gear, hip protector

STEP	RATIONALE

ASSESSMENT

1. Identify patient using at least two identifiers (e.g., name and birthday or name and medical record number) according to agency policy.	Ensures correct patient. Complies with The Joint Commission standards and improves patient safety (TJC, 2023).
2. Review electronic health record (EHR) and determine if patient has a recent history of a fall and risks for injury (ABCs) (Institute for Healthcare Improvement [IHI], 2017): • Age over 85 • Bone disorders (e.g., metastasis, osteoporosis, previous leg/hip fractures) • Coagulation disorders (e.g., leukemia, thrombocytopenia, anticoagulant use) • Surgery (specifically thoracic or abdominal surgery or lower limb amputation)	Conditions increase likelihood of serious injury from a fall, such as fracture or internal hemorrhage.
3. Assess patient's/family caregiver's health literacy.	Determines degree to which individuals have the ability to find, understand, and use information and services to make informed health-related decisions and actions for themselves and others (CDC, 2023).

STEP	RATIONALE
4. Perform hand hygiene. Assess for fall risks using a validated fall risk assessment tool. Compute fall risk score.	Reduces transmission of microorganisms. A variety of intrinsic physiological factors predispose patients to falls. Fall risk tools based on the risk factors of a population (e.g., elderly, oncological, or neurological patient) are more sensitive for predicting falls.

Clinical Judgment *Implement a standardized cognitive assessment tool and integrate into fall risk assessment if cognitive assessment is not included in the fall risk assessment tool (HRET, 2016).*

STEP	RATIONALE
5. Continue with a comprehensive individualized patient assessment and consider patient's unique intrinsic fall risks (TJC, 2022a) (see Table 14.1). Perform a fall risk assessment in general acute care settings on admission, on transfer from one unit to another, with a significant change in a patient's condition, or after a fall (AHRQ, 2013).	Reveals all factors placing patient at a fall risk.
6. Perform the Banner Mobility Assessment Tool (BMAT) (Matz et al., 2019) or the Timed Up and Go (TUG) test (CDC, 2017; Kiel, 2022) if patient is able to ambulate (see Chapter 11). At a minimum, observe an ambulatory patient walking in room (with or without help).	The BMAT assesses four functional tasks to identify the level of mobility a patient can achieve, revealing if assistance is needed (Matz et al., 2019). The TUG test measures the progress of balance, sit to stand, and walking.

Clinical Judgment *It is important to assess both what patients perceive regarding their ability to ambulate and what your objective assessments reveal. Do not rely only on what the patient tells you. Patients, especially older adults, often overestimate their ability to walk due to not recognizing their declining motor performance (Kawasaki & Tozawa, 2020; Caffier et al., 2019).*

STEP	RATIONALE
7. Assess patient's pain severity (use rating scale ranging from 0 to 10).	Pain, especially when it is associated with lower extremities (e.g., arthritis, injury), is a fall risk factor.
8. Ask patient or family caregiver if patient has a history of recent falls or other injuries within the home. Assess previous falls using the acronym SPLATT (Ritchey et al., 2022). • Symptoms at time of fall • Previous fall • Location of fall • Activity at time of fall • Time of fall • Trauma after fall	Symptoms are helpful in identifying cause for fall. Onset, location, and activity offer details on how to prevent future falls.
9. Review patient's medications (including over-the-counter [OTC] medications and herbal products) for drugs that create risk for falls (e.g., benzodiazepines, antipsychotics, antidepressants, opioids and barbiturates, anticonvulsants). Compare those drugs with ones on the Beers Criteria® lists (American Geriatrics Society [AGS], 2019; Greenberg, 2019).	These drugs commonly cause drowsiness. The AGS Beers Criteria® include lists of certain medications worth discussing with patients because the medications may not be the safest or most appropriate options for older adults (AGS, 2019). The five lists included in the AGS Beers Criteria® describe medications with scientific evidence suggesting they should be: • Avoided by most older people (outside of hospice and palliative care settings) • Avoided by older people with specific health conditions • Avoided in combination with other treatments because of the risk for harmful "drug-drug" interactions • Used with caution because of the potential for harmful side effects • Dosed differently or avoided in people with reduced kidney function, which affects how the body processes medicine
10. Assess for polypharmacy (unnecessary use of multiple [five or more] and/or redundant medications in management of the same condition and drugs inappropriate for condition).	A study has shown that the prevalence of patients who fell and were admitted to a hospital increased according to the number of medications taken, from 1.5% of falls for people reporting no medications to 4.7% of falls among those taking 1 to 4 medications, 7.9% of falls among those with polypharmacy, and 14.8% among those reporting heightened polypharmacy (Zaninotto et al., 2020).
11. As needed, assess patient's fear of falling using the Falls Efficacy Scale (FES-1) or the Activities-specific Balance Confidence (ABC) scale, which measures a patient's confidence with doing specific activities of daily living without falling or losing balance (Soh, 2021).	Fear of falling is significantly associated with falls in community-dwelling older adults, especially in individuals with more than 1 fall in the past year (Asai et al., 2022).

STEP	RATIONALE
12. Assess for orthostatic hypotension (OH) in patients who are 65 and older, have a history of a fall, and/or take multiple medications.	OH is common in older patients due to age-related changes within the nervous and vascular systems. Polypharmacy, immobility, decreased activity levels, frailty, and cognitive impairment are also associated with OH (Dani et al., 2021).
13. Assess condition of any assistive devices or equipment used by patient (e.g., legs on bedside commode, end tips on a walker).	Equipment in poor repair increases risk for falls.
14. If patient is in a wheelchair, assess level of comfort, fatigue, boredom, mental status, and level of engagement with others.	These factors can cause patient to attempt to exit a wheelchair without help.
15. Use patient-centered approach to determine what patient already knows about risks for falling. Show patient and family caregiver results of fall risk assessment and explain significance of risk factors. Explain how a plan for fall prevention will be developed.	Allows you to determine content to include in fall prevention education (Dykes & Hurley, 2021).
16. Assess patient's knowledge, prior experience with fall prevention, and feelings about these measures.	Reveals need for patient instruction and/or support.
17. Assess patient's goals or preferences for how to implement fall prevention strategies.	Matching your approach with patient goals will likely improve patient's participation. Initial commitment from learners is critical. Learners process information just collected from the assessment and articulate their own plan (Chinai et al., 2018).
18. If patient has a fall risk, apply color-coded wristband (see illustration). Some agencies institute fall risk signs on doors; others may use color-coded socks or gowns.	Color-coded yellow bands, socks, and gowns are easily recognizable.

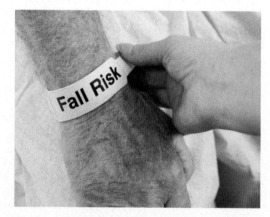

STEP 18 Fall risk armband alerts health care staff to patient's risk of falling.

PLANNING

1. Expected outcomes following completion of procedure:	
• Patient's environment is free of hazards.	Hazards predispose to tripping and falls.
• Patient and/or family caregiver is able to identify fall risks.	Awareness of risks promotes cooperation and understanding of fall prevention plan.
• Patient and/or family caregiver verbalizes understanding of fall interventions planned.	Patient-centered approach involves mutual decision making.
• Patient demonstrates adherence to select fall prevention interventions.	Demonstrates patient and family caregiver learning.
• Patient does not experience a fall or injury.	Lowers patient's fall risk.
2. Provide privacy by closing room curtains or door. Be sure patient is comfortable.	Fall precautions successfully prevent a fall.
	Protects patient privacy; reduces anxiety; promotes cooperation.
3. Perform hand hygiene. Prepare equipment at bedside, making sure all is functional.	Reduces transmission of microorganisms. A well-equipped room with functioning equipment promotes safety.
4. Explain individual safety measures as they pertain to patient's specific fall risks. Also plan for time to discuss fall prevention in the home. *Option:* Some agencies use a patient acknowledgment form for patients to personally acknowledge their fall risks (HRET, 2016; Bargmann & Brundrett, 2020).	Clear, concise information with explanations for purpose, benefits, and expectations results in increased patient participation.

STEP	RATIONALE

5. Educate patients and family caregivers on medication side effects that increase risk for falls (HRET, 2016). | Patients on multiple medications are often unaware of risk factors.

IMPLEMENTATION

1. Conduct hourly purposeful rounds on all patients to determine status of pain, be proactive in offering assistance to toilet, assess comfort of position, and assess need to relocate personal items for easy reach; provide pain-relief intervention. | Hourly rounding has been shown to improve patient satisfaction and reduce falls relating to patients performing activities without assistance (Manges et al., 2020). Patients who fall have been shown to not seek help while toileting (HRET, 2016).

2. Implement early mobility protocols within health care agency (see Chapter 12). Follow protocols to ensure patient increases level of mobility progressively. | Hospital-associated physical deconditioning is related to a significant increase in disability and dependency after hospitalization (Chen et al., 2022). Physical deconditioning is a risk for hospitalized patients who spend most of their time in bed, even when they are able to walk.

3. Implement Universal Fall Precautions.
 a. Adjust bed to low position with wheels locked (see illustration) (AHRQ, 2013). | Height of bed allows ambulatory patient to get in and out of bed easily and safely.
 b. Encourage use of properly fitted skid-proof footwear (AHRQ, 2013). | Prevents falls from slipping on floor.
 c. Orient patient to surroundings. Explain nurse call system and routines to expect in plan of care (AHRQ, 2013; HRET, 2016). | Orientation to room and plan of care provides familiarity with environment and activities to anticipate.

Clinical Judgment *Agencies with successful fall prevention programs have implemented a patient agreement form to use nurse call system for all ambulation (HRET, 2016). Be sure agreement has been signed.*

 (1) Provide patient's hearing aid and glasses. Be sure that each is functioning and clean (AHRQ, 2013). If patient complains of visual or hearing problems, refer to appropriate health care provider. | Enables patient to remain alert to conditions in environment.

 (2) Place nurse call system in an accessible location within patient's reach (see illustrations). Explain and demonstrate how to use system at bedside and in bathroom. Have patient perform return demonstration. | Knowledge of location and use of nurse call system is essential for patient to be able to call for help quickly. Reaching for an object when in bed can lead to an accidental fall.

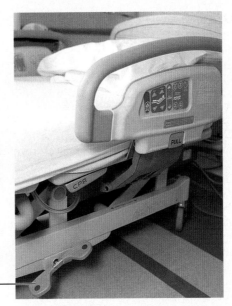

Brake lock

STEP 3a Hospital bed should be kept in lowest position with wheels locked and side rails up (as appropriate). *Option:* Place a floor mat on floor alongside bed.

STEP	RATIONALE

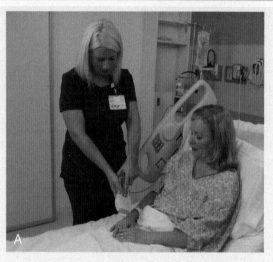
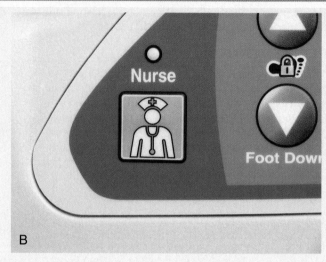

STEP 3c(2) **(A)** Nurse demonstrates use of nurse call system to patient. **(B)** Nurse call system within bed.

(3) Explain to patient/family caregiver when and why to use nurse call system (e.g., report pain, assistance needed to get out of bed or go to bathroom) (HRET, 2016). Provide clear instructions regarding mobility restrictions.	Increases likelihood that patient/family caregiver will call for help and of staff being able to respond to patient's needs in a timely way.
d. Safe use of side rails:	
(1) Explain to patient and family caregiver reason for patient to use side rails: moving and turning self in bed, comfort and security, easy access to nurse call system (U.S. Food and Drug Administration [FDA], 2017).	Promotes a feeling of comfort and security. Aids in turning and repositioning and provides easy access to bed controls (FDA, 2017).
(2) Check agency policy regarding side rail use.	
(a) Dependent, less mobile patients: In two–side rail bed, keep both rails up. (**NOTE:** Rails on newer hospital beds allow for room at foot of bed for patient to safely exit bed.) In four–side rail bed, only leave two upper rails up.	Side rails are restraint devices if they restrict a patient's freedom of movement and therefore do not promote the individual's independent functioning (TJC, 2022b).
(b) Patient able to get out of bed independently: In four–side rail bed, leave two upper side rails up. In two–side rail bed, keep only one rail up.	Allows for safe exit from bed.
e. Make patient's environment safe (see Fig. 14.1).	
(1) Remove excess equipment, supplies, and furniture from rooms and halls.	Reduces likelihood of falling or tripping over objects.
(2) Keep floors free of clutter and obstacles (e.g., intravenous [IV] pole, electrical cords), particularly path to bathroom (AHRQ, 2013).	Reduces likelihood of falling or tripping over objects.
(3) Coil and secure excess electrical, telephone, and any other cords or tubing.	Reduces risk of entanglement.
(4) Clean all spills on floors promptly (AHRQ, 2013). Post sign indicating wet floor. Remove sign when floor is dry (usually done by housekeeping).	Reduces risk of falling on slippery, wet surfaces.
(5) Ensure adequate glare-free lighting; use a night-light at night.	Glare may be problem for older adults because of vision changes.
(6) Have assistive devices (e.g., cane, walker, bedside commode) on exit side of bed. Have chair back of a bedside commode placed against wall of room if possible.	Provides added support when transferring out of bed. Stabilizes commode.
(7) Arrange personal items (e.g., water pitcher, telephone, reading materials, dentures) within patient's easy reach and in logical way (AHRQ, 2013).	Facilitates independence and self-care; prevents falls related to reaching for hard-to-reach items.
(8) Secure locks on beds, stretchers, and wheelchairs (AHRQ, 2013).	Prevents accidental movement of devices during patient transfer.

STEP	RATIONALE
4. Use a proper-size mattress or mattress with raised foam edges (FDA, 2017).	Prevent patients from being trapped between the mattress and rail.
a. Reduce the gaps between the mattress and side rails (FDA, 2017).	Prevent patient entrapment.
5. Provide comfort measures; offer ordered analgesics for patients experiencing pain, preferably around-the-clock.	Pain can cause patients to exit bed or reduce out-of-bed activity. Knee pain has been shown to double the risk of multiple falls in older community-dwelling people (Hicks et al., 2020). Be cautious, as opioids further increase fall risk.
6. Interventions for patients at moderate to high risk for falling (based on fall risk assessment):	
a. Prioritize nurse call system responses to patients at high risk; use a team approach, with all staff knowing responsibility to respond.	Ensures rapid response by care provider when patient calls for help; decreases chance of patient trying to get out of bed on own.
b. Establish elimination schedule; use bedside commode when appropriate.	Proactive toileting keeps patients from being unattended with sudden urge to use toilet.

Clinical Judgment *Toileting is a common event leading to a patient's fall (Berry & Kiel, 2022).*

STEP	RATIONALE
c. Stay with patient during toileting (standing outside bathroom door). Increase availability and use of raised toilet seats and toilet safety frames/grab bars (VA Healthcare, 2015).	Patients often try to get up to stand and walk back to their beds from the bathroom without help. Raised seats make it easier to sit on or stand up from toilet. Toilet frames and grab bars can be grasped to provide support when standing and sitting.
d. Place patient in a geri chair or wheelchair. Use wheelchair only for transport, not for sitting an extended time. Consult with therapy services when considering the use of a wedge cushion.	Maintains alignment and comfort and makes it difficult to exit chair. A wedge cushion tilts the pelvis toward the back of the chair, resulting in increased pressure on the sacrum and coccyx, which can place patient at increased risk of pressure injury development.
e. Provide hip protectors, which are padded shorts or underwear that is worn over or in place of underwear (used more often in long-term care settings).	Prevent fractures by distributing the force of a fall on the hip to the softer tissue around the buttocks and thigh (U.S. Department of Veterans Affairs, 2019).
f. Consider use of a low bed that has lower height than standard hospital bed. Apply nonskid floor mats (U.S. Department of Veterans Affairs, 2019).	Low beds may reduce fall-related injuries by making it difficult for patients with lower extremity weakness or pain in lower joints to exert effort needed to stand. Mats prevent fall injuries when a patient falls from the bed.
g. Activate a bed alarm or surveillance system, such as a camera monitoring system for patient (VA Healthcare, 2015).	Alarm activates when patient rises off sensor. Alarm sounds alert to staff. Continuous video monitoring provides surveillance of multiple patients simultaneously. Camera can detect an unassisted bed exit and alert staff (Jones et al., 2021).

Clinical Judgment *Use judgment when considering use of a bed or chair alarm. Avoid overreliance on an alarm as a fall prevention measure. Research has shown that alarms may be disruptive, especially to cognitively impaired patients. Determine if use of a bed or chair alarm is restricting patient mobility and independence (LeLaurin & Shorr, 2019). The use of multiple alarm devices (e.g., IV pump, bed alarm, electrocardiographic monitor) can result in sound dispersion and alarm fatigue among health care providers.*

STEP	RATIONALE
h. Confer with PT about gait training, strength and balance training, and regular weight-bearing activities.	Exercise can reduce falls, fall-related fractures, and several risk factors for falls in individuals with low bone density and older adults. Strength and balance training reduces the rate of falls in older adults (Sherrington et al., 2019).
i. Use sitters or restraints only when alternatives are exhausted.	A sitter is a nonprofessional staff member who stays in a patient room to closely observe patients who are at risk for falling. Restraints should be used only as a final option (see Skill 14.2).
j. Consider having patient wear head protective gear (e.g., oncology patient or patients at risk for bleeding).	Contains impact-resistant material within the hat that surrounds the head and protects against head injury.
7. When ambulating a patient, have patient wear a gait belt or use a walking sling, and walk alongside patient (see Chapters 11 and 12).	Safe patient-handling techniques allow for safe patient ambulation and prevention of injury to you and patient. Using a gait belt during an assisted fall has been shown to decrease the potential for fall injury (Venema et al., 2019).
8. Safe use of wheelchair:	
a. Be sure that wheelchair is correct fit for patient: Patient thighs are level while sitting, feet flat on floor; back of chair comes up to mid shoulder, elbows rest on armrests without leaning over or tucking arms in, and two finger widths of space between patient and side of chair.	Correctly fitted chair promotes comfort, making it less likely for patient to try to exit it.
b. Transfer patient to wheelchair by using safe handling techniques (see Chapter 12).	Cushion prevents patient from slipping out of chair.

STEP	RATIONALE

c. Back wheelchair into and out of elevator or door, leading with large rear wheels first (see illustration).

Prevents smaller front wheels from catching in crack between elevator and floor, causing chair to tip.

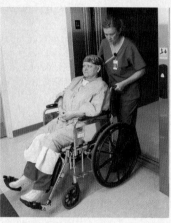

STEP 8c Nurse backing wheelchair into elevator.

d. Manage patient's pain, and do not allow patient to sit in wheelchair for an extended amount of time; provide alternative sitting option.

Reduces restlessness and discomfort that can lead to wheelchair exit.

9. Schedule oral medication administration for at least 2 hours prior to "bedtime" (HRET, 2016).

Reduces risk created by medications that can cause patients to have to use bathroom during night, such as diuretic medications.

10. After implementing safety strategies, help patient to a comfortable position.

Reduces restlessness and desire to exit bed. Restores comfort and sense of well-being.

11. Raise side rails (as appropriate) and lower bed to lowest position, locking into position (FDA, 2017).

Ensures patient safety and prevents falls.

12. Place nurse call system in an accessible location within patient's reach.

Ensures patient can call for assistance if needed.

13. Remove and dispose of supplies and perform hand hygiene.

Reduces transmission of microorganisms.

EVALUATION

1. Ask patient/family caregiver to identify patient's fall risks.

Demonstrates learning.

2. Ask patient/family caregiver to describe fall prevention interventions to implement.

Demonstrates learning.

3. Evaluate patient's ability to use assistive devices such as walker or bedside commode at different times during the day.

Adjustments in devices may become necessary. Evaluating at different times can help identify strengths and weaknesses.

4. Evaluate for changes in motor, sensory, and cognitive status and review if any falls or injuries have occurred.

May require different interventions to be added. Fall outcomes determine success of plan.

5. Evaluate patient's character and level of pain using a pain rating scale.

Determines if patient's pain (if present) is under adequate control.

6. Evaluate patient adherence with fall prevention interventions (e.g., use of nurse call system, footwear, mobility restrictions).

Patients often overestimate their ability despite fall prevention education given by health care providers (Dabkowski et al., 2022).

7. Continue hourly purposeful rounding.

Reduces patient anxiety, lessens need for patient to exit bed independently.

8. Use Teach-Back: "I want to be sure I explained clearly to you why you are at risk to fall. Tell me some of those reasons." Revise your instruction now or develop a plan for revised patient/family caregiver teaching if patient/family caregiver is not able to teach back correctly.

Teach-back is a technique for health care providers to ensure that they have explained medical information clearly so that patients and their families understand what you communicated to them (AHRQ, 2023).

Unexpected Outcomes	Related Interventions
1. Patient/family caregiver unable to identify fall risks or fall prevention strategies or does not adhere to recommended fall prevention measures.	• Reinforce identified risks and review safety measures with patient and family caregiver. Enlist other health care team members to reinforce measures with patient/family caregivers. • Consider using other instructional options.

STEP	RATIONALE
2. Patient found on floor after falling.	• Call for assistance. • Assess patient for injury and stay with patient until help arrives. • Notify primary health care provider and family caregiver. • Complete an agency occurrence or sentinel event report (see agency policy). • Conduct a postfall huddle/debrief as soon as possible after the fall. Involve staff at all levels and the patient if possible. Discuss whether appropriate interventions were in place, considerations as to why fall occurred, staffing at time of fall, which environment of care factors were in place, and how care plan will change (VA Healthcare, 2015; HRET, 2016).

Documentation

- Document in the plan of care specific fall prevention interventions. Use whiteboards in patient rooms to communicate patient fall risks to all staff (HRET, 2016).
- Document what patient is able to explain or not explain about fall risks and interventions taken.
- If fall occurs, complete an agency safety event or incident report, noting objective details of a fall (time, location, patient's condition, treatment, treatment response, patient or witness account of the fall, environmental conditions). Do not place the report in patient's EHR.
- Document evaluation of patient/family caregiver learning and adherence to the plan of care.

Hand-Off Reporting

- Use a hand-off communication tool that includes specific patient risks for falls and falls with injury between caregivers (include assistive personnel). Discuss patient-specific interventions taken (HRET, 2016).
- Report immediately to the health care provider if patient sustains a fall or an injury.

Special Considerations

Patient Education

- The website for the Centers for Disease Control and Prevention STEADI (Stopping Elderly Accidents, Deaths, and Injuries) program offers educational materials for older adults and family caregivers at https://www.cdc.gov/steadi/index.html.
- Encourage patients to have annual vision and hearing examinations. Adaptive devices such as a hearing aid or glasses are sometimes necessary or need modification.
- Emphasize to patients the need to always look ahead when ambulating and to use good posture.
- Teach patients how to use assistive devices and keep them in good repair.

Pediatrics

- Encourage parents to follow these safety recommendations (Safe Kids Worldwide, 2015):
  - *Window safety:* Install window guards or window stops to prevent unintentional falls from the window; keep furniture away from windows.
  - Keep babies and young children strapped into highchairs, infant carriers, shopping carts, swings, or strollers. Place carriers on the floor, not on top of a table or furniture; do not leave child alone in a shopping cart.
  - Use a stationary activity center rather than a baby walker to prevent falls due to rolling down the stairs and to prevent reaching unsafe objects such as window cords or hot appliances.
  - *Playground safety:* Supervise children on playgrounds; use playgrounds that have shock-absorbing surfaces.
  - Use safety gates attached to the wall at the top and bottom of stairs. Ensure the right gate is used for the top of the stairs.
  - Consider antislip rugs for floors, decals, or mats in the bathtub to prevent falls that can result in a fracture or head injury.
  - *Keep sports safe.* Be sure that child wears protective gear such as wrist guards, knee and elbow pads, and a helmet for biking or skating when playing active sports.
  - Secure TVs and furniture to the wall to prevent tip overs.
- Keep side rails of hospital beds down to allow toddlers and preschoolers easy exit and decrease the need to crawl over the rails (Hockenberry et al., 2022).
- When caring for infants, keep a hand on child when you turn away from the bedside.

Older Adults

- A study has shown that of men in their 50s, 60s, and 70s, 77% did not use the nurse call system. By talking with patients, it was discovered that although independence was part of the issue for older male patients not using the nurse call system, a bigger issue was they did not feel comfortable being helped by young nurses, who reminded them of their daughters and granddaughters. In an effort to increase nurse call system usage, have male caregiver (when available) assist (HRET, 2016).
- Reliably educate patients who are anticoagulated about what to do after a fall (e.g., call health care provider, go to emergency department if profusely bleeding from injury). Patients on anticoagulation with repeat falls have significantly higher rates of death with a bleeding injury (Chiu et al., 2018). Patients need to know risks of being on anticoagulants and risks when anticoagulants are discontinued.
- Educate patients who have osteoporosis about bone health and use of hip protectors in the home (U.S. Department of Veterans Affairs, 2019).
- Interventions to improve balance confidence have shown benefits, including multicomponent behavioral group interventions and exercise (including tai chi), which increases lower body strength and dynamic balance.
- The BEERS Criteria® lists identify drugs that place the elderly at increased risk for injury and falls (https://www.americangeriatrics.org/media-center/news/older-people-medications-are-common-updated-ags-beers-criteriar-aims-make-sure).

Populations With Disabilities

- Another area of fall risk includes wheelchair-related falls involving people with disabilities. Patients fall from wheelchairs as a result of unlocked brakes, overreaching, sliding, tipping the chair, and unassisted transfers. Wheelchair-related injuries from falls include fractures, concussions, dislocations, amputations, and serious head and spinal injuries. An example of a wheelchair characteristic that increases risk for falls is having smaller and harder front wheels that cause a chair to tip when striking uneven terrain. Caregivers are also at risk for injury by not handling patients correctly or not asking for help. Injuries can occur while caregivers transfer patients who are agitated,

fearful, unsteady, or too weak to transfer. Tripping over the front foot or leg rest and leaning over the back of the wheelchair to engage or disengage the wheel lock are common sources of injury.

Home Care
- See Chapter 42.

✦ SKILL 14.2 | **Designing a Restraint-Free Environment**

 Video Clip

A restraint-free environment is the first goal of care for all patients. A restraint is any method (chemical or physical) of restricting individuals' freedom of movement, including physical activity or normal access to their bodies that (1) is not a usual part of a medical diagnostic or treatment procedure, (2) is not indicated to treat the individuals' medical conditions, or (3) does not promote the individuals' independent functioning (TJC, 2022b). Serious and often fatal complications can result from the use of restraints (Sharifi et al., 2021) (Box 14.1). Because of the risks associated with the use of restraints, current legislation emphasizes reducing this use.

The Centers for Medicare and Medicaid Services (CMS) set the standard that restraint or seclusion may be imposed only to ensure the immediate physical safety of a patient and must be discontinued at the earliest possible time (CMS, 2020). In trying to create a restraint-free environment, patients at risk for falling or

wandering present safety challenges and require special precautions. Wandering is aimless pacing, attempts at elopement, or getting lost on one's own. Consequences of wandering vary from minor to severe injury and death (Agrawal et al., 2021). Wandering is common among patients who are confused or disoriented (e.g., delirium) or have dementia. Interrupting a wandering patient can increase the patient's distress.

Delegation

The skills of assessing patient behaviors and orientation to the environment and determining the type of restraint-free interventions to use cannot be delegated to assistive personnel (AP). Actions that provide a safe environment can be delegated to AP. Direct the AP about:
- Using specific diversional or activity-based measures for making the environment safe
- Applying appropriate monitoring or alarm devices
- Reporting patient behaviors and actions (e.g., confusion, getting out of bed unassisted) to the nurse

Interprofessional Collaboration
- In the long-term care setting, the AP and case managers may observe patient behavior and recognize signs of wandering.
- Consult with physical, speech, occupational, and activity therapists for exercise options and activities that provide meaningful stimulation.

BOX 14.1

Risks Associated With Application of Physical Restraints

- Bruises
- Decubitus ulcers
- Respiratory complications
- Urinary incontinence and constipation
- Undernutrition
- Increased dependence in activities of daily living
- Impaired muscle strength and balance
- Decreased cardiovascular endurance
- Increased agitation
- Increased risk for mortality caused by strangulation or as a consequence of serious injuries—for example, fracture, head trauma

Equipment
- Visual or auditory stimuli meaningful to patient (e.g., photos, music, streaming devices, calendar, piece of art)
- Activity-based interventions (e.g., puzzles, games, arts and crafts)
- Wraparound belt
- *Options:* Electronic bracelet, continuous video monitoring system, or pressure pad alarm sensor

---

STEP	RATIONALE

ASSESSMENT

1. Identify patient using at least two identifiers (e.g., name and birthday or name and medical record number) according to agency policy.

2. Review electronic health record (EHR) for patient's medical history for memory impairment and underlying causes of agitation and cognitive impairment (e.g., delirium, dementia, depression). Also assess for the following: considered dangerous to self or others, gravely disabled as result of mental disorder, lacking cognitive ability (either permanently or temporarily) to make relevant decisions, alcohol or substance withdrawal, fluid and electrolyte imbalance, physical limitations that increase risk.

Ensures correct patient. Complies with The Joint Commission standards and improves patient safety (TJC, 2023).

Causes of agitation and wandering are commonly associated with these conditions (Berry & Kiel, 2022).

STEP	RATIONALE
3. In patients with known dementia, assess for signs of restlessness: pacing, fidgeting, repetitive motor movements, and repetitive questioning (Alzheimer's Association, 2023a).	Being able to distinguish restlessness from other behaviors may assist in recognition and appropriate treatment (Regier & Gitlin, 2017).

Clinical Judgment *In a patient with dementia, restlessness is not (1) the disordered locomotion that is the hallmark of wandering behavior, (2) associated with attempts to elope or leave without permission of caregivers from an institution or home, (3) the physiological effects of a substance (e.g., neuroleptic medication, withdrawal from benzodiazepines) or another medical condition (e.g., hypoglycemia), (4) a mental disorder other than dementia (e.g., generalized anxiety disorder) or movement disorder (e.g., restless legs syndrome, essential tremor, Parkinson disease) (Regier & Gitlin, 2017).*

STEP	RATIONALE
4. Review patient's medications for over-the-counter (OTC) and prescribed medications (see Table 14.1) that pose risk for falling (compare with medications on Beers Criteria® lists [AGS, 2019]). Assess for interactions and untoward effects.	Medication interactions or side effects often contribute to falling or altered mental status.
5. Perform hand hygiene. Assess patient's behavior (e.g., orientation, level of consciousness, ability to understand and follow directions, combative behaviors), balance, gait, vision, hearing, bowel/bladder routine, level of pain, electrolyte and blood count values, and presence of orthostatic hypotension.	Reduces transfer of microorganisms. Accurate assessment identifies patients with safety risks and the physiological causes for patient behaviors that prompt caregivers to use restraints. Ensures proper selection of nonrestraint interventions.
6. For patients who wander or have known dementia, screen for cognitive decline using a validated patient assessment tool, such as the General Practitioner Assessment of Cognition (GPCOG), the Memory Impairment Screen (MIS), or the Mini-Cog™ (Alzheimer's Association, 2023b). Assess patient during time of day when cognition normally decreases (e.g., end of the day or at night) (see Chapter 6).	Findings aid in determining presence of a cognitive impairment. Tools can be administered by trained medical staff members who are not physicians; however, a diagnosis of a cognitive impairment must be conducted by a physician (Alzheimer's Association, 2023b).
7. Assess degree of wandering behavior using Algase Wandering Scale (Version 2) (AWS-V2) (Martin et al., 2015; Nelson & Algase, 2007).	The AWS-V2 is a valid and reliable measure overall and for persistent walking, spatial disorientation, and eloping behavior subscales.
8. Assess patient and family caregiver's health literacy.	Determines degree to which individuals have the ability to find, understand, and use information and services to make informed health-related decisions and actions for themselves and others (CDC, 2023).
9. Assess patient's or family caregiver's knowledge of condition and risks for falls or wandering.	Reveals need for patient instruction and/or support.
10. For patients with dementia, ask family about their usual communication style and cues to indicate pain, fatigue, hunger, and need to urinate or defecate.	Enables you to use best method to determine patient needs, which often prompt wandering or agitation when needs are unmet.
11. Inspect condition of any therapeutic medical devices.	Patients who become restless, agitated, or confused will attempt to remove medical devices and then become candidates for physical restraint.
12. Assess daily to determine if a medical device is necessary or can be discontinued. Consider alternative therapy (e.g., oral medications instead of intravenous [IV]) when possible.	Patients who are agitated often try to remove medical devices.

PLANNING

1. Expected outcomes following completion of procedure: • Patient is injury free and/or does not inflict injury on others while in restraint-free environment. • Patient does not remove a therapeutic medical device.	Restraint alternatives are successful in reducing agitation and preventing injury. Maintains continuity of care and prevents injury to patient.
2. Provide privacy, be sure patient is comfortable, and prepare room environment.	Reduces patient anxiety/restlessness and facilitates an organized procedure.
3. Explain procedure to patient and family caregiver.	Promotes patient cooperation.
4. Perform hand hygiene and gather any necessary supplies.	Reduces transmission of microorganisms.

STEP	RATIONALE

IMPLEMENTATION

1. Orient patient and family caregiver to surroundings, introduce to staff, and explain all treatments and procedures. Be sure that patient is able to read your name badge.

Builds trust; promotes patient understanding and cooperation.

2. Assign same staff to care for patient as often as possible. Encourage family and friends to stay with patient. In some agencies, volunteers are effective companions.

Increases familiarity with individuals in patient's environment, decreasing anxiety and restlessness. Companions are helpful and prevent patient from being alone.

3. Place patient in room that is easily accessible to care providers and close to nurses' station.

Allows for frequent observation to reduce falls in high-risk patients.

4. Follow all Universal Fall Precautions (see Skill 14.1) to create a safe environment (AHRQ, 2013; Dykes & Hurley, 2021).

Reduces environmental risks for falls/injuries.

5. Be sure that patient is wearing glasses, hearing aid, or other sensory-aid devices and that all are functioning.

Improves patient's level of orientation to environment.

6. Provide visual and auditory stimuli meaningful to patient (e.g., watch/clock, calendar, streaming devices [with patient's choice of music], television, and family pictures).

Orients patient to day, time, and physical surroundings. You must individualize stimuli for this to be effective.

7. Anticipate patient's basic needs (e.g., toileting, relief of pain, relief of hunger) as quickly as possible; conduct hourly rounds (Gliner et al., 2022).

Providing basic needs in a timely fashion decreases patient discomfort, anxiety, restlessness, and incidence of falls.

8. Provide scheduled ambulation, chair activity, and toileting (e.g., ask patient every hour during rounds about toileting needs). Organize treatments so patient has uninterrupted periods throughout the day. Consider using a bedside commode for patients who are weak, unsteady, or unsafe to ambulate to the bathroom (insist that patient be assisted out of bed).

Early mobility is essential for all patients (see Chapter 12). Regular opportunity to void lowers risk of patient trying to reach bathroom alone. Constant activity overstimulates patients. Commode makes toileting safer and more accessible to patients who are unsafe to ambulate to the bathroom unassisted.

Clinical Judgment *Caution: A bedside commode can sometimes encourage patients to get up unassisted. However, it is important to reinforce to patient and family caregiver that assistance is required and to use the nurse call system.*

9. Position IV catheters, urinary catheters, and tubes/drains out of patient view. Use commercial tube holders, camouflage by wrapping IV site with bandage or stockinette, and use long-sleeved robes and commercial sleeves over arms (Boltz et al., 2020). Place undergarments on patient with urinary catheter, or cover abdominal feeding tubes/drains with loose abdominal binder.

Maintains medical treatment while reducing patient access to tubes/lines needed for treatment delivery.

10. Implement strategies to decrease wandering:
    a. Eliminate stressors from environment such as cold at night, changes in daily routines, and extra visitors.

    Reduced stress allows patient's energy to be channeled more appropriately.

    b. Use stress-reduction techniques such as back rub, massage, and guided imagery (see Chapter 16).

    Reduces level of anxiety and restlessness.

    c. Use activity-based interventions: puzzles, games, music therapy, doll therapy, pet therapy, art therapy, mirrors in front of exit doors, activity apron, and the integration of purposeful activities such as chores (folding towels) and crafts (Lourida et al., 2020). Be sure that it is an activity in which patient has interest. Involve family caregiver (if appropriate).

    Activity-based interventions individualized to the patient with dementia have shown improvement in patient engagement, mood, and agitating behaviors (Lourida et al., 2020).

11. Position patient comfortably in chair or wheelchair with a wraparound safety belt. Place chair alarm pad, wedge cushion, and/or nonstick matting in place under patient.

Wraparound belt offers security but allows patient to lift flap for self-release. Pad and mat prevent patient from slipping down, which could cause strangulation.

STEP	RATIONALE
12. Use motion or bed occupancy alarm system for unsteady patients who forget to or do not call for assistance when getting out of bed or chair (Dykes & Hurley, 2021). See manufacturer's directions and agency policy. Another option is a chair pad with alarm.	Alarms alert staff to patient who is standing or rising from bed or chair without help.
a. Explain use of device to patient and family caregiver.	Promotes patient and family cooperation.
b. When patient is in chair, position pad correctly, ensuring it is under patient's buttocks.	System responds to a change in pressure, requiring accurate placement.
c. Test alarm by applying and releasing pressure.	Ensures that alarm is audible through nurse call system.
13. Use available locating technology (i.e., Global Positioning System [GPS], radio frequency, Bluetooth, and Wi-Fi) for patients who wander. Follow manufacturer's directions.	Tag in bracelet or wearable device contains radio frequency circuit that communicates with detection sensor usually installed at an exit door or elevator. Distance between tag and monitor is constantly measured with an alarm, which sounds when predetermined distance is exceeded.
14. Minimize invasive treatments (e.g., tube feedings, blood sampling) as much as possible.	Stimuli increase patients' restlessness.
15. Assist patient to a comfortable position.	Restores comfort and sense of well-being.
16. Raise side rails (as appropriate) and lower bed to lowest position, locking into position (FDA, 2017).	Ensures patient safety and prevents falls.
17. Place nurse call system in an accessible location within patient's reach.	Ensures patient can call for assistance if needed.
18. Dispose of supplies and perform hand hygiene.	Reduces transmission of microorganisms.

EVALUATION

1. Monitor patient's behavior routinely and check condition of medical devices.	Will determine if agitation, wandering, or attempt to remove medical devices has been prevented.
2. Observe patient for any injuries.	Patient should be injury free.
3. Observe patient's behavior toward staff, visitors, and other patients.	Ensures that patient's behavior does not cause injury to others.
4. **Use Teach-Back:** "We've talked about what we are doing to reduce your husband's wandering. Tell me ways you can help. I want to be sure you understand." Revise your instruction now or develop a plan for revised family caregiver teaching if family caregiver is not able to teach back correctly.	Teach-back is a technique for health care providers to ensure that they have explained medical information clearly so that patients and their families understand what is communicated to them (AHRQ, 2023).

Unexpected Outcomes

1. Patient displays behaviors that increase risk for injury to self or others.

2. Patient sustains injury or is agitated and places others at risk for injury.

3. Patient wanders away from health care agency.

Related Interventions

- Review episodes for pattern (e.g., activity, time of day) that indicates alternatives that would eliminate behavior.
- Discuss alternative interventions with all health care providers and family caregivers.
- Notify health care provider. Complete incident or occurrence report according to agency policy.
- Identify alternative measures for safety or behavioral control.
- Apply physical restraint (see Skill 14.3) only after all other interventions have been unsuccessful.
- Be prepared to follow agency policy, which should include whom to notify; who will search for patient; which areas will be searched and their priority; who will notify authorities, if necessary; who will notify family members; and who will coordinate search efforts.

Documentation

- Document all behaviors that relate to cognitive status and ability to maintain safety: orientation to time, place, and person; ability to follow directions; mood and emotional status; understanding of condition and treatment plan; medication effects related to behaviors; restraint alternatives used; and patient response to your interventions.
- Document evaluation of patient/family caregiver learning.

Hand-Off Reporting

- Report to other health care providers all interventions being used to prevent agitation or wandering and any occurrences of wandering or other behavior that place the patient at risk for injury.
- Report any patient injury from a fall to health care provider immediately.

Special Considerations

Patient Education

- Teach family caregivers ways to involve patient in their visits, keeping patient appropriately stimulated.
- Teach the family caregiver how to adapt the home environment (see Chapter 41) to minimize wandering.

Older Adults

- Keep older adults active and ambulatory to increase endurance and function.
- Reminiscence helps older adults remain oriented.

Home Care

- Patients at risk for violence to others need intensive supervision. Family members and home health caregivers need to recognize this and take appropriate preventive measures. Here are some tips:
  - Some home care staff members have immediate access to their agency or an emergency responder by pressing an access button inserted on their identification badge.
  - Nurses should always be on the alert and watch for signals of violence, such as substance abuse, threats, or the presence of weapons.
  - Defuse anger by displaying a calm and caring demeanor.
  - Avoid behaviors that may be interpreted as aggressive—getting close, speaking loudly, moving quickly.
  - Have family caregiver set up an area in the home where it is safe for an older adult to wander.

✦ SKILL 14.3   Applying Physical Restraints

 Video Clip

Three forms of restraints are used in health care settings: physical restraints, chemical restraints, and seclusion. CMS defines physical restraints as any manual method, physical or mechanical device, material, or equipment that immobilizes or reduces the ability of a patient to move the arms, legs, body, or head freely (CMS, 2020). Physical restraint may involve:

- Applying a wrist, elbow, ankle, or waist restraint
- Preventing a patient in a recliner, wheelchair, or enclosed bed from freely exiting on their own
- Tucking in a sheet very tightly so the patient cannot move
- Keeping all side rails up to prevent the patient from voluntarily getting out of bed (TJC, 2022b)

A chemical restraint is the use of a drug to restrict a patient's movement or behavior when the drug or dosage used is not an approved standard of treatment for the patient's condition (CMS, 2020). Seclusion is commonly used in emergency departments and psychiatric inpatient units. CMS defines seclusion as involuntary confinement of a patient alone in a room or place from which the patient is physically prevented from leaving (CMS, 2020).

The focus of this skill is the use of physical restraints. Physical restraints are commonly used in health care agencies to protect the integrity of medically necessary devices (e.g., drainage tubes, catheters, intravenous [IV] catheters), to prevent ambulation when it is unsafe to do so, or when patients are physically aggressive toward caregivers or others. The use of restraints is most common in the critical care setting where patients who are acutely ill often unknowingly try to remove their endotracheal tubes or other life-sustaining medical devices (Perez et al., 2019). Unplanned removal of endotracheal tubes is commonly seen in patients with agitation, delirium, inadequate sedation, and reduced patient surveillance by health care staff (Devlin et al., 2018). The process of using restraints requires continuous assessment by all health care providers to determine the appropriateness of use and the type of restraint or safety device to use.

CMS (2020) has a standard citing that all patients have the right to be free from restraint or seclusion, in any form, im-

posed as a means of coercion, discipline, convenience, or retaliation by staff. In addition, CMS emphasizes that restraint or seclusion may be used only to ensure the immediate physical safety of a patient, a staff member, or others and must be discontinued at the earliest possible time. When the use of a restraint is necessary, the least restrictive method must be used to ensure a patient's safety (CMS, 2020). It is important to note that CMS does not consider the use of restraints as a routine part of a fall prevention protocol. CMS standards note that there is no evidence that the use of physical restraint (including, but not limited to, raised side rails) will prevent or reduce falls (CMS, 2020).

When patients are at risk of harming themselves, you have a duty to act to promote patient safety (American Nurses Association [ANA], 2020). Properly and cautiously applied physical restraints may enhance patient safety and reduce the risk of patient injury or even death. You play a key role in identifying when a patient's safety or behavior creates risks indicating the use of restraints. Interprofessional collaboration is critical in determining whether restraints should be used and, once used, managed safely. The Joint Commission (TJC, 2022a) has standards for reducing use of restraints in health care settings (see Skill 14.2).

Remember that restraints are only a temporary way to keep patients safe. There are approaches to use to better secure medical devices and prevent accidental removal without using restraints (Box 14.2). Research has shown that patients sustain fewer injuries if left unrestrained (Berry & Kiel, 2022). Know your agency's policies for the use of restraints. A licensed health care provider's order, based on a thorough face-to-face assessment, is needed to implement use of restraints. A patient's or family caregiver's informed consent is necessary in the long-term care setting.

The use of restraints is associated with serious complications, including pressure injuries, hypostatic pneumonia, constipation, incontinence, and death. The U.S. Food and Drug Administration (FDA) regulates restraints as medical devices and requires manufacturers to label them "prescription only." Most patient deaths in the past have resulted from strangulation from a vest or jacket

Strategies for Reducing Accidental Removal of Medical Devices

Endotracheal Tube
- Verification of security of system used to anchor tube (see Chapter 24).
- Appropriate sedation and analgesia protocols to reduce agitation.
- Document and mark position of the tube at lip and teeth. Confirm mark stays constant.

Nasogastric Tube
- If being used for feeding, consult with nutritionist and speech therapist for swallow evaluation to consider gastrostomy feeding or other appropriate feeding measures.
- Anchor tubing by taping technique or commercial holder (see Chapter 32).
- Mark exit point of tube at time of x-ray placement confirmation and check at regular intervals.

Intravenous (IV) Lines
- Use commercial holder for anchoring.
- Tape or secure IV line.
- Keep IV bag out of visual field.

Bladder Indwelling Catheter
- Consider intermittent catheterization (see Chapter 33).
- Ensure catheter is secured on leg to reduce tension.

Adapted from Boltz M, et al: Evidence-based geriatric nursing protocols for best practice, ed 6, New York, 2020, Springer; and Harding M, et al: Lewis's medical-surgical nursing: assessment and management of clinical problems, ed 11, St. Louis, 2020, Elsevier.

restraint. Numerous agencies no longer use vest restraints. For these reasons this text does not describe their use.

Delegation

The skill of assessing a patient's behavior, orientation to the environment, need for restraints, and appropriate use of restraints cannot be delegated to assistive personnel (AP). The application and routine checking of a restraint can be delegated to AP. CMS (2020) requires training of all direct care staff who monitor restrained patients and apply and/or remove restraints. Instruct the AP about:
- Appropriate restraint to use and correct placement of restraint
- When and how to change patient's position and provide range-of-motion exercises, hydration, toileting, skin care, and time for socialization
- When to report signs and symptoms of patient not tolerating restraint and what to do

Interprofessional Collaboration
- Inform direct care staff such as physical or occupational therapists and IV nurses regarding the patient behavior leading to use of restraints and how the patient reacts when restraint is removed for therapy.
- Inform health care providers regarding the patient's behavior to determine if restraints can be discontinued or a less restrictive alternative device can be used.

Equipment
- Proper-size restraint
- Padding (if needed)

STEP	RATIONALE

ASSESSMENT

1. Identify patient using at least two identifiers (e.g., name and birthday or name and medical record number) according to agency policy.

   Ensures correct patient. Complies with The Joint Commission standards and improves patient safety (TJC, 2023).

2. Review the electronic health record (EHR) for underlying cause(s) of agitation and cognitive impairment that may lead to patient-initiated medical device removal (Boltz et al., 2020).

   Physiological alterations might lead to accidental patient-initiated medical device removal (Boltz et al., 2020). Identification of conditions might lead to more appropriate medical or pharmacological treatment, eliminating need for restraints.

   a. If there is an abrupt change in patient perception, attention, or level of consciousness, perform hand hygiene. Assess for respiratory and neurological alterations, fever and sepsis, hypoglycemia and hyperglycemia, alcohol or substance withdrawal, and fluid and electrolyte imbalance.

   Reduces transmission of microorganisms. Factors can develop quickly that affect patient cognition.

   b. Notify health care provider of change in mental status and compromised physiological status.

   Health care provider must determine if change in status results in behavior that necessitates temporary use of restraint.

3. Obtain baseline or premorbid cognitive function from family caregivers.

   Excellent sources of information for patient's behavior patterns and past history.

4. Establish whether patient has history of wandering behavior, dementia, or depression (Boltz et al., 2020).

   Cognitively impaired patients are at risk for exiting bed without asking for assistance.

5. Review medications that can cause risk for falling (Boltz et al., 2020; AGS, 2019) and changes in mental status (see Table 14.1).

   Medications can alter cognition, cause drowsiness and postural hypotension, and create other risks.

6. Review EHR for current laboratory values (e.g., electrolytes, blood glucose, blood culture, urinalysis).

   May reveal a fluid and electrolyte imbalance or other problems such as a blood glucose imbalance, infection, or stroke, all of which can cause sudden confusion in the elderly (National Health Service [NHS], 2021).

STEP	RATIONALE
7. Assess patient's current behavior (e.g., confusion, disorientation, agitation, restlessness, combativeness, inability to follow directions, or repeated removal of therapeutic devices). Does patient create a risk to other patients?	If patient's behavior continues despite treatment or restraint alternatives, use of least restrictive restraint might be indicated.

Clinical Judgment *In the case of alcohol withdrawal, resistance against restraints can increase temperature, produce rhabdomyolysis, and cause physical injury (Hoffman & Weinhouse, 2023).*

STEP	RATIONALE
8. If restraint alternatives failed earlier, confer with health care provider. Review agency policies and state laws regarding restraints. Obtain current health care provider's order for restraint, including purpose, type, location, and time or duration of restraint. Determine if signed consent for use of restraint is necessary (long-term care). For nonviolent/non–self-destructive patients, orders are renewed per hospital policy.	A restraint order that is being used for violent or self-destructive behavior has a definite time limit (e.g., every 4 hours for adults, every 2 hours for children and adolescents ages 9–17); these orders may be renewed according to the prescribed time limits for a maximum of 24 consecutive hours (CMS, 2020). A health care provider's order for least restrictive type of restraint is required (CMS, 2020).

Clinical Judgment *A licensed independent health care provider responsible for the care of the patient evaluates the patient in person within 1 hour of the initiation of restraint used for the management of violent or self-destructive behavior that jeopardizes the physical safety of the patient, staff, or others. A registered nurse, an advanced practice nurse, or a physician assistant may conduct the in-person evaluation if trained in accordance with the requirements and if consultation with the aforementioned health care provider occurs after the evaluation as determined by hospital policy (CMS, 2020).*

STEP	RATIONALE
9. Review manufacturer's instructions for restraint application. Determine most appropriate size restraint. Be familiar with all devices.	Incorrect sizing and application of restraint device can result in patient injury or death.
10. Assess patient and family caregiver health literacy.	Determines degree to which individuals have the ability to find, understand, and use information and services to make informed health-related decisions and actions for themselves and others (CDC, 2023).
11. Assess patient's/family caregiver's knowledge, prior experience with restraints, and feelings about their use.	Reveals need for patient instruction and/or support.

PLANNING

STEP	RATIONALE
1. Expected outcomes following completion of procedure: • Patient maintains intact skin integrity, pulses, temperature, color, and sensation of restrained body part. • Patient is free from injury. • Patient's therapy (e.g., endotracheal tube, IV catheter, feeding tube) is uninterrupted. • Patient maintains self-esteem and sense of dignity. • Restraint discontinued as soon as possible.	Restraints applied and monitored correctly. Restraints applied correctly and removed in a timely manner. Disruption of therapy causes patient injury, delay in treatment, and possibly pain and increased risk of infection. Physical restraints have a negative psychological impact on patients, creating feelings of fear, anger, embarrassment, and loss of dignity (de Bruijn et al., 2020). Complies with standards, limiting time patient is at risk for injury.
2. Perform hand hygiene. Prepare restraint, being sure it is intact.	Reduces transmission of microorganisms. Ensures restraint is in condition for correct use.
3. Provide patient privacy and drape as appropriate for comfort.	Promotes patient comfort.
4. Explain to patient and family caregiver the choice of restraint and why it is needed, how it will be applied, length of time to be used, procedure for ongoing assessment, and criteria for discontinuation.	Promotes patient/family cooperation and helps to minimize any anxiety.

IMPLEMENTATION

STEP	RATIONALE
1. Adjust bed to proper height and lower side rail on side of patient contact. Be sure that patient is comfortable and in proper body alignment.	Allows you to reposition patient during restraint application without injuring self or patient. Proper alignment prevents contracture formation when restraints are in place.
2. Inspect area where restraint is to be placed. Note if there is any nearby tubing or device. Assess condition of skin, sensation, adequacy of circulation, and range of joint motion.	Restraints sometimes compress and interfere with functioning of devices or tubes. Assessment provides baseline to monitor patient's response to restraint, condition of patient's skin, and presence of pressure injuries.

STEP	RATIONALE

3. Pad skin and bony prominences (as necessary) that will be under restraint.

Reduces friction and pressure from restraint to skin and underlying tissue.

4. Apply proper-size restraint. **NOTE:** Refer to manufacturer's directions.

   a. *Mitten restraint:* Thumbless mitten device restrains patient's hands. Place hand in mitten, being sure that Velcro strap is around wrist and not forearm (see illustration).

Prevents patient from dislodging or removing medical device, removing dressings, or scratching. Hand mitts are considered a restraint if (TJC, 2022b):

(1) The mitts are pinned or otherwise attached to the bed/bedding, or wrist restraints are also used, and/or

(2) The mitts are applied so tightly that the patient's hands or fingers are immobilized, and/or

(3) The mitts are so bulky that the patient's ability to use the hands is significantly reduced, and/or

(4) The mitts cannot be easily removed intentionally by the patient in the same manner it was applied by staff, considering the patient's physical condition.

Clinical Judgment *Mittens are considered a restraint alternative if untethered and patient is physically and cognitively able to remove the mitten.*

   b. *Elbow restraint (freedom splint):* Restraint consists of rigidly padded device that wraps around arm and is closed with Velcro. The upper end has a clamp that hooks to sleeve of patient's gown or shirt (see illustration). Center splint over elbow with opening facing away from patient. Secure splint by threading hook and loop strap through buckle and back onto itself. Ensure Velcro straps are positioned away from the patient.

The restraint makes it difficult to remove or disrupt a medical device near the face or neck. It does not impede removing abdominal or urinary medical devices. With freedom splints, patients have difficulty bending their arms. Their use may not prevent a patient from removing IV lines.

   c. *Self-releasing roll belt restraint* (see illustration).

   (1) While patient is out of bed, center belt on bed at patient's waist level with belt label facing head of bed.

Eases eventual application of belt.

   (2) Position the long straps so they hang off each side of the mattress. Attach straps to each side of the bed frame by using quick-release ties or a quick-release buckle.

Moveable part allows patient to be raised and lowered in bed without causing pressure to abdomen.

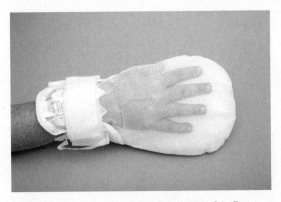

STEP 4a Mitten restraint. (*From Sorrentino SA, Remmert LN: Mosby's textbook for nursing assistants, ed 10, St. Louis, 2021, Elsevier.*)

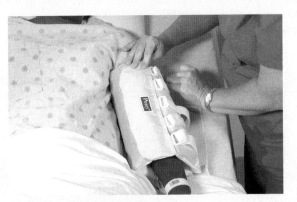

STEP 4b Freedom elbow restraint. (*Copyright © Mosby's Clinical Skills: Essentials Collection.*)

STEP	RATIONALE

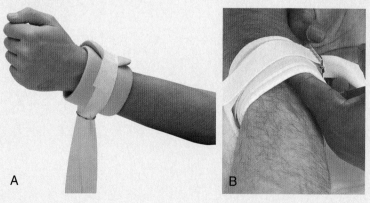

STEP 4c Properly applied self-releasing roll belt restraint allows patient to turn in bed. (*From Sorrentino SA, Remmert LN:* Mosby's textbook for nursing assistants, *ed 10, St Louis 2021, Elsevier.*)

(3) Reconnect the QR buckle and pull on the strap end to tighten strap to bed; repeat on other side of bed.

(4) To attach belt to patient, open the QR buckle and the belt; place patient on bed with belt at waist level. Bring belt around patient waist and secure hook and loop fastener and QR buckle.

(5) Ensure belt is snug but does not restrict breathing. Ensure bed frame straps are snug to the mattress and will not slide or move if bed is adjusted.

d. *Option:* Place patient in an enclosure bed. Bed is less restrictive in that it allows the patient to freely move within the bed (Harris, 2015).

Bed may be appropriate for a patient at high risk for falling or a fall injury and for patients who are impulsive, agitated, or unsteady or who wander (Harris, 2015).

Clinical Judgment *An enclosure bed is a restraint in that it restricts a patient from voluntarily getting out of bed. Bed should not be used solely for prevention of falls (TJC, 2022b). Refer to manufacturer's instructions and agency policy prior to placing a patient in the bed. Do not use other restraint devices (e.g., body, wrist) in the bed. The bed is not intended for use with patients with multiple lines or tubes; patients who are violent, combative, self-destructive, suicidal, or claustrophobic; or patients who do not meet weight requirements. Reevaluate use of the bed if patient becomes agitated or distraught. Ensure that all staff are fully trained on how to use the bed. Inform family and caregivers about the bed and reason for use.*

e. *Soft extremity (ankle or wrist) restraint:* Restraint made of soft quilted material or sheepskin with foam padding. Wrap limb restraint around wrist or ankle with soft part toward skin and secure snugly (not tightly) in place with Velcro strap (see illustration A). Insert two fingers under secured restraint (see illustration B).

May be appropriate for patients who are becoming increasingly agitated, cannot be redirected with distraction, and keep trying to remove needed medical devices. Restraint designed to immobilize one or all extremities. Tight application interferes with circulation and potentially causes neurovascular injury.

A B

STEP 4e **(A)** Extremity restraint. **(B)** Check restraint for constriction by inserting two fingers under restraint.

STEP	RATIONALE

Clinical Judgment *Patient with wrist and ankle restraints is at risk for aspiration if positioned supine. Place patient in lateral position or with head of bed elevated rather than supine.*

5. Attach restraint straps to part of bedframe that moves when raising or lowering head of bed. Be sure that straps are secure. *Do not attach to side rails.* Attach restraint to chair frame for patient in chair or wheelchair, being sure that buckle is out of patient's reach. (Exception: Freedom restraint not secured to bed frame.)

Properly positioned strap does not tighten and restrict circulation when bed is raised or lowered.

6. Secure restraints on bedframe with quick-release buckle (see illustration). Do not tie strap in a knot. Be sure that buckle is out of patient reach.

Allows for quick release in emergency.

7. Double-check and insert two fingers under secured restraint one more time. Assess proper placement of restraint, including skin integrity, pulses, skin temperature and color, and sensation of restrained body part. Raise siderails (as appropriate) and place bed in lowest position after restraint(s) applied.

Provides baseline to later evaluate if injury develops from restraint. Provides safest environment in which to leave a patient who is restrained.

8. Perform hand hygiene. Follow agency policies regarding frequency of restraint removal, monitoring and assessment, and assessment content (TJC, 2022b; CMS, 2020). More frequent monitoring may be required based on type of restraint used, cognitive status, and individual needs of the patient. Reposition patient, provide comfort and toileting measures, and evaluate patient condition each time. If patient is agitated, violent, or nonadherent, remove one restraint at a time and/or have staff assistance while removing restraints.

Provides opportunity to attend to patient's basic needs and determine need for continuation of restraints. A temporary, directly supervised release of a restraint that occurs for the purpose of caring for a patient's needs (e.g., vital signs, toileting, feeding, or range-of-motion exercises) is not considered a discontinuation of the restraint (CMS, 2020).

Clinical Judgment *Restraints cannot be ordered on an as-needed basis (PRN). If a patient was recently released from restraint and exhibits behavior that can be handled only through the reapplication of restraint or seclusion, a new order is required (CMS, 2020).*

Clinical Judgment *Do not leave a patient who is violent or aggressive unattended while restraints are off. Monitoring of violent/self-destructive patients placed in restraints and in seclusion is continuous (by way of video and audio) versus every 2 hours for nonviolent patients (CMS, 2020).*

9. Place nurse call system in an accessible location within patient's reach.

Allows patient or family caregiver to get help quickly.

10. Leave bed or chair with wheels locked. Raise side rails (as appropriate) and lower bed to lowest position, locking into position (FDA, 2017).

Prevents bed or chair from moving if patient tries to get out. If patient falls with bed in lowest position, this reduces chance of injury.

11. Remove and dispose of any supplies. Perform hand hygiene.

Reduces transmission of microorganisms.

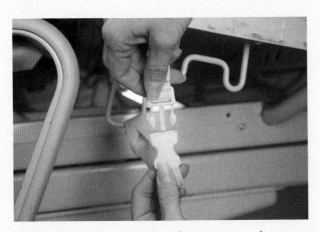

STEP 6 Quick-release buckle makes it easier to disconnect and evacuate patients in an emergency.

STEP	RATIONALE

EVALUATION

1. After restraint application, evaluate patient's response to restraints:

   a. Nonviolent patients: Conduct evaluation for signs of injury (e.g., circulation, range of motion, vital signs, skin condition), behavior and psychological status, and readiness for discontinuation (frequency based on agency policy) (TJC, 2022a; CMS, 2020).

Frequent evaluation prevents injury to patient and ensures removal of restraint at earliest possible time. Frequency of monitoring guides staff in determining appropriate intervals for evaluation based on patient's needs and condition, type of restraint used, risk associated with use of chosen intervention, and other relevant factors.

   b. Violent/self-destructive patients: Conduct same evaluation per agency policy. Perform visual checks if patient is too agitated to approach (TJC, 2022a; CMS, 2020).

Frequency of evaluation is based on patient need and situational factors (e.g., every 15 minutes, every 30 minutes, or continually).

2. Evaluate patient's need for toileting, nutrition and fluids, hygiene, and elimination, and release restraint at least every 2 hours.

Prevents injury to patient and attends to basic needs.

3. Evaluate patient for any complications of immobility.

Early detection of skin irritation, restricted breathing, or reduction in mobility prevents serious adverse events.

4. Renewal of restraints (CMS, 2020):

Ensures that restraint application continues to be medically appropriate.

   a. Nonviolent patients may have renewal of restraints based on hospital policy. However, the restraint must be discontinued at the earliest possible time, regardless of the scheduled expiration of the order.

   b. Violent/self-destructive patients may have restraints renewed within the following limits:
- 4 hours for adults 18 years of age or older
- 2 hours for children and adolescents 9 to 17 years of age
- 1 hour for children under 9 years of age

   Orders may be renewed according to the time limits for a maximum of 24 consecutive hours.

5. Observe IV catheters, urinary catheters, and drainage tubes to determine that they are positioned correctly and that therapy remains uninterrupted.

Reinsertion is uncomfortable and increases risk for infection or interrupts therapy.

6. Use Teach-Back: "We've talked about the reason we're using restraints on your father. Tell me that reason. I want to be sure you understand." Revise your instruction now or develop a plan for revised family caregiver teaching if family caregiver is not able to teach back correctly.

Teach-back is a technique for health care providers to ensure that they have explained medical information clearly so that patients and their families understand what you communicated to them (AHRQ, 2023).

Unexpected Outcomes	Related Interventions
1. Patient experiences impaired skin integrity.	• Evaluate need for continued use of restraint and if alternatives can be used. • If restraint is still needed, be sure that it is applied correctly and provide adequate padding. • Check skin under restraint for abrasions and remove restraints more often. Provide appropriate skin care and change wet or soiled restraints.
2. Patient becomes more confused or agitated.	• Determine cause of behavior and eliminate if possible; consult with health care provider. • Determine need for more or less sensory stimulation and make any stimulation meaningful. • Reorient as needed and try restraint-free options.
3. Patient has neurovascular injury (e.g., cyanosis, pallor, and coldness of skin, or patient complains of tingling, pain, or numbness).	• Remove restraint immediately, stay with patient, and have health care provider notified. • Protect extremity from further injury.

Documentation

- Document restraint alternatives used and patient's response, patient's current behavior and medical condition, level of orientation, and patient or family member's statement of understanding of the purpose of restraint and consent for application (if required by agency).
- Document placement and purpose for restraint, type and location of restraint, time applied, time restraint ended, and all routine assessments.
- Document patient's behavior after restraint application. Document times patient was assessed, attempts to use alternatives to restraint and patient's response, times restraint was released (temporarily and permanently), and patient's response when restraint was removed.
- Document evaluation of patient/family caregiver learning.

Hand-Off Reporting

- Report any injury resulting from a restraint to registered nurse in charge and health care provider immediately.
- During hand-off report, note the location and type of restraint, last time assessment was conducted, and findings.

Special Considerations

Patient Education

- Explain thoroughly to patient and family caregiver the use of restraints. Caution family caregiver against removing, repositioning, or retying restraint.

Pediatrics

- Limit the use of restraints to clinically appropriate and adequately justified situations (e.g., examination or treatment that involves the head and neck) after using all appropriate alternatives. Remain with infant while restrained and remove restraint immediately after treatment is completed.

- A staff member picking up, redirecting, or holding an infant, toddler, or preschool-age child to comfort the patient is not considered a restraint (CMS, 2020).
- When a child needs to be restrained for a procedure, it is best if the person applying the restraint is not the child's parent or guardian.
- When an infant or small child requires a restraint, a mummy wrap using a blanket or sheet effectively controls the child's movements (Hockenberry et al., 2022). Have parents stand by to support the child when the wrap is applied. Do not cover the child's face, obstruct the airway, or impair circulation.

Older Adults

- Restrained older adults are more prone to sustain adverse consequences of restraints and often respond with anger, fear, depression, humiliation, demoralization, discomfort, and resignation (de Bruijn, 2020).
- Consider the risks associated with restraints (e.g., pressure injuries, impaired strength and balance) for older adults (Touhy & Jett, 2023). All of the complications of immobility are amplified, leading to greater risk for functional decline.

Populations With Disabilities

- In general, patients who have intellectual and developmental disabilities (IDDs) can be restrained only to control behaviors that create an emergency or crisis situation.

Home Care

- Do not send a patient home with intent of restraining unless a device is necessary to protect patient from injury. If patient's family wishes to use restraints at home, a physician's order is required, and you need to give clear instructions regarding proper application, care needed while in restraints, and complications for which to observe. Carefully assess the family for competency and understanding of intent for using a restraint.

PROCEDURAL GUIDELINE 14.1 *Fire, Electrical, and Chemical Safety*

U.S. fire departments responded to an estimated 5750 structural fires in health care facilities per year from 2011 to 2015, resulting in over $50 million in property damage (National Fire Protection Association [NFPA], 2017). Almost half of the fires occurred in nursing homes, followed by mental health facilities, hospitals or hospices, and clinics or doctor's offices. Fortunately, most of the fires were very small. The leading causes of fires in health care facilities involve cooking equipment in cafeterias, electrical distribution and lighting equipment, intentional causes, and smoking materials (NFPA, 2017). Smoking-related fires pose a significant risk because of unauthorized smoking in beds or bathrooms by patients and visitors. Health care agencies routinely check and maintain all electrical devices. Every biomedical device (e.g., suction machine, infusion pump) must have a safety inspection sticker with an expiration date applied to it. Electrical equipment in good working order requires a three-prong electrical plug for proper grounding. If a patient brings an electrical device to a hospital, an engineer must inspect the device for safe wiring and function before use. Prevention is the key to fire safety. Always adhere to agency smoking policies, use equipment correctly, and keep combustible materials away from heat sources.

Chemicals in medications (e.g., chemotherapy drugs), anesthetic gases, cleaning solutions, and disinfectants are potentially toxic. They injure the body after skin or mucous membrane (e.g., eyes) contact, ingestion, or vapor inhalation. Health care agencies provide employees access to a safety data sheet (SDS) (previously called material safety data sheet) for each hazardous chemical in the workplace (Occupational Safety and Health Administration [OSHA], 2016). An SDS form contains information about the properties of each chemical and how to handle the substance safely (Box 14.3).

Delegation

The skill of fire, electrical, and chemical safety can be delegated to assistive personnel (AP). You lead the health care team in an emergency response. Direct the AP to:
- Identify patients requiring the most help to evacuate or protect
- Be aware of any risks for chemical exposure

Interprofessional Collaboration

- In the event of fire, collaborate with the fire department.
- In the event of an electrical or chemical event, the team collaborates with the safety officer of the health care agency. Knowing the location of all staff and patients is essential during these types of emergencies in case of need for evacuation.

Continued

PROCEDURAL GUIDELINE 14.1 *Fire, Electrical, and Chemical Safety—cont'd*

BOX 14.3

Information Required on OSHA Safety Data Sheets

- **Identification**—Product identifier; manufacturer or distributor name, address, phone number; emergency phone number; recommended use; restrictions on use
- **Hazard(s)**—All hazards regarding the chemical; required label element
- **Composition/information on ingredients**—Chemical ingredients; trade secret claims
- **First-aid measures**—Symptoms/effects, acute, delayed; required treatment
- **Fire-fighting measures**—Suitable extinguishing techniques, equipment; chemical hazards from fire
- **Accidental release measures**—Emergency procedures; protective equipment; proper methods of containment and cleanup
- **Handling and storage**—Precautions for safe handling and storage, including incompatibilities
- **Exposure controls/personal protection**—OSHA's Permissible Exposure Limits (PELs) and any other exposure limit used or recommended by the chemical manufacturer, importer, or employer and appropriate engineering controls; personal protective equipment (PPE)
- **Physical and chemical properties**—Lists characteristics of chemical
- **Stability and reactivity**—Lists chemical stability and possibility of hazardous reactions
- **Toxicological information**—Routes of exposure; related symptoms, acute and chronic effects; numerical measures of toxicity

OSHA, Occupational Safety and Health Administration.
Adapted from U.S. Department of Labor: *OSHA quickcard: hazard communication safety data sheets,* 2016. https://www.osha.gov/Publications/HazComm_QuickCard_SafetyData.html. Accessed November 17, 2023.

Equipment
Fire
Appropriate fire extinguisher for fire: type A, B, C, or ABC

Chemical
Appropriate personal protective equipment: clean gloves, mask, gown; SDS form; hazardous drug/chemotherapy spill kit (e.g., chemotherapy gloves, chemotherapy gown, face/eye protection, N95 respirator, and shoe covers)

Steps
1. Review agency policies for rapid response to fire, electrical, and chemical emergency. Know your responsibilities, such as initiating fire alarm and patient evacuation.
2. Know the location of fire alarms, emergency equipment (e.g., fire extinguishers), SDS forms, emergency eyewash stations, and emergency exit routes on your work unit.
3. Be alert to situations that increase the risk of fire (e.g., a patient on oxygen charging a cell phone while in bed). Regularly check patient rooms for electrical or fire hazards.

4. Know which patients are on oxygen. Oxygen delivery may be shut off in the event of a severe fire; be aware of location and who has access to the shut-off valve.
5. Inspect equipment for current maintenance sticker. Check electrical equipment for basic safety features (e.g., intact cords and plugs, intact casing). Know agency process for tagging and reporting broken or unsafe equipment.
6. Know your patient's mental status and ability to ambulate, transfer, or move so that if a fire occurs you can anticipate the procedures needed for evacuation.
7. Fire safety:
   a. Follow the acronym **RACE.**
      (1) **R**escue patient from immediate injury by removing from area or shielding from fire to avoid burns.
      (2) **A**ctivate fire alarm immediately. Follow agency policy for alerting staff to respond. In many situations perform Steps (1) and (2) simultaneously by using call system to alert staff while you help patients at risk.
      (3) **C**ontain the fire by:
         (a) Closing all doors and windows.
         (b) Turning off oxygen and electrical equipment.
         (c) Placing wet towels along base of doors.
      (4) **E**vacuate patients:
         (a) Direct ambulatory patients to walk by themselves to a safe area. Know the fire exits and emergency evacuation route.
         (b) If patient is on life support, maintain respiratory status manually (Ambu bag) until you remove patient from fire area.
         (c) Move bedridden patients by stretcher, bed, or wheelchair.
         (d) For patients who cannot walk or ambulate, use these options:
            (i) Place on blanket and drag patient out of area of danger.
            (ii) *Use two-person swing:* Place patient in sitting position and have two staff members form a seat by clasping forearms together. Lift patient into "seat" and carry out of area of danger (see illustrations).

Clinical Judgment *Consider the patient's weight and size when choosing an evacuation carry. Use safe patient-handling techniques. Have a staff member help to avoid injury.*

         (e) If fire department personnel are on the scene, they will help with evacuation of patients.
   b. Extinguish fire using appropriate fire extinguisher: **type A** for ordinary combustibles (e.g., wood, cloth, paper, most plastics), **type B** for flammable liquids (e.g., gasoline, grease, paint, anesthetic gas), **type C** for electrical equipment, **type ABC** for any type of fire (most common extinguisher in use). To use an extinguisher, follow the acronym **PASS.**
      (1) **P**ull the pin (see illustration A).
      (2) **A**im nozzle at base of fire (see illustration B).

PROCEDURAL GUIDELINE 14.1 *Fire, Electrical, and Chemical Safety—cont'd*

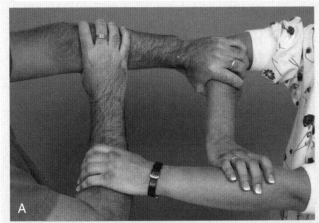

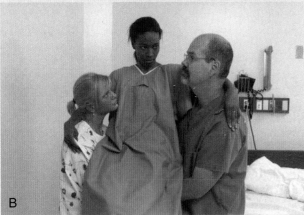

STEP 7a(4)(d)(ii) **(A)** Hands positioned to form two-person evacuation swing. **(B)** Patient seated firmly on swing and holding shoulders of nurses for evacuation.

    (3) <u>S</u>queeze extinguisher handles (see illustration C).
    (4) <u>S</u>weep from side to side to coat area evenly.
  c. Most agencies have fire doors that are held open by magnets and close automatically when a fire alarm sounds. Fire doors should never be blocked.
8. Once patient has been evacuated, make the patient comfortable. Keep locks on wheelchairs or beds locked. Perform hand hygiene.
9. Electrical safety:
  a. If patient receives an electrical shock, immediately turn off power to electrical source and assess for presence of a pulse. *Caution:* When disengaging electrical source, check for presence of water on floor.

Clinical Judgment *Do not touch a person who is being shocked while still engaged with the electrical source. If unable to turn off power, call agency emergency number for help.*

  b. Once the source of electricity is disconnected, provide appropriate assistance. If patient is pulseless, institute emergency resuscitation (see Chapter 25).
  c. Notify emergency personnel and patient's health care provider.

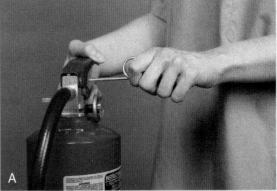

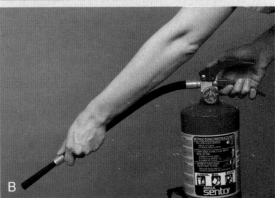

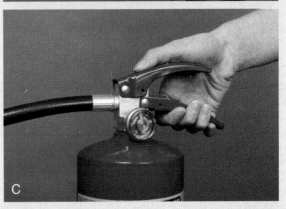

STEP 7b(1–3) **(A)** Pull safety pin from fire extinguisher. **(B)** Aim nozzle of hose at base of fire. **(C)** Squeeze handle while sweeping side to side with nozzle.

  d. If patient has a pulse and remains alert and oriented, obtain vital signs and assess the skin for signs of thermal injury.
10. Chemical safety for liquid hazardous drugs (HD):
  a. Refer to health care agency specific policies and/or SDS when cleaning up an HD spill. Obtain an HD spill kit if available. Commercially available HD/chemotherapy spill kits typically include two pairs of chemotherapy gloves; chemoresistant gown and shoe covers; absorbent pads; scoop, brush, and puncture-proof container for collecting glass fragments; goggles and respirator masks; hazardous waste disposal bags; and labels for bags (Oncology Nursing Society [ONS, 2018]).

Continued

PROCEDURAL GUIDELINE 14.1 *Fire, Electrical, and Chemical Safety—cont'd*

  b. If you or a work colleague are exposed to an HD/chemotherapy drug (ONS, 2018):

    (1) Remove both sets of contaminated gloves and/or clothing immediately.

    (2) Dispose of gloves and clothing in hazardous drug waste bag for placement in a container designated for hazardous drugs.

    (3) Wash hands thoroughly with soap and water for at least 15 minutes.

    (4) If contamination of skin or eyes is suspected, seek medical attention as soon as possible.

    (5) Treat chemical splashes to the eyes immediately. Flush eyes with water using clean, lukewarm tap water for 15 to 20 minutes. Remove contact lenses if flushing does not remove them (see Chapter 19).

    (6) Treat skin exposure by standing under a shower or place exposed area under faucet with running lukewarm tap water for 15 to 20 minutes.

  c. Notify people in the immediate area of a spill and evacuate all nonessential personnel from area.

  d. Refer to SDS; if spilled material is flammable, turn off electrical and heat sources.

  e. Avoid breathing vapors of spilled material; apply appropriate respirator.

  f. Dispose of any materials used in cleanup as hazardous waste.

11. Documentation: Usually made as a sentinel event report and not in electronic health record (EHR).

12. Hand-off reporting; follow agency policy for reporting a sentinel event.

✦ SKILL 14.4   Seizure Precautions

A seizure is a sudden, abnormal, electrical discharge in the brain causing alterations in behavior, sensation, or consciousness. Anything that interrupts the normal connections between neurons in the brain can cause a seizure, including a high fever, low blood sugar, high blood sugar, alcohol or drug withdrawal, or a brain concussion (Johns Hopkins Medicine, n.d.). Anyone can have one or more seizures; however, a person who has two or more seizures over 24 hours is considered to have epilepsy (Sawaf et al., 2023). The two broad categories of epileptic seizures are generalized seizures (involving both sides of the brain) and focal/ partial seizures (involving one or more areas of one side of the brain) (Box 14.4). Status epilepticus is a neurological and medical emergency defined as 5 or more minutes of either continuous seizure activity or repetitive seizures with no intervening recovery of consciousness (Cruickshank, 2022). It is a medical and neurological emergency requiring prompt treatment (Drislane, 2022). Status epilepticus can be convulsive (shown by rhythmic jerking of the extremities) or nonconvulsive (seizure activity shown on an electroencephalogram [EEG]). The National Institute for Health and Care Excellence (NICE) released practice guidelines for patients with status epilepticus (NICE, 2022). Within the first 2 minutes, establishing and protecting the airway when a patient loses consciousness is a priority. Noninvasive airway protection and gas exchange with head positioning should be done immediately, keeping the airway patent and administering oxygen. Intubation (insertion of an artificial airway) is attempted only if gas exchange is compromised, if seizures last 30 minutes or more, or if urgent brain imaging is needed (Drislane, 2022). Seizure precautions are guidelines that health care providers follow to minimize injury to a patient during any type of seizure. Observation during a seizure is critical.

Delegation

The skill of assessing a patient's risk for seizures cannot be delegated to assistive personnel (AP). However, the interventions for making a patient's environment safe and the ongoing care of patients on seizure precautions can be delegated. Instruct the AP about:

- The patient's prior seizure history and factors that may trigger a seizure

---

BOX 14.4

Possible Precipitating Factors or Causes for Seizures

Acute Processes

- Photosensitivity (e.g., flashing lights, video games)
- Metabolic disturbances: electrolyte abnormalities, hypoglycemia, renal failure
- Sepsis
- Central nervous system (CNS) infection: meningitis, encephalitis, abscess
- Stroke: ischemic, intracerebral, or subarachnoid hemorrhage; cerebral sinus thrombosis
- Head trauma with or without epidural or subdural hematoma
- Drug issues/toxicity: withdrawal from opioid, benzodiazepine, barbiturate, or alcohol; nonadherence with antiepileptic drug (AED) regimen
- Hypoxia, cardiac arrest
- Encephalopathy

Chronic Processes

- Preexisting epilepsy: breakthrough seizures or discontinuation of AEDs
- Chronic alcohol abuse; ethanol intoxication or withdrawal
- CNS tumors

Factors in Children

- Prolonged febrile seizures are the most frequent cause of status epilepticus in children
- CNS infections, especially bacterial meningitis, inborn errors of metabolism, and ingestion are frequent causes of status epilepticus

Adapted from Brophy GM, et al: Guidelines for the evaluation and management of status epilepticus. *Neurocrit Care* 17(1):3, 2012; Lesser RP, Johnson E: Status epilepticus. *BMJ Best Pract* 2018. https://bestpractice.bmj.com/topics/en-us/464. Accessed November 17, 2023.

- Taking immediate action in the event of a seizure by protecting the patient from falling or injury
- Not restraining the patient or placing anything into patient's mouth
- Informing the nurse immediately when seizure activity develops
- Observing the patient's behaviors during a seizure

Interprofessional Collaboration

- All health care providers should be aware of patient being placed on seizure precautions.

Equipment

- Seizure pads for side rails and headboard
- Suction machine, oral Yankauer suction catheter, oral airway (see Chapter 24)
- Oxygen via nasal cannula or face mask
- Equipment for vital signs (VS), pulse oximetry, and blood glucose testing (see Chapters 5 and 7)
- Equipment for intravenous (IV) line insertion (see Chapter 28); bag of 0.9% normal saline solution
- Emergency antiepileptic medications (NICE, 2022):
  - Status epilepticus seizures (Drislane, 2022):
    - Initial therapy (given within the first 5 minutes): benzodiazepine (lorazepam, midazolam, diazepam)

- Second therapy: nonbenzodiazepine (e.g., levetiracetam, fosphenytoin, phenytoin, valproate)
- Epileptic seizures (Nevitt et al., 2022):
  - First-line treatment (tried first and usually used on its own):
    - Focal/partial seizure—carbamazepine, lamotrigine
    - Generalized seizures—sodium valproate, lamotrigine
  - Alternative first-line treatment (added to a first-line treatment [so are used in combination]):
    - Focal/partial seizure: levetiracetam, oxcarbazepine, sodium valproate
    - Generalized seizures—carbamazepine, oxcarbazepine
- Clean gloves
- *Option:* Protective headgear

STEP	RATIONALE

ASSESSMENT

1. Identify patient using at least two identifiers (e.g., name and birthday or name and medical record number) according to agency policy.

2. Review electronic health record (EHR) for medical and surgical conditions that may contribute to or be a cause of a seizure (see Box 14.4) and for any bleeding tendencies.

3. Assess EHR for patient's seizure history (e.g., new diagnosis, seizure within last year), previous precipitating factors (see Box 14.4), frequency of seizures, presence and type of aura (e.g., reduced vision, visual illusions, noises, metallic taste, noxious odor) (Sawaf et al., 2023), symptoms during a seizure, and phases of seizure events known (Box 14.5). Use a family caregiver as resource if needed.

Ensures patient safety. Complies with The Joint Commission standards and improves patient safety (TJC, 2023).

Common conditions that lead to seizures or worsen existing seizure condition. Bleeding conditions predispose patient to injury during a seizure.

Allows you to eliminate triggers that can cause seizure, anticipate onset of seizure activity, and take appropriate safety precautions.

BOX 14.5

Phases of a Seizure

- Aura—The start of a partial seizure. If an aura is the only phase a patient experiences, the patient has had a simple partial seizure. If the seizure spreads and affects consciousness, it is a complete partial seizure. If the seizure spreads to the rest of the brain, it is a generalized seizure.

- Ictus—"Attack." Ictus is another word for the physical seizure involving a series of muscle contractions, called tonic and clonic contractions.
- Postictal—After the attack. Postictal refers to the aftereffects of a seizure (e.g., arm numbness, altered consciousness, partial paralysis, loss of memory).

STEP	RATIONALE

4. Assess patient's/family caregiver's health literacy.

5. Assess medication history (e.g., antidepressants and antipsychotics). Ask patient to describe schedule used to adhere to anticonvulsants and review therapeutic drug levels if laboratory test results available.

6. Inspect patient's environment for potential safety hazards (e.g., extra furniture or equipment). Keep bed in low position with side rails up at head of bed (FDA, 2017).

Determines degree to which individuals have the ability to find, understand, and use information and services to make informed health-related decisions and actions for themselves and others (CDC, 2023).

Certain medications lower seizure threshold. Seizure medications must be taken as prescribed and not stopped suddenly; doing otherwise may precipitate seizure activity. Nonadherence to seizure medication regimen is associated with increased risk of premature death (NICE, 2022).

Protects patient from injury sustained by striking head or body on furniture or equipment.

STEP	RATIONALE
7. Assess patient's individual and cultural perspective about the meaning of seizures/epilepsy and treatment.	Research has shown that in low- and middle-income countries, traditional beliefs about the causes of epilepsy lead to stigma; people may not be aware that their seizures can be prevented with medications and therefore seek help through alternative drugs or healers (Espinosa-Jovel et al., 2018).
8. Assess patient's knowledge, prior experience with seizure precautions, and feelings about these measures.	Reveals need for patient instruction and/or support.

PLANNING

1. Expected outcomes following completion of procedure:	
• Patient remains free of traumatic injury while experiencing seizure.	Seizure precautions prevent patients from incurring injury from a fall or seizure.
• Patient's airway remains patent during seizure activity.	Airway occlusion and aspiration are potential complications of seizure activity.
• Patient does not experience lowered sense of self-esteem following seizure episode.	Loss of bowel or bladder control is common in generalized seizures, causing patient to feel embarrassed.
• Patient or family caregiver can identify triggers that lead to patient having a seizure.	Knowledge can help in preventing seizure activity.
2. Perform hand hygiene and prepare equipment.	Reduces transmission of microorganisms.
3. Be sure patient is in a comfortable position. Reduce lighting in room and try to control for any sudden, loud, unexpected noise.	Startle seizures are most often precipitated by an unexpected stimulus such as a fire alarm or car backfiring (National Epilepsy Training, 2019).
4. Inform patient and appropriate family caregiver that patient is on seizure precautions and what these precautions entail. Discuss the possible triggers that result in patient's seizure activity. Include discussion of approaches to adopt seizure precautions in the patient's home environment.	May help to relieve patient and family caregiver anxiety and aid in their participation in patient care.

IMPLEMENTATION

STEP	RATIONALE
1. For patients with history of seizures, keep bed in lowest position with side rails up (see agency policy). Pad rails if patient is at risk for head injury and, as an option, offer protective headgear. Have oral suction and oxygen equipment ready for use.	Modifications to environment minimize risk of injury from seizure activity or related fall. Use padded side rails and headgear only when patient is at risk for head injury (see illustration).

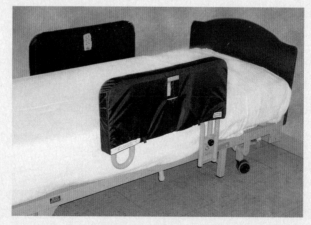

STEP 1 Padded side rails for patients at risk for head injury.

Clinical Judgment *When a patient is placed on seizure precautions and all side rails are raised, the use of side rails would not be considered restraint. The use of padded side rails in this situation should protect the patient from harm, including falling out of bed should the patient have a seizure (CMS, 2020).*

2. Place patient with history of seizures in room close to nurse's station or room with video monitor (if available).	Improves likelihood of quick identification of seizure and response with emergency equipment.

STEP	RATIONALE
3. Focal/partial or general seizure response: **a.** Position patient safely.	Position protects patient from aspiration and traumatic injury, especially head injury.
(1) Guide a patient who is standing or sitting to the floor, and protect head by cradling in your lap or place pillow under head. Position patient so as to keep head tilted to maximize breathing (if able). Try to position patient on side *but do not force*. Do not lift patient from floor to bed during seizure.	
(2) If in bed, turn patient onto side *(do not force)* and raise side rails.	
b. Note time the seizure began. Stay with patient and call for help immediately to have staff member bring emergency cart to bedside and clear surrounding area of furniture. Provide airway protection and gas exchange by positioning head. Have health care provider and Rapid Response Team notified immediately.	Initial management requires immediate supportive care to maintain ABCs (airway, breathing, circulation) and prompt administration of antiseizure medications (Drislane, 2022).

Clinical Judgment *Activate your agency's Rapid Response Team. When a patient demonstrates signs of imminent clinical deterioration, a team of providers is summoned to the bedside to immediately assess and treat the patient with the goal of preventing intensive care unit transfer, cardiac arrest, or death (AHRQ, 2019b).*

STEP	RATIONALE
c. Keep patient in side-lying position (if possible), supporting head and keeping it flexed slightly forward.	Position prevents tongue from blocking airway and promotes drainage of secretions, reducing risk of aspiration.
d. Do not restrain patient; if patient is flailing limbs, hold them loosely. Loosen restrictive clothing/gown to aid breathing.	Prevents musculoskeletal injury. Promotes free ventilatory movement of chest and abdomen.
e. *Never force any object into patient's mouth* such as fingers, medicine, tongue depressor, or airway when teeth are clenched.	Prevents injury to mouth and possible aspiration.

Clinical Judgment *Injury can result from forcible insertion of a hard object into the mouth. Soft objects break and become aspirated. Insert a bite block or oral airway in advance if you recognize the possibility of a generalized seizure.*

STEP	RATIONALE
f. If possible, provide privacy. Have staff control flow of visitors in area.	Embarrassment is common after a seizure, especially if others witnessed it.
g. Observe sequence and timing of seizure activity. Note type of seizure activity (tonic, clonic, staring, blinking); whether more than one type of seizure occurs; sequence of seizure progression; level of consciousness; character of breathing; presence of incontinence; presence of autonomic signs of lip smacking, mastication, or grimacing; and rolling of eyes.	Continued observation helps to document, diagnose, and treat seizure disorder.
h. As patient regains consciousness, assess VS, reorient, and reassure. Explain what happened and answer patient's questions. Stay with patient until fully awake.	Informing patients of type of seizure activity experienced helps them to participate knowledgeably in their care. Some patients remain confused for a period of time after seizure or become violent.
4. Status epilepticus is a medical and neurological emergency.	
a. Follow Steps 3a to 3e to protect patient, and call Rapid Response Team.	Ensures rapid management of airway and breathing.
b. Assist health care provider with oropharyngeal or nasopharyngeal airway insertion (see Chapter 24) if oxygen saturation is compromised or if seizure lasts ≥30 minutes. (**NOTE:** Apply clean gloves if timing allows.) Physician on team will intubate patient when jaw is relaxed (between seizure activity).	Airway establishes oxygenation (Drislane, 2022).
c. Access and administer oxygen; turn on suction equipment; keep airway patent with oral suctioning (if possible).	Maintains oxygenation.

STEP	RATIONALE

Clinical Judgment *Never place hands in patient's mouth during a seizure. The patient may accidentally bite your fingers. Do not force any type of airway into mouth.*

d. Have another nurse on team measure blood pressure, heart rate, respirations, and oxygen saturation immediately and then every 2 minutes, and have team member perform fingerstick to check blood glucose (Sawaf et al., 2023).	Necessary to monitor and support baseline VS and determine if patient is hypoglycemic (common cause of seizure).
e. Member of team will prepare for and insert IV catheter (if one is not in place) with 0.9% sodium chloride infusing and administer IV antiseizure medications (see Chapter 22).	Provides route for IV medication to stop seizure, for fluid resuscitation, and to collect samples for electrolytes, hematology, toxicology screen, and anticonvulsant levels (Sawaf et al., 2023).
f. As seizure subsides, suction patient's airway if secretions have accumulated. If oral airway was inserted, be sure that it remains in correct position (see Chapter 24). Continue oxygen administration.	Maintains open airway, decreases chance of aspiration, and promotes oxygenation.
g. Keep patient in side-lying position of comfort in bed with side rails up and bed in lowest position and locked in place (FDA, 2017).	Provides for continued safety to reduce risk of aspiration of secretions as patient regains consciousness and lessens risk of fall with injury if patient tries to exit bed.
5. As patient regains consciousness, reorient and reassure. Explain what happened and provide quiet, nonstimulating environment (e.g., lights low, minimal care interruptions).	Provides for continued safety. Patients are often confused and lethargic following seizure (postictal). Patients are at risk for falls if they attempt to get out of bed.
6. Place nurse call system in an accessible location within patient's reach. Instruct patient not to get out of bed without help.	Ensures patient can call for assistance if needed.
7. Clean up patient care area; remove and dispose of gloves and used supplies. Perform hand hygiene.	Reduces transmission of microorganisms.

EVALUATION

1. Check VS and oxygen saturation every 15 minutes during postictal phase and maintain patent airway.	Determines patient's cardiopulmonary status and response to seizure episode.
2. Recheck blood glucose per health care provider order or agency protocol.	Determines if normal blood glucose level has been reached.
3. Examine patient for injury, including oral cavity (broken teeth, laceration of tongue or mucosa) and extremities.	Determines presence of any traumatic injuries resulting from seizure activity.

Clinical Judgment *If onset of seizure was not witnessed and you suspect that patient fell and struck head, treat as a closed head injury or spinal injury. Place a cervical collar on patient before attempting to turn or reposition. If patient is on anticoagulants, there is a high risk of intracranial bleeding if head injury occurred.*

4. Evaluate patient's mental status after seizure (level of consciousness, confusion, hallucinations). Encourage patient to verbalize feelings and describe an awareness of seizure triggers.	Temporary mental status changes are common following seizure. Therapeutic interaction enables patient to recognize feelings associated with having a seizure disorder and minimizes lowering of self-esteem.
5. Assist health care provider while conducting thorough neurological examination of patient and collect any ordered blood test specimens (see Chapter 7).	Evaluates for any head trauma and life-threatening metabolic condition (Sawaf et al., 2023).
6. **After return to level of consciousness where patient can be attentive, use Teach-Back:** "We talked about what your family should do if you have a seizure at home. Tell me what steps you would take (include family caregiver)." Revise your instruction now or develop a plan for revised patient/family caregiver teaching if patient/family caregiver is not able to teach back correctly.	Teach-back is a technique for health care providers to ensure that they have explained medical information clearly so that patients and their families understand what you communicated to them (AHRQ, 2023).

Unexpected Outcomes	Related Interventions
1. Patient sustains traumatic injury.	• Continue to protect patient from further injury. • Notify health care provider immediately. • Administer prescribed treatments. • Reassess patient's environment and eliminate any safety hazards. • Complete agency occurrence report.
2. Patient aspirates oral secretions.	• Turn onto side, insert oral airway, and apply suction to remove material in oral pharynx and maintain patent airway (see Chapter 24). • Administer oxygen as needed per order.

Documentation

- Document what you observed before, during, and after seizure by providing a detailed description of the type of seizure activity and sequence of events (e.g., presence of aura [if any], level of consciousness, VS and oxygen saturation, color, movement of extremities, incontinence, patient's status immediately following seizure, and time frame of events).
- Document treatments administered for the seizure, establishment of IV line, fluid infusing, and stabilization of airway.
- Document evaluation of patient/family caregiver learning.

Hand-Off Reporting

- When a patient has had a seizure, report to oncoming staff a detailed description of seizure and patient's response to therapy.
- Alert health care provider immediately as seizure begins. Status epilepticus is an emergency situation requiring immediate medical therapy.

Special Considerations

Patient Education

- Ensure that patients and caregivers understand that epilepsy is synonymous with seizure disorder and other culturally appropriate terms. This helps optimize adherence with treatment, disease management instructions, and use of other resources targeted at persons with epilepsy.
- Education and awareness campaigns aimed at improving access to care, reducing stigma, and increasing awareness of adverse events, such as sudden unexpected death from epilepsy (SUDEP), should include a more diverse definition of epilepsy in their messages (Epilepsy Foundation, 2019).
- Encourage patients to keep diaries of when seizures happen to help show if there is a pattern to a patient's seizures and whether any situations trigger the seizures (like being tired or stressed). A diary might also be useful to see how well medication is working to control seizures (Epilepsy Foundation, 2022).
- Inform patients that they should never stop medications suddenly because this precipitates seizures or could cause withdrawal symptoms (Epilepsy Foundation, n.d.b).
- Advise patients to confer with a health care provider about concerns with their seizure medications. Nonadherence to anticonvulsant regimens is a leading cause of breakthrough seizures (Sawaf et al., 2023).
- Advise patients to avoid alcohol, which is often incompatible with anticonvulsive medications and intensifies central nervous system depression.
- Inform patients with epilepsy to discuss with a pharmacist or health care provider before taking any over-the-counter medications that may cause seizures or interact with seizure medications (Epilepsy Foundation, n.d.c).
- Advise patients who take hormonal contraceptives or hormone replacement medications that some antiseizure medications can impair their effectiveness (NICE, 2022).
- Proper oral hygiene and frequent dental care are necessary when patient takes phenytoin long-term because gingival hyperplasia is a side effect.
- Encourage patient to wear a medical alert bracelet or carry identification card noting presence of seizure disorder and listing medications taken.
- Fatigue, stress, and illness can potentiate seizures. Teach patients to eat a balanced diet regularly, get adequate sleep, and consult their health care provider promptly when ill.
- A seizure disorder usually imposes driving limitations. It is recommended that a waiting period of 1 seizure-free year elapse before patient attempts to drive or operate dangerous equipment (see individual state law).

Pediatrics

- Teach parents what to observe in their child's seizure.
- Encourage children with severe atonic seizures (abrupt loss of muscle tone, often dropping to floor) to wear helmets to protect them when they fall.
- The Epilepsy Foundation (n.d.a) offers tips on keeping children with epilepsy safe. These tips include:
  - Have your child take medication as prescribed at the same times every day. Use alarms, schedules, or pill boxes to help.
  - Make sure your child gets enough sleep to help lower the risk for seizures.
  - Encourage parents to make a seizure action plan. This helps organize seizure information and tells others (e.g., teachers, coaches, babysitter) what to do when a seizure occurs.
  - Maximize their social, physical, and psychological well-being while maintaining safety. Limiting normal childhood activities such as sports and getting together with friends fosters low self-esteem and can do more harm than good. Always make sure a responsible adult knows what to do if a seizure happens.
  - Set clear rules and limits. Some activities can be dangerous for children, especially those whose seizures are not well controlled. Never swim alone; wear appropriate safety gear when riding a bike or when participating in a sport; play, ride, or exercise with a buddy when possible.

Older Adults

- Older adults often have symptoms that make it difficult to recognize a seizure disorder. Confusion lasting several days, receptive and expressive speech problems, and unusual behaviors are often the result of a seizure.
- Older adults metabolize some antiseizure medications more slowly, allowing drugs to accumulate and possibly result in toxicity. Consult a pharmacist for specific information.
- If patient has dentures, do not try to remove them during a seizure. If they loosen, tilt head slightly forward and remove after seizure.

Home Care

- Instruct family caregiver about steps to take when patient experiences a seizure.
- Assess patient's home for environmental hazards that could increase the risk of injury in the event of a fall.
- Assist family to eliminate any sources of triggers in the home that are unique to precipitating a patient's seizures.
- Until a seizure condition is well controlled (usually for at least 1 year), make sure that patient does not take a tub bath or engage in activities such as swimming unless a knowledgeable family member is present.
- Refer patient to the Epilepsy Foundation or a community resource for support groups.

♦ CLINICAL JUDGMENT AND NEXT-GENERATION NCLEX® EXAMINATION–STYLE QUESTIONS

The night-shift nurse is caring for an 85-year-old woman with mild dementia. During hourly rounding, the nurse finds the patient lying on the bathroom floor, incontinent of urine. She is rubbing her hip but is not crying or groaning in pain. She says, "I just got a little confused when I was going to the bathroom, and I fell. I think I'm alright." The patient has a history of cancer, type 2 diabetes, and hypertension. She is scheduled for chemotherapy in the morning and also is taking a biguanide drug, an antihypertensive drug, and a diuretic drug.

1. Complete the following sentence by selecting from the list of word choices below.

   The nurse must first address the patient's **1 [Select]** followed by the patient's **2 [Select]**.

Options for 1	Options for 2
Blood pressure	Hip
Cognitive status	Urinary status
Oxygen saturation	Blood glucose level

2. Once the patient is stabilized, the nurse reevaluates precautions that can reduce the risk for falls. Which intervention will the nurse plan to institute at this time?
   1. Provide a sitter in the room to keep patient in bed.
   2. Place in a geri chair to continuously monitor.
   3. Apply a hip protector to pad the area in case of falls.
   4. Request order to give diuretic in the morning.

3. The next morning, the patient is observed walking down the hallway and attempting to enter the supply room. The nurse puts additional precautions into place. Which of the following tasks will be delegated to assistive personnel (AP)? **Select all that apply.**
   1. Determine the patient's level of orientation.
   2. Place a pad alarm device onto the patient's chair.
   3. Report if patient tries to get out of bed without assistance.
   4. Select type of restraint-free intervention to use.
   5. Use music as a diversion for patient.

4. The patient's daughter visits that evening. Which question will the nurse **prioritize** when talking with the daughter about ways to keep the patient safe?
   1. What is the patient's usual communication style?
   2. Does the patient have a specific bedtime routine?
   3. Have you noticed cues that indicate the patient is hungry?
   4. What activities did the patient enjoy doing at home?

5. The next day, the patient will receive chemotherapy. While preparing the chemotherapy, the nurse notes that a portion of the liquid medication is spilled on the floor. Which action will the nurse take **first**?
   1. Obtain spill kit.
   2. Remove both sets of gloves immediately.
   3. Wash hands thoroughly with soap and water for 15 minutes.
   4. If contamination of skin is suspected, seek medical attention.

Visit the Evolve site for Answers to the Clinical Judgment and Next-Generation NCLEX® Examination–Style Questions.

REFERENCES

Aboumatar HJ, et al: Promising practices for achieving patient-centered hospital care: a national study of high-performing US hospitals, *Med Care* 53(9): 758–767, 2015.

Agency for Healthcare Research and Quality (AHRQ): *Preventing falls in hospitals: a tookit for improving quality of care*, Rockville, MD, 2013, AHRQ. https://www.ahrq.gov/professionals/systems/hospital/fallpxtoolkit/fallpxtk3.html#3-2. Accessed November 17, 2023.

Agency for Healthcare Research and Quality (AHRQ): *Culture of safety*, 2019a. https://psnet.ahrq.gov/primers/primer/5/Culture-of-Safety. Accessed November 28, 2023.

Agency for Healthcare Research and Quality (AHRQ): *Rapid response systems*, 2019b. https://psnet.ahrq.gov/primers/primer/4/rapid-response-systems. Accessed November 17, 2023.

Agency for Healthcare Research and Quality (AHRQ): *Teach-Back: intervention*, 2023. https://www.ahrq.gov/patient-safety/reports/engage/interventions/teachback.html.

Agrawal A, et al: Approach to management of wandering in dementia: ethical and legal issues, *Indian J Psychol Med* 43(Suppl 5):S53, 2021.

Alzheimer's Association: *Alzheimer's disease facts and figures*, 2023a. https://www.alz.org/media/Documents/alzheimers-facts-and-figures.pdf. Accessed March 2023.

Alzheimer's Association: *Cognitive assessment tools*, 2023b. https://www.alz.org/professionals/health-systems-medical-professionals/clinical-resources/cognitive-assessment-tools. Accessed March 2023.

American Geriatrics Society (AGS): *For older people, medications are common; updated AGS Beers Criteria® Aims to Make Sure They're Appropriate, Too*, 2019. https://www.americangeriatrics.org/media-center/news/older-people-medications-are-common-updated-ags-beers-criteriar-aims-make-sure. Accessed November 17, 2023.

American Nurses Association (ANA) Center for Ethics and Human Rights: *ANA position statement: the ethical use of restraints: balancing dual nursing duties of patient safety and personal safety*, 2020. https://www.nursingworld.org/~48f80d/globalassets/practiceandpolicy/nursing-excellence/ana-position-statements/nursing-practice/restraints-position-statement.pdf. Accessed November 17, 2023.

Asai T, et al: The association between fear of falling and occurrence of falls: a one-year cohort study, *BMC Geriatr* 22:393, 2022.

Bargmann A, Brundrett S: Implementation of a multicomponent fall prevention program: contacting with patients for fall safety, *Mil Med* 185(Suppl 2):28–34, 2020.

Berry S, Kiel D: Falls: prevention in nursing care facilities and the hospital setting, 2022. *UpToDate*. https://www.uptodate.com/contents/falls-prevention-in-nursing-care-facilities-and-the-hospital-setting?search5falls-prevention-in-nursing-care-facilities-and-the-hospital-setting.%20Accessed%20July%209&source5search_result&selectedTitle53,150&usage_type5default&display_rank53. Accessed November 17, 2023.

Betancourt J, et al: The patient's culture and effective communication, *UpToDate*, 2021. https://www.uptodate.com/contents/cross-cultural-care-and-communication. Accessed November 17, 2023.

Boltz M, et al: *Evidence-based geriatric nursing protocols for best practice*, ed 6, New York, 2020, Springer.

Caffier D, et al: Do older people accurately estimate the length of their first step during gait initiation? *Exp Aging Res* 45(4):357–371, 2019.

Callis N: Falls prevention: identification of predictive fall risk factors, *Appl Nurs Res* 29:53–58, 2016.

Centers for Disease Control and Prevention (CDC): *The timed up and go test (TUG)*, 2017. https://www.cdc.gov/steadi/pdf/TUG_Test-print.pdf. Accessed November 17, 2023.

Centers for Disease Control and Prevention (CDC): *STEADI—Older adult fall prevention*, 2021. https://www.cdc.gov/steadi/index.html. Accessed November 17, 2023.

Centers for Disease Control and Prevention (CDC): *What is health literacy?* 2023. https://www.cdc.gov/healthliteracy/learn/index.html.

Centers for Medicare and Medicaid Services (CMS): *Survey protocol, regulations, and interpretive guidelines for hospitals*, 2020. https://www.cms.gov/Regulations-and-Guidance/Guidance/Manuals/downloads/som107ap_a_hospitals.pdf. Accessed March 2023.

Chen Y, et al: Hospital-associated deconditioning: not only physical but cognitive, *Int J Geriatr Psychiatry* 37(3):1–13, 2022.

Chinai SA, et al: Taking advantage of the teachable moment: a review of learner-centered clinical teaching models, *West J Emerg Med* 19(1):28–34, 2018.

Chiu AS, et al: Recurrent falls among elderly patients and the impact of anticoagulation therapy, *World J Surg* 42(12):3932–3938, 2018.

Cruickshank M, et al: *Pre-hospital and emergency department treatment of convulsive status epilepticus in adults: an evidence synthesis.* Southampton (UK), 2022, NIHR Journals Library. (Health Technology Assessment, No. 26.20.) Available from: https://www.ncbi.nlm.nih.gov/books/NBK579010/.

Dani M, et al: Orthostatic hypotension in older people: considerations, diagnosis and management, *Clin Med* 21(3):e275–e282, 2021.

de Bruijn W, et al: Physical and pharmacological restraints in hospital care: protocol for a systematic review, *Front Psychiatry* 10:921, 2020.

Devlin J, et al: Clinical practice guidelines for the prevention and management of pain, agitation/sedation, delirium, immobility, and sleep disruption in adult patients in the ICU, *Crit Care Med J* 46(9):e825–e873, 2018.

Dabkowski E, et al: Adult inpatients' perceptions of their fall risk: a scoping review. *Healthcare* 10(6):995, 2022.

Drislane FW: Convulsive status epilepticus in adults: management, 2022, UpToDate, http://www.uptodate.com/contents/convulsive-status-epilepticus-in-adults-management#H232906673. Accessed November 17, 2023.

Dykes PC, et al: Evaluation of a patient-centered fall prevention tool kit to reduce falls and injuries: a nonrandomized controlled trial. *JAMA Netw Open* 3(11):e2025889, 2020. doi:10.1001/jamanetworkopen.2020.25889.

Dykes PC, Hurley AC: Patient-centered fall prevention, *Nurs Manage* 52(3):51–54, 2021.

Epilepsy Foundation: *Epilepsy for parents and caregivers: kids*, n.d.a. https://www.epilepsy.com/parents-and-caregivers/kids. Accessed November 17, 2023.

Epilepsy Foundation: *Missed medicines as a seizure trigger*, n.d.b. https://www.epilepsy.com/what-is-epilepsy/seizure-triggers/missed-medicines. Accessed November 17, 2023.

Epilepsy Foundation: *Over counter medications and epilepsy*, n.d.c. https://www.epilepsy.com/what-is-epilepsy/seizure-triggers/over-counter-medications. Accessed November 17, 2023.

Epilepsy Foundation: *Sudden Unexpected Death from Epilepsy (SUDEP)*, 2019. https://www.epilepsy.com/learn/early-death-and-sudep/sudep. Accessed November 17, 2023.

Epilepsy Foundation: *Using seizure diaries*, https://www.epilepsy.com/ living-epilepsy/epilepsy-foundation-my-seizure-diary. Accessed November 17, 2023.

Espinosa-Jovel C, et al: Epidemiological profile of epilepsy in low income populations, *Seizure* 56:67–72, 2018.

Fehlberg EA, et al: Impact of the CMS no-pay policy on hospital-acquired fall prevention related practice patterns, *Innov Aging* 1(3):igx036, 2017.

Gliner M, et al: Patient falls, nurse communication and hourly rounding in acute care: linking patient experience and outcomes, *J Public Health Manag Pract* 28(2):e462–e470, 2022. doi:10.1097/PHH.0000000000001387.

Greenberg SA: *The 2019 American Geriatrics Society Updated Beers Criteria® for Potentially Inappropriate Medication Use in Older Adults*, (16), 2019. https://hign.org/sites/default/files/2020-06/Try_This_General_Assessment_16.pdf. Accessed November 17, 2023.

Harris JL: Enclosure bed: a protective and calming restraint, *Am Nurse Today*, 10(1):30–31, 2015. https://myamericannurse.com/wp-content/uploads/2015/01/ant1-Restraints-1218-ENCLOSURE.pdf. Accessed November 17, 2023.

Health Research and Educational Trust (HRET): *Preventing patient falls: a systematic approach from the Joint Commission Center for Transforming Healthcare project*, Chicago, IL, 2016, Health Research and Educational Trust (HRET). http://www.hpoe.org/Reports-HPOE/2016/preventing-patient-falls.pdf. Accessed November 17, 2023.

Hicks C, et al: Reduced strength, poor balance and concern about falls mediate the relationship between knee pain and fall risk in older people, *BMC Geriatr* 20(94):1–8, 2020.

Hockenberry MJ, et al: *Wong's essentials of pediatric nursing*, ed 11, St. Louis, 2022, Mosby.

Hoffman RS, Weinhouse GL: Management of moderate and severe alcohol withdrawal syndromes, 2023, *UpToDate*. https://www.uptodate.com/contents/management-of-moderate-and-severe-alcohol-withdrawal-syndromes. Accessed November 17, 2023.

Institute for Healthcare Improvement (IHI): *The ABCs of reducing harm from falls*, 2017. http://www.ihi.org/resources/Pages/ImprovementStories/ABCsofReducingHarmfromFalls.aspx. Accessed November 17, 2023.

Institute for Patient- and Family-Centered Care (IPFCC): *Patient-and-family-centered care*, n.d. Ipfcc.org/about/pfcc.html. Accessed November 17, 2023.

International Council of Nurses (ICN): *The ICN code of ethics for nurses*, 2021. https://www.icn.ch/sites/default/files/2023-06/ICN_Code-of-Ethics_EN_Web.pdf. Accessed November 17, 2023.

Johns Hopkins Medicine: *Seizures*, https://www.hopkinsmedicine.org/health/conditions-and-diseases/epilepsy. Accessed November 17, 2023.

Jones KJ, et al: Evaluation of automated video monitoring to decrease the risk of unattended bed exits in small rural hospitals, *J Patient Saf* 17(8):e716–e726, 2021.

Johnston M, Magnan MA: Using a fall prevention checklist to reduce hospital falls: results of a quality improvement project, *Am J Nurs* 119(3):43–49, 2019.

Kawasaki T, Tozawa R: Motor function relating to the accuracy of self-overestimation error in community-dwelling older adults, *Front Neurol* 11:1–6, 2020.

Kiel DP: Falls in older persons: risk factors and patient evaluation, 2022, *UpToDate*. https://www.uptodate.com/contents/falls-in-older-persons-risk-factors-and-patient-evaluation. Accessed November 17, 2023.

Kwame A, Petrucka P: A literature-based study of patient-centered care and communication in nurse-patient interactions: barriers, facilitators, and the way forward, *BMC Nursing* 20:158, 2021.

LeLaurin J, Shorr R: Preventing falls in hospitalized patients: state of the science, *Clin Geriatr Med* 35(2):273–283, 2019.

Lourida I, et al: Activity interventions to improve the experience of care in hospital for people living with dementia: a systematic review, *BMC Geriatr* 20:131, 2020.

Manges M, et al: Hourly rounding and medical-surgical patient falls: a review of the literature, *Int J Sci Res Methodol* 17(2):85–95, 2020.

Martin E, et al: French validation of the revised Algase wandering scale for long-term care, *Am J Alzheimers Dis Other Demen* 30(8):762, 2015.

Matz M, et al: *Patient handling and mobility assessments*, ed 2, 2019, The Facility Guidelines Institute. http://www.fgiguidelines.org/wp-content/uploads/2019/10/FGI-Patient-Handling-and-Mobility-Assessments_191008.pdf. Accessed November 17, 2023.

Miake-Lye IM, et al: Inpatient fall prevention programs as a patient safety strategy: a systematic review, *Ann Intern Med* 158(5 Pt 2):390–396, 2013.

Montero-Odasso MM, et al: Evaluation of clinical practice guidelines on fall prevention and management for older adults: a systematic review, *JAMA Netw Open* 4(12):e2138911, 2021.

National Epilepsy Training: *Startle epilepsy*, 2019. https://www.nationalepilepsy-training.co.uk/startle-epilepsy. Accessed November 17, 2023.

National Fire Protection Association (NFPA): *Structure fires in health care facilities*, 2017. https://www.nfpa.org//-/media/Files/News-and-Research/Fire-statistics-and-reports/Building-and-life-safety/oshealthcarefacilities.pdf. Accessed November 17, 2023.

National Health Service (NHS): *Sudden confusion (delirium)*, 2021. https://www.nhs.uk/conditions/confusion/. Accessed November 28, 2023.

National Institute for Health and Care Excellence (NICE): *Epilepsies in children, young people and adults*, 2022. http://www.nice.org.uk/guidance/ng217. Accessed November 17, 2023.

National Institute on Aging (NIA): *Exercise and physical activity for healthy aging: get fit for life*, 2020. https://order.nia.nih.gov/sites/default/files/2021-02/exercise-physical-activity-get-fit4-life.pdf. Accessed November 17, 2023.

Nelson AL, Algase DL: *Evidence-based protocols for managing wandering behavior*, New York, 2007, Springer Publishing.

Nevitt SJ, et al: Antiepileptic drug monotherapy for epilepsy: a network meta-analysis of individual participant data. *Cochrane Database Syst Rev* 4(4):CD011412, 2022.

Occupational Safety and Health Administration (OSHA): *OSHA quickcard: hazard communication safety data sheets*, 2016. https://www.osha.gov/Publications/HazComm_QuickCard_SafetyData.html. Accessed November 17, 2023.

Oncology Nursing Society (ONS): *Toolkit for safe handling of hazardous drugs for nurses in oncology*, 2018. https://www.ons.org/sites/default/files/2018-06/ONS_Safe_Handling_Toolkit_0.pdf. Accessed November 17, 2023.

Perez D, et al: Physical restraints in intensive care-an integrative review, *Aust Crit Care* 32(2):165–174, 2019.

Quality and Safety Education for Nurses (QSEN) Institute: *QSEN competencies*, 2020. http://qsen.org/competencies/pre-licensure-ksas/. Accessed November 20, 2023.

Regier NG, Gitlin LN: Towards defining restlessness in individuals with dementia, *Aging Ment Health* 21(5):543–552, 2017.

Ritchey KC, et al: "Falls" in Handbook of Physical Medicine and Rehabilitation, edited by Marlis Gonzales-Fernandez and Stephen Schaaf, New York, 2022, Springer Publishing Co, p 399.

Rogers S, et al: CDC STEADI: *Best practices for developing an inpatient program to prevent older adult falls after discharge*, Atlanta, GA, 2021, National Center for Injury Prevention and Control, Centers for Disease Control and Prevention.

Safe Kids Worldwide: *Fall prevention tips: everything you need to know to keep your kids safe from falls*, 2015. https://www.safekids.org/sites/default/files/documents/falls_prevention_tips_2015.pdf. Accessed November 17, 2023.

Sawaf A, et al: Seizure precautions, In Stat Pearls, 2023, StatPearls Publishing. https://www.ncbi.nlm.nih.gov/books/NBK536958/?report=printable. Accessed November 17, 2023.

Sharifi A, et al: The principles of physical restraint use for hospitalized elderly people: an integrated literature review, *Syst Rev* 10(1):129, 2021.

Sherrington C, et al: Exercise for preventing falls in older people living in the community, *Cochrane Database Syst Rev* 1(1):CD012424, 2019. https://doi.org/10.1002/14651858.CD012424.pub2.

Soh SL, et al: Falls efficacy: extending the understanding of self-efficacy in older adults towards managing falls, *J Frailty Sarcopenia Falls* 6(3):131–138, 2021. https://www.ncbi.nlm.nih.gov/pmc/articles/PMC8419849/pdf/JFSF-6-131.pdf. Accessed November 20, 2023.

Stevens JA, Burns ER: *A CDC compendium of effective fall interventions: what works for community-dwelling older adults*, ed 3, Atlanta, GA, 2015, Centers for Disease Control and Prevention, National Center for Injury Prevention and Control. https://www.cdc.gov/falls/pdf/cdc_falls_compendium-2015-a.pdf. Accessed November 17, 2023.

Szanton S, et al: Pilot outcomes of a multicomponent fall risk program integrated into daily lives of community-dwelling older adults, *J Appl Gerontol* 40(3): 320–327, 2021.

The Joint Commission (TJC): *Most commonly reviewed sentinel event types*, 2021. https://www.jointcommission.org/-/media/tjc/documents/resources/patient-safety-topics/sentinel-event/most-frequently-reviewed-event-types-2020.pdf. Accessed November 17, 2023.

The Joint Commission (TJC): *Sentinel Event Alert 55: preventing falls and fall-related injuries in health care facilities*, September 28, 2015. https://www.jointcommission.org/assets/1/18/SEA_55.pdf. Accessed November 17, 2023.

The Joint Commission (TJC): *Speak up about your care*, 2019. https://www.jointcommission.org/resources/for-consumers/speak-up-campaigns/about-your-care/. Accessed November 17, 2023.

The Joint Commission (TJC): *2022 Comprehensive accreditation manual for hospitals: the official handbook*, Oakbrook Terrace, IL, 2022a, The Joint Commission.

The Joint Commission (TJC): *Provision of care, treatment and services (Hospital and Hospital Clinics/Hospitals) - restraint and seclusion - enclosure beds, side rails and mitts*, July 20, 2022b. https://www.jointcommission.org/standards/standard-faqs/critical-access-hospital/provision-of-care-treatment-and-services-pc/000001668/. Accessed November 17, 2023.

The Joint Commission (TJC): *2023 National patient safety goals*, Oakbrook Terrace, IL, 2023, The Joint Commission. https://www.jointcommission.org/standards/national-patient-safety-goals/.

Touhy T, Jett K: *Toward healthy aging*, ed 11, St. Louis, 2023, Elsevier.

U.S. Department of Veterans Affairs (VA): *VA National center for patient safety – falls toolkit*, 2019. https://www.patientsafety.va.gov/professionals/onthejob/falls.asp. Accessed November 17, 2023.

U.S. Food and Drug Administration (FDA): *A guide to bed safety bed rails in hospitals, nursing homes and home health care: the facts*, 2017. https://www.fda.gov/medical-devices/hospital-beds/guide-bed-safety-bed-rails-hospitals-nursing-homes-and-home-health-care-facts. Accessed November 17, 2023.

VA Healthcare: *Implementation guide for fall injury reduction*, 2015, VA National Center for Patient Safety Reducing Preventable Falls and Fall-Related Injuries. https://www.patientsafety.va.gov/docs/fallstoolkit14/falls_implementation_%20guide%20_02_2015.pdf. Accessed November 17, 2023.

Venema DM, et al: Patient and system factors associated with unassisted and injurious falls in hospitals: an observational study, *BMC Geriatr* 19(348):1–10, 2019.

World Health Organization (WHO): *Patient safety*, 2023. https://www.who.int/news-room/fact-sheets/detail/patient-safety. Accessed November 17, 2023.

Zaninotto P, et al. Polypharmacy is a risk factor for hospital admission due to a fall: evidence from the English Longitudinal Study of Ageing, *BMC Public Health* 20:1804, 2020. https://doi.org/10.1186/s12889-020-09920-x. Accessed November 20, 2023.

15 | Disaster Preparedness

SKILLS AND PROCEDURES

Skill 15.1 **Care of a Patient After Biological Exposure, p. 424**

Skill 15.2 **Care of a Patient After Chemical Exposure, p. 430**

Skill 15.3 **Care of a Patient After Radiation Exposure, p. 434**

Skill 15.4 **Care of a Patient After a Natural Disaster, p. 438**

OBJECTIVES

Mastery of content in this chapter will enable you to:
- Outline elements of emergency preparedness and response.
- Explain the characteristics of different types of disasters.
- Identify actions to take in the event of biological, chemical, or radiation exposure.
- Outline guidelines for patient care in the event of a mass casualty incident (MCI).
- Explain psychosocial effects of disasters on patients.
- Identify psychosocial effects of disasters on nurses and other health care providers.

MEDIA RESOURCES

- http://evolve.elsevier.com/Perry/skills
- Review Questions
- Audio Glossary
- Answers to Clinical Judgment and Next-Generation NCLEX® Examination–Style Questions
- Skills Performance Checklists
- Printable Key Points

PURPOSE

The terrorist attacks on the World Trade Center and Pentagon on September 11, 2001, forever changed the reality and sense of security felt by citizens of the United States. These attacks also brought attention to possible biological, chemical, and radiation exposure disasters that remain a concern today. The Centers for Disease Control and Prevention (CDC) has identified categories of natural disasters and severe weather: earthquakes, landslides/mudslides, volcanoes, extreme heat, lightning, wildfires, floods, tornadoes, winter weather, hurricanes, and tsunamis (CDC, 2022a). Because of the more frequent occurrence of natural disasters, most people who live in areas of risk know basic emergency response measures. Another type of disaster that changed the reality for citizens across the world was the pandemic outbreak of coronavirus disease identified in 2019 (COVID-19). A pandemic is the worldwide spread of a new disease (Healthdirect.gov, 2022). COVID-19 is an infectious disease caused by the SARS-CoV-2 virus (World Health Organization [WHO], 2022a). The recent pandemic has demonstrated the importance of both the general public and health care providers understanding the implications of any form of disaster and how to respond.

Individuals and communities need to understand what risks to prepare for in any emergency and how to prepare for them (Federal Emergency Management Agency [FEMA], 2019). All emergency events increase the demand for disaster preparedness of health care providers who will educate the public and deliver care to diverse populations at times of crisis. Nurses play a key role in the coordination and implementation of an interprofessional approach to prepare for and respond to disasters. In addition, nurses and other professionals are also at risk for the physical and psychological effects of disasters.

An example is the response of health care professionals to the experience of caring for COVID-19 patients. A survey of 1257 nurses and physicians caring for patients with the disease in China found that these providers (41.5% of respondents) had significantly more depression, anxiety, insomnia, and distress than providers who did not care directly for patients (Lai et al., 2020). Information gathered from the many postdisaster evaluations that have occurred in recent years has provided a considerable body of knowledge and experience to improve the response of an entire health care team and the agencies and individuals involved in a disaster response.

PRACTICE STANDARDS

- American Red Cross, 2022: How to Prepare for Emergencies
- Centers for Disease Control and Prevention (CDC), 2021a: Public Health Emergency Preparedness and Response Capabilities: National Standards for State, Local, Tribal, and Territorial Public Health
- Federal Emergency Management Agency (FEMA), 2019: National Threat and Hazard Identification and Risk Assessment (THIRA): Overview and Methodology

SUPPLEMENTAL STANDARDS

- Centers for Disease Control and Prevention (CDC), 2022a: Natural Disasters and Severe Weather
- Federal Emergency Management Agency (FEMA), 2022: Make a Plan
- National Center for Disaster Medicine & Public Health, 2022: Core competencies In Disaster Health

Disaster Definitions and Types

- **Disaster:** A catastrophic and/or destructive event (e.g., tsunamis, terrorist attacks) that disrupts normal functioning; may include any anticipated or unexpected event, the effects of which lead to significant destruction and/or adverse consequences
- **Mass casualty incident or event (MCI):** Any event or situation (e.g., bombing of a public area) that results in multiple casualties and/or deaths; exists when health care needs exceed health care resources
- **All-hazards event:** Multiple man-made or natural events with destructive capacity to cause multiple casualties
- **All-hazards preparedness:** The comprehensive preparedness necessary to manage casualties resulting from a disaster, regardless of etiology
- **Casualty:** Any individual who is ill, injured, missing, or killed as a result of an MCI
- **Medical disasters:** Catastrophic events (e.g., mass shootings) that result in human casualties that overwhelm the available health care resources
- **Natural/environmental disasters:** Catastrophic events that result from an ecological event that exceeds the capacity of the community (e.g., the impact of hurricanes or tornados on a community)
- **Man-made disasters:** Catastrophic events (e.g., wildfires), the principal direct cause of which is attributable to human action
- **Pandemic:** Worldwide spread of a new disease
- **Technological disasters:** Catastrophic events in which people, property, community infrastructure, and economic welfare are adversely affected by the disruption of technology (e.g., industrial accidents, unplanned release of nuclear waste)

PRINCIPLES FOR PRACTICE

- A disaster is any unexpected event, the effect of which leads to significant destruction and/or adverse consequences (Box 15.1).
- Surveillance of the public by the World Health Organization (2020b) focuses on current public health threats, such as outbreaks of measles, COVID-19, and Ebola virus disease (EVD) (Boxes 15.2, 15.3, and 15.4).
- The most common forms of disaster are natural or man-made. If the public is not adequately protected, the spread of natural-borne disease can create a natural disaster.
- The CDC strategic plan Public Health Emergency Preparedness and Response Capabilities: National Standards for State, Local, Tribal, and Territorial Public Health focuses on the sustainability of public health resources and infrastructure (CDC, 2021a).
- In the event of a biological, chemical, or radiation attack, the CDC strategic plan includes preparedness and prevention, detection and surveillance, diagnosis and characterization of agents, response, and communication.
- Detection and surveillance focus on an awareness of the environment, recognizing what is unusual or different, and knowing what these differences possibly mean for the purpose of mitigation or prevention (Department of Homeland Security [DHS], n.d.).
- Traditional modes of communication will likely be interrupted in the event of a mass casualty incident (MCI); part of disaster preparedness involves backup plans such as the use of two-way radios and satellite phones.
- Through the clinician outreach and communication activity (COCA) resource, the CDC helps health care providers respond to emergencies by communicating relevant and timely information (CDC, 2022a).

Measles Outbreaks

- Measles outbreaks continue to spread rapidly around the world, with millions of people globally at risk of the disease.
- COVID-19 is increasing the risk of measles outbreaks. Almost 41 countries delayed their measles campaigns for 2020 or 2021 due to the COVID-19 pandemic. This increased the risk of bigger outbreaks around the world, including the United States.
  - Although measles was declared eliminated in the United States in 2000, almost 1300 cases of measles were reported in 31 states in the United States in 2019—the greatest number since 1992.
  - Measles is caused by a virus in the paramyxovirus family and is normally passed through direct contact and air. The virus infects the respiratory tract and then spreads throughout the body. Measles is a human disease and is not known to occur in animals.
- Outbreaks are straining health care systems and leading to serious illness, disability, and deaths in many parts of the world.
- Measles is almost entirely preventable with two doses of the measles vaccine. High rates of vaccination coverage—95% nationally and within communities—are needed to ensure that measles is unable to spread.
- Reasons for people not being vaccinated vary and include lack of access to high-quality health care or vaccination services, conflict and displacement, misinformation about vaccines, and low awareness about the need to vaccinate. In a number of countries, measles is spreading among older children, youth, and adults who have not received vaccination in the past.

Data adapted from Centers for Disease Control (CDC): *Global measles outbreaks,* 2023. https://www.cdc.gov/globalhealth/measles/data/global-measles-outbreaks.html. Accessed November 3, 2023.

Ebola Virus Disease (EVD)

- *Ebolavirus* is transmitted to people from wild animals (e.g., fruit bats, porcupines, nonhuman primates) and then spreads in the human population through direct contact with the blood, secretions, organs, or other bodily fluids of infected people and with surfaces and materials (e.g., bedding, clothing) contaminated with these fluids.
- The average EVD case fatality rate is around 50%. Case fatality rates have varied from 25% to 90% in past outbreaks.
- EVD was first discovered in 1976. Recent outbreaks: North Kivu, Democratic Republic of the Congo, October–December 2021; North Kivu, Democratic Republic of the Congo, February–May 2021; N'Zerekore, Guinea, February–June 2021; Équateur, Democratic Republic of the Congo, June–November 2020.
- The incubation period is 2 to 21 days; humans are not infectious until they develop symptoms.
- Early symptoms include sudden onset of fever, fatigue, muscle pain, headache, and sore throat, followed by vomiting, diarrhea, rash, symptoms of impaired kidney and liver function, and in some cases both internal and external bleeding.
- Treatment includes supportive care; two vaccines currently are under trial in humans.
- Prevention and control focus on reducing the risk of transmission and engaging in outbreak containment measures.
- Health care providers use Standard Precautions and apply extra infection control measures when caring for a patient with EVD.

Data from World Health Organization (WHO): *Ebola virus disease,* 2022. https://www.who.int/health-topics/ebola/#tab=tab_1. Accessed November 20, 2023.

- The American Red Cross (2022) advocates preparedness and coordination of prompt, effective emergency efforts. This includes outreach to other agencies or groups through mutual aid agreements (e.g., willingness of an agency to provide shelter

BOX 15.4

COVID-19

- Coronavirus disease (COVID-19) is an infectious disease caused by a newly discovered coronavirus SARS-CoV-2 in 2019.
- Most people infected with the COVID-19 virus will experience mild to moderate gastrointestinal or respiratory illness and recover without requiring special treatment. Older adults and those with underlying medical problems such as cardiovascular disease, diabetes mellitus, chronic respiratory disease, and cancer are more likely to develop serious illness.
- COVID-19 symptoms include cough, fever or chills, shortness of breath or difficulty breathing, muscle or body aches, sore throat, new loss of taste or smell, diarrhea, headache, fatigue, nausea or vomiting, and congestion or runny nose. COVID-19 can be severe, and some cases have caused death.
- The best way to prevent and slow down transmission is to be well informed about the COVID-19 virus, the disease it causes, and how it spreads. Get vaccinated when it's your turn and follow local guidance.
- Public health and social measures (PHSM) have proven critical to limiting transmission of COVID-19 and reducing deaths. PHSMs include personal protective measures (e.g., physical distancing, avoiding crowded settings, hand hygiene, respiratory etiquette, mask-wearing); environmental measures (e.g., cleaning, disinfection, ventilation); surveillance and response measures (e.g., testing, genetic sequencing, contact tracing, isolation, quarantine); physical distancing measures (e.g., regulating the number and flow of people attending gatherings, maintaining distance in public or workplaces,

domestic movement restrictions); and international travel-related measures.
- The COVID-19 virus spreads primarily through aerosolized droplets of saliva or discharge from the nose when an infected person coughs or sneezes, so it is important that you also practice respiratory etiquette (e.g., by coughing into a flexed elbow).
- There are two types of tests for COVID-19:
  - Viral or diagnostic test: checks specimens from your nose or your mouth to find out if you are currently infected with the virus that causes COVID-19. Viral tests do not detect antibodies, which would suggest a previous infection, and they do not measure your level of immunity. Viral tests can be performed in a laboratory, at a testing site, and at home.
  - Antibody or serology tests: look for antibodies in your blood that fight the virus that causes COVID-19. Antibodies are made after you have been infected or have been vaccinated against an infection. Vaccination is a safe, effective way to teach your body to create antibodies. Antibody tests should generally not be used to diagnose a current infection with the virus that causes COVID-19. An antibody test may not show if you have a current infection because it can take 1 to 3 weeks after the infection for your body to make antibodies. An antibody test can show if a person was previously exposed to or infected with the virus and if the body has created antibodies in an attempt to defend itself. It takes at least 12 days after exposure for the body to make enough antibodies to show up on a test.

Adapted from World Health Organization: *Coronavirus*. https://www.who.int/health-topics/coronavirus#tab=tab_1, 2022. Accessed September 28, 2023; and Johns Hopkins: *Coronavirus health information*. https://www.hopkinsmedicine.org/coronavirus/health-articles.html#symptoms. Accessed September 28, 2023.

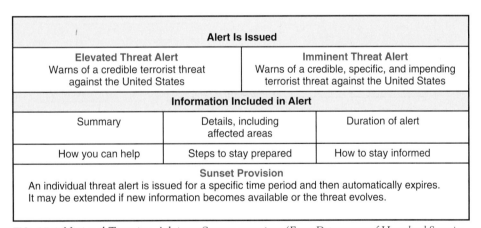

Alert Is Issued		
Elevated Threat Alert Warns of a credible terrorist threat against the United States		**Imminent Threat Alert** Warns of a credible, specific, and impending terrorist threat against the United States
Information Included in Alert		
Summary	Details, including affected areas	Duration of alert
How you can help	Steps to stay prepared	How to stay informed
Sunset Provision An individual threat alert is issued for a specific time period and then automatically expires. It may be extended if new information becomes available or the threat evolves.		

FIG. 15.1 National Terrorism Advisory System overview. (*From Department of Homeland Security—adapted from data available*. http://www.dhs.gov/xlibrary/assets/ntas/ntas-public-guide.pdf. *Accessed September 28, 2023.*)

[school or church]), clothing (e.g., department store, Salvation Army), or care for the deceased (funeral homes).
- Disaster planning is an interprofessional and multiagency task. Average citizens, government agencies, and other health care workers play a vital role in addition to nurses in disaster preparedness.
- Disaster preparedness: Some states have laws that now require disaster training as part of the continuing education requirement for licensure (American Nurses Association [ANA], 2019).
- Nurses may deliver care during emergencies in states where they are not licensed. The ANA (2019) is continually working to create laws to protect providers.
- The National Terrorism Advisory System (NTAS) facilitates public awareness of disasters. The system provides government

officials, first responders, and public citizens with information regarding the nature and degree of terrorist threat (Fig. 15.1) (DHS, 2021).
- Detection is the first goal in an MCI and includes (1) determining the presence of an MCI or public health emergency (PHE), (2) recognizing the cause of the incident, and (3) becoming aware of the environment or, more specifically, changes in the environment (e.g., an unusual pattern of patient presentation or unusual smells).
- Although many events have a clear cause, others have an insidious onset. Detection is sometimes simply the awareness of an unusual health care situation.
- Incident command is the need for an emergency system to be activated when a threat or hazard is suspected. For most individuals this means activating the 9-1-1 system.

- An incident command system (ICS) is used by all disciplines to help respond to an emergency situation (FEMA, 2019). See Fig. 15.2 for an example of a hospital ICS.
- Support is for the victims of disaster and all health care providers involved. Support is holistic, encompassing the body, mind, and spirit. Health care providers (including nurses, first responders, and physicians) are at risk for posttraumatic stress disorder (PTSD).
- Once local and federal authorities confirm the need for medicine and supplies, the CDC's strategic national stockpile (SNS) is accessed and items are delivered to the state in need. Each state has a plan to receive and distribute SNS (DHHS, 2021).

- Health care providers care for the worried well (those injured and able to transport themselves to a health care agency and those frightened by the events) and the sick and injured individuals already admitted to the hospital or emergency department (ED).
- First responders quickly distinguish between actual victims with exposure to the weapon of mass destruction (chemical, biological, or nuclear) that led to the MCI and the worried well.
- Health care providers offer a valuable resource and cannot spend time maintaining the security of a health care agency.
- Nurses provide public health education to empower resilience in communities by focusing on individual self-accountability and responsibility and knowing how to access community, state, and federal resources.

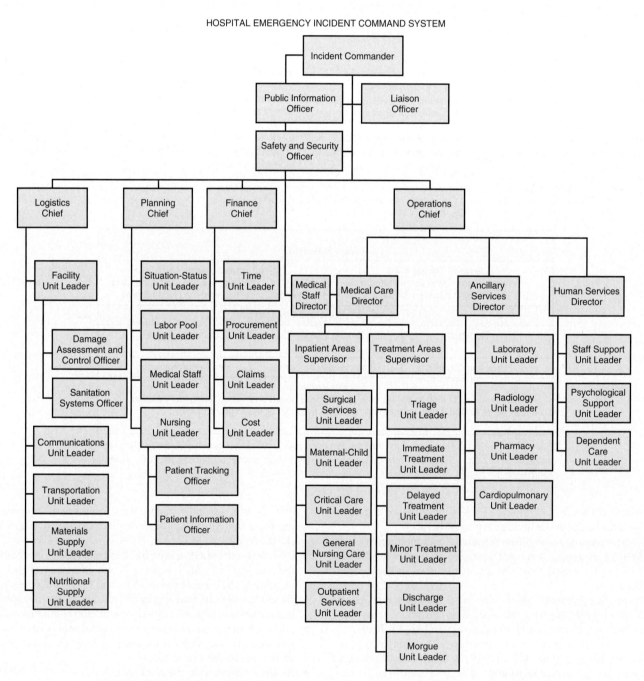

FIG. 15.2 The hospital emergency incident command system prepares all response teams to work smoothly in a disaster situation.

PERSON-CENTERED CARE

- Triage, treat, and evacuate: Triage is the process of sorting individuals by the seriousness of their condition and the likelihood of their survival (Box 15.5). Apply compassion and respect in this process. Learn your patients' concerns and fears.

- Disaster triage can be accomplished with the START (Simple Triage and Rapid Treatment) triage system (Fig. 15.3).
- START uses clinical parameters to evaluate patients: ability to walk; presence or absence of spontaneous breathing; respiratory rate greater or less than 30 per minute; perfusion assessment using either the palpable radial pulse or visible capillary refill rate; and

---

BOX 15.5

IDME—Triage Categories

Immediate (Red)
- Unconscious or unresponsive
- Altered mental status
- Experiencing hypoxia or near-hypoxia
- Chest pain
- Chest wounds
- Full-thickness burns over 20%–60% of the body
- Uncontrollable bleeding
- Amputations above elbow or knee
- Rapid or weak pulse
- Open abdominal wounds

Delayed (Yellow)
- Deep lacerations
- Open fractures with controlled bleeding and strong pulses
- Multiple fractures
- Finger amputations
- Abdominal injuries with stable vital signs
- Closed head injuries without altered level of consciousness

Minimal (Green)
- Abrasions
- Contusions
- Sprains
- Minor lacerations
- No apparent injuries
- Other injuries of similar severity

Expectant (Black)
- Victims still alive but so severely injured as to have little chance of survival
- Victims who have died

IDME, Immediate, delayed, minimal, expectant.

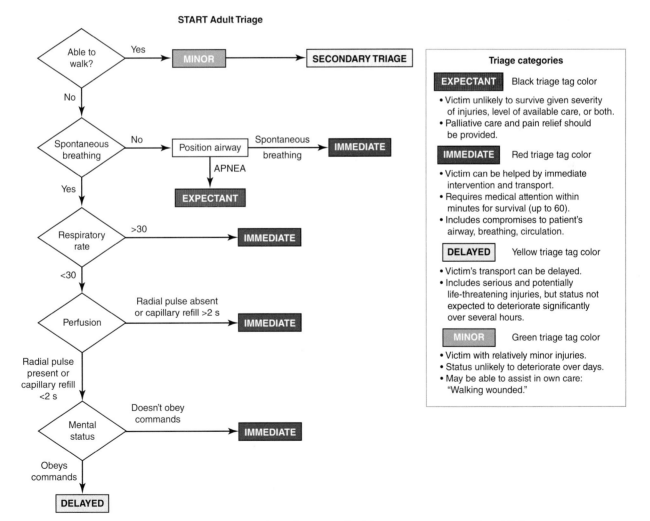

FIG. 15.3 START *(Simple Triage and Rapid Treatment)* adult triage assessment. *(From US Department of Health and Human Services, Chemical Hazards Emergency Medical Management, 2021. https:// chemm.hhs.gov/startadult.htm. Accessed September 28, 2023.)*

mental status as assessed by ability to obey commands (Chemical Hazards Emergency Medical Management [CHEMM], 2021a).

- START triage should take between 30 and 60 seconds per patient. The intention is to identify patients who will benefit most from the resources available, with the goal of decreasing the number of patients who die from survivable injuries (CHEMM, 2021a).
- In an epidemic situation, triage is also used to prevent secondary spread of the disease.
- During triage the focus may shift to psychological support of survivors or transport to specific facilities.
- Remain calm and assess a patient's immediate psychological response. Some patients present with dissociative symptoms such as disorientation, depression, anxiety, psychosis, and an inability to care for themselves.
- Community engagement is key to successfully controlling people's responses during disasters; establishing trust is essential.
- A lack of cultural considerations of victims leads to the impression of insensitivity and biases toward patients who are different racially, sexually, or ethnically.
- Regardless of cultural differences and perhaps language difficulties, it is important to convey compassion and work closely with people within the community for disaster recovery. Professional interpreters become an important resource.
- Some disaster events result in a changed culture for individuals, families, and communities. Once a disaster has struck, there can be a sense of vulnerability that causes increased fear and a sense of insecurity.

EVIDENCE-BASED PRACTICE

Lessons Learned From a Pandemic

The recent COVID-19 pandemic raised awareness of the importance for all nurses to receive proper education in order to prepare and respond to a disaster and lead at times of crisis. The COVID-19 pandemic highlighted the lack of preparation most nurses had and the struggles they faced, especially at the height of the pandemic. Disasters create a sudden and unexpected demand for health care services that can compromise nurses' and a health care agency's ability to function under normal circumstances (Cariaso-Sugay et al., 2021). In light of the pandemic, nurses have strongly expressed a need for better education and preparedness, and recent research has given the profession some insights as to how to address these needs:

- Understanding basic emergency management principles that form an organization's emergency operations plan is essential for nurse leaders; this was achieved through a quality improvement (QI) education program. The program included an overview of Federal Emergency Management Agency (FEMA) standards of care, the health system's emergency and department operations plans, and the American Organization of Nurse Leaders (AONL) guiding principles for nurse leaders in crisis management (Cariaso-Sugay et al., 2021).
- Offering the QI program at continued intervals and adding simulation and interactive training were suggestions from participants to better sustain knowledge and skills over time (Cariaso-Sugay et al., 2021).
- Undergraduate nursing curriculum often includes theory on disaster management but is missing specific education on psychological preparedness, assessment of disaster risks, or comprehensive disaster response planning. There is also a need for education to physically and psychologically prepare nurses to respond to disasters and other crises in not only the present but also long term (Karnjuš et al., 2021).

- Using the International Council of Nurses (ICN) Framework of Disaster Nursing Competencies can be helpful because disasters are often not bound by country borders; therefore, the international assistance of health care professionals, such as during the COVID-19 crisis in the most-affected countries, can be particularly needed (Karnjuš et al., 2021).
- In 2019, the ICN published a new revised Framework of Disaster Nursing Competencies describing what a nurse should be capable of doing, depending on expertise level, and outlining eight domains of nurse competence in disaster situations: preparation and planning, communication, incident management systems, safety and security, assessment, intervention, recovery, and law and ethics (Karnjuš et al., 2021).
- ICN further describes three different levels of nurses' expertise regarding competencies and disaster-preparedness skills, namely competencies (1) for all registered nurses, (2) for nurses who are or aspire to be a designated disaster responder within an organization, and (3) for nurses who respond to a wide range of disasters and emergencies. The same level of preparedness in disaster cases is not needed or expected for all nurses (Karnjuš et al., 2021).
- Nurses are first responders to disasters, caring for people with different types and levels of trauma. They have to be well prepared skillwise and able to provide appropriate psychological support for the victims and nurses themselves (Said et al., 2020).
- Psychological preparedness training and predisaster planning can strengthen a nurse's ability to respond. Completion of PTSD assessment and trait anxiety in the nurses involved in disaster response can assist in providing support and consultations to those who may experience such symptoms (Said et al., 2020).
- Appropriate training could influence self-efficacy, dispositional optimism, and self-esteem and reduce anxiety and PTSD symptoms (Said et al., 2020).

SAFETY GUIDELINES

When considering all forms of disaster, there are basic safety guidelines for a nurse or other health care provider to follow:

- The first priority at any disaster scene is to protect yourself and other team members. The second priority is to protect the injured, public, and environment (Box 15.6).
- It is essential that rescue and health care workers avoid becoming victims. This may go against your initial instinct to help others, but first responders must wait until a disaster scene has been secured and all safety precautions have been taken.

BOX 15.6

Safety and Security

- Trained emergency personnel (e.g., firefighters and police) are responsible for the safety and security of a disaster scene.
- Nurses stay out of a disaster scene unless well trained and invited. Call 9-1-1 if emergency personnel have not already been notified.
- Do not disturb the scene; key evidence could be lost or contaminated.
- A health care agency becomes a secondary disaster site when contaminated by the agent from the original disaster scene. For example, a patient has been exposed to mustard gas, an oily chemical that is difficult to remove from a patient's body. If not properly decontaminated, the victim contaminated by the mustard gas will inadvertently contaminate health care providers and others (CDC, 2022b).

Potential Hazards at the Scene of a Disaster

- Downed power lines
- Smoke and toxic gases
- Debris that can result in trauma
- Fractured or leaking gas lines
- Fire resulting in burns
- Structural collapse
- Blood and other body fluids
- Inclement weather
- Hazardous materials
- Nuclear, biological, or chemical exposure

- Flooding and the threat of drowning
- Radiation exposure
- Explosion, particularly secondary explosions
- Snipers
- Darkness
- Infection
- High-velocity projectiles and the pressure wave after an explosion
- Becoming incapacitated and unable to protect yourself or your patient

---

- Assessing hazards is more important than knowing the exact cause of a disaster; MCI can result in secondary hazards that come in many forms (Box 15.7).
- The potential for public alarm and major disruption of everyday life is enormous. Know crisis intervention and stress-management techniques.
- In an MCI the majority of people, whether contaminated, exposed, or not, will self-triage and go directly to a local hospital, bypassing triage and treatment. Plans are needed to transfer patients to other medical facilities.
- Personal protective equipment (PPE) minimizes the risk for contact with contaminated materials or individuals. Proper use of advanced forms of PPE requires training, fitting, and an understanding that not all PPE protects against all potential hazards (FDA, 2021).
- When used inappropriately, PPE becomes a hazard (e.g., dehydration; decreased vision, mobility, ability to communicate). Some of these hazards result because, while using advanced forms of PPE, the user is unable to eat, drink, or go to the bathroom.
- PPE is categorized by levels A to D for the level of safety provided.
  - Level A—Maximum protection selected when the greatest level of skin, respiratory, and eye protection is required. It provides a self-contained breathing apparatus, total encapsulating chemical-protective suit, coveralls, undergarments, chemical-resistant boots and gloves, hard hat, and disposable protective suit worn over the encapsulating suit (Fig. 15.4). Highly trained personnel use level A protection in heavily contaminated areas. Practical limitations include limited air supply (20–50 minutes) and heat stress. If you are not wearing this type of protection and you are near an area where level A PPE is being used, get out or do not enter.
  - Level B—Provides the highest level of respiratory protection but lower level of skin protection. Used by trained responders, this PPE includes a self-contained breathing apparatus; a hooded chemical-resistant suit; and face, boot, and glove protection. Level B protection also requires training and fitting.
  - Level C—First responders (emergency personnel first on the scene) and hospital personnel are trained and fitted to use level C protection, which involves knowing the concentration and type of airborne substance(s) and the criteria for using air-purifying respirators. Level C constitutes the use of half-mask air-purifying respirators (National Institute for Occupational Safety and Health [NIOSH] approved), hooded chemical-resistant clothing, and protective gloves and boots. Because of the garment protection worn with levels A, B, and C, the user is at risk for dehydration and hyperthermia.
  - Level D—Standard work uniforms or work clothes are appropriate and used for nuisance contamination only. The

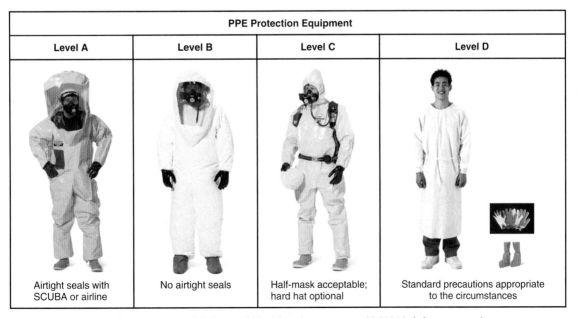

PPE Protection Equipment			
Level A	**Level B**	**Level C**	**Level D**
Airtight seals with SCUBA or airline	No airtight seals	Half-mask acceptable; hard hat optional	Standard precautions appropriate to the circumstances

FIG. 15.4 The Occupational Safety and Health Administration (OSHA) defines personal protective equipment for the four levels of hazardous exposure. *PPE,* Personal protective equipment; *SCUBA,* self-contained underwater breathing apparatus.

users must wear coveralls and chemical-resistant shoes; and, depending on the contaminant, gloves, goggles, masks, face shields, and hard hats may also be worn. There is no respiratory protection. It is important to take standard precautions when using level D protection (Chapter 9). Depending on the circumstances, some health care providers also choose to use a fluid-impermeable gown, cap, eye protection, mask, gloves, and shoe covers (US Food and Drug Administration [FDA], 2021).

- The most recently labeled level of protection is BioPPE, which requires the use of standard work clothes along with contact and respiratory protection. Double gloving and an N95 mask (see Chapter 9) or a better respirator are recommended. BioPPE protection is not adequate when caring for patients exposed to toxic chemicals; however, it provides adequate protection against radiological and biological agents (Lynch et al., 2021).
- Hand hygiene that includes washing with soap and water followed by use of an alcohol gel is important at all levels.

◆ SKILL 15.1   Care of a Patient After Biological Exposure

Bioterrorism is the deliberate release of viruses, bacteria, toxins, or fungi with the goal of causing panic, mass casualties, or severe economic disruption (Rathjen & Shahbodaghi, 2021). The use of biological agents is a considerable terrorist threat because they are easy to disperse and affect large numbers of people at a relatively low cost (Box 15.8). Incubation periods and common initial clinical symptoms make detection of a biological attack difficult. Some biological attacks are unannounced or covert, and the onset of symptoms is delayed by an incubation period (i.e., the time between exposure and onset of symptoms). Differing biological agents have incubation periods from 1 or 2 days to several weeks, during which some of these agents may be transmitted as an infected patient exposes others. The mode of transmission of the biological agent determines the severity

of the disaster. Recognition of bioterrorism is a challenge because early signs and symptoms mimic the flu or produce a rash mistaken for a viral illness (Fig. 15.5). Sometimes several biological agents are disseminated at the same time, further confusing the issue. To understand how to protect yourself from becoming a victim, you need to understand the mode of transmission and precautions to take for biosafety (Table 15.1).

Delegation

The skill of assessing a patient exposed to a biological agent cannot be delegated to assistive personnel (AP). Direct the AP to:

- Use appropriate PPE to prevent exposure during care activities
- Use proper techniques for handling a body after death to prevent contamination

---

BOX 15.8

Potential Bioterrorism Agents/Diseases

- Highest priority agents include organisms that pose a risk to national security because they can be easily disseminated or transmitted from person to person, result in high mortality rates, and have the potential for major public health impact:
  - Anthrax (*Bacillus anthracis*)
  - Botulism (*Clostridium botulinum* toxin)
  - Plague (*Yersinia pestis*)
  - Smallpox
  - Tularemia (*Francisella tularensis*)
  - Viral hemorrhagic fevers (filoviruses [Ebola, Marburg], arenaviruses [Lassa])
- Second highest priority agents include those that are moderately easy to disseminate and result in moderate morbidity rates and low mortality rates:
  - Brucellosis (*Brucella* species)
  - Epsilon toxin of *Clostridium perfringens*
  - Food safety threats (*Salmonella* species, *Escherichia coli* O157:H7, *Shigella*)
  - Glanders (*Burkholderia mallei*)
  - Melioidosis (*Burkholderia pseudomallei*)
  - Psittacosis (*Chlamydia psittaci*)
  - Q fever (*Coxiella burnetii*)
  - Ricin toxin from *Ricinus communis* (castor beans)
  - Staphylococcal enterotoxin B
  - Typhus fever (*Rickettsia prowazekii*)
  - Water safety threats (e.g., *V. cholerae, Cryptosporidium parvum*)
- Third highest-priority agents include emerging pathogens that could be engineered for mass dissemination in the future because of availability, ease of production and dissemination, and potential for high morbidity and mortality rates and major health impact:
  - Emerging infectious diseases such as Nipah virus and hantavirus

Data from Centers for Disease Control and Prevention (CDC): *Bioterrorism,* 2018. https://emergency.cdc.gov/agent/agentlist-category.asp. Accessed September 28, 2023.

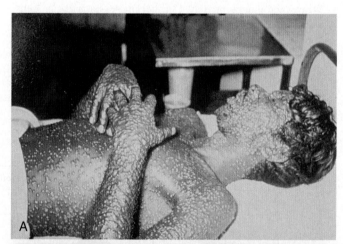

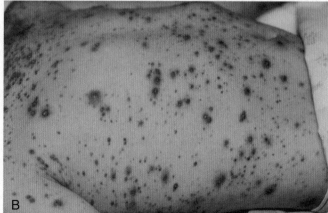

FIG. 15.5 Differences in distribution of smallpox versus chickenpox. (A) Man with smallpox. (B) Chickenpox covering patient torso. (*A courtesy CDC/NIP/Barbara Rice. B courtesy David Effron, M.D.*)

TABLE 15.1

Summary of Selected Class A Biological Warfare Agents

Disease and Infectious Agent	Form and Incubation (Time to Onset of Symptoms)	Untreated Course of Disease		Probable Route of Contamination for Use as Biological Warfare Agent	Treatment of Mass Casualties	Prophylaxis or Vaccine
		Early-Onset Symptoms	Late-Onset Symptoms			
Bacterial Biological Agents						
Anthrax *Bacillus anthracis,* a gram-positive bacillus that can remain stable in spore form	Inhalation or pulmonary (usually within 48 h but may incubate for up to 60 days)	Febrile flulike symptoms (malaise, low-grade fever, dry cough, and headache)	Severe respiratory distress, hemodynamic failure, and death	Aerosol; no person-to-person transmission	Ciprofloxacin or doxycycline	Ciprofloxacin or, if susceptible, doxycycline; vaccine available but in short supply
	Cutaneous (1–12 days)	Local urticaria; painless papular lesions usually located on head, forearms, or hands	Papular lesions become vesicular, later developing black eschar and edema	Person-to-person transmission with direct contact with skin lesions		
	Gastrointestinal (1–7 days)	Abdominal pain, nausea, vomiting, and diarrhea	Gastrointestinal bleeding, fever; usually followed by toxic sepsis and death	Contaminated food and/or water		
Plague Acute, severe bacterial infection secondary to gram-negative bacillus, *Yersinia pestis*	Bubonic Onset of symptoms dependent on route of transmission (1–6 days)	Swollen, tender lymph nodes (most notable femoral and inguinal), high fever, rapid pulse	Hypotension, extreme exhaustion, death	Aerosol and then human to human by droplet inhalation	Ciprofloxacin or doxycycline	Ciprofloxacin or doxycycline; no vaccine available at present time
	Pneumonic (1–6 days)	High fever, chills, tachycardia, headache	Fulminate pneumonia (foamy hemoptysis, tachypnea, and dyspnea), sepsis, and death			
Botulism (*Clostridium botulinum* toxin) Anaerobic gram-positive bacillus that produces a potent muscle-paralyzing neurotoxin	Foodborne (12–36 hours)	Nausea, vomiting, diarrhea	Symmetrical cranial nerve paralysis, descending flaccid paralysis (progressive paralysis of arms, respiratory muscles, and legs), and death	Contaminated food	Passive immunization (antitoxin); supportive care	Passive immunization (antitoxin); antitoxin available in short supply
	Inhalational (2 h to 8 days)	No fever, no changes in mental status	Symmetrical cranial nerve paralysis, descending flaccid paralysis (progressive paralysis of arms, respiratory muscles, and legs), and death	Inhalation of aerosolized toxin		
Typhoidal tularemia *Francisella tularensis,* an extremely infectious bacteria	Contaminated water or food or via aerosol distribution (1–14 days)	Flulike symptoms (headache, cough, fever and chills, malaise)	Pharyngeal ulcers, pleuritic chest pain, pneumonia, pericarditis, respiratory failure, sepsis, and death	Inhalation of aerosolized bacteria	Ciprofloxacin or doxycycline	Ciprofloxacin or doxycycline; vaccine available, only limited supply; vaccine offers incomplete protection

Continued

TABLE 15.1

Summary of Selected Class A Biological Warfare Agents—cont'd

Disease and Infectious Agent	Form and Incubation (Time to Onset of Symptoms)	Untreated Course of Disease		Probable Route of Contamination for Use as Biological Warfare Agent	Treatment of Mass Casualties	Prophylaxis or Vaccine
		Early-Onset Symptoms	Late-Onset Symptoms			
Major Viral Biological Agent of Concern—Smallpox						
Smallpox variola virus	Distribution via airborne droplets, aerosols, and fomites (7–17 days; weaponized smallpox when delivered in aerosolized form has an incubation period of only 3–5 days)	Acute viral symptoms (high fever, myalgia, headache, and backache)	Continued viral symptoms, high fever, prostration, synchronous onset of rash progressing from macules to papules to vesicles, and eschar formation Vesicles more abundant on extremities and face, and all develop at the same time; pustules appear on palms of hands and soles of feet (unlike chickenpox)	Transmitted person to person by large droplets; therefore spread may be by inhalation of aerosolized virus, oral secretions, infected human vector exposure, or exposure to contaminated objects	Supportive therapy only (ventilator)	None; vaccine available in short supply

Interprofessional Collaboration

- Disasters can cause a public health emergency (PHE). You will collaborate with first responders and the health care team (e.g., infection control specialists) in the assessment and treatment of these patients and to ensure the safety of all providers.

Equipment

Choice of equipment depends on the route of transmission of the infectious agent. The following is a general list of supplies that might be used in the event of release of the most contagious biological agents:
- Biohazard bags with label
- Soap and water
- 0.5% diluted bleach or Environmental Protection Agency (EPA)–approved germicidal agent
- Negative-pressure room (high-efficiency particulate air [HEPA] filtration may be required) with anteroom

- Clean gloves
- Gown
- Shoe covers
- Head covers
- Mask
- Standard face mask
- N95 mask
- Face shield
- Equipment for physical examination and vital signs (including pulse oximeter)
- Oxygen therapy (see Chapter 23)
- Airway maintenance supplies
- Intravenous therapy supplies

STEP	RATIONALE

ASSESSMENT

1. Perform hand hygiene. Don proper PPE.

2. Identify patient using at least two identifiers (e.g., name and birthday or name and medical record number) according to agency policy.

3. Conduct focused health history and physical examination (e.g., skin assessment; pulmonary assessment—oxygen saturation, lung sounds, sputum character; cardiac—heart sounds; gastrointestinal [GI]—nausea, vomiting, diarrhea; neurological—movement of extremities, Glasgow Coma Scale, reflexes). Review history of patient's presenting symptoms and determine if pattern exists (see Chapter 6).

Proper PPE provides safety to personnel and helps prevent spread of infectious agent to health care provider (FDA, 2021).

Ensures correct patient. Complies with The Joint Commission standards and improves patient safety (TJC, 2023).

Symptom identification and clustering data help to accurately determine exposure to type of biological agent and patient's response.

STEP	RATIONALE
4. Measure patient's vital signs (including SpO_2) and assess the character of pain, rating severity on a scale of 0 to 10.	Provides baseline to later evaluate patient's response to therapy.
5. Assess patient's/family caregiver's health literacy.	Determines degree to which individuals have the ability to find, understand, and use information and services to make informed health-related decisions and actions for themselves and others (CDC, 2023).
6. Review results of diagnostic tests and consult with health care provider.	Initial signs and symptoms of exposure to biological agent suggest common disorders (e.g., flu). Further review of diagnostic findings helps to rule out other common disorders.
7. Assess patient for health risks (e.g., history of heart disease, pulmonary disease, cancer) that complicate effects of exposure to biological agent.	Patients with preexisting medical conditions often require additional treatment or are at greater risk for death.
8. Stay calm. Listen and assess patient's immediate psychological response after exposure. Some patients present with dissociative symptoms (e.g., feeling as though "not there" or sensing that everything is outside of the person): disorientation, depression, anxiety, psychosis, and inability to care for self. Even without direct exposure to a biological agent, many individuals, spurred by feelings of fear and doom, present for emergency services.	Aids in providing appropriate crisis intervention and stress management. Remaining calm and projecting confidence while assessing individuals for clinical symptoms reduce anxiety of the ill and worried well as people experience the general sense of panic associated with a biological event (Steele, 2023).
9. Identify all patient contacts and gather names, addresses, and phone numbers before the patient leaves the emergency department (ED).	All patient contacts need to be identified for proper follow-up by public health department. Often patients will self-triage and transport to ED.
10. Identify agency resources available (e.g., critical-incident stress-debriefing teams, counselors, psychiatric/mental health nurse practitioners).	Expert resources help to assess extent of psychological impact of disaster.

Clinical Judgment *Consider that a biological event has occurred when large numbers of ill persons present who have unexplained yet similar symptoms; when there are unexplained deaths, particularly among young and healthy populations; when there is an unusual pattern associated with the symptoms (e.g., geographical, seasonal, patient population); when a patient fails to respond to traditional therapy; or when a single patient presents with symptoms suggestive of an uncommon agent (e.g., anthrax or smallpox). Once you suspect a biological event, notify incident command immediately.*

PLANNING

1. Expected outcomes following completion of procedure: • Patient reports reduction in pain acuity.	In some cases, care is only palliative, with comfort as the focus. Do not underestimate the value of *comfort as care*.
• Patient's vital signs (including O_2 saturation) return to baseline.	When there are no underlying medical conditions and if the patient's disease process is responsive to treatment (when available), vital signs will normalize. However, this may take days or weeks.
• Patient's work of breathing decreases.	Indicates improved gas exchange and cardiac output.
• Patient's skin integrity returns to baseline.	Antibiotic and antitoxin therapy will aid in resolution/healing of lesions over time.
• Patient's level of consciousness (LOC) returns to baseline.	Treatment measures restore neurological function and oxygenation status.
• Patient's mental health status returns to pretrauma level of functioning.	Crisis intervention successfully reduces patient's anxiety, fear, and dissociative symptoms (Steele, 2023).
2. Provide timely and accurate information: accurate description of agent to which patient is exposed and implications for patient and family.	Information relieves anxiety and fear.
3. Organize and set up any equipment needed.	Ensures efficiency.
4. Close door to room or bedside curtains.	Provides for patient privacy.

IMPLEMENTATION

1. Continue wearing PPE applied before assessment. Follow transmission-based isolation precautions (see Chapter 9). (See Table 15.1 for route of contamination.) Use strict isolation with smallpox because of its communicability from person to person. Use Airborne Precautions, Contact Precautions, and a negative-pressure room for patients suspected of having smallpox.	Reduces transmission of microorganisms and the likelihood of additional secondary sites of contamination.

STEP	RATIONALE
2. Decontaminate (see emergency policies). If you suspect anthrax, have patient remove clothing and place in labeled plastic biohazard bag. *Caution: Do not pull over patient's head; instead, cut garments off.* Instruct patient to shower thoroughly with soap and water.	Handle clothing minimally to avoid agitation. Showering with soap and water helps decontaminate and reduce exposure.
3. Administer appropriate antibiotics and/or antitoxins.	Various biological agents are commonly treated with ciprofloxacin and/or doxycycline.
4. Administer immunizations (in the event of smallpox).	The best treatment is prevention by immunization with vaccine before onset of symptoms. Historically, the vaccine has been effective in preventing smallpox infection in 95% of those vaccinated (CDC, 2021b).
5. Administer fluid and nutrition therapy.	Biological agents commonly cause GI disturbances that sometimes result in dehydration.
6. Administer oxygen therapy.	Various biological agents (e.g., pulmonary anthrax) commonly cause respiratory symptoms that result in altered gas exchange.
7. Provide supportive care (e.g., comfort measures, including pain management).	Some victims of a biological attack will not survive; palliative care is essential (see Chapter 17).
8. Counsel patient and family caregiver about acute and potential long-term psychological effects of exposure. Offer access to trained counselors. Support survivors of a disaster by identifying resources available.	Reactions of patients will include shock, fear, and immobilization. Long-term psychological effects can arise without proper counseling. Social support networks foster coping in the days following a disaster (Steele, 2023).
9. Raise side rails (as appropriate) and lower bed to lowest position, locking into position.	Ensures patient safety and prevents falls.
10. Dispose of any used supplies in appropriate receptacle.	Reduces transmission of microorganisms.
11. Place nurse call system in an accessible location within patient's reach.	Ensures patient can call for assistance if needed.
12. After leaving patient area, remove most heavily contaminated items first. Peel off gown and gloves, roll inside out, and dispose of them. Perform hand hygiene. Remove face shield from behind and dispose of safely. Remove goggles and mask from behind. Place goggles in container for reprocessing; dispose of mask safely. Perform hand hygiene.	Avoids contamination of self, others, and environment. Reduces transmission of microorganisms.

Clinical Judgment *Collaborate with the health care provider and other rescue workers for an interprofessional ongoing plan for managing patients exposed to a biological agent while caring for other patients who are already present in the health care agency seeking care for illness unrelated to the current mass casualty incident (MCI).*

EVALUATION

1. Observe for improved airway maintenance, breathing, circulation, LOC, and neurological functioning.	Evaluates patient's response to available treatment and/or supportive care.
2. Evaluate vital signs and character of pain.	Evaluates patient's response to treatment.
3. Inspect condition of patient's skin; note character of remaining lesions.	Evaluates patient's response to antibiotic therapy.
4. **Use Teach-Back:** "I want to be sure you know the resources you have to help support you through this illness. Tell me about the counseling resources we discussed." Revise your instruction now or develop a plan for revised patient/family caregiver teaching if patient/family caregiver is not able to teach back correctly.	Teach-back is a technique for health care providers to ensure that they have explained medical information clearly so that patients and their families understand what is communicated to them (AHRQ, 2023).

Unexpected Outcomes	Related Interventions
1. Patient's physical or psychological symptoms progress.	• Notify health care provider. • Notify mental health treatment team. • Remain calm, offer reassurance, and protect self and others from physical harm. • Continue to provide comfort care.
2. Patient death occurs.	• When handling bodies, take into account continued risk for contamination; make sure that everyone is fully informed regarding proper procedure.
3. Secondary contamination of rescue workers.	• Rescue workers immediately report symptoms to a health care provider or nursing supervisor.

Documentation

- Use disaster checklists to quickly document specific data regarding patient status, treatment administered, and response to treatment and/or comfort measures. Document patient/family caregiver's response to instruction.

Hand-Off Reporting

- Report any unexpected outcome to health care provider in charge.
- Report suspected cases of a biological incident to health care provider or ED officer. In the event of an ED exposure to a communicable disease, the department will be locked down immediately. Public health officials (e.g., emergency officer) will determine if the health care agency should be locked down.

Special Considerations

Patient Education

- Preparation for an MCI goes a long way toward preventing casualties and chaos. Public education regarding the likelihood of a mass casualty biological event is necessary and includes information about types of biological agents, mode of transmission, symptoms, treatment, and locations of shelters and disaster treatment sites.
- Preparedness includes teaching individuals, families, and communities about resilience and the ability to care for themselves when support services are not available or are inaccessible.
- Health care providers need an opportunity to debrief after a disaster to help avoid psychological complications such as posttraumatic stress disorder (PTSD).
- Encourage families to prepare for the unexpected (see Home Care).

Pediatrics

- Children are one of the most vulnerable populations, and many facets influence the impact of disaster on children. These facets often include age, sex, family dynamics, and the level of and direct exposure to disaster (Hockenberry et al., 2022).
- Children have both physical and emotional needs during disasters. They often show stress-related symptoms and may have temporary changes in behavior after a disaster (Hockenberry et al., 2022).
- Many disasters result in the need to relocate, which creates stress and unique challenges in children. Stress may increase by changes in children's cultural, psychological, and social environment. Reactions of parents and other family members contribute to how well the child will cope with relocation and whether or not the child will be able to stay connected with friends and familiar activities (Hockenberry et al., 2022).
- Children are vulnerable to the adverse effects of environmental chemicals and toxins because (1) pound for pound, children take in larger doses of toxins through food, water, and air; (2) their organ systems are less mature and unable to remove some of the toxins; and (3) their life expectancy is longer, and long-term effects of exposure to toxins is unknown (Hockenberry et al., 2022).
- Disasters disrupt infrastructure and may cause large-scale displacement, leading to unsafe water, lack of access to health care, and decreases in vector control and infectious agents. Outbreaks of communicable diseases have been reported after natural disasters, and children are more likely to develop infections secondary to immature immune systems (Hockenberry et al., 2022).
- Keep families together after a disaster. Family togetherness offers reassurance to a child and lessens fears of being abandoned and unprotected (Hockenberry et al., 2022).

- Media have an enormous influence over children and may affect development and behavior. Encourage parents to limit their children's exposure to media reports of the disaster and to watch television with them whenever possible to clarify information and answer questions (Hockenberry et al., 2022).
- The death of a child is always traumatic. Parents may have a compelling need to be present during pediatric resuscitation and at the time of death; ideally you should allow it. It is important for a nurse to be present to explain what is happening and facilitate the grieving process (Hockenberry et al., 2022).

Older Adults

- Under disaster conditions, triage older adults according to injuries, not age.
- Because older adults often have several concurrent illnesses, exposure to a biological agent often worsens these conditions and results in the need for more immediate care than an initial triage may suggest.
- Older adults have a greater prevalence of chronic conditions, multimorbidity, cognitive impairment, and medication concerns during disasters (American Academy of Nursing [AAN], 2021).
- Older adults have a greater dependence on assistive devices (i.e., walkers, glasses) supplies and support requirements (from family caregivers and others) during disasters (AAN, 2021).
- Greater issues of social isolation make older persons more vulnerable (AAN, 2021).

Populations With Disabilities

- Collaboration with governmental organizations is critical for developing strategies to make emergency communications and related announcements accessible to people with disabilities (Kim & Zakour, 2018).

Home Care

- Assemble a disaster kit before disaster strikes. The American Red Cross (2022) offers free literature on establishing home care preparedness (Boxes 15.9 and 15.10).
- Individuals with special needs (e.g., hearing impairment, impaired mobility, special diets) and individuals without vehicles require additional planning to be prepared for a disaster.
- Post emergency telephone numbers by the telephone and teach children how and when to call 9-1-1.
- Family members need to establish a meeting place away from home in case they cannot stay in it or cannot reach home during a disaster.
- Remain isolated and advise friends and relatives not to visit if family members are symptomatic.
- Instruct family to use the appropriate PPE needed to protect the family; this can include sheltering in place.
- Maintain strict hand hygiene for both well and symptomatic family members after using the bathroom, before eating and drinking, and after contact with pets.
- When a sick individual's symptoms worsen, transport to the nearest designated health care agency.
- Change a sick person's clothing and bed linens frequently; wash them separately from those of other family members, using any commercial detergent.
- Disinfect surfaces with which the symptomatic person comes in contact. Use an appropriate disinfectant (e.g., Lysol), especially when soiled by blood or other body fluids.
- Family caregivers need to get plenty of rest, drink fluids frequently, and eat a healthy diet. If the caregiver develops symptoms, obtain appropriate medical care immediately.

BOX 15.9

Basic Disaster Supply Kit

- Water: 1 gallon of water per person per day (minimum of 3-day supply for evacuation/2-week supply for home)
- Food: minimum of 3-day supply for evacuation/2-week supply for home
- Flashlight
- Battery-powered or hand-crank radio (NOAA Weather Radio, if possible)
- Extra batteries (similar item available in the Red Cross Store)
- Deluxe family first aid kit
- Medications (7-day supply) and medical items
- Multipurpose tool
- Sanitation and personal hygiene items
- Copies of personal documents (medication list and pertinent medical information, proof of address, deed/lease to home, passports, birth certificates, insurance policies)
- Cell phone with chargers (similar item available in the Red Cross Store)
- Family and emergency contact information
- Extra cash
- Emergency blanket
- Map(s) of the area

Consider the needs of all family members and add to your kit:
- Medical supplies (hearing aids with extra batteries, glasses, contact lenses, syringes, etc.)
- Baby supplies (bottles, formula, baby food, diapers)
- Games and activities for children
- Pet supplies (collar, leash, ID, food, carrier, bowl)
- Two-way radios
- Extra set of car keys and house keys
- Manual can opener

Additional supplies to keep at home or in your survival kit based on the types of disasters common to your area:
- Whistle
- N95 or surgical masks
- Matches
- Rain gear
- Towels
- Work gloves
- Tools/supplies for securing your home
- Extra clothing, hat and sturdy shoes
- Plastic sheeting
- Duct tape
- Scissors
- Household liquid bleach
- Entertainment items
- Blankets or sleeping bags

Data from American Red Cross: *How to prepare for emergencies*, 2022. https://www.redcross.org/get-help/how-to-prepare-for-emergencies.html. Accessed September 28, 2023.

BOX 15.10

Guidelines for a Food Disaster Supply Kit

- Store at least a 3-day supply of nonperishable food.
- Choose foods your family will eat.
- Remember special dietary needs.
- Avoid foods that will make you thirsty.
- Suggested foods to include in the emergency kit:
  - Ready-to-eat canned meats, fruits, and vegetables, and a can opener
  - Protein or fruit bars

- Dry cereal or granola
- Peanut butter
- Dried fruit
- Canned juices
- Nonperishable pasteurized milk
- High-energy foods
- Food for infants
- Comfort/stress foods

Data from Department of Homeland Security: *Food: Suggested emergency food supplies,* 2022. https://www.ready.gov/food. Accessed September 28, 2023.

◆ SKILL 15.2   Care of a Patient After Chemical Exposure

A chemical disaster is the dispersal of a toxic chemical agent into the environment, most commonly a result of a chemical plant explosion or freight car derailment. The mechanism of dispersal is not always known. In fact, the dispersal mechanism such as an explosion or fire can be a secondary terrorist attack designed to create more fatalities. Explosions spread a toxic chemical in uncontrolled directions, creating more victims. Symptoms from chemical exposure are usually apparent within minutes, but some are delayed up to 24 hours. Early recognition of a chemical event is a priority because you will need to administer many chemical antidotes quickly. Toxic chemical incidents such as biological events are often unannounced or overt. Terrorists often intend for chemical agents to cause mass casualties and induce fear and/or mass hysteria.

Chemical events usually are confined to small areas, although larger dispersal of these agents may occur (e.g., via a crop duster). The nature and scale of contamination depends on the state of the

agent used (e.g., gas versus liquid), characteristics of the chemical used (e.g., heavy or lighter than air), and where the event occurs (e.g., indoors, where ventilation systems affect dispersal; or outdoors, where wind and velocity affect speed and direction of dispersal). For safety reasons, rescue workers should be upwind and uphill from a toxic chemical disaster scene to avoid exposure. The exception is when cyanide gas has been released. Cyanide is lighter than air and thus will travel uphill. It has the unique smell of bitter almonds. If you detect the smell, evacuate the area immediately, although exposure may have already occurred (CDC, 2022b).

Because symptoms are almost immediate, evacuate victims as quickly as possible from a contaminated zone to a decontamination zone. Special respiratory and skin personal protective equipment (PPE) protects rescue workers (FDA, 2021). Before decontamination, victims are a potential source of contamination for rescue workers. Protect yourself against toxic chemical contamination when in contact with a contaminated patient. Secondary contamination is high

TABLE 15.2

Summary of Selected Chemical Warfare Agents

Chemical Agent	Onset of Symptoms	Untreated Course of Chemical Exposure
"Lethal" agents—nerve agents (tabun, sarin, soman, and VX)	Symptoms are generally immediate.	Pinpoint pupils and shortly thereafter salivation, runny nose, dyspnea, chest tightness, nausea, muscle twitching, coma, seizures, and death
"Blood" agents—hydrogen cyanide	Rapid onset of symptoms; cyanide poisoning is often associated with the smell of bitter almonds.	Death caused by asphyxiation
"Blister" agents—mustard and lewisite	Symptoms may be immediate or delayed.	Skin irritation and blistering
"Choking" agents—phosgene and chlorine	Symptoms can be immediate or delayed up to 24 hours.	Coughing, choking, and disruption in pulmonary function that can lead to death

with toxic chemical incidents. Table 15.2 summarizes chemical warfare agents, presenting symptoms, and untreated course of exposure.

The rapid chemical decontamination of victims of a toxic chemical incident is more important than determining the exact chemical. When rapid decontamination is needed, trained personnel are required. Decontamination is either gross or technical, which generally occurs at a scene. A hospital provides decontamination when a contaminated individual presents for treatment. Nurses and all other health care personnel need to use appropriate precautions to avoid becoming victims.

Delegation

The skill of assessing a patient exposed to a chemical agent cannot be delegated to assistive personnel (AP). Assistive personnel can provide supportive care. Direct the AP to:
- Use appropriate PPE to prevent chemical exposure
- Use techniques for handling a body after death to prevent contamination

Interprofessional Collaboration

- First responders and local and federal law enforcement will be part of the interprofessional team.

Equipment

- Decontamination room or area (adult decontamination rooms may not meet the needs of children requiring decontamination; decontamination areas for ambulatory victims will not meet the needs of those who are not ambulatory)

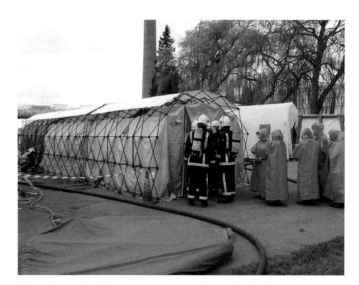

FIG. 15.6 Inflatable decontamination shower for ambulatory victims. *(Courtesy Professional Protection Systems, Ltd.)*

- Scissors or a tool to cut off clothing
- Biohazard bags with labels
- Large volumes of water, decontamination shower (Fig. 15.6)
- Appropriate PPE
- Equipment for physical examination and vital signs
- Equipment for supportive care

STEP	RATIONALE

ASSESSMENT

1. Perform hand hygiene. Don proper PPE.

Provides safety to personnel and helps prevent spread of infectious agent to health care provider.

2. Identify patient using at least two identifiers (e.g., name and birthday or name and medical record number) according to agency policy.

Ensures correct patient. Complies with The Joint Commission standards and improves patient safety (TJC, 2023).

3. Conduct focused physical assessment (see Chapter 6) (e.g., skin assessment; pulmonary assessment—oxygen saturation, lung sounds; cardiac—heart sounds; gastrointestinal [GI]—nausea, vomiting) (see Skill 15.1). Observe for presence of liquid on patient's skin, mucous membranes, or clothing and odor (e.g., chlorine), assessing the condition of skin to determine severity of exposure.

Common conditions present when chemical exposure has occurred. Symptoms vary, depending on type of chemical used.

STEP	RATIONALE
4. Measure patient's vital signs (including SpO2) and include assessment of character of pain, rating severity on a scale of 0 to 10.	Establishes patient baseline to later determine response to therapies.
5. Assess patient's/family caregiver's health literacy.	Determines degree to which individuals have the ability to find, understand, and use information and services to make informed health-related decisions and actions for themselves and others (CDC, 2023).
6. Assess patient for preexisting medical conditions that will complicate effects of toxic chemical exposure.	These patients will likely require additional treatment and sometimes are at greater risk for death.

Clinical Judgment *Consider a toxic chemical event when large numbers of ill persons present who have unexplained yet similar symptoms. The primary objective for initial care is decontamination (i.e., the removal of harmful contaminants from the skin surface). You achieve this by removing clothing; scrubbing the skin; and hydrolysis, a process of chemical dilution using large volumes of water.*

STEP	RATIONALE
7. Remain calm. Listen and assess patient's immediate psychological response after chemical exposure. Some patients present with dissociative symptoms: disorientation, depression, anxiety, psychosis, and inability to care for self. Even without direct exposure to a chemical agent, many individuals, spurred by feelings of fear and doom, will present for emergency services and quickly overwhelm available emergency services.	Remaining calm and projecting confidence reduces anxiety of the ill and worried well as they experience the general sense of panic associated with chemical exposure. Compassionate engagement helps those who are faced with a natural disaster by allowing individuals to know that the first responder's purpose is to provide safety and emotional comfort (Steele, 2023).
8. Identify agency resources available (e.g., critical-incident stress-debriefing teams, counselors, psychiatric/mental health nurse practitioners).	Expert resources assess extent of psychological impact of disorders.

PLANNING

1. Expected outcomes following completion of procedure:	
• Patient reports less pain with reduction in severity on a 0-to-10 scale.	Because of the fatal nature of many chemical agents, the only care available may be palliative.
• Patient's vital signs return to baseline.	When there are no underlying medical conditions and *if* patient's condition is responsive to treatment (when available), vital signs will return to normal within days or weeks.
• Patient's work of breathing decreases.	Indicates improved gas exchange and cardiac output.
• Patient's skin integrity returns to baseline, or no new injury develops.	Minimizing exposure of skin to chemical agent reduces severity and extent of lesions.
• Patient's level of consciousness (LOC) returns to baseline.	Neurological stability is achieved by minimizing exposure to chemical and giving antitoxin quickly.
• Patient's mental health status returns to a pretrauma level of functioning.	Crisis intervention successfully reduces patient's anxiety, fear, and dissociative symptoms (Steele, 2023).
2. Provide privacy and explain care to patient and family caregivers, including decontamination and treatment. Explain your role, orient to location and activities to perform, explain what patient has experienced, and ask, "How are you feeling right now?" Assure them that a medical professional will see them shortly.	Protects patient's privacy; reduces anxiety. Promotes cooperation.
3. Obtain and organize equipment for decontamination.	Prevents discomfort and embarrassment when clothing is removed. Ensures more efficiency when completing a procedure.

IMPLEMENTATION

1. Continue wearing PPE applied during assessment. Prepare for decontamination.	Reduces transmission of and injury from toxic chemicals. Reduces likelihood of secondary toxic chemical contamination to untrained personnel attempting decontamination.

Clinical Judgment *Only trained personnel using required PPE may decontaminate patients with toxic chemical contamination. Hold victim outside decontamination area until preparations are completed for decontamination. If patient is grossly contaminated, consider decontamination before entry into building.*

2. Decontaminate patient:	
a. Act quickly; avoid touching contaminated parts of clothing as much as possible.	Prevents your own contamination.

STEP	RATIONALE
b. Remove all of patient's clothing. **Caution:** *Do not pull over patient's head; instead, cut garments off.*	Cutting off clothing prevents contamination of head and hair.
c. Use large amounts of soap and water to wash patient thoroughly.	Leads to chemical dilution and in some cases prevents patient death.
d. If eyes are burning or vision is blurred, rinse eyes with plain water for 10 to 15 minutes. If patient wears contacts, remove and place with contaminated clothing; do not reinsert in eyes. Wash eyeglasses with soap and water; reapply when completed.	Flushes toxins from eye.
3. Dispose of patient's contaminated clothing in appropriate biohazard bag and seal. Place bag in another plastic bag and seal (see agency policy).	Reduces likelihood of secondary chemical contamination.
4. Initiate treatment for chemical agent using appropriate chemical agent protocol (see agency policy).	Appropriate chemical agent protocol varies with patient exposure (e.g., mustard, nerve agent, chlorine, lewisite).

Clinical Judgment *For mustard-specific triage, keep in mind that patients arriving directly from the scene of potential exposure (within 30–60 minutes) will rarely have symptoms. The sooner after exposure that symptoms occur, the more likely they are to progress and become severe. The triage priority categories are:* **Immediate** (<4 up to 12 hours postexposure): *lower respiratory signs (dyspnea);* **Delayed** (>4 hours [eye and skin] or >12 hours [respiratory] postexposure): *eye lesions with impaired vision, skin lesion covering 2% to 50% of body surface area for liquid exposure or any body surface burn for vapor exposure, lower respiratory symptoms (e.g., cough with sputum production, dyspnea); and* **Minimal** (>4 hours postexposure): *minor eye lesion, no visual impairment, skin lesion <2% body surface in noncritical areas, minor respiratory (CHEMM, 2021b).*

STEP	RATIONALE
5. Establish airway if needed; administer oxygen therapy (see Chapter 23).	Various chemical agents commonly cause respiratory problems that will result in altered gas exchange.
6. Control bleeding.	Various chemical agents cause extensive bleeding.
7. Establish intravascular access. Administer fluid and nutrition therapy (see Chapters 28 and 32).	Various chemical agents commonly cause GI disturbances that can result in dehydration.
8. Provide supportive care (e.g., comfort measures, including hygiene and pain management) (see Chapters 16–18).	Some victims will not survive; it is essential for a nurse to provide palliative symptom control.
9. Counsel patient and family on both acute and potential long-term psychological effects of exposure. Offer access to trained counselors.	Reaction of patients to exposure includes shock, immobilization, and fear. Long-term psychological effects can arise without proper counseling.
10. Raise side rails (as appropriate) and lower bed to lowest position, locking into position.	Ensures patient safety and prevents falls.
11. Dispose of any used supplies in appropriate receptacle.	Reduces transmission of microorganisms.
12. Place nurse call system in an accessible location within patient's reach.	Ensures patient can call for assistance if needed.
13. Remove most heavily contaminated items first. Peel off gown and gloves, roll inside out, and dispose of them. Perform hand hygiene. Remove face shield from behind and dispose of safely. Remove goggles and mask from behind. Place goggles in container for reprocessing; dispose of mask safely. Perform hand hygiene.	Avoids contamination of self, others, and environment. Reduces transmission of microorganisms.

Clinical Judgment *Collaborate with the health care provider and other rescue workers for an interprofessional ongoing plan to manage patients exposed to a toxic chemical agent. You will need to do this while also caring for other patients who are already present in the health care agency seeking care for illness unrelated to the current mass casualty incident (MCI).*

EVALUATION

1. Observe status of airway maintenance, breathing, circulation, LOC, and neurological functioning. Assess vital signs.	Evaluates patient's physical response to available treatment and/or supportive care.
2. Assess character of patient's pain and rate acuity on a pain scale of 0 to 10.	Determines if comfort measures are effective.
3. Inspect condition of skin; note extent of blistering.	Determines extent of healing.
4. Evaluate patient's level of orientation, ability to problem solve, and perception of condition.	Evaluates patient's psychological status and ability to make decisions.
5. **Use Teach-Back:** "I want to be sure I explained to you the focus of our treatment for your spouse. Tell me what you recall about the treatment plan." Revise your instruction now or develop a plan for revised patient/family caregiver teaching if patient/family caregiver is not able to teach back correctly.	Teach-back is a technique for health care providers to ensure that they have explained medical information clearly so that patients and their families understand what is communicated to them (AHRQ, 2023).

STEP	RATIONALE

Unexpected Outcomes

1. Secondary contamination of rescue workers occurs.

2. Patient's physical symptoms progress despite appropriate treatment.

3. Patient's psychological symptoms progress despite appropriate treatment. Patient exhibits anxiety, disorientation, and suicidal ideation.

4. Patient death occurs.

Related Interventions

- Rescue workers immediately remove their clothing, scrub their bodies, and use copious amounts of soap and water.
- Contain clothes in appropriate biohazard bags.
- Provide clean clothes.
- Notify health care provider in charge.
- Continue to provide comfort care.
- Notify mental health treatment team.
- Remain calm, offer reassurance, and protect self and others from physical harm.
- Continue to provide comfort measures.
- When handling bodies, there is continued risk for contamination; make sure that everyone is fully informed regarding proper procedures (see Skill 17.3) and follow agency procedures for specific chemical exposures. When delegating preparation of the deceased, always take into account the level of training of those managing the body.

Documentation

- Document patient's status, decontamination and treatment procedures, and response to treatment and/or comfort measures. Document patient/family caregiver's response to instruction.

Hand-Off Reporting

- Report any unexpected outcome to health care provider in charge.
- Report suspected cases of a toxic chemical event to health care provider or emergency officer.

Special Considerations
Patient Education

- See Skill 15.1 for public education considerations.

Pediatrics

- To avoid becoming a secondary victim, emergency responders need to consider potential contamination before picking up and holding children. Often decontamination consists of providing fresh air and a large volume of low-pressure warm water. Because children are more susceptible to hypothermia, observe for potential signs.

- Adult decontamination facilities are not always appropriate to meet the needs of children. The special PPE worn by rescue workers may frighten young children. The cleaning process and possible separation from uncontaminated parents will likely cause considerable stress and anxiety. Additional health care workers are often necessary to ensure that adequate decontamination has taken place. Verbal encouragement and praise are effective in facilitating the process.
- See Skill 15.1 for additional pediatric considerations.

Older Adults

- See Skill 15.1 for gerontological considerations.

Populations With Disabilities

- See Skill 15.1 for disabled considerations.

Home Care

- Keep upwind and uphill from the release of the toxic chemical unless it is cyanide.
- Use appropriate PPE to protect the family; this includes sheltering in place.
- See Skill 15.1 for additional home care considerations.

✦ SKILL 15.3   Care of a Patient After Radiation Exposure

People are exposed to radiation from many sources including rocks and soil, food, water, air, airline travel, medical procedures, fallout from past nuclear weapons testing, and radiation emergencies. Radiological events differ from nuclear events. A radiological event is the dispersal of radioactive material via a "dirty bomb," by deliberate contamination of food or water supplies, or over the terrain. A nuclear event involves a device that releases nuclear energy in an explosive manner as a result of a nuclear chain reaction. Radiation affects the body in many ways, depending on the level of exposure. High levels of radiation exposure cause a person to develop acute radiation syndrome (ARS) with symptoms of nausea, vomiting, and diarrhea (Mayo Clinic, 2022).

Radiation comes in a variety of forms. Alpha particles are the least dangerous, traveling only a few centimeters. They do not penetrate materials easily and are harmful only if ingested. An

individual's clothing blocks alpha particles from reaching the skin. Beta particles penetrate a short distance into the skin. Protective clothing is necessary for protection. Gamma rays pose the greatest health risk because the waves penetrate deeply, causing severe burns and internal injury. Lead shielding protects against gamma rays. Blasts caused by a nuclear explosion cause not only injury from radiation exposure but also traumatic injuries and burns. Some victims will present with many combined forms of injury requiring treatment. The sooner symptoms begin to appear, the greater a patient's exposure to the radiation. Early symptoms (i.e., within a few hours) suggest that an individual has received a lethal dose of radiation.

Nuclear incidents usually result in wide destruction requiring specialized equipment and resources at the scene to assess structural damage and levels of radioactivity. Radiological events usually cover much smaller areas, but they are often difficult to define. Specialized equipment and training are required to assess the source of radioactivity, determine the scope of contamination, and perform decontamination. The principles to follow to protect individuals from exposure include **get inside, stay inside, and stay tuned** (Mayo Clinic, 2022).

Delegation

The skill of assessment and care of a patient exposed to a radiological agent cannot be delegated to assistive personnel (AP). Direct the AP to:

- Use appropriate PPE to prevent exposure.
- Use techniques for handling a body after death to prevent contamination.

Interprofessional Collaboration

- You will work with an interprofessional team, including specialists in the field of radiation exposure, to care for these patients and limit exposure to others.

Equipment

- Decontamination room or area (adult decontamination rooms do not always meet the needs of children requiring decontamination; decontamination of ambulatory victims will not meet the needs of those who are not ambulatory)
- Scissors or some other tool to cut off clothing
- Clothing containers; type depends on the kind of radiological exposure
- Appropriate PPE for use by personnel in area of radiation release
- Appropriate PPE for health care workers in health care agency setting (i.e., surgical masks, N95 masks recommended if available)
- Radiation meter to survey hands and clothing at frequent intervals
- Equipment for select specimen collection
- Equipment for physical examination and vital signs

STEP	RATIONALE

ASSESSMENT

STEP	RATIONALE
1. Perform hand hygiene. Don proper PPE.	Provides safety to personnel and helps prevent spread of infectious agent to health care provider.
2. Identify patient using at least two identifiers (e.g., name and birthday or name and medical record number) according to agency policy.	Ensures correct patient. Complies with The Joint Commission standards and improves patient safety (TJC, 2023).

Clinical Judgment *Before assessment, a specially trained technician conducts a radiation survey of the patient, initially scanning the face, hands, and feet with a radiation survey instrument. If meter results are positive, a thorough survey (5–8 minutes per person) is conducted.*

STEP	RATIONALE
3. Assess patient's symptoms by performing a focused physical examination (see Skill 15.1).	Symptom identification and clustering data are first steps to determine patient's condition and response to radiation.
4. Measure patient's vital signs (including SpO$_2$) and include assessment of the character of pain, rating severity on a scale of 0 to 10.	Provides baseline to later evaluate patient's response to therapy.

Clinical Judgment *Do not touch a wound if you suspect that radioactive fragments are present.*

STEP	RATIONALE
5. Assess patient's/family caregiver's health literacy.	Determines degree to which individuals have the ability to find, understand, and use information and services to make informed health-related decisions and actions for themselves and others (CDC, 2023).
6. Assess patient for preexisting medical conditions that will complicate effects of the radiological exposure. Symptoms of acute radiation exposure include nausea, vomiting, headache, and diarrhea (Mayo Clinic, 2022).	Patients with preexisting medical conditions can require additional treatment or are at greater risk for death.
7. Review results of diagnostic tests and consult with health care provider.	Determines extent of changes to immune system (e.g., CBC results).
8. Determine patient's allergies, specifically allergy to iodine. Be sure patient has allergy identification wristband.	Patients with iodine sensitivity need to avoid taking potassium iodide, the treatment of choice for radioactive iodine exposure.
9. Assess individual psychological response to radiological event. Some patients present with dissociative symptoms (e.g., feeling as though "not there," sensing that experiences are outside the person): disorientation, depression, anxiety, psychosis, and an inability to care for self. Ask patient, "How do you feel now?" Determine level of orientation and ability to follow conversation.	Allows you to provide appropriate crisis intervention and stress management (Steele, 2023). Remaining calm and projecting confidence while assessing individuals for clinical symptoms versus feeling of panic goes a long way toward reducing the anxiety of the ill and worried well while experiencing the general sense of panic associated with a radiological event.
10. Identify agency resources available (e.g., critical-incident stress-debriefing teams, counselors, psychiatric/mental health nurse practitioners).	Expert resources assess extent of psychological impact of disaster.

STEP	RATIONALE

Clinical Judgment *A radiological event is the event most feared by most individuals. Many are uneducated regarding the dangers of and differences among radiation materials. Health care agencies will likely have many anxious, frightened individuals who can potentially create a danger to the environment. Assess individual for signs of psychological distress. Early identification of symptoms and stress-management interventions can help prevent an individual or mass panic response (Mayo Clinic, 2022).*

PLANNING

1. Expected outcomes following completion of procedure:	
• Patient reports reduced pain and nausea.	In some cases the only care that is available is palliative.
• Patient is successfully decontaminated.	Decontamination procedures remove radioactive materials from patient's skin.
• Patient's vital signs return to baseline.	When there are no underlying medical conditions and *if the patient's disease process is responsive to treatment (when available), vital signs will return to normal within days or weeks.*
• Patient is free of nausea and diarrhea.	Gastrointestinal (GI) alterations following radiation exposure typically respond to antidiarrheal and antiemetic medications.
• Patient's skin integrity returns to baseline.	Radiological burns are minimized through successful decontamination procedures.
• Patient's immune system (e.g., complete blood count [CBC]) returns to baseline.	Exposure to radiation is minimized successfully.
• Patient's work of breathing decreases.	Indicates improved gas exchange and cardiac output.
2. Provide privacy and explain care to patient and family. Explain your role, orient to location and activities to perform, explain what patient has experienced, and ask, "How are you feeling right now?" Assure them that medical personnel will see them shortly.	Protects patient's privacy; reduces anxiety. Promotes cooperation. Crisis intervention reestablishes patient's orientation and sense of reality (Steele, 2023).
3. Obtain and organize equipment for decontamination.	Ensures more efficiency when completing a procedure.

IMPLEMENTATION

1. Perform hand hygiene. Apply clean gloves.	Reduces transmission of microorganisms.
2. Continue wearing PPE applied during assessment. Prepare for decontamination. Only trained personnel use required PPE to decontaminate patients with radiological contamination.	Reduces likelihood of secondary radiological contamination to untrained personnel attempting decontamination.
3. Decontaminate patient:	
a. Remove patient's clothing.	Normally eliminates up to 90% of contamination.
b. Wash patient's skin thoroughly with water and soap, taking care not to abrade or irritate the skin.	Use of large amounts of water is critical in decontamination.
c. Use tepid decontamination water. Cover wounds with waterproof dressings to avoid spread of radioactivity (Radiation Emergency Medical Management [REMM], 2022a).	Water that is too cold will close pores, and water that is too hot enhances absorption of radioactive materials (REMM, 2022a).
d. Have radiation technician resurvey patient after washing using dosimeter. Rewash as needed.	Determines if residual radiation is present. Used to measure an absorbed dose of ionizing radiation.
e. Isolate and cover any area of skin that is still positive for radiation by using plastic bag or wrap.	Area is washed until no further reduction in contamination is achieved (verified by survey instrumentation) and then covered to reduce exposure of health care workers.
4. Bag and tag patient's contaminated clothing for further evaluation and place in appropriate biohazard container.	Reduces likelihood of secondary contamination when you use containers designed to contain radiological particles.

Clinical Judgment *Collaborate with the health care provider and other rescue workers for an interprofessional ongoing plan to manage patients exposed to radiological materials. You will need to do this while also caring for other patients who are already present in the health care agency seeking care for illness unrelated to the current nuclear or radiological event.*

5. Prepare for possibly obtaining a CBC, urinalysis, fecal specimen, and swabs of body orifices (see Chapter 7).	CBC establishes baseline to determine patient's immunological status over time. A health care provider who suspects internal contamination will order collection of urine, feces, and body orifice swabs to analyze for radionuclides.
6. Treat symptoms according to ordinary treatment practices: provide intravenous fluid support, antidiarrheal therapies, antiemetic medications, and potassium iodide tablets.	Patient exposed to radiation is at risk for GI alterations and fluid imbalance (Mayo Clinic, 2022).

STEP	RATIONALE
7. Counsel patient and family on both acute and potential long-term psychological effects of exposure. Offer access to trained counselors.	Reaction of patients to exposure includes shock, immobilization, and fear. Long-term psychological effects can arise without proper counseling (Steele, 2023).
8. Raise side rails (as appropriate) and lower bed to lowest position, locking into position.	Ensures patient safety and prevents falls.
9. Dispose of any used supplies in appropriate receptacle.	Reduces transmission of microorganisms.
10. Place nurse call system in an accessible location within patient's reach.	Ensures patient can call for assistance if needed.
11. Remove most heavily contaminated items first. Peel off gown and gloves, roll inside out, and dispose of them. Perform hand hygiene. Remove face shield from behind and dispose of safely. Remove goggles and mask from behind. Place goggles in container for reprocessing; dispose of mask safely. Perform hand hygiene.	Avoids contamination of self, others, and environment. Reduces transmission of microorganisms.

EVALUATION

1. Observe skin integrity, fluid balance, respiratory and GI status, level of consciousness (LOC), and neurological functioning. Look for improvement of other radiological agent–specific symptoms. Evaluate vital signs.	Evaluates patient's physical response to available treatment and/or supportive care.
2. Monitor CBC and other laboratory tests.	Determines patient's immune response.
3. Evaluate patient's LOC, orientation, and ability to relate events. Ask if patient remembers what has occurred; observe affect.	Determines if psychological status has improved.
4. **Use Teach-Back:** "I want to talk again with you about radiation sickness and what you can do to make your family member more comfortable. Tell me how you would do this in the home." Revise your instruction now or develop a plan for revised patient/family caregiver teaching if patient/family caregiver is not able to teach back correctly.	Teach-back is a technique for health care providers to ensure that they have explained medical information clearly so that patients and their families understand what is communicated to them (AHRQ, 2023).

Unexpected Outcomes	Related Interventions
1. Secondary contamination of rescue workers occurs.	• Institute appropriate decontamination of worker.
2. Patient's symptoms progress despite appropriate treatment.	• Notify health care provider in charge. • Continue to provide comfort care.
3. Patient's psychological state deteriorates with development of disorientation, suicidal ideation, violence toward others.	• Notify mental health treatment team. • Remain calm, offer reassurance, and protect self and others from physical harm. • Continue to provide comfort care (see Chapter 17).
4. Patient death occurs.	• When handling bodies, take into account continued risk for contamination; make sure that everyone is fully informed about proper procedure. • If the deceased is known or suspected to be contaminated, all people handling the body will wear PPE and a personal dosimeter. A Disaster Mortuary Operational Response Team (DMORT) may need to be called to assist (REMM, 2022b). • When delegating preparation of the deceased, take into account the level of training of those managing the body.

Documentation

- Document treatments provided and patient's physical and psychological response. Document patient and family caregiver response to instruction.

Hand-Off Reporting

- Report presence of open wound and any suspected radioactive fragment to health care provider in charge immediately.
- Report any unexpected outcomes to health care provider.

Special Considerations

Patient Education

- See Skill 15.1 for patient education considerations.

Pediatrics

- Children are vulnerable to radiation because (1) their organ systems are more sensitive than those of adults, and (2) they have more years of life expectancy over which to develop complications from the radiological exposure.
- See Skills 15.1 and 15.2 for additional pediatric considerations.

Older Adults

- Because some older adults have many concurrent illnesses, radiological agents can worsen these conditions and result in an older adult needing more immediate care than an initial triage had indicated.
- See Skill 15.1 for additional gerontological considerations.

Populations With Disabilities

- See Skill 15.1.

Home Care

- When a radiological or nuclear event occurs, listen to the radio or television for special instructions, including appropriate means for maintaining a safe shelter.
- Keep upwind and uphill from the release of the radioactive materials.
- See Skill 15.1 for additional home care considerations.

✦ SKILL 15.4   Care of a Patient After a Natural Disaster

Each natural disaster is unique and can range from a local community fire to a Category 5 hurricane that affects a large geographical area. As a result, the type of injuries patients may experience will differ. Common injuries during a hurricane are cuts caused by flying glass or other debris, as well as back injuries experienced during the event or cleanup. Other injuries include puncture wounds resulting from exposed nails, metal, or glass, and bone fractures. Flooding can easily occur, putting persons at risk for drowning, physical trauma, heart attacks, electrocution, carbon monoxide poisoning, or fire associated with flooding (WHO, 2022c). Floods can also have medium- and long-term health impacts including water- and vector-borne diseases, such as cholera, typhoid, or malaria; injuries such as lacerations or punctures; mental health effects associated with emergency situations and disrupted health care services; and damaged basic infrastructure, such as food and water supplies (WHO, 2022c). The Occupational Safety and Health Administration (n.d.) notes that in the case of earthquakes, most earthquake-related injuries result from collapsing walls, flying glass, and falling objects as a result of the ground shaking or from people trying to move more than a few feet during the shaking.

Unlike with other disasters, planning can begin far in advance to prepare for a natural disaster, depending on the geographical area where the patient lives and the associated natural disaster risks. People who live in areas prone to earthquakes, for example, benefit from practice drills for what to do when shaking begins (Fig. 15.7), and people who live in areas at risk for wildfires can plan ahead to have a room to close off air from the outside, reduce smoke exposure, and learn how to evacuate safely (CDC, 2021a). Severe weather conditions can also cause harm, with temperature and conditions of extremes of hot and cold that affect everyday life, travel, and numerous health conditions.

Delegation

The skill of assessing a patient exposed to a natural disaster cannot be delegated to assistive personnel (AP). Direct the AP to:
- Use appropriate PPE to prevent exposure during care activities.

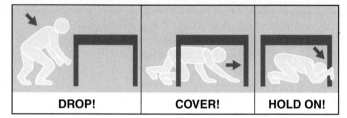

FIG. 15.7 Actions to take to remain safe and healthy in the event of an earthquake. (*From Centers for Disease Control and Prevention [CDC]: Natural disasters and severe weather. www.cdc.gov/disasters. Accessed September 28, 2023.*)

Interprofessional Collaboration

- Natural disasters are very different, and the interprofessional team will change roles and responsibilities to meet the needs of the particular patients.

Equipment

Choice of equipment depends on the type of natural disaster that occurred and subsequent injuries and health care concerns. Following is a general list of supplies that might be used:
- Biohazard bags with label
- Soap and water
- Clean gloves
- Gown
- Shoe covers
- Head covers
- Mask
- Standard face mask
- N95 mask
- Face shield
- Equipment for physical examination and vital signs
- Oxygen therapy
- Airway maintenance supplies
- Intravenous therapy supplies
- Vital signs equipment

STEP	RATIONALE

ASSESSMENT

1. Perform hand hygiene. Don proper PPE.

2. Identify patient using at least two identifiers (e.g., name and birthday or name and medical record number) according to agency policy.

Proper PPE provides safety to personnel and helps prevent spread of infectious agent to health care provider.

Ensures correct patient. Complies with The Joint Commission standards and improves patient safety (TJC, 2023).

STEP	RATIONALE
3. Conduct focused health history and physical examination depending on area of injury (e.g., skin assessment, pulmonary assessment [oxygen saturation, lung sounds], musculoskeletal integrity and movement of extremities, neurological [Glasgow Coma Scale]). Review history of patient's presenting symptoms and determine if pattern exists (see Chapter 6).	Symptom identification and clustering data help to accurately determine injuries sustained. Physical symptoms will greatly vary depending on type of disaster (i.e., fire, hurricane, severe hot or cold weather).
4. Measure patient's vital signs and include assessment of character of pain, rating severity on a scale of 0 to 10.	Provides baseline to later evaluate patient's response to therapy.
5. Assess patient's/family caregiver's health literacy.	Determines degree to which individuals have the ability to find, understand, and use information and services to make informed health-related decisions and actions for themselves and others (CDC, 2023).
6. Assess patient for health risks (e.g., history of heart disease, pulmonary disease, cancer, pregnancy) that complicate effects of exposure to the natural disaster.	Patients with preexisting medical conditions often require additional treatment or are at greater risk for death. Frail older adults will require additional assessment (Alaska Nurses Association, 2019).
7. Review results of diagnostic tests and consult with health care provider.	Provides baseline to measure change in patient's status.
8. Stay calm. Listen and assess patient's immediate psychological response after experience. Some patients present with dissociative symptoms (e.g., feeling as though "not there" or sensing that everything is outside of the person): disorientation, depression, anxiety, psychosis, and inability to care for self.	Aids in providing appropriate crisis intervention and stress management (Steele, 2023). Remaining calm and projecting confidence while assessing individuals for clinical symptoms reduce anxiety of the ill and worried well while experiencing the general sense of panic associated with a natural disaster event.
9. Identify agency resources available (e.g., critical-incident stress-debriefing teams, counselors, psychiatric/mental health nurse practitioners).	Expert resources help to assess extent of psychological impact of disaster.

Clinical Judgment *Cleaning and sanitizing the household after an emergency is important to help prevent the spread of illness and disease. The CDC (2021a) offers recommendations to clean and sanitize household items and surfaces, including ways to prevent mold from water contamination.*

PLANNING

1. Expected outcomes following completion of procedure:
   - Patient reports reduced pain.

   - Patient's vital signs return to baseline.

   - Patient has normal ROM and strength in injured extremity.
   - Patient's skin integrity returns to baseline.

   - Patient's level of consciousness (LOC) returns to baseline.

   - Patient's mental health status returns to pretrauma level of functioning.
2. Dispense timely and accurate information: accurate description of the disaster to which patient is exposed and implications for patient and family caregiver.
3. Provide for patient privacy and explain procedure.
4. Obtain and organize equipment for decontamination.

In some cases, care is only palliative, with comfort as the focus. Do not underestimate the value of comfort as care.

When there are no underlying medical conditions and if the patient's injury is responsive to treatment (when available), vital signs will normalize.

Indicates healing of muscle strain or other musculoskeletal injury.

Antibiotic and antitoxin therapy will aid in resolution/healing of lacerations over time. Burns will require long-term treatment.

Treatment measures restore neurological function and oxygenation status.

Crisis intervention successfully reduces patient's anxiety, fear, and dissociative symptoms (Steele, 2023).

Information relieves anxiety and fear.

Protects patient's privacy; reduces anxiety. Promotes cooperation.
Ensures more efficiency when completing a procedure.

IMPLEMENTATION

1. Continue wearing PPE applied before assessment. Follow transmission-based isolation precautions (see Chapter 9). (See Table 15.1 for route of contamination.)	Reduces transmission of microorganisms and the likelihood of additional secondary sites of contamination.
2. Administer appropriate antibiotics as indicated.	Prevents infection.
3. Administer fluid and nutrition therapy (Chapters 28 and 32).	Patient may be dehydrated owing to long period between impact and rescue time.

STEP	RATIONALE
4. Administer appropriate wound care (Chapter 38).	Protects wound and promotes healing.
5. Provide supportive care (e.g., comfort measures, including pain management).	Some victims will not survive; palliative care is essential (see Chapter 17).
6. Counsel patient and family caregiver about acute and potential long-term psychological effects of experiencing disaster. Offer access to trained counselors. Support survivors of a disaster by identifying resources available (e.g., Red Cross, Salvation Army).	Patients may no longer have housing or a safe home to live in. Social support networks foster coping in the days after a disaster.
7. Raise side rails (as appropriate) and lower bed to lowest position, locking into position.	Ensures patient safety and prevents falls.
8. Dispose of any used supplies in appropriate receptacle.	Reduces transmission of microorganisms.
9. Place nurse call system in an accessible location within patient's reach.	Ensures patient can call for assistance if needed.
10. After leaving patient area, remove most heavily contaminated items first. Peel off gown and gloves, roll inside out, and dispose of them. Perform hand hygiene. Remove face shield from behind and dispose of safely. Remove goggles and mask from behind. Place goggles in container for reprocessing; dispose of mask safely. Perform hand hygiene.	Avoids contamination of self, others, and environment. Reduces transmission of microorganisms.

Clinical Judgment *Collaborate with the health care provider and other rescue workers for an interprofessional ongoing plan for managing patients while caring for other patients who are already present in the health care agency seeking care for illness unrelated to the current mass casualty incident (MCI).*

EVALUATION

1. Observe for improved airway maintenance, breathing, circulation, LOC, and neurological functioning.	Evaluates patient's response to available treatment and/or supportive care.
2. Evaluate vital signs and level of pain.	Evaluates patient's response to treatment.
3. Inspect condition of patient's skin; note character of any wounds.	Evaluates patient's response to antibiotic therapy.
4. Query patient: "Tell me how you feel right now." Check level of orientation and ability to conduct conversation.	Evaluates patient for changes that suggest either improvement or deterioration of psychological status.
5. **Use Teach-Back:** "I want to discuss your wound care when you return home. We discussed the steps earlier; tell me how you are going to care for your wound." Revise your instruction now or develop a plan for revised patient/family caregiver teaching if patient/family caregiver is not able to teach back correctly.	Teach-back is a technique for health care providers to ensure that they have explained medical information clearly so that patients and their families understand what is communicated to them (AHRQ, 2023).

Unexpected Outcomes	Related Interventions
1. Patient's physical or psychological symptoms progress.	• Notify health care provider. • Notify mental health treatment team. • Remain calm, offer reassurance, and protect self and others from physical harm. • Continue to provide comfort care.
2. Patient death occurs.	• When handling bodies, consider continued risk for contamination; make sure that everyone is fully informed regarding proper procedure.

Documentation

• Document patient's status, treatments provided, and response. Document patient and family caregiver response to teaching.

Hand-Off Reporting

• Report presence of new wounds and injuries to health care provider in charge.
• Report any unexpected outcomes to health care provider.

Special Considerations
Patient Education

• Preparedness for natural disasters can occur well before a disaster is expected and imminent.

• For the specific risks, educate patients and families how to best respond and how to access emergency services.
• For expectant parents, teach them to prepare an emergency kit including prenatal vitamins and prescription medications along with contact information for all health care providers. Emergency birth supplies including clean towels, sharp scissors, an infant bulb syringe, medical gloves, two white shoelaces, sheets, sanitary pads, blankets, and infant and maternity clothing are also good items to include (Alaska Nurses Association, 2019).

Pediatrics

• Regardless of a child's age, the child may feel upset or have other strong emotions after a disaster. Some children react right away, whereas others may show signs of difficulty much later. How a child reacts and the common signs of distress can vary according to the child's age, previous experiences, and how the child typically copes with stress (CDC, 2021a).

- Children need help from adults in an emergency. They do not fully understand how to keep themselves safe, may not be able to explain what hurts or bothers them, and understand less about the situation than adults do (Alaska Nurses Association, 2019).

Older Adults

- Chronic conditions (e.g., arthritis) can affect the ability to walk several blocks, reach overhead, or move quickly; plan for assistive devices and assistance in evacuation or rescue (Alaska Nurses Association, 2019).
- Patients with dementia will require more time and resources to deal with effects of a natural disaster and might become disoriented (Schnitker et al., 2019).
- See Skill 15.1 for additional gerontological considerations.

Populations With Disabilities

- Collaboration with governmental organizations is critical for developing strategies to make emergency communications and related announcements accessible to people with disabilities (Kim & Zakour, 2018).

Home Care

- Be aware of risks of natural disasters, paying attention to radio and television warnings.
- Give patient and family caregivers list of shelter and support services for immediate and long-term help. Include national resources such as Ready.gov; the Disaster Distress Helpline (www.samhsa.gov/find-help/disaster-distress-helpline); and the Emergency Prescription Assistance Program (www.phe.gov/Preparedness/planning/epap).

✦ CLINICAL JUDGMENT AND NEXT GENERATION NCLEX® EXAMINATION–STYLE QUESTIONS

Two parents, a young child, and a 70-year-old grandparent were brought to the emergency department after being rescued by first responders. A tornado hit the neighborhood, destroying the house. The father has a large laceration on the left thigh, which is bleeding through the bandage applied by first responders. The 8-year-old child has a wound to the left foot and right arm. The mother reports no injuries yet is concerned about the grandparent. The grandparent reports mild left-sided chest pain, nausea, and dizziness but insists the symptoms are related to being upset about the tornado destroying the house. The nurse documents a history and physical for the grandparent.

1. Highlight the findings that require **immediate** follow-up by the nurse.

Body System	Findings
Neurological	PERRLA; reports feeling dizzy and says, "I'm sure it's because I'm so anxious about losing our home."
Pulmonary	Lungs clear to auscultation bilaterally
Cardiovascular	Pulses 2+ in all extremities; capillary refill 2 seconds; reports left-sided chest pain that is "sharp"
Gastrointestinal	Bowel sounds present x 4 quadrants; abdomen soft and round, nontender to touch; reports mild nausea

2. Using the START triage system, how will the nurse tag the grandparent?
1. Green
2. Yellow
3. Red
4. Black

3. The nurse prepares to care for the 8-year-old child. Which action will the nurse take?
1. Take the child to be examined alone.
2. Complete a head-to-toe assessment.
3. Speak directly only to the parents.
4. Allow the child time to voice fears.
5. Ask social service to be present during the assessment.

4. The nurse has provided education to the father about how to take medication and care for the leg laceration at home. Which statement by the father indicates that teaching from the nurse was effective?
1. "I should leave this bandage on for about a week until my leg heals."
2. "I plan to use sterile gloves and sterile technique when I care for the wound."
3. "I am supposed to clean the laceration several times daily with alcohol."
4. "I will take all of the antibioti cs the provider gave me even if my leg looks better."

5. As the parents and child prepare for discharge, the nurse is asked which resources should be accessed to better prepare for any future disaster. Which resource will the n urse recommend? **Select all that apply.**
1. Ready.gov
2. American Nurses Association
3. American Medical Association
4. Nearest local community health center
5. Centers for Disease Control and Prevention website

Visit the Evolve site for Answers to the Clinical Judgment and Next Generation NCLEX® Examination–Style Questions.

REFERENCES

Agency for Healthcare Research and Quality (AHRQ): *Teach-Back: intervention*, 2023. https://www.ahrq.gov/patient-safety/reports/engage/interventions/teach-back.html.

Alaska Nurses Association: Disaster preparedness: considerations for specific groups, *Alaska Nurse* 70(1):8, 2019.

American Academy of Nursing (AAN): *American Academy of Nursing and American Red Cross issue recommendations on disaster preparedness, response, and recovery for older adults*, 2021. https://www.wahpetondailynews.com/news/coronavirus/american-academy-of-nursing-and-amercan-red-cross-issue-disaster-prep-recommendations/article_07c8bed6-7b8d-11ea-9ac5-bb2662692be7.html. Accessed September 28, 2023.

American Nurses Association (ANA): *Disaster preparedness*, 2019. https://www.nursingworld.org/practice-policy/work-environment/health-safety/disaster-preparedness/. Accessed September 28, 2023.

American Red Cross: *How to prepare for emergencies*, 2022. https://www.redcross.org/get-help/how-to-prepare-for-emergencies.html. Accessed May 17, 2022.

Cariaso-Sugay J, et al: Nurse leaders' knowledge and confidence managing disasters in the acute care setting, *Nurs Admin Q* 45(2):142–151, 2021.

Centers for Disease Control and Prevention (CDC): *Public health emergency preparedness and response capabilities: national standards for state, local, tribal, and territorial public health*, 2021a. https://www.cdc.gov/cpr/readiness/capabilities.htm. Accessed September 28, 2023.

Centers for Disease Control and Prevention (CDC): *History of smallpox*, 2021b. https://www.cdc.gov/smallpox/history/history.html. Accessed September 28, 2023.

Centers for Disease Control and Prevention (CDC): *Natural disasters and severe weather*, 2022a. https://www.cdc.gov/disasters/. Accessed September 28, 2023.

Centers for Disease Control and Prevention (CDC): *Chemical emergencies*, 2022b. https://www.cdc.gov/chemicalemergencies/. Accessed September 28, 2023.

Centers for Disease Control and Prevention (CDC): *What is health literacy?* 2023. https://www.cdc.gov/healthliteracy/learn. Accessed September 28, 2023.

Chemical Hazards Emergency Medical Management (CHEMM): *START adult triage algorithm*, 2021a. https://chemm.hhs.gov/startadult.htm. Accessed September 28, 2023.

Chemical Hazards Emergency Medical Management (CHEMM): *Mustard acute management overview*, 2021b. https://chemm.hhs.gov/mustard_prehospital_mmg.htm#:~:text=Immediate%20-%20mustard%20casualties%2C%20especially%20those%20with%20eye,decontamination%20may%20limit%20the%20severity%20of%20the%20lesions. Accessed September 28, 2023.

Department of Homeland Security (DHS): *If you see something, say something*, n.d. https://www.dhs.gov/see-something-say-something. Accessed September 28, 2023.

Department of Homeland Security (DHS): *National Terrorism Advisory System*, 2021. https://www.dhs.gov/ntas-frequently-asked-questions. Accessed September 28, 2023.

Federal Emergency Management Agency (FEMA): *2019 National Threat and Hazard Identification and Risk Assessment (THIRA): Overview and methodology*, 2019. https://www.fema.gov/sites/default/files/2020-06/fema_national-thira-overview-methodology_2019_0.pdf. Accessed September 28, 2023.

Federal Emergency Management Agency (FEMA): *Make a plan*, 2022. https://www.ready.gov/plan. Accessed September 28, 2023.

Healthdirect.gov: *What is a pandemic?* 2022. https://www.healthdirect.gov.au/what-is-a-pandemic. Accessed September 28, 2023.

Hockenberry M, et al: *Wong's essentials of pediatric nursing*, ed 11, St. Louis, 2022, Elsevier.

Kim HJ, Zakour M: Exploring the factors associated with the disaster preparedness of human service organizations serving persons with disabilities, *Hum Serv Organ Manag Leadersh Gov* 42(1):19, 2018.

Karnjuš I, et al: *Nurses' core disaster-response competencies for combating COVID-19—a cross-sectional study*, 2021. https://journals.plos.org/plosone/article?id=10.1371/journal.pone.0252934. Accessed September 28, 2023.

Lai J, et al: Factors associated with mental health outcomes among health care workers exposed to coronavirus disease, *JAMA Netw Open* 3:e20397, 2020.

Lynch JB, et al: *Infectious Diseases Society of America guidelines on infection prevention for healthcare personnel caring for patients with suspected or known COVID-19*, 2021. https://www.jointcommission.org/-/media/tjc/documents/covid19/idsa-ppe-recommendations-11-22-2021.pdf. Accessed April 7, 2023.

Mayo Clinic: *Radiation sickness*, 2022. https://www.mayoclinic.org/diseases-conditions/radiation-sickness/symptoms-causes/syc-20377058. Accessed September 28, 2023.

National Center for Disaster Medicine & Public Health: *Core competencies in disaster health*. https://ncdmph.usuhs.edu/education. Accessed September 28, 2023.

Occupational Safety and Health Administration (OSHA), US Dept of Labor: *Earthquakes Guide*, n.d. https://www.osha.gov/emergency-preparedness/guides/earthquakes. Accessed September 28, 2023.

Radiation Emergency Medical Management (REMM): *Procedures for radiation decontamination*, 2022a. https://remm.hhs.gov/ext_contamination.htm. Accessed September 28, 2023.

Radiation Emergency Medical Management (REMM): *Management of the deceased in radiation emergencies*, 2022b. https://remm.hhs.gov/deceased.htm. Accessed September 29, 2023.

Rathjen NA, Shahbodaghi SD: Bioterrorism, *Am Fam Physician* 104,4:376, 2021.

Said NB, et al: Psychological preparedness for disasters among nurses with disaster field experience: An international online survey, *Int J Disaster Risk Reduct* 46:101533, 2020.

Schnitker L, et al: A national survey of aged care facility managers' views of preparedness for natural disasters relevant to residents with dementia, *Australas J Ageing* 38(3):182, 2019.

Steele D: *Keltner's Psychiatric nursing*, ed 9, St. Louis, 2023, Elsevier.

The Joint Commission (TJC): *2023 National patient safety goals*, Oakbrook Terrace, IL, 2023, The Joint Commission. https://www.jointcommission.org/standards/national-patient-safety-goals/.

US Department of Health and Human Services (DHHS): *Strategic National Stockpile*, 2021. https://www.phe.gov/about/sns/Pages/default.aspx. Accessed September 28, 2023.

US Food and Drug Administration (FDA): *Personal protective equipment for infection control*, 2021. https://www.fda.gov/medical-devices/general-hospital-devices-and-supplies/personal-protective-equipment-infection-control. Accessed September 28, 2023.

World Health Organization (WHO): *Coronavirus*, 2022a. https://www.who.int/health-topics/coronavirus#tab=tab_1. Accessed September 28, 2023.

World Health Organization (WHO): *Ebola virus disease*, 2022b. https://www.who.int/health-topics/ebola/#tab=tab_1. Accessed September 28, 2023.

World Health Organization (WHO): *Floods*, 2022c. https://www.who.int/health-topics/floods#tab=tab_1. Accessed September 28, 2023.

16 | Pain Management

SKILLS AND PROCEDURES

Skill 16.1 **Pain Assessment and Basic Comfort Measures, p. 446**

Skill 16.2 **Nonpharmacological Pain Management, p. 453**

Skill 16.3 **Pharmacological Pain Management, p. 460**

Skill 16.4 **Patient-Controlled Analgesia, p. 466**

Skill 16.5 **Epidural Analgesia, p. 472**

Skill 16.6 **Local Anesthetic Infusion Pump for Analgesia, p. 479**

Skill 16.7 **Moist and Dry Heat Applications, p. 482**

Skill 16.8 **Cold Application, p. 489**

OBJECTIVES

Mastery of content in this chapter will enable you to:
- Assess a patient's level of pain.
- Assess a patient's level of sedation.
- Explain how a comprehensive pain assessment allows you to provide patient appropriate comfort measures.
- Examine the nursing implications for using evidence-based nonpharmacological pain interventions.
- Discuss the potential side effects following administration of pharmacological therapies.
- Explore the nursing interventions associated with pharmacological side effects of analgesics.

- Explain the process for safe use of a patient-controlled analgesia (PCA) device.
- Assess and manage a patient receiving epidural analgesia or a local anesthetic infusion pump.
- Compare and contrast the physiological effects of heat and cold therapies.
- Discuss safety measures to follow when applying heat and cold therapies.
- Evaluate the effectiveness of pain-management techniques.

MEDIA RESOURCES

- http://evolve.elsevier.com/Perry/skills
- Review Questions
- Case Studies

- ▶ Video Clips
- Audio Glossary
- Answers to Clinical Judgment and Next-Generation NCLEX® Examination–Style Questions

PURPOSE

Pain is the most common reason that people seek health care, and it is also a common reason why people turn to complementary and integrative health approaches (National Institutes of Health [NIH], 2022). Pain is often underrecognized, misunderstood, and inadequately treated. It is also a major health problem across the world, in part due to the rising opioid crisis. A person in pain often feels distress or suffering and seeks relief. One of the major challenges with pain is that nurses and health care providers may find it difficult to understand the level of pain that patients experience. There are objective signs and symptoms used for assessing pain, yet nurses often rely only on patients' subjective self-reports. No two people experience pain in the same way, and no two painful events create identical responses or feelings in a person. In 1995 the American Pain Society urged that pain assessment become the fifth vital sign. As a result, health care agencies incorporated numerical rating scales (NRSs) to ensure that pain would be assessed in all patients. However, a large body of evidence indicates that measuring pain intensity only, using unidimensional tools such as an NRS, has not

improved pain outcomes (Scher et al., 2018). Instead a comprehensive pain assessment is recommended (Scher et al., 2018).

A patient is the one who knows whether pain is present and what the experience is like. However, over recent years health care providers have become overly reliant on using only patients' self-reports of pain intensity to assess their level of pain. Routinely you will see nurses within hospital settings ask patients to rate their pain on a pain scale (e.g., "On a scale of 0 to 10, how is your pain today?"). Prescribing based on a pain score alone is not advocated by The Joint Commission (TJC) (Baker, 2017). Nurses can screen for pain by using pain scales, but when pain is present, they must perform a more comprehensive assessment. A plan of treatment needs to include a patient's clinical condition and past medical history (TJC, 2022). In the update of a position statement by the American Society for Pain Management Nursing (ASPMN), there is a warning about the risks associated with assessment and treatment based solely on pain-intensity measurement (Quinlan-Cowell et al., 2022):
- Overreliance on pain-intensity scores and use of pain scales is correlated with inappropriate analgesic prescription (North Carolina Institute of Medicine [NCIOM], 2020).

- Patient reports of pain intensity are influenced by many biopsychosocial factors, including but not limited to anxiety, fear, worry, depression, and lack of sleep, as well as performance of activities of daily living (ADLs) (Quinlan-Colwell, 2020; Adeboye et al., 2021; Sturgeon et al., 2021).
- There is no evidence that a particular medication or dose will relieve pain in a given individual reporting a specific pain intensity (Pasero et al., 2016).
- The practice of dosing to numbers prevents essential nursing pain assessment and critical thinking, which involve more than hearing and documenting pain intensity (Pasero et al., 2016).
- Your role as a nurse is to be a patient advocate and to recognize the unique nature of pain for each patient, thoroughly assess the character of the pain, use clinical judgment to identify the nature of the patient's associated health problems, and help select appropriate therapies. Part of clinical judgment is to consider the pharmacological and nonpharmacological therapies needed to achieve optimum patient outcomes.

PRACTICE STANDARDS

- Centers for Disease Control and Prevention (CDC), 2016: CDC Guideline for Prescribing Opioids for Chronic Pain—Opioid administration
- Centers for Disease Control and Prevention (CDC), 2022: About CDC's Opioid Prescribing Guideline—Opioid administration
- Chou R et al., 2016: Management of Postoperative Pain: A Clinical Practice Guideline From The American Pain Society, The American Society of Regional Anesthesia and Pain Medicine, and the American Society of Anesthesiologists' Committee on Regional Anesthesia, Executive Committee, And Administrative Council—Management of postoperative pain
- Gorski et al., 2021: Infusion Therapy Standards of Practice, 8th ed—Epidural analgesia
- Pasero C et al., 2016: American Society for Pain Management Nursing (ASPMN) Position Statement: Prescribing and Administering Opioid Doses Based Solely on Pain Intensity—Opioid administration
- The Joint Commission (TJC), 2018: Pain Assessment and Management Standards for Hospitals—Assessment standards
- The Joint Commission (TJC), 2023: National Patient Safety Goals—Patient identification

SUPPLEMENTAL STANDARDS

- Cooney MF, 2016: Postoperative Pain Management: Clinical Practice Guidelines—Postoperative pain
- The Royal College of Anaesthetists (RCoA), 2020: Best Practice in the Management of Epidural Analgesia in the Hospital Setting—Management of epidural infusions
- World Health Organization (WHO), 2019: WHO Revision of Pain Management Guidelines

PRINCIPLES FOR PRACTICE

- The TJC (2018) pain assessment and management standards outline a multilevel approach to pain management to help frontline nurses at the bedside and other health care providers deliver safe, individualized pain care (TJC, 2018; TJC, 2022).
- Patients' cognitive impairments represent special challenges to pain assessment. Carefully observe patients' behaviors and nonverbal responses to pain when they are unable to self-report. Use valid pain-assessment tools (e.g., Pain Assessment

in Advanced Dementia Scale [PAINAD], Pain Assessment in Impaired Cognition [PAIC]) that are designed for nonverbal patients (e.g., those with advanced dementia) (GeriatricPain.org, 2023; Tapp et al., 2019).
- Types of pain include neuropathic (pain caused by a lesion or disease affecting the somatosensory system, such as peripheral diabetic neuropathy), nociceptive (pain clearly associated with tissue damage or inflammation experienced after trauma or surgery), and mixed pain states. Either type can be acute or become chronic. A patient may present with more than one type of pain. Knowing the pathophysiology of pain and common pain descriptors improves your ability to make informed clinical decisions.
- The most effective pain management combines pharmacological and nonpharmacological strategies, described as a multimodal approach.
- The current pharmacological approach to acute and chronic pain management is to provide multimodal analgesia, which combines drugs with at least two different mechanisms of action so pain control can be optimized.
- There are three types of analgesics: (1) nonopioids, including acetaminophen and nonsteroidal antiinflammatory drugs (NSAIDs); (2) opioids (traditionally called narcotics); and (3) adjuvants or coanalgesics, a variety of medications that have primary indications other than pain but may provide analgesic properties (Portenoy, 2000).
- Although there is a priority among health care providers to limit prescription of opioids because of concern about risk for addiction, there is another key issue: opioids do not actually work well for chronic pain in many patients. In some cases, research shows that opioids can actually increase the feeling of pain, described as hyperalgesia (NIH, 2020).
- Timely analgesic administration before a patient's pain becomes severe is crucial for optimal relief. Pain is easier to prevent than to treat. Be proactive in managing a patient's pain, not reactive.
- In many clinical situations, administration of pharmacological agents "around the clock" (ATC) rather than on an "as-needed" (prn) basis is preferable (Inoue et al., 2021; Brant et al., 2017).
- Make every effort to provide complementary/integrative pain-management methods (e.g., music therapy, massage), which generally do not require a health care provider's order (check agency policy). This provides patients the opportunity to assume an active role in achieving a higher level of comfort and in some instances freedom from pain.
- Be willing to use more than one type of pain-relief measure as appropriate, and use measures that a patient believes are effective when possible. Provide education to patients and family caregivers if their choice of pain control may pose risks.
- Keep an open mind about ways to relieve pain.
- Keep trying. When efforts at pain relief fail, do not abandon the patient, but reassess the situation. Persistent pain is treatable, with improvement anticipated, but it is not curable (Galicia-Castillo & Weiner, 2023).
- Although pain may not be totally eliminated, substantial improvement in function is realistic (Galicia-Castillo & Weiner, 2023).

PERSON-CENTERED CARE

- Living in an ethnically and culturally diverse society requires health care providers to respect and consider the particular cultures from which their patients come. Health care providers who learn the nuances of culture are rewarded with the knowledge they have been more effective in managing their patients' pain, and are better able to help family caregivers and friends of their patients adjust to the dying process (Givler et al., 2023). Recognize all factors influencing a patient's pain and integrate them into a patient-centered treatment plan for pain management.

- Pain management should be patient centered, with nurses practicing patient advocacy, patient empowerment, compassion, and respect. Caring for patients in pain requires recognition that pain can and should be relieved.
- Language barriers often result in inadequate pain assessment and treatment because the health care provider cannot communicate the treatment risks and benefits. If the patient's English skills are limited, the patient should be offered a professional interpreter. The use of professional interpreters decreases communication errors, improves clinical outcomes, and increases patient satisfaction (Givler et al., 2023).
- Recognize variations in patients' subjective responses to pain. Undertreatment or overtreatment might occur if nurses are not aware of cultural norms associated with pain and pain expression because pain is subjective.
- Distinct cultural norms regarding pain and pain management exist for religious; lesbian, gay, bisexual, transgender, or queer (LGBTQ); deaf; disabled; and socioeconomic communities that influence perceptions of health care, including concepts of pain (Narayan, 2017).
- Be sensitive to variations in communication styles. Some cultures believe that nonverbal expression of pain is sufficient to describe the pain experience. For example, all individuals are different, but research has shown that some cultures are stoic regarding pain and may maintain a neutral facial expression despite being in severe pain (Givler et al., 2023). Others who are not apt to verbalize that they are in pain may assume that if pain medication is appropriate, the nurse will bring it and that asking would therefore be inappropriate.
- Understand that expression of pain is unacceptable within certain cultures. Some patients believe that asking for help indicates a lack of respect, whereas others believe acknowledging pain is a sign of weakness.
- Teaching your patient and their family caregiver about pain treatment and having an attitude of dignity and caring will help patients realize that achieving good pain control promotes healing.
- All patients with substance abuse disorders need to be treated with empathy and acceptance, using a holistic approach (St. Marie & Broglio, 2020).

EVIDENCE-BASED PRACTICE

Evidence-Based Pain Management: State of the Science

The Palliative and Supportive Care Cochrane Review Group conducts systematic reviews that focus on health care interventions in chronic and acute pain, palliative and supportive care, and headaches and migraines. A review group headed by Aldington and Eccleston (2019) reviewed all of the systematic reviews conducted by Cochrane across the age range, with reviews on pain at the start and end of life, in youths, and in seniors (Aldington & Eccleston, 2019):

- Few of the systematic reviews of interventions for acute pain showed clinically significant differences at a meaningful level when experimental interventions were compared with standard treatments. Clinicians expect a clinically significant response in acute pain to be one in which the experimental

treatment reduces pain to 50% or less of the patients' maximum, or results in at least a 30% reduction from baseline. This was not the case.
- Among the over 50,000 patients included in acute pain treatment studies, only slightly more than 50% of patients randomized to a treatment group achieved at least a 50% pain reduction after 4 to 6 hours who would not have done so with placebos.
- In terms of chronic pain, there is no evidence to support the use of high-dose (200 mg or more morphine equivalent daily) opioids in chronic noncancer pain. Researchers do not have strong evidence for how to tailor interventions to individuals or even to subgroups of individuals.
- The review of the Cochran reviews by Aldington and Eccleston (2019) did not include examination of nonpharmacological interventions used by nurses in daily practice. Skelly and others (2018) conducted a systematic review of 202 studies of noninvasive nonpharmacological treatments for five common chronic pain conditions (chronic low back pain; chronic neck pain; osteoarthritis of the knee, hip, or hand; fibromyalgia; and tension headache). As a result, exercise, multidisciplinary rehabilitation, acupuncture, cognitive behavioral therapy, and mind-body practices were most consistently associated with slight to moderate improvements in function and pain control for specific chronic pain conditions. Nursing implications to consider from this systematic review include:
  - Apply evidence that is relevant to everyday practice for each individual patient based on the unique condition and the patient variables affecting the pain experience.
  - Complete comprehensive pain assessments (see Skill 16.1) to understand each patient's unique pain experience in order to tailor interventions.
  - Partner with patients to use nonpharmacological interventions (see Skill 16.2) in addition to pharmacological and medical treatment measures. Use nonpharmacological interventions that patients perceive as potentially helpful.

SAFETY GUIDELINES

- Consider a patient's cognitive status and other factors that may interfere with accurate pain assessment. When the patient is cognitively alert, use the patient's subjective report of pain as the benchmark for measurement of the effectiveness of pain therapies.
- Monitor patients who receive opioids (by any route) for signs and symptoms of oversedation and respiratory depression. Oversedation (patient is difficult to arouse) precedes respiratory depression, especially in opioid-naïve patients (i.e., patients who *are not* chronically receiving opioid analgesics on a daily basis) (Rosenquist, 2023). Using standardized sedation scales such as the *Pasero Opioid Sedation Scale* (POSS), the *Richmond Agitation-Sedation Scale*, and the *Sedation-Agitation Scale* can alert you to early signs of respiratory depression and improve observation and intervention for oversedation (Hall & Stanley, 2019). The POSS is an effective tool for the measurement of opioid sedation and is recommended for use in adult patients (Hall & Stanley, 2019) (see agency policy for tool to use).
- Assist patients receiving opioids with standing, ambulation, and transfers. Research shows an increased risk of falls, fall injuries, and fractures among older adults who use opioids (Yoshikawa et al., 2020).
- Monitor vital signs (VS) and assess patients for adverse effects of epidural analgesia, such as hypotension; changes in lower

extremity sensation; patient stating "metallic taste" in mouth; increased pain at insertion site; decreased bladder tonicity necessitating catheterization; and venous pooling, which may precipitate deep vein thrombosis (DVT).

- Know agency policy for frequency of pain assessment and timing for follow-up assessments. For the first 24 hours on opioids, patients require frequent assessment—at least every 4 hours.
- Older adults are more at risk for tissue damage because of altered responses to changes in body temperature; therefore they need frequent skin assessment during cold and heat treatments (Touhy & Jett, 2023).

✦ SKILL 16.1 Pain Assessment and Basic Comfort Measures

Registered nurses, licensed practical nurses, and assistive personnel (AP) routinely assess for the presence and severity of patients' pain through the process of screening. Screening involves assessment of the possible presence of a problem. However, a comprehensive pain assessment gathers more detailed information through collection and synthesis of data from observation, interviewing a patient, and physical examination (TJC, 2022). An accurate and comprehensive pain assessment by a registered nurse is necessary to identify the nature of a patient's pain. It is recommended that nurses conduct comprehensive pain assessments that guide sound clinical decision making.

- Patient-specific, key factors to consider include age, quality of pain, sedation level, respiratory status, functional status, and physical and psychiatric co-morbidities (Quinlan-Cowell et al., 2022).
- Consider self-reported pain-intensity ratings and behavioral pain scores within a context of multiple factors, including clinical history, patient preferences, response to previous treatments, and current respiratory status and sedation level (Cooney & Quinlan-Cowell, 2020; Drew & Peltier, 2018).
- Use pain-assessment tools that are valid, reliable, and individualized to the patient's needs and characteristics, and that reflect your patient's understanding of pain (Karcioglu et al., 2018; Cooney & Drew, 2021; Quinlan-Colwell et al., 2022).
- Do not use pain-intensity ratings or descriptors or behavioral pain scores alone to dose analgesics. This simplistic approach negates the complexity of clinical decision making that is needed to provide safe and effective analgesia (Cooney & Quinlan-Colwell, 2020).

A thorough assessment allows you to arrive at proper nursing diagnoses and select appropriate pain-relief therapies. Effectively managing a patient's pain does not necessarily mean eliminating it, but it is important to reduce pain to a level that is acceptable to the patient. Developing an effective plan of care for pain management requires ongoing education and evaluation of your assessment skills and the application of principles of interprofessional pain management (American Nurses Association [ANA], 2018). Nursing attitudes about pain management play an important role in improving the patient experience in successful pain management, so it is important to examine your own attitudes regarding pain and understand how ethnicity, cultural differences, and religious beliefs reflect on nursing practice (ANA, 2018). Patient-centered care, involving family caregivers and the accurate assessment and interpretation of a patient's pain experience, is essential to successful pain-management outcomes. Because pain is subjective, patient self-report is currently the standard for assessment.

Delegation

The skill of pain assessment cannot be delegated to assistive personnel (AP); however, the AP may screen patients for pain and provide selected nonpharmacological strategies (e.g., backrubs, hygiene comfort measures) as instructed by a nurse. Direct the AP to:

- Report if a patient screens for an increase in pain or requests pharmacological treatment.
- Eliminate environmental conditions that worsen pain (e.g., an excessively warm, noisy room).
- Provide maximum rest periods for patients; a written schedule for family caregivers to follow is ideal.
- Turn and place patients in a position of comfort at least every 2 hours or remind patients to turn themselves. Encourage the patient to use a pillow for splinting if needed.
- Observe for and report behavioral signs of pain for patients who are unable to self-report.
- Report in a timely manner any patient reports of pain intensity above the predetermined goal and nonverbal behaviors suggestive of pain.

Interprofessional Collaboration

- An advanced practice nurse or member of an interprofessional pain team can assess patients who present with chronic, intractable pain; pain that is not responding to treatment; and cases of multiple pain sources.

Equipment

- Pain rating scales (check agency policy)

STEP	RATIONALE

ASSESSMENT

1. Identify patient using at least two identifiers (e.g., name and birthday or name and medical record number) according to agency policy.

Ensures correct patient. Complies with The Joint Commission standards and improves patient safety (TJC, 2023).

2. Obtain data from patient's electronic health record (EHR): patient demographics, pain history, recent invasive procedures (e.g., tests, surgery), patient condition and co-morbidities, patient's previous response to pain medications, laboratory test results (e.g., kidney and liver function).

Comprehensive data are needed to allow you to focus your pain assessment, to guide safe and effective dosing of pain medication, and for implementing nonpharmacological pain-management interventions (Quinlan-Colwell et al., 2022).

STEP	RATIONALE
3. Assess patient's/family caregiver's health literacy.	Determines degree to which individuals have the ability to find, understand, and use information and services to make informed health-related decisions and actions for themselves and others (CDC, 2023a).
4. Assess patient's knowledge, prior experience with pain management, and feelings about procedure.	Reveals need for patient instruction and/or support.
5. If patient can self-report, ask if the patient is in pain. Ask family caregivers if they believe the patient is in pain (Gélinas, 2016). Pain measures must be selected according to the patient's ability to communicate. Use a comprehensive approach for patients who are nonverbal (Box 16.1). Older adults and patients from various cultures may not admit to having pain. Use terms such as *hurt* or *discomfort*, or use a professional interpreter if language difference exists.	Patient's self-report of pain should be accepted, but when used as the sole assessment, it prohibits a complete pain assessment and application of critical thinking. Pain-intensity ratings are completely subjective, cannot be measured objectively, are dynamic (as the experience of pain is dynamic), and may be describing a construct other than intensity (i.e., suffering) (Quinlan-Colwell et al., 2022). Cross-cultural comparisons differ in defining pain management and perceptions of successful pain control (Botti et al., 2015).
6. Perform hand hygiene and apply gloves. Have patient point to area of discomfort. Examine area: inspect for discoloration, swelling, or drainage; palpate gently for change in temperature, area of altered sensation, pain, or areas that trigger pain; assess range of motion (ROM) of involved joints. Auscultation can help to identify abnormalities (e.g., lung crackles) and determine cause of pain (see Chapter 6). When assessing abdomen, always auscultate first and then inspect and palpate.	Reduces transmission of infection. Reveals nature of pain, which will direct you to making clinical judgments needed for appropriate interventions.

7. When patient self-reports pain, assess physical, behavioral, and emotional signs and symptoms, including nonverbal indicators of pain:
  a. Moaning, crying, whimpering, groaning, vocalizations
  b. Decreased activity
  c. Facial expressions (e.g., grimace, clenched teeth)
  d. Change in usual behavior (e.g., less active, irritable)
  e. Abnormal gait (e.g., shuffling) and posture (e.g., bent, leaning)
  f. Guarding a body part; functional impairment such as decreased ROM
  g. Depression, hopelessness, anger, fear, social withdrawal
	Signs and symptoms may reveal source and nature of pain. Nonverbal responses to pain are useful in assessing pain in patients who are cognitively impaired or unable to self-report (Gallagher et al., 2017). Experiencing pain may decrease opportunities to engage in activities, experiences, or relationships, causing a negative effect that contributes to feelings of depression, hopelessness, anger, fear, and social withdrawal. Patients guard a painful body part to reduce pain severity.

BOX 16.1

Pain Assessment in Nonverbal Patients: Recommended Assessment Approaches

- Individuals with dementia are at particular risk of untreated pain because their ability to recognize, evaluate, and verbally communicate their pain gradually decreases across the course of dementia (Kunz & Lautenbacher, 2019).
- When assessing self-report of pain in patients with dementia, take these precautions (International Association for the Study of Pain [IASP], 2021):
  - Use simple scales (e.g., verbal descriptor scales, numerical rating scales) or one requiring a yes-or-no response (Herr et al., 2019).
  - Repeat each question and the instructions on how to use the scale.
  - Leave adequate time to respond.
- Observational pain behavior rating scales for individuals with dementia have been developed (e.g., Pain Assessment Checklist for Seniors with Limited Ability to Communicate [PACSLAC], Pain Assessment in Impaired Cognition [PAIC] scale, Doloplus, Pain Assessment in Advanced Dementia Scale [PAINAD]). These scales usually include observational items related to facial expressions, vocalization, and body movements. Complete an observational scale

when a patient is at rest (after some minutes of observation) or when the patient is performing daily life activities.
- Assess for the potential cause of pain through physical examination (e.g., palpation).
- Assume that pain is present after ruling out other causes (infection or constipation).
- Identify pathological conditions or procedures that may cause pain.
- Ask family or usual caregivers as to whether patients' current behaviors (e.g., crying out, restlessness) are different from customary behaviors. Changes in behavior may signal pain.
- Vital signs are not sensitive indicators for the presence of pain.
- An electronic pain-assessment tool (ePAT) app has been developed to provide point-of-care facial recognition technology for detecting facial microexpressions indicative of pain, as well as the presence of pain-related behaviors (voice, movement, behavior, activity, and body) (Atee, 2017). ePAT was shown to have clinical usefulness for identifying pain in patients with moderate to severe dementia (Hoti et al., 2018).

Data from Herr K, et al: Pain assessment in the patient unable to self-report: clinical practice recommendations in support of the ASPMN 2019 position statement, *Pain Manag Nurs* 20(5):404–417, 2019; and Horgas A: *Try this: assessing pain in older adults with dementia, from the Hartford Institute for Geriatric Nursing, New York University Rory Meyers College of Nursing, and the Alzheimer's Association, Issue Number D2, revised 2018.* https://hign.org/sites/default/files/2020-06/Try_This_Dementia_2.pdf.

STEP	RATIONALE
8. Assess for decreased gastrointestinal (GI) motility, constipation, nausea, and vomiting.	Constipation can occur with most pain medications; however, it is most common with opioid therapy. Opioid-induced constipation (OIC) develops when GI tract opioid receptors are activated. The GI tract is sensitive to low doses of opioids and, as a result, intestinal motility is inhibited (Yan et al., 2021).
9. Assess for insomnia, anorexia, and fatigue.	Co-occurrence of pain and insomnia or fatigue is common and is strongly associated with reduced functional ability (Baker et al., 2017). Lack of sleep and the presence of fatigue influence pain-intensity self-reports (Quinlan-Colwell et al., 2022).
10. Assess the character and quality of pain (acute or chronic), location(s) of the pain, pain history, pain quality, pain type, pain duration (intermittent, constant, or breakthrough), and pain intensity (Quinlan-Colwell et al., 2022). Follow agency policy regarding frequency of assessment. Use the PQRSTU pain-assessment format as a guide in collecting complete information about a patient's pain.	The PQRSTU mnemonic is useful for assessing pain and other patient symptoms (Lapum et al., n.d.).
a. *Provocative/palliative factors* (e.g., "What makes your pain better or worse?"): Consider patient's experience with over-the-counter (OTC) drugs (including herbals, marijuana and topicals), exercises, and cognitive behavioral therapies that have helped to reduce pain in the past.	Identifies nature and source of pain and what patient uses to reduce discomfort.
b. *Quality:* Use open-ended questions such as "Tell me what your pain feels like."	Helps determine underlying pain mechanism (e.g., nociceptive, inflammatory, or neuropathic pain).
c. *Region/radiation* (e.g., "Show me everywhere your pain is."). Have patient use finger (if possible) to point out areas of pain.	Identifies location of pain, which may reveal possible causative factors for acute/transient pain.
d. *Severity:* Use valid pain rating scale appropriate to patient's age, language skills, developmental level, and comprehension (see illustration) (Karcioglu et al., 2018). There are three categories of scales: Numerical rating scales (NRSs) use numbers to rate pain; visual analogue scales (VAS) typically ask patients to mark a place on a scale that matches their level of pain; categorical scales use words or pictures and may also incorporate numbers, colors, or relative location to communicate pain. Examples include the Universal Pain Scale and Critical-Care Pain Observation Tool [CPOT] (Wojnar-Gruszka et al, 2022). Ask patient to rate pain at rest, before any intervention, and when moving or engaging in care activity. In the case of patients with dementia, those who have no verbal skills, or patients who are sedated or intubated, use observational pain-assessment scales such as the Behavioral Pain Scale (BPS), PAINAD, and Adult Nonverbal Pain Scale (GeriatricPain.org, 2023; Kotfis et al., 2017).	The official position of the American Society for Pain Management Nursing (ASPMN) is that the practice of prescribing doses of opioid analgesics based solely on a patient's pain intensity should be prohibited; it disregards the relevance of other essential elements of assessment and may contribute to untoward patient outcomes, such as excessive sedation and respiratory depression as a result of overmedication (Quinlan-Cowell et al., 2022; Jungquist & Quinlan-Colwell, 2020). A clinically useful pain-assessment tool should be multidimensional to capture the complexity of patients' pain experience.
e. *Timing:* Ask patient how long pain has been present and how often it occurs. Is it constant, intermittent, continuous, or a combination? Does pain increase during specific times of day, with particular activities, or in specific locations?	Timing of pain may reveal if pain is acute or chronic and source of pain.
f. *U:* How is pain affecting "**U**" (patient) regarding activities of daily living (ADLs), work, relationships, and enjoyment of life?	Provides baseline information to later gauge effectiveness of interventions.

STEP	RATIONALE

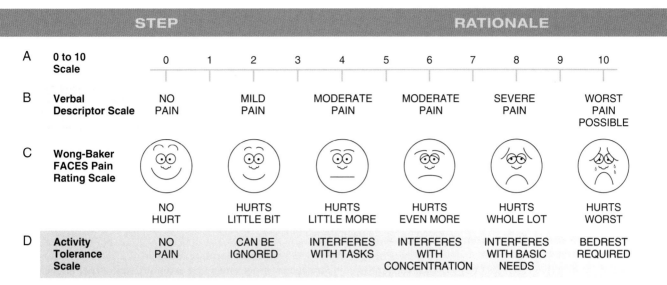

STEP 10d (A–D) Universal pain rating scales. (*From Hollen CJ, Stein LNM. Concept-based clinical nursing skills: fundamental to advanced, St. Louis, 2021, Elsevier. Copyright ©1983 Wong-Baker FACES Foundation. www.WongBaker FACES.org. Used with permission. Originally published in Whaley and Wong's nursing care of infants and children. Copyright © Elsevier, Inc.*)*

11. Assess patient's response to previous pharmacological interventions, especially ability to function (e.g., sleeping, eating, and other ADLs). Determine if any analgesic side effects are likely based on medication and patient's previous responses (e.g., itching or nausea).	Determines extent to which therapies have or have not been successful in the past. Some side effects, especially itching, can occur with morphine, are often poorly tolerated by patients, and indicate the need to identify another analgesic.
12. Assess for allergies with focus on medications. Apply allergy band if an allergy is identified.	Aspirin and nonsteroidal antiinflammatory drugs (NSAIDs) are associated with a wide variety of allergic symptoms (Mayo Clinic, 2022).

PLANNING

1. Expected outcomes following completion of procedure: • Patient verbalizes symptoms of pain relief.	Providing patient-centered interventions increases likelihood of pain control.
• Patient displays nonverbal behaviors such as relaxed face and absence of squinting.	Nonverbal indicators of pain will decline with pain relief.
• Patient reports improvement in sleep, nutritional intake, physical activity, and personal relationships.	Adequate pain relief usually permits patient to become more functional and to participate in usual ADLs.
2. Set pain-intensity goal with patient (when appropriate).	Pain is unique to each person; therefore patient is helped to set individual goal for tolerable pain severity (ANA, 2018).
3. Provide privacy by closing room door or bedside curtains.	Privacy during conversation and pain-relief measures may enhance pain relief.
4. Prepare patient's environment. • Temperature suited to patient	Temperature and sound extremes can enhance patient's perception of pain.
• Sound	Loud or sudden noises may contribute to anxiety and exacerbate pain.
• Lighting	Bright or very dim lighting can aggravate pain sensation.
• Eliminate unnecessary interruptions and coordinate care activities; allow for rest	Fatigue increases pain perception.
5. Explain procedures to be used for pain relief and how patient can be involved.	Ensures patient understanding.
6. Provide educational materials to patient and family caregiver (TJC, 2018; TJC, 2022).	Pain-assessment and pain-relief measures may be needed at home. Education will improve patient and caregiver adherence.

STEP	RATIONALE

IMPLEMENTATION

1. Perform hand hygiene and apply clean gloves (if indicated).

   Reduces transmission of microorganisms.

2. Teach patient how to use appropriate pain rating scale available in health care agency. Explain range of intensity scores and how they relate to measuring pain.

   Accurate reporting by patient or family caregiver improves ongoing pain screening. (Determine if family caregiver can learn to assess pain in more depth.)

3. Prepare and administer appropriate pain-relieving medications (nonopioids, opioids, coanalgesic or multimodal combination) per health care provider's order (see Chapter 20). Choice of medication depends on patient's condition.

   Nonopioids are effective for mild to moderate pain. Patients with chronic pain are typically prescribed multimodal analgesics for pain relief.

4. Remove or reduce painful stimuli:

   Reduction of pain stimuli and pressure receptors maximizes responses to pain-relieving interventions.

   a. Help patient turn and reposition to comfortable position in good body alignment.

   Reduces stress on musculoskeletal system.

   b. Smooth wrinkles in bed linens.

   Reduces pressure and irritation to skin.

   c. Loosen constrictive bandages (if appropriate to purpose of bandage) or loosen, reposition, or remove devices (e.g., blood pressure cuff, sequential stockings).

   Bandage or device encircling extremity can restrict circulation and movement and cause pain.

   d. Reposition underlying tubes or equipment.

   Removes pressure on skin. Allows patient to reposition more freely on own.

   e. Use pillows as needed for alignment and positioning support (see illustration).

   Helps maintain position that reduces strain on muscles and pressure areas.

5. Teach patient how to splint over painful site (e.g., surgical incision) using either a pillow or hand (see Chapter 36).

   Splinting reduces pain by minimizing muscle movement at time of stress (e.g., coughing).

   a. Explain purpose of splinting.

   Promotes patient's cooperation.

   b. Place pillow or blanket over site of discomfort and help patient place hands firmly over area of discomfort (see illustration). *Option:* May also splint using hands only.

   Splinting immobilizes painful incisional area.

   c. Have patient splint area firmly while coughing, deep breathing, and turning.

   Splinting decreases movement and subsequent pain during activity.

6. Reduce or eliminate emotional factors that increase pain experiences (see Skill 16.2). Use biopsychosocial treatments.

   A variety of mind-body techniques, such as relaxation, guided imagery, therapeutic suggestion, and meditation, enhance the mind's ability to lessen pain symptoms (Houzé et al., 2017; National Center for Complementary and Integrative Health [NCCIH], 2019a; Garland et al., 2020).

   a. Offer information that reduces anxiety (e.g., explaining cause of pain if known).

   Anxiety is a common condition that accompanies chronic pain; pain triggers apprehension and distress (Institute for Chronic Pain, 2021).

   b. Offer patient opportunity to pray or read spiritual writings (if appropriate).

   Serves as form of distraction and provides spiritual comfort.

   c. Spend time to allow patient to talk about pain and answer questions. Listen attentively.

   Conveys a sense of caring and interest in patient's welfare.

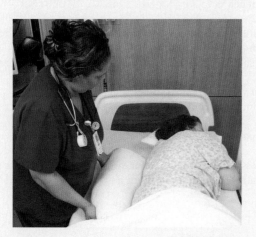

STEP 4e Positioning patient in side-lying lateral position with pillow for comfort.

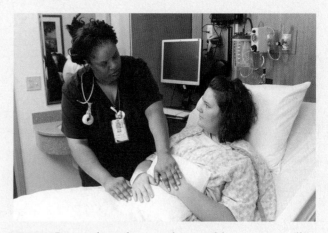

STEP 5b Patient shown how to splint painful area using a pillow.

STEP	RATIONALE
7. Before leaving, make sure patient is in a comfortable position.	Restores comfort and sense of well-being. Positioning is a nonpharmacological intervention for pain relief.
8. Raise side rails (as appropriate) and lower bed to lowest position, locking into position.	Ensures patient safety and prevents falls.
9. Place nurse call system in an accessible location within patient's reach.	Ensures patient can call for assistance if needed.
10. If used, remove and dispose of gloves. Perform hand hygiene.	Reduces transmission of microorganisms.

EVALUATION

1. Based on agency reassessment criteria (e.g., 30–60 minutes after intervention), reassess patient's pain after comfort measures.	Evaluates effectiveness of pain-relieving interventions in timely manner.
2. Compare patient's current pain with personally set pain-intensity goal.	Helps determine appropriate changes to pain-management plan and can reveal need for further assessment. Makes patient active participant in care.
3. Compare patient's ability to function and perform ADLs before and after pain interventions. Initiate a nurse-patient dialogue about the effectiveness of pain-relieving interventions on function and ability to perform ADLs.	Pain-intensity ratings are not necessarily a reflection of pain relief for chronic pain; therefore, preintervention and postintervention assessment of function should be incorporated to determine effectiveness (Chou et al., 2016).
4. Observe patient's nonverbal behaviors after pain interventions using observational pain-assessment tool with patients who are unable to self-report (patients who are critically ill and/or intubated, cognitively impaired, or sedated). Current research shows that the two tools best validated for critically ill patients unable to self-report pain are the Behavioral Pain Scale (BPS) and the Critical-Care Pain Observation Tool (CPOT) (Kotfis et al., 2017).	Determines effectiveness of pain-relieving interventions and improves pain assessment and management (Varndell et al., 2017).
5. **Use Teach-Back:** "We discussed how splinting and relaxation can relieve your pain. Explain to me when you can use these approaches at home." Revise your instruction now or develop a plan for revised patient/family caregiver teaching if patient/family caregiver is not able to teach back correctly.	Teach-back is a technique for health care providers to ensure that they have explained medical information clearly so that patients and their families understand what is communicated to them (Agency for Healthcare Research and Quality [AHRQ], 2023).

Unexpected Outcomes

1. Patient verbalizes continued pain that shows a worsening of pain qualities, including pain intensity, or displays nonverbal behavior reflecting worsening pain.

2. Patient experiences unexpected or adverse reaction to medication.

Related Interventions

- Repeat complete pain assessment; rule out if there is another complication or developing medical problem causing pain.
- Implement different nonpharmacological pain-relief measures.
- Ask patient and family caregivers which alternatives might be helpful.
- Notify health care provider.

- Assess unexpected effects on patient.
- Notify health care provider immediately.
- Be prepared to administer antidote if indicated (e.g., antiemetic, antihistamine, opioid-reversing agent such as naloxone).
- Be prepared to administer oxygen and monitor SpO_2 or capnography.
- Monitor for effectiveness of antidote; antidote may have shorter half-life than opioid; repeat dose of antidote may be needed.
- Complete adverse reaction documentation according to agency policy.

Documentation

- Document character of pain before and after an intervention, the pain-relief therapies used, whether pain relief was achieved, any patient or family education provided, and patient response to interventions.
- Document your evaluation of patient learning.

Hand-Off Reporting

- Report to health care provider inadequate pain relief, a reduction in patient function, and side effects and adverse effects of both pharmacological and nonpharmacological pain interventions.

Special Considerations
Patient Education

- Explain to family caregiver and patient the pain-management plan, side effects of treatment (and how to act), impact expected of pain on ADLs, safe use of analgesics, and storage and disposal of opioids when prescribed (TJC, 2018; TJC, 2022).

TABLE 16.1

Misconceptions: Barriers to the Assessment and Treatment of Pain

Misconception	Correction
The best judge of the existence and severity of a patient's pain is the health care provider or nurse caring for the patient.	The patient's self-report is the most reliable indicator of the existence and perceived intensity of pain.
Clinicians should use their personal opinions and beliefs about the truthfulness of a patient to determine true pain status.	Allowing each clinician to act on personal beliefs presents the potential for different pain assessments by different clinicians, leading to different interventions from each clinician. This results in inconsistent and often inadequate pain management. A patient's self-report of pain is the standard for pain assessment.
Visible signs, either physiological or behavioral, always accompany pain and can be used to verify its existence and severity.	Even with severe pain, periods of physiological and behavioral adaptation occur, leading to periods of minimal or no observable signs of pain. Lack of pain expression does not necessarily mean lack of pain.
Cognitively impaired older adults are unable to use pain rating scales.	When an appropriate pain rating scale is used and a patient is given sufficient time to process information and respond, many cognitively impaired older adults can use a pain rating scale.
If patients hurt enough, they will tell you.	Patients are often hesitant to report pain for fear of being labeled as complainers, hypochondriacs, or addicts.
Psychosocial interventions alone reduce or alleviate pain.	Nonpharmacological interventions are synergistic with medications but are not a substitute for pharmacological management of pain.
Pain is a natural side effect of aging.	As we age, some "nuisance pain" from physical wear and tear is normal. That differs, however, from chronic pain, which is not a part of aging.
It's better to tough it out and just live with pain.	Ignoring pain can have serious consequences, especially if patients self-medicate in unhealthy ways rather than see a health care professional.

Adapted from Pasero C, McCaffery M: *Pain: assessment and pharmacological management,* St. Louis, 2011, Mosby; and Cleveland Clinic: *7 common myths about chronic pain,* 2020, https://health.clevelandclinic.org/7-common-myths-of-chronic-pain/.

- Review patient's and family caregiver's understanding of how to use the pain rating scale and ability to assess/report pain more thoroughly when providing pain therapies.
- Explain to patient and family caregiver about the behavioral changes that may result from pain (e.g., change in activity level or decreased social interaction).
- Ask patient and family caregiver about fear of addiction, a common primary concern, or other misconceptions that could undermine the patient's pain relief (Table 16.1).

Pediatrics
- For children younger than 6 years, use behavioral pain scales to assess pain. For children older than 6 years, pain assessment is based on a self-report. These tools have been shown to be easy and quick to use for screening (Brand, 2022): Wong-Baker FACES pain scale, Pieces of Hurt, multiple-sized poker chips, visual analogue scales, and the Adolescent Paediatric Pain Tool.
- The International Children's Palliative Care Network (ICPCN) has developed the ICPCN Pain Assessment App with three different pain scales that are immediately available on a user's phone. The scale provides the option of a faces, numerical, or hand pain scale to use with children from 3 years of age upward and documents the child's responses to allow monitoring of the type and level of pain the child is experiencing (ICPCN, 2022).
- The absolute value of a pain-intensity score is not as important as the changes in scores in each individual child. In clinical use with individual patients, a change in pain of 2 of 10 (i.e., a change of one face on the FACES scale) represents the least change that can be considered clinically significant when using a faces scale (Birnie et al., 2019).
- Infants and children respond to pain differently than adults. For example, they cry and thrash about, have sleep disturbances,

suck or rock, refuse to eat or play, show expressions of anger or frustration, or are quiet and withdrawn. Variations in pain response are related to the child's personality, developmental level, and previous pain experiences (Hockenberry et al., 2022).
- The accurate assessment of pain in children, as in adults, is multifactorial and requires a systematic approach. One approach is called QUESTT (Brand, 2022):
  - Question the child.
  - Use the age and developmentally appropriate pain rating scales.
  - Observe behavior and assess physiological changes.
  - Secure parental involvement.
  - Take the cause of pain into account.
  - Take actions and evaluate results.
- QUESTT initiates a structured approach to pain assessment. In an ideal situation, a child should be questioned before the painful episode occurs to establish the child's expectations, perceptions, and previous experiences of pain (Brand, 2022).

Older Adults
- Older adults who are able to express themselves can use self-report pain scales. In addition, your assessment should include how the pain is affecting function, sleep, appetite, activity, mood, and relationships with others (Touhy & Jett, 2023).
- Encourage older adults to describe previous experiences with pain and pain management (Touhy & Jett, 2023).
- Some older adults may require more time (than younger adults) for you to explain a pain-assessment scale.
- It is often difficult or impossible to assess pain in patients who are endotracheally intubated, sedated, or unresponsive; or in older adults with communication and cognitive impairments (Booker & Haedtke, 2016). This is especially true in palliative care patients, who have pain at any point during their disease

trajectory and are often unable to self-report the presence, location, severity, or impact of their pain (McGuire, 2016). There is the risk of these patients not receiving adequate analgesia. Use a behavioral pain scale recommended by your agency, but recognize the need for a comprehensive assessment.

- Older adults have the highest incidence of disease and undergo more surgery, procedural interventions, injury, and hospitalization than younger adults (Schofield & Gibson, 2021). Common causes of pain in older adults include osteoarthritis (back, knees, hips); night-time leg cramps; claudicating or limping from pain usually caused by poor blood circulation; neuropathies or damage to nerves of the peripheral nervous system; shingles; trauma from falls; and postsurgery pain (Schofield & Gibson, 2021).

Populations With Disabilities

- Diagnostic error can occur when signs and symptoms of pain are mistakenly attributed to an individual's intellectual and developmental disability. Creating personal profiles (e.g., hospital passports) to describe individuals' common signs of pain can assist health care providers in recognizing pain behaviors (Barney et al., 2020).
- Facial and behavioral expressions of pain are often shaped by individual factors such as probable, often unknown, differences in central nervous system structure and function associated with a person's disability, as well as situational factors such as

the immediate surroundings, caregiver behavior, and culture (Barney et al., 2020).

- Various behavioral scales exist for assessing pain in patients with intellectual and developmental disabilities. There is no broad consensus as to which scales should be used in routine practice (Barney et al., 2020).
- For adults with severe cognitive impairment, Pain Assessment in Advanced Dementia (PAINAD) and Doloplus-2 are recommended pain scales (Schofield, 2018). PAINAD requires observing patients for 5 minutes before scoring their behaviors in five behavioral dimensions. The Doloplus-2 tool is performed by a proxy rater who observes the subject and evaluates the presence of 10 pain-related behaviors on a scale from 0 to 3, representing increasing presence of the behavior (Rajan & Behrends, 2019).

Home Care

- Consider home conditions such as type of bed and environmental stimuli. A supportive bed and quiet environment enhance sleep and promote pain management.
- Family caregivers are often the main support for older adults. Educate them about causes of painful conditions, common misconceptions about use of analgesics, type of pain medicines appropriate for the patient, how to safely store and dispose of medications, and how to support adherence to medication regimen (see Chapter 41).

✦ SKILL 16.2 Nonpharmacological Pain Management

 Video Clip

Nonpharmacological therapies in most cases can be delivered independently by a nurse. These therapies administered together with conventional pharmacological therapy make them complementary (NCCIH, 2021). When nonpharmacological therapies are used in place of conventional pharmacological or other medical procedures, they are considered alternative therapies (NCCIH, 2021). Integrative health care brings conventional and complementary approaches together in a coordinated way (NCCIH, 2021). The mission of the National Center for Complementary and Integrative Health (NCCIH) is to determine, through rigorous scientific investigation, the fundamental science, usefulness, and safety of complementary and integrative health approaches and their roles in improving health and health care (NCCIH, 2022a). There are four classifications of complementary therapies:

- Nutritional (e.g., special diets, diet supplements, herbs, and probiotics)
- Psychological (e.g., mindfulness, meditation, progressive relaxation, guided imagery, spirituality and reflection)
- Physical (e.g., massage, Pilates)
- Combinations such as psychological and physical (e.g., yoga; tai chi; acupuncture; music, dance, or art therapies) or psychological and nutritional (e.g., mindful eating)

Complementary approaches are recommended as nonpharmacological interventions in multimodal approaches to pain management (Chou et al., 2016; Houzé et al., 2017). It is important for patients to be full participants in complementary or alternative

therapies to increase the likelihood of relaxation occurring. As a nurse you will require special training to assist patients with techniques such as meditation, therapeutic touch, or tai chi.

Delegation

Assessment of a patient's pain cannot be delegated to assistive personnel (AP). The skill of nonpharmacological pain management strategies can be delegated to AP who are trained in their use. Direct the AP by:

- Identifying and explaining which nonpharmacological measures work best for the patient
- Explaining how to adapt strategies to patient restrictions (e.g., massage in side-lying versus prone position)
- Instructing to immediately report a worsening of the patient's pain

Interprofessional Collaboration

- An interprofessional pain management team member is the best resource for alternative therapies to use.

Equipment

- Appropriate pain rating scales
- *Distraction:* Patient's (all ages) preference (e.g., reading material, video game, puzzles, music, 3D immersions [e.g., virtual reality, Google Cardboard, smartphone applications]). *Option:* If using music, have patient's earbuds available.
- *Relaxation:* Patient's music preference for relaxation
- *Massage:* Lotion or oil (consider lavender aromatherapy lotion [non–alcohol based]), sheet, bath towel

STEP	RATIONALE

ASSESSMENT

1. Identify patient using at least two identifiers (e.g., name and birthday or name and medical record number) according to agency policy.

Ensures correct patient. Complies with The Joint Commission standards and improves patient safety (TJC, 2023).

2. Assess patient's/family caregiver's health literacy.

Determines degree to which individuals have the ability to find, understand, and use information and services to make informed health-related decisions and actions for themselves and others (CDC, 2023a).

3. Assess patient's knowledge, prior experience with nonpharmacological pain management, and feelings about procedure.

Reveals need for patient instruction and/or support.

4. Identify descriptive terms that you will use when guiding patient through relaxation or guided imagery.

Establishes connection with patient to enhance your ability to guide relaxation.

5. Perform hand hygiene. Perform complete pain assessment (see Skill 16.1).

Reduces transmission of microorganisms. A complete pain assessment guides safe and effective dosing of pain medication and implementation of complementary nonpharmacological interventions (Pasero et al., 2016).

6. Assess character of patient's respirations.

Establishes baseline. Relaxation techniques focus on breathing.

7. Review health care provider's orders for pain-relief therapies (if required by agency).

In some acute care settings, a medical order is necessary to perform certain nonpharmacological therapies (e.g., heat application).

8. Assess patient's understanding of pain and willingness to receive nonpharmacological pain-relief measures.

Participation increases effectiveness of pain-relief measure. If patient is reluctant to try activity, provide information about suggested therapy.

9. Assess preferred patient pastime activities (e.g., reading, crocheting, game on electronic device, board games, music).

Improves likelihood of distraction being effective.

10. Assess type of image patient would prefer to use in guided imagery (e.g., nature scene, interaction with friends, joyful moment).

Prevents use of image that could frighten patient.

11. Review any restrictions in patient's mobility or positioning.

Determines whether massage is appropriate and the position to have patient assume.

PLANNING

1. Expected outcomes following completion of procedures:
   - Patient demonstrates and describes pain-relief measures.
   - Patient is relaxed and comfortable after technique as evidenced by slow, deep respirations; calm facial expressions; calm tone of voice; relaxed muscles; and relaxed posture.
   - Patient reports pain relief on an intensity or behavioral scale.

Demonstrates patient understanding and learning.

The use of complementary and integrative therapies helps patients relax and experience less discomfort.

Patient's subjective report is most reliable indicator of presence/relief of pain.

2. Provide privacy by closing room door or bedside curtains.

Promotes patient's ability to relax.

3. Perform hand hygiene. Organize equipment at bedside.

Reduces transmission of infection. Promotes efficient procedure.

4. Explain purpose of nonpharmacological technique and what you expect of patient during activity. Explain how to use pain rating scale (see Skill 16.1).

Proper explanation of activity enhances patient participation. Accurate reporting of pain by patient improves your evaluation and treatment.

5. Set mutual pain-intensity goal with patient (when able) for rest and during routine care activities.

Pain is unique to each person; therefore help the patient set individual goal for tolerable pain severity (ANA, 2018).

6. Plan time to perform technique when patient can concentrate (e.g., after voiding, awakening from nap).

Increases opportunity for success.

7. Administer an ordered analgesic 30 minutes before implementing a nonpharmacological therapy.

Patient is able to gain a level of comfort needed to perform nonpharmacological therapies.

8. Position the patient and drape if needed.

Promotes comfort.

9. Prepare environment: Make room temperature suited to patient. Control level of sound and lighting. Minimize interruptions and coordinate care activities; allow time for rest.

Temperature and sound extremes can enhance patient's perception of pain.

Bright or very dim lighting can aggravate pain sensation. Fatigue increases pain perception.

STEP	RATIONALE

IMPLEMENTATION

1. Perform hand hygiene

2. Massage:

Reduces transmission of microorganisms.

The NCCIH (2019b) reports that massage has been shown to be helpful for stress reduction, anxiety, depression, fatigue, and quality of life in breast cancer patients. In addition, massage therapy has potential as part of supportive care in lung cancer patients whose anxiety or pain is not adequately controlled by usual care.

Clinical Judgment *Massage is contraindicated in cases of undiagnosed pain; lumps; muscle, bone, or joint injury; and bruised, swollen, or inflamed areas. As a nurse you are not a professional massage therapist. Follow this procedure carefully, using only pressure requested by patient and recognizing risks associated with patient's condition. For example, when working with cancer patients, modify how you massage tissues; you may have to use less pressure than usual in areas that are sensitive because of cancer or cancer treatments (NCCIH, 2019b).*

a. Place patient in comfortable position such as prone or side lying. Have patients with difficulty breathing lie on side of bed with head of bed elevated.

Positioning enhances relaxation and exposes areas to be massaged.

b. Adjust bed to comfortable position for you; lower upper side rail on side where you are standing. Drape patient to expose only area that you will massage.

Ensures proper body mechanics and prevents strain on back.

c. Turn on music to patient's preference.

Promotes relaxation.

d. Ensure that patient is not allergic to lotion and accepts using it; warm lotion in your hands or in a basin of warm water. **NOTE:** If you massage head and scalp, delay use of lotion until completed.

Warm lotion is soothing, and warmth helps produce local muscle relaxation. Patient participates in approach to care.

e. Choose stroke technique based on desired effect or body part (Acupuncture Massage College [AMC, 2022]). Ask patient to identify the type of touch preferred (light touch, firm pressure).

Ensures fuller relaxation of body part. Eases any anxiety patient might have.

Clinical Judgment *Use gentle massage with patients who are unable to communicate, and monitor nonverbal behavior closely because they cannot tell you if massage becomes uncomfortable.*

(1) *Effleurage:* set of stroking movements that consist of a series of long, gliding or circular massage strokes applied using different degrees of pressure (see illustration) (AMC, 2022).

Light, gliding stroke used without manipulating deep muscles promotes relaxation, extends muscles, increases nutrient absorption, and improves lymphatic and venous circulation.

(2) *Pétrissage:* manually compressing soft tissues of an area through rhythmic kneading and/or rolling (see illustration) (AMC, 2022).

Gently kneading tense muscle groups promotes relaxation and stimulates local circulation.

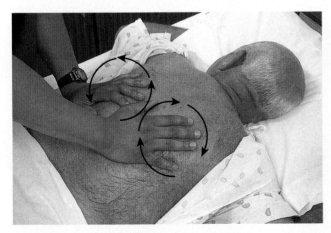

STEP 2e(1) Effleurage.

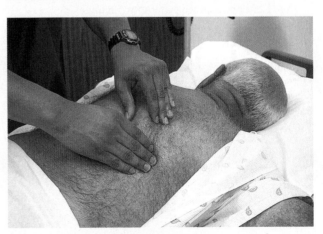

STEP 2e(2) Pétrissage.

STEP	RATIONALE
(3) *Friction:* firm and focused rubbing technique that is applied to a specific area, usually using just with fingers or thumbs (AMC, 2022).	Circular strokes bring blood to surface of skin, increasing local circulation and loosening tight muscle groups.
f. Encourage patient to breathe deeply in and out (consciously allowing pelvic muscles to relax) during massage.	Promotes parasympathetic response for relaxation.
g. Stand behind patient; stimulate scalp and temples.	Your position increases effectiveness of massage and facilitates proper body mechanics.
h. Supporting patient's head, use your fingers to apply gentle friction, rubbing muscles at base of head.	Stimulates local circulation and relaxation.
i. Reposition if needed. With patient in supine position, massage hands and arms.	Hand massage therapy may decrease muscle tension.
(1) Support hand and gently apply friction to palm using both thumbs.	
(2) Support base of finger and massage each finger in corkscrew motion, then massage back of hand.	
(3) Use pétrissage to knead muscles of forearm and upper arm between thumb and forefinger.	Encourages relaxation; enhances circulation and venous return.
j. If patient has no neck injury or condition that contraindicates neck manipulation, gently massage neck:	Massage is contraindicated after spinal cord injuries or surgery to head and neck because of risk for further injury.
(1) Place patient prone unless contraindicated. Otherwise, use side-lying position.	Provides access to neck muscles.
(2) Use pétrissage over each neck muscle between thumb and forefinger.	Reduces tension that often localizes in neck muscles.
(3) Gently stretch neck by placing one hand on top of shoulders and other at base of head. Gently move hands away from each other.	Helps relax body of muscle.
k. Massage back:	Patient with back injury, surgery, or epidural infusion should not receive back massage.
(1) Assist patient to prone position unless contraindicated; side-lying position is an option.	Provides access to muscle groups in back.
(2) Do not allow hands to leave patient's skin.	Continuous contact with surface of skin is soothing and stimulates circulation to tissues. Breaking contact with skin can startle patient.
(3) Apply hands first to sacral area; use effleurage to stroke upward from buttocks to shoulders. Massage over scapulae with smooth, firm stroke. Continue in one smooth stroke to upper arms and laterally along sides of back down to iliac crest (see illustration). Continue massage pattern for 3 minutes.	General, firm pressure applied to all muscle groups promotes relaxation.

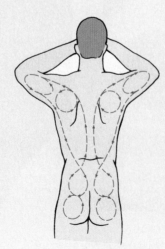

STEP 2k(3) Circular massage of the back.

STEP	RATIONALE
(4) Use effleurage along muscles of spine in upward and outward motion.	Massage follows distribution of major muscle groups.
(5) Use pétrissage on muscles of each shoulder toward front of patient.	Area often tightens because of tension.
(6) Use palms in upward and outward circular motion from lower buttocks to neck.	Brings blood to surface of skin.
(7) Knead muscles of upper back and shoulder.	These muscles are thick and can be massaged vigorously.
(8) Use both hands to knead muscles up one side of back and then the other.	
(9) End massage with long, stroking effleurage movements.	Most soothing of massage movements.
l. Massage feet:	
(1) Place patient in supine position.	Returns patient to comfortable anatomical position.
(2) Hold foot firmly. Support ankle with one hand or support sides of foot with each hand while performing massage.	Maintains joint stability during massage (Hatcher, 2017).
(3) Make circular motions with thumb and fingers around bones of ankle and top of foot.	All massage strokes help to relax muscles.
(4) Massage sides and top of each toe.	
(5) Use friction to make circular motions on bottom of foot.	Note if patient becomes ticklish, which is uncomfortable.
(7) Knead sides of foot between index finger and thumb.	
(8) Conclude with firm, sweeping motions over top and bottom of foot.	Strokes that are too light may tickle.
m. Tell patient that you are ending massage.	Informs and prepares patient to inhale and exhale deeply.
n. When procedure is complete, instruct patient to inhale deeply and exhale. Caution to move slowly after resting a few minutes.	Returns patient to more awake and alert state. When deeply relaxed, patient may experience dizziness on raising head too rapidly and need time for vessels to redistribute blood supply.
o. Wipe excess lotion or oil from patient's body with bath towel.	Excess lotion or oil can irritate skin and lead to breakdown.
3. Progressive relaxation with slow, deep breathing:	Research involving healthy subjects has shown that slow deep breathing can be a meaningful intervention for patients with stress-related diseases (Lee et al., 2021).
	Maximizes ability to relax.
a. Have patient assume comfortable sitting position: sit with feet uncrossed or lie in supine position with small pillow under head.	
b. Instruct patient to take several slow, deep breaths, relaxing lower pelvic muscles. It may help to have patients close their eyes.	Increased oxygen lessens anxiety and prevents shortness of breath with relaxation. Avoids hyperventilation. Eye closure maintains patient focus on exercise.
c. Explain as follows: "Let the air coming in through your nose move downward into your lower belly. Let your belly expand fully. Now breathe slowly out through your mouth or nose. Let the muscles in your pelvis and lower belly relax. Alternate normal and deep breaths several times. Pay attention to how you feel when you breathe in and breathe out normally and when you breathe deeply. Shallow breathing makes you feel tense and constricted, while deep breathing helps you relax."	Patient able to focus on exercise with your coaching. Becoming mindful of how body feels can enhance relaxation.
d. Continue the exercise: "To practice, put one hand on your abdomen, just below your belly button. Feel your hand rise about an inch each time you breathe in, and fall about an inch each time you breathe out. Your chest will rise slightly, too, along with your belly. Remember to relax your belly so that each time you breathe in, it expands fully. As you breathe out slowly, let yourself sigh out loud."	Allows patient to master slow, deep breathing.
e. Observe patient and caution against hyperventilation.	Causes patient to exhale more carbon dioxide than is produced and thus results in respiratory alkalosis and an elevated blood pH. Patient becomes dizzy and light-headed.

STEP	RATIONALE
f. Coach patient to locate any area of muscle tension and alternate tightening and relaxing all muscle groups for 6 to 7 seconds, beginning at feet and working upward toward head.	Relaxation is an integrated response associated with diminished sympathetic nervous system arousal; decreased muscle tension is desired outcome.
(1) Instruct patient to tighten muscles during inhalation and relax muscles during exhalation.	Deep breathing has been reported to reduce stress through relaxation (Perciavalle et al., 2017).
(2) As each muscle group relaxes, ask patient to enjoy relaxed feeling and allow mind to drift and think how nice it is to be relaxed. Have patient breathe deeply.	Allows opportunity to enjoy feelings of relaxation.
(3) Calmly explain during exercise that patient may feel sensations of tingling, heaviness, floating, or warmth as relaxation occurs.	Prevents anxiety if sensation occurs without warning.
(4) Have patient continue slow, deep breaths throughout exercise.	
(5) When finished, have patient inhale deeply, exhale, and then initially move about slowly after resting a few minutes.	Returns patient to more awake and alert state. Rising too rapidly can cause dizziness.
4. Guided imagery:	
a. Direct patient through exercise by having the patient focus on an image. Example is as follows:	
(1) Instruct patient to imagine that inhaled air is a ball of healing energy.	Developing specific images helps remove pain perception.
(2) Imagine that inhaled air travels to area of pain.	Patient's ability to concentrate decreases pain perception.
b. Alternatively, you may direct imagery:	
(1) Ask patient to imagine a pleasant place such as a beach or mountains. Give examples, but make sure that it is an image and experience that the patient chooses.	Directs imagery after selection of restful place.
(2) Direct patient to experience all sensory aspects of the restful place (e.g., for beach: warm breeze, warm sand between toes, warmth of sunshine, rhythmic sound of waves, smell of salt air, gulls gliding and swooping in air).	Helps patient concentrate and relax through stimulation of numerous senses to achieve clinical outcomes of interest (e.g., decrease in pain, anxiety, and stress) (Patricolo et al., 2017).
(3) Direct patient to continue deep, slow, rhythmic breathing.	Promotes relaxation through muscle relaxation.
(4) Direct patient to count to three, inhale, and open eyes. Suggest that patient move about slowly initially.	Slowly resuming movement and upright positioning is recommended due to state of relaxation and possible orthostatic changes in blood pressure.
(5) Provide patient time to practice exercise without interruption. Practice relaxation tapes are available almost everywhere; libraries are an excellent source.	Guided imagery requires an intense level of concentration that takes time to achieve.
5. Distraction:	Mental distractions block pain signals from the body before they ever reach the brain. Pain sensations compete for attention with other forms of sensory input (Keane, 2021).
a. Direct patient's attention away from pain. Involve patient in a distraction technique.	Redirection of attention with music therapy, for example, has been reported to have a positive effect on pain and anxiety reduction (Li et al., 2017).
b. Music: Play selection for approximately 30 minutes in location where patient is comfortable. Set volume or loudness at comfortable level. Use music of patient's choosing. Emphasize listening to rhythm, and adjust volume as pain increases or decreases.	Music therapy has become a common therapy in palliative care and has been shown to achieve pain management; relaxation; happiness and hope; reduced anxiety and depression; enhanced spirituality; and improved quality of life (Nyashanu et al., 2021).
c. Direct patient to give detailed account of an event or story; describe pleasant memories.	Stress details of event to enhance distraction from painful stimulus.
d. Provide activity (e.g., puzzle, music, virtual reality headset program, video game, reading material) at time when patient is relaxed.	Engagement in activity requires level of comfort for participation.
e. Engage patient in meaningful conversation; encourage participation of family members and visitors.	Visitors can help direct attention away from mild to moderate pain. Rarely is someone in severe pain able to use distraction.

STEP	RATIONALE
6. Help patient to a comfortable position.	Restores comfort and sense of well-being.
7. Raise side rails (as appropriate) and lower bed to lowest position, locking into position.	Ensures patient safety and prevents falls.
8. Appropriately dispose of supplies and equipment. Remove and dispose of gloves and perform hand hygiene.	Reduces transmission of microorganisms.
9. Place nurse call system in an accessible location within patient's reach.	Ensures patient can call for assistance if needed and promotes safety and prevents falls.

EVALUATION

1. Observe character of respirations, body position, facial expression, tone of voice, mood, mannerisms, and verbalization of discomfort.

   Determines effectiveness of procedure, level of relaxation, degree of pain relief achieved, and which procedures were most effective.

2. Ask patient to describe character of pain and use pain rating scale; compare score with patient's goal.

   Measures change in nature and intensity of pain.

3. Observe patient perform pain-control measures.

   Confirms learning.

4. **Use Teach-Back:** "I want to be sure I explained some of the ways you can reduce your pain without using medication. Tell me what technique you might want to try." Revise your instruction now or develop a plan for revised patient/family caregiver teaching if patient/family caregiver is not able to teach back correctly.

   Teach-back is a technique for health care providers to ensure that they have explained medical information clearly so that patients and their families understand what is communicated to them (AHRQ, 2023).

Unexpected Outcomes

1. Patient is not able to concentrate on nonpharmacological technique because pain intensity is unchanged or escalating or patient demonstrates nonverbal behaviors indicative of pain.

Related Interventions

- Evaluate character of pain and determine if further analgesia is necessary.
- Ensure that environment is conducive to learning and using technique.
- Consult with health care provider on increase in current analgesic dose or consider alternate medication.
- Consider different technique or combination of complementary strategies.

Documentation

- Document patient's assessment findings before and after procedure, nonpharmacological technique(s) used, preparation and instruction given to patient/family caregiver, patient's response, change in pain character and intensity, and further comfort needs required. Incorporate pain-relief technique into nursing care plan.
- Document your evaluation of patient and family caregiver learning.

Hand-Off Reporting

- Report any unusual responses to techniques (e.g., uncontrolled or aggravated pain or anxiety) to nurse in charge or health care provider.
- Report inadequate pain relief, a reduction in patient function, and side effects or adverse effects from pain interventions to health care provider.
- Report patient's response to nonpharmacological interventions to the staff at change of shift and in care plan meetings.

Special Considerations

Pediatrics

- Adapt distraction and relaxation strategies to the developmental level of the child (e.g., use a pacifier for an infant, offer reading or playing a recording of a favorite story for a preschooler, encourage a teenager to watch a favorite movie or listen to music). Play therapists are usually available at large pediatric hospitals and are good resources for appropriate distraction techniques (Hockenberry et al., 2022).
- Many complementary approaches are used but have not been tested for safety in children. Biofeedback, guided imagery, hypnosis, mindfulness, and yoga are some of the mind and body practices that have the best evidence of being effective for children for various symptoms (such as anxiety and stress) and are low risk. Diet supplements are used frequently for children,

but children's small size, developing organs, and immature immune system make them more vulnerable than adults to having allergic or other adverse reactions to dietary supplements (NCCIH, 2017).

- Parents may be helpful in providing pain relief. For example, they provide comfort by their presence, conversation, and holding and cuddling their child (Hockenberry et al., 2022).

Older Adults

- Visual, hearing, cognitive, and motor impairments make it difficult for older adults to be able to effectively use procedures such as distraction, relaxation, or guided imagery. Make certain that glasses, hearing aids, and other assistive devices are in place.
- Mind and body practices, including relaxation techniques and meditative exercise forms such as yoga, tai chi, and qi gong, are being widely used by older adults for fitness and relaxation. A number of systematic reviews point to the potential benefit of mind and body approaches for symptom management, particularly for pain. Although the research on these approaches is not conclusive, they may help older adults maintain motivation to incorporate relaxation, meditation, and physical exercise into their regular activities (NCCIH, 2022b).

Populations With Disabilities

- Cognitive behavioral strategies may not be appropriate for patients with intellectual or developmental disabilities (Boltz et al., 2020).
- Many adults and children use complementary health approaches such as omega-3 fatty acids, melatonin, herbs and other dietary supplements, special diets, neurofeedback, and several mind and body practices including meditation to control attention deficit/hyperactivity disorder (ADHD) symptoms (NCCIH, 2023). Many of these complementary health approaches have been studied for ADHD, but none have been conclusively shown to be more effective than conventional therapies (NCCIH, 2023).

Home Care

- Family members need to collaborate on planning time to reduce noise and other stimuli in the home to promote a patient's ability to perform relaxation and other nonpharmacological techniques.

✦ SKILL 16.3 Pharmacological Pain Management

Analgesics are the most common and effective method of pain relief. Opioid analgesics have been a mainstay for the adequate treatment of moderate and severe cancer pain. Newer options that are quite effective, yet opioid sparing, are now available using multimodal treatments. However, suboptimal pain management often results due to the absence of a comprehensive pain assessment and analysis of a patient's pain experience. Health care providers often do not assess pain thoroughly, may access incorrect drug information, and have unjustified concerns about patient addiction. Nonverbal patients are especially vulnerable to being undertreated. For example, undertreatment often occurs in critically ill patients who are on ventilators and thus have difficulty or are unable to self-report pain-related symptoms, creating uncertainty with nurses regarding effective pain management (Rababa, 2017). The World Health Organization (WHO, 2018) and Oncology Nursing Society (ONS, 2022) address guidelines for the pharmacological management of cancer pain. These guidelines have great utility for other painful, progressive conditions.

- The goal of optimum pain management is to reduce pain to levels that allow for an acceptable quality of life.
- A comprehensive assessment should guide treatment, recognizing that individuals experience and express pain differently. Assessment includes the use of evidence-based, reliable assessment tools with a goal of capturing and documenting patient-reported pain outcomes.
- A pain-management plan includes pharmacological treatment and interventions to address the physical, psychological, spiritual, and sociocultural elements of the pain experience.
- Analgesics, including opioids, must be accessible—both available and affordable
- Nursing clinical judgment is critical to the safe use and management of analgesics for all patients to ensure the best approach for pain management.

Opioids

In the late 1990s, pharmaceutical companies reassured the medical community that patients would not become addicted to opioid pain relievers, and health care providers began to prescribe them at greater rates (U.S. Department of Health and Human Services [USDHHS], 2022). Increased prescription of opioid medications led to widespread misuse of both prescription and nonprescription opioids before it became clear that these medications could indeed be highly addictive. The USDHHS declared the opioid crisis a public health emergency (USDHHS, 2022). Every day, more than 130 people in the United States die after overdosing on opioids and over 2 million Americans live with addiction to opioids (NIH, 2023). As the National Institute on Drug Abuse (NIDA, 2023) has reported, "Nearly 92,000 persons in the U.S. died from drug-involved overdose in 2020, including illicit drugs and prescription opioids. More than 68% of overdose deaths involving heroin also involved synthetic opioids other than methadone (primarily fentanyl)."

The opioid crisis is a major public health concern worldwide. Abuse is a pattern of drug use that exists despite adverse consequences or risk of consequences. Abuse of a prescription medication involves its use in a manner that deviates from accepted medical, legal, and social standards, generally to achieve a euphoric state ("high"), or that is other than the purpose for which the medication was prescribed (Federation of State Medical Boards, 2017). As of 2019, prescription opioids were a factor in 32% of opioid overdose deaths (National Center for Drug Abuse Statistics, 2022). Health care providers must assess patients' risks for addiction and dependency before prescribing opioids and use multimodal approaches to managing pain. It is essential that nurses educate patients and family caregivers about safe use of opioids. Remember, opioids are the preferred analgesic for maintenance of pain relief related to cancer, depending on clinical assessment and pain severity, in order to sustain effective and safe pain control (WHO, 2018). The correct dose of opioid for cancer-related pain is the dose that relieves the patient's pain to an acceptable level.

Patients who receive opioids for chronic pain often require higher doses of analgesics to alleviate new or increased pain; this is tolerance, not an early sign of addiction (Box 16.2). The Centers

BOX 16.2

Terminology Related to the Use of Opioids in Pain Treatment

The American Society for Pain Management Nursing and the International Nurses Society on Addictions believe that individuals with co-occurring pain and substance use disorder have the right to be treated with dignity and respect. In addition, they should receive evidence-based, high-quality assessment and management using an integrated and holistic approach (Sowicz et al., 2022). Common conditions involving use of opioids include the following:

- *Physical dependence:* A state of adaptation that is manifested by a drug class–specific withdrawal syndrome produced by abrupt cessation, rapid dose reduction, decreasing blood level of an opioid, and/or administration of a drug that can act as an antagonist.
- *Addiction:* A primary, chronic disease of brain reward, motivation, memory, and related neurocircuitry (Federation of State Medical Boards, 2017). Dysfunction in these circuits leads to characteristic biological, psychological, social, and spiritual manifestations. Addictive behaviors include one or more of the following: impaired control over drug use, compulsive use, continued use despite harm, diminished recognition of problems related to one's behavior, and craving.
- *Drug tolerance:* A state of adaptation in which exposure to a drug induces changes that result in a diminution of one or more of the effects of the drug over time.

Approved by the Boards of Directors of the American Academy of Pain Medicine, The American Pain Society, and American Society of Addiction Medicine, American Pain Society.

BOX 16.3

How to Administer Naloxone in an Emergency Setting

When you find an individual who is suspected of overdosing:
- Attempt to wake patient. If no response, common signs of opioid overdose are constricted pupils; slow or no breathing; snoring sound; and blue, gray, or pale skin color.
- Check for pulse and respirations. Call 911.
- Ventilate patient (following CPR guidelines) for a few quick breaths (if the person is not breathing).
- Naloxone will not reverse other sedating substances, and frequently a repeat dose of naloxone may be needed.
- Options:
  - Affix a nasal atomizer to the needleless syringe and then assemble the cartridge of naloxone (according to package directions).
  - Inspect the patient for any obstruction of nares from blood or mucous plug. If clear, tilt the individual's head back and spray the full dose (2 mL) into the naris.
  - Inject 1 mL (100 units) of naloxone intramuscularly using autoinjector.
- If there is no breathing or breathing continues to be shallow, continue to perform ventilation while waiting for the naloxone to take effect. Continue to monitor respiratory rate.
- If there is no change in 3–5 minutes, administer another dose of naloxone and continue to ventilate the patient and initiate CPR if needed. Stay with patient.

CPR, Cardiopulmonary resuscitation.

for Disease Control and Prevention (CDC, 2016; CDC, 2022) issued guidelines for prescribing opioids for chronic pain. The guidelines also cover issues for acute pain and are not intended for patients who are in active cancer treatment, palliative care, or end-of-life care, as these patients may require higher-than-normal doses:

- Use immediate-release opioids when starting opioids.
- Start with the lowest effective dosage and carefully reassess evidence of individual benefits and risks before increasing dosages. Determine if patient is opioid naïve or has had experience taking opioids, as this affects choice of analgesic and dose.
- When opioids are needed for acute pain, prescribe no more than needed. Three or fewer days will often be sufficient; more than 7 days will rarely be needed.
- Do not prescribe extended-release or long-acting opioids for acute pain.
- Follow up and reevaluate risk of harm; reduce dose or taper and discontinue if needed.

Opioids have commonly been prescribed for the relief of postoperative pain. However, the use of opioids in the perioperative period is decreasing as a result of opioid prescription limitation laws and health care agency policies regulating the number of days and amounts of analgesics prescribed and promotion of the use of enhanced recovery after surgery (ERAS) protocols (which limit opioid use), multimodal pain regimens, epidural analgesia, and ultrasound-guided peripheral nerve blocks (Berardino et al., 2021). Chronic opioid use for continued pain management once patients return home from surgery is a health problem (Hinther et al., 2021). As a nurse, be prepared to explain thoroughly to patients and family caregivers the importance of following ordered prescriptions and taking less potent analgesics after discharge (see Chapter 41).

Nurses must know the signs and symptoms of opioid addiction, as well as the association between opioids and respiratory depression. Assessment and nursing knowledge of interventions in pain management, including the use of opioid-reversing agents (naloxone), are crucial in preventing and acting quickly in life-threatening situations. Box 16.3 describes steps for naloxone administration. Also monitor for potential side effects of opioid analgesics and recommend or institute supportive measures (e.g., addition of stool softener for common side effect of constipation).

Delegation

The skill of analgesic administration cannot be delegated to assistive personnel (AP). Instruct the AP by:
- Explaining the behaviors and physical changes associated with the specific patient's pain and to report their occurrence immediately
- Reviewing specific comfort measures to use to support patient's pain relief

Interprofessional Collaboration

- Consult with health care provider and/or pharmacist if you have concerns about patient's response to an analgesic.

Equipment

- Prescribed medication
- Pain scale (numerical or visual and behavioral)
- Necessary medication administration device (see Chapters 21, 22, 41)
- Medication administration record (MAR) or computer printout
- Controlled substance record (for opioids only)
- Clean gloves (optional depending on dose form of medication administered)
- Antiseptic swab
- Sharps needle disposal container
- Stethoscope, sphygmomanometer, pulse oximeter

STEP	RATIONALE

ASSESSMENT

1. Review patient's electronic health record (EHR) for medical and medication history, including history of allergies.
   a. Patients with characteristics/conditions that may cause them to be sensitive to opioid effects (U.S. Department of Labor, n.d.) include adults 65 years and older and patients with respiratory conditions (sleep apnea, asthma, or chronic obstructive pulmonary disease); wasting syndrome (cachexia); or impaired energy or strength (debilitated patients).
   b. Patients with health conditions or characteristics that place them at higher risk of misuse (U.S. Department of Labor, n.d.) include adults 18 to 25 years old and patients with a history of mental health disorders (depression, anxiety, posttraumatic stress disorder [PTSD]) or a history of alcohol or substance abuse.

Determines need for medication or possible contraindications to medication administration. Sensitivity to opioid effects may lead to overdose. Screens patient for risk of allergic reaction. Patients with risk of misuse of opioids will be at risk for overdose (U.S. Department of Labor., n.d.)

2. Assess patient's risks for receiving analgesics:
   a. History of gastrointestinal [GI] bleeding or renal insufficiency
   b. History of obstructive or central sleep apnea
   c. History of being opioid naïve or opioid experienced

Risk factor may contraindicate use of nonsteroidal antiinflammatory drugs (NSAIDs).
Risk factor may contraindicate use of opioids.
Individual who has not used opioids consistently in the past may be at risk for complications.

3. Identify patient using two identifiers (e.g., name and birthday or name and medical record number) according to agency policy. Compare identifiers with information on the patient's medication administration record (MAR) or electronic health record (EHR).

Ensures correct patient. Complies with The Joint Commission standards and improves patient safety (TJC, 2023).

4. Assess patient's/family caregiver's health literacy.

Determines degree to which individuals have the ability to find, understand, and use information and services to make informed health-related decisions and actions for themselves and others (CDC, 2023a).

5. Assess patient's knowledge, prior experience with pharmacological pain management, and feelings about procedure.

Reveals need for patient instruction and/or support.

6. Perform hand hygiene and complete a thorough pain assessment (see Skill 16.1), including patient's previous response to ordered analgesic.

Reduces transmission of infection. Provides baseline for type and nature of pain condition to determine efficacy of analgesic. Assists in selection of type of analgesic to administer and choice of dose to administer within a range order.

7. For patients going to surgery or undergoing procedure requiring sedation, complete an assessment of patient's risk for obstructive sleep apnea (OSA) by using the STOP-Bang screening tool, which checks for:
   • Snoring
   • Tiredness, fatigue, or sleepiness during the day
   • Patient has been Observed to stop breathing or choke during sleep
   • Being treated for high blood Pressure
   • Body mass index >35 kg/m²
   • Age older than 50
   • Neck circumference >40 cm (16 inches)
   • Male Gender

Required in most hospitals before surgery. Identifies patients at risk for OSA, who then may require adjustments to typical opioid pain management postoperatively. Opioid use can increase incidence of OSA. The standard STOP-Bang scoring classifies patients with any three positive responses from eight questions as having risk of OSA (Kawada, 2019; Olson et al., 2022).

8. Assess the anticipated time of onset, time to peak effect, duration of action, and side effects of the analgesic to be administered (review pharmacology reference). For example, intravenous [IV] medications act very quickly and can bring pain relief within 15 to 30 minutes; oral extended-release preparations may take 2 hours to be effective.

Allows for planning pain-relief measures with patient activities, anticipating peak and duration of analgesic, and evaluating effectiveness of analgesic.

9. Consider the type of activities patient is scheduled to undergo (e.g., rehabilitation, scheduled tests, ambulation).

Allows you to time administration of analgesic early enough to gain maximal pain relief during the time of the activity.

STEP	RATIONALE

BOX 16.4

The Pasero Opioid Sedation Scale (POSS)[a]

S = Sleep, easy to arouse
1 = Awake and alert
2 = Slightly drowsy, easily aroused
3 = Frequently drowsy, arousable, drifts off to sleep during conversation
4 = Somnolent, minimal or no response to physical stimulation
Remember: Sedation precedes respiratory depression.

[a]Many institutions will include nursing actions to be taken for each level of sedation.
From Pasero C, McCaffery M: *Pain assessment and pharmacological management*, St. Louis, 2011, Mosby.

STEP	RATIONALE
10. Check last time medication was administered (including dose and route) and degree of relief experienced. Verify the appropriateness of the dose and the dosing interval for the current situation. Consult with health care provider about an around-the-clock (ATC) dose. ATC administration with multimodal use of pain medications (opioids and nonopioids) should be incorporated into the pain-management nursing care plan (Chou et al., 2016; Coluzzi et al., 2017).	Determines if next dose can be administered and whether dose adjustment is necessary. ATC maintains medication at therapeutic blood level.
11. Assess patient's respiratory rate and sedation level (as appropriate) by using the Pasero Opioid Sedation Scale (POSS) (Box 16.4).	Provides baseline for respiratory status.
12. Know the comparative potencies of analgesics given by different routes (e.g., oral, transdermal, sublingual, IV). Refer to an equianalgesic chart or pharmacist.	If nurses on succeeding shifts choose different routes for the same doses, a patient will not receive the same level of pain control.

PLANNING

STEP	RATIONALE
1. Expected outcomes following completion of procedure:	
• Patient reports pain relief and achieves a self-report of pain intensity at or below personal pain-intensity goal.	Patient achieves acceptable level of comfort.
• Patient experiences a reduction in pain behaviors (e.g., guarding, moaning, restlessness).	Pain relief achieved.
• Patient is able to function adequately and perform activities of daily living (ADLs; e.g., walking, working, eating, sleeping, interacting).	A return to performing ADLs has a positive impact on reducing psychological and physiological stress.
• Patient does not experience intolerable or unmanageable drug side effects.	Safe effective dose of medication administered.
• Patient understands the pain-management plan and actively participates in the decision-making process.	Teaches patient how to make medication choices effectively after discharge or independently at home.
2. Talk with patient and determine an individualized pain-management strategy with a pain-relief goal that is agreeable to the patient (ANA, 2018). Use the wipe-off whiteboard in patient's room to write the plan for administration times. Identify strategies such as staggering prn acetaminophen and ibuprofen between doses of prn opioids (Chou et al., 2016).	Gives patient a sense of ownership and control of drug schedule without need to rely on memory. Teaches patient how to make medication choices effectively after discharge or independently at home.
3. Provide privacy by closing room door or bedside curtain.	Promotes sense of comfort.
4. Set up equipment at bedside.	Organizes the work area in preparation for the procedure.
5. Position and drape patient if needed.	Ensures patient's comfort.
6. Explain medication to be administered, anticipated effects, and what patient should report.	Proper explanation enhances patient participation. Accurate reporting of pain by patient improves your evaluation and treatment.
7. Provide educational information to patient and family caregiver. If the patient will need opioid therapy at home, education and a prescription for naloxone and training in the administration of naloxone should be given. Naloxone (8 mg) has been approved in the form of a nasal spray and an injectable form (U.S. Food and Drug Administration [FDA], 2021; CDC, 2023b).	Pain-management education may be needed when managing symptoms at home, including information about adverse reactions. Nasal spray administration of naloxone provides an easy route of administration.

STEP	RATIONALE

IMPLEMENTATION

1. Check accuracy and completeness of each MAR or computer printout with health care provider's written medication order. Check patient's name, medication name and dosage, route of administration, and frequency (e.g., one time, range order, prn) or time of administration. Reprint on computer any part of MAR that is difficult to read.

   The order sheet is the most reliable source and only legal record of medications that patient is to receive. Ensures that patient receives the correct medications (Palese et al., 2019). Transcription errors are a source of medication errors (Zhu & Weingart, 2022).

2. Perform hand hygiene. Prepare selected analgesic, following the "seven rights" for medication administration (see Chapters 20, 21, and 22).

   Reduces transmission of microorganisms. Ensures safe and appropriate medication administration. This is the first and second check for accuracy.

3. Recheck patient's identity at bedside using two identifiers (e.g., name and birthday or name and medical record number) according to agency policy. Compare identifiers with information on the patient's MAR or electronic health record (EHR).

   Ensures correct patient. Complies with The Joint Commission standards and improves patient safety (TJC, 2023).

4. At the bedside, compare MAR or computer printout with the name of the medication on the medication label and patient name (armband). Recheck and ask if patient has allergies.

   Timely administration improves pain management. Final check of medication ensures that right patient receives right medication. Confirms patient's allergy history. This is the third check for accuracy.

5. Reassess patient's pain/sedation level and respiratory status before administering the medication.

   Ensures appropriateness of medication administration. Safe patient monitoring requires assessing a patient's level of sedation and respiratory status at baseline and ongoing interval assessments (Pasero et al., 2016).

6. Perform hand hygiene and apply gloves (if needed based on route of medication).

   Reduces transmission of infection.

Clinical Judgment *If a patient is unable to swallow or has a gastrostomy or jejunostomy tube in place, remember that, with the exception of methadone, the extended-release opioid formulations* **may not be crushed for administration.** *Some capsules may be opened and the contents mixed in applesauce or other soft food, but they may not be crushed. Transdermal patches cannot be cut in half before application.*

7. Administer analgesic, following these guidelines:

   Ensures safe medication administration.

   a. Administer as soon as pain occurs or ATC as ordered.

   Pain is easier to prevent than to treat. The ATC schedule avoids the low plasma concentrations that permit breakthrough pain. This is especially important for the first 24 to 48 hours postoperatively to control pain.

   b. Administer prn or one-time dose 30 to 60 minutes, depending on route, before pain-producing procedures or activities.

   Allows you to anticipate timing of analgesic to coordinate with procedures or activities that might be painful.

Clinical Judgment *Patients receiving around-the-clock (ATC) opioids should also receive laxatives. Opioids decrease intestinal propulsion (peristalsis) but not intestinal motility (churning), so stool softeners alone are ineffective. The most common regimen is a stimulant (senna/bisacodyl) with or without a stool softener (docusate), or daily administration of an osmotic laxative (polyethylene glycol) (Sizar et al., 2023).*

8. Provide basic (e.g., positioning, hygiene) and nonpharmacological comfort measures in addition to analgesics (see Skill 16.2).

   Increases effectiveness of pharmacological agents; treats nonphysiological aspects of pain.

9. Administer nursing care measures during times of peak effects of analgesics. Explain after giving medication (for example): "I will return in 30 minutes after the medicine reduces your pain to do the dressing change." Consider duration of action of analgesics when planning activities.

   Effects vary depending on the type of medication used; allows for anticipation of next dose; permits evaluation of analgesic effects; maximizes effectiveness of nursing measures to prevent complications.

10. Help patient to a comfortable position.

    Restores comfort and sense of well-being.

11. Raise side rails (as appropriate) and lower bed to lowest position, locking into position.

    Ensures patient safety and prevents falls.

12. Remove and dispose of gloves (if used) and perform hand hygiene.

    Prevents spread of microorganisms.

13. Place nurse call system in an accessible location within patient's reach.

    Ensures patient can call for assistance if needed and promotes safety and prevents falls.

STEP	RATIONALE

EVALUATION

1. Have patient self-report PQRSTU aspects of pain (see Skill 16.2) and pain intensity using appropriate pain scale both at rest and with activity (Karcioglu et al., 2018). Use nonverbal scale as needed.

   Evaluates effectiveness of pain-management regimen.

2. Monitor for adverse medication effect and perform vital sign (VS) measurement, note signs of opioid-induced sedation and respiratory depression (OSRD).

   Use a valid sedation scale (POSS) to detect early opioid-induced respiratory depression (see Box 16.4). Monitoring sedation levels may be more effective for detection than a decreased respiratory rate because hypoxemic episodes may occur in the absence of a low respiratory rate; therefore the use of both pulse oximetry and capnography is recommended (Meisenberg et al., 2017; Nagappa et al., 2017).

3. Observe patient's position; mobility; relaxation; and ability to rest, sleep, eat, and participate in usual activities.

   Provides nonverbal and behavioral information for evaluation of patient response to analgesic.

4. When opioids are used, evaluate for opioid-induced constipation (OIC). A recommended tool is the Bowel Function Index (BFI) (Crockett et al., 2019). Patients are asked to score the following three parameters on a scale of 1 to 100 over the previous 7-day period (Yoon & Bruner, 2017):
   - Ease of defecation
   - Feeling of incomplete defecation
   - Personal judgment of patient regarding constipation during the past 7 days

   Early identification of constipation enables timely prescription of appropriate laxative.

5. **Use Teach-Back:** "I want to be sure you understand when to ask for medication to relieve your pain. Give me an example of when you would ask for pain medication." Revise your instruction now or develop a plan for revised patient/family caregiver teaching if patient/family caregiver is not able to teach back correctly.

   Teach-back is a technique for health care providers to ensure that they have explained medical information clearly so that patients and their families understand what is communicated to them (AHRQ, 2023).

Unexpected Outcomes

1. Patient reports no pain relief, including pain intensity is greater than desired or shows nonverbal behaviors reflecting pain.

Related Interventions

- Discuss current pain-control regimen with the patient.
- Determine what has worked best to provide relief. If the medication has failed, document the result and inform the patient that you will notify the health care provider that the treatment is not effective and options will be discussed.
- Evaluate the dose of medication administered with the health care provider and consider an alternative dose or an adjuvant.
- Try alternative nonpharmacological interventions (see Skill 16.2).
- Reassure patient you will do everything you can to solve the problem of inadequate pain control. Discomfort that is unrelieved or worse may indicate need for additional diagnostic, medical, or surgical intervention or a change in pain management.

2. Patient develops respiratory depression.

- Do not give additional dose of analgesic. Stay with patient, monitor respirations, and protect airway.
- Notify health care provider and be prepared to administer an opioid-reversing agent per health care provider order, such as naloxone. Naloxone quickly reverses opioid overdose and can restore normal breathing within 2 to 3 minutes in a person whose breath has slowed, or even stopped, as a result of opioid overdose (CDC, 2023b; Kampman & Jarvis, 2015). More than one dose of naloxone may be required when stronger opioids such as fentanyl are involved.
- Continue to monitor VS (especially respirations) and pulse oximetry.

Documentation

- Document patient's pain rating (15–30 minutes before and after IV medication and 30–60 minutes before and after oral medication), other self-report descriptions, behavioral and physiological response to analgesic, and additional comfort measures given. Incorporate pain-relief techniques in nursing care plan.
- Document medication, indication for the medication, dose, route, and time given in MAR or computer printout.
- Document your evaluation of patient and family caregiver learning.

Hand-Off Reporting

- Report unsuccessful or untoward patient response to analgesics to health care provider.

Special Considerations

Patient Education

- Determine if patient or family caregiver has concerns about opioid use (e.g., fear of addiction or side effects [constipation, nausea, vomiting]). Many patients fear constipation if taking an opioid and will not take it due to that fear or concern. Provide education regarding these issues, along with appropriate prophylactic bowel regimen and dietary needs.
- Give instructions during pain-free or pain-reduced states and before initiating therapy. Instruct surgical patients before surgery or procedures about pain management (see agency policy).
- Inform patient of nonpharmacological pain-management strategies (see Skill 16.2).
- The CDC (2023b) encourages education of the general public about the signs of opioid overdose. Recognizing an opioid overdose can be difficult. Here are a few signs and symptoms for family and friends to look out for:
  - Falling asleep or losing consciousness; unresponsiveness
  - Shallow breathing or no breathing
  - Choking or gurgling sounds with breaths
  - Pinpoint pupils
- If a family member suspects patient overdosing or in distress, explain that it is important that the family member call 911 immediately, stay with patient, give naloxone if available, try to keep patient awake and breathing, and turn patient on side to prevent choking and aspiration (CDC, 2023b).

Pediatrics

- The American Academy of Pediatrics published guidelines on the management of iatrogenically (health care associated) induced opioid dependence and withdrawal in children (McKeown, 2022):
  - Children exposed to opioids for longer than 14 days usually need to be weaned with a gradual reduction in dose over time.
  - Pain status should be assessed at the time of weaning.
  - Monitor for withdrawal symptoms using the Sophia Observation Withdrawal Symptoms Scale.
- There is little guidance on opioid prescription for the pediatric population, causing medication safety concerns for pain management in children and adolescents (Matson et al., 2019).
- Educate parents and family caregivers on safe administration, storage, and disposal of all medications, especially analgesics; emphasize that medications should not be shared, and caregivers should always give the medication dose prescribed.

Older Adults

- Older patients sometimes appear more sensitive to analgesics and experience more opioid side effects. Older adults' reduced renal and liver function slows opioid metabolism and excretion. This causes a faster peak effect and a longer duration of action of the opioid.
- Health care providers should avoid the concurrent use of opioids with either benzodiazepines or gabapentinoids in all populations due to the increased risk of overdose and severe sedation-related adverse events such as respiratory depression and death (Rochon, 2023). Older adults are particularly likely to have these medications prescribed.

Populations With Disabilities

- O'Dwyer and colleagues (2018) report that people with intellectual disabilities (IDs) are at risk of medication-related harm relating to appropriateness and safety of medicine use. Polypharmacy is prevalent, and some prescribing practices may not be appropriate. There may also be underutilization of clinically needed therapies. With the growing older population of people with IDs, health care providers must be vigilant for adverse effects of medicines that may not manifest at younger ages. In particular, the use of multiple psychotropic agents should be frequently evaluated to assess benefits and risks.

Home Care

- Underutilization of prescribed analgesics by caregivers is a common barrier to effective pain management in the home hospice environment.
- See Chapter 42 for safe medication administration in the home.

✦ SKILL 16.4   Patient-Controlled Analgesia

 Video Clip

Patient-controlled analgesia (PCA) is used to treat acute, chronic, postoperative, and labor pain (Pastino & Lakra, 2022). A benefit of PCA is that it is interactive, giving patients pain control through self-administration of analgesics. A variety of medications can be used for PCA and are administered intravenously, through an epidural, or a peripheral nerve catheter (they are placed adjacent to the nerve and block pain continuously) (Pastino & Lakra, 2022). As their pain increases, patients receive analgesic doses through use of a small, computerized pump to deliver a prescribed dose of medication with a push of a button (Box 16.5). The three most common medications used in PCA are the opioids morphine, hydromorphone, and fentanyl.

BOX 16.5

Patient-Controlled Analgesia Dosing

- A loading dose is an optional clinician bolus given postoperatively or during a pain crisis to bring the pain down to an acceptable level.
- An on-demand bolus dose is initiated by a patient when pain severity increases. It should provide clinically significant analgesia.
- A lockout interval prevents repeat bolus administration until a predetermined period of time has elapsed.
- A basal rate provides a continuous "background" infusion.

Adapted from Pastino A, Lakra A: Patient Controlled Analgesia, NIH, National Library of Medicine, *Stat Pearls*, 2022, https://www.ncbi.nlm.nih.gov/books/NBK551610/.

Patient safety is critical during PCA administration. Patient risk factors for oversedation and respiratory depression when using PCA include an opioid-naïve status; obesity; age (infants and small children or older adults); confusion; obstructive sleep apnea syndrome (OSAS); multiple co-morbid conditions, such as lung, renal, and hepatic diseases; smoking; and use of certain medications (e.g., opioids, muscle relaxants, sleeping medications) (Meisenberg et al., 2017). Because patients depress a button on a PCA device to deliver a regulated dose of analgesic, they must be able to understand how, why, and when to self-administer medication and be able to depress the device physically. A safety mechanism on PCA pumps has a lockout interval that prevents patients from overmedicating. Family caregivers must understand the purpose of PCA and why they cannot push the PCA button for a patient. Doing so is called PCA by proxy, a phenomenon that has been documented to lead to respiratory depression (Pastino & Lakra, 2022). Patients, family caregivers, and visitors need to be educated so that they understand, before PCA treatment begins, the dangers of someone besides the patient pressing the button.

Delegation

The skill of PCA administration cannot be delegated to assistive personnel (AP). Direct the AP to:

- Notify a nurse if the patient complains of change in status, including unrelieved pain or difficulty awaking.

- Notify a nurse if the patient has questions about the PCA process or equipment.
- Never administer a PCA dose for the patient, and notify a nurse if anyone other than the patient is observed administering a dose for the patient.

Interprofessional Collaboration

- An interprofessional team (including nurses, advanced practice nurses, physicians, pharmacists) should collaborate to ensure appropriate conversion of PCA to oral or intravenous (IV) medication administration, adjuvant medications, opioid reversal, and management of adverse effects.

Equipment

- PCA pump system and tubing
- Analgesic cartridge or syringe with identification label and time tape (may already be attached and completed by pharmacy)
- Needleless connector
- Antiseptic swab
- Adhesive tape
- Clean gloves (when applicable)
- Opioid-reversal agent (e.g., naloxone)
- Equipment for measuring vital signs (VS), pulse oximetry, and capnography
- Medication administration record (MAR)

STEP	RATIONALE

ASSESSMENT

1. Review electronic health record (EHR) to assess patient's medical and medication history, including drug allergies.	Determines need for medication or possible contraindications for medication administration.

Clinical Judgment *When assessing allergies, be aware that nausea is not an allergic reaction and can be treated; pruritus alone is not an allergic reaction and is common to opioid use. Pruritus is treatable and does not contraindicate the use of PCA (Hirabayashi et al., 2017).*

2. Review medication information in drug reference manual or consult with pharmacist if uncertain about any PCA medications to be administered.	Understanding medications before administering them prevents medication errors (Pasero et al., 2016).
3. Identify patient using at least two identifiers (e.g., name and birthday or name and medical record number) according to agency policy. Compare identifiers with information on patient's medication administration record (MAR) or electronic health record (EHR).	Ensures correct patient. Complies with The Joint Commission standards and improves patient safety (TJC, 2023).
4. Assess patient's/family caregiver's health literacy.	Determines degree to which individuals have the ability to find, understand, and use information and services to make informed health-related decisions and actions for themselves and others (CDC, 2023a).
5. Assess patient's knowledge, prior experience with previous pain-management strategies, including PCA, and feelings about procedure.	Reveals need for patient instruction and/or support.
6. Assess patient's ability to manipulate PCA control and cognitive status for ability to understand purpose of PCA and how to use control device.	Determines patient's ability to use PCA safely and correctly.
7. Assess environment for factors that could contribute to pain (e.g., noise, room temperature).	Elimination of irritating stimuli may help to reduce pain perception (see Skill 16.1).
8. Assess for presence of known, untreated, or unknown OSAS; condition poses a significant risk for respiratory depression (Kawada, 2019; Olson et al., 2022). Use the STOP-Bang questionnaire to assess the patient for OSAS (see agency policy) (Kawada, 2019; Olson et al., 2022).	Assessment should be completed before surgery by anesthesia provider (see agency policy). Identification allows treatment teams (surgeon, respiratory therapy, anesthesia provider) to take appropriate precautions, such as making continuous positive airway pressure (CPAP) or bi-level positive airway pressure (BiPAP) ventilation devices available.

STEP	RATIONALE
9. Perform hand hygiene. Apply clean gloves. Assess patency of IV access and surrounding tissue for inflammation or swelling (see Chapter 29). Remove and dispose of gloves; perform hand hygiene.	Reduces transmission of microorganisms. IV line needs to be patent for safe administration of pain medication. Confirmation of placement of IV catheter and integrity of surrounding tissues ensures that medication is safely administered.

PLANNING

1. Expected outcomes following completion of procedure:	
• Patient reports pain relief and achieves a self-report of pain intensity at or below personal pain-intensity goal.	Patient achieves acceptable level of comfort.
• Patient exhibits relaxed facial expression and body position.	Nonverbal cues of pain relief.
• Patient remains alert and oriented.	Indicates freedom from overly sedating effects of opioids. Sleepiness is usually from fatigue and not necessarily a sign of oversedation.
• Patient increasingly participates in self-care activities.	Suggests successful pain relief.
• Patient correctly operates PCA device.	Demonstrates patient has learned safe and appropriate use of PCA.
2. Talk with patient and determine a mutual pain-relief goal (ANA, 2018).	Gives patient a sense of ownership and control of pain management.
3. Provide privacy by closing room door or bedside curtains.	Promotes patient's comfort.
4. Organize equipment at bedside.	Organizes the work area in preparation for the procedure.
5. Position and drape patient comfortably if needed.	Ensures patient's comfort.
6. Provide patient and family caregiver with individually tailored education, including information on procedure for administration and treatment options for management of postoperative pain with PCA. If the patient will need opioid therapy at home, education and a prescription for naloxone and training in the administration of naloxone should be given. Naloxone is available as a nasal spray and autoinjector (CDC, 2023b). This is particularly important with patients who have a history of opioid addiction (Kampman & Jarvis, 2015).	It is important that the patient and family caregiver understand pain management with PCA and establish realistic pain-control goals.

IMPLEMENTATION

1. Check accuracy and completeness of each MAR or computer printout with health care provider's written medication order. Check patient's name, medication name and dosage, route of administration, lockout period, and frequency of medication (demand, continuous, or both). Reprint on computer any part of MAR that is difficult to read.	The order sheet is the most reliable source and only legal record of medications that patient is to receive. Ensures that patient receives the correct medications (Palese et al., 2019). Transcription errors are a source of medication errors (Zhu & Weingart, 2022).
2. Perform hand hygiene. Follow the "seven rights" for medication administration (see Chapter 20). Obtain PCA analgesic in module prepared by pharmacy. Check label of medication two times: when removed from storage and when preparing for assembly.	Reduces transmission of microorganisms. Ensures safe and appropriate medication administration. *This is the first and second check for accuracy.*
3. Recheck patient's identity at bedside, using at least two identifiers (e.g., name and birthday or name and medical record number) according to agency policy. Compare identifiers with information on patient's MAR or electronic health record (EHR).	Ensures correct patient. Complies with The Joint Commission standards and improves patient safety (TJC, 2023).
4. At bedside, compare MAR or computer printout with name of medication on drug cartridge. Have second registered nurse (RN) confirm health care provider's order and the correct setup of PCA. Second RN should check order and the device independently and not just look at existing setup.	Ensures that correct patient receives right medication. *This is the third check for accuracy.*
5. Before initiating analgesia: a. Explain again the purpose of PCA and demonstrate function of PCA to patient and family caregiver. Give verbal and written instruction warning against anyone other than the patient pressing the PCA button (Cooney, 2016).	It is important that the patient and family members understand how to use PCA safely before patient becomes sedated. Allows for patient-centered care and improved patient outcomes with pain control (Shindul-Rothschild, 2017).
b. Explain type of medication and method of delivery.	Informs patient of therapy to be received.

STEP	RATIONALE

Clinical Judgment *Background basal infusion of opioids has been associated with increased risk of nausea, vomiting, and respiratory depression. However, in opioid-tolerant patients, a background basal infusion may be necessary due to the potential for undertreatment and possible opioid withdrawal (Chou et al., 2016).*

c. If a background basal rate is used, explain that device safely administers continuous medication, but a self-initiated on-demand small, frequent amount of medication can be administered for unrelieved pain when patient pushes the PCA button.

A background basal infusion delivers a continuous dose of analgesic medication. The PCA pump is programmed to allow additional patient-controlled doses for pain that is not relieved by the continuous infusion (breakthrough pain) (Pastino & Lakra, 2022).

d. Explain that self-dosing is desirable as it aids patient in repositioning, walking, and coughing or deep breathing.

Promotes patient's participation in care; pain relief encourages early ambulation.

Clinical Judgment *Patient on patient-controlled analgesia (PCA) who ambulates should have a nurse assist to prevent chances of a fall.*

e. Explain that device is programmed to deliver ordered type and dose of pain medication, lockout interval, and 1- to 4-hour dosage limits. Explain how lockout time prevents overdose.

Relieves anxiety in patients who might be concerned about overdosing.

f. Demonstrate to patient how to push medication demand button (see illustrations). Instruct family caregiver to not push PCA button to give medication.

Administration by proxy is not recommended in adults (Chou et al., 2016; TJC, 2018).

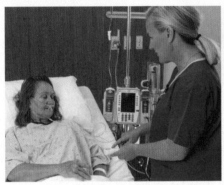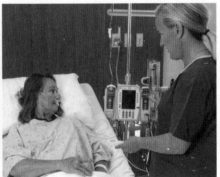

STEP 5f Patient learns how to press PCA device button.

g. Instruct patient to notify nurse for possible side effects: problems in gaining pain relief, changes in severity or location of pain, alarm sounding, or questions.

Engages patient as partner in care.

6. Apply clean gloves. Check infuser and patient-control module for accurate labeling or evidence of leaking.

Reduces transmission of infection. Avoids medication error and injury to patient.

7. Position patient to be sure that venipuncture or central-line site is accessible.

Ensures unimpeded flow of infusion.

8. Insert drug cartridge into infusion device (see illustration) and prime tubing (see Chapter 23).

Locks system and prevents air from infusing into IV tubing.

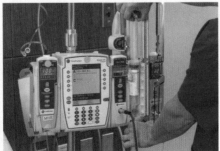

STEP 8 Nurse inserting drug cartridge into PCA device.

9. Attach needleless adapter to tubing adapter of patient-controlled module.

Needed to connect with IV line.

STEP	RATIONALE
10. Wipe injection port of maintenance IV line vigorously with antiseptic swab for 15 seconds and allow to dry.	Minimizes entry of surface microorganisms during needle insertion, reducing risk of catheter-related bloodstream infection.
11. Insert needleless adapter into injection port nearest patient (at Y-site of peripheral IV, port on saline lock or port on central line). There should not be a chance to use PCA tubing for administering IV push with another drug.	Establishes route for medication to enter main IV line. Needleless systems prevent needlestick injuries. Prevents medication interaction and incompatibility.
12. Secure connection and anchor PCA tubing onto patient's arm with tape. Label PCA tubing.	Prevents dislodging of needleless adapter from port. Facilitates patient's ability to ambulate. Label prevents error from connecting tubing from different device to PCA.
13. Program computerized PCA pump as ordered to deliver prescribed medication dose and lockout interval. Have second RN check setting. (**NOTE:** Recheck with oncoming RN during shift hand-off to ensure line reconciliation.)	Ensures safe, therapeutic drug administration. With appropriate dose intervals (e.g., 10 minutes), usually an appreciable analgesic effect and/or mild sedation is achieved before patient can access the next dose; thus there is lower chance for oversedation and respiratory depression. A second nurse check reduces risk for medication error (Kane-Gill et al., 2017).
14. Administer loading dose of analgesia as prescribed. Manually give one-time dose or turn on pump and program dose into pump.	Establishes an initial level of analgesia.
15. Remove and discard gloves and used supplies in appropriate containers. Dispose of empty cassette or syringe in compliance with institutional policy. Perform hand hygiene.	Reduces transmission of microorganisms. The federal Controlled Substances Act regulates control and dispensation of opioids for all institutions.
16. If patient is experiencing pain, have patient demonstrate use of PCA system; if not, have patient repeat instructions given earlier.	Repeating instructions reinforces learning. Checking patient's understanding through return demonstration determines patient's level of understanding and ability to manipulate device.
17. Be sure that IV access site is protected, and recheck infusion rate before leaving patient.	Ensures patency of IV line.
18. Help patient to a comfortable position.	Restores comfort and sense of well-being.
19. Raise side rails (as appropriate) and lower bed to lowest position, locking into position.	Ensures patient safety and prevents falls.
20. Place nurse call system in an accessible location within patient's reach.	Ensures patient can call for assistance if needed and promotes safety and prevents falls.
21. To discontinue PCA:	
a. Identify patient using at least two identifiers (TJC, 2023). Check health care provider order for discontinuation. Obtain necessary PCA information from pump for documentation; note date, time, amount infused, and amount of drug wasted and reason for wastage.	Ensures correct documentation of a Schedule II drug. Two RNs must witness wastage of opioids (narcotics) and sign record to meet requirements of the Controlled Substances Act for scheduled drugs.
b. Perform hand hygiene and apply clean gloves. Turn off pump. Disconnect PCA tubing from the IV access site but maintain IV access.	Reduces transmission of microorganisms. Follow health care provider order or agency policy and procedure for maintenance of IV site.
c. Dispose of empty cartridge, tubing, and soiled supplies according to agency policy. Remove and dispose of gloves and perform hand hygiene.	Reduces transmission of microorganisms.
d. Help patient to a comfortable position.	Restores comfort and sense of well-being.
e. Raise side rails (as appropriate) and lower bed to lowest position, locking into position.	Ensures patient safety and prevents falls.
f. Place nurse call system in an accessible location within patient's reach.	Ensures patient can call for assistance if needed and promotes safety and prevents falls.

STEP	RATIONALE

EVALUATION

1. Ask patient if pain is relieved. Then use pain rating scale to evaluate patient's pain intensity following ambulation, treatments, and procedures according to agency policy.
2. Observe patient for nausea or pruritus.
3. Monitor patient's level of sedation. The Pasero Opioid Sedation Scale (POSS) (see Box 16.4) is a valid tool for monitoring unintended patient sedation (Hall & Stanley, 2019; Pasero & McCaffery, 2011). Also use VS, pulse oximetry, and capnography for monitoring; however, study findings report nurse observation and administration of the POSS as superior in earlier identification of respiratory depression and oversedation (Chou et al., 2016). Monitor every 1 to 2 hours for first 12 hours for the first 24-hour period after surgery (see agency policy). Monitor more often at start, during first 24 hours, and at night when hypoventilation and hypoxia tend to occur during sleep.
4. Have patient demonstrate dose delivery.
5. According to agency policy, evaluate number of attempts (number of times patient pushed button), delivery of demand doses (number of times drug actually given and total amount of medication delivered in particular time frame), and basal dose if ordered.
6. Observe patient initiating self-care.
7. **Use Teach-Back:** "I want to be sure I explained how PCA will help with your pain and how you should use the device. Tell me when you should press the button to activate the PCA." Revise your instruction now or develop a plan for revised patient/family caregiver teaching if patient/family caregiver is not able to teach back correctly.

Determines subjectively and objectively patient's response to PCA dosing. Documenting "PCA in use" or "PCA effective" is not an adequate record of patient's pain level.

Common treatable side effects of opioids.

Patient is at highest risk for opioid-induced sedation and respiratory depression (OSRD) during the first 24 hours of PCA administration. Although there is low sensitivity for detecting hypoventilation with pulse oximetry when supplemental oxygen is used, and evidence is insufficient to firmly recommend capnography (Chou et al., 2016), these interventions are used in monitoring for OSRD and provide important clinical information in your assessment. Excess sedation (patient is difficult to arouse) precedes respiratory depression. Differences in ventilation are observed between wakefulness and sleep, which correlates with states of brain arousal. Opioid-induced respiratory depression is also regulated by sleep-wake mechanisms (Nagappa et al., 2017).

Confirms skill in use of PCA.

Evaluates effectiveness of PCA dose and frequency in relieving pain. Maintains compliance with Controlled Substances Act.

Demonstrates pain relief.

Teach-back is a technique for health care providers to ensure that they have explained medical information clearly so that patients and their families understand what is communicated to them (AHRQ, 2023).

Unexpected Outcomes	Related Interventions
1. Patient verbalizes continued or worsening discomfort and/or displays nonverbal behaviors indicative of pain.	• Perform complete pain reassessment. • Assess for possible complications other than pain. • Inspect IV site for possible catheter occlusion or infiltration. • Evaluate number of attempts and deliveries initiated by patient. • Evaluate pump for operational problems. • Consult with health care provider.
2. Patient is sedated and not easily aroused.	• Stop PCA and notify health care provider immediately. • Monitor VS, oxygen saturation, and/or capnography every 10 minutes or more often. • Elevate head of bed 30 degrees unless contraindicated. • Instruct patient to take deep breaths (if able). • Apply oxygen at 2 L/min per nasal cannula (if ordered). • Evaluate amount of opioid delivered within past 4 to 8 hours. • Ask family members if they pressed button without patient's knowledge. • Review MAR for other possible sedating drugs. • Prepare to administer an opioid-reversing agent (e.g., naloxone).
3. Patient unable to manipulate PCA device to maintain pain control.	• Consult with health care provider regarding alternative medication route or possibly a basal (continuous) dose.

Documentation

- Document on MAR appropriate drug, concentration, dose (basal and demand), time started, lockout time, and amount of solution infused and remaining per agency policy. Many agencies have a separate flow sheet for PCA documentation.
- Document assessment of patient's response to analgesic. Also include VS, oximetry and capnography results, sedation status, pain rating, and status of vascular access device.

- Calculate and document infused dose: add demand and continuous doses together.
- Document your evaluation of patient learning.

Hand-Off Reporting

- Include information regarding VS, pulse oximetry and capnography, pain-assessment scores, STOP-Bang score for OSAS if done, POSS sedation scores, level of consciousness, anxiety level, and activity level (Chou et al., 2016; Cooney, 2016; Meisenberg et al., 2017).

- During a hand-off report, the oncoming and outgoing nurse should inspect and agree with PCA pump programming as a means of medication reconciliation (Kane-Gill et al., 2017).
- Report signs of oversedation to health care provider immediately.

Special Considerations
Patient Education
- Give instruction during pain-reduced state when possible. Instruct surgical patients before surgery.
- Encourage patients to activate PCA at the earliest indication of pain (Elhage et al., 2021).
- Inform patient of nonpharmacological therapies that can enhance pain relief (see Skill 16.2).

Pediatrics
- Consult with pharmacy about the proper dilutions to use for opioids in children.
- If a child is unable to understand the concept of PCA or does not want to control the device, a nurse-controlled opioid infusion would be more suitable.

- It is important that a child's parents understand the concept of PCA so that they can support their child in its use.

Older Adults
- In a study involving elderly postoperative patients, the patients were knowledgeable about how to use the PCA device but not about how often they could receive PCA medication. This lack of knowledge may influence how often they request pain medication. In the study, almost 90% of patients received less than 25% of the PCA allowable medication dose (Brown et al., 2015). Ongoing reinstruction may be necessary with this age-group.

Home Care
- PCA can be used at home by people who are in hospice or who have moderate to severe pain caused by cancer (Johns Hopkins Medicine, 2023).
- Before implementing PCA in a home setting, thoroughly assess patient's and family caregiver's ability to understand its use, safety measures to follow, and proper dosing approach.

✦ SKILL 16.5   Epidural Analgesia

The administration of analgesics into the epidural space is an efficient and effective intervention to manage acute pain during labor (Sng & Sia, 2017; American Society of Anesthesiologists, 2021); after surgery (Hernandez & Singh, 2022); following trauma to the chest, abdomen, pelvis, or lower limbs (Bouzat et al., 2017; University of California, San Francisco [UCSF], 2022); and for chronic cancer pain (Meghani & Vapiwala, 2018). The spinal cord is approximately 45 cm (17.7 inches) shorter than the spinal canal in the adult and ends at the first lumbar vertebra (L1) in 50% of adults and second lumbar vertebra (L2) in about 40% (Hernandez & Singh, 2022). The spinal cord is suspended in cerebrospinal fluid (CSF) and surrounded by the arachnoid membrane. The arachnoid (and subarachnoid space) extends caudally in the adult to S2 to

S3. The arachnoid is close to the dura mater. The spinal epidural space contains CSF, fatty and connective tissues, and vessels and lymph channels (Fig. 16.1). The distance between the skin and the epidural space is variable depending on factors such as age and weight (Hernandez & Singh, 2022).

An anesthesia provider, using sterile technique, inserts a needle to place a temporary short-term or long-term catheter into the epidural space below the first and second lumbar vertebra, where the spinal cord ends. The needle passes through the skin, subcutaneous tissue, supraspinous and interspinous ligaments, and spinal ligament. The provider will feel a loss of resistance on the syringe that indicates the epidural space has been entered (UCSF, 2022). The syringe is then removed from the needle and a catheter is

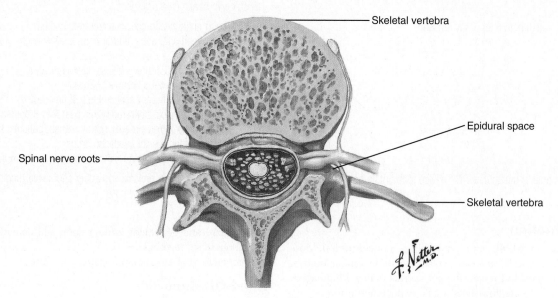

Skeletal vertebra

Epidural space

Spinal nerve roots

Skeletal vertebra

FIG. 16.1 Anatomical drawing of epidural space. (*Reprinted from www.netterimages.com. Copyright © Elsevier, Inc. All rights reserved.*)

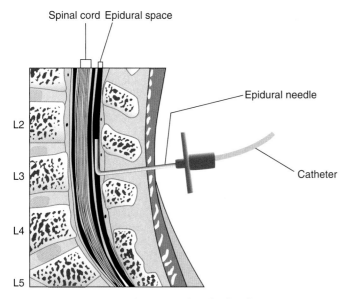

Spinal cord   Epidural space

L2

L3

L4

L5

Epidural needle

Catheter

FIG. 16.2 Placement of epidural catheter.

threaded through the needle, and 4 to 6 cm (1.5–2.3 inches) of the catheter is left within the epidural space (UCSF, 2022) (Fig. 16.2). The procedure for insertion of an epidural catheter requires a patient's informed consent.

Benefits of epidural analgesia include higher patient satisfaction (Sng & Sia, 2017) and a reduction in complications (e.g., oversedation, nausea and vomiting, and respiratory depression) (Bouzat et al., 2017). With proper management techniques and patient monitoring, benefits outweigh complications, which can include hypotension, nausea, vomiting, postpuncture headache after dural perforation, transient neurological syndrome (symmetrical back pain radiating to the buttocks and legs), and epidural hematoma (Hernandez & Singh, 2022). Common opioids given epidurally include hydromorphone, fentanyl, and sufentanil, which require safe, effective interprofessional management. Opioids may be given alone or in combination with dilute local anesthetics (balanced analgesia). The infusion of both an opioid plus a local anesthetic requires careful monitoring because in addition to the risks associated with opioids, there is also risk of local anesthetic toxicity. You must know what an infusion contains in order to properly monitor and administer a safe infusion. Morphine is used for inpatient epidural infusions, but it is unsuitable when used as an anesthetic (Sivevski et al., 2018) for ambulatory surgery because of its slow onset time (30–60 minutes), dose-related duration of analgesia (13–33 hours), and side effects, particularly the delayed onset of respiratory depression.

Analgesic dosing with epidural anesthesia includes (Sanchez & Perez, 2022; Kwak, 2019):

- *Manual intermittent bolus*—Intermittent injection of analgesic by a health care provider offers a better area of distribution when compared with continuous infusion. Intermittent boluses result in fluctuations between pain and analgesia with adequate pain management after bolus administration and increasing pain levels after analgesics start to wear off.
- *Continuous epidural infusion* (CEI)—Continuous infusion of local anesthetics and opioids is practical and can achieve stable analgesia. However, it has been associated with increased local

anesthetic consumption and therefore can lead to profound and sustained motor blockade.

- *Patient-controlled epidural analgesia* (PCEA)—Patient adjusts the time of local anesthetic dosing to pain episodes (e.g., labor contractions). PCEA has shown lower total dose usage of bupivacaine and ropivacaine compared with CEI.
- *Programmed intermittent epidural bolus* (PIEB)—Technique provides better maintenance of epidural analgesia compared with CEI owing to less local anesthetic consumption. It involves administration of automatic intermittent epidural boluses with high-pressure injection, which allows a wider and more uniform spread of the epidural solution

Agencies typically require a registered nurse (RN) to be certified in managing and monitoring epidural anesthesia (Sanchez & Perez, 2022). Follow agency policy and procedure for appropriate patient assessment and ongoing monitoring, infusion line maintenance and care using sterile technique, dose management, and precautions for safe patient ambulation.

Delegation

The skill of managing epidural analgesia cannot be delegated to AP. Direct the AP to:

- Observe the dressing over the insertion site when repositioning or ambulating patients to prevent catheter disruption.
- Avoid pulling patient up in bed while lying flat on the back; this can dislodge the epidural catheter.
- Report any catheter disconnection or leakage from dressing immediately.
- Immediately report to the nurse any change in patient status, comfort level, or loss of sensation or movement.

Interprofessional Collaboration

- Consult with physician who inserted catheter if you have questions about catheter placement and whether patient may be at risk for unexpected complications.
- Pharmacists are resources for information regarding analgesic agents.

Equipment

- Clean gloves
- Sterile gloves (if removing epidural dressing)
- Prediluted preservative-free opioid as prescribed by health care provider for use in intravenous (IV) infusion pump (This is prepared by pharmacy.)
- Epidural infusion pump and compatible International Organization for Standardization (ISO) tubing: NRFit is the name for ISO-compliant neuraxial connectors (Institute for Safe Medication Practices [ISMP], 2021). Most neuraxial connectors compliant with ISO standards are yellow and have an NRFit logo. (Do not use Y-ports for infusions.) NRFit tubing connects directly to epidural infusion line (ISMP, 2021).
- 0.2-micron, surfactant-free, particulate-retentive, and air-eliminating filter (Gorski et al., 2021)
- Antiseptic wipe: aqueous chlorhexidine solution or povidone-iodine solution (Gorski et al., 2021)
- Tape
- Label (for injection port)
- Equipment for measuring vital signs (VS) and pulse oximetry or capnography (see agency policy)
- Medication administration record (MAR) or computer printout

STEP	RATIONALE

ASSESSMENT

1. Identify patient using at least two identifiers (e.g., name and birthday or name and medical record number) according to agency policy if you are preparing infusion. Compare identifiers with information on patient's medical administration record (MAR) or electronic health record (EHR).

Ensures correct patient. Complies with The Joint Commission standards and improves patient safety (TJC, 2023).

2. Review EHR to assess patient's medical and medication history, including drug allergies.

Determines need for medication or possible contraindications to medication administration.

3. Check EHR to see if patient is receiving anticoagulants (Gorski et al., 2021). (**NOTE:** This should be checked by a health care provider before catheter insertion.):

   a. Obtain dosage, route, date, and time of last anticoagulant administration.

   b. Review coagulation lab results.

   c. Consult with provider regarding how long to withhold anticoagulants before the planned insertion.

Anticoagulants must be withheld before intraspinal insertion and before removal due to risk for epidural hematoma and paralysis (Gorski et al., 2021). Recent anticoagulation contraindicates the placement of epidural catheter because of inability to apply pressure at insertion site and risk for bleeding (Hernandez & Singh, 2022).

4. Assess patient's/family caregiver's health literacy.

Determines degree to which individuals have the ability to find, understand, and use information and services to make informed health-related decisions and actions for themselves and others (CDC, 2023a).

5. Assess if patient routinely takes herbal medications; document complete list.

Some herbal medications (e.g., ginkgo biloba, ginseng, ginger) interfere with clotting. However, there is no contraindication to their use when receiving epidural medication (Hernandez & Singh, 2022).

6. Assess patient for presence of any allergies or history of reactions to opioids or anesthetics. Have patient describe allergic response.

History of allergies may contraindicate a certain medication for epidural infusion. Allows you to identify allergic response early if one develops.

7. Perform hand hygiene and complete a pain assessment (see Skill 16.1).

Reduces transmission of microorganisms. Assessment data guide safe and effective dosing of pain medication and establish baseline to evaluate epidural efficacy and patient response.

8. Assess patient's sedation level by using Pasero Opioid Sedation Scale (POSS), assessing level of wakefulness or alertness, ability to follow commands, and level of drowsiness/responsiveness (see Box 16.4).

Establishes baseline before first dose. Assessment of sedation level is more reliable for detecting early opioid-induced respiratory depression than decreased respiratory rate. Sedation always precedes respiratory depression from opioids.

9. Assess rate, pattern, and depth of respirations; pulse oximetry or capnography; blood pressure; and temperature (see Chapter 5).

Establishes baseline of circulatory and oxygenation status. Capnography measures ventilation. Opioids can cause hypotension. Infection is a complication of an epidural, reflected by fever.

10. Assess initial motor and sensory function of lower extremities (see Chapter 6). Test sensation to touch in lower extremities. Have patient flex both feet and knees and raise each leg off bed. Pay special attention to patients with preexisting sensory or motor abnormalities.

Establishes baseline. Ongoing monitoring of motor and sensory status ensures that neural blockage is not affecting function (Lourens, 2016).

Clinical Judgment *For all patients on patient-controlled epidural anesthesia (PCEA), assess for sensory and motor function before ambulation or transfer (Goldberg et al., 2017).*

11. Apply clean gloves. Inspect epidural catheter insertion site for redness, warmth, tenderness, swelling, and drainage. A sterile semipermeable transparent dressing is recommended for site visualization and should be clean, dry, and intact over the insertion site and secure (Gorski et al., 2021).

Catheter sites are at risk for local infections. Purulent drainage is sign of infection. Clear drainage may indicate CSF leaking from punctured dura. Bloody drainage may indicate that catheter entered blood vessel (Lourens, 2016).

12. Follow epidural catheter tubing and verify that catheter is secured to patient's skin from back, side, or front.

Prevents catheter dislodgement or migration.

Clinical Judgment *Note that pharmacies in most health care settings prepare and provide the medication/infusion bag.*

13. Patient will usually also have a peripheral IV infusing. Check condition of IV site and patency of IV tubing (see Chapter 28).

Provides access to deliver emergency medications and other therapeutic medications as needed.

STEP	RATIONALE

Clinical Judgment *Infusion pumps should be configured specifically for epidural analgesia with preset limits for maximum infusion rate and bolus size; lockout time should be standardized if used for patient-controlled epidural analgesia (PCEA) (Mattox, 2017).*

14. Remove and dispose of gloves. Perform hand hygiene.	Reduces transmission of infection.
15. Assess patient's knowledge, prior experience with epidural analgesia, and feelings about procedure.	Reveals need for patient instruction and/or support.

PLANNING

1. Expected outcomes following completion of procedure:	
• Patient verbalizes pain relief, and score on pain scale is less than baseline prior to epidural initiation.	Indicates that drug and dose are effective in relieving pain.
• Patient has no headache during epidural infusion or after discontinuation.	Catheter is positioned correctly in the epidural space. Headache (worsening when patient sits up) is an indication of a postdural puncture headache in which there is CSF leakage from the puncture site and usually occurs between 12 and 72 hours after catheter insertion (Lourens, 2016).
• Patient remains normotensive, and heart rate remains at or above baseline.	Indicates absence of circulatory side effects of epidural opioids.
• Patient is alert, oriented, and easily aroused.	Indicates absence of excessive sedation/oversedation.
• Patient's respirations are regular, of adequate depth, and equal to or greater than 8 breaths/min. Pulse oximetry SpO_2 95% or greater; capnography end-tidal CO_2 5% or 35 to 37 mm Hg.	Indicates adequate ventilation and reduced risk for respiratory depression from opioids.
• Patient voids without difficulty; averages a minimum of 30 mL/h.	Indicates absence of urinary retention (potential opioid side effect).
• Patient has no or minimal pruritus and no paresthesia of lower extremities.	Indicates absence of potential side effects of epidural medications.
• Epidural system remains intact and functioning.	Infusion system is patent; no interruption in medication delivery to epidural space.
2. Talk with patient and determine a mutual pain-relief goal (ANA, 2018).	Gives patient a sense of ownership and control of pain management.
3. Place patients receiving epidural analgesia close to the nurses' station.	Ensures close supervision during infusion.
4. Provide privacy by closing room door or bedside curtains.	Promotes patient comfort.
5. Set up equipment.	Organizes the work area in preparation for the procedure.
6. Educate patient and family caregiver with individually tailored education: purpose of epidural and treatment options such as PCEA. If the patient will need opioid therapy at home, education and a prescription for naloxone and training in the administration of naloxone should be given. Naloxone is available as a nasal spray and autoinjector (CDC, 2023b). This is important with patients who have a history of opioid addiction (Kampman & Jarvis, 2015).	It is important that the patient and family caregiver understand pain management with PCEA and establish pain-control goals.

IMPLEMENTATION

1. Check accuracy and completeness of each MAR or computer printout with health care provider's written medication order. Check patient's name, medication name and dosage, route of administration, and frequency (e.g., one time, range order, prn) or time of administration. Reprint on computer any part of MAR that is difficult to read.	The order sheet is the most reliable source and only legal record of medications that patient is to receive. Ensures that patient receives the correct medications (Palese et al., 2019). Transcription errors are a source of medication errors (Zhu & Weingart, 2022).
2. Perform hand hygiene and follow the "seven rights" for medication administration (see Chapter 20). **NOTE:** *Pharmacy prepares medication for pump.* Check label of medication carefully with MAR or computer printout two times.	Reduces transmission of microorganisms. Ensures safe and appropriate medication administration. *This is the first and second check for accuracy.*
3. Recheck patient's identity at bedside using at least two identifiers (e.g., name and birthday or name and medical record number) according to agency policy if you are preparing infusion. Compare identifiers with information on patient's MAR or EHR.	Ensures correct patient. Complies with The Joint Commission standards and improves patient safety (TJC, 2023).

STEP	RATIONALE
4. At the bedside, compare MAR or computer printout with name of medication on drug cassette/container. Perform an independent double check with another qualified RN, pharmacist, or physician prior to administration (including when syringe/medication container, rate, and/or concentration is changed) (Gorski et al., 2021). See agency policy.	*This is the third check for accuracy* and ensures that right patient receives right medication.

Clinical Judgment *Other routine opioid medications ordered for the patient should be avoided when the patient is using an opioid epidural infusion.*

STEP	RATIONALE
5. Apply clean gloves. Administer infusion. *Anesthesia provider typically starts or administers first dose.* Thereafter, nurse maintains infusion, gives boluses.	Prevents transmission of infection.
a. Continuous epidural infusion (CEI):	
(1) Infusion pump: Insert cassette/container of diluted preservative-free medication into pump. Then connect pump to NRFit infusion tubing and prime tubing (see Chapter 22).	Use an electronic infusion pump with anti–free-flow protection to administer continuous infusions (Gorski et al., 2021). Tubing filled with solution and free of air bubbles avoids air embolus.

Clinical Judgment *Incidents with catastrophic consequences have been reported due to inappropriate medication, enteral feeding liquid, or air being mistakenly administered into epidural space (Mattox, 2017). The International Organization for Standardization (ISO) NRFit tubing and connectors prevent tubing misconnections between small-bore catheters used for different applications including intravenous (IV), enteral, and neuraxial (ISMP, 2021).*

STEP	RATIONALE
(2) Insert NRFit tubing into infusion pump and attach distal end of tubing to antibacterial filter; then wipe off hub of epidural catheter thoroughly with antiseptic swab, then dry. Using aseptic technique, connect end of NRFit tubing to hub of catheter.	Pump propels fluid through tubing. Filter reduces entrance of microorganisms into infusion line. Do not use alcohol to wipe off hub, as it is neurotoxic and can enter closed system when tubings are connected.

Clinical Judgment *NRFit epidural tubing for neuraxial application will not connect with medical device connectors for respiratory, enteral, urological, limb cuff, or intravenous (IV) routes of administration, thus preventing wrong route errors.*

STEP	RATIONALE
(3) Check infusion pump for proper calibration, setting, and operation. Many agencies have two nurses independently check settings.	Ensures that patient is receiving proper dosing.
(4) Tape tubing and hub connections. Epidural infusion system between pump and patient should be considered closed, with no injection or Y-ports. Epidural infusions should be labeled "For Epidural Use Only." Start infusion.	Taping maintains secure closed system to prevent infection. Labeling adds extra security to ensure that analgesic is administered into correct line and the epidural space (Mattox, 2017).
b. Bolus dose via infusion pump:	
(1) While helping anesthesia provider, perform Steps 5a(1)–(4) above. Adjust infusion pump setting for preset limit for maximum bolus size (volume of medication) and interval. Initiate pump to deliver ordered bolus.	Prevents accidental infusion of an overdose.
c. PCEA bolus dose on demand:	
(1) While helping anesthesia provider, perform Steps 5a(1)–(4) above. Set pump for bolus size and lockout time (as ordered).	Gives patient control over administration of analgesia. Prevents overdosing.
(2) Have patient initiate demand dose as needed to relieve pain.	When patient anticipates pain before it becomes severe, analgesic is most effective.
6. Assess and monitor patients after initiating or restarting an epidural infusion for at least the first 24 hours; assess every 1 to 2 hours until stable, then every 4 hours or with each home visit (Gorski et al., 2021). Explain procedure to patient and also instruct patient on signs or problems to report to nurse (e.g., pruritus, inability to pass urine, change in sensation).	Builds trust to encourage patient to be partner in care.
7. Help patient to a comfortable position.	Restores comfort and sense of well-being.
8. Raise side rails (as appropriate) and lower bed to lowest position, locking into position.	Ensures patient safety and prevents falls.
9. Dispose of supplies and equipment.	Maintains clean and organized workspace.

STEP	RATIONALE
10. Remove and dispose of gloves. Perform hand hygiene.	Reduces transmission of microorganisms.
11. Place nurse call system in an accessible location within patient's reach.	Ensures patient can call for assistance if needed and promotes patient safety and prevents falls.
12. Postanalgesia:	
a. Keep a peripheral IV line patent for 24 hours after epidural analgesia has ended.	Provides route for any emergency medications, especially naloxone administration in the event of respiratory depression (Gorski et al., 2021).
b. Before removal of epidural catheter, consult with provider regarding how long to withhold therapeutic anticoagulants before the planned procedure (Gorski et al., 2021). Check agency policy for removal of epidural catheter and extra precautions if patient is receiving anticoagulation therapy.	Removal of epidural catheter while patient is anticoagulated increases risk for spinal hematoma due to inability to compress area. Anesthesia provider will remove catheter.

EVALUATION

1. Evaluate pain character and measure severity using a valid pain rating scale of 0 to 10. Compare with patient's desired goal.	Evaluates effectiveness of epidural analgesia.
2. Evaluate blood pressure and heart rate; respiratory rate, rhythm, depth, and pattern; pulse oximetry or capnography; and sedation level based on patient's clinical condition. Generally measured more frequently in first 12 hours of infusions (e.g., hourly; see agency policy), after bolus infusions or changes of infusion rate, and in periods of cardiovascular or respiratory instability (Nagappa et al., 2017).	Oversedation occurs before respiratory depression and should be monitored closely to prevent respiratory depression. Postural hypotension, vasodilation, and heart rate changes may occur from pain or medication side effects (Mattox, 2017).

Clinical Judgment *Help patient when changing positions. This protects patient who is at risk for postural hypotension.*

3. Evaluate catheter insertion site every 2 to 4 hours for redness, warmth, tenderness, swelling, or drainage. Note character of drainage (e.g., bloody, clear, or purulent).	Observations are made to detect onset of infection at infusion site. Bloody drainage may occur if catheter has migrated into a vessel. Report immediately and treat as emergency (Lourens, 2016).
4. Inspect epidural site for disruption or displacement of catheter.	Could lead to infusion of medication into higher level of spinal cord.

Clinical Judgment Do **not** *place patient in Trendelenburg position, as gravity will displace infusion solution further upward and may result in more respiratory depression or cardiac effects.*

5. Observe for pruritus, especially of face, head, neck, and torso. Inform patient that this is a side effect but is often not an allergic response.	Pruritus *alone* is rarely the result of an allergy to opioids (Hirabayashi et al., 2017).
6. Ask if patient has nausea and vomiting and presence of headache. Note any nonverbal signs of headache (grimacing, massaging head). Monitor for patient sensing a metallic taste in mouth.	Nausea from epidural analgesia worsens with movement. Headache and CSF leakage may occur from a dural puncture. Taste sensitivity may indicate toxic response to local anesthetic.
7. Monitor intake and output. Evaluate for bladder distention and urinary frequency or urgency. Consult with health care provider for possible need for intermittent catheterization.	Prevents urinary retention.
8. Evaluate for motor weakness or numbness and tingling of lower extremities (paresthesias).	Reducing epidural dose (per order) may help eliminate unwanted motor and sensory deficits (Goldberg et al., 2017).
9. **Use Teach-Back:** "We discussed the side effects or problems that you might have from the epidural medicine that you are receiving. Which effects should you tell me about?" Revise your instruction now or develop a plan for revised patient/family caregiver teaching if patient/family caregiver is not able to teach back correctly.	Teach-back is a technique for health care providers to ensure that they have explained medical information clearly so that patients and their families understand what is communicated to them (AHRQ, 2023).

Unexpected Outcomes

1. Patient states that pain is still present or has increased. Primary causes to look for include insufficient drug dose delivery.

Related Interventions

- Check all tubing for kinking, connections, medication doses, and pump settings.
- Confer with health care provider on adequacy of medication dose.

STEP	RATIONALE
2. Patient is sedated or not easily aroused and/or experiences periods of apnea or respirations <8 breaths/min.	• Stop epidural infusion immediately and elevate patient's head of bed 30 degrees (unless contraindicated). Stay with patient and call for help. • Notify health care provider and prepare to administer naloxone per health care provider's order (agency procedure manual may have protocol). • Monitor all VS, pulse oximetry, capnography, and sedation level continuously until patient is easily aroused and respiratory rate is 8 to 10 breaths/min with adequate depth for 2 hours.
3. Patient reports sudden headache. Clear drainage is present on epidural dressing, or more than 1 mL of fluid is aspirated from catheter.	• Stop infusion or bolus dosing. Stay with patient and call for help. • Notify health care provider.
4. Patient experiences minimal urinary output, urinary frequency or urgency, bladder distention, pruritus, or nausea and vomiting.	• Consult with health care provider about reducing dose of opioid and discuss treatment for side effects.

Documentation

- Document drug name, dose, method of infusion (bolus, demand, or continuous), and time given (if bolus) or time begun and ended (if continuous or demand infusion) on appropriate MAR. Specify concentration and diluent.
- With continuous or demand infusion, obtain and document pump readout hourly for first 24 hours after infusion begins and then every 4 hours.
- Document regular assessments of patient's status: VS, SpO$_2$ or end-tidal carbon dioxide, intake and output (I&O), sedation level, pain character and severity, neurological status, appearance of epidural site, presence or absence of side effects or adverse reactions to medication, and presence or absence of complications.
- Document your evaluation of patient and family caregiver learning.

Hand-Off Reporting

- Report the patient's pain-management plan, changes in infusion, patient response, and most recent dose to aid in reducing medication errors (Sadule-Rios et al., 2017).
- The oncoming and outgoing RNs should inspect and agree with infusion pump programming/settings as a means of medication reconciliation (Kane-Gill et al., 2017).
- Report detailed information regarding VS, pulse oximetry and capnography, pain assessment, STOP-Bang score for obstructive sleep apnea syndrome (OSAS) if appropriate (see Skill 16.3), POSS sedation scores, level of consciousness, anxiety level, and activity level.

Special Considerations

Patient Education

- Explain to patient/family caregiver catheter placement and purpose (drawing or showing pictures often helps). Also explain action and signs and symptoms of adverse reactions to opioid. Teach when and which signs and symptoms to report to a nurse.
- Inform patient of other pain-management strategies that supplement or enhance pharmacological intervention (e.g., imagery, distraction, relaxation).
- Some patients may attempt to ambulate while connected to infusion pump without help or overdo other activities. Assist all of these patients with ambulation; have patient always call for help with any activity. Caution them to begin walking slowly to avoid injury. Explain that the first attempt to ambulate may feel strange secondary to decreased sensation, but motor (leg) function should be unaffected.

Pediatrics

- Most pediatric patients receive epidural analgesia in conjunction with a general anesthetic; the main purpose of the epidural catheter is to deliver enough local anesthetic solution for effective intraoperative and postoperative analgesia (Belen et al., 2022).
- Bupivacaine, ropivacaine, and levobupivacaine given in diluted forms are the most commonly used local anesthetics for neuraxial anesthesia in children. Lidocaine is not commonly used in children (Belen et al., 2022).
- Hourly assessments are recommended, especially in the first 12 hours of an infusion. There should be regular review of the need for infusion, especially after 48 hours.
- A dedicated pediatric acute pain team consisting of anesthesiologists and nurses is vital to ensure standardized assessments of pain, vigilant patient monitoring, and the proper treatment of adverse effects for support of children (Belen et al., 2022).
- Tips for parents to support children on patient controlled epidural analgesia include (Intermountain Primary Children's Hospital, 2018):
  - Notice when your child is in pain (restless, crying, or refusing to eat or sleep) and tell the child's nurse.
  - Watch for other signs that your child is uncomfortable.
  - Encourage your child to press the pain medicine pump button if the child feels that the pain is getting worse and not to wait until the pain is strong.
  - Have your child press the pump button before doing things that may hurt, such as coughing, moving, doing physical therapy, or having bandages changed.

Older Adults

- Epidural infusion is a well-accepted option to minimize perioperative side effects in geriatric patients (Sivevski et al., 2018).
- Older adults are at the same risk for complications and medication adverse effects as other adult patients.

Home Care

- Patients needing long-term therapy are discharged with a tunneled catheter. Before considering PCEA in the home, assess the patient's fine-motor skills, cognitive ability, and degree of involvement of family caregiver.
- Teach patient and family caregiver proper dosage and administration of medication via an epidural ambulatory infusion pump. Evaluating the patient's technique for catheter care, administering medication, and reinforcing instructions are priorities.

- Instruct patient and family caregiver on common side effects—constipation, nausea, vomiting, dry mouth, itching, drowsiness, dizziness, confusion, weakness, numbness, or tingling in the arms or legs, difficulty urinating—and what to report.
- Teach patient and family caregiver strict aseptic technique for medication administration as needed and for all catheter care

procedures, including dressing changes. Instruct patient to change dressing every week (policy varies with home care agency). Teach signs and symptoms of infection and instruct patient to report to nurse or health care provider immediately.
- Give patient and family caregiver phone numbers of health care providers to contact in emergency and resources in the community.

✦ SKILL 16.6   Local Anesthetic Infusion Pump for Analgesia

Local infiltration and continuous infusion of a surgical wound with anesthetic is part of a multimodal analgesia approach for postoperative pain control (Paladini et al., 2020). The insertion of a small one-way catheter into a surgical wound site may be used for delivering a local anesthetic to maintain analgesia during and after surgery (Rawal, 2016). The catheter is secured to the skin with a surgical dressing such as Tegaderm and then attached to a portable infusion system (Fig. 16.3). The system delivers a local anesthetic agent (e.g., bupivacaine, lidocaine, or ropivacaine) so that it constantly "bathes" the specific nerve or nerve plexus responsible for pain at the surgical site. There are a variety of infusion pump systems, with most offering targeted pain relief (e.g., up to 5 days) with variable flow-rate settings. A variety of continuous delivery methods can be chosen, including patient-controlled analgesia, continuous infusion, or intermittent bolus (Paladini et al., 2020).

Use of local anesthetic pumps is designed to decrease the amount of early postoperative pain; patients may still require oral analgesics, but the total oral dosage is often reduced (Chou et al., 2016). Studies have shown that patients with local anesthetic infusions have lower pain scores with rest or mobilization at 24 and 48 hours compared with patients who receive placebos (Zhang et al., 2017). A review of studies has shown that local anesthesia infusion reduces pain intensity and opioid consumption with continuous wound infiltration (Paladini et al., 2020).

Local infusion pumps are for one-time use only and usually remain in for a few days, allowing patients to control their postoperative pain at home. Patients and their family caregivers learn how to remove the catheter at home. The elastomeric pumps used for local anesthetic analgesia do not have alarms and should be monitored closely for failure, such as early emptying of medication. All staff, patients, and family caregivers should be given education on signs and symptoms and emergency management of local anesthetic toxicity (Chou et al., 2016). Nursing care also involves assessment of the catheter site and connections and evaluation of local anesthetic side effects.

Delegation

The skill of managing local anesthetic infusion pump analgesia cannot be delegated to assistive personnel (AP). Direct the AP to:
- Pay close attention to the insertion site when providing care to avoid dislocation.
- Report if the dressing becomes moist; report any catheter disconnection immediately.
- Notify nurse immediately of a change in patient's status or level of comfort.

Interprofessional Collaboration

- Consult with health care provider if patient is not reporting local pain relief.

Equipment

- Infusion pump with catheter placed during surgery

Home Catheter Removal

- Clean gloves
- Sterile 4 × 4–inch gauze pads
- Adhesive bandage
- Tape
- Plastic bag

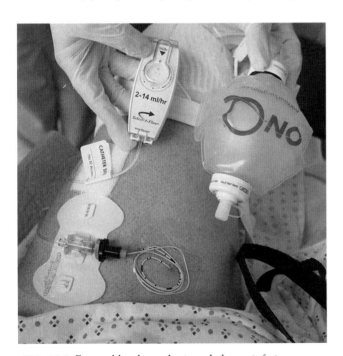

FIG. 16.3 External local anesthetic ambulatory infusion pump.

STEP	RATIONALE

ASSESSMENT

1. Identify patient using two identifiers (e.g., name and birthday or name and medical record number) according to agency policy. Compare identifiers with information on the patient's medication administration record (MAR) or electronic health record (EHR). | Ensures correct patient. Complies with The Joint Commission standards and improves patient safety (TJC, 2023).

STEP	RATIONALE
2. Review surgeon's operative report for position of catheter.	Confirms catheter location with your own observation. Provides baseline to determine if catheter ever becomes dislodged.
3. Assess patient's/family caregiver's health literacy.	Determines degree to which individuals have the ability to find, understand, and use information and services to make informed health-related decisions and actions for themselves and others (CDC, 2023a).
4. Assess patient's knowledge, prior experience with local infusion pump for analgesia, and feelings about procedure.	Reveals need for patient instruction and/or support.
5. Perform hand hygiene, apply clean gloves, and assess surgical dressing and site of catheter insertion. Dressing should be dry and intact.	Determines if catheter is securely positioned.
6. Be sure that catheter tubing is correctly labeled, and then assess catheter connection. Be sure that it is secure. If catheter becomes detached, do *not* reattach or reinsert; instead, notify surgeon immediately.	Reattachment could lead to infection. Tubing misconnections could lead to infusion of inappropriate agents into surgical wound site.
7. Assess for presence of blood backing up in tubing. If blood is present, stop infusion and notify health care provider. Remove and dispose of gloves and perform hand hygiene.	Indicates possible displacement of catheter into blood vessel. Reduces transmission of microorganisms.
8. Perform a complete pain assessment (see Skill 16.1).	Provides baseline to determine efficacy of analgesia.
9. Read medication label on device and compare with MAR or health care provider's order.	Provides information regarding type of anesthetic being infused, concentration, volume, flow rate, and date and time prepared.
10. Determine level of activity that patient can perform per health care provider's orders.	Excessive activity can cause catheter displacement.
11. Confirm patient's allergies (should be initially completed preoperatively and intraoperatively). Assess for early signs of local anesthetic toxicity: tinnitus, blurred vision, dizziness, tongue paresthesias, and circumoral numbness. Excitatory central nervous system (CNS) signs such as nervousness, agitation, restlessness, and muscle twitching are the result of blockade of inhibitory pathways (Open Anesthesia, 2023).	Early identification of toxicity prevents or lessens possibility of complications. Although local anesthetic systemic toxicities are rare, systemic toxicity can occur in five categories: CNS, cardiovascular, hematologic, allergic, and local tissue responses. Signs and symptoms of toxicity usually involve the CNS or the cardiovascular system and can be potentially fatal (Wadlund, 2017; Open Anesthesia, 2023).

PLANNING

1. Expected outcomes following completion of procedure:	
• Patient achieves self-report of pain relief; severity at or below baseline.	Patient achieves acceptable level of comfort.
• Patient achieves reduction of nonverbal behaviors such as grimacing, clenching teeth, and rocking.	In the case of cancer patients, nonverbal behaviors are valid and reliable indicators of pain in absence of self-report (Gallagher et al., 2017).
• Patient moves about in bed, sleeps and eats better, is more active, and communicates easily.	Adequate pain relief allows patient to participate in activities of daily living (ADLs).
• Catheter is removed without injury to patient.	Patient and family caregiver correctly follow instructions for catheter removal.
2. Talk with patient and determine a mutual pain-relief goal (ANA, 2018).	Gives patient a sense of ownership and control of pain management.
3. Provide privacy by closing door or bedside curtains. Set up equipment.	Promotes patient comfort. Organizes the work area in preparation for the procedure.
4. Position and drape patient as needed so that catheter insertion site is visible.	Ensures patient's comfort.
5. Instruct patients on purpose of infusion pump and how it provides pain relief. In cases of bolus delivery, instruct patient on how and when to use. Instruct family members to *not* deliver a bolus to patient. Let patients know they might still require a safe oral analgesic.	Proper delivery of medication enhances success of pain relief.

IMPLEMENTATION

1. Perform hand hygiene.	Reduces transmission of microorganisms.
2. While patient is still an inpatient, routinely check:	Routine monitoring ensures pump is infusing without blockage and that analgesic is effective.
• Pump functioning	
• Catheter insertion site in wound	
• Effects of the nerve block	

STEP	RATIONALE
• Patient's self-report of pain control • Overall skin condition • Muscle strength	
3. Use caution when you reposition or ambulate patient. Do not pull on catheter.	Avoids catheter dislodgement.
4. Prepare patient for discharge: Depending on type of pump, it may be necessary for you to connect the catheter to a smaller pump for use at home. See manufacturer's directions.	Easier pump management and visualization of medication infusion; smaller pumps are used when smaller drug reservoirs are sufficient in the home setting.
5. Teach the patient or family caregiver what to observe and how to remove catheter at home (may also be done by home health nurse). Provide educational materials (e.g., printed brochures, DVD, phone app accessibility). It is rare that the catheter and pump are removed in the hospital. Instructions for removal are as follows:	Visual and auditory materials help with comprehension and retention and serve as a review for patient and family caregiver when providing catheter care and monitoring for local anesthetic toxicity.
a. Explain how to perform hand hygiene and apply clean gloves.	Decreases transmission of microorganisms.
b. Have patient assume relaxed position in bed or chair with lower extremity in normal alignment.	Relaxes joint muscles, reducing traction from muscle tension, and provides distraction.
c. Apply clean gloves. Have patient or family caregiver gently lift adhesive dressing covering catheter insertion site and remove any remaining tape.	Exposes catheter insertion site.
d. Direct the patient or family caregiver to place 4 × 4–inch gauze over site, grasp catheter as close as possible to where it enters skin, and gently pull it out with steady motion. This should cause little discomfort or resistance; a small amount of blood or fluid drainage is normal.	Prevents breakage of catheter.
e. Have patient or family caregiver look for mark on end of catheter tip. Hold new sterile gauze using pressure over the site for at least 2 minutes.	Indicates complete removal of catheter. Achieves hemostasis.

Clinical Judgment *Patients receiving anticoagulants may require pressure to be applied longer (5 minutes).*

f. Wash skin to remove any surgical soap or adhesive near the site. Apply clean adhesive bandage.	Cleanses insertion site.
g. Place catheter in plastic bag using Standard Precautions. Remind patient to bring to health care provider's office at first follow-up visit. Remove and dispose of gloves; perform hand hygiene.	Catheter will be inspected by health care provider to ensure that no breakage occurred. Reduces transmission of microorganisms.
h. Explain to patient that any remaining numbness should go away within 24 hours after catheter is removed.	Allows patient and caregiver to anticipate progress and recognize problems.
6. Remind patient or family caregiver of follow-up appointment with surgeon.	Increases patient adherence.
7. Discharge per health care provider order and agency policy.	Verifies that all discharge planning steps were completed and that there is appropriate equipment for the patient at home.

EVALUATION

1. Inpatient setting:	
a. Ask patient to describe character of pain and rate severity using a pain scale both at rest and with activity (Karcioglu et al., 2018).	Determines patient response to local infusion of medication.
b. Observe for signs of adverse drug reaction.	Local analgesics can result in systemic adverse effects if absorbed in circulation (Wadlund, 2017).
c. Observe patient's position, mobility and strength, relaxation, participation in ADLs, and any nonverbal behaviors.	Indicates successful pain management.
d. Inspect condition of skin and surgical dressing.	Wet dressing indicates possible catheter migration out of wound, especially if drainage is clear. Skin should not become inflamed.
2. During follow-up visit, inspect catheter exit site.	Determines if area has healed without infection.

STEP	RATIONALE
3. **Use Teach-Back:** "It is important for you to remove the catheter at home correctly. Explain to me the steps to take to remove the catheter." Revise your instruction now or develop a plan for revised patient/family caregiver teaching if patient/family caregiver is not able to teach back correctly.	Teach-back is a technique for health care providers to ensure that they have explained medical information clearly so that patients and their families understand what is communicated to them (AHRQ, 2023).

Unexpected Outcomes	Related Interventions
1. Patient verbalizes pain intensity greater than previously determined goal or demonstrates nonverbal behaviors indicative of pain.	• Check reservoir for presence of medication. • Check patency of tubing. • Notify health care provider.
2. Patient reports symptoms of local anesthetic adverse reaction (bleeding, arrhythmias, weakness or numbness of affected area, seizure, confusion, infection, drowsiness, ringing in ears); possible hypersensitivity to local anesthetic; displacement of catheter into vein; or pump failure (releasing too much drug into site).	• Stop infusion (Wadlund, 2017). • Notify health care provider.

Documentation

- Document drug, concentration, dose administered, type of demand feature (continuous or demand), additional analgesics needed to control pain, and any side effects or adverse reactions to epidural opioid or local anesthetic.
- Document location of catheter, patient's pain character and rating, condition of insertion site and dressing, response to anesthetic, additional comfort measures, and date catheter removed (if still inpatient).
- Document your evaluation of patient and family caregiver learning.

Hand-Off Reporting

- Report damp dressing or displaced catheter to surgeon.
- Report to oncoming nurse the location of catheter, type of pump, type of medication, concentration, dose and time local analgesia initiated, patient bolus administration history, patient response, and any side effects or adverse reactions to local anesthetic (Wadlund, 2017).
- Report patient's pain-management plan, including additional comfort measures.

Special Considerations
Patient Education

- Provide preoperative teaching about purpose and use of device before patient goes to operating room. Explain that the pump has safety features built into it. The patient cannot administer too much medication.
- If device is on demand (not continuous), instruct patient to depress button on pump at the frequency ordered by health care provider. The machine is programmed to give a certain amount of medication.
- Instruct patient to inform nurse if pain exceeds pain-intensity goal because additional oral and/or intravenous analgesics are usually available for breakthrough pain.

Pediatrics

- Local continuous infusion pumps have been used for children undergoing orthopedic surgery. Instruct parents and the child in proper use, including precautions for not dislodging catheter.

Older Adults

- Continuous dosing is sometimes administered, but demand doses require a mentally competent adult. In addition, take special precautions to protect the catheter.
- Anesthetic infusion may provide for more than just optimal pain management but could be beneficial due to its indirect effects following surgery (e.g., help the older adult to reduce the incidence of muscle wasting with earlier and more active postoperative physical therapy).

Home Care

- Instruct patient and family caregiver on proper care of insertion site and pump and the possible side effects to monitor and report (excessive fluid or bleeding on the dressing occurs; patient has signs of local anesthetic toxicity or develops signs of infection [redness and tenderness at catheter site, drainage, or fever]. Provide written copy of instructions.
- Provide verbal and written instructions regarding how and when to discontinue device at home. Remind patient to place catheter in a plastic bag and bring it to first follow-up visit with health care provider.
- Provide instructions regarding any restrictions to extremity movement after surgery.
- Home-health nurse may be ordered to remove pump via health care provider's order.
- Provide patient with information about using nonpharmacological therapies to aid pain relief.
- Teach patient to rest between periods of activity at home and hospital because fatigue increases pain perception.

◆ SKILL 16.7 Moist and Dry Heat Applications

Moist heat applications are beneficial in increasing skeletal muscle and ligament relaxation and flexibility; promoting healing; and relieving spasms, joint stiffness, and pain (Table 16.2). Because there is poor skin penetration (less than 1 cm), superficial heat generally affects only cutaneous blood flow and cutaneous nerve receptors (Chen, 2021). In addition to increasing local blood flow by applying heat, the higher cutaneous temperature also has an analgesic effect. Moist heat is most commonly used after the acute phase of a musculoskeletal injury and during and after childbirth, surgery, and superficial thrombophlebitis (Petrofsky et al., 2017a;

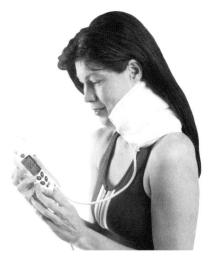

TABLE 16.2

Physiological Effects of Hot and Cold Applications

	Heat	Cold
Pain	↓	↓
Muscle spasm	↓	↓
Metabolism	↑	↓
Blood flow	↑	↓
Inflammation	↑	↓
Edema	↑	↓
Extensibility	↑	↓

FIG. 16.4 Digital moist heat pack. (*Image used with permission from Theratherm, Chattanooga, TN, a DJO Company. All rights reserved.*)

Szekeres et al., 2018). Moist local heat applications include warm compresses and commercial moist heat packs. Immersion in moist heat involves use of warm baths, soaks, and sitz baths. Newer electronic digital moist heat packs allow patients to control the temperature of the heat application (Fig. 16.4).

Dry heat is also used to reduce pain and increase healing by increasing blood flow in tissues and can be used at a low level for a longer period with less chance of tissue injury (Petrofsky et al., 2016). A water-flow pad (e.g., aquathermia pad), electric heating pads, and commercial dry heat packs are common forms of dry heat therapy. Both types of heat applications are advantageous to patients in relieving pain, improving range of motion (ROM), and facilitating healing. A nurse's primary responsibility is to know if a patient is at risk for injury from a heat application and how to apply and monitor a heat application safely (Table 16.3).

Delegation

The skill of applying dry or moist heat can be delegated to assistive personnel (AP). However, in most settings a nurse applies any sterile applications. The nurse assesses and evaluates the condition of the skin and tissues in the area that is to be treated and explains the purpose of the treatment. If there are risks or expected complications, this skill cannot be delegated. Instruct the AP about:
- Proper temperature of the application
- Skin changes to immediately report (e.g., burning, blistering, or excessive redness)

- Specific patient complaints and changes in vital signs (VS) to immediately report to the nurse (e.g., pain, dizziness or lightheadedness, increased or decreased pulse, decreased blood pressure)
- Specific requirements for positioning and application time (see agency policy and manufacturer's instructions)
- Reporting when treatment is complete so that an evaluation of the patient's response can be made

Interprofessional Collaboration

- Consult with physical therapist for use of moist or dry heat applications when appropriate.

Equipment

All Moist Heat Applications
- Prescribed analgesia (if ordered)
- Dry bath towel, bath blanket
- Warmed prescribed solution (i.e., normal saline) or commercially prepared compress
- Biohazard waste bag
- Clean gloves

TABLE 16.3

Characteristics of Heat and Cold Application

	Examples of Conditions	Precautions and Contraindications	Adverse Outcomes
Cold application	Immediately after direct trauma such as a sprain, strain, fracture, muscle spasm; after superficial lacerations or puncture wounds; after minor burns; chronic pain from arthritis, joint trauma; delayed-onset muscle soreness; inflammation	Circulatory insufficiency Raynaud phenomenon Cold hypersensitivity Existing area of skin numbness (neuropathy) Diabetes mellitus Frostbite	• Impedes the transport of inflammatory chemicals and cells to the injured site, delaying normal inflammatory response (Wang & Ni, 2021) • Cardiovascular effects (bradycardia) • Urticaria • Tissue death and nerve damage
Heat application	Inflamed or edematous body part; new surgical wound; infected wound; arthritis; degenerative joint disease; localized joint pain, muscle pain, muscle strains; low back pain; menstrual cramping; hemorrhoid, perianal, and vaginal inflammation; local abscess	Pregnancy Laminectomy site Malignancy Vascular insufficiency Neuropathy Open lesion (e.g., shingles, postherpetic neuralgia) Eyes, testes, heart	• Burns • Infections • Increased pain • Increased inflammation

- Clean basin
- Waterproof pad
- Ties or cloth tape
- Clean gauze or towel for compress
- Equipment for measuring blood pressure
- Options for moist heat application, depending on health care provider's order:
  - Sterile compress, sterile basin, sterile gauze, and sterile gloves

- Disposable sitz bath: prescribed solution and any topical medication after the soak

Dry Heat Applications
- Aquathermia pad and control unit or commercial chemical heat pack
- Distilled water (for aquathermia pad)
- Bath towel or pillowcase
- Ties, tape, or gauze roll

STEP	RATIONALE

ASSESSMENT

1. Identify patient using at least two identifiers (e.g., name and birthday or name and medical record number) according to agency policy.

Ensures correct patient. Complies with The Joint Commission standards and improves patient safety (TJC, 2023).

2. Refer to health care provider's order for type of heat application, location and duration of application, and desired temperature. Check agency policies regarding temperature.

Ensures safe practice by verifying specific location for therapy and type and duration of heat application. Agency policy usually sets recommended temperature for aquathermia pad.

3. Refer to patient's electronic health record (EHR) for history of unstable cardiac conditions; experienced side effects of cardiac, antihypertensive, or vasoactive medications; active bleeding; receiving nitroglycerin or other therapeutic medicinal skin patch; acute inflammatory reactions; recent (<72 hours) musculoskeletal injury; vascular disease; paralysis; peripheral neuropathy; multiple sclerosis, with patient sensitive to heat; and skin conditions such as eczema (see Table 16.3) (Ratliff, 2017).

May reveal contraindications to therapy. Patients with cardiovascular conditions and who exhibit side effects of cardiac, antihypertensive, and vasoactive medications may be at risk for sudden changes in blood pressure and blood flow caused by vasodilation. Heat causes vasodilation, which aggravates active bleeding and can increase hemorrhage or bleeding into soft tissues adjacent to musculoskeletal injury (Petrofsky et al., 2017b). Vasodilation increases rate of medication absorption when direct heat is applied over a medication patch.

4. Review EHR for history of diabetes mellitus with neuropathy and for history of open skin lesions, especially active shingles and/or postherpetic neuralgia.

Reduced sensation may contraindicate application of heat and increases risk of skin injury from application.

5. Assess patient's/family caregiver's health literacy.

Determines degree to which individuals have the ability to find, understand, and use information and services to make informed health-related decisions and actions for themselves and others (CDC, 2023a).

6. Assess patient's knowledge, prior experience with moist or dry heat application, and feelings about procedure.

Reveals need for patient instruction and/or support.

7. Perform hand hygiene, apply gloves, and assess condition of skin around area to be treated. Perform neurovascular assessments for sensitivity to temperature and pain by measuring light touch, pinprick, and temperature sensation (see Chapter 6).

Certain conditions alter conduction of sensory impulses that transmit temperature and pain, predisposing patients to injury from heat applications. Patients with diminished sensation to heat or cold must be monitored closely during treatment. Reduced sensitivity may contraindicate application.

8. When treating a wound (see Implementation Step 2c), assess it for size, color, drainage type and volume, and odor (this assessment may be deferred until dressing is removed and heat is applied). Remove and discard gloves; perform hand hygiene.

Provides baseline to determine change in wound following heat application. Provides baseline for patient's comfort level.

9. Assess patient's level of consciousness and responsiveness (e.g., confusion, disorientation, dementia).

Patients with reduced level of consciousness are unable to sense or report reduced sensation or discomfort from therapy, which may necessitate more frequent monitoring.

10. Ask patient to describe character of pain and rate intensity on a pain scale (Karcioglu et al., 2018).

Provides baseline to determine level of pain relief.

11. Assess patient's blood pressure and pulse.

Establishes baseline to determine response to therapy.

12. Assess patient's mobility: ROM, ability to align extremity for aquathermia pad application, and ability to position self in sitz bath and sit up from bath.

Determines level of help needed to position patient for treatment.

13. Check electrical plugs and cords of aquathermia pad for obvious fraying or cracking.

Prevents injury from accidental electrical shock.

STEP	RATIONALE

PLANNING

1. Expected outcomes following completion of procedure:
- Affected area is pink and warm to touch immediately after heat application.
- After multiple moist heat applications, wound shows signs of healing (e.g., tissue granulation; reduced edema, drainage, inflammation).
- Patient denies burning sensation during application.
- Patient achieves a self-report of pain relief and severity at or below personal pain-intensity goal.

Vasodilation increases blood flow to site.

Moist heat increases blood flow, enhances white blood cell infiltration, and removes waste products from cells (Chatterjee, 2017).

Indicates temperature applied appropriately.
Patient achieves acceptable level of comfort.

Clinical Judgment *Note that in some situations, heat applications cause pain signals to be overridden and decrease pain perception in the cerebral cortex (Wu et al., 2017).*

- Patient demonstrates increased mobility in ROM.

Superficial heat increases joint mobility by increasing connective tissue extensibility and reducing pain and tissue viscosity (Petrofsky et al., 2017a; Szekeres et al., 2018). Heat used in conjunction with physical therapy and/or exercise improves function and mobility (Szekeres et al., 2018).

- Blood pressure and pulse are within patient's normal range.

No systemic vascular changes occur. Goal of therapy is to achieve localized vascular response.

- Patient or family caregiver correctly explains how to apply warm therapy and provides demonstration.

Measures level of learning; necessary for home care.

2. Talk with patient and determine a mutual pain-relief goal (ANA, 2018).

Gives patient a sense of ownership and control of pain management.

3. Provide privacy by closing room door or bedside curtains.

Promotes patient comfort.

4. Prepare and organize equipment at bedside.

Prevents unnecessary delays in procedure.

5. Position patient in bed, keeping affected body part in proper alignment. Expose body part to be covered with heat application and drape patient with bath blanket or towel as needed.

Limited mobility in uncomfortable position causes muscular stress. Draping prevents cooling.

6. Place waterproof pad under patient. (*Exception:* Do not do this with sitz bath or commercial heat pad.)

Protects bed linen from moisture and soiling.

7. Explain steps of procedure and purpose to patient. Describe sensation that patient will feel, such as warmth and wetness. Explain precautions to prevent burning.

Minimizes patient's anxiety and promotes relaxation during procedure.

8. Provide patient and family caregiver with educational materials regarding heat therapy.

Educational materials guide patients and family caregivers when using heat therapy at home.

IMPLEMENTATION

1. Perform hand hygiene and apply clean gloves.

Reduces transmission of microorganisms.

2. Apply moist sterile compress:

  a. Heat prescribed solution to desired temperature by immersing closed bottle of solution into a basin of warmed water. **Do not use a microwave to warm solution.**

Prevents burns by ensuring proper temperature of solution.

  b. Prepare aquathermia pad if it is to be placed over compress. Temperature is usually preset by manufacturer or bioengineering.

Prevents burning by using proper temperature.

  c. Remove any existing dressing covering wound. Inspect condition of wound and surrounding skin. Inflamed wound appears reddened, but surrounding skin is less red in color. Remove and place gloves and soiled dressing in biohazard bag and dispose per agency policy.

Reduces transmission of microorganisms. Provides baseline to measure wound healing.

Clinical Judgment *If skin surrounding wound is inflamed, reddened, has active bleeding or drainage, moist heat application may be contraindicated. Verify with health care provider.*

  d. Perform hand hygiene.

Reduces transmission of microorganisms.

STEP	RATIONALE
e. Moisten compress.	Appropriate aseptic technique keeps gauze compress clean or sterile. Sterile compress is needed when applied to open wound. Reduces transmission of microorganisms.
(1) Pour warmed solution into container. **If sterile asepsis is required,** use sterile container (see Chapter 10).	
(2) Open gauze. **If applying sterile technique,** open and lay on sterile wrapper. Then immerse sterile gauze into sterile solution.	Sterile compress is needed when applied to open wound.
(3) **If sterile technique is NOT required,** immerse gauze into container of solution using clean aseptic technique.	
(4) If using commercially prepared compress, follow manufacturer's instructions for warming.	Reduces chance of accidental burning.

Clinical Judgment *To avoid injury to a patient, test temperature of sterile solution by applying a drop to your inner forearm (without contaminating solution). It should feel warm to the skin without burning.*

STEP	RATIONALE
f. Apply sterile gloves if compress is sterile; otherwise apply clean gloves.	Allows you to manipulate sterile dressing and touch open wound.
g. Pick up one layer of immersed gauze, wring out any excess solution, and apply it lightly to wound; avoid surrounding unaffected skin. *Option:* Apply commercial compress or heat pack over wound only; use only with clean wounds.	Excess moisture macerates skin and increases risk for burns and infection. Skin is sensitive to sudden change in temperature.
h. After a few seconds, lift edge of gauze to assess for skin redness or other injuries.	Increased redness indicates burn. Burns and injuries from warm therapies are preventable events.
i. If patient tolerates compress, pack gauze snugly against wound. Be sure to cover all wound surfaces with warm compress.	Packing compress prevents rapid cooling from ambient air currents.
j. Cover moist compress with dry sterile dressing and bath towel. If necessary, pin or tie in place. Remove and dispose of gloves and perform hand hygiene.	Dry sterile dressing prevents transfer of microorganisms to wound via capillary action caused by moist compress. Towel insulates compress to prevent heat loss.
k. *Option:* Apply aquathermia pad, commercial heat pack, or waterproof heating pad over towel. Keep it in place for desired duration of application (see Step 4).	Provides constant temperature to compress.
l. Leave compress in place for 15 to 20 minutes or less (per order or agency policy) and change warm compress using sterile technique every 5 to 10 minutes (observing condition of skin) or as ordered during duration of therapy.	Maintains constant temperature for best therapeutic benefit. Moist heat promotes transfer of heat to underlying subcutaneous tissues, which helps reduce thermal injury to skin (Petrofsky et al., 2017b). Time limits with higher temperatures prevent risk of overexposure and injury to underlying skin.
m. After prescribed time, perform hand hygiene and apply clean gloves. Remove pad, towel, compress, and heating device. Evaluate wound and condition of skin and replace dry sterile dressing (using sterile gloves) as ordered (see Chapter 40).	Continued exposure to moisture macerates skin. Prevents entrance of microorganisms into wound site.
3. Sitz bath or warm soak:	
a. Remove any existing dressing covering wound. Inspect condition of wound and surrounding skin. Pay particular attention to suture line.	Provides baseline to determine response to warm soak.
b. Remove and dispose of gloves and dressings in proper receptacle and perform hand hygiene.	Reduces transmission of microorganisms.
c. When exudate or drainage is present, apply a new pair of clean gloves and clean intact skin around open area with clean cloth and soap and water. Sterile gloves and gauze may be needed to clean open wound (check agency policy). Remove and dispose of gloves and perform hand hygiene.	Cleaning removes organisms so that bath solution does not spread infection.
d. Fill sitz bath or bathtub in bathroom with warmed solution (see illustration). Check temperature (check agency policy). *Option:* If using bag of normal saline, warm per agency policy.	Ensures proper temperature and reduces risk for burns.

STEP	RATIONALE
e. Assist patient to bathroom to immerse body part in sitz bath, bathtub, or basin. Cover patient with bath blanket or towel once position is achieved.	Prevents falls. Covering patient prevents heat loss through evaporation and maintains constant temperature.
f. Assess heart rate. Make sure that patient does not feel light-headed or dizzy and that nurse call system is within reach. Check every 5 minutes for patient tolerance.	Provides baseline to determine if vascular response to vasodilation occurs during treatment. Prevents injury.
g. Apply clean gloves. After 15 to 20 minutes, remove patient from soak or bath; dry body parts thoroughly.	Avoids chilling. Enhances patient's comfort.
h. Assist patient to preferred comfortable position.	Maintains patient's comfort.
i. Drain solution from basin or tub. Clean and place in proper storage area according to agency policy. Dispose of soiled linen. Remove and discard gloves; perform hand hygiene.	Reduces transmission of microorganisms.
4. Aquathermia heating pad for dry application:	
a. Cover or wrap area to be treated with single layer of bath towel or enclose pad with pillowcase.	Prevents heated surface from touching patient's skin directly and increasing risk for skin injury.

Clinical Judgment *Do not pin wrap to pad because this may cause a leak in the device.*

STEP	RATIONALE
b. Place pad over affected area and secure with tape, tie, or gauze as needed (see illustration).	Pad delivers dry, warm heat to injured tissues. Pad should not slip onto different body part.
c. Turn on aquathermia unit and check temperature setting. **NOTE:** Agency's bioengineering department sets temperature of unit. Remove gloves and perform hand hygiene.	Prevents exposure of patient to temperature extremes. Reduces transmission of microorganisms.
d. Monitor condition of skin over site every 5 minutes and ask patient about sensation of burning.	Determines if heat exposure is causing any burn, blistering, or injury to underlying skin.
e. After no more than 20 minutes (or time ordered by health care provider), perform hand hygiene, apply new pair of clean gloves, and remove pad and store.	Heat therapy may reduce pain and spasm and increase blood flow and compliance of soft tissue structures (Petrofsky et al., 2017a).
5. Apply commercially prepared heat pack.	
a. Break pouch inside larger pack (follow manufacturer's guidelines). Apply to affected area.	Activates chemicals within pack to warm outer surface.

Clinical Judgment *Never position patient to lie directly on a heating device. This position prevents dissipation of heat and increases risk for burns.*

STEP	RATIONALE
b. Monitor condition of skin over site every 5 minutes; observe underlying skin for injury and ask patient about any sensation of burning. Remove gloves and perform hand hygiene.	Determines if heat exposure is causing any burn, blistering, or injury to underlying skin. Reduces transmission of infection.

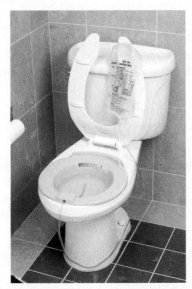

STEP 3d Disposable sitz bath. (Used with permission, Briggs Corporation.)

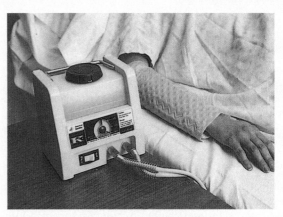

STEP 4b Aquathermia pad.

STEP	RATIONALE
c. After no more than 20 minutes (or time ordered by health care provider), perform hand hygiene, apply new pair of clean gloves, and remove pad and store.	Heat therapy may reduce pain and spasm and increase blood flow and compliance of soft tissue structures (Petrofsky et al., 2017a).
6. Remove and dispose of any remaining equipment and gloves; perform hand hygiene.	Reduces transmission of microorganisms.
7. Help patient return to preferred comfortable position.	Restores comfort and sense of well-being.
8. Raise side rails (as appropriate) and lower to lowest position, locking into position.	Ensures patient safety and prevents falls.
9. Place nurse call system in an accessible location within patient's reach.	Ensures patient can call for assistance if needed and promotes safety and prevents falls.

EVALUATION

1. Inspect condition of body part or wound; observe skin integrity, color, and temperature, and note any dryness, edema, blistering, drainage, or sensitivity to touch. In case of sitz bath, inspect perineal area.	Evaluates effectiveness of heat application and whether there is presence of injury.
2. Obtain blood pressure and pulse; compare with baseline.	Determines if systemic vascular response to vasodilation has occurred.
3. Ask patient to describe character of pain and severity of pain using a pain scale (Karcioglu et al., 2018). Ask about any sensation of burning following treatment.	Determines if patient was exposed to temperature extreme, resulting in burn. Evaluates patient's subjective response to therapy.
4. Evaluate ROM of affected body part.	Determines if edema or muscle spasm is relieved.

Clinical Judgment *Do not have patient immediately exercise muscle to evaluate results of therapy. Active exercise can aggravate muscle strain. Heat in conjunction with exercise as a form of therapy is beneficial.*

5. **Use Teach-Back:** "I want to be sure you understand how to apply a warm moist compress so that you can do this at home. Show me how you would apply this compress at home." Revise your instruction now or develop a plan for revised patient/family caregiver teaching if patient/family caregiver is not able to teach back correctly.	Teach-back is a technique for health care providers to ensure that they have explained medical information clearly so that patients and their families understand what is communicated to them (AHRQ, 2023).

Unexpected Outcomes	Related Interventions
1. Patient's skin is reddened, tender, swollen, and sensitive to touch during/after moist heat application, or patient complains of burning.	• Discontinue moist application immediately. • Verify proper temperature or check aquathermia device for proper functioning. • Notify health care provider and, if there is a burn, complete an incident or adverse occurrence report (see agency policy).
2. Body part remains painful and is difficult to move after heat application.	• Discontinue aquathermia pad, compress, or heat pack use. • Observe for localized swelling or skin breakdown. • Notify health care provider.
3. Patient or family caregiver applies heat incorrectly or is unable to explain precautions.	• Reinstruct patient or family caregiver as needed. Consider possible home health referral (if patient is eligible).

Documentation

• Document type of application (compress, pad, bath, or pack); location and duration of application; condition of body part, wound, or skin before and after treatment; and patient's response to therapy.
• Document your evaluation of patient and family caregiver learning.

Hand-Off Reporting

• During hand-off to next shift, report the location and type of heat therapy, medication used (if ordered), duration and time of therapy, skin assessment, VS, pain assessment before and after therapy, patient response to therapy, and any adverse reactions.

• Report patient's heat therapy management plan to oncoming nurse.

Special Considerations
Patient Education

• Instruct family caregivers and patients on how to assess patients with reduced sensation to determine if temperature of heat application is too hot.
• After using moist heat, caution patient against rubbing the wound with a towel, as it may irritate a surgical site and cause it to bleed. Pat the area dry instead.
• Instruct patient and family caregiver to not use highest setting on any external heat device and to check the patient's skin frequently for redness or blistering on the skin exposed to the heat.

Pediatrics

- The skin of infants and children is thin and fragile and therefore easily damaged. Take extra care to verify temperature and temperature settings. Use special caution in applying any heat therapy (Hockenberry et al., 2022). Remain with child during procedure.
- It is helpful to incorporate play into the time a child is required to use a heat soak. Placing items with which the child can interact in the basin is helpful. Place clean boats or other water toys in the bath. Adult supervision is required.

Older Adults

- As a result of chronic diseases, malnourishment, or use of long-term steroid use, patients may have impaired circulation, fragility of the skin, or impaired sensation to temperature.

- Older adults who have lost subcutaneous tissue and fat have no insulation and may be at increased risk of injury from heat application (Touhy & Jett, 2023).

Populations With Disabilities

- Any patient with cognitive impairment should not be allowed to apply a heat therapy independently.

Home Care

- When necessary, assess availability of family caregiver to help patient apply moist heat and to not leave patient unattended.
- Patient may need assistive devices to get in or out of a sitz bath or tub.
- Patients may use bathtub at home for sitz baths. Before making the sitz bath, make sure that the tub is cleansed thoroughly and then rinsed thoroughly of dirt and cleaning agents used.

✦ SKILL 16.8   Cold Application

Cold therapy refers to the superficial application of cold to the surface of the skin, with or without compression or with a mechanical recirculating device to maintain cold temperatures (Chou et al., 2016). Cold therapy treats the localized inflammatory response of an injured body part by reducing edema, hematoma formation, and pain; reducing muscle spasm; reducing the inflammatory reaction to trauma; decreasing tissue metabolism; and reducing enzymatic activity (see Table 16.3) (Wang & Ni, 2021). Cold therapy most commonly is used immediately after soft tissue and musculoskeletal injuries such as sprains or strains; however, it has been widely used in the postoperative setting with patients who have undergone orthopedic surgical procedures (e.g., joint replacements, spinal fusion, and lumbar discectomy) (Quinlan et al., 2017). One form of cold therapy (specifically ice application) is used regularly as an immediate treatment to induce analgesia following acute soft tissue injuries when there is pronounced edema; however, a prolonged ice application has proved to delay the start of the healing and lengthen the recovery process (Wang & Ni, 2021). It can also take 15 to 30 minutes to achieve temperatures low enough to produce local analgesia (Wang & Ni, 2021). Cold therapy should be used judiciously and only for the short term. Any cold therapy that reduces inflammation also delays healing, because the process of inflammation is an essential aspect of recovery itself (Wang & Ni, 2021). Although cold therapy typically slows the soft tissue swelling to some extent, it does not hasten the recovery process (Wang & Ni, 2021).

Although stronger evidence is needed, use of ice is still common in medicine and physical therapy. The most common cold therapy methods include cold compresses, ice packs, electronically controlled continuous-flow devices, and cold-water immersion athletic therapy (Chatterjee, 2017; Rigby & Dye, 2017). The most important nursing responsibilities in applying cold therapy include knowing a patient's risk for injury, understanding normal body responses to cold, assessing the integrity of the body part to be treated, determining a patient's ability to sense temperature variations, and ensuring proper function of equipment.

Delegation

The skill of applying cold applications can be delegated to assistive personnel (AP) (see agency policy). The nurse assesses and evaluates the patient and explains the purpose of the treatment. If there are risks or possible complications, this skill is not delegated. Instruct the AP to:

- Keep the application in place for only the length of time specified in the health care provider's order.
- Immediately report any excessive redness of the skin, increase in pain, or decrease in sensation.
- Report when treatment is complete so that a nurse can evaluate the patient's response.

Interprofessional Collaboration

- Physical therapists often use cold therapy as a form of longer-term treatment.

Equipment

All Compresses, Bags, and Packs

- Clean gloves (if blood or body fluids are present)
- Cloth tape or ties or elastic wrap bandage
- Soft cloth cover: towel, pillowcase, or stockinette
- Bath towel or blanket and waterproof absorbent pad

Cold Compress

- Absorbent gauze (clean or sterile) folded to desired size
- Basin
- Prescribed solution at desired temperature

Ice Bag or Gel Pack

- Ice bag
- Ice chips and water *or*
- Reusable commercial gel pack (cold pack)
- Disposable commercial chemical cold pack

Electronically Controlled Cooling Device

- Cool-water flow pad or cooling pad and electrical pump
- Gauze roll or elastic wrap

STEP	RATIONALE

ASSESSMENT

1. Identify patient using at least two identifiers (e.g., name and birthday or name and medical record number) according to agency policy.

   Ensures correct patient. Complies with The Joint Commission standards and improves patient safety (TJC, 2023).

2. Refer to health care provider's order for type, location, and duration of application. Temperature of a cooling pad will be ordered or preset.

   Health care provider's order is required for all cold applications.

3. Consider time elapsed since injury occurred. If this is an acute injury, follow these principles:
   Protect—Protect injured area to reduce further tissue damage. Immobilize with splint, sling, or brace.
   Rest—Reduce activity until cold can be applied.
   Ice—When applied in a timely manner, provides physiological benefits (see Table 16.2).
   Compress—Mild compression reduces the edema that forms following an injury by promoting vasoconstriction.
   Elevate—Raising affected extremity promotes venous return, reducing edema.

   Apply cold therapy as soon as possible after injury to reduce swelling, inflammation, tissue bleeding, and pain (Chatterjee, 2017; Quinlan et al., 2017).

Clinical Judgment *Do not apply ice directly to the skin. Always have a light covering on skin or be sure ice is enclosed in a cloth cover before applying ice.*

4. Review electronic health record (EHR) for any contraindications or precautionary conditions (see Table 16.3).

   These conditions contraindicate use of cold therapy because they increase the risk for skin and tissue injury when exposed to cold.

5. Assess patient's/family caregiver's health literacy.

   Determines degree to which individuals have the ability to find, understand, and use information and services to make informed health-related decisions and actions for themselves and others (CDC, 2023a).

6. Perform hand hygiene and apply clean gloves. Inspect condition of injured or affected part. Gently palpate area for edema (apply clean gloves if there is risk of exposure to body fluids).

   Reduces transmission of microorganisms. Provides baseline for determining change in condition of injured tissues.

7. Perform neurovascular check and inspect surrounding skin for integrity, circulation (presence of pulses), color, temperature, and sensitivity to touch (see Chapter 6). Remove and dispose of gloves. Perform hand hygiene.

   Determines if patient is insensitive to cold extremes, which increases risk for injury and may contraindicate use of therapy. Reduces transmission of microorganisms.

Clinical Judgment *Keep injured part in alignment and immobilized. Movement can cause further injury to strains, sprains, or fractures.*

8. Assess patient's level of consciousness and responsiveness.

   Patients with reduced level of consciousness are unable to sense or report reduced sensation or discomfort.

9. Ask patient to describe character of pain and rate severity on a valid pain scale (Karcioglu et al., 2018). Assess range of motion (ROM) of an affected extremity.

   Provides baseline for determining pain relief and ROM with therapy.

10. Assess patient's knowledge, prior experience with cold application, and feelings about procedure.

    Reveals need for patient instruction and/or support.

PLANNING

1. Expected outcomes following completion of procedure:
   - Affected area is slightly pale and cool to touch.

     Result of vasoconstriction from cold.
   - There is decreased edema and/or bleeding in tissues at site of injury.

     Cold reduces blood flow to affected part by reducing protein extravasation from vasculature and subsequent edema formation (Quinlan et al., 2017).
   - Patient achieves a self-report of pain relief and pain severity at or below personal pain-intensity goal.

     Patient achieves acceptable level of comfort. Cold decreases local swelling, reduces inflammatory response, and decreases nerve conduction and subsequent pain, creating localized analgesic effect (Codding & Getz, 2017).
   - Patient's ROM increases.

     Cold reduces swelling.
   - Patient or family caregiver correctly states how to apply cold therapy and provides demonstration.

     Documents learning for home care.

STEP	RATIONALE
2. Talk with patient and determine a mutual pain-relief goal (ANA, 2018).	Gives patient a sense of ownership and control of pain management.
3. Provide privacy by closing room door or curtain.	Promotes comfort.
4. Perform hand hygiene. Prepare equipment at bedside.	Promotes efficiency of procedure.
5. Position patient in bed, keeping affected body part in proper alignment. Expose body part to be covered with cold application, and drape other body parts with bath blanket or towel as needed.	Limited mobility in uncomfortable position causes muscular stress. Draping avoids unnecessary exposure of body parts, maintaining patient's comfort and privacy.
6. Explain procedure and precautions.	Improves likelihood of patient's adherence to therapy.
7. Provide patient and family caregiver with educational materials regarding how to use cold therapy safely at home.	Educational materials guide patients and family caregivers in using therapy correctly and avoiding patient injury.

IMPLEMENTATION

1. Perform hand hygiene and apply clean gloves.	Reduces transmission of microorganisms.
2. Place towel or absorbent pad under area that you will treat.	Prevents soiling of bed linen.
3. Apply cold compress:	
a. Place ice and water in basin and test temperature on inner aspect of your arm.	Extreme temperature can cause tissue damage.
b. Submerge gauze into basin filled with cold solution; wring out excess moisture.	Dripping gauze is uncomfortable to patient.
c. Apply compress to affected area, molding it gently but firmly over site.	Ensures that cold is directed over site of injury. Compression applied.
d. Remove, remoisten, and reapply to maintain temperature as needed for a total time of 15 to 20 minutes (ACE, 2019).	
4. Apply ice pack or bag:	
a. Fill bag with water, secure cap, and invert.	Ensures that there are no leaks.
b. Empty water and fill bag two-thirds full with small ice chips and water.	Bag is easier to mold over body part when it is not full.
c. Express excess air from bag, secure bag closure, and wipe bag dry.	Excess air interferes with cold conduction. Allows bag to conform to area and promotes maximum contact.
d. Squeeze or knead commercial ice pack according to manufacturer's directions.	Releases alcohol-based solution to create cold temperature.
e. Wrap pack or bag with single layer of towel, pillowcase, or stockinette. Apply over injury. Secure with tape as needed. Always place a barrier (e.g., towel, pillowcase, ice pack covering) between cooling device and the patient's skin to avoid tissue injury. Keep in place 15 to 20 minutes. Repeat 4 to 8 times daily or as ordered (ACE, 2019).	Protects patient's tissue and absorbs condensation. Prevents direct exposure of cold against patient's skin.
5. Apply commercial gel pack:	
a. Remove from freezer.	
b. Wrap pack with towel, pillowcase, or stockinette. Apply pack directly over injury.	Protects patient's tissue and absorbs condensation. Prevents direct exposure of cold against patient's skin.
c. Secure with gauze, cloth tape, or ties as needed. Keep in place 15 to 20 minutes. Repeat 4 to 8 times daily or as ordered (ACE, 2019).	

Clinical Judgment *Do not reapply ice pack to red or bluish areas; continual use of ice pack makes ischemia worse.*

6. Apply electronically controlled cooling device:	
a. Prepare device following manufacturer's directions. Some devices are gravity fed and require you to manually fill with ice water.	Motorized units circulate chilled water.
b. Make sure that all connections are intact and temperature, if adjustable, is set (see agency policy).	Ensures safe temperature application.
c. Wrap cool-water flow pad in single layer of towel or pillowcase.	Prevents adverse reactions from cold such as burn or frostbite.
d. Wrap cool pad around body part.	Ensures even application of cold temperature.

STEP	RATIONALE
e. Turn device on and check correct temperature. (**NOTE:** Temperature is usually preset in health care settings [check agency policy]).	Ensures effective therapy. Preset temperature reduces risk of skin and tissue injury.
f. Secure with elastic wrap bandage, gauze roll, or ties. Keep in place 15 to 20 minutes. Repeat 4 to 8 times daily or as ordered (ACE, 2019).	Ensures cold is distributed to correct body part.
7. Remove and dispose of gloves in proper container. Perform hand hygiene.	Reduces transmission of microorganisms.
8. Check condition of skin every 5 minutes for duration of application.	Determines if there are adverse reactions to cold (e.g., mottling, redness, burning, blistering, numbness).
a. If area is edematous, sensation may be reduced; use extra caution during cold therapy and assess site more often.	Prevents injury to skin and tissues.
b. Some numbness and tingling are common sensations with cold applications and indicate adverse reactions only when severe and coupled with other symptoms. Stop treatment when patient complains of burning sensation or increased sensation of numbness in the area of treatment.	When applying cold, skin will initially feel cold, followed by relief of pain. As cold continues, patient will feel burning sensation, then pain in skin, and finally numbness.
9. After 15 to 20 minutes (or as ordered by health care provider), perform hand hygiene, apply clean gloves, remove cold application, and gently dry off any moisture.	Drying prevents maceration of skin.

Clinical Judgment *Areas with little body fat (e.g., knee, ankle, and elbow) do not tolerate cold as well as fatty areas (e.g., thigh and buttocks) do. For bony areas, decrease time of cold application to lower range.*

STEP	RATIONALE
10. Assist patient to a comfortable position.	Restores comfort and sense of well-being.
11. Raise side rails (as appropriate) and lower bed to lowest position, locking into position.	Ensures patient safety and prevents falls.
12. Dispose of soiled linen, supplies, and equipment. Remove gloves and perform hand hygiene.	Reduces transmission of microorganisms.
13. Place nurse call system in an accessible location within patient's reach.	Ensures patient can call for assistance if needed and promotes safety and prevents falls.

EVALUATION

1. Inspect affected area for integrity, color, skin temperature, and sensitivity to touch. Reevaluate 30 minutes after procedure.	Determines reaction to cold application.
2. Apply clean gloves. Palpate affected area gently and note any edema, bruising, and bleeding. Remove and dispose of gloves; perform hand hygiene.	Reduces transmission of microorganisms. Determines level of improvement.
3. Ask patient to report level of pain and rate severity on a pain rating scale (Karcioglu et al., 2018).	Determines if pain has been relieved.
4. Measure ROM of affected body part.	Determines if edema or muscle spasm is relieved.
5. **Use Teach-Back:** "Let's review together how to apply an ice pack to your ankle correctly. Show me how to apply the ice pack." Revise your instruction now or develop a plan for revised patient/family caregiver teaching if patient/family caregiver is not able to teach back correctly.	Teach-back is a technique for health care providers to ensure that they have explained medical information clearly so that patients and their families understand what is communicated to them (AHRQ, 2023).

Unexpected Outcomes	Related Interventions
1. Skin appears mottled, reddened, or bluish as a result of exposure to cold.	• Stop treatment. • Notify health care provider.
2. Patient complains of burning pain and numbness.	• Stop therapy. • Notify health care provider.
3. Patient or family caregiver is unable to describe or demonstrate therapy.	• Provide further instruction and/or demonstration.

Documentation

- Document location of treatment site; pain level; appearance and condition of skin before and after treatment; type, location, and duration of application; and patient's response to therapy.
- Document your evaluation of patient and family caregiver learning.

Hand-Off Reporting

- Report any sensations of burning, numbness, or unrelieved pain or skin color changes to health care provider.
- During hand-off to next shift, report the location and type of cold therapy, medication used (if ordered), duration and time of therapy, skin assessment, vital signs (VS), pain assessment before and after therapy, patient response to therapy, and any adverse reactions.
- Report patient's cold therapy management plan and patient and family caregiver's understanding of therapy.

Special Considerations

Patient Education

- Injuries requiring cold therapies usually occur outside of acute care settings. Patients active in sports should know steps to take for applying cold therapies correctly.
- Stress to patients and family caregivers the importance of not applying any cold therapy for too long a time (no longer than 20 minutes) to reduce chance of injury to the skin and soft tissues.

- Instruct patients and family caregivers on how to observe the skin and perform pain assessment.

Pediatrics

- Cool soaks decrease itching with some skin lesions. Use the same precautions and play therapy techniques as for warm soaks (Hockenberry et al., 2022).

Older Adults

- Older adults are more at risk for tissue damage because of altered responses to change in body temperature; therefore they need frequent skin assessment during treatment (Touhy & Jett, 2023).

Populations With Disabilities

- Any patient with an intellectual or development disability should not be allowed to apply a cold therapy independently.

Home Care

- To apply a cold pack at home (Oregon Ear, Nose and Throat, 2023):
  - Bags of frozen peas or corn are inexpensive, last 10 to 20 minutes, and mold well to the body.
  - Mix 710 mL (3 cups) water and 235 mL (1 cup) rubbing alcohol in a freezer bag. Seal the bag and place it in the freezer until slush forms. Refreeze the bag when the slush melts.
  - Buy cold packs that can be reused. Store them in the freezer. Some of them are designed to wrap around an injured area, such as an arm or knee.

✦ CLINICAL JUDGMENT AND NEXT-GENERATION NCLEX® EXAMINATION–STYLE QUESTIONS

A 73-year-old patient was admitted through the emergency department (ED) after having fallen down steps at a movie theatre near home. An ambulance brought the patient to the ED. Emergency medical technicians (EMTs) report that the patient was found lying on the left side reporting moderate pain at the hip, with a superficial abrasion and small laceration over the left eye. Current vital signs include blood pressure 138/78 mm Hg, pulse 82 beats/min, respirations 18 breaths/min, temperature 37.1°C (98.8°F) and oxygen saturation 98% on room air. The patient denies being on any medication aside from metformin, 500 mg twice daily, for type 2 diabetes. While performing the assessment, the patient says to the nurse, "I'm more worried about what happened to my wife. She was with me at the theater and can't drive." The transport staff arrives to take the patient to x-ray; as the patient is moved to the stretcher, the patient cries out in pain and then rates the pain as 9 on a 0-to-10 scale.

1. The patient's pain is unrelieved after returning from x-ray. The nurse observes the patient visibly crying and repeating, "My hip hurts terribly." Choose the *most likely* options for the information missing from the statement below by selecting from the lists of options provided. The patient most likely has a(n) **1 [Select]** as evidenced by **2 [Select]**.

Options for 1	Options for 2
Broken hip	Taking metformin
Panic attack	Concern about his wife
Elevated blood glucose	Abrasions and lacerations
Infection	Excruciating pain

2. For each system below, click to specify the potential nursing intervention that would be appropriate for care of the patient at this time. Each body system supports only 1 potential nursing intervention.

System	Potential Nursing Intervention
Constitutional (pain)	○ Massage the affected hip ○ Administer IV morphine as prescribed ○ Remind patient that pain will pass and is not serious
Integumentary	○ Gently cleanse abrasion and laceration with saline ○ Place an occlusive dressing over the abrasion and laceration ○ Prioritize care for abrasion and laceration over other patient needs
Psychosocial	○ Tell the patient that their spouse is likely fine ○ Offer to call the patient's spouse and check in ○ Tell the patient the focus should be on their own health problems currently

3. The patient's x-ray is positive for a left hip fracture. Following surgery, patient-controlled analgesia (PCA) is implemented with a programmed on-demand dosage. Which of the following assessment data will the nurse gather? **Select all that apply.**
   1. Cognition
   2. Pain rating on a 0-to-10 scale
   3. Patency of IV catheter
   4. Review of electronic health record for history of obstructive sleep apnea
   5. Ability of family caregivers to initiate PCA dose

4. The patient asks the nurse, "Can I get addicted to morphine from this PCA pump?" Which nursing response is appropriate?
1. "Addiction is unlikely, as you will soon be switched to a nonopioid drug to manage pain."
2. "Since you have never had drug addiction problems, there is nothing to worry about."
3. "Try not to push the button too often to avoid becoming addicted."
4. "Why would you think you could become addicted from using morphine after surgery?"

5. Several days later, the patient is to be discharged to home. What medication teaching will the nurse provide prior to discharge?
1. Only take medication if pain is unbearable.
2. Take medication about 30 minutes before walking.
3. Double the amount of medication prescribed if pain is not controlled.
4. There are very few side effects associated with pain medication.

Visit the Evolve site for Answers to Clinical Judgment and Next-Generation NCLEX® Examination–Style Questions.

REFERENCES

ACE: Hot or Cold Therapy: What's Right for Your Injury? ACE 3M 2019. https://www.acebrand.com/3M/en_US/ace-brand/tips-how-to/full-story/?storyid=0b614a19-46f8-4e54-8c1f-920603862b6d.

Adeboye A, et al: Assessment of functional pain score by comparing to traditional pain scores, *Cureus* 13(8):e16847, 2021.

Acupuncture Massage College (AMC): *Swedish massage techniques*, 2022. https://www.amcollege.edu/blog/5-techniques-of-swedish-massage-amc-miami. Accessed August 30, 2023.

Agency for Healthcare Research and Quality (AHRQ): *Teach-back: intervention*, 2023. https://www.ahrq.gov/patient-safety/reports/engage/interventions/teach-back.html.

Aldington D, Eccleston C: Evidence-based pain management: building on the foundations of Cochrane systematic reviews, *Am J Public Health* 109(1):46–49, 2019.

American Nurses Association (ANA): *The ethical responsibility to manage pain and the suffering it causes*, 2018. https://www.nursingworld.org/~495e9b/globalassets/docs/ana/ethics/theethicalresponsibilitytomanagepainandthesufferingitcauses2018.pdf. Accessed August 30, 2023.

American Society of Anesthesiologists (ASA): *Guidelines for neuraxial analgesia or anesthesia in obstetrics, committee on obstetrics and anesthesia*, October 13, 2021, American Society of Anesthesiologists. https://www.asahq.org/standards-and-guidelines/guidelines/guidelines-for-neuraxial-anesthesia-in-obstetrics. Accessed August 30, 2023.

Atee M, et al: Pain assessment in dementia: evaluation of a point-of-care technological solution, *J Alzheimers Dis* 60(1):137–150, 2017.

Baker DW: History of The Joint Commission pain standards: lessons for today's prescription opioid epidemic, *JAMA* 317(11):1117–1118, 2017.

Baker S, et al: Musculoskeletal pain and co-morbid insomnia in adults: a population study of the prevalence and impact on restricted social participation, *BMC Fam Pract* 18(1):17, 2017.

Barney CC, et al: Challenges in pain assessment and management among individuals with intellectual and developmental disabilities, *Pain Rep* 5(4):e821, 2020. https://journals.lww.com/painrpts/Fulltext/2020/08000/Challenges_in_pain_assessment_and_management_among.1.aspx.

Belen BD, et al: *Pediatric epidural and spinal anesthesia and analgesia*, New York School of Regional Anesthesia (NYSORA): https://www.nysora.com/topics/sub-specialties/pediatric-anesthesia/pediatric-epidural-spinal-anesthesia-analgesia/. Accessed August 30, 2023.

Berardino K, et al: An update on postoperative opioid use and alternative pain control following spine surgery, *Orthop Rev (Pavia)* 13(2):24978, 2021.

Birnie K, et al: Recommendations for selection of self-report pain intensity measures in children and adolescents: a systematic review and quality assessment of measurement properties, *Pain* 160(1):5–18, 2019.

Boltz M, et al: *Evidence-based geriatric nursing protocols for best practice*, ed 6, New York, 2020, Springer.

Booker SQ, Haedtke C: Assessing pain in nonverbal older adults, *Nursing* 46(5):66–69, 2016. https://journals.lww.com/nursing/Fulltext/2016/05000/Assessing_pain_in_nonverbal_older_adults.19.aspx.

Botti M, et al: Cross-cultural examination of the structure of the revised American Pain Society Patient Outcome Questionnaire (APS-POQ-R), *J Pain* 16(8):727, 2015.

Bouzat P, et al: Chest trauma: first 48 hours management, *Anaesth Crit Care Pain Med* 36(2):135, 2017.

Brand K: Pain assessment in children, *Anaesth Intensive Care Med* 23(5):260–263, 2022.

Brant J, et al: Breakthrough cancer pain: a systematic review of pharmacologic management, *CJON* 21(3):71–80, 2017.

Brown A, et al: Do elderly patients use patient-controlled analgesia medication delivery systems correctly? *Orthop Nurs* 34(4):203–208, 2015.

Centers for Disease Control and Prevention (CDC): *CDC Guideline for prescribing opioids for chronic pain — United States, 2016.* https://www.cdc.gov/mmwr/volumes/65/rr/rr6501e1.htm?CDC_AA_refVal=https%3A%2F%2Fwww.cdc.gov%2Fmmwr%2Fvolumes%2F65%2Frr%2Frr6501e1er.htm. Accessed August 30, 2023.

Centers for Disease Control and Prevention (CDC): *CDC's clinical practice guideline for prescribing opioids for pain, 2022.* https://www.cdc.gov/opioids/healthcare-professionals/prescribing/guideline/index.html?s_cid=DOP_Clinician_Search_Paid_001&gclid=EAIaIQobChMIp_KU5NaEgQMV1QbnCh2twwD-CEAAYASAAEgJaA_D_BwE. Accessed August 30, 2023.

Centers for Disease Control and Prevention (CDC): *What is health literacy?* 2023a. https://www.cdc.gov/healthliteracy/learn/index.html.

Centers for Disease Control and Prevention (CDC): *Lifesaving naloxone*, 2023b, CDC. https://www.cdc.gov/stopoverdose/naloxone/index.html.

Chatterjee R: Elbow pain: the 10-minute assessment, *Co-Kinetic J* 73:18, 2017.

Chen W: Physical agent modalities. In Cifu DX, editor: *Braddom's rehabilitation care: a clinical handbook*, ed 6, 2021, Elsevier.

Chou R, Gordon DB, de Leon-Casasola OA, et al: Management of postoperative pain: a clinical practice guideline from the American Pain Society, the American Society of Regional Anesthesia and Pain Medicine, and the American Society of Anesthesiologists' Committee on Regional Anesthesia, Executive Committee, and Administrative Council, *J Pain* 17(2):131, 2016.

Codding J, Getz C: Pain management strategies in shoulder arthroplasty, *Orthop Clin North Am* 49:81, 2017.

Coluzzi F, et al: The challenge of perioperative pain management in opioid-tolerant patients, *Ther Clin Risk Manag* 13:1163, 2017.

Cooney MF: Postoperative pain management: clinical practice guidelines, *J Perianesth Nurs* 31(5):445, 2016.

Cooney M, Drew D: Pain assessment in cognitively intact adults. In *Assessment and multimodal management of pain: an integrative approach*, St. Louis, 2021, Elsevier, pp 73–119.

Cooney MF, Quinlan-Colwell A: Basic concepts involved with administration of analgesic medications. In Cooney MF, Quinlan-Colwell A, editors: *Assessment and multimodal management of pain: an integrative approach*, St. Louis, MO, 2020, Elsevier, pp 163–194.

Crockett S, et al: American Gastroenterological Association Institute guideline on the medical management of opioid-induced constipation, *AGA* 156(1):218-226, 2019.

Drew D, Peltier C: Pain assessment. In Czarnecki ML, Turner HN, editors: *Core curriculum for pain management nursing*, ed 3, St. Louis, MO, 2018, Elsevier, pp 67–82.

Elhage SA, et al: Preoperative patient opioid education, standardization of prescriptions, and their impact on overall patient satisfaction, *Surgery* 169(3):655–659, 2021. Accessed August 30, 2023.

Federation of State Medical Boards (FSMB): *Guidelines for the chronic use of opioid analgesics*, 2017. https://www.fsmb.org/siteassets/advocacy/policies/opioid_guidelines_as_adopted_april-2017_final.pdf. Accessed August 30, 2023.

Galicia-Castillo C, Weiner DK: *Treatment of persistent pain in older adults*, 2023, UpToDate. https://www.uptodate.com/contents/treatment-of-persistent-pain-in-older-adults. Accessed August 30, 2023.

Gallagher E, et al: Cancer-related pain assessment: monitoring the effectiveness of interventions, *Clin J Oncol Nurs* 21(3):8, 2017.

Garland EL, et al: Mind-body therapies for opioid-treated pain: a systematic review and meta-analysis, *JAMA Intern Med* 180(1):91–105, 2020.

Gélinas C: Pain assessment in the critically ill adult: recent evidence and new trends, *Intensive Crit Care Nurs* 34:1, 2016.

GeriatricPain.org: *Pain Assessment IN Advanced Dementia (PAINAD)*, University of Iowa, 2023. https://geriatricpain.org/painad. Accessed August 30, 2023.

Givler A, et al: *The importance of cultural competence in pain and palliative care*, 2023, National Center for BioTechnology Information (NCBI). https://www.ncbi.nlm.nih.gov/books/NBK493154/. Accessed August 30, 2023.

Goldberg SF, et al: Practical management of a regional anesthesia-driven acute pain service, *Adv Anesth* 35:191, 2017.

Gorski LA, et al: *Infusion therapy standards of practice*, ed 8, Norwood, MA, 2021, Infusion Nurses Society.

Hall KR, Stanley AY: Literature review: assessment of opioid-related sedation and the Pasero Opioid Sedation Scale, *J Perianesth Nurs* 34(1):132–142, 2019. https://pubmed.ncbi.nlm.nih.gov/29709268/. Accessed August 30, 2023.

Hatcher J: Manual therapy student handbook: assessment and treatment of the ankle and foot, *Co-Kinetic J* 71:34, 2017.

Hernandez AN, Singh P: Epidural Anesthesia, NIH- National Library of Medicine. In *Stat Pearls* [Internet], Last Update: March 9, 2022. https://www.ncbi.nlm.nih.gov/books/NBK542219/. Accessed August 30, 2023.

Herr K, et al: Pain assessment in the patient unable to self-report: Clinical practice recommendations in support of the ASPMN 2019 position statement, *Pain Manag Nurs* 20(5):404–417, 2019.

Hinther A, et al: *Efficacy of multimodal analgesia for postoperative pain management in head and neck cancer patients,* 2021, Semantic Scholar. https://www.semantic-scholar.org/paper/Efficacy-of-Multimodal-Analgesia-for-Postoperative-Hinther-Nakoneshny/67a0e661fe2270bc568eaebfa80cdeb23446b669.

Hirabayashi M, et al: Prophylactic pentazocine reduces the incidence of pruritus after cesarean delivery under spinal anesthesia with opioids: a prospective randomized clinical trial, *Anesth Analg* 124(6):1930, 2017.

Hockenberry MJ, et al: *Wong's essentials of pediatric nursing,* ed 11, St. Louis, 2022, Mosby.

Hoti K, et al: Clinimetric properties of the electronic Pain Assessment Tool (ePaT) for aged-care residents with moderate to severe dementia, *J Pain Res* 11:1037–1044, 2018.

Houzé B, et al: Efficacy, tolerability, and safety of non-pharmacological therapies for chronic pain: an umbrella review on various CAM approaches, *Prog Neuropsychopharmacol Biol Psychiatry* 79(Pt B):192, 2017.

Inoue S: Postoperative around-the-clock administration of intravenous acetaminophen for pain control following robot-assisted radical prostatectomy, *Sci Rep* 11:5174, 2021.

Institute for Chronic Pain (ICP): *Anxiety,* 2021. https://instituteforchronicpain.org/understanding-chronic-pain/complications/anxiety. Accessed November 16, 2023.

Institute for Safe Medication Practices (ISMP): *NRFit: A global "fit" for neuraxial medication safety,* 2021, https://www.ismp.org/resources/nrfit-global-fit-neuraxial-medication-safety. Accessed November 16, 2023.

Intermountain Primary Children's Hospital: *Let's talk about patient-controlled epidural analgesia (PCEA),* 2018. https://intermountainhealthcare.org/ckr-ext/Dcmnt?ncid=520408199. Accessed August 30, 2023.

International Association for the Study of Pain (IASP): *Pain assessment in dementia,* 2021. https://www.iasp-pain.org/resources/fact-sheets/pain-assessment-in-dementia/. Accessed August 30, 2023.

International Childrens' Palliative Care Network (ICPCN): *The ICPCN pain assessment app for children and young people,* 2022. https://icpcn.org/resources/icpcn-pain-app/. Accessed August 30, 2023.

Johns Hopkins Medicine: *Patient-controlled analgesia pumps,* 2023. https://www.hopkinsmedicine.org/health/treatment-tests-and-therapies/patientcontrolled-analgesia-pumps. Accessed August 30, 2023.

Jungquist CR, Quinlan-Colwell A: Preventing opioid-induced advancing sedation and respiratory depression. In Cooney MF, Quinlan-Colwell A, editors: *Assessment and multimodal management of pain: an integrative approach.* St. Louis, MO, 2020, Elsevier, pp 337–359.

Kampman K, Jarvis M: American Society of Addiction Medicine (ASAM) national practice guideline for the use of medications in the treatment of addiction involving opioid use, *J Addict Med* 5:358, 2015.

Kane-Gill SL, et al: Clinical practice guideline: safe medication use in the ICU, *Crit Care Med* 45(9):e877, 2017.

Karcioglu O, et al: A systematic review of the pain scales in adults: which to use? *Am J Emerg Med* 36(4):707–714, 2018.

Kawada T: Screening ability of STOP-Bang questionnaire for obstructive sleep apnea, *Anesth Analg* 128(3):e48, 2019.

Keane K: What is distraction therapy (for pain)? *Arthritis New South Wales,* 2021. https://www.arthritisnsw.org.au/what-is-distraction-therapy-for-pain/. Accessed August 30, 2023.

Kotfis K, et al: Methods of pain assessment in adult intensive care unit patients— Polish version of the CPOT (Critical Care Pain Observation Tool) and BPS (Behavioral Pain Scale), *Anaesthesiol Intensive Ther* 49(1):66–72, 2017.

Kunz M, Lautenbacher S: Assessing pain in patients with dementia, *Anaesthesist* 68(12):814–820, 2019. doi:10.1007/s00101-019-00683-8.

Kwak K: Need for an optimal regimen of programmed intermittent epidural bolus administration for maintenance of labor analgesia, *Korean J Anesthesiol* 72(5):407–408, 2019.

Lapum JL, et al: *The complete subjective health assessment: the PQRSTU assessment,* n.d. eCampus Ontario. https://ecampusontario.pressbooks.pub/healthassessment/chapter/the-pqrstu-assessment/. Accessed August 30, 2023.

Lee Su-Ha, et al: Effects of deep and slow breathing on stress stimulation caused by high-intensity exercise in healthy adults, *Psychol Health Med* 26(9):1079–1090, 2021

Li J, et al: The effects of music intervention on burn patients during treatment procedures: a systematic review and meta-analysis of randomized controlled trials, *BMC Complement Altern Med* 17(1):158, 2017.

Lourens GB: Complications associated with epidural catheter analgesia, *Nurse Pract* 41(10):12, 2016.

Matson KL, et al: Opioid use in children, *J Pediatr Pharmacol Ther* 24(1):72–75, 2019.

Mattox E: Complications of peripheral venous access devices: prevention, detection, and recovery strategies, *Crit Care Nurse* 37(2):e1, 2017.

Mayo Clinic: *Aspirin allergy: what are the symptoms?* 2022. https://www.mayoclinic.org/diseases-conditions/drug-allergy/expert-answers/aspirin-allergy/faq-20058225. Accessed August 30, 2023.

McGuire DB: Pain assessment in non-communicative adult palliative care patients, *Nurs Clin North Am* 51(3):397–431, 2016.

McKeown NK: *Withdrawal syndromes: treatment and management,* 2022, Medscape. https://emedicine.medscape.com/article/819502-treatment#d11. Accessed August 30, 2023.

Meghani SH, Vapiwala N: Bridging the critical divide in pain management guidelines from the CDC, NCCN, and ASCO for cancer survivors, *JAMA Oncol* 4(10):1323–1324, 2018. https://jamanetwork.com/journals/jamaoncology/article-abstract/2682591. Accessed August 30, 2023.

Meisenberg B, et al: Implementation of solutions to reduce opioid-induced oversedation and respiratory depression, *Am J Health Syst Pharm* 74(3):162, 2017.

Nagappa M, et al: Opioids, respiratory depression, and sleep-disordered breathing, *Best Pract Res Clin Anaesthesiol* 31(4):469, 2017.

Narayan MC: Strategies for implementing the national standards for culturally and linguistically appropriate services (CLAS) in home health care, *Home Health Care Manag Pract* 29(3):168, 2017.

National Center for Drug Abuse Statistics (NCDAS): *Opioid epidemic: addiction statistics,* 2022d, NCDAS. https://drugabusestatistics.org/opioid-epidemic/#:~:text=Prescription%20opioids%20are%20a%20factor%20in%2032%25%20of,prescriptions%20for%2046.7%25%20of%20Americans%20to%20receive%20one. Accessed August 30, 2023.

National Center for Complementary and Integrative Health (NCCIH): *Children and the use of complementary health approaches,* 2017, NIH. https://www.nccih.nih.gov/health/children-and-the-use-of-complementary-health-approaches. Accessed August 30, 2023.

National Center for Complementary and Integrative Health (NCCIH): *Complementary, alternative, or integrative health: what's in a name?* 2021, NIH. https://www.nccih.nih.gov/health/complementary-alternative-or-integrative-health-whats-in-a-name. Accessed August 30, 2023.

National Center for Complementary and Integrative Health (NCCIH): *NCCIH Clinical Digest for Health Professionals: Mind and body approaches for chronic pain: what the science says,* 2019a, NCCIH. https://www.nccih.nih.gov/health/providers/digest/mind-and-body-approaches-for-chronic-pain. Accessed August 30, 2023.

National Center for Complementary and Integrative Health (NCCIH): *Massage therapy: what you need to know,* 2019b, NCCIH. https://www.nccih.nih.gov/health/massage-therapy-what-you-need-to-know. Accessed August 30, 2023.

National Center for Complementary and Integrative Health NCCIH): *About NCCIH,* 2022a. https://www.nccih.nih.gov/about. Accessed August 30, 2023.

National Center for Complementary and Integrative Health (NCCIH): *NCCIH Clinical Digest: Mind and body practices for older adults,* 2022b. https://www.nccih.nih.gov/health/providers/digest/mind-and-body-practices-for-older-adults. Accessed August 30, 2023.

National Center for Integrative Health (NCCIH): *NCCIH clinical digest: ADHD and complementary health approaches,* 2023. https://nccih.nih.gov/health/providers/digest/adhd. Accessed August 30, 2023.

National Institute on Drug Abuse (NIDA): *Drug overdose death rates,* 2023. https://nida.nih.gov/research-topics/trends-statistics/overdose-death-rates. Accessed August, 30, 2023.

National Institutes of Health (NIH): How integrative health research tackles the pain management crisis, *NIH Medline Plus Magazine,* 2020. https://magazine.medlineplus.gov/article/how-integrative-health-research-tackles-the-pain-management-crisis. Accessed August 30, 2023.

National Institutes of Health (NIH), National Center for Complementary and Integrative Health (NCCIH): *Pain,* 2022. https://www.nccih.nih.gov/health/pain. Accessed August 30, 2023.

National Institutes of Health (NIH): *HEAL initiative research plan,* 2023. https://www.nih.gov/research-training/medical-research-initiatives/heal-initiative/heal-initiative-research-plan. Accessed August 30, 2023.

North Carolina Institute of Medicine (NCIOM): *Healthy North Carolina 2030: a path toward health,* 2020. https://nciom.org/wp-content/uploads/2020/01/HNC-REPORT-FINAL-Spread2.pdf. Accessed August 30, 2023.

Nyashanu M, et al: Exploring the efficacy of music in palliative care: a scoping review, *Palliat Support Care* 19(3):355–360, 2021.

O'Dwyer M, et al: Medication use and potentially inappropriate prescribing in older adults with intellectual disabilities: a neglected area of research, *Ther Adv Drug Saf* 9(9):535–557, 2018.

Olson E, et al: Surgical risk and the preoperative evaluation and management of adults with obstructive sleep apnea, *UpToDate,* 2022. https://www.uptodate.com/contents/surgical-risk-and-the-preoperative-evaluation-and-management-of-adults-with-obstructive-sleep-apnea. Accessed August 30, 2023.

Oncology Nursing Society (ONS): *Cancer Pain Management*, 2022, ONS. https://www.ons.org/make-difference/ons-center-advocacy-and-health-policy/position-statements/cancer-pain-management Accessed August 30, 2023.

Open Anesthesia: *Local anesthetics: systemic toxicity*, 2023. https://www.openanesthesia.org/keywords/local-anesthetic-systemic-toxicity/. Accessed August 30, 2023.

Oregon Ear, Nose, and Throat: *Patient education—using ice and cold packs*, 2023. http://oregon-ent.com/patient-education/hw-view.php?DOCHWID=sig43888spec. Accessed August 30, 2023.

Paladini G, et al: Continuous wound infiltration of local anesthetics in postoperative pain management: safety, efficacy and current perspectives, *Pain Res* 13: 285–294, 2020.

Palese A, et al: "I am administering medication-please do not interrupt me": Red tabards preventing interruptions as perceived by surgical patients, *J Patient Saf* 15(1):30, 2019.

Pasero C, McCaffery M: *Pain assessment and pharmacological management*, St. Louis, 2011, Mosby.

Pasero C, et al: American Society for Pain Management Nursing position statement: prescribing and administering opioid doses based solely on pain intensity, *Pain Manag Nurs* 17(3):170, 2016.

Pastino A, Lakra A: *Patient Controlled Analgesia, NIH, National Library of Medicine*, 2023. Stat Pearls. https://www.ncbi.nlm.nih.gov/books/NBK551610/. Accessed August 30, 2023.

Patricolo GE, et al: Beneficial effects of guided imagery or clinical massage on the status of patients in a progressive care unit, *Crit Care Nurse* 37(1):62, 2017.

Perciavalle V, et al: The role of deep breathing on stress, *Neurol Sci* 38:451, 2017.

Petrofsky JS, et al: Use of low level of continuous heat as an adjunct to physical therapy improves knee pain recovery and the compliance for home exercise in patients with chronic knee pain: a randomized controlled trial, *J Strength Cond Res* 30(11):3107, 2016.

Petrofsky J, et al: The efficacy of sustained heat treatment on delayed-onset muscle soreness, *Clin J Sport Med* 27(4):329, 2017a.

Petrofsky JS, et al: Use of low level of continuous heat and ibuprofen as an adjunct to physical therapy improves pain relief, range of motion and the compliance for home exercise in patients with nonspecific neck pain: a randomized controlled trial, *J Back Musculoskelet Rehab* 30(4):889, 2017b.

Portenoy RK: Current pharmacotherapy of chronic pain, *J Pain Symptom Management* 19(Suppl 1):S16–S20, 2000.

Quinlan P, et al: Effects of localized cold therapy on pain in postoperative spinal fusion patients: a randomized control trial, *Orthop Nurs* 36(5):344, 2017.

Quinlan-Colwell A: Importance of multimodal pain management. In Cooney MF, Quinlan-Colwell A, editors: *Assessment and multimodal management of pain: an integrative approach*, St. Louis, MO, 2020, Elsevier, pp 19–27.

Quinlan-Colwell A, et al: Prescribing and administering opioid doses based solely on pain intensity: update of a position statement by the American Society for Pain Management Nursing, *Pain Manag Nurs* 23(3):265–266, 2022. https://www.sciencedirect.com/science/article/pii/S152490422100240X. Accessed August 30, 2023.

Rababa M: The association of nurses' assessment and certainty to pain management and outcomes for nursing home residents in Jordan, *Geriatr Nurs* 39(1):66, 2017.

Rajan, J, Behrends M: Acute pain in older adults: recommendations for assessment and treatment, *Anesthesiology Clin* 37:507–520, 2019.

Ratliff CR: Descriptive study of the frequency of medical adhesive–related skin injuries in a vascular clinic, *J Vasc Nurs* 35(2):86, 2017.

Rawal N: Current issues in postoperative pain management, *Eur J Anaesthesiol* 33(3):160, 2016.

Rigby J, Dye S: Effectiveness of various cryotherapy systems at decreasing ankle skin temperatures and applying compression, *Int J Athl Ther Train* 22(6):32, 2017.

Rochon PA: *Drug prescribing for older adults*, 2023, UpToDate. https://www.uptodate.com/contents/drug-prescribing-for-older-adults?topicRef=16525&source=see_link. Accessed August 30, 2023.

Rosenquist R: *Use of opioids in the management of chronic non-cancer pain*, 2023, UpToDate. https://www.uptodate.com/contents/use-of-opioids-in-the-management-of-chronic-non-cancer-pain. Accessed August 30, 2023.

Sadule-Rios N, et al: Off to a good start: bedside report, *Medsurg Nurs* 26(5):343, 2017.

Sanchez MG, Perez ER: *NIH, National Library of Medicine*, 2022, Stat Pearls. https://www.ncbi.nlm.nih.gov/books/NBK554550/. Accessed August 30, 2023.

Scher C, et al: Moving beyond pain as the fifth vital sign and patient satisfaction scores to improve pain care in the 21st century, *Pain Manag Nurs* 19(2): 125–129, 2018.

Schofield P: The assessment of pain in older people: UK national guidelines, *Age Ageing* 47(Suppl 1):i1–i22, 2018.

Schofield P, Gibson S: *Pain in Older Adults: Pain and suffering often make the afflicted individual more vulnerable and this is especially true in the case of older adults*, 2021, International Association for the Study of Pain (IASP). https://www.iasp-pain.org/resources/fact-sheets/pain-in-older-adults/. Accessed August 30, 2023.

Shindul-Rothschild J, et al: Beyond the pain scale: provider communication and staffing predictive of patients' satisfaction with pain control, *Pain Manag Nurs* 18(6):401, 2017.

Sivevski AG, et al: Neuraxial anesthesia in the geriatric patient, *Front Med (Lausanne)* 5:254, 2018.

Sizar O, et al: *Opioid induced constipation, NIH, National Library of Medicine*, 2023, Stat Pearls. https://www.ncbi.nlm.nih.gov/books/NBK493184/. Accessed August 30, 2023.

Skelly AC, et al: *Noninvasive nonpharmacological treatment for chronic pain: a systematic review. Comparative Effectiveness Review No. 209. (Prepared by the Pacific Northwest Evidence-based Practice Center under Contract No. 290-2015-00009-1.) AHRQ Publication No 18-EHC013-EF*. Rockville, MD, June 2018, Agency for Healthcare Research and Quality.

Sng B, Sia A: Maintenance of epidural labour analgesia: the old, the new and the future, *Best Pract Res Clin Anaesthesiol* 31:15, 2017.

Sowicz T, et al: Pain management and substance use disorders, *Pain Manag Nurs* 23(6): 691-692, 2022.

St. Marie B, Broglio K: Managing pain in the setting of opioid disorder, *Pain Manag Nurs* 21:26–34, 2020.

Sturgeon JA, et al: Pain intensity as a lagging indicator of patient improvement: longitudinal relationships with sleep, psychiatric distress, and function in multidisciplinary care, *J Pain* 22(3):313, 2021.

Szekeres M, et al: The short-term effects of hot packs vs therapeutic whirlpool on active wrist range of motion for patients with distal radius fracture: a randomized controlled trial, *J Hand Ther* 31(3):276–281, 2018.

Tapp D, et al: Observational pain assessment instruments for use with nonverbal patients at the end-of-life: a systematic review, *J Palliat Care* 34(4):255–266, 2019.

The Joint Commission (TJC): New and revised standards related to pain assessment and management, January 1, 2018, *The Joint Commission Perspectives*, 37(7): 1-4, 2017. https://www.ashp.org/-/media/C230BF8CAC50442D87BF2DAA8998DAFA.ashx.

The Joint Commission (TJC): *Pain assessment and management standards for hospitals*, R3 Report, 2018. https://www.jointcommission.org/-/media/tjc/documents/standards/r3-reports/r3_report_issue_11_2_11_19_rev.pdf. Accessed August 30, 2023.

The Joint Commission (TJC): *What are the key concepts organizations need to understand regarding the pain management requirements in the Leadership (LD) and Provision of Care, Treatment, and Services (PC) chapters?* 2022. https://www.jointcommission.org/standards/standard-faqs/hospital-and-hospital-clinics/provision-of-care-treatment-and-services-pc/000002161/. Accessed August 30, 2023.

The Joint Commission (TJC): *2023 National patient safety goals*, Oakbrook Terrace, IL, 2023, The Joint Commission. https://www.jointcommission.org/standards/national-patient-safety-goals/.

The Royal College of Anaesthetists: *Best practice in the management of epidural analgesia in the hospital setting*, London, 2020, The Faculty of Pain Medicine of the Royal College of Anaesthetist. https://www.fpm.ac.uk/sites/fpm/files/documents/2020-09/Epidural-AUG-2020-FINAL.pdf.

Touhy T, Jett K: *Toward healthy aging*, ed 11, St. Louis, 2023, Mosby.

University of California, San Francisco (UCSF): *Epidural anesthesia: mechanism of action and indications*, 2022, UCSF. https://pain.ucsf.edu/neuraxial-anesthesia/epidural-anesthesia-mechanism-action-and-indications. Accessed August 30, 2023.

U.S. Department of Health and Human Services (USDHHS): *Opioid facts and statistics*, 2022. https://www.hhs.gov/opioids/statistics/index.html. Accessed August 30, 2023.

U.S. Department of Labor: *Risk factors for opioid misuse, addiction, and overdose*, n.d. Office of Workers Compensation Programs, Department of Labor. https://www.dol.gov/agencies/owcp/opioids/riskfactors.

U.S. Food and Drug Administration (FDA): *FDA approves higher dosage of naloxone nasal spray to treat opioid overdose*, 2021, US Food and Drug administration. https://www.fda.gov/news-events/press-announcements/fda-approves-higher-dosage-naloxone-nasal-spray-treat-opioid-overdose. Accessed August 30, 2023.

Varndell W, et al: A systematic review of observational pain assessment instruments for use with nonverbal intubated critically ill adult patients in the emergency department: an assessment of their suitability and psychometric properties, *J Clin Nurs* 26(1–2):7, 2017.

Wadlund D: Local anesthetic systemic toxicity, *AORN J* 106(5):367, 2017.

Wang Zi-Rue, Ni Guo-Xin: Is it time to put traditional cold therapy in rehabilitation of soft-tissue injuries out to pasture? *World J Clin Cases* 9(17):4116–4122, 2021.

Wojnar-Gruszka K, et al: Pain assessment with the BPS and CCPOT behavioral pain scales in mechanically ventilated patients requiring analgesia and sedation. *Int J Environ Res Public Health* 19(17):10894, 2022.

World Health Organization (WHO): *WHO guidelines for the pharmacological and radiotherapeutic management of cancer pain in adults and adolescents*, Geneva, 2018, World Health Organization. Licence: CC BY-NC-SA 3.0 IGO.

World Health Organization (WHO): *WHO revision of pain management guidelines*, 2019. https://www.who.int/news/item/27-08-2019-who-revision-of-pain-management-guidelines. Accessed August 30, 2023.

Wu Y, et al: Characterizing human skin blood flow regulation in response to different local skin temperature perturbations, *Microvasc Red* 111:96, 2017.

Yan Y, et al: The effect of opioids on gastrointestinal function in the ICU, *Crit Care* 25:370, 2021.

Yoon SC, Bruner HC: Naloxegol in opioid-induced constipation: a new paradigm in the treatment of a common problem, *Patient Prefer Adherence* 11:1265, 2017.

Yoshikawa A, et al: Opioid use and the risk of falls, fall injuries and fractures among older adults: a systematic review and meta-analysis, *J Gerontol A Biol Sci Med Sci* 75(10):1989–1995, 2020.

Zhang Y, et al: Local anesthetic infusion pump for pain management following total knee arthroplasty: a meta-analysis, *BMC Musculoskelet Disord* 18:32, 2017.

Zhu J, Weingart S: Prevention of adverse drug events in hospitals, *UpToDate*, 2022. https://www.uptodate.com/contents/prevention-of-adverse-drug-events-in-hospitals. Accessed August 30, 2023.

17 | End-of-Life Care

SKILLS AND PROCEDURES

Skill 17.1 **Supporting Patients and Families in Grief, p. 500**

Skill 17.2 **Symptom Management at the End of Life, p. 504**

Skill 17.3 **Care of the Body After Death, p. 510**

OBJECTIVES

Mastery of content in this chapter will enable you to:
- Discuss principles of palliative care.
- Explain hospice care.
- Examine approaches to physical symptom management at the end of life.
- Examine approaches to spiritual symptom management at the end of life.

- Explain physiological changes in impending death.
- Explain a nurse's role in assisting patients and families in grief and at the end of life.
- Discuss the process of postmortem care.
- Discuss a nurse's role in facilitating autopsy and organ and tissue donation requests.

MEDIA RESOURCES

- http://evolve.elsevier.com/Perry/skills
- Review Questions
- Audio Glossary
- Case Studies

- Answers to Clinical Judgment and Next-Generation NCLEX® Examination-Style Questions
- Skills Performance Checklists
- Printable Key Points

PURPOSE

Nurses have historically played a vital role in the care of patients and family caregivers facing serious, life-limiting illness and death. The World Health Organization (2020) defines palliative care as an approach that "improves the quality of life of patients and their families facing the problems associated with life-threatening illness, through the prevention and relief of suffering by means of early identification and impeccable assessment and treatment of pain and other problems, physical, psychosocial and spiritual." Palliative care may be provided in any setting by any clinician caring for the seriously ill (National Consensus Project for Quality Palliative Care [NCP], 2018). The goals of palliative care (Box 17.1) include comprehensive management of pain and other symptoms and psychosocial and spiritual support provided by an interprofessional team composed of physicians, nurses, therapists, social workers, chaplains, and dietitians (National Consensus Project for Quality Palliative Care [NCP], 2018). To be successful, it is important to provide a caring presence and apply therapeutic communication principles (Fig. 17.1).

At the end of life, palliative care may transition to hospice care. Hospice, an interprofessional, patient- and family-centered program of care, helps people live as well as possible through the dying process. Patients are eligible for hospice care as a Medicare or Medicaid benefit during the final phase of a terminal illness, usually the last 6 months of life. Because hospice is a philosophy of care, the services can be provided at home; in freestanding hospice agencies; or in nursing home, extended care, or acute care settings.

At the time of death, nurses provide compassionate patient-centered care to patients and family caregivers by offering information, guidance, and support and facilitating communication. In addition, nurses provide postmortem care (e.g., care of the body after death) in a dignified manner, consistent with a patient's religious and cultural beliefs.

PRACTICE STANDARDS

- National Consensus Project for Quality Palliative Care (NCP), 2018: *Clinical Practice Guidelines for Quality Palliative Care—*Palliative care principles and practice
- The Joint Commission (TJC), 2023: National Patient Safety Goals—Patient identification
- World Health Organization (WHO), 2020: Palliative Care—Principles of palliative care.

PRINCIPLES FOR PRACTICE

- Expert palliative care involves helping patients reach peaceful deaths at the end of life (HFA, 2022a).
- An interprofessional team collaboratively discusses and documents patient status, patient and family needs, treatment options, and symptom management (NCP, 2018).
- Coordination of palliative care is an important element of care, especially when patients receive community-based palliative care (NCP, 2018).
- Providing palliative care requires holistic assessment of a patient, management of physical signs and symptoms, and

BOX 17.1

Goals of Palliative Care

- Improve the quality of life of patients (adults and children) and family caregivers who are facing problems associated with life-threatening illness.
- Prevent and relieve suffering through the early identification, correct assessment, and treatment of pain and other physical, psychosocial, or spiritual problems.
- Affirm life and regard dying as a normal process; can reduce unnecessary hospitalizations.
- Aim to neither hasten nor postpone death.
- Address pain and difficulty in breathing—two of the most frequent and serious symptoms experienced by patients in need of palliative care.
- Offer a support system to help patients live as actively as possible until death.
- Offer a support system to help the family cope during the patient's illness and in bereavement.
- Enhance quality of life and positively influence the course of illness.

Adapted from World Health Organization (WHO): *Palliative care,* 2020. https://www.who.int/news-room/fact-sheets/detail/palliative-care/. Accessed October 7, 2023.

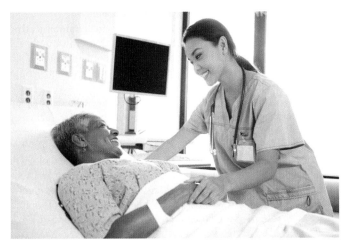

FIG. 17.1 Nurses use their presence and therapeutic communication to assess how symptoms affect a patient's life. *(From iStock.com/monkeybusinessimages.)*

provision of psychosocial and spiritual support to patients and their family caregivers (Touhy & Jett, 2022).

- Symptoms are experienced by a patient and can be reported only by the patient. Signs that may accompany a patient's symptoms are observed by the nurse.
- Management of physical symptoms at the end of life can decrease psychosocial distress, thus improving overall quality of life (American Cancer Society [ACS], 2019b).
- To receive hospice care at home, a family caregiver must be available and willing to provide care when a patient is no longer able to function alone. Hospice team members offer 24-hour accessibility and coordinate care between the home and inpatient settings.
- As the time of a patient's death approaches, the hospice team provides intensive support to the patient and family caregivers. Hospice benefits include respite for family caregivers, limited hospitalization for acute symptom management, and bereavement

care after death. The Hospice Foundation of America (2022a) offers numerous resources.

- To nurture your capacity to remain empathically engaged with patients and family caregivers, you must also care for yourself physically, spiritually, and emotionally.
- Recognize your own attitudes, feelings, values, and expectations about death and the individual, cultural, and spiritual diversity existing in these beliefs and customs.

PERSON-CENTERED CARE

- A patient-centered approach to palliative and end-of-life care engages a patient and family caregivers with an interprofessional team that provides education and supports the patient and family caregivers, helping them to be informed and make autonomous decisions regarding the patient's treatment (or discontinuation of treatment) (NCP, 2018).
- Listen carefully to understand the significance of a loss to a patient or family caregiver, identify concerns, and assess the patient's ability to sustain hope and move forward in life (NCP, 2018).
- Talk with patients about their perception of time. Conversations regarding experience of time may help to find daily activities best fitting the patient's wishes, aiming at making the most of their remaining time (Rovers et al., 2019).
- Patients are encouraged to set realistic goals and help identify ways to achieve them so that they can maintain their usual routines and a sense of normalcy.
- When patients with advanced illness are no longer able to participate in making decisions, they can communicate their values and preferences in an advance directive. Advance directives are legal documents that explain how patients want their medical decisions to be made if they cannot make the decisions themselves (ACS, 2019c).
- An advance directive lets the health care team and family caregivers know what kind of health care patients want or who patients want to make decisions when they cannot. An advance directive also helps patients think ahead of time about the kind of care they want (ACS, 2019c).
- If a patient has an advance directive, place a copy in the electronic health record (EHR) and instruct the patient to give copies to their health care provider and family caregivers (see agency policy). Know that some states have specific forms that must be used (ACS, 2019c).
- Cardiopulmonary resuscitation (CPR) (see Chapter 27) is used in cases of cardiac and/or pulmonary arrest. Adults in consultation with the health care team may consent to a "do not resuscitate" (DNR) status verbally or in writing. Assure patients who choose not to be resuscitated that they will continue to receive full palliative care and symptom relief.
- Communication impacts family caregivers' experience during and after inpatient care, including after death. Involvement of family caregivers in decision making can be limited during times of crisis (e.g., COVID-19 pandemic); family caregivers may have limited access to a patient and may not be able to have face-to-face conversations regarding patient preferences for end-of-life care (Robert et al., 2020).
- Use strategies to reinforce communication including facilitating written, audio, and video messages between the patient and family caregivers; flexible visitation during end-of-life care; and providing end-of-life family caregiver meetings, in person or virtual (Robert et al., 2020).

EVIDENCE-BASED PRACTICE

Caregiver Needs

- Caregiver burden has been defined as the level of multifaceted strain perceived by the caregiver from caring for a family member and/or loved one over time (Liu et al., 2020). This burden can strain their physical, psychological, and spiritual health and also strain relationships; support needs vary greatly, and there is no "one size fits all" (Bijnsdorp et al., 2020). The caregiver may not recognize the impact this strain is having on them, and they may not realize there are resources to help them and their loved one. It is essential that nurses understand the needs of caregivers so that they can provide strategies and resources to assist caregivers to hopefully prevent or minimize strain and burden.
- Some caregivers report positive experiences but find it difficult to set boundaries. Caregivers may begin to feel like an extension of the person receiving care and feel undervalued. Caregivers need someone to listen and talk with while debating and making tough decisions, setting boundaries, and getting advice when needed (Bijnsdorp et al., 2020).
- Having supportive relationships from other family members allows for sharing tasks and responsibilities. Those in nonsupportive relationships often feel that health care providers do not provide enough time, sufficiently answer questions, or honor wishes. All caregiver relationships need to be assessed to ensure proper support during the day and night (Bijnsdorp et al., 2020).
- Caregivers need a sense of security in the care situation: they want to be better prepared for what to expect in the future in order to respond better to situations. Caregivers also need some time away from the caring situation (e.g., respite options of daycare or involving volunteers) to avoid the effects of strain and assistance in looking at alternative support options (e.g., courses, peer support or support groups) (Bijnsdorp et al., 2020).
- Insufficient financial resources, multiple responsibility conflict, and lack of social activities can lead to caregiver burden. Higher levels of support have been found to lessen burden; family, community, and social support are important sources of support for caregivers. Organizations that offer emotional support and counseling and community day care centers can help ease the caregiver's burden by allowing the caregiver to take adequate rest (Liu et al., 2020).
- The Family Caregivers Alliance recommends (1) an assessment of family caregiver needs that leads to a care plan with support services; (2) caregiver education and support programs; (3) respite to reduce caregiver burden; (4) financial support to alleviate the economic stress of caregiving; and (5) primary care interventions that address caregiver needs. Look for local services that are low cost or free and assist caregivers in applying for programs (Blater, 2020).

SAFETY GUIDELINES

- Patients who are seriously ill experience decreased muscle strength and limited endurance. However, patients may prefer to get out of bed for meals or to walk to the bathroom as long as possible. Have patients sit for a minute before getting out of bed. Guard against falls by having patients use appropriate assistive devices for walking. Remain until patients are safely seated or lying down (see Chapter 12).
- Place a patient who wants to eat or drink in an upright position and offer small bites of food or sips of water slowly to avoid aspiration (see Chapter 30). Be sure that the nurse call system is in an accessible location within the patient's reach at all times and consider calls as a high priority.
- Proper patient identification, especially in communicating a patient's DNR or CPR status, ensures that unwanted and unhelpful medical interventions are not implemented (TJC, 2023a). Know the methods of your agency for designating a patient's resuscitation status.
- Patients approaching end of life are more prone to diminished skin perfusion, limited mobility, incontinence, and decreased nutrition; all of these can contribute to the development of pressure injuries (see Chapter 39) (HFA, 2022b; Samuriwo, 2019).
- Nonpharmacological therapy and nonopioid pharmacological therapy are preferred for chronic pain. Before starting and routinely during opioid therapy, discuss with patients and family caregivers the known risks and realistic benefits of opioid therapy (Centers for Disease Control and Prevention [CDC], 2022).

◆ SKILL 17.1   Supporting Patients and Families in Grief

Grief experiences in situations of serious illness and at the end of life have profound physical, psychological, social, and spiritual effects on dying people, family members, friends, and family caregivers. The grief associated with serious illness or death may arise from fear of the unknown, pain, sadness about leaving loved ones behind, loss of control, or unresolved guilt.

Hospitalization, chronic illness, and disability involve multiple losses. Hospitalized patients lose privacy and control over normal routines. With chronic illness, a person's body no longer functions as it once did, leading to a loss of self-esteem and social roles. Disability and threat of end of life creates financial insecurity and often threatens interpersonal relationships. Death separates people from the physical presence of a person in their lives.

Grief

Grief is a natural and normal response to loss; it is universal but also a personal reaction (HFA, 2022a). Grief is based on personal experiences, psychological makeup, cultural expectations, and family and spiritual beliefs. Losses at the end of life may be financial, physical, emotional, social, or spiritual. Examples of these losses include role changes, altered self-image, loss of income, or emotional distress. The depth and duration of grief (e.g., one's inner emotional response to loss) depend on the type of loss and the person's perception of it. Coping with grief involves a period of mourning (e.g., the outward, social expressions of grief and the behavior associated with loss). Mourning behaviors and rituals help grieving individuals adapt to loss, receive social support, adjust expectations, and go forward in life. Most mourning rituals are culturally influenced, learned behaviors. Bereavement includes grief and mourning (e.g., the inner emotional responses and outward behaviors in response to loss).

Help patients by understanding types of grief. Normal or uncomplicated grief is evidenced by feelings, behaviors, and reactions associated with loss such as sadness, anger, crying, resentment, and loneliness. Families may feel the presence of and yearn for the lost person. It may be difficult to resume life as it was before the loss. An uncomplicated grief experience often helps a person mature and develop life perspective. Anticipatory grief occurs before an actual loss or death and involves gradual disengagement from what is being lost. For example, if a dying process is lengthy, the patient and family caregiver prepare for death before it occurs and sometimes, but not always, display fewer common grief responses at the time of death. Complicated grief (symptoms lasting 6 months or longer) occurs when a person experiences significant distress related to the loss. Criteria for a person experiencing complicated grief may include an inability to accept the death of the loved one; emotional numbness, bitterness, or anger; excessive avoidance of loss reminders; difficulty trusting others; and expressing the feeling that life is meaningless (Parisi et al., 2019).

People do not experience grief in the same way. Some people do not report feeling distressed or depressed, and others feel distressed for a lifetime without negative consequences. Not all people want to process the emotional experience of grief and focus instead on resilience, growth, or positive outcomes after a loss.

Use basic knowledge of grief responses to support patients and family caregivers and to address other common psychosocial and spiritual symptoms at the end of life. Patients and family caregivers may talk openly about a patient's approaching death, and others choose not to acknowledge it. Health care providers, depending on personal and cultural understandings of grief and death, often avoid initiating conversations on these difficult topics. Provide opportunities for discussion, paying close attention to a patient's response and indications of a desire to talk further. Educating a patient and family caregiver about what to expect during the final days or hours can alleviate anxiety and promote a more positive death experience for all involved (NCP, 2018).

Delegation

The skills of assessing patients' or family caregivers' grief reactions and designing appropriate interventions cannot be delegated to assistive personnel (AP). Direct the AP to:

- Inform the nurse when a patient or family caregiver exhibits behavior commonly associated with grief (e.g., crying, anger, withdrawal)
- Form supportive relationships with patients and family caregivers and inform the nurse when patients or family caregivers have questions or concerns
- Alert the nurse to the arrival of family caregivers so that the nurse can discuss the plan of care and offer support

Interprofessional Collaboration

- The interprofessional palliative care team, consisting of health care providers, social workers, religious support, and bereavement specialists, support the patient and family caregivers.
- The interprofessional team provides family caregivers a list of resources for postloss support and grief support (e.g., Substance Abuse and Mental Health Services Administration [SAMHSA]; local community hospice and palliative care organizations and grief counselors; the American Cancer Society [ACS]).

STEP	RATIONALE

ASSESSMENT

1. Identify patient using at least two identifiers (e.g., name and birthday or name and medical record number) according to agency policy.

Ensures correct patient. Complies with The Joint Commission standards and improves patient safety (TJC, 2023a).

2. Sit near patient in a quiet, private location. Center yourself and establish a quiet presence. Establish eye contact. Be aware that use of eye contact in some cultures conveys disrespect or discomfort.

Presence expresses caring and creates healing moments (Steele, 2023). Privacy protects confidentiality and promotes a sense of safety for a patient when expressing thoughts and emotions.

3. Consider the influence of patient's cultural background on communication. Apply principles of plain language and health literacy during assessment (NCP, 2018).

Individual differences influence patient's grief response and communication style.

4. Assess patient's/family caregiver's health literacy.

Determines degree to which individuals have the ability to find, understand, and use information and services to make informed health-related decisions and actions for themselves and others (CDC, 2023).

5. Listen carefully to patient's story. Observe patient responses. Use open communication. Encourage questions.

Develops trust in a caring relationship. Actively listening to patient's concerns and verbalizing patient's needs conveys empathy and compassion (Steele, 2023).

6. Determine meaning of the loss to patient: its type, suddenness, and when it occurred. Use open-ended questions such as:
   - "Tell me how your loss affects your family."
   - "You said your illness was unexpected. Describe how that made you feel."

The type, meaning, suddenness, and time elapsed since the loss influence the grief experience and coping methods.

7. Combine knowledge of grief theory with observation of patient behaviors. Validate observations by sharing them with patient; paraphrase, clarify, or summarize, as in the following examples:
   - "You've mentioned several times that you feel hopeless."
   - "It seems that this is hard for you to talk about."
   - "You look sad. Is there something in particular that brought on your tears?"

Use information about type and stage of grief to guide discussion, not to judge patient's responses (Steele, 2023). Confirms accuracy of your observations and validates patient's feelings. Prompts patient to continue.

STEP	RATIONALE
8. Encourage patient to describe the loss and its impact on daily life (e.g., "You said your diagnosis changed your life forever. Tell me more.").	Listening to patient's description helps to minimize assumptions.
9. Ask patient to describe the coping strategies used most often in difficult times (e.g., "What or who helps you when you are having a difficult time or difficulty coping?").	Familiar, effective coping strategies are often helpful in the current crisis, loss, or grief experience.
10. Assess family caregivers' unique needs and resources. Note if patient receives care at home and who gives the care.	Illness significantly affects family relationships. Family caregivers need support and guidance to aid in processing emotions and any fears related to end-of-life care (HFA, 2022a).
11. Assess patient's spiritual needs, beliefs, and resources. Focus on needs such as trust, life purpose, faith/belief, and hope.	Identifies patient's spiritual beliefs and values. Enables patient autonomy by identifying beliefs and preferences for care or rituals related to faith and/or spirituality. Offers a greater understanding of patient's culture and values, leading to patient-centered care.

PLANNING

1. Expected outcomes following completion of procedures:	
• Patient maintains relationships with significant people.	Patient in grief or loss benefits from connections with social network.
• Patient expresses grief in keeping with cultural and religious practices.	Patient receives support necessary to retain cherished values and ways of being.
• Patient uses effective coping strategies.	Use of strategies will be reflected in patient's ability to identify sense of relief.
• Patient maintains normal life routines.	Patient adjusts to life-changing circumstances and maintains sense of control.
2. Close room door and bedside curtain.	Provides patient privacy.

IMPLEMENTATION

1. Show an empathetic understanding of patient's strengths and needs.	Promotes nurse-patient trust, caring, compassion, and empathy.
2. Offer information about patient's illness and treatment. Clarify misunderstandings or misinformation. Use culturally appropriate language, simple terms, and appropriate instructional material.	Misunderstanding adds to patient's uncertainty, anxiety, and suffering (Steele, 2023).
3. Encourage patient to sustain relationships with others to help maintain independence and receive necessary help. Include patient-identified family caregivers and support people in discussions.	Affiliation with others offers support and helps patient stay engaged in life.
4. Help patient achieve short-term goals (e.g., symptom relief, task completion, resolution of relational problems).	Helping patients identify and meet personal goals contributes to their quality of life.
5. Provide frequent opportunities for patient and family caregivers to express fears and concerns. Be attentive to expressions of intense emotions.	Emotions change quickly and frequently during stress and complicate communication for nurses and patients (Steele, 2023).
6. Educate and support patient and family caregivers. Discuss procedures, plan of care, and anticipated changes. Use interprofessional team to support patient's needs and preferences.	Provides emotional support and comfort, decreases anxiety, and allows patient to rest. Advocating for patient encourages patient autonomy and incorporates patient preferences into plan of care.
7. Instruct patient in relaxation strategies: mindfulness-based stress reduction, guided imagery, meditation, hand massage, healing touch (see Chapter 16).	Complementary therapies have been shown in select cases to relieve anxiety and effectively reduce stress, thus providing useful coping strategies (National Center for Complementary and Integrative Health [NCCIH], 2022).
8. Encourage visits with loved ones, life review with stories or photographs, or projects such as organizing photo albums or journal writing.	Reviewing positive and negative events in one's life allows a person to find meaning in experiences, resolve conflicts, and come to a place of acceptance.
9. Facilitate patient's religious/spiritual practices and connections with religious community. Use prayer or music and provide a listening presence. Make a referral to a spiritual care provider if appropriate.	Spiritual interventions help patients maintain hope and connect with core identity. Spiritual interventions can decrease anxiety, promote a sense of peace, and help patient find meaning in life (O'Brien et al., 2019).
10. At end of discussion, help patient to comfortable position.	Promotes patient comfort and safety.

STEP	RATIONALE
11. Place nurse call system in an accessible location within patient's reach.	Ensures patient can call for assistance if needed.
12. Raise side rails (as appropriate) and lower bed to lowest position, locking into position.	Ensures patient safety and prevents falls.

EVALUATION

1. Note patient descriptions of relationships and activities with others.	Provides information on extent to which patient retains relational ties.
2. Observe patient's behaviors during ongoing interactions.	Demonstrates patient's ability to express grief and coping.
3. Elicit patient perceptions of benefit or outcomes gained from use of coping interventions.	Evaluates efficacy of interventions.
4. Discuss progress toward performing routine activities at home.	Evaluates patient's achievement of desired goals or need for goal revision.
5. **Use Teach-Back:** "I want to be sure I explained clearly how to perform guided imagery. In your own words, tell me ways you can use this technique." Revise your instruction now or develop plan for revised patient/family caregiver teaching if patient/family caregiver is not able to teach back correctly.	Teach-back is a technique for health care providers to ensure that they have explained medical information clearly so that patients and their families understand what is communicated to them (Agency for Healthcare Research and Quality [AHRQ], 2023).

Unexpected Outcomes

1. Patient does not acknowledge loss and shows signs of extreme sorrow, anger, withdrawal, or denial.
2. Family caregiver and patient relationships do not give patient needed support.

Related Interventions

- Consider referral to grief specialist professional (e.g., nurse practitioner, psychologist, spiritual care provider).
- Share and validate observations of family caregiver strain or patient concern over interactions.
- Consider family caregiver-patient discussion with health care team.

Documentation

- Document interventions used to support patient coping and note patient's verbal and nonverbal responses.

Hand-Off Reporting

- Report patient's grief reactions to members of the interprofessional team, noting behaviors that affect health outcomes such as treatment refusals or prolonged inactivity.

Special Considerations

Patient Education

- Give family caregivers basic information about common grief responses and how to offer support. Coach caregivers on ways to provide physical, emotional, and spiritual support to patient and one another (e.g., providing basic hygiene, listening attentively, avoiding false reassurances, allowing for the expression of difficult emotions, reminiscing and talking about normal family activities).

Maternal-Child Health

- Because of the lack of understanding, miscarriage has been called "the silent loss," often unrecognized by others. Guilt is a normal grief reaction. Encourage the family to gather together to share expressions of loss. Self-help groups and private therapists can assist in dealing with grief; patients often blame themselves for the miscarriage and need to be able to share feelings with those who will truly listen (HFA, 2022c).

Pediatrics

- Children's understanding of death, influenced by age and developmental level, differs from that of adults. Respect parents' wishes about when and what to tell children about illness or death. When discussing sensitive topics with children, encourage parents to offer caring explanations at a level a child is able to understand.
- Play therapy or drawing helps children express thoughts, emotions, or fears about illness or death.
- Be alert to all family members' grief reactions because there may be feelings of guilt, resentment, or helplessness with the illness or death of a sibling, child, or grandchild. Facilitate communication with family members who must be separated from the child.
- Surrogate decision makers, usually the parents, need to make health care decisions for infants and young children. Some decisions are difficult because outcomes in children are often unpredictable.
- Parents value obtaining adequate information and communication, being physically present with their child, and children receiving adequate pain management, social support, and empathy from health care providers at end of life (Hockenberry et al., 2022).

Older Adults

- Losing a partner after a long and satisfying relationship is difficult and essentially a loss of self. The mourning is as much for oneself as for the individual (Touhy & Jett, 2022).
- Intense grief may cause a temporary decrease in cognitive function that can manifest as confusion (Touhy & Jett, 2022).
- Many older adults have coexisting medical conditions that add to the symptom burden. These people have also lived long enough to have experienced cumulative losses, including

family and support group members, which complicates the grief experience.

Populations With Disabilities

- When working with patients with cognitive and/or communication impairment or incapacity, the interprofessional team identifies the availability and willingness of a surrogate decision-maker and supports that individual with education related to signs and symptoms of psychological and psychiatric distress, as well as techniques to help alleviate distress (NCP, 2018).

Home Care

- Follow up with the grieving family caregivers a few weeks after the death to offer support and check in to see if any other services are needed.

✦ SKILL 17.2   Symptom Management at the End of Life

High-quality palliative care offers vigilant symptom management while avoiding futile treatment. To promote ethical practice environments, the American Nurses Association (ANA) states that nurses must learn about end-of-life treatment policies, including those that minimize unwarranted, unwanted, or unnecessary medical treatment (ANA, 2021). It is crucial to have an interprofessional team approach to symptom assessment and treatment as pain and symptom management are complicated processes (NCP, 2018) (see Chapter 16).

Patients living with life-limiting illness experience multiple, complex physical, emotional, and spiritual symptoms. Relief of symptoms is balanced with the possible side effects of medication (HFA, 2022b). Managing patients' symptoms at the end of life begins by understanding the impact that these symptoms have on patients' and their family caregiver's lives from their shared and individual point of view (Fig. 17.2). Ethnicity and culture are strongly related to attitudes toward life-sustaining treatments during terminal illness and the use of hospice services. Consider these factors when you assess all symptoms and concerns thoroughly because a patient's fear of not being heard or believed compounds the magnitude of symptoms. Patients identify pain as the most common and severe symptom (see Chapter 16). In addition to the psychological and spiritual interventions discussed in Skill 17.1, nurses manage physiological symptoms at the end of life.

Delegation

Supportive care for symptom management can be delegated to assistive personnel (AP). However, the nurse must conduct the initial assessments of symptoms and determination of therapies. Direct the AP to:

- Notify the nurse if patient reports new symptoms or if existing symptoms worsen or change
- Provide basic comfort care such as positioning, room temperature control, hygiene, and mouth care
- Report possible adverse effects of drug therapy as instructed by the nurse

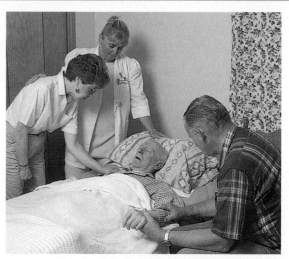

FIG. 17.2 A patient-centered approach involves family and patients as partners in care. (*From Williams PA:* deWit's fundamental concepts and skills for nursing, *ed 5, St. Louis, 2018, Elsevier.*)

- Speak to unconscious or dying patients because hearing is the last sense to diminish

Interprofessional Collaboration

- Symptom management at end-of-life requires an interprofessional approach as nurses work with health care providers and seek complementary strategies to enhance a patient's comfort.

Equipment

- Personal care items most preferred by patient
- Comfort and hygiene products
- Stethoscope
- Clean gloves

STEP	RATIONALE

ASSESSMENT

1. Identify patient using at least two identifiers (e.g., name and birthday or name and medical record number) according to agency policy.	Ensures patient safety. Complies with The Joint Commission standards and improves patient safety (TJC, 2023a).
2. Assess patient's and family caregiver's health literacy, level of understanding, and experience with symptoms.	Determines degree to which individuals have the ability to find, understand, and use information and services to make informed health-related decisions and actions for themselves and others (CDC, 2023).

STEP	RATIONALE
3. Ask patients to describe symptoms in their own words. Use open-ended prompts such as "Describe your leg pain to me" or "Tell me about how you are sleeping since you started taking this medicine."	Symptoms are personal perceptions and experienced only by the patient.
4. Allow sufficient time for patients to describe symptoms and encourage saying more: • "Is there anything else bothering you?" • "You've told me about your _____ pain. Do you have pain anywhere else?"	Ensures a more complete assessment. Prevents making assumptions about patient's symptoms, prematurely stopping the assessment process.
5. Assess patient's emotional health. Does the patient feel anxious, sad, depressed, bored, or understimulated? Use standardized tool to assess anxiety if available (Steele, 2023).	Emotional conditions have potential to worsen fatigue in patients with cancer (ACS, 2019a).
6. Assess character of patient's pain and rate severity on a pain scale of 0 to 10 (see Chapter 16). If patient cannot self-report pain, observe for these symptoms (ACS, 2019a; HFA, 2022b):	Pain "screening" is a process for assessing/evaluating the possible presence of pain, whereas an "assessment" gathers more detailed information through collection of data, observation, and physical examination (TJC, 2023b). Consistent use of a standard pain scale helps assess changes in patient pain severity and evaluates effectiveness of pain interventions. Using a pain scale is recommended by the American Cancer Society (ACS, 2019b) for describing patients' responses to pain-relief measures. Pain scales such as the Pain Assessment in Advanced Dementia (PAIAD) can be used for patients with dementia. Patients unable to report or verbalize pain show nonverbal signs of pain.
• Noisy breathing—labored, harsh, or rapid breaths • Mandibular breathing • Making pained sounds—including groaning, moaning, or expressing hurt • Facial expressions—looking sad, tense, or frightened; frowning or crying • Body language—tension, clenched fists, knees pulled up, inflexibility, restlessness, or looking like they are trying to get away from the hurt area • Body movement—changing positions to get comfortable but cannot	
7. Perform hand hygiene. Apply clean gloves.	Reduces transmission of microorganisms.
8. Assess for feeling of breathlessness (does patient feel they are getting enough air?), respiratory rate, breathing patterns, and lung sounds. Assess for presence of airway secretions.	Dyspnea, air hunger, or shortness of breath results from metabolic or respiratory changes. Near the end of life, Cheyne-Stokes respirations are common and are characterized by alternating periods of apnea and hyperpnea.
9. Observe condition of skin, especially dependent areas such as the back, heels, and buttocks (see Chapters 6 and 39).	Decreased peripheral circulation and activity level contribute to skin breakdown (Samuriwo, 2019).
10. Inspect patient's oral cavity, including mucosa, tongue, and teeth (see Chapter 6).	Dehydration, difficulty swallowing, and inflammation of mouth are common at end of life.
11. Assess bowel function (see Chapter 34).	Patients experience constipation because of decreased oral intake, immobility, and medications such as opioids (CDC, 2022). Patients who have diarrhea are at risk for dehydration.
a. Determine usual bowel elimination pattern (frequency, character, usual time of day) and effectiveness of usual bowel management routines.	
b. If patient is passing liquid stool, assess for presence of fecal impaction (see agency policy). Remove and dispose of gloves, perform hand hygiene, and reapply clean gloves.	Watery stool leaking around blockage indicates fecal impaction. Reduces transmission of microorganisms.
c. Review medication regimens, prescriptions, and over-the-counter drugs known to cause constipation (e.g., opioids, antacids).	Medications can alter bowel elimination patterns. Diarrhea results from infections, diseases, or medications (e.g., antibiotics or chemotherapy). Change in therapy might be necessary.
d. Identify typical food and fluid intake over 1 week and patient's activity levels.	Oral intake and activity levels influence bowel elimination patterns.

STEP	RATIONALE
12. Assess urinary elimination (see Chapter 33) and ability to control urination. If incontinent, assess for skin breakdown around perineum and dependent areas and for patient discomfort.	Urinary incontinence results from patient's disease process, altered level of consciousness, or medications (diuretics, anticholinergics, opioids).
13. Remove and dispose of gloves. Perform hand hygiene.	Reduces transmission of microorganisms.
14. Assess patient's appetite, ability to swallow, and for presence of nausea or vomiting. Use standardized tool for assessment if available.	Medications, pain, depression, disease progression, or decreased blood flow to digestive organs near death often contribute to nausea, vomiting, and decreased appetite (HFA, 2022b).
15. Assess daily food and fluid intake in relation to patient's condition and preferences.	Nutrition screening helps to identify deficits and allows for interventions to be carried out to improve nutritional status if patient is tolerating eating (see Chapter 30).
16. Use descriptive scale to assess fatigue (e.g., scale with descriptors none, moderate, severe). Ask if fatigue limits patient's ability to perform desired activities.	Metabolic demands of a disease, anemia as a result of chemotherapy, treatments, and cumulative effects of other symptoms cause weakness and fatigue (ACS, 2019a).
17. Assess for terminal delirium in patient near death (e.g., confusion, restlessness, and/or agitation, with or without day-night reversal) (HFA, 2022b).	Allows you to identify this condition and implement interventions to keep patient safe and decrease patient anxiety.
a. Consider if patient has pain, nausea, dyspnea, full bladder or bowel, poor sleep patterns, anxiety, or joint pain from immobility.	Risk factors for presence of delirium are common physical problems that need to be treated or ruled out as causative factors.
b. Review electronic health record (EHR) for hypercalcemia, hypoglycemia, hyponatremia, or dehydration.	Metabolic imbalances cause restlessness or delirium.
c. Review patient's medications.	Unintended responses to medications result in changed activity states.
d. Determine if patient has unresolved emotional or spiritual issues.	Spiritual distress contributes to restlessness or increased pain.
18. Assess patient's or family caregiver's goals for symptom management.	Ensures patient or family caregiver are able to make decisions about symptom management.

PLANNING

1. Expected outcomes following completion of procedure:	
• Patient reports acceptable level of pain.	Indicates pain control.
• Patient reports feeling warm and comfortable.	Warming interventions help reverse effects of reduced peripheral circulation.
• Patient reports comfortable eating and drinking patterns.	Optimal food and fluid intake are based on patient preferences and comfort.
• Patient has soft, formed bowel movements.	Indicates adequate bowel function and peristaltic activity.
• Skin remains free of irritation or breakdown.	Interventions to protect skin from bowel or urinary incontinence are effective.
• Patient is not restless.	Therapies have calming effect.
• Patient reports less distress from fatigue.	Energy conservation methods are effective; patient adjusts to changes in activity level.
• Patient experiences less shortness of breath and labored breathing.	Patient is less apprehensive and breathes easily.
2. Close room door and bedside curtain.	Provides patient privacy.
3. Obtain and organize equipment at bedside.	Ensures more efficient procedure.
4. Arrange for extra personnel as needed.	Patient may need extra assistance.

IMPLEMENTATION

1. Perform hand hygiene.	Reduces transmission of microorganisms.
2. Provide pain relief. Use multimodal interventions.	Management of symptoms should be multimodal (ANA, 2018; NCP, 2018).
a. Administer ordered analgesics and adjuvants. Confer with health care provider and recommend an around-the-clock (ATC) dosing schedule, especially if pain is anticipated for majority of day. A variety of extended- or controlled-release oral opioid formulations (dosing intervals of 8, 10, 12, or 24 h) and transdermal patches (72 h) are effective.	Opioids should be given on a fixed dosage schedule ATC rather than "as needed" (prn), with doses given before pain returns (Burchum & Rosenthal, 2022). An ATC medication lessens the severity of end-of-dose pain, allowing a patient to sleep through the night and reducing "clock watching" for the next dose. Extended-release medications maintain constant serum opioid concentration, minimizing toxic and subtherapeutic concentrations (Burchum & Rosenthal, 2022).

STEP	RATIONALE
b. Provide nonpharmacological interventions such as mindfulness-based stress reduction, music therapy, relaxation exercises, and guided imagery (see Chapter 16).	Nonpharmacological measures supplement pain medication and can increase patient comfort (CDC, 2022). Music interventions have been found to decrease pain, anxiety, nausea, shortness of breath, and feelings of depression, along with providing significant increases in feelings of well-being (Peng et al., 2019).
c. Educate patient and family caregiver on causes and patterns of pain and safety of opioid use and explain interventions.	Encourages patient autonomy and reduces emotional distress, clarifying misinformation about opioid therapies.
d. Reassess patient's pain 1 hour after administration of pain medication or alternative therapy. If pain medication was administered via IV push route, reassess in 15–30 minutes.	To determine if desired effect of medication or alternative treatment was achieved; if patient has reduced pain level. IV push route of medication administration acts more quickly than alternative routes.
3. Provide general comfort measures.	
a. Provide bath and skin care based on patient's preferences and hygiene needs (see Chapter 18). **NOTE:** Daily baths are not always desired or necessary at end of life if they cause discomfort, fatigue, or increased pain (see agency policy).	Clean skin promotes comfort.
b. Provide eye care and use artificial tears in patients with decreased consciousness (see Chapter 19).	Eye irritation causes pain. Blink reflex diminishes near death, causing drying of cornea.
c. Reposition frequently; do not position on tubes or other objects.	Prolonged, even slight pressure from weight of patient's body or objects causes skin injury.
4. Provide oral hygiene after meals and at bedtime while awake and more frequently in mouth-breathing or unconscious patients (see Chapter 18).	Oral mucosa integrity is needed for normal swallowing and to minimize anorexia and malnutrition. Mouth rinses remove oral debris and clean the mouth. Dehydration develops as patient experiences metabolic changes and fluid intake declines.
a. Use antifungal oral rinses as prescribed or sodium bicarbonate or normal saline rinses.	Patients near death breathe through the mouth, drying oral mucosa.
b. Moisten lips with nonpetroleum balm.	Prevents skin breakdown.
5. Initiate bowel management regimen to reduce risk for constipation or diarrhea:	Interventions improve peristalsis in constipation, soften fecal mass, and decrease abdominal discomfort.
a. Give patient whatever fluids are enjoyable if medically tolerated. Near end of life, patient may refuse fluids. Do not force fluid intake.	Decreased blood flow to intestines at end of life causes anorexia.
b. Encourage regular physical activity (e.g., walking) if desired or tolerated.	Terminal care should be focused on patient preferences and physical abilities.
c. Administer daily stool softener or laxative, especially in patients using opioids for pain management.	Reduces risk of constipation.
d. In case of diarrhea, provide low-residue diet; treat infections or discontinue medications if possible. Administer antidiarrheal medications. Patients with chronic diarrhea require rigorous skin care to promote comfort. Option: a fecal management system can be used if indicated for patients with chronic diarrhea.	Treatments reduce incidence and severity of diarrhea, which can lead to dehydration and moisture-associated skin damage (MASD). If untreated, MASD can rapidly lead to excoriation and skin breakdown (Voegeli & Hillery, 2021).
6. Manage urinary incontinence with intervention appropriate for patient's conditions (e.g., condom catheter, adult incontinence pads [see Chapter 33]).	Urinary output declines near death, making it possible to manage incontinence without an indwelling catheter (HFA, 2022b).

Clinical Judgment *Consider an indwelling catheter only if skin integrity, patient preference, or fatigue from bed changes becomes an issue.*

STEP	RATIONALE
7. Offer patient favorite foods in amount and at time desired. Do not overly encourage patient to eat.	Patients may be experiencing gastrointestinal (GI) distress, dry mouth, or other symptoms related to their disease process, which may contribute to decreased oral intake. In addition, patients nearing final hours of life decrease their oral intake as a result of slowing of bodily functions and/or altered level of consciousness (HFA, 2022b).
a. Treat nausea by administering antiemetics intravenously or rectally as prescribed. As nausea subsides, offer clear liquids and ice chips if able to swallow. Avoid caffeinated liquids, milk, and fruit juices.	GI mucosa tolerates clear liquids more readily. Certain liquids increase stomach acidity.

STEP	RATIONALE
8. Manage fatigue.	Taking rest breaks during activity will help conserve energy. Tired patients need help and monitoring to ensure patient safety.
a. Help patient identify valued or desired tasks (e.g., grooming, reading) and preferred time of day to perform tasks, and determine how to conserve energy for only those tasks. Help with activities of daily living as appropriate. Eliminate extra steps in activities.	
b. Explain care activities before performing and include patient in setting daily schedule.	Minimizes anxiety and maintains patient's autonomy and involvement.
c. Discuss with patient easy ways to incorporate gentle movement (e.g., yoga, walking, and ROM exercises) into daily activities.	Research has shown that even for people with advanced-stage cancer, exercise can lessen pain and decrease anxiety, stress, depression, shortness of breath, and fatigue.
9. Support patient's breathing efforts.	Promotes comfort and reduces fatigue.
a. Position for comfort in semi-Fowler or Fowler position.	Promotes maximal ventilation, lung expansion, and drainage of secretions.

Clinical Judgment *Elevating head of bed above 30 degrees increases risk of pressure injury formation. If patient requires Fowler position to breathe comfortably, turn often and increase frequency of skin monitoring.*

STEP	RATIONALE
b. Elevate head to facilitate postural drainage. Turn from side to side to mobilize and drain secretions. Suction only if necessary.	Deep airway suctioning causes discomfort and is not effective in reducing airway noise or secretion clearance (HFA, 2022b).
c. Provide ordered antimuscarinic medications.	Anticholinergic medications reduce saliva and excessive secretions, thus decreasing noisy respirations.
d. Stay with patients experiencing dyspnea or air hunger. Use interventions that patients perceive as relieving shortness of breath (choice of oxygen-delivery modes, fan near face, body position). Administer opioids or anxiolytics as prescribed. Benzodiazepines may also be administered for anxiety related to dyspnea. Keep room cool with low humidity.	Sharing control with patients reduces anxiety that contributes to feelings of air hunger. Morphine is the drug of choice for dyspnea, decreasing respiratory rate, and decreasing anxiety. Use of oxygen has little benefit unless patient feels better using it.
10. Manage restlessness.	
a. Keep patient's room quiet with soft lighting and at comfortable temperature. Offer family caregivers opportunities to maintain close contact. Encourage use of soft music, prayer, or reading from patient's favorite book.	Reduces unnecessary external stimulation and provides comforting space. Privacy allows family caregivers chance to provide verbal assurances and touch. Presence of a family caregiver to hold a hand provides a calming effect.
b. Use least-sedating pharmacological options to control restlessness. Consult with interprofessional team about titrating a medication (e.g., lorazepam). Discontinue all nonessential medication. Use subcutaneous, transdermal, sublingual, or rectal medication delivery routes.	Reduce delirium without making patient unconscious. Control of restlessness relieves family's concern that patient is in pain or distress. Determine cause of delirium, if possible, to decrease use of medication (HFA, 2022b).
11. Manage anxiety.	
a. Provide counseling and supportive therapy. Consult with prescribing health care provider for benzodiazepines, the drugs of choice. Offer available counseling services (e.g., pastoral care, psychologist, social work).	Counseling improves patient/family caregiver understanding of the disease and its expected course and identifies strengths and coping strategies (Steele, 2023).

Clinical Judgment *Caution: The use of benzodiazepines in very elderly patients can result in a paradoxical agitation.*

STEP	RATIONALE
12. Remove and dispose of gloves. Perform hand hygiene.	Reduces transmission of microorganisms.
13. Raise side rails (as appropriate) and lower bed to lowest position, locking into position.	Ensures patient safety and prevents falls.
14. Place nurse call system in an accessible location within patient's reach.	Ensures patient can call for assistance if needed.
15. Perform hand hygiene.	Reduces transmission of microorganisms.

EVALUATION

1. Ask patient to describe character of pain and rate severity on scale of 0 to 10 (see Chapter 16); evaluate for change in pain characteristics and note behavior in nonverbal patients.	Determines extent of pain relief.
2. Ask patient to describe mouth comfort and inspect oral cavity.	Evaluates condition of oral cavity and ability to chew or swallow.

STEP	RATIONALE
3. Evaluate frequency of defecation; after patient defecates, inspect feces.	Determines status of bowel function and character of stool.
4. Observe skin condition.	Determines if skin tears or areas of pressure or maceration are present.
5. Ask patient to rate fatigue (scale from none to moderate to severe) and compare with baseline. Observe for fatigue or shortness of breath when patient performs activities.	Determines if patient is less distressed with activity.
6. Observe patient's respiratory patterns and ask if breathing is easy and comfortable.	Determines if respiratory distress is relieved.
7. Observe patient's behavior or ask family to report on it. Note level of restlessness.	Determines level of comfort and extent of restlessness.
8. **Use Teach-Back:** "I want to be sure I explained that we want to control your pain, and this requires you to describe it. Tell me what the numbers on the pain scale mean. Tell me when it is a good time to let me know about your pain before it gets too severe." Revise your instruction now or develop a plan for revised patient/family caregiver teaching if patient/family caregiver is not able to teach back correctly.	Teach-back is a technique for health care providers to ensure that they have explained medical information clearly so that patients and their families understand what is communicated to them (AHRQ, 2023).

Unexpected Outcomes

1. One or several symptoms remain unresolved, with patient reporting little or no relief.
2. Patient becomes anxious, fearful, or exhausted as a result of continued symptoms.

Related Interventions

- Increase frequency of or change an intervention.
- Try combination therapies.
- Give patients therapy choices and try different interventions.
- Explain desired outcomes of therapies and possible reasons for symptoms.
- Answer call lights quickly and explain plan of care throughout the day.

Documentation

- Document detailed description of patient symptoms, related interventions, and patient response. Use consistent descriptors for comparison over time.
- Document your evaluation of patient and family caregiver learning.
- Document successful symptom interventions in the care plan.

Hand-Off Reporting

- Report unexpected new symptoms or uncontrolled existing symptoms to health care provider.

Special Considerations

Patient Education

- Involve family caregivers in the patient's care (see Fig. 17.2). With proper instruction they can perform most symptom-management interventions, deliver personal care (e.g., bathing, oral hygiene), and administer medications in the home setting.
- Recognize a patient's transition to the active dying phase and communicate to the patient and family caregiver the expectation of imminent death. Educate the patient and family caregivers about signs of imminent death (NCP, 2018).

Pediatrics

- Allow young children to visit a dying parent or grandparent if desired. Encourage parents to express concerns about how to talk about death and loss with a child.
- Teach parents how to recognize and assess pain in a nonverbal child.
- Encourage involvement of siblings of a child who is dying on the basis of needs and readiness (Hockenberry et al., 2022).

Older Adults

- Include older adults in conversations and accommodate communication limits (e.g., hearing and visual deficits).
- Older adults need companionship and maintenance of self-esteem. Detached family caregiver behaviors such as being slow to respond to physical discomforts, failing to keep room odor free, and speaking in hushed tones of voice are often perceived by the person as abandonment. Encourage a family caregiver, friend, sitter, or hospice volunteer to stay with the patient during the night. Some older adults who have developed a lifestyle around aloneness prefer solitude. Be sensitive to the patient's preferences (Touhy & Jett, 2022).
- Assessing and addressing pain in an older adult who is cognitively impaired or nonverbal is sometimes difficult and involves proactive symptom management.

Populations With Disabilities

- Address the patient directly; use the patient's preferred communication method and tools; slow down communication; involve family caregivers but be attentive to inappropriate taking over of decision making (Sullivan et al., 2018).
- Support the patient to assure health care needs, concerns, and perspectives are understood (Sullivan et al., 2018).

Home Care

- Recommend that family caregivers self-monitor energy levels and request respite care when needing relief. Suggest resources for help with meals, shopping, or staying with the patient while the family goes out.

Nurses provide postmortem care in patients' homes and institutional settings. If possible, ask in advance if the family caregiver needs you to make any special accommodations with respect to culture or religion, and seek assistance as needed with someone familiar with that culture or religion. Treat the body after death with respect according to the cultural and religious practices of the family caregivers and in accordance with local law (NCP, 2018).

Two legal considerations arise at the time of death. First, the 1986 Omnibus Budget Reconciliation Act (OBRA) legally requires that a patient's survivors be made aware of the option of organ and tissue donation. In most states citizens can sign the back of driver's licenses if being an organ or tissue donor is desired. However, a family caregiver still usually gives consent for donation at the time of death. Patients may indicate the wish to donate organs and tissue in an advance directive.

In the case of vital organ donation (e.g., heart, lungs, liver, pancreas, kidneys), a patient must remain on life support until the organs are surgically removed. Often your role in organ procurement includes helping to identify potential organ donors, providing care for the donor's body, and caring for the family throughout the donation process (Tocher, 2019). Family caregivers often need help understanding what "brain death" (i.e., the irreversible absence of all brain function, including the brainstem) means for a person who has died. Patients appear to still be alive because life support keeps the deceased's organs functioning until they can be retrieved. Tissues such as eyes, bone, and skin are retrieved from deceased patients not on life support. Because of the sensitive nature of making requests for organ donation, professionals educated in organ procurement often assume that responsibility. These experts inform family caregivers of the options for donation, provide information about costs (no cost to the family), and explain that donation does not delay funeral arrangements.

Nurses also play a role in the donation request process. Facilitate the conversation by providing a private place and helping to identify the surrogate to be involved in the request. Sometimes you notify the local donor registry to determine if a patient qualifies for organ donation because certain medical conditions prohibit donation. Reinforce explanations of the procedure and inform the family caregiver about how you will care for the deceased's body. Above all, honor cultural and religious practices and support family caregiver's final decision. Donor families often report that donating organs helped them grieve and that it was a positive experience.

The second procedure of legal and medical significance often performed after a death is an autopsy, or postmortem examination. An autopsy, the surgical dissection of a body after death, helps determine the exact cause and circumstances of a death, discovers the pathway of a disease, or provides research data. It is not performed in every death. State laws determine when autopsies are required, but they are usually performed in circumstances of unusual death (e.g., violent trauma, unexpected death in the home) and when death occurs within 24 hours of hospital admission. Be available to answer questions and support the family's choices. Autopsies normally do not delay burial or change the appearance of the deceased, but there may be a cost to families.

Delegation

The skill of care of a body after death can be delegated to assistive personnel (AP). However, it is often easier for the nurse and AP to work together in providing postmortem care. Direct the AP to:
- Follow agency policy in cases of autopsy or organ and tissue donation
- Honor cultural or religious rituals when performing postmortem care
- Handle the body with dignity and respect for privacy

Interprofessional Collaboration
- Health care providers and support services assist family caregivers during this time of death, ensuring that the body is cared for with dignity and family caregivers are supported.

Equipment
- Clean gloves and isolation gown
- Plastic bag for hazardous waste disposal
- Washbasin, washcloth, warm water, and bath towel
- Clean gown or disposable gown for body as indicated by agency policy
- Shroud kit with name tags
- Syringes for removing urinary catheter
- Scissors
- Small pillow or towel
- Paper tape, gauze dressings
- Paper bag, plastic bag, or other suitable receptacle for patient's belongings to be returned to family members
- Valuables envelope

STEP	RATIONALE

ASSESSMENT

1. Identify patient using at least two identifiers (e.g., name and birthday or name and medical record number) according to agency policy.

2. Ask health care provider to establish time of death and determine if an autopsy is being requested. If an autopsy is planned or a possible crime is involved, use special precautions to preserve evidence (see agency policy).

3. Determine if family caregivers or significant others are present and have been informed of the death. Identify patient's surrogate (next of kin or durable power of attorney [DPOA]).

Ensures correct patient. Complies with The Joint Commission standards and improves patient safety (TJC, 2023a).

Certifies patient's death. Autopsy can determine cause of death and reveal more about a disease. Patient's legal representative and the health care provider or designated requester must sign an autopsy consent form.

Verifies that family has been notified of patient's death to avoid inappropriate communication of this sensitive information (Touhy & Jett, 2022).

STEP	RATIONALE
4. Determine if patient's surrogate has been asked about organ and tissue donation and validate that donation request form has been signed. Notify organ request team per agency policy.	Federal guidelines require documentation that request has been made.
5. Provide family caregivers and friends a private place to gather. Allow time to ask questions (including those about medical care) or discuss grief.	Creates safe environment for grieving family. Questions provide information about how coping with loss is going and what one's needs might be.
6. Ask family caregivers if they have requests for preparation or viewing of the body (e.g., washing the body, position of body, special clothing, shaving). Determine if they wish to be present or help with care of the body.	Respects individuality of patient and family caregiver and supports their right to having cultural or religious values and beliefs upheld. Provides closure for those who wish to help with body preparation.
7. Contact support person (e.g., pastoral care, social work) to stay with family caregivers not helping to prepare the body. Implement in timely manner a bereavement care plan after patient's death when family caregiver remains the focus of care (NCP, 2018).	Provides family caregiver support during an emotional time.
8. Consult health care providers' orders for special care directives or specimens that are to be collected.	Specimens may be used in determining cause of death.
9. Perform hand hygiene; apply clean gloves, gown, or protective barriers.	Reduces transmission of microorganisms.
10. Assess general condition of the body and note presence of dressings, tubes, and medical equipment.	Validates if tissue damage was present before postmortem care.
11. If leaving room at this time, remove personal protective equipment and perform hand hygiene. Otherwise keep PPE on. Close room door for privacy.	Reduces transmission of microorganisms.

PLANNING

1. Expected outcomes following completion of procedure:	
• Body is free of new skin damage.	Careful handling of body prevents lacerations, bruises, or abrasions during postmortem care.
• Significant others able to express grief.	Significant others feel supported through their loss.

Clinical Judgment *Position the patient supine using the appropriate equipment, as per agency policy. It is important to straighten the limbs before rigor mortis begins (National Institute on Aging [NIA], 2022).*

2. With patient supine in bed, place arms at side. A private room for postmortem care is preferred, but if patient has a roommate, explain and move this person to another location temporarily. Remove and dispose of gloves and other PPE and perform hand hygiene.	Provides staff with larger area for postmortem care and for family caregivers to gather in a private setting. Reduces transmission of microorganisms.
3. As soon as possible, a patient's death must be "pronounced" by someone in authority (e.g., physician in hospital or nursing agency, hospice nurse). This person completes forms certifying the cause, time, and place of death. The legal form is necessary for life insurance and financial and property issues. If hospice is helping, a plan for what happens after death is already in place (NIA, 2022).	These steps make it possible for an official death certificate to be prepared.
4. Direct AP to gather needed equipment and arrange at bedside.	Because this is often an emotional time for family members, organized efficient care is important.

IMPLEMENTATION

1. Help family caregivers notify others of the death. Promptly notify the chosen mortuary and discuss plans for postmortem care.	Following a death, grieving persons have difficulty focusing on details and often need guidance. Being informed increases a sense of control.
2. If patient has made tissue donation, consult agency policy for guidelines regarding care of the body.	Retrieval of tissues (e.g., eyes, bone, skin) may require special procedures.
3. Prepare body. Perform hand hygiene; apply clean gloves, gown, or other PPE. Close room door.	Reduces transmission of microorganisms.

Clinical Judgment *Have family caregivers helping in postmortem care wear a gown and gloves to protect against body fluids.*

STEP	RATIONALE
4. Remove indwelling devices (e.g., urinary catheter, endotracheal tube). Disconnect and cap off (no need to remove) intravenous lines. *Do not remove indwelling devices in cases of autopsy* (follow agency policy).	Creates normal appearance for family viewing of body. Removing intravenous catheters allows fluids to leak. Removal of tubes and lines is contraindicated if an autopsy is planned.
5. Clean the mouth and clean and replace dentures as soon as possible. If dentures cannot be replaced, send them with body in clearly labeled denture cup and transport with body to mortuary. If culturally appropriate, close mouth with rolled-up towel under chin.	Gives face more natural appearance. If dentures are not replaced, it can be difficult later for workers at funeral home to place dentures.
6. Place small pillow under head or position according to cultural preferences. Do not tie hands together on top of body. Check agency policy regarding need to secure hands and feet. Use only circular gauze bandaging on body.	Patient appears natural. Weight of limp arms causes skin damage and discoloration if hands are tied. Some agencies require securing appendages to prevent tissue damage when body is being moved.
7. Close the eyes by applying light pressure for 30 seconds. Use saline-moistened gauze if corneal or eye donation is to take place. Some cultures prefer that eyes remain open.	Closed eyes convey to some people a more peaceful and natural appearance. Gauze prevents corneal drying.
8. Groom and arrange hair into preferred style, if known. Remove any clips, hairpins, or rubber bands. **Do not shave patient**. Some cultures and faith groups prohibit shaving.	Hard objects damage or discolor face and scalp.

Clinical Judgment *Shaving a recently deceased person is not recommended because the skin is still warm and bruising and marking may appear days later.*

STEP	RATIONALE
9. Wash soiled body parts. Some cultural practices require that family members clean the body.	Prepares body for viewing and reduces odors. Mortuary personnel provide complete bath.
10. Remove soiled dressings and replace with clean dressings, using paper tape or circular gauze bandaging.	Changing dressings controls odors and creates more acceptable appearance. Paper tape minimizes skin damage when tape is removed.

Clinical Judgment *Turning a recently dead body to the side sometimes causes the flow of exhaled air. This is a normal event and not a sign of life.*

STEP	RATIONALE
11. Place absorbent pad under buttocks.	Relaxation of sphincter muscles at time of death causes release of urine or feces (HFA, 2022b). Use appropriate disposal for urine, bowel, or emesis if patient is taking hazardous drugs.
12. Place clean gown on body. Some agencies require gown removal before placing body in shroud.	Provides privacy and prepares body for viewing.
13. Identify personal belongings that stay with body and those to be given to family.	Prevents loss of valuable or meaningful property.
14. If family caregiver requests viewing, respect individual cultural practices. Otherwise, place clean sheet over body up to chin with arms outside covers. Remove medical equipment from room. Provide soft lighting and chairs.	Maintains respect for patient and those viewing body. Prevents exposure of body parts. Removing medical equipment provides more peaceful, natural setting.
15. Allow family caregiver time alone with body and encourage saying goodbye with religious rituals in a culturally appropriate manner. Some families want time to sit quietly with the body, console each other, and share memories (NIA, 2022). Some cultural practices include maintaining silence at the time of death, whereas in other cultures grief is expressed with intense emotional displays, loud wailing, or "falling out." Do not rush any grieving process.	Compassionate care provides family caregivers with meaningful experience during early phase of grief. Ensure privacy and a safe environment. Provide chair at bedside for family member who might collapse.
16. After viewing, remove linens and gown per agency policy. Place body in shroud provided by the agency (see illustration).	Shroud protects injury to skin, avoids exposure of body, and provides barrier against potentially contaminated body fluids.
17. Place identification label on outside of shroud if required by agency policy. Follow agency policy for marking a body that poses an infectious risk to others. Remove and dispose of personal protective equipment and perform hygiene.	Ensures proper identification of body (TJC, 2023a). Reduces exposure of morgue and mortuary staff to contamination.
18. Arrange prompt transportation of body to the mortuary. If you anticipate a delay, transport body to the morgue.	Mortuary personnel get best results if embalming occurs before full rigor mortis (i.e., stiffening of body after death) occurs.

STEP	RATIONALE

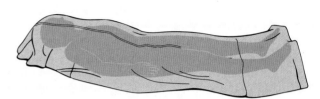

STEP 16 Body in shroud.

EVALUATION

1. Observe family caregivers', friends', and significant others' response to the loss.
2. Note appearance and condition of patient's skin during preparation of the body.

The need for referral or help is based on evaluation of person's unique response to loss.

Validates condition of skin and provides information for postmortem care documentation should any inquiries come later.

Unexpected Outcomes

1. A family caregiver becomes immobilized with grief and has difficulty functioning.

2. A grieving person becomes agitated and threatens or strikes out against others.

Related Interventions

- Enlist the help of a family caregiver or trusted friend to provide direction and support.
- Determine if family would like pastoral care.
- Call for assistance from a psychiatric nurse practitioner, spiritual care provider, or social worker who has a relationship with the family (Steele, 2023).
- Enlist help from security staff or crisis intervention professional if safety is a concern.

Documentation

- Document time of death, describe any resuscitative measures taken (if applicable), and note the name of the professional certifying the death.
- Document any special preparation of the body for autopsy or organ/tissue donation. Note whom you called and who made the request for organ/tissue donation.
- Document name of mortuary and names of family caregivers notified at the time of death and their relationship to the deceased.
- Document on appropriate form personal articles left on the body (e.g., teeth, glasses), jewelry taped to skin, or tubes and lines left in place. Note how valuables and personal belongings were handled and who received them. Secure signatures as required by agency policy.
- Document time the body was transported and its destination. Note the location of body identification tags.

Special Considerations

Pediatrics

- Offer family caregivers, especially parents, the opportunity to be with the child throughout the dying process and to help with body preparation.

- Parents frequently want to hold the child's body after death. Parents of deceased newborns often want a memento (e.g., picture, article of clothing, footprint, lock of hair). Make every effort to honor parent requests.

Older Adults

- Some older adults have small families and surviving circles of friends. Nurses and other care providers are sometimes the only human presence during death. Arrange for someone to be with the person when death is imminent.

Home Care

- Educate family caregivers caring for a patient dying at home about what to expect at the time of death (Table 17.1).
- Consider the type of support that family caregivers will need at the time of death and make arrangements.
- After death in the home, follow agency guidelines for body preparation and transfer and for disposal of durable medical equipment (e.g., tubing, needles, syringes), soiled dressings or linens, and medications. Instruct family caregivers in safe and proper handling and disposal of medical waste.
- Ensure that family caregivers have resources for support while grieving, such as local counselors or hospice organizations as needed (HFA, 2022a).

Physical Signs and Symptoms in the Final Stages of Dying

Physical Signs and Symptoms	Rationale	Intervention
Coolness, color, and temperature change in hands, arms, feet, and legs; mottling of legs; perspiration	Peripheral circulation diminished as blood shunts to vital organs Patient may feel cool to touch, but core temperature normal	Place socks on feet. Cover with light blanket. Do not use electric blanket because person is unable to report excess heat.
Increased sleeping	Decreased energy, psychological withdrawal, medications	Spend time with person; hold hands. Speak to person, even if no response.
Disorientation, confusion of time, place, person	Metabolic changes, medications, changing sleep/wake cycles, decreased oxygenation	Identify self by name; reorient person to time and place. Decrease environmental stimuli.
Incontinence of urine and/or bowel	Decreased muscle tone and consciousness	Change bedding as appropriate. Use bed pads; try not to use indwelling catheters.
Upper airway secretions; noisy respirations	Decreased cough reflex, mandibular breathing, inability to expectorate secretions or clear throat, relaxation of glottis, decreased muscle tone	Elevate head with pillow or raise head of bed; turn head to side to drain secretions. Suction minimally.
Restlessness	Metabolic changes and decrease in oxygen to brain	Calm patient by speech and action; reduce light, rub back, stroke arms, or read aloud. Do not use restraints.
Decreased intake of food and fluids, nausea	Blood shunted away from gastrointestinal (GI) tract, causing decreased GI motility and anorexia; ketosis	Do not force patient to eat or drink; give ice chips or popsicles if desired. Provide mouth care.

Adapted from Touhy TA, Jett KF: *Ebersole and Hess' gerontological nursing and healthy aging,* ed 6, St. Louis, 2022, Elsevier.

✦ CLINICAL JUDGMENT AND NEXT GENERATION NCLEX® EXAMINATION–STYLE QUESTIONS

The nurse is caring for an 89-year-old patient admitted for palliative care who has a history of metastatic bone cancer. Current pain is rated at "7" on a 0–10 scale. The patient is alert and oriented, although she says, "I am just so tired." She expresses to the nurse and family, "I do not want any aggressive therapy—just make me comfortable." VS: BP 110/66 mm Hg, HR 86 beats/min, RR 22 breaths/min, T 37.3°C (99.2°F), and SPO₂ 96% on RA. The patient tells the nurse, "I have had a good life. I'm ready to die peacefully." The patient is surrounded by several family members in the room who are crying and arguing about what kind of care they believe the patient should receive if she continues to decline. The patient does not have an advance directive on file in the electronic health record.

1. Highlight the findings that concern the nurse at this time. (Highlight: Highlight Text)

Health History	Nurses' Notes	Vital Signs	Laboratory Results

1634: Patient in bed, reporting pain of 7 on a 0–10 scale, which she says is "about what it always is." Height: 163 cm (64 in); weight: 45.8 kg (101 lb). VS: T 37.3°C (99.2°F); HR 86 beats/min; RR 22 beats/min; BP 110/66 mm Hg; SpO₂ 96% on RA. No advance directives on file. Patient expresses desire to forego any aggressive therapy; states, "Just make me comfortable." Family in the room expressing various viewpoints on which kind of care should be given if the patient declines.

2. The nurse is explaining palliative care to the patient's family. Which statements will the nurse make to express ways that palliative care is administered? **Select all that apply.**
1. "Provide the patient with relief from pain and other symptoms."
2. "Create a therapeutic environment for the patient's well-being."
3. "Attempt to hasten the disease progression."
4. "Help family cope with the patient's current situation."
5. "Enhance patient's quality of life at this time."

3. While providing care, the patient reports trouble breathing. Which symptoms will the nurse anticipate on assessment? **Select all that apply.**
1. Increased respirations
2. Warm skin on touch
3. Decreased blood pressure
4. Quiet inspiration and exhalation
5. Restlessness

4. The family asks questions about an advance directive. Which information will the nurse provide?
1. "The health care provider will decide which interventions are necessary."
2. "An advance directive ensures that all health care providers know the patient's specific wishes."
3. "A 'do not resuscitate' (DNR) order means that nurses will stop giving pain medication and all other treatment."
4. "An advance directive is a legal document that the patient can change at any time if they are oriented."
5. "If the patient with an advance directive becomes unconscious, the family can change the plan of care."

5. Several days later, the patient dies while the granddaughter and nurse are at the bedside. The granddaughter says, "I am so glad my grandmother isn't suffering anymore." Which response by the nurse is appropriate at this time?
1. "It is not right to be joyful when someone dies."
2. "I felt the same way when my grandmother died."
3. "Thank you for the privilege of caring for her."
4. "Can you leave the room so that I can prepare the body?"

Visit the Evolve site for Answers to Clinical Judgment and Next Generation NCLEX® Examination2Style Questions.

REFERENCES

Agency for Healthcare Research and Quality (AHRQ): *Teach-back: intervention*, 2023. https://www.ahrq.gov/patient-safety/reports/engage/interventions/teach-back.html.

American Cancer Society (ACS): *Physical changes as you near the end of life*, 2019a. https://www.cancer.org/treatment/end-of-life-care/nearing-the-end-of-life/physical-symptoms.html. Accessed October 7, 2023.

American Cancer Society (ACS): *Developing a pain control plan*, 2019b. https://www.cancer.org/treatment/treatments-and-side-effects/physical-side-effects/pain/developing-a-pain-control-plan.html. Accessed October 7, 2023.

American Cancer Society (ACS): *What is an Advance Directive?* 2019c. https://www.cancer.org/treatment/finding-and-paying-for-treatment/understanding-financial-and-legal-matters/advance-directives/what-is-an-advance-health-care-directive.html. Accessed October 7, 2023.

American Nurses Association (ANA): *The ethical responsibility to manage pain and the suffering it causes*, 2018. https://www.nursingworld.org/practice-policy/nursing-excellence/official-position-statements/id/the-ethical-responsibility-to-manage-pain-and-the-suffering-it-causes/. Accessed October 7, 2023.

American Nurses Association (ANA): *Nurses' professional responsibility to promote ethical practice environments*, 2021. https://www.nursingworld.org/~4ab6e6/globalassets/practiceandpolicy/nursing-excellence/ana-position-statements/nursing-practice/nurses-professional-responsibility-to-promote-ethical-practice-environments-2021-final.pdf. Accessed October 7, 2023.

Bijnsdorp FM, et al: Profiles of family caregivers of patients at the end of life at home: a Qualitative methodological study into family caregiver's support needs, *BMC Palliative Care* 19:51, 2020.

Blater AH: Addressing unpaid family caregiver burden with supportive services, *NCMJ* 81(4):270, 2020.

Burchum JR, Rosenthal LD: *Lehne's pharmacology for nursing care*, ed 11, St. Louis, 2022, Elsevier.

Centers for Disease Control and Prevention (CDC): *CDC Guideline for prescribing opioids for chronic pain — United States*, 2022. https://www.cdc.gov/opioids/guideline-update/. Accessed October 7, 2023.

Centers for Disease Control and Prevention (CDC): *What is health literacy?* 2023. https://www.cdc.gov/healthliteracy/learn/index.html.

Hockenberry MJ, et al: *Wong's essentials of pediatric nursing*, ed 11, St. Louis, 2022, Elsevier.

Hospice Foundation of America (HFA): *What is hospice?* 2022a. https://hospicefoundation.org/Hospice-Care/Hospice-Services. Accessed October 7, 2023.

Hospice Foundation of America (HFA): *Signs of approaching death*, 2022b. https://hospicefoundation.org/Hospice-Care/Signs-of-Approaching-Death. Accessed October 7, 2023.

Hospice Foundation of America (HFA): *Mourning a miscarriage*, 2022c. https://hospicefoundation.org/End-of-Life-Support-and-Resources/Grief-Support/Journeys-with-Grief-Articles/Mourning-a-Miscarriage. Accessed October 7, 2023.

Liu J, et al: Caregiver burden: a concept analysis, *Int J Nurs Sci* 7:438–445, 2020.

National Center for Complementary and Integrative Health (NCCIH): *Relaxation techniques: what you need to know*, 2022. https://nccih.nih.gov/health/stress/relaxation.htm. Accessed October 7, 2023.

National Consensus Project for Quality Palliative Care (NCP): *Clinical practice guidelines for quality palliative care*, ed 4, 2018. https://www.nationalcoalitionhpc.org/wp-content/uploads/2020/07/NCHPC-NCPGuidelines_4thED_web_FINAL.pdf. Accessed November 19, 2023.

National Institute on Aging (NIA): *End of life: what to do after someone dies*, 2020. https://www.nia.nih.gov/health/what-do-after-someone-dies. Accessed October 7, 2023.

O'Brien MR, et al: Meeting patients' spiritual needs during end-of-life care: a qualitative study of nurses' and healthcare professionals' perceptions of spiritual care training, *J Clin Nurs* 28(1-2):182, 2019.

Parisi A, et al: The relationship between substance misuse and complicated grief: a systematic review, *J Subst Abuse Treat* 103:43, 2019.

Peng CS, et al: Music intervention as a tool in improving patient experience in palliative care, *Am J Hosp Palliat Care* 36(1):45, 2019.

Robert R, et al: Ethical dilemmas due to the Covid-19 pandemic, *Ann Intensive Care* 10:84, 2020.

Rovers JJE, et al: Living at the end-of-life: experience of time of patients with cancer, *BMC Palliat Care* 18(1):40, 2019.

Samuriwo R: Enhancing end-of-life skin care to prevent pressure ulcers in primary care, *J Community Nurs* 33(3):56, 2019.

Steele D: *Keltner's psychiatric nursing*, ed 9, St. Louis, 2023, Elsevier.

Sullivan WF, et al: Primary care of adults with intellectual and developmental disabilities: 2018 Canadian consensus guidelines, *Can Fam Physician* 64:254, 2018.

The Joint Commission (TJC): *2023 National patient safety goals*, Oakbrook Terrace, IL, 2023a, The Joint Commission. https://www.jointcommission.org/standards/national-patient-safety-goals/.

The Joint Commission (TJC): *Pain assessment and management—understanding the requirements: What are the key concepts organizations need to understand regarding the pain management requirements in the Leadership (LD) and Provision of Care, Treatment, and Services (PC) chapters?* 2023b, TJC. https://www.jointcommission.org/standards/standard-faqs/hospital-and-hospital-clinics/provision-of-care-treatment-and-services-pc/000002161/. Accessed April 13, 2023.

Tocher J, et al: The role of specialist nurses for organ donation: a solution for maximizing organ donation rates? *J Clin Nurs* 28(9-10):2020, 2019.

Touhy TA, Jett KF: *Ebersole and Hess' gerontological nursing and healthy aging*, ed 6, St. Louis, 2022, Elsevier.

Voegeli D, Hillery S: Prevention and management of moisture-associated skin damage, *Br J Nurs* 30(15):S40–S46, 2021.

World Health Organization: *Palliative care*, 2020. https://www.who.int/news-room/fact-sheets/detail/palliative-care. Accessed October 7, 2023.

Safety and Comfort: Next-Generation NCLEX® (NGN)–Style Unfolding Case Study

PHASE 1

QUESTION 1.

A building collapsed in a local community after it caught fire. A disaster was declared, and an incident command center was established. The triage nurse was sent into an area to assess victims.

Select the individuals who will be issued a red tag by the triage nurse.

- 19-year-old who is walking around and hysterically looking for their sister
- 24-year-old with a displaced fracture of the femur
- 36-year-old with first-degree injuries to 50% of the body
- 40-year-old with a tourniquet around a traumatic leg amputation
- 58-year-old who is sitting upright and appears confused

QUESTION 2.

The client with the red tag is brought to the emergency department by squad.

Complete the following sentence by selecting from the lists of options below.

The emergency nurse anticipates that the client is at high risk for **1 [Select]** due to **2 [Select]**.

Options for 1	Options for 2
Hypoventilation	Oxygen saturation 95%
Hypertension	Screaming
Hemorrhage	Presence of a tourniquet
Fluid overload	Multiple lacerations

PHASE 2

QUESTION 3.

The client is now in the emergency department awaiting evaluation.

Complete the following sentence by selecting from the list of options below.

The nurse will **1 [Select]** and **2 [Select]** to increase client safety at this time.

Options for 1	Options for 2
Administer hypotonic IV fluids	Delegate monitoring to assistive personnel (AP)
Page the trauma surgery team	Attempt to locate family member information
Remove the tourniquet	Stay with the client

QUESTION 4.

The client was taken to surgery and then sent to a surgical intensive care unit (SICU). The nurse in the SICU is planning care for the client, who has regained consciousness after the surgery but is very sleepy and lethargic.

Select whether the potential nursing actions are indicated or not indicated for the plan of care.

Potential Nursing Action	Indicated	Not Indicated
Delegate fall risk assessment to assistive personnel (AP).		
Apply restraints prophylactically.		
Arrange for a sitter to be present in the room.		
Administer morphine per health care provider's "prn–as needed" order every 2–4 hours.		
Monitor vital signs every 15 minutes for the first hour.		

PHASE 3

QUESTION 5.

The client has awakened from surgery and is crying while reporting pain in the operative extremity. Select 3 actions the nurse would take at this time.

○ Remove surgical dressings to facilitate comfort.
○ Reassure the client that postsurgical pain of this intensity is normal.
○ Assess character of pain and ask client to rate severity on a scale of 0 to 10.
○ Prepare to administer pain medication as ordered and on time.
○ Evaluate the medication record for regular and PRN pain medication.
○ Tell the client to try to relax to regain control, as crying will exacerbate the pain level.
○ Ask family members whether the client would like to have a chaplain come to the room.

QUESTION 6.

During the inpatient stay following surgery, diagnostic testing revealed that the client had an inoperable brain tumor. The client was discharged to hospice care and has been cared for by a hospice nurse in the home.

Which of the following client statements would show that interventions undertaken by the hospice nurse have provided comfort at the end of life? **Select all that apply.**

○ "I have lived a wonderful life."
○ "My pain level is an 8 on a 0-to-10 scale."
○ "I am sure that if I have enough faith, I will be cured."
○ "The family and I have spent a lot of time together lately."
○ "My spouse and I made funeral arrangements earlier this week."
○ "I have been using aromatherapy to decrease my pain levels."
○ "My priest stops by several times a week to see how I am doing."

Adequate and complete hygiene is important for a patient's health and level of comfort. Hygiene is a basic human need that requires a patient's participation in the selection of hygiene approaches and choosing when to provide care. Before providing any hygiene, assess your patient's hygiene practices and preferences (e.g., specific products, time preferences). Recognize cultural considerations regarding personal hygiene practices or the need for gender congruent caregivers. Asking your patients or their family caregiver about hygiene practices promotes hygiene and also provides person-centered care.

All of the skills associated with bathing are intimate and at times can be embarrassing for a patient. Before initiating hygiene care, assess your patient and identify cues that indicate any embarrassment or discomfort in having someone provide this care. Take this time to explain how you will maintain patient privacy and confidentiality and why it is important that a health care professional provide the care.

When providing hygiene, take the opportunity to fully assess your patient's skin, mobility status, and independent functioning. For example, during bathing, use your clinical judgment to conduct focused skin assessments to determine any risk for or actual pressure injuries, including medical adhesive−related skin injuries (MARSIs) and medical device−related pressure injuries (MDRPIs). Analyze any assessment cues to determine what skin care protocols are needed or if you need to use an agency's skin care/wound care nurse as a resource. Also focus your assessment on your patient's comfort and mobility. If your patient is in pain, administer an analgesic 20 to 30 minutes before bathing. Determine if your patient can physically assist with bathing or if it is difficult for them to change positions. This information will help you plan for the type of bath to provide and future position changes or transfer.

Bathing provides an opportunity to perform nail and foot care. Know what type of nail care requires a health care provider's order (e.g., patients with diabetes mellitus and other peripheral vascular diseases). Before implementing any nail or foot care, use clinical judgment to assess and analyze data about any existing or at-risk nail or foot problems. Assess the skin on the feet for any pressure or tissue injuries. Identify cues, such as the inability to perceive sensation or decreased pulses, which could indicate impaired circulation, which also increases your patient's risk for skin or tissue injuries. Do not overlook cues that indicate poorly fitting shoes, such as blisters or calluses.

Oral hygiene promotes good oral health and prevents complications associated with other health conditions. When you care for unconscious or debilitated patients, recognize the risk for infection and/or aspiration to guide your assessment. These patients need regular and specific oral hygiene practices. Clinical judgment will allow you to adapt a skill to meet the patient's needs. For example, if a patient cannot fully expectorate mucus from the mouth, do you offer an oral suction device the patient can use, or do you have a family caregiver learn how to provide suctioning? Analyze any assessment cues to determine frequency and type of oral hygiene.

Hair care supports a patient's comfort, appearance, and sense of well-being. Before implementing any hair care, it is important to assess for any cultural considerations because cutting or shaving any hair may be forbidden. Assess your patient's hair and scalp for any cues that indicate a problem (e.g., dandruff, head lice, hair loss). When problems are identified, plan and implement measures to reduce or treat the problem. For example, men's facial hair needs to be kept free of food and secretions. Brushing and combing a patient's hair reduces matting and tangling. Blood, dressings, and diaphoresis leave a sticky residue and oil on the hair that must be removed. Hair care interventions may seem basic, but they are important in promoting your patient's comfort and sense of well-being.

18 | Personal Hygiene and Bed Making

SKILLS AND PROCEDURES

Skill 18.1 **Complete or Partial Bed Bath, p. 524**

Procedural Guideline 18.1 **Perineal Care, p. 534**

Procedural Guideline 18.2 **Bathing With Use of Chlorhexidine Chloride Gluconate (CHG) Disposable Washcloths, Tub, or Shower, p. 536**

Skill 18.2 **Oral Hygiene, p. 538**

Procedural Guideline 18.3 **Care of Dentures, p. 542**

Skill 18.3 **Performing Mouth Care for an Unconscious or Debilitated Patient, p. 544**

Procedural Guideline 18.4 **Hair Care—Combing and Shaving, p. 547**

Procedural Guideline 18.5 **Hair Care—Shampooing Using Disposable Dry Shampoo Cap, p. 550**

Skill 18.4 **Performing Nail and Foot Care, p. 551**

Procedural Guideline 18.6 **Making an Occupied Bed, p. 557**

Procedural Guideline 18.7 **Making an Unoccupied Bed, p. 561**

OBJECTIVES

Mastery of content in this chapter will enable you to:
- Outline factors that influence personal hygiene practices.
- Discuss how a nurse applies clinical judgment when assessing patients' hygiene problems.
- Discuss precautions for minimizing transmission of infection during hygiene care.
- Identify clinical guidelines to use for providing personal hygiene procedures to patients.
- Assess a patient's total hygiene needs.
- Discuss conditions that place patients at risk for impaired skin integrity.
- Discuss factors that influence the condition of the nails and feet.
- Explain the importance of foot care for the patient with diabetes mellitus.
- Discuss conditions that place patients at risk for impaired oral mucous membranes.
- Summarize common hair and scalp problems and their related interventions.
- Discuss how to adapt hygiene care for a patient who is cognitively impaired.
- Demonstrate hygiene procedures for the care of the skin, perineum, feet and nails, mouth, eyes, ears, and nose.

MEDIA RESOURCES

- http://evolve.elsevier.com/Perry/skills
- Review Questions
- Case Studies
- ▶ Video Clips
- Audio Glossary
- Answers to Clinical Judgment and Next-Generation NCLEX® Examination–Style Questions
- Printable Key Points
- Skills Performance Checklists

PURPOSE

Proper hygiene care requires an understanding of the anatomy and physiology of the skin, nails, oral cavity, eyes, ears, and nose. For example, the skin and mucosal cells exchange oxygen, nutrients, and fluids with underlying blood vessels. The cells require adequate nutrition, hydration, and circulation to resist injury and disease. It is also important to understand how patients' health conditions alter the anatomy or physiology of these tissues. Clinical decision making involves anticipating how you can protect patients with proper hygiene techniques. Good, evidence-based hygiene techniques promote the normal structure and function of these tissues.

Hygiene is also important for promoting and preserving mental health. When you deliver hygiene to a patient, it is an excellent time to discuss health-related concerns, perform a physical assessment, and provide patient education. Providing personal hygiene is necessary for an individual's comfort, safety, and sense of well-being.

PRACTICE STANDARDS

- Agency for Healthcare Research and Quality (AHRQ), 2013: Universal ICU Decolonization: An Enhanced Protocol
- European Pressure Ulcer Advisory Panel (EPUAP), National Pressure Injury Advisory Panel (NPIAP), and Pan Pacific Pressure

Injury Alliance, 2019a: Treatment of Pressure Ulcers/Injuries: Clinical Practice Guideline. The International Guideline
- Institute for Healthcare Improvement (IHI), 2023: Ventilator-Associated Pneumonia, Oral Care for Critically Ill Patients
- The Joint Commission (TJC), 2023: National Patient Safety Goals—Patient identification

SUPPLEMENTAL STANDARDS

- European Pressure Ulcer Advisory Panel (EPUAP), National Pressure Injury Advisory Panel (NPIAP), and Pan Pacific Pressure Injury Alliance, Emily Haesler (editor), 2019b: Treatment of Pressure Ulcers/Injuries: Quick Reference Guide
- Centers for Disease Control and Prevention (CDC), 2023—Oral Health in Healthcare Settings to Prevent Pneumonia Toolkit
- American Diabetes Association (ADA), 2023: Foot Complications

PRINCIPLES FOR PRACTICE

- Regular bathing of all patients is essential to maintain skin integrity by promoting circulation and hydration.
- Providing personal hygiene for people with cognitive issues or dementia is a complicated process. It involves identifying physical, emotional, and environmental factors that affect the patient's unique needs and limitations to promote a safe, acceptable, and comfortable personal hygiene process for a patient's skin, mouth, hair, and teeth (Marchini et al., 2019; Mendes, 2018).
- Assess patient's exposure to medical adhesives and risk for medical adhesive–related skin injury (MARSI), which increases risk for pressure injuries (Fumarola et al., 2020).
- Assess for patient's risk for moisture-associated skin damage (MASD). Prolonged exposure to moisture from urinary or fecal incontinence, wound drainage, diaphoresis, vomitus, etc. results in inflamed skin with irregular borders, rash, or changes in skin color (Earlam & Woods, 2022).
- Assess patient's potential risk for incontinence-associated dermatitis (IAD), which is a form of MASD. This includes patients who are incontinent of urine and/or stool and have poor skin condition, impaired mobility, impaired nutritional intake, prolonged fever, and diaphoresis (Earlam & Woods, 2022; Thayer & Nix, 2022).
- When you provide patient hygiene, maintain a patient's privacy and comfort and encourage patients to participate in their hygiene care.
- Bathing the patient is an excellent opportunity to perform a complete skin assessment.

PERSON-CENTERED CARE

- Ask the patient about personal care practices before initiating a hygiene measure.
- Always convey sensitivity and respect for a patient's personal cultural beliefs and habits in the way you provide hygiene.
- Maintain privacy, especially for women from cultures that value female modesty, and provide gender congruent caregivers as requested (Giger & Haddad, 2021).
- Recognize that some cultures prohibit or restrict touching. Incorporate awareness that people from different cultural backgrounds have differing preferences regarding personal space. In some cases, touch is considered magical and healing; others view it as evil or anxiety producing (Giger & Haddad, 2021).

- Depending on cultural considerations and the ability of a patient to help with care, it may be beneficial to involve a family member or significant other in the patient's hygiene so that complete, culturally sensitive, patient-centered care is provided.
- Recognize cultural hair practice and do not cut or shave hair without prior discussion with patient or family (Bowen & O'Brien-Richardson, 2017).
- Skin problems cause changes that affect a patient's appearance and body image. Be sensitive to a patient's feelings while caring for skin problems.
- Be sure to take each patient's preferences into consideration when providing hygiene. Simply asking patients about their preferences (e.g., products to use, best time to perform aspects of hygiene) can create a more trusting and nurturing environment.
- Preserve the dignity of patients with dementia or cognitive or developmental disabilities by shifting the focus of care from tasks of bathing to the needs and abilities of the person, with emphasis on comfort, safety, autonomy, and self-esteem (Bobbette et al., 2020; Sullivan et al., 2018).

EVIDENCE-BASED PRACTICE

Chlorhexidine Gluconate Bathing and Reduction of Health Care–Associated Infections

Health care–associated infections (HAIs) exist as one of the most common adverse events during hospitalization (see Procedural Guideline 18.2). Although the critically ill might be most susceptible, all hospitalized patients are at risk (Frost et al., 2018; Johns Hopkins Medicine, 2023; Knobloch et al., 2021). The proper use of chlorhexidine gluconate (CHG) during bathing has been shown to reduce skin colonization with potential pathogens and can therefore lessen the risk of central venous catheter (CVC)-associated bloodstream infection and the risk of surgical wound infections. Evidence-based interventions for CHG bathing include:
- CHG bathing for preoperative skin antisepsis is associated with fewer surgical site infections (Mohan et al., 2019). A CHG scrub/shower is used preoperatively in the home setting or in a hospital setting.
- Daily bathing with CHG substantially reduces patients' cutaneous microbial burden (Chapman et al., 2021; Knobloch et al., 2021), thus reducing a patient's risk for bloodstream HAIs, including methicillin-resistant *Staphylococcus aureus* (MRSA) and vancomycin-resistant *Enterococcus* (VRE) infections (Frost et al., 2018; Tien et al., 2021).
- Daily bathing with 2% (CHG) (cloths or in bath water) is effective against a wide spectrum of gram-positive and gram-negative bacteria bloodstream infections (Dray et al., 2019) and central line–associated bloodstream infections (CLABSIs) (Jusino-Leon et al., 2019).
- When using CHG solution in bath water, it is important to reserve a bath basin for only bathing and not storage.
- CHG bathing reduces HAI exposure to infected or colonized roommates and prior room occupants (Wu et al., 2019).

SAFETY GUIDELINES

- Patients who are totally dependent on someone else require help with personal hygiene or must learn or adapt to new hygiene techniques. When providing personal hygiene, important safety principles to follow are prevention of infection and patient injury.

- To reduce the risk of infection, always perform hygiene measures moving from cleanest to less clean or dirty areas. (**NOTE:** This often requires you to change gloves and perform hand hygiene during care activities).
- Continence issues in people with impaired cognition or dementia are difficult to manage and pose threats to a patient's skin integrity, increase the risk of falls, and increase social isolation (Wilson, 2018).
- Use clean gloves when you anticipate contact with nonintact skin or mucous membranes or when there is or may likely be contact with drainage, secretions, excretions, or blood. Additional precautions requiring other personal protective equipment (PPE) may be necessary depending on the patient's condition (see Chapter 9).
- Keep all personal-hygiene care items within a patient's reach. When the head of the bed is raised, the bedside stand is usually not within easy reach and must be moved forward. If a patient must leave the bed to go to the bathroom, be sure that there is a clear pathway to prevent falls.
- When using water or solutions for hygiene care, be sure to test the solution temperature to prevent burn injury. This is especially important for patients with reduced sensation, such as those with diabetes mellitus, peripheral neuropathy, or spinal cord injury.
- Monitor laboratory findings such as coagulation studies and patient's medical history of coagulopathies before shaving a patient or administering oral care to prevent bleeding.

THE SKIN

The skin serves several functions, including protection, secretion, excretion, body temperature regulation, and cutaneous sensation.

The layers of the skin include the epidermis, dermis, and subcutaneous tissue (also known as the *hypodermis*), which shares some of the protective functions of the skin. The skin is the largest organ in the human body; it protects the body from heat, light, injury, and infection. It serves to (1) help regulate body temperature; (2) store water, vitamin D, and fat; (3) help sense pain and other stimuli; and (4) prevent the entry of bacteria.

The epidermis, or outer skin layer, is the first line of defense against external injury and infection. Sebum, secreted from hair follicles from sebaceous glands, provides an acidic coating. This acidic coating protects the epidermis against penetration by chemicals and microorganisms. It also minimizes loss of water and plasma proteins.

Two types of sweat glands, the eccrine and apocrine glands, are distributed over the surface of the skin. Eccrine glands secrete a watery fluid (sweat) that helps control temperature through evaporation. The apocrine glands secrete sweat in the axillary and genital areas. Bacterial decomposition of sweat from the apocrine glands causes body odor.

The subcutaneous tissue functions as a heat insulator, supports upper skin layers in withstanding stresses and pressure, and anchors the skin loosely to underlying structures such as muscle. The subcutaneous tissue layer contains blood vessels, nerves, lymph tissue, and loose connective tissue filled with fat cells. Little subcutaneous tissue underlies the oral mucosa.

Bacteria reside on the outer surface of the skin. The resident bacteria are normal flora that do not cause disease but prevent disease-causing microorganisms from reproducing. Because a part of the skin is usually exposed to environmental irritants and is an active organ sensitive to physiological changes within the body, some skin problems commonly occur (Table 18.1).

TABLE 18.1			
Common Skin Problems			
Problem	**Characteristics**	**Implications**	**Interventions**
Dry skin 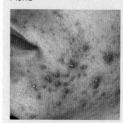	Flaky, rough texture caused by lack of moisture in outer stratum corneum, resulting in less pliable epidermis; most common on anterior surfaces of lower legs, knees, elbows, and backs of hands	Skin may crack, bleed, and become inflamed. As a result, redness, pruritus, and discomfort may develop.	Effective treatment of dry skin does not include limiting frequency of bathing but lies in bathing with warm, not hot, water and use of moisturizers (nonpetroleum). Use super-fatted soap for cleaning. Rinse body of all soap well because residue left can cause irritation and breakdown. Add moisture to air through use of humidifier. Increase fluid intake when skin is dry.
Acne	Inflammatory, papulopustular skin eruption, usually involving bacterial breakdown of sebum; appears on face, neck, shoulders, and back	Infected material within pustule can spread if area is squeezed or picked. Permanent scarring can result.	Wash hair and skin each day with warm water and soap to remove oil. Use cosmetics sparingly because oily cosmetics or creams accumulate in pores and tend to make condition worse. Implement necessary dietary restrictions by eliminating foods found to aggravate condition. Use prescribed topical antibiotics for severe acne.

(From James WD, et al: *Andrew's diseases of the skin: clinical dermatology*, ed 10, Philadelphia, 2007, Saunders.)

TABLE 18.1

Common Skin Problems—cont'd

Problem	Characteristics	Implications	Interventions
Hirsutism 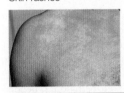 *(From Goyal D, et al: Coffin-Siris syndrome with Mayer-Rokitanksy-Küster-Hauser syndrome: a case report, J Med Case Report 4:354, 2010.)*	Excessive growth of body and facial hair, especially in women	May cause negative body image by giving female a male appearance.	Shaving is safest method to remove hair. Electrolysis and laser permanently remove hair. Tweezing and bleaching are temporary.
Skin rashes 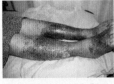	Skin eruption that results from overexposure to sun or moisture or from allergic reaction; may be flat or raised, localized or systemic, pruritic or nonpruritic	If skin is continually scratched, inflammation and infection may occur. Rashes also cause discomfort.	Wash area thoroughly and apply antiseptic spray or lotion to prevent further itching and aid healing process. Warm or cold soaks may relieve inflammation.
Contact dermatitis 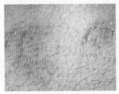 *(From Morison MJ: Chronic wound care: a problem-based approach, Edinburgh, Scotland, 2004, Elsevier Limited.)*	Acute or chronic eczematous rash characterized by abrupt onset with well-defined geometric margins of erythema, pruritus, pain, and appearance of scaly, oozing lesions; appears on head, neck, scalp, hands, legs, dorsum of feet, and trunk	Dermatitis is often difficult to eliminate because person is usually in continual contact with substance causing skin reaction. Substance may be hard to identify.	Identify and avoid contributing agents (e.g., cleaners, poison ivy or oak, cosmetics, latex, shoes/rubber). Treatment consists of removing contributing agent, if identified, and applying over-the-counter topical steroids or calamine lotion. In some cases, prescription steroids may be ordered. Patients may also find comfort with tepid baths.
Abrasion *(From Cottran SR et al: From the teaching collection of the Department of Dermatology, Dallas, University of Texas, Southwestern Medical School.)*	Scraping or rubbing away of epidermis may result in localized bleeding and later weeping of serous fluid	Infection occurs easily as result of loss of protective skin layer.	Nurses should always be careful not to scratch patients with their jewelry or fingernails. Wash abrasions with mild soap and water. Dressing or bandage could increase risk for infection because of retained moisture.

THE ORAL CAVITY

The oral cavity consists of the lips surrounding the opening of the mouth, the cheeks running along the sidewalls of the cavity, the tongue and its muscles, and the hard and soft palate. The mucous membrane, continuous with the skin, lines the oral cavity. The floor of the mouth and the undersurface of the tongue are richly supplied with blood vessels. Normal oral mucosa glistens and is pink, soft, moist, smooth, and without lesions. Ulcerations or trauma frequently results in significant bleeding. Several glands within and outside the oral cavity secrete saliva. Saliva cleanses the mouth, dissolves food chemicals to promote taste, moistens food to facilitate bolus formation, and contains enzymes. Medications, exposure to radiation, dehydration, and mouth breathing may impair salivary secretion in the mouth, which increases the patient's risk for **xerostomia**, or dry mouth. Saliva provides a means for removing cellular and bacterial

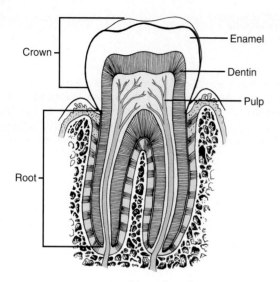

FIG. 18.1 Normal tooth.

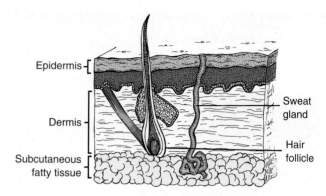

FIG. 18.2 Cross section of hair follicle and supporting structures.

debris that can cause infection, particularly fungal infection. Hyposalivation results in dry mouth, or xerostomia. It affects taste, swallowing, digestion, nutrition, and denture fit and can increase the risk for oral ulcerations and trauma (VonStein et al., 2019).

The gums, or gingivae, are mucous membranes with underlying supportive fibrous tissue. They encircle the necks of erupted teeth to hold them firmly in place. The gums are normally pink, moist, firm, and relatively inelastic.

The teeth are organs of chewing, or mastication. Dentin, a hard, ivorylike substance that surrounds the pulp cavity, forms a major part of the tooth (Fig. 18.1). A layer of enamel, visible in the oral cavity, covers the upper part of the tooth, or crown. The periodontal membrane, just below the gum margins, surrounds the tooth root and holds it firmly in place. A tooth receives its blood, lymph, and nerve supply from the base of the tooth socket within the jaw. Healthy teeth are smooth, shiny, and properly aligned. Difficulty in chewing develops when surrounding gum tissues become inflamed or infected or when teeth are lost or become loosened.

THE HAIR

Hair grows from follicles located within the dermis of the skin (Fig. 18.2). Tiny blood vessels supply nourishment for each

follicle for normal hair growth. Each hair has a shaft extending from the follicle. Sebaceous glands secrete the oily substance (i.e., sebum) into each follicle, which lubricates the hair and scalp. The hair shaft is normally shiny and pliant and is not excessively oily, dry, or brittle. The primary function of hair is to act as the first line of protection. For example, hair protects the scalp from injury. Eyebrows and eyelashes protect the eyes from foreign particles.

Special hair-care practices focus on care for scalp, axilla, and pubic areas. Hair growth, distribution, and pattern are indicators of a person's health status. Hormonal changes, emotional and physical stress, aging, intake of toxins (e.g., arsenic, cocaine), gender, race, nutrition, infection, and certain diseases affect hair characteristics. A person's appearance and sense of well-being often depend on the way the hair looks and feels. Illness or disability sometimes prevents patients from maintaining daily hair care.

THE NAILS

The nails are epithelial tissues that grow from the root of the nail bed, located in the skin at the nail groove. A normal, healthy nail is transparent, smooth, and convex, with a pink nail bed and translucent white tip. A normal color indicates adequate oxygenation to peripheral tissues. Pigment deposits or bands are common in nail beds of patients with dark skin. The feet and nails require special care to prevent infection, odor, and injury. Problems typically result from abuse or poor care. Foot pain can often change a walking gait, causing strain on different muscle groups.

◆ **SKILL 18.1**   **Complete or Partial Bed Bath**

 Video Clip

Bathing removes sweat, oil, dirt, and microorganisms from the skin. It also stimulates circulation and provides a refreshed and relaxed feeling. For some patients a bath is a time for socialization and pleasure, especially for those who are bedridden or seriously disabled. It is essential to regularly offer baths to hospitalized patients to prevent infection and promote comfort.

The European Pressure Ulcer Advisory Panel (EPUAP), National Pressure Injury Advisory Panel (NPIAP), and Pan Pacific Pressure Injury Alliance National Pressure Ulcer Advisory Panel provide guidelines for the stages of pressure injuries and skin care measures to reduce pressure injury risk (EPUAP, NPIAP, PPPIA, 2019a; 2019b). Although these guidelines are intended for pressure injury prevention, they provide sound principles for skin assessment and good bathing techniques.

- Clean the skin at the time of soiling and at routine intervals (see agency policy). Individualize frequency of cleaning according to patient need and preference. Problems such as incontinence, incontinence-associated dermatitis (IAD), moisture-associated skin damage (MASD), wound drainage, or excessive diaphoresis require frequent skin assessment and bathing several times a day. Older adults and infants should be bathed only once or twice a week to prevent removal of protective skin oils.
- IAD is the most common form of moisture-associated skin damage. It is characterized by erythema and edema on the skin surface and can evolve into erosion and secondary cutaneous infection (Thayer & Nix, 2022).
- Avoid hot or excessively cold water and use a mild cleansing agent to minimize skin and tissue irritation.

- Avoid use of force and friction on the skin when bathing patients. Do not massage reddened areas, especially over bony prominences. Massaging causes breaks in surface capillaries, which can promote pressure injury formation.
- Minimize environmental factors that lead to skin drying such as low humidity (less than 40%) and exposure to cold. Depending on a patient's age and physical condition, maintain room temperature between 20°C and 23°C (68°F and 74°F). Infants, older adults, and acutely ill patients may need a warmer temperature. However, certain critically ill patients require cooler room temperatures to lower the metabolic demands of the body. Controlling drafts and eliminating lingering odors from draining wounds, vomitus, bedpans, or urinals also improve a patient's comfort.
- Use bathing as a time to interact with and perform a physical assessment of the patient's skin and other relevant body systems and discuss issues of concern for a patient.
- During bathing, help patients through normal joint range-of-motion (ROM) exercises to promote circulation and joint integrity.
- For patients who tire easily, consider giving a partial versus complete bed bath.

There are two categories of baths: cleansing and therapeutic. Cleansing baths include the bed bath, tub bath, sponge bath at the sink, shower, and prepackaged disposable bed bath (Box 18.1). The type of cleansing bath to use depends on the assessment of a patient's physical capabilities and degree of hygiene required. When a person is unable to perform personal care because of illness or disability, you are responsible for helping with bathing. You can also clean and groom hair, shave a patient, and clean the nails during or immediately after a bath.

Health care providers generally order therapeutic baths for a specific effect, such as soothing the skin or promoting the healing process. Types of therapeutic baths include the following:
- Sitz bath (see Chapter 16): Cleans and reduces pain and inflammation of perineal and anal areas.
- Medicated bath (addition of over-the-counter, herbal, or health care provider–ordered ingredient to bath): Relieves skin irritation and creates an antibacterial and drying effect.

Perineal care (see Procedural Guideline 18.1) involves thorough cleaning of a patient's external genitalia and surrounding skin. A patient routinely receives perineal care during a bath. However, patients at risk for acquiring an infection need more frequent perineal care, such as those who have IAD or an indwelling Foley catheter or who are postpartum or recovering from rectal or genital surgery.

Delegation

Assessment of the patient's skin, pain level, and ROM cannot be delegated to assistive personnel (AP). The skill of bathing can be delegated to AP. Instruct the AP to:
- Not massage reddened skin areas during bathing (EPUAP, NPIAP, PPPIA, 2019b).
- Not soak patient's feet unless directed by nurse.
- Report any signs of impaired skin integrity to the nurse.

BOX 18.1

Types of Baths

- **Complete bed bath:** Bath administered to totally dependent patient in bed.
- **Partial bed bath:** Bed bath that consists of bathing only body parts that would cause discomfort if left unbathed, such as the hands, face, axilla, and perineal area. Partial bath also includes washing back and providing back rub. Dependent patients in need of partial hygiene or self-sufficient bedridden patients who are unable to reach all body parts receive a partial bed bath.
- **Sponge bath at the sink:** Involves bathing from a bath basin or sink with patient sitting in a chair. Patient can perform part of the bath independently. Nurse helps with hard-to-reach areas.
- **Tub bath:** Involves immersion in a tub of water that allows more thorough washing and rinsing than a bed bath. Patients may require nurse's help. Some agencies have tubs equipped with lifting devices that facilitate positioning dependent patients in the tub.
- **Shower:** Patient sits or stands under a continuous stream of water. The shower provides more thorough cleaning than a bed bath but can be tiring.
- **Disposable bed bath/travel bath:** The bag bath contains several soft, nonwoven cotton cloths that are premoistened in a solution of no-rinse surfactant cleaner and emollient. The bag bath offers an alternative because of the ease of use, reduced time bathing, and patient comfort.
- **Chlorhexidine gluconate (CHG) bath:** Antimicrobial agent used to reduce incidence of hospital-acquired infections on skin, invasive lines, and catheters (Dray et al., 2019; Frost et al., 2018).

- Properly position a patient with musculoskeletal limitations or an indwelling Foley catheter or other equipment (e.g., intravenous [IV] tubing).

Interprofessional Collaboration

Wound Care Ostomy Nurse (WOCN) or skin care nurses are able to identify specific bathing and skin care interventions when patients have a pressure injury or are at increased risk for a pressure injury (see Chapter 39).

Equipment

- Washcloths and bath towels
- Bath blanket
- Bar or liquid soap, or 4-oz bottle of 4% CHG (dispensed in a single bath-size bottle)
- Toiletry items (deodorant, lotion). **NOTE:** If using CHG, use an agency-approved body lotion.
- Disposable wipes
- Warm water
- Clean hospital gown or patient's own pajamas or gown
- Laundry bag
- Clean gloves
- Wash basin
- Eye patch/shield and nonallergenic tape (for unconscious patient)

STEP	RATIONALE

ASSESSMENT

1. Identify patient using at least two identifiers (e.g., name and birthday or name and medical record number) according to agency policy.	Ensures patient safety. Complies with The Joint Commission standards and improves patient safety (TJC, 2023).

STEP	RATIONALE
2. Review patient's electronic health record (EHR) for orders for specific precautions concerning patient's movement or positioning and whether there is an order for a therapeutic bath.	Prevents accidental injury to patient during bathing activities. Determines level of help that patient needs.
3. Review patient's EHR for allergy or sensitivity to CHG.	When allergy or sensitivity is present, select another cleansing solution.
4. Review prior nurses' notes to determine patient's tolerance for bathing: activity tolerance, comfort level, musculoskeletal function, and presence of shortness of breath.	Determines patient's ability to perform or tolerate bathing and type of bath to administer (e.g., tub bath, bed bath).
5. Review EHR to determine patient's risk for developing a medical adhesive–related skin injury (MARSI): using adhesive devices or tape on skin, moisture-associated skin damage (MASD), incontinence-associated dermatitis (IAD), age, dehydration, malnutrition, exposure to radiation therapy, underlying chronic conditions (e.g., diabetes mellitus, immunosuppression) and edema of skin, and the presence of erythema, blistering, or excoriation or erosion of skin or rash under or adjacent to adhesive's securing dressing.	Common risk factors for medical adhesive–related skin injury (MARSI) (Fumarola et al., 2020). Erythema, blistering, and excoriation are signs of MARSI and are related to the skin's reaction to an adhesive (Hitchcock et al., 2021; Thayer et al., 2022). Erosion of underlying or superficial periwound skin or periwound area or rash are indication of moisture-associated skin damage (MASD) and IAD (Earlam & Woods, 2022).
6. Assess patient's/family caregiver's health literacy.	Determines degree to which individuals have the ability to find, understand, and use information and services to make informed health-related decisions and actions for themselves and others (CDC, 2023b).
7. Note and confirm with patient any allergies or sensitivities to bath products.	Prevents allergic reactions to hygiene products during bathing.
8. Assess patient's fall risk status (if partial bathing out of bed or self-bath is to be performed) (see Chapter 14).	Allows you to anticipate needed precautions, such as having patient sit on chair in front of basin.
9. Assess patient's cognitive (Mini-Mental State Examination) and functional status (e.g., Barthel index or the index of activities of daily living [ADLs] to measure self-care ability). For patients with suspected dementia, observe for agitation and changes in behavior, especially after telling patient it is bath time.	Functional status assesses a patient's capacity for self-bathing and how much supervision/help is needed to accomplish daily ADL tasks.

Clinical Judgment *Patients with dementia may become agitated and aggressive during bathing activities. Consider using alternative bathing procedures such as bath bag or cloth wipes with these patients (Bobbette et al., 2020; Scales et al., 2018).*

STEP	RATIONALE
10. Perform hand hygiene and apply clean gloves (if contacting body fluids). Assess patient's visual status, ability to sit without support, hand grasp, and ROM of extremities (see Chapter 6).	Reduces transmission of microorganisms. Further determines degree of help needed for bathing.
11. Assess for presence and position of external medical device/equipment (e.g., IV line or oxygen tubing). Inspect condition of skin under devices.	Directs skin assessment to identify potential pressure injury areas from medical devices and affects how you will position patient and plan bathing activities.
12. Assess patient's bathing preferences: frequency and time of day preferred, type of hygiene products used, and other factors related to preferences.	Allows patient to participate in plan of care. Promotes patient's comfort and willingness to cooperate. Using a patient's established routine may reduce agitation in a patient with dementia (Scales et al., 2018).
13. Ask whether patient has noticed any problems related to condition of skin and genitalia: excess moisture, inflammation, drainage or excretions from lesions or body cavities, rashes, or other skin lesions.	Provides information to direct physical assessment of skin and genitalia during bathing. Also influences selection of skin care products.
14. Identify risks for skin impairment: older age, immobilization, reduced sensation, nutrition and hydration, excess skin moisture or drainage, shear or friction on skin, vascular insufficiencies, presence of external devices. *Option:* Use a pressure injury assessment tool (e.g., Braden Scale; see Chapter 39).	Risk factors increase the likelihood of injury to the skin because of pressure, impaired tissue synthesis, softening of or friction on tissues, and impaired circulation (EPUAP/NPIAP/PPPIA, 2019b).
15. Before or during bath, assess condition of patient's skin. Note presence of dryness (indicated by flaking, redness, scaling, and cracking), excessive moisture, inflammation, presence of any drainage, or pressure injuries (see Chapter 39).	Provides baseline for comparison of skin integrity over time.

STEP	RATIONALE
16. Remove and dispose of gloves (if worn) and perform hand hygiene.	Reduces transmission of microorganisms.
17. Assess character of patient's pain (if present) and have patient rate pain severity on a 0-to-10 pain scale (see Chapter 16).	Provides baseline measure. A bath can soothe and comfort patient.
18. Assess patient's knowledge and prior experience with skin hygiene in terms of its importance, preventive measures to take, and common problems and feelings about procedure. (see Table 18.1).	Reveals need for patient instruction and/or support.

PLANNING

1. Expected outcomes following completion of procedure:	
• Skin is free of excretions, drainage, or odor.	Skin is clean.
• Skin shows decreased redness, cracking, flaking, and scaling.	Indicates reduction in skin dryness.
• Joint ROM remains same or improves from previous measurement.	Repeated ROM exercise during bathing helps prevent contractures and promotes joint movement.
• Patient expresses sense of comfort and relaxation.	Bath relaxes patient and removes sources of discomfort.
• Patient tolerates bath without fatigue or chilling.	Fatigue during bathing indicates worsening of chronic cardiopulmonary conditions.
• Patient describes benefits and techniques of proper hygiene and skin care.	Demonstrates learning with ability to repeat back to demonstrate understanding.
2. Provide privacy and explain procedure. Ask patient for suggestions on how to prepare supplies. If partial bath, ask how much of bath patient wishes to complete.	Protects patient's privacy; reduces anxiety, promotes cooperation and self-care as appropriate.
3. Adjust room temperature and ventilation, close room doors and windows, and draw room divider curtain.	Warm room that is free of drafts prevents rapid loss of body heat during bathing. Privacy provides for patient's mental and physical comfort.
4. Organize and prepare equipment on bedside table. If it is necessary to leave room, be sure that nurse call system is within patient's reach, bed is in low position, and wheels are locked.	Ensures more efficiency when completing bathing. Organized work area avoids interrupting procedure or leaving patient unattended to retrieve missing equipment. Provides for patient safety.

Clinical Judgment *Never leave the bedside without ensuring that appropriate number of side rails have been raised (see agency policy). The number of side rails depends on the patient's fall risk assessment; however, having all side rails raised is considered a restraint.*

IMPLEMENTATION

1. Perform hand hygiene and apply clean gloves. Offer bedpan or urinal. Provide toilet tissue and dispose of any excrement properly. Dispose of gloves and perform hand hygiene. Provide patient towel and moist washcloth.	Reduces transmission of microorganisms. Patient feels more comfortable after voiding. Prevents interruption of bath.
2. If patient has nonintact skin or skin is soiled with drainage, excretions, or body secretions, apply new pair of clean gloves before beginning bath.	Reduces transmission of microorganisms.
3. Raise bed to comfortable working height. Lower side rail closest to you and help patient assume comfortable supine position, maintaining body alignment. Bring patient toward side closest to you (staying supine).	Aids access to patient. Maintains patient's comfort throughout procedure. Uses proper body mechanics, thus minimizing strain on back muscles. If patient is overweight, use other caregiver or lift device for positioning (see Chapter 11).
4. Place bath blanket over patient. Have patient hold top of bath blanket and remove top sheet from under bath blanket without exposing patient. Place soiled linen in laundry bag.	Blanket provides warmth and privacy. Take care to avoid linen contacting uniform.
5. Remove patient's gown or pajamas.	Provides full exposure of body parts during bathing.
a. If gown has snaps on sleeves, simply unsnap and remove gown without pulling IV tubing (if present).	
b. If gown has no snaps and if an extremity is *injured* or has reduced mobility, begin removal from *unaffected* side first.	Undressing unaffected side first allows easier manipulation of gown over body part with reduced ROM.

STEP	RATIONALE

c. If patient has an IV line and gown with no snaps at shoulders and sleeve, remove gown from arm *without* IV line first. Then remove gown from arm with IV line (see illustration A). Pause IV fluid infusion by pressing appropriate sensor on IV pump. Remove IV tubing from pump; use regulator to slow IV infusion. Remove IV bag from pole (see illustration B) and slide IV bag and tubing through arm of patient's gown (see illustration C). Rehang IV bag (see illustration D), reconnect tubing to pump, open regulator clamp, and restart IV fluid infusion by pressing appropriate sensor on IV pump. If IV fluids are infusing by gravity, check IV flow rate and regulate if necessary. *Do not disconnect IV tubing to remove gown.*

Manipulation of IV tubing and bag can disrupt IV infusion flow rate. **Do not delegate regulation of IV flow rate to AP.**

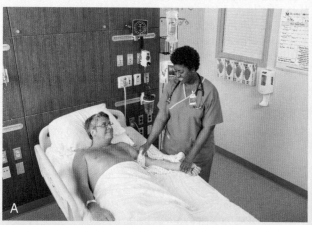
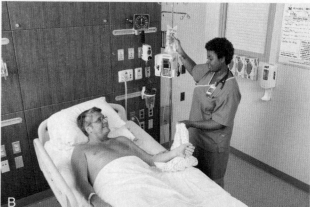
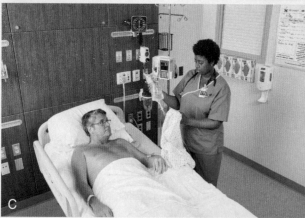
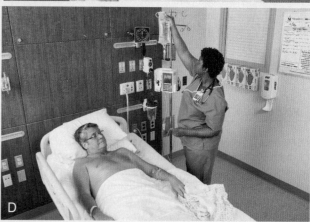

STEP 5c **(A)** Remove patient's gown. **(B)** Remove IV bag from pole. **(C)** Slide IV tubing and bag through arm of patient's gown. **(D)** Rehang IV bag.

6. Raise side rail. Lower bed temporarily to lowest position and raise on return after you fill wash basin two-thirds full with warm water. Place basin along with supplies on over-bed table and position over patient's bed. Check water temperature and have patient place fingers in water.

7. Lower side rail. Remove pillow (if tolerated). Raise head of bed 30 to 45 degrees if allowed. Place bath towel under patient's head. Place second bath towel over patient's chest.

Raising side rail and lowering bed maintains patient's safety. Warm water promotes comfort, relaxes muscles, and prevents unnecessary chilling. Use of over-bed table allows you to move to opposite side of bed without having to move equipment. Tests water temperature to prevent burns to skin.

Removal of pillow makes it easier to wash patient's ears and neck. Placement of towels prevents soiling of bed linen and bath blanket.

STEP	RATIONALE

8. Wash face.

Clinical Judgment *Do not use bath water with 4% liquid CHG added or 2% CHG bathing cloths (see Procedural Guideline 18.2) on the eyes or face (AHRQ, 2013; Chapman et al., 2021).*

a. Ask if patient is wearing contact lenses. You may choose to remove at this time.

Prevents accidental injury to eyes.

b. Form a mitt with washcloth (see illustration); immerse in water and wring thoroughly.

Mitt retains water and heat better than loosely held washcloth; keeps cold edges from brushing against patient and prevents splashing.

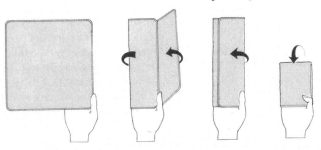

STEP 8b Steps for folding washcloth to form a mitt.

c. Wash patient's eyes with plain warm water, using a clean area of cloth for each eye and bathing from inner to outer canthus (see illustrations). Soak any crusts on eyelid for 2 to 3 minutes with warm, damp cloth before attempting removal. Dry around eyes thoroughly but gently.

Soap irritates eyes. Use of separate sections of mitt reduces infection transmission. Bathing eye gently from inner to outer canthus prevents secretions from entering nasolacrimal duct. Pressure causes internal injury.

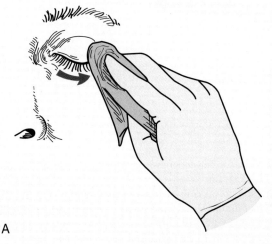
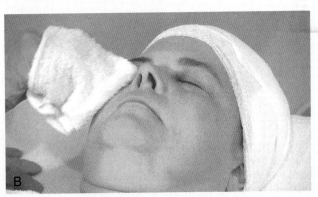

STEP 8c Wash eye from inner to outer canthus. **(A)** Direction for cleaning eye. **(B)** Washing eye from inner to outer canthus.

d. Ask if patient wants to use soap on face. Otherwise wash, rinse, and dry forehead, cheeks, nose, neck, and ears without using soap. Ask men if they want to be shaved (see Procedural Guideline 18.4).

Soap tends to dry face, which is exposed to air more than other body parts.

e. Provide eye care for unconscious patient (see Skill 18.3).

Patients who are unconscious have lost the normal protective corneal reflex of blinking, increasing the risk for corneal drying, abrasions, and eye infection (Kaye et al., 2019; Morris et al., 2018).

(1) Instill eyedrops or ointment per health care provider's order (see Chapter 19).

(2) In the absence of blink reflex, keep eyelids closed. Close eye gently, using back of your fingertip, before placing eye patch or shield. Place tape over patch or shield. Do not tape eyelid.

When blink reflex is absent, patient loses a protective mechanism. Keeping eyelids closed maintains eye moisture and prevents injury (Kocaçal Güler et al., 2018).

STEP	RATIONALE

9. Wash upper extremities and trunk. *Option:* Change bath water at this time. Obtain new 6-quart basin and mix contents of a 4-ounce bottle of 4% CHG with warm water (Dray et al., 2019).

Evidence shows that CHG use in daily bathing can reduce incidence of hospital-acquired infections (Dray et al., 2019). CHG reduces bacteria for up to 24 hours and prevents infection (AHRQ, 2013).

Clinical Judgment *When using CHG in a bath basin of water, use one washcloth for washing each major body part. Then dispose of cloth and use a new cloth for the next body part (Martin et al., 2017). Dipping cloth back into basin contaminates solution and makes CHG less effective. Do not rinse after bathing with CHG solution. Allow CHG to dry on the skin to achieve antimicrobial effects.*

a. Remove bath blanket from patient's arm that is closest to you. Place bath towel lengthwise under arm using long, firm strokes from distal to proximal (fingers to axilla).

b. Raise and support arm above head (if possible) to wash axilla, rinse, and dry thoroughly (see illustration). Apply deodorant to underarms as needed or desired.

Towel prevents soiling of bed. Soap lowers surface tension and facilitates removal of debris and bacteria when friction is applied during washing. Long, firm strokes stimulate circulation; moving distal to proximal promotes venous return.

Movement of arm exposes axilla and exercises normal ROM of joint. Alkaline residue from soap discourages growth of normal skin bacteria. Drying prevents excess moisture, which can cause skin maceration or softening. Respect patient's preference for use of hygiene products.

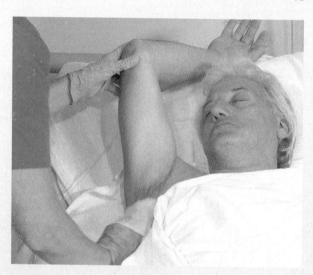

STEP 9b Position of patient's arm for washing axilla.

c. Move to other side of bed and repeat steps with other arm.

d. Cover patient's chest with bath towel and fold bath blanket down to umbilicus. Bathe chest with long, firm strokes. Take special care with skin under female patient's breasts, lifting breast upward if necessary while bathing underneath breast. Rinse if using soap and water and dry well.

10. Wash hands and nails.

a. Fold bath towel in half and lay it on bed beside patient. Place basin on towel. Immerse patient's hand in water. Allow hand to soak for 3 to 5 minutes before cleaning fingernails (see Skill 18.4). Repeat for other hand.

Provides for better access to patient and reduces risk for back strain.

Draping prevents unnecessary exposure of body parts. Towel maintains warmth and privacy. Secretions and dirt collect easily in areas of tight skinfolds. Skin under breasts is vulnerable to excoriation if not kept clean and dry.

Soaking softens cuticles and calluses of hand, loosens debris beneath nails, and enhances feeling of cleanliness. Thorough drying removes moisture from between fingers.

Clinical Judgment *Do not soak fingers of patient with diabetes. Soaking hands of patient with diabetes mellitus can lead to maceration and risk for infection. When a patient has diabetes, gently clear any dirt from under the nails and file across (see Skill 18.4, Implementation, Step 9).*

11. Check temperature of bath water and change water if necessary; otherwise continue. **NOTE:** If using CHG solution in bath water, do not discard water. One bottle of CHG soap is sufficient for a complete bath.

Warm water maintains patient's comfort.

Clinical Judgment *Be sure that both side rails are up before obtaining fresh water. In addition, lower bed when it is necessary to leave bedside.* **NOTE:** *Having all side rails raised is considered a restraint. Check agency policy.*

STEP	RATIONALE

12. Wash abdomen.
   a. Place bath towel lengthwise over chest and abdomen. (You may need two towels.) Fold bath blanket down to just above pubic region. Bathe, rinse, and dry abdomen with special attention to umbilicus and skinfolds of abdomen and groin. Keep abdomen covered between washing and rinsing. Dry well.

Keeping skinfolds clean and dry helps prevent odor and skin irritation. Moisture and sediment that collect in skinfolds predispose skin to maceration.

   b. Apply clean gown or pajama top on affected side first. *Option:* You may omit this step until completion of bath.

Maintains patient's warmth and comfort. Allows easier manipulation of gown over body part with reduced ROM.

Clinical Judgment *If one extremity is injured or immobilized, always dress affected side first.*

13. Wash lower extremities.
   a. Cover chest and abdomen with top of bath blanket. Expose near leg by folding blanket toward midline. Be sure that other leg and perineum remain draped. Place bath towel under leg as you support patient's knee and ankle.

Prevents overexposure. Method of placement supports patient's joint.

   b. Wash leg using long, firm strokes from ankle to knee and knee to thigh (see illustration). Assess condition of extremities. Rinse and dry well. Remove and discard towel.

Promotes circulation and venous return. Assessment is key to identifying signs and symptoms of venous thrombosis.

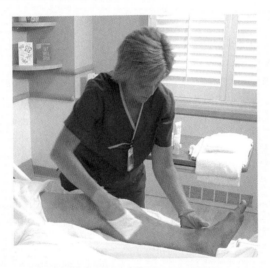

STEP 13b Washing patient's leg.

Clinical Judgment *When bathing lower extremities, assess for signs of warmth, redness, swelling, tenderness, and pain in the lower extremities because these might be early signs of deep vein thrombosis (DVT).*

   c. Clean foot, making sure to bathe between toes. Clean and file nails as needed (check agency policy) (see Skill 18.4). Dry toes and feet completely.

Secretions and moisture are often present between toes, predisposing patient to maceration and skin breakdown. Do not cut nails of a patient with diabetes. See agency policy for podiatrist care.

   d. Raise side rail; remove towel; move to opposite side of bed, lower side rail, place dry towel under second leg, and repeat Steps 13b and c for other leg and foot. Apply light layer of moisturizing lotion to both feet. When finished, remove used towel.

Moisturizers are effective in reducing dry skin; however, in excess they can cause maceration.

   e. Cover patient with bath blanket, raise side rail for patient's safety, remove and dispose of soiled gloves, and perform hand hygiene. Change bath water and/or CHG solution and water.

Decreased bath water temperature causes chilling. Clean water reduces microorganism transmission.

14. Wash back.
   a. Apply clean gloves (if not already applied). Lower side rail. Help patient assume prone or side-lying position using safe patient-handling techniques (see Chapter 11) (as applicable). Place towel lengthwise along patient's side.

Exposes back and buttocks for bathing.

STEP	RATIONALE

b. If fecal material is present, enclose in fold of underpad or toilet tissue and remove with disposable wipes.

Skinfolds near buttocks and anus may contain fecal secretions and microorganisms.

c. Keep patient draped by sliding bath blanket over shoulders and thighs during bathing. Wash, rinse, and dry back from neck to buttocks with long, firm strokes. Pay special attention to folds of buttocks and anus.

Maintains warmth and prevents unnecessary exposure.

d. Clean buttocks and anus, washing front to back (see illustration). Clean, rinse, and dry area thoroughly. If needed, place clean, absorbent pad under patient's buttocks. Remove and dispose of gloves. Perform hand hygiene.

Cleaning buttocks after back prevents contamination of water. Reduces transmission of microorganisms.

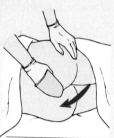

STEP 14d Clean buttocks and anus, washing back to front.

15. While patient is supine, provide perineal care (see Procedural Guideline 18.1). Perform hand hygiene.

Clinical Judgment *At end of bath, if you have used 4% CHG solution, skin may feel sticky for a few minutes. Do not wipe off. Allow to air dry.*

16. Massage back if patient desires (see Chapter 16). — Promotes patient relaxation.
17. Apply body lotion to skin and topical moisturizing agents to dry, flaky, reddened, or scaling areas. — Dry skin results in reduced pliability and cracking. Moisturizers help to prevent skin breakdown.

Clinical Judgment *Massage is contraindicated in the presence of redness and inflammation and where there is the possibility of damaged blood vessels or fragile skin (EPUAP, NPUAP, PPPIA, 2019a; 2019b). Massaging the legs is also contraindicated because of the possible presence of a blood clot, which could become dislodged.*

18. Help patient to a comfortable position. — Restores comfort and sense of well-being.
19. Help patient complete grooming (e.g., combing hair, shaving). — Promotes patient's body image.
20. Check function and position of external devices (e.g., indwelling catheters, nasogastric tubes, IV tubes, braces). — Ensures that bathing activities did not disrupt systems. Verifying position of medical devices helps reduce the risk for medical device–related pressure injuries (MDRPI) (EPUAP, NPIAP, PPPIA, 2019b).

21. Replace top bed linen by pulling sheet and bedspread from foot of bed to cover patient before removing bath blanket. Apply clean gloves if linen is soiled. Assist patient to a comfortable position. *Option:* Make occupied bed at this time (see Procedural Guideline 18.6). — Maintains patient's warmth, comfort, and privacy.

22. Raise side rails (as appropriate) and lower bed to lowest position, locking into position. — Ensures patient safety and prevents falls.

23. Place nurse call system in an accessible location within patient's reach. — Ensures patient can call for assistance if needed.

24. Apply clean gloves and disinfect/rinse and dry bed basin according to agency policy. This is especially important if using CHG solution. Remove and dispose of gloves and perform hand hygiene. — Reduces transmission of microorganisms. Evidence has shown that basins are frequently contaminated with microbes, and some have found that bacteria grew in up to 98% of the basins (Donskey & Deshpande, 2016; Ruiz et al., 2017).

STEP	RATIONALE

EVALUATION

1. Observe skin; pay particular attention to areas that were previously soiled, reddened, flaking, scaling, or cracking or that showed early signs of breakdown. Inspect areas normally exposed to pressure.

Bathing should leave skin clean and clear. If there are signs of skin irritation (e.g., redness, blistering), take steps to reduce pressure.

2. Observe how patient moves extremities during bathing. If necessary, ask patient to move specific extremities.

Provides information about changes in patient's joint mobility.

3. Ask patient to describe if pain relieved (when appropriate) and rate level of comfort (on a scale of 0–10).

Determines changes in level of comfort during bathing and any range of motion (ROM) activities.

4. Ask if patient feels tired (on a scale of 0–10).

Measures tolerance to bathing activity.

5. **Use Teach-Back:** "I want to be sure I explained the importance of keeping your skin clean and dry, especially while in the hospital. Tell me why we want to bathe you daily." Revise your instruction now or develop a plan for revised patient/family caregiver teaching if patient/family caregiver is not able to teach back correctly.

Teach-back is a technique for health care providers to ensure that they have explained medical information clearly so that patients and their families understand what is communicated to them (AHRQ, 2023)

Unexpected Outcomes

1. Areas of excessive dryness, rashes, irritation, MARSI, MASD, IAD, or pressure injury appear on skin.

Related Interventions

- Review agency skin care policy regarding special cleansing and moisturizing products.
- If using CHG soap, it may become necessary to reduce frequency of bathing. Sensitivity to CHG is rare.
- Limit frequency of complete baths.
- In presence of MARSI, use the correct adhesive product based on clinical assessment, prepare the skin, apply adhesive product correctly, and remove the adhesive product correctly (Thayer et al., 2022). Increase frequency of skin assessment. For patients at high risk for infection, use sterile skin barriers and adhesive removers (Fumarola et al., 2020).
- In presence of IAD, immediately cleanse the perineum with a no-rinse, pH balanced, water-based skin care product that contains "surfactants" to reduce surface tension and allow cleansing with a minimum of "friction." When available, use urine and fecal containment systems (Thayer & Nix, 2022).
- Complete pressure injury assessment (see Chapter 39).
- Ensure patient is not positioned over pressure points and medical devices.
- Institute turning and positioning measures to keep patient off pressure injury.
- Consult WOCN or wound care specialist about revised skin care practices, wound care, and/or the need for a support surface bed (Chapter 13) if patient is at risk for skin breakdown.

2. Patient becomes excessively tired and unable to cooperate or participate in bathing.

- Reschedule bathing to a time when patient is more rested.
- Patients with cardiopulmonary conditions and breathing difficulties require pillow or elevated head of bed during bathing.
- Notify health care provider about changes in patient's fatigue level.
- Perform hygiene measures in stages between scheduled rest periods.

3. Patient seems unusually restless or complains of discomfort.

- Use less stressful method of bathing such as a disposable bath (see Procedural Guideline 18.2).
- Consider administering as needed (PRN) analgesic or antianxiety medication before bathing.
- Schedule rest periods before bathing.

Documentation

- Document procedure, observations (e.g., breaks in skin, inflammation, or areas of pressure injury), level of patient participation, and how the patient tolerated procedure.
- Document your evaluation of patient and family caregiver learning.

Hand-Off Reporting

- Report evidence of alterations in skin integrity, break in suture line, or increased wound secretions to nurse in charge or health care provider. Patient may require special skin care.

Special Considerations

Patient Education

- Teach patients and/or family caregiver how to inspect surfaces between skinfolds and explain the signs of irritation or breakdown. Use simple language.
- Include a family caregiver in learning the bathing process. Plan for a return demonstration.

Pediatrics

- Some adolescents require and/or prefer more frequent bathing as a result of more active sebaceous glands (Hockenberry et al., 2022).
- Young adolescent girls should learn basic perineal hygiene measures and know why they are predisposed to urinary tract infections.

Older Adults

- Older adults with incontinence need meticulous skin care to reduce IAD and the risk of infection. The use of barrier creams is sometimes recommended to keep the skin intact and free from infections.

Populations With Disabilities

- When patients are intellectually or developmentally disabled or have dementia, they require specialized preparatory interventions. Avoid actions that trigger restlessness, agitation, or confusion (e.g., sudden change in hygiene time or plan; touching feet, axilla, or perineal area; non–bath-related communications; and failing to prepare the resident for the bath) (Mendes, 2018; Scales et al., 2018). When giving a patient with dementia a bath, follow these guidelines:
  - Do not rush, and speak in a low, pleasant voice, giving information before and all through the bathing process (Rokstad et al., 2017).
  - If agitation occurs, use distraction; bring up a pleasant topic or use other distraction, such as music, singing, holding an object, or eating.
  - Concentrate on the person's feelings and reactions. Pay attention and do not converse with others (Villar et al, 2018; Yevchak et al., 2017).

Home Care

- Type of bath chosen depends on assessment of the home, availability of running water, and condition of bathing facilities.
- In the home, set up equipment according to patient's established routines.
- Patients at risk for falls may benefit from the following:
  - Installation of grab bars in shower
  - Adhesive strips applied to shower or tub floor
  - Addition of a shower chair or placement of a chair or stool

---

PROCEDURAL GUIDELINE 18.1 *Perineal Care*

Perineal care is the thorough cleaning of the patient's external genitalia and surrounding skin. A patient routinely receives perineal care during a complete bed bath (see Skill 18.1). However, patients at risk for acquiring an infection need more frequent perineal care, such as those who have moisture-associated skin damage (MASD) or incontinence-associated dermatitis (IAD), have an indwelling Foley catheter, are postpartum, or are recovering from rectal or genital surgery.

Regular perineal care is especially important for patients with indwelling Foley catheters in the effort to reduce catheter-associated urinary tract infection (CAUTI) (see Chapter 33). Wear clean gloves during perineal care because of the risk of contact with infectious organisms present in fecal, urinary, or vaginal secretions. To avoid embarrassment, always act in a professional and sensitive manner, ask patient's permission before providing care, and provide patient privacy at all times.

Delegation

The skill of perineal care can be delegated to assistive personnel (AP). Instruct the AP to:

- Avoid any physical restriction that affects proper positioning of patient.
- Properly position a patient with an indwelling Foley catheter.
- Inform the nurse of any perineal drainage, excoriation, or rash or other skin damage.
- Inform the nurse if character of urine draining from Foley catheter changes.

Interprofessional Collaboration

- For patients who have skin tears, injury, or IAD, consult with a WOCN or skin care specialist for individualized skin care interventions.

Equipment

Washing perineum: Clean gloves, washcloths, cleaning product, bath basin with warm water, bath towels, bath blanket, waterproof pad, laundry bag, *option:* bedpan (patient may be positioned on pan with cleansing performed after voiding)

Perineal/catheter care: Cleaning product for bath water, CHG cloths (which can be used for perineal and catheter care) or disposable antiseptic wipes, clean gloves (**NOTE:** Some agencies do not use CHG because of concern over risk of mucosal irritation [see agency policy]).

Additional supplies when perineal care is provided other than during a bath: cotton balls or swabs, solution bottle or container filled with warm water or prescribed rinsing solution, bedpan, waterproof bag

Steps

1. Identify patient using at least two identifiers (e.g., name and birthday or name and medical record number), according to agency policy (TJC, 2023).
2. Assess environment for safety (e.g., check room for spills, make sure that equipment is working properly and that bed is in locked, low position).
3. Assess patient's/family caregiver's health literacy.
4. Assess patient's knowledge, prior experience with perineal care, and feelings about procedure.
5. Provide privacy and explain procedure and importance in preventing infection.
6. Gather and organize supplies needed for procedure.
7. Perform hand hygiene. Apply clean gloves. Place basin with warm water and cleansing solution on over-bed table.
8. Perineal care for a female:
   a. If patient is able to maneuver and handle washcloth, allow to clean perineum on own.

PROCEDURAL GUIDELINE 18.1 *Perineal Care—cont'd*

b. If patient has limited mobility, help to assume dorsal recumbent position. Note restrictions or a limitation in patient's positioning. Position waterproof pad under patient's buttocks.

c. Drape patient with bath blanket placed in shape of a diamond.

Clinical Judgment *If patient is unable to assume the dorsal recumbent position, gather three towels. Drape the front of each leg with a towel, and place the third towel over the patient's perineum.*

d. Fold both outer corners of bath blanket up around patient's legs onto abdomen and under hip (see illustration). Lift lower tip of bath blanket when you are ready to expose the perineum.

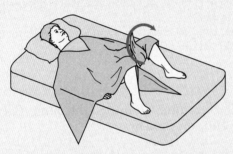

STEP 8d Drape patient for perineal care.

e. Inspect buttock and entire perineum for signs of IAD from urine or stool. Assessment findings include erythema, which can range from red to dark red; blistering or pustules; or skin that is warm or firm on palpation due to underlying inflammation (Thayer & Nix, 2022).

f. Inspect perineum for any urethral or vaginal discharge. When a catheter is present, observe for any discharge on the catheter.

g. Wash and dry patient's upper thighs. (**NOTE**: If agency uses CHG solution for perineal care, do not rinse; allow to dry.)

h. Wash labia majora. Use nondominant hand to gently retract labia from thigh. Use dominant hand to wash carefully in skinfolds. Wipe in direction from perineum to rectum (front to back). Repeat on opposite side using separate section of washcloth or new washcloth. Rinse and dry area thoroughly.

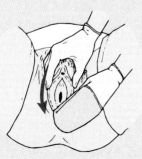

STEP 8i Clean from perineum to rectum (front to back).

i. Gently separate labia with nondominant hand to expose urethral meatus and vaginal orifice. With dominant hand, wash downward from pubic area toward rectum in one smooth stroke (see illustration). Use separate section of cloth for each stroke. Clean thoroughly over labia minora, clitoris, and vaginal orifice. Avoid tension on indwelling catheter if present, and clean area around it thoroughly.

Clinical Judgment *Avoid tension on indwelling catheter if present and clean area around it thoroughly. Follow agency policy regarding perineal care when an indwelling catheter is in place. Currently, cleaning periurethral area with antiseptics is not recommended for prevention of CAUTI, but routine perineal care is currently the standard (CDC, 2019).*

j. Rinse and dry area thoroughly using front-to-back method.

k. If patient uses bedpan, pour warm water over perineal area and dry thoroughly. (Exception: Do not rinse if using CHG.)

l. Fold lower corner of bath blanket back between patient's legs and over perineum. Ask patient to lower legs and assume comfortable position.

9. Perineal care for a male:

a. If patient is able to maneuver and handle washcloth, allow him to clean perineum on his own.

b. Help patient to supine position. Note restriction in mobility.

c. Fold lower half of bath blanket up to expose upper thighs. Wash and dry thighs.

d. Cover thighs with bath towels. Raise bath blanket to expose genitalia. Gently raise penis and place bath towel underneath. Gently grasp shaft of penis. If patient is uncircumcised, retract foreskin. If patient has an erection, defer procedure until later.

e. Inspect the perineum. Observe for any drainage or irritation. Inspect buttock and entire perineum for signs of IAD from urine or stool. Assessment findings include erythema, which can range from red to dark red: blistering or pustules, or skin may be warm or firm on palpation due to underlying inflammation (Thayer & Nix, 2022).

f. Wash tip of penis at urethral meatus first. Using circular motion, clean from meatus outward (see illustration). Discard washcloth and repeat with clean cloth until penis is clean. Rinse and dry gently and thoroughly. (Exception: Do not rinse if using CHG.)

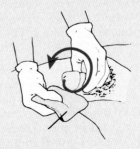

STEP 9f Use circular motion to clean tip of penis.

Continued

PROCEDURAL GUIDELINE 18.1 *Perineal Care—cont'd*

g. Return foreskin to its natural position.

Clinical Judgment *After administering male perineal care for uncircumcised males, make sure that foreskin is in its natural position. This is extremely important in patients with decreased sensation in their lower extremities. Tightening foreskin around shaft of penis causes local edema and discomfort and, if not corrected, may cause permanent urethral damage.*

h. Take a new washcloth and gently clean shaft of penis and scrotum by having patient abduct legs. Pay special attention to underlying surface of penis. Lift scrotum carefully and wash underlying skinfolds. Rinse and dry thoroughly. (Exception: Do not rinse if using CHG.)

i. Fold bath blanket back over patient's perineum and help him to comfortable position.

10. For both female and male patients, avoid placing tension on an indwelling catheter, if present, and clean it thoroughly during procedure (see Chapter 33).

11. Observe perineal skin for any irritation, redness, or drainage that persists after perineal hygiene.

12. Remove and dispose of gloves and used supplies in proper receptacles and perform hand hygiene.

13. Help patient to a comfortable position.

14. Raise side rails (as appropriate) and lower bed to lowest position, locking into position.

15. Place nurse call system in an accessible location within patient's reach.

16. **Use Teach-Back:** "We talked about how to wash your genital area to reduce the chance of infection. Describe for me how to wash your genital area." Revise your instruction now or develop a plan for revised patient/family caregiver teaching if patient/family caregiver is not able to teach back correctly.

17. Document perineal skin assessment and patient tolerance of procedure.

18. Provide hand-off report to health care provider for changes in perineal skin integrity.

PROCEDURAL GUIDELINE 18.2 *Bathing With Use of Chlorhexidine Chloride Gluconate (CHG) Disposable Washcloths, Tub, or Shower*

The use of disposable washcloths impregnated with an antiseptic solution such as CHG is common in acute care hospitals, especially critical care settings. Daily bathing with some form of CHG is more of a standard practice across health care agencies to prevent HAIs.

CHG in the cloths is fast acting, has broad-spectrum microorganism coverage, continues antimicrobial activity up to 24 hours after application, and is rinse free and disposable. Research documents that CHG bathing is particularly effective for ICU patients (Johns Hopkins Medicine, 2023; Ruiz et al., 2017). The cloths are used in many settings and for all bathing purposes, including once-a-day full-body bathing, incontinence care, preoperative antisepsis, or any reason for additional cleaning (AHRQ, 2013). Daily bathing with 2% CHG-impregnated cloths versus nonantimicrobial washcloths reduces cross-contamination and colonization of multidrug-resistant organisms (MDROs) (Martin et al., 2017; Ruiz et al., 2017). Patients often describe their skin as feeling a bit sticky. Explain to patients the importance of using CHG to protect them against serious infection. When using CHG-impregnated cloths, use a clean CHG washcloth/cloth for each area of the body. Disposable cloths reduce the risk of HAIs and multidrug resistant organism (MDRO) contamination of wash basins (Martin et al., 2017).

Although showers are available to patients in acute care, you will see tub and shower bathing more commonly in long-term care settings. When patients use a tub or shower, follow guidelines to maintain patient safety to prevent falls.

Delegation
The skill of bathing in a tub or shower or using disposable cloths for bathing can be delegated to assistive personnel (AP). Instruct the AP to:
- Not massage reddened skin areas during bathing.
- Properly position patients with musculoskeletal limitations or an indwelling Foley catheter or other equipment (e.g., intravenous tubing).

- Report any changes in patient balance and mobility before ambulating patient to tub or shower.
- Report changes in skin or perineal area or signs of impaired skin integrity to the nurse.

Interprofessional Collaboration
- A WOCN nurse or skin care specialist can individualize care for patients when the skin has blistering or redness or is nonintact.

Equipment
Prepackaged disposable CHG impregnated cloths; washcloths, cleaning product, and bath towels (for tub or shower); bath blanket, toiletry items (deodorant, lotion), disposable wipes, clean hospital gown or patient's own pajamas or gown, laundry bag, clean gloves

Steps
1. Identify patient using at least two identifiers (e.g., name and birthday or name and medical record number) according to agency policy (TJC, 2023).
2. Assess environment for safety (e.g., check room for spills; make sure that equipment is working properly and that bed is in locked, low position) and provide privacy.
3. Assess degree of help patient will need for bathing, risk for falling (e.g., ability to stand, get into a tub), patient's risk for skin breakdown, and presence of allergy or sensitivity to bathing solution (e.g., CHG) (see Skill 18.1).
4. Assess patient's/family caregiver's health literacy.
5. Assess patient's knowledge, prior experience with bathing, and feelings about procedure.
6. Provide privacy and explain procedure.
7. Arrange supplies and toiletry items at bedside if using CHG-impregnated cloths; otherwise, prepare supplies and equipment in patient's bathroom or a shower room.
8. Perform hand hygiene and apply clean gloves.

PROCEDURAL GUIDELINE 18.2 *Bathing With Use of Chlorhexidine Chloride Gluconate (CHG) Disposable Washcloths, Tub, or Shower—cont'd*

9. **Bathing cloths:** (This procedure follows the AHRQ [2013] universal bathing protocol for decolonization, used commonly in critical care and acute care hospitals.)
   a. Adjust room temperature and ventilation, close room doors and windows, and draw room divider curtain.
   b. Position patient supine or in a position of comfort. Use a bath blanket to drape areas of body not being cleaned as bath proceeds (see Skill 18.1).
   c. Help patient remove old gown (see Skill 18.1).
   d. *Option:* Warm package of bathing cloths in a microwave, following package directions. Do not use a microwave that is used for food preparation. The cleaning pack contains multiple premoistened cloths. Check the amount before beginning to ensure you have enough.

Clinical Judgment *Check temperature of cloth after warming and have patient check as well to prevent burns to the skin.*

   e. Wash patient's face and eyes with plain warm water (see Skill 18.1).

Clinical Judgment *Do not use bath water with 4% CHG solution or 2% CHG bathing cloths on the eyes or face. Only use clear water or mild soap and water on the face (AHRQ, 2013).*

   f. Use all six bathing cloths in the following order (see illustration), positioning and using drapes as described in Skill 18.1:
      (1) Cloth 1: Neck, shoulders, and chest
      (2) Cloth 2: Both arms, both hands, web spaces, and axilla
      (3) Cloth 3: Abdomen and groin/perineum
      (4) Cloth 4: Right leg, right foot, and web spaces
      (5) Cloth 5: Left leg, left foot, and web spaces
      (6) Cloth 6: Back of neck, back, and buttocks

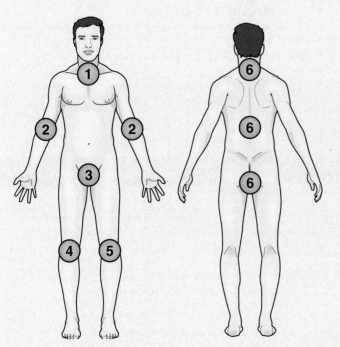

STEP 9f Order for use of six bathing cloths.

   g. Firmly cleanse skin with CHG cloth. Tell patient that the skin may feel sticky for a few minutes.
   h. Ensure thorough cleaning of soiled areas, such as the neck, skinfolds, and perineal areas. CHG is safe to use on perineal areas, including external mucosa. It is also safe for superficial wounds, including stage 1 and stage 2 decubitus pressure injuries (AHRQ, 2013).

Clinical Judgment *If there is excessive soiling (e.g., in perineal region), use an extra cloth or conventional washcloths, soap, water, and towels.*

   i. Do NOT rinse, wipe off, or dry with another cloth. Allow to air dry (AHRQ, 2013).
   j. After application of cloth to each body site, use separate cloths for cleaning tubing from Foleys, drains, G-tube/J-tubes, rectal tubes, or chest tubes within 6 inches of the patient (AHRQ, 2013).
   k. CHG cloths have built-in moisturizers. Tell patient skin may feel sticky for a few minutes.
   l. If additional moisturizer is needed, use only CHG-compatible products (check agency policy).
   m. Dispose of leftover cloths, help patient to a comfortable position, and assist in applying clean gown.

10. **Tub bath or shower:**

Clinical Judgment *Before delegation to AP for a tub bath or shower, assess patient's fall risk status; consider patient's physical ability to stand, get into tub, and review orders for precautions concerning movement or positioning. A health care provider's order is usually needed for tub bath or shower.*

   a. Schedule use of shower or tub.
   b. Check tub or shower for cleanliness. Use cleaning techniques outlined in agency policy. Place rubber mat on tub or shower bottom. Place skid-proof disposable bath-mat or towel on floor in front of tub or shower.
   c. Place hygiene and toiletry items within easy reach of tub or shower.
   d. Help patient to bathroom if necessary. Have patient wear robe and skid-proof slippers to bathroom.
   e. Demonstrate how to use nurse call signal for help. Place "occupied" sign on bathroom door. Close door.
   f. Fill bathtub halfway with warm water. Check temperature of bath water, have patient test it, and adjust it if it is too warm or too cold. Explain which faucet controls hot water.

Clinical Judgment *Do not use bath oil in tub water because this can cause slipping and resultant fall.*

   g. If patient is taking shower, turn shower on and adjust water temperature before the patient enters shower stall. Use shower seat or tub chair if available.
   h. Explain that patient cannot remain in tub longer than 20 minutes. Check on patient every 5 minutes. Remove and dispose of gloves; perform hand hygiene.
   i. Apply clean gloves. Return to bathroom when patient signals and knock before entering.

Continued

PROCEDURAL GUIDELINE 18.2 *Bathing with Use of Chlorhexidine Chloride Gluconate (CHG) Disposable Washcloths, Tub, or Shower—cont'd*

j. For patient who is unsteady, drain tub of water before patient attempts to get out. Place bath towel over patient's shoulders. Help patient get out of tub as needed and help with drying. If possible, have a shower chair available for patient to sit.

k. Help patient as needed to don clean gown or pajamas, slippers, and robe. (In home, extended care, or rehabilitation setting, encourage patient to wear regular clothing.)

l. Help patient to room and to a comfortable position in bed or chair.

m. If patient is in bed, raise side rails (as appropriate) and lower bed to lowest position, locking into position.

n. Place nurse call system in an accessible location within patient's reach.

o. Clean tub or shower according to agency policy. Remove soiled linen and place in dirty laundry bag. Discard disposable equipment in proper receptacle.

Place "unoccupied" sign on bathroom door. Return supplies to storage area.

p. Remove and dispose of gloves and used supplies in proper receptacles and perform hand hygiene.

11. Observe condition of patient's skin. Pay attention to areas that were previously soiled, reddened, flaking, scaling, or showing signs of breakdown.

12. Ask patient to rate level of fatigue and comfort.

13. **Use Teach-Back:** "I want to be sure I explained clearly the need for frequent bathing when you have a fever. Tell me why this is important." Revise your instruction now or develop a plan for revised patient/family caregiver teaching if patient/family caregiver is not able to teach back correctly.

14. Document the type of bathing and patient tolerance and any changes to the patient's skin.

15. Provide hand-off report about any changes in skin integrity to health care provider.

✦ SKILL 18.2 Oral Hygiene

Maintenance of daily oral hygiene, including brushing, flossing, and rinsing, is essential for the prevention and control of plaque-associated oral diseases. In addition to preventing inflammation and infection, oral hygiene in general promotes comfort, ease of swallowing for better food intake, and verbal communication. Brushing cleans the teeth of food particles, plaque (the cause of dental caries), and bacteria; massages the gums; and relieves discomfort from unpleasant odors and tastes. Flossing removes tartar that collects at the gum line. Rinsing removes dislodged food particles and excess toothpaste.

Delegation

The skill of oral hygiene (including toothbrushing, flossing, and rinsing) can be delegated to assistive personnel (AP). However, the nurse is responsible for assessing the patient's gag reflex to determine if the patient is at risk for aspiration. Instruct the AP to:

- Be aware of specific types of changes in oral mucosa (e.g., presence of lesions or open sores) to report to the nurse
- Position the patient to avoid aspiration and keep head of bed (HOB) raised 30 to 45 degrees
- Immediately report to the nurse excessive patient coughing or choking during or after oral hygiene

- Report bleeding of oral mucosa or gums, patient report of pain, and any changes in oral mucosa (e.g., open areas or lesions)

Equipment

- Soft-bristled toothbrush (hard toothbrush damages enamel and gums)
- Nonabrasive fluoride toothpaste or dentifrice
- Dental floss
- Chlorhexidine gluconate (CHG) 0.12% (optional, see agency policy)
- Tongue depressor
- Penlight
- Water glass with cool water, straw
- Normal saline or an essential oil–antiseptic mouth rinse (optional)
- Emesis basin
- Bath towels to place over patient's chest; paper towels
- Clean gloves
- *Option:* Moisturizing lubricant for lips

STEP	RATIONALE

ASSESSMENT

1. Identify patient using at least two identifiers (e.g., name and birthday or name and medical record number) according to agency policy.

2. Review patient's electronic health record (EHR, including health care provider's order and nurses' notes, and identify presence of common oral hygiene problems: dental caries—chalky white discoloration of tooth or presence of brown or black discoloration; gingivitis—inflammation of gums; periodontitis—receding gum lines, inflammation, gaps between teeth; halitosis—bad breath; cheilitis—cracked lips; dry, cracked, and coated tongue.

Ensures patient safety. Complies with The Joint Commission standards and improves patient safety (TJC, 2023).

Conditions may indicate a need for more frequent or specialized oral care with antiseptic or CHG mouth wash.

STEP	RATIONALE
3. Review EHR and assess patient's risk for oral hygiene problems:	Certain conditions and medications increase likelihood of impaired oral cavity integrity and need for preventive care.
a. Dehydration: Inability to take fluids or food by mouth; health care provider's order prohibiting food or fluids by mouth (NPO) for a procedure or because of patient's condition	Causes excess drying and fragility of mucous membranes and lips; increases accumulation of thick secretions on tongue and gums.
b. Presence of nasogastric or oxygen tubes; mouth breathers	Causes drying of mucosa.
c. Chemotherapeutic drugs	Drugs kill rapidly multiplying cells, including sloughing of normal cells lining oral cavity. Mucositis with ulcers and inflammation can develop.
d. Radiation therapy to head and neck	Reduces salivary flow and lowers pH of saliva; leads to stomatitis and tooth decay (NCI, 2019).
e. Presence of artificial airway (e.g., endotracheal tube)	Tube irritates gums and mucosa. Excess secretions accumulate on teeth and tongue.
f. Blood-clotting disorders (e.g., leukemia, aplastic anemia)	Predisposes to inflammation and bleeding of gums.
g. Oral surgery, trauma to mouth	Break in mucosa increases risk for infection. Vigorous brushing can disrupt suture lines.
h. Chemical injury	Results from irritants such as alcohol, tobacco, acidic foods, or side effects of medications (e.g., antibiotics, steroids, antidepressants).
i. Diabetes mellitus	Prone to dryness of mouth, gingivitis, periodontal disease, and loss of teeth.
j. Mucositis: Inflammation of oral mucous membrane	Can occur during chemotherapy and with severe infections.
4. Assess patient's/family caregiver's health literacy.	Determines degree to which individuals have the ability to find, understand, and use information and services to make informed health-related decisions and actions for themselves and others (CDC, 2023b).
5. Ask patient about routine oral hygiene practices.	Identifies errors in patient's technique, deficiencies in preventive oral hygiene, and patient's level of knowledge regarding dental care.
a. Frequency of toothbrushing and flossing	American Dental Association (2022) recommends brushing teeth at least twice a day with ADA-accepted fluoride toothpaste and once-a-day flossing.
b. Type of toothpaste, dentifrice, and mouth rinse used (assess if chlorhexidine is indicated for use)	Antimicrobial mouth rinses and toothpastes decrease bacteria and stop bacterial growth in dental plaque, which can cause an early, reversible form of gum disease called *gingivitis* (ADA, 2023).
c. Last dental visit and frequency of visits	The ADA recommends regular dental visits; however, frequency of visits can vary for each patient and should be determined by the dentist (ADA, 2023).
6. Assess patient's ability to grasp and manipulate toothbrush.	Determines level of help required from nurse. Some older patients or people with musculoskeletal or nervous system alterations are unable to hold toothbrush with firm grip or manipulate brush. Large-handled toothbrushes or a toothbrush handle pushed through a small rubber ball may be of help.
7. Perform hand hygiene and apply clean gloves.	Reduces transmission of microorganisms.
8. Using tongue depressor and penlight, inspect integrity of lips, teeth, buccal mucosa, gums, palate, and tongue; also, assess for gag reflex and ability to swallow (see Chapter 6). Remove and dispose of gloves and perform hand hygiene.	Provides opportunity to visually assess oral cavity and palpate areas of inflammation or swelling. Reduces transmission of microorganisms.
9. Assess patient's knowledge, prior experience with oral hygiene, and feelings about procedure.	Reveals need for patient instruction and/or support.

PLANNING

1. Expected outcomes following completion of procedure:	
• Patient expresses feeling of mouth cleanliness.	Hygiene measures remove secretions and thickened mucosa.
• Oral cavity structures have normal characteristics:	Hygiene measures maintain integrity of teeth and healthy oral mucosa.
• Oral mucosa is moist, intact, and of normal color.	
• Gums are pink, firm, and adherent to neck of teeth.	
• Teeth are clean, smooth, and shiny.	
• Tongue is pink and without secretions or coating.	

STEP	RATIONALE
• Patient describes correct oral hygiene techniques.	Demonstrates understanding of instruction.
• Patient makes choices regarding hygiene procedure and helps by flossing and brushing.	Patient is able to manage self-care.
2. Provide privacy and explain procedure to patient and discuss preferences regarding use of hygiene aids.	Protects patient's privacy, reduces anxiety, and promotes cooperation.
3. Organize and set up any equipment and supplies at bedside.	Ensures more efficiency when completing the procedure.
4. Raise bed to a comfortable working height. Raise HOB to at least semi-Fowler position (unless contraindicated) and lower side rail. Move patient or help patient move close to side from which you choose to work. A side-lying position can be used.	Raising bed and positioning patient promote good body mechanics and prevent nurse from muscle strain. Semi-Fowler position helps prevent patient from choking or aspirating. **NOTE:** If patient is overweight, use safe handling techniques (see Chapter 11).

IMPLEMENTATION

STEP	RATIONALE
1. Place towel over patient's chest.	Prevents soiling of patient's gown.
2. Perform hand hygiene. Apply clean gloves if you provide brushing.	Prevents transmission of microorganisms in body fluids.
3. Apply toothpaste to brush bristles. Hold brush over emesis basin. Pour small amount of water over toothpaste.	Moisture distributes toothpaste over tooth surfaces.
4. Patient may help by brushing. Hold toothbrush bristles at 45-degree angle to gum line (see illustration). Be sure that tips of bristles rest against and penetrate under gum line. Brush inner and outer surfaces of upper and lower teeth by brushing from gum to crown of each tooth. Clean biting surfaces of teeth by holding top of bristles parallel with teeth and brushing gently back and forth (see illustration). Brush sides of teeth by moving bristles back and forth (see illustration).	Angle allows brush to reach all tooth surfaces and clean under gum line where plaque and tartar accumulate. Back-and-forth motion loosens food particles caught between teeth and along chewing surfaces.
5. Have patient hold brush at 45-degree angle and lightly brush over surface and sides of tongue (see illustration). Avoid initiating gag reflex.	Microorganisms collect and grow on surface of tongue and contribute to bad breath. Gagging may cause aspiration of toothpaste.

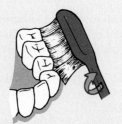 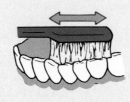 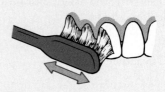

STEP 4 Directions of brush for toothbrushing.

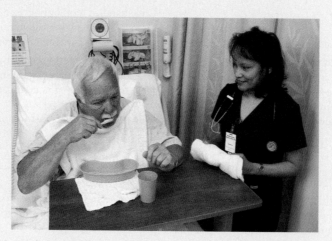

STEP 5 Nurse observes patient's toothbrushing technique, including brushing of tongue.

STEP	RATIONALE
6. Have patient rinse mouth thoroughly with water by taking several sips of water (may use straw), swishing water across all tooth surfaces, and spitting into emesis basin. Use this time to observe patient's brushing technique and teach importance of brushing teeth twice a day.	Rinsing removes food particles.
7. Have patient rinse teeth with antiseptic mouthwash for 30 seconds. Then have patient spit rinse into emesis basin.	An antiseptic mouthwash is effective in helping to prevent or control tooth decay, reduce plaque, prevent or reduce gingivitis, reduce the speed that tartar forms on the teeth, or produce a combination of these effects (ADA, 2023). Avoid using commercial brands of mouthwash that contain alcohol, which is drying to oral mucosa.
8. Help to wipe patient's mouth.	Promotes sense of comfort.
9. *Option:* Allow patient to floss. Floss between all teeth. Hold floss against tooth while moving it up and down sides of teeth. Instruct patient in importance of daily flossing.	Flossing once daily removes plaque and decay-causing bacteria between teeth and under gum line, preventing gum disease. Immunocompromised patients are sometimes on precautions that prohibit use of floss or Waterpik because of dislodging bacteria and possible bleeding of gums.
10. Wipe off bedside table, discard soiled linen in dirty laundry bag, and return equipment to proper place.	Proper disposal of soiled equipment prevents spread of infection.
11. Help patient to a comfortable position.	Restores comfort and sense of well-being.
12. Raise side rails (as appropriate) and lower bed to lowest position, locking into position.	Ensures patient safety and prevents falls.
13. Remove and dispose of supplies and gloves (if worn) and perform hand hygiene.	Prevents transmission of microorganisms.
14. Place nurse call system in an accessible location within patient's reach.	Ensures patient can call for assistance if needed.

EVALUATION

1. Ask patient if any area of oral cavity feels uncomfortable or irritated.	Pain indicates need for further inspection for possible breaks in oral mucosa or identification of stomatitis or infection.
2. Apply clean gloves and inspect condition of oral cavity. Remove and dispose of gloves and perform hand hygiene.	Determines effectiveness of hygiene and rinsing. Prevents transmission of microorganisms.
3. Observe patient brushing and flossing.	Evaluates patient's ability to demonstrate correct technique.
4. **Use Teach-Back:** "We discussed what is important for taking proper care of your teeth and gums. Tell me how often you should brush your teeth and what to use." Revise your instruction now or develop a plan for revised patient/family caregiver teaching if patient/family caregiver is not able to teach back correctly.	Teach-back is a technique for health care providers to ensure that they have explained medical information clearly so that patients and their families understand what is communicated to them (AHRQ, 2023).

Unexpected Outcomes	Related Interventions
1. Mucosa is dry and inflamed. Tongue has thick coating.	• Increase patient's hydration (if not contraindicated). • Increase frequency of oral care, focusing on tongue brushing.
2. Cheilosis—dry, cracked lips	• Apply moisturizing lubricant to patient's lips.
3. Gum margins are retracted from teeth, with localized areas of inflammation. Bleeding occurs around gum margins.	• Report findings because patient may have an underlying bleeding tendency. • Switch to softer-bristled toothbrush or sponge toothette. • Avoid vigorous brushing and flossing.

4. Mucosa becomes inflamed from repeated chemotherapy administration, and a lesion from sloughing of tissue develops. These conditions can also be caused by radiation therapy used to treat head and neck cancers.	• Determine best-practice oral regimen for mucositis and stomatitis. Common regimens used to promote healing and comfort include:
	 • Use fluoride toothpaste.
	 • Rinse 4 to 6 times a day using the following rinses (NCI, 2019):
	  • ½ teaspoon of salt and ½ teaspoon of baking soda in 1 cup of warm water.
	  • Salvia substitutes as ordered by dentist or other health care provider.
	 • If dry mouth (xerostomia) and hyposalivation occur, additional rinses to increase moisture may be used. Brushing and gentle flossing should be continued as well.

Documentation

- Document procedure on basic care checklist.
- Document condition of oral cavity.
- Document your evaluation of patient and family caregiver learning.

Hand-Off Reporting

- Report bleeding, pain, or presence of lesions to nurse in charge or health care provider.

Special Considerations

Patient Education

- Educate patients about methods to prevent tooth decay (e.g., reduce intake of carbohydrates, especially sweet, sticky snacks between meals; brush within 30 minutes of eating sweets; rinse mouth thoroughly with water or alcohol-free antiseptic mouth rinse; use fluoride toothpaste). Use simple language and available teaching materials at proper literacy level.
- Educate patients to visit a dentist regularly (based on dentist's recommendations) for professional cleaning and oral examination; frequency of visits varies for each patient and should be determined by the dentist (ADA, 2023).
- When teaching special oral-care regimens, include family caregiver.
- Avoid mints if conditions of the mouth are associated with ulcerations of the oral mucosa.

Pediatrics

- Every infant should receive an oral-health risk assessment from a primary health care provider or qualified health care professional by 6 months of age (American Academy of Pediatrics [AAP], 2022; AAPD, 2021).
- Have parents start oral hygiene measures no later than the time of eruption of the first primary tooth and perform toothbrushing twice daily. Have them use a soft toothbrush of age-appropriate size and the correct amount of fluoridated toothpaste (AAPD, 2021).
- Teach parents to not place infants in bed with a bottle; this causes tooth decay and ear infections. Choose drinks and foods that do not contain a lot of sugar (AAP, 2022).

Older Adults

- A number of normal age-related changes occur in the oral cavity. Thinning of the oral mucosa and decreased vascularity of the gingivae predispose older adults to injury and periodontal disease. Loss of tissue elasticity and decreased mass and strength of the muscles make chewing more difficult. Loss of the alveolar bone can loosen natural teeth (Touhy & Jett, 2022).
- Some older adults may find it difficult to maintain good oral hygiene with flossing and brushing because of decreased dexterity and decreasing eyesight.
- Meticulous oral care for patients in hospitals or nursing homes with acute illnesses reduces the risk for and death from HAIs (Sjögren et al., 2016; Zimmerman et al., 2020).

Populations With Disabilities

- Oral hygiene may be difficult to complete in some patients with an intellectual or developmental disability including dementia. Establish and stick to consistent oral care practices (e.g., times of day, duration of procedure, products used) (Marchini et al., 2019).
- If patient becomes resistive, stop procedure and return after a rest period (Jablonski et al., 2018).

Home Care

- During the initial admission, document the condition of a patient's mouth, teeth, and gums, thus providing a baseline for assessing the patient's ability to adhere to special diets and fluid intake and carry out oral hygiene practices.

PROCEDURAL GUIDELINE 18.3 *Care of Dentures*

 Video Clip

Denture care removes food and debris from and around dentures. In addition, routine denture care reduces the risk for gingival infection. Denture stomatitis is a common form of candidiasis and is also caused by other oral bacteria (Lodi, 2022). Encourage patients who wear dentures to continue to care for them as frequently as with natural teeth. Loose dentures can cause discomfort and make it difficult for patients to chew food and speak clearly. Offer dental care after every meal and before a patient goes to bed. Some patients are unable to care for their dentures, and nurses become responsible for providing denture and oral care. Dentures are a patient's personal property; thus be sure to handle them with care because they are easy to break.

Delegation

The skill of denture care can be delegated to assistive personnel (AP). Instruct the AP to:

- Not use hot or excessively cold water when caring for dentures.
- Inform the nurse if the patient has any oral discomfort or if there are cracks in dentures.

Interprofessional Collaboration

When poor-fitting dentures cause mouth lesions and interfere with oral nutrition, encourage patient and/or family caregiver to contact a dentist.

Equipment

Soft-bristled toothbrush or denture toothbrush; denture dentifrice or toothpaste; denture adhesive (optional); glass of water; emesis basin or sink; 4 × 4–inch gauze; washcloth; denture cup (for storage); clean gloves; tongue blade (optional)

Steps

1. Identify patient using at least two identifiers (e.g., name and birthday or name and medical record number) according to agency policy (TJC, 2023).
2. Assess environment for safety (e.g., check room for spills; make sure that bed is in locked, low position).
3. Assess patient's/family caregiver's health literacy.
4. Assess patient's knowledge, prior experience with denture care, and feelings about procedure.
5. Perform hand hygiene.

PROCEDURAL GUIDELINE 18.3 *Care of Dentures—cont'd*

6. Ask patient whether dentures fit and whether there is any gum or mucous membrane tenderness or irritation. Ask patient about denture care and product preferences.
7. Determine whether patient has necessary dexterity to clean dentures independently or requires help.
8. Lower side rail. Position patient comfortably sitting up in bed or help patient walk from bed to chair placed in front of sink.
9. Fill emesis basin with tepid water. (If using sink, place washcloth in bottom of sink and fill sink with approximately 2.5 cm [1 inch] of water.)
10. Perform hand hygiene again and apply clean gloves.
11. Ask patient to remove dentures. If patient is unable to do this independently, grasp upper plate at front with thumb and index finger wrapped in gauze and pull downward. Gently lift lower denture from jaw and rotate one side downward to remove from patient's mouth. Place dentures in emesis basin or sink lined with washcloth and 2.5 cm (1 inch) of water.
12. Inspect oral cavity, paying attention to gums, tongue, and upper palate. Observe for lesions, plaques, and areas of irritation. Palpate areas as needed. You may need a tongue blade to see any suspected problem areas more clearly.

Clinical Judgment *Oral mucosal lesions are common in older adults, especially in patients living in long-term care homes. These lesions are associated with local and systemic factors (e.g., ill-fitting dentures, infection). Lesions can occur anywhere in the oral cavity.*

13. Apply cleaning agent to brush and brush surfaces of dentures (see illustration). Hold dentures close to water. Hold brush horizontally and use back-and-forth motion to clean biting surfaces. Use short strokes from top of denture to biting surfaces to clean outer teeth surfaces. Hold brush vertically and use short strokes to clean inner teeth surfaces. Hold brush horizontally and use back-and-forth motion to clean undersurface of dentures (see Skill 18.2).

14. Rinse thoroughly in tepid water. If water is too cold, dentures can crack. If it is too hot, dentures can become warped and no longer fit.
15. When necessary, apply a thin layer of denture adhesive to undersurface before inserting.
16. Reinsert dentures as soon as possible. If patient needs help with inserting dentures, moisten upper denture and press firmly to seal it in place. Insert moistened lower denture (if applicable). Ask whether denture(s) feels comfortable. **NOTE:** It is common for patients to choose not to wear their dentures during an acute illness.
17. Some patients prefer to store their dentures to give gums a rest and reduce risk for infection. Store in tepid water in enclosed, labeled denture cup. Keep denture cup in a secure place labeled with patient's name to prevent loss when not worn (e.g., at night, during surgery).

Clinical Judgment *Dentures are expensive. Help prevent the potential loss of dentures by giving them to a family member, when possible (e.g., when a patient goes to surgery). A patient may not always return to the same preoperative room; giving the dentures to a family member helps avoid misplacement of the dentures.*

18. **Use Teach-Back:** "I want to be sure I explained clearly how to clean your dentures. Show me how you would brush your lower denture." Revise your instruction now or develop a plan for revised patient/family caregiver teaching if patient/family caregiver is not able to teach back correctly.
19. Return patient to a comfortable position. Raise side rails (as appropriate) and lower bed to lowest position, locking into position.
20. Remove and dispose of supplies and gloves (if worn) and perform hand hygiene.
21. Place nurse call system in an accessible location within patient's reach.
22. Document and report any abnormalities noted involving oral mucosa.
23. Provide hand-off report to health care provider regarding any oral sores, oral lesions, or poor-fitting dentures.

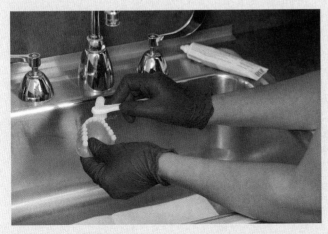

STEP 13 Brushing surface of dentures.

✦ SKILL 18.3   Performing Mouth Care for an Unconscious or Debilitated Patient

Special oral care is needed for unconscious or debilitated patients because they are more susceptible to infection due to the change in normal flora of the oral cavity, increased plaque formation from dryness of the mouth, and decreased salivation. Dryness of the oral mucosa is also caused by mouth breathing and oxygen therapy (Cuthbertson & Dale, 2021). Respiratory secretions are often thick and place patients at risk for ineffective airway clearance, requiring oral suction (see Chapter 24). Secretions in the oral cavity change rapidly to gram-negative pneumonia-producing bacteria, which places patients at risk if aspiration occurs.

Because many debilitated patients have either a reduced or absent gag reflex, providing oral care requires protection of patients from choking and aspiration. The safest technique is to have two nurses provide care. You provide oral care while another nurse or AP suctions oral secretions as needed with a Yankauer suction tip (see Chapter 24). You can also delegate oral care to two APs with proper instructions. Evaluate the level and frequency of oral care needed daily during assessment of the oral cavity.

Delegation

The skill of providing oral hygiene to an unconscious or debilitated patient can be delegated to AP. The nurse is responsible for assessing a patient's gag reflex. Instruct the AP to:
- Have another AP help and properly position patient for mouth care.
- Be aware of special precautions such as aspiration precautions.
- Use an oral suction catheter for clearing oral secretions (see Skill 25.1).

- Report signs of impaired integrity of oral mucosa, including any bleeding of mucosa or gums or excessive coughing or choking to the nurse.

Interprofessional Collaboration

- When there are signs of excessive coughing or choking or an increase in respiratory secretions, consult with the health care provider to determine if patient has aspirated or if respiratory condition is worsening.

Equipment

- Small pediatric, soft-bristled toothbrush, toothette sponges, or suction toothbrushes for patients for whom brushing is contraindicated
- Antibacterial solution per agency policy (e.g., CHG 0.12%)
- Fluoride toothpaste
- Water-based mouth moisturizer
- Tongue blade
- Penlight
- Oral suction equipment
- Oral airway (uncooperative patient or patient who shows bite reflex)
- Water-soluble lip lubricant
- Water glass with cool water
- Face and bath towel
- Emesis basin
- Clean gloves

STEP	RATIONALE

ASSESSMENT

1. Identify patient using at least two identifiers (e.g., name and birthday or name and medical record number) according to agency policy.	Ensures patient safety. Complies with The Joint Commission standards and improves patient safety (TJC, 2023).
2. Review patient's EHR, including health care provider's order and nurses' notes. Note condition of oral cavity, previous suctioning, and any antiseptic solutions used.	Health care provider's order is needed for antiseptic solutions used for mouth care.
3. Review patient's EHR to assess patient's risk for oral hygiene problems (see Skill 18.2).	Certain conditions increase likelihood of alterations in integrity of oral cavity mucosa and structures, necessitating more frequent care.
4. Assess patient's/family caregiver's health literacy.	Determines degree to which individuals have the ability to find, understand, and use information and services to make informed health-related decisions and actions for themselves and others (CDC, 2023b).
5. Perform hand hygiene and apply clean gloves.	Reduces transmission of microorganisms in blood or saliva.
6. Assess for presence of gag reflex by placing tongue blade on back half of tongue.	Helps in determining aspiration risk.

Clinical Judgment *Patients with impaired gag reflex are unable to clear airway secretions and often accumulate secretions in the back of the oral cavity and have a higher risk for aspiration. Keep suction equipment available at patients' bedside.*

7. Inspect condition of oral cavity. Inspect lips, teeth, gums, buccal mucosa, palate, and tongue using tongue blade and penlight if necessary. Observe for color, moisture, lesions, injury, ulcers, and condition of teeth or dentures (see Chapter 6).	Determines condition of oral cavity and need for hygiene. Establishes baseline to show improvement following oral care.

Clinical Judgment *The critically ill patient with an artificial airway and who is on mechanical ventilation is at risk for ventilator-associated pneumonia (VAP). Once intubated, the artificial airway bypasses normal airway defenses, which also causes a rapid change in the normal oral flora (de Lacerda Vidal et al., 2017; IHI, 2023; Zhao, 2020). Studies have shown daily brushing and use of CHG to significantly reduce incidence of VAP (Singh et al., 2022; Cooper 2021) and were effective in preventing nosocomial pneumonia among adult populations in intensive care units (ICUs) (Cooper, 2021; Rabello et al., 2018).*

STEP	RATIONALE
8. Assess patient's respirations or oxygen saturation.	Assists in early recognition of aspiration.
9. Remove and dispose of gloves. Perform hand hygiene.	Reduces transmission of microorganisms.
10. Assess patient's or family caregiver's knowledge, prior experience with mouth care, and feelings about procedure.	Reveals need for patient instruction and/or support.

PLANNING

1. Expected outcomes following completion of procedure: • Oral cavity structures have normal characteristics (see Chapter 6).	Degree of improvement in condition of oral cavity following oral hygiene depends on extent of secretions or changes that existed before care.
• Debilitated patient expresses feeling of mouth cleanliness.	Comfort achieved.
• Oropharynx remains clear of secretions.	Secretions removed, thus avoiding aspiration.
2. Provide privacy and explain procedure to patient or family caregiver if present.	Protects patient's privacy; reduces anxiety. Promotes cooperation.
3. Gather equipment and supplies and organize at bedside. Have AP assist if needed.	Ensures more efficiency when completing the procedure.

IMPLEMENTATION

1. Perform hand hygiene and apply clean gloves.	Reduces transmission of microorganisms.
2. Place towel on over-bed table and arrange equipment. If needed, turn on suction machine and connect tubing to suction catheter.	Prevents soiling of tabletop. Equipment prepared in advance ensures smooth, safe procedure. Supplies within reach create organized workspace.
3. Raise bed to appropriate working height, lower side rail.	Use of good body mechanics with bed in high position prevents injury.
4. Unless contraindicated (e.g., head injury, neck trauma), position patient in side-lying position. Turn patient's head toward mattress in dependent position with HOB elevated at least 30 degrees.	Allows secretions to drain from mouth instead of collecting in back of pharynx. Prevents aspiration. If patient is overweight, follow safe handling techniques for positioning (see Chapter 11).
5. Place second towel under patient's head and emesis basin under chin.	Prevents soiling of bed linen.
6. Remove dentures or partial plates if present.	Allows for thorough cleaning of prosthetics later. Provides clearer access to oral cavity.
7. If patient is uncooperative or having difficulty keeping mouth open, insert an oral airway. Insert upside down and turn airway sideways and over tongue to keep teeth apart (see Chapter 24). Insert when patient is relaxed if possible. Do not use force.	Prevents patient from biting down on nurse's fingers and provides access to oral cavity.

Clinical Judgment *Never place fingers into the mouth of an unconscious or debilitated patient. This could occlude the airway. Also, the normal response is to bite down and possibly cause injury to caregiver.*

8. Clean mouth using brush moistened in water. Apply toothpaste or use antibacterial solution to loosen crusts. Hold toothbrush bristles at 45-degree angle to gum line. Be sure that tips of bristles rest against and penetrate under gum line. Brush inner and outer surfaces of upper and lower teeth by brushing from gum to crown of each tooth; clean biting surfaces of teeth by holding top of bristles parallel with teeth and brushing gently back and forth (see Skill 18.2). Brush sides of teeth by moving bristles back and forth. Use toothette sponge if patient has bleeding tendency or use of toothbrush is contraindicated. Suction any accumulated secretions. Moisten brush with clear water or CHG solution to rinse. Clean lips and mucosa with toothette (see illustration). Use brush or toothette to clean roof of mouth, gums, and inside cheeks. Gently brush tongue but avoid stimulating gag reflex (if present). Repeat rinsing several times and use suction to remove secretions. Use towel to dry off lips.	Brushing action mechanically removes plaque, the sticky biofilm of bacteria that collects above and below the gum line. Tooth brushing used in conjunction with a CHG protocol reduces VAP and other respiratory infections in nonventilated patients (Cuthbertson & Dale, 2021; Singh et al., 2022). The use of CHG oral hygiene protocol is part of daily oral care to reduce the incidence of VAP and should not be omitted (de Lacerda Vidal et al., 2017). The Institute for Healthcare Improvement (IHI, 2023) recommends the use of 0.12% CHG as part of daily oral care in critically ill patients. Repeated rinsing removes all debris and aids in moistening mucosa. Suction removes secretions and fluids that collect in posterior pharynx, thus reducing aspiration risk.

Clinical Judgment *Oral care for debilitated or unconscious patients requires mechanical tooth and tongue brushing and CHG oral hygiene. Patients require the benefits of both oral hygiene measures to reduce risk of VAP, dental caries, and halitosis (Cooper, 2021; Cuthbertson & Dale, 2021).*

STEP	RATIONALE

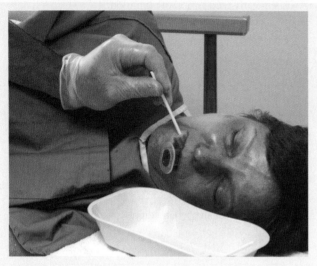

STEP 8 Cleaning lips and mucosa around oral airway with toothette.

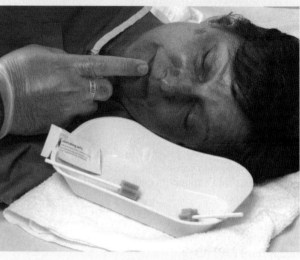

STEP 9 Application of water-soluble moisturizer to lips.

9. Apply thin layer of water-soluble moisturizer to lips (see illustration).	Lip moisturizing is necessary to protect the gums from drying and cracking (Cuthbertson & Dale, 2021).
10. Inform patient that procedure is completed. Help patient to a comfortable position.	Provides meaningful stimulation to unconscious or less responsive patient.
11. Clean equipment and return to its proper place. Place soiled linen in dirty laundry bag.	Proper disposal of soiled equipment prevents spread of infection.
12. Remove and dispose of supplies and gloves and perform hand hygiene.	Reduces transmission of microorganisms.
13. When suction equipment is used, be sure to have a clean suction catheter ready and attached to the suction source.	In case of an emergency, suction equipment is clean and ready to use to clear patient's airway.
14. Raise side rails (as appropriate) and lower bed to lowest position, locking into position.	Ensures patient safety and prevents falls.
15. Place nurse call system in an accessible location within patient's reach.	Ensures patient can call for assistance if needed.

EVALUATION

1. Apply clean gloves and use tongue blade and penlight to inspect oral cavity.	Determines efficacy of cleaning. Once thick secretions are removed, underlying inflammation or lesions may be revealed.
2. Ask alert, debilitated patient if mouth feels clean.	Evaluates level of comfort.
3. **Use Teach-Back:** "I explained what is needed to reduce your partner's risk of choking on secretions in the throat. Tell me the ways you will prevent choking when you give mouth care at home." Revise your instruction now or develop a plan for revised patient/family caregiver teaching if patient/family caregiver is not able to teach back correctly.	Teach-back is a technique for health care providers to ensure that they have explained medical information clearly so that patients and their families understand what is communicated to them (AHRQ, 2023).

Unexpected Outcomes	Related Interventions
1. Secretions or crusts remain on mucosa, tongue, or gums.	• Provide more frequent oral hygiene.
2. Localized inflammation or bleeding of lips, gums, or mucosa is present.	• Provide more frequent oral hygiene with toothette sponges.
	• Apply water-based mouth moisturizer to provide moisture and maintain integrity of oral mucosa.
	• Chemotherapy and radiation can cause mucositis (inflammation of mucous membranes in mouth) because of sloughing of epithelial tissue. Room temperature saline rinses, bicarbonate and sterile water rinses, and oral care with a soft-bristled toothbrush decrease severity and duration of mucositis.
3. Patient aspirates secretions.	• Suction oral airway as secretions accumulate to maintain airway patency (see Chapter 24).
	• Elevate patient's HOB to facilitate breathing.
	• If aspiration is suspected, notify health care provider. Prepare patient for chest x-ray film examination.

Documentation

- Document procedure, appearance of oral cavity, presence of gag reflex, and patient's response to procedure.
- Document your evaluation of patient and family caregiver learning.

Hand-Off Reporting

- Report any unusual findings (e.g., bleeding, ulceration, choking response) to nurse in charge or health care provider.

Special Considerations

Patient Education

- Family members may care for a debilitated patient in the home. Explain to family caregiver how to position patient and perform both manual toothbrushing and CHG oral hygiene if CHG is ordered. Instruction in how to perform mouth care is necessary so that the family caregiver understands how to protect the patient from aspirating while thoroughly cleaning the oral cavity. Use the teach-back technique by observing family caregiver perform mouth care procedure effectively or asking them to describe the procedure.

Pediatrics/Older Adults/Populations With Disabilities

- See Skill 18.2.

Home Care

- Suction the oral cavity with a bulb syringe; if unavailable, substitute a gravy baster or large syringe. Caution family caregiver against instilling a large amount of water or rinsing agent in the oral cavity because of the risk of aspiration. Observe the caregiver using a baster.
- If the patient breathes through the mouth, a soft-bristled toothbrush moistened and used every 1 to 2 hours will keep the mouth moist and fresh.

PROCEDURAL GUIDELINE 18.4 *Hair Care—Combing and Shaving*

A person's comfort, appearance, and sense of well-being are influenced by how the hair looks and feels. Brushing, combing, and shaving are basic hygiene measures for all patients unable to provide self-care. Most long-term care agencies have beauty shops where patients can go for professional hair care. An immobilized patient's hair soon becomes tangled if not brushed or combed regularly. Dressings may leave sticky adhesive, blood, or antiseptic solutions on the hair. Diaphoresis leaves hair oily and unmanageable. Proper hair care is important to a person's body image.

Certain chemotherapy agents and radiation therapy cause loss of hair (alopecia). Many patients choose to wear a wig; however, some choose to wear hair scarves or turbans. Table 18.2 describes common hair and scalp conditions and nursing interventions.

Dependent patients with beards or mustaches need help keeping facial hair clean, especially after eating. Shaving facial hair is a task most men prefer to do for themselves daily. Because some religions and cultures forbid cutting or shaving any body hair, be certain to obtain consent from these patients. Be sure to assess before shaving if patients are on anticoagulants or conditions that create risk for bleeding.

TABLE 18.2

Hair and Scalp Problems

Characteristics	Implications	Interventions
Dandruff—Scaling of scalp accompanied by itching; in severe cases dandruff on eyebrows	Dandruff causes embarrassment; if it enters eyes, conjunctivitis may develop.	Shampoo regularly with medicated shampoo; in severe cases obtain health care provider's advice.
Ticks—Small gray-brown parasites that burrow into skin and suck blood	Ticks transmit several diseases, including Rocky Mountain spotted fever, Lyme disease, and tularemia.	Do not pull ticks from skin because sucking apparatus remains and may become infected; placing drop of oil on tick or covering it with petrolatum eases removal; oil suffocates tick.
Pediculosis capitis (head lice)—Tiny gray brown–white parasitic insects that attach to hair strands; about size of a sesame seed; nits or eggs look like oval particles attached at an angle to hair shaft; bites or pustules may be observed behind ears and at hairline	Head lice are difficult to remove and, if not treated, may spread to furniture and other people.	Check entire scalp. Use medicated shampoo for eliminating lice or permethrin (Nix), available as a cream rinse. *Caution against use of products containing lindane because the ingredient is toxic and known to cause adverse reactions* (National Pediculosis Association, 2023). Remove patient's clothing before treatment and apply new clothing following treatment. Repeat treatment according to product directions. Check hair for nits and comb with nit comb for 2 to 3 days until sure all lice and nits have been removed. Manual removal of lice is best option when treatment has failed. Vacuum infested areas of home. Wash linens in hot water and dry for at least 30 minutes.
Pediculosis corporis (body lice)—Tend to cling to clothing, thus may not be easily seen; suck blood and lay eggs on clothing and furniture	Patient itches constantly; scratches on skin may become infected; hemorrhagic spots may appear on skin where lice are sucking blood. It may spread to other people.	Patient should bathe or shower thoroughly; after skin is dried, apply lotion for eliminating lice; after 12 to 24 hours another bath or shower should be taken; bag infested clothing or linen until laundered. Vacuum items that cannot be washed.

Continued

PROCEDURAL GUIDELINE 18.4 *Hair Care—Combing and Shaving—cont'd*

TABLE 18.2

Hair and Scalp Problems–cont'd

Characteristics	Implications	Interventions
Pediculosis pubis (crab lice)—Found in pubic hair; gray-white with red legs	Lice may spread through bed linen, clothing, furniture, or sexual contact.	Shave hair of affected area; clean as for body lice; if lice were sexually transmitted, partner must be notified.
Hair loss (alopecia)—Balding patches in periphery of hairline; hair becomes brittle and broken; caused by diseases, medication side effects, and improper use of hair-care products and hair-styling devices	Patches of uneven hair growth and loss alter patient's appearance.	Offer patients access to scarves, hairpieces, or wigs. Stop hair-care practices that damage hair.

Delegation

The skills of combing and shaving can be delegated to assistive personnel (AP). Instruct the AP to:

- Properly position a patient with head or neck mobility restrictions.
- Apply knowledge of care for lice, stressing steps to take to prevent transmission to other patients.
- Report how the patient tolerated the procedure and any concerns (e.g., neck pain).
- Use an electric razor for any patient at risk for bleeding tendencies.

Equipment
Hair Care
Wide-tooth comb and hairbrush (Black patients' hair often requires use of a ceramic comb [AADA, 2023])

Mustache Care
Scissors, brush or comb, bath towel, gooseneck lamp, or overhead light

Steps
1. Identify patient using at least two identifiers (e.g., name and birthday or name and medical record number) according to agency policy (TJC, 2023).
2. Review patient's EHR to determine that there are no contraindications to procedure. Check agency policy for health care provider order as needed. Certain medical conditions such as head and neck injuries, spinal cord injuries, and arthritis place patient at risk for injury during hair care, shaving, or mustache care because of positioning and manipulation of patient's head and neck.
3. Assess patient's/family caregiver's health literacy.
4. Assess patient's hair care and shaving product preferences (e.g., shampoo, aftershave lotion, skin conditioner).

Clinical Judgment *According to the American Academy of Dermatology Association (AADA) (2023), Black hair is unique in appearance and structure. It is especially fragile and prone to injury and damage. Braids, cornrows, or weaves do not require combing or brushing but should not be too tight.*

5. Assess if patient has bleeding tendency. Review medical history, medications, and laboratory values (e.g., platelet count,

anticoagulation studies). Bleeding tendency contraindicates shaving with a straight razor.

Clinical Judgment *Have any patient on anticoagulants or who has low platelets use an electric razor.*

6. Assess patient's knowledge, prior experience with hair care, and feelings about procedure.
7. Assess patient's ability to manipulate comb, brush, or razor.
8. Provide privacy and explain your intent to provide hair/beard care. Ask patient to explain during procedure the steps used to comb hair and/or shave. Ask patient to indicate if there is any discomfort during procedure.
9. Gather equipment and arrange supplies at patient's bedside.
10. Position patient sitting in chair or up in bed with head elevated 45 to 90 degrees (as tolerated).
11. Perform hand hygiene. Inspect condition of hair and scalp (this can also be done just before starting shampoo or combing). Inspect for presence of any infestation (e.g., pediculosis). Inspect for drainage from any head wounds. **NOTE:** Apply clean gloves if drainage or infestation is suspected. Apply a gown if infestation is suspected (National Pediculosis Association, 2023).
12. Perform hand hygiene, dispose of gloves (if worn), and apply clean gloves if necessary.
13. Combing and brushing hair:
    a. Part hair into two sections and then separate it into two more sections (see illustrations).
    b. Brush or comb from scalp toward hair ends.
    c. Moisten hair lightly with water, conditioner, or alcohol-free detangle product before combing.
    d. Move fingers through hair to loosen any larger tangles.
    e. Using a wide-tooth comb, start on either side of head and insert comb with teeth upward to hair near scalp. Comb through hair in circular motion by turning wrist while lifting up and out. Continue until all hair is combed through and comb into place to shape and style.
14. Shaving with disposable razor:
    a. Place bath towel over patient's chest and shoulders.
    b. Run warm water in wash basin. Check water temperature.
    c. Place washcloth in basin and wring out thoroughly. Apply cloth over patient's entire face for several seconds.

PROCEDURAL GUIDELINE 18.4 *Hair Care—Combing and Shaving—cont'd*

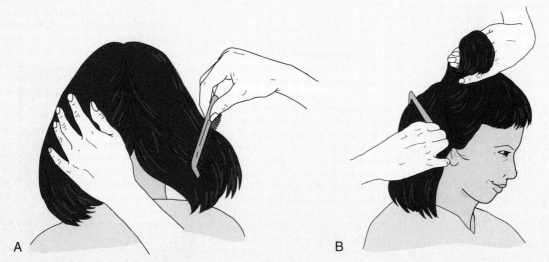

STEP 13a Parting hair. (A) Part hair down the middle and divide it into two main sections. (B) Part main section into two smaller sections.

d. Apply approximately ¼ inch shaving cream or soap to patient's face. Smooth cream evenly over sides of face, on chin, and under nose.

e. Hold razor in dominant hand at 45-degree angle to patient's skin. Begin by shaving across one side of patient's face using short, firm strokes in direction that hair grows (see illustration). Use nondominant hand to gently pull skin taut while shaving. Ask if patient feels comfortable.

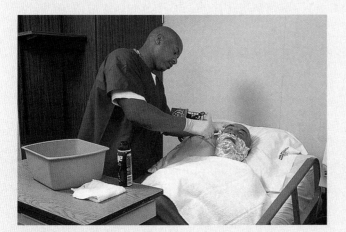

STEP 14e Shaving patient using short, firm strokes.

f. Dip razor blade in water because shaving cream accumulates on edge of blade.

g. After all facial hair is shaved, rinse face thoroughly with warm, moistened washcloth.

h. Dry face thoroughly and apply aftershave lotion if desired. Remove towel.

15. Shaving with electric razor:
a. Place bath towel over patient's chest and shoulders.
b. Apply skin conditioner or preshave preparation.

c. Turn razor on and begin by shaving across side of face. Gently hold skin taut while shaving over surface of skin. Use gentle downward stroke of razor in direction of hair growth.

d. After completing shave, remove towel and apply aftershave lotion as desired unless contraindicated.

16. Mustache and beard care:
a. Place bath towel over patient's chest and shoulders.
b. If necessary, gently comb mustache or beard.
c. Allow patient to use mirror and direct areas to trim with scissors.
d. After completing, remove towel.

17. Discard soiled linen in dirty laundry bag. Remove and dispose of gloves. Perform hand hygiene.

18. Help patient to a comfortable position.

19. Raise side rails (as appropriate) and lower bed to lowest position, locking into position.

20. Return reusable equipment to proper place.

21. Inspect condition of shaved area and skin underneath beard or mustache. Look for areas of localized bleeding from cuts and areas of dryness. If there is an area of bleeding, take a tissue and apply direct pressure for a minute.

22. Ask patient how hair and scalp feel, and if patient was shaved, ask if face feels clean and comfortable.

23. Place nurse call system in an accessible location within patient's reach.

24. **Use Teach-Back:** "I want to be sure I explained to you the risks of using a regular razor at home. Tell me what type of razor you should use and why this is important. Tell me the things to watch for with a bleeding tendency." Revise your instruction now or develop a plan for revised patient/family caregiver teaching if patient/family caregiver is not able to teach back correctly.

25. Document procedure and patient tolerance of procedure.

26. Provide hand-off report to health care provider for an intolerance to procedure or bleeding that continues over a minute.

PROCEDURAL GUIDELINE 18.5 *Hair Care—Shampooing Using Disposable Dry Shampoo Cap*

Sometimes when bed-bound patients need a shampoo, a disposable shampoo cap system is effective. The frequency of shampooing depends on the condition and soiling of the hair. You can use the shampoo cap if the patient is able to sit in a chair or up in bed (check agency policy).

Delegation

The skill of shampooing the hair of bed-bound patients with a disposable dry shampoo cap product can be delegated to assistive personnel (AP). Instruct the AP to:

- Position a patient properly with a head or neck mobility restriction
- Care for lice according to agency policy, stressing steps to take to prevent transmission to other patients

Equipment

Bath towels, clean gloves, clean gown (optional) (if patient has known head lice), clean comb and brush

Disposable Shampoo

Disposable shampoo cap product

Steps

1. Identify patient using at least two identifiers (e.g., name and birthday or name and medical record number) according to agency policy (TJC, 2023).
2. Review patient's EHR to ensure there are no contraindications to procedure. Make sure that a patient's condition does not contraindicate neck hyperextension. Check agency policy for health care provider order as needed.

   Clinical Judgment *Certain medical conditions such as head and neck injuries, spinal cord injuries, and arthritis place patient at risk for injury during shampooing because of positioning and manipulation of patient's head and neck. In addition, patients with positional vertigo are not able to tolerate neck hyperextension as it might increase dizziness.*

3. Assess patient's/family caregiver's health literacy.
4. Assess patient's knowledge, prior experience with a disposable shampoo cap, and feelings about procedure.
5. Perform hand hygiene and apply clean gloves. Inspect condition of hair and scalp before beginning shampoo. This determines if special hair care or treatments are necessary (e.g., dandruff, lice, removal of blood). In trauma patients, inspect for draining head wounds. If lice are present, wear disposable gown in addition to gloves (National Pediculosis Association, 2023). Remove and dispose of gloves. Perform hand hygiene.
6. Provide privacy and explain procedure and what the patient needs to do during the procedure.
7. Gather and assemble equipment at bedside, including pitcher with warm water, shampoo, and extra towels.
8. Raise bed to a comfortable working height and lower side rail on side on which you will stand.
9. Shampooing with disposable shampoo product using a cap:
   a. Position patient supine with head and shoulders at top edge of bed or patient can be sitting on chair or in bed. Apply clean gloves.

   b. Comb hair to remove any tangles or debris.
   c. Open package, apply cap, and secure all hair beneath cap (see illustration).

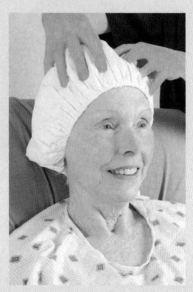

STEP 9c Patient wearing disposable shampoo cap.

   d. Massage head through cap. Check fitting around head to maintain correct fit.
   e. Massage 2 to 4 minutes according to directions on package; additional time may be required for longer hair or hair matted with blood.
   f. Discard cap in trash; do not dispose of in toilet because it may clog plumbing.
   g. If patient desires, towel dry hair. Place patient in a comfortable position to brush or comb patient's hair.
10. Remove and dispose of gloves and used supplies in proper receptacles and perform hand hygiene. Store reusable supplies.
11. Inspect condition of hair and scalp.
12. Raise side rails (as appropriate) and lower bed to lowest position, locking into position.
13. Place nurse call system in an accessible location within patient's reach.
14. **Use Teach-Back:** "During the shampoo we discussed ways to reduce risk of getting exposed to lice in your home. Tell me three ways to reduce the chance of exposing yourself and others to lice." Revise your instruction now or develop a plan for revised patient/family caregiver teaching if patient/family caregiver is not able to teach back correctly.
15. Document procedure and patient's tolerance on appropriate checklist or nurses' notes.
16. Report to health care provider any episodes of extreme dizziness or discomfort in the neck during shampooing.

✦ SKILL 18.4   Performing Nail and Foot Care

Routine nail and foot care involves soaking the hands and feet to soften cuticles and layers of horny cells, thorough cleaning, drying, and proper nail trimming. The one exception is patients with diabetes mellitus or peripheral vascular disease. Soaking is contraindicated in these cases because of the risk for tissue ulceration or infection; soaking causes skin softening or **maceration** of tissue.

When providing nail care, the patient can remain in bed or sit in a chair. In some settings, such as long-term care, or with specific patients, such as a person with diabetes mellitus or peripheral vascular disease, you need a health care provider's order to trim toenails. The risk of accidentally cutting skin around a nail and predisposing a patient to infection is the reason orders are required. Check agency policy to determine whether an order is necessary.

Feet and nails often require special care to prevent infection, odors, pain, and injury to soft tissues. Often people are unaware of foot or nail problems until discomfort or pain occurs. Common foot and nail problems are presented in Table 18.3. For proper foot and nail care, instruct patients to protect the feet from injury, keep them clean and dry, and wear appropriate footwear. Instruct patients how to properly inspect the feet for lesions, dryness, or signs of infection.

Patients most at risk for developing serious foot problems are those with diabetes mellitus, peripheral neuropathy, and peripheral vascular disease (PVD). These disorders cause a reduction in blood flow to the extremities and a loss of sensory, motor, and autonomic nerve function (Manickum et al., 2021). As a result, a patient is unable to feel heat and cold, pain, pressure, and positioning of the foot or feet. The reduction in blood flow impairs

TABLE 18.3
Common Foot and Nail Problems

Condition	Characteristics	Implications	Interventions
Callus 	Thickened portion of epidermis, consisting of mass of horny, keratotic cells; usually flat and painless; found on undersurface of foot or on palm of hand; caused by local friction or pressure	Foot calluses often cause discomfort when wearing tight-fitting shoes.	Refer patient to podiatrist; do not self-treat. The use of orthotic devices cushions and redistributes weight to relieve pressure on calluses.
Corns  *From Weston WL, Lane AT: Color textbook of pediatric dermatology, ed 4, St Louis, 2007, Mosby.*	Keratosis caused by friction and pressure from shoes; mainly on toes, over bony prominence; usually cone shaped, round, and raised; calluses with painful core	Conical shape compresses underlying dermis, making it thin and tender. Tight shoes aggravate pain. Tissue attaches to bone if allowed to grow. Patient may experience alteration in gait because of pain.	Refer patient to podiatrist. Avoid use of oval corn pads, which increase pressure on toes. Use wider, softer shoes.
Plantar warts *From Weston WL, Lane AT: Color textbook of pediatric dermatology, ed 4, St Louis, 2007, Mosby.*	Fungating lesions on sole of foot caused by papillomavirus	Warts are sometimes contagious, are painful, and make walking difficult.	Refer patient to podiatrist.
Athlete's foot (tinea pedis)	Fungal infection of foot; scaliness and cracking of skin between toes and on soles of feet; small blisters containing fluid may appear, apparently induced by constricting footwear (e.g., sneakers)	Athlete's foot can spread to other body parts, especially hands. It is contagious and frequently recurs.	Feet should be well ventilated. Drying feet well after bathing and applying powder help prevent infection. Wearing clean socks or stockings reduces incidence. Health care provider orders application of griseofulvin, miconazole nitrate, or tolnaftate.

Continued

TABLE 18.3

Common Foot and Nail Problems—cont'd

Condition	Characteristics	Implications	Interventions
Ingrown nails *From Habif TP: Clinical dermatology: a color guide to diagnosis and therapy, ed 2, St Louis, 1990, Mosby.*	Toenail or fingernail growing inward into soft tissue around nail; results from improper nail trimming, poor shoe fit, or heredity	Ingrown nails cause localized swelling and pain at the lateral nail; some become infected.	Treatment is frequent warm soaks (exception: patient with diabetes mellitus or other vascular diseases, such as Buerger disease) in antiseptic solution and removal of part of nail that has grown into skin. Teach patient proper nail-trimming techniques. Refer to podiatrist.
Paronychia 	Inflammation of tissue surrounding nail after hangnail or other injury; occurs in people who frequently have their hands in water; common in patients with diabetes mellitus	Area can become infected.	Treatment is warm compresses or soaks *(exception: patient with diabetes)* and local application of antibiotic ointments. Paronychia can be prevented by careful manicuring.
Foot odors	Result of excess perspiration promoting microorganism growth and possibly faulty foot hygiene or improper footwear	Odor frequently embarrasses patient. Excess perspiration causes discomfort.	Frequent washing, use of foot deodorants and powders, and clean footwear prevent or reduce this problem.

healing and promotes risk for infection. The development of diabetic foot ulcers has three contributing factors: (1) peripheral neuropathy (changes in the function and efficiency of the nerves), (2) ischemia (decrease in the blood flow related to plaque formation in arteries), and (3) a pivotal event (trauma caused by banging the toe or stepping on a foreign object). If foot ulcers do not heal, they can become infected quickly and lead to gangrene and subsequent amputation.

People with peripheral vascular disease and diabetes develop many types of foot complications associated with nerve damage and poor blood flow to the lower extremities. Foot injuries in these patients can quickly turn into a serious problem with slow healing, infection, and the possibility of amputation. Advise patients to follow the American Diabetic Association (2022) guidelines in a routine foot and nail care program (see Patient Education section following Skill 18.4).

Delegation

The skill of nail and foot care of patients *without diabetes mellitus, peripheral vascular disease*, or *circulatory compromise* can be delegated to assistive personnel (AP). Instruct the AP to:
- Not trim patient's nails (unless permitted by agency or health care provider).

- Use special considerations for patient positioning.
- Report any breaks in skin, redness, numbness, swelling, or pain to the nurse.

Interprofessional Collaboration

A podiatrist or diabetic foot care specialist can recommend patient-specific foot care assessments and treatments for patients with PVD, diabetes mellitus, and foot ulcers.

Equipment

- Wash basin
- Emesis basin
- Washcloth and towel
- Nail clippers (check agency policy)
- Soft nail or cuticle brush
- Plastic applicator stick
- Emery board or nail file
- Body lotion
- Disposable bathmat
- Clean gloves

STEP	RATIONALE

ASSESSMENT

1. Identify patient using at least two identifiers (e.g., name and birthday or name and medical record number) according to agency policy.	Ensures patient safety. Complies with The Joint Commission standards and improves patient safety (TJC, 2023).
2. Review patient's EHR, including health care provider's order and nurses' notes. Verify health care provider's order for cutting nails (check agency policy).	Many agencies require a health care provider's order before you can trim nails. A podiatrist should assess and develop a regular schedule for nail care for patients with vascular insufficiency or peripheral neuropathy.

STEP	RATIONALE
3. Review EHR for patient's risk for foot or nail problems.	Certain conditions increase likelihood of foot or nail problems because of circulatory changes or patient's ability to perform self-care (Beuscher, 2022).
a. Older adult	Normal physiological changes such as poor vision, lack of coordination, or inability to bend over contribute to difficulty in performing foot and nail care (Touhy & Jett, 2022). Normal physiological changes of aging can result in brittle nails. Discolored, extremely thickened, and deformed nails can indicate infection, fungus, or disease (Beuscher et al., 2021).
b. Diabetes mellitus, peripheral vascular disease (PVD)	Vascular changes reduce blood flow to peripheral tissues and reduces sensation to the feet. Break in skin integrity places patient with diabetes mellitus and PVD at high risk for skin infection (ADA, 2023).
c. Heart failure, renal disease	Both conditions increase tissue edema, particularly in dependent areas (e.g., feet). Edema reduces blood flow to neighboring tissues.
d. Cerebrovascular accident (stroke)	Presence of residual foot or leg weakness or paralysis results in altered gait and walking patterns, both of which increase friction and pressure on feet.
e. History of lower extremity arterial disease and leg pain	Claudicating pain is related to ischemia with diabetic and neuropathic disorders.
f. Immunosuppression, such as HIV or a result of chemotherapy	Immunosuppression reduces body's ability to fight infection. Poorly fitting shoes, infected toenails, and injury to the skin of a patient's foot increase the risk for severe infection and mobility issues (Beuscher, 2022).
4. Assess environment for safety (check room for spills, make sure equipment is working properly, bed is locked and in low position).	Reduces risk for falls.
5. Assess patient's/family caregiver's health literacy.	Determines degree to which individuals have the ability to find, understand, and use information and services to make informed health-related decisions and actions for themselves and others (CDC, 2023b).
6. Assess patient's foot and nail care practices for existing foot problems (e.g., home remedies such as cutting corns with razor blade or scissors, applying adhesive tape on foot, or using oval corn pads on toes). Use this time to instruct patients about foot care.	Identifies self-care practices that place patient at risk for foot injuries.
7. Assess type of home remedies that patient uses for existing foot problems:	Certain preparations or applications cause more injury to soft tissue than initial foot problem.
a. Over-the-counter liquid preparations to remove corns	Liquid preparations cause burns and ulcerations.
b. Cutting corns or calluses with razor blade or scissors	Cutting corns or calluses sometimes results in infection caused by a break in skin integrity. The patient with diabetes or any patient with decreased peripheral circulation has an increased risk for infection secondary to a break in skin integrity (Beuscher, 2021).
c. Use of oval corn pads	Oval pads exert pressure on toes, thereby decreasing circulation to surrounding tissues.
d. Application of adhesive tape	Skin of older adult is thin and delicate and prone to tearing when adhesive tape is removed.
8. Ask patients whether they use nail polish and polish remover frequently.	Chemicals in these products cause excessive drying of nails.
9. Assess type of footwear patient wears: Does patient wear socks? Compression hose? Are shoes tight or ill fitting? Are garters or knee-high nylons worn? Is footwear clean?	Properly fitting shoes reduce patients' risks for foot and nail problems (e.g., infection, areas of friction, ulcerations). These conditions decrease mobility and increase risk for amputation in patients with diabetes (Beuscher, 2021; Chapman, 2017).
10. If possible, observe patients walking to assess their gait.	Alterations in bony structures of the foot, excessive nail growth, or sores often cause pain, imbalance, and unsteady gait.

STEP	RATIONALE
11. Perform hand hygiene. Apply clean gloves if drainage present. Inspect all surfaces of fingers, toes, feet, and nails. Pay particular attention to areas of dryness, inflammation, or cracking. Also inspect areas between toes, heels, and soles of feet.	Reduces transmission of microorganisms. Integrity of feet and nails determines frequency and level of hygiene required. Heels, soles, and sides of feet are prone to irritation from ill-fitting shoes.
12. Assess color and temperature of toes, feet, and fingers. Assess capillary refill of nails. Palpate radial and ulnar pulse of each hand and dorsalis pedis pulse of foot; note character of pulses (see Chapter 6). Remove and dispose of gloves (if worn). Perform hand hygiene.	Assesses adequacy of blood flow to extremities. Circulatory alterations often change integrity of nails and increase patient's chance of localized infection when break in skin integrity occurs. Reduces transmission of microorganisms.

Clinical Judgment *Patients with PVD or diabetes mellitus, older adults, and patients with a suppressed immune system often require nail care from a specialist to reduce the risk of tissue injury and infection. Defer care other than washing the feet in these cases until patient has an evaluation by a foot specialist.*

STEP	RATIONALE
13. Assess patient or family caregiver's ability to care for nails or feet: visual alterations, fatigue, and musculoskeletal weakness.	Extent of patient's ability to perform self-care determines degree of help required from nurse and need to educate family caregiver.
14. Assess patient's knowledge, prior experience with nail and foot care, and feelings about procedure.	Reveals need for patient instruction and/or support.

PLANNING

1. Expected outcomes following completion of procedure:	
• Nails are smooth. Cuticles and tissues surrounding nail are clear and of normal color. Surfaces of feet are smooth.	Excess skin layers are removed. Nail integrity and cleanliness are maintained.
• Patient walks freely, without pain or unusual gait.	Foot care removes excess skin layers or shortens nails so that patient can walk more comfortably.
• Patient explains or demonstrates nail care correctly.	Patient learns self-care skill.
2. Provide privacy and explain procedure to patient, including fact that proper soaking of nails on hands requires several minutes in warm water. **Exception:** Patients with diabetes mellitus do not soak hands or feet.	Protects patient's privacy, reduces anxiety, and promotes cooperation. Patient must be willing to place fingers in basin up to 10 minutes. Patient may become anxious or tired.
3. Gather and organize equipment and supplies at bedside on over-bed table.	Avoids interrupting procedure or leaving patient unattended to retrieve missing equipment.

IMPLEMENTATION

1. Help ambulatory patient sit in chair and place disposable bathmat on floor under patient's feet. Help bedfast patient to supine position with head of bed elevated 45 degrees and place waterproof pad on mattress (keep side rail up until ready to begin).	Sitting in chair facilitates immersing feet in basin. Bathmat or towel protects feet from exposure to soil or microorganisms on floor; towel lessens chance of splashing water on floor or bed.
2. Fill wash basin with warm water. Test water temperature. Place basin on floor or lower the side rail and place basin on pad on mattress. Be sure patient can bend knees and place one foot in basin at a time. If patient has diabetes mellitus, peripheral neuropathy, or PVD, go to Step 11 to begin foot care.	Prevents accidental burns to patient's skin.

Clinical Judgment *Do not soak the feet of patients with diabetes mellitus or peripheral vascular disease or it may lead to maceration (excessive softening of the skin) and drying of the skin (ADA, 2023; Beuscher, 2021), leading to tissue breakdown and infection.*

3. Adjust over-bed table to low position and place it over patient's lap.	Easy access prevents accidental spills.
4. Instruct patient to place fingers in emesis basin and arms in a comfortable position.	Prolonged positioning causes discomfort unless normal anatomical alignment is maintained.
5. Allow feet and fingernails to soak 3 to 5 minutes. If patient has diabetes mellitus, peripheral neuropathy, or PVD, skip soaking and go straight to Step 11.	Goal is to soften debris beneath nails so that it can be removed easily.
6. Perform hand hygiene and apply clean gloves. Clean gently under fingernails with end of plastic applicator stick while fingers are immersed (see illustration).	Removes debris under nails that harbors microorganisms.

STEP	RATIONALE

Clinical Judgment *Check agency policy for appropriate process for cleaning beneath nails. Do not use an orange stick or end of cotton swab; these splinter and can cause injury.*

7. Use soft cuticle brush or nailbrush to clean around cuticles to decrease overgrowth.

Nailbrush helps to prevent inflammation and injury to cuticles. The cuticle slowly grows over the nail and must be pushed back with a soft nail brush regularly.

8. Remove emesis basin and dry fingers thoroughly.

Thorough drying impedes fungal growth and prevents maceration of tissues.

9. File fingernails straight across and even with tops of fingers. If permitted by agency policy, use nail clippers and clip fingernails straight across and even with tops of fingers (see illustration) and then smooth nail using file. Use disposable emery board and file nail to ensure that there are no sharp corners.

Filing nail straight across to eliminate sharp nail edges minimizes risk that nail can injure the adjacent tissue (Beuscher, 2021).

Shaping corners of nails damages tissues, which increases the risk for infection (Jeffcoate et al., 2018).

Clinical Judgment *Check agency policy on nail care regarding filing and trimming. When a patient has thickened or misshaped nails, a podiatrist, wound care nurse, or nurse who specializes in nail care should provide foot and toenail care (Beuscher, 2022).*

10. Move over-bed table away from patient.
11. Perform hand hygiene and apply clean gloves. Begin foot care by scrubbing callused areas of feet with washcloth. Clean between toes with washcloth.

Provides easier access to feet. Friction removes dead skin layers.

12. Dry feet thoroughly and clean under toenails (see Step 6).

Nails harbor debris and dirt and are a source of potential infection from poor care habits (Ball et al., 2023).

13. Trim toenails using procedures in Step 9. Do not file corners of toenails. Check agency policy for trimming patient's nails.

Shaping corners of toenails damages tissues, which increases the risk for infection (Beuscher, 2022; Jeffcoate et al., 2018).

14. Apply lotion to feet and hands. Rub in thoroughly. Do not leave excess lotion between toes.

Lotion lubricates dry skin by helping to retain moisture.

15. Help patient to a comfortable position in bed.

Restores comfort and sense of well-being.

16. Raise side rails (as appropriate) and lower bed to lowest position, locking into position.

Ensures patient safety and prevents falls.

17. Place nurse call system in an accessible location within patient's reach.

Ensures patient can call for assistance if needed.

18. Clean equipment according to organizational policy and return equipment to proper place. Remove and dispose of supplies and gloves and perform hand hygiene.

Reduces transmission of microorganisms.

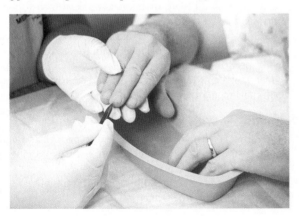

STEP 6 Clean under fingernails.

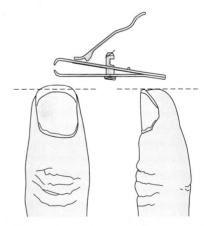

STEP 9 Trim nails straight across when using nail clipper.

EVALUATION

1. Inspect nails, areas between fingers and toes, and surrounding skin surfaces.

Inspection enables you to evaluate condition of skin and nails and allows you to note any remaining rough nail edges.

2. If possible, have patient stand and walk and describe any discomfort.

Evaluates if nail care removed excess skin or uneven nail surfaces that can cause discomfort.

3. Observe patient's walk after foot and nail care.

Evaluate level of comfort and mobility achieved.

STEP	RATIONALE
4. **Use Teach-Back:** "We discussed how to prevent infection in the skin around your nails. This is important because you have diabetes. Tell me the tips you should follow to protect your feet from infection." Revise your instruction now or develop a plan for revised patient/family caregiver teaching if patient/family caregiver is not able to teach back correctly.	Teach-back is a technique for health care providers to ensure that they have explained medical information clearly so that patients and their families understand what is communicated to them (AHRQ, 2023).

Unexpected Outcomes	Related Interventions
1. Cuticles and surrounding tissues are inflamed and tender to touch.	• Repeat nail care. • Evaluate need for antifungal cream.
2. Localized areas of tenderness occur on feet with calluses or corns at point of friction.	• Change in footwear or corrective foot surgery may be needed for permanent improvement in calluses or corns. • Refer patient to podiatrist.
3. Ulcerations involving toes or feet may remain.	• Institute wound care policies (see Chapters 39 and 40). • Consult with wound care specialist and/or podiatrist. • Increase frequency of assessment and hygiene.

Documentation

- Document procedure and observations of condition of nails and skin around nails.
- Document your evaluation of patient and family caregiver learning.

Hand-Off Reporting

- Report any areas of discomfort, breaks in skin, or ulcerations to nurse in charge or health care provider.

Special Considerations

Patient Education

- Use a variety of teaching formats regarding foot and nail care (e.g., brochures, videos, DVDs) that are consistent with patient's health literacy level. Instruct patient not to walk barefoot or use corn or callus products. Include family caregiver in foot and nail care education.
- Instruct a patient with diabetes mellitus, peripheral neuropathy, or PVD to do the following (American Diabetes Association [ADA], 2023):
  - Check your feet every day. Look at your bare feet for red spots, cuts, swelling, and blisters. If you cannot see the bottoms of your feet, use a mirror or ask someone for help.
  - Be more active. Plan a physical activity program with your health care team.
  - Ask your doctor about Medicare coverage for special shoes.
  - Wash your feet every day. Dry them carefully, especially between the toes. Keep your skin soft and smooth. Rub a thin coat of skin lotion over the tops and bottoms of your feet but not between your toes.
  - If you can see and reach your toenails, trim them when needed.
  - Wear shoes and socks at all times. Never walk barefoot.
  - Wear comfortable shoes that fit well and protect your feet. Check inside your shoes before wearing them. Make sure that the lining is smooth and there are no objects inside.
  - Protect your feet from hot and cold. Wear shoes at the beach or on hot pavement.
  - Do not put your feet into hot water. Test water before putting your feet in it just as you would before bathing a baby.

- Never use hot water bottles, heating pads, or electric blankets. You can burn your feet without realizing it.
- Put your feet up when sitting. Wiggle your toes and move your ankles up and down for 5 minutes 2 or 3 times a day. Do not cross your legs for long periods of time.
- Do not smoke.

Pediatrics

- Teach a parent how to assess a child's nails and trim them to prevent the child from scratching the skin.
- Use appropriate-size clippers for infants and small children (check agency policy). *Do not use scissors.*

Older Adults

- Changes in aging skin include thinning of epidermis and subcutaneous fat and dryness because of decreased activity of oil and sweat glands. These changes are often evident in the feet. In addition, nails become discolored, thickened, deformed, and brittle.
- PVD, peripheral neuropathy, and long periods of limited exercise or bed rest impact balance, stability, and sensory impairment, resulting in impaired mobility.
- Older adults may lose the dexterity and coordination needed to trim nails regularly.

Populations With Disabilities

- Carefully explain nail care procedure to patient and family. In many instances, family presence can assist in keeping patient calm and cooperative during procedure.
- If patient becomes confused or agitated, stop nail care, and reinitiate care at another time.

Home Care

- Assess the home for any areas where a person could accidentally injure the feet such as rugs, objects that block pathways, or uneven walks or flooring.
- Encourage patients to not go barefoot or wear open-toed shoes.
- Place contact information of podiatrist, health care provider, and home care nurse close by for easy access.

PROCEDURAL GUIDELINE 18.6 *Making an Occupied Bed*

The hospital bed is the piece of equipment a patient uses the most. It should be comfortable and safe, as well as adaptable to various positions. The typical hospital bed consists of a firm mattress on a metal frame that you can raise or lower horizontally. The frame is divided into three sections so that the operator can raise and lower the head and foot of the bed separately and incline the entire bed with the head up or down to change the bed position (Table 18.4). Four casters allow you to move the bed easily. Each caster has a brake to make sure the bed is stationary. Beds have side rails that you can raise or lower by pushing or

TABLE 18.4		
Common Bed Positions		
Position	**Description**	**Uses**
Fowler 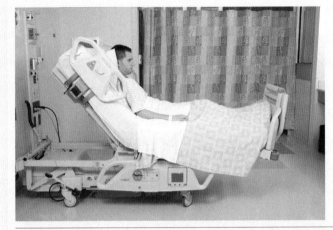	Head of bed raised to angle of 45 to 90 degrees; semisitting position; foot of bed may also raise at knee	Preferred while patient eats; used during nasogastric tube insertion and nasotracheal suction; promotes lung expansion
Semi-Fowler 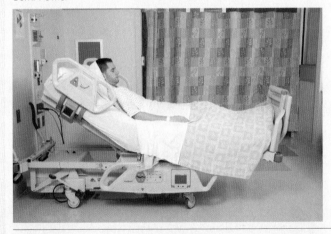	Head of bed raised approximately 30 to 45 degrees; incline less than Fowler position; foot of bed may also raise at knee	Promotes lung expansion; relieves strain on abdominal muscles Used when patients receive gastric feedings to reduce risk for aspiration
Trendelenburg 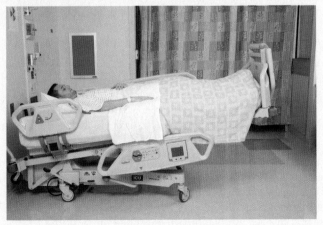	Entire bedframe tilted with head of bed down	For postural drainage, facilitates venous return in patients with poor peripheral perfusion

Continued

PROCEDURAL GUIDELINE 18.6 *Making an Occupied Bed—cont'd*

TABLE 18.4

Common Bed Positions—cont'd

Position	Description	Uses
Reverse Trendelenburg 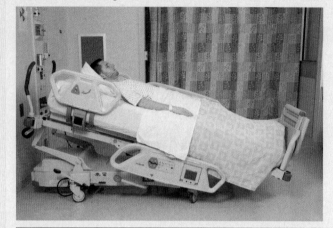	Entire bedframe tilted with foot of bed down	Used infrequently; promotes gastric emptying and prevents esophageal reflux
Supine or flat 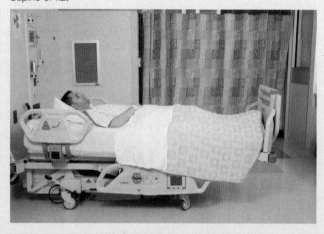	Entire bedframe horizontally parallel with floor	For patients with vertebral injuries and in cervical traction; position used for patients who are hypotensive and generally preferred by patients for sleeping

pulling a knob located on both sides of the bed. Research shows that the risk for patient falls is greater when side rails on both sides of a bed are raised because patients try to climb over the rails to exit the bed. Elevated bed rails are considered a restraint and increase the potential for injury if a fall occurs. Check agency policy on use of bed rails.

Making an occupied bed is required when a patient cannot tolerate being out of bed. If a patient is confined to bed, you should make the bed in a way that conserves time and the patient's energy. A patient's weight, mobility status, pain acuity, and restrictions related to clinical condition or treatment all affect the number of individuals needed to make an occupied bed. Identify the number of additional personnel needed and use safe patient-handling techniques when you turn and position a patient over bed linen (see Chapter 11). In cases in which a patient experiences severe pain, an analgesic administered 30 minutes before making a bed can control pain and maintain comfort.

Even though a patient is unable to get out of bed, encourage self-help as much as possible. For example, if patients can turn, help in moving up in bed, or hold top sheets during application, have them do so. These activities help maintain a patient's strength and mobility and allow participation in hygiene care.

Delegation

The skill of making an occupied bed can be delegated to assistive personnel (AP). Instruct the AP to:
- Avoid positioning patient in specific position and follow activity restrictions that apply.
- Look for wound drainage or loosened equipment that might be found in the bed linens.
- Obtain help from other caregivers for positioning a patient during linen change and the importance of using good body mechanics and supporting patient alignment.

Interprofessional Collaboration

- Consult with respiratory therapy or a registered dietitian nutritionist when using special precautions (e.g., aspiration precautions [see Chapter 30] or positioning for tube-feeding infusion [see Chapter 31]) when positioning a patient during bed making.

Equipment

Linen bags: mattress pad (change only when soiled); bottom sheet (fitted or flat); draw sheet (optional); top sheet, blanket, bedspread, pillowcases; waterproof pads (optional); clean gloves (if linen is soiled or there is risk of exposure to body fluids); antiseptic cleanser; washcloth (see illustration on next page)

PROCEDURAL GUIDELINE 18.6 *Making an Occupied Bed—cont'd*

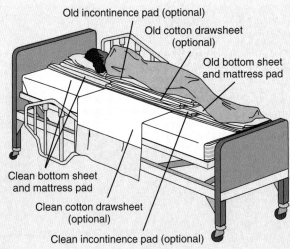

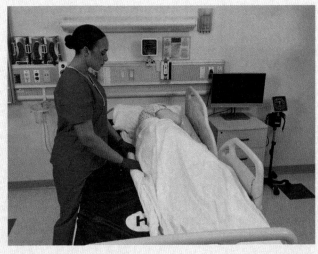

STEP 11 Tuck all soiled linen from one side of bed alongside patient's back.

Steps

1. Review EHR and assess restrictions in mobility/positioning of patient.
2. Organize supplies and close room door or divider curtain to provide privacy.
3. Assess environment for safety (e.g., check room for spills; make sure that equipment is working properly and that bed is in locked position and appropriate number of side rails are raised).
4. Perform hand hygiene. Apply clean gloves if patient has been incontinent or if drainage is present on linen.
5. Explain procedure to patient, noting that patient will be asked to turn over layers of linen.
6. Raise bed to a comfortable working height; lower HOB as tolerated, keeping patient comfortable. Remove nurse call system (if separate from bed rails).

Clinical Judgment *If patient is on aspiration precautions or receiving tube feeding, always keep HOB 30 degrees or higher.*

7. Lower side rail on side where you are standing. Loosen all top linen. Remove bedspread and blanket separately, leaving patient covered with top sheet. If blanket or spread is soiled, place in linen bag. If to be reused, fold into square and place over back of chair.
8. Cover patient with clean bath blanket by unfolding it over top sheet. Have patient hold top edge of bath blanket or tuck blanket under shoulders. Grasp top sheet under bath blanket at patient's shoulders and bring sheet down to foot of bed. Remove sheet and discard in dirty laundry bag.
9. Position patient on far side of bed, turned onto side and facing away from you. **Note:** This is when another caregiver can help you by standing at bedside across from you. Encourage patient to use side rail to turn. Adjust pillow under patient's head.
10. Assess to make sure that there is no tension on any external medical devices.
11. Loosen bottom linens, moving from head to foot. Fanfold or roll any cloth incontinence pads, drawsheet (if present), and bottom sheet (in that order) toward patient. Tuck edges of old linen just under patient's buttocks, back, and shoulders (see illustration). Do not fanfold mattress pad (if it is to be reused). Remove any disposable pads and discard in receptacle.

12. Clean, disinfect, and dry mattress surface if it is soiled or has moisture (see agency policy).
13. Apply clean linens to the exposed half of bed in separate layers. When needed, start with a new mattress pad by placing it lengthwise with center crease in middle of bed. Fanfold pad to center of bed alongside patient. Repeat process with bottom sheet.
14. If bottom sheet is fitted, pull corners of new sheet smoothly over mattress corner at top and bottom of bed. Fold remaining portion of sheet across bed surface, toward patient's back.
15. If bottom sheet is flat, place over mattress. Allow edge of sheet closest to you to hang about 25 cm (10 inches) over mattress edge on side and at HOB. Be sure that lower hem of bottom sheet lies seam down along bottom edge of mattress. Spread remaining portion of sheet over mattress toward patient's back.
16. For a flat sheet, miter the top corner at HOB.
    a. Face HOB diagonally. Place hand away from HOB under top corner of mattress, near mattress edge, and lift.
    b. With other hand, tuck top edge of bottom sheet smoothly under mattress so that side edges of sheet above and below mattress meet when brought together.
    c. To miter a corner, pick up top edge of sheet at about 45 cm (18 inches) from top end of mattress (see illustration).

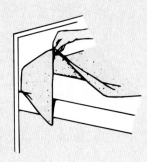

STEP 16c Top edge of sheet picked up.

Continued

PROCEDURAL GUIDELINE 18.6 *Making an Occupied Bed—cont'd*

d. Lift sheet and lay it on top of mattress to form a neat triangular fold with lower base of triangle even with mattress side edges (see illustration).

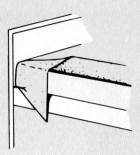

STEP 16d Sheet on top of mattress in a triangular fold.

e. Tuck lower edge of sheet, which is hanging free below the mattress, under the mattress. Tuck with palms down without pulling triangular fold.

f. Hold part of sheet covering side of mattress in place with one hand. With other hand, pick up top of triangular linen fold and bring it down over side of mattress (see illustrations). Tuck under mattress with palms down without pulling fold (see illustration).

17. Tuck remaining part of sheet under side of mattress, moving toward foot of bed. Keep linen smooth.

18. Place new drawsheet along middle of bed lengthwise. Fanfold or roll drawsheet on top of clean bottom sheet. Tuck under patient's buttocks and torso without touching old linen.

19. Add waterproof pad (absorbent side up) over drawsheet with seam side down. Fanfold toward patient. Continue to keep clean and soiled linen separate. Also keep linen under patient as flat as possible because patient will need to roll over old and new layers of linen when you are ready to make other side of bed.

20. Explain that the patient will be rolling over a thick layer of linens. Keeping patient covered, ask patient to log roll toward you slowly over layers of linen and to not raise the hips (see illustration). Stress the need to roll while staying aligned.

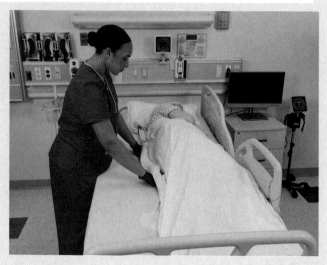

STEP 20 Patient begins rolling over layers of linen.

21. You will now raise side rail and move to opposite side of bed. *Option:* The caregiver helping you will help position patient. Have patient roll away from you toward other side of bed, over all of the folds of linen. Again, have patient keep hips still.

22. Lower side rail. Loosen edges of soiled linen from under mattress. Remove soiled linen by folding into a bundle or square.

23. Hold linen away from your body and place it in laundry bag.

24. Clean, disinfect, and dry other half of mattress as needed.

25. Pull clean, fanfolded or rolled mattress pad; sheet; drawsheet; and incontinence pad out from beneath patient toward you. Smooth all linen out over mattress from head to foot of bed. Help patient roll back to supine position and reposition pillow.

26. If bottom sheet is fitted, pull corners over mattress edges. Smooth out sheet.

27. If flat sheet is used, miter top corner of bottom flat sheet (see Steps 16a–f).

28. Facing side of bed, grasp remaining edge of bottom flat sheet. Lean back slightly, keep back straight, and pull while tucking excess linen under mattress from HOB to foot of bed. Avoid lifting mattress during tucking.

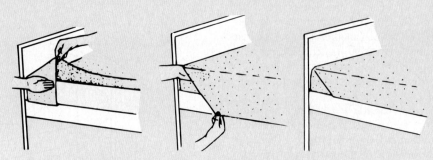

STEP 16f Triangular fold placed over side of mattress; sheet tucked under mattress.

PROCEDURAL GUIDELINE 18.6 *Making an Occupied Bed—cont'd*

29. Smooth fanfolded drawsheet over bottom sheet (tucking is optional). Smooth waterproof incontinence pads, making sure that bed surface is wrinkle free.
30. Place top sheet over patient with vertical centerfold lengthwise down middle of bed and with seam side of hem facing up. Open sheet out from head to foot and unfold over patient. Be sure that top edge of sheet is even with top edge of mattress.
31. Place clean or reused bed blanket on bed over patient. Make sure that top edge is parallel with top edge of sheet and 15 to 20 cm (6 to 8 inches) from edge of top sheet. Raise side rail.
32. Go to other side of bed. Lower side rail. Spread sheet and blanket out evenly.
33. Have patient hold onto sheet and blanket while you remove bath blanket; discard in linen bag.
34. Make cuff by turning edge of top sheet down over top edge of blanket.
35. Make horizontal toe pleat; stand at foot of bed and fanfold in sheet and blanket 5 to 10 cm (2 to 4 inches) across bed. Pull sheet and blanket up from bottom to make fold approximately 15 cm (6 inches) from bottom edge of mattress.
36. Standing at side of bed, tuck in remaining part of sheet and blanket under foot of mattress. Tuck top sheet and blanket together. Be sure that toe pleats are not pulled out.
37. Make modified mitered corner with top sheet and blanket. (Follow Steps 16a–f.) After making triangular fold, do not tuck tip of triangle (see illustration).
38. Go to other side of bed. Repeat Steps 35 and 37.
39. Change pillowcase. Have patient raise head. While supporting neck with one hand, remove pillow. Allow patient to lower head. Remove soiled case and place in linen bag. Grasp clean pillowcase at center of closed end. Gather

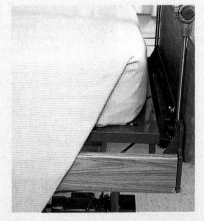

STEP 37 Mitered corner.

case, turning it inside out over the hand holding it. With the same hand, pick up middle of one end of pillow. Pull pillowcase down over pillow with other hand. Do not hold pillow against your uniform. Be sure that pillow corners fit evenly into corners of case. Reposition pillow under patient's head.
40. Help patient to a comfortable position.
41. Raise side rails (as appropriate), and lower bed to lowest position, locking into position.
42. Place nurse call system in an accessible location within patient's reach.
43. Place all linen in dirty laundry bag. Remove and dispose of gloves.
44. Arrange and organize patient's room and perform hand hygiene.
45. During procedure inspect skin for areas of irritation. Observe patient for signs of fatigue, dyspnea, pain, or other sources of discomfort.

PROCEDURAL GUIDELINE 18.7 *Making an Unoccupied Bed*

In some settings, bed linen is not changed every day; however, you always need to change any wet or soiled linen promptly. Moisture on bed linen can easily lead to skin breakdown. A completed, unoccupied bed is one left open with the top sheets fanfolded down. One example is a postoperative surgical bed prepared for patients returning from the operating room (OR) or procedural area. The bed is left with the top sheets fanfolded lengthwise and not tucked in to facilitate a patient's transfer from a stretcher. A closed bed, which is made with the top sheets pulled up to the head of the bed, is made by the housekeeping department after a patient is discharged and the bed is cleaned.

Delegation

The skill of making an unoccupied bed can be delegated to assistive personnel (AP). Instruct the AP to:
- Follow positioning or activity restrictions that apply to patient's ability to get out of and back into bed.
- Use special linen if patient is on an airflow mattress.

Equipment

Linen bag, mattress pad (change only when soiled), bottom sheet (fitted or flat), drawsheet (optional), top sheet, blanket, bedspread, waterproof pads (optional), pillowcases, bedside chair or table, clean gloves (if linen is soiled), washcloth or paper towel, and antiseptic cleanser.

Steps

1. Perform hand hygiene. If patient has been incontinent or if excess drainage is on linen, apply clean gloves.
2. Assess activity orders or restrictions in mobility in planning whether patient can get out of bed for procedure. Help patient to bedside chair or recliner.
3. Lower side rails on both sides of bed, and raise bed to a comfortable working position.
4. Remove soiled linen and place in laundry bag. Avoid shaking or fanning linen.

Continued

PROCEDURAL GUIDELINE 18.7 *Making an Unoccupied Bed—cont'd*

5. Reposition mattress, and wipe off any moisture with a washcloth or paper towel moistened in antiseptic solution. Dry thoroughly.
6. Apply all bottom linen on one side of bed (before moving to opposite side):
   a. To apply a fitted sheet, pull corners over ends of mattress, being sure it is placed smoothly over mattress.
   b. To apply a flat unfitted sheet, allow about 25 cm (10 inches) to hang over sides of mattress edges (along sides and head of bed). Make sure that lower hem of sheet lies seam down, even with bottom edge of mattress. Pull remaining top part of sheet over top edge of mattress.
7. While standing at head of bed, miter top corner of flat bottom sheet (see Procedural Guideline 18.6 Steps 16a-f).
8. Tuck remaining part of unfitted sheet under mattress from head to foot of bed.
9. *Optional:* Apply drawsheet and waterproof incontinence pad, laying centerfolds along middle of bed lengthwise. Smooth drawsheet and pad over mattress and tuck excess edge of drawsheet under mattress, keeping palms down. Center position of pad over bottom sheet.
10. Move to opposite side of bed and pull corners of fitted sheet over ends of mattress, and then spread it smoothly over edge of mattress from head to foot of bed.
11. For an unfitted sheet, miter top corner of bottom sheet (see Step 7), making sure that corner is taut.
12. Grasp remaining edge of unfitted bottom sheet and tuck tightly under mattress while moving from head to foot of bed.
13. Smooth folded drawsheet over bottom sheet and tuck under mattress, first at middle, then at top, and then at bottom.

14. If needed, apply single waterproof pad over bottom sheet or drawsheet.
15. Place top sheet over bed with vertical centerfold lengthwise down middle of bed. Open sheet out from head to foot, being sure that top edge of sheet is even with top edge of mattress.
16. Make horizontal toe pleat: stand at foot of bed and make fanfold in sheet 5 to 10 cm (2–4 inches) across bed. Pull sheet up from bottom to make fold approximately 15 cm (6 inches) from bottom edge of mattress.
17. Tuck in remaining part of sheet under foot of mattress. Place blanket over bed with top edge parallel to top edge of sheet and 15 to 20 cm (6–8 inches) down from edge of sheet. (*Optional:* Apply additional spread over bed.)
18. Make cuff by turning edge of top sheet down over top edge of blanket and spread.
19. Standing on one side at foot of bed, lift mattress corner slightly with one hand; with other hand tuck top sheet, blanket, and spread under mattress. Be sure that toe pleats are not pulled out.
20. Make modified mitered corner with top sheet, blanket, and spread. After making triangular fold, do not tuck tip of triangle (see Procedural Guideline 18.6, Step 37).
21. Go to other side of bed. Spread sheet and blanket, and spread out evenly. Make cuff with top sheet and blanket. Make modified corner at foot of bed.
22. Apply clean pillowcase.
23. Place nurse call system in an accessible location within patient's reach. Return bed to low position, allowing for patient transfer. Lock wheels. Help patient to bed to assume a comfortable position.
24. Arrange patient's room. Remove and discard supplies. Perform hand hygiene.

♦ CLINICAL JUDGMENT AND NEXT GENERATION NCLEX® EXAMINATION–STYLE QUESTIONS

The nurse is caring for a patient who is 78 years old with a 13-year history of type 1 diabetes mellitus and hypertension. The patient is to be discharged after 3 days of hospitalization following an admission for diabetic ketoacidosis. The patient has a healing right-heel ulcer that requires foot care instructions and help with daily dressing changes. The patient lives alone and will need help performing most routine activities of daily living (ADLs) during the initial recovery period. A home care nurse has been obtained.

1. When the patient is sitting in a chair, which action will the home care nurse take to make an unoccupied bed? **Select all that apply.**
   1. Raise bed to working height.
   2. Place used, soiled linens on the floor.
   3. Apply all bottom linen on one side of bed before moving to opposite side.
   4. Tuck top sheet and blanket in at bottom of bed using a modified mitered corner.
   5. Fanfold top blankets to the end of the bed when the procedure is complete.

2. The nurse is assisting the patient with hygiene. Which of the following actions are appropriate when providing male perineal care? **Select all that apply.**
   1. Leave the foreskin of an uncircumcised patient retracted after cleaning.
   2. Cleanse tip of penis at urethral meatus using a circular motion.
   3. Cleanse the shaft and scrotum before cleansing the urethral meatus.
   4. Avoid placing tension on an indwelling catheter if one is present.
   5. Lift scrotum and wash the underlying skin folds.

3. Which action will the nurse perform **first** when helping the patient with oral care?
   1. Remove dentures or partial plates if present.
   2. Perform hand hygiene and apply clean gloves.
   3. Brush inner and outer surfaces of upper and lower teeth.
   4. Clean the biting surface of each tooth.

4. Which foot care instructions will the nurse provide to the patient? Select whether the teaching is indicated, not indicated, or non-essential.

Health Teaching	Indicated	Not Indicated	Non-Essential
Observe your bare feet daily for red spots, cuts, swelling, and blisters.			
Never walk barefoot.			
Use a heating pad to relax aching feet.			
Get measured for well-fitting shoes, especially exercise shoes.			
Move your toes and ankles up and down several times a day.			
Avoid nail polish on toes.			
Use alcohol wipes or cotton balls saturated with alcohol on feet before foot care.			
Trim toenails weekly.			

5. Which assessment data lead the nurse to determine that the patient is at risk for incontinence-associated dermatitis (IAD)?
   1. Occasional incontinence of urine
   2. Decreased mobility
   3. Ongoing fever
   4. Impaired tissue integrity
   5. Reduced nutrition intake

Visit the Evolve site for Answers to Clinical Judgment and Next Generation NCLEX® Examination–Style Questions.

REFERENCES

Agency for Healthcare Research and Quality (AHRQ): *Universal ICU decolonization: an enhanced protocol*, 2013. https://www.ahrq.gov/hai/universal-icu-decolonization/index.html. Accessed September 10, 2023.

Agency for Healthcare Research and Quality (AHRQ): *Teach-back: intervention*, 2023. https://www.ahrq.gov/patient-safety/reports/engage/interventions/teachback.html.

American Academy of Dermatology Association (AADA): *African American hair: tips for everyday care*, 2023. https://www.aad.org/public/diseases/hair-loss/hair-care/african-american. Accessed September 10, 2023.

American Academy of Pediatric Dentistry (AAPD): *Perinatal and infant oral health care*, 2021. https://www.aapd.org/globalassets/media/policies_guidelines/bp_perinataloralhealthcare.pdf. Accessed September 10, 2023.

American Academy of Pediatrics (AAP): *Oral health starts early: AAP policy explained*, 2023. https://www.healthychildren.org/English/healthy-living/oral-health/Pages/Brushing-Up-on-Oral-Health-Never-Too-Early-to-Start.aspx#:~:text=Oral%20health%20starts%20early.,months%20of%20their%20first%20tooth. Accessed September 10, 2023.

American Dental Association (ADA): *Brushing your teeth*, 2022. http://www.mouthhealthy.org/en/az-topics/b/brushing-your-teeth. Accessed September 10, 2023.

American Diabetes Association (ADA): *Foot complications*, 2023. https://www.diabetes.org/diabetes/complications/foot-complications. Accessed September 2022. Accessed September 10, 2023.

Ball J, et al: *Seidel's guide to physical examination*, ed 10, St. Louis, 2023, Mosby.

Beuscher T, et al: Expanding a foot care education program for nurses: a quality improvement survey, *J WOCN* 46(5):441, 2021.

Beuscher T: Foot and nail care. In *Wound ostomy continence nurses' society: core curriculum wound management*, ed 2, Philadelphia, 2022, Wolters Kluwer.

Bobbette N, et al: Adults with intellectual and developmental disabilities and interprofessional, team-based primary health care: a scoping review, *JBI Evid Synth* 18(7):1470, 2020.

Bowen F, O'Brien-Richardson P: Cultural hair practices, physical activity, and obesity among urban African-American girls, *J Am Assoc Nurse Pract* 29(12):754, 2017.

Centers for Disease Control and Prevention (CDC): *Guideline for prevention of catheter associated urinary tract infections 2009, Updated 2019*, Healthcare Infection Control Practices Advisory Committee, 2019, CDC. https://www.cdc.gov/infectioncontrol/pdf/guidelines/cauti-guidelines-H.pdf. Accessed September 10, 2023.

Centers for Disease Control and Prevention (CDC): *Oral health in healthcare settings to prevent pneumonia toolkit*, 2023a, https://www.cdc.gov/hai/prevent/oral-health-toolkit.html. Accessed November 10, 2023.

Centers for Disease Control and Prevention (CDC): *What is health literacy?* 2023b. https://www.cdc.gov/healthliteracy/learn/index.html.

Chapman S: Foot care for people with diabetes: prevention of complications and treatment, *Br J Community Nurs* 22(5):226, 2017.

Chapman L, et al: Chlorhexidine gluconate bathing program to reduce health care–associated infections in both critically Ill and non–critically Ill patients, *Crit Care Nurse* 41(5):e1–e8, 2021.

Cooper AS: Cochrane Review Summary: Oral hygiene care to prevent ventilator-associated pneumonia in critically ill patients, *Crit Care Nurse* 41(4):80–82, 2021.

Cuthbertson BH, Dale CM: Less daily oral hygiene is morn in the ICU: yes, *Intensive Care Med* 46(3):331, 2021.

de Lacerda Vidal CF, et al: Impact of oral hygiene involving toothbrushing versus chlorhexidine irrigation in the prevention of ventilator-associated pneumonia: a randomized study, *BMC Infect Dis* 17:112, 2017.

Donskey CJ, Deshpande A: Effect of chlorhexidine bathing in preventing infections and reducing skin burden and environmental contamination: a review of the literature, *Am J Infect Control* 44:e17, 2016.

Dray S, et al: What's new in the prevention of healthcare-associated infections using chlorhexidine gluconate-impregnated washcloths, *Intensive Care Med* 45(2):249, 2019.

Earlam AS, Woods L: Moisture-associated skin damage: The basics, *Am Nurse J* 17(10):6, 2022.

European Pressure Ulcer Advisory Panel (EPUAP) and National Pressure Injury Advisory Panel (NPIAP), and Pan Pacific Pressure Injury Alliance: *Treatment of pressure ulcers/injuries: Clinical Practice Guideline. The International Guideline*, Emily Haesler (ED), 2019a, EPUAP/NPIAP/PPPIA.

European Pressure Ulcer Advisory Panel (EPUAP) and National Pressure Injury Advisory Panel (NPIAP), and Pan Pacific Pressure Injury Alliance: *Treatment of pressure ulcers/injuries: Quick Reference Guide*, Emily Haesler (ED), 2019b, EPUAP/NPIAP/PPPIA.

Frost SA, et al: Evidence for the effectiveness of chlorhexidine bathing and health care-associated infections among adult intensive care patients: a trial sequential meta-analysis, *BMC Infect Dis* 18(1):1474, 2018.

Fumarola S, et al: Overlooked and underestimated: medical adhesive-related skin injuries. Best practice consensus document on prevention, *J Wound Care* 29(Suppl 3c):S1–S24, 2020.

Giger J, Haddad L: *Transcultural nursing assessment and intervention*, ed 8, St. Louis, 2021, Mosby.

Hitchcock J, et al: Preventing medical adhesive-related skin injury (MARSI), *Br J Nurs* 12;30(15), 2023.

Hockenberry ML, et al: *Essentials of pediatric nursing*, ed 11, St. Louis, 2022, Elsevier.

Institute for Healthcare Improvement (IHI): *Ventilator-associated pneumonia*, 2023. http://www.ihi.org/Topics/VAP/Pages/default.aspx. Accessed September 10, 2023.

Jablonski RA, et al: Randomised clinical trial: efficacy of strategies to provide oral hygiene activities to nursing home residents with dementia who resist mouth care, *Gerodontology* 35(4):365, 2018.

Johns Hopkins Medicine: *CHG bathing to prevent healthcare-associated infections*, 2023. https://www.hopkinsmedicine.org/health/treatment-tests-and-therapies/chg-bathing-to-prevent-healthcareassociated-infections. Accessed September 10, 2023.

Jeffcoate WJ, et al: Current challenges and opportunities in the prevention and management of diabetic foot ulcers, *Diabetes Care* 41:645, 2018.

Jusino-Leon, et al: Chlorhexidine Gluconate baths: supporting daily use to reduce central line–associated infections affecting immunocompromised patients, *Clin J Oncol Nurs* 23(2):E32–E38, 2019.

Kaye AD, et al: Postoperative management of corneal abrasions and clinical implications: a comprehensive review, *Curr Pain Headache Rep* 23(7):1, 2019.

Knobloch MJ, et al: Implementing daily chlorhexidine gluconate (CHG) bathing in VA settings: The human factors engineering to prevent resistant organisms (HERO) project, *Am J Infec Cont* 40:775, 2021.

Kocaçal Güler E, et al: Nurses can play an active role in the early diagnosis of exposure keratopathy in intensive care patients, *J Nurs Sci* 15(1):31, 2018.

Lodi G: *Oral lesions*, 2022, UpToDate. https://www.uptodate.com/contents/oral-lesions. Accessed September 10, 2023.

Manickum P, et al: Knowledge and practice of diabetic foot care-a scoping review, *Diabetes Metab Syndr* 15(3):783–793, 2021.

Marchini L, Ettinger R, Caprio T, et al: Oral health care for patients with Alzheimer's disease: an update, *Spec Care Dentist* 39(3):262, 2019.

Martin ET, et al: Bathing hospitalized dependent patients with prepackaged disposable washcloths instead of traditional bath basins: a case-crossover study, *Am J Infect Control* 45(9):990, 2017.

Mendes A: Meeting the care needs of a person with dementia who is distressed, *Br J Nurs* 27(4):219, 2018.

Mohan S, et al: Preoperative chlorhexidine gluconate scrub shower for inpatient vascular patients: a quality improvement project, *Ann Vasc Surg* 57:174–176, 2019.

Morris A, et al: Effectiveness of corneal abrasion prevention interventions for adults undergoing general anesthesia for more than one hour: a systematic review protocol, *JBI Database System Rev Implement Rep* 16(9):1785, 2018.

National Cancer Institute (NCI): *Oral complications of chemotherapy and head/neck radiation (PDQ)*, 2019. http://www.cancer.gov/cancertopics/pdq/supportivecare/oralcomplications/Patient. Accessed September 10, 2023.

National Pediculosis Association: *Welcome to HeadLice.org*, 2023. https://www.headlice.org/comb/. Accessed September 10, 2023.

Rabello F, et al: Effectiveness of oral chlorhexidine for the prevention of nosocomial pneumonia and ventilator-associated pneumonia in intensive care units: overview of systematic reviews, *Int J Dent Hyg* 16(4):441, 2018.

Rokstad AMM, et al: The impact of the dementia ABC educational programme on competence in person-centered dementia care and job satisfaction of care staff, *Int J Older People Nurs* 12(2), 2017.

Ruiz J, et al: Daily bathing strategies and cross-contamination of multidrug-resistant organisms: impact of chlorhexidine-impregnated wipes in a multidrug-resistant gram-negative bacteria endemic intensive care unit, *Am J Infect Control* 45(10):1069, 2017.

Scales K, et al: Evidence-based nonpharmacological practices to address behavioral and psychological symptoms of dementia, *Gerontologist* 58:S88, 2018.

Singh P, et al: Efficacy of oral care protocols in the prevention of ventilator-associated pneumonia in mechanically ventilated patients, *Cureus* 14(4):e23750, 2022. doi:10.7759/cureus.23750.

Sjögren P, et al: Oral care and mortality in older adults with pneumonia in hospitals or nursing homes: systematic review and meta-analysis, *J Am Geriatr Soc* 64(10):2109–2115, 2016.

Sullivan WF, et al: Primary care of adults with intellectual and developmental disabilities: 2018 Canadian Consensus Guidelines, *Can Fam Physician* 64:254, 2018.

Thayer D, et al: Prevention and management of moisture-associated skin damage (MASD), medical adhesive-related skin injury (MARSI), and skin tears. In McNichol LL, et al: *WOCN Core curriculum wound management*, ed 2, Philadelphia, 2022, Wolters Kluwer.

Thayer D, Nix D: Incontinence-associated dermatitis. In McNichol LL, et al., editors: *WOCN Core Curriculum Wound Management*, ed 2, Philadelphia, 2022, Wolters Kluwer.

The Joint Commission (TJC): *2023 National patient safety goals*, Oakbrook Terrace, IL, 2023, The Joint Commission. https://www.jointcommission.org/standards/national-patient-safety-goals/.

Tien KL, et al: Chlorhexidine bathing to prevent healthcare-associated vancomycin-resistant enterococcus infections: a cluster quasi experimental controlled study at intensive care units, *J Formos Med Assoc* 120:1014, 2021.

Touhy T, Jett K: *Ebersole and Hess' Gerontological nursing & healthy aging*, ed 6, St. Louis, 2022, Mosby.

Villar F, et al: Involving institutionalised people with dementia in their care-planning meetings: lessons learnt by the staff, *Scand J Caring Sci* 32(2):567, 2018.

VonStein M, et al: Effect of a scheduled nurse intervention on thirst and dry mouth in intensive care patients, *Am J Crit Care* 28(1):41, 2019.

Wilson M: Skin care for older people living with dementia, *Nurs Resid Care* 20(3):151, 2018.

Wu YL, et al: Exposure to infected/colonized roommates and prior room occupants increases the risks of healthcare-associated infections with the same organism, *J Hosp Infect* 101(2):231, 2019.

Yevchak A, et al: Implementing nurse-facilitated person-centered care approaches for patients with delirium superimposed on dementia in the acute care setting, *J Gerontol Nurs* 43(12):21, 2017.

Zhao T, et al: Oral hygiene care for critically ill patients to prevent ventilator-associated pneumonia, *Cochrane Database Syst Rev* 12(12):CD008367, 2020. https://www.cochrane.org/CD008367/ORAL_oral-hygiene-care-critically-ill-patients-prevent-ventilator-associated-pneumonia. Accessed September 10, 2023.

Zimmerman S: Effectiveness of a mouth care program provided by nursing home staff vs standard care on reducing pneumonia incidence: a cluster randomized trial, *JAMA Netw Open* 3(6):e204321, 2020.

19 | Care of the Eye and Ear

SKILLS AND PROCEDURES

Procedural Guideline 19.1 **Eye Care for Comatose Patients, p. 566**

Procedural Guideline 19.2 **Taking Care of Contact Lenses, p. 567**

Skill 19.1 **Eye Irrigation, p. 570**

Skill 19.2 **Ear Irrigation, p. 573**

Skill 19.3 **Care of Hearing Aids, p. 577**

OBJECTIVES

Mastery of content in this chapter will enable you to:
- Explain safety guidelines used in the care of eye and ear prostheses.
- Summarize patient-centered care guidelines used in caring for eye and ear prostheses.
- Demonstrate the correct method to remove, store, clean, and insert a contact lens.
- Demonstrate the correct method to perform eye and ear irrigations.
- Discuss techniques that determine whether a hearing aid functions properly.
- Demonstrate the correct method to remove, clean, and reinsert a hearing aid.

MEDIA RESOURCES

- http://evolve.elsevier.com/Perry/skills
- Review Questions
- Audio Glossary
- Answers to Clinical Judgment and Next-Generation NCLEX® Examination–Style Questions
- Skills Performance Checklists
- Printable Key Points

PURPOSE

Vision and hearing are two special senses that help people carry out all activities of daily and recreational living. Risks to a patient's eye or ear structures or function can alter independence, safety, body image, and self-confidence. The skills in this chapter demonstrate how to help patients protect their vision and hearing and use artificial sensory devices correctly to replace or restore sensory function.

PRACTICE STANDARDS

- American Optometric Association, 2023a: Healthy Vision and Contact Lenses, 2022a—Care of Contact Lenses
- Horton GA et al., 2020: Cerumen Management: An Updated Clinical Review and Evidence-Based Approach for Primary Care Physicians— Patient assessment for ear irrigation
- The Joint Commission (TJC), 2023: National Patient Safety Goals—Patient identification

PRINCIPLES FOR PRACTICE

- Meaningful sensory stimuli help people learn about their environment.
- Receiving and understanding environmental stimuli promote healthy functioning.
- Alteration in a patient's vision and hearing affects health literacy, independence, and adherence to medical and pharmacological therapies.
- Artificial sensory aids can restore some vision and hearing loss. However, these aids must fit and work properly for patients to function optimally in their environments.
- When caring for patients who use aids to help with visual or auditory loss, it is important that you and the health care team, along with the patient and family, understand how to clean and care for these aids. Breakage or loss of a sensory aid is expensive.

PERSON-CENTERED CARE

- When a patient with visual or auditory impairment is without visual or hearing devices, communication is altered and the patient becomes more dependent on staff (Webb, 2022).
- The noises within health care agencies including hospitals, rehabilitation centers, and skilled nursing facilities make hearing difficult. The hard flooring surfaces, medical equipment, electronic entertainment devices, and constant need to speak with other health care professionals all produce noise.
- When a patient has auditory impairments, the increased background noise in an unfamiliar environment often makes a patient more anxious and decreases the ability to adjust to new surroundings.
- At times you use touch to get the attention of a patient with severe visual loss or decreased hearing. Remember to ask patients if touch is permitted. Some patients may prefer a same-sex caregiver before touch can be used.

- Understand the cause of a person's sensory loss and then determine the patient's own perception of the reason for the loss and how it is affecting life.
- Identify a patient's usual practices in using and maintaining sensory assistive devices.

EVIDENCE-BASED PRACTICE

Impact of Dual Sensory Impairment

Vision and hearing impairment occurring together are referred to as dual sensory impairment (DSI). DSI has the potential to cause difficulty with activities of daily living, reduce physical activity, and impair social interactions (Kwan et al., 2022). The condition affects patients' mental health and contributes to greater levels of anxiety and depression than in those with only hearing or vision impairment (Guillermo et al., 2021; Pardhan et al., 2021). Furthermore, DSI diminishes communication and socialization (Kwan et al., 2022). A longitudinal study found that DSI was a predictor of mortality in older adults, causing cognitive declines at a rate greater than that of either vision loss only or hearing loss alone (Kwan et al., 2022). Guidelines for the management of patients with DSI include the following:

- Early identification and treatment of sensory impairments is essential to optimize patients' health status and improve quality of life (Morandi et al., 2021).
- Woman with DSI are at higher risk for depression and anxiety (Guillermo et al., 2021).
- Patients with DSI identified communication, mobility, relationships, and recreation and leisure as important aspects of their life (Jaiswal et al., 2021).
- Provide DSI assistive technology (e.g., hearing aids, cochlear implants, magnifiers, and braille displays) and rehabilitation services (Jaiswal et al., 2021).

- There is a risk of cognitive impairment and decline in DSI (Morandi et al., 2021). Combined impairments in vision, hearing, and cognition are associated with greater difficulty in function and communication (Kwan et al., 2022).

SAFETY GUIDELINES

- Safety is a priority whenever you care for patients with sensory alterations. Anticipate how the sensory alteration potentially places a patient at risk for injury (e.g., ability to maneuver through home, climb stairs, and respond to alarms) and assess risk with patient.
- Select interventions on the basis of the type of sensory loss, patient preference, and patient safety.
- Orient patient to any new environment or changes within an existing environment to minimize safety hazards (e.g., visual loss affects a patient's ability to see the edge of the stairs). In addition, educate family caregivers about the best way to help a patient adapt to sensory loss.
- When patients have visual impairments, they may have difficulty with tasks requiring visual detail (e.g., reading prescriptions or syringe scales). This increases the risk of improper administration of medications in the home setting. In addition, certain eye conditions such as cataracts and macular degeneration cause a patient difficulty when adjusting to changes in contrast and brightness.
- Provide additional time for patients with hearing loss to ask repeated questions about their care or upcoming procedure.
- If a patient must sign a consent form for a procedure or surgery, be sure to have a method to verify that the patient read, heard, and understood the procedure.

PROCEDURAL GUIDELINE 19.1 *Eye Care for Comatose Patients*

Comatose patients do not have the natural protective mechanisms of blinking and eye lubrication to protect the cornea. Ocular surface disease is common in the intensive care population, with more than 24% of patients developing corneal defects (Ay & Alay, 2022; Lahiji et al., 2021). Critically ill patients are often on mechanical ventilators and thus heavily sedated, which alters the normal blinking reflex.

Blinking flushes debris out of the eye. When patients are heavily sedated or in a coma, tear production is reduced, thus decreasing the normal lubrication of the corneal surface. In the intensive care unit (ICU) patient population, normal eye protective mechanisms can be impaired by use of mechanical ventilation, muscle relaxants, and sedatives; quick evaporation of tears and endotracheal tube fixators can increase intraocular pressure (Lahiji et al., 2021).

Tears maintain a moist environment, lubricate the eyes, wash away foreign material and cell debris, prevent organisms from adhering to the ocular surface, and transport oxygen to the outer eye surface. When a patient's normal protective eye mechanisms are ineffective, eye care is vital. Left unprotected, damage to the cornea can occur. This damage ranges from corneal scarring, infection, premature cataract formation, or vision changes. Simple eye hygiene measures such as eye ointment, moisture chambers, eyedrop lubrication, and corneal surface protection are

the best interventions to decrease the risk for or prevent damage to the cornea (Ay & Alay, 2022; Lahiji et al., 2021).

Delegation

The skill of providing basic eye care for a comatose patient can be delegated to assistive personnel (AP). However, it is the nurse's responsibility to assess a patient's eyes and administer the sterile lubricant. Direct the AP to:

- Adapt the skill for specific patients (e.g., using skin-sensitive tape to affix eye pads for patients with sensitive skin)
- Immediately report any eye drainage or irritation to the nurse for further assessment

Interprofessional Collaboration

- The health care provider, optometry services, and rehabilitation services should all be included in the management of eye care for the comatose patient.

Equipment

Clean gloves; warm water; normal saline solution; clean washcloth; cotton balls; eye pads or patches; paper tape; eyedropper bulb syringe; sterile ointment (e.g., Lacrilube, VitA-POS) or eyedrop preparations as ordered

PROCEDURAL GUIDELINE 19.1 *Eye Care for Comatose Patients—cont'd*

Option: A moisture chamber (e.g., polyethylene covers or polyacrylamide hydrogel dressings that seal off the eye from the environment) may also be used; verify with agency policy.

Steps

1. Identify patient using at least two identifiers (e.g., name and birthday or name and medical record number) according to agency policy (TJC, 2023).
2. Review patient's electronic health record (EHR) to identify any preadmission eye conditions and current treatments that may pose a risk for reduced blink reflex (e.g., sedation; muscle relaxants limiting lid closure; poststroke status, with paralysis of facial nerve).
3. Assess patient's/family caregiver's health literacy.
4. Perform hand hygiene.
5. Apply clean gloves if drainage is present. Inspect patient's eyes for drainage, corneal dullness, irritation, redness of conjunctiva, and lesions.
6. Continually explain each step of the assessment procedure. It is unknown how much a comatose patient can hear; thus it is important to continually orient a patient to any procedure. Have an interpreter available, if possible, when you know a patient does not speak English.
7. Remove eye patch (if present). Assess for blink reflex (see Chapter 6).
8. Examine the pupils; determine if pupils are equal and round and react to light and accommodation (PERRLA) (see Chapter 6).
9. Observe patient's eye movements, noting symmetry of movement. Remove and dispose of gloves (if worn) and perform hand hygiene. Apply new pair of gloves.
10. Arrange supplies at bedside. Lower side rails and place bed in working position.
11. Provide privacy and explain procedure to patient and family caregivers.
12. Position patient in supine position.
13. Use clean washcloth or cotton balls moistened with warm water or sterile saline and gently wipe each eye from inner to outer canthus. Use a separate, clean cotton ball or corner of the washcloth for each eye.

Clinical Judgment *Be sure water is warm and not hot to avoid damaging eye.*

14. Apply lubricant to eye.
    a. Ointment: Pull the lower eyelid down with finger and apply the ointment over the top of the lower lid into the gap between the lid and the conjunctiva (see Chapter 21). Twist tube slightly to release ointment.
    b. Eyedrops: Use eyedropper to instill the prescribed lubricant (e.g., sterile saline, methylcellulose, liquid tears) into conjunctival sac, wiping away any excess lubricant (see Chapter 21).
15. Be sure the lashes are positioned clear of the cornea to prevent iatrogenic corneal abrasion.
16. If the blink reflex is absent, gently close patient's eyes and apply eye patches or pads. Secure patch, being careful not to tape a patient's eyes. If eye patches or pads are soiled, replace with fresh ones to decrease risk of infection.
17. Dispose of used supplies; remove and dispose of gloves. Perform hand hygiene.
18. Help patient to a comfortable position.
19. Place nurse call system in an accessible location within patient's reach.
20. Raise side rails (as appropriate) and lower bed to lowest position, locking into position.
21. Remove eye pads or patches every 4 hours or as ordered, and observe condition of patient's eyes for drainage, irritation, redness, and lesions.
22. **Use Teach-Back:** "I want to be sure you understand what I explained about why I'm giving you these eyedrops. Tell me why the eyedrops are important." Revise your instruction now or develop a plan for revised patient/family caregiver teaching if patient/family caregiver is not able to teach back correctly.
23. Document eye examination findings, administration of ointment or drops, and family caregiver learning.
24. Notify health care provider about signs of irritation or infection.

PROCEDURAL GUIDELINE 19.2 *Taking Care of Contact Lenses*

A contact lens is a thin, concave disk that fits directly over the cornea of the eye. It is transparent and it covers at least the pupil and may be colorless or tinted. Contact lenses correct refractive errors of the eye or abnormalities in the shape of the cornea that distort vision. They are relatively easy to apply and remove by an individual wearer.

Today, soft contact lenses and rigid gas permeable (RGP) lenses are available. Most disposable soft contact lenses are made of a flexible hydrogel plastic and cover the entire cornea and a small rim of the sclera. The flexible plastics allow oxygen to pass through to the cornea. Newer soft lens materials offer the user simplified cleaning and disinfection (American Optometric Association, 2023b). Extended wear contact lenses, usually soft lenses, are available for overnight or continuous wear ranging from 1 to 6 nights or up to 30 days. RGP lenses are smaller than the soft lens, and initial awareness of the lens is present but total comfort usually occurs within a couple of weeks. RGP lenses are removed at the end of each day. Contact lenses must accommodate patient needs for comfort, vision correction, and convenience and must be prescribed by an eye care professional (American Optometric Association, 2023b).

It is important to remember that all lenses must be removed periodically to prevent infection and corneal damage and that proper cleaning and safe handling are necessary before reinserting a lens (American Optometric Association, 2023a). Patient education prepares patients for how to clean and store, insert, and remove lenses correctly. The frequency for lens care varies with the type of lenses worn. Patients should consult with their ophthalmologist for specific care recommendations.

Continued

PROCEDURAL GUIDELINE 19.2 *Taking Care of Contact Lenses—cont'd*

It is important to determine in emergency or critical care settings whether patients are wearing contact lenses, particularly when they are admitted. These patients are often unable to remove lenses independently. The same is true for an unresponsive or confused patient who is in any setting. If a seriously ill patient is wearing contact lenses and this fact goes undetected, severe corneal injury can result if the lens is not removed.

Delegation
The skill of educating patients about caring for contact lenses cannot be delegated. The skill of removing a contact lens in an emergency cannot be delegated. Direct the AP to:
- Report immediately to the nurse any eye pain or discomfort, redness, swelling, tearing, or drainage for further assessment
- Assist patients with equipment setup when patients perform lens care

Interprofessional Collaboration
- Optometry services should be involved in the education of a patient with contact lenses.

Equipment
Bath towels or waterproof pads; sterile saline solution; sterile lens care solution(s) for cleaning, disinfecting, and rinsing; sterile wetting or conditioning solution (depends on care regimen); sterile enzyme solution (depends on care regimen); flashlight or penlight; clean lens storage container; suction cup (optional); powder-free, clean gloves; instructional materials

Steps
1. Identify patient using at least two identifiers (e.g., name and birthday or name and medical record number) according to agency policy (TJC, 2023).
2. Assess patient's/family caregiver's health literacy.
3. Perform hand hygiene. Inspect patient's eyes or ask patient if contact lens is in place.

Clinical Judgment *If a patient is unconscious or confused, you must examine the eye for the presence of contact lenses, which are often difficult to detect if they are colorless (untinted).*

4. Determine if patient is able to manipulate and hold contact lenses and if glasses are available for periods when contacts are not in use.
5. If patient has worn lenses, assess knowledge about usual routine for wearing, cleaning, and storing lenses.
6. Ask if patient has experienced any unusual visual signs/symptoms (e.g., change in visual acuity, blurred vision, halos, photophobia).
7. Review types of medication prescribed for patient: sedatives, hypnotics, muscle relaxants, antihistamines, or another medication that decreases blink reflex and subsequent lubrication of cornea.
8. Provide privacy and explain procedure to patient. Prepare equipment at bedside, including any written materials or photo images to complement instruction.
9. Have patient sit in bed or chair with a mirror available.
10. Encourage patient to keep fingernails short and smooth and instruct to perform hand hygiene before lens care.

11. Have patient verify expiration date of all solutions.
12. Instruct patient on lens removal:
    a. Removal of soft lens: Have patient follow Steps (1) through (6) for each eye.
       (1) Look at the contact lens in the eye. It is usually over the cornea. Shining a penlight or flashlight sideways onto the eye may help locate the position of the lens.
       (2) Instill 2 or 3 drops of sterile saline solution into the eye.
       (3) Look straight ahead, retract the lower eyelid with the nondominant hand, and expose lower edge of lens.
       (4) Use the pad of the index finger of the dominant hand and slide lens off cornea down onto lower sclera (white of the eye).
       (5) While pulling the upper eyelid down gently with thumb of nondominant hand, compress lens lightly between thumb and index finger.
       (6) By gently pinching the lens, lift the lens out without allowing edges to stick together. Place lens in storage case.

Clinical Judgment *If lens edges stick together, place lens in palm and soak thoroughly with sterile saline solution. Gently roll lens with index finger in back-and-forth motion. If necessary, soak lens in storage solution, which may return lens to normal shape.*

    b. Removal of hard lenses: Have patient follow Steps (1) through (6) for each eye.
       (1) Look at the contact lens in the eye. It is normally positioned directly over the cornea. Shining a penlight or flashlight sideways onto the eye may help locate the position of the lens.

Clinical Judgment *If lens is not positioned directly over the cornea, have patient close eyelid, place index and middle fingers of one hand on eyelid just beside the lens and beneath, and gently attempt to massage lens back into place. If lens cannot be repositioned, an immediate referral to an ophthalmologist is needed.*

       (2) Place index finger of dominant hand on outer corner of the eye and gently draw skin back toward ear.
       (3) Blink while being careful to not release pressure on corner of eye.

Clinical Judgment *For patients unable to open eye or blink on command, nurse will remove lens using a lens suction cup to remove lens from eye. Gently apply suction cup to lens surface and lift out.*

       (4) If lens does not dislodge, gently retract eyelid beyond edge of lens. Press lower eyelid gently against lower edge of lens to dislodge it.
       (5) Allow both eyelids to close slightly and grasp lens as it rises from the eye. Cup lens in hand.
       (6) Always look at the lens to be sure that it is intact. Place it in storage container.
13. Cleaning and storage: Typical cleaning and disinfecting of contact lenses (verify specific method for lenses):
    a. Discuss with patient the risk for infection if lenses are not properly cleaned on a regular basis and stored between use.

PROCEDURAL GUIDELINE 19.2 *Taking Care of Contact Lenses—cont'd*

b. Have patient apply 1 or 2 drops of cleaning solution to lens in palm of hand. Using index finger (soft lenses) or little finger (rigid lenses), rub lens gently but thoroughly on both sides for 20 to 30 seconds.

c. Holding lens over emesis basin, have patient rinse thoroughly with recommended rinsing solution.

Clinical Judgment *Caution patients against use of tap water or homemade saline for cleaning, rinsing, or storage (American Optometric Association, 2023c). Periodic cleaning may be part of the prescribed regimen. Follow manufacturer's instructions and schedules.*

d. Have patient place lens in proper storage case compartment: "R" for right lens and "L" for left. Rigid lenses are placed inside up.

e. Fill the storage case with recommended disinfectant or storage solution.

f. Instruct patient to secure cover(s) over storage case. (If lenses are to be stored at a patient's bedside in health care agency, label case with patient's name, identification number, and room number.)

14. Inserting lenses:

a. Inserting a soft lens: Instruct patient to follow Steps (1) through (6) for each eye.

(1) Remove right lens from storage case and rinse with recommended rinsing solution; inspect lens for foreign materials, tears, and other damage.

(2) Hold lens on tip of index finger of dominant hand with concave side up.

(3) Look at lens from side at eye level to ensure that it is not inverted (see illustration).

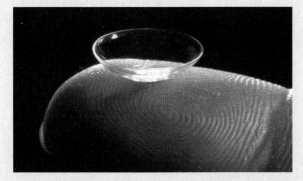

STEP 14a(3) Correct position of soft lens before insertion.

(4) Take index finger of nondominant hand and retract upper eyelid until iris is exposed. Using thumb of nondominant hand, pull down lower lid.

(5) Look straight ahead and focus on an object in the distance while gently tipping and placing lens directly on cornea and releasing lids slowly, starting with lower lid.

(6) Close the eyes briefly and avoid blinking.

b. Inserting a rigid lens: Instruct patient to follow Steps (1) through (7) for each eye.

(1) Remove right lens from storage case; try to lift lens straight up.

(2) Hold lens on tip of index finger of dominant hand with concave side up.

(3) Look at the lens to ensure that it is moist, clean, clear, and free of chips or cracks.

(4) Wet the lens surfaces with a few drops of prescribed wetting solution.

(5) Take index finger of nondominant hand and retract upper eyelid until iris is exposed. Use thumb of nondominant hand and pull down lower lid.

(6) Look straight ahead and focus on an object in the distance. Gently place lens directly on cornea and release lids slowly, starting with lower lid (see illustration).

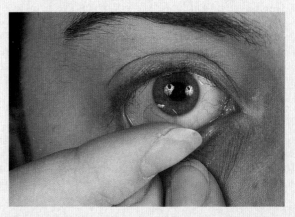

STEP 14b(6) Instruct patient to look straight ahead and focus on an object in the distance.

(7) Close the eyes briefly and avoid blinking.

15. Inspect eye to ensure that patient has placed lens on cornea.

Clinical Judgment *If lens is on sclera rather than cornea, ask patient to slowly close eye and look toward the lens. Gentle pressure on the eyelid may help to center the lens on the cornea. Ask patient to blink a few times.*

16. Ask patient to cover other eye with hand and report if vision is clear and lens is comfortable.

17. Dispose of supplies in appropriate container and have patient perform hand hygiene.

18. Help patient to a comfortable position.

19. Place nurse call system in an accessible location within patient's reach.

20. Raise side rails (as appropriate) and lower bed to lowest position, locking into position. Perform hand hygiene.

21. Ask patient if lens feels comfortable after removal and reinsertion of lenses.

22. Ask patient if there is blurred vision, pain, or foreign body sensation.

23. Teach patient to inspect the eyes for redness, pain, or swelling of eyelids or conjunctiva after lens removal. Also look for discharge or excess tearing.

24. **Use Teach-Back:** "I want to be sure you understand how to clean your contact lenses. Show me the way to clean your lenses." Revise your instruction now or develop a plan for revised patient/family caregiver teaching if patient/family caregiver is not able to teach back correctly.

✦ SKILL 19.1   Eye Irrigation

Chemical injuries to the eye can be work related or occur at home, caused by common household cleaning solutions or exposure to other fumes and aerosols. Burns from acids such as bleach, toilet cleaners, and battery fluid cause a haze on the cornea, which often clears, and there is a good chance of recovery. Burns from alkalis such as lye, ammonia, and dishwasher detergent cause ocular surface damage and vision impairment. Extensive anterior eye injury occurs with alkaline substances, which can be more severe than acid burns (Claassen et al., 2021). A chemical injury to the eye is an emergency and requires flushing it with copious amounts of irrigation fluid. Although irrigating solutions are usually normal saline, cool tap water is recommended during the emergent phase because it is effective, is immediately available for first aid, and initially helps to dilute the concentration of the chemical. Tap water irrigation is also used in emergency situations when a foreign object has entered the eye. If the person wears contact lenses and they do not wash out with the irrigation, have the person try to remove the lenses. The goal in treating ocular chemical injury is to prevent or reduce visual loss caused by the burn (Claassen et al., 2021).

Delegation

The skill of eye irrigation cannot be delegated to the AP. Direct the AP to:

- Report any patient complaint of discomfort or excess tearing following irrigation

Interprofessional Collaboration

- The health care provider should be involved in the care of the patient needing eye irrigation.

Equipment

- Emergency: Cool tap water
- Nonemergent: Prescribed irrigating solution, volume usually 30 to 180 mL at 32°C to 38°C (90°F to 100°F) (For chemical flushing, use normal saline or lactated Ringer solution in large volume to provide continuous irrigation over 15–30 minutes.)
- pH test strip
- Sterile basin or bag of solution
- Curved emesis basin
- Waterproof pad or towel
- 4 × 4–inch gauze pads
- Soft bulb syringe, eyedropper, or intravenous (IV) tubing
- Clean gloves
- Penlight
- Medication administration record (MAR)

STEP	RATIONALE

ASSESSMENT

1. Acute emergent situations: Perform hand hygiene and prepare to use copious amounts of clear, cool water (normal saline or lactated Ringer solution if quickly available) to flush eyes until secretions are cleared. **NOTE:** Irrigation for at least 15 minutes is recommended; 30 minutes is preferable (Solim et al., 2021). Follow irrigation steps in Implementation section later.	Minimizes corneal damage, visual impairment, and permanent loss of vision (Claassen et al., 2021).

Clinical Judgment *Eye irrigation is the immediate treatment for a chemical burn. When possible, determine the chemical. Do not wait if the preferred solution is not available. Delays in irrigation have been associated with more severe injury. Instead, use plain tap water for irrigation (Claassen et al., 2021; Solim et al., 2021).*

When eye irrigation is an emergency treatment for a chemical burn, do not stop to obtain a comprehensive assessment of the eye. Perform a brief assessment to ensure the patient does not have a contraindication for eye irrigation.

2. Nonemergent situations: Identify patient using at least two identifiers (e.g., name and birthday or name and medical record number) according to agency policy.	Ensures patient safety. Complies with The Joint Commission standards and improves patient safety (TJC, 2023).
3. Review health care provider's medication order, including solution to be instilled and affected eye(s) (right, left, or both) to receive irrigation.	Ensures safe and correct administration of irrigant.
4. Assess patient/family caregiver's health literacy.	Determines degree to which individuals have the ability to find, understand, and use information and services to make informed health-related decisions and actions for themselves and others (CDC, 2023).
5. Obtain history of the injury to assess reason for eye irrigation (e.g., type of injury, when it occurred).	Determines amount and type of solution and immediacy of need for treatment.
6. Perform hand hygiene. Apply gloves if drainage is present. Determine the patient's ability to open the affected eye. If the patient is unable to open the eye, hold eyelids open manually or with an eye speculum. *Option*: Apply local anesthetic.	Reduces transmission of microorganisms. Spasm of the eyelid or pain makes opening the eye difficult. Local anesthetics such as proparacaine or tetracaine cause topical numbness and are used before eye examination procedures.

STEP	RATIONALE
7. If time permits, do a complete eye examination, including determining if pupils are equal and round and react to light and accommodation (PERRLA) (see Chapter 6). Have patient look in all directions to determine if there are any visible foreign bodies.	Provides baseline information and determines presence of any foreign bodies.
8. Observe eye for redness, excessive tearing, discharge, and swelling. Ask patient about symptoms of itching, burning, pain, blurred vision, or photophobia. Remove and dispose of gloves; perform hand hygiene.	Establishes baseline signs and symptoms. Reduces transmission of microorganisms.
9. When chemical contamination is suspected, assess pH of the patient's tears. Insert a folded end of a universal pH strip into the conjunctival sac and read results after 30 seconds (Gwenhure, 2020). Compare pH in both eyes.	pH measures the acidity or alkalinity of a solution on a scale of 1 to 14, with 7 as neutral. Normal pH of tears is between 7.0 and 7.4 (Corbett & Bizrah, 2018). If one eye is unaffected, pH provides baseline for normal.
10. Ask patient to rate level of eye pain. Use scale of 0 to 10.	Establishes baseline for level of pain.
11. Assess patient's knowledge, prior experience with eye irrigation, and feelings about procedure.	Reveals need for patient instruction and/or support.

PLANNING

1. Expected outcomes following completion of procedure:	
• Patient demonstrates minimal anxiety during and after irrigation.	Potential for anxiety and pain is high during emergency.
• Patient verbalizes reduced pain, burning, or itching and improved visual acuity after irrigation.	Reflects effectiveness of procedure in removing irritant.
• Patient maintains normal pupillary reaction and eye movement after irrigation.	Reflects effectiveness of procedure in minimizing exposure to irritant and preventing eye damage.
2. Check accuracy and completeness of each MAR with health care provider's written medication or procedure order. Check patient's name, irrigation solution name and concentration, route of administration, and time for administration. Compare MAR with label of eye irrigation solution.	The order sheet is the most reliable source and only legal record of drugs or procedure that patient is to receive. Ensures that patient receives correct medication.
3. Provide privacy and explain procedure to patient.	Protects patient's privacy; reduces anxiety. Promotes cooperation.
4. Organize and set up any equipment needed to perform procedure.	Ensures more efficiency when completing the procedure.

IMPLEMENTATION

1. Perform hand hygiene. Apply clean gloves.	Reduces transmission of microorganisms. Protects hands from chemical irritants.
2. Remove any contact lens if possible (see Procedural Guideline 19.2). Remove and dispose of gloves after contact lens is removed. Perform hand hygiene and apply new gloves.	Prompt removal of lenses is needed to safely and completely irrigate foreign substances from patient's eyes. Removal of gloves following contact lens removal prevents reintroduction of chemical transferred from lens to glove.

Clinical Judgment *In an emergency such as first aid for a chemical burn, irrigation is the immediate treatment. Flush eye from the inner to outer canthus with cool tap water.* **Do not delay treatment** *by removing a patient's contact lenses unless rapid swelling is occurring.*

3. Explain to patient that eye can be closed periodically and that no object will touch it.	Informing patients what to expect decreases anxiety and reassures them.
4. With patient in supine or semi-Fowler position in bed, place towel or waterproof pad under patient's face and curved emesis basin just below patient's cheek on side of affected eye. Turn head toward affected eye. If both eyes are affected, keep patient supine for simultaneous irrigation of both eyes.	Position facilitates flow of solution from inner to outer canthus, preventing contamination of unaffected eye and nasolacrimal duct.
5. Using gauze moistened with health care provider's ordered solution (or normal saline), gently clean visible secretions or foreign material from eyelid margins and eyelashes, wiping from inner to outer canthus.	Minimizes transfer of material into eye during irrigation. Prevents secretions from entering nasolacrimal duct.
6. Explain next steps to patient and encourage relaxation:	Retraction minimizes blinking and allows irrigation of conjunctiva.
a. With gloved finger gently retract upper and lower eyelids to expose conjunctival sacs.	
b. To hold lids open, apply gentle pressure to lower bony orbit and bony prominence beneath eyebrow. Do not apply pressure over eye.	
7. Hold irrigating syringe, dropper, or IV tubing approximately 2.5 cm (1 inch) from inner canthus.	Direct contact with irrigation equipment may injure eye.

STEP	RATIONALE

8. Ask patient to look in all directions while maintaining irrigation. Gently irrigate with steady stream toward lower conjunctival sac, moving from inner to outer canthus (see illustration).

Minimizes force of stream on patient's cornea. Flushes irritant out and away from the other eye and nasolacrimal duct.

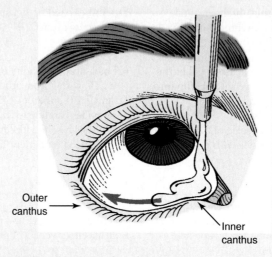

Outer
canthus

Inner
canthus

STEP 8 Irrigation of eye from inner to outer canthus.

9. Reinforce importance of procedure and encourage patient by using calm, confident, soft voice.

Reduces anxiety.

10. Allow patient to blink periodically.

Lid closure moves secretions from upper conjunctival sac.

11. Continue irrigation with prescribed solution volume or time or until secretions are cleared.

Assessment of eye secretion pH may be necessary if eye was exposed to an acidic or basic solution during injury (Solim et al., 2021).

12. Blot excess moisture from eyelids and face with gauze or towel.

Promotes patient comfort.

13. Dispose of soiled supplies; remove and dispose of gloves. Perform hand hygiene.

Reduces transmission of microorganisms.

14. Help patient to a comfortable position.

Gives patient a sense of well-being.

15. Raise side rails (as appropriate) and lower bed to lowest position, locking into position.

Ensures patient safety and prevents falls.

16. Place nurse call system in an accessible location within patient's reach.

Ensures patient can call for assistance if needed.

EVALUATION

1. Observe for verbal and nonverbal signs of anxiety during irrigation.

Verifies that patient is adequately comforted.

2. Assess patient's comfort level after irrigation.

Verifies effective removal of irritant.

3. Inspect eye for movement and determine if pupils are equal, round, and react to light and accommodation (PERRLA).

Impaired reaction to light, accommodation, or movement may indicate injury.

4. Ask patient about improved visual acuity. Have patient read written material.

Corneal damage from irritant can result in altered visual acuity (e.g., blurred vision, cloudiness).

5. **Use Teach-Back:** "I want to be sure I explained why it is important to understand eye safety at work. Tell me what you should do if you accidentally have a solution splash into your eyes." Revise your instruction now or develop a plan for revised patient/family caregiver teaching if patient/family caregiver is not able to teach back correctly.

Teach-back is a technique for health care providers to ensure that they have explained medical information clearly so that patients and families understand what is communicated (Agency for Healthcare Research and Quality [AHRQ], 2023).

STEP	RATIONALE

Unexpected Outcomes

1. Patient is anxious.

2. Patient complains of pain or foreign body sensation in eye following irrigation, excessive tearing, or photophobia.

Related Interventions

- Reinforce rationale for irrigation.
- Allow patient to close eye periodically during irrigation.
- Instruct patient to take slow, deep breaths.
- Advise patient to close eye and avoid eye movement.
- Immediately notify health care provider or eye care practitioner.

Documentation

- Document reason for irrigation, condition of eye before and after irrigation, patient's report of pain and visual symptoms, type and amount of irrigation solution, and length of time irrigation performed.
- Document your evaluation of patient and family caregiver learning.

Hand-Off Reporting

- Use agency's standardized hand-off communication to communicate reason for irrigation, type and amount of irrigation solution, and length of time irrigation performed.
- Report patient's condition of eye, symptoms, and tolerance of eye irrigation.
- Report immediately to the health care provider if patient complains of increased pain, blurred vision, or other visual changes.

Special Considerations

Patient Education

- Encourage patient to see eye care professional to determine if exposure to chemical caused permanent eye damage.

- Help patients and family identify potential hazards at home and work. Instruct them about measures to reduce the risk for eye injuries, such as personal protective eyewear (goggles, face shield, safety glasses). The eye protection device depends on the type of hazard, the circumstances of exposure, other protective equipment used, and individual vision needs (American Optometric Association, 2023d).
- Instruct patients on the signs and symptoms of an eye injury and what to do if another eye injury occurs.
- Inform patients about the cleaning and safe handling of contact lenses.

Pediatrics

- A child with a foreign body or chemical in the eye may panic. It may be necessary to safely restrain the child to safely and quickly irrigate the eye.

Home Care

- See Patient Education section.

◆ SKILL 19.2   Ear Irrigation

Common indications for irrigation of the external ear canal are the presence of foreign bodies and buildup of cerumen (earwax) in the canal. The procedure is not without potential hazards and is not indicated for an ear infection. Usually irrigations are performed with water warmed to body temperature to avoid vertigo or nausea in patients. The greatest danger during ear irrigation is trauma to the tympanic membrane by forcing an irrigant into the ear canal under pressure (Meyer et al., 2020). Damage to the external auditory meatus may occur by scratching the lining of the canal if a patient suddenly moves or if there is inadequate control of the irrigating syringe. Drying the ear improperly may lead to acute otitis externa (infection of the outer ear).

Ear emergencies can include the presence of foreign bodies, insect bites, or percussion injuries. In addition, a patient can also have damage from inside the ear, which includes blood and drainage. Sometimes the cause of bloody or clear-to-tan drainage may be the result of a head or neck injury. If a head or neck injury is suspected, immobilize the patient. Cover the outside of the ear with a sterile dressing (if available), get medical help immediately, and **do not irrigate the ear**. In addition, **do not irrigate** the ear if the patient has anatomical abnormalities of the ear or a history of surgery of the ear or ear canal, including myringotomy tubes (Sevy et al., 2023).

Delegation

The skill of administering ear irrigation cannot be delegated to assistive personnel (AP). Direct the AP to:

- Immediately report any potential side effects following an ear irrigation (e.g., pain, drainage, dizziness)
- Help a patient when ambulating because some light-headedness may be present, which increases a patient's risk for falling

Interprofessional Collaboration

- The health care provider and audiology services (as appropriate), are involved in the care and follow-up of the patient who requires ear irrigation.

Equipment

- Clean gloves
- Otoscope (optional)
- Irrigation or bulb syringe
- Basin for irrigating solution (Use sterile basin if sterile irrigating solution is used [when tympanic membrane is ruptured].)
- Emesis basin for drainage or irrigating solution exiting the ear
- Towel
- Cotton balls or 4 × 4–inch gauze
- Water warmed to body temperature
- *Option*: Mineral oil, 1% sodium docusate solutions, and carbamide peroxide solutions for softening cerumen before irrigation (Schumann et al., 2022)

STEP	RATIONALE

ASSESSMENT

1. Identify patient using at least two identifiers (e.g., name and birthday or name and medical record number) according to agency policy.

Ensures patient safety. Complies with The Joint Commission standards and improves patient safety (TJC, 2023).

2. Review health care provider's irrigation order, including solution to be instilled and affected ear(s): right (AD), left (AS), or both (AU) to receive irrigation.

Ensures safe and correct administration of solution.

3. Review EHR for history of diabetes mellitus, eczema, or other skin problem in the ear canal; a weakened immune system; or ruptured tympanic membrane (Horton et al., 2020).

These conditions contradict irrigation.

4. Assess patient's/family caregiver's health literacy.

Determines degree to which individuals have the ability to find, understand, and use information and services to make informed health-related decisions and actions for themselves and others (CDC, 2023).

5. Perform hand hygiene and inspect pinna and external auditory meatus for redness, swelling, drainage, abrasions, and presence of cerumen or foreign objects. (Apply clean gloves if drainage present.)

Findings provide baseline to monitor effects of medication or solution.

  a. Always attempt to remove foreign objects in ear by first simply straightening ear canal.

Straightening the ear canal may cause the object to fall out.

Clinical Judgment *If vegetable matter such as a dried bean or pea is occluded in the canal, do not perform irrigation. The material can swell on contact with water and cause further damage to the canal (Hockenberry et al., 2024).*

6. Use otoscope to inspect deeper parts of auditory canal and tympanic membrane. *Caution:* If you visualize an object, do not push it farther into the ear canal.

When auditory canal is unobstructed, this inspection verifies if tympanic membrane is intact.

7. Ask if patient is having earache or fullness in the ear, partial hearing loss, tinnitus (ringing in the ear), itching or discharge in ear, or coughing (Horton et al., 2020).

Common symptoms of cerumen impaction.

8. Using a scale of 0 to 10, ask patient to rate severity of ear discomfort. Remove and dispose of gloves (if worn). Perform hand hygiene.

Provides baseline assessment. Pain is symptomatic of external ear infection or inflammation.

9. Assess patient's hearing acuity (see Chapter 6).

Occlusion of auditory canal by cerumen or foreign object can impair hearing.

10. Assess patient's knowledge, prior experience with ear irrigation, and feelings about procedure.

Reveals need for patient instruction and/or support.

PLANNING

1. Expected outcomes following completion of procedure:
  - Patient denies pain during instillation.
  - Patient demonstrates hearing conversation more clearly in affected ear.
  - Patient is able to discuss purpose of irrigation and describe correct ear-care techniques.
  - Patient's canal is clear of cerumen, foreign material, and discharge.

Fluid is properly instilled.
Obstruction in ear canal is resolved.

Feedback reflects patient's learning.

Inflammation, irritation, and occlusion of canal are relieved.

2. If patient is found to have impacted cerumen, instill 1 or 2 drops of cerumen softener into ear twice a day for 2 to 3 days before irrigation.

Loosens cerumen and ensures easier removal during irrigation.

3. Provide privacy and explain procedure. Inform patients that irrigation may cause sensation of dizziness, ear fullness, and warmth.

Protects patient's privacy; reduces anxiety. Promotes cooperation.

4. Organize and set up any equipment needed to perform procedure.

Ensures more efficiency when completing the procedure.

STEP	RATIONALE

5. Assist patient into a sitting or lying position with head turned toward affected ear. Place towel under patient's head and ear. When possible, have patient hold emesis basin.

Positioning minimizes leakage of fluids around neck and facial area. Solution will flow from ear canal to basin.

IMPLEMENTATION

1. Perform hand hygiene. Pour warmed water into basin. Check temperature of solution by pouring small drop on your inner forearm. **NOTE:** If sterile irrigating water is used, sterile basin is required.

   Reduces transfer of microorganisms; helps you perform procedure smoothly.

2. Apply clean gloves. Gently clean auricle and outer ear canal with gauze or cotton balls. Do *not* force drainage or cerumen into ear canal. Remove and dispose of gloves. Perform hand hygiene. Reapply clean gloves.

   Prevents infected material from reentering ear canal. Forceful instillation of solution into occluded canal can cause injury to eardrum. Reduces transmission of microorganisms.

3. Fill irrigating syringe with solution (approximately 50 mL).

4. For adults and children older than 3 years old, gently pull pinna up and back. In children 3 years or younger, pinna should be pulled down and back (Hockenberry et al., 2024). Adults can lie supine. Place tip of irrigating device just inside external meatus. Leave space around irrigating tip and canal.

   Enough fluid is needed to provide a steady irrigating stream. Pulling pinna straightens external ear canal. Prevents obstruction of canal with device, which can lead to increased pressure on tympanic membrane.

5. Slowly instill irrigating solution by holding tip of syringe 1 cm (½ inch) above opening to ear canal. Direct fluid toward superior aspect of ear canal. Allow it to drain out into basin during instillation. Continue until canal is cleaned or solution is used (see illustration).

   Slow instillation prevents buildup of pressure in ear canal and ensures contact of solution with all canal surfaces.

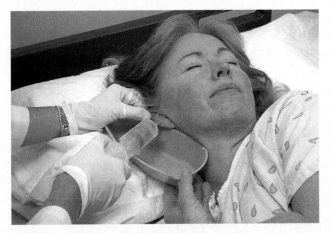

STEP 5 Tip of syringe does not occlude ear canal during irrigation.

6. Maintain flow of irrigation in steady stream until pieces of cerumen or exudate flow from canal.

   Constant flow of fluid loosens cerumen.

7. Periodically ask if patient is experiencing pain, nausea, or vertigo.

   Symptoms indicate that irrigating solution is too hot or too cold or instilled with too much pressure.

8. Drain excessive fluid from ear by having patient tilt head toward affected side.

   Excess fluid may promote microorganism growth if not drained.

9. Dry outer ear canal gently with cotton ball. Leave cotton ball in place for 5 to 10 minutes.

   Drying prevents buildup of moisture that can lead to otitis externa.

10. Help patient to a comfortable position.

   Gives patient a sense of well-being.

STEP	RATIONALE
11. Remove and dispose of gloves. Perform hand hygiene.	Reduces transmission of microorganisms.
12. Raise side rails (as appropriate) and lower bed to lowest position, locking into position.	Ensures patient safety and prevents falls.
13. Place nurse call system in an accessible location within patient's reach.	Ensures patient can call for assistance if needed.

EVALUATION

1. Ask patient if discomfort is noted during instillation of solution.	Water instilled improperly under pressure causes discomfort.
2. Ask patient about sensations of light-headedness or dizziness.	Instillation of fluid can cause these symptoms, which can put patient at risk for falling.
3. Reinspect condition of meatus and canal.	Determines if solution reduces inflammation and removes foreign materials.
4. Assess patient's level of pain and hearing acuity, and assess for presence of preirrigation symptoms.	Determines if cerumen has been removed and hearing is improved.
5. **Use Teach-Back:** "I want to be sure you understand how I showed you to insert the syringe for an ear irrigation. Show me how you would do this for your mother." Revise your instruction now or develop a plan for revised patient/family caregiver teaching if patient/family caregiver is not able to teach back correctly.	Teach-back is a technique for health care providers to ensure that they have explained medical information clearly so that patients and their families understand what is communicated (AHRQ, 2023).

Unexpected Outcomes	Related Interventions
1. Patient complains of increased ear pain during irrigation. Rupture of eardrum may have occurred.	• Stop irrigations and notify health care provider immediately.
2. Ear canal remains occluded with cerumen.	• Repeat irrigation.
3. Foreign body remains in ear canal.	• Refer patient to otolaryngologist if foreign object remains after irrigation.

Documentation

- Document indication for ear irrigation, symptoms of cerumen buildup or infection, condition of the tympanic membrane and ear canal before and after irrigation, characteristics of cerumen or other material removed, and patient's hearing acuity before and after procedure.
- Document the type and amount of solution, time of administration, and the ear receiving the irrigation.
- Document adverse effects and patient response to ear irrigation.
- Document your evaluation of patient and family caregiver learning.

Hand-Off Reporting

- Report indication for ear irrigation, which ear was irrigated, any adverse effects, and any change in hearing acuity.
- Report patient response to procedure and outcome of irrigation (e.g., cerumen plug removed).

Special Considerations

Patient Education

- Instruct patient that cerumen has an antibacterial effect that maintains an acid pH in the auditory canal.
- Instruct patients to clean ears daily with a washcloth, soap, and warm water.
- Warn patients against inserting objects (e.g., cotton swabs, hairpins) into ear canal.

Pediatrics

- When cleaning the ear of a small child, be certain that child's head is immobilized to prevent puncturing eardrum. It may be necessary to have child's parent or staff participate (Hockenberry et al., 2024).

Older Adults

- Irrigation of the ear can trigger a cough during the procedure and lead to tinnitus and vertigo. Perform irrigation according to agency policy and be attentive to patient safety.
- Assess the patient's mental state and physical dexterity (Touhy & Jett, 2022). Both can impact ear hygiene and otic medication adherence. Ask the patient to demonstrate the skill and assist the patient with self-administration, as appropriate.

Populations With Disabilities

- Patient groups that are vulnerable or unlikely to complain about earwax or loss of hearing, such as people with cognitive impairment, need to have their ears and hearing regularly assessed.

Home Care

- Instruct patient to use a clean bulb syringe for irrigation. Cerumen softener preparations can help with removal of cerumen.

✦ SKILL 19.3   Care of Hearing Aids

Hearing is vital for normal communication and orientation to sounds in the environment. Hearing impairment is most common in older adults. Many patients do not seek professional help for this impairment, nor do they consistently wear aids. According to the World Health Organization (WHO), more than 5% of people worldwide have disabling hearing loss (WHO, 2023). Nonuse of hearing aids has been shown to be related to poor hearing aid care and maintenance, concerns about the value of a hearing aid, speech clarity, poor hearing aid fit or discomfort, and negative attitude toward usage (Alicea & Doherty, 2021).

Initially a person with hearing loss may deny the condition or think that there is a stigma attached to the actual hearing loss or need for a hearing aid (Alicea & Doherty, 2021). Any hearing loss has social implications, and the person may not engage in social activities. There are also many safety considerations. Not only do people with hearing loss have difficulty hearing car horns and emergency sirens, they also have difficulty understanding interactions with health care providers and educational instruction and, as a result, may not manage the symptoms or therapies safely.

When your patient has a hearing aid, your role is to understand how it functions and how to help the patient care for it. It is the role of a hearing professional to recommend the type of aid the patient needs, provide fitting, and establish the best auditory settings for individual patients (American Speech-Language-Hearing Association, n.d.). For people with hearing loss, a proper hearing aid improves the ability to hear and understand spoken words. Several styles of hearing aids are available, including new programmable aids (Table 19.1). Hearing aids amplify sound so it is heard at a more effective level. All hearing aids have four basic components:

1. A microphone, which receives and converts sound into electrical signals
2. An amplifier, which increases the strength of the electrical signal
3. A receiver, which converts the strengthened signal back into sound
4. A power source (batteries)

TABLE 19.1

Types of Hearing Aids

Type	Advantages	Disadvantages	Cautions
In-the-ear (ITE) hearing aids fit completely in the outer ear and are used for mild-to-severe hearing loss. 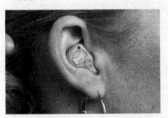	Design of the aid can improve sound transmission through telephone calls. Some ITEs have a *telecoil*, which is a magnetic circuit that allows users to receive sound through the circuitry of the hearing aid versus the microphone.	ITE aids are damaged by earwax and ear drainage, and their small size can cause adjustment problems and feedback.	Not usually worn by children because the casings need to be replaced as the ear grows.
Behind-the-ear (BTE) hearing aids are worn behind the ear and are connected to a plastic ear mold that fits inside the outer ear. 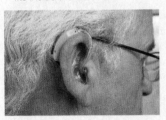	Sound travels through the ear mold into the ear. People of all ages wear BTE aids for mild to profound hearing loss.	Poorly fitting BTE ear molds can cause feedback, a whistling sound caused by the fit of the hearing aid.	May not be appropriate for children or adults who are active in sports because of potential for damage of the device.
Completely-in-canal (CIC) aids are customized to fit the size and shape of the ear canal. 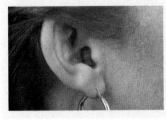	Canal aids are used for mild to moderately severe hearing loss and are largely concealed in the ear canal.	Because of their small size, canal aids may be difficult for the user to adjust and remove and may not be able to hold additional devices such as a telecoil.	Expensive and not recommended for children. Can also be damaged by earwax and ear drainage.

Data from Food and Drug Administration: *Hearing aids*, U.S. Food and Drug Administration, 2023. https://www.fda.gov/medical-devices/consumer-products/hearing-aids. Accessed October 3, 2023.

All hearing aids do not work the same. The two main types of electronic hearing aids are analog and digital. Analog technology converts sound waves into electrical waves, which are amplified. These are custom built to meet the needs of the user and programmed by the manufacturer according to the specifications of an audiologist. Digital technology converts sound waves into numerical codes. The aid is programmed to amplify some frequencies more than others. Digital aids give the audiologist more flexibility in fine-tuning the aid to meet the patient's needs. They can also be programmed to focus on sounds from a specific direction (Alicea & Doherty, 2021).

An alternate to traditional hearing aids is the use of a cochlear implant. A cochlear implant (CI) is a surgically implanted electronic device that bypasses damaged portions of the inner ear to deliver sound signals to the auditory nerve through electrodes placed in the cochlea of the inner ear. An implant includes the internal component and an external sound processor that fits behind the ear. CIs have been successful in restoring a sense of hearing for many individuals with moderate to profound hearing loss. Adults with moderate-to-profound sensorineural hearing loss may be candidates for a CI when more traditional approaches to amplification have not provided adequate speech recognition and improvement in access to sound (Schafer et al., 2021).

Cochlear implants allow for improved speech development, restoration of hearing, and the potential for increased earning potential. Hearing aids are customizable after successful implantation. The audiology team works with the patient to adjust implant settings to achieve the best quality in daily living needs (Krogmann & Khalili, 2022).

It is a challenge to adjust one's communication style to accommodate a patient with a hearing impairment. Use the patient as a resource for identifying the communication techniques that are generally helpful. Be sure that a patient can see your face, speak slowly in a normal tone, and rephrase rather than repeat if the person cannot understand you. Also remember that a patient is unable to hear alerts such as fire alarms or overhead announcements.

Delegation
This skill of caring for a hearing aid can be delegated to assistive personnel (AP). Direct the AP to:
- Report ear pain, inflammation, drainage, odor, or changes in hearing
- Identify alternative ways to communicate with a patient while the aid is not in use
- Learn how to carefully handle the aid to prevent damage or injury

Interprofessional Collaboration
- The health care provider, audiology services, and rehabilitation services are involved in the management of care for a patient with a hearing impairment

Equipment
- Soft towel and washcloth
- Facial tissues
- Brush or wax loop
- Storage case
- Warm water and soap
- Spare battery, size depends on aid (optional)
- Clean gloves (if drainage present)

STEP	RATIONALE
ASSESSMENT	
1. Identify patient using at least two identifiers (e.g., name and birthday or name and medical record number) according to agency policy.	Ensures patient safety. Complies with The Joint Commission standards and improves patient safety (TJC, 2023).
2. Review patient electronic health record (EHR) for type of hearing aid and patient's hearing acuity.	Ensures safe and appropriate care.
3. Determine whether patient can hear clearly with hearing aid by talking slowly and clearly in normal tone of voice.	Inability to hear may indicate a problem with the hearing aid or battery or that the particular model is no longer effective for patient.
4. Assess patient's/family caregiver's health literacy.	Determines degree to which individuals have the ability to find, understand, and use information and services to make informed health-related decisions and actions for themselves and others (CDC, 2023).
5. Ask patient to demonstrate (if able) manipulation and holding of hearing aid.	Determines level of assistance required in care.
6. Assess if hearing aid is working by removing from patient's ear. Close battery case and turn volume slowly to high. Cup hand over hearing aid. If you hear a squealing sound (feedback), it is working. If no sound is heard, replace batteries and test again.	May indicate malfunctioning of hearing aid.
7. Determine patient's usual hearing aid–care practices. *Option:* Observe patient clean hearing aid.	Provides information as to how patient cares for device and identifies patient preferences.
8. Perform hand hygiene. If drainage is present, apply clean gloves. Assess patient for any unusual physical or auditory signs/symptoms (pain, itching, redness, discharge, odor, tinnitus, decreased acuity). If hearing is reduced, ask: When did this start? Is it present all the time? Does the quality of hearing acuity change with male versus female voices or adult versus children's voices?	Reduces transmission of microorganisms. May indicate injury, infection, or cerumen accumulation.

STEP	RATIONALE
9. Remove and dispose of gloves (if worn). Perform hand hygiene.	Reduces transmission of microorganisms.
10. Assess hearing aid for cracks, rough edges, or accumulation of cerumen around aid, which can block sound.	Poorly fitting hearing aids cause irritation and/or discomfort to external ear canal. Cerumen can block the ear canal and contribute to hearing loss.
11. Assess patient's and family caregiver's knowledge, prior experience with cleaning and maintaining hearing aid, and feelings about procedure.	Reveals need for patient instruction and/or support.

PLANNING

1. Expected outcomes following completion of procedure: • Patient verbalizes comfort after removal and reinsertion of hearing aid. • Patient responds appropriately to normal conversation and environmental sounds. • Patient demonstrates proper care of hearing aid.	Hearing aid is removed or inserted properly and positioned correctly. Hearing aid and batteries are operational. Aid is secure and unobstructed. Learning is achieved.
2. Provide privacy and explain procedure with patient and family caregiver (if present). Explain all steps before removing aid.	Protects patient's privacy; reduces anxiety. Promotes cooperation.
3. Organize and set up any equipment needed to perform procedure.	Ensures more efficiency when completing the procedure.
4. Have patient assume supine, side-lying, or sitting position in bed or chair.	Provides easy access to ear. Promotes patient comfort.

IMPLEMENTATION

1. Perform hand hygiene. Apply clean gloves if patient has ear drainage.	Reduces transmission of microorganisms.
2. **Removing and cleaning hearing aid(s)** a. Patient or nurse turns hearing aid(s) volume off, usually by turning volume control to left or toward patient's nose. Then grasp aid securely and gently remove device following natural ear contour.	Prevents feedback (whistling) during removal. Prevents dropping hearing aid. Prevents injury to ear.

Clinical Judgment *Some hearing aids such as the completely-in-canal (CIC) device do not have a volume control but are turned off by opening the battery door. Other aids have the volume control located on a remote device. Be sure that your patient knows the importance of having the volume turned off when the aid is not in use.*

b. Hold aid over towel and wipe exterior with tissue to remove cerumen.	Prevents breakage or damage if aid is dropped. Cerumen may irritate canal and interfere with fit.
c. Inspect ear mold for cracks or rough edges, any fray in cords, or accumulation of cerumen around aid, which can block sound.	May irritate ear canal.
d. Inspect all openings in aid for accumulated cerumen. Carefully remove cerumen with wax loop or other device supplied with hearing aid.	Cerumen may block sound from receiver. It may also block pressure equalization channel and create feeling of ear pressure.

Clinical Judgment *The pressure equalization channel is a tiny hole through the entire length of the ear mold and should be clear for the entire length. The receiver points into the ear through another opening. It is easily damaged. NEVER insert anything into the receiver port!*

e. Open battery door, place hearing aid in labeled storage container, and allow it to air dry.	Allows drying of internal components. Protects against breakage and loss.
f. Place towel beneath patient's ear(s). Wash ear canal(s) with washcloth moistened in soap and water. Rinse with moistened cloth and then dry.	Absorbs excess water. Removes cerumen from external ear canal. Removes soap residue and water that may harbor microbes or damage aid.
g. Assess ear canal for redness, tenderness, discharge, or odor.	Signs may indicate injury or infection.
h. Repeat procedure for other hearing aid if bilateral.	
i. If storing hearing aid(s), place each in dry storage case with desiccant material. Label case with patient's name and room number. If more than one aid, note right or left. Indicate in patient's EHR where aid is stored.	Protects hearing aid against damage, moisture, and breakage. Documents how and where hearing aid is stored.
j. Dispose of towels, remove and dispose of gloves, and perform hand hygiene.	Reduces transmission of microorganisms.

STEP	RATIONALE
3. Inserting hearing aid(s)	
a. Remove hearing aid(s) from storage case and check battery (see Assessment section). Check that volume is off.	
b. Identify hearing aid as either right (marked "R" or red color coded) or left (marked "L" or blue color coded).	Proper orientation prevents damage to device and patient injury.
c. When possible, allow patient to insert aid. Otherwise, hold hearing aid with thumb and index finger of dominant hand so that canal (long part with holes) is at bottom. Insert pointed end of ear mold into ear canal. Follow natural ear contours to guide aid into place.	Prevents dropping. Proper positioning prevents injury. Pulling on ear may distort canal and make insertion more difficult.
d. Anchor any separate pieces, as in case of behind-the-ear (BTE) aid or body aid.	Prevents pieces from falling and breaking.
e. Adjust or have patient adjust volume gradually to comfortable level for talking to patient in regular voice 3 to 4 feet away. For BTE device, rotate volume control toward nose to increase volume and away from nose to decrease volume.	Gradual adjustment prevents discomfort and injury to ear.
f. Repeat insertion for other hearing aid, if bilateral.	
g. Close and store case. Remove and dispose of gloves if worn.	Preserves desiccant. Prevents loss. Reduces transmission of microorganisms.
h. Assist patient to a comfortable position.	Gives patient a sense of well-being.
i. Raise side rails (as appropriate) and lower bed to lowest position, locking into position.	Ensures patient safety and prevents falls.
j. Place nurse call system in an accessible location within patient's reach.	Ensures patient can call for assistance if needed.
k. Perform hand hygiene.	Reduces transmission of microorganisms.

EVALUATION

1. Ask patient to rate level of comfort after removal or insertion.
2. Observe patient during normal conversation and in response to environmental sounds.
3. **Use Teach-Back:** "I want to be sure you understand what I showed you to remove, clean, and reinsert your father's hearing aid. Let's take time now and show me how to do it." Revise your instruction now or develop a plan for revised patient/family caregiver teaching if patient/family caregiver is not able to teach back correctly.

Verifies proper technique and positioning.

Verifies the aid is operational, correctly positioned, unobstructed, and effective.

Teach-back is a technique for health care providers to ensure that they have explained medical information clearly so that patients and their families understand what is communicated to them (AHRQ, 2023).

Unexpected Outcomes

1. Patient is unable to hear conversations or environmental sounds. Patient's verbal responses are inappropriate.

2. Patient experiences discomfort or pain, inflammation, drainage, or odor from affected ear.

Related Interventions

- Check function, type, and placement of battery and replace it if indicated.
- Increase volume if adjustable.
- Inspect aid and ear canal for cerumen blockage.
- Refer to audiologist for reassessment.
- Remove aid and inspect for sharp or rough edges. Refer to provider for repair.
- Assess ear for signs of injury or infection.
- Confirm correct R or L placement. Reposition hearing aid.

Documentation

- Document appearance of external ear, symptoms of cerumen buildup, and patient's hearing acuity before and after procedure.
- Document removal of hearing aid, storage location if not reinserted after cleaning, and patient's preferred communication techniques. If family takes aid home, be sure that this information is documented.
- Document your evaluation of patient and family caregiver learning.

Hand-Off Reporting

- Report any sudden changes in hearing to health care provider.

Special Considerations

Patient Education

- Instruct family that batteries are toxic if swallowed, and keep them away from pets and children.
- Instruct patient to insert the aid after the hair is dried and any hair spray applied. Heat from the hair dryer or perfumes and hair spray can damage the aid.
- Dogs in particular and cats are attracted to the smell of used hearing aids. Advise patient to protect the hearing aids and their pets by properly storing the aids out of reach.
- Encourage patients to identify helpful communication tips and teach them to others. Many patients find facial cues informative. Speakers must:
  1. Face patient, stay within 3 to 4 feet away, and keep hands away from mouth.
  2. Get patient's attention before speaking.
  3. Rephrase rather than repeat when a patient cannot understand.
  4. Reduce background noise or move to a quiet area.

Pediatrics

- Children are more often fitted with BTE hearing aids because the ear canal is still growing.
- The aid is made less conspicuous with hair styling or becomes a statement of fashion and personality with a brightly colored or transparent case.

- Children need help to prevent acoustic feedback (whistling), which they are unable to hear.

Older Adults

- Advise patient to protect the hearing aid from water, alcohol, hair spray or cologne, perspiration, rain, and snow and to avoid exposing it to extremes of temperature.
- Encourage patient to store hearing aids and batteries with desiccant or in an electronic dryer to prolong life, minimize repairs, and preserve batteries.
- The small size of some hearing aids may make them difficult to manipulate, particularly for individuals with decreased dexterity or visual acuity. Consult an audiologist to identify an aid that accommodates a patient's particular need.

Patients With Disabilities

- People with disabilities, including hearing loss and deafness, can benefit from social support. Assist patient in the identification of community programs that promote involvement of people with disabilities (WHO, 2023).

Home Care

- Determine presence and willingness of family caregiver to perform necessary care of hearing aid.
- Assess patient's home and determine need for special precautions given patient's limited hearing.

◆ CLINICAL JUDGMENT AND NEXT GENERATION NCLEX® EXAMINATION–STYLE QUESTIONS

The outpatient nurse is assessing an 82-year-old patient who is hard of hearing and has been experiencing blurry vision lately. The patient's spouse came to the appointment. The patient states, "I don't know what happened. I was driving home and looked over to turn up the radio. I didn't see an upcoming stop sign, so I hit the car in front of me." The patient goes on to tell you, "I was not wearing my hearing aid, and I am supposed to have cataract surgery soon for my right eye."

1. Which approach will the nurse use to communicate with the patient? **Select all that apply.**
   1. Speak much more loudly than usual
   2. Talk slowly in a normal tone
   3. Stand so that the patient can see the nurse's face
   4. Obtain the use of an interpreter
   5. Address only the spouse when talking

2. The nurse checks the hearing aid to make sure it is working. After washing hands and applying clean gloves, which action will the nurse take **next**?
   1. Place hearing aid in storage case
   2. Wash the patient's ear canal
   3. Use brush to gently clean holes in the device
   4. Replace the battery

3. When further assessing the patient's sight, which questions will the nurse ask? **Select all that apply.**
   1. "Why did you decide to drive when you know that you will have eye surgery soon?"
   2. "Have you noticed new changes in your vision recently?"
   3. "Do you normally wear corrective lenses like glasses or contact lenses?"
   4. "Are your eyes drier than usual?"
   5. "Have you experienced any eye injuries lately?"

4. Which statement by the patient requires further nursing intervention?
   1. "I clean my eyes from the inner corner to the outside of each eye."
   2. "I use eye drops to lubricate my eyes like my optometrist directed me."
   3. "I have an appointment with my doctor next week regarding cataract surgery."
   4. "I feel like my left eye is starting to get blurry like my right eye."

5. When providing education to the patient regarding hearing aids and hearing, which information will the nurse provide? **Select all that apply.**
   1. Tell your family ways that help you hear the best.
   2. Stay at least 5 feet away from someone to hear more clearly.
   3. Protect your hearing aids by storing them out of reach of children and pets.
   4. It is normal for hearing aids to cause discomfort.
   5. Heat from a hair dryer can damage hearing aids.
   6. Reduce background noise or move to a quiet area when talking with others.
   7. You will need to change the batteries in the hearing aids every few days.
   8. Once the hearing aids have been inserted, do not remove them.

Visit the Evolve site for Answers to Clinical Judgment and Next Generation NCLEX® Examination2Style Questions.

REFERENCES

Agency for Healthcare Research and Quality (AHRQ): *Teach-back: intervention*, 2023. https://www.ahrq.gov/patient-safety/reports/engage/interventions/teachback.html.

Alicea C, Doherty K: Targeted re-instruction for hearing aid use and care skills, *Am J Audiol* 30:590–601, 2021.

American Optometric Association: *Healthy vision and contact lenses*, 2023a. https://www.aoa.org/healthy-eyes/vision-and-vision-correction/healthy-vision-and-contact-lenses?sso=y. Accessed October 3, 2023.

American Optometric Association: *Types of contact lenses*, 2023b. https://www.aoa.org/healthy-eyes/vision-and-vision-correction/types-of-contact-lenses?sso=y. Accessed October 3, 2023.

American Optometric Association: *Contact lens care*, 2023c. https://www.aoa.org/healthy-eyes/vision-and-vision-correction/contact-lens-care?sso=y. Accessed October 3, 2023.

American Optometric Association: *Protecting your eyes at work*, 2023d. https://www.aoa.org/healthy-eyes/caring-for-your-eyes/protecting-your-vision?sso=y. Accessed October 3, 2023.

American Speech-Language-Hearing Association: *Audiologist roles and responsibilities*, n.d. https://www.asha.org/Students/Audiologist-Roles-and-Responsibilities/. Accessed October 3, 2023.

Ay E, Alay D: Ophthalmic findings in COVID-19 intensive care prospective study: frequency of ophthalmic findings, relationship with inflammation markers, and effect on prognosis in patients treated in the COVID-19 intensive care unit, *Turk J Ophthalmol* 52:6–13, 2022.

Centers for Disease Control and Prevention (CDC): *What is health literacy?* 2023. https://www.cdc.gov/healthliteracy/learn/index.html.

Claassen K, et al. Current status of emergency treatment of chemical eye burns in workplaces, *Int J Ophthalmol* 14(2):306–309, 2021.

Corbett MC, Bizrah M: Chemical injuries of the ocular surface, *Focus: The Royal College of Opthalmologists Quarterly Magazine*, April 2018. https://www.rcophth.ac.uk/wp-content/uploads/2018/04/College-News-April-2018-Focus.pdf.

Food and Drug Administration (FDA): *Hearing aids*, 2023, U.S. Food and Drug Administration. https://www.fda.gov/medical-devices/consumer-products/hearing-aids. Accessed October 3, 2023.

Guillermo S, et al: Visual, hearing, and dual sensory impairment are associated with higher depression and anxiety in women, *Arch Physical Med Rehabil* 102(10):e104, 2021.

Gwenhure T: Procedure for eye irrigation to treat ocular chemical injury. *Nursing Times [online]* 116(2):46-48, 2020.

Hockenberry MJ, et al: *Wong's nursing care of infants and children*, ed 12, St. Louis, 2024, Elsevier.

Horton GA, et al: Cerumen management: an updated clinical review and evidence-based approach for primary care physicians, *J Prim Care Community Health* 11:1–5, 2020.

Krogmann R, Khalili Y: *Cochlear implants*. Treasure Island: FL: StatPearls Publishing, 2022.

Kwan C, et al: Cognitive decline, sensory impairment, and the use of audio-visual aids by long-term care facility residents, *BMC Geriatr* 22:216, 2022.

Jaiswal A, et al: What can be done differently to enable the social participation of individuals with deafblindness or dual sensory impairment? *Arch Phys Med Rehabil Assoc* 102(10):e104, 2021.

Lahiji P, et al: The effect of implementation of evidence-based eye care protocol for patients in the intensive care units on superficial eye disorders, *BMC Ophthalmol* 21:275, 2021.

Morandi A, et al: Visual and hearing impairment are associated with delirium in hospitalized patients: results of a multisite prevalence study, *J Am Med Dir Assoc* 22(6):1162–1167, 2021.

Meyer F, et al: Cerumen impaction removal in general practices: a comparison of approved standard products, *J Prim Care Community Health* 11:1–5, 2020.

Schafer E, et al: Meta-analysis of speech recognition outcomes in younger and older adults with cochlear implants, *Am J Audiol* 30:481–496, 2021.

Schumann JA, et al: Ear irrigation. *Stat Pearls* [Internet], National Library of Medicine, September 26, 2022. https://www.ncbi.nlm.nih.gov/books/NBK459335/.

Sevy J, et al: *Cerumen impaction removal*. Treasure Island: FL: StatPearls Publishing, 2023.

Solim M, et al: Clinical outcomes and safety of Diphoterine® irrigation for chemical eye injury: A singlecentre experience in the United Kingdom, *Ther Adv Ophthalmol* 13:1–8, 2021.

The Joint Commission (TJC): *2023 National patient safety goals*, Oakbrook Terrace, IL, 2023, The Joint Commission. https://www.jointcommission.org/standards/national-patient-safety-goals/.

Touhy TA, Jett KF: *Ebersole and Hess' gerontological nursing and healthy aging*, ed 6, St. Louis, 2022, Elsevier.

Webb A: Effective communication in medical settings; your rights under the law, *Hearing Life* 43(2):16–17, 2022.

World Health Organization: *Deafness and hearing loss*, 2023. https://www.who.int/news-room/fact-sheets/detail/deafness-and-hearing-loss. Accessed October 3, 2023.

Hygiene: Next-Generation NCLEX® (NGN)–Style Unfolding Case Study

PHASE 1

QUESTION 1.

The oncoming nurse is reviewing the previous nurse's documentation regarding a newly admitted client.

Highlight the information that indicates to the oncoming nurse that the client would benefit from a full bed bath.

History and Physical	Nurses' Notes	Vital Signs	Laboratory Results

1544: Client admitted after a 3-day stay on the intensive care unit (ICU) for diabetic ketoacidosis. History of type 1 diabetes mellitus and glaucoma. Client is very weak; awakes when hearing name and then falls back asleep quickly. Lung sounds clear. S_1S_2 present without murmur. Bowel sounds present × 4 quadrants. Strength diminished and weak, yet equal in all extremities. No skin breakdown noted. Upon assessment, the client has been incontinent of urine. Blood glucose 1 hour after last meal is 140 mg/dL. Vital signs: T 37.6°C (99.6°F); HR 68 beats/min; RR 12 breaths/min; BP 108/72 mm Hg; SpO_2 99% on RA.

QUESTION 2.

Nursing assessment noted that the client was incontinent of urine.

Complete the following sentence by selecting from the lists of options below.

The nurse identifies that the client is at high risk for <u>1 [Select]</u> due to <u>2 [Select]</u>.

Options for 1	Options for 2
Skin breakdown	Blood glucose 140 mg/dL
Urinary tract infection	Incontinence
Ongoing diabetes ketoacidosis	Type 1 diabetes
Sepsis	Temperature 37.6°C (99.6°F)

PHASE 2

QUESTION 3.

The clients is incontinent of urine and at risk for skin breakdown.

Complete the following sentence by selecting from the lists of options below.

The nurse will <u>1 [Select]</u> and <u>2 [Select]</u> as the priorities of care at this time.

Options for 1	Options for 2
Obtain a temperature	Auscultate the lungs
Change the bed	Place an absorbent pad beneath the client
Perform a subsequent blood glucose test	Provide the client with a bath

QUESTION 4.

The nurse is planning care.

Determine whether the following potential nursing actions are indicated or not indicated for the plan of care.

Potential Nursing Actions	Indicated	Not Indicated
Perform a full skin assessment during the bed bath.		
Delegate a full bed bath and linen change to assistive personnel (AP).		
Have the client sit in a chair while the linens are changed.		
Contact the health care provider.		
Determine whether the client uses eyedrops for glaucoma.		

PHASE 3

QUESTION 5.

The nurse is at the bedside ready to administer eyedrops for glaucoma to the client.

Select the **3** actions the nurse would take at this time.

- ○ Don sterile gloves prior to administration.
- ○ Identify the client with one form of identification.
- ○ Wipe each eye from the outer to the inner canthus.
- ○ Assess the eyes for redness, drainage, irritation, and lesions.
- ○ Stabilize the eyedropper against the inner canthus of each eye.
- ○ Explain the procedure to the client before administering eyedrops.
- ○ Observe the pupils for equality in reaction to light and accommodation.

QUESTION 6.

Which of the following client statements show that interventions undertaken by the nurse were effective? **Select all that apply.**

- ○ "My skin feels rough and dry."
- ○ "I feel like sitting up in bed at this time."
- ○ "I haven't experienced skin breakdown since I was hospitalized."
- ○ "All of the movement I had to do during my bath made me nauseated."
- ○ "I noticed that I have some little blisters on the backs of both of my heels."
- ○ "My spouse and I are planning to make a healthy menu plan when I am discharged."

Safe medication administration is a complex process that requires sound clinical judgment. You apply knowledge of patients' conditions, pharmacological concepts, types of medication actions, expected therapeutic and possible adverse effects, and unexpected reactions when deciding how to properly prepare and administer medications. Each patient will present clinical conditions, physical risk factors, and a knowledge level that will require you to adapt your approach in how you educate the patient about medications. When you perform one of the medication administration skills in this unit, you will apply critical thinking in making clinical judgments about how to safely and accurately prepare, administer, and evaluate medications for your patients.

Administration of medications is a time-sensitive and time-pressured nursing action. Safe medication preparation practices include having a quiet, uninterrupted environment to review and prepare all medication orders. In addition to having a thorough pharmacological knowledge base, you must know the nursing implications for each medication. Carefully read the label on a medication container and compare with the health care provider's order; accurately calculate and double-check dosages, especially for high-risk medications; and review the need for any preadministration assessments. When you prepare any medication for a patient, you are the individual responsible for administering that medication.

There are standards to use when assessing a patient to determine if a medication order is accurate and appropriate for your patient. You also apply clinical judgment to ensure that you practice the seven rights of medication administration: (1) the right medication is given; (2) the right dose is available; (3) the medication is administered to the right patient, (4) by the right route, (5) and at the right time; (6) following administration, there is the right documentation of the medication administration; and (7) the right indication for the medication ordered.

Prior to administering any medications, assess your patient and use clinical judgment to determine if any modifications are needed. For example, a patient with facial paralysis may have difficulty swallowing a pill but can safely handle the medication when mixed in a soft food. Use clinical judgment to determine whether the tablet can be safely crushed, if the contents of a capsule containing the same medication can be removed, or if the medication comes in a liquid form. Then obtain an order from the health care provider to administer the medication in the modified format.

In another example, you assess your patient's skin prior to administering a topical analgesic patch. You note that the area underneath the existing patch is excessively dry, blistered, and slightly red. These cues indicate that you need to select a different site for patch placement and provide skin care to the area of tissue injury. This is necessary because topical medications are absorbed through the patient's skin, and impairments to the patient's skin and/or underlying tissue can impede the therapeutic effect.

Inhaled medications are absorbed through a patient's respiratory tract. Inhalation is an effective drug delivery system because it places the medication at the site of action. However, the success of inhaled medications depends on patients' proper use of inhalers. For positive patient outcomes, use clinical judgment in observing how your patients use their inhalers, and identify cues to determine if they are using the inhaler devices properly or whether further patient education is necessary.

Administering any parenteral medication is an invasive procedure. In addition to safe medication practices, you apply knowledge from basic skin, musculoskeletal, and venous system anatomy in order to safely administer parenteral medications. Use your assessment skills to identify the correct injection site and condition of the skin. Observe and analyze patient data cues, such as edema, injury, rash, and so on, that determine whether the site is acceptable for an injection. Your assessment should also lead to clinical judgments regarding patient positioning. Can the patient assist with positioning, or is another health care provider needed to assist?

Safe medication practices are essential to ensuring successful medication therapies, improving patient outcomes, and reducing medication errors. These practices rely on critical thinking, which involves applying knowledge and experience, coupled with competent medication administration skills. Patients can change quickly, environmental factors add to the complexity of any task, and new medications become available, but the one condition that ensures safe medication practice is the use of clinical judgment. When administering and preparing medications, apply critical thinking to make appropriate patient assessments, analyze cues derived from the assessment data to identify any problem areas, and then form clinical judgments needed to plan and implement safe medication practices. Once medications have been given, evaluate the patient's response to all types of medications.

20 Safe Medication Preparation

OUTLINE

Practice Standards, p. 587

Supplemental Standards, p. 587

Principles for Practice, p. 587

Pharmacological Concepts, p. 587

Medication Dose Responses, p. 588

Types of Medication Action, p. 589

Medication Tolerance and Dependence, p. 591

Medication Misuse, p. 591

Routes of Administration, p. 591

Medication Distribution, p. 593

Systems of Medication Measurement, p. 595

Person-Centered Care, p. 596

Safe Medication Administration, p. 596

Medication Preparation, p. 600

Evidence-Based Practice, p. 603

Preventing Medication Errors, p. 603

Safety Guidelines, p. 603

Nursing Process, p. 603

Reporting Medication Errors, p. 605

Patient and Family Caregiver Teaching, p. 605

OBJECTIVES

Mastery of content in this chapter will enable you to:
- Discuss nursing roles and responsibilities in medication administration.
- Discuss National Patient Safety Goals for medication administration.
- Explain factors that contribute to medication errors.
- Compare and contrast different types of medication actions.
- List and discuss the seven rights of medication administration.

- Identify the system of measurement for a given prescribed medication.
- Make use of selected method to calculate medication doses.
- Demonstrate the safety features of medication delivery systems.
- Identify guidelines for safe administration of medications.
- Identify nursing actions to prevent medication errors.
- Discuss methods used to educate patients about prescribed medications.

MEDIA RESOURCES

- http://evolve.elsevier.com/Perry/skills
- Review Questions
- Case Studies
- Audio Glossary

- **NSO** Nursing Skills Online
- Answers to Clinical Judgment and Next-Generation NCLEX® Examination–Style Questions
- Printable Key Points

Safe and accurate medication administration is a challenging and important nursing responsibility. You are responsible for having a full understanding of medication therapy and the related nursing implications. Nurses play an essential role in assessing for factors that place patients at risk when receiving medications and in preparing, administering, and evaluating the effects of medications. Nurses are also responsible for teaching a patient and family caregiver about medications and their side effects and evaluating a patient's and family caregiver's ability to administer medications at home.

PRACTICE STANDARDS

- Institute for Safe Medication Practices (ISMP), 2021: List of error-prone abbreviations—ISMP's list of error-prone abbreviations, symbols, and dose designations
- Institute for Safe Medication Practices (ISMP), 2022: ISMP targeted medication safety best practices for hospitals
- The Joint Commission (TJC), 2023: National Patient Safety Goals—Patient identification
- U.S. Department of Health and Human Services (USDHHS), Centers for Medicare and Medicaid Services (CMS), 2020: Updated Guidance on Medication Administration, Hospital Appendix A of State Operations Manual

SUPPLEMENTAL STANDARDS

- U.S. Food and Drug Administration (FDA), 2022: MedWatch: The FDA Safety Information and Adverse Event Reporting Program

PRINCIPLES FOR PRACTICE

Pharmacological Concepts
Medication Names

Some medications have as many as three different names. The chemical name of a medication provides an exact description of its composition and molecular structure. Nurses rarely use chemical names in clinical practice. An example of a chemical name is N-acetyl-para-aminophenol, which is commonly known as Tylenol. The manufacturer that first develops the medication gives the generic or nonproprietary name, with United States Adopted Names (USAN) Council approval (American Medical Association [AMA], 2022). Acetaminophen is an example of the generic name for Tylenol. The generic name becomes the official name listed in official publications such as the United States Pharmacopeia (USP). The trade name, brand name, or proprietary name is the name under which a manufacturer markets a medication. The trade name has the symbol (^{TM}) at the upper right of the name, indicating that the manufacturer has trademarked the name of the medication (e.g., Panadol and Tempra).

Manufacturers typically choose trade names that are easy to pronounce, spell, and remember. Many companies produce the same medication, and similarities in trade names are often confusing. Be careful to obtain the exact name and spelling for each medication before administering to your patients. Because similarities in medication names are a common cause of medication errors, the Institute for Safe Medication Practices (ISMP, 2021) publishes a list of medications that are frequently confused with one another. The ISMP recommends the use of FDA-approved tall-man or mixed-case letters when possible (e.g., aMILoride versus amLODIPine) to help health care providers easily recognize the difference between these commonly confused medications.

The physical appearances of some drugs with similar color, size, and shape have led to medication errors. For example, St. Joseph's aspirin and Crestor, a lipid-lowering agent, have a similar peach color, size, and circular shape. Generic drugs are often prescribed as a more cost-efficient substitution for brand-name medications. However, there may be dramatic differences in appearance of generic drugs, depending on the manufacturer (FDA, 2021). Patients may be confused as to why their medications have different colors or shapes when the prescription is refilled. Generic medications may be made by different manufacturers, so they may differ in appearance.

Classification

Medication classification indicates the effect of a medication on a body system, the symptoms a medication relieves, or its desired effect. Usually each class contains more than one medication that is used for the same type of health problem. For example, patients who have asthma often take a variety of medications to control their illness, such as beta$_2$-adrenergic agonists. The beta$_2$-adrenergic classification contains more than 15 different medications (Burchum & Rosenthal, 2022). Some medications are in more than one class; for example, aspirin is an analgesic, an antipyretic, and an antiinflammatory medication.

Medication Forms

Medications are available in a variety of forms or preparations. The form of the medication determines its route of administration. The composition of a medication influences its absorption and metabolism. Many medications are made in several forms such as tablets, caplets, or suppositories. When administering a medication, be certain to use the proper form (Table 20.1).

Pharmacokinetics

A medication must enter a patient's body; be absorbed and distributed to cells, tissues, or a specific organ; and then alter physiological function to be therapeutic. Pharmacokinetics is the study of how medications enter the body, reach their site of action, are metabolized, and exit the body. Understanding pharmacokinetics allows you to properly time medication administration, select an administration route, and judge a patient's response to medications. Absorption is the passage of medication molecules into the blood from the site of administration. Factors that influence the rate of absorption include the administration route, ability of a medication to dissolve, blood flow to the administration site, body surface area (BSA), and lipid solubility of a medication (Table 20.2). After a medication is absorbed, it is distributed to tissues and organs and finally to the site of drug action. The rate and extent of distribution depend on circulation, cell membrane permeability, and protein binding. Poor perfusion (e.g., heart failure and edema of the skin) alters medication distribution. A medication must pass through biological membranes to reach certain organs. Some membranes are barriers to the passage of medications. For example, the blood-brain barrier allows only fat-soluble medications to pass into the brain and cerebrospinal fluid. The degree to which oral medications bind to serum proteins such as albumin affects distribution. Even though a drug can bind with albumin, only some molecules will be bound at any moment (Burchum & Rosenthal, 2022). Bound molecules of medication cannot reach their sites of action or undergo metabolism or excretion until the bond is broken. This increases a drug's half-life (Burchum & Rosenthal, 2022). Only the unbound, or "free," medication is active. Older adults and patients with liver disease or malnutrition have reduced albumin, which increases the amount of unbound medication and increases their risk for medication toxicity.

After a medication reaches its site of action, it is metabolized into a less active or inactive form. Biotransformation occurs under the influence of enzymes that detoxify, degrade (break down), and remove biologically active chemicals. Most biotransformation occurs in the liver, although the lungs, kidneys, blood, and intestines also play a role. Patients (e.g., older adults and those with chronic disease) are at risk for medication toxicity if their organs cannot metabolize medications effectively.

The final aspect of pharmacokinetics is excretion, the process by which medications exit the body through the lungs, exocrine glands, bowel, kidneys, and liver (Burchum & Rosenthal, 2022).

TABLE 20.1

Forms of Medication

Form	Description
Medication Forms Commonly Prepared for Administration by Oral Route	
Solid Forms	
Caplet	Shaped like a capsule and coated for ease of swallowing
Capsule	Medication encased in a gelatin shell
Tablet	Powdered medication compressed into a hard disk or cylinder; in addition to primary medication, contains binders (adhesive to allow powder to stick together), disintegrators (to promote tablet dissolution), lubricants (for ease of manufacturing), and fillers (for convenient tablet size)
Enteric coated	Coated tablet that does not dissolve in stomach; coating dissolves in intestine, where medication is absorbed
Liquid Forms	
Elixir	Clear fluid containing water and alcohol; often sweetened
Extract	Concentrated medication form made by removing the active part of the medication from its components; extracts are prepared as a syrup or dried form of pharmacologically active medication, usually made by evaporating solution
Aqueous solution	Substance dissolved in water and syrups
Aqueous suspension	Finely dissolved drug particles in liquid medium must be shaken; when left standing, particles settle to bottom of container
Syrup	Medication dissolved in concentrated sugar solution
Tincture	Alcohol extract from plant or vegetable
Other Oral Forms and Terms Associated With Oral Preparations	
Troche (lozenge)	Flat, round tablet that dissolves in mouth to release medication; not meant for ingestion
Aerosol	Aqueous medication sprayed and absorbed in mouth and upper airway; not meant for ingestion
Sustained release	Tablet or capsule that contains small particles of a medication coated with material that requires a varying amount of time to dissolve
Medication Forms Commonly Prepared for Administration by Topical Route	
Ointment (salve or cream)	Semisolid, externally applied preparation, usually containing one or more medications
Liniment	Usually contains alcohol, oil, or soapy emollient applied to skin
Lotion	Semiliquid suspension that usually protects, cools, or cleans skin
Paste	Medication preparation that is thicker than ointment; absorbed through skin more slowly than ointment; often used for skin protection
Transdermal patch or disk	Medicated disk or patch embedded with medication that is applied to skin. Drug absorbed through skin over a designated period of time (e.g., 24 hours)
Medication Forms Commonly Prepared for Administration by Parenteral Route	
Solution	Sterile preparation that contains water/normal saline with one or more dissolved compounds
Powder	Sterile particles of medication that are dissolved in a sterile liquid (e.g., water, normal saline) before administration
Medication Forms Commonly Prepared for Instillation Into Body Cavities	
Suppository	Solid dosage form mixed with gelatin and shaped in form of a pellet for insertion into body cavity (rectum or vagina) (Suppository melts when it reaches body temperature and is then absorbed.)
Intraocular disk	Small, flexible oval (similar to a contact lens) consisting of two soft outer layers and a middle layer containing medication; slowly releases medication when moistened by ocular fluid

The chemical makeup of a medication determines the organ of excretion. For example, gaseous and volatile compounds such as nitrous oxide exit through the lungs. The site of excretion poses implications for nursing care. For example, when medications exit through sweat glands, you provide skin care to reduce irritation. You must know if a medication is excreted through the intestines because the administration of laxatives or enemas increases peristalsis, accelerates excretion, and thus lessens the time for medication effects. When patients have reduced renal function, they are at risk for medication toxicity because the kidneys are the main organs for medication excretion.

Medication Dose Responses

A medication undergoes absorption, distribution, metabolism, and excretion after administration. Medications take time to enter the bloodstream, except when administered intravenously (IV). When a medication is prescribed, the goal is a continual blood level within a safe therapeutic range. The minimum effective concentration (MEC) is the plasma level of a medication below which the effect of the medication does not occur. The toxic concentration is the level at which toxic effects occur. The safe therapeutic range is between the MEC and the toxic concentration (Fig. 20.1). When a medication is administered repeatedly,

TABLE 20.2

Medication Absorption

Absorption Factor	Physiological Effects
Route of administration	Topical applications on skin absorb slowly. Medications applied to mucous membranes and respiratory airways absorb quickly. Oral medications pass through the gastrointestinal tract and absorb slowly. The intravenous route produces the most rapid absorption. Medication is available immediately when it enters the systemic circulation.
Ability to dissolve	Solutions and liquid suspensions absorb more readily than tablets or capsules. Acidic medications pass through the gastric mucosa rapidly and absorb rapidly, whereas basic medications (pH greater than 7.0) do not absorb before reaching the small intestine.
Blood flow	When the administration site contains a rich blood supply, medications absorb rapidly.
Body surface area	A medication in contact with a large surface area (e.g., small intestine) absorbs faster than one in contact with smaller surface area (e.g., stomach).
Lipid solubility	Medications that are highly lipid soluble absorb more readily.

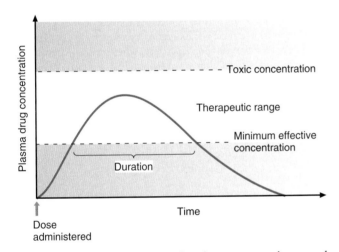

FIG. 20.1 The therapeutic range of medication occurs between the minimum effective concentration and the toxic concentration. (*From Burchum J, Rosenthal L: Lehne's pharmacology for nursing care, ed 10, St Louis, 2019, Elsevier.*)

its serum level fluctuates between doses. The highest level is called the *peak concentration,* and the lowest level is called the *trough concentration.* After peaking, the serum concentration falls progressively. With IV infusions, the peak concentration occurs quickly, but the serum level also begins to fall immediately. Some medication doses (e.g., vancomycin or gentamicin) are based on peak and trough serum levels. A patient's trough level is drawn as a blood sample 30 minutes before the drug is administered, when the drug should be at its lowest serum level, and the peak level is drawn whenever the drug is expected to reach its peak concentration. The results of the blood test reveal if the drug is reaching its therapeutic blood level.

All medications have a biological half-life, which is the time it takes for excretion processes to lower the serum medication concentration by half. To maintain a therapeutic plateau, a patient needs to receive regular fixed doses. For example, pain medications are most effective for some cancer patients when they are given around the clock (ATC) rather than when a patient intermittently reports pain because the body maintains an almost constant level of pain medication (Burchum & Rosenthal, 2022). After an initial medication dose, the patient receives each successive dose when the previous dose reaches its half-life. The patient and nurse need to follow regular dosage schedules and administer prescribed doses at correct intervals. Know the following time intervals of medication action to anticipate the effect of a medication:

- Onset of medication action: Time it takes after a medication is administered for it to produce a response
- *Peak action:* Time it takes for a medication to reach its highest effective peak concentration
- *Trough:* Minimum blood serum concentration of medication reached just before the next scheduled dose
- *Duration of action:* Length of time during which a medication is present in a concentration great enough to produce a therapeutic effect
- *Plateau:* Blood serum concentration reached and maintained after repeated, fixed doses

Types of Medication Action

Medications vary in the way they act and their types of action. Patients do not always respond in the same way to each successive dose of a medication. Sometimes the same medication causes very different responses in different patients. Therefore it is essential to understand all the effects that medications have on patients.

Therapeutic Effects

Each medication has a therapeutic effect (i.e., the intended or desired physiological response of a medication). For example, you administer morphine sulfate, an analgesic, to relieve a patient's pain. Sometimes a single medication has many therapeutic effects. For example, aspirin relieves pain and reduces fever and tissue inflammation. Knowing the desired therapeutic effect for each medication allows you to provide patient education and accurately evaluate its desired effect.

Adverse Drug Reactions

An adverse drug reaction (ADR) or event (ADE) is defined by the World Health Organization (WHO) as a noxious and unintended response to a drug that occurs at doses normally used in humans for the prophylaxis, diagnosis, or treatment of disease or for the modifications of physiological function (WHO, 2020). These unpredictable events harm patients (Centers for Disease Control and Prevention [CDC], 2019). Although sometimes they are apparent immediately, unfortunately they often take weeks or months to develop. Early clinical recognition of ADRs is the important first step in identification. ADRs range from mild (e.g., rashes or photosensitivity to light) to potentially fatal (anaphylaxis). An ADR will usually require the drug to be discontinued or the dose reduced immediately (WHO, 2020).

When drugs are used properly, many ADRs can be avoided or minimized (Burchum & Rosenthal, 2022). Prompt recognition and reporting of ADRs prevent serious injury to patients. The drug classes most commonly responsible for ADRs in adults are adrenal corticosteroids, antibiotics, anticoagulants, antineoplastic and immunosuppressive drugs, cardiovascular drugs, nonsteroidal antiinflammatory drugs, and opiates (WHO, 2020). Always assess patients who may be at high risk for an ADR, such as pregnant women and patients with chronic disorders (e.g., hypertension, epilepsy, heart disease, psychoses) (Burchum & Rosenthal, 2022). Health care providers report adverse events to the FDA using the MedWatch program (FDA, 2022).

Allergic Reactions. Allergic reactions are a type of ADR that results from exposure to an initial dose of a medication causing a patient to become sensitized immunologically. The medication acts as an antigen, which causes antibodies to be produced. With repeated administration, a patient develops an allergic response to the drug, its chemical preservatives, or a metabolite. Allergic reactions range from mild to severe, depending on the patient and the medication (Table 20.3).

Among the different classes of medications, antibiotics cause a high incidence of allergic reactions. Severe or anaphylactic reactions, which are life threatening, are characterized by sudden constriction of bronchiolar muscles, edema of the pharynx and larynx, severe wheezing, and shortness of breath. Some patients become severely hypotensive, necessitating emergency resuscitation measures. Antibiotic hypersensitivity is common leading to adverse reactions such as diarrhea, nausea, vomiting, rashes, and gastrointestinal distress (Jourdan et al., 2020). A hypersensitivity is not an allergy. Accurate documentation of antibiotic-reported adverse reactions, the reactions and context associated with these adverse reactions, and whether these reactions confer a true allergy

must be documented (Jourdan et al., 2020). Patients who do not have true allergies may not be given first-line antibiotics, which are often more effective than second- or third- line antibiotics. First-line antibiotics have fewer side effects, are narrower in therapeutic range, and are more cost efficient (Jourdan et al., 2020).

It is common practice for hospitalized patients with known drug allergies to have their allergy information in a clearly identifiable place. This allows all caregivers to be aware of each patient's allergies. In many agencies this information is documented in a special section of the electronic health record (EHR), on the front of a patient's hard-copy medical record, in the medication administration record (MAR), or on a specially designed label that is applied to the front of a patient's chart. Patients also receive color-coded allergy identification bands to wear around the wrist. *Always document a patient's allergies in the MAR.* Patients who are cared for in other settings (e.g., home or community clinics) and have a known history of an allergy to a medication or substance should wear an identification bracelet or medal, which alerts all health care providers to the allergies in case a patient is found unconscious or is unable to communicate (Fig. 20.2). It is often common that patients list having an allergy to a drug when it is not a true allergy but rather a hypersensitivity or side effect. It is important for the nurse to be able to recognize the difference between a true allergy and a side effect. For example, a patient who has nausea is more likely to have a hypersensitivity, whereas the occurrence of hives may indicate an allergic reaction. Ask patients to describe the common effects they experience from medications.

Side Effects

Every medication has the potential to cause harm. No medication is totally safe and absolutely free of nontherapeutic effects. *Side effect* is a term often used interchangeably with ADR. Side effects are any effects caused by a drug other than the intended therapeutic

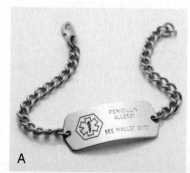
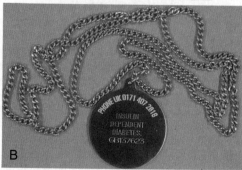

FIG. 20.2 Identification bracelet (A) and medal (B). (*A from iStock.com/monkeybusinessimages; B from Scully C: Scully's medical problems in dentistry, ed 7, St Louis, 2014, Elsevier.*)

TABLE 20.3

Mild Allergic Reactions

Symptom	Description
Angioedema	Acute, painless, dermal, subcutaneous, or submucosal swelling involving the face, neck, lips, larynx, hands, feet, or genitalia
Eczema (rash)	Small, raised vesicles that are usually reddened; often distributed over the entire body
Pruritus	Itching of the skin; accompanies most rashes
Rhinitis	Inflammation of mucous membranes lining the nose, causing swelling and clear watery discharge
Urticaria (hives)	Raised, irregularly shaped skin eruptions with varying sizes and shapes; eruptions have reddened margins and pale centers

effect, whether beneficial, neutral, or harmful (WHO, 2020). They are predictable and often unavoidable secondary effects produced at a usual therapeutic drug dose level. The intensity of side effects is often dose dependent. If the side effects are serious enough to outweigh the benefits of the therapeutic action of a medication, the health care provider will likely discontinue the medication. Patients commonly stop taking medications because of side effects such as anorexia, nausea, vomiting, dizziness, drowsiness, dry mouth, constipation, and diarrhea. Report any side effect to the health care provider to ensure that it is not incorrectly interpreted as a more serious ADR.

Toxic Effects

The WHO (2020) defines drug toxicity as the adverse effects of a drug that occur because the dose or plasma concentration has risen above the therapeutic range, either unintentionally or intentionally (drug overdose). Toxic effects develop after prolonged intake of a medication or when a medication accumulates in the blood because of impaired metabolism or excretion. Excess amounts of a medication within the body sometimes have lethal effects, depending on the action of the medication. For example, toxic levels of morphine, an opioid, cause severe respiratory depression and death. Antidotes are available to treat specific types of medication toxicity. For example, naloxone, an opioid antagonist, reverses the effects of opioid toxicity.

Idiosyncratic Reactions

An idiosyncratic reaction is an unpredictable effect in which a patient overreacts or underreacts to a medication or has a reaction different from normal. Predicting which patients will have an idiosyncratic response is impossible. For example, lorazepam is an antianxiety medication that may cause agitation and delirium when given to an older adult.

Medication Interactions

When one medication modifies the action of another medication, a medication interaction occurs. Medication interactions are common in individuals who take many medications. Some medications increase or diminish the action of other medications and alter the way in which another medication is absorbed, metabolized, or eliminated from the body. When two medications have a synergistic effect, their combined effect is greater than the effect of one drug given separately. For example, alcohol is a central nervous system depressant that has a synergistic effect with antihistamines, antidepressants, and narcotic analgesics. Sometimes a medication interaction is the desired effect. Health providers often combine medications to create an interaction that has a therapeutic effect. For example, a patient with hypertension may receive several medications such as diuretics and vasodilators, which act together to control the blood pressure when one medication alone is not effective.

Medication Tolerance and Dependence

Medication tolerance is the diminished response to a medication with repeated use and occurs over time. A patient receives the same medication for long periods of time and then requires higher doses to produce the same desired effect. Patients taking various pain medications may develop tolerance over time. It may take a month or longer for tolerance to occur.

Medication tolerance is not the same as medication dependence. Two types of medication dependence exist: psychological (or addiction) and physical. In psychological dependence, the patient desires the medication for a benefit other than the intended effect.

Physical dependence implies that a patient will experience withdrawal effects if the medication is stopped abruptly. When patients receive medications for a short time, such as for postoperative pain, dependence is rare. However, prescribed opioids increase a patient's risk for addiction. To reduce this risk, the CDC (n.d.) has developed evidence-based guidelines for health care providers who prescribe opioids.

Nurses and other health care professionals play an important role in the care of patients with drug addiction. Patients need to be approached with positive attitudes so that the patient may be more open to learning about treatment options. Using the newest evidence-based treatment options can help patients with addictions receive the care and treatment they need.

Medication Misuse

Misuse of medication includes overuse, underuse, and nonadherence. Patients of all ages misuse medications. Older adults are at greatest risk because of polypharmacy (taking 5 or more pills a day or currently taking medications for five or more conditions [Okoli et al., 2020]). The incidence of prescription and over-the-counter (OTC) drug misuse and abuse is increasing. The most commonly abused prescription medications are opioids, stimulants, tranquilizers, and sedatives. Common OTC medications that patients misuse or abuse include antihistamines, cough syrup, and cold medication containing dextromethorphan (Schifano et al., 2021). A thorough patient assessment can reveal factors contributing to nonadherence and overuse or underuse of medications. You are ethically and legally responsible to understand the problems of persons using medications improperly. When caring for patients with suspected medication abuse or dependence, be aware of your values and attitudes about the willful use of harmful substances.

Routes of Administration

The route prescribed for administering a medication (Table 20.4) depends on its properties and desired effect and on a patient's physical and mental condition. Because of what you know about each patient, you need to collaborate with a health care provider in determining the best route for a patient's medical condition. Table 20.5 summarizes the factors that influence the choice of administration routes.

TABLE 20.4

Routes of Medication Administration

Route	Description
Nonparenteral	
Oral, buccal	By mouth/mucous membrane
Sublingual	Under the tongue
Topical	On the skin (as a cream or patch) and eyedrops/eardrops
Suppository	Into the rectum or vagina
Inhaled	In through the respiratory system
Parenteral	
Intramuscular (IM)	Into a muscle
Subcutaneous	Into the subcutaneous tissue of the skin
Intradermal (ID)	Into the dermis of the skin
Epidural	Into the epidural space
Intravenous (IV)	Into a vein

TABLE 20.5

Factors Influencing Choice of Administration Routes

Advantages	Disadvantages/Contraindications
Oral, Buccal, Sublingual Routes	
Routes are easy and comfortable to administer, convenient, economical; may produce local or systemic effects; and rarely cause anxiety for patient.	Gastric secretions destroy some medications. Oral administration is contraindicated in patients who are NPO and unable to swallow (e.g., patients with neuromuscular disorders, esophageal strictures, and mouth lesions). Routes are avoided when patient has alterations in GI function (e.g., nausea and vomiting), with reduced GI motility (after general anesthesia or bowel inflammation), and with surgical resection of part of GI tract. Do not give oral medications when patient has gastric suction or before certain diagnostic tests or surgery. An unconscious or confused patient is unable or unwilling to swallow or hold sublingual medication under tongue or buccal medication in cheek. Oral medications sometimes irritate lining of GI tract, discolor teeth, or have an unpleasant taste.
Subcutaneous, Intramuscular, Intravenous, Intradermal, Epidural Routes	
Routes provide means of administration when oral medications are contraindicated. More rapid absorption occurs than with topical or oral routes.	There are risks for introducing infection, and medications are expensive. Some patients experience pain from repeated needlesticks. Avoid subcutaneous, IM, and ID routes in patients with bleeding tendencies. There is risk for tissue damage with subcutaneous injections.
IV infusion provides medication delivery when patient is critically ill or long-term therapy is necessary. If peripheral perfusion is poor, IV route is preferred over injections.	IV and IM routes have higher absorption rates, thus placing patients at higher risk for reactions.
Epidural provides excellent pain control (see Chapter 16).	It limits mobility during administration, and there is risk for infection.
Skin	
Topical	
Topical skin applications provide primarily local effect. Route is usually painless. Limited side effects occur.	Extensive applications often require dressings that are bulky for a patient when maneuvering. Do not apply to skin if abrasions are present, unless that is the reason for order. Avoid placing over areas of skin with excessive hair growth, as absorption and adherence may be decreased. Medications can be absorbed by person applying them if gloves are not worn.
Transdermal	
Transdermal applications provide prolonged systemic effects with limited side effects.	Application leaves oily or pasty substance on skin and may soil clothing. Some patients have sensitivity to adhesive.
Mucous Membranes (Includes Eyes, Ears, Nose, Vaginal, Rectal, Buccal, and Sublingual Routes)	
Therapeutic effects are provided by local application to involved sites. Aqueous solutions are readily absorbed and capable of causing systemic effects.	Mucous membranes are highly sensitive to some medication concentrations. Insertion of rectal and vaginal medications often causes embarrassment.
Mucous membranes provide route of administration when oral medications are contraindicated.	Rectal suppositories are contraindicated if patients have had rectal surgery or if active rectal bleeding is present. If eardrum is ruptured, otic medications are usually contraindicated.
Inhalation	
Inhalation provides rapid relief for local respiratory problems. An inhaled form of insulin is also available. Route provides easy access for introduction of general anesthetic gases.	Some local agents cause serious systemic effects. If patients are unable to administer inhaler correctly, medication is ineffective. Inhalation is difficult to learn for older adults and children.
Intraocular Disk	
Route is advantageous in that it does not require frequent administration (e.g., as for eyedrops). Patient can also wear disk when sleeping or swimming. Dry eyes do not affect medication delivery.	Local reactions such as tearing, itching, or redness of the eyes occur. Patient needs to know how to insert disk into and remove from eye. Medication is often expensive. Medication is contraindicated in patients with eye infections.

GI, Gastrointestinal; *ID*, intradermal; *IM*, intramuscular; *IV*, intravenous; *NPO*, nothing by mouth.

Medication Distribution

Health care providers write medication orders, pharmacists dispense medications, and nurses verify and deliver medications to patients. Verification is the three-system check to ensure safe medication administration. The first check is performed by the health care provider—ordering the right drug for the right purpose. The pharmacist performs the second check to ensure that the drug is appropriate and ordered correctly and then provided to the unit correctly. Finally, the nurse verifies the drug before administration with the *three checks* for accuracy to be sure that it is appropriate and ordered correctly.

Several technologies for medication distribution have the potential for reducing medication errors and ADRs. The technologies include computerized provider order entry (CPOE), automated medication dispensing systems (AMDSs), and bar-coding (Batson et al., 2021; Keenan et al., 2021).

Computerized Provider Order Entry

CPOE is a system that allows health care providers to enter orders for medications electronically, eliminating the need for written orders. CPOE increases the accuracy and legibility of medication orders, updates the heath care provider of any drug interactions or reactions, and provides a means of timely communication within the interprofessional team (Keenan et al., 2021). Decision support software integrated into a CPOE system allows for automatic drug allergy checks, dosage indications, baseline laboratory result checks, and identification of potential drug interactions. For example, if the health system determines that an increase or decrease in serum potassium values of 1 mEq/L in a 24-hour period is significant, a patient whose serum potassium falls from 4 mEq/L to 3 mEq/L will be included in the lab report that goes into the CPOE. The pharmacist or other health care provider can then examine the medication profile to determine whether the drop in the potassium occurred because of an ADR (e.g., a diuretic) (WHO, 2020). When a health care provider enters an order through CPOE, the information about the order immediately transmits to the pharmacy and ultimately to the nurses' MAR without the need for written transcription.

Distribution Systems

Systems for storing and distributing medications vary. Agencies providing nursing care have special areas for stocking and dispensing medications. Special medication rooms, portable locked carts, computerized medication cabinets, and individual storage units next to patients' rooms are examples of storage areas used. Medication storage areas must be locked when unattended.

Unit Dose

The standard for medication distribution is the unit-dose system. The system uses an AMDS or a cart containing a drawer with a 24-hour supply of medications for each patient. Each drawer has a label with the name of the patient in each designated room. The unit dose is the ordered dose of medication that the patient receives at one time. Each medication form is wrapped separately. At a designated time each day, the drawers in the cart are refilled by a pharmacy technician. A cart also contains limited amounts of as-needed (prn) and stock medications for special situations. The unit-dose system is designed to reduce the number of medication errors and saves steps in dispensing medications.

Automated Medication Dispensing Systems

AMDSs (Fig. 20.3) within a health care agency are networked with one another and with other computer systems in the agency (e.g., the computerized EHR). AMDSs control the dispensing of all medications, including opioids. Each nurse has a personal security code,

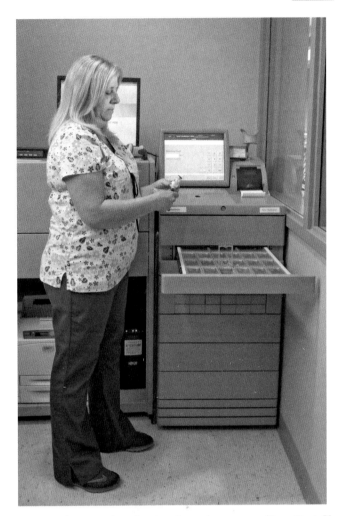

FIG. 20.3 Automated medication dispensing system. *(From Davis K, Guerra T: Mosby's pharmacy technician: principles and practice, ed 5, St Louis, 2019, Elsevier.)*

allowing access to the system. If your agency uses a system that requires bioidentification, you must place your finger on a screen to access the computer. Once logged onto the AMDS, select the patient's name and medication profile. Then select the medication, dosage, and route from the medication administration record (MAR) on the computer screen. The system opens the medication drawer or dispenses the medication, records the event, and charges it to the patient. If the system is connected to the patient's MAR, information about the medication (e.g., name, dose, time) and the name of the nurse who retrieved the medication from the AMDS is documented in the patient's record. Some systems require nurses to scan bar codes before documenting this information in the patient's MAR. AMDS and barcode scanning improve accuracy of patient identification and correct medication administration and medical record keeping, reducing the chance of medication errors (Batson et al., 2021; Keenan et al., 2021).

Special Handling of Controlled Substances

You are responsible for following legal regulations when administering controlled substances (medications with potential for abuse). Controlled substances must be properly stored to prevent diversion. Diversion occurs when prescription medicines are obtained or used illegally by health care providers. Violations of the Controlled Substances Act may result in fines, imprisonment, and loss of license. Health care agencies have policies for the proper storage and distribution of controlled substances, including opioids (Box 20.1). In addition, there are new tamper-evident syringes available for opioids that do not need any assembly and feature bar-coding on both the packaging and label (e.g., hydromorphone). Most agencies use computerized systems for medication access and distribution (Fig 20.4).

BOX 20.1

Guidelines for Safe Opioid (Narcotic) Administration and Control

- Store all opioids in a locked, secure cabinet or container (e.g., computerized, locked cabinets are preferred).
- Use tamper-evident syringes when available (e.g., hydromorphone).
- Maintain a running count of opioids by counting them whenever dispensing them. If you find a discrepancy, report it immediately and correct the discrepancy.
- Use a special inventory record each time an opioid is dispensed. Records are often kept electronically and provide an accurate ongoing count of opioids used, wasted, and remaining.
- Use the record to document the patient's name, date, time of medication administration, name of medication, and dosage. If the agency keeps a paper record, the nurse dispensing the medication signs the record. If the agency uses a computerized system, the computer records the nurse's name.
- A second nurse witnesses disposal of the unused part if a nurse gives only part of a dose of a controlled substance. Computerized systems record the nurses' names electronically. If paper records are kept, both nurses sign their names on the form.
- Follow agency policy for appropriate waste of unused portions of opioids. Do not place wasted parts of medications in sharps containers.

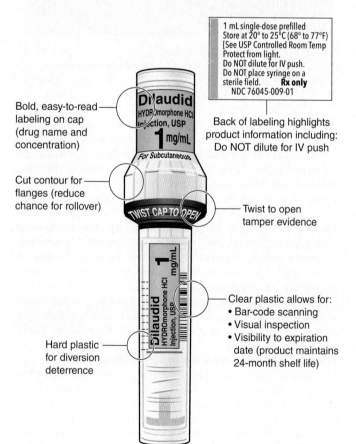

FIG. 20.4 Tamper-evident syringe (e.g., hydromorphone).

Handling Chemotherapy Medications

A common treatment for cancer is chemotherapy—antineoplastic drugs that act by killing cells that divide rapidly, one of the main properties of most cancer cells. Chemotherapy is administered in both IV and oral forms. In 2019 the Hematology/Oncology Pharmacy Association, in conjunction with the Oncology Nursing Society (ONS), updated the chemotherapy administration standards to improve both patient and nurse safety related to administration of these medications (ONS, 2018; ONS, 2022). Nurses must undergo certification to administer IV chemotherapy. However, oral chemotherapy is becoming more common and can be administered by any registered nurse (RN).

Oral chemotherapy has the same exposure risks to health care providers, patients, and their family caregivers as IV forms (Pardhan et al., 2021). Physically touching a chemotherapy tablet is dangerous. Chemotherapy is highly toxic not only to cancer cells but also to normal cells. Chemotherapy drugs cause DNA damage, leading to cell death or cell growth arrest. The damage to others may not be known for months or years because the injuries could include cancer, birth defects, or immune dysfunction. It is critical for health care providers, patients, and family caregivers to use proper protective techniques to avoid exposure to oral chemotherapy tablets.

A patient excretes chemotherapy chemicals through urine, stool, vomit, sweat, and saliva. When patients self-administer chemotherapy at home, families should be warned of the dangers of exposure. For example, patients' toilets should be double-flushed after use, during, and for 48 hours after discontinuation of chemotherapy. Toilets are a hazard for children and pets.

Accidental exposure to oral chemotherapeutic agents can occur during handling (Pardhan et al., 2021). Guidelines for health care providers, patients, and family caregivers to handle these drugs safely and appropriately are essential:

- In health care agencies, cytotoxic agents should be stored in a designated area per the manufacturer's instructions and separate from noncytotoxic agents.
- Use gloves that have been tested for chemotherapy or hazardous medication use, and double glove when indicated when preparing and handling chemotherapy medications and after handling agent or bodily secretions (Gorski et al., 2021; ONS, 2022).
- Perform thorough hand hygiene before and after glove application.
- Do not crush, cut, or split chemotherapy drugs.
- Use separate equipment to prepare chemotherapy and regular medications. Nurses must now use closed-system transfer devices when administering IV chemotherapy (Fig. 20.5) (Gorski et al., 2021).
- The health care agency must have a spill policy in place (Gorski et al., 2021).
- All disposable protective clothing is considered a single use item (Gorski et al., 2021). Dispose of protective clothing as well as any disposable materials used while handling chemotherapeutic agents as cytotoxic waste according to the local waste disposal regulatory guidelines.
- Wash any clothes or sheets that have body fluids on them in a washing machine—not by hand. Wash them twice in hot water with regular laundry detergent. Do not wash them with other clothes. If they cannot be washed right away, seal them in a plastic bag.

Bar-Coding

Bar-code labels are required on all medications, vaccines, and OTC drugs used in health care agencies. EHR technology improves patient care quality and coordination by providing health

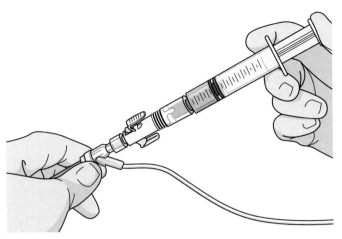

FIG. 20.5 Closed-system transfer device.

care providers easier access to patient information in a secure format. The use of electronic bar codes on medication labels and packaging has the potential to improve patient safety in several ways. Bar codes electronically link with a health care agency computer system. A patient's MAR entered into the computer database and encoded in the patient's wristband is accessible to a nurse through a handheld device. The device scans the patient's wristband and then displays the MAR. When administering a medication, the nurse scans the bar code on the drug and the patient's medical record number on the wristband. The computer processes the scanned information, charts it, and updates the patient's MAR record appropriately. The use of bar codes improves accuracy of patient identification, provides alerts to potential medication errors, and improves medical record keeping (Tolley et al., 2022).

Systems of Medication Measurement

Safely administering medications requires the ability to compute medication doses accurately and measure medications correctly. A careless mistake in placing a decimal point or adding a zero to a dose can lead to a fatal error. **Check every dose carefully before giving a medication.**

The health care industry in the United States primarily uses the metric system of measurement for medication therapy. Globally, most nations use the metric system as their standard of measurement. The Institute for Safe Medication Practices does not recommend use of a household teaspoon or tablespoon to give liquid medicines. They are inaccurate and may deliver more or less medicine than prescribed. Most over-the counter (OTC) liquid medicines almost always come with their own measuring devices using metric measures(Consumer Med Safety, 2023). Health care providers rarely use the apothecary measurement system, which includes ounces, pounds, and pints.

Metric System

As a decimal system, the metric system is the most logically organized of the measurement systems. Metric units are easy to convert and compute through simple multiplication and division. Each basic unit of measure is organized into units of 10. Multiplying or dividing by 10 forms secondary units. In multiplication the decimal point moves to the right; in division the decimal moves to the left. For example:

$$10 \text{ mg} \times 10 = 100 \text{ mg}$$
$$10 \text{ mg} \div 10 = 1 \text{ mg}$$

The basic units of measure in the metric system are the meter (length), the liter (volume), and the gram (weight). For drug calculations, you will primarily use volume and weight units. In the metric system, lowercase or capital letters designate the basic units:

$$\text{Gram} = \text{g or Gm}$$
$$\text{Liter} = \text{l or L}$$

Use only lowercase letters for abbreviations for subdivisions of major units:

$$\text{Milligram} = \text{mg}$$
$$\text{Milliliter} = \text{mL}$$

A system of Latin prefixes designates subdivision of the basic units: *deci-* (1/10 or 0.1), *centi-* (1/100)or 0.01), and *milli-* (1/1000 or 0.001). Greek prefixes designate multiples of the basic units: *deka-* (10), *hecto-* (100), and *kilo-* (1000). When writing medication dosages in metric units, health care providers and nurses use either fractions or multiples of a unit. Convert fractions to decimals:

$$500 \text{ mg or } 0.5 \text{ g, not } ½ \text{ g}$$
$$10 \text{ mL or } 0.01 \text{ L, not } 1/100 \text{ L}$$

Many actual or potential medication errors happen with the use of fractions or decimal points. For example, to make the decimal point more visible, a leading zero is *always* placed in front of a decimal (e.g., use 0.25, *not* .25). *Never* use a trailing zero (i.e., a zero after a decimal point) because if a health care worker does not see the decimal point, the patient may receive 10 times more medication than prescribed (e.g., use 5, *not* 5.0) (ISMP, 2021).

Household Measurement

Most people are familiar with household measures such as drops, teaspoons, tablespoons, cups, and quarts. Even though household measurements are convenient and familiar, they are inaccurate. Dose errors have occurred when household measures are used (ISMP, 2022; Consumer Med Safety, 2023). As a result, the ISMP recommends a best practice for all oral liquids that are not commercially available as unit-dose products. The liquids should be dispensed by the pharmacy in an oral syringe using metric measurement (ISMP, 2022). The ISMP also recommends that patients or family caregivers purchase oral liquid dosing devices (oral syringes, cups, droppers) that display only the metric scale. Encourage patients to never use household measuring devices with liquid medications (Table 20.6). Today's OTC liquid medications almost always have their own measuring devices (Consumer Med Safety, 2023).

Solutions

Solutions of various concentrations are used for injections, irrigations, and infusions. A solution is a given mass of solid substance dissolved in a known volume of fluid or a given volume of liquid dissolved in a known volume of another fluid. Solutions are available in units of mass per units of volume (e.g., g/mL or g/L). You can also express the concentration of a solution as a percentage. A 10% solution is 10 g of solid dissolved in 100 mL of solution. A proportion also expresses concentrations. A 1/1000 solution represents a solution containing 1 g of solid in 1000 mL of liquid or 1 mL of liquid mixed with 1000 mL of another liquid.

TABLE 20.6

TABLE 20.6

Equivalents of Measurement

Metric	Household
1 mL	15 drops (gtt)
5 mL	1 teaspoon (tsp)
15 mL	1 tablespoon (tbsp)
30 mL	2 tablespoon (tbsp)
240 mL	1 cup (c)
480 mL (approximately 500 mL)	1 pint (pt)
960 mL (approximately 1 L)	1 quart (qt)
3840 mL (approximately 4 L)	1 gallon (gal)

PERSON-CENTERED CARE

- A nurse's responsibility when administering medications safely must include effective communication with staff, pharmacy, patients, and family caregivers.
- Patients are an important resource for understanding the knowledge they have about their medications, their perceptions about the effects of medications, and their expectations for treatment.
- Consider factors that influence patients' abilities to communicate effectively such as anxiety, pain, hearing, or their cultural background. Therapeutic communication is essential to nursing practice and critical in safe medication administration.
- A new scientific field, pharmacogenetics, involves the study of the genetic influence on drug response that occurs from inherited metabolic defects or deficiencies. The most common mechanism of genetic influence on medications is the alteration in drug metabolism. The outcome is either a reduced benefit or increased toxicity of the medication (Burchum & Rosenthal, 2022). As a nurse you cannot detect a genetic abnormality. However, you can learn to become aware of cultural differences in drug responses to better monitor drug therapy.
- A patient's level of education, experience with medication therapy, and the family's influence on actions significantly influence medication adherence. For example, in some groups it is not acceptable to complain about gastrointestinal problems; therefore it is common for patients not to report nausea, vomiting, and bowel changes related to medication use.
- Assess cultural beliefs, attitudes, and values when administering medications and teaching patients about self-administration.
- Establish trust with patients and resolve conflicts between medication issues and cultural beliefs to achieve optimal patient outcomes (Ball et al., 2023).
- Assess whether the patient practices any alternative therapies or takes any herbal preparations (Krau, 2021). Herbal and homeopathic remedies may alter the response to a medication.
- Consider cultural influences on medication response, metabolism, and side effects if a patient is not responding to medication therapy as expected. Confer with the health care provider, because a change in the patient's medication is sometimes necessary.
- Assess food preferences that may interfere with patients' medication therapy (Krau, 2021).

Safe Medication Administration

Standards are actions that help ensure safe nursing practice. Standards for medication administration are set by health care agencies, nursing professional organizations, and other agencies. The Joint Commission (TJC, 2023) has specific safety implications for ad-

BOX 20.2

The Joint Commission 2023 Hospital National Patient Safety Goals: Implications for Medication Administration

- Identify patient correctly. Use at least two patient identifiers (neither can be patient's room number) when providing care, treatment (e.g., medications), or services.
- Improve the effectiveness of communication among caregivers.
- Standardize a list of abbreviations, acronyms, symbols, and dose designations that are not to be used throughout an agency.
- Improve the safety of using medications.
- Before a procedure, label all medications and medication containers (e.g., syringes, medicine cups, and basins) that are not labeled. Do this in areas where medicines and supplies are set up, such as on and off the sterile field in perioperative and other procedural settings. Labels include drug name, strength, amount, expiration date when not used within 24 hours, and expiration time when expiration occurs in less than 24 hours.
- Take extra care with patients who take anticoagulants. Use only oral unit-dose products and premixed infusions. When heparin is administered intravenously and continuously, use programmable infusion pumps.
- Maintain and communicate accurate patient medication information.
- Accurately and completely reconcile medications across the continuum of care.
- There is a process for comparing the patient's current medications with those ordered for the patient while under the care of the health care agency.
- Communicate a complete list of the patient's medications to the next provider of service when a patient is referred or transferred to another setting, service, or level of care. Also provide the complete list to the patient on discharge from the agency.
- Encourage patients' active involvement in their own care as a patient safety strategy.

Adapted from The Joint Commission (TJC): *2023 National Patient Safety Goals Effective 2023 for the Hospital Program,* Oakbrook Terrace, IL, 2023. https://www.jointcommission.org/-/media/tjc/documents/standards/national-patient-safety-goals/2023/npsg_chapter_hap_jul2023.pdf. Accessed April 23, 2023.

ministering medications (Box 20.2). In addition, most agencies have procedure manuals that contain policies about which medications nurses can and cannot administer. The types and dosages that nurses may administer often vary from unit to unit within an agency. Professional standards such as *Nursing: Scope and Standards of Practice* (American Nurses Association [ANA], 2021) apply to safe medication administration. In some states and health care agencies, assistive personnel (AP) and medical technicians with specialized training can administer a limited set of medications. Refer to state nurse practice acts and agency policy regarding the roles and responsibilities of licensed practical nurses (LPNs), licensed vocational nurses (LVNs), AP, and medical technicians in medication administration. There are five traditional rights of medication administration that have been added to over time (Hanson & Haddad, 2022). To prevent medication errors, follow the seven rights of medication administration consistently every time you prepare and administer medications. Many medication errors are linked in some way to an inconsistency in adhering to the seven rights:

1. Right medication
2. Right dose
3. Right patient
4. Right route
5. Right time
6. Right documentation
7. Right indication

Right Medication

TJC has included medication reconciliation as a National Patient Safety Goal for 2023 (TJC, 2023). When a patient enters a health care setting, a complete list of the patient's current medications must be reviewed and documented with the patient involved. You will compare the medications that health care providers order with the medications on a patient's list. When the patient is transferred to another service or health care setting, you again must reconcile the patient's current list of medications. The goal of medication reconciliation is to ensure that there is only one list of medications and to address or correct any discrepancies before discharge from the health care setting (TJC, 2023).

In 2004 TJC created its "do not use" list of abbreviations in partnership with the ISMP (2022) as part of the requirements for meeting a National Patient Safety Goal to reduce errors in medication administration. The list of unacceptable abbreviations contains abbreviations that have been found to increase the incidence of errors in medication administration (e.g., q.d. or QD, which can be mistaken as q.i.d., especially if the period after the "q" or the tail of the "q" is misunderstood as an "i"). You are responsible for using correct abbreviations and verifying that an order was accurately transcribed. Electronic medical records using CPOE now incorporate the "do not use" abbreviations. Many agencies have a policy that requires nurses on a specific shift to verify the accuracy of MAR forms printed for each patient each day. Whenever new orders are handwritten on the MAR, the nurse adding the orders must verify that they are added accurately. When verification is complete, you initial and sign the order.

During medication administration, you compare a health care provider's order with the MAR when a medication is ordered initially. Nurses verify information whenever new MARs are written or distributed or when patients transfer from one nursing unit to another or to a different health care setting. At the time of medication administration, you compare the label of a medication with the MAR three times: (1) when removing the medication from the storage bin, (2) before placing the medication in the medication cup or before taking the medication to the patient's room, and (3) again at the bedside before giving the medication to the patient. *These are the three checks for accuracy.* If the medication is ordered by trade name and dispensed from the pharmacy by generic name, verify that there is no discrepancy.

Medication Orders. You must have a medication order before administering medications to a patient. Written orders or those entered electronically through a CPOE system are preferred to minimize transcription errors or errors in visual interpretation. Verbal and telephone orders are optional forms of orders when written or electronic communication between the health care provider and nurse is not possible. When you receive a verbal or telephone order, you write or enter the order clearly on the health care provider's order sheet. You then read back the order for verification and document the read-back. The name of the health care provider and your signature are included. The health care provider will countersign the order later, usually within 24 hours after making it (see agency policy). Box 20.3 provides guidelines for safely taking verbal or telephone orders for medications.

Five common types of orders based on frequency and/or urgency of medication administration are standing orders; prn orders; and single (one-time) orders, which include STAT orders and now orders. Each order needs to include the patient's name, the drug ordered, dosage, route of administration, and time(s) of administration.

Guidelines for Verbal and Telephone Orders

- Only authorized staff receives and documents telephone or verbal orders. Agency identifies in writing the staff who are authorized.
- Clearly identify patient's name, room number, and diagnosis.
- Read back all orders to health care provider (TJC, 2022).
- Use clarification questions to avoid misunderstandings.
- Write "TO" (telephone order) or "VO" (verbal order), including date and time, name of patient, and complete order; sign the name of the health care provider and nurse.
- Follow agency policies; some facilities require documentation of the "read-back" or require two nurses to review and sign telephone or verbal orders.
- Health care provider co-signs the order within the time frame required by the agency (usually 24 hours; verify agency policy).

You carry out a *standing order* until a health care provider cancels it by issuing another order or until a prescribed number of days elapse. A standing order sometimes indicates a final day or number of doses. Many agencies have a policy for automatically discontinuing standing orders.

A medication can be ordered to be given only when a patient requires or requests it. This is a prn (as-needed) order. You assess patients thoroughly to determine their need for the medications. A prn order usually has a minimum interval set for the time between medication administration (e.g., every 4h prn)

Single (one-time) orders are common for preoperative medications or medications given before diagnostic procedures. The medication is ordered to be given only once at a specified time. A STAT order means that you give a single dose of medication immediately and only once. STAT orders are used for emergencies when a patient's condition changes suddenly. A now order is more specific than a one-time order and is used when a patient needs a medication quickly but not as soon as a STAT order. When you receive a now order, you have up to 90 minutes to give the drug (see agency policy).

Although TJC allows the use of range orders, there continue to be concerns about providing enough guidance to nurses while still allowing them to address the individual needs of patients. An example of a poorly written range order is "give morphine sulfate 2 to 6 mg IV push every 4h prn for pain." This order is not specific about guidelines needed to give a correct dose. A range order must provide objective measures for nurses to use to determine the correct dose. An example of a good order is "give Lortab 1–2 by mouth q 4 hours prn pain. For pain rating of 1–5, 1 tab; for pain rating of 5–10, 2 tabs." A range order should include specific indications such as a pain rating score or temperature level, especially for use of a medication indicated for more than one reason (e.g., ibuprofen, which could be indicated for pain or fever). Health care agencies should allow prn range orders for opioid analgesics to meet the patient needs for safe and effective pain management. There should be clear processes in place to ensure health care provider competency in the writing, nursing interpretation, and implementation of these orders.

Once you determine that the information on the patient's MAR is accurate, use the MAR to prepare and administer medications. When preparing medications from bottles or containers, *compare the label of the medication container with the MAR 3 times:*

1. Before removing the container from the supply drawer or shelf
2. As the amount of medication ordered is removed from the container

3. At the patient's bedside before administering the medication to the patient

Never prepare medications from unmarked containers or containers with illegible labels (TJC, 2023). With unit-dose prepackaged medications, check the label with the MAR when taking medications out of the medication dispensing system. Finally, verify all medications at the patient's bedside with the patient's MAR and use at least two identifiers before giving the patient any medications (TJC, 2023).

If a patient questions a medication, stop and recheck to be certain that there is no mistake. An alert patient or family caregiver will know whether a medication is different from those received before. In most cases the medication order has been changed, or the drug is manufactured by a different company than the drug the patient has been using at home. However, attention to a patient's question is how errors are identified and prevented.

Right Dose

The unit-dose system is designed to minimize errors. When a medication is prepared from a larger volume or strength than needed or when the health care provider orders a medication with a system of measurement different from what the pharmacist supplies, the chance of error increases. After calculating a dose of a high-risk medication such as insulin or warfarin, compare the calculation with one done independently by a second nurse. This verification is especially important if it is an unusual calculation or involves a potentially toxic drug.

Prepare medications accurately by using standard measurement devices such as graduated cups, syringes, and scaled droppers. Educate patients to use similar measurement devices at home, such as measuring spoons with metric calibrations rather than household teaspoons and tablespoons, which are inaccurate.

Medication errors occur when pills need to be split. Studies show that the accuracy of split tablets is questionable, even if a tablet is scored (Ingram et al., 2018). In addition, in the home setting patients may assume that tablets in containers have already been split when they have not or may split them again when they have been split already (Ingram et al., 2018).

To promote patient safety in some inpatient settings, pharmacists split medications, label and package them, and return them to the nurse for administration. Because pill splitting can be problematic in the home, determine if a patient has the manual dexterity or visual acuity to split tablets. The FDA (2020) developed suggestions to help patients split pills. They include ensuring that the tablet is designed to be split, using a tablet splitter, and not splitting the entire prescription at one time. If possible, health care providers need to avoid ordering medications that require splitting.

Tablets are sometimes crushed and mixed with food. Verify with a pharmacist to *determine whether a medication can be crushed*. Be sure to clean the crushing device completely before crushing the tablet. Remnants of previously crushed medications increase concentration of the medication or result in a patient receiving part of an unprescribed medication. Mix crushed medications with very small amounts of food or liquid. Do not use a patient's favorite foods or liquids because medications alter their taste and decrease the patient's desire for them. This is especially a concern for pediatric patients. *Always check to determine whether a medication can be crushed.* Medications that are enteric-coated or slow-release formulations have special coatings to prevent them from being absorbed too quickly. These medications should not be crushed. Refer to the "Do Not Crush List" (ISMP, 2020) to ensure that a medication is safe to crush.

Right Patient

Medication errors often occur because one patient gets a drug intended for another patient. Therefore a key step in administering medications safely is being sure that you give the right medication to the right patient. It is difficult to remember every patient's name and face. Before giving a medication to a patient, always use at least two patient identifiers (TJC, 2023). Acceptable patient identifiers include the patient's name, an identification number assigned by a health care agency such as the medical record number, or date of birth. Do not use a patient's room number as an identifier. The required identification process mandates collecting patient identifiers reliably when a patient is first admitted to a health care agency. Once identifiers are assigned to a patient (e.g., putting identifiers on an armband and placing the armband on the patient), a nurse uses them to match the patient with the patient name on the MAR.

To identify a patient correctly in an acute care setting, at the patient's bedside compare the patient identifiers on the MAR with those on the identification bracelet (Fig. 20.6). Asking patients to state their full names and identification information provides a third way to verify that you are giving medications to the right patient. If an identification bracelet becomes smudged or illegible or is missing, get a new one for the patient. In health care settings that are non–acute care settings (e.g., long-term care agency), TJC does not require the use of armbands for identification. However, nurses must use a system to verify the patient's identification with at least two identifiers, such as resident picture, before administering medications.

In addition to using two identifiers, some agencies use a wireless bar-code scanner to identify the right patient (Fig. 20.7). This system requires you to scan a personal bar code that is commonly placed on your name tag first. Then you scan a bar code on the single-dose medication package. Finally, you scan the patient's armband prior to medication administration. This information is stored in a computer for documentation purposes.

Right Route

The health care provider's order must designate a route of administration. If the route of administration is missing or if the specified

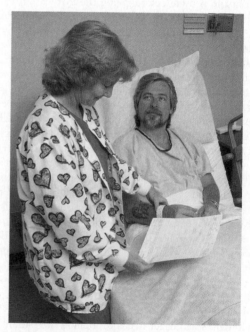

FIG. 20.6 Before administering any medications, check patient's identification and allergy bracelets.

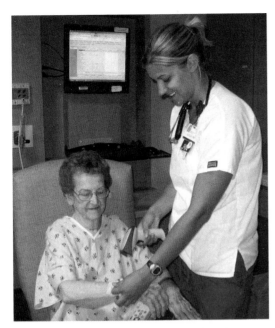

FIG. 20.7 Nurse using bar-code scanner to identify patient during medication administration.

route is not the recommended route, you must consult the health care provider immediately to verify a prescribed route. When it is necessary to prepare oral medications in syringes, use syringes intended for oral medication use. These syringes reduce the risk of giving a medication through the parenteral route. When injections are administered, use only preparations intended for parenteral use. The accidental IV injection of a liquid intended for oral use produces local complications (e.g., sterile skin abscess) or systemic effects (e.g., a fatality). Medication companies label parenteral medications "for injectable use only." The ISMP (2022) recommends that pharmacists, *not nurses*, prepare all oral medications as a unit product to ensure patient safety. Medications prepared commercially are an exception.

If you work in a setting that requires you to prepare oral medications for enteral administration (e.g., via a tube feeding), use only enteral syringes (e.g., ENFit) when you prepare oral medications. Enteral syringes use a color different from that of parenteral syringes and are clearly labeled for oral or enteral use. The syringe tips of enteral syringes will not connect with parenteral medication administration systems. Needles do not attach to enteral syringes, and the syringes cannot be inserted into any type of IV line. Label the syringe after preparing the medication and be sure to remove any caps from the tip of an oral syringe before administering the medication (see Chapter 21).

Right Time

Safe medication administration involves adherence to prescribed doses and dosage schedules. Some agencies set schedules for medication administration. However, nurses can alter this schedule based on knowledge about a medication. For example, at some agencies medications that are taken once a day are given at 9:00 a.m. However, if a medication works best when given at bedtime, the nurse administers it before the patient goes to sleep. In addition, acute care agencies use guidelines from the ISMP and Centers for Medicaid and Medicare Services (USDHHS, 2020) to determine safe, effective, and timely administration of scheduled medications. According to USDHHS (2020) guidelines, agencies

need to determine which medications are not eligible for scheduled dosing times and instead must be given at precise times (e.g., STAT doses, first-time or loading doses, one-time doses). In addition, agencies must determine which medications are time-critical scheduled and which are non–time-critical scheduled. With time-critical medications (e.g., antibiotics, anticoagulants, insulin, immunosuppressants), early or delayed administration of maintenance doses of more than 30 minutes before or after the scheduled dose will most likely cause harm or result in subtherapeutic responses in a patient. Non–time-critical medications include medications in which the timing of administration most likely will not affect the desired effect of the medication if the medication is given 1 to 2 hours before or after its scheduled time. Therefore you administer time-critical scheduled medications at a precise time or within 30 minutes before or after the scheduled time. You administer medications identified as non–time-critical within 1 to 2 hours of their scheduled time. Know your agency policies about the timing of medications to ensure that you administer medications at the right time (USDHHS, 2020).

Always know why a medication is ordered for a certain time of the day and whether you are able to alter the time schedule. For example, two medications are ordered, one q8h (every 8 hours) and the other 3 times per day. Both medications are scheduled 3 times a day over 24 hours. The health care provider intends for you to give the q8h medication ATC to maintain its therapeutic blood levels. In contrast, you need to give the other medication during the waking hours. Each agency has a recommended time schedule for medications ordered at frequent intervals. You can alter these recommended times if necessary or appropriate.

Give priority to medications that must act at certain times. For example, give insulin at a precise interval before a meal. Give antibiotics on time ATC to maintain therapeutic blood levels. All medications require your clinical judgment to determine the proper time for administration. Administer a prn sleeping medication when the patient is ready for bed. You always document whenever there is a call to the patient's health care provider to obtain a change in a medication order.

When preparing patients for discharge, help them plan schedules based on preferred medication intervals, pharmacokinetics of the medication, and the patient's daily schedule. For patients who have difficulty remembering when to take medications, make a chart that lists the times when they should take each medication or prepare a special container to hold each timed dose.

Right Documentation

Many medication errors result from inaccurate documentation. Therefore always document medications accurately at the time of administration and identify any inaccurate documentation before you give medications.

Before you administer a medication, ensure that the MAR clearly shows:
- The patient's full name
- The full name of the ordered medication (without abbreviations of medication names)
- The time the medication is to be administered
- The dosage, route, and frequency of administration

Do not give medications that have incomplete or illegible orders. Verify inaccurate orders before giving medications. It is better to give the correct medication later than to give your patient the wrong medication. Document the administration of each medication on the MAR as soon as you give it. Never document a medication before giving it. Document the name of the medication, the dose, the time of administration, and the route. Also document the site of any injections you give. Document the patient's response to the medication in the nurses' notes.

Right Indication

ISMP (2019) added a seventh right of medication administration that would enhance the safety of every medication order: the *right indication*. Indication-based prescribing narrows medication choices, dosage forms, and dosing regimens, which reduces the risk of a wrong medication being chosen (Grissinger, 2019). In addition, indication-based prescribing empowers and educates patients, which can improve medication adherence. Communication improves between the interprofessional team and the patients and family caregivers. Medication reconciliation also improves because indication-based prescribing aids in preventing re-prescribing.

Medication Preparation

It is legally advisable to administer only the medications that you prepare. Administering a medication prepared by another nurse increases the opportunity for errors. You must perform several steps before actual administration of medications, including interpreting medication labels, converting measurement units within a system or between systems, and calculating medication doses. The importance of checking similar names and verifying the correct drug cannot be overemphasized.

Interpreting Medication Labels

Medication labels include several basic pieces of information: the trade name of the drug in large letters, the generic name in smaller letters, the form of the drug, the dosage, the expiration date, the lot number, and the name of the manufacturer (Fig. 20.8). The trade name given by the manufacturer suggests the action of the drug, and the generic name is the chemical name.

Dosage Calculations

To administer medications safely, use your mathematics skills to calculate medication dosages and mix solutions. The ability to calculate doses safely is important because you will not always dispense medications in the unit of measure in which they are ordered. Medication companies package and bottle medications using certain standard equivalents. You are responsible for converting available units of volume and weight to the prescribed doses. Be aware of approximate equivalents in all major measurement systems and use conversion tables. An example follows:

The order reads: vancomycin (Vancocin) 1 g IV.

The pharmacy supplies vancomycin in 500-mg vials.

Because the dose on the medication label is in milligrams, conversion should be from grams to milligrams; 1 g = 1000 mg.

In addition to medication administration, nurses use volume and weight conversions in a variety of other nursing activities, including converting fluid ounces to milliliters to measure intake and output (I&O) or converting volume equivalents to calculate IV flow rates.

Conversions Within One System. Converting measurements within one system is relatively easy; simply divide or multiply in the metric system. For example, to change milligrams to grams, divide by 1000 or move the decimal three points to the left.

$$1000 \text{ mg} = 1 \text{ g}$$
$$350 \text{ mg} = 0.35 \text{ g}$$

To convert liters to milliliters, multiply by 1000 or move the decimal three points to the right.

$$1 \text{ L} = 1000 \text{ mL}$$
$$0.25 \text{ L} = 250 \text{ mL}$$

To convert units of measurement within the household system, consult an equivalency table. For example, when converting fluid ounces to quarts, you first need to know that 32 ounces is the equivalent of 1 quart. To convert 8 ounces to a quart measurement, divide 8 by 32 to get the equivalent: ¼ or 0.25 quart.

Conversion Between Systems. Conversion between systems is becoming less common because of the ISMP (2022) recommendations for use of the metric system for liquid medication dosing. Even though health care providers are encouraged to order using the metric system, you may encounter a situation in which you calculate the correct dose of a medication by converting weights or volumes from one system of measurement to another. For example, metric units are sometimes converted to equivalent household measures for medication administration at home. To convert from one

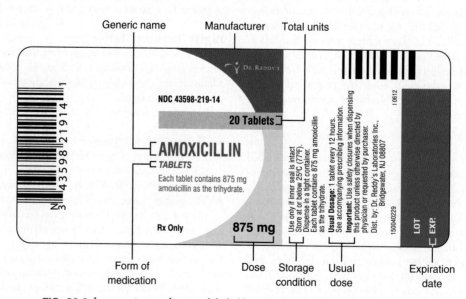

FIG. 20.8 Interpreting medication label. (Courtesy Dr. Reddy's Laboratories, Inc.)

BOX 20.4

Formula Method

$$\frac{D}{H} = V = \text{Amount to give}$$

D is the ordered or desired dose, ordered by the health care provider for the patient (e.g., 250 mg of penicillin PO 4 times daily).

H is the drug dose on hand or available for use. The dose is on the drug label (e.g., penicillin tablets 250 mg each).

V is the volume (liquid) or vehicle (number of tablets, capsules) that delivers the available dose, the amount to give.

NOTE: The desired dose *(D)* and the on-hand dose *(H)* must be in the same unit of measurement. If they are in different units, you must convert before completing the formula.

BOX 20.5

Dimensional Analysis

Use the following steps to solve medication problems using dimensional analysis:

1. Identify the unit of measure that you need to administer. For example, if you are giving a pill, you will usually be giving a tablet or a capsule; for parenteral or oral medications, the unit is milliliters.
2. Estimate the answer in your mind.
3. Place the name or appropriate abbreviation for *x* on the left side of the equation (e.g., *x* tab, *x* mL).
4. Place available information from the problem in a fraction format on the right side of the equation. Place the abbreviation or unit that matches what you are going to administer (determined in Step 1) in the numerator.
5. Look at the medication order and add other factors into the problem. Set up the numerator so that it matches the unit in the previous denominator.
6. Cancel out like units of measurement on the right side of the equation. You should end up with only one unit left in the equation, and it should match the unit on the left side of the equation.
7. Reduce to the lowest terms if possible and solve the problem or solve for *x*. Label your answer.
8. Compare your estimate from Step 1 with your answer in Step 2.

measurement system to another, always use equivalent measurements. Tables of equivalent measurements are available in all health care agencies. The pharmacist is also a good resource.

The liquids should be dispensed by the pharmacy in an oral syringe using metric measurement (ISMP, 2022). The ISMP (2022) also recommends that patients or family caregivers purchase oral liquid dosing devices (oral syringes, cups, droppers) that display only the metric scale. Encourage patients to never use household measuring devices with liquid medications.

Dosage Calculations. Dosage calculation methods include the formula method (Box 20.4), dimensional analysis (Box 20.5), and ratio and proportion (Box 20.6). Use the method that is the most logical and comfortable for you. Use this same method consistently. Before you begin any calculation, make a mental estimate of the approximate and reasonable dosage. If your estimate does not closely match the answer you calculate, you need to recheck your math before preparing and administering the medication. To enhance your accuracy, use your clinical judgment about the steps you go through in calculating medications. Most health care agencies require a nurse to double-check calculations with another nurse before giving medications, especially when the risk for giving the wrong medication dose is high

BOX 20.6

The Ratio-and-Proportion Method

1. The numbers in a ratio are separated by a colon (:).
2. A proportion is an equation that has two ratios of equal value.
3. The first and last numbers are called the *extremes*. The second and third numbers are called the *means*.
4. Write a proportion in one of three ways:
   a. 1:2 = 5:10
   b. 1:2::5:10
   c. ½ = ⁵⁄₁₀
5. Make sure that all the terms are in the same unit or system of measurement.
6. Label all the terms in the proportion.
7. Place the ratio you know (e.g., information on the drug label) first.
8. Put the terms of the ratio in the same sequence (e.g., mg:mL = mg:mL).
9. Cross-multiply the means and the extremes and then divide both sides by the number for the *x* to obtain the dosage.
10. Always label the answer.

(e.g., heparin, chemotherapy drug, or insulin). Always have another nurse or health care provider double-check your work if the answer to a medication calculation seems unreasonable or inappropriate.

Formula Method

Dose ordered: Demerol 50 mg IM
Medication available: 100 mg in 1 mL

Step 1.

$$\frac{\text{Dose ordered}}{\text{Dose on hand}} \times \text{Amount on hand} = \text{Amount to give}$$

Step 2. Calculate your answer:

$$\frac{50\,\text{mg}}{100\,\text{mg}} \times 1\,\text{mL} \times = 0.5\,\text{mL}$$

Dimensional Analysis Method. This method is used when the dose ordered has the same label as the dose available.

Dose ordered: 0.5 g
Tablets available: 0.25 g per tablet

Step 1. The starting factor is 0.5 g.
The answer label is tablets (i.e., How many tablets should be given?).

Step 2. Formulate the conversion equation:
The equivalent needed is 1 tablet = 0.25 g.

$$\frac{0.5\,\text{g}}{1} \times \frac{1\,\text{tab}}{0.25\,\text{g}} = \text{tabs}$$

Cancel labels (g). **NOTE:** If properly written, all labels except the answer label will cancel.

Step 3. Solve the equation. Reduce the numerical values and multiply the numerators and denominators.

Cross multiply the equation:

$$\frac{0.5\,\text{g}}{1} \times \frac{1\,\text{tab}}{0.25\,\text{g}} = \text{tabs}$$

Divide both sides by the number before *x*:

$$x \times \frac{0.5 \text{ tab}}{0.25 \text{ g}} = \text{tabs}$$
$$x = 2 \text{ tabs}$$

Ratio-and-Proportion Method. A ratio indicates the relationship between two numbers.

Dose ordered: Phenytoin solution 100 mg by mouth

Medication available: 125 mg/5 mL

Step 1. Set up the proportion:

$$\frac{125 \text{ mg}}{5} = \frac{100 \text{ mg}}{x \text{ mL}}$$

Step 2. Cross multiply the equation:

$$125x = 100 \times 5$$
$$125x = 500$$

Step 3. Divide both sides by the number before *x*:

$$\frac{125x}{125} = \frac{500}{125}$$
$$x = \frac{500}{125}$$
$$x = 4 \text{ mL}$$

Pediatric Doses. Calculating children's medication doses requires caution (Hockenberry et al., 2022). Evidence shows that children are at risk for experiencing an ADR as a result of their metabolic rate (Burchum & Rosenthal, 2022). Medication errors can be prevented in children by (Marufu et al., 2022):
- Involving the interprofessional team, including pharmacist
- Reducing distractions during medication calculations and preparation
- Using smart pumps hands-on demonstration
- Providing education

The child's age, weight, and maturity of body systems all affect the ability to metabolize and excrete medication. Other factors that influence medication dosages in children include the difficulty in evaluating the desired effect and the hydration status of the child. In most cases the health care provider will calculate the dose for a child before ordering the medication. However, it is your responsibility to be aware of the safe dosage range for any medication administered, and you should recheck/recalculate to confirm the correct dose.

Different formulas and methods are used to calculate medication dosages in children. Most of the time you calculate medications based on a child's weight. You can use the ratio-and-proportion method, the formula method, or dimensional analysis to calculate a pediatric dose using body weight (see above). Although used less often, a child's body surface area (BSA) is used to determine chemotherapy doses. Refer to a pediatric or pharmacology resource and consult with the patient's health care provider or the pharmacist if you must calculate a medication based on BSA.

Dosages in Older Adults. Adverse drug reactions occur 4 times more often in older-adult patients than in younger patients when presenting to health care agencies (Ruscin & Linnebar,

Safe Medication Administration in Older Adults

- Consult with the health care provider to keep the medication plan as simple as possible (Burchum & Rosenthal, 2022). Ensure that patients have an accurate list of all their medications (Ruscin & Linnebar, 2021).
- Assess functional status (including vision, hand grasp, fine-motor skills) to determine whether patient will require assistance in taking medications (Touhy & Jett, 2022).
- Some older adults have a greater sensitivity to medications, especially those that act on the central nervous system. Carefully monitor patients' responses to medications and anticipate dosage adjustments as needed (Touhy & Jett, 2022).
- Keep instructions clear and simple and provide written materials in large print (Burchum & Rosenthal, 2022).
- Minimize distractions and make sure that older adult is comfortable (Touhy & Jett, 2022).
- Teach the complications and interactions of all over-the counter medications (Touhy & Jett, 2022).
- Teach the older adult to set up a daily or weekly schedule for medications using memory aids such as a calendar (Touhy & Jett, 2022). Have a family caregiver help with medication administration as needed.
- Monitor patient's response to medications to assess for overuse or underuse of the medication and anticipate possible dosage modifications (Ruscin & Linnebar, 2021; Touhy & Jett, 2022).
- Reduce the chance of errors by educating the patient and family caregiver on each medication during each encounter (Ruscin & Linnebar, 2021).
- Include patient's family caregiver or key support person in any type of instruction.
- Evaluate teaching by having patient repeat back instructions.

2021). The most common serious manifestations include falls, orthostatic hypotension, heart failure, sedation, and delirium. Older adults require special nursing considerations during medication administration (Box 20.7). Be vigilant when administering medications and know the physiological changes of aging so that you can anticipate ADRs. Nurses collaborate with health care providers to minimize adverse medication reactions in older adults by evaluating the indication for each drug, considering age-related changes and their relationship to dosing, starting with the lowest effective dose, and frequently reconciling medications (Ruscin & Linnebar, 2021).

A common problem for older adults is polypharmacy. There is no consensus definition for polypharmacy, although the common definitions include five or more concurrent drugs or the mixing of nutritional or herbal supplements with medications (Burchum & Rosenthal, 2022; Touhy & Jett, 2022). Older adults experience polypharmacy when they seek relief from a variety of symptoms (e.g., constipation, insomnia, pain) and see multiple health care providers. When determining polypharmacy, review all older adults' prescribed medications and all other supplements and OTC medications. Polypharmacy increases the risk of adverse effects and interactions with other medications.

Safety precautions are needed to reduce or eliminate the risk factors associated with medication regimens for older adults, including assessing a patient's health status, current medication regimen (including OTC drugs and herbal products), the reason for existing and proposed medications, and any environmental factors that influence accurate and safe medication administration by the patient and family caregiver(s). The American Geriatrics Society (AGS) has established the Beers Criteria®, which include criteria for medications that may be inappropriate to administer to older adults (AGS, 2019).

EVIDENCE-BASED PRACTICE

Preventing Medication Errors

ADRs account for the largest number of adverse events patients experience in health care facilities. Often, they occur when a wrong dosage or medication is delivered to patients. ADRs can occur prior to admission, during the stay, or after discharge. A multisystem approach including the provider, nurse, and health care system should be used to prevent medication errors (Batson et al., 2021).

- Everyone administering medications should review the medication list at each patient encounter.
- Be vigilant when handling and administering high-risk medications.
- Consider medications as the cause of any new symptoms.
- Use CPOE when possible, to (Keenan et al., 2021):
  - Standardize practice
  - Improve legibility of orders
  - Alert and update health care providers on side effects, drug-drug interactions, and new orders
- The healthcare system should use an EHR that interfaces with CPOE if available to improve communication and alert all providers to administration times (Keenan et al., 2021).
- Research has shown that 90% of medication errors occurred at the ordering and transcribing steps of the medication process (Agency for Healthcare Research and Quality [AHRQ], 2019). The use of CPOE is a strategy to reduce medication errors that occur from ordering the wrong medication, medication dose, or frequency, as well as errors from transcription of poorly hand-written medication orders (AHRQ, 2019).
- Bar-coding medications linked to patient identification bracelets improves safety and provides one last opportunity to identify a medication error.
- Medication reconciliation identifies medication discrepancies and prevents errors.
- Address nonadherence issues for patients such as fear of addiction.
- Patient, family caregiver, and provider education can be used to prevent medication errors.

SAFETY GUIDELINES

Medication administration safety is a priority goal for safe nursing practice. It begins by having a thorough understanding of the medications you administer, the rationale for why patients are prescribed the medications, and whether patients have any drug allergies. It is then important for you to follow safe preparation and administration standards, which are part of the seven rights of medication administration and are designed to prevent medication errors (Box 20.8). Medication safety also requires you to understand the principles of pharmacokinetics, growth and development, nutrition, and mathematics. TJC (2023) has specific National Patient Safety Goals for using medications safely (see Box 20.2).

NURSING PROCESS

Application of the nursing process ensures that clinical reasoning and clinical judgment are integrated into a patient's care. As a nurse your role extends beyond simply giving drugs to a patient. You are also responsible for understanding why your patient is receiving the medication therapy; monitoring patients' responses to medications; providing education to patients and family caregivers; and informing health care providers when medications are effective, ineffective, or no longer necessary.

BOX 20.8

Steps to Prevent Medication Errors

- Follow the seven rights of medication administration.
- Only prepare medications for one patient at a time.
- Be sure to read labels at least 3 times (comparing MAR with label): when removing medication from storage, before taking to patient's room, before giving medication. These are the *three checks* for accuracy.
- Use at least two patient identifiers every time you administer medications (e.g., patient name, birthday, hospital number) whenever administering a medication.
- Do not allow any other activity to interrupt administration of medication to a patient (e.g., phone call, pager, discussion with other staff).
- Double-check all calculations and other high-risk medication administration processes (e.g., patient-controlled analgesia) and verify with another nurse.
- Do not interpret illegible handwriting; clarify with the health care provider.
- Question unusually large or small doses.
- Document all medications as soon as they are given.
- When you have made or discovered an error, reflect on what went wrong and ask how you could have prevented it. Complete an occurrence report per agency policy.
- Evaluate the context or situation in which a medication error occurred. This helps to determine if nurses have the necessary resources for safe medication administration.
- When repeated medication errors occur within a work area, identify and analyze the factors that may have caused the errors and take corrective action.
- Attend in-service programs on the medications you commonly administer.
- Ensure that you are well rested when caring for patients. Nurses make more errors when they are tired.
- Involve and educate patients when administering medications. Address patients' concerns about medications before administering them (e.g., concerns about their appearance or side effects).
- Follow established agency policies and procedures when using technology to administer medications (e.g., automated medication dispensing system [AMDS] and bar-code scanning). Medication errors occur when nurses "work around" the technology (e.g., override alerts without thinking about them).

MAR, Medication administration record.

Assessment

Begin your assessment by reviewing a patient's medical history and performing a focused physical assessment (for obvious problems); this will yield information about the patient's presenting signs and symptoms and any indications for or contraindications to medication therapy. Certain diseases or illnesses (e.g., liver or kidney disease) place patients at risk for adverse medication effects. For example, if a patient has a gastric ulcer, forms of aspirin increase the chance of bleeding. Long-term health problems require specific medications. This knowledge helps you anticipate the medications that your patient requires.

Include an assessment of patient allergies. Determine if a patient has actual allergic reactions or drug sensitivities, which are uncomfortable side effects. *Never give a patient a medication when there is a known allergy.* Many medications have ingredients found in food sources. For example, if your patient is allergic to shellfish, the patient may be sensitive to products containing iodine such as Betadine or dyes used in radiological testing. In an acute care setting, patients with allergies wear identification bands that list each medication allergy. All allergies and the types of reactions are noted on the patient's admission notes, in medication records, and in history and physical examination findings.

Your assessment also involves identifying all medications that the patient takes every day at home, including prescriptions, OTC preparations, and herbal supplements. To ensure you do this accurately, be sure to assess a patient's health literacy level, which will influence how well a patient might be able to understand and explain a medication regimen. Determine how long the patient has taken each medication, the current dosage schedule, and whether the patient has had any adverse effects to any of the medications. The patient should know the name, purpose, dosage, route, and side effects of medications and supplements that are being taken. Often patients take many medications and carry a list that includes this information. Patients have different levels of understanding. One patient may describe a diuretic as a "water pill," whereas another may describe it as a drug to minimize swelling and lower blood pressure. Still another may describe it as "the little white pill I take in the morning." By assessing the patient's level of knowledge, you determine the need for teaching. If a patient is unable to understand or remember pertinent information, it may be necessary to involve a family caregiver.

Depending on a medication's action, also assess vital signs and laboratory data. It is important to have a baseline assessment to be able to determine adverse effects from medication versus an existing condition (e.g., a skin rash can be a first indicator of a serious reaction or could be an existing skin condition unrelated to medication). If assessment data contraindicate medication administration, hold the drug and notify the health care provider.

Planning

During planning, organize nursing activities to ensure the safe administration of medications. Evidence shows that distractions or hurrying during medication preparation administration increases the risk of medication errors (Wang et al., 2021). Suggestions to reduce distraction include signage identifying the medication administration area and wearing some identifying clothing (e.g., vest) when preparing medications (Wang et al., 2021). The following are general goals of medication administration:

1. Patient achieves therapeutic effect of the prescribed medication.
2. Patient complications related to the prescribed medication are absent.
3. Patient and family caregivers understand medication therapy.
4. Patient and family caregivers administer medication safely (when appropriate).

Implementation

Nursing interventions focus on safe and effective drug administration. This includes careful medication preparation, accurate and timely administration, and patient education.

Preadministration Activities

1. Identify the medication action, purpose, side effects, and nursing implications for administering and monitoring. Ensure that the medication order has not expired.
2. Minimize distractions (e.g., discussion with staff, phone call, use of pager), close the door of medication room, and post "do not disturb" signage. Do not perform other tasks while preparing medications.
3. Make sure the information on the electronic MAR or printed MAR corresponds exactly with the health care provider's order and with the medication container label. Clarify orders that are unclear or illegible.

4. Calculate medication doses accurately and use appropriate measuring devices. Verify that the dose prescribed is within a safe dosage range and is appropriate for the patient situation.
5. Take medications to patient at correct time (see seven rights of medication administration), including time-critical and non–time-critical medications (see agency policy).
6. Review any preadministration assessment findings (e.g., vital signs, laboratory test results).
7. Use thorough hand hygiene technique. Avoid touching tablets and capsules. Wear chemotherapy-approved gloves if you are administering oral chemotherapy agents.
8. Use sterile technique for preparing parenteral medications. Wear clean gloves when administering parenteral medications and certain topical medications.
9. Keep medications secure. Administer only medications that you personally prepare. Do not ask another nurse to administer medications that you prepare.
10. When preparing medications, be sure that the label is clear and legible and that the drug is properly mixed; has not changed in color, clarity, or consistency; and has not expired.
11. Keep tablets and capsules in their wrappers and open them at the patient's bedside. This allows you to review each medication with the patient. If a patient refuses medication, there is no question about which one is withheld.
12. TJC (2023) has a standard for labeling syringes, including labeling all unlabeled medicines (e.g., medicines in syringes, cups, and basins) before a procedure. This should be done in the area where medicines and supplies are prepared.

Medication Administration

1. Follow the seven rights of medication administration (see agency policy).
2. Inform the patient of the name, purpose, action, and common side effects of each medication. Evaluate the patient's knowledge of the medication, and provide appropriate teaching using teach-back technique.
3. Stay with the patient until the medication is taken. Provide assistance as necessary. Do not leave medication at the bedside without a health care provider's order. For example, some patients may take their own vitamins while in the agency.
4. Respect the patient's right to refuse a medication. If the medication wrapper remains intact, return the medication to the patient's unit-dose drawer. When medication is refused, determine the reason and act accordingly. For example, if the patient has unpleasant side effects, it may be possible to eliminate them by giving the pills with food or using a different time schedule.

Postadministration Activities

1. Properly document medications administered (see seven rights of medication administration).
2. Document data pertinent to a patient's response; this is especially important when giving medications ordered prn. Include ability of patient and family caregiver to teach-back the education provided.
3. If a medication is refused, document that it was not given, the reason for the refusal, and when the health care provider was notified.

Evaluation

After you administer a medication, consider how the medication is expected to affect the patient and evaluate the patient's condition and response to it. This includes measurement of vital signs when appropriate. Look for therapeutic and adverse effects. If adverse effects develop, you need to recognize the clinical signs and respond quickly:

1. Monitor for evidence of therapeutic effects, side effects, and adverse reactions. This includes monitoring physical response (e.g., heart rhythm, blood pressure, skin integrity, urine output, or laboratory results). Minimize side effects whenever possible (e.g., offer lozenge for dry mouth or provide an antiemetic as ordered to prevent nausea with chemotherapy medications).
2. When a medication is given for relief of symptoms, ask the patient to report if symptoms have diminished or been relieved after medication is administered (e.g., 30 minutes after medicating for pain).
3. Observe injection sites for bruises, inflammation, localized pain, numbness, or bleeding.
4. Evaluate that patient and family caregiver understand purpose of medication therapy, dose regimens, and ability to self-administer medication by using teach-back techniques.

REPORTING MEDICATION ERRORS

Medication errors often harm patients because of inappropriate medication use. Errors include inaccurate prescribing; administering the wrong medication, by the wrong route, and in the wrong time interval; and administering extra doses or failing to administer a medication. Medication errors are related to professional practice, health care product design, or procedures and systems such as product labeling and distribution. When an error occurs, the patient's safety and well-being become the top priority. A nurse assesses and examines the patient's condition and notifies the health care provider of the incident as soon as possible. Once the patient is stable, the nurse reports the incident to the appropriate person in the agency (e.g., manager or supervisor).

As a nurse, you are responsible for preparing a written incident or occurrence report that must be filed usually within 24 hours of an incident (see agency policy). The incident report is an internal audit tool and not a permanent part of the medical record. To legally protect the health care professional and agency, do not mention that an incident report was completed in the nurses' notes in the EHR or chart. Agencies use incident reports to track incident patterns and initiate performance improvement programs as needed. Depending on the circumstances and the severity of the outcome, the nurse or agency may be responsible for reporting the incident to TJC, MedWatch (the FDA's medical product safety reporting program), or the ISMP's National Medication Errors Reporting Program.

It is good risk management to report all medication errors, including mistakes that do not cause obvious or immediate harm or near misses. You should feel comfortable in reporting an error and not fear repercussions from managerial staff. Even when a patient suffers no harm from a medication error, the agency can still learn why the mistake occurred and what to do in the future to avoid similar errors. There are strategies that you can implement to prevent medication errors (see Box 20.8).

PATIENT AND FAMILY CAREGIVER TEACHING

A well-informed patient is more likely to take medications correctly. However, many patients and family caregivers have limited health literacy, meaning that they do not understand how to read medication labels and calculate doses. You will also care for patients who do not speak English. Therefore any patient education requires a thorough assessment of a patient's learning needs and abilities. It is legally mandated by the National Standards for Culturally and Linguistically Appropriate Services in Health and Health Care (the National CLAS Standards) to provide easy-to-understand print and multimedia materials in the languages commonly used by the populations in a service area (U.S. Department of Health and Human Services Office of Minority Health, 2021).

Many patients do not adhere to their medication regimens due to drug sensitivities, inadequate resources to purchase medications, or patients' perceptions of the medication's value. A patient must understand the value of a specific medication and the implications that might arise if the medication is not taken regularly. Patients may also have cognitive limitations, affecting their ability to prepare medications or remember drug schedules. Adapt any teaching approach to the patient's values and lifestyle. There are times a medication dosage schedule can be adjusted to match patient routines.

Provide an individualized approach to teaching, using visual aids, instructional booklets written in simple language or the patient's language, or even online videos or DVDs. When teaching patients about their medications, include people identified as being significant to the patient's recovery (e.g., family caregivers or home care providers).

Begin instruction as soon as possible so you can have several teaching sessions. It is ideal to use instructional materials written at no higher than a sixth-grade reading level. Provide instructions written in the patient's language if available. If the patient speaks another language, have a professional interpreter available during instruction. Do not use a family member as the interpreter. When providing instruction, have the patient or family caregiver repeat the name and use for each medication plus the dosing instructions. Current recommendations suggest the use of teach-back as a method to confirm patient learning and improve health care provider education (Geum et al., 2021). For example, have the patient explain for you the dosage schedule of a medication that you taught so you can confirm understanding. Have the patient demonstrate preparation of each medication. Provide time to discuss problem scenarios (e.g., side effects develop, a syringe becomes contaminated) to test the patient's knowledge of what to do should something go wrong. Determine if the patient requires an adherence aid or memory cue. This is especially important in older adults. Medication dose containers organized by the hours and days of the week are very useful. Pill boxes with times displayed and electronic dispensers are also available. If patients miss a dose of medication, they need to know how to adjust their medication schedule safely.

Evaluating the effectiveness of teaching ensures that a patient or family caregiver can administer medications in a safe manner. One method of evaluating patient or family caregiver understanding is to create medication cards with the generic and trade names of the medication on the front of the card and all pertinent medication information on the back of the card. Another method is to have patients read labels on prepared medications. Remember that medication bottles often have fine print and are difficult to read for the patient with impaired vision. Have the pharmacy prepare medications for such patients with large-print labels. If the patient correctly identifies the name of the medication, ask the following questions:

- Tell me the reason you are taking this medication?
- How often do you take this medication and at what time of day?
- What side effects can occur with this medication?
- If this side effect occurs, what are you going to do about it?

Be sure to also assess the patient's sensory, motor, and cognitive functions (e.g., ability to open medication bottles). Impairments may affect the patient's ability to safely self-administer medications, and family caregivers or home health aides may need to help with medication administration.

✦ CLINICAL JUDGMENT AND NEXT-GENERATION NCLEX® EXAMINATION–STYLE QUESTIONS

A 72-year-old patient visits the medical clinic 2 weeks after a myocardial infarction. The patient denies any chest pain since having an angioplasty. He states, "I feel pretty good, but I've had some weakness and dizziness over the past week." Regular medications the patient takes include sertraline, levothyroxine, and docusate. The health care provider recently added metoprolol. The patient says, "I got the metoprolol refilled last week; I'm supposed to take 75 mg, but the pharmacy only had 150 mg tablets." The health record also indicates that the patient takes melatonin and an herbal preparation for sleep.

1. Which medication would the nurse anticipate is **most likely** to have caused the patient to have dizziness and weakness?
   1. Sertraline
   2. Levothyroxine
   3. Docusate
   4. Metoprolol

2. To further assess the patient regarding dizziness and weakness, which of the following questions would the nurse ask? **Select all that apply.**
   1. "How many tablets of metoprolol are you taking at a time?"
   2. "How many times have you had dizziness and weakness over the past week?"
   3. "How long do the episodes of dizziness and weakness last?"
   4. "Have you noticed how long after taking metoprolol that you feel weak and dizzy?"
   5. "What kind of ingredients are in the herbal preparation you take for sleep?"

3. After seeing the health care provider, several changes are made to the patient's medication regimen. Which of the following orders would the nurse need to clarify before teaching the patient about safely taking these drugs? **Select all that apply.**
   1. Timoptic .25% solution 1 drop OD BID
   2. Metoprolol 12.50 mg QD
   3. Insulin glargine 6 u SC twice a day
   4. Enalapril 2.5 mg. PO 3 times a day; hold for systolic blood pressure <100
   5. Baby aspirin, 81 mg, one chewable tablet by mouth one time daily each morning

4. The patient states, "I don't like having to take medicine because the labels on the bottles are too small for me to see." Which of the following actions would the nurse take? **Select all that apply.**
   1. Set up a pill-dispensing system to prepare medications for each day of the week.
   2. Talk with the pharmacy to request larger, easier-to-read labels on medication bottles.
   3. Tell the patient there is nothing that can be done other than using a magnifying glass.
   4. Explain that a home health care nurse will have to come daily to dispense medicine.
   5. Use teach-back to ensure that the patient knows how to safely take each medication.

5. The nurse is preparing to teach the patient about taking multiple medications. Select 2 topics that the nurse would include in the teaching.
   1. Set a smartphone alarm for each dose of medication that must be taken.
   2. Any time you miss a dose of medication, double the following dose.
   3. It can be helpful to color-code medication bottles so you recognize them easily.
   4. Rely on caregivers to administer all of your medications.
   5. You will need to get all of your medication information from the pharmacy.
   6. If you are confused about a medication, search online for how to take it.
   7. Take all of your medications at one time so you do not forget any of them.

Visit the Evolve site for Answers to Clinical Judgment and Next-Generation NCLEX® Examination–Style Questions.

REFERENCES

Agency for Healthcare Research and Quality (AHRQ): *Computerized provider order entry,* 2019. https://psnet.ahrq.gov/primer/computerized-provider-order-entry. Accessed September 12, 2023.

American Geriatrics Society (AGS): 2019 Updated AGS Beers Criteria® for Potentially Inappropriate Medication Use in Older Adults, American Geriatrics Society Beers Criteria® Update by the 2019 Expert Panel, *J Am Geriatr Soc* 67(4):674, 2019. doi:10.1111/jgs.15767.

American Nurses Association (ANA): *Nursing scope and standards of practice,* ed 4, Silver Springs, MD, 2021, The Association.

American Medical Association (AMA): *Procedure for USAN name selection,* 2022. https://www.ama-assn.org/procedure-usan-name-selection. Accessed September 12, 2023.

Ball J, et al: *Seidel's guide to physical examination: an interprofessional approach,* ed 10, St. Louis, MO, 2023, Elsevier.

Batson S, et al: Automation of in-hospital pharmacy dispensing: a systematic review, *Eur J Hosp Pharm* 28(2):58, 2021.

Burchum J, Rosenthal L: *Lehne's pharmacology for nursing care,* ed 11, St. Louis, 2022, Saunders.

Centers for Disease Control and Prevention (CDC): *Adverse drug events from specific medicines,* 2019. https://www.cdc.gov/medicationsafety/adverse-drug-events-specific-medicines.html. Accessed September 12, 2023.

Centers for Disease Control and Prevention (CDC): *CDC guideline for prescribing opioids for chronic pain,* n.d. https://www.cdc.gov/drugoverdose/pdf/guidelines_at-a-glance-a.pdf.

Consumer Med Safety: *Over the counter O-T-C medicines: safety tips when measuring doses,* 2023, Institute for Safe Medicine Practices. https://www.consumermed-safety.org/over-the-counter-medicines/measuring-the-dose-of-liquid-medicines/safety-tips-when-measuring-doses-of-liquid-medicines. Accessed April 22, 2023.

Geum E, et al: Effectiveness of discharge education with the teach-back method on 30-day read mission: a systematic review, *J Patient Saf* 17(4):305–310, 2021.

Gorski L, et al: *Infusion therapy standards of practice,* ed 8, Norwood: Mass, 2021, Infusion Nurses Society (INS).

Grissinger M: Is an indication-based prescribing system in our future? *P & T* 44(5):232–266, 2019.

Hanson A, Haddad L: *Nursing rights of medication administration,* Treasure Island, FL, 2022, StatPearls.

Hockenberry MJ, et al: *Wong's essentials of pediatric nursing,* ed 11, St. Louis, 2022, Mosby.

Ingram V et al: The breakup: errors when altering oral solid dosage forms. *Pa Patient Saf Advis* 15(3):1-20, 2018.

Institute for Safe Medication Practices (ISMP): *Overcoming barriers to indication based prescribing,* 2019. https://www.ismp.org/news/overcoming-barriers-indication-based-prescribing. Accessed September 12, 2023.

Institute for Safe Medication Practices (ISMP): *Oral dosage forms that should not be crushed,* 2020. https://www.ismp.org/recommendations/do-not-crush. Accessed September 12, 2023.

Institute for Safe Medication Practices (ISMP). *List of error-prone abbreviations,* 2021. https://www.ismp.org/recommendations/error-prone-abbreviations-list. Accessed September 12, 2023.

Institute for Safe Medication Practices (ISMP): *ISMP targeted medication safety best practices for hospitals*, 2022. https://www.ismp.org/guidelines/best-practices-hospitals. Accessed September 13, 2023.

Jourdan A, et al: Antibiotic hypersensitivity and adverse reactions: management and implications in clinical practice, *Allergy Asthma Clin Immunol* 16:6, 2020.

Keenan R, et al: Computerized provider order entry and patient safety: a scoping review, *Knowl Manag E-Learning* 13(4):452–476, 2021.

Krau SD, editor: Complementary and alternative medicine, part II. Herbal supplements and vitamins, *An Issue of Nursing Clinics* 56(1), 2021. Elsevier Health Sciences.

Okoli C, et al: Relationship between polypharmacy and quality of life among people in 24 countries living with HIV, *Prev Chronic Dis* 17:190359, 2020.

Oncology Nursing Society (ONS): *Toolkit for safe handling of hazardous drugs for nurses in oncology*, 2018. https://www.ons.org/sites/default/files/2018-06/ONS_Safe_Handling_Toolkit_0.pdf.

Oncology Nursing Society (ONS): *Ensuring healthcare worker safety when handling hazardous drugs*, 2022. https://www.ons.org/make-difference/ons-center-advocacy-and-health-policy/position-statements/ensuring-healthcare. Accessed September 12, 2023.

Marufu T, et al: Nursing interventions to reduce medication errors in paediatrics and neonates: systematic review and meta-analysis, *J Pediatr Nurs* 62:e139–e147, 2022.

Pardhan A, et al: Evolving best practice for take home cancer drugs, *JCO Oncol Pract* 17:(4):e526–e536, 2021.

Ruscin J, Linnebar S: *Drug related problems in older adults*, Kenilworth, NJ, 2021, Merck and the Merck Manuals.

Schifano F, et al: Focus on over-the-counter drugs' misuse: a systematic review on antihistamines, cough medicines, and decongestants, *Front Psychiatry* 12:657397, 2021.

The Joint Commission (TJC): *2023 National patient safety goals effective 2023 for the hospital program*, Oakbrook Terrace, IL, 2023, The Joint Commission (TJC). https://www.jointcommission.org/-/media/tjc/documents/standards/national-patient-safety-goals/2023/npsg_chapter_hap_jul2023.pdf. Accessed April 23, 2023.

Tolley C, et al: The impact of a novel medication scanner on administration errors in the hospital setting: a before and after feasibility study, *BMC Med Inform Decis Mak* 22:86, 2022.

Touhy T, Jett K: *Ebersole and Hess' gerontological nursing and health aging*, ed 6, St. Louis, 2022, Elsevier.

U.S. Department of Health and Human Services (USDHHS), Centers for Medicare and Medicaid Services (CMS): *Updated guidance on medication administration, Hospital Appendix A of State Operations Manual*, Baltimore, 2020, Department of Health and Human Services.

U.S. Department of Health and Human Services Office of Minority Health: *Think cultural health*, 2021. https://minorityhealth.hhs.gov/omh/browse.aspx?lvl=2&lvlid=53. Accessed September 12, 2023.

U.S. Food and Drug Administration (FDA): *Generic drug facts*, 2021. https://www.fda.gov/drugs/generic-drugs/generic-drug-facts. Accessed September 13, 2023.

U.S. Food and Drug Administration (FDA): *MedWatch: the FDA safety information and adverse event reporting program*, 2022. https://www.fda.gov/safety/medwatch/default.htm. Accessed September 13, 2023.

U.S. Food and Drug Administration (FDA): *Tablet scoring: nomenclature, labeling, and data for evaluation*, 2020. https://www.fda.gov/regulatory-information/search-fda-guidance-documents/tablet-scoringnomenclature-labeling-and-data-evaluation. Accessed September 12, 2023.

Wang W, et al: Current status and influencing factors of nursing interruption events, *Am J Manag Care* 27(6):e188–e194, 2021.

World Health Organization (WHO): *A adverse drug reaction definition by the World Health Organization*, 2020. https://www.publichealth.com.ng/adverse-drug-reaction-definition-by-world-health-organization/. Accessed September 12, 2023.

21 | Nonparenteral Medications

SKILLS AND PROCEDURES

Skill 21.1 **Administering Oral Medications, p. 610**

Skill 21.2 **Administering Medications Through a Feeding Tube, p. 618**

Skill 21.3 **Applying Topical Medications to the Skin, p. 623**

Skill 21.4 **Administering Ophthalmic Medications, p. 629**

Skill 21.5 **Administering Ear Medications, p. 635**

Skill 21.6 **Administering Nasal Instillations, p. 638**

Skill 21.7 **Using Metered-Dose Inhalers (MDIs), p. 642**

Skill 21.8 **Using Small-Volume Nebulizers, p. 649**

Procedural Guideline 21.1 **Administering Vaginal Medications, p. 653**

Procedural Guideline 21.2 **Administering Rectal Suppositories, p. 655**

OBJECTIVES

Mastery of content will enable you to:

- Explain the principles to follow in the administration of nonparenteral medications.
- Discuss patient-centered practices to use to improve a patient's medication adherence.
- Identify guidelines for administering oral, enteral, and topical medications.
- List factors to assess before administering medications.
- Demonstrate safe and correct administration of a medication by oral, enteral, and topical routes.

- Compare and contrast types of topical administrations that require sterile technique and those that require clean medical aseptic technique.
- Identify conditions contraindicating the administration of medications by various oral and topical routes.
- Develop a teaching plan regarding medication use for a selected patient.
- Take part in instructing patients in the proper use of a metered-dose inhaler (MDI), a dry powder inhaler (DPI), and small-volume nebulizer.

MEDIA RESOURCES

- http://evolve.elsevier.com/Perry/skills
- Review Questions
- Audio Glossary
- ▶ Video Clips

- **NSO** Nursing Skills Online
- Answers to Clinical Judgment and Next-Generation NCLEX® Examination–Style Questions
- Printable Key Points
- Skills Performance Checklists

PURPOSE

Nonparenteral medications include medications that are administered orally, topically, and by inhalation, such as oral and enteral medications, topical skin preparations, eyedrops, and eardrops. Nonparenteral medications are not administered by injection. This chapter also includes enteral medications administered via a feeding tube.

The route chosen depends on the properties and desired effects of the medication and the physical and mental condition of the patient. There are many reasons why it may be necessary to change from one route to another. When this occurs, you are responsible for consulting with a health care provider for an order or conferring with the pharmacist to safely meet a patient's needs.

PRACTICE STANDARDS

- Institute for Safe Medication Practices, 2023: ISMP's List of Confused Drug Names
- ISMP, 2022: Targeted Medication Safety Best Practices for Hospitals—Correct equipment, pill splitting
- ISMP, 2021: ISMP's List of Error-Prone Abbreviations, Symbols, and Dose Designations
- The Joint Commission (TJC), 2023: National Patient Safety Goals—Patient identification
- U.S. Department of Health and Human Services (USDHHS), Centers for Medicare and Medicaid Services, 2020: Updated Guidance on Medication Administration, Hospital Appendix A of State Operations Manual—Time-critical medications

SUPPLEMENTAL STANDARDS

- National Institute on Aging, 2022: Taking Medications Safely as You Age

PRINCIPLES FOR PRACTICE

- Patient safety is the major principle of practice with nonparental and enteral medication administration (see Safety Guidelines).
- The oral route (by mouth) is the easiest and most desirable way to administer medications.
- Topical administration of medications involves applying drugs directly to skin or mucous or tissue membranes. See Box 21.1 for examples of topical medication routes.
- Apply medications to the skin by spraying, painting, or spreading medication over a localized area. Transdermal patches (adhesive-backed medicated disks), which are applied to the skin, provide a continuous release of medication over several hours or days.
- Medications applied to membranes such as the cornea of the eye or the rectal mucosa are absorbed quickly because of the vascularity of the membrane and can have systemic effects. In addition, you can experience systemic effects of a topical medication if you do not wear clean gloves.

PERSON-CENTERED CARE

- An excellent time to provide patient teaching is during medication administration.
- The goal of patient teaching is to improve patient adherence to medication regimens. Patients fail to adhere to medication regimens because of patient, medication, and provider issues. Patient adherence improves when patient education programs and techniques are matched to patients' and family caregivers' health literacy (Delavar et al., 2020).
- Through patient-centered health education, health literacy is improved and adherence and self-management with medications and illness improve (Tan et al., 2019).
- Medication issues also include complex medication regimens and medication discrepancies. Health care provider issues include poor instruction, inappropriate prescriptions, and lack

---

BOX 21.1

Examples of Topical Medication Routes

- *Sublingual:* medication placed under the tongue; is dissolvable
- *Buccal:* medication placed between the upper or lower molar teeth and cheek area; is dissolvable
- *Direct application to skin or mucosa:* lotion, ointment, cream, powder, foam, spray, patch, and disk
- *Direct application to mucous membrane:* eyedrops, gargling, swabbing the throat
- *Spraying:* instillation into nose or throat
- *Inhalation of medicated aerosol spray:* distributes medication throughout the nasal passages and the tracheobronchial airway; two types of devices designed for this purpose: metered-dose inhalers (MDIs) and small-volume nebulizers
- *Inhalation of dry powder medication:* distributes medication in powder form throughout the tracheobronchial airway; device designed for this purpose: dry powder inhaler (DPI)
- *Inserting drug into a body cavity:* rectal or vaginal suppositories, vaginal creams, or foams

---

of provider knowledge about adherence. Patients need explanations about the purpose of medications, benefits, expected effects, and how to plan a daily schedule.
- Health beliefs vary by culture and influence how patients manage and respond to medication therapy. It is important to consider cultural influences on drug response, metabolism, and side effects if a patient is not responding to drug therapy as expected.
- Differences in values, attitudes, and beliefs affect a patient's adherence to medication therapy.
- Herbal remedies and alternative therapies may be common practice in some cultures and can interfere with prescribed medications.
- Certain food preferences may have food-drug interactions. Vegetarian and vegan diets can affect warfarin or medications for glycemic control.
- Printed materials used for instruction should be written at an appropriate reading level (6th to 8th grade) and delivered in a manner that meets individual patient needs such as visual impairment or hearing or cognitive impairments. Involve family caregivers in the education sessions because they may be the ones administering medications.

EVIDENCE-BASED PRACTICE

Enhanced Nebulizer Designs

New technology for nebulizer design addresses issues of medication loss and speed of medication delivery, and it allows delivery of a bolus dose of nebulized aerosol medication (Gardner & Wilkinson, 2019). In addition, enhanced jet nebulizers provide predictable and reliable drug delivery while avoiding the effects of active humidification and humidifier contamination when used during mechanical ventilation (Ashraf et al., 2020).
- Some of the benefits and cautions of newer enhanced nebulizer designs include:
  - Breath-enhanced nebulizers minimize waste and produce more aerosolized medication during inhalation (Gardner & Wilkinson, 2019).
  - Faster nebulization rate due to the production of small particles in the aerosol.
  - Continuously nebulizes medication into a holding chamber, using a system of one-way valves to direct exhaled air away from the holding chamber and the aerosolized medication (Gardner & Wilkinson, 2019).
  - Breath-enhanced nebulizers ensure better control of drug delivery (Ashraf et al., 2020).
- Ongoing assessment of patient outcomes following use of enhanced nebulization is crucial because some patients may do better with conventional jet nebulizers, especially children with acute asthma (Gardner & Wilkinson, 2019).

SAFETY GUIDELINES

- Safe medication administration requires you to follow the seven rights of medication administration for all nonparenteral and enteral medications: Right Medication, Right Dose, Right Patient, Right Route, Right Time, Right Documentation, and Right Indication. Also know the ISMP and TJC guidelines, confusing drug names (ISMP, 2023), drug actions and interactions, potential side effects and adverse effects, and how to safely administer medication through various nonparenteral routes.
- Know your state's Nurse Practice Act with regard to the roles and responsibilities of licensed practical/vocational nurses (LPNs/LVNs), certified nurse assistants, and medication technicians regarding drug administration. Many states allow specially

trained assistive personnel (AP) and medication technicians to give medications such as select oral medications, topical agents, eye drops, eardrops, and rectal and vaginal suppositories. Also check agency policy.

- Be vigilant during medication administration. Avoid distractions while preparing a parenteral medication. No-Interruption Zones (NIZs) have been recommended to reduce distractions during medication preparation and administration (Palese et al., 2019; Wang et al., 2021).

- Clarify unclear medication orders and ask for help whenever you are uncertain about an order or calculation. Consult with your peers, pharmacists, and other health care providers, and be sure that you have resolved all concerns related to medication administration before preparing and giving medications.

- Use at least two identifiers before administering medications and check against the medication administration record (MAR). Follow agency policy for patient identification.

- Follow best practices for calculating medication doses, double-check the calculations, and *do not* administer if the dosage appears incorrect. Follow agency policy for drug calculations for the very young or high-risk medications (e.g., cardiotonics, some opioid medications).

- Best-practice guidelines for safe medication administration require clinical judgment, clinical decision making competency, and theoretical and clinical practice competency. Medication administration is not a routine nursing action. You must critically think about the medications you are giving. Ask yourself: "Is the medication still appropriate for the patient's condition, or do I need to contact the health care provider?" "This pill looks different. I need to verify with pharmacy" (Billstein-Leber et al., 2018).

- Assess a patient's sensory function, including sight, hearing, touch, and physical coordination and dexterity. Sensory function and coordination deficits impair a patient's ability to see medications, read labels at home, and discriminate one medication from another. Coordination and dexterity impairments hinder a patient's ability to open prescription bottles and dispense the correct dosage.

- Patients often receive more than one oral medication at a time. Evaluate each medication for potential drug-drug or drug-food interactions. When unsure, consult with a pharmacist to clarify the risk of an interaction and determine the measure to reduce it.

- Always assess for drug allergies. If a patient reports having an allergy, ask about the type of reaction that occurred.

- Evaluate if a patient can take oral medication with food. In most cases the presence of food in the stomach delays drug absorption. However, some medications must be taken before meals, and others may need to be taken with meals. Some drugs irritate the stomach lining and need to be taken with food.

- For all medications administered, review the order for patient's name, drug, dosage, route, and time of administration.

- Use the technology (e.g., bar scanning, eMARs) available in your agency when preparing and giving medications. Follow all policies related to use of the technology, and do not use work-arounds.

- Use the correct equipment for administering all medications. For example, when delivering liquid medications, use only unit dose containers dispensed by the pharmacy (ISMP, 2022).

- For all medications administered, gather information pertinent to the drug(s) ordered: purpose, normal dosage and route, common side effects, time of onset and peak, contraindications, and nursing implications.

- Determine if medications require any specific nursing actions (e.g., obtaining vital signs, drug levels, or electrolytes) before administration.

- If patients are mentally and physically able, prepare them for discharge by instructing them in self-administration techniques. Include family caregivers if possible.

- Check the expiration date for all medications.

- Before medication administration, it is critical to ensure that all information is correct. You should check for accuracy three times:
  1. The first check is when the medications are pulled or retrieved from the automated dispensing machine, the medication drawer, or whatever system is in place at the agency.
  2. The second check is when preparation of the medications for administration takes place.
  3. The final check occurs at the patient's bedside just before medications are given.

◆ SKILL 21.1 Administering Oral Medications

 Video Clip

Patients are usually able to ingest or self-administer oral medications with few problems. If oral medications are contraindicated (e.g., inability to swallow, gastric suction), take precautions to protect patients from aspiration (see Skill 31.3). Nurses usually prepare medications in areas designed for medication preparation or at unit-dose carts.

The form or preparation of an oral medication affects how well it is absorbed after it is ingested. Liquids are absorbed faster than tablets or capsules and are usually absorbed in the stomach. Give an oral medication with a meal if its absorption is enhanced by food in the stomach. Some medications must be taken between meals, 2 to 3 hours later (Burchum & Rosenthal, 2022).

Some oral medications are absorbed in the intestinal tract. Enteric-coated preparations resist being dissolved by gastric juices. The enteric coating protects the stomach lining from irritation by the medication. These preparations are absorbed in the small intestine. Never crush or split an enteric-coated medication. Crushing or splitting these preparations causes the medication to be released too early; the medication may become inactive in the stomach or fail to reach the intended site of action.

Delegation

The skill of administering oral medications cannot be delegated to assistive personnel (AP). Direct the AP to:

- Report occurrence of potential side effects of medications to the nurse.
- Inform the nurse if patient condition changes or worsens (e.g., pain, itching, or rash) after medication administration.

Interprofessional Collaboration

- A speech pathologist can assist patients who have impaired swallowing by teaching swallowing techniques.

Equipment

- Automated, computer-controlled drug-dispensing system or medication cart
- Disposable medication cups (mL-only cups); oral use syringes
- Glass of water, juice, or preferred liquid and drinking straw
- Pill-crushing device (optional)

- Paper towels
- Medication administration record (MAR) (electronic or printed)
- Clean gloves (if handling an oral medication) **NOTE:** Gloves must be worn when administering an oral chemotherapy drug.

STEP	RATIONALE

ASSESSMENT

1. Check accuracy and completeness of each MAR or computer printout with health care provider's written medication order. Check patient's name, medication name and dosage, route of administration, and time of administration. Clarify incomplete or unclear orders with health care provider before administration.

The order sheet is the most reliable source and only legal record of medications that patient is to receive. Ensures that patient receives the correct medications (Palese et al., 2019). Transcription errors are a source of medication errors (Zhu & Weingart, 2022).

2. Review medication reference for pertinent information related to medication, including action, purpose, normal dose and route, side effects, time of onset and peak action, indication, and nursing implications.

Allows you to anticipate effects of drug and observe patient's response.

3. Review electronic health record (EHR) for any contraindications to patient receiving oral medication, including being on nothing by mouth (NPO) status, inability to swallow, nausea/vomiting, bowel inflammation, reduced peristalsis, recent GI surgery, gastric suction, and decreased level of consciousness (LOC). Notify health care provider if any contraindications are present.

Alterations in GI function can interfere with medication absorption, distribution, and excretion. Patients with GI suction do not receive actions of oral medications because the medications are suctioned from the GI tract before they are absorbed.

4. Assess patient's medical and medication history and history of allergies. List medication allergies on each page of the MAR and prominently display on the patient's EHR. When allergies are present, patient should wear an allergy bracelet.

These factors influence how certain medications act. Information reveals previous problems with medication administration. Allergy alert helps prevent adverse effects.

5. Check date of expiration for medication.

Dose potency can increase or decrease when outdated.

6. Assess patient's/family caregiver's health literacy.

Determines degree to which individuals have the ability to find, understand, and use information and services to make informed health-related decisions and actions for themselves and others (Centers for Disease Control and Prevention [CDC], 2023).

7. Perform hand hygiene and assess for any contraindications to patient receiving oral medication, including inability to swallow, nausea/vomiting, reduced peristalsis, and decreased level of consciousness (LOC). Notify health care provider if any contraindications are present.

Alterations can interfere with drug absorption, distribution, and excretion. Giving oral medications to patients with impaired swallowing, impaired cognition, decreased LOC, patients who required oral secretion suctioning, and those who had cough reflex at rest had increased risk for aspiration (Suzuki et al., 2022).

8. Assess risk for aspiration using a dysphagia screening tool if available (see Skill 31.3). Protect patient from aspiration by assessing swallowing ability (Box 21.2).

Aspiration occurs when food, fluid, or medication intended for GI administration is inadvertently administered into the respiratory tract. Patients with altered ability to swallow, impaired gag reflex, and who have a tracheostomy are at risk for aspiration (Forough et al., 2018; Nativ-Zeltzer et al., 2022).

9. Ask patient to confirm history of allergies: known type of allergies and allergic reaction.

Confirms patient's allergies. Communication of allergies is essential for safe, effective care.

10. Gather and review physical assessment findings and laboratory data that influence drug administration, such as vital signs and results of renal and liver function studies.

Data may reveal need to contraindicate drug administration. Renal and liver function status affects metabolism and excretion of medications (Burchum & Rosenthal, 2022).

STEP	RATIONALE

BOX 21.2

Protecting the Patient From Aspiration

- Allow patient to self-administer medications if possible.
- Know the signs of dysphagia (difficulty swallowing): cough, change in voice tone or quality after swallowing, delayed swallowing, incomplete oral clearance or pocketing of food, regurgitation.
- Assess patient's ability to swallow and cough by checking for presence of gag reflex and then offering 50 mL of water in 5-mL allotments. Stop if patient begins to cough.
- Prepare oral medication in form that is easiest to swallow.
- Position the patient in an upright seated position at a 90-degree angle with feet on the floor, hips and knees at 90 degrees, head midline, and back erect if possible and if not contraindicated by the patient's condition.
- Suggest that the patient slightly flex the head in a chin-down position before swallowing.
- Prepare oral medications in the form that is easiest to swallow.
- If patient has unilateral (one-sided) weakness, place medication in stronger side of mouth.

- Administer pills one at a time, ensuring that each medication is properly swallowed before next one is introduced.
- Thicken regular liquids or offer fruit nectars if patient cannot tolerate thin liquids.
- Some medications can be crushed and mixed with pureed foods if necessary. Refer to a medication reference to identify medications that are safe to crush.
- Avoid straws because they decrease the control the patient has over volume intake, which increases risk of aspiration.
- Have patient hold and drink from a cup if possible.
- Time medications, if possible, to coincide with mealtimes or when patient is well rested and awake.
- Administer medications using another route if risk of aspiration is severe (see agency policy).

---

11. Assess patient's preference for fluids and determine if medications can be given with these fluids. Maintain fluid restrictions as prescribed.

Some fluids interfere with medication absorption (e.g., dairy products affect tetracycline). Offering fluids during drug administration is an excellent way to increase patient's fluid intake. Fluids ease swallowing and facilitate absorption from the GI tract. However, fluid restrictions exist; skillful planning of fluid intake must coordinate with medication times and type of medications.

12. Assess patient's knowledge, prior experience regarding health and medication use, medication schedule, and ability to prepare medications.

Reveals need for patient instruction about specific medication and support to achieve drug adherence (e.g., involvement of family caregiver).

PLANNING

1. Expected outcomes following completion of procedure:
   - Patient responds appropriately to desired medication effect.
   - Patient denies any GI discomfort or symptoms of alterations.
   - Patient explains purpose of medication and drug dosage schedule.

Drug has exerted its therapeutic action.
Oral medications have been given appropriately to avoid irritation of GI mucosa.
Demonstrates understanding of drug therapy.

2. Provide privacy and explain procedure to patient. Discuss purpose and side effects of each medication. If applicable, teach patient how to report any side effects. Be specific if patient wishes to self-administer medications. Allow sufficient time for patient to ask questions.

Protects patient's privacy; reduces anxiety. Promotes cooperation.
Makes patient a participant in care, which minimizes anxiety. Patient's understanding of each medication improves adherence with drug therapy. Prepares patient to self-administer drug, which increases feelings of independence.

3. Plan preparation to avoid interruptions. Create a quiet environment. Do not take phone calls or talk with others. Follow agency "No-Interruption Zone (NIZ)" policy. Keep all pages of MARs or computer printouts for one patient together or look at only one patient's electronic MAR at a time.

Interruptions contribute to medication errors (Palese et al., 2019; Wang et al., 2021).

4. Collect and organize appropriate equipment and MAR.

Ensures more efficiency when completing a procedure.

IMPLEMENTATION

1. Perform hand hygiene. Prepare medications for one patient at a time, avoiding distractions.

Ensures that medication is sterile.

   a. Arrange medication tray and cups in medication preparation area or move medication cart to position outside patient's room.

Organization of equipment saves time and reduces error.

STEP	RATIONALE

b. Log on to automated medication dispensing system (AMDS) or unlock medicine drawer or cart.

Medications are safeguarded when locked in cabinet, cart, or AMDS.

c. Prepare medications by following the seven rights of medication administration. Keep all pages of MARs or computer printouts for one patient together or look at only one patient's medication administration computer screen.

Prevents preparation errors.

d. Select correct medication from AMDS, unit-dose drawer, or stock supply. Compare name of medication on label with medication administration record (MAR) or computer printout (see illustration). Exit AMDS after removing drug(s).

Reading label and comparing it against transcribed order reduces errors. Exiting AMDS ensures that no one else can remove medications using your identity. *This is the first check for accuracy and ensures safe administration.*

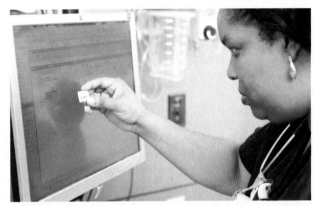

STEP 1d Nurse compares label of medication with transcribed medication order on computerized medication administration record.

e. Check or calculate medication dose as needed. Double-check any calculation. Check expiration date on all medications and return outdated medication to pharmacy.

Double-checking pharmacy calculations reduces risk for error. Agency policy may require you to check calculations of certain medications with another nurse (ISMP, 2022). Expired medications may be inactive or harmful to patient.

f. If preparing a controlled substance, check record for previous medication count and compare current count with available supply. Controlled drugs may be stored in computerized locked cart (see Chapter 20).

Controlled substance laws require nurses to carefully monitor and count dispensed narcotics.

g. Prepare solid forms of oral medications.

(1) To prepare unit-dose tablets or capsules, place packaged tablet or capsule directly into medication cup without removing wrapper. Administer medications only from containers with labels that are clearly marked.

Wrappers maintain cleanliness and identify drug name and dose, which can facilitate teaching.

(2) When using a blister pack, "pop" medications through foil or paper backing into a medication cup.

Packs provide a 1-month supply, with each "blister" usually containing a single dose.

(3) When preparing tablet or capsule from a floor stock bottle, pour required number into bottle cap and transfer to medication cup. Do not touch medication with fingers. Return unused medication to container.

Avoids contamination and waste of medication.

(4) If it is necessary to give half the dose of medication, pharmacy should split, label, package, and send medication to unit. If you must split medication, use clean, gloved hand to cut with clean pill-cutting device. Only cut tablets that are prescored by the manufacturer (line traverses the center of the tablet).

Reduces contamination of the tablet. In health care agencies, only pharmacy should split tablets to ensure patient safety (ISMP, 2022). If a tablet is FDA approved to be split, this information will be printed in the "HOW SUPPLIED" section of the manufacturer's package insert.

STEP	RATIONALE
(5) Place all tablets or capsules in unit dose individual packets that patient will receive in one medicine cup, except for those requiring preadministration assessments (e.g., pulse rate or blood pressure). Place those medications in separate additional cup with wrapper intact.	Keeping medications that require preadministration assessments separate from others serves as a reminder and makes it easier to withhold drugs as needed.
(6) If patient has difficulty swallowing and liquid medications are not an option, use a pill-crushing device. Clean device before using. Place medicine between two cups, and grind and crush (see illustration). Mix ground tablet in small amount (teaspoon) of soft food (custard or applesauce).	Large tablets are often difficult to swallow. Ground tablet mixed with palatable soft food is usually easier to swallow.

Clinical Judgment *Not all medications can be crushed safely. Consult with a pharmacist.*

h. Prepare liquids.	
(1) Use unit-dose container with correct amount of medication. Gently shake container. Administer medication packaged in a single-dose cup directly from the single-dose cup. Do not pour medicine into another cup.	Using unit-dose container with correct dosage of medication provides most accurate dose of medication (ISMP, 2021). Shaking container ensures that medication is mixed before administration.

Clinical Judgment *On the basis of current best practice (ISMP, 2021), liquid medications that are not available or are not in correct dose in a unit-dose container should be dispensed by the pharmacy in special oral syringes marked "Oral Use Only." These syringes do not connect to any type of parenteral (e.g., intravenous [IV]) tubing. In addition, current evidence shows that liquid measuring devices on patient care units result in inaccurate dosing. Having oral medications prepared in the pharmacy ensures that you give the most accurate dose of a medication possible and prevents parenteral administration of oral medications.*

(2) Administer medications only in oral use syringes, which in some agencies are prepared by the pharmacy (see illustration). Do not use hypodermic syringe or syringe with needle or syringe cap (see Chapter 20).	Only use syringes specifically designed for oral use when administering liquid medications. Allows more accurate measurement of small amounts.
	If using hypodermic syringes, the medication may be administered parenterally accidentally; or the syringe cap or needle, if not removed from the syringe before administration, may become dislodged and accidentally aspirated during administration of oral medications (ISMP, 2022).

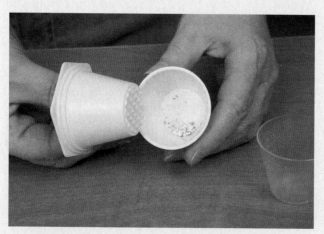

STEP 1g(6) Crushing tablet with pill-crushing device.

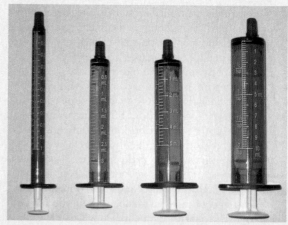

STEP 1h(2) Use special oral medication syringes to prepare small amounts of liquid medications.

STEP	RATIONALE
i. Return stock containers or unused unit-dose medications to shelf or drawer. Label medication cups and poured medications with patient's name before leaving medication preparation area. Do not leave drugs unattended.	Ensures that correct medications are prepared for correct patient.
j. Before going to patient's room, compare patient's name and name of medication on label of prepared medications with MAR.	*This is the second check for accuracy and ensures safe administration.*
2. Administer medications.	
a. Take medication to patient at correct time (see agency policy). Medications that require exact timing include STAT doses, first-time or loading doses, and one-time doses. Give time-critical scheduled medications (e.g., antibiotics, anticoagulants, insulin, anticonvulsants, or immunosuppressive agents) at exact time ordered (no more than 30 minutes before or after scheduled dose). Give non–time-critical scheduled medications within a range of 1 or 2 hours of scheduled dose (CMS, 2023). During administration, apply seven rights of medication administration. Perform hand hygiene.	Hospitals must adopt medication administration policy and procedure for timing of medication administration that considers nature of the prescribed medication, specific clinical application, and patient needs (CMS, 2023; USDHHS, 2020). Time-critical scheduled medications are those for which early or delayed administration of maintenance doses of greater than 30 minutes before or after the scheduled dose may cause harm or result in substantial suboptimal therapy or pharmacological effect. Non–time-critical medications are those for which early or delayed administration within a specified range of either 1 or 2 hours should not cause harm or result in substantial suboptimal therapy or pharmacological effect (CMS, 2023; USDHHS, 2020).
b. Identify patient using at least two identifiers (e.g., name and birthday or name and medical record number) according to agency policy. Compare identifiers with information on patient's MAR or EHR.	Ensures correct patient. Complies with The Joint Commission standards and improves patient safety (TJC, 2023). Some agencies are now using a bar-code system to help with patient identification (check agency policy).
c. At patient's bedside, again compare MAR or computer printout with names of medications on medication labels and patient name. Ask patient again about any allergies.	*This is the third check for accuracy* and ensures that patient receives correct medication. Confirms patient's allergy history.
d. Close curtains or room door. Perform hand hygiene. Perform necessary preadministration assessment (e.g., blood pressure, pulse) for specific medications.	Provides patient privacy. Reduces transmission of microorganisms. Determines whether specific medications should be withheld at that time.
e. Help patient to sitting or Fowler position. Use side-lying position if the patient is unable to sit. Have patient stay in this position for 30 minutes after administration.	Decreases risk for aspiration during swallowing.

Clinical Judgment *If patient expresses concern regarding accuracy of a medication, do not give the medication. Explore patient's concern and verify health care provider's order before administering. Listening to patient's concerns may prevent a medication error.*

f. For tablets: Patient may want to hold solid medications in hand or cup before placing in mouth. Offer water or preferred liquid to help patient swallow medications.	Patient can become familiar with medications by seeing each drug. Choice of fluid can improve fluid intake.

Clinical Judgment *If administering an oral chemotherapy medication, you can administer it from the cup directly into the patient's mouth or apply gloves before handling pill or tablet. Never use bare hands to touch a chemotherapy medication as residue can be absorbed through your skin (OSHA, n.d.).*

g. For orally disintegrating formulations (tablets or strips): Remove medication from packet just before use. Do not push tablet through foil. Place medication on top of patient's tongue. Caution against chewing it.	Orally disintegrating formulations begin to dissolve when placed on tongue. Water is not needed. Careful removal from packaging is necessary because tablets and strips are thin and fragile.
h. For sublingually administered medications: Have patient place medication under tongue and allow it to dissolve completely (see illustration). Caution patient against swallowing tablet.	Drug is absorbed through blood vessels of undersurface of tongue. If swallowed, it is destroyed by gastric juices or rapidly detoxified by liver, preventing therapeutic blood level.
i. For buccal-administered medications: Have patient place medication in mouth against mucous membranes of cheek and gums until it dissolves (see illustration).	Buccal medications act locally or systemically as they are swallowed in saliva.

STEP	RATIONALE

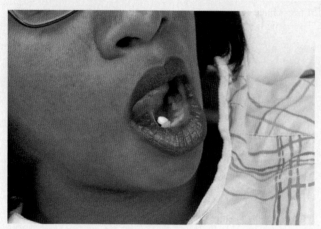

STEP 2h Proper placement of sublingual tablet in sublingual pocket.

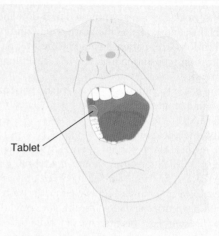

Tablet

STEP 2i Buccal administration of tablet.

Clinical Judgment *Avoid administering anything by mouth until orally disintegrating buccal or sublingual medication is completely dissolved.*

j. For powdered medications: Mix with liquids at bedside and give to patient to drink.	When prepared in advance, powdered drugs thicken; some even harden, making swallowing difficult.
k. For crushed medications mixed with food: Give each medication separately in teaspoon of food.	Ensures that patient swallows all of the medicine.
l. For lozenge: Caution patient against chewing or swallowing lozenges.	Lozenges act through slow absorption through oral mucosa, not gastric mucosa.
m. For effervescent medication: Add tablet or powder to glass of water. Administer immediately after dissolving.	Effervescence improves unpleasant taste and often relieves GI problems.
n. If patient is unable to hold medications, place medication cup or oral syringe to lips and gently introduce each medication into mouth one at a time. Administer each tablet or capsule one at a time. Inject liquid from oral syringe slowly. A spoon can also be used to place pill in patient's mouth. Do not rush or force medications.	Administering a single tablet or capsule eases swallowing and decreases risk for aspiration. Slow injection of liquid prevents aspiration.

Clinical Judgment *If tablet or capsule falls to the floor, discard it and repeat preparation. Drug is contaminated.*

o. Stay until patient swallows each medication completely or takes it by the prescribed route. Ask patient to open mouth if uncertain whether medication has been swallowed.	Ensures that patient receives ordered dose. If left unattended, patient may not take dose or may save drugs, causing health risks.
p. For highly acidic medications (e.g., aspirin), offer patients a nonfat snack (e.g., crackers) if not contraindicated by their condition.	Reduces gastric irritation. Fat content of foods may delay drug absorption.
3. Help patient return to position of comfort.	Maintains patient's comfort.
4. Raise side rails (as appropriate) and lower bed to lowest position, locking into position.	Ensures patient safety and prevents falls.
5. Place nurse call system in an accessible location within patient's reach.	Ensures patient can call for assistance if needed.
6. Dispose of all contaminated supplies in appropriate receptacle, remove and dispose of gloves, and perform hand hygiene.	Reduces transmission of microorganisms. Use appropriate disposal receptacle if patient on hazardous drugs (ONS, 2018, 2022).
7. Replenish stock such as cups and straws, return cart to medication room, and clean work area.	Enhances efficiency and reduces transfer of microorganisms.

STEP	RATIONALE

EVALUATION

1. Return to bedside to evaluate patient's response to medications at times that correlate with onset, peak, and duration of the medication.

Evaluates therapeutic benefit of medication and helps to detect onset of side effects or allergic reactions. Sublingual medications act in 15 minutes; most oral medications act in 30 to 60 minutes.

2. Ask patient or family caregiver to identify medication name and explain purpose, action, dose schedule, and potential side effects.

Determines level of knowledge gained by patient and family caregiver.

3. **Use Teach-Back:** "I want to be sure I showed you how to use your sublingual nitroglycerin. Show me where you will place the tablet in your mouth." Revise your instruction now or develop a plan for revised patient/family caregiver teaching if patient/family caregiver is not able to teach back correctly.

Teach-back is a technique for health care providers to ensure that they have explained medical information clearly so that patients and their families understand what is communicated to them (Agency for Healthcare Research and Quality [AHRQ], 2023).

Unexpected Outcomes

1. Patient exhibits adverse effects (e.g., side effect, toxic effect, allergic reaction).

Related Interventions

- Notify health care provider and pharmacy immediately.
- Withhold further doses.
- Assess vital signs.
- Symptoms such as urticaria, rash, pruritus, rhinitis, and wheezing may indicate an allergic reaction and need for emergency medications.
- Add allergy information to patient's EHR.

2. Patient refuses medication.

- Assess why patient is refusing medication.
- Provide further instruction.
- Do not force patient to take medications.
- Notify health care provider.

3. Patient is unable to explain drug information.

- Further assess patient's or family caregiver's knowledge of medications and guidelines for drug safety.
- Further instruction or different approach to instruction is necessary.

Documentation

- Document drug, dose, route, and time administered immediately after administration, not before. Include initials or signature.
- Document patient's response and any adverse effects to medication.
- Document your evaluation of patient learning.
- If drug is withheld, document reason and follow agency policy for noting withheld doses.

Hand-Off Reporting

- Report adverse effects/patient response and/or withheld drugs to nurse in charge or health care provider. Depending on medication, immediate health care provider notification may be required.

Special Considerations

Patient Education

- Instruct patient and family caregiver about specific information pertaining to drug regimen (purpose, action, dose, dosage intervals, side effects, foods to avoid or take with drugs). If patient is taking multiple medications, consider recommending a dose organizer.
- All patients should learn the basic guidelines for drug safety in the home (see Skill 43.3).

Pediatrics

- Liquid forms of medication are safer to swallow to avoid aspiration of small pills.

- Children refuse bitter or distasteful oral preparations. Mix the drug with a small amount (about 1 tsp) of a sweet-tasting substance such as jam, applesauce, sherbet, ice cream, or fruit puree. Do not use honey for infants because of the risk of botulism. Offer the child juice or a flavored ice pop after medication administration. Do not place medication in an essential food item such as milk or formula; the child may refuse the food at a later time.
- Measure the liquid medications with a plastic calibrated oral dosing syringe or a spoon. Calibrated spoons have proven to be most accurate for the pediatric population (Hockenberry et al., 2022).

Older Adults

- Physiological changes of aging influence how oral medications are distributed, absorbed, and excreted. Common changes include loss of elasticity in oral mucosa; reduction in parotid gland secretion, causing dry mouth; delayed esophageal clearance; impaired swallowing; reduction in gastric acidity and stomach peristalsis; increased susceptibility to highly acidic drugs; reduced liver function, resulting in altered drug metabolism; and reduced renal function and colon motility, slowing drug excretion (Touhy & Jett, 2022). Both altered drug metabolism and excretion may lead to drug toxicity (Burchum & Rosenthal, 2022).
- Give medications with a full glass of water (unless restricted) to aid passage of the drug. Give patient time to swallow.
- Patients may have several health problems or chronic conditions requiring the use of multiple drugs, often prescribed by

different health care providers. Polypharmacy creates a high risk for drug interactions and adverse reactions (Burchum & Rosenthal, 2022).

Populations With Disabilities

- Cognitive impairment and depression interact with health literacy. Individualized patient teaching techniques that simplify tasks and patient roles may help to overcome cognitive load and suboptimal performance in self-medication administration (Sullivan et al., 2018).

- When possible and practical, patients with delirium may benefit by having a family caregiver present during oral medication administration (Yevchak et al., 2017).

Home Care

- When measuring liquid medications at home, instruct patients and family caregivers how to accurately use a dosing cup to administer medications in the home (see Chapter 20).
- See Skills 42.3 and 43.6.

♦ SKILL 21.2 Administering Medications Through a Feeding Tube

Patients who have enteral feeding tubes are unable to receive food or medications by mouth. Nasogastric feeding tubes generally are small-bore tubes that are inserted into the stomach via one of the nares (see Chapter 31). For long-term enteral feedings, a percutaneous endoscopic gastrostomy (PEG) tube or a jejunostomy tube may be inserted surgically. Never administer medications into nasogastric tubes that are inserted for decompression.

Special consideration is needed when administering medications to patients with enteral or small-bore feeding tubes. Failing to follow current evidence-based recommendations from the American Society for Parenteral and Enteral Nutrition (ASPEN) can result in tube obstruction, reduced medication effectiveness, and increased risk of medication toxicity (Boullata et al., 2017). Tubing misconnections continue to cause patient injury because tubes with different functions can be connected with Luer connectors (Ayers, 2020; Malone et al., 2019). In response to this issue, the International Organization for Standardization (IOS, 2020) has developed tubing connector standards in which the enteral connector will no longer be Luer compatible (ISMP, 2022). An enteral-only connection system (ENFit) is available, and health care agencies have changed enteral nutrition practices, policies, procedures, and processes per the new guidelines. Before giving a medication by this route, verify that the location of the tube (e.g., stomach or jejunum) is compatible with medication absorption. For example, iron dissolves in the stomach and is mostly absorbed in the duodenum. If it is administered through a jejunal tube, it has poor bioavailability.

Preferably, medications administered by enteral tubes should be in liquid form. However, when the liquid form of the medication is not available, check with a pharmacist to determine if you can use the oral medication tablet or capsule by crushing or dissolving it or piercing the gel capsule. However, do not crush sublingual, sustained-release, chewable, long-acting, or enteric-coated medications. Hospital pharmacies may be able to provide the prescribed medication in a liquid suspension, which does not affect its effectiveness (ISMP, 2022). Always verify correct placement of a nasogastric tube before administering medications (see agency policy; see Skill 31.2).

Delegation

The skill of administering medications by enteral feeding tubes cannot be delegated to assistive personnel (AP). Direct the AP to:
- Keep the head of the bed elevated a minimum of 30 degrees (preferably 45 degrees) for 1 h after medication administration; follow agency policy.
- Report immediately to the nurse coughing, choking, gagging, or drooling of liquid.

- Report to the nurse the occurrence of possible medication side effects (specific to medication).

Interprofessional Collaboration

- A pharmacist will advise you if a medication can be crushed or dissolved for enteral administration.

Equipment

- Medication administration record (MAR) (electronic or printed)
- Appropriate medication syringe or 60-mL Asepto syringe for large-bore tubes only
- ENFit connection system designed to fit the specific enteral tube (Fig. 21.1)
- Gastric pH test strip (scale of 0 to 11.0)
- Graduated container
- Medication to be administered (usually prepared in the medication syringe)
- Pill crusher if medication in tablet form
- Water or sterile water for immunocompromised patients
- Tongue blade or straw to stir dissolved medication
- Clean gloves
- Stethoscope and pulse oximeter (for evaluation)

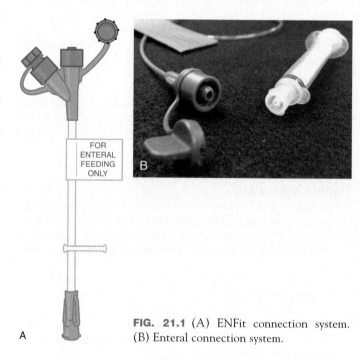

FOR ENTERAL FEEDING ONLY

A

FIG. 21.1 (A) ENFit connection system. (B) Enteral connection system.

STEP	RATIONALE

ASSESSMENT

1. Check accuracy and completeness of MAR or computer printout with health care provider's original medication order. Check patient's name, medication name and dosage, route of administration, and time of administration. Reprint on computer any part of MAR that is difficult to read.

The order sheet is the most reliable source and only legal record of medications that patient is to receive. Ensures that patient receives the correct medications (Palese et al., 2019; Wang et al., 2021). Transcription errors are a source of medication errors (Zhu & Weingart, 2022).

2. Review medication reference information related to medication, including action, purpose, normal dose and route, side effects, time of onset and peak action, and nursing implications.

Allows you to anticipate effects of medication while observing patient's response.

   a. Determine if there is any type of interaction between medications delivered via feeding tube and contact pharmacist if there is any question (Boullata, 2021).

The risk for drug-drug interactions is high when two or more medications are given via this route because they can interact together as soon as they are administered. When medications interact with one another, timing of administration may need to change or a new medication may need to be prescribed.

3. Assess patient's medical and medication history and history of allergies. List food and medication allergies on each page of the MAR and prominently display on the patient's electronic health record (EHR). When allergies are present, patient should wear an allergy bracelet.

Factors influence how certain medications act. Reveals patient's need for medication.

Allergy alert helps prevent adverse effects.

4. Review EHR to determine patient's age and history of dehydration, malnutrition, exposure to radiation therapy, underlying chronic conditions (e.g., diabetes mellitus, immunosuppression), and edema of the skin.

Common risk factors for medical adhesive–related skin injury (MARSI). Patients with enteral tubes have some type of adhesive device (e.g., adhesive tape, commercial securement device) to reduce the risk for dislodgment of the enteral tube and are at risk for MARSI (Fumarola et al., 2020).

5. Assess patient's/family caregiver's health literacy.

Determines degree to which individuals have the ability to find, understand, and use information and services to make informed health-related decisions and actions for themselves and others (CDC, 2023).

6. Review EHR for any contraindications to receiving enteral medications, including presence of bowel inflammation, reduced peristalsis, recent gastrointestinal (GI) surgery, and gastric suction that cannot be turned off.

Alterations in GI function can interfere with drug absorption, distribution, and excretion. Patients with GI suction do not benefit from medication because it may be suctioned from the GI tract before it is absorbed.

7. Ask patient to confirm allergies: known allergies and allergic response.

Confirms patient's allergies.

8. For postoperative patient, review postoperative orders for type of enteral tube care.

Manipulation and irrigation of tube or instillation of medications may be contraindicated.

9. Perform hand hygiene. Gather and review physical assessment data (e.g., bowel sounds, abdominal distention), observe patient's skin around feeding tube and tape or securement devices for irritation or signs of MARSI, and review laboratory data (e.g., renal and liver function) that may influence drug administration.

Reduces transmission of microorganisms. Physical examination findings or laboratory data may contraindicate drug administration.

10. Check with pharmacy for availability of liquid preparation for patient's medications. Prescriber may need to change dosage form.

When possible, liquid formulation of the medication is the best option. The agency pharmacy may have the ability to provide a liquid preparation that is compatible with the enteral nutrition formula (Boullata et al., 2017).

11. Avoid complicated medication schedule that interrupts enteral feedings. Check with health care provider and use alternative medication route when possible.

Ensures proper medication administration route. Avoids medication interactions.

   a. Determine where medication is absorbed and ensure that point of absorption is not bypassed by feeding tube. For example, some antacids are absorbed in the stomach. If the enteral tube is placed in the intestine, medication may not be absorbed.

   b. Determine whether medication interacts with enteral feedings (Boullata, 2021). If there is a risk of interaction, stop feeding for at least 20 minutes before administering medication (check agency policy).

12. Assess patient's knowledge, prior experience with enteral medication, and feelings about procedure.

Reveals need for patient instruction and/or support.

STEP	RATIONALE

PLANNING

1. Expected outcomes following completion of procedure:
   - Patient experiences desired medication effect within period of onset of medication.

   - Patient's feeding tube remains patent after administration of medication.

   - Patient does not aspirate during or after medication administration.
2. Provide privacy and explain procedure to patient. Discuss purpose of each medication, indication, action, and possible adverse effects. Allow patient to ask any questions.
3. Plan preparation to avoid interruptions. Create a quiet environment. Do not take phone calls or talk with others. Follow agency "No-Interruption Zone" policy. Keep all pages of MARs or computer printouts for one patient together or look at only one patient's electronic MAR at a time.
4. Collect and organize appropriate equipment and MAR for administering enteral medications at bedside.

Drug has exerted its therapeutic action.

Patent enteral tube indicates passage of medication into stomach, ensuring proper absorption. If tube becomes blocked, administration of other medications and feedings are not possible.
Patient safety in medication administration is maintained.

Protects patient's privacy; reduces anxiety. Promotes cooperation.
Patient has right to be informed, and patient's understanding of each medication improves adherence to drug therapy.
Interruptions contribute to medication errors (Palese et al., 2019; Wang et al., 2021).

Ensures more efficiency when completing the procedure.

IMPLEMENTATION

1. Perform hand hygiene. Prepare medications for instillation into feeding tube (see Skill 21.1). Check medication label against MAR 2 times. Fill graduated container with 50 to 100 mL of tepid water. Use sterile water for immunocompromised or critically ill patients (Boullata, 2017).

These are the first and second checks for accuracy and ensure that correct medication is administered. Preparation process ensures that right patient receives right medication. Tepid water prevents abdominal cramping, which can occur with cold water.

Clinical Judgment *Whenever possible, use liquid medications instead of crushed tablets. If you have to crush tablets, flush the tubing before and after the medication administration to prevent the drug from adhering to the inside of the tube. In addition, make sure that concentrated medications are thoroughly diluted. Never add crushed medications directly to a tube feeding (Boullata, 2021; Lord, 2018; Spilios et al., 2021).*

   a. Tablets: Crush each tablet into a fine powder using pill-crushing device or two medication cups (see Skill 21.1). Dissolve each tablet in separate cup of 30 mL of warm water.
   b. Capsules: Ensure that contents of capsule (granules or gelatin) can be expressed from covering (consult with pharmacist). Perform hand hygiene, apply gloves, and open capsule or pierce gel cap with sterile needle and empty contents into 30 mL of warm water (or solution designated by drug company). Gel caps dissolve in warm water, but this may take 15 to 20 minutes.
   c. Prepare liquid medication according to Skill 21.1.
2. Never add medications directly to a container or bag of tube feeding. Sometimes tube feeding needs to be held. Verify this and the amount of time that you hold a feeding with agency policy.
3. Take medication(s) to patient at correct time (see agency policy). Medications that require exact timing include STAT, first-time or loading doses, and one-time doses. Give time-critical scheduled medications (e.g., antibiotics, anticoagulants, insulin, anticonvulsants, immunosuppressive agents) at exact time ordered (no later than 30 minutes before or after scheduled dose). Give non–time-critical scheduled medications within a range of 1 or 2 hours of scheduled dose (CMS, 2023). During administration, apply seven rights of medication administration. Perform hand hygiene.

Fine powder dissolves more easily, reducing chance of occluding feeding tube.

Ensures that contents of capsules are in solution to prevent occlusion of tube.

Prevents feeding tube occlusion and ensures timely administration of full dose.

Hospitals must adopt medication administration policy and procedure for timing of medication administration that considers nature of the prescribed medication, specific clinical application, and patient needs (CMS, 2023; USDHHS, 2020). Time-critical scheduled medications are those for which early or delayed administration of maintenance doses of greater than 30 minutes before or after the scheduled dose may cause harm or result in substantial suboptimal therapy or pharmacological effect. Non–time-critical medications are those for which early or delayed administration within a specified range of either 1 or 2 hours should not cause harm or result in substantial suboptimal therapy or pharmacological effect (CMS, 2023; USDHHS, 2020).

STEP	RATIONALE
4. Identify patient using at least two identifiers (e.g., name and birthday or name and medical record number) according to agency policy. Compare identifiers with information on patient's MAR or EHR.	Ensures correct patient. Complies with The Joint Commission standards and improves patient safety (TJC, 2023).
5. At patient's bedside, again compare MAR or computer printout with names of medications on medication labels and patient name. Ask patient again about any allergies.	*This is the third check for accuracy* and ensures that patient receives correct medication. Confirms patient's allergy history.
6. Provide privacy. Assist patient to sitting position. Elevate head of bed to minimum of 30 degrees and preferably 45 degrees (unless contraindicated) or sit patient up in a chair (Boullata et al., 2017).	Provides patient privacy. Reduces risk for aspiration, keeping head above stomach.
7. If continuous enteral tube feeding is infusing, adjust infusion pump setting to hold tube feeding.	Feeding solution should not infuse while residuals are checked or medications are administered. The presence of a feeding solution may impede drug absorption (Boullata, 2017; Boulatta, 2021).
8. Perform hand hygiene and apply clean gloves. Auscultate for presence of bowel sounds. Verify placement of feeding tube (see Skill 31.2) by observing gastric contents and checking pH of aspirate contents. Gastric pH less than 5.0 is a good indicator that the tip of the tube is correctly placed in stomach (Boullata et al., 2017; Judd, 2020; Lyman et al., 2020).	Presence of bowel sounds indicates gastric peristalsis. Verification of feeding tube placement ensures proper tube position and reduces risk of introducing fluids into respiratory tract and subsequent aspiration.

Clinical Judgment *Assess for signs of MARSI (e.g., blistering, redness, irritation around the feeding tube site while verifying feeding tube placement or checking for gastric residual volume).*

STEP	RATIONALE
9. Check for gastric residual volume (GRV). Draw up 10 to 30 mL of air into a 60-mL syringe and connect syringe to feeding tube. Flush tube with air and pull back slowly to aspirate gastric contents. Determine GRV using either scale on syringe or a graduate container. Return aspirated contents to stomach unless a single GRV exceeds 500 mL (see agency policy). When GRV is excessive, hold medication and contact health care provider (Boullata et al., 2017). Some agencies prohibit GRV for small bore feeding tubes (see agency policy) (Judd, 2020).	GRV categories have been identified in studies as significant when patients have two or more GRVs exceeding 500 mL (Boullata et al., 2017). Large residuals indicate delayed gastric emptying and put patient at increased risk for vomiting and/or aspiration (Boullata et al., 2017; Burchum & Rosenthal, 2022).
10. Irrigate the tubing.	
a. Pinch or clamp enteral tube and remove syringe. Draw up 30 mL of water into syringe. Reinsert tip of syringe into tube, release clamp, and flush tubing. Clamp tube again and remove syringe.	Pinching or clamping tubing prevents leakage or spillage of stomach contents. Flushing ensures that tube is patent.
b. Using the appropriate enteral connector (see Fig. 21.1), attach to enteral tube.	Standardization of connector tubing improves patient safety. Tubing standards are designed to reduce tubing misconnections that result in patient injury (Boullata et al., 2017; TJC, 2022).

Clinical Judgment *Verify that the enteral connector meets the ISO tubing connector standards (Boullata et al., 2017; IOS, 2020). Do not attach the enteral tubing to a standardized Luer syringe or needleless device (FDA, 2022; IOS, 2020).*

STEP	RATIONALE
11. Attach medication syringe to connector port on the enteral feeding tube. Ensure there is an airtight connection between the syringe and enteral tube and administer medication slowly.	Ensures delivery of medications.
12. *Option:* For a large-bore feeding tube, attach Asepto syringe to ENFit connector. Administer dose liquid or dissolved medication by pouring into syringe. Allow to flow by gravity.	

Clinical Judgment *If medication does not flow freely, raise the height of the syringe to increase the rate of flow or try having the patient change position slightly because the end of the feeding tube may be against the gastric mucosa. If these measures do not improve the flow, a gentle push with the bulb of an Asepto syringe or plunger of the syringe may facilitate the flow of fluid.*

STEP	RATIONALE
a. After giving only one dose of medication, flush tubing with 30 to 60 mL of water after administration.	Maintains patency of enteral tube and ensures that medication passes through tube to stomach (Boullata et al., 2017).

STEP	RATIONALE
b. To administer more than one medication, give each separately and flush between medications with 15 to 30 mL of water.	Allows for accurate identification of medication if dose is spilled. In addition, some medications may be incompatible, and giving medication separately followed by a flush solution decreases the risk for medication incompatibilities (Boullata et al., 2017).
c. Follow last dose of medication with 30 to 60 mL of water.	Maintains patency of enteral tube and ensures passage of medication into stomach (Boullata et al., 2017).
13. Clamp proximal end of feeding tube if tube feeding is not being administered and cap end of tube.	Prevents air from entering stomach between medication doses.
14. When continuous tube feeding is being administered by infusion pump, disconnect infusion pump and administer medication as ordered, followed by at least 15 mL of water, and then immediately reattach infusion pump. When medications are not compatible with feeding solution, hold feeding for an additional 30 to 60 minutes as ordered (Boullata et al., 2017; Burchum & Rosenthal, 2022).	Optimizes enteral medication delivery and allows for adequate absorption of medication and avoids potential drug-food interaction between medication and enteral feeding (Boullata et al., 2017; Boullata, 2021).
15. Remove and dispose of gloves.	Reduces transmission of microorganisms.
16. Help patient to comfortable position and keep head of bed elevated for 1 h (see agency policy).	Reduces risk of aspiration.
17. Raise side rails (as appropriate) and lower bed to lowest position, locking into position.	Ensures patient safety and prevents falls.
18. Place nurse call system in an accessible location within patient's reach.	Ensures patient can call for assistance if needed.
19. Dispose of all contaminated supplies in appropriate receptacle and perform hand hygiene.	Reduces transmission of microorganisms. Use appropriate disposal receptacle if patient on hazardous drugs (ONS, 2018; 2022).

EVALUATION

1. Observe patient for signs of aspiration, such as choking, gurgling, gurgling speech, breath sounds, and difficulty breathing.	Provides for prompt intervention if aspiration has occurred.
2. Return within 30 minutes to evaluate patient's response to medications.	Monitoring patient's response evaluates therapeutic benefit of drug and helps detect onset of side effects or allergic reactions.
3. Use Teach-Back: "I want to be sure I explained clearly why your father must take his medications through his feeding tube. Tell me why he is receiving his medications through his feeding tube." Revise your instruction now or develop a plan for revised patient/family caregiver teaching if patient/family caregiver is not able to teach back correctly.	Teach-back is a technique for health care providers to ensure that they have explained medical information clearly so that patients and their families understand what is communicated to them (AHRQ, 2023).

Unexpected Outcomes	Related Interventions
1. Patient exhibits signs of aspiration, including respiratory distress, changes in vital signs, or changes in oxygen saturation.	• Stop all medications/fluids through feeding tube. • Elevate head of bed and stay with patient. • Assess vital signs and breath sounds while another staff member notifies health care provider.
2. Patient does not receive medication because of blocked enteral tube.	• For newly inserted tube, notify health care provider and obtain x-ray film confirmation of placement. • Requires interventions to unclog tube to ensure drug delivery (Box 21.3).
3. Patient exhibits adverse effects (side effect, toxic effect, allergic reaction).	• Withhold further doses. • Notify health care provider and pharmacy immediately. • Symptoms such as urticaria, rash, pruritus, rhinitis, and wheezing indicate allergic reaction. • Enter patient allergy in EHR.

BOX 21.3

Unclogging a Blocked Feeding Tube

- Prevent tube from becoming blocked by flushing it with at least 15 to 30 mL of tepid water before and after administering each dose of medication, 30 to 60 mL after last dose of medication, before and after checking gastric residual volumes, and every 4 to 12 hours around the clock (refer to agency policies).
- Gently flush tube with large-bore syringe and warm water. Do not use small-bore syringe because this exerts too much pressure and may rupture tube.
- If irrigation with water is not effective, obtain an order for a pancrelipase tablet and follow manufacturer guidelines for tube irrigation. In addition, a declogging stylus may be used (see agency policy).
- The tube may need to be removed and a new one inserted if the medication is urgent.

Modified from Boullata J, et al: ASPEN safe practices for enteral nutrition therapy, *JPEN J Parenter Enteral Nutr* 41(1):15, 2017.

Documentation

- Document method used to check for tube placement, GRV, and pH of aspirate. Document drug, dose, route, and time administered immediately *after* administration, not before.
- Document your evaluation of patient learning.
- Document total amount of water used for medication administration.

Hand-Off Reporting

- Report adverse effects or patient response and withheld drugs to nurse in charge or health care provider.

Special Considerations

Patient Education

- Teach patient or family caregiver how to store medications and tube-feeding supplements (see Chapter 20).
- Demonstrate to family caregiver how to prepare medications, including crushing them if appropriate.
- Demonstrate to patient or family caregiver how to verify correct placement of tube.
- Teach family caregiver the importance of consistent flushing of feeding tube before and after medication administration.

Pediatrics

- Volumes for instillation of medications or for irrigation of enteral tubes should be small enough to clear tubing (Hockenberry et al., 2022).

Older Adults

- Older adults have a slower gastrointestinal absorption, and it is important that gastric residual volumes be assessed before administering medications through a feeding tube (Touhy & Jett, 2022).

Populations With Disabilities

- Plan for extra time for medication administration in patients with cognitive impairments and limited communication skills because of the potential for difficulty understanding the need for and the procedure of administering medications through a feeding tube (Mendes, 2018; Sullivan et al., 2018).

◆ SKILL 21.3 Applying Topical Medications to the Skin

 Video Clip

Topical administration of medication involves applying drugs locally to the skin, mucous membranes, or tissues. Topical drugs such as lotions, patches, pastes, and ointments primarily produce local effects, but they can create systemic effects if absorbed through the skin. Systemic effects are more likely to occur if the skin is thin, drug concentration is high, contact with the skin is prolonged, or the drug is applied to skin that is not intact. In addition, skin hydration and environmental humidity affect percutaneous absorption of a medication. An increase in skin hydration increases absorption. Last, skin encrustations and dead tissue harbor microorganisms and block contact of medications with the affected tissue or membrane.

Never apply new medication over a previously applied medication because it will decrease the therapeutic benefit to a patient. Always clean the skin or wound thoroughly before applying a new dose of a topical medication. Apply each type of medication, whether an ointment, a lotion, a powder, or a patch, according to directions to ensure proper penetration and absorption. Because many locally applied medications such as lotions, pastes, and ointments create systemic and local effects, apply these medications with gloves and applicators.

Delegation

The skill of administering most topical medications, including transdermal skin patches, cannot be delegated to assistive personnel

(AP). However, some agencies (e.g., long-term care) may allow specially trained AP to apply some forms of topical agents. Check agency policies. Direct the AP to:
- Report immediately to the nurse any skin irritation, burning, blistering, or increased itching over site of application.
- Not apply any dressing over the topical medication unless instructed to by the nurse.

Interprofessional Collaboration

- A dermatologist or skin care specialist can assist to determine future medication when a patient develops a new skin condition or an existing condition worsens.

Equipment

- Clean gloves (for intact skin) or sterile gloves (for nonintact skin)
- Cotton-tipped applicators or tongue blades (optional)
- Ordered medication (powder, cream, lotion, ointment, spray, patch)
- Basin of warm water, washcloth, towel, nondrying soap
- Sterile dressing, tape
- Felt-tip pen (optional)
- Medication administration record (MAR) (electronic or printed)
- Plastic wrap, transparent dressing (if ordered) (optional)

STEP	RATIONALE

ASSESSMENT

1. Check accuracy and completeness of each MAR or computer printout with health care provider's written medication order. Check patient's name, medication name and dosage, route of administration, and time of administration. Clarify incomplete or unclear orders with health care provider before administration.

The order sheet is the most reliable source and only legal record of medications that patient is to receive. Ensures that patient receives the correct medications (Palese et al., 2019; Wang et al., 2021). Transcription errors are a source of medication errors (Zhu & Weingart, 2022).

2. Review medication reference information related to medication, including action, purpose, normal dose and route, side effects, time of onset and peak action, and nursing implications.

Allows you to anticipate effects of drug and observe patient's response.

3. Assess patient's medical and medication history and history of allergies (including latex and topical agent). List drug allergies on each page of the MAR and prominently display on the patient's electronic health record (EHR) per agency policy. When patient has allergy, provide allergy bracelet.

Information reflects patient's need for and potential responses to medications. Allergic contact dermatitis is relatively common and can worsen dermatological (skin) condition. In addition, some patients may be allergic to preservatives or fragrances in topical medications. Latex allergy requires use of nonlatex gloves. Communication of allergies is essential for safe and effective care.

4. Review EHR to determine patient's age and history of dehydration, malnutrition, exposure to radiation therapy, underlying chronic conditions (e.g., diabetes mellitus, immunosuppression), and edema of the skin.

Common risk factors for medical adhesive–related skin injury (MARSI) (Fumarola et al., 2020). Adhesive may be present on skin patches.

5. Assess patient's/family caregiver's health literacy.

Determines degree to which individuals have the ability to find, understand, and use information and services to make informed health-related decisions and actions for themselves and others (CDC, 2023).

6. Ask patient to confirm history of allergies: known allergies and allergic response.

Confirms patient's allergies.

7. Perform hand hygiene and assess condition of skin or membrane where medication is to be applied (see Chapter 6). If there is an open wound or drainage, apply clean gloves. First wash site thoroughly with mild, nondrying soap and warm water; rinse; and dry. Be sure to remove any previously applied medication or debris. Also remove any blood, body fluids, secretions, or excretions. Assess for symptoms of skin irritation such as pruritus or burning. Remove gloves when finished. Perform hand hygiene.

Reduces transmission of microorganisms. Cleaning site thoroughly promotes proper assessment of skin surface. Assessment provides baseline to determine change in condition of skin after therapy or any signs of skin irritation or MARSI from any dressing adhesive. Application of certain topical agents can lessen or aggravate these symptoms.

Cleaning removes any residual medication from the previous dose, which reduces potential adverse medication reactions or skin irritation (Burchum & Rosenthal, 2022; Fumarola et al., 2020).

8. Determine amount of topical agent required for application by assessing skin site, reviewing health care provider's order, and reading application directions carefully (a thin, even layer is usually adequate).

An excessive amount of topical agent can irritate skin chemically, negate effectiveness of drug, and/or cause adverse systemic effects such as decreased white blood cell (WBC) counts.

9. Determine if patient or family caregiver is physically able to apply medication by assessing grasp, hand strength, reach, and coordination.

Necessary if patient is to self-administer drug at home.

10. Assess patient's knowledge, prior experience with topical medications, and feelings about the procedure.

Reveals need for patient instruction and/or support.

PLANNING

1. Expected outcomes following completion of procedure:
- Patient can identify drug and describe action, purpose, dose, side effects, and schedule of medication.
- Patient can apply medication without help on prescribed schedule.
- With repeated applications, skin becomes clear, without inflammation or drainage from lesions.

Demonstrates learning.

Demonstrates learning and adherence.

Existing lesions heal and/or disappear as result of therapeutic action of medication.

STEP	RATIONALE
2. Provide privacy and explain procedure to patient. Discuss purpose and side effects of each medication. If applicable, teach patient how to report any side effects. Be specific if patient wishes to self-administer medications. Allow sufficient time for patient to ask questions.	Protects patient's privacy; reduces anxiety. Promotes cooperation. Patient's understanding of each medication improves adherence to drug therapy. Prepares patient to self-administer drug, which increases feelings of independence.
3. Plan preparation to avoid interruption. Create a quiet environment. Do not take phone calls or talk with others. Follow agency "No-Interruption Zone" policy. Keep all pages of MAR or computer printout for one patient together or look at only one patient's electronic MAR at a time.	Interruptions contribute to medication errors (Palese et al., 2019; Wang et al., 2021).
4. Obtain and organize supplies for topical medication administration at bedside	Ensures more efficiency when completing procedure.

IMPLEMENTATION

1. Perform hand hygiene. Prepare medications for application. Check label of medication against MAR 2 times (see Skill 21.1). Preparation usually involves taking bottle or tube of lotion, cream, ointment, or patch out of storage and to patient's room. Check expiration date on container.	Reduces transmission of infection. *These are the first and second checks for accuracy* and ensure that correct medication is administered.
2. Take medication(s) to patient at correct time (see agency policy). Medications that require exact timing include stat, first-time or loading doses, and one-time doses (e.g., nitroglycerin). During administration, apply seven rights of medication administration. Perform hand hygiene.	Hospitals must adopt medication administration policy and procedure for timing of medication administration that considers nature of the prescribed medication, specific clinical application, and patient needs (CMS, 2023; USDHHS, 2020). Time-critical scheduled medications are those for which early or delayed administration of maintenance doses of greater than 30 minutes before or after the scheduled dose may cause harm or result in substantial suboptimal therapy or pharmacological effect. Non–time-critical medications are those for which early or delayed administration within a specified range of either 1 or 2 hours should not cause harm or result in substantial suboptimal therapy or pharmacological effect (CMS, 2023; USDHHS, 2020).
3. Identify patient using at least two identifiers (e.g., name and birthday or name and medical record number) according to agency policy. Compare identifiers with information on patient's MAR or EHR.	Ensures correct patient. Complies with The Joint Commission standards and improves patient safety (TJC, 2023).
4. At patient's bedside, again compare MAR or computer printout with names of medications on medication labels and patient name. Ask patient again about any allergies.	*This is the third check for accuracy* and ensures that patient receives correct medication. Confirms patient's allergy history.
5. Help patient to comfortable position. Organize and arrange supplies at bedside.	Allows easy access to application site.
6. Perform hand hygiene. If patient's skin is broken, apply sterile gloves. Otherwise, apply clean gloves.	Reduces transmission of microorganisms.
7. Apply topical creams, ointments, and oil-based lotions.	
a. Move patient gown to expose affected area while keeping unaffected areas covered.	Provides visualization for application and protects privacy.
b. Wash, rinse, and dry affected area before applying medication if not done earlier (see Assessment, Step 7).	Cleaning removes microorganisms from remaining debris and any surface medication (Burcham & Rosenthal, 2022).
c. If skin is excessively dry and flaking, apply topical agent while skin is still damp.	Increased skin hydration and surface humidity enhance absorption of topical medication (Burcham & Rosenthal, 2022).
d. After washing, remove gloves, perform hand hygiene, and apply new clean or sterile gloves.	Sterile gloves are used when applying agents to open, noninfectious skin lesions. Changing gloves prevents cross-contamination of infected or contagious lesions. Gloves also protect you from topical absorption of the medication and subsequent drug effects.
e. Place required amount of medication in palm of gloved hand and soften by rubbing briskly between hands.	Softening topical agent makes it easier to spread on skin.

STEP	RATIONALE
f. Tell patient that initial application of agent may feel cold. Once medication is softened, spread it evenly over skin surface, using long, even strokes that follow direction of hair growth. Do not vigorously rub skin. Apply to thickness specified by manufacturer instructions.	Ensures even distribution and sufficient dosage of medication. Technique prevents irritation of hair follicles.
g. Explain to patient that skin may feel greasy after application.	Ointments often contain oils.
8. Apply antianginal (nitroglycerin) ointment.	
a. Remove previous dose paper. Fold used paper containing any residual medication with used sides together and dispose of it in biohazard trash container. Wipe off residual medication with tissue.	Prevents overdose that can occur with multiple-dose papers left in place. Proper disposal protects you and others from accidental exposure to medication.
b. Write date, time, and your initials on new application paper.	Label provides reference to prevent missing doses.
c. Antianginal (nitroglycerin) ointments are usually ordered in inches and can be measured on small sheets of paper marked off in 1.25 cm (½-inch) markings. Unit-dose packages are available. Apply desired number of inches of ointment using paper-measuring guide (see illustration).	Ensures correct dose of medication.

Clinical Judgment *Unit-dose packages are available.* **NOTE:** *One package equals 2.5 cm (1 inch); smaller amounts should not be measured from this package.*

d. Select new application site: Apply nitroglycerin to chest area, back, abdomen, or anterior thigh (Burchum & Rosenthal, 2022). Do not apply on nonintact skin or hairy surfaces or over scar tissue.	Application sites are rotated to reduce skin irritation. Application on nonintact skin may result in increased absorption of medication. Application on hairy surfaces or scar tissue may decrease absorption (Burchum & Rosenthal, 2022).
e. Apply ointment to skin surface by holding edge or back of paper-measuring guide and placing ointment and paper directly on skin (see illustration). Do not rub or massage ointment into skin.	Minimizes chance of ointment covering gloves and later touching nurse's hands. Medication is designed to absorb slowly over several hours; massaging increases absorption rate.
f. Secure ointment and paper with transparent dressing or strip of tape. Apply dressing or plastic wrap only when instructed by pharmacy (Burchum & Rosenthal, 2022).	Prevents staining of clothing or inadvertent removal of medication. Covering topical medications with dressing or plastic wrap increases heat and skin humidity and rate of absorption of medication (Goldstein & Goldstein, 2023; Burchum & Rosenthal, 2022)

Clinical Judgment *Medication patches with adhesive borders can cause medical adhesive–related skin injuries (Fumarola et al., 2020). Consider patient's risk for a skin injury (e.g., age, edema, dehydration, malnutrition). Assess for local signs of irritation or damaged skin at application site.*

9. Apply transdermal patches (e.g., analgesic, nicotine, nitroglycerin, estrogen).	
a. If old patch is present, remove it and clean area. Be sure to check between skinfolds for patch.	Failure to remove old patch can result in overdose. Many patches are small, clear, or flesh colored and can be easily hidden between skinfolds. Cleaning removes residual medication traces of previous patch.

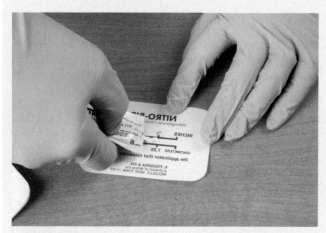

STEP 8c Ointment spread in inches over measuring guide.

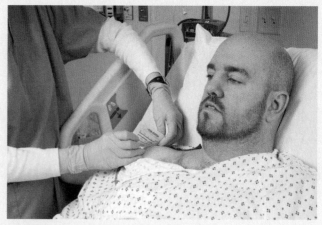

STEP 8e Nurse applies wrapper with medication to patient's skin.

STEP	RATIONALE
b. Dispose of old patch by folding in half with sticky sides together. Some facilities require patch to be cut before disposal (see agency policy). Dispose of it in biohazard trash bag. Remove and dispose of gloves and perform hand hygiene.	Proper disposal prevents accidental exposure to medication. Reduces transmission of microorganisms.
c. Use soft-tip or felt-tip pen to date and initial outer side of new patch before applying it and note time of administration.	Visual reminder prevents missing or extra doses. Ballpoint pen damages patch and alters medication delivery.
d. Choose a new site that is clean, intact, dry, and free of hair. Some patches have specific instructions for placement locations (e.g., Testoderm patches are placed on scrotum; a scopolamine patch is placed behind the ear; *never apply* an estrogen patch to breast tissue or waistline). Do not apply patch on skin that is oily, burned, cut, or irritated in any way.	Ensures complete medication absorption. Estrogen patches should never be placed on the breast, genitals, or other reproductive organs. There is a risk for systemic absorption of the hormone, which can increase patient's risk for breast, testicular, or ovarian cancers (Burchum & Rosenthal, 2022).
e. Apply clean gloves. Carefully remove patch from its protective covering by pulling off liner. Hold patch by edge without touching adhesive edges.	Touching only edges ensures that patch will adhere and that medication dose has not changed. Removing protective covering allows medication to be absorbed through skin.
f. Apply patch. Hold palm of one hand firmly over patch for 10 seconds. Make sure that it sticks well, especially around edges. Apply overlay if provided with patch.	Adequate adhesion prevents loss of patch, which results in decreased dose and effectiveness.

Clinical Judgment *Never apply heat such as with a heating pad over a transdermal patch because this results in an increased rate of absorption with potentially serious adverse effects.*

g. Do not apply patch to previously used sites for at least 1 week.	Rotation of site reduces skin irritation from medication and adhesive (Burchum & Rosenthal, 2022).
h. Instruct patient that transdermal patches are never to be cut in half; a change in dose would require prescription for new strength of transdermal medication.	Cutting transdermal patch in half would alter intended medication delivery of transdermal system, resulting in inadequate or altered drug levels.

Clinical Judgment *It is recommended to have a daily "patch-free" interval of 10 to 12 hours because tolerance develops if patches are used 24 hours a day every day (Burchum & Rosenthal, 2022). Apply a new patch each morning, leave in place for 12 to 14 hours, and remove in the evening.*

i. Instruct patient to always remove old patch and clean skin before applying new one. Patients should not use alternative forms of medication when using patches. For example, patients should not apply nitroglycerin ointment in addition to patch unless specifically ordered to do so by a health care provider.	Use of patch with additional or alternative drug preparation can result in toxicity or other side effects.
10. Administer aerosol sprays (e.g., local anesthetic sprays).	
a. Shake container vigorously. Read container label for distance recommended to hold spray away from area, usually 15 to 30 cm (6–12 inches).	Mixing ensures delivery of fine, even spray. Proper distance ensures that fine spray hits skin surface. Holding container too close results in thin, watery distribution.
b. Ask patient to turn face away from spray or briefly cover face with towel while spraying neck or chest.	Prevents inhalation of spray.
c. Spray medication evenly over affected site (in some cases, time spray for a period of seconds).	Ensures that affected area of skin is covered with thin spray.
11. Apply suspension-based lotion.	
a. Shake container vigorously.	Mixes powder throughout liquid to form well-mixed suspension.
b. Apply small amount of lotion to small gauze dressing or pad and apply to skin by stroking evenly in direction of hair growth.	Method of application leaves protective film of powder on skin after water base of suspension dries. Technique prevents irritation to hair follicles.
c. Explain to patient that area will feel cool and dry.	Water evaporates to leave thin layer of powder.
12. Apply powder.	
a. Be sure that skin surface is thoroughly dry. With your nondominant hand, fully spread apart any skinfolds such as between toes or under axilla and dry with towel.	Minimizes caking and crusting of powder. Fully exposes skin surface for application.
b. If area of application is near face, ask patient to turn face away from powder or briefly cover face with towel.	Prevents inhalation of powder.
c. Dust skin site lightly with dispenser so that area is covered with fine, thin layer of powder. *Option:* Cover skin area with dressing if ordered by health care provider.	Thin layer of powder has slight lubricating properties, which reduces friction and promotes drying (Burchum & Rosenthal, 2022).

STEP	RATIONALE
13. Help patient to comfortable position, reapply gown, and cover with bed linen as desired.	Gives patient a sense of well-being.
14. Raise side rails (as appropriate) and lower bed to lowest position, locking into position.	Ensures patient safety and prevents falls.
15. Place nurse call system in an accessible location within patient's reach.	Ensures patient can call for assistance if needed.
16. Dispose of all contaminated supplies in appropriate receptacle, remove and dispose of gloves, and perform hand hygiene.	Reduces transmission of microorganisms. 

EVALUATION

1. Inspect condition of skin between applications.

   Determines if skin condition is improving or verifies that skin is intact and not irritated.

2. Have patient keep diary of doses taken.

   Confirms adherence to prescribed therapy.

3. Observe patient or family caregiver apply topical medication.

   Return demonstration measures learning.

4. **Use Teach-Back:** "I want to be sure I explained how the medication you are taking works and the side effects of the cream. In your own words, tell me how the drug works, your correct amount, and any side effects." Revise your instruction now or develop a plan for revised patient/family caregiver teaching if patient/family caregiver is not able to teach-back correctly.

   Teach-back is a technique for health care providers to ensure that they have explained medical information clearly so that patients and their families understand what is communicated to them (AHRQ, 2023).

Unexpected Outcomes	Related Interventions
1. Skin site appears inflamed and edematous with blistering and oozing of fluid from lesions. These signs indicate subacute inflammation or eczema that can develop if skin lesions are getting worse.	• Hold medication. • Notify health care provider; alternative therapies may be needed.
2. Patient is unable to explain information about drug or does not administer as prescribed.	• Identify possible reasons for nonadherence and explore alternative approaches or options.

Documentation

• Document drug, dose or strength, site of application, and time administered immediately after administration, not before.

• Document your evaluation of patient learning.

• Describe condition of skin before each topical application of medication.

Hand-Off Reporting

• Report adverse effects or changes in appearance and condition of skin lesions to health care provider.

Special Considerations

Patient Education

• Instruct patient and family caregiver to:

  • Not apply to irritated or damaged skin.

  • Not use heating pads, hot water bottle, or warm compresses over medication.

  • Only use a bandage or plastic wrap if instructed by a pharmacist.

  • Use medication exactly as prescribed.

• Contact health care provider if medication comes in contact with eyes or other mucous membranes such as the mouth.

• Instruct patients to use only warm-water rinse without soap for cleaning inflamed skin.

• If a transdermal patch begins to peel off before the next dose is due, remove it, clean the skin, and apply a new patch to a different area rather than taping over the patch (Burchum & Rosenthal, 2022).

Older Adults

• Changes in the skin of an older-adult patient include increased fragility, wrinkling, dryness, flaking, and increased tendency to bruise. Be aware of these changes when applying topical medications to ensure proper application.

Home Care

• Instruct patient to wrap applicators, used patches, and similar materials and dispose of them into cardboard or plastic disposable containers. Careful disposal is necessary to ensure the safety of patient, other adults, pets, and children.

✦ SKILL 21.4   Administering Ophthalmic Medications

 Video Clip

Common eye (ophthalmic) medications are in the form of drops and ointments, including over-the-counter preparations such as artificial tears and vasoconstrictors. However, many patients receive prescribed ophthalmic drugs for eye conditions such as glaucoma and infection and following cataract extraction. In addition, there is a third type of delivery system, the intraocular disk. Medications delivered by disk resemble a contact lens, but the disk is placed in the conjunctival sac, not on the cornea, and it remains in place for up to 1 week.

The eye is the most sensitive organ to which you apply medications. The cornea is richly supplied with sensitive nerve fibers. Care must be taken to prevent instilling medication directly onto the cornea. The conjunctival sac is much less sensitive and thus a more appropriate site for medication instillation.

Any patient receiving topical eye medications should learn correct self-administration of the medication, especially patients with glaucoma, who must often undergo lifelong medication administration for control of this disease. You can easily instruct patients while administering medications. Family caregivers often administer eye medications when patients are unable to manipulate applicators (e.g., arthritis, neurologic condition), immediately after eye surgery, and when a patient's vision is so impaired that it is difficult to assemble needed supplies and handle applicators correctly.

Delegation

The skill of administering ophthalmic medications cannot be delegated to assistive personnel (AP). Direct the AP about:

- Specific potential side effects of medications and to report their occurrence.
- Potential for temporary burning or blurring of vision after administration of eye medications.

Interprofessional Collaboration

- An ophthalmologist assists if patient's eye condition worsens or different symptoms develop.

Equipment

- Appropriate medication (eyedrops with sterile eyedropper, ointment tube, medicated intraocular disk)
- Clean gloves
- Medication administration record (MAR) (electronic or printed)
- Eyedrops/ointment
- Cotton ball or tissue
- Wash basin filled with warm water and washcloth
- Eye patch and tape (optional)

STEP	RATIONALE

ASSESSMENT

1. Check accuracy and completeness of each MAR or computer printout with health care provider's written medication order. Check patient's name, medication name and dosage, route of administration, and time of administration. Clarify incomplete or unclear orders with health care provider before administration.

   The order sheet is the most reliable source and only legal record of medications that patient is to receive. Ensures that patient receives the correct medications (Palese et al., 2019; Wang et al., 2021). Transcription errors are a source of medication errors (Zhu & Weingart, 2022).

2. Review medication reference information about medication, including action, purpose, normal dose and route, side effects, time of onset and peak action, and nursing implications.

   Allows you to anticipate effects of drug and observe patient's response.

3. Assess patient's medical and medication history and history of allergies (including latex). List drug allergies on each page of the MAR and prominently display on the patient's electronic health record (EHR) per agency policy. When patient has allergy, provide allergy bracelet.

   Factors influence how certain drugs act. Reveals patient's need for and likely response to medication. Communication of allergies is essential for safe and effective care.

4. Assess patient's/family caregiver's health literacy.

   Determines degree to which individuals have the ability to find, understand, and use information and services to make informed health-related decisions and actions for themselves and others (CDC, 2023).

5. Ask patient to confirm history of allergies: known allergies and allergic response.

   Confirms patient's allergies.

6. Perform hand hygiene and apply clean gloves (if drainage is present). Assess condition of external eye structures (see Chapter 6). This may also be done just before drug instillation.

   Provides baseline to determine if local response to medications occurs. Also indicates need to clean eye before drug application.

7. Determine whether patient has any symptoms of eye discomfort or visual impairment (e.g., blurred vision, burning, itching).

   Certain eye medications act to either lessen or increase these symptoms.

8. Assess patient's level of consciousness (LOC) and ability to follow directions.

   If patient becomes restless or combative during procedure, there is greater risk for patient to move head and cause accidental eye injury.

9. Assess patient's and family caregiver's ability to manipulate and hold dropper or ocular disk.

   Reflects patient's ability to learn to self-administer drug.

STEP	RATIONALE
10. Assess patient's and family caregiver's knowledge, prior experience with eye medications, and feelings about procedure.	Reveals need for patient instruction and/or support.

PLANNING

1. Expected outcomes following completion of procedure:	
• Patient experiences desired effect of medication.	Drug is administered correctly without injury to patient.
• Patient denies eye discomfort.	Drug is administered correctly without injury to patient.
• Patient experiences no side effects, and symptoms (e.g., irritation) are relieved.	Drug is distributed and absorbed properly.
• Patient is able to discuss information about medication and technique correctly.	Demonstrates learning.
• Patient demonstrates self-instillation of eyedrops.	Demonstrates learning.
2. Provide privacy and explain the purpose of each medication, action, indication, and possible adverse effects. Allow sufficient time for patient to ask any questions. Patients who self-instill medications may be allowed to give drops under your supervision (check agency policy).	Protects patient's privacy; reduces anxiety. Promotes cooperation. Patient's understanding of each medication improves adherence to drug therapy. Prepares patient to self-administer drug, which increases feelings of independence.
3. Plan preparation to avoid interruption. Create a quiet environment. Do not take phone calls or talk with others. Follow agency "No-Interruption Zone" policy. Keep all pages of MAR or computer printout for one patient together or look at only one patient's electronic MAR at a time.	Interruptions contribute to medication errors (Palese et al., 2019; Wang et al., 2021).
4. Obtain and organize equipment for ophthalmic medication administration at bedside.	Ensures more efficiency when completing procedure.
5. Preparation usually involves taking eyedrops out of refrigerator and rewarming to room temperature before administering to patient. Check expiration date on container.	Eye medications should be room temperature, unless specifically directed otherwise.

Clinical Judgment *Prepare patients who are receiving eyedrops that dilate pupils (mydriatics) that vision will be blurred temporarily and the eyes will be sensitive to light.*

IMPLEMENTATION

1. Perform hand hygiene. Prepare medications for one patient at a time using aseptic technique and avoiding distractions (see Skill 21.1). Check label of medication against MAR two times, when removing medication from unit dose or AMDS and before leaving preparation area (see Skill 21.1).	Ensures that medication is sterile. *These are the first and second checks for accuracy* and ensure that correct medication is administered.

Clinical Judgment *Verify that medication preparations are at room temperature.*

2. Take medication(s) to patient at correct time (see agency policy). Medications that require exact timing include STAT, first-time or loading doses, and one-time doses. Give time-critical scheduled medications (e.g., antibiotics) at exact time ordered (no later than 30 minutes before or after scheduled dose). Give non–time-critical scheduled medications within a range of 1 or 2 hours of scheduled dose (CMS, 2023). During administration, apply seven rights of medication administration. Perform hand hygiene.	Hospitals must adopt medication administration policy and procedure for timing of medication administration that considers nature of the prescribed medication, specific clinical application, and patient needs (CMS, 2023; USDHHS, 2020). Time-critical scheduled medications are those for which early or delayed administration of maintenance doses of greater than 30 minutes before or after the scheduled dose may cause harm or result in substantial suboptimal therapy or pharmacological effect. Non–time-critical medications are those for which early or delayed administration within a specified range of either 1 or 2 hours should not cause harm or result in substantial suboptimal therapy or pharmacological effect (CMS, 2023; USDHHS, 2020).
3. Identify patient using at least two identifiers (e.g., name and birthday or name and medical record number) according to agency policy. Compare identifiers with information on patient's MAR or EHR.	Ensures correct patient. Complies with The Joint Commission standards and improves patient safety (TJC, 2023).
4. At patient's bedside, again compare MAR or computer printout with names of medications on medication labels and patient name. Ask patient about any allergies.	*This is the third check for accuracy* and ensures that patient receives correct medication. Confirms patient's allergy history.
5. Provide privacy and help patient to comfortable sitting position. Arrange supplies at bedside.	Provides patient privacy. Ensures an organized procedure.

STEP	RATIONALE

Clinical Judgment *Reinforce to patients receiving eyedrops (mydriatics) that vision will be blurred temporarily and sensitivity to light may occur. Patient should not drive or operate machinery or perform any activity that requires clear vision until vision and sensitivity to light return to normal.*

6. Administer eye medications.

   a. Perform hand hygiene and apply clean gloves. Ask patient to lie supine or sit back in chair with head slightly hyperextended, looking up.

Position provides easy access to eye for medication instillation and minimizes drainage of medication into tear duct.

Clinical Judgment *Do not hyperextend the neck of a patient with cervical spine injury.*

   b. If drainage or crusting is present along eyelid margins or inner canthus, gently wash away. Soak any dried crusts with warm, damp washcloth or cotton ball over eye for several minutes. Always wipe clean from inner to outer canthus (see illustration). Remove and dispose of gloves and perform hand hygiene.

Soaking allows easy removal of crusts without applying pressure to eye. Cleaning from inner to outer canthus avoids entrance of microorganisms into lacrimal duct (Burchum & Rosenthal, 2022). Reduces transmission of microorganisms.

   c. Explain that there might be temporary burning sensation from drops.

Corneas are highly sensitive.

   d. Instill eyedrops.

     (1) Apply clean gloves. Hold clean cotton ball or tissue in nondominant hand on patient's cheekbone just below lower eyelid.

Prevents transmission of microorganisms.
Cotton or tissue absorbs medication that escapes eye.

     (2) With tissue or cotton ball resting below lower lid, gently press downward with thumb or forefinger against bony orbit, exposing conjunctival sac. Never press directly against patient's eyeball.

Prevents pressure and trauma to eyeball and prevents fingers from touching eye.

     (3) Ask patient to look at ceiling. Rest dominant hand on patient's forehead; hold filled medication eyedropper approximately 1 to 2 cm (¼–½ inch) above conjunctival sac.

Action moves cornea up and away from conjunctival sac and reduces blink reflex. Prevents accidental contact of eyedropper with eye and reduces risk of injury and transfer of microorganisms to dropper (ophthalmic medications are sterile).

     (4) Drop prescribed number of drops into lower conjunctival sac (see illustration).

Conjunctival sac normally holds 1 or 2 drops. Provides even distribution of medication across eye.

     (5) If patient blinks or closes eye, causing drops to land on outer lid margins, repeat procedure.

Therapeutic effect of drug is obtained only when drops enter conjunctival sac.

     (6) When administering drops that may cause systemic effects, apply gentle pressure to patient's nasolacrimal duct with clean tissue for 30 to 60 seconds over each eye, one at a time (see illustration). Avoid pressure directly against patient's eyeball.

Prevents overflow of medication into nasal and pharyngeal passages. Prevents absorption into systemic circulation (Burchum & Rosenthal, 2022).

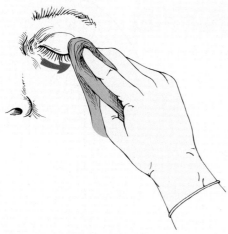

STEP 6b Clean eye, washing from inner to outer canthus before administering drops or ointment.

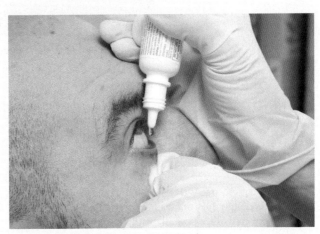

STEP 6d(4) Hold eyedropper over lower conjunctival sac.

STEP	RATIONALE

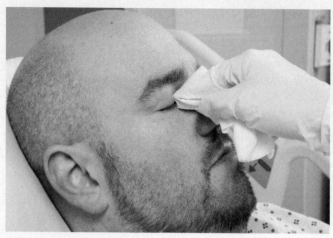

STEP 6d(6) Apply gentle pressure against nasolacrimal duct after giving eye medications.

STEP	RATIONALE
(7) After instilling drops, ask patient to close eyes gently.	Helps distribute medication. Squinting or squeezing eyelids forces medication from conjunctival sac (Burchum & Rosenthal, 2022).
e. Instill ophthalmic ointment.	
(1) Apply clean gloves. Holding applicator above lower lid margin, apply thin ribbon of ointment evenly along inner edge of lower eyelid on conjunctiva (see illustration) from inner to outer canthus.	Reduces transmission of microorganisms. Distributes medication evenly across eye and lid margin.

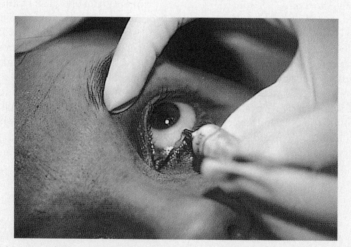

STEP 6e(1) Nurse applies ointment along inner edge of lower eyelid from inner to outer canthus.

STEP	RATIONALE
(2) Have patient close eye and rub lid lightly in circular motion with cotton ball if not contraindicated. Avoid placing pressure directly against patient's eyeball.	Further distributes medication without traumatizing eye.
(3) If excess medication is on eyelid, gently wipe it from inner to outer canthus.	Promotes comfort and prevents trauma to eye.
(4) If patient needs an eye patch, apply clean one by placing it over affected eye so that entire eye is covered. Tape securely without applying pressure to eye.	Clean eye patch reduces risk of infection.

STEP	RATIONALE

f. Insert intraocular disk.

(1) Apply clean gloves. Open package containing disk. Gently press your fingertip against disk so that it adheres to your finger. It may be necessary to moisten gloved finger with sterile saline. Position convex side of disk on your fingertip.

Allows you to inspect disk for damage or deformity.

(2) With your other hand, gently pull patient's lower eyelid away from eye. Ask patient to look up.

Prepares conjunctival sac for receiving medicated disk and moves sensitive cornea away.

(3) Place disk in conjunctival sac so that it floats on sclera between iris and lower eyelid (see illustration).

Ensures delivery of medication.

(4) Pull patient's lower eyelid out and over disk (see illustration). You should not be able to see disk at this time. Repeat if you can see disk.

Ensures accurate medication delivery.

7. After administering eye medications, remove and dispose of gloves and soiled supplies; perform hand hygiene.

Reduces spread of microorganisms. Use appropriate disposal receptacle if patient is on hazardous drugs (ONS, 2018, 2022).

8. Remove intraocular disk.

a. Perform hand hygiene and apply clean gloves. Gently pull downward on lower eyelid using your nondominant hand.

Exposes disk.

b. Using forefinger and thumb of your dominant hand, pinch disk and lift it out of patient's eye (see illustration).

c. Remove and dispose of gloves and perform hand hygiene.

Reduces transmission of microorganisms. Use appropriate disposal receptacle if patient is on hazardous drugs (ONS, 2018, 2022).

9. Help patient to comfortable position.

Gives patient a sense of well-being.

10. Raise side rails (as appropriate) and lower bed to lowest position, locking into position.

Ensures patient safety and prevents falls.

11. Place nurse call system in an accessible location within patient's reach.

Ensures patient can call for assistance if needed.

12. Perform hand hygiene.

Reduces transmission of microorganisms.

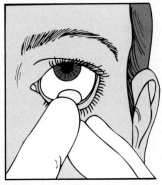

STEP 6f(3) Place intraocular disk in conjunctival sac between iris and lower eyelid.

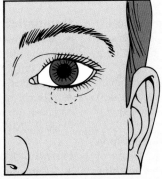

STEP 6f(4) Gently pull patient's lower eyelid over disk.

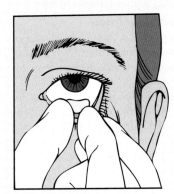

STEP 8b Carefully pinch disk to remove it from patient's eye.

STEP	RATIONALE

EVALUATION

1. Observe response to medication by assessing visual changes, asking if symptoms are relieved, and noting any side effects or discomfort felt.

Evaluates effects of medication.

2. Ask patient to discuss purpose of drug, action, side effects, and technique of administration.

Determines patient's level of understanding.

3. **Use Teach-Back:** "I want to be sure I showed you how to insert the intraocular disk. Show me how to insert it into your left eye." Revise your instruction now or develop a plan for revised patient/family caregiver teaching if patient/family caregiver is not able to teach back correctly.

Teach-back is a technique for health care providers to ensure that they have explained medical information clearly so that patients and their families understand what is communicated to them (AHRQ, 2023).

Unexpected Outcomes

Related Interventions

1. Patient complains of burning or pain or experiences local side effects (e.g., headache, bloodshot eyes, local eye irritation). Drug concentration and patient's sensitivity both influence chances of side effects developing. Eyedrops may have been instilled onto cornea, or dropper touched surface of eye.

- Dim room lights to reduce glare and associated discomfort.
- Notify health care provider for possible adjustment in medication type and dosage.

2. Patient experiences systemic effects from drops (e.g., increased heart rate and blood pressure from epinephrine, decreased heart rate and blood pressure from timolol).

- Notify health care provider immediately.
- Remain with patient. Assess vital signs.
- Withhold further doses.

3. Patient or family caregiver is unable to explain drug information or steps for taking eyedrops and/or has trouble manipulating dropper.

- Repeat instructions and include family caregiver as appropriate. Include return demonstration.

Documentation

- Document drug, concentration, dose or strength, number of drops, site of application (left, right, or both eyes), and time of administration immediately after administration, not before. Include initials or signature.
- Document your evaluation of patient learning.
- Document objective data related to tissues involved (e.g., redness, drainage, irritation), any subjective data (e.g., pain, itching, altered vision), and patient's response to medications. Note evidence of any side effects.

Hand-Off Reporting

- Report adverse effects/patient response and/or withheld drugs to nurse in charge or health care provider. Depending on medication, immediate health care provider notification may be required.

Special Considerations

Patient Education

- Warn patients that mydriatics (agent used to dilate the pupils) temporarily blur vision. Wearing sunglasses reduces photophobia. If necessary, make arrangements for someone to drive patient home from an office or clinic visit.
- Patients who receive medications that paralyze the ciliary muscles of the eye (e.g., scopolamine, atropine, cycloplegics) should not drive or attempt to perform any activity that requires acute vision after receiving medication.
- Instruct patient or family caregiver to avoid instilling any form of eye medications directly onto the cornea. The cornea of the eye has many pain fibers and thus is sensitive to anything applied to it.
- Instruct patient or family caregiver to avoid touching the eyelids or other eye structures with eyedroppers or ointment tubes.

The risk of transmitting infection from one eye to the other is high.
- Use eye medication only for the patient's affected eye.

Pediatrics

- Infants often clench the eyes tightly to avoid eyedrops. Place the drops at the nasal corner where the lids meet with the infant supine. When the infant opens the eye, the medication will flow into it.
- If the eye ointment is to be given once a day, administer at bedtime because it will blur the child's vision (Hockenberry et al., 2022).

Older Adults

- Evaluate patient's and/or family caregiver's ability to perform all the necessary steps for the administration of eyedrops and ointments.

Populations With Disabilities

- When instilling eye medications in the eyes of a patient with severe visual impairment or who is blind, tell the patient when the drops are going to be administered. This can assist the patient in controlling the blink reflex.
- Always inform a cognitively impaired patient about the instillation of an eye medication before administration (Yevchak et al., 2017).

Home Care

- When using over-the-counter (OTC) eyedrops, patients should not share medications with other family caregivers. Risk for infection transmission is high. In addition, instruct patients to follow manufacturer instructions carefully for dosing.

✦ SKILL 21.5 Administering Ear Medications

 Video Clip

Ear (otic) medications are usually in a solution and instilled by drops. When administering ear medications, be aware of certain safety precautions. Internal ear structures are sensitive to temperature extremes; administer eardrops at room temperature. Instilling cold drops can cause vertigo (severe dizziness) or nausea and debilitate a patient for several minutes. Although structures of the outer ear are not sterile, use sterile drops and solutions in case the eardrum is ruptured. The entrance of nonsterile solutions into middle ear structures often results in infection. A final safety precaution is to avoid forcing any solution into the ear. Do not occlude the ear canal with a medicine dropper because this can cause pressure within the canal during instillation and subsequent injury to the eardrum. If you follow these precautions, instillation of eardrops is a safe and effective therapy.

Equipment
- Medication administration record (MAR) (electronic or printed)
- Medication bottle with dropper
- Cotton-tipped applicator, cotton balls
- Clean gloves if drainage is present

Delegation
The skill of administering ear medications cannot be delegated to assistive personnel (AP). Direct the AP about:
- Potential side effects of medications and to report their occurrence.
- The potential for dizziness or irritation after administration of ear medications.

Interprofessional Collaboration
- An ear-nose-throat specialist can remove impacted ear wax before administering ear drops.

STEP	RATIONALE

ASSESSMENT

1. Check accuracy and completeness of each MAR or computer printout with health care provider's written medication order. Check patient's name, medication name and dosage, route of administration, and time of administration. Clarify incomplete or unclear orders with health care provider before administration.	The order sheet is the most reliable source and only legal record of medications that patient is to receive. Ensures that patient receives the correct medications (Palese et al., 2019; Wang et al., 2021). Transcription errors are a source of medication errors (Zhu & Weingart, 2022).
2. Review medication reference for pertinent information related to medication, including action, purpose, normal dose and route, side effects, time of onset and peak action, indication, and nursing implications.	Knowledge of expected and adverse reactions to ear medication helps you determine which symptoms to monitor (and how frequently) and when to reassess patient.
3. Assess patient's medical and medication history and history of allergies (including latex). List drug allergies on each page of the MAR and prominently display on the patient's electronic health record (EHR) per agency policy. When patient has allergy, provide allergy bracelet.	Factors influence how certain drugs act. Reveals patient's need for and likely response to medication. Communication of allergies is essential for safe and effective care.
4. Assess patient's/family caregiver's health literacy.	Determines degree to which individuals have the ability to find, understand, and use information and services to make informed health-related decisions and actions for themselves and others (CDC, 2023).
5. Ask patient to confirm history of allergies: known allergies and allergic response.	Confirms patient's allergies.
6. Perform hand hygiene and assess condition of external ear structures (see Chapter 6). This may be done just before drug instillation (if drainage is present, apply clean gloves).	Provides baseline to determine if local response to medications occurs. Also indicates need to clean ear before drug application.
7. Determine whether patient has any symptoms of ear discomfort or hearing impairment.	Certain ear medications act to either lessen or increase these symptoms. Occlusion of external ear canal by swelling, drainage, or cerumen can impair hearing acuity and cause pain.
8. Assess patient's level of consciousness (LOC) and ability to follow directions. Perform hand hygiene.	If patient becomes restless or combative during procedure, greater risk for accidental ear injury exists.
9. Assess patient's or family caregiver's ability to manipulate and hold ear dropper.	Reflects patient's ability to learn to self-administer drug.
10. Assess patient's knowledge, prior experience with ear medications, desire to self-administer medication, and feelings about procedure.	Reveals need for patient instruction and/or support. Motivation influences teaching approach.

STEP	RATIONALE

PLANNING

1. Expected outcomes following completion of procedure:
   - Patient experiences desired effect of medication. (e.g., reduced irritation, less dizziness).
   - Patient denies discomfort.
   - Patient experiences no side effects.
   - Patient is able to discuss information about medication and technique correctly.
   - Patient demonstrates self-instillation of eardrops.
2. Provide privacy and explain purpose of each medication, action, indication, and possible adverse effects. Allow sufficient time for patient to ask any questions. Patients who self-instill medications may be allowed to give ear medications under nurse's supervision (check agency policy).
3. Plan preparation to avoid interruption. Create a quiet environment. Do not take phone calls or talk with others. Follow agency "No-Interruption Zone" policy. Keep all pages of MAR or computer printout for one patient together or look at only one patient's electronic MAR at a time.
4. Obtain and organize equipment for eardrop installation at bedside.
5. Preparation usually involves taking eardrops out of refrigerator and rewarming to room temperature before administering to patient. Check expiration date on container.

Drug is administered correctly without injury to patient.

Drug is administered correctly without injury to patient.
Drug is distributed and absorbed properly.
Demonstrates learning.

Demonstrates learning.
Protects patient's privacy; reduces anxiety. Promotes cooperation. Patient's understanding of each medication improves adherence to drug therapy. Prepares patient to self-administer drug, which increases feelings of independence.

Interruptions contribute to medication errors (Palese et al., 2019; Wang et al., 2021).

Ensures more efficiency when completing the procedure.
Ear structures are sensitive to temperature extremes. Cold may cause vertigo and nausea. Warming eardrops reduces risks for vertigo and nausea.

IMPLEMENTATION

1. Perform hand hygiene. Prepare medications for one patient at a time using aseptic technique and avoiding distractions (see Skill 21.1). Check label of medication carefully with MAR or computer printout 2 times (see Skill 21.1) when preparing medication.

2. Take medication(s) to patient at correct time (see agency policy). Medications that require exact timing include STAT, first-time or loading doses, and one-time doses. Give time-critical scheduled medications (e.g., antibiotics) at exact time ordered (no later than 30 minutes before or after scheduled dose). Give non–time-critical scheduled medications within a range of 1 or 2 hours of scheduled dose (CMS, 2023). During administration, apply seven rights of medication administration. Perform hand hygiene.

3. Identify patient using at least two identifiers (e.g., name and birthday or name and medical record number) according to agency policy. Compare identifiers with information on patient's MAR or EHR.

4. At patient's bedside, again compare MAR or computer printout with names of medications on medication labels and patient name. Ask patient again about any allergies.

5. Perform hand hygiene. Position patient on side (if not contraindicated) with ear to be treated facing up, or patient may sit in chair or at bedside. Stabilize patient's head with their own hand. *Option:* Apply clean gloves if ear drainage present.

6. Straighten ear canal by pulling pinna up and back to 10 o'clock position (adult or child older than age 3) (see illustration) or down and back to 6 to 9 o'clock position (child younger than age 3).

7. If cerumen or drainage occludes outermost part of ear canal, wipe out gently with cotton-tipped applicator (see illustration). Take care not to force cerumen into canal.

Ensures that medication is sterile.
These are the first and second checks for accuracy and ensure that correct medication is administered.

Hospitals must adopt medication administration policy and procedure for timing of medication administration that considers nature of the prescribed medication, specific clinical application, and patient needs (USDHHS, 2020; CMS, 2023). Time-critical scheduled medications are those for which early or delayed administration of maintenance doses of greater than 30 minutes before or after the scheduled dose may cause harm or result in substantial suboptimal therapy or pharmacological effect. Non–time-critical medications are those for which early or delayed administration within a specified range of either 1 or 2 hours should not cause harm or result in substantial suboptimal therapy or pharmacological effect (CMS, 2023; USDHHS, 2020).

Ensures correct patient. Complies with The Joint Commission standards and improves patient safety (TJC, 2023).

This is the third check for accuracy and ensures that patient receives correct medication. Confirms patient's allergy history.
Facilitates distribution of medication into ear.

Straightening ear canal provides direct access to deeper ear structures. Anatomical differences in younger children and infants necessitate different methods of positioning canal (Hockenberry et al., 2022).

Cerumen and drainage harbor microorganisms and can block distribution of medication into canal. Occlusion blocks sound transmission.

STEP	RATIONALE

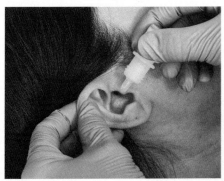
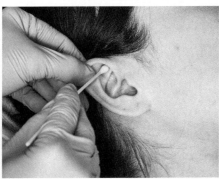
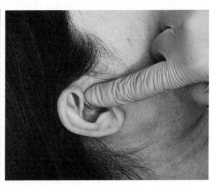

STEP 6 Pull pinna up and back for adults and children older than 3 years.

STEP 7 Always clean only outer canal. Do not push cerumen or secretions into ear.

STEP 9 Nurse applies gentle pressure to tragus of ear after instilling drops.

8. Instill prescribed drops holding dropper 1 cm (½ inch) above ear canal.

Avoiding contact with external ear canal prevents contamination of dropper, which could contaminate medication in container.

9. Ask patient to remain in side-lying position for a few minutes. Apply gentle massage or pressure to tragus of ear with finger (see illustration).

Allows complete distribution of medication. Pressure and massage move medication inward.

10. If ordered, gently insert part of cotton ball into outermost part of canal. Do not press cotton into canal.

Prevents escape of medication when patient sits or stands.

11. Remove cotton after 15 minutes. Help patient to comfortable position after drops are absorbed.

Allows time for drug distribution and absorption.

12. Raise side rails (as appropriate) and lower bed to lowest position, locking into position.

Ensures patient safety and prevents falls.

13. Place nurse call system in an accessible location within patient's reach.

Ensures patient can call for assistance if needed.

14. Dispose of all contaminated supplies in appropriate receptacle, remove and dispose of gloves, and perform hand hygiene.

Reduces transmission of microorganisms.

EVALUATION

1. Observe response to medication by assessing hearing changes, asking if symptoms are relieved, and noting any side effects or discomfort felt.

Evaluates effects of medication.

2. Ask patient to discuss purpose of drug, action, side effects, and technique of administration.

Determines patient's level of understanding.

3. **Use Teach-Back:** "I want to be sure I clearly showed you how to administer eardrops. Let's take this time we have to show me how to place eardrops in your right ear." Revise your instruction now or develop a plan for revised patient/family caregiver teaching if patient/family caregiver is not able to teach back correctly.

Teach-back is a technique for health care providers to ensure that they have explained medical information clearly so that patients and their families understand what is communicated to them (AHRQ, 2023).

STEP	RATIONALE

Unexpected Outcomes

1. Ear canal remains inflamed, swollen, tender to palpation. Drainage is present.

2. Patient's hearing acuity does not improve.

Related Interventions

- Hold next dose.
- Notify health care provider for possible adjustment in medication type and dosage.
- Notify health care provider.
- Cerumen may be impacted, requiring ear irrigation.

Documentation

- Document drug, concentration, dose or strength, number of drops, site of application (left, right, or both ears), and time of administration immediately after administration, not before. Include initials or signature.
- Document objective data related to tissues involved (e.g., drainage, tenderness, irritation), any subjective data (e.g., ear pain, ringing in ears, change in hearing acuity), and patient's response to medications. Note any side effects experienced.
- Document your evaluation of patient learning.

Hand-Off Reporting

- Report adverse effects/patient response and/or withheld drugs to nurse in charge or health care provider. Depending on

medication, immediate health care provider notification may be required.

Special Considerations
Pediatrics

- Insert cotton pledgets loosely into ear canal to prevent medication from flowing out. To prevent cotton from absorbing medication, premoisten it with a few drops of medication (Hockenberry et al., 2022).

Populations With Disabilities

- Always inform a cognitively impaired patient about the instillation of an ear medication before administration (Yevchak et al., 2017).

✦ SKILL 21.6   Administering Nasal Instillations

Patients with nasal sinus problems may receive drugs by spray, drops, or tampons. The most commonly administered form of nasal instillation is a decongestant spray or drops used to relieve sinus congestion and cold symptoms. Many over-the-counter (OTC) nasal preparations contain sympathomimetic drugs (e.g., Neo-Synephrine). These drugs are relatively safe when administered nasally because only small doses are needed. However, the drugs can enter the systemic circulation via the nasal mucosa or gastrointestinal tract if an excess amount is swallowed, causing restlessness, nervousness, tremors, or insomnia in some patients. Long-term use of decongestant nasal spray can actually worsen nasal congestion because of a rebound effect. Nasal sprays are easy for a patient to self-administer. Health care providers treat severe nosebleeds by placing nasal packing or tampons, which are treated with epinephrine to slow bleeding.

Delegation

The skill of administering nasal instillations cannot be delegated to assistive personnel (AP). Direct the AP about:
- Potential side effects of medications and to report their occurrence to the nurse.
- Reporting any bloody nasal drainage to the nurse.

Interprofessional Collaboration

- An ENT specialist can order new medications or interventions when nasal congestion is not resolved or worsens.

Equipment

- Prepared medication with clean dropper or spray container
- Facial tissue
- Small pillow (optional)
- Washcloth (optional)
- Clean gloves
- Medication administration record (MAR) (electronic or printed)

STEP	RATIONALE

ASSESSMENT

1. Check accuracy and completeness of each MAR or computer printout with health care provider's written medication order. Check patient's name, medication name and dosage, route of administration, and time of administration. Clarify incomplete or unclear orders with health care provider before administration.

2. Review medication reference information for medication action, purpose, normal dose, side effects, time and peak of onset, how slowly to give medication, and nursing implications.

The order sheet is the most reliable source and only legal record of medications that patient is to receive. Ensures that patient receives the correct medications (Palese et al., 2019; Wang et al., 2021). Transcription errors are a source of medication errors (Zhu & Weingart, 2022).

Allows you to administer medication safely and monitor patient's response to therapy.

STEP	RATIONALE
3. Assess patient's medical history (e.g., hypertension, heart disease, diabetes, hyperthyroidism), medication history, and history of allergies. List drug allergies on each page of the MAR and prominently display on the patient's electronic health record (EHR) per agency policy. When patient has allergy, provide allergy bracelet.	These conditions contraindicate use of decongestants that stimulate central nervous system. Communication of allergies is essential for safe and effective care.
4. Assess patient's/family caregiver's health literacy.	Determines degree to which individuals have the ability to find, understand, and use information and services to make informed health-related decisions and actions for themselves and others (CDC, 2023).
5. Ask patient to confirm history of allergies: known allergies and allergic response.	Confirms patient's allergies.
6. Perform hand hygiene. When drainage is present, apply clean gloves. Use penlight and inspect condition of nose and sinuses (see Chapter 6). Palpate sinuses for pain or tenderness. Note type of drainage if present. Remove gloves and perform hand hygiene.	Provides baseline to monitor effects of medication. Presence of discharge interferes with drug absorption. Clear nasal discharge indicates sinus problem. Yellow or greenish discharge indicates infection. Reduces transmission of microorganisms.
7. Assess patient's knowledge, prior experience regarding use of nasal instillations, technique for instillation, willingness to learn self-administration, and feelings about procedure.	Reveals need for patient instruction and/or support.

PLANNING

1. Expected outcomes following completion of procedure: • Patient is able to breathe without difficulty through nose. • Patient's nasal sinuses are clear, moist, pink, and without drainage after repeated instillations (applies to anti-infective medications). • Patient is able to explain purpose of medication and administers nasal instillations correctly.	Nasal congestion has been relieved. Inflammation of mucosa has been relieved. Feedback reflects patient's learning.
2. Provide privacy and explain procedure to patient. Discuss purpose and side effects of each medication. If applicable, teach patient how to report any side effects. Be specific if patient wishes to self-administer medications. Allow sufficient time for patient to ask questions.	Protects patient's privacy; reduces anxiety. Promotes cooperation. Patient's understanding of each medication improves adherence to drug therapy. Prepares patient to self-administer drug, which increases feelings of independence.
3. Plan preparation to avoid interruption. Create a quiet environment. Do not take phone calls or talk with others. Follow agency "No-Interruption Zone" policy. Keep all pages of MAR or computer printout for one patient together or look at only one patient's electronic MAR at a time.	Interruptions contribute to medication errors (Palese et al., 2019; Wang et al., 2021).
4. Obtain and organize equipment for nasal instillation of medication at bedside.	Ensures more efficiency when completing procedure.
5. Preparation usually involves taking nasal spray out of storage and to patient's room. Check expiration date on container.	Allows for sufficient time for ear medications to attain room temperature.

IMPLEMENTATION

1. Perform hand hygiene. Prepare medications for one patient at a time using aseptic technique and avoiding distractions (see Skill 21.1). Check label of medication carefully with MAR or computer printout two times (see Skill 21.1).	Ensures that medication is sterile. *These are the first and second checks for accuracy* and ensure that correct medication is administered.
2. Take medication(s) to patient at correct time (see agency policy). Medications that require exact timing include STAT, first-time or loading doses, and one-time doses. Give time-critical scheduled medications (e.g., antibiotics) at exact time ordered (no later than 30 minutes before or after scheduled dose). Give non–time-critical scheduled medications within a range of 1 or 2 hours of scheduled dose (CMS, 2023). During administration, apply seven rights of medication administration. Perform hand hygiene.	Hospitals must adopt medication administration policy and procedure for timing of medication administration that considers nature of the prescribed medication, specific clinical application, and patient needs (CMS, 2023; USDHHS, 2020). Time-critical scheduled medications are those for which early or delayed administration of maintenance doses of greater than 30 minutes before or after the scheduled dose may cause harm or result in substantial suboptimal therapy or pharmacological effect. Non–time-critical medications are those for which early or delayed administration within a specified range of either 1 or 2 hours should not cause harm or result in substantial suboptimal therapy or pharmacological effect (CMS, 2023; USDHHS, 2020).

STEP	RATIONALE
3. Identify patient using at least two identifiers (e.g., name and birthday or name and medical record number) according to agency policy. Compare identifiers with information on patient's MAR or EHR.	Ensures correct patient. Complies with The Joint Commission standards and improves patient safety (TJC, 2023).
4. At patient's bedside, again compare MAR or computer printout with names of medications on medication labels and patient name. Ask patient again about any allergies.	*This is the third check for accuracy* and ensures that patient receives correct medication. Confirms patient's allergy history.
5. Help patient to comfortable position.	Allows easy access to application site.
6. Perform hand hygiene. Arrange supplies and medications at bedside. Apply clean gloves (if drainage is present).	Reduces spread of microorganisms; ensures smooth, orderly procedure.
7. Gently roll or shake container. Instruct patient to clear or blow nose gently unless contraindicated (e.g., risk of increased intracranial pressure or nosebleed).	Ensures distribution of medication. Allows medication to reach sinuses.
8. Administer nose drops.	
a. Help patient to supine position and position head properly (Burchum & Rosenthal, 2022).	Proper positioning provides access to specific nasal passages.
(1) For access to posterior pharynx, tilt patient's head backward.	
(2) For access to ethmoid or sphenoid sinus, tilt head back over edge of bed or place small pillow under patient's shoulder and tilt head back (see illustration).	
(3) For access to frontal and maxillary sinus, tilt head back over edge of bed or pillow with head turned toward side to be treated (see illustration).	Position allows medication to drain into affected sinus.
b. Support patient's head with nondominant hand.	Prevents straining neck muscles.
c. Instruct patient to breathe through mouth.	Mouth breathing reduces chance of aspirating nasal drops into trachea and lungs.
d. Hold dropper 1 cm (½ inch) above nares and instill prescribed number of drops toward midline of ethmoid bone.	Avoids contamination of dropper. Instilling toward ethmoid bone facilitates distribution of medication over nasal mucosa.
e. Have patient remain in supine position 5 minutes.	Prevents premature loss of medication through nares.
f. Offer facial tissue to blot runny nose, but caution patient against blowing nose for several minutes.	Provides comfort but allows for absorption of medication.
9. Administer nasal spray.	
a. Help patient into upright position with head tilted slightly forward.	Proper positioning permits medication spray to reach nasal passages.

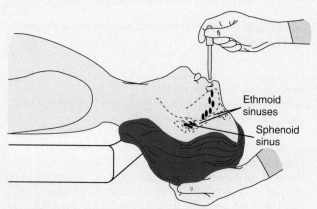

STEP 8a(2) Position for instilling nose drops into ethmoid or sphenoid sinus.

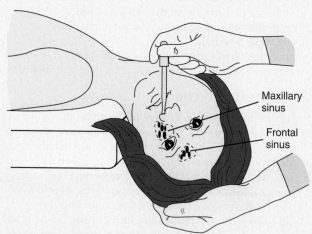

STEP 8a(3) Position for instilling nose drops into frontal and maxillary sinus.

STEP	RATIONALE

b. Instruct or assist patient to insert tip of nasal spray into appropriate nares and occlude other nostril with finger (see illustration). Point spray tip toward side and away from center of nose (Burchum & Rosenthal, 2022).

Allows for proper administration of medication.

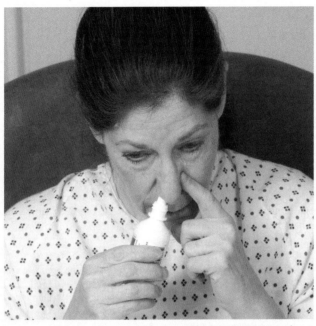

STEP 9b Occlude other nostril before self-administering nasal spray.

c. Have patient spray medication into nose while inhaling. Help to remove nozzle from nose and instruct to breathe out through mouth.

Allows for proper administration and distribution of nasal medication as high into nasal passages as possible.

d. Offer facial tissue to blot runny nose, but caution patient against blowing nose for several minutes.

Provides comfort but allows for absorption of medication.

Clinical Judgment *Some medications are designed for one spray per dose. Examples include calcitonin, desmopressin, and sumatriptan. It is essential to ensure that the patient understands the correct number of sprays to use per dose to prevent overdosing.*

10. Help patient to a comfortable position after medication is absorbed.

Restores comfort and sense of well-being.

11. Raise side rails (as appropriate) and lower bed to lowest position, locking into position.

Ensures patient safety and prevents falls.

12. Place nurse call system in an accessible location within patient's reach.

Ensures patient can call for assistance if needed.

13. Dispose of all contaminated supplies in appropriate receptacle, remove and dispose of gloves, and perform hand hygiene.

Reduces transmission of microorganisms.

EVALUATION

1. Observe patient for onset of side effects 15 to 30 minutes after administration.

Drugs absorbed through mucosa can cause systemic reaction.

2. Ask if patient is able to breathe through nose after decongestant administration. May be necessary to have patient occlude one nostril at a time and breathe deeply.

Determines effectiveness of decongestant medication.

3. Reinspect condition of nasal passages between instillations.

Condition of mucosa reveals response to medication.

4. Ask patient to describe risks of overuse of decongestants and methods for administration.

Feedback ensures that patient can self-administer drugs properly.

5. Have patient demonstrate self-medication.

Feedback demonstrates learning.

STEP	RATIONALE
6. Use Teach-Back: "I want to be sure I explained the importance to not overuse your nasal spray. Explain to me why it is important not to overuse nasal sprays." Revise your instruction now or develop a plan for revised patient/family caregiver teaching if patient/family caregiver is not able to teach back correctly.	Teach-back is a technique for health care providers to ensure that they have explained medical information clearly so that patients and their families understand what is communicated to them (AHRQ, 2023).

Unexpected Outcomes	Related Interventions
1. Patient is unable to breathe easily through nasal passages. Mucosa appears swollen, and congestion is unrelieved, possibly because of rebound effect.	• Stop medication use. • Notify health care provider and consider alternative therapy.
2. Nasal mucosa remains inflamed and tender, with discharge from nares.	• Consider alternative therapy.
3. Patient complains of sinus headache. Sinuses remain congested.	• Consider alternative therapy, such as nasal irrigation.

Documentation

- Document drug name, concentration, number of drops, nares into which drug was instilled, and actual time of administration immediately after administration, not before. Include initials or signature.
- Document patient's response to medication.
- Document your evaluation of patient learning.

Hand-Off Reporting

- Report any unusual systemic or adverse effects/patient response and/or withheld drugs to nurse in charge or health care provider.

Special Considerations

Patient Education

- Instruct patients that each family caregiver should have a different dropper or spray applicator. Instruct patients to wash or rinse applicators after each use.

- Use OTC nasal sprays or nose drops for only one illness; bottles easily become contaminated with bacteria.
- Overuse of nasal sprays and drops can cause rebound sinus congestion, resulting in sinus pain and headache.

Pediatrics

- Infants are nose breathers, and the possible congestion caused by nasal medications may inhibit their sucking. Administer nose drops if ordered 20 to 30 minutes before feedings (Hockenberry et al., 2022).

Populations With Disabilities

- Administering nasal medications may cause patients with dementia or cognitive impairment to become more distressed. If the patient becomes distressed, stop and give some time to calm down. Do not restrain patient to administer nasal medications (Mendes, 2018).

◆ SKILL 21.7 Using Metered-Dose Inhalers (MDIs)

Medications administered with handheld inhalers are dispersed through an aerosol spray, mist, or powder that penetrates the airways. Pressurized metered-dose inhalers (pMDIs), soft mist inhalers, and dry powder inhalers (DPIs) deliver medications that produce local effects such as bronchodilation. Some of these medications are absorbed rapidly through the pulmonary circulation and can cause systemic side effects (e.g., albuterol may cause palpitations, tremors, tachycardia). Patients who receive drugs by inhalation frequently experience asthma and chronic respiratory disease. Drugs administered by inhalation provide control of airway hyperactivity or bronchial constriction. Because patients depend on these medications for disease control, patient teaching is vital for correct use of inhalers and to ensure effectiveness of inhaled medications.

A pMDI is a small, handheld device that disperses medication into the airways through an aerosol spray or mist by activation of a propellant. Dosing is usually achieved with 1 or 2 puffs. DPIs deliver inhaled medication in a fine powder formulation to the respiratory tract (see Procedural Guideline 21.1). Soft mist inhalers (SMIs) turn liquid medicine into a fine mist when inhaled. SMIs are thought to deposit less medication on the back of the throat, meaning that more of it reaches the lungs. The deeper passages of the

respiratory tract provide a large surface area for drug absorption, and the alveolar-capillary network absorbs medication rapidly.

A pMDI requires coordination during the breathing cycle. Many patients spray only the back of their throats and fail to receive a full dose. The inhaler must be depressed to expel medication just as the patient inhales. This ensures that medication reaches the lower airways.

Sometimes patients use a spacer with the pMDI. A spacer is a 10.16 to 20.32 cm (4–8 inches) long tube that attaches to the pMDI and allows the particles of medication to slow down and break into smaller pieces. This helps the medication get deeper into the lungs and enhances absorption. Spacers are helpful when a patient has difficulty coordinating the steps involved in self-administering medications. However, patients who do not use their spacers correctly do not receive the full effect of the medication. DPIs and soft mist inhalers do not use spacers. A patient with poor coordination may need to use a spacer device or soft mist inhaler to administer the medication properly (Burchum & Rosenthal, 2022). Box 21.4 summarizes common problems that occur when using an inhaler.

DPIs hold dry powder medication and create an aerosol when the patient inhales through a reservoir that contains a dose of

BOX 21.4

Common Problems in Using an Inhaler

- *Not taking the medication as prescribed:* Taking either too much or too little.
- *Incorrect activation:* This usually occurs through pressing the canister *before* taking a breath. These actions should be done simultaneously so that the drug can be carried down to the lungs with the breath.
- *Forgetting to shake the inhaler:* The drug is in a suspension, so particles may settle. If the inhaler is not shaken, it may not deliver the correct dose of the drug.
- *Not waiting long enough between puffs:* A delay between puffs is needed before taking a second puff; otherwise, an incorrect dose may be delivered or the drug may not penetrate into the lungs.
- *Failure to clean the valve:* Particles may jam the valve in the mouthpiece unless it is cleaned occasionally. This is a frequent cause of failure to get 200 puffs from one inhaler.
- *Failure to observe whether the inhaler is actually releasing a spray:* If it is not, this should be checked with the pharmacist.
- *Failure to recognize when the canister is empty:* This occurs when the metered-dose inhaler has no built-in dose counter or instructions in dose counting.

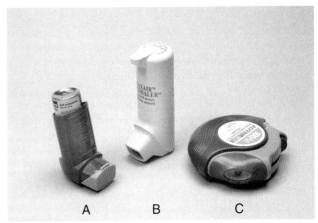

FIG. 21.2 Types of inhalers. (A) Metered-dose inhaler (MDI). (B) Breath-actuated dry powder inhaler (DPI). (C) Dry powder inhaler (DPI).

the medication. Some DPIs are breath-actuated, so breath-dose coordination is unnecessary, and they are easier to use. Compared with MDIs, DPIs deliver more medication to the lungs (Burchum & Rosenthal, 2019). Some DPIs are unit dosed. These inhalers require patients to load a single dose of medication into the inhaler with each use. Other DPIs hold enough medication for 1 month.

Delegation

The skill of administering metered-dose inhalers cannot be delegated to assistive personnel (AP). Direct the AP about:
- Potential side effects of medications and to report their occurrence to the nurse.

- Reporting breathing difficulty (e.g., paroxysmal or sustained coughing, audible wheezing) to the nurse.

Interprofessional Collaboration

- A respiratory therapist can guide the patient and family caregiver when either has difficulty manipulating and correctly using an MDI

Equipment

- Inhaler device with medication canister (MDI, SMI, or DPI) (Fig. 21.2A–C)
- Spacer device such as AeroChamber or InspirEase (optional)
- Facial tissues (optional)
- Stethoscope
- Medication administration record (MAR) (electronic or printed)
- Peak flowmeter (optional)

STEP	RATIONALE

ASSESSMENT

1. Check accuracy and completeness of each MAR or computer printout with health care provider's written medication order. Check patient's name, medication name and dosage, route of administration, and time of administration. Clarify incomplete or unclear orders with health care provider before administration.

2. Review medication reference for pertinent information related to medication, including action, purpose, normal dose and route, side effects, time of onset and peak action, indication, and nursing implications.

3. Assess patient's medical and medication history and history of allergies. List drug allergies on each page of the MAR and prominently display on the patient's electronic health record (EHR) per agency policy. When patient has allergy, provide allergy bracelet.

4. Assess patient's/family caregiver's health literacy.

5. Ask patient to confirm history of allergies: known allergies and allergic response.

The order sheet is the most reliable source and only legal record of medications that patient is to receive. Ensures that patient receives the correct medications (Palese et al., 2019; Wang et al., 2021). Transcription errors are a source of medication errors (Zhu & Weingart, 2022).

Allows you to anticipate effects of drug and observe patient's response.

Determines need for medication or possible contraindications for medication administration.
Communication of allergies is essential for safe and effective care.

Determines degree to which individuals have the ability to find, understand, and use information and services to make informed health-related decisions and actions for themselves and others (CDC, 2023).
Confirms patient's allergies.

STEP	RATIONALE
6. Perform hand hygiene and assess respiratory pattern and auscultate breath sounds (see Chapter 6). Also assess exercise tolerance; does patient develop shortness of breath easily?	Establishes baseline of airway status for comparison during and after treatment.
7. Measure the patient's peak expiratory flow rate using a peak flowmeter. Have patient measure if doing so at home. Use patient's peak flowmeter if available (see Chapter 23, PG 23.1).	A peak flowmeter is used to measure air flow or peak expiratory flow rate and aids in monitoring airway status of patients with chronic asthma (American Academy of Allergy, Asthma, and Immunology [AAAAI], 2020).
8. Assess patient's symptoms before initiating medication therapy.	Provides information to evaluate desired effect of medication.
9. Assess patient's ability to hold, manipulate, and depress canister and inhaler.	Any impairment of grasp or presence of hand tremors interferes with patient's ability to depress canister within inhaler. Spacer device is often necessary.
10. If patient was previously instructed in self-administration, have them demonstrate how to use the device. Perform hand hygiene.	Patients who have adequate understanding of how to use an inhaler may forget the procedure. Ongoing assessment of inhaler technique identifies areas for further education and reinforcement (AAAAI, 2020). Reduces transmission of microorganisms.
11. Assess patient's readiness and ability to learn (e.g., asks questions about medication; is alert; participates in own care; is not fatigued, in pain, or in respiratory distress).	When selecting an aerosol delivery device, consider several factors, such as medication availability and administration time, patient age and ability to use the device correctly, portability of device, convenience in both outpatient and inpatient settings, and costs, as well as health care provider and patient preference (AAAAI, 2020).

Clinical Judgment *In some situations, mental or physical limitations affect patient's ability to learn and methods used for instruction.*

12. Assess patient's knowledge, prior experience, understanding of disease and purpose and action of prescribed medications, and feelings about procedure.	Reveals need for patient education and/or support. Knowledge of disease is essential for patient to realistically understand use of inhaler.

PLANNING

1. Expected outcomes following completion of procedure: • Patient correctly self-administers a metered dose. • Patient describes proper time during respiratory cycle to inhale and spray and number of inhalations for each administration. • Respirations regular, without wheezing, and lung sounds indicate that airways are less restrictive.	Demonstrates learning. Demonstrates learning and ensures correct administration of medication. Demonstrates therapeutic effect of medication in improving gas exchange.
2. Provide privacy and explain procedure to patient. Discuss purpose of each medication, action, and possible adverse effects. Allow patient to ask any questions about the drugs. Explain what a metered dose is and how to administer. Warn about overuse of inhaler and side effects. Be specific if patient wishes to self-administer drug. Explain where and how to set up at home.	Protects patient's privacy; reduces anxiety. Promotes cooperation. Patient's understanding of each medication improves adherence to drug therapy. Prepares patient to self-administer drug, which increases feelings of independence.
3. Plan preparation to avoid interruption. Create a quiet environment. Do not take phone calls or talk with others. Follow agency "No-Interruption Zone" policy. Keep all pages of MAR or computer printout for one patient together or look at only one patient's electronic MAR at a time.	Interruptions contribute to medication errors (Palese et al., 2019; Wang et al., 2021).
4. Organize and set up any equipment for MDI administration at bedside.	Ensures more efficiency when completing the procedure.

IMPLEMENTATION

1. Perform hand hygiene and prepare medications for inhalation. Check label of medication against MAR 2 times (see Skill 21.1). Preparation usually involves taking inhaler device out of storage and into patient's room. Check expiration date on container.	*These are the first and second checks for accuracy.* Process ensures that right patient receives right medication.

STEP	RATIONALE

2. Take medication to patient at correct time (see agency policy). Medications that require exact timing include STAT dose, first-time or loading doses, and one-time doses. Give time-critical scheduled medications (e.g., bronchodilator) at exact time ordered (no more than 30 minutes before or after scheduled dose). Give non–time-critical scheduled medications within a range of 1 or 2 hours of scheduled dose (CMS, 2023). During administration, apply seven rights of medication administration. Perform hand hygiene.

Hospitals must adopt medication administration policy and procedure for timing of medication administration that considers nature of the prescribed medication, specific clinical application, and patient needs (CMS, 2023; USDHHS, 2020). Time-critical scheduled medications are those for which early or delayed administration of maintenance doses of greater than 30 minutes before or after the scheduled dose may cause harm or result in substantial suboptimal therapy or pharmacological effect. Non–time-critical medications are those for which early or delayed administration within a specified range of either 1 or 2 hours should not cause harm or result in substantial suboptimal therapy or pharmacological effect (CMS, 2023; USDHHS, 2020). Reduces transmission of microorganisms.

3. Identify patient using at least two identifiers (e.g., name and birthday or name and medical record number) according to agency policy. Compare identifiers with information on patient's MAR or EHR.

Ensures correct patient. Complies with The Joint Commission standards and improves patient safety (TJC, 2023).

4. At patient's bedside, again compare MAR or computer printout with names of medications on medication labels and patient name. Ask patient about any allergies.

This is the third check for accuracy and ensures that patient receives correct medication. Confirms patient's allergy history.

5. Help patient to sit up in a chair or high-Fowler position if in bed. Allow adequate time for patient to manipulate inhaler, canister, and spacer device (if provided). Explain and demonstrate how canister fits into inhaler.

Position facilitates use of inhaler.
Manipulating the equipment helps the patient become familiar with the inhaler, canister, and spacer device.

6. Perform hand hygiene. Explain and demonstrate steps for administering MDI without spacer.

Reduces transmission of microorganisms. Simple one-on-one instruction and demonstration of step-by-step administration allows patient to ask questions at any point during procedure and increases patient adherence to inhaler use (Schmitz et al., 2019).

   a. Insert MDI canister into holder. Then remove mouthpiece cover from inhaler.

Clinical Judgment *If using an MDI that is new or has not been used for several days, push a "test spray" into the air to prime the device before using. This ensures that the MDI is patent and the metal canister is positioned properly.*

   b. Shake inhaler well for 2 to 5 seconds (five or six shakes).

Aerosolizes fine particles of medication.

   c. Hold inhaler in dominant hand.

   d. Have patient stand or sit and instruct how to position inhaler in one of two ways:

     (1) Have patient place the mouthpiece in the mouth between the teeth and over the tongue, aimed toward back of throat, with lips closed tightly around it. Do not block the mouthpiece with the teeth or tongue (see illustration).

Proper positioning of inhaler is essential for correctly administering medication.

     (2) Position mouthpiece 2 to 4 cm (1–2 inches) in front of widely opened mouth (see illustration), with opening of inhaler toward back of throat. Lips should not touch inhaler.

Directs aerosol spray toward airway. This is best way to deliver medication without a spacer.

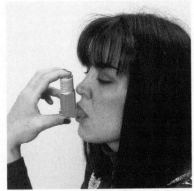

STEP 6d(1) Patient opens lips and places inhaler mouthpiece in mouth with opening toward back of throat.

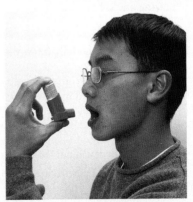

STEP 6d(2) Patient positions inhaler mouthpiece 2 to 4 cm (1–2 inches) from widely open mouth. This is considered the best way to deliver medication without a spacer.

STEP	RATIONALE
e. While holding the mouthpiece away from the mouth, have patient take deep breath and exhale completely.	Empties lung volume and prepares airway to receive medication.
f. With inhaler positioned, have patient hold it with thumb at mouthpiece and index and middle fingers at top. This is a three-point or bilateral hand position.	MDIs are easier to activate when patients use a three-point or lateral hand position to activate canister (Burchum & Rosenthal, 2022).
g. Instruct patient to tilt head back slightly and inhale slowly and deeply through mouth for 3 to 5 seconds while depressing canister fully.	Medication is distributed to airways during inhalation.
h. Have patient hold breath for about 10 seconds.	Facilitates delivery of aerosol spray droplets to deeper branches of airways.
i. Have patient remove MDI from mouth before exhaling and exhale slowly through nose or pursed lips.	Keeps small airways open during exhalation.
7. Explain and demonstrate steps to administer MDI using spacer device.	Simple one-on-one instruction and demonstration of step-by-step administration allows patient to ask questions at any point during procedure and increases patient adherence to inhaler use (Schmitz et al., 2019).
a. Remove mouthpiece cover from MDI and mouthpiece of spacer device.	Inhaler fits into end of spacer device.
b. Shake inhaler well for 2 to 5 seconds (five or six shakes).	Ensures mixing of medication in canister.
c. Insert MDI into end of spacer device.	Spacer device traps medication released from MDI; patient then inhales drug from device. These devices improve delivery of correct dose of inhaled medication (Burchum & Rosenthal, 2022).
d. Instruct patient to place spacer device mouthpiece in mouth and close lips. Do not insert beyond raised lip on mouthpiece. Avoid covering small exhalation slots with lips.	Medication should not escape through mouth.
e. Have patient take a deep breath, exhale, and then breathe normally through spacer device mouthpiece (see illustration).	Allows patient to relax before delivering medication.

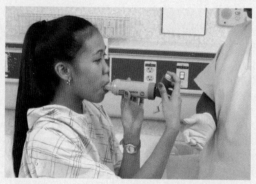

STEP 7e Using spacer device with an MDI.

STEP	RATIONALE
f. Instruct patient to depress medication canister one (1) time, spraying one (1) puff into spacer device.	Space contains fine spray and allows patient to inhale more medication. The spacer increases drug delivery and deposition of the medication on the oropharyngeal mucosa (Burchum & Rosenthal, 2022).
g. Patient breathes in slowly and fully through the mouth for 5 seconds.	Ensures that particles of medication are distributed to deeper airways.
h. Instruct patient to hold full breath for 10 seconds.	Ensures full drug distribution.
i. Have patient remove MDI and spacer and then exhale.	
8. Explain steps to administer a DPI.	
a. If DPI has an external counter, note number indicated.	Determines doses remaining.
b. Remove mouthpiece cover. Do not shake inhaler.	
c. Prepare medication. Some DPIs require loading medication before administration, some require rotation of a lever to load medication or insertion of a capsule, and some require insertion of a disk into inhaler device. Follow manufacturer's specific instructions.	Primes inhaler, ensuring that medication is delivered to patient effectively.

STEP	RATIONALE

d. Have patient take a breath and exhale away from the inhaler.

Prevents loss of powder.

e. Have patient position mouthpiece of DPI between lips and inhale quickly and deeply through mouth (see illustration).

Keeps medication from escaping through mouth. Forceful inhalation creates an aerosol.

f. Have patient hold breath for 5 to 10 seconds.

Distributes medication.

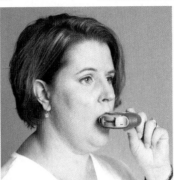

STEP 8e Have patient place mouthpiece of dry powder inhaler (DPI) between lips.

9. Explain steps to administer a soft mist inhaler:
  a. Prepare inhaler. Follow package directions
  b. Prime inhaler. Point the inhaler toward the ground and press the dose-release button before closing the cap. With the cap closed, turn the clear base half a turn in the same direction as the arrows on the label until the base clicks. Then fully open the cap and once again point the inhaler at the ground and press the dose-release button. Repeat this process until a cloud of mist is visible. Once a cloud is visible, repeat the process three more times. The SMI is then ready to use with 60 puffs (30 doses) available.

Priming required to have a dose ready for inhalation.

  c. Load one puff of medication by keeping the cap closed and turning the clear base half a turn in the same direction as the arrows on the label until the base clicks.
  d. Open the cap until it snaps fully open. Stand or sit up straight and breathe out slowly and fully.

Position promoting full ventilation along with slow breathing improves delivery of full dose to airways.

  e. Do not breathe out over the inhaler.
  f. Seal lips around the mouthpiece of the inhaler without covering the air vents on the sides, and point the inhaler toward the back of the throat.
  g. Take a slow, deep breath in through the mouthpiece and press the dose-release button. Breathe in slowly for as long as is comfortable, then hold breath for 10 seconds before slowing exhaling.
  h. Repeat the process to deliver the second puff (two puffs equals one dose).
  i. Close the cap and store inhaler.
10. Instruct patient to wait 20 to 30 seconds between inhalations (if same medication) or 2 to 5 minutes between inhalations (if different medications). Be sure patient inhales correct number of prescribed puffs.

Medications must be inhaled sequentially. Always administer bronchodilators before steroids so that dilators can open airway passages (Burchum & Rosenthal, 2022).

11. Instruct patient to not repeat inhalations before next scheduled dose.

Medications are prescribed at intervals during day to provide constant drug levels and minimize side effects. Beta-adrenergic medications are used either on an "as needed" basis or regularly every 4 to 6 hours.

12. Warn patients that they may feel gagging sensation in throat caused by droplets of medication on pharynx or tongue.

This occurs when medication is sprayed and inhaled incorrectly.

STEP	RATIONALE
13. About 2 minutes after last dose, instruct patient to rinse mouth with warm water and spit water out.	Steroids may alter normal flora of oral mucosa and lead to development of fungal infection. Rinsing out patient's mouth reduces risk of fungal infection (Burchum & Rosenthal, 2022).
14. Instruct patient how to clean the inhaler.	Demonstration supports patient learning and proper care of device at home. Removes residual medication and reduces spread of microorganisms.
a. Once a day, remove MDI canister and cap from the mouthpiece. Do not wash the canister or immerse it in water. Run warm tap water through the top and bottom of the plastic mouthpiece for 30 to 60 seconds. Make sure that inhaler is completely dry before reusing. Do not get valve mechanism of canister wet.	Water damages valve mechanism of canister. Accumulation of medication around mouthpiece interferes with proper medication distribution during use.
b. Instruct patient to clean mouthpiece twice a week with a mild dishwashing soap, rinse thoroughly, and dry completely before storage.	Provides better antimicrobial removal. Pressurized metered-dose inhalers (pMDIs) are potential reservoirs for bacteria.
c. Clean an SMI once a week by wiping the mouthpiece (inside and outside) with a clean, damp cloth.	Removes residue where microorganisms reside.
15. Ask if patient has any questions.	Clarifies misconceptions or misunderstanding and provides opportunity for further patient teaching.
16. Help patient to comfortable position.	Restores comfort and sense of well-being.
17. Raise side rails (as appropriate) and lower bed to lowest position, locking into position.	Ensures patient safety and prevents falls.
18. Place nurse call system in an accessible location within patient's reach.	Ensures patient can call for assistance if needed.
19. Dispose of all contaminated supplies in appropriate receptacle, remove and dispose of gloves, and perform hand hygiene.	Reduces transmission of microorganisms.

EVALUATION

1. Auscultate patient lungs, listen for abnormal breath sounds, and obtain peak flow measures if ordered.	Determines patient response to medication.
2. Have patient explain and demonstrate steps in use of inhaler and cleaning of inhaler.	Return demonstration provides feedback for measuring patient's learning.
3. Ask patient to explain drug schedule and dose of medication.	Improves likelihood of adherence to therapy.
4. Ask patient to describe side effects of medication and criteria for calling health care provider.	Allows patient to recognize signs of overuse and need to seek medical support when drugs are ineffective.
5. **Use Teach-Back:** "I want to be sure I clearly showed you how to use your inhaler. Let's take this time; show me how you will use the inhaler to take your medicine." Revise your instruction now or develop a plan for revised patient/family caregiver teaching if patient/family caregiver is not able to teach back correctly.	Teach-back is a technique for health care providers to ensure that they have explained medical information clearly so that patients and their families understand what is communicated to them (AHRQ, 2023).

Unexpected Outcomes	Related Interventions
1. Patient's respirations are rapid and shallow; breath sounds indicate wheezing.	• Evaluate vital signs and respiratory status. • Notify health care provider. • Reassess type of medication and/or delivery method.
2. Patient needs bronchodilator more than every 4 hours (may indicate respiratory problem).	• Reassess type of medication and delivery methods needed. • Notify health care provider.
3. Patient experiences cardiac dysrhythmias (light-headedness, syncope), especially if receiving beta-adrenergic medications.	• Withhold all further doses of medication. • Evaluate cardiac and pulmonary status (see Chapter 6). • Notify health care provider for reassessment of type of medication and delivery method.

Documentation

• Document drug, dose or strength, number of inhalations, and time administered immediately after administration, not before. Include initials or signature.

• Document patient's response to MDI (e.g., respiratory rate and pattern, breath sounds), evidence of side effects (e.g., arrhythmia, patient's feelings of anxiety), and patient's ability to use MDI.
• Document your evaluation of patient learning.

BOX 21.5

Counting Doses in a Metered-Dose Inhaler

Most metered-dose inhalers (MDIs) currently do not have automatic dose counters. Patients need to keep careful track of the number of inhalations used in their MDIs. Failure to do so may result in patients using an empty inhaler during an acute exacerbation of a respiratory problem. To track doses:

- Note first day of use on a calendar.
- Note number of inhalations in the canister (e.g., 200 inhalations per MDI).
- Note number of inhalations used per day (e.g., 2 inhalations a day 3 times a day equals 6 inhalations per day).
- Divide the total number of inhalations in the canister by the number of inhalations needed per day to determine the number of days that the inhaler should last (e.g., 200 inhalations divided by 6 inhalations per day equals approximately 33 days of 3 times–a-day dosing).
- Mark on a calendar the date the inhaler will be empty, and obtain a refill of the inhaler a few days before this target date.

BOX 21.6

How to Use a Peak Flowmeter

1. Instruct patient to hold meter horizontally, ensuring that fingers do not impede the gauge.
2. Have patient take a deep breath through the mouth, filling the lungs completely.
3. Have the patient place the lips tightly around the mouthpiece of the flowmeter.
4. Instruct patient to blow as hard through meter as fast as possible with a single breath.
5. Note the final position of the marker. This is the patient's peak flow rate.
6. Have the patient repeat the steps blowing into the peak flowmeter two more times. Document the highest reading of the three.

Adapted from Hill B: Measuring peak expiratory flow in adults with asthma, *Br J Nurs* 28(14):924, 2019.

Hand-Off Reporting

- Report any side effects of medication to health care provider.

Special Considerations

Patient Education

- Allow for one-on-one supervised practice of the procedures. Patients may have difficulty timing an inhalation with activation of medication canister without repeated instruction (Schmitz et al., 2019).
- Teach patient to keep track of the number of inhalations in the MDI (Box 21.5).
- Teach patients to use small, handheld peak flowmeters to monitor response to therapy when inhalers are prescribed. A peak flowmeter measures the peak expiratory flow rate (PEFR), which is a person's maximum speed of expiration (Box 21.6).

Pediatrics

- A spacer is of benefit to young children because they have difficulty coordinating inhaler activation and inhaling (Hockenberry et al., 2022).

- Educate child and parent about the need to use the inhaler during school hours. Help family find resources within the school or day care facility. Many school systems do not permit self-administration of MDIs. Follow school policy regarding having the MDI available for use during school hours. A health care provider's order may be necessary (Schmitz et al., 2019).

Older Adults

- Older adults may be unable to depress medication canisters because of weakened grasp or inability to coordinate actuation of the canister with inhalation. The use of a spacer device may be helpful (O'Conor et al., 2015).

Populations With Disabilities

- For patients with cognitive impairments, it is necessary to instruct a family caregiver how to use an MDI and remind caregiver that when patient becomes distressed, stop and give the patient time to calm down (Mendes, 2018).

Home Care

- Remind patients to carry prescribed inhalers at all times to use as immediate treatment in case of an acute asthma attack.

◆ SKILL 21.8 Using Small-Volume Nebulizers

Nebulization is a process of adding medications or moisture to inspired air by mixing particles of various sizes with air. Adding moisture to the respiratory system through nebulization improves clearance of pulmonary secretions. Medications such as bronchodilators, mucolytics, and corticosteroids are often administered by nebulization.

Small-volume nebulizers convert a drug solution into a mist that is then inhaled by a patient into the tracheobronchial tree. A nebulized medication is designed to create a local effect, but it can be absorbed into the bloodstream through the alveoli. As a result, systemic effects from the medication may occur.

Delegation

In many health care agencies, a respiratory therapist performs the skill of administering medications by nebulizer. The nurse must be aware of the type and actions of the inhaled medication that the patient is receiving. The skill of administering medications by nebulizer cannot be delegated to assistive personnel (AP). Direct the AP about:

- Potential side effects of medications and to report their occurrence to the nurse.

- Reporting paroxysmal coughing, ineffective breathing patterns, and other respiratory difficulties to the nurse.

Interprofessional Collaboration

- A pharmacist supplies and prepares the medication needed for a nebulizer treatment. A respiratory therapist usually administers medications by nebulizer.

Equipment

- Medication ordered and diluent (if needed)
- Medicine dropper or syringe
- Nebulizer bottle and tubing assembly
- Small-volume nebulizer machine (often called *handheld nebulizer* or *nebulizer*)
- Pulse oximeter and peak flow device
- Stethoscope
- Medication administration record (MAR) (electronic or printed)
- *Option:* nose clip

STEP	RATIONALE

ASSESSMENT

1. Check accuracy and completeness of each MAR or computer printout with health care provider's written medication order. Check patient's name, medication name and dosage, route of administration, and time of administration. Clarify incomplete or unclear orders with health care provider before administration.

The order sheet is the most reliable source and only legal record of medications that patient is to receive. Ensures that patient receives the correct medications (Palese et al., 2019; Wang et al., 2021). Transcription errors are a source of medication errors (Zhu & Weingart, 2022).

2. Review medication reference for pertinent information related to medication, including diluent, action, purpose, normal
dose and route, side effects, time of onset and peak action, indication, and nursing implications.

Allows you to anticipate effects of drug and observe patient's response.

3. Assess patient's medical and medication history and history of allergies. List medication allergies on each page of the MAR and prominently display on the patient's electronic health record (EHR). When allergies are present, patient should wear an allergy bracelet.

These factors influence how certain medications act. Information reveals previous problems with medication administration. Allergy alert helps prevent adverse effects.

4. Assess patient's/family caregiver's health literacy.

Determines degree to which individuals have the ability to find, understand, and use information and services to make informed health-related decisions and actions for themselves and others (CDC, 2023).

5. Ask patient to confirm history of allergies: known allergies and allergic response.

Confirms patient's allergies.

6. Perform hand hygiene. Assess pulse, respirations, breath sounds, pulse oximetry, and peak flow measurement (if ordered) before beginning treatment.

Establishes baseline for comparison during and after treatment.

7. Assess patient's grasp and ability to assemble, hold, and manipulate nebulizer mouthpiece and tubing; identify any mobility restrictions (e.g., casts, hemiplegia).

Any impairment of cognition or grasp or the presence of hand tremors affects patient's ability to use equipment. Presence of mobility restrictions indicates need for assistance.

8. Assess patient's knowledge, prior experience with nebulizers and nebulizer medication, and feelings about procedure.

Reveals need for patient instruction and/or support.

9. Assess patient's readiness to learn. Patient should not be fatigued, in pain, or in respiratory distress.

Determines best time to provide instruction and techniques to use.

PLANNING

1. Expected outcomes following completion of procedure:
   - Respirations are regular without wheezing.
   - Patient's peak expiratory flow and oxygen saturation level are normal or at patient's target.
   - Patient describes side effects of medication and criteria for calling health care provider (e.g., low peak flow rate).
   - Patient demonstrates self-administration of nebulized dose of medication correctly.

Demonstrates therapeutic effect of medication.
Demonstrates therapeutic effect of medication.

Increases likelihood of adherence to therapeutic regimen.

Demonstrates proper administration of medication and documents learning.

2. Provide privacy and explain procedure to patient. Be specific if patient wishes to self-administer drug. Discuss purpose of each medication, action, and possible adverse effects. Allow patient to ask any questions about the drugs. Explain how to assemble nebulizer and proper use.

Helps patient be a participant in care, which minimizes anxiety. Patient's understanding of each medication improves adherence to drug therapy. Prepares patient to self-administer drug, which increases feelings of independence.

3. Plan preparation to avoid interruption. Create a quiet environment. Do not take phone calls or talk with others. Follow agency "No-Interruption Zone" policy. Keep all pages of MAR or computer printout for one patient together or look at only one patient's electronic MAR at a time.

Begins patient teaching regarding medications.
Interruptions contribute to medication errors (Palese et al., 2019; Wang et al., 2021).

4. Organize and set up any equipment for nebulizer treatment at bedside.

Ensures more efficient procedure.

STEP	RATIONALE

IMPLEMENTATION

1. Perform hand hygiene and prepare medications for inhalation. Check label of medication against MAR two times (see Skill 21.1). Preparation usually involves taking medication vial out of storage and taking to patient's room. Check expiration date on container.

   These are the first and second checks for accuracy. Process ensures that right patient receives correct medication.

2. Take medication to patient at correct time (see agency policy). Medications that require exact timing include STAT dose, first-time or loading doses, and one-time doses. Give time-critical scheduled medications (e.g., bronchodilator, corticosteroid) at exact time ordered (no more than 30 minutes before or after scheduled dose). Give non–time-critical scheduled medications within a range of 1 or 2 hours of scheduled dose (CMS, 2023). During administration, apply seven rights of medication administration. Perform hand hygiene.

   Hospitals must adopt medication administration policy and procedure for timing of medication administration that considers nature of the prescribed medication, specific clinical application, and patient needs (CMS, 2023; USDHHS, 2020). Time-critical scheduled medications are those for which early or delayed administration of maintenance doses of greater than 30 minutes before or after the scheduled dose may cause harm or result in substantial suboptimal therapy or pharmacological effect. Non–time-critical medications are those for which early or delayed administration within a specified range of either 1 or 2 hours should not cause harm or result in substantial suboptimal therapy or pharmacological effect (CMS, 2023; USDHHS, 2020). Reduces transmission of microorganisms.

3. Identify patient using at least two identifiers (e.g., name and birthday or name and medical record number) according to agency policy. Compare identifiers with information on patient's MAR or EHR.

   Ensures correct patient. Complies with The Joint Commission standards and improves patient safety (TJC, 2023).

4. At patient's bedside, again compare MAR or computer printout with names of medications on medication labels and patient name. Ask patient again if they have any allergies.

   This is the third check for accuracy and ensures that patient receives correct medication. Confirms patient's allergy history.

5. Perform hand hygiene and apply clean gloves (if risk of exposure to secretions). Assemble nebulizer equipment per manufacturer directions.

   Assembly may vary slightly with different manufacturers. Proper assembly ensures safe delivery of medication.

6. Add prescribed medication by pouring medicine into nebulizer cup. (*Option:* You may use a medicine dropper or syringe to instill medication.)

   Ensures proper dose and delivery of ordered medication.

7. Attach top to nebulizer cup and be sure that it is secure. Then connect cup to mouthpiece or face mask.

   Prevents loss of medication.

8. Connect tubing to both aerosol compressor and nebulizer cup.

   Ensures aerosol delivery to mouthpiece.

9. Assist patient to sitting or semi-Fowler position. Have patient hold mouthpiece between lips with gentle pressure, but be sure lips are sealed (see illustration).

   Position promotes maximal ventilation. Prevents escape of nebulized medication.

Clinical Judgment *If patient is an infant, child, or tired adult or unable to follow instructions, use face mask. Use of face mask does not require patient to remember to hold mouthpiece correctly.*

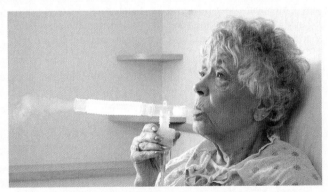

STEP 9 Nebulizer mouthpiece placed between patient's lips.

STEP	RATIONALE

Clinical Judgment *Use special adapters for patients with tracheostomy, which promotes greater deposition of medication in airways.*

10. Turn on small-volume nebulizer machine and ensure that a sufficient mist begins to flow.	Verifies that equipment is working properly during delivery of medication.
11. Instruct patient to take deep breath, slowly, to a volume slightly greater than normal. Encourage brief, end-inspiratory pause for about 2 to 3 seconds, and then have patient exhale passively. *Option:* If needed, use a nose clip so that patient breathes only through the mouth.	Improves effectiveness of medication.
a. If patient is dyspneic, encourage holding every fourth or fifth breath for 5 to 10 seconds.	Maximizes effectiveness of medication.
b. Remind patient to repeat breathing pattern until drug s completely nebulized. This usually takes about 10 to 15 minutes.	Maximizes effectiveness of medication.
(1) Some health care providers set time limit as length of treatment rather than waiting for medication to completely nebulize.	
c. Tap nebulizer cup occasionally during and toward end of treatment.	Releases droplets that are clinging to side of cup, thus allowing for renebulization of solution.
d. Monitor patient's pulse during procedure, especially if beta-adrenergic bronchodilators are used.	Enables you to observe for tachycardia, a potential side effect of medications.
12. When medication is completely nebulized, turn off machine. Rinse nebulizer cup per agency policy. Dry completely and store tubing assembly per agency policy.	Proper storage reduces transfer of microorganisms.
13. If steroids are nebulized, instruct patient to rinse mouth and gargle with warm water after nebulizer treatment. Have patient spit out solution.	Removes medication residue from oral cavity and helps to prevent oral candidiasis, a possible adverse effect of inhaled steroid therapy.
14. After nebulizer treatment is complete, have patient take several deep breaths and cough to expectorate mucus.	Nebulized medication is often ordered to open airways and promote expectoration of mucus.
15. Help patient to comfortable position.	Restores comfort and sense of well-being.
16. Raise side rails (as appropriate) and lower bed to lowest position, locking into position.	Ensures patient safety and prevents falls.
17. Place nurse call system in an accessible location within patient's reach.	Ensures patient can call for assistance if needed.
18. Dispose of all contaminated supplies in appropriate receptacle, remove and dispose of gloves, and perform hand hygiene.	Reduces transmission of microorganisms.

EVALUATION

1. Assess patient's respirations, breath sounds, cough effort, sputum production, pulse oximetry, and peak flow measures if ordered.	Determines status of breathing pattern and adequacy of ventilation/gas exchange. Allows comparison with baseline data and evaluation of effectiveness of procedure.
2. Ask patient to explain drug schedule.	Improves likelihood of adherence to therapy.
3. Ask patient to describe side effects of medication and criteria for calling health care provider.	Allows patient to recognize signs of overuse and need to seek medical support when drugs are ineffective.
4. **Use Teach-Back:** "I want to be sure I was clear about how to put together the nebulizer and add medications. Show me the steps for assembling the nebulizer and adding medications." Revise your instruction now or develop a plan for revised patient/family caregiver teaching if patient/family caregiver is not able to teach back correctly.	Teach-back is a technique for health care providers to ensure that they have explained medical information clearly so that patients and their families understand what is communicated to them (AHRQ, 2023).

Unexpected Outcomes	Related Interventions
1. Patient's respirations are rapid and shallow; breath sounds indicate wheezing, and peak flow reading is below target.	• Reassess patient's ability to self-administer nebulizer. • Reassess type of medication and/or delivery method. • Notify health care provider.
2. Patient experiences paroxysms of coughing. Aerosolized particles can irritate posterior pharynx.	• Reassess type of medication and/or delivery method. • Notify health care provider.
3. Patient experiences cardiac dysrhythmias (light-headedness, syncope), especially if receiving a beta-adrenergic.	• Withhold all further doses of medication. Assess vital signs. • Notify health care provider for reassessment of type of medication and delivery method.

Documentation

- Document drug, dose and strength, route, length of treatment, and time administered immediately after administration, not before.
- Document patient's response to treatment.
- Document your evaluation of patient learning.

Hand-Off Reporting

- Report adverse effects/patient response and/or withheld drugs to nurse in charge or health care provider.

Special Considerations

Patient Education

- Teach patient not to store medication in nebulizer for later use.
- Advise patients taking long-acting beta-agonists about possible adverse effects, including nervousness, restlessness, tremor, headache, nausea, rapid or pounding heart rate, and dizziness.
- Teach patients how to use small, handheld peak flowmeters to monitor response to therapy when inhaled drugs are prescribed (see Box 21.6).

Pediatrics

- Use a mask for the nebulizer treatment if child is too young to hold mouthpiece correctly for the duration of the treatment (Hockenberry et al., 2022).

- Instruct child to breathe normally with mouth open to provide a direct route to the airways for the medication.
- Educate child and parent about the need to use the nebulizer during school or day care hours. Help family find resources within the school or day care facility. Follow school policy regarding having the nebulizer and medication available for use during school hours. A health care provider's order may be necessary.

Older Adults

- Older adults with a weak grasp, hand tremors, or coordination problems may not be able to manipulate or hold a nebulizer, and a face mask may be needed.

Populations With Disabilities

- Patients with cognitive impairments or dementia often have greater success with small-volume nebulizers with a face mask versus MDI (Sullivan, 2018; Yevchak et al., 2017).

Home Care

- When at home, rinse nebulizer parts after each use with clear water and air dry.

PROCEDURAL GUIDELINE 21.1 *Administering Vaginal Medications*

Female patients who develop vaginal infections often require topical application of antiinfective agents. Vaginal medications are available in foam, jelly, cream, or suppository form. Medicated irrigations or douches can also be given. However, their excessive use can lead to vaginal irritation.

Vaginal suppositories are oval shaped and come individually packaged in foil wrappers. They are larger and more oval than rectal suppositories (Fig. 21.3). Storage in a refrigerator prevents the solid suppositories from melting. You insert a suppository into the vagina with an applicator or a gloved hand. After insertion, body temperature causes the suppository to melt for effective medication distribution. You can insert foam, jellies, and creams with an inserter or applicator. Patients often prefer administering their own vaginal medications, and you should give them privacy to do so.

Delegation

The skill of administering vaginal medications cannot be delegated to assistive personnel (AP). Direct the AP about:

- Potential side effects of medications and to report their occurrence to the nurse.
- Reporting any change in comfort level or new or increased vaginal discharge or bleeding to the nurse.

Interprofessional Collaboration

- A gynecological specialist can prescribe treatments and medications if vaginal infection persists or discharge changes in color or amount.

Equipment

Medication administration record (MAR) (electronic or printed); vaginal cream, foam, jelly, tablet, suppository (see Fig. 21.3), or irrigating solution; applicators (see Fig. 21.4) (if needed); clean

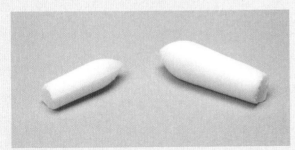

FIG. 21.3 Vaginal suppositories (right) are larger and more oval than rectal suppositories (left).

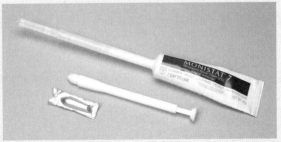

FIG. 21.4 From top: Vaginal cream with applicator, applicator, and vaginal suppository.

Continued

PROCEDURAL GUIDELINE 21.1 *Administering Vaginal Medications—cont'd*

gloves; tissues; towels and/or washcloths; perineal pad; drape or sheet; water-soluble lubricants; bedpan; irrigation or douche container (if needed); gooseneck lamp (optional)

Steps

1. Check accuracy and completeness of each MAR or computer printout with health care provider's written medication order. Check patient's name, medication name and dosage, route of administration, and time of administration. Clarify incomplete or unclear orders with health care provider before administration.

2. Review pertinent information related to medication, including action, indication, purpose, normal dose and route, side effects, time of onset and peak action, and nursing implications.

3. Assess patient's medical and medication history and history of allergies. List drug allergies on each page of the MAR and prominently display on the patient's electronic health record (EHR) per agency policy. When patient has allergy, provide allergy bracelet.

4. Assess patient's/family caregiver's health literacy.

5. Ask patient to confirm history of allergies: known allergies and allergic response.

6. Ask if patient is experiencing any symptoms of pruritus, burning, or discomfort.

7. Assess patient's knowledge and prior experience with vaginal suppository insertion.

8. Perform hand hygiene and apply clean gloves. During perineal care, inspect condition of vaginal tissues; note if irritation or drainage is present. Remove gloves and perform hand hygiene.

9. Assess patient's ability to manipulate applicator, suppository, or irrigation equipment and to properly position self to insert medication (may be done just before insertion).

10. Discuss purpose of each medication, action, and possible adverse effects. Allow patient to ask any questions.

11. Perform hand hygiene and prepare medication using aseptic technique. Prepare medications for one patient at a time, avoiding distractions during preparation. Keep all pages of MARs or computer printouts for one patient together or look at only one patient's electronic MAR at a time. Check label of medication carefully with MAR or computer printout two times (see Skill 21.1) when preparing medication. *This is the first and second check for accuracy.*

12. Take medication(s) to patient at correct time (see agency policy). Give non–time-critical scheduled medications within a range of 1 or 2 hours of scheduled dose (CMS, 2023; USDHHS, 2020). During administration, apply seven rights of medication administration. Perform hand hygiene.

13. Identify patient using at least two identifiers (e.g., name and birthday or name and medical record number) according to agency policy. Compare identifiers with information on patient's MAR or EHR (TJC, 2023).

14. At patient's bedside, again compare MAR or computer printout with names of medications on medication labels and patient name. *This is the third check for accuracy.* Ask patient again about any allergies.

15. Close room door or bedside curtains. Arrange supplies at bedside. Have patient void (using bathroom facilities or

bedpan). Help patient lie in dorsal recumbent position. Patients with restricted mobility in knees or hips may lie supine with legs abducted.

16. Keep abdomen and lower extremities draped.

17. Be sure that vaginal orifice is well illuminated by room light. Otherwise, position portable gooseneck lamp.

18. Perform hand hygiene and apply clean gloves.

19. Insert vaginal suppository.

    a. Remove suppository from wrapper and apply liberal amount of water-soluble lubricant to smooth or rounded end (see illustration). Be sure that suppository is at room temperature. Lubricate gloved index finger of dominant hand.

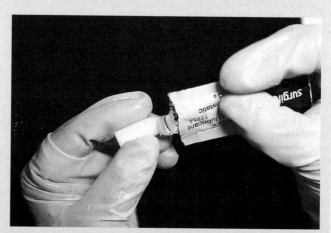

STEP 19a Lubricate tip of suppository.

    b. With nondominant gloved hand, gently separate labial folds in front-to-back direction.

    c. With dominant gloved hand, insert rounded end of suppository along posterior wall of vaginal canal the entire length of finger (7.5–10 cm [3–4 inches]) (see illustration).

    d. Withdraw finger and wipe away remaining lubricant from around orifice and labia with tissue or cloth.

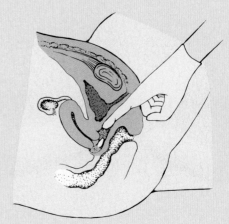

STEP 19c Angle of vaginal suppository insertion.

PROCEDURAL GUIDELINE 21.1 *Administering Vaginal Medications—cont'd*

20. Apply cream or foam.
    a. Fill cream or foam applicator following package directions.
    b. With nondominant gloved hand, gently separate labial folds.
    c. With dominant gloved hand, gently insert applicator approximately 5 to 7.5 cm (2–3 inches). Push applicator plunger to deposit medication into vagina (see illustration).

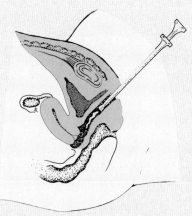

STEP 20c Applicator inserted into vaginal canal. Plunger pushed to instill medication.

    d. Withdraw applicator and place on paper towel. Wipe off residual cream from labia or vaginal orifice with tissue or cloth.
21. Administer irrigation or douche.
    a. Place patient on bedpan with absorbent pad underneath.
    b. Be sure that irrigation or douche fluid is at body temperature. Run fluid through container nozzle (priming the tubing).
    c. Gently separate labial folds and direct nozzle toward sacrum, following floor of vagina.
    d. Raise container approximately 30 to 50 cm (12–20 inches) above level of vagina. Insert nozzle 7 to 10 cm (3–4 inches). Allow solution to flow while rotating nozzle. Administer all irrigating solution.
    e. Withdraw nozzle and help patient to comfortable sitting position.
    f. Allow patient to remain on bedpan for a few minutes. Clean perineum with soap and water.
    g. Help patient off bedpan. Dry perineal area. Return patient to a comfortable position.
22. Instruct patient who received suppository, cream, or tablet to remain on her back for at least 10 minutes.
23. If using an applicator, wash with soap and warm water, rinse, air dry, and then store for future use.
24. Remove and dispose gloves and soiled supplies. Perform hand hygiene.
25. Offer perineal pad when patient resumes ambulation.
26. Raise side rails (as appropriate) and lower bed to lowest position, locking into position.
27. Place nurse call system in an accessible location within patient's reach.
28. Thirty minutes after administration, return to patient's room. Perform hand hygiene and apply gloves. Inspect condition of vaginal canal and external genitalia between applications. Assess vaginal irritation or discharge if present. Remove and dispose of gloves and perform hand hygiene.
29. **Use Teach-Back:** "I want to be sure I explained how to use the vaginal cream applicator. Show me how you will draw the correct amount of cream into the applicator." Revise your instruction now or develop a plan for revised patient/family caregiver teaching if patient/family caregiver is not able to teach back correctly.
30. Document drug (or vaginal irrigating solution), dose, type of installation, and time administered. Document patient response and your evaluation of patient learning.
31. Report to health care provider if symptoms do not improve or worsen.

PROCEDURAL GUIDELINE 21.2 *Administering Rectal Suppositories*

A rectal suppository is a form of medication that acts when it melts and is absorbed into the rectal mucosa. Rectal medications exert either local effects on gastrointestinal (GI) mucosa (e.g., promoting defecation) or systemic effects (e.g., relieving nausea or providing analgesia).

Rectal suppositories are thinner and more bullet shaped than vaginal suppositories (see Fig. 21.3). The rounded end prevents anal trauma during insertion. When you administer a rectal suppository, placing it past the internal anal sphincter and against the rectal mucosa is important. Improper placement can result in expulsion of the suppository before the medication dissolves and is absorbed into the mucosa. The rectal route is not as reliable as oral or parenteral routes in terms of drug absorption and distribution. However, the medications are relatively safe because they rarely cause local irritation or side effects. Rectal medications are contraindicated in patients with recent surgery on the rectum,
bowel, or prostate gland; rectal bleeding or prolapse; and low platelet counts (Burchum & Rosenthal, 2022).

Delegation
The skill of rectal suppository administration cannot be delegated to assistive personnel (AP). Direct the AP about:
- Reporting expected fecal discharge or bowel movement to the nurse.
- Potential side effects of medications and to report their occurrence to the nurse.
- Informing nurse of any rectal pain or bleeding.

Equipment
Rectal suppository; water-soluble lubricating jelly; clean gloves; tissue; drape; bed pan (optional); medication administration record (MAR) (electronic or printed)

Continued

PROCEDURAL GUIDELINE 21.2 *Administering Rectal Suppositories—cont'd*

Steps

1. Check accuracy and completeness of each MAR or computer printout with health care provider's written medication order. Check patient's name, medication name and dosage, route of administration, and time of administration. Reprint on computer any part of MAR that is difficult to read.
2. Review pertinent information related to medication, including action, indication, purpose, normal dose and route, side effects, time of onset and peak action, and nursing implications.
3. Assess patient's medical and medication history and history of allergies. List drug allergies on each page of the MAR and prominently display on the patient's electronic health record (EHR) per agency policy. When patient has allergy, provide allergy bracelet.
4. Assess patient's/family caregiver's health literacy.
5. Ask patient to confirm history of allergies: known allergies and allergic response.
6. Review any presenting signs and symptoms of GI alterations (e.g., constipation or diarrhea).
7. Assess patient's ability to hold suppository and position self to insert medication.
8. Assess patient's knowledge and experience with rectal suppository insertion.
9. Discuss purpose of each medication, action, indication, and possible adverse effects. Allow patient to ask any questions.
10. Perform hand hygiene and prepare medication using aseptic technique. Prepare medications for one patient at a time, avoiding distractions. Keep all pages of MARs or computer printouts for one patient together or look at only one patient's electronic MAR at a time. Check label of medication carefully with MAR or computer printout (see Skill 21.1) two times when preparing medication. *This is the first and second check for accuracy.*
11. Take medication(s) to patient at correct time (see agency policy). Give non–time-critical scheduled medications within a range of 1 or 2 hours of scheduled dose (CMS, 2023). During administration, apply seven rights of medication administration. Perform hand hygiene.
12. Identify patient using at least two identifiers (e.g., name and birthday or name and medical record number) according to agency policy. Compare identifiers with information on patient's MAR or EHR (TJC, 2023).
13. At patient's bedside, again compare MAR or computer printout with names of medications on medication labels and patient name. Ask patient if they have any allergies. *This is the third check for accuracy.*
14. Provide privacy and prepare environment. Perform hand hygiene and apply clean gloves.
15. Help patient assume left side-lying position with upper leg flexed upward.
16. If patient has mobility impairment, help into lateral position. Obtain help to turn patient and use pillows under upper arm and leg.
17. Keep patient draped with only anal area exposed.
18. Examine condition of anus externally. *Option:* Palpate rectal walls as needed (e.g., if impaction is suspected) (see Chapter 8). If you palpate rectal walls, dispose of gloves by turning them inside out and placing them in proper receptacle if they become soiled. Otherwise, keep gloves on your hands and proceed to Step 20.

Clinical Judgment *Do not palpate patient's rectum if there is a recent history of rectal surgery. A suppository is contraindicated in the presence of active bleeding and diarrhea (Burchum & Rosenthal, 2022).*

19. If previous gloves were soiled or discarded, perform hand hygiene and apply new pair of clean gloves.
20. Remove suppository from foil wrapper and lubricate rounded end with water-soluble lubricant. Lubricate gloved index finger of dominant hand. If patient has hemorrhoids, use liberal amount of lubricant and touch area gently.
21. Ask patient to take slow, deep breaths through mouth and relax anal sphincter.
22. Retract patient's buttocks with nondominant hand. With gloved index finger of dominant hand, insert suppository gently through anus, past internal sphincter, and against rectal wall, 10 cm (4 inches) in adults (see illustration) or 5 cm (2 inches) in infants and children. You should feel rectal sphincter close around your finger.

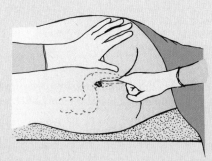

STEP 22 Insert rectal suppository past sphincter and against rectal wall.

Clinical Judgment *Do not insert suppository into a mass of fecal material; this will reduce effectiveness of medication.*

23. *Option:* A suppository may be given through a colostomy (not ileostomy) if ordered. Patient should lie supine. Use small amount of water-soluble lubricant for insertion.
24. Withdraw finger and wipe patient's anal area.
25. Ask patient to remain flat or on side for 5 minutes.
26. Discard gloves by turning them inside out and dispose of them and used supplies in appropriate receptacle. Perform hand hygiene. Use appropriate disposal receptacle if patient is on hazardous drugs (ONS, 2018, 2022).
27. If suppository contains laxative or fecal softener, place call light within reach so that patient can obtain help to reach bedpan or toilet.
28. If suppository was given for constipation, remind patient *not* to flush commode after bowel movement.
29. Return to bedside within 5 minutes to determine if suppository was expelled.
30. Help patient to a comfortable position.
31. Raise side rails (as appropriate) and lower bed to lowest position, locking into position.

PROCEDURAL GUIDELINE 21.2 *Administering Rectal Suppositories—cont'd*

32. Place nurse call system in an accessible location within patient's reach.

33. Evaluate character of stool if passed.

34. **Use Teach-Back:** "I want to be sure I explained clearly to you how to insert a rectal suppository. Describe the steps you take to insert the suppository." Revise your instruction now or develop a plan for revised patient/family caregiver teaching if

patient/family caregiver is not able to teach back correctly.

35. Document the drug, dosage, route, and actual time and date of administration on MAR immediately after administration, not before. Document patient response to medication. Document your evaluation of patient learning.

36. Report adverse effects/patient response and/or withheld drugs to nurse in charge or health care provider.

◆ CLINICAL JUDGMENT AND NEXT GENERATION NCLEX® EXAMINATION–STYLE QUESTIONS

A 75-year-old patient was recently discharged to home following an admission for dehydration and gastroenteritis. The patient has a history of hypertension, asthma, angina, and osteoarthritis. The patient also has an abscess on the right calf that was caused by an infected bug bite. Medications include:

- Hydrochlorothiazide 25 mg every morning by mouth (PO) (diuretic)
- Diltiazem SR capsule, 120 mg once a day PO (calcium channel blocker)
- Albuterol MDI 2 puffs 4 times a day (inhaled bronchodilator)
- Bacitracin topical ointment (500 units/g) applied topically to wound twice a day (antibiotic)
- Nitroglycerin transdermal patch, 0.2 mg/h, one each morning topically (nitrate)
- Nitroglycerin sublingual tablets, 0.4 mg, as needed for chest pain (nitrate)

1. The home health care nurse visits the patient 3 days after discharge. Highlight the assessment findings that require follow-up by the nurse:

   The patient reports feeling dizzy, having a cough, and chest soreness upon inspiration. The patient also states, "I'm not really hungry and I don't feel much like eating." While listening to breath sounds, which include rhonchi, the nurse notes that there are three nitroglycerin transdermal patches on the patient's chest. VS: T 38.6°C (101.4°F); HR 90 beats/min; RR 20 breaths/min; BP 170/98 mm Hg; SpO₂ 92% on RA.

2. While inspecting the right calf abscess, the nurse finds that there is a thick crust of old medication on the wound. The patient explains, "I don't like to waste the medication that is already there, so I just put the new medicine on top of it." Which nursing response is appropriate?
   1. "The potential for more infection increases when layering medication."
   2. "That is a good way to save money on medication."
   3. "We will need to clean this off with alcohol and hot water."
   4. "This is the way the wound looks when healing."

3. When providing more education about the patient's medication regimen, which information will the nurse convey about the use of nitroglycerin ointment? **Select all that apply.**
   1. Clean skin thoroughly before applying the next dose of medication.
   2. Apply gloves before applying the ointment.
   3. Allow your caregiver to apply medication without gloves.
   4. Attend all laboratory appointments to test for therapeutic drug values.
   5. Wear gloves to discard used ointment wrappers.

4. The patient is readmitted to the hospital with dehydration and sepsis. The nurse notes that the health care provider has ordered medications through a small-bore nasogastric feeding. Which nursing actions are appropriate? **Select all that apply.**
   1. Verifying tube placement after medications are given
   2. Mixing all medications together and giving all at once
   3. Using an enteral tube syringe to administer medications
   4. Flushing tube with 30 to 60 mL of water after the last dose of medication
   5. Ensuring that a chest radiograph has been done to confirm tube placement before medicating

5. During hospitalization, the patient is to receive medication via a pressurized metered-dose inhaler (pMDI) with a spacer. Which action will the nurse take first when it is time to receive this medication?
   1. Perform a respiratory assessment.
   2. Place spacer mouthpiece into patient's mouth and instruct patient to close lips around it.
   3. Shake inhaler for 2 to 5 seconds.
   4. Instruct patient to breathe in slowly through mouth for 3 to 5 seconds.

Visit the Evolve site for Answers to Clinical Judgment and Next Generation NCLEX® Examination-Style Questions.

REFERENCES

Agency for Healthcare Research and Quality (AHRQ): *Teach-back: intervention,* 2023. https://www.ahrq.gov/patient-safety/reports/engage/interventions/teachback.html.

American Academy of Allergy Asthma & Immunology (AAAI): *Peak flow meter,* 2020. https://www.aaaai.org/tools-for-the-public/conditions-library/asthma/peak-flow-meter. Accessed November 20, 2023.

Ashraf A, et al: Comparison of vibrating mesh, jet, and breath-enhanced nebulizer during mechanical ventilation, *Respir Care* 65(10):1419, 2020.

Ayers P, editor: *ASPEN enteral nutrition handbook,* ed 3, Silver Spring, MD, 2020, ASPEN.

Billstein-Leber M, et al: ASHP guidelines on preventing medication errors in hospitals, *Am J Health Syst Pharm* 75:1493, 2018.

Boullata J: Enteral medication for the tube-fed patient: making this route safe and effective, *Nutr Clin Pract* 36(1):111, 2021.

Boullata J, et al: ASPEN safe practices for enteral nutrition therapy?, *JPEN J Parenter Enteral Nutr* 41(1):15, 2017.

Burchum JR, Rosenthal LD: *Lehne's pharmacology for nursing care,* ed 11, St. Louis, 2022, Elsevier.

Centers for Disease Control and Prevention (CDC): *What is health literacy?* 2023. https://www.cdc.gov/healthliteracy/learn/index.html.

Centers for Medicare & Medicaid Services (CMS): *State operations manual appendix a–survey protocol, regulations and interpretive guidelines for hospitals,* 2023. https://www.cms.gov/regulations-and-guidance/guidance/manuals/downloads/som107ap_a_hospitals.pdf. Accessed November 20, 2023.

Delavar F, et al: The effects of self-management education tailored to health literacy on medication adherence and blood pressure control among elderly people with primary hypertension: a randomized controlled trial, *Patient Educ Couns* 103:336, 2020.

Forough A, et al: Nurses' experiences of medication administration to people with swallowing difficulties in aged care agencies: a systematic review protocol, *JBI Database System Rev Implement Rep* 15(4):932, 2018.

Fumarola S, et al: Overlooked and underestimated: medical adhesive-related skin injuries. Best practice consensus document on prevention, *J Wound Care* 29 (Suppl 3c):S1–S24, 2020.

Gardner M, Wilkinson MH: Randomized clinical trial comparing breath-enhanced to conventional nebulizers in the treatment of children with acute asthma, *J Pediatr* 204:425, 2019.

Goldstein BG, Goldstein AO: *Topical corticosteroids: use and adverse effects*, 2023, Up-to-Date. https://www.uptodate.com/contents/topical-corticosteroids-use-and-adverse-effects. Accessed May 2023.

Hill B: Measuring peak expiratory flow in adults with asthma, *Br J Nurs* 28(14):924, 2019.

Hockenberry M, et al: *Essentials of pediatric nursing*, ed 11, St. Louis, 2022, Mosby.

Institute for Safe Medication Practices (ISMP): *ISMP's list of error-prone abbreviations, symbols, and dose designations*, 2021. https://www.ismp.org/recommendations/error-prone-abbreviations-list. Accessed November 12, 2023.

Institute for Safe Medication Practices (ISMP): *Targeted medication safety best practices for hospitals*, 2022. https://www.ismp.org/recommendations/error-prone-abbreviations-list. Accessed November 12, 2023.

Institute for Safe Medication Practices (ISMP): *ISMP's list of confused drug names*, 2023, https://www.ismp.org/recommendations/confused-drug-names-list. Accessed November 12, 2023.

International Organization for Standardization (IOS): *Enteral feeding systems: design and testing*, 2020. https://www.iso.org/obp/ui/#iso:std:iso:20695:ed-1:v1:en. Accessed November 12, 2023.

Judd M: Confirming nasogastric tube placement in adults, *Nursing* 50(4):43, 2020.

Lord L: Enteral access devices: types, function, care, and challenges, *Nutr Clin Pract* 33(1):16–38, 2018.

Lyman B, et al: *Actionable patient safety solutions (APSS) #15: nasogastric tube (NGT) placement and verification*, 2020, Patient Safety Movement Foundation, pp 1–16. https://patientsafetymovement.org/wp-content/uploads/2017/10/APSS-15-4.pdf. Accessed November 12, 2023.

Malone A, et al: *ASPEN enteral nutrition handbook*, ed 2, Silver Spring, MD, 2019, ASPEN.

Mendes A: Meeting the care needs of a person with dementia who is distressed, *Br J Nurs* 27(4):219, 2018.

National Institute on Aging: *Taking medications safely as you age*, 2022, https://www.nia.nih.gov/health/taking-medicines-safely-you-age. Accessed November 12, 2023.

Nativ-Zeltzer N, et al: Predictors of aspiration pneumonia and mortality in patients with dysphagia, *Laryngoscope* 132:1172, 2022.

Occupational Safety and Health Administration (OSHA): *Safety and health topics: hazardous drugs*, n.d. https://www.osha.gov/SLTC/hazardousdrugs/controlling_occex_hazardousdrugs.html. Accessed November 12, 2023.

O'Conor R, et al: Health literacy, cognitive function, proper use and adherence in inhaled asthma controller medications among older adults, *Chest* 147(5):1307, 2015.

Oncology Nurses Society (ONS): *Toolkit for safe handling of hazardous drugs for nurses in oncology*, 2018. https://www.ons.org/sites/default/files/2018-06/ONS_Safe_Handling_Toolkit_0.pdf. Accessed November 12, 2023.

Oncology Nurses Society (ONS): *Ensuring healthcare worker safety when handling hazardous drugs*, 2022. https://www.ons.org/make-difference/ons-center-advocacy-and-health-policy/position-statements/ensuring-healthcare. Accessed November 12, 2023.

Palese A, et al: "I am administering medication—please do not interrupt me": red tabards preventing interruptions as perceived by surgical patients, *J Patient Safe* 15(1):30, 2019.

Schmitz D, et al: Imperative instruction for pressurized metered-dose inhalers: provider perspectives, *Respir Care* 64(3):292, 2019.

Spilios M, et al: Safety and feasibility of crushing sevelamer tablets for enteral feeding tube administration, *J Clin Pharm Ther* 46:369. 2021.

Sullivan W, et al: Primary care of adults with intellectual and developmental disabilities: clinical practice guidelines, *Can Fam Physician* 64:254, 2018.

Suzuki T, et al: Relationship between survival and oral status, swallowing function, and oral intake level in older patients with aspiration pneumonia, *Dysphagia* 37:558, 2022.

Tan JP, et al: A systematic review and meta-analysis on the effectiveness of education on medication adherence for patients with hypertension, hyperlipidaemia, and diabetes, *J Adv Nurs* 75:2478, 2019.

The Joint Commission (TJC): *2023 National patient safety goals*, Oakbrook Terrace, IL, 2023, The Joint Commission. https://www.jointcommission.org/standards/national-patient-safety-goals/.

Touhy T, Jett K: *Ebersole and Hess' gerontological nursing & health aging*, ed 6, St. Louis, 2022, Elsevier.

U.S. Department of Health and Human Services, Centers for Medicare & Medicaid (USDHHS): *Updated guidance on medication administration, Hospital Appendix A of State Operations Manual*, Baltimore, 2020, Department of Health and Human Services.

U.S. Food and Drug Administration (FDA): *Reducing risks through standards developments for medical device connectors*, 2022. https://www.fda.gov/medical-devices/medical-device-connectors/reducing-risks-through-standards-development-medical-device-connectors. Accessed May 2023.

Wang W, et al: Current status and influencing factors of nursing interruption events, *Am J Manag Care* 27(6):e1ii–e194, 2021.

Yevchak A, et al: Implementing nurse-facilitated person-centered care approaches for patients with delirium superimposed on dementia in the acute care setting, *J Gerontol Nurs* 43(12):21, 2017.

Zhu J, Weingart S: *Prevention of adverse drug events in hospitals*, 2022, UpToDate. https://www.uptodate.com/contents/prevention-of-adverse-drug-events-in-hospitals. Accessed November 12, 2023.

22 | Parenteral Medications

SKILLS AND PROCEDURES

Skill 22.1 **Preparing Injections: Ampules and Vials, p. 664**

Procedural Guideline 22.1 **Mixing Parenteral Medications in One Syringe, p. 670**

Skill 22.2 **Administering Intradermal Injections, p. 673**

Skill 22.3 **Administering Subcutaneous Injections, p. 677**

Skill 22.4 **Administering Intramuscular Injections, p. 685**

Skill 22.5 **Administering Medications by Intravenous Push, p. 692**

Skill 22.6 **Administering Intravenous Medications by Piggyback and Syringe Pumps, p. 699**

Skill 22.7 **Administering Medications by Continuous Subcutaneous Infusion, p. 705**

OBJECTIVES

Mastery of content in this chapter will enable you to:

- Apply principles of correct preparation of injectable medications from a vial and an ampule.
- Identify advantages, disadvantages, and risks of administering medications by each parenteral route.
- Evaluate the effectiveness and expected outcomes of administering medications by each parenteral route.
- Understand the importance of selecting the proper-size syringe and needle for an injection.
- Analyze factors to consider when selecting injection sites.

- Understand ways to promote patient comfort while administering an injection.
- Apply correct technique for administration of intradermal, subcutaneous, and intramuscular injections.
- Evaluate the risks of three different intravenous routes.
- Apply correct techniques for administration of intravenous medication by intravenous piggyback, intermittent infusion, or syringe pump.
- Apply learned principles of initiation, maintenance, and discontinuation of a continuous subcutaneous infusion.

MEDIA RESOURCES

- http://evolve.elsevier.com/Perry/skills
- Review Questions
- Audio Glossary
- ▶ Video Clips

- **NSO** Nursing Skills Online
- Answers to Clinical Judgment and Next-Generation NCLEX® Examination–Style Questions
- Skills Performance Checklists
- Printable Key Points

PURPOSE

The route of medication administration is the path by which a drug comes in contact with the body. Medications administered by the *parenteral* route enter body tissues and the circulatory system by injection using a needle. Injected medications are thus more quickly absorbed than oral medications. Examples of situations where parenteral routes are used include when patients are vomiting, cannot swallow, or are restricted from taking oral fluids or require intravenous (IV) medications. A specific set of skills is required for each type of injection to ensure that the medication reaches the proper location. There are four routes for parenteral administration:

1. *Subcutaneous injection:* Injection into tissues just under the dermis of the skin
2. *Intramuscular (IM) injection:* Injection into the body of a muscle

3. *Intradermal (ID) injection:* Injection into the dermis just under the epidermis
4. *IV injection or infusion:* Injection into a vein

PRACTICE STANDARDS

- Gorski et al., 2021: Infusion Therapy Standards of Practice—Practice guidelines for intravenous infusions
- Institute for Safe Medication Practices (ISMP), 2022: ISMP Targeted Medication Safety Best Practices for Hospitals—Best practices for preventing medication errors
- Fumarola S et al., 2020: Best Practice Consensus Document on Prevention—Prevention of medical adhesive–related skin injuries—Risk factors and signs and symptoms of medical adhesive–related skin injuries
- The Joint Commission (TJC), 2023: National Patient Safety Goals—Patient identification

- U.S. Department of Health and Human Services (USDHHS), Centers for Medicare and Medicaid Services, 2020: Updated Guidance on Medication Administration, Hospital Appendix A of State Operations Manual

SUPPLEMENTAL STANDARDS

- Centers for Disease Control and Prevention (CDC), n.d.b: CDC Guideline for Prescribing Opioids for Chronic Pain
- Institute for Safe Medication Practices (ISMP): ISMP's List of Error-Prone Abbreviations, Symbols, and Dose Designations, 2021

PRINCIPLES FOR PRACTICE

- When managing a patient's medications, communicate clearly with the interprofessional team and assess and incorporate the patient's preferences and priorities of care, using the best evidence when making decisions about patient care.
- While administering medications, educate patients and family caregivers about each of their prescribed medications. Patients can often identify medications that they are unfamiliar with, have not taken before, or are contraindicated. Make sure that all questions have been answered for the patient before administering medications. Educate family caregivers as appropriate.
- To minimize a patient's discomfort when giving an injection:
  - Use sharp, beveled needles of the shortest length and smallest gauge possible.
  - Change the needle if liquid medication coats the shaft of the needle.
  - Position and flex a patient's limbs to reduce muscular tension.
  - Divert the patient's attention away from the injection procedure.
  - Apply a vapocoolant spray (e.g., Fluori-Methane spray or ethyl chloride) or topical anesthetic (e.g., 5% topical lidocaine-prilocaine emulsion) to an injection site before giving a medication when possible, or place wrapped ice on the site for a minute before injection.

PERSON-CENTERED CARE

- Research shows that several cultural factors can influence drug response, pharmacokinetics, and pharmacodynamics, as well as patient adherence and education, including race ethnicity, genetic factors, diet, environment, and weight (Burchum & Rosenthal, 2022; Giger & Haddad, 2021; Ramamoorthy et al., 2022).
- Knowledge about variations in therapeutic dose and adverse effects is essential in administering medications to different ethnic groups. Some patients experience a therapeutic response at a different dosage than recommended and require careful monitoring (Ramamoorthy et al., 2022).
- Use communication skills when assessing and educating diverse patient populations. Use open-ended questions to determine comfort level and preferences regarding any procedures to be performed.
- An assessment of preferences that may be related to culture can also yield information about dietary preferences, tobacco and alcohol use, and use of herbal remedies that affect drug action and response. The nurse should not make assumptions about cultural preferences, but rather ask the patient about preferences related to care and health management.
- Cultural context is essential in planning education for patients and families (Burchum & Rosenthal, 2022).

- During medication reconciliation, nurses, pharmacists, and other health care providers compare the patient's current medications with any newly ordered medications prescribed for the patient. Throughout this process, identification and resolution of orders that are duplicated, as well as the evaluation of the risk for unintended medication interactions, can occur. Creating and maintaining an accurate list of all patient medications helps to ensure safe and effective patient care.

EVIDENCE-BASED PRACTICE

Subcutaneous Injection Technique

Evidence and research about best practices for patient assessment and site selection regarding insulin administration over the past several years have led to modifications in suggested practice. Evidence-based guidelines for the administration of insulin injections include the following:

- Use the same technique for both insulin syringes and insulin pens.
- Select an injection site where there is a body area where 2.5 cm (1 inch) of subcutaneous fat can be pinched.
- Smart insulin pens have been linked to improved glycemic control and lower health care costs (Sperling & Laffel, 2022).
- Insert a $1/2$- or $5/16$-inch (28- to 31-gauge) needle, perpendicular (90 degrees) to the pinched skin.
- If the patient is receiving a small dose (less than 5 units) of insulin, a pen injector should not be used because there is a 50% chance of dose errors (Weinstock, 2022).
- Do not aspirate the injection. Hold the needle in place for several seconds. This is especially important with insulin pens to prevent leakage of medication.
- Insulin is absorbed rapidly through the abdominal wall, so this should be the first choice for an injection site.
- Several factors influence optimal insulin therapy including subcutaneous injection technique (Weinstock, 2022).

SAFETY GUIDELINES

Patient safety in administering medication involves following the seven rights of medication administration (see Chapter 20). Follow these guidelines to ensure safe medication administration:

- Be vigilant during medication administration. Avoid distractions while preparing a parenteral medication. No-Interruption Zones (NIZs) have been recommended to reduce distractions during medication preparation and administration (Palese et al., 2019; Wang et al., 2021). NIZs are created by placing signs, red tape, or tile borders on the floor around medication carts or areas. Some agencies now require nurses preparing medications to wear a brightly colored vest (e.g., orange) to prevent interruptions. **Nurses standing in these zones are not to be interrupted**.
- Be sure that patients receive the appropriate medications. Know why the patient is receiving each medication; plan what should be done before, during, and after medication administration; and evaluate the effectiveness of medications and any adverse effects.
- Verify that medications have not expired by checking labels.
- Use at least two identifiers before administering medications and check against the medication administration record (MAR) (TJC, 2023). Follow agency policy for patient identification.
- Before administering medication, it is critical to ensure that all information is correct; accuracy should be checked 3 times:
  1. The first check is when the medications are pulled or retrieved from the automated dispensing machine (ADM), the medication drawer, or whatever system is in place at the agency.

2. The second check is when preparation of the medications for administration takes place.
3. The third and final check occurs at the patient's bedside just before medications are given.
- Clarify unclear medication orders and ask for help whenever there is uncertainty about an order or calculation. Consult with peers, pharmacists, and other health care providers and ensure that all concerns are resolved related to medication administration before preparing and giving medications.
- Use the technology (e.g., bar scanning, electronic MARs) available in your agency when preparing and giving medications. Follow all policies related to use of the technology, and do not use "workarounds." A *workaround* bypasses a procedure, policy, or problem in a system. Nurses who use "workarounds" fail to follow agency protocols, policies, or procedures during medication administration, often in order to more quickly complete the medication administration process.
- Use strict aseptic technique during parenteral medication preparation and administration (Table 22.1).
- Educate patients and family caregivers about each medication that is taken while you are administering medications. It is important for a patient to know each medication with respect to purpose, daily dose and when to take the medications, the most common side effects, and the problems to report to the health care provider. Make sure that you answer all patient questions before administering medications. Educate family caregivers if appropriate.
- Most of the time you cannot delegate medication administration. Ensure that you follow standards set by the State's Nurse Practice Act and guidelines established by your agency. Licensed practical nurses or licensed vocational nurses can often administer medications via the oral (PO), subcutaneous, IM, and ID routes. Sometimes they can give medications intravenously if they have had special training and if the medications are not high-alert medications. Some states also allow certified medical assistants to administer some types of medications (e.g., oral and topical medications) in long-term care agencies.
- During an injection, insert the needle at the proper angle (based on type of injection), smoothly and quickly (Fig. 22.1). Do not hesitate, and slowly push the needle into tissue.
- Inject the medication slowly but smoothly.
- Hold the syringe steady once the needle is in the tissue to prevent tissue damage.
- Withdraw the needle smoothly at the same angle used for insertion.
- Gently apply an antiseptic pad (e.g., chlorhexidine, alcohol) or dry, sterile gauze pad to the site.
- Apply gentle pressure at the injection site unless administering an anticoagulation medication. When giving an anticoagulant, or if patient is receiving anticoagulants, apply firm pressure for 1 to 2 minutes
- Rotate injection sites to prevent the formation of indurations and abscesses.

Needlestick Prevention

The most frequent route of exposure to bloodborne disease for health care workers is from needlestick injuries (Occupational Safety and Health Administration [OSHA], n.d.). These injuries occur when health care workers inappropriately recap needles, mishandle IV lines and needles, or leave needles at a patient's bedside. However, the implementation of safe needle devices can prevent needlestick injuries (OSHA, n.d.). The Needlestick Safety and Prevention Act is a federal law mandating that health care agencies use safe needle devices to reduce the frequency of needlestick injury. Employers are required to maintain a current exposure

TABLE 22.1

Preventing Infection During an Injection

Principle	Technique
Prevent contamination of solution	Ampules should not sit open, and medication should be removed quickly.
Prevent needle contamination	Do not let needle touch contaminated surface (e.g., outer edges of ampule or vial, outer surface of needle cap, your hands, countertop, or table surface). Do not touch length of plunger or inner part of barrel. Keep tip of syringe covered with cap or needle.
Prepare skin	Wash skin soiled with dirt, drainage, or feces with soap and water. Use friction and a circular motion while cleaning with an antiseptic swab. Swab from center of site and move outward in a 5-cm (2-inch) radius.
Reduce transfer of microorganisms	Perform hand hygiene for a minimum of 20 seconds.

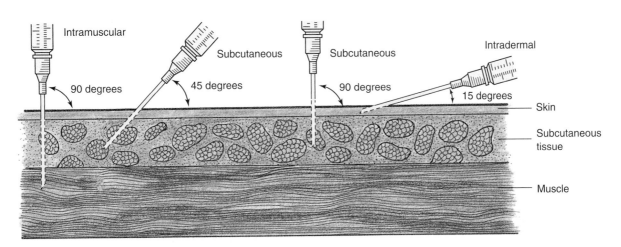

FIG. 22.1 Comparison of angles of insertion for intramuscular (90 degrees), subcutaneous (45 or 90 degrees), and intradermal (15 degrees) injections.

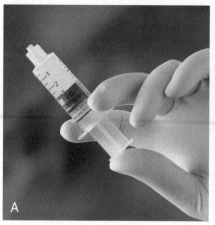
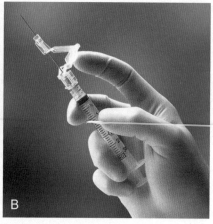
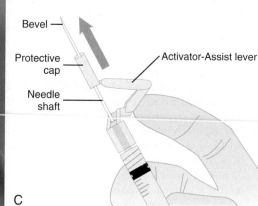

FIG. 22.2 (A) Needleless system. (B) Safety needle system. (C) Detail of safety needle system. (A and B Courtesy © Becton, Dickinson and Company.)

BOX 22.1

Recommendations for the Prevention of Needlestick Injuries

- Avoid using needles when effective needleless systems or SESIP safety devices are available.
- Do not recap any needle after medication administration.
- Plan safe handling and disposal of needles before beginning a procedure.
- Immediately dispose of needles, needleless systems, and SESIP into puncture-proof and leak-proof sharps disposal containers.
- Maintain a sharps injury log that documents the following: type and brand of device involved in the incident; location of the incident (e.g., department or work area); and description of the incident. Maintain the privacy of the employee who has had a sharps injury.
- Attend education offerings on bloodborne pathogens, and follow recommendations for infection prevention, including receiving the hepatitis B vaccine.
- Participate in the selection and evaluation of SESIP devices with safety features within your agency whenever possible.

SESIP, Sharp with engineered sharps injury protection.
Data from Occupational Safety and Health Administration (OSHA): *Bloodborne pathogens and needlestick prevention*, n.d. https://www.osha.gov/SLTC/bloodbornepathogens/index.html.

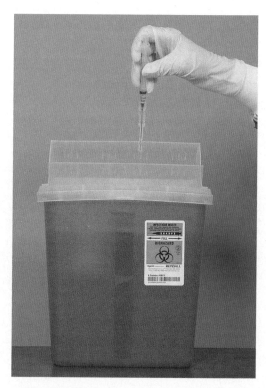

FIG. 22.3 Sharps disposal using only one hand.

---

control plan and seek employee input when considering changing medical devices (OSHA, n.d.).

A sharp with engineered sharps injury protection (SESIP) is a device effective in preventing needlesticks. One type of SESIP is a blunt-end cannula (Fig. 22.2A); another is a safety syringe equipped with a plastic guard or sheath that slips over the needle as it is withdrawn from the skin (see Fig. 22.2B–C). The guard immediately covers the needle, eliminating the chance for a needlestick injury. A variety of other SESIP devices are found in needleless IV connection systems (see Chapter 28). Box 22.1 lists recommendations for health care workers to reduce their risk of needlestick injuries.

Special puncture-proof and leak-proof containers are available in agencies for the disposal of sharps. Containers are made so that only one hand needs to be used when disposing of uncapped needles. In addition, containers must stand upright, have features that prevent overfilling, and be colored red or labeled with a biohazard symbol (Fig. 22.3). The one-hand scoop method should be used only if or when SESIP is not available.

Equipment

Determine the appropriate size of a syringe and length and gauge of a needle on the basis of the volume of solution ordered, medication route, type of medication prescribed, and depth of the patient's injection site based on body size. Syringes come with needleless systems or safety needles that help prevent needlestick injuries. A variety of electronic infusion pumps deliver IV or continuous subcutaneous infusions. Infusion pumps ensure a constant and accurate delivery of medication.

Syringes

Syringes are single use, disposable, and either Luer-Lok or non–Luer-Lok. The design of the syringe tip influences the name. Syringes are packaged separately in a paper wrapper or rigid plastic container. Syringes come with or without a sterile needle and with

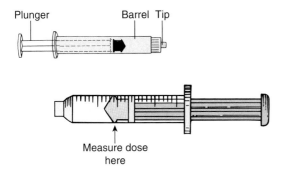

FIG. 22.4 Parts of a syringe.

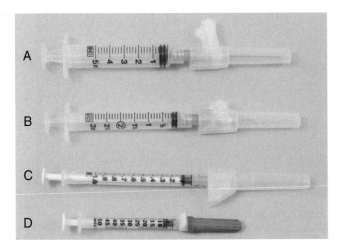

FIG. 22.5 Examples of types of syringes. (A) A 5-mL syringe. (B) Tuberculin syringe marked in increments of 0.01 for doses of less than 1 mL. (C) Insulin syringe marked in units (100). (D) Insulin syringe marked in units (50).

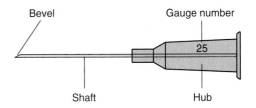

FIG. 22.6 Parts of a needle.

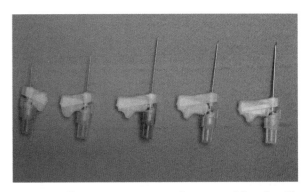

FIG. 22.7 Needles come in a variety of gauges and lengths. Choose correct needle, gauge, and length for the injection ordered.

a needleless SESIP device. The parts of a syringe are shown in Figure 22.4. Non–Luer-Lok syringes use needles or needleless devices that slip onto the tip. Luer-Lok syringes (Fig. 22.5A) use standard needles or needleless devices that are twisted onto the tip and lock themselves in place. The Luer-Lok design prevents the accidental removal of a needle from the syringe.

Syringes come in a variety of sizes, from 0.5 to 60 mL. It is unusual to use a syringe larger than 5 mL for an injection (see Fig 22.5A). A syringe with a volume of 1 to 3 mL is usually adequate for a subcutaneous or IM injection (see Fig. 22.5B). A larger volume creates discomfort. Use larger syringes to administer certain IV medications and irrigate wounds or drainage tubes. Syringes often come prepackaged with a needle attached. However, sometimes the needle is changed on the basis of the route of administration and size of a patient.

The tuberculin syringe (see Fig. 22.5C) is calibrated in sixteenths of a minim and hundredths of a milliliter and has a capacity of 1 mL. Use a tuberculin syringe to prepare small amounts of medications (e.g., ID or subcutaneous injections). A tuberculin syringe is also useful when preparing small, precise doses for infants or young children.

Insulin syringes (see Fig. 22.5D) hold 0.3 to 1 mL, and low-dose insulin syringes (30 units per 0.3 mL or 50 units per 0.5 mL) hold 0.3 to 1 mL. Both come with preattached needles and are calibrated in units. Most insulin syringes are U-100s, designed for use with U-100–strength insulin. Each milliliter of solution contains 100 units of insulin.

Use a larger syringe to administer certain IV medications. Some syringes are packaged with the needle attached, and some syringes require changing the needle based on the viscosity of the medication, route of administration, and size of the patient. Before use, carefully examine the syringe to determine the measurement scale and ensure that you use the correct syringe for preparing the ordered medication.

Needles

Some needles come packaged in individual sheaths, allowing flexibility in choosing the appropriate needle for a patient situation, whereas others are preattached to standard-size syringes. Needles are disposable, and most are made of stainless steel. A needle has three parts: the hub, which fits onto the tip of a syringe; the shaft, which connects to the hub; and the bevel, or slanted tip (Fig. 22.6). The needle hub, shaft, and bevel must always remain sterile. To prevent contamination, use gentle force to place the needle onto the syringe with the cap intact. Some needles come with filters for preparation of medications. Never use filters when administering a medication.

The tip of a needle, or the bevel, is always slanted. When the needle is injected into tissue, the bevel creates a narrow slit that quickly closes after the needle is removed to prevent leakage of medication, blood, or serum. Longer beveled tips are sharper and narrower, which minimizes tissue discomfort during a subcutaneous or IM injection.

Most needles vary in length from ¼ to 3 inches (Fig. 22.7). Choose the needle length according to a patient's size, weight, and the type of tissue into which the medication is to be injected. Current evidence suggests that needle length should be based on a patient's body mass index (BMI) (Holliday et al., 2019). There should be a 5-mm depth of muscle penetration for an IM injection (Sebro, 2022). Children or slender adults generally require shorter needles (⅜–⅝ inch) such as those used for subcutaneous injections. Individuals of average or above average weight require use of longer needles (1–1½ inch) such as those used for IM injections. As the needle gauge becomes smaller, the diameter becomes larger. The selection of a gauge depends on the viscosity of fluid to be injected or infused.

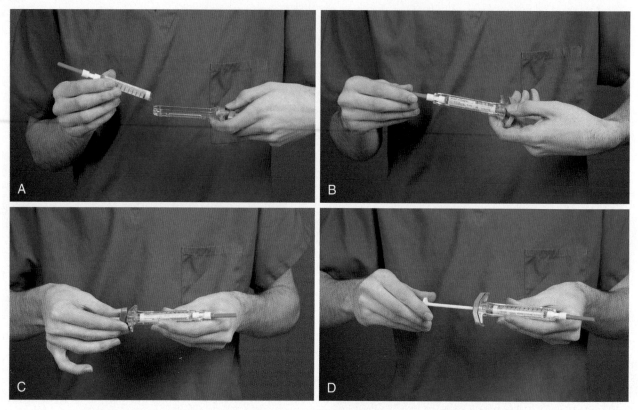

FIG. 22.8 (A) Carpuject syringe holder and prefilled sterile cartridge with needle. (B) Assembling the Carpuject. (C) Cartridge slides into syringe barrel, turns, and locks at needle end. (D) Plunger screws into cartridge end.

Disposable Injection Units

Single-dose, prefilled, disposable syringes are available for some medications. Preparation of medication doses in these syringes is not needed, except perhaps to expel unneeded parts of medication or air. However, it is important to check the medication and concentration carefully because prefilled syringes appear to be similar. Prefilled unit-dose systems such as Tubex and Carpuject injection systems include reusable plastic syringe holders and disposable, prefilled, sterile, glass cartridge units. A newer option is the iSecure Syringe System, a one-piece, prefilled syringe designed to fit in ADMs.

To assemble a prefilled system, place the cartridge, barrel first, into the plastic syringe holder (Fig. 22.8A). Following manufacturer instructions, turn the plunger rod to the left (counterclockwise) (see Fig. 22.8B) and then lock to the right (clockwise) until it "clicks" (see Fig. 22.8C). Finally, remove the needle guard and advance the plunger (see Fig. 22.8D) to expel air and any excess medication, as with a regular syringe. The cartridge may be used with SESIP needles. After giving a medication, dispose of the glass cartridge safely in a puncture- and leak-proof container. This design reduces the risk for needlestick injury.

Injection Pens

Insulin pens are pen-shaped injector devices that contain a reservoir for insulin or an insulin cartridge. A pen is designed to permit self-injection and is intended for single-person use. In health care settings, these devices are often used by health care personnel to administer insulin to patients. The devices are designed to be used multiple times by a single person, using a new needle for each injection (CDC, n.d.a).

✦ SKILL 22.1 Preparing Injections: Ampules and Vials

Ampules contain single doses of injectable medication in a liquid form and are available in sizes from 1 to 10 mL or more. An ampule is made of glass with a constricted, prescored neck that is snapped off to allow access to a medication (Fig. 22.9A). A colored ring around the neck indicates where the ampule is prescored to be broken easily. Medication is easily withdrawn from the ampule by aspirating with a filter needle and syringe. Use filter needles when preparing medication from a glass ampule to prevent glass particles from being drawn into the syringe (Unahalekhaka & Nuthong, 2022). *Do not* use the filter needle to administer the medication.

For injectable medications, place an appropriate-size needle on the syringe after withdrawing the medication.

A vial is a single-dose or multidose plastic or glass container with a rubber seal at the top (see Fig. 22.9B). After opening a single-dose vial, discard it, regardless of the amount of medication used (Institute for Safe Medication Practices [ISMP], 2022). A multidose vial contains several doses of a medication and thus can be used several times, although only for a single patient. When using a multidose vial, write the date on which the vial is opened on the vial label. Verify agency policy regarding the length of time

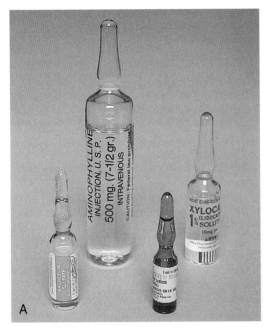

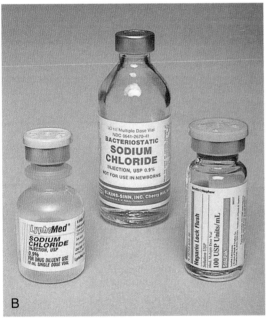

FIG. 22.9 (A) Medication in ampules. (B) Medication in vials.

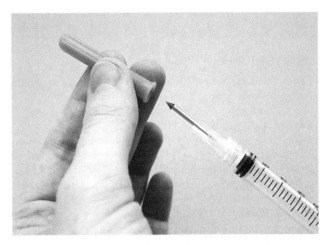

FIG. 22.10 Syringe with needleless vial access adapter.

Unlike an ampule, a vial is a closed system. You must inject air into the vial to permit easy withdrawal of the solution. Some medications, even when in a vial, may need to be drawn up with a filter needle because of the nature of the medication. Agency policies and package inserts from the manufacturer indicate drugs that should be prepared with a filter needle.

Occasionally the health care provider orders an injectable medication that must be reconstituted because it comes in a powdered form. This frequently occurs with a time-sensitive injectable medication, which must be administered within a specific time period to guarantee full drug effectiveness.

Delegation

The skill of preparing injections from ampules and vials cannot be delegated to assistive personnel (AP).

Interprofessional Collaboration

- The agency pharmacist prepares medication prior to delivery to nursing unit. Collaborate to discuss safe dosage and issues regarding medication route.

Equipment

Medication in an Ampule

- Syringe, needle, and filter needle
- Small sterile gauze pad or unopened antiseptic swab

Medication in a Vial

- Syringe and two needles
- Needles:
  - Needleless blunt-tip vial access cannula (Fig. 22.10) or needle (with safety sheath) for drawing up medication (if needed)
  - Filter needle if indicated
- Small, sterile gauze pad or antiseptic swab
- Diluent (e.g., 0.9% sodium chloride or sterile water if indicated)

Both

- Medication administration record (MAR) or computer printout
- Sharp with engineered sharps injury protection (SESIP) safety needle for injection
- Medication in vial or ampule
- Puncture-proof container for disposal of syringes, needles, and glass

an opened multidose vial may be used. Properly discard a multidose vial when the allowed time has expired.

A metal or plastic cap protects a rubber seal of a vial. Remove the cap when you first prepare a vial for use. Vials may contain liquid or dry forms of medications; medications that are unstable in solution are packaged in dry form. The vial label specifies the solvent or diluents used to dissolve the medication and the amount needed to prepare a desired medication concentration. Normal saline and sterile distilled water are the most common solutions.

Some vials have two chambers separated by a rubber stopper. One chamber contains the diluent solution; the other contains the dry medication. Before preparing the medication, push on the upper chamber to dislodge the rubber stopper and allow the powder and the diluent to mix. Gently roll the vial to mix the diluent and medication powder; do not shake.

STEP	RATIONALE

ASSESSMENT

1. Check accuracy and completeness of each MAR or computer printout with health care provider's written medication order. Check patient's name, medication name and dosage, route of administration, and time of administration. Clarify incomplete or unclear orders with health care provider before administration.

The order sheet is the most reliable source and only legal record of medications that patient is to receive. Ensures that patient receives correct medications (Palese et al., 2019). Transcription errors are a source of medication errors (Zhu & Weingart, 2022).

2. Review medication reference for pertinent information related to medication, including action, purpose, normal dose and route, side effects, time of onset and peak action, indication, and nursing implications.

Allows you to anticipate effects of medication while observing patient response.

3. Assess patient's medical and medication history and history of allergies. List medication allergies on each page of the MAR and prominently display on the patient's electronic health record (EHR). When allergies are present, patient should wear an allergy bracelet.

Factors influence how certain medications act. Reveals patient's need for medication.
Allergy alert helps prevent adverse effects.

4. Perform hand hygiene. Assess patient's body build, muscle size, and weight/BMI (if giving subcutaneous or IM medication).

Prevents transmission of microorganisms. Determines type and size of syringe and needle for injection.

PLANNING

1. Expected outcomes following completion of procedure:
   • Proper dose is prepared. No air bubbles are in syringe barrel.

Ensures right dose. Air bubbles displace medication. Elimination of air ensures accuracy of medication dose.

2. Perform hand hygiene.

Prevents transmission of microorganisms.

3. Plan preparation to avoid interruptions. Create a quiet environment. Do not accept phone calls or talk with others. Follow agency "No-Interruption Zone" policy. Keep all pages of MARs or computer printouts for one patient together, or look at only one patient's electronic MAR at a time.

Interruptions contribute to medication errors (Palese et al., 2019; Wang et al., 2021).

IMPLEMENTATION

1. Prepare medications.
   a. If using a medication cart, move it outside patient's room.
   b. Unlock medication drawer or cart or log on to automated dispensing machine (ADM).

Organization of equipment saves time and reduces error.
Medications are safeguarded when locked in cabinet, cart, or ADM.

   c. Select correct medication from stock supply or unit-dose drawer. Compare label of medication with MAR computer printout or computer screen.

Reading label and comparing it with transcribed order reduces errors. *This is the first check for accuracy.*

   d. Check expiration date on each medication, one at a time.

Medications used past their expiration date are sometimes inactive, less effective, or harmful to patients.

   e. Calculate medication dose as needed. Double-check your calculations. In the case of high-risk medications, ask another nurse to perform an independent double check of dosage (see agency policy).

Double checking may help reduce error. Independent double checks should be used only for selective high-alert medications (not all medications) that most warrant their use (ISMP, 2022).

   f. If preparing a controlled substance, check record for previous medication count and compare with supply available.

Controlled substance laws require careful monitoring of dispensed narcotics.

   g. Do not leave medications unattended.

Nurse is responsible for safekeeping of medications.

   h. If in a perioperative or procedural area, label the syringe with the name of the medication and dose.

Syringe needs to be labeled before medication is placed in the syringe to prevent any possible mix-up with a syringe filled with something other than the medication (TJC, 2023).

NOTE: It is not necessary to label a medication prepared for an individual patient if it is immediately administered by an authorized staff member, taken directly to a patient, and administered to that patient without any break in the process (TJC, 2023).

2. Prepare ampule.
   a. Tap top of ampule lightly and quickly with finger until fluid moves from its neck (see illustration).

Dislodges any fluid that collects above neck of ampule. All solution moves into lower chamber.

STEP	RATIONALE
b. Place small gauze pad around neck of ampule (see illustration).	Protects fingers from trauma as glass tip is broken off. Do not use opened alcohol swab to wrap around top of ampule because alcohol may leak into ampule.
c. Snap neck of ampule quickly and firmly away from hands (see illustration).	Protects your fingers and face from shattering glass.
d. Hold ampule upside down or set it on flat surface. Insert filter needle into center of ampule opening. Do not allow needle tip or shaft to touch rim of ampule.	Broken rim of ampule is considered contaminated. When ampule is inverted, solution dribbles out if needle tip or shaft touches rim of ampule.
e. Filter needle should be long enough so tip is at bottom of ampule. Draw up medication quickly.	System is open to airborne contaminants. Filter needles filter out any fragments of glass (Unahalekhaka & Nuthong, 2022).
f. Aspirate medication into syringe by gently pulling back on plunger (see illustration).	Withdrawal of plunger creates negative pressure within syringe barrel, which pulls fluid into syringe.
g. Keep needle tip under surface of liquid. Tip ampule to bring all fluid within reach of needle.	Prevents aspiration of air bubbles.
h. If you aspirate air bubbles, do not expel air into ampule.	Air pressure forces fluid out of ampule, and medication will be lost.

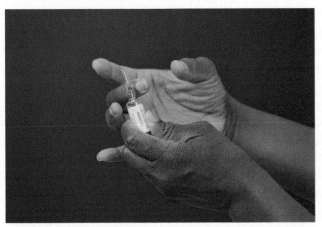

STEP 2a Tapping ampule moves fluid down neck.

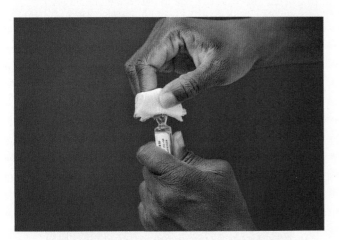

STEP 2b Gauze pad placed around neck of ampule.

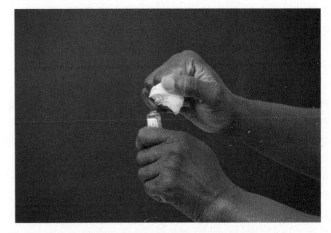

STEP 2c Neck snapped away from hands.

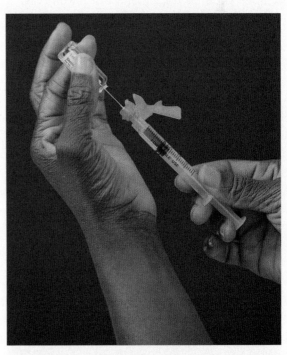

STEP 2f Medication aspirated with ampule inverted.

STEP	RATIONALE
i. To expel excess air bubbles, remove needle from ampule. Hold syringe vertically with needle pointing up. Tap side of syringe to cause bubbles to rise toward needle. Draw back slightly on plunger and push plunger upward to eject air. Do not eject fluid.	Withdrawing plunger too far removes it from barrel. Holding syringe vertically allows fluid to settle in bottom of barrel. Pulling back on plunger allows fluid within needle to enter barrel so that fluid is not expelled. You then expel air at top of barrel and within needle.
j. If syringe contains excess fluid, use sink for disposal. Hold syringe vertically with needle tip up and slanted slightly toward sink. Slowly eject excess fluid into sink. Recheck fluid level in syringe by holding it vertically.	Safely disperses excess medication into sink. Position of needle allows you to expel medication without having it flow down needle shaft. Rechecking fluid level ensures proper dose.
k. Cover needle with its safety sheath or cap. Replace filter needle with regular SESIP needle.	Minimizes needlesticks. Filter needles cannot be used for injection.
3. Prepare vial containing a solution.	
a. Remove cap covering top of unused vial to expose sterile rubber seal. If a multidose vial has been used before, the cap is already removed. Firmly and briskly wipe surface of rubber seal with antiseptic swab and allow it to dry.	Vial comes packaged with cap that cannot be replaced after seal removal. Not all drug manufacturers guarantee that rubber seals of unused vials are sterile. Swabbing reduces transmission of microorganisms. Allowing antiseptic to dry prevents it from coating needle and mixing with medication.
b. Pick up syringe and remove needle cap or cap covering needleless access device. Pull back on plunger to draw amount of air into syringe equivalent to volume of medication to be aspirated from vial.	Injecting air into vial prevents buildup of negative pressure in vial when aspirating medication.

Clinical Judgment *Some medications and agencies require use of a filter needle when preparing medications from vials. Check agency policy or medication reference. If you use a filter needle to aspirate medication, you need to change it to a regular SESIP needle of the appropriate size to administer medication (Antoszyk, 2018).*

STEP	RATIONALE
c. With vial on flat surface, insert tip of needle, needleless device, or blunt filled needle through center of rubber seal (see illustration). Apply pressure to tip of needle during insertion.	Center of seal is thinner and easier to penetrate. Using firm pressure prevents dislodging rubber particles that could enter vial or needle.
d. Inject air into air space of vial, holding onto plunger. Hold plunger firmly; plunger is sometimes forced backward by air pressure within vial.	Injection of air creates vacuum needed to get medication to flow into syringe. Injecting into air space of vial prevents formation of bubbles and an inaccurate dose.
e. Invert vial while keeping firm hold on syringe and plunger. Hold vial between thumb and middle fingers of nondominant hand (see illustration). Grasp end of syringe barrel and plunger with thumb and forefinger of dominant hand to counteract pressure in vial.	Inverting vial allows fluid to settle in lower half of container. Position of hands prevents forceful movement of plunger and permits easy manipulation of syringe.

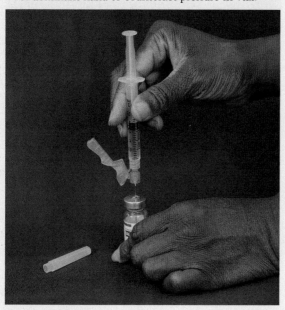

STEP 3c Insert safety needle through center of vial diaphragm (with vial flat on table).

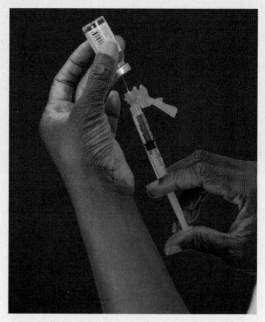

STEP 3e Withdraw fluid with vial inverted.

STEP	RATIONALE
f. Keep tip of needle, or needleless device below fluid level. Blunt-tip needles are now available and are different from needleless devices.	Prevents aspiration of air. Blunt-tip needles are used for preparing and administering medications to patients through an intravenous (IV) device rather than injecting directly into the patient.
g. Allow air pressure from vial to fill syringe gradually with medication. If necessary, pull back slightly on plunger to obtain correct amount of medication.	Positive pressure within vial forces fluid into syringe.
h. When you obtain desired volume, position needle or needleless device into air space of vial; tap side of syringe barrel gently to dislodge any air bubbles (see illustration). Eject any air remaining at top of syringe into vial.	Forcefully striking barrel while needle is inserted in vial may bend needle. Accumulation of air displaces medication and causes dose errors.

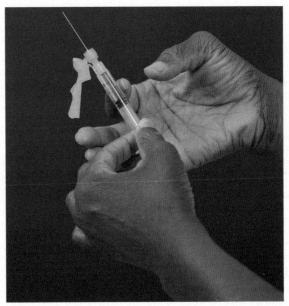

STEP 3h Hold syringe upright; tap barrel to dislodge air bubbles.

STEP	RATIONALE
i. Remove needle or needleless access device from vial by pulling back on barrel of syringe.	Pulling plunger rather than barrel causes plunger to separate from barrel, resulting in loss of medication.
j. Hold syringe at eye level at 90-degree angle to ensure correct volume and absence of air bubbles. Remove any remaining air by tapping barrel to dislodge any air bubbles. Draw back slightly on plunger; then push it upward to eject air. Do not eject fluid. Recheck volume of medication.	Holding syringe vertically allows fluid to settle in bottom of barrel. Tapping dislodges air to top of barrel. Pulling back on plunger allows fluid within needle to enter barrel so that fluid is not expelled. You then expel air at top of barrel and within needle.

Clinical Judgment *When preparing medication from single-dose vial, do not assume that volume listed on label is total volume in vial. Some manufacturers provide small amount of extra liquid, expecting loss during preparation. Be sure to draw up only desired volume.*

STEP	RATIONALE
k. Before you need to inject medication into patient's tissue, change needle with regular SESIP to appropriate gauge and length according to route of medication administration.	Inserting needle through rubber stopper dulls beveled tip. New needle is sharper and, because no fluid is along shaft, does not track medication through tissues. Filter needles cannot be used for injection.
l. Cover needle with its safety sheath or cap following agency safety guidelines.	Minimizes needlesticks.
m. For multidose vial, make a label that includes date of opening, concentration of drug per milliliter, and your initials.	Ensures that nurses can prepare future doses correctly. You discard some drugs within a certain time frame after mixing.
4. Prepare vial containing powder (reconstituting medications).	
a. Remove cap covering vial of powdered medication and cap covering vial of proper diluent. Firmly swab both rubber seals with antiseptic swab and allow it to dry.	Allowing antiseptic to dry prevents it from coating needle and mixing with medication.
b. Draw up manufacturer suggestion for volume and type of diluent into syringe following Steps 3b through 3j.	Prepares diluent in syringe for injection into vial containing powdered medication.

STEP	RATIONALE
c. Insert tip of needle or needleless device through center of rubber seal of vial of powdered medication. Inject diluent into vial. Remove needle.	Diluent begins to dissolve and reconstitute medication.
d. Mix medication thoroughly. Roll in palms. Do not shake.	Ensures proper dispersal of medication throughout solution and prevents formation of air bubbles.
e. Reconstituted medication in vial is ready to be drawn into new syringe. Read label carefully to determine dose after reconstitution.	Once you add diluent, concentration of medication (mg/mL) determines dose you give. Reading medication label carefully decreases medication errors.
f. Draw up reconstituted medication into syringe. Insert needleless device/needle into vial. Do not add air. Then follow Steps 3e through 3j.	Prepares medication for administration.

Clinical Judgment *Some agencies require that doses of certain medications (e.g., insulin, heparin) be checked using an independent double check by another nurse (ISMP, 2022). Check policies and procedures before administering medication.*

5. Compare label of medication with MAR, computer screen, or computer printout.	*This is the second check for accuracy.*
6. Both the vials and/or ampules and the syringe may be barcoded. Both will go to the bedside and be bar coded at the bedside before administration (see later skills related to parenteral administration of medication). If medication prepared in syringe is not given immediately, label syringe.	Prevents medication errors (ISMP, 2022; TJC, 2023) (see Chapter 20).
7. Dispose of soiled supplies. Place broken ampule and/or used vials and used needle or needleless device in puncture- and leak-proof container. Clean work area and perform hand hygiene.	Controls transmission of infection. Proper disposal of glass and needle prevents accidental injury to staff.

EVALUATION

1. Just before administering drug to patient, compare MAR with label of prepared drug and compare dose in syringe with desired dose.	Ensures that dose is accurate. *This is the third check for accuracy.*

Unexpected Outcomes	Related Interventions
1. Air bubbles remain in syringe.	• Expel air from syringe and add medication to it until you prepare correct dose.
2. Incorrect dose of medication is prepared.	• Discard prepared dose. • Prepare correct new dose.

PROCEDURAL GUIDELINE 22.1 *Mixing Parenteral Medications in One Syringe*

Some medications need to be mixed from two vials or from a vial and an ampule. Mixing compatible medications avoids the need to give a patient more than one injection. Most patient care units have medication compatibility charts. Compatibility charts are in drug reference guides, posted within patient care unit medication rooms, or available electronically. If you have any questions about compatibility of medications, contact the pharmacist. When mixing medications, you must correctly aspirate fluid from each type of container. When using multidose vials, do not contaminate the contents of the vial with medication from another vial or ampule.

When mixing medications from a vial and an ampule, prepare medications from the vial first. Then withdraw medication from the ampule using the same syringe and a filter needle. When mixing medications from two vials, do not contaminate one medication with another, ensure that the final dose is accurate, and maintain aseptic technique.

Give special consideration to the proper preparation of insulin, which comes in vials and prefilled pens. Patients with type 1 diabetes

mellitus may receive any number of injectable insulins for managing blood glucose. The types of insulin vary by the rate of action, including rapid-acting, short-acting, intermediate-acting, long-acting, and ultra–long-acting (ADA, n.d.). In many cases patients receive single injections that include premixed solutions (combinations of insulin that are already prepared in mixtures). Examples of these mixtures include Humalog Mix 50/50, 70/30, and 75/25, which contain mixtures of short- and intermediate-acting insulins (ADA, n.d.). To provide safe and effective care, you need to know the onset, peak, and duration for each of your patients' ordered insulin doses. Refer to a medication reference or consult with a pharmacist if you are unsure of this information. Regular insulin is the only type of insulin that can be given intravenously.

In some situations, patients who are ordered a combination of different types of insulin will need to mix insulins from two different vials. Although this is becoming less common, it is important to learn how to mix insulins properly. Before drawing up insulin doses, gently roll a cloudy insulin preparation between the palms

PROCEDURAL GUIDELINE 22.1 *Mixing Parenteral Medications in One Syringe—cont'd*

of the hands to resuspend the insulin. Do not shake insulin vials because shaking causes bubbles to form. Bubbles take up space in the syringe and alter the dose (Burchum & Rosenthal, 2022).

When more than one type of insulin is required to manage a patient's diabetes, you can mix them into one syringe *if* they are compatible. Consult a pharmacist or drug package instructions to determine insulin compatibilities. Always prepare the short- or rapid-acting insulin first to prevent it from being contaminated with the longer-acting insulin (Burchum & Rosenthal, 2022). In most settings insulin is not mixed. Box 22.2 lists recommendations for mixing insulins. Confirmation of accurate insulin preparation requires a second nurse to verify accurate insulin and accurate dose.

Delegation
The skill of mixing medications in one syringe cannot be delegated to assistive personnel (AP).

Interprofessional Collaboration
- Consult with an agency pharmacist for information about insulin onset, peak, and duration if it is not available.

Equipment
Single-dose or multidose vials and ampules containing medication; syringe and two needles; needles (needleless blunt-tip vial access cannula or needle for drawing up medication; filter needle if indicated; sharp with engineered sharps injury protection

BOX 22.2

Recommendations for Mixing Insulins

- Patients whose blood glucose levels are well controlled on a mixed-insulin dose need to maintain their individual routine when preparing and administering their insulin.
- Do not mix insulin with any other medications or diluents unless approved by the health care provider.
- Never mix insulin glargine or insulin detemir with other types of insulin.
- Inject rapid-acting insulins mixed with NPH insulin within 15 minutes before a meal.
- Verify insulin doses with another nurse *while* you are preparing the injection.

Modified from American Association of Diabetes Educators: *Insulin injection*, 2020. https://www.diabeteseducator.org/docs/default-source/legacy-docs/_resources/pdf/general/Insulin_Injection_How_To_AADE.pdf, BD Diabetes care.

[SESIP] needle for injection); antiseptic swab; puncture-proof container for disposing of syringes, needles, and glass; medication administration record (MAR) or computer printout; medication in vial or ampule; medication label

Steps
1. Check accuracy and completeness of MAR or computer printout with health care provider's written medication order. Check patient's name, medication name and dosage, route of administration, and time of administration. Clarify incomplete or unclear orders with health care provider before administration.
2. Review medication reference for pertinent information related to medication, including action, purpose, side effects, and nursing implications.
3. Perform hand hygiene. Assess patient body build, muscle size, and weight/BMI if giving subcutaneous or IM medication.
4. Consider compatibility of medications to be mixed and type of injection.
5. Check expiration date of medication printed on vial or ampule.
6. Perform hand hygiene.
7. Prepare medication for one patient at a time following the seven rights of medication administration (see Chapter 20). Select an ampule or vial from the unit-dose drawer or automated dispensing system. Compare the label of each medication with the MAR or computer printout. In the case of insulin, ensure that correct type(s) of insulin are prepared. *This is the first check for accuracy.*
8. Mixing medications from two vials (see illustration):
   a. Take syringe with needleless device or filter needle and aspirate volume of air equivalent to first medication dose (vial A).
   b. Inject air into vial A, making sure that needle or needleless device does not touch solution (see illustration A).
   c. Holding onto plunger, withdraw needle or needleless device and syringe from vial A. Aspirate air equivalent to second medication dose (vial B) into syringe.
   d. Insert needle or needleless device into vial B, inject volume of air into vial B, and withdraw medication from vial B into syringe (see illustration B).
   e. Withdraw needle or needleless device and syringe from vial B. Ensure that proper volume has been obtained.

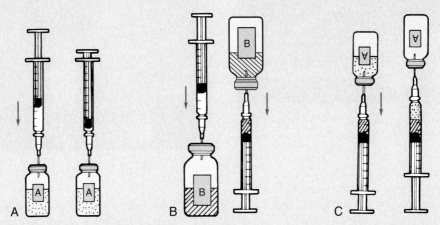

STEP 8 (A) Inject air into vial A. (B) Inject air into vial B and withdraw dose. (C) Withdraw medication from vial A; medications are now mixed.

Continued

PROCEDURAL GUIDELINE 22.1 *Mixing Parenteral Medications in One Syringe—cont'd*

f. Determine by viewing syringe scale the appropriate combined volume of medications.

g. Insert needle or needleless device into vial A, being careful not to push plunger and expel medication within syringe into vial. Invert vial and carefully withdraw the desired amount of medication from vial A into syringe (see illustration C).

h. Withdraw needle or needleless device and expel any excess air from syringe. Check fluid level in syringe for proper dose. Medications are now mixed.

Clinical Judgment *If too much medication is withdrawn from second vial, discard syringe and start over. Do not push medication back into either vial.*

i. Change needle or needleless device for appropriate-size needle if medication is being injected. Keep needle or needleless device capped until administration time.

9. Mixing insulin:
   a. If cloudy insulin is being administered, roll bottle of insulin between hands to resuspend insulin preparation.
   b. Wipe off tops of both insulin vials with antiseptic swab.
   c. Verify insulin dose against MAR.

Clinical Judgment *If long-acting insulin glargine (Lantus) is ordered, note that it should not be mixed with other insulin preparations.*

d. If mixing rapid- or short-acting insulin with intermediate- or long-acting insulin, take insulin syringe and aspirate volume of air equivalent to dose to be withdrawn from intermediate- or long-acting insulin first (see illustration). If two intermediate- or long-acting insulins are mixed, either vial can be prepared first as order is not important in this case.

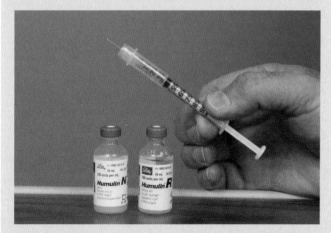

STEP 9d Aspirate air equivalent to dose to be withdrawn from intermediate insulin.

e. Insert needle and inject air into vial of intermediate- or long-acting insulin. Do not let tip of needle touch solution.

f. Remove syringe from vial of insulin without aspirating medication.

g. With the same syringe, inject air equal to the dose of rapid- or short-acting insulin into vial and withdraw correct dose into syringe (see illustration).

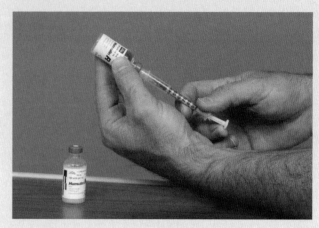

STEP 9g Withdraw short-acting insulin.

h. Remove syringe from rapid- or short-acting insulin and remove any air bubbles to ensure accurate dose.

i. Verify short-acting insulin dosage with MAR and verify insulin prepared in syringe with another nurse to ensure that correct dosage of insulin was prepared. Determine which point on syringe scale the combined units of insulin should measure by adding the number of units of both insulins together (e.g., 4 units Regular + 10 units NPH = 14 units total). Verify combined dosage. A second nurse confirms.

j. Place needle of syringe back into vial of intermediate- or long-acting insulin. Be careful not to push plunger and inject insulin in syringe into vial.

k. Invert vial and carefully withdraw desired amount of insulin into syringe (see illustration).

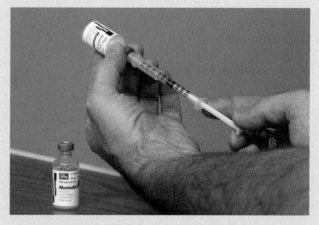

STEP 9k Withdraw intermediate insulin.

l. Withdraw needle and check fluid level in syringe. Verify with another nurse that correct total dose was prepared. Keep needle of prepared syringe sheathed or capped until ready to administer medication.

PROCEDURAL GUIDELINE 22.1 *Mixing Parenteral Medications in One Syringe—cont'd*

10. Mixing medications from a vial and an ampule:
   a. Prepare medication from vial first, following Skill 22.1, Step 3.
   b. Determine on syringe scale the combined volume of medications that should be measured.

Clinical Judgment *If needleless access device was used in preparing medication from vial, change needleless system to a filter needle to remove medication from ampule.*

   c. Next, using the same syringe, prepare second medication from ampule, following Step 2 in Skill 22.1.
   d. Withdraw filter needle from ampule and verify fluid level in syringe. Change filter needle to appropriate SESIP needle. Keep device or needle sheathed or capped until administering medication.

   e. Check syringe carefully for total combined dose of medications.
11. Compare MAR, computer screen, or computer printout with prepared medication and labels on vials/ampules. *This is the second check for accuracy.*
12. The vial and/or ampules and syringes must be saved if barcoding is required (ISMP, 2022). The labeled syringe (when indicated) is placed next to the vial, and both are barcoded at the bedside.
13. Dispose of soiled supplies. Place used ampules and/or vials and needle or needleless device in puncture- and leak-proof container.
14. Clean work area and perform hand hygiene.
15. Check syringe again carefully for total combined dose of medications.
16. *The third check for accuracy* occurs at patient's bedside.

✦ SKILL 22.2 Administering Intradermal Injections

 Video Clip

Intradermal (ID) injections are typically administered for skin testing (e.g., tuberculosis [TB] screening and allergy tests). Because such medications are concentrated, they are injected into the dermis, where blood supply is reduced, and drug absorption occurs slowly. A patient may have an anaphylactic reaction if a medication enters the circulation too rapidly. Health care providers perform skin testing in patients with histories of numerous allergies. Skin testing often requires you to inspect the test site visually; you need to ensure that ID sites are free of lesions and injuries and are relatively hairless. The inner forearm and upper back are ideal locations.

To administer an ID injection, use a tuberculin or small syringe with a short (³⁄₈- to ⁵⁄₈-inch), fine-gauge (25- to 27-gauge) needle. The angle of insertion for an ID injection is 5 to 15 degrees (see Fig. 22.1). Inject only small amounts of medication (0.01–0.1 mL) intradermally. If a bleb does not appear or if the site bleeds after needle withdrawal, the medication may have entered subcutaneous tissues. In this situation, skin test results will not be valid.

Delegation

The skill of administering ID injections cannot be delegated to assistive personnel (AP). Direct the AP about:
- Potential medication side effects or allergic response signs/symptoms and to report their occurrence to the nurse
- Reporting any change in the patient's vital signs or condition to the nurse

Interprofessional Collaboration

- Consult with infection control department if TB is suspected to provide guidelines for isolation.

Equipment

- Syringe: 1-mL TB syringe with preattached 25- or 27-gauge needle, ³⁄₈ to ⁵⁄₈ inch
- Small gauze pad
- Antiseptic swab
- Vial or ampule of medication
- Clean gloves
- Medication administration record (MAR) or computer printout
- Puncture-proof container

STEP	RATIONALE

ASSESSMENT

1. Check accuracy and completeness of MAR or computer printout with health care provider's original medication order. Check patient's name, medication name and dosage, route of administration, and time of administration. Clarify incomplete or unclear orders with health care provider before administration.

The order sheet is the most reliable source and only legal record of medications that patient is to receive. Ensures that patient receives the correct medications (Palese et al., 2019). Transcription errors are a source of medication errors (Zhu & Weingart, 2022).

2. Review medication reference information about expected reaction/anticipated effects when testing skin with specific allergen and appropriate time to interpret injection site results.

Type of reaction depends on patient's ability to mount a cell-mediated immune response. Knowledge of expected and adverse reactions to skin testing helps you determine for which symptoms to monitor, how frequently, and when to reassess patient.

STEP	RATIONALE
3. Assess patient's/family caregiver's health literacy.	Determines degree to which individuals have the ability to find, understand, and use information and services to make informed health-related decisions and actions for themselves and others (CDC, 2023).
4. Ask patient to describe history of allergies: known type of allergies and normal allergic reaction. Compare information with health history. Place allergy band on patient's wrist if allergy is identified.	You do not administer any medication if there is a known patient allergy. Medications are potent and can cause severe anaphylaxis.
5. Perform hand hygiene. Inspect skin to assess for contraindication to ID injections such as reduced local tissue perfusion. Assess for history of severe adverse reactions or necrosis that happened after previous ID injection.	Decreased perfusion reduces absorption of medication. Prior history of severe reactions increases the risk for future severe reactions.
6. Check date of expiration for medication.	Dose potency can increase or decrease when outdated.
7. Assess patient's knowledge, prior experience with ID injections, test being conducted, and feelings about procedure.	Reveals need for patient instruction and/or support.

PLANNING

1. Expected outcomes following completion of procedure:	
• Patient experiences mild burning sensation during injection but no discomfort after injection.	Normal reaction to medication deposited in dermis.
• Small, light-colored bleb approximately 6 mm (¼ inch) in diameter forms at site and gradually disappears. Minimal bruising may be present.	Medication is in dermis and eventually absorbed. Bruising is result of minor bleeding from capillaries.
2. Patient can identify signs of skin reaction and their significance.	Demonstrates learning.
3. Provide privacy and explain test and procedure to patient. Discuss signs and symptoms of ID reaction. If applicable, teach patient how to report any side effects from injection.	Protects patient's privacy; reduces anxiety. Promotes cooperation.
4. Plan preparation to avoid interruptions. Create a quiet environment. Do not accept phone calls or talk with others. Follow agency "No-Interruption Zone" policy. Keep all pages of MARs or computer printouts for one patient together or look at only one patient's electronic MAR at a time.	Interruptions contribute to medication errors (Palese et al., 2019; Wang et al., 2021).
5. Obtain and organize equipment for ID injection at bedside.	Ensures more efficiency when completing a procedure.

IMPLEMENTATION

1. Perform hand hygiene. Prepare medications for one patient at a time using aseptic technique and avoiding distractions (see Skill 22.1). Check label of medication carefully with MAR or computer printout when removing medication from storage and after preparing medication (see Skill 22.1 or Procedural Guideline 22.1).	Ensures that medication is sterile. *These are the first and second checks for accuracy* and ensure that correct medication is administered.
2. Take medication(s) to patient at correct time (see agency policy). Give non–time-critical scheduled medications within a range of 1 to 2 hours of scheduled dose (CMS, 2020). During administration, apply seven rights of medication administration.	Hospitals must adopt medication administration policy and procedure for timing of medication administration that considers nature of the prescribed medication, specific clinical application, and patient needs (CMS, 2020; U.S. Department of Health and Human Services [USDHHS], 2020).
3. Identify patient using at least two identifiers (e.g., name and birthday or name and medical record number) according to agency policy. Compare identifiers with information on patient's MAR or EHR.	Ensures correct patient. Complies with The Joint Commission standards and improves patient safety (TJC, 2023). Some agencies use a bar-code system as a method of patient identification.
4. At patient's bedside, again compare MAR or computer printout with names of medications on medication labels and patient name. Ask patient about any allergies.	*This is the third check for accuracy* and ensures that patient receives correct medication. Confirms patient's allergy history.
5. Perform hand hygiene and apply clean gloves. Keep sheet or gown draped over body parts not requiring exposure.	Reduces transmission of infection. Provides privacy.
6. Help patient to a comfortable position. Have patient extend elbow, and support elbow and forearm on flat surface.	Positions arm for selection of injection site.

STEP	RATIONALE
7. Select appropriate injection site on inner aspect of forearm. Note lesions or discolorations of skin. If possible, select a site three to four finger widths below antecubital space and one hand width above wrist. If you cannot use forearm, inspect upper back. If necessary, use sites appropriate for subcutaneous injections (see Fig. 22.11).	The skin of the forearm produces a smaller wheal than using the back (CDC, n.d.c.).
8. Instruct patient to keep forearm stable. Clean site with antiseptic swab. Apply swab at center of site and rotate outward in circular direction for about 5 cm (2 inches). *Option:* Use vapocoolant spray (e.g., ethyl chloride) before injection.	Mechanical action of swab removes secretions containing microorganisms. Decreases pain at injection site.
9. Hold swab or gauze between third and fourth fingers of nondominant hand.	Gauze or swab remains readily accessible when withdrawing needle.
10. Remove needle cap from needle by pulling it straight off.	Preventing needle from touching sides of cap prevents contamination.
11. Hold syringe between thumb and forefinger of dominant hand with bevel of needle pointing up.	Smooth injection requires proper manipulation of syringe parts. With bevel up, you are less likely to deposit medication into tissues below dermis.
12. Administer injection.	
a. With nondominant hand, stretch skin over site with forefinger or thumb.	Needle pierces tight skin more easily.
b. With needle almost against patient's skin, insert it slowly at 5- to 15-degree angle until resistance is felt. Advance needle through epidermis to approximately 3 mm (⅛ inch) below skin surface. You will see bulge of needle tip through skin (see illustration).	Ensures that needle tip is in dermis. You obtain inaccurate results if you do not inject needle at correct angle and depth.
c. Inject medication slowly. Normally you feel resistance. If not, needle is too deep; remove and begin again.	Slow injection minimizes discomfort at site. Dermal layer is tight and does not expand easily when you inject solution.

Clinical Judgment   *It is not necessary to aspirate because dermis is relatively avascular.*

STEP	RATIONALE
d. While injecting medication, note that small wheal (approximately 6 to 10 mm [¼–⅜ inch]) resembling mosquito bite appears on skin surface (see illustration).	The wheal should appear as a pale, raised area with distinct edges and an orange-peel appearance that does not disappear immediately.
(1) If no wheal forms or if the wheal is less than 6 mm of induration, the test should be repeated immediately, approximately 5 cm (2 inches) from original site or on the other arm.	Small wheal indicates inadequate fluid or injection done incorrectly.
e. After withdrawing needle, apply antiseptic swab or gauze gently over site.	Do not massage site. Apply bandage if needed.
13. Discard uncapped needle or needle enclosed in safety shield and attached syringe in puncture- and leak-proof receptacle.	Prevents injury to patients and health care personnel. Recapping needles increases risk for a needlestick injury (OSHA, n.d.).

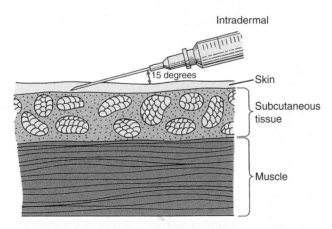

STEP 12b Intradermal needle tip inserted into dermis.

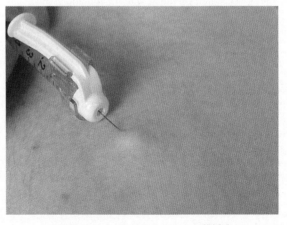

STEP 12d Injection creates small bleb.

STEP	RATIONALE
14. Help patient to a comfortable position.	Restores comfort and sense of well-being.
15. Place nurse call system in an accessible location within patient's reach.	Ensures patient can call for assistance if needed.
16. Raise side rails (as appropriate) and lower bed to lowest position, locking into position.	Ensures patient safety and prevents falls.
17. Dispose of all contaminated supplies in appropriate receptacle, remove and dispose of gloves, and perform hand hygiene.	Reduces transmission of microorganisms.
18. Stay with patient for several minutes and observe for any allergic reactions.	Dyspnea, wheezing, and circulatory collapse are signs of severe anaphylactic reaction and are likely to occur immediately after injection.

EVALUATION

1. Return to room in 15 to 30 minutes and ask if patient feels any acute pain, burning, numbness, or tingling at injection site.

   Continued discomfort could indicate injury to underlying tissues.

2. Ask patient to discuss implications of skin testing and signs of hypersensitivity.

   Patient's ability to recognize signs of skin testing helps to ensure timely reporting of results.

3. Inspect bleb. *Option:* Use skin pencil and draw circle around perimeter of injection site. Read TB test site between 48 and 72 hours after injection; look for induration (hard, dense, raised area) of skin around injection site of:

   Determines if reaction to antigen occurs; indication positive for TB or tested allergens.

   Site must be read at various intervals to determine test results. Mark site according to agency policy; this makes site easy to find. Results of skin testing are determined at various times on the basis of the type of medication used or type of skin testing completed. Manufacturer directions determine when to read test results.

   - 15 mm or more in patients with no known risk factors for TB

     Degree of reaction varies on the basis of patient condition.

   - 10 mm or more in patients who have recently immigrated from countries with high infection rates; injection drug users; residents and employees of high-risk settings; patients with certain chronic illnesses; children younger than 4 years; and infants, children, and adolescents exposed to high-risk adults (Pahal & Sharma, 2022)
   - 5 mm or more in patients who are human immunodeficiency virus (HIV) positive, have fibrotic changes on chest x-ray film consistent with previous TB infection, have had organ transplants, or are immunosuppressed

4. **Use Teach-Back:** "I want to be sure I explained to you the purpose of TB skin testing and what you might see on your arm after the test. Explain to me what the injection site might look like in 2 to 3 days." Revise your instruction now or develop a plan for revised patient/family caregiver teaching if patient/family caregiver is not able to teach back correctly.

   Teach-back is a technique for health care providers to ensure that they have explained medical information clearly so that patients and their families understand what is communicated to them (Agency for Healthcare Research and Quality [AHRQ], 2023).

STEP	RATIONALE

Unexpected Outcomes

1. Patient complains of localized pain or continued burning at injection site, indicating potential injury to nerve or vessels.
2. Raised, reddened, or hard zone (induration) forms around ID test site.

3. Patient has adverse reaction with signs of urticaria, pruritus, wheezing, and dyspnea.

Related Interventions

- Assess injection site.
- Notify patient's health care provider.

- Notify patient's health care provider.
- Document sensitivity to injected allergen or positive test result if tuberculin skin testing was completed.

- Notify patient's health care provider.
- Follow agency policy for appropriate response to drug reactions (e.g., administration of antihistamine such as diphenhydramine or epinephrine).
- Add allergy information to patient's record.

Documentation

- Document drug, dose, route, site, time, and date on MAR immediately after administration. Correctly sign MAR according to agency policy.
- Document area of ID injection and appearance of skin.
- Document patient teaching, validation of understanding, and patient's response to medication (including adverse effects).

Hand-Off Reporting

- Report any undesirable effects from medication to patient's health care provider.
- Report the location, time, and date on which a final reading for a reaction is required.

Special Considerations
Patient Education

- Instruct patient not to squeeze medication out of injection site.
- Teach patient that negative skin test results may not rule out allergies, especially when low concentrations of medication are used.
- Instruct the patient that even if the injection site looks normal, a final reading by a nurse or health care provider is required.

- Patient should wear medical identification band listing all allergies.
- Caution patient not to wash off markings around injection site.
- Explain to patient how to observe for skin reactions.

Pediatrics
- Children with ongoing exposure to high-risk individuals (e.g., infection with HIV, homeless, incarcerated) should be tested for TB every 2 to 3 years (Hockenberry et al., 2022).

Older Adults
- The skin of the older adult is less elastic and must be held taut to ensure that ID injection is administered correctly. Caution is required to prevent skin tears, especially in those treated with long-term steroid therapy (Touhy & Jett, 2023).
- There is a gradual decline in response to the test after age 50, but skin testing can still produce accurate results.

Populations With Disabilities
- Patients on tricyclic antidepressants may have a weak or negative response due to medication interference.

✦ SKILL 22.3   Administering Subcutaneous Injections

 Video Clip

Subcutaneous injections involve depositing medication into the loose connective tissue underlying the dermis. Because subcutaneous tissue does not contain as many blood vessels as muscles, medications are absorbed more slowly than with intramuscular (IM) injections. Physical exercise or application of hot or cold compresses influences the rate of drug absorption by altering local blood flow to tissues. Any condition that impairs blood flow is a contraindication for subcutaneous injections. Because subcutaneous tissue contains pain receptors, a patient often experiences slight discomfort.

Subcutaneous tissue is sensitive to irritating solutions and large volumes of medications. Thus, you only administer small volumes (0.5–1.5 mL) of water-soluble medications subcutaneously to adults. In children, you give smaller volumes up to 0.5 mL (Hockenberry et al., 2022). Examples of subcutaneous medications include epinephrine, insulin, allergy medications, opioids, and heparin.

The best subcutaneous injection sites include the outer aspect of the upper arms, the abdomen from below the costal margins to the iliac crests, and the anterior aspects of the thighs (Fig. 22.11).

These areas are easily accessible and are large enough to allow rotating multiple injections within each anatomical location.

Choose an injection site that is free of skin lesions, bony prominences, and large underlying muscles or nerves. A patient's body weight and adipose tissue indicate the depth of the subcutaneous layer. Choose the needle length and angle of insertion on the basis of a patient's weight and an estimation of the amount of subcutaneous tissue (Rahamimov et al., 2021). Typically, a 25-gauge, ⅝-inch (16-mm) needle inserted at a 45-degree angle or a ½-inch (12-mm) needle inserted at a 90-degree angle is used to administer subcutaneous medications to a normal-size adult patient. Some children require a ½-inch needle. If the patient is obese, pinch the tissue and use a needle long enough to insert through fatty tissue at the base of the skinfold. Thin patients often do not have enough tissue for subcutaneous injections; the upper abdomen is usually the best site in this case. To ensure that a subcutaneous medication reaches the subcutaneous tissue, follow this rule: If you can grasp 2 inches (5 cm) of tissue, insert the needle at a 90-degree angle; if you can grasp 2.5 cm (1 inch) of tissue, insert the needle at a 45-degree angle.

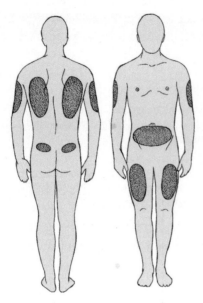

FIG. 22.11 Common sites for subcutaneous injections.

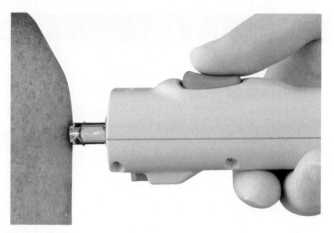

FIG. 22.13 Jet injection system is held perpendicular to skin. (*Courtesy Pharmajet. All rights reserved.*)

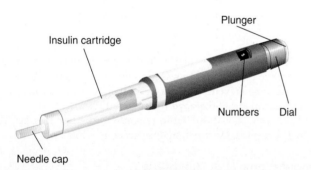

FIG. 22.12 Insulin injection pen. (*From Lewis SL, Bucher L, Heitkemper MM: Medical-surgical nursing: assessment and management of clinical problems, ed 10, St Louis, 2017, Mosby.*)

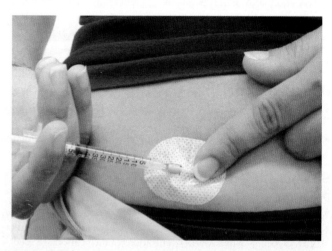

FIG. 22.14 Subcutaneous device. (*Courtesy IntraPump Infusion Systems. All rights reserved.*)

Newer research in insulin administration shows that insulin needles that are 5/16 inch (8 mm) or longer often enter the muscles of men and people with a BMI of 25 or less. Shorter (3/16-inch or 4- to 5-mm) needles were associated with less pain, adequate control of blood sugars, and risk of bleeding and bruising (Gorska-Ciebiada et al., 2020). Therefore when administering insulin you should use needles of 3/16 inch (4–5 mm) administered at a 90-degree angle to reduce pain and achieve adequate control of blood sugars with minimal adverse effects for people of all BMIs, including children (Gorska-Ciebiada et al., 2020; Weinstock, 2022).

Several new technologies are available for administration of subcutaneous injections. *Injection pens* are a technology that patients can use to self-administer medications (e.g., epinephrine, insulin, interferon) subcutaneously (Fig. 22.12). A new generation of injection pens includes a smart insulin pen (e.g., InPen), a reusable injector pen with a smartphone app that can assist patients in managing insulin delivery. This smart system calculates doses, tracks each dose, and provides reminders and alerts. They are available as an add-on to an existing insulin pen or in a reusable form, which requires prefilled cartridges. In many health care settings, nurses administer insulin using pens. They offer a convenient delivery method using prefilled, disposable cartridges. The patient pinches the skin, inserts the needle, and injects a predetermined medication dose. Teaching is essential to ensure that patients use

the correct injection technique and deliver the correct dose of medication. Patients need to be taught the importance of purging the pen before a dose is given. The disadvantages of this technology include the inability to mix compatible types of insulin, which may increase the number of injections required, as well as patient inconvenience and pain (Najmi et al., 2021). One new technology is a *needleless jet injection system* that administers subcutaneous medications without the use of needles. Needle-free injections use high pressure to penetrate the skin with the medication into the subcutaneous tissue (Fig. 22.13). Another new advance in subcutaneous injection is the *subcutaneous injection device* (e.g., insuflon) (Fig. 22.14), which is inserted into the subcutaneous tissue; the needle is then removed, leaving the cannula in the tissue to provide an avenue for administering medications for up to 3 days without having to puncture the skin with each injection.

Special Considerations for Administration of Insulin

Most patients manage type 1 diabetes mellitus with insulin injections. Anatomical injection site rotation is no longer necessary because newer human insulins carry a lower risk for skin hypertrophy and lipoatrophy. At one time, patients would rotate to different anatomical areas. Now patients choose one anatomical area (e.g., the abdomen) and systematically rotate sites within that region,

TABLE 22.2

Comparison of Insulin Preparations

Insulin Type	Onset (Min)	Peak Effect (Hours)	Duration of Action (Hours)
Rapid-Acting			
Insulin lispro (Humalog)	15–30	0.5–2.5	3–6
Insulin aspart (NovoLog)	10–20	1–3	3–5
Insulin glulisine (Apidra)	10–15	1–1.5	3–5
Short-Acting			
Regular insulin (e.g., Humulin R, Novolin R)	30–60	1–5	6–10
Intermediate-Acting			
Isophane insulin suspension (NPH)	60–120	6–14	16–24
Long-Acting			
Insulin glargine (Lantus)	70	None	18–24
Insulin detemir (Levemir)	60–120	None	12–24
Ultra-Long-Acting			
Insulin glargine (Toujeo)	360	None	>24
Insulin degludec (Tresiba)	30–90	None	>24
Insulin Combinations			
Humulin 70/30	30–60	1.5–16	10–16
Novolin 70/30	30–60	2–12	10–16
Novolog Mix 70/30	10–20	1–4	15–18

Data from Burchum J, Rosenthal L: *Lehne's pharmacology for nursing care*, ed 11, St. Louis, 2022, Elsevier.

which maintains consistent insulin absorption from day to day. Absorption rates of insulin vary on the basis of the injection site. Insulin is most quickly absorbed in the abdomen and most slowly in the thighs (Burchum & Rosenthal, 2022; Weinstock, 2022).

The timing of injections is critical to correct insulin administration. Health care providers plan insulin injection times on the basis of blood glucose levels and when a patient will eat (because of the associated rise in glucose). Knowing the peak action and duration of the insulin is essential when developing an effective diabetes management plan. Table 22.2 compares a variety of insulin preparations. Box 22.3 provides general guidelines for insulin administration.

Special Considerations for Administration of Heparin

Heparin therapy provides therapeutic anticoagulation to reduce the risk for thrombus formation by suppressing clot formation. Therefore patients receiving heparin are at risk for bleeding, including bleeding gums, hematemesis, hematuria, or melena. Results from coagulation blood tests (e.g., activated partial thromboplastin time [aPTT] and partial thromboplastin time [PTT]) allow health care providers to monitor the desired therapeutic range for heparin therapy.

Before administering heparin, assess for any new conditions that contraindicate its use, including cerebral or aortic aneurysm, cerebrovascular hemorrhage, severe hypertension, and blood dyscrasias. In addition, assess for conditions in which increased risk for hemorrhage is present: recent childbirth; severe diabetes and renal disease; liver disease; severe trauma; and active ulcers or lesions of the gastrointestinal (GI), genitourinary (GU), or respiratory tract. Assess the patient's current medication regimen, including use of over-the-counter (OTC) and herbal medications (e.g., garlic, ginger, ginkgo, horse chestnut, feverfew), for possible interaction with heparin. Other medications that interact with

BOX 22.3

General Guidelines for Insulin Administration

- Store vials of insulin in the refrigerator, not the freezer. Keep vials currently being used at room temperature. Do not inject cold insulin.
- Inspect vials before each use for changes in appearance (e.g., clumping, frosting, precipitation, change in clarity or color), indicating lack of potency.
- Do not substitute/interchange insulin types unless approved by the patient's health care provider.
- Preferred injection sites include the abdomen (avoiding a 5-cm [2-inch] radius around the umbilicus) and the outer aspect of the thighs.
- Have patient self-administer insulin whenever possible.
- Patients who take insulin need to self-monitor their blood glucose.
- Patients with insulin pumps can use a pump technology known as sensor-augmented insulin pump therapy wherein the pump is synchronized to the patient's glucometer, allowing for a more sensitive approach to blood glucose monitoring (Weinstock, 2022).
- All patients who take insulin should carry at least 15 g carbohydrate (e.g., 4 ounces of fruit juice, 4 ounces of regular soft drink, 8 ounces of skim milk, 6–10 hard candies) in the event of a hypoglycemic reaction.

Adapted from American Diabetes Association (ADA): Diabetes care in the hospital: standards of medical care in diabetes—2019, *Diabetes Care* 42(S1): S173, 2019.

heparin include aspirin, nonsteroidal antiinflammatory drugs (NSAIDs), cephalosporins, antithyroid agents, probenecid, and thrombolytics.

Heparin is administered subcutaneously or intravenously. Low-molecular-weight heparins (LMWHs) (e.g., enoxaparin) are more effective than unfractionated heparin in some patients. The anticoagulant effects are more predictable (Burchum & Rosenthal, 2022). LMWHs have a longer half-life and require less laboratory monitoring but are expensive. To minimize the pain and bruising associated with LMWH, it is given subcutaneously on the right or left side of the abdomen, at least 5 cm (2 inches) away from the umbilicus (or in the patient's "love handles"). Administer LMWH in its prefilled syringe with the attached needle and do not expel the air bubble in the syringe before giving the medication. New evidence supports a slower injection rate of 30 seconds to reduce bruising and pain.

Delegation

The skill of administering subcutaneous injections cannot be delegated to assistive personnel (AP). Direct the AP about:
- Potential medication side effects and to immediately report their occurrence to the nurse
- Reporting any change in the patient's condition to the nurse

Interprofessional Collaboration

- The diabetes nurse educator and the endocrinologist participate in the management of patient-specific diabetes mellitus educational and insulin needs.

Equipment

- Proper-size syringe and sharp with engineered sharps injury protection (SESIP) needle:
  - Subcutaneous: syringe (1–3 mL) and needle (25–27 gauge, ⅛ to ⅝ inch)
  - Immunizations: 23- to 25-gauge, ⅝-inch needle (CDC, 2022)
  - Subcutaneous U-100 insulin: insulin syringe (1 mL) with preattached needle (28–31 gauge [5/16–3/16 inch])
  - Subcutaneous U-500 insulin: 1 mL tuberculin (TB) syringe with needle (25–27 gauge, ½ to ⅝ inch)
  - Insulin prefilled pen
- Small gauze pad (optional)
- Antiseptic swab
- Medication vial
- Clean gloves
- Medication administration record (MAR) or computer printout
- Puncture-proof container
- *Option:* Moist ice pack and towel

STEP	RATIONALE

ASSESSMENT

1. Check accuracy and completeness of each MAR or computer printout with health care provider's written medication order. Check patient's name, medication name and dosage, route of administration, and time of administration. Clarify incomplete or unclear orders with health care provider before administration.

The order sheet is the most reliable source and only legal record of medications that patient is to receive. Ensures that patient receives the correct medications (Palese et al., 2019). Transcription errors are a source of medication errors (Zhu & Weingart, 2022).

2. Review EHR to assess patient's medical and medication history. If patient is in circulatory shock, subcutaneous injection is withheld and a different route is chosen.

Determines need for medication or possible contraindications for medication administration. Reduces absorption of medication.

3. Review medication reference information for medication action, purpose, normal dose, side effects, time and peak of onset, and nursing implications.

Allows you to administer medication safely and monitor patient's response to therapy.

4. Assess relevant laboratory results (e.g., blood glucose, partial thromboplastin).

Provides baseline for measuring drug response.

5. Assess patient's/family caregiver's health literacy.

Determines degree to which individuals have the ability to find, understand, and use information and services to make informed health-related decisions and actions for themselves and others (CDC, 2023).

6. Ask patient to describe history of allergies: known type of allergies and normal allergic reaction. Compare information with health history. Place allergy band on patient's wrist if allergy is identified.

Do not prepare medication if there is known patient allergy.

7. Check date of expiration for medication on vial/pen.

Dose potency can increase or decrease when outdated.

8. Observe patient's previous verbal and nonverbal responses toward injection (Does patient have a fear of needles?).

Anticipating patient's anxiety allows use of distraction techniques to reduce pain awareness.

9. Perform hand hygiene. Assess condition of skin at potential sites for contraindication to subcutaneous injections such as reduced local tissue perfusion.

Reduced tissue perfusion interferes with drug absorption and distribution.

10. Assess patient's symptoms before initiating medication therapy.

Provides information to evaluate desired effect of medication.

11. Assess condition (amount) of patient's adipose tissue. Perform hand hygiene.

Adipose tissue influences methods for administering injections. Reduces transmission of microorganisms.

12. Assess patient's knowledge, prior experience with subcutaneous injections, medication to receive, and feelings about procedure.

Reveals need for patient instruction and/or support.

STEP	RATIONALE

PLANNING

1. Expected outcomes following completion of procedure:
   - Patient experiences no pain or mild burning at injection site.
   - Patient achieves desired effect of medication with no signs of allergies or undesired effects.
   - Patient explains purpose, dosage, and effects of medication.
2. Provide privacy and explain medication and procedure to patient. Discuss rationale and expected sensations related to the subcutaneous injection. If applicable, teach patient how to report any side effects.
3. Plan preparation to avoid interruptions. Create a quiet environment. Do not accept phone calls or talk with others. Follow agency "no-interruption zone" policy. Keep all pages of MARs or computer printouts for one patient together or look at only one patient's electronic MAR at a time.
4. Obtain and organize equipment for subcutaneous injection at bedside.

Medications may cause minor tissue irritation.
Medication administered without patient injury.

Demonstrates learning.
Protects patient's privacy; reduces anxiety. Promotes cooperation.

Interruptions contribute to medication errors (Palese et al., 2019; Wang et al., 2021).

Ensures more efficiency when completing a procedure.

IMPLEMENTATION

1. Perform hand hygiene. Prepare medications for one patient at a time using aseptic technique and avoiding distractions (see Skill 22.1). Check label of medication carefully with MAR or computer printout when removing medication from storage and after preparation (see Skill 22.1 or Procedural Guideline 22.1).
2. Take medication(s) to patient at correct time (see agency policy). Give non–time-critical scheduled medications within a range of 1 to 2 hours of scheduled dose (CMS, 2020). During administration, apply seven rights of medication administration.

Ensures that medication is sterile.
These are the first and second checks for accuracy and ensure that correct medication is administered.

Hospitals must adopt medication administration policy and procedure for timing of medication administration that considers nature of the prescribed medication, specific clinical application, and patient needs (CMS, 2020; USDHHS, 2020)

Clinical Judgment *The timing of insulin injections is critical. A patient must eat immediately after injecting fast-acting insulin. Short-acting insulin begins to work within half an hour, so you need to inject half an hour before eating. Insulin combinations can be taken before a meal to provide a stable level of insulin that continues for an extended time after the meal (ADA, 2022).*

3. Identify patient using at least two identifiers (e.g., name and birthday or name and medical record number) according to agency policy. Compare identifiers with information on patient's MAR or EHR.
4. At patient's bedside, again compare MAR or computer printout with names of medications on medication labels and patient name. Ask patient about any allergies.
5. Perform hand hygiene and apply clean gloves. Keep sheet or gown draped over body parts not requiring exposure.
6. Position patient comfortably for site assessment. Select appropriate injection site. Inspect skin surface over sites for bruises, inflammation, or edema. Do not use an area that is bruised or has signs associated with infection.

Ensures correct patient. Complies with The Joint Commission standards and improves patient safety (TJC, 2023).
Some agencies use a bar-code system as a method for patient identification.
This is the third check for accuracy and ensures that patient receives correct medication. Confirms patient's allergy history.

Reduces transmission of infection. Respects dignity of patient while exposing injection area.
Injection sites are free of abnormalities that interfere with drug absorption. Sites used repeatedly become hardened from lipohypertrophy (increased growth in fatty tissue).

Clinical Judgment *Applying ice or a cold pack to the injection site for 1 minute before the injection may decrease the patient's perception of pain (Hockenberry et al., 2022).*

7. Palpate sites and avoid those with masses or tenderness. Be sure that needle is correct size by grasping skinfold at site with thumb and forefinger. Measure fold from top to bottom. Make sure that needle is one-half length of fold.
   a. When administering insulin or heparin, abdominal injection sites are preferred, followed by thigh injection site.
   b. When administering LMWH subcutaneously, choose site on right or left side of abdomen, at least 5 cm (2 inches) away from umbilicus.

You can mistakenly give subcutaneous injections in muscle, especially in abdomen and thigh sites. Appropriate size of needle is needed to reach subcutaneous tissue (Gorska-Ciebiada et al., 2020).
Risk for bruising is not affected by site.

Injecting LMWH on side of abdomen helps decrease pain and bruising at injection site.

STEP	RATIONALE
c. Rotate insulin site within an anatomical area (e.g., abdomen) and systematically rotate sites within that area.	Rotating injection sites within same anatomical site maintains consistency in day-to-day insulin absorption.
8. Keep patient in a comfortable position. Have patient relax arm, leg, or abdomen, depending on site selection.	Relaxation of site minimizes discomfort.
9. Relocate site using anatomical landmarks.	Injection into correct anatomical site prevents injury to nerves, bone, and blood vessels.
10. Clean site with antiseptic swab. Apply swab at center of site and rotate outward in circular direction for about 5 cm (2 inches) (see illustration).	Mechanical action of swab removes secretions containing microorganisms.
11. Hold swab or gauze between third and fourth fingers of nondominant hand.	Swab or gauze remains readily accessible for use when withdrawing needle after the injection.
12. Remove needle cap or protective sheath by pulling it straight off.	Preventing needle from touching sides of cap prevents contamination.
13. Hold syringe between thumb and forefinger of dominant hand; hold as dart (see illustration).	Quick, smooth injection requires proper manipulation of syringe parts.
14. Administer injection (via syringe):	
a. For average-size patient, hold skin across injection site or pinch skin with nondominant hand.	Needle penetrates tight skin more easily than loose skin. Pinching elevates subcutaneous tissue and desensitizes area.
b. Inject needle quickly and firmly at 45- to 90-degree angle (see illustration). Release skin if pinched. *Option:* When using injection pen or giving heparin, continue to pinch skin while injecting medicine.	Quick, firm insertion minimizes discomfort. (Injecting medication into compressed tissue irritates nerve fibers.) Correct angle prevents accidental injection into muscle.
c. For obese patient, pinch skin at site and inject needle at 90-degree angle below tissue fold.	Obese patients have fatty layer of tissue above subcutaneous layer.

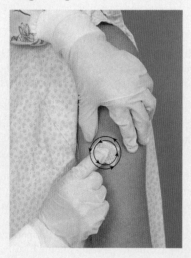

STEP 10 Clean site with circular motion.

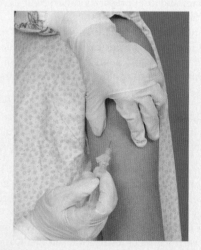

STEP 13 Hold syringe as if grasping a dart.

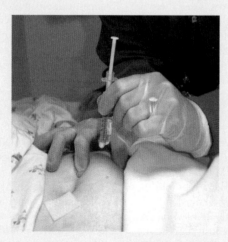

STEP 14b Subcutaneous injection. Angle and needle length depend on thickness of skinfold.

STEP	RATIONALE
d. After needle enters site, grasp lower end of syringe barrel with nondominant hand to stabilize. Move dominant hand to end of plunger and slowly inject medication over several seconds (see illustration). When giving heparin, inject over 30 seconds. Avoid moving syringe.	Movement of syringe may displace needle and cause discomfort. Slow injection of medication minimizes discomfort.

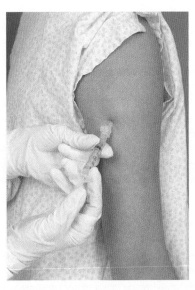

STEP 14d Inject medication slowly.

Clinical Judgment *Aspiration after injecting a subcutaneous medication is not necessary. Piercing a blood vessel in a subcutaneous injection is rare. Aspiration after injecting heparin and insulin is not recommended (CDC, 2022; Lilley et al., 2020).*

STEP	RATIONALE
e. Withdraw needle quickly while placing antiseptic swab or gauze gently over site.	Supporting tissues around injection site minimizes discomfort during needle withdrawal. Dry gauze may minimize patient discomfort associated with antiseptic on nonintact skin.
f. *Option:* When administering heparin, apply a moist ice pack over injection site and leave in place for 3 to 5 minutes.	Cold application can be an effective intervention to prevent the occurrence and reduce size of bruising in patients receiving subcutaneous heparin (Amaniyan et al., 2020).
15. Administer injection (via injection pen):	
a. Prime the insulin pen, which removes air bubbles from the needle. The pen must be primed before each injection.	Ensures that the needle is open and working.
b. To prime the insulin pen, turn the dosage knob to the 2 units indicator. With the pen pointing upward, push the knob all the way. At least one drop of insulin should appear. You may need to repeat this step until a drop appears.	
c. Select the dose of insulin that has been prescribed by turning the dosage knob.	A clicking sound is heard when the dial is turned.
d. Remove the pen cap. Insert the needle with a quick motion into the skin at a 90-degree angle. The needle should go all the way into the skin.	Safety pen needle has a removable outer cover, but the inner cover is a fixed safety shield that is not removed. The shield will be pushed back, exposing the needle as the injector is pressed against the injection site.
e. Slowly push the knob of the pen all the way in to deliver the full dose. Hold the pen at the site for 6 to 10 seconds, and then pull the needle out. Place antiseptic swab or gauze gently over site.	Supporting tissues around injection site minimizes discomfort during needle withdrawal. Dry gauze may minimize patient discomfort associated with antiseptic on nonintact skin.
f. Replace the pen cap and store at room temperature.	
16. Apply gentle pressure to site. *Do not massage site.* (If heparin is given, or if patient is on an oral anticoagulant, hold antiseptic swab or gauze to site for 30 to 60 seconds and apply ice pack.)	Aids absorption. Massage can damage underlying tissue. Time interval prevents bleeding at site. Cold pack reduces bruising.

STEP	RATIONALE

17. Discard uncapped needle or needle enclosed in safety shield and attached syringe (see illustrations) in puncture- and leak-proof receptacle.

Prevents injury to patients and health care personnel. Recapping needles increases risk for a needlestick injury (OSHA, n.d.).

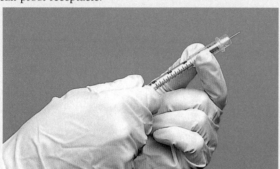 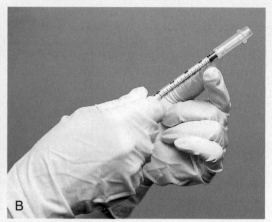

STEP 17 Needle with plastic guard to prevent needlesticks. (A) Position of guard before injection. (B) After injection, guard locks in place, covering needle.

18. Help patient to a comfortable position.

Restores comfort and sense of well-being.

19. Place nurse call system in an accessible location within patient's reach.

Ensures patient can call for assistance if needed.

20. Raise side rails (as appropriate) and lower bed to lowest position, locking into position.

Ensures patient safety and prevents falls.

21. Dispose of all contaminated supplies in appropriate receptacle, remove and dispose of gloves, and perform hand hygiene.

Reduces transmission of microorganisms.

22. Stay with patient for several minutes and observe for any allergic reactions.

Dyspnea, wheezing, and circulatory collapse are signs of severe anaphylactic reaction.

EVALUATION

1. Return to room in 15 to 30 minutes and ask if patient feels any acute pain, burning, numbness, or tingling at injection site.

Continued discomfort may indicate injury to underlying bones or nerves.

2. Inspect site, noting bruising or induration. Provide warm compress to site.

Bruising or induration indicates complication associated with injection.

3. Observe patient's response to medication at times that correlate with onset, peak, and duration of medication. Review laboratory results as appropriate (e.g., blood glucose, partial thromboplastin).

Adverse effects of parenteral medications develop rapidly. Evaluate effect of medication on basis of onset, peak, and duration of action.

4. Use Teach-Back: "I want to be sure I explained to you the reason for this subcutaneous injection. Tell me why you are receiving this injection." Revise your instruction now or develop a plan for revised patient/family caregiver teaching if patient/family caregiver is not able to teach back correctly.

Teach-back is a technique for health care providers to ensure that they have explained medical information clearly so that patients and their families understand what is communicated to them (AHRQ, 2023).

STEP	RATIONALE
Unexpected Outcomes	**Related Interventions**
1. Patient complains of localized pain, numbness, tingling, or burning at injection site.	• Assess injection site; may indicate potential injury to nerve or tissues. • Notify patient's health care provider and do not reuse site.
2. Patient displays adverse reaction with signs of urticaria, eczema, pruritus, wheezing, and dyspnea.	• Monitor patient's heart rate, respirations, blood pressure, and temperature. • Follow agency policy or guidelines for appropriate response to allergic reactions (e.g., administration of antihistamine such as diphenhydramine or epinephrine) and notify patient's health care provider immediately. • Add allergy information to patient's record.
3. Hypertrophy of skin develops from repeated subcutaneous injection.	• Do not use same anatomical area for future injections. • Instruct patient not to use site for 6 months.

Documentation

- Immediately after administration, document medication, dose, route, site, time, and date given. Sign MAR according to agency policy.
- Document any undesirable effects from the injection.
- Document patient teaching, validation of understanding, and patient's response to medication.

Hand-Off Reporting

- Report any undesirable effects from medication to patient's health care provider.

Special Considerations

Patient Education

- Instruct patient to wear medical identification bracelet indicating important medical information, including bleeding tendencies, illnesses (e.g., diabetes mellitus), and allergies.
- Patients who require daily injections need to learn techniques of self-administration (see Skill 42.6). Teach injection techniques to a family caregiver.

Pediatrics

- Clean and rotate sites in children every 48 to 72 hours or at the first sign of inflammation (Hockenberry et al., 2022).
- Provide appropriate distraction to decrease the stress of the injection.

Older Adults

- Aging patients have less elastic skin and reduced subcutaneous skinfold thickness. The upper abdominal site is the best site to use when the patient has little subcutaneous tissue.
- Oral antihyperglycemics may be of more value to the patient older than 80 years or older adults in long-term care because this population is at double the risk of insulin-related hypoglycemia.

Populations With Disabilities

- Pain can present atypically in patients with limited communication and can be difficult to recognize. When administering an injection, monitor vital signs, appearance, and behavior (Sullivan et al., 2018).
- Provide diabetes education that is adapted for patients with intellectual and developmental disabilities and their family caregivers (Sullivan et al., 2018).

Home Care

- Improper disposal of used needles and sharps in the home setting poses a health risk to the public and waste workers. Several options for safe sharps disposal at home exist, including allowing patients to transport their own sharps containers from home to collection sites (e.g., doctor's office, a hospital, a pharmacy); mailing their used syringes to a collection site (mail-back programs); syringe exchange programs; and special devices that destroy the needle on the syringe, rendering it safe for disposal (see Chapter 41).

◆ SKILL 22.4   Administering Intramuscular Injections

 Video Clip

The intramuscular (IM) injection route deposits medication into deep muscle tissue, which has a rich blood supply, allowing medication to absorb faster than by the subcutaneous route. There is an increased risk for injecting drugs directly into blood vessels when the IM route is used. Any factor that interferes with local tissue blood flow affects the rate and extent of drug absorption. In addition, if a medication is not injected correctly into a muscle, complications can arise such as abscess, hematoma, ecchymosis, pain, and vascular and nerve injury (Vicdan et al., 2019).

Nurses must use clinical judgment in determining the site, depth, needle, volume to use for a medication or vaccine, and method of administration (i.e. whether to bunch or stretch muscle tissue), according to evidence-based practice. Nurses should continue their ongoing education on IM injection practices to ensure safe injection practices (Demir & Aydin, 2021).

The viscosity of a medication, injection site, a patient's body mass index (BMI), weight, gender, and amount of adipose tissue influence needle size selection (CDC, 2022). Determine needle gauge according to the medication to be administered. Some medications, such as hepatitis B and tetanus, diphtheria, and pertussis (Tdap) immunizations, are given only intramuscularly. Use a longer and heavier-gauge needle to pass through subcutaneous tissue and penetrate deep muscle tissue (see Fig. 22.1). The choice of needle length and site of injection must be made on the basis of the size of the muscle, thickness of adipose tissue at the injection site, volume to be administered, injection technique, and depth below the muscle surface to be injected (CDC, 2022). Investigate other medication routes, especially when IM injections are ordered for patients with obesity. Note that the most common IM injections are immunizations.

Many needles available in health care settings are not long enough to reach the muscle, especially in female patients and those who are obese (Chhabria & Standford, 2022). Because most agencies have needles that range in length from only ⅜ to 1½ inches, investigate different medication routes, especially when IM injections are ordered for obese female patients.

The angle of insertion for an IM injection is 90 degrees. Muscle is less sensitive to irritating and viscous medications. An adult patient of average development tolerates 3 mL of medication into a larger muscle without severe muscle discomfort (Lilley et al., 2020). However, larger volumes of medication (4–5 mL) are unlikely to be absorbed properly. Children, older adults, and patients with a lower BMI tolerate only 2 mL of an IM injection, depending on the site. Do not give more than 1 mL to small children and older infants, and do not give more than 0.5 mL to smaller infants (Hockenberry et al., 2022).

Rotate IM injection sites to decrease the risk for hypertrophy. Emaciated or atrophied muscles absorb medication poorly, and their use should be avoided when possible. The **Z-track** method, a technique for pulling the skin during an injection, is recommended for IM injections (Ayinde et al., 2021). It prevents leakage of medication into subcutaneous tissues, seals medication in the muscle, and minimizes irritation. To use the **Z-track** method, apply the appropriate-size needle to the syringe and clean and select an IM site, preferably in a large, deep muscle (such as the ventrogluteal). Pull the overlying skin and subcutaneous tissues approximately 2.5 to 3.5 cm (1–1½ inches) laterally to the side with the ulnar side of the nondominant hand. Hold the skin in this position until you have administered the injection (Fig. 22.15A). Inject the needle deeply into the muscle, aspirate for blood return, and then inject the medication slowly for 10 seconds. **EXCEPTION:** To reduce injection site discomfort when *administering vaccines or toxoids,* the CDC (2022) guidelines state that there is no longer a need to aspirate after the needle is injected. However, follow agency policy regarding aspirating after injecting an IM needle for vaccines. Keep the needle inserted for 10 seconds to allow the medication to disperse evenly. Release the skin after withdrawing the needle. This leaves a zigzag path that seals the needle track wherever tissue planes slide across one another (see Fig. 22.15B). The medication is sealed in the muscle tissue.

Injection Sites

When selecting an IM site, determine that the site is free of pain, infection, necrosis, bruising, and abrasions. Also consider the location of underlying bones, nerves, and blood vessels and the volume of medication that you will administer. Because of the sciatic nerve location, the dorsogluteal muscle is not recommended as an injection site.

Ventrogluteal Site

The ventrogluteal muscle involves the gluteus medius; it is situated deep and away from major nerves and blood vessels. This site is the preferred and safest site for all adults, children, and infants, especially for medications that have larger volumes and are more viscous and irritating (Hockenberry et al., 2022; Vicdan et al., 2019).

Locate the ventrogluteal muscle by positioning the patient in a supine or lateral position. One way to locate the ventrogluteal muscle is by the "V" method. You position a patient in a supine or lateral position with the knee and hip flexed to relax the muscle. Use your right hand for the left hip and your left hand for the right hip. For example, if you are administering the injection into the patient's left hip, place the palm of your right hand over the greater trochanter of the patient's hip with your wrist perpendicular to the femur. Then move your thumb toward the patient's groin and your index finger toward the anterior superior iliac spine. Extend or open your middle

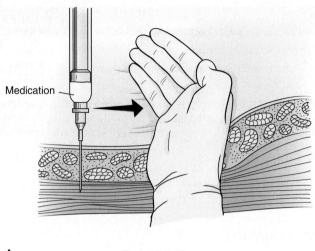

Medication

A   During injection

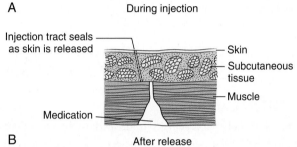

Injection tract seals as skin is released

Medication

B   After release

Skin
Subcutaneous tissue
Muscle

FIG. 22.15 (A) Pulling on overlying skin with dorsum of hand during intramuscular injection moves tissue to prevent later tracking. (B) Z-track left after injection prevents deposit of medication through sensitive tissue.

finger back along the iliac crest toward the patient's buttock. The index finger, middle finger, and iliac crest form a **V**-shaped triangle, with the injection site in the center of the triangle (Fig. 22.16A) (Larkin et al., 2018a). To relax this muscle, help patients lie on the side or back, flexing the knee and hip (see Fig. 22.16B).

Some evidence suggests that the "V" technique is not always reliable because of differences in nurses' hand structure and patients' body structure, especially when a patient has obesity (Güllu & Akgün, 2021). Therefore the "G" method, or geometric method, is another option for identifying the correct ventrogluteal site. With a patient in the side-lying position, you reference three bone prominences and draw imaginary lines between the ends of the bones. You imagine lines drawn from the patient's greater trochanter to the iliac crest, and then to the anterosuperior iliac spine, and from the greater trochanter to the anterosuperior iliac spine. Thus, a triangle is created by the imaginary lines. After that, draw median lines from every single corner of triangle to the opposite side. The convergence point of the three median lines is the center for the triangle, the needle entry point for IM injections.

Vastus Lateralis Muscle

The vastus lateralis muscle is another injection site used in adults and is an alternate site for administration of medication or biologics (e.g., immunizations) to infants, toddlers, and children (Hockenberry et al., 2022). The muscle is thick and well developed; it is located on the anterior lateral aspect of the thigh. It extends in an adult from a hand breadth above the knee to a hand breadth below the greater trochanter of the femur (Fig. 22.17A). Use the middle third of the muscle for injection. The width of the muscle usually extends from the midline of the thigh to the midline of the outer side of the thigh. With young children or frail patients, it helps to grasp the body of the

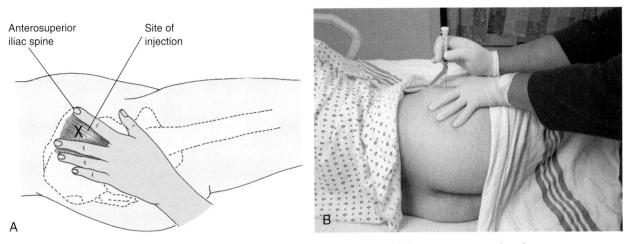

FIG. 22.16 (A) Anatomical view of ventrogluteal injection site. (B) Injection at ventrogluteal site avoids major nerves and blood vessels.

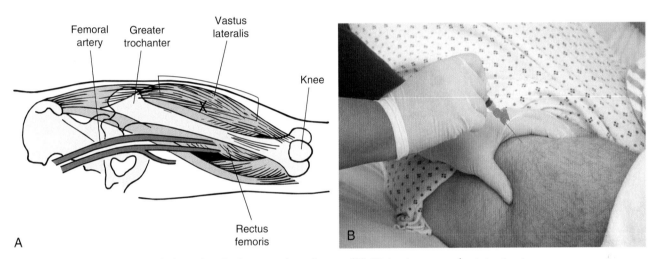

FIG. 22.17 (A) Landmarks for vastus lateralis site. (B) Giving intramuscular injection in vastus lateralis site.

muscle during injection to be sure that the medication is deposited in muscle tissue. To help relax the muscle, ask the patient to lie flat with the knee slightly flexed and foot externally rotated or to assume a sitting position (see Fig. 22.17B).

Deltoid Muscle

Although the deltoid site is easily accessible, the muscle is not well developed in many adults. There is potential for injury because the axillary, radial, brachial, and ulnar nerves and the brachial artery lie within the upper arm under the triceps and along the humerus. Use this site for small medication volumes (2 mL or less) (CDC, 2022). *Carefully assess the condition of the deltoid muscle, consult medication references for suitability of medication, and carefully locate the injection site using anatomical landmarks.* Use this site for small medication volumes; for administration of routine immunizations in toddlers, older children, and adults; or when other sites are inaccessible because of dressings or casts.

Locate the deltoid muscle by fully exposing the patient's upper arm and shoulder and asking the patient to relax the arm at the side or by supporting the patient's arm and flexing the elbow. Do not roll up any tight-fitting sleeve. Allow the patient to sit, stand, or lie down. Palpate the lower edge of the acromion process, which forms the base of a triangle in line with the midpoint of the lateral

aspect of the upper arm. The injection site is in the center of the triangle, about 3 to 5 cm (1.2–2 inches) below the acromion process (Fig. 22.18A). Locate the apex of the triangle by placing four fingers across the deltoid muscle with the top finger along the acromion process. The injection site is three finger widths below the acromion process (see Fig. 22.18B).

Delegation

The skill of administering IM injections cannot be delegated to assistive personnel (AP). Direct the AP about:
- Potential medication side effects and to immediately report their occurrence to the nurse
- Reporting any change in the patient's condition to the nurse

Interprofessional Collaboration

- The agency pharmacist can determine the smallest volume in which the medication for IM injection can be provided.

Equipment

- Proper-size syringe and sharp with engineered sharps injury protection (SESIP) needle:
  - IM: Syringe 2 to 3 mL for adult, 0.5 to 1 mL for infants and small children

- Needle length corresponding to site of injection, age, gender, and BMI of patient (see immunization guidelines below)
- Antibiotics and hormonal agents: All injection sites can be used. Child: ⅝–1¼ inch (16–32 mm); Adult: ⅝–1½ inches (16-38 mm)

NEEDLE LENGTH FOR IMMUNIZATIONS (BASED ON CDC 2022 GUIDELINES)

Site	Child	Adult
Ventrogluteal	Not recommended	1½ inches (38 mm)
Vastus lateralis (on anterolateral thigh)	⅝–1¼ inch (16–32 mm)	⅝–1 inch (16–25 mm)
Deltoid	⅝–1 inch (16–25 mm)	1½ inches (38 mm)

Gender—Male	Gender—Female	Needle Length
<60 kg (130 lb)	<60 kg (130 lb)[a]	1 inch (25 mm)
60–70 kg (130–152 lb)	60–70 kg (130–152 lb)[a]	1 inch (25 mm)
70–118 kg (152–260 lb)	70–90 kg (152–200 lb)	1-1½ inches (25–38 mm)
>118 kg (260 lb)	>90 kg (200 lb)	1½ inches (38 mm)

Age Group	Needle Length	Site
Neonates[b]	⅝ inch (16 mm)[c]	Vastus lateralis (on anterolateral thigh)
Infants, 1–12 months	1 inch (25 mm)	Vastus lateralis (on anterolateral thigh)
Toddlers, 1–2 years	1–1¼ inch (25–32 mm)	Vastus lateralis[d] (on anterolateral thigh)
	⅝[b]–1 inch (16–25 mm)	Deltoid muscle of arm
Children, 3–10 years	⅝[b]–1 inch (16–25 mm)	Deltoid muscle of arm[c]
	1–1¼ inches (25–32 mm)	Vastus lateralis (on anterolateral thigh)
Children, 11–18 years	⅝[c]-1 inch (16–25 mm)	Deltoid muscle of arm[d]
	1–1½ inches (25–38 mm)	Vastus lateralis (on anterolateral thigh)

[a]Some experts recommend a ⅝-inch needle for men and women who weigh <60 kg. If used, skin must be stretched tightly (do not bunch subcutaneous tissue).
[b]First 28 days of life.
[c]If skin is stretched tightly and subcutaneous tissues are not bunched.
[d]Preferred site.

- Needle gauge often depends on length of needle; administer antibiotics, hormones, and biological material in aqueous solution with a 22- to 25-gauge needle.

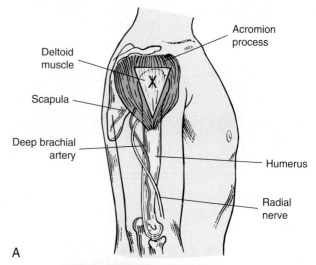

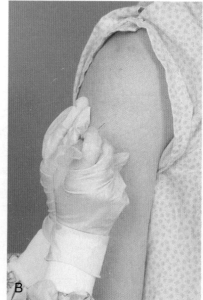

FIG. 22.18 (A) Landmarks for deltoid site. (B) Giving intramuscular injection in deltoid site.

All Injections

- Small gauze pad
- Antiseptic swab
- Vial or ampule of medication
- Clean gloves
- Medication administration record (MAR) (electronic or printed)
- Puncture-proof container for sharps

STEP	RATIONALE

ASSESSMENT

1. Check accuracy and completeness of each MAR or computer printout with health care provider's written medication order. Check patient's name, medication name and dosage, route of administration, and time of administration. Clarify incomplete or unclear orders with health care provider before administration.

The order sheet is the most reliable source and only legal record of medications that patient is to receive. Ensures that patient receives the correct medications (Palese et al., 2019). Transcription errors are a source of medication errors (Zhu & Weingart, 2022).

STEP	RATIONALE
2. Review EHR to assess patient's medical and medication history. If patient is in circulatory shock, intramuscular injection is withheld and a different route is chosen.	Determines need for medication or possible contraindications for medication administration. Reduces absorption of medication.
3. Review medication reference information for medication action, purpose, normal dose, side effects, time of peak onset, and nursing implications.	Allows you to administer medication safely and monitor patient's response to therapy.
4. Assess patient's/family caregiver's health literacy.	Determines degree to which individuals have the ability to find, understand, and use information and services to make informed health-related decisions and actions for themselves and others (CDC, 2023).
5. Ask patient to describe history of allergies: known type of allergies and normal allergic reaction. Compare information with health history. Place allergy band on patient's wrist if allergy is identified.	Do not prepare medication if there is a known patient allergy.
6. Check date of expiration for medication.	Dose potency increases or decreases when outdated.
7. Observe patient's previous verbal and nonverbal responses regarding injection (e.g., regarding fear of needles).	Anticipating patient's anxiety allows use of distraction techniques to reduce pain awareness.
8. Perform hand hygiene. Assess condition of skin at potential sites for contraindication to IM injections such as muscle atrophy, bruising, or reduced blood flow. Assess adequacy of adipose tissue.	Atrophied muscle absorbs medication poorly. Factors interfering with blood flow to muscles impair drug absorption.
9. Assess patient's symptoms before initiating medication therapy.	Provides information for you to evaluate desired effects of medication.

Clinical Judgment *Because of the documented adverse effects of IM injections, other routes of medication injection are preferred. Consider contacting health care provider for alternative route of medication administration.*

STEP	RATIONALE
10. Assess patient's knowledge, prior experience with IM injections, type of medication to receive, and feelings about procedure.	Reveals need for patient instruction and/or support.

PLANNING

STEP	RATIONALE
1. Expected outcomes following completion of procedure:	
• Patient experiences no pain or mild burning at injection site.	Medications may cause minor tissue irritation.
• Patient achieves desired effect of medication with no signs of allergies or undesired effects.	Medication administered without patient injury.
• Patient explains purpose, dosage, and effects of medication.	Demonstrates learning.
2. Provide privacy and explain medication and procedure to patient. Discuss need for and experience of receiving an IM injection. If applicable, teach patient how to report side effects.	Protects patient's privacy; reduces anxiety. Promotes cooperation.
3. Plan preparation to avoid interruptions. Create a quiet environment. Do not accept phone calls or talk with others. Follow agency "no-interruption zone" policy. Keep all pages of MARs or computer printouts for one patient together or look at only one patient's electronic MAR at a time.	Interruptions contribute to medication errors (Palese et al., 2019; Wang et al., 2021).
4. Obtain and organize equipment for IM injection at bedside.	Ensures more efficiency when completing a procedure.

IMPLEMENTATION

STEP	RATIONALE
1. Perform hand hygiene. Prepare medications for one patient at a time using aseptic technique and avoiding distractions (see Skill 22.1). Check label of medication carefully with MAR or computer printout when removing drug from storage and after preparation (see Skill 22.1 or Procedural Guideline 22.1).	Ensures that medication is sterile. *These are the first and second checks for accuracy* and ensure that correct medication is administered.
2. Take medication(s) to patient at correct time (see agency policy). Give non–time-critical scheduled medications within a range of 1 to 2 hours of scheduled dose (CMS, 2020). During administration, apply seven rights of medication administration.	Hospitals must adopt medication administration policy and procedure for timing of medication administration that considers nature of the prescribed medication, specific clinical application, and patient needs (CMS, 2020; USDHHS, 2020).

STEP	RATIONALE
3. Identify patient using at least two identifiers (e.g., name and birthday or name and medical record number) according to agency policy. Compare identifiers with information on patient's MAR or EHR.	Ensures correct patient. Complies with The Joint Commission standards and improves patient safety (TJC, 2023). Some agencies use a bar-code system as a method of patient identification.
4. At patient's bedside, again compare MAR or computer printout with names of medications on medication labels and patient name. Ask patient about allergies.	*This is the third check for accuracy* and ensures that patient receives correct medication. Confirms patient's allergy history.
5. Perform hand hygiene and apply clean gloves. Keep sheet or gown draped over body parts not requiring exposure.	Reduces transmission of infection. Respects patient's dignity while exposing injection site.
6. Position patient comfortably to access site. Select an appropriate site. Note integrity and size of muscle. Palpate for tenderness or hardness. Avoid these areas. If patient receives frequent injections, rotate sites. Use ventrogluteal if possible.	Ventrogluteal is preferred injection site for adults. It is also preferred site for children of all ages except for immunizations (Hockenberry et al., 2022; Vicdan et al., 2019).
7. Have patient maintain a comfortable position depending on chosen site (e.g., sit, lie flat, on side, or prone).	Reduces strain on muscle and minimizes injection discomfort.

Clinical Judgment *Ensure that medical condition (e.g., circulatory shock, orthopedic surgery, traumatic injury) does not contraindicate patient's position for injection.*

STEP	RATIONALE
8. Relocate site using anatomical landmarks.	Injection into correct anatomical site prevents injury to nerves, bone, and blood vessels.
9. Clean site with antiseptic swab. Apply swab at center of site and rotate outward in circular direction for about 5 cm (2 inches).	Mechanical action of swab removes secretions containing microorganisms.
a. *Option:* Apply 5% topical lidocaine-prilocaine emulsion on injection site at least 1 hour before IM injection or use vapocoolant spray (e.g., ethyl chloride) just before injection.	Decreases pain at injection site. A 5% topical lidocaine-prilocaine emulsion does not interfere with response to vaccines (CDC, 2022).
10. Hold swab or gauze between third and fourth fingers of nondominant hand.	Swab or gauze remains readily accessible for use when withdrawing needle after injection.
11. Remove needle cap or sheath by pulling it straight off.	Preventing needle from touching sides of cap prevents contamination.
12. Hold syringe between thumb and forefinger of dominant hand; hold as dart, palm down.	Quick, smooth injection requires proper manipulation of syringe parts.
13. Administer injection using Z-track method:	
a. Position ulnar side of nondominant hand just below site and pull skin laterally approximately 2.5 to 3.5 cm (1–1½ inches). Hold position while medication is injected. With dominant hand, inject needle quickly at 90-degree angle into muscle (see Fig. 22.15A).	Z-track creates zigzag path through tissues that seals needle track to avoid tracking medication. A quick dartlike injection reduces discomfort. Use Z-track for all IM injections (Ayinde et al., 2021).
b. *Option:* If patient's muscle mass is small, grasp body of muscle between thumb and forefingers.	Ensures that medication reaches muscle mass (CDC, 2022; Hockenberry et al., 2022).
c. After needle pierces skin, still pulling on skin with nondominant hand, grasp lower end of syringe barrel with fingers of nondominant hand to stabilize it. Move dominant hand to end of plunger. Avoid moving syringe.	Smooth manipulation of syringe reduces discomfort from needle movement. Skin remains pulled until after medication is injected to ensure Z-track administration.
d. Pull back on plunger 5 to 10 seconds. *Exception:* aspiration not required with administration of immunizations (CDC, 2022). If no blood appears, inject medication slowly at rate of 10 sec/mL.	Aspiration of blood into syringe indicates possible placement into a vein. Slow injection rate reduces pain and tissue trauma and reduces chance of leakage of medication back through needle track (Hockenberry et al., 2022).

Clinical Judgment *If blood appears in syringe, remove needle, dispose of medication and syringe properly, and prepare another dose of medication for injection to prevent injection of medication directly into the bloodstream.*

STEP	RATIONALE
e. Once medication is injected, wait 10 seconds, then smoothly and steadily withdraw needle, release the skin, and apply gauze with gentle pressure over site (see Fig. 22.15B). If patient is taking anticoagulants, hold antiseptic swab or gauze to site for 30 to 60 seconds. Do not massage site.	Allows time for medication to absorb into muscle before removing syringe. Dry gauze minimizes discomfort associated with antiseptic on nonintact skin. Massage damages underlying tissue.
14. Help patient to a comfortable position.	Restores comfort and sense of well-being.

STEP	RATIONALE
15. Discard uncapped needle or needle enclosed in safety shield and attached syringe into puncture- and leak-proof receptacle.	Prevents injury to patients and health care personnel. Recapping needles increases risk for needlestick injury (OSHA, n.d.).
16. Place nurse call system in an accessible location within patient's reach.	Ensures patient can call for assistance if needed.
17. Raise side rails (as appropriate) and lower bed to lowest position, locking into position.	Ensures patient safety and prevents falls.
18. Dispose of all contaminated supplies in appropriate receptacle, remove and dispose of gloves, and perform hand hygiene.	Reduces transmission of microorganisms.
19. Stay with patient for several minutes and observe for any allergic reactions.	Dyspnea, wheezing, and circulatory collapse are signs of severe anaphylactic reaction.

EVALUATION

1. Return to room in 15 to 30 minutes and ask if patient feels any acute pain, burning, numbness, or tingling at injection site.

Continued discomfort may indicate injury to underlying bones or nerves.

2. Inspect site; note any bruising or induration. *Option:* Apply warm compress to site.

Bruising or induration indicates complication associated with injection. Warm compress promotes comfort and promotes drug absorption. Document findings and notify health care provider.

3. Observe patient's response to medication at times that correlate with onset, peak, and duration of medication.

IM medications are absorbed rapidly. Adverse effects of parenteral medications develop rapidly. Evaluate effect of medication based on onset, peak, and duration of actions of medication.

4. Use Teach-Back: "I want to be sure I explained to you the things to observe for after your injection. Explain to me why you are receiving the medication/vaccine and what you might expect to happen if you have a reaction." Revise your instruction now or develop a plan for revised patient/family caregiver teaching if patient/family caregiver is not able to teach back correctly.

Teach-back is a technique for health care providers to ensure that they have explained medical information clearly so that patients and their families understand what is communicated to them (AHRQ, 2023).

Unexpected Outcomes

1. Patient complains of localized pain or continued burning at injection site, indicating potential injury to nerve or vessels.

2. During injection, blood is aspirated.

3. Patient displays adverse reaction with signs of urticaria, eczema, pruritus, wheezing, and dyspnea.

Related Interventions

- Assess injection site.
- Notify patient's health care provider.

- Immediately stop injection and remove needle.
- Prepare and administer new syringe of medication at different site.

- Follow agency policy or guidelines for appropriate response to allergic reactions (e.g., administration of antihistamine such as diphenhydramine or epinephrine).
- Notify patient's health care provider immediately.
- Add allergy information to patient's record.

Documentation

- Immediately after administration, document medication, dose, route, site, time, date given, and any adverse effects.
- Document any undesirable effects from the injection.
- Document patient teaching, validation of understanding, and patient's response to medication.

Hand-Off Reporting

- Report any undesirable effects from medication to patient's health care provider.

Special Considerations

Patient Education

- Patients who require regular injections (e.g., vitamin B_{12}) need to learn techniques of self-administration. Teach a family caregiver injection technique and the importance of rotating sites to decrease the risk for hypertrophy.
- Instruct patient and family caregiver to observe injection sites for complications and immediately report complications to the health care provider.

692 CHAPTER 22 PARENTERAL MEDICATIONS

- Instruct patient and family caregiver to observe for effectiveness of medication and adverse reactions and report ineffectiveness of medication and adverse reactions to the health care provider.
- Have patient perform several return demonstrations of medication preparation to validate that learning has taken place.

Pediatrics

- Children can be anxious or fearful of needles. Help with proper positioning and holding the child is sometimes necessary. Distraction such as blowing bubbles or a toy horn, giving the child something to hold and feel in the hands, and applying pressure over the site can be helpful in reducing anxiety (Hockenberry et al., 2022).
- Use of 5% topical lidocaine-prilocaine emulsion to reduce pain is beneficial in pediatric patients.

Older Adults

- Older patients may have decreased muscle mass, which reduces drug absorption from IM injections (Touhy & Jett, 2023). In addition, older adults may have loss of muscle tone and strength that impairs mobility, placing them at high risk for falls if they attempt to hold or guard a painful injection site.

Populations With Disabilities

- Patients with intellectual disabilities have lower rates of screening for infectious disease if they are living in residential group homes. Include this population in routine immunization programs (Sullivan et al., 2018).

Home Care

- Self-administration of an IM injection is difficult, especially in the ventrogluteal site. Teach a family caregiver to identify and administer injections in this site.
- Instruct adult patients who require frequent injections to apply 5% topical lidocaine-prilocaine emulsion to the injection site before administration.

◆ SKILL 22.5 Administering Medications by Intravenous Push

Several potential patient safety risks (e.g., incorrect dose calculation, aseptic technique, incorrect labeling, electronic pump programming errors, lack of medication knowledge, and mix-up with another medication) can occur when nurses are required to prepare medications in IV containers on patient care units (Gorski, 2023). Consequently, safety standards and evidence-based practice no longer support the practice of nurses mixing IV medications on a routine basis (Gorski, 2023; Infusion Nurses Society [INS], 2021). There are several current best practices for preparation and administration of IV medication (Box 22.4).

BOX 22.4

Best Practices for Administration of Intravenous Solutions and Medications

- Review medication orders for standardized concentrations and dosages of medication.
- Use standardized procedures for ordering, preparing, and administering IV medications.
- Administer solutions and medications prepared and dispensed from the pharmacy or as commercially prepared when possible.
- Never prepare high-alert medications (e.g., heparin, dopamine, dobutamine, nitroglycerin, potassium, antibiotics, or magnesium) on a patient care unit.
- Review medication order for use of standardized infusion concentrations of "high-alert" medications.
- Standardize the storage of IV medications.
- To help remember safety checks for administering IV medications, use the mnemonic *CATS PRRR: C*, compatibilities; *A*, allergies; *T*, tubing correct; *S*, site checked; *P*, pump safety checked; *R*, right rate; *R*, release clamps; *R*, return and reassess the patient.
- Use standardized label practices. Bold patient name, generic drug name, and patient-specific dose.
- Correctly use technology such as intelligent-infusion devices, bar code–assisted medication administration, and electronic medication administration record.

Adapted from Gorski L, et al: *Infusion therapy standards of practice*, ed 8, Norwood: Mass, 2021, Infusion Nurses Society (INS); Gorski L: *Phillips's manual of I.V. therapeutics: evidence-based practice for infusion therapy*, ed 8, Philadelphia, 2023, FA Davis; and The Joint Commission: *2022 National Patient Safety Goals hospital program*, 2022, https://www.jointcommission.org/standards/national-patient-safety-goals/.

Nurses only mix medications into IV fluids in emergency situations. The nurse *never* prepares high-alert medications (e.g., heparin, dopamine, dobutamine, nitroglycerin, potassium, antibiotics, magnesium) on a patient care unit. Check with a pharmacist before mixing a medication in an IV container. If a pharmacist confirms that you need to prepare the medication, ask another nurse to verify your medication calculations and have that nurse watch you during the entire procedure to ensure that you prepare the medication safely. First ensure that the IV fluid and medication are compatible. Then prepare the medication in a syringe using strict aseptic technique. *Do not* add medications to IV bags that are already hanging because there is no way to determine the exact concentration of the medication. Add medications *only* to new IV bags.

An IV push is a method of medication administration that introduces a concentrated dose of a medication directly into a vein by way of an existing IV access. An IV push usually requires small volumes of fluid, which is an advantage for patients who are at risk for fluid overload. Agencies have policies and procedures that identify the medications that nurses can administer by IV push and other IV routes. These policies are based on the medication, compatibility and availability of staff, and type of monitoring equipment available. There are advantages and disadvantages to administering IV push medications (Box 22.5).

An IV push poses an increased risk to the patient because it allows no time to correct errors. Administering an IV push medication too quickly can cause death. Therefore be careful in calculating the correct amount of the medication to give and the rate of administration (see agency policy or manufacturer directions). In addition, a push may cause direct irritation to the lining of blood vessels; thus placement of an IV catheter or needle should always be confirmed. Never give an IV push if the insertion site appears edematous or reddened or if the IV fluids do not flow at the ordered rate. Accidental injection of some medications into tissues surrounding a vein can cause pain, sloughing of tissues, and abscesses.

Verify the rate of administration of IV push medication using agency guidelines or a medication reference guide. Follow these strategies to reduce harm from rapid IV push medications (Gorski, 2023; Spencer, 2020):

- Use commercially available or pharmacy-prepared IV push medication whenever possible.

Advantages and Disadvantages of the Intravenous Push Method

Advantages	Disadvantages
• Barriers of absorption are bypassed. • There is rapid onset of medication effects, which is useful in patients experiencing critical or emergent health problems. • Medications can be prepared quickly and given over a shorter time than by intravenous (IV) piggyback. • Doses of short-acting medications can be titrated based on patient's needs and responses to the drug therapy. This is important for infants, children, and older patients. • Method provides a more accurate dose of medication delivered because no medication is left in intravenously.	• Not all medications can be delivered by IV push. • There is higher risk for infusion reactions; some are mild to severe because the medication action peaks quickly. • When giving medication quickly (e.g., in less than 1 minute), there is little opportunity to stop the injection if an adverse reaction occurs. • Risk for infiltration and phlebitis is increased, especially if a highly concentrated medication, a small peripheral vein, or a short venous access device is used. • Hypersensitivity reaction can cause an immediate or delayed systemic reaction to a medication, necessitating supportive measures.

- Do not dilute IV push medications unless recommended by the manufacturer, agency policy, or reference literature.
- IV push medications should be administered at the rate recommended by the manufacturer, agency policy, or reference literature.
- Appropriately label clinically prepared syringes if medication is not immediately administered by the clinician who prepares it (TJC, 2023).
- Determine the rate needed and amount of time involved to administer the medication.
- Identify all incompatibilities (i.e., drug or solution) with existing infusions.
- Review the amount of medication that a patient will receive each minute, the recommended concentration, and rate of administration. For example, if a patient is to receive 6 mL of a medication over 3 minutes, give 2 mL of the IV push medication every minute.
- Understand the purpose of the medication and any potential adverse reactions related to the rate and route of administration. Some IV medications can only be given by IV push safely when a patient is being monitored continuously for dysrhythmias, blood pressure changes, or other adverse effects. Therefore you can push some medications only in specific areas within a health care agency (e.g., critical care unit). Confirm agency guidelines regarding requirements for special monitoring.

- Develop an interprofessional agency plan for an IV push medication process improvement committee that includes nursing and pharmacy.
- Standardize terminology such as the rate in which specific IV push medications should be infused.
- Standardize where that information can be immediately found (e.g., in the medication administration record [MAR]).
- Collaborate with the pharmacy to create a "virtual kit," in which medication and the appropriate diluent, if needed, are available at the same time from the automated medication dispensing system (AMDS).
- Incorporate ISMP best practices into agency nursing policies and practice.

IV push medications are given through either an existing continuous IV infusion or an intermittent venous access (commonly called a *saline lock*). A saline lock is an IV catheter with a small "well" or chamber covered by a rubber cap. An IV catheter can be converted into a lock by inserting a special rubber-seal injection cap into the end of the catheter (see Chapter 28). Use of a lock saves time by eliminating constant monitoring of an IV line. It also offers better mobility, safety, and comfort for patients by eliminating the need for a continuous IV line. After you administer an IV push through an intermittent venous access, flush with a normal saline solution to keep it patent.

Delegation

The skill of administering medications by IV push cannot be delegated to assistive personnel (AP). Direct the AP about:
- Potential medication actions and side effects of the medications and to immediately report their occurrence to the nurse
- Reporting any patient complaints of moisture or discomfort around IV insertion site
- Obtaining any required vital signs and reporting them to the nurse

Interprofessional Collaboration

- The agency pharmacist can identify medications that require mixing/preparation by the nurse.

Equipment

- Watch with second hand
- Clean gloves
- Antiseptic swab
- Medication in vial or ampule
- Proper-size syringes for medication and saline flush with needleless device or sharp with engineered sharps injury protection (SESIP) needle (21–25 gauge)
- IV lock: Vial of normal saline flush solution (saline recommended [Gorski, 2023]); if agency continues to use heparin flush, the most common concentration is 10 units/mL; check agency policy
- Medication administration record (MAR) or computer printout
- Puncture-proof container

STEP	RATIONALE

ASSESSMENT

1. Check accuracy and completeness of each MAR or computer printout with health care provider's written medication order. Check patient's name, medication name and dosage, route of administration, and time of administration. Clarify incomplete or unclear orders with health care provider before administration.	The order sheet is the most reliable source and only legal record of medications that patient is to receive. Ensures that patient receives the correct medications (Palese et al., 2019). Transcription errors are a source of medication errors (Zhu & Weingart, 2022).

STEP	RATIONALE
2. Review EHR to assess patient's medical and medication history.	Identifies need for medication.
3. Assess relevant laboratory results (e.g., blood urea nitrogen [BUN], creatinine).	Provides baseline for measuring drug response.
4. Review medication reference information for medication action, purpose, side effects, normal dose, time of peak onset, how slowly to give medication, and nursing implications such as need to dilute medication or administer through a filter.	Knowledge of medication allows safe administration and monitoring of patient's response to therapy.
5. If you give medication through an existing IV line, determine compatibility of medication with IV fluids and any additives within IV solution.	IV medication is not always compatible with IV solution and/or additives, and a new site may need to be initiated (Gorski, 2023).
6. Perform hand hygiene. Assess condition of IV needle insertion site for signs of infiltration or phlebitis.	Do not administer medication if site is edematous or inflamed.
7. Assess patency of patient's existing IV infusion line or saline lock (see Chapter 28). Perform hand hygiene.	For medication to reach venous circulation effectively, IV line must be patent and fluids must infuse easily.
8. Assess patient's/family caregiver's health literacy.	Determines degree to which individuals have the ability to find, understand, and use information and services to make informed health-related decisions and actions for themselves and others (CDC, 2023).
9. Ask patient to describe history of allergies: known type of allergies and normal allergic reaction. Compare information with health history. Place allergy band on patient's wrist if allergy is identified.	IV push delivers medication rapidly. Allergic response, if present, is immediate.
10. Assess patient's symptoms before initiating medication therapy.	Provides information to evaluate desired effects of medication.
11. Assess patient's knowledge, prior experience with IV push administration, the medication to be received, and feelings about procedure.	Reveals need for patient instruction and/or support.

PLANNING

1. Expected outcomes following completion of procedure:	
• Patient experiences no medication side effects or adverse reactions.	Medication administered safely with desired therapeutic effect achieved.
• IV site remains intact, without signs of swelling or inflammation or symptoms of tenderness at site.	Medication infuses without complications to IV site and surrounding tissues.
• Patient explains purpose and side effects of medication.	Demonstrates learning.
2. Provide privacy and explain medication and procedure to patient. Discuss need for and sensations expected with IV push. If applicable, teach patient how to report any side effects.	Protects patient's privacy; reduces anxiety. Promotes cooperation.
3. Plan preparation to avoid interruptions. Create a quiet environment. Do not accept phone calls or talk with others. Follow agency "No-Interruption Zone" policy. Keep all pages of MARs or computer printouts for one patient together or look at only one patient's electronic MAR at a time.	Interruptions contribute to medication errors (Palese et al., 2019; Wang et al., 2021).
4. Close room door and bedside curtain.	Provides patient privacy.
5. Obtain and organize equipment for IV push infusion at bedside.	Ensures more efficiency when completing a procedure.

IMPLEMENTATION

1. Perform hand hygiene. Prepare medications for one patient at a time using aseptic technique and avoiding distractions (see Skill 22.1). Check label of medication carefully with MAR or computer printout when removing medication from storage and after preparation (see Skill 22.1 or Procedural Guideline 22.1).	Reduces transmission of microorganisms. Ensures that medication is sterile. *These are the first and second checks for accuracy* and ensure that correct medication is administered.

Clinical Judgment *Some IV medications require dilution before administration. Verify with agency policy or pharmacy if dilution is permitted. If a small amount of medication is given (e.g., less than 1 mL), dilute medication in small amount (e.g., 5 mL) of normal saline or sterile water so that it does not collect in the "dead spaces" (e.g., Y-site injection port, IV cap) of the IV delivery system.*

STEP	RATIONALE

2. Take medication(s) to patient at correct time (see agency policy). Give non–time-critical scheduled medications within a range of 1 to 2 hours of scheduled dose (CMS, 2020). During administration, apply seven rights of medication administration.

Hospitals must adopt medication administration policy and procedure for timing of medication administration that considers nature of the prescribed medication, specific clinical application, and patient needs (CMS, 2020; USDHHS, 2020)

3. Identify patient using at least two identifiers (e.g., name and birthday or name and medical record number) according to agency policy. Compare identifiers with information on patient's MAR or EHR.

Ensures correct patient. Complies with The Joint Commission standards and improves patient safety (TJC, 2023).
Some agencies use a bar-code scanning system as a method of patient identification.

4. At patient's bedside, again compare MAR or computer printout with names of medications on medication labels and patient name. Ask patient about allergies.

This is the third check for accuracy and ensures that patient receives correct medication. Confirms patient's allergy history.

5. Perform hand hygiene and apply clean gloves.

Reduces transmission of infection.

6. Administer IV push (existing IV line):

   a. Select injection port of IV tubing closest to patient. Use needleless injection port.

Follows provisions of Needlestick Safety and Prevention Act of 2001 (OSHA, n.d.).

Clinical Judgment *Never administer IV medications through tubing that is infusing blood, blood products, or parenteral nutrition solutions.*

   b. Clean injection port with antiseptic swab. Allow to dry.

Prevents transfer of microorganisms during blunt cannula insertion.

   c. *Connect syringe to IV line:* Insert needleless tip of syringe containing drug through center of port (see illustration).

Prevents introduction of microorganisms. Prevents damage to port diaphragm and possible leakage from site.

   d. Occlude IV line by pinching tubing just above injection port (see illustration). Pull back gently on plunger of syringe to aspirate for blood return.

Final check ensures that medication is being delivered into bloodstream.

Clinical Judgment *In the case of smaller-gauge IV needles, blood return sometimes is not aspirated even if IV line is patent. If IV site does not show signs of infiltration and IV fluid is infusing without difficulty, administer IV push.*

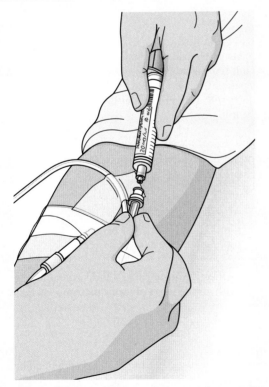

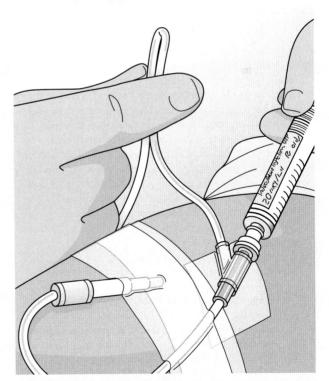

STEP 6c Connect syringe to intravenous line with needleless blunt cannula tip.

STEP 6d Occlude intravenous tubing above injection port.

STEP	RATIONALE

e. Release tubing and inject medication within amount of time recommended by agency policy, pharmacist, or medication reference manual. Use watch to time administrations (see illustration). You can pinch IV line while pushing medication and release it when not pushing medication. Allow IV fluids to infuse when not pushing medication.

Ensures safe medication infusion. Most medications are delivered slowly, between 1 and 10 minutes; for example, morphine IV push delivery of 15 mg is recommended over 4 to 5 minutes (Gorski, 2023). Rapid injection of IV drug can be fatal. Allowing IV fluids to infuse while pushing IV drug enables medication to be delivered to patient at prescribed rate.

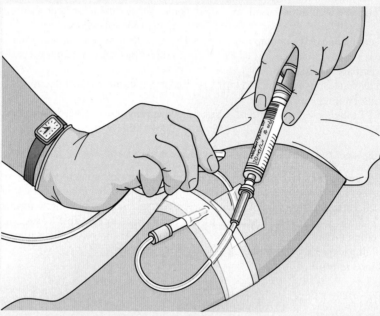

STEP 6e Use watch to time intravenous push medication.

f. After injecting medication, withdraw syringe and recheck IV fluid infusion rate.

Injection of an IV push may alter rate of fluid infusion. Rapid fluid infusion can cause circulatory fluid overload.

g. If IV medication is incompatible with IV fluids, stop IV fluids, clamp IV line, and flush with 10 mL of normal saline or sterile water (see agency policy). Then give IV push medication over appropriate amount of time and flush with another 10 mL of normal saline or sterile water at *same rate* as medication was administered.

Allows IV push to be administered without risks associated with IV incompatibilities. Ensure that agency guidelines permit flushing lines with incompatible medications. A new site may need to be initiated.

h. If current IV line is infusing a medication, disconnect it and administer IV push medication only as outlined in Step 7 below. Verify agency policy for stopping IV fluids or continuous IV medications. If unable to stop IV infusion, start new IV site (see Chapter 28) and administer medication using IV push (IV lock) method.

Avoids giving patient sudden bolus of medication in existing IV line.

7. Administer IV push (IV lock):

a. Prepare flush solutions according to agency policy.

(1) *Saline flush method (preferred method):* If current agency does not provide prefilled normal saline syringes for flushing IV lines, prepare two syringes filled with 2 to 3 mL of normal saline (0.9%). Label syringe to distinguish it from the syringe containing the medication that is being administered.

Normal saline is effective in keeping IV locks patent and is compatible with a wide range of medications (Gorski, 2023).

(2) Heparin flush method (refer to agency policy).

Many agencies no longer use heparin flush for peripheral lines (Gorski, 2023).

b. Administer medication:

(1) Clean injection port with antiseptic swab.

Prevents transfer of microorganisms during needle insertion.

(2) Insert needleless tip of syringe containing the normal saline 0.9% (or heparin if required by agency) through center of injection port of IV lock.

STEP	RATIONALE
(3) Pull back gently on syringe plunger and check for blood return.	Indicates if needle or catheter is in vein.
(4) Flush IV site by pushing slowly on plunger.	Clears needle and reservoir of blood. Flushing without difficulty indicates patent IV line.

Clinical Judgment *Carefully observe the area of skin above the IV catheter. Note any puffiness or swelling as the IV site is flushed, which could indicate infiltration into the vein, requiring removal of catheter.*

STEP	RATIONALE
(5) Remove saline-filled syringe.	
(6) Clean injection port with antiseptic swab. Allow to dry.	Prevents transmission of microorganisms.
(7) Insert needleless tip of syringe containing prepared medication through injection port of IV lock.	Allows administration of medication.
(8) Inject medication within amount of time recommended by agency policy, pharmacist, or medication reference manual. Use watch to time administration.	Many medication errors are associated with IV push medications being administered too quickly. Following guidelines for IV push rates promotes patient safety.
(9) After administering IV push, withdraw syringe.	
(10) Clean injection port with antiseptic swab. Allow to dry.	Prevents transmission of microorganisms.
(11) Flush injection port.	
(a) Attach syringe with normal saline and inject flush at same rate that medication was delivered.	Flushing IV line with saline prevents occlusion of IV access device and ensures that all medication is delivered. Flushing IV site at same rate as medication ensures that any medication remaining within IV needle is delivered at the correct rate.
8. Ensure that IV continues to run at proper hourly rate after administering medication.	Prevents fluid infusion error.
9. Dispose of SESIP covered needles and syringes in puncture- and leak-proof container.	Prevents accidental needlestick injuries and follows CDC guidelines for disposal of sharps (OSHA, n.d.).
10. Help patient to a comfortable position.	Restores comfort and sense of well-being.
11. Place nurse call system in an accessible location within patient's reach.	Ensures patient can call for assistance if needed.
12. Raise side rails (as appropriate) and lower bed to lowest position, locking into position.	Ensures patient safety and prevents falls.
13. Dispose of all contaminated supplies in appropriate receptacle, remove and dispose of gloves, and perform hand hygiene.	Reduces transmission of microorganisms. Use appropriate disposal receptacle if patient receiving hazardous drugs (Kennedy et al., 2023).
14. Stay with patient for several minutes and observe for any allergic reactions.	Dyspnea, wheezing, and circulatory collapse are signs of anaphylactic reaction.

EVALUATION

1. Observe patient closely for adverse reactions during administration and for several minutes thereafter.	IV medications act rapidly.
2. Observe IV site during injection for sudden swelling and for 48 hours after IV push.	Swelling indicates infiltration into tissues surrounding vein. Signs of infiltration may not occur for 48 hours.
3. Assess patient's status, including relevant lab test results, after giving medication to evaluate effectiveness of the medication.	Some IV medications can cause rapid changes in patient's physiological status. Some medications require careful monitoring and assessment and possibly future laboratory testing (e.g., vasopressors and antiarrhythmics require blood pressure and heart rate monitoring, and heparin requires laboratory studies after administration to determine therapeutic levels).
4. **Use Teach-Back:** "I want to be sure I explained to you why you are receiving this IV push medication. Can you explain to me what the medication is for and when to call the nurse?" Revise your instruction now or develop a plan for revised patient/family caregiver teaching if patient/family caregiver is not able to teach back correctly.	Teach-back is a technique for health care providers to ensure that they have explained medical information clearly so that patients and their families understand what is communicated to them (AHRQ, 2023).

STEP	RATIONALE
Unexpected Outcomes	**Related Interventions**
1. Patient develops adverse reaction to medication.	• Stop delivering medication immediately and follow agency policy or guidelines for appropriate response to allergic reaction (e.g., administration of antihistamine such as diphenhydramine or epinephrine) and reporting of adverse drug reactions. • Notify patient's health care provider of adverse effects immediately. • Add allergy information to patient's record.
2. IV medication is incompatible with IV fluids (e.g., IV fluid becomes cloudy in tubing) (see agency policy).	• Stop IV fluids and clamp IV line. • Flush IV line with 10 mL of 0.9% sodium chloride or sterile water. • Give IV push over appropriate amount of time. • Flush with another 10 mL of 0.9% sodium chloride or sterile water at same rate as medication was administered. • Restart IV fluids with new tubing at prescribed rate. • If unable to stop IV infusion, start new IV site (see Chapter 28) and administer medication using IV push (IV lock) method.
3. IV site shows symptoms of infiltration or phlebitis (see Chapter 28).	• Stop IV infusion immediately or discontinue access device and restart in another site. • Determine how much damage IV medication has produced in subcutaneous tissue. • Provide IV extravasation care (e.g., injecting phentolamine around IV infiltration site) as indicated by agency policy, use a medication reference, and consult pharmacist to determine appropriate follow-up care.

Documentation

- Immediately document medication administration, including drug, dose, route, time instilled, and date and time administered on MAR.
- Document patient teaching, validation of understanding, and patient's response to medication.

Hand-Off Reporting

- Report any adverse reactions to patient's health care provider. Patient response sometimes indicates need for additional medical therapy.

Special Considerations

Patient Education

- Teach patient and/or family caregiver that effects of IV push medications occur rapidly. Explain reasons for giving medication quickly and teach purpose of medication and signs of adverse effects.

Pediatrics

- The therapeutic dose of IV push medications for infants and children is often small and difficult to prepare accurately, even with a tuberculin syringe. Infuse these medications slowly and in small volumes because of the risk for fluid-volume overload (Hockenberry et al., 2022). To maintain pediatric safety, carefully follow agency guidelines when administering IV push medication.

Older Adults

- The renal and metabolic systems do not function as efficiently because of the aging process. To reduce the risk for adverse effects of IV push medications, consult appropriate references as needed to ensure knowledge regarding adverse drug effects and interactions. Older patients may tolerate IV push medications if they are given over longer periods of time.

Populations With Disabilities

- In patients with intellectual disabilities, pain may manifest atypically and be difficult to recognize. Work with the family caregiver and use adaptive tools (e.g., Noncommunicating Adult Pain Scale Checklist) to monitor for signs of pain and other symptoms (Sullivan et al., 2018).

Home Care

- IV push medications are frequently given in the home. Nurses, pharmacists, and health care providers need to collaborate closely in the care of these patients. Patients and family caregivers who are independently responsible for managing IV medications need to understand all aspects of administration safety. Adequate eyesight and manual dexterity are necessary to manipulate a syringe. Patients need to understand their venous access device, the rate at which to give medications, and how to flush their access device and maintain it.
- Educate patients and family caregivers about how to store their medications safely within their home environment, dispose of their IV supplies, and whom to contact in case of an emergency.

◆ **SKILL 22.6**   **Administering Intravenous Medications by Piggyback and Syringe Pumps**

One method of administering intravenous (IV) medications uses small volumes (25–250 mL) of IV fluids that are compatible with existing IV fluids and infused over a desired time frame. This method reduces the risk for rapid dose infusion and provides independence for patients. Patients must have an established IV line that is kept patent by either a continuous infusion or intermittent flushes of normal saline. You can administer intermittent infusion of medication with any of the following methods:

- *Piggyback.* A piggyback is a small (25- to 250-mL) IV bag or bottle connected to a short tubing line that connects to the *upper* Y-port of a primary infusion line or to an intermittent venous access such as a saline lock. The IV container that holds the medication is labeled following the IV piggyback medication format. The piggyback tubing is a microdrip or macrodrip system (see Chapter 28). The set is called a *piggyback* because the small bag or bottle is set *higher* than the primary infusion bag or bottle. In the piggyback setup, the main line does not infuse when a compatible piggybacked medication is infusing. The port of the primary IV line contains a back-check valve that automatically stops the flow of the primary infusion once the piggyback infusion flows. After the piggyback solution infuses and the solution within the tubing falls below the level of the primary infusion drip chamber, the back-check valve opens and the primary infusion starts to flow again.
- *Volume-control administration.* Volume-control administration sets (e.g., Volutrol, Buretrol, Pediatrol) are small (50- to 150-mL) containers that attach just below the primary infusion bag or bottle. The set is attached and filled in a manner similar to that used with a regular IV infusion. However, the priming filling of the set is different, depending on the type of filter (floating valve or membrane) within the set. Follow package directions for priming sets.
- *Syringe pump.* The mini-infusion pump is battery operated and delivers medication in small amounts of fluid (5–60 mL) within controlled infusion times using standard syringes.

Delegation

The skill of administering IV medications by piggyback and syringe pumps cannot be delegated to assistive personnel (AP). Direct the AP about:

- Potential medication actions and side effects and to immediately report their occurrence to the nurse
- Reporting any patient complaints of moisture or discomfort around IV insertion site
- Reporting any change in patient's condition or vital signs to the nurse

Interprofessional Collaboration

- Collaborate with agency pharmacist to ensure IV medications are properly labeled and administered.

Equipment

- Adhesive tape (optional)
- Antiseptic swab
- Clean gloves
- IV pole
- Medication administration record (MAR) or computer printout
- Puncture-proof container
- Labels—all tubing, IV bags, medications

Piggyback or Syringe Pump

- Medication prepared in 5- to 250-mL labeled infusion bag or syringe
- Prefilled syringe of normal saline flush solution (for saline lock only)
- Short microdrip, macrodrip, or mini-infusion IV tubing set with blunt-end needleless cannula attachment
- Needleless device
- Syringe pump if indicated

Volume-Control Administration Set

- Volutrol or Buretrol
- Infusion tubing with needleless system attachment
- Syringe (1–20 mL)
- Vial or ampule of ordered medication

STEP	RATIONALE

ASSESSMENT

STEP	RATIONALE
1. Check accuracy and completeness of each MAR or computer printout with health care provider's written medication order. Check patient's name, medication name and dosage, route of administration, and time of administration. Clarify incomplete or unclear orders with health care provider before administration.	The order sheet is the most reliable source and only legal record of medications that patient is to receive. Ensures that patient receives the correct medications (Palese et al., 2019). Transcription errors are a source of medication errors (Zhu & Weingart, 2022).
2. Review EHR to assess patient's medical and medication history (e.g., intake and output).	Determines need for medication or possible contraindications to medication administration.
3. Assess relevant laboratory results (e.g., blood urea nitrogen [BUN], creatinine, liver function test results).	Provides baseline for measuring drug response.
4. Review medication reference information for medication action, purpose, normal dose, side effects, time and peak of onset, how slowly to give medication, and nursing implications (e.g., need to dilute medication, administer through filter).	Allows safe medication administration and monitoring of patient's response to therapy.

STEP	RATIONALE
5. Assess patient's/family caregiver's health literacy.	Determines degree to which individuals have the ability to find, understand, and use information and services to make informed health-related decisions and actions for themselves and others (CDC, 2023).
6. Assess patient's history of allergies: known type of allergens and normal allergic reaction. Apply allergy band to patient's wrist if allergy identified.	IV administration of medication may cause rapid response. Allergic response is immediate.
7. If you give medication through existing IV line, determine compatibility of medication with IV fluids and any additional additives within IV solution.	IV medication is sometimes not compatible with IV solution and/or additives.

Clinical Judgment *Never administer IV medications through tubing that is infusing blood, blood products, or parenteral nutrition solutions.*

STEP	RATIONALE
8. To reduce the risks for administration set misconnections: **a.** Perform hand hygiene. Trace all catheters/administration sets/add-on devices between the patient and container.	Reduces transmission of microorganisms. Misconnections can occur when all connections are not checked before connecting or reconnecting infusion/device at each care transition (Gorski et al., 2021).
9. Assess patency and placement of patient's existing IV infusion line or saline lock (see Chapter 28).	Infusion line must be patent. Do not administer medication if site is edematous or inflamed.

Clinical Judgment *If patient's IV site is saline locked, clean the port with antiseptic and assess the patency of the IV line by flushing it with 2 to 3 mL of sterile sodium chloride.*

STEP	RATIONALE
10. Assess patient's symptoms before initiating medication therapy.	Provides information to evaluate desired effects of medication.
11. Assess patient's knowledge of medication, prior experience with IV piggyback or syringe pump medication, and feelings about procedure.	Reveals need for patient instruction and/or support.

PLANNING

STEP	RATIONALE
1. Expected outcomes following completion of procedure: • Patient experiences no adverse reactions. • Medication infuses within desired time frame. • IV site remains intact without signs of swelling, inflammation, or symptoms of tenderness at site. • Patient explains medication purposes, action, side effects, and dosage.	Medication was administered safely with desired therapeutic effect. IV line remains patent. Fluid infuses into vein, not tissues. Demonstrates learning.
2. Provide privacy and explain medication and procedure to patient. Discuss purpose and side effects of IV piggyback or syringe pump medications. If applicable, teach patient how to report any side effects.	Protects patient's privacy; reduces anxiety. Promotes cooperation.
3. Plan preparation to avoid interruptions. Create a quiet environment. Do not accept phone calls or talk with others. Follow agency "No-Interruption Zone" policy. Keep all pages of MARs or computer printouts for one patient together or look at only one patient's electronic MAR at a time.	Interruptions contribute to medication errors (Palese et al., 2019; Wang et al., 2021).
4. Close room door and bedside curtain.	Provides patient privacy.
5. Obtain and organize equipment for IV piggyback or syringe pump medications at bedside.	Ensures more efficient procedure.

IMPLEMENTATION

STEP	RATIONALE
1. Perform hand hygiene. Prepare medications for one patient at a time using aseptic technique and avoiding distractions (see Skill 22.1). Check label of medication carefully with MAR or computer printout at time medication is removed from storage and after preparation (see Skill 22.1 or Procedural Guideline 22.1).	Reduces transmission of microorganisms. Ensures that medication is sterile. *These are the first and second checks for accuracy* and ensure that correct medication is administered.
2. Take medication(s) to patient at correct time (see agency policy). Give non–time-critical scheduled medications within a range of 1 to 2 hours of scheduled dose (CMS, 2020). During administration, apply seven rights of medication administration.	Hospitals must adopt medication administration policy and procedure for timing of medication administration that considers nature of the prescribed medication, specific clinical application, and patient needs (CMS, 2020; USDHHS, 2020).

STEP	RATIONALE

3. Identify patient using at least two identifiers (e.g., name and birthday or name and medical record number) according to agency policy. Compare identifiers with information on patient's MAR or EHR.

Ensures correct patient. Complies with The Joint Commission standards and improves patient safety (TJC, 2023).

Some agencies use a bar-code system as a method of patient identification.

4. At patient's bedside, again compare MAR or computer printout with names of medications on medication labels and patient name. Ask patient if they have allergies.

This is the third check for accuracy and ensures that patient receives correct medication. Confirms patient's allergy history.

5. Administer infusion. Perform hand hygiene. Apply clean gloves.

Reduces transmission of microorganisms.

  a. Piggyback infusion:

    (1) Connect infusion tubing to piggyback medication bag (see Chapter 28). Fill tubing by opening regulator flow clamp. Once tubing is full, close clamp and cap end of tubing.

Filling infusion tubing with solution and freeing air bubbles prevent air embolus.

    (2) Hang piggyback (see illustration) medication bag above level of primary fluid bag. (*Option:* Use hook to lower main bag.)

Height of fluid bag affects rate of flow to patient.

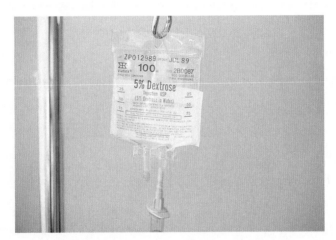

STEP 5a(2) Small-volume minibag for piggyback infusion.

(3) Connect tubing of piggyback infusion to appropriate connector on upper Y-port of primary infusion line:

Connection allows IV medication to enter main IV line.

(a) Continuous Infusion: Wipe off needleless port of main IV line with antiseptic swab and allow to dry. Then insert needleless cannula tip of piggyback infusion tubing into port (see illustrations).

Use needleless connections to prevent accidental needlestick injuries (Gorski et al., 2021; OSHA, n.d.).

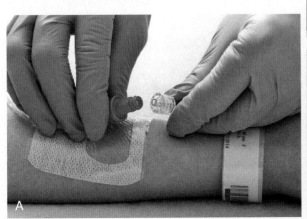 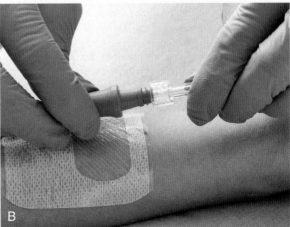

STEP 5a(3)(a) (A) Needleless lock cannula system. (B) Blunt-ended cannula inserts into port and locks.

STEP	RATIONALE
(b) *Option:* Connect tubing of piggyback infusion to normal saline lock: Follow Steps 7a(1) through 7b(6) in Skill 22.5 to flush and prepare lock. Wipe off port with antiseptic swab, let dry, and insert tip of piggyback infusion tubing into port via needleless access.	Flushing of lock ensures patency.
(4) Regulate flow rate of medication solution by adjusting regulator clamp or IV pump infusion rate. Infusion times vary. Refer to medication reference or agency policy for safe flow rate.	Provides slow, safe, intermittent infusion of medication and maintains therapeutic blood levels.
(5) Label all tubing and IV bags with your initials, patient initials, date, and time the drug was hung and when it is due to be infused.	Prevents medication errors (ISMP, 2022).
(6) Once medication has infused:	
(a) Check flow rate of primary infusion. Primary infusion automatically begins after piggyback solution is empty.	Back-check valve on piggyback prevents flow of primary infusion until medication infuses. Checking flow rate ensures proper administration of IV fluids.
(b) Check normal saline lock: Disconnect piggyback tubing, clean port of lock with antiseptic swab, and flush IV line with 2 to 3 mL of sterile 0.9% sodium chloride. Maintain sterility of IV tubing between intermittent infusions.	Prevents buildup of medication in saline lock device.
(7) Regulate continuous main infusion line to ordered rate.	Infusion of piggyback sometimes interferes with main line infusion rate.
(8) Leave IV piggyback and tubing in place for future drug administration (see agency policy) or discard in puncture- and leak-proof container.	Establishing secondary line produces route for microorganisms to enter main line. Repeated changes in tubing increase risk for infection transmission.
b. Volume-control administration set (e.g., Volutrol):	
(1) Fill Volutrol with desired amount of IV fluid (50–100 mL) by opening clamp between Volutrol and main IV bag.	Small volume of fluid dilutes IV medication and reduces risk of fluid infusing too rapidly.
(2) Close clamp and check to be sure that clamp on air vent Volutrol chamber is open.	Prevents additional leakage of fluid into Volutrol. Air vent allows fluid in Volutrol to exit at regulated rate.
(3) Clean injection port on top of Volutrol with antiseptic swab.	Prevents introduction of microorganisms during needle insertion.
(4) Remove needle cap or sheath and insert needleless tip or syringe needle of medication syringe through port and inject medication. Gently rotate Volutrol between hands.	Rotating mixes medication with solution to ensure equal distribution in Volutrol.
(5) Regulate IV infusion rate to allow medication to infuse in time recommended by agency policy, pharmacist, or medication reference manual.	For optimal therapeutic effect, medication should infuse in prescribed time interval.
(6) Label Volutrol with name of medication; dosage and total volume, including diluent; and time of administration, following ISMP (2019) safe-medication label format.	Alerts nurses to medication being infused. Prevents other medications from being added to Volutrol.
(7) If patient is receiving continuous IV infusion, check infusion rate after Volutrol infusion is complete.	Ensures appropriate rate of administration.
(8) Dispose of uncapped needle or needle enclosed in safety shield and syringe in puncture- and leak-proof container.	Prevents accidental needlesticks (OSHA, n.d.). Reduces transmission of microorganisms.
c. Syringe pump administration:	
(1) Connect prefilled syringe to mini-infusion tubing; remove end cap of tubing.	Special tubing designed to fit syringe delivers medication to main IV line.
(2) Carefully apply pressure to syringe plunger, allowing tubing to fill with medication.	Ensures that tubing is free of air bubbles to prevent air embolus.
(3) Place syringe into mini-infusion pump (follow product directions) and hang on IV pole. Be sure that syringe is secured (see illustration).	Secure placement is needed for proper infusion.

STEP	RATIONALE

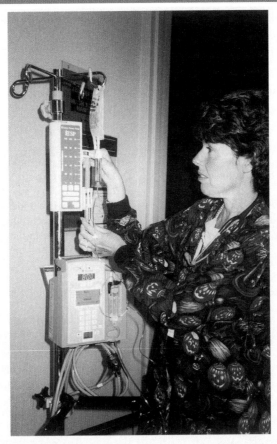

STEP 5c(3) Syringe pump. (*Courtesy and © Becton, Dickinson and Company.*)

STEP	RATIONALE
(4) Connect end of mini-infusion tubing to main IV line or saline lock:	Establishes route for IV medication to enter main IV line.
(a) *Existing IV line:* Wipe off needleless port on main IV line with antiseptic swab, allow to dry, and insert tip of mini-infusion tubing through center of port.	Needleless connections reduce risk for accidental needlestick injuries (OSHA, n.d.).
(b) *Normal saline lock:* Follow Steps 7a(1) through 7b(6) in Skill 22.5 to flush and prepare lock. Wipe off port with antiseptic swab, allow to dry, and insert tip of mini-infusion tubing.	
(5) Set pump to deliver medication within time recommended by agency policy, pharmacist, or medication reference manual. Press button on pump to begin infusion.	Pump automatically delivers medication at safe, constant rate based on volume in syringe.
(6) Once medication has infused:	
(a) *Main IV infusion:* Check flow rate. Infusion automatically begins to flow once pump stops. Regulate infusion to desired rate as needed.	Maintains patent line for primary IV fluids.
(b) *Normal saline lock:* Disconnect tubing, clean port with antiseptic swab, and flush IV line with 2 to 3 mL of sterile 0.9% sodium chloride. Maintain sterility of IV tubing between intermittent infusions.	Prevents buildup of medication in lock device.
6. Help patient to a comfortable position.	Restores comfort and sense of well-being.
7. Place nurse call system in an accessible location within patient's reach.	Ensures patient can call for assistance if needed.

STEP	RATIONALE
8. Raise side rails (as appropriate) and lower bed to lowest position, locking into position.	Ensures patient safety and prevents falls.
9. Dispose of all contaminated supplies in appropriate receptacle, remove and dispose of gloves, and perform hand hygiene.	Reduces transmission of microorganisms. Use appropriate disposal receptacle if patient is receiving hazardous drugs (Kennedy et al., 2023).
10. Stay with patient for several minutes and observe for any allergic reactions.	Dyspnea, wheezing, and circulatory collapse are signs of severe anaphylactic reaction.

EVALUATION

1. Observe patient for signs or symptoms of adverse reaction.	IV medications act rapidly.
2. During infusion, periodically check infusion rate and condition of IV site.	IV must remain patent for proper drug administration. Infiltration of IV site requires discontinuing infusion.
3. Ask patient to explain purpose and side effects of medication.	Evaluates patient's understanding of instruction.
4. **Use Teach-Back:** "I want to be sure I explained to you the reason for this IV medication. Can you explain to me why you are receiving the medication and what problems to report to the nurse?" Revise your instruction now or develop a plan for revised patient/family caregiver teaching if patient/family caregiver is not able to teach back correctly.	Teach-back is a technique for health care providers to ensure that they have explained medical information clearly so that patients and their families understand what is communicated to them (AHRQ, 2023).

Unexpected Outcomes	Related Interventions
1. Patient develops adverse or allergic reaction to medication.	• Stop medication infusion immediately. • Follow agency policy or guidelines for appropriate response to allergic reaction (e.g., administration of antihistamine such as diphenhydramine or epinephrine) and reporting of adverse medication reactions. • Notify patient's health care provider of adverse effects immediately. • Add allergy information to patient's electronic health record (EHR) per agency policy.
2. Medication does not infuse over established time frame.	• Determine reason (e.g., improper calculation of flow rate, poor positioning of IV needle at insertion site, infiltration). • Take corrective action as indicated.
3. IV site shows signs of infiltration or phlebitis (see Chapter 28).	• Stop IV infusion and discontinue access device. • Treat IV site as indicated by agency policy. • Insert new IV catheter if therapy continues. • For infiltration, determine how harmful IV medication has been to subcutaneous tissue. Provide IV extravasation care (e.g., injecting phentolamine around IV infiltration site) as indicated by agency policy or consult pharmacist to determine appropriate follow-up care.

Documentation

• Immediately document medication, dose, route, infusion rate, and date and time administered in MAR.
• Document volume of fluid in medication bag or Volutrol on intake and output (I&O) form.
• Document patient teaching, validation of understanding, and patient's response to medication.

Hand-Off Reporting

• Report any adverse reactions to patient's health care provider.

Special Considerations

Patient Education

• Review all IV medications with patient and family caregivers, including why patient is receiving the medication and potential adverse effects, including allergic responses.
• Teach patient and/or family caregivers not to alter the ordered rate of infusion without consulting the health care provider.

IV medications need to be infused at a specified rate to achieve their desired effect and avoid adverse effects.
• Teach patient and/or family caregiver to report any adverse effects immediately.

Pediatrics

• Infants and young children are more vulnerable to alterations in fluid balance and do not adjust quickly to changes. Therefore, to assess fluid balance, monitor I&O carefully when infusing IV medications (Hockenberry et al., 2022).

Older Adults

• Altered pharmacokinetics of medications and the effects of polypharmacy place older adults at risk for medication toxicity. Carefully monitor the response of older adults to IV medications, including review of renal and hepatic function laboratory data as needed (Touhy & Jett, 2023).

- Older adults are at risk for developing fluid volume overload and require careful assessment for signs of overload and heart failure.

Populations With Disabilities

- For patients with an intellectual disability, it is important to provide enough time to ensure that individuals can make their specific health concerns understood (Sullivan et al., 2018).

Home Care

- Patients or family caregivers who administer IV medications at home require education about the steps of medication administration. The patient or family caregiver needs to perform several return demonstrations of IV medication administration before performing this skill independently. In addition, patients and family caregivers need to know signs of IV medication administration complications such as phlebitis and infiltration and what to do if problems occur.

✦ SKILL 22.7 Administering Medications by Continuous Subcutaneous Infusion

The continuous subcutaneous infusion (CSQI or CSCI) route of medication administration is used for selected medications (e.g., opioids, insulin, and meds used to stop preterm labor [e.g., terbutaline] and to treat pulmonary hypertension [treprostinil sodium]). The benefits of this route include providing a route for patients with poor venous access, providing pain relief to patients who are unable to tolerate oral pain medications, and allowing patients greater mobility and better pain control (than IM injections) (Khoury et al., 2022). A medication administered by CSQI usually has a faster onset of action than oral routes. One factor that determines the infusion rate of CSQI is the rate of medication absorption. Most patients can absorb up to 5 mL/h of medication, but the rate of absorption is more dependent on osmotic pressure than rate of administration (Gorski et al, 2021).

Patients with diabetes mellitus who use CSQI for management of blood glucose levels receive intense diabetes self-management education from qualified diabetes educators and insulin pump trainers. A new system, Medtronic MiniMed, integrates an insulin pump with real-time continuous glucose monitoring (Fig. 22.19). Patients with diabetes mellitus who use insulin pumps generally require less insulin because it is absorbed and used more efficiently (Weinstock, 2022). Box 22.6 lists criteria for selecting insulin pumps for patient use.

The procedure to initiate and discontinue CSQI therapy is similar, regardless of the type of medication being delivered. Use a small-gauge (25–27) winged butterfly intravenous (IV) needle or special commercially prepared Teflon cannula to deliver medications. Although Teflon cannulas generally are more expensive, they are more comfortable for the patient and have lower rates of complications than winged IV needles. The cannulas are associated with fewer needlestick injuries. Base the choice of needle type on agency guidelines or patient preference. Use the needle with the shortest length and the smallest gauge necessary to establish and maintain the infusion.

The upper, anterior chest wall above the breast, away from the axilla or the abdomen, is the preferred site for CSQI therapy (Griffin, 2021). Site selection depends on a patient's activity level and the type of medication delivered. For example, pain medications given to ambulatory patients are best delivered in the upper chest, which allows a patient to move freely. Insulin is absorbed most consistently in the abdomen; in this case choose a site in the abdomen away from the waistline. Always avoid sites where the tubing of the pump could be disturbed. Rotate sites used for medication administration at least every 2 to 7 days or whenever complications, such as leaking, occur (Gorski et al, 2021).

The CSQI route requires a computerized pump with safety features, including lockout intervals and warning alarms. Ideally,

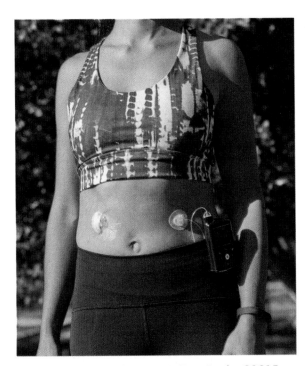

FIG. 22.19 MiniMed Paradigm REAL-Time Insulin CSQI Pump and Continuous Glucose Monitoring System. (*Copyright © 2023 Medtronic. All rights reserved. Used with the permission of Medtronic.*)

BOX 22.6

Patient Selection Criteria for Use of Insulin Pumps

- Possesses strong motivation and commitment to use diabetes management skills
- Requires or desires improved control of blood glucose levels
- Requires greater flexibility than allowed by traditional insulin injection schedules
- Is willing and able to participate in a formal diabetes education program
- Possesses strong critical thinking and problem-solving skills
- Accepts responsibilities associated with the self-management of diabetes
- Can perform self–blood glucose monitoring and operate the insulin pump
- Displays evidence of effective coping patterns
- Has family support systems available
- Secures financial resources to cover costs associated with CSQI

CSQI, Continuous subcutaneous infusion.
Data from American Diabetes Association (ADA): Diabetes care in the hospital: standards of medical care in diabetes—2019, *Diabetes Care* 42(S1):S173, 2019.

medication pumps are individualized on the basis of the medication being delivered and a patient's needs. You also need to consider the availability and cost of the pump and its supplies. When possible, have patients select the pump that fits their individual and home needs and is easiest to use.

Delegation

The skill of administering CSQI medications cannot be delegated to assistive personnel (AP). Direct the AP about:

- Potential medication side effects or reactions and to immediately report their occurrence to the nurse
- Reporting complications (e.g., leaking, redness, discomfort) at the CSQI needle insertion site to the nurse
- Obtaining any required vital signs and reporting them to the nurse

Interprofessional Collaboration

- The agency pharmacist, diabetes educator, and pain specialist should be involved in the management of CSQI.

Equipment

Initiation of CSQI

- Clean gloves
- Antiseptic swab
- CSQI-designed catheter/needle (e.g., Quick-Set, Saf-T-Intima, Auto Soft) with adhesive disk or small (25- to 27-gauge) winged IV catheter with attached tubing
- Infusion pump
- Occlusive, transparent dressing
- Tape
- Medication in appropriate syringe or container
- Medication administration record (MAR) or computer printout

Discontinuing CSQI

- Clean gloves
- Small, sterile gauze dressing
- Tape or adhesive bandage
- Antiseptic swab
- Puncture-proof container

STEP	RATIONALE

ASSESSMENT

1. Check accuracy and completeness of each MAR or computer printout with health care provider's written medication order. Check patient's name, medication name and dosage, route of administration, and time of administration. Clarify incomplete or unclear orders with health care provider before administration.

The order sheet is the most reliable source and only legal record of medications that patient is to receive. Ensures that patient receives the correct medications (Palese et al., 2019). Transcription errors are a source of medication errors (Zhu & Weingart, 2022).

2. Review EHR to assess patient's medical and medication history.

Determines need for medication or possible contraindications for medication administration.

3. Assess for contraindications to CSQI (e.g., history of thrombocytopenia or reduced local tissue perfusion).

Any existing coagulation disorder contraindicates heparin infusion. Reduced tissue perfusion interferes with medication absorption and distribution.

4. Review EHR for the following factors: neonates and older adults; dry skin; dehydration; malnutrition; certain medications, such as long-term use of corticosteroids, chemotherapeutic agents, and antiinflammatory agents; dermatological conditions; and underlying medical conditions that affect the skin (e.g., diabetes, immunosuppression).

Risk factors for developing medical adhesive–related skin injuries (MARSIs) from transparent dressing and/or adhesive patch (Fumarola et al., 2020). Presence of factors requires diligent monitoring of skin.

5. Collect drug reference information necessary to administer drug safely, including action, purpose, side effects, normal dose, time of peak onset, rate setting for pump, and nursing implications.

Knowledge of medication allows safe medication administration and monitoring of patient response to therapy.

6. Assess patient's/family caregiver's health literacy.

Determines degree to which individuals have the ability to find, understand, and use information and services to make informed health-related decisions and actions for themselves and others (CDC, 2023).

7. Assess patient's history of allergies: known type of allergens and normal allergic reaction. Place allergy band on patient's wrist if allergy is identified.

CSQI administration of medications may cause rapid response. Allergic response is immediate.

8. Assess patient's previous verbal and nonverbal response to needle insertion (Does patient fear needles?).

Anticipating patient's anxiety allows use of distraction techniques to reduce pain awareness.

9. If an analgesic is being administered, assess character of patient's pain and rate severity on a pain scale (i.e., from 0 to 10, with 0 being no pain and 10 being the worst pain ever experienced).

Provides an objective measure of pain severity.

10. Perform hand hygiene. Assess adequacy of patient's adipose tissue to determine appropriate infusion site. If previous insertion site exists, assess for redness, maceration, or skin tear.

Physiological changes of aging or patient illness influence amount of subcutaneous tissue, which affects choice of catheter insertion site. Signs of MARSI (Fumarola et al., 2020).

STEP	RATIONALE
11. Assess patient's knowledge, prior experience with CSQI, and feelings about procedure.	Reveals need for patient instruction and/or support.

PLANNING

STEP	RATIONALE
1. Expected outcomes following completion of procedure: • Needle insertion site remains free from infection.	Risk for infection at needle insertion site is potential complication of CSQI therapy.
• Patient achieves desired effect of medication with no signs of adverse reactions.	Medication is delivered safely with desired therapeutic effect achieved.
• Patient explains purpose, dosage, and effects of medication and verbalizes understanding of CSQI therapy.	Demonstrates learning.
2. Provide privacy and explain procedure to patient. Discuss need for and what to anticipate with the initiation of CSQI. If applicable, teach patient how to perform cannula insertion.	Protects patient's privacy, reduces anxiety, promotes cooperation.
3. Plan preparation to avoid interruptions. Create a quiet environment. Do not accept phone calls or talk with others. Follow agency "No-Interruption Zone" policy. Keep all pages of MARs or computer printouts for one patient together or look at only one patient's electronic MAR at a time.	Interruptions contribute to medication errors (Palese et al., 2019; Wang et al., 2021).
4. Review manufacturer directions for how to use pump.	Ensures proper use of equipment.
5. Obtain and organize equipment for CSQI at bedside.	Ensures more efficiency when completing a procedure.

IMPLEMENTATION

STEP	RATIONALE
1. Review manufacturer directions for how to use pump and infusion set. **NOTE:** Insertion steps for infusion set will vary by type of device used.	Ensures proper use of equipment.
2. Perform hand hygiene. Check label of medication carefully with MAR or computer printout when removing medication from storage and after preparation. **NOTE:** You will prepare the medication by either a syringe or reservoir transfer device (see Step 7a) that comes with a commercial infusion set.	*These are the first two checks for accuracy* ensuring that correct medication is administered.
3. At bedside, identify patient using at least two identifiers (e.g., name and birthday or name and medical record number) according to agency policy. Compare identifiers with information on patient's MAR or EHR.	Ensures correct patient. Complies with The Joint Commission standards and improves patient safety (TJC, 2023). Some agencies use a bar-code system as a method of patient identification.
4. At patient's bedside, again compare MAR or computer printout with name of medication on label of syringe and patient name. Ask patient again about allergies.	*This is the third check for accuracy* and ensures that patient receives correct medication. Confirms patient's allergy history.
5. Position patient comfortably, supine or sitting. Drape extremities.	Respects patient's dignity.
6. Perform hand hygiene. Program infusion pump. If not using a commercial infusion set device, prepare infusion tubing of needle by priming with syringe filled with medication.	Ensures that medication dose administered is accurate. Reduces transmission of microorganisms. Prevents air from entering subcutaneous tissue.
7. Prepare commercial infusion set: a. For a commercial device such as a Quik Set, use the transfer device and reservoir that comes with the set. Fill reservoir with the prescribed medication per device directions.	Reservoir holds a dose of medication that will usually last 2 to 3 days (e.g., insulin).
b. Once reservoir is full, remove the transfer device used to fill the reservoir. Discard in appropriate receptacle.	Reduces transmission of microorganisms.
c. Connect reservoir to the tubing of the infusion pump. Most pumps contain a compartment for the reservoir. Turn on pump and fill tubing following manufacturer's guidelines or directions shown on pump screen. Most pumps will show a message when pump is successfully filled.	Priming of tubing prevents air from entering subcutaneous tissue. Ensures proper pump function.
d. Prepare cannula/needle insertion device per manufacturer's directions. Most cannulas/needles come in an insertion device.	Insertion device ensures ease of cannula/needle insertion without contamination.

STEP	RATIONALE

8. Initiate CSQI:

a. Perform hand hygiene and apply clean gloves. Select appropriate injection site free of irritation and away from bony prominences and waistline. Most common sites used are the subclavicular area and abdomen. Choose site that patient can access. Note condition of skin around proposed insertion site.

Ensures proper medication absorption. Provides baseline for condition of skin.

b. Clean injection site with antiseptic swab. Apply swab at center of site and rotate outward in a circular direction for about 5 cm (2 inches). Allow to dry.

Reduces risk for infection at insertion site.

c. Commercial device (see illustration):

(1) Remove guard to expose cannula/needle in insertion device. (**NOTE:** Some devices also require removal of adhesive backing from disk that will secure cannula/needle.)

Prepares needle for insertion. Ensures needle will enter subcutaneous tissue.

(2) Hold insertion device against the prepared site on patient's skin.

Delivers cannula/needle into subcutaneous tissue.

(3) Follow manufacturer's directions and push down on device, inserting cannula/needle into the skin.

(4) Once cannula/needle is in place, pull inserter away from the body and press adhesive disk surrounding the cannula/needle against the skin.

Secures cannula/needle.

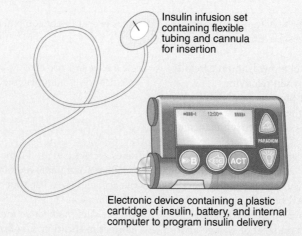

Insulin infusion set containing flexible tubing and cannula for insertion

Electronic device containing a plastic cartridge of insulin, battery, and internal computer to program insulin delivery

STEP 8c Insulin pump with a disposable reservoir for insulin (inside the pump) and a disposable infusion set (with tubing and a cannula for subcutaneous insertion). (*From Hobson RP, Ralston SH, Penman ID, Strachan MWJ: Davidson's principles and practice of medicine, ed 23, St. Louis, 2018, Elsevier.*)

d. Winged needle:

(1) If using a winged needle attached to prepared pump and tubing, pinch skin at insertion site, and then gently and firmly insert needle at a 45- to 90-degree angle. Refer to manufacturer's directions.

Decreases pain related to insertion of needle. Angle ensures subcutaneous tissue placement.

(2) Release skinfold and apply gentle pressure around adhesive disk. *Option:* Cover with transparent semipermeable membrane (TSM).

Secures needle.

9. Initiate medication infusion:

a. Commercial device: Be sure cannula/needle is secure. Turn on pump and check infusion rate.

Ensures correct dose administration.

b. Winged needle: Attach tubing from needle to tubing from infusion pump and turn on pump. Check infusion rate.

10. Inspect site before leaving patient and instruct patient to inform you if site becomes red or swollen or begins to leak.

Initiate new site with new needle whenever erythema or leaking occurs. If site is free from complications, rotate needle every 2 to 7 days (Gorski et al, 2021). Adhesive may cause MARSI (Fumarola et al., 2020).

STEP	RATIONALE
11. Help patient to a comfortable position.	Restores comfort and sense of well-being.
12. Place nurse call system in an accessible location within patient's reach.	Ensures patient can call for assistance if needed.
13. Raise side rails (as appropriate) and lower bed to lowest position, locking into position.	Ensures patient safety and prevents falls.
14. Dispose of all contaminated supplies in appropriate receptacle, remove and dispose of gloves, and perform hand hygiene.	Reduces transmission of microorganisms.
15. Discontinue CSQI:	
a. Verify order and establish alternative method for medication administration if applicable.	If medication will be required after discontinuing CSQI, a different medication and/or route is often necessary to continue to manage patient's illness or pain.
b. Stop infusion pump.	Prevents medication from spilling.
c. Perform hand hygiene and apply clean gloves.	Follows CDC recommendations to prevent accidental exposure to blood and body fluids (OSHA, n.d.).
d. Remove disk: Gently loosen a corner of the dressing. Lift off disk while removing needle from skin at same angle it was inserted.	
e. Remove tape from wings of needle or remove transparent dressing without dislodging or removing needle and without pulling skin. *Option:* Remove nonbordered transparent membrane dressing by loosening a corner of the dressing and stretching it horizontally in the opposite direction of the wound (stretch and relax technique). Walk fingers under the dressing to continue stretching it. One hand should continuously support the skin adhered to the dressing. The process can be repeated around the dressing (Fumarola et al., 2020). Discard tape/dressing in appropriate receptacle. Pull needle out at same angle at which it was inserted.	Exposes needle. Minimizes risk of MARSI during removal. Minimizes patient discomfort.
f. Apply gentle pressure at site until no fluid leaks out of skin.	Dressing adheres to site if skin remains dry.
g. Apply small sterile gauze dressing or adhesive bandage to site.	Prevents bacterial entry into puncture site.
h. Help patient to a comfortable position.	Restores comfort and sense of well-being.
i. Place nurse call system in an accessible location within patient's reach.	Ensures patient can call for assistance if needed.
j. Raise side rails (as appropriate) and lower bed to lowest position, locking into position.	Ensures patient safety and prevents falls.
k. Dispose of all contaminated supplies in appropriate receptacle, remove and dispose of gloves, and perform hand hygiene.	Reduces transmission of microorganisms. Use appropriate disposal receptacle if patient is on hazardous drugs (Kennedy et al., 2023).

EVALUATION

1. Evaluate patient's response to medication.	Determines effect of therapy. Decreased or absent response to medication may indicate that patient is not receiving medication into subcutaneous tissue (e.g., pump malfunction, medication leaking at site).
2. Assess site at least every 4 hours for redness, pain, drainage, or swelling.	Indicates infection at insertion site. Inflammation and maceration can be result of medical adhesive–related skin injury (Fumarola et al., 2020).
3. **Use Teach-Back:** "I want to be sure you understand how the continuous infusion of the medication into your skin works and benefits you. Tell me in your own words why you have a continuous infusion and what to look for if a problem develops." Revise your instruction now or develop a plan for revised patient/family caregiver teaching if patient/family caregiver is not able to teach back correctly.	Teach-back is a technique for health care providers to ensure that they have explained medical information clearly so that patients and their families understand what is communicated to them (AHRQ, 2023).

STEP	RATIONALE
Unexpected Outcomes	**Related Interventions**

1. Patient complains of localized pain or burning at insertion site; or site appears red or swollen or is leaking, indicating potential infection, MARSI, or needle dislodgement.	• Remove needle and place new needle in different site.
	• Continue to monitor original site for signs of infection and notify health care provider if you suspect infection.
	• Provide good skin care (Fumarola et al., 2020):
	  • Avoid washing the skin too much and use a pH-balanced soap substitute to avoid drying the skin.
	  • Hydrate the skin to ensure the patient drinks enough water to prevent dehydration.
	  • Use emollient as a moisture barrier.

2. Patient displays signs of allergic reaction to medication.	• Stop delivering medication immediately and follow agency policy or guidelines for appropriate response to allergic reaction (e.g., administration of antihistamine such as diphenhydramine or epinephrine) and reporting of adverse drug reactions. • Notify patient's health care provider of adverse effects immediately. • Add allergy information to EHR.
3. CSQI cannula becomes dislodged.	• Stop infusion, apply pressure at site until no fluid leaks out of skin, cover site with gauze dressing or adhesive bandage, and initiate new site. • Assess patient to determine effects of not receiving medication (e.g., assess patient's pain level using age-appropriate pain scale, obtain blood glucose level).

Documentation

• After initiating CSQI, immediately document medication, dose, route, site, time, date, and type of medication pump.
• If medication is an opioid, follow agency policy to document waste.
• Document patient's response to medication and appearance of site every 4 hours or according to agency policy.
• Document patient teaching, validation of understanding, and patient's response to medication.

Hand-Off Reporting

• Report any adverse effects from medication or infection or MARSI at insertion site to patient's health care provider, and document according to agency policy. Patient's condition often indicates need for additional medical therapy.

Special Considerations

Patient Education

• Instruct patient to wear medical alert bracelet along with medical information, including disease (e.g., diabetes), allergies, and a contact phone number for the pump manufacturer for technical support.
• Instruct patients to carry backup batteries and extra medication if they are going to be away from home.
• Patients receiving insulin require intensive diabetes management education (Box 22.7).
• Never immerse pumps in water or expose them to x-rays or magnetic resonance imaging.

Pediatrics

• Insulin pumps offer flexibility for adolescents, allowing them to assume the responsibility of diabetes management. Extensive patient and family education is needed in using CSQI (Hockenberry et al., 2022).

BOX 22.7

Education Topics for Patients Receiving Insulin With Continuous Subcutaneous Infusion (CSQI)

• Blood glucose monitoring
• Meal planning and food choices
• Incorporating exercise into daily routine
• How to program and use the insulin pump
• Illness guidelines and management
• Management of hypoglycemia
• Prevention and management of hyperglycemia
• Prevention of infection, especially at CSQI infusion site
• Problem-solving and decision-making skills when pump malfunctions
• Special considerations and precautions (e.g., what to do with pump when showering and sleeping)

Adapted from American Diabetes Association (ADA): Diabetes care in the hospital: standards of medical care in diabetes—2019, *Diabetes Care* 42(S1): S173, 2019; Griffin, K: *Guidelines for subcutaneous infusion device management in palliative care and other settings,* ed 3, Queensland, Australia, 2021, Queensland Health, Centre for Palliative Care Research and Education.

• Clean and rotate sites in children every 48 to 72 hours or at the first sign of inflammation (Hockenberry et al., 2022).

Older Adults

• Hypodermoclysis (the subcutaneous infusion of fluids) is an easy-to-use, safe, and cost-effective alternative to IV hydration for older adults (Touhy & Jett, 2023).

Populations With Disabilities

• Patients with cognitive impairment experienced less agitation when receiving CSQI than traditional IV therapy (Caccialanza et al., 2018).

Home Care

- Patients in the home using CSQI need a responsible family caregiver if available. Educate the patient or family caregiver about the desired effect of the medication, side effects and adverse effects of the medication, operation of the pump, how to evaluate the effectiveness of the medication, when and how to assess and rotate insertion sites, and when to call a health care provider if problems occur. Patients need to know where and how to obtain and dispose of all required supplies.
- Patients managing CSQI at home may use an antibacterial soap (e.g., Hibiclens, pHisoHex) instead of alcohol or chlorhexidine to cleanse the insertion site.

◆ CLINICAL JUDGMENT AND NEXT-GENERATION NCLEX® EXAMINATION–STYLE QUESTIONS

The nurse is developing a plan of care for a patient with type I diabetes, an infection, and thrombophlebitis who is receiving antibiotics and heparin every 8 hours. The heparin comes prepared from the pharmacy in a single-dose vial.

1. Which aspect of the patient's care can the nurse delegate to assistive personnel (AP)?
   1. Report any noted signs of bleeding.
   2. Assess response to heparin.
   3. Compare medication orders with pharmacy-dispensed heparin.
   4. Draw up medication to prepare for injection.
2. While hospitalized, the patient is to receive the Mpox vaccine intradermally (ID). After cleaning the site, which action will the nurse take **next**?
   1. Watch for creation of a bleb upon injection.
   2. Advance needle through epidermis to 3 mm.
   3. Using nondominant hand, stretch skin over site with forefinger.
   4. Insert needle at a 5- to 15-degree angle into skin until resistance is felt.
3. The experienced nurse is watching a new nurse prepare to give the patient an injection with a medication that comes in an ampule. Which of the following actions by the new nurse requires the experienced nurse to intervene? **Select all that apply.**
   1. Prepares to use the filter needle for administration
   2. Checks the ampule against the medication administration record
   3. Breaks the ampule at the colored, prescored ring around the neck
   4. Uses filter needle to prepare medication from a glass ampule
   5. Applies a separate needle to the syringe after withdrawing medication
   6. Identifies patient by bar-coded arm band and medical record number before injection
   7. Returns ampule to medication bin after drawing up dose for administration
4. The nurse is preparing to administer an IV push medication to the patient who has a compatible IV fluid running through IV tubing. Which action will the nurse take **next** after cleaning the injection port site?
   1. Release tubing and inject medication.
   2. Pull back gently on syringe plunger to aspirate blood return.
   3. Connect syringe to port of IV line.
   4. Occlude IV line by pinching tubing just above injection port.
5. When the patient is to be discharged, the nurse provides teaching about taking heparin at home. Which information will the nurse provide?
   1. If minimal bruising occurs, seek emergency care.
   2. Periodic laboratory work will need to be performed.
   3. Use a hard toothbrush to remove all plaque, which can lead to infection.
   4. Most supplements available over the counter can be used while on heparin therapy.

Visit the Evolve site for answers to Clinical Judgment and Next-Generation NCLEX® Examination–Style Questions.

REFERENCES

Agency for Healthcare Research and Quality (AHRQ): *Teach-back: intervention*, 2023. https://www.ahrq.gov/patient-safety/reports/engage/interventions/teach-back.html.

American Diabetes Association (ADA): *Insulin basics*, n.d., https://diabetes.org/health-wellness/medication/insulin-basics. Accessed October 12, 2023.

American Diabetes Association (ADA): *Insulin routines*, 2022. https://www.diabetes.org/healthy-living/medication-treatments/insulin-other-injectables/insulin-routines. Accessed October 12, 2023.

Amaniyan S: Cold application on bruising at the subcutaneous heparin injection site: a systematic review and meta-analysis, *SAGE Open J* 6:2377960820901370, 2020. https://journals.sagepub.com/doi/full/10.1177/2377960820901370. Accessed May 16, 2023.

Antoszyk A, et al: Usability of the ranibizumab 0.5 mg prefilled syringe: human factors studies to evaluate critical task completion by healthcare professionals, *PDA J Pharm Sci Technol* 72:411, 2018.

Ayinde O, et al: The effect of intramuscular injection technique on injection associated pain; a systematic review and meta-analysis, *PLoS One* 16(5):e0250883, 2021.

Burchum J, Rosenthal L: *Lehne's pharmacology for nursing care*, ed 11, St. Louis, 2022, Elsevier.

Caccialanza R, et al: Subcutaneous infusion of fluids for hydration or nutrition: a review, *J Parenter Enteral Nutr* 42(2):296, 2018.

Centers for Disease Control and Prevention (CDC): *CDC Clinical Reminder – Insulin pens must never be used for more than one person*, n.d.a. https://www.cdc.gov/injectionsafety/PDF/Clinical-Reminder-insulin-pen.pdf.

Centers for Disease Control and Prevention (CDC): *CDC guideline for prescribing opioids for chronic pain*, n.d.b. https://www.cdc.gov/drugoverdose/pdf/guidelines_at-a-glance-a.pdf.

Centers for Disease Control (CDC): *Mantoux tuberculin skin test*, n.d.c. https://www.cdc.gov/tb/education/mantoux/pdf/mantoux_tb_skin_test.pdf. Accessed October 12, 2023.

Centers for Disease Control and Prevention (CDC): *Vaccine recommendations and guidelines of the Advisory Committee on Immunization Practices (ACIP)*, 2022. https://www.cdc.gov/vaccines/hcp/acip-recs/general-recs/administration.html.

Centers for Disease Control and Prevention (CDC): *What is health literacy?* 2023. https://www.cdc.gov/healthliteracy/learn/index.html.

Centers for Medicare & Medicaid Services (CMS): *State operations manual appendix a–survey protocol, regulations and interpretive guidelines for hospitals*, 2020. https://www.cms.gov/Regulations-and-Guidance/Guidance/Manuals/downloads/som107ap_a_hospitals.pdf. Accessed May 15, 2023.

Chhabria S, Stanford F: A long shot: the importance of needle length in vaccinating patients with obesity against COVID-19, *Vaccine* 40(1):9–10, 2022.

Demir, SO, Aydin AK: Investigation of nurses' knowledge of intramuscular injections and factors affecting injection site preference: a case-based survey, *Int J Caring Sci* 13(3):1578, 2021.

Fumarola S, et al: Overlooked and underestimated: medical adhesive-related skin injuries. Best practice consensus document on prevention, *J Wound Care* 29(Suppl 3c):S1–S24, 2020.

Giger JN, Haddad L: *Transcultural nursing: assessment and intervention*, ed 8, St. Louis, 2021, Mosby.

Gorska-Ciebiada M, et al: Improved insulin injection technique, treatment satisfaction and glycemic control: Results from a large cohort education study, *J Clin Transl Endocrinol* 4(19):100217, 2020.

Gorski L: *Phillips's manual of I.V. therapeutics: evidence-based practice for infusion therapy*, ed 8, Philadelphia, PA, 2023, FA Davis.

Gorski L, et al: *Infusion therapy standards of practice*, ed 8, Norwood: Mass, 2021, Infusion Nurses Society (INS), Journal of Infusion Nursing.

Griffin K: *Guidelines for subcutaneous infusion device management in palliative care and other settings*, ed 3, Queensland, Australia, 2021, Queensland Health, Centre for Palliative Care Research and Education.

Güllu A, Akgün S: The effect of training on the "V" and "G" techniques used in the ventrogluteal site and injection application to this site on the knowledge level of nurses, *IAIM* 8(8):15–33, 2021.

Hockenberry MJ, et al: *Wong's essentials of pediatric nursing*, ed 11, St. Louis, 2022, Elsevier.

Holliday RM, et al: Body mass index: a reliable predictor of subcutaneous fat thickness and needle length for ventral gluteal intramuscular injections, *Am J Ther* 26(1):e72–e78, 2019.

Institute for Safe Medication Practices (ISMP): *ISMP safety enhancements every hospital must consider in wake of another tragic neuromuscular blocker event*, 2019. https://www.ismp.org/resources/safety-enhancements-every-hospital-must-consider-wake-another-tragic-neuromuscular.

Institute for Safe Medication Practices (ISMP). *ISMP targeted medication safety best practices for hospitals*, 2022. https://www.ismp.org/search/node?keys=ISMP+target ed+medication+safety+best+practices+for+hospitals%2C+. Accessed October 12, 2023.

Institute for Safe Medication Practices (ISMP): *ISMP's list of error-prone abbreviations, symbols, and dose designations*, 2021. https://www.ismp.org/recommendations/error-prone-abbreviations-list.

Kennedy K, et al: Safe handling of hazardous drugs. *J Oncol Pharm Prac* 29(2): 401–412, 2023.

Khoury J, et al: Evaluation of efficacy and safety of subcutaneous acetaminophen in geriatrics and palliative care, BMC *Palliat Care* 21:42, 2022.

Larkin T, et al: Comparison of the V and G methods for ventrogluteal site identification: muscle and subcutaneous fat thickness and considerations for successful intramuscular injection, *Int J Ment Health Nurs* 27(2):631, 2018a.

Larkin T, et al: Influence of gender, BMI, and body shape on theoretical injection outcome at the ventrogluteal and dorsogluteal sites, *J Clin Nurs* 27(1-2):E242, 2018b.

Lilley LL, et al: *Pharmacology and the nursing process*, ed 9, St. Louis, 2020, Mosby.

Najmi U, et al: Inpatient insulin pen implementation, waste, and potential cost savings: a community hospital experience, *J Diabetes Sci Technol* 15(4): 741–747, 2021.

Occupational Safety and Health Administration (OSHA): *Bloodborne pathogens and needlestick prevention*, n.d. https://www.osha.gov/SLTC/bloodbornepathogens/index.html.

Pahal P, Sharma S: *PPD skin test*, Treasure Island (FL), 2022, StatPearls Publishing.

Palese A, et al: "I am administering medication-please do not interrupt me": red tabards preventing interruptions as perceived by surgical patients, *J Patient Safe* 15(1):30, 2019.

Rahamimov N, et al: Inadequate deltoid muscle penetration and concerns of improper COVID mRNA vaccine administration can be avoided by injection technique modification, *Vaccine* 39(37):5326–5330, 2021.

Ramamoorthy A, Kim H, Shah-Williams E, Zhang L: Racial and ethnic differences in drug disposition and response: review of New molecular entities approved between 2014 and 2019, *J Clin Pharmacol* 62(4):486–493, 2022.

Sebro R: Statistical estimation of deltoid subcutaneous fat pad thickness: implications for needle length for vaccination, *Sci Rep* 12:1069, 2022.

Spencer C: I.V. Push medication administration: bridging education and practice through standardization, *Am Nurse J*: ANA, 2020. https://www.myamericannurse.com/i-v-push-medication-administration-bridging-education-and-practice-through-standardization/. Accessed October 9, 2023.

Sperling M, Laffel L: Current management of glycemia in children with Type 1 diabetes mellitus, *N Engl J Med* 386:1155–1164, 2022.

Sullivan W, et al: Primary care of adults with intellectual and developmental disabilities: clinical practice guidelines, *Can Fam Physician* 64:254, 2018.

The Joint Commission (TJC): *2023 National patient safety goals*, Oakbrook Terrace, IL, 2023, The Joint Commission. https://www.jointcommission.org/standards/national-patient-safety-goals/.

Touhy TA, Jett KF: *Ebersole and Hess' toward healthy aging*, ed 11, St. Louis, 2023, Elsevier.

Unahalekhaka A, Nuthong P: Glass particulate adulterated in single dose ampoules: a patient safety concern, *J Clin Nurs* 32:1135–1139, 2023.

U.S. Department of Health and Human Services, Centers for Medicare & Medicaid (USDHHS): *Updated guidance on medication administration, Hospital Appendix A of State Operations Manual*, Baltimore, 2020, Department of Health and Human Services.

Vicdan A, et al: Evaluation of the training given to the nurses on the injection application to the ventrogluteal site: a quasi-experimental study, *Int J Caring Sci* 12(3):1467, 2019.

Wang W, et al: Current status and influencing factors of nursing interruption events, *Am J Manag Care* 27(6):e188–e194, 2021.

Weinstock R: *General principles of insulin therapy in diabetes mellitus*, 2022, UpToDate. http://www.uptodate.com/contents/general-principles-of-insulin-therapy-in-diabetes-mellitus. Accessed May 13, 2023.

Zhu J, Weingart S: *Prevention of adverse drug events in hospitals*, 2022. https://www.uptodate.com/contents/prevention-of-adverse-drug-events-in-hospitals. Accessed October 12, 2023.

UNIT 8
Medication Administration:
Next-Generation NCLEX® (NGN)–Style
Unfolding Case Study

PHASE 1

QUESTION 1.

A 65-year-old client underwent left hip replacement surgery yesterday and is currently recovering on the surgical unit. The client has an intravenous (IV) solution running in the left hand of D5 ½NS at 75 mL/hr and has a left hip soft silicone dressing in place. VS: T 37°C (98.6°F); HR 88 beats/min: RR 18 breaths/min. Pain assessment is currently 8 on a 0-to-10 scale. The client has a long history of insulin-dependent diabetes mellitus.

Select the **3** assessment findings that require follow-up by the nurse:

o Has no history of chronic health problems except diabetes mellitus
o Small amount of serosanguineous drainage present on surgical dressing
o Reports left hip pain of 8 on a 0-to-10 pain intensity scale
o Easily arousable
o Heart rate = 88 beats/min
o Blood pressure = 152/90 mm Hg
o Current blood sugar is 140 mg/dL

QUESTION 2.

A 65-year-old client underwent left hip replacement surgery yesterday and is currently recovering on the surgical unit. The client has an intravenous (IV) solution running in the left hand of D5 ½NS at 75 mL/hr and has a left hip soft silicone dressing in place. VS: T 37°C (98.6°F); HR 88 beats/min; RR 18 breaths/min. Pain assessment is currently 8 on a 0-to-10 scale after being moved in bed. Morphine 2 mg subcutaneously is ordered for pain and glargine 10 units subcutaneously once per day. The client has a long history of insulin-dependent diabetes mellitus. The nurse documents the following assessment findings:

• Has no history of chronic health problems except diabetes mellitus
• Client is familiar with taking glargine at home
• Small amount of serosanguineous drainage present on surgical dressing
• Reports left hip pain of 8 on a 0-to-10 pain intensity scale
• Easily arousable
• Heart rate = 88 beats/min
• Blood pressure = 152/90 mm Hg
• Current blood sugar is 140 mg/dL

Complete the following sentences by selecting from the lists of options below.

Based on the client's assessment data, the nurse determines that the client's vital sign findings are due to **1 [Select]** and **1 [Select]**. The client's blood sugar reading is caused by **2 [Select]** and the blood pressure reading is due to **3 [Select]**.

Options for 1	Options for 2	Options for 3
Incisional infection	Morphine	Postoperative pain
Anxiety	Incisional pain	Glargine
Recent movement in bed	IV D5 ½NS	Immobility
Postoperative stress	Glargine	Morphine
Blood sugar changes	Age	Age
Anesthesia side effects	Blood pressure reading	Anesthesia side effects

PHASE 2

QUESTION 3.

A 65-year-old client underwent left hip replacement surgery yesterday and is currently recovering on the surgical unit; the client has a history of diabetes mellitus. An hour after receiving morphine subcutaneously, the client states that pain in hip is a 4 on a 0-to-10 pain intensity scale when moving in bed with assistance. A repeat blood sugar reading is now 162 mg/dL, and client is to receive a supplemental dose of 10 units of regular insulin subcutaneously now. The health care provider has ordered low molecular weight heparin (LMWH) 5000 units subcutaneously now and every 12 hours.

When planning care for this client, for which **priority** potential complications would the nurse monitor? **Select all that apply.**

o Deep vein thrombosis
o Incisional infection
o Hypoglycemia
o Bleeding
o Hypotension
o Constipation
o Urinary tract infection
o Anxiety
o Hyperglycemia

QUESTION 4.

A 65-year-old client underwent left hip replacement surgery yesterday and is currently recovering on the surgical unit; the client has a history of diabetes mellitus. An hour after receiving morphine subcutaneously, the client states that pain in hip is a 4 on a 0-to-10 pain intensity scale when moving in bed with assistance. A repeat blood sugar reading is now 162 mg/dL, and client is to receive a supplemental dose of 10 units of regular insulin subcutaneously now. The health care provider has ordered low molecular weight heparin (LMWH) 5000 units subcutaneously now and every 12 hours. Client states being confused about the need for so many injections for the hip repair, and the client has several questions about the care.

Indicate which nursing response listed in the far left column is appropriate for each client question. Note that not all responses will be used.

Nurse's Responses	Client Questions	Appropriate Nurse's Response for Each Client Question
1 "Since you are not yet up and walking, you need to keep your blood moving in your body."	"How long am I going to need this injection in my stomach?"	
2 "You need to move and exercise your hip to help prevent clots."	"Will I need to have these injections at home?"	
3 "You will not need any medications to prevent clots at home as long as you are able to move and walk and remain mobile."	"My neighbor had a broken leg and stayed in bed to prevent clots from moving from her legs. So why do I need to move?"	
4 "You will be able to move and walk with a walker for a while until the physical therapist tells you not to use it any longer."	"Can I take a bath when I get home?"	
5 "You may bathe or shower when you are up to it as long as you cover your incision to prevent moisture."	"When will I be able to bear weight on this hip?"	
6 "You will not be able to bear weight on your surgical hip side for several weeks."		
7 "You will not be able to get out of bed for several weeks"		
8 "Clients on this medication might need to remain on it for a lifetime."		

PHASE 3

QUESTION 5.

A 65-year-old client underwent left hip replacement surgery 3 days ago and is currently recovering on the surgical unit; the client has a history of diabetes mellitus. The client continues on the ordered glargine subcutaneously once per day but now must use supplemental regular insulin subcutaneously until they see the surgeon in 6 weeks. The client is also going home on warfarin orally for 4 weeks. The nurse provides health teaching for the client and family in preparation for discharge.

Determine whether the health teaching items are indicated, not indicated, or non-essential before the client's discharge at this time.

Health Teaching	Indicated	Not Indicated	Non-Essential
"Do not mix the glargine and regular insulin in the same syringe."			
"You may store the insulin in the refrigerator if not in use."			
"Inject the insulin when it is cold from the refrigerator."			
"Rotate the insulin injection sites between the abdomen and outer thigh."			
"There is no need to check your urine or stool for blood."			
"Be careful with OTC medications such as aspirin and herbal additions such as garlic and ginger."			
"Inspect your injection sites every day for increased redness, heat, or drainage; if any of these are present, call your surgeon immediately."			

QUESTION 6.

A 65-year-old client underwent left hip replacement surgery 3 days ago and is currently recovering on the surgical unit; the client has a history of diabetes mellitus. The client continues on ordered glargine subcutaneously once per day but now must use supplemental regular insulin subcutaneously until they see the surgeon in 6 weeks. The client is also going home on warfarin 5 mg orally for 4 weeks. The nurse provides health teaching for the client and family in preparation for discharge.

Determine whether the interventions were effective, not effective, or unrelated.

Evaluation Finding	Effective	Not Effective	Unrelated
Injection sites show no sign of infection			
Reports increased pain in left hip			
Draws up both insulin glargine and regular in same syringe			
Uses different sites for insulin injections			
Reports having periods of anxiety			
States that cannot see the markings on the insulin syringe			

UNIT 9
Oxygenation

The skills commonly used to support oxygenation are those that improve either ventilation or respiratory gas exchange. Clinical judgment in the care of patients with impaired oxygenation involves assessing patient data, analyzing clinical cues, identifying the patients' problems, and determining the appropriate nursing interventions to improve the patient's oxygenation status. Knowledge of a patient's clinical condition, how it affects the physiology of normal gas exchange and ventilation, and experience in caring for patients with similar alterations will assist not only in knowing what to assess but also in selecting appropriate interventions. Experience is vital in knowing how to adapt skills to meet a patient's unique needs. For example, when conditions such as abdominal surgery or traumatic rib fracture occur, you will learn that the associated pain of these conditions reduces lung expansion and ventilation. With less air moving through airways, oxygenation is also reduced. Interventions for maximizing ventilation (e.g., positioning) and pain control (analgesia) become care priorities. When a patient's condition directly affects gas exchange (e.g., pneumonia, bronchitis, flu), potential interventions for maximizing oxygenation include administration of oxygen therapy, airway management (e.g., suctioning, coughing exercises, chest physiotherapy), and fluid hydration to thin secretions.

The following example illustrates impaired oxygenation. Your patient has pneumonia, and you are told that the patient is diaphoretic and tachycardic, has a fever and thick sputum, and has difficulty coughing. Use critical thinking to reflect on your knowledge about normal lung function and the pathophysiology of pneumonia causing inflammation and accumulation of airway secretions. Focus your assessment and collect data to confirm reported findings. Look for additional cues, such as temperature 38.9°C (102°F), respiratory rate 26 breaths/min, pulse 110 beats/min, SpO_2 85%, blood pressure 100/80 mm Hg, pallor, inability to clear airway with coughing, and abnormal lung sounds. Analysis of these cues indicates that the patient has poor airway clearance and reduced gas exchange. Based on the patient's problems, use clinical judgment to identify individualized nursing interventions to improve oxygenation (e.g., oxygen therapy) and airway management (e.g., suctioning).

The clinical condition of patients with impaired oxygenation can change very quickly. Thorough ongoing focused assessment is critical to monitoring a patient closely and knowing the physiological changes to expect so as to conduct correct and timely assessments. In addition, any respiratory problem can have consequences that affect a patient's cardiac status. Sometimes the consequences can be life threatening, necessitating knowledge and skill in implementing emergency life-support measures.

23 | Oxygen Therapy

SKILLS AND PROCEDURES

Skill 23.1 **Applying an Oxygen-Delivery Device, p. 720**

Skill 23.2 **Administering Oxygen Therapy to a Patient With an Artificial Airway, p. 727**

Skill 23.3 **Using Incentive Spirometry, p. 730**

Skill 23.4 **Care of a Patient Receiving Noninvasive Positive Pressure Ventilation, p. 734**

Procedural Guideline 23.1 **Use of a Peak Flowmeter, p. 739**

Skill 23.5 **Care of a Patient on a Mechanical Ventilator, p. 742**

OBJECTIVES

Mastery of content in this chapter will enable you to:
- Discuss indications for oxygen therapy.
- Compare and contrast the different types of oxygen therapy.
- Discuss safe practices when administering oxygen therapy.
- Demonstrate the application of an oxygen-delivery device.
- Demonstrate how to obtain peak expiratory flow rate (PEFR) measurements.
- Demonstrate how to properly use incentive spirometry.
- Demonstrate how to properly care for a patient receiving noninvasive positive pressure ventilation (NIPPV).
- Demonstrate how to properly care for a patient receiving invasive mechanical ventilation.

MEDIA RESOURCES

- http://evolve.elsevier.com/Perry/skills
- Review Questions
- Audio Glossary
- ▶ Video Clips
- Case Studies
- Answers to Clinical Judgment and Next-Generation NCLEX® Examination–Style Questions
- Skills Performance Checklists
- Printable Key Points

PURPOSE

Oxygen is necessary for the body's organs and tissues to function properly. When there is a disturbance in oxygenation resulting from ineffective gas exchange or ventilation, hypoxia and hypoxemia develop. When patients show signs of hypoxia or hypoxemia, such as dyspnea, tachypnea, tachycardia, or anxiety, use clinical judgment. This involves assessing the patient's physical condition as well as medical history, medications, and physiology of the pulmonary system to identify nursing diagnoses and choosing interventions that treat the cause of decreased oxygenation. Apply the skills in this chapter that are most appropriate for the nature of the patient's oxygenation problem.

PRACTICE STANDARDS

- American Association of Critical Care Nurses (AACN), 2018: AACN Practice Alert: Prevention of Aspiration in Adults, 2018 Update
- Restrepo R, Walsh B, 2022update: American Association for Respiratory Care (AARC) Clinical Practice Guideline: Humidification During Invasive and Noninvasive Mechanical Ventilation

- The Joint Commission (TJC), 2023: National Patient Safety Goals—Patient identification, infection prevention

SUPPLEMENTAL STANDARDS

- American Thoracic Society (ATS), 2020: Oxygen Therapy
- Lewarski, 2021: Brief Review of the ATS CPG: Home Oxygen Therapy for Adults with Chronic Lung Disease

PRINCIPLES FOR PRACTICE

- Oxygen therapy is used in a variety of conditions to treat hypoxia, which is a condition in which there is insufficient oxygen to meet the metabolic demands of the tissues (Box 23.1).
- Hemoglobin is the carrier of respiratory gases: oxygen (O_2) and carbon dioxide (CO_2). Hemoglobin combines with the gas to carry it to and from the cells. Decreased hemoglobin levels reduce the amount of oxygen transported to the cells and carbon dioxide transported away from the cells, which can lead to hypoxia and hypercarbia (increased concentration of CO_2 in blood).
- Hemoglobin levels and acid-base status directly affect oxygenation. Acidemia increases the ability of hemoglobin to release

Signs and Symptoms Associated With Acute Hypoxia

- Apprehension, anxiety, behavioral changes
- Decreased level of consciousness, confusion, drowsiness, altered concentration
- Increased pulse rate (**NOTE:** In patients with late-stage cardiac disease, the pulse rate may not increase.)
- Cardiac dysrhythmias
- Elevated blood pressure, evolving to decreased blood pressure
- Increased rate and depth of respiration or irregular respiratory patterns
- Increased work of breathing, use of accessory muscles of respiration, retractions, nasal flaring
- Increased fatigue
- Decreased lung sounds, adventitious lung sounds (e.g., crackles, wheezes)
- Pulse oximetry (SpO_2) less than 90%
- Dyspnea
- Pallor, cyanosis (Cyanosis is a late sign associated with acute hypoxia.)
- Dizziness

oxygen to the tissues. Alkalemia decreases the ability of hemoglobin to release oxygen to the tissues.

- Pain and anxiety increase a patient's oxygen needs. Therefore assess patient's pain, character of respirations, pulse oximetry (SpO_2) values, level of consciousness (LOC), and observed behaviors reflecting anxiety (Hockenberry et al., 2024; Harding et al., 2023).
- Fever increases the body's metabolic rate and, in turn, oxygen demand.
- Treat oxygen as a medication. As with any drug, continuously monitor the dosage or concentration of oxygen and routinely check the health care provider's orders to verify that the patient is receiving the prescribed oxygen concentration. Follow the seven rights of medication administration when administering oxygen (see Chapter 20).
- Oxygen therapy must be carefully administered in certain patients to reduce the risk for respiratory failure. For example, patients with obstructive respiratory diseases require a low supplemental oxygen to avoid decreasing the normal respiratory drive and elevated carbon dioxide levels, which leads to respiratory failure; and in patients with certain types of congenital heart defects, oxygen affects blood flow through the heart and lungs.

PERSON-CENTERED CARE

- Take time to explain to a patient and family caregiver the oxygen setup and necessary safety precautions needed when oxygen is in use.
- Ensure that patients and visitors understand signs posted in the room or hallway about the presence of oxygen therapy.
- Safely accommodate valued practices of cultural groups when caring for patients with disturbances in oxygenation. For example, some cultures burn incense to promote healing of ill members. However, the smell of the incense can induce bronchospasm in certain patients. Oxygen is highly flammable, but members of some cultures who light candles to celebrate or honor holidays may accept the use of battery-operated candles while in a hospital. When oxygen is used in the home, designate areas where patients can safely burn incense or light candles. Collaborate with family caregivers and religious leaders about how to accommodate these practices during illness and recovery.

EVIDENCE-BASED PRACTICE

High-Flow Nasal Cannula

High-flow nasal cannula (HFNC) is a relatively new method of oxygen delivery. It provides humidified oxygen through a nasal cannula at flow rates as high as 60 L/min while an air-oxygen blender allows for the titration of the FiO_2. The cannula is typically larger in diameter than the standard nasal cannula (see Skill 23.1). HFNC is used to treat respiratory failure and exacerbations of chronic pulmonary disease; early evidence also indicates that there is less need for invasive ventilation in patients who are initially treated with HFNC (Li et al., 2023; Xia et al., 2022; Xu et al., 2018). In addition, HFNC can improve hypoxemia in patients after esophagectomy (Xia et al., 2021).

HFNC used for the treatment of acute respiratory failure with hypoxemia and/or hypercapnia has increased over the past decade, particularly in intensive care units (Rochwerg et al., 2019). Some patients who had severe respiratory failure associated with COVID-19 received oxygen therapy via HFNC. The results of HFNC as a treatment for COVID-19 yielded mixed results, and analysis is ongoing. Some patients improved, but there was little or no change in length of intubation and hospital stay (Beran et al., 2022).

HFNC provides an inspired oxygen concentration (FiO_2) from 21% to 100% at flow rates up to 60 L/min. Recent evidence suggests that the use of HFNC is a safe treatment for respiratory failure and decreases the need for tracheal intubation (Kim et al., 2018; Li et al., 2023; Rochwerg et al., 2019). Its use also shows higher patient satisfaction and comfort when compared with noninvasive ventilation (NIV) (Li et al., 2023; Renda et al., 2018). Nursing care for patients with HFNC includes:

- Prongs should not completely occlude the nares of the patient.
- When using heated high-flow nasal cannula (HHFNC), the temperature of the oxygen should be set at 37°C.
- Individualize flow settings during HFNC treatment and titrate flow based on clinical findings such as oxygenation, respiratory rate (RR), and patient comfort (Kim et al, 2018; Li et al., 2023).
- Heart rate, respiratory rate, and oxygen saturation levels should be continuously monitored.

SAFETY GUIDELINES

- Treat supplemental oxygen therapy as a medication.
- Know a patient's baseline range of vital signs and pulse oximetry (SpO_2) values. Patients with sudden changes in their vital signs, LOC, or behavior are possibly experiencing profound hypoxemia. Patients who demonstrate subtle changes over time have worsening of a chronic or existing condition or a new medical condition.
- Know a patient's most recent hemoglobin values and past and current arterial blood gas (ABG) values.
- Identify conditions that increase a patient's risk for aspiration of gastric contents into the lung, resulting in airway obstruction or pneumonia. These include the presence of enteral feeding tubes or nasal and oral gastric tubes, a decreased LOC, and a decreased swallowing ability (AACN, 2018).
- Be aware of environmental conditions. Patients with chronic respiratory diseases have difficulty maintaining optimal oxygen levels in polluted environments.
- Document a patient's smoking history. Smoking damages the mucociliary clearance mechanism of the lungs and paralyzes the ciliary action, resulting in a decreased ability to clear mucus from the airways.

- Chronic lung diseases, such as obstructive pulmonary diseases, are often caused by smoking and result in pooling of mucus in the airways, creating an environment for infections. Ultimately, long-term chronic lung diseases result in hypoxia.
- Have working suction equipment available to help clear airway secretions, particularly in patients with artificial airways such as an endotracheal (ET) tube or tracheostomy.
- Most agencies require that a self-inflating resuscitation bag and appropriate-size mask be available in patient rooms, particularly for patients requiring mechanical ventilation.
- If a patient is to receive home oxygen therapy, complete an environmental assessment to determine respiratory hazards in the home, such as the use of gas stoves or kerosene space heaters or the presence of smokers in the home (see Chapter 41).
- Provide education to patient and family about safe home oxygen therapy so they understand proper use of the equipment (Box 23.2). Stress the importance of home safety measures for oxygen use (see Chapter 41).

◆ SKILL 23.1 Applying an Oxygen-Delivery Device

 Video Clip

Various diseases (e.g., pneumonia, chronic lung diseases such as bronchitis and chronic obstructive pulmonary disease [COPD]) require the use of oxygen therapy. Pneumonia results in impaired gas exchange because of fluid and secretions in the lung, which decreases the diffusion of oxygen from the lungs to the arterial blood supply. Patients with chronic lung diseases often require home oxygen therapy. These patients may require oxygen 24 hours a day; therefore care is taken to plan administration around patient needs (ATS, 2020; Huether et al., 2020).

Oxygen therapy is inexpensive, widely available, and used in a variety of settings. Selection of the type of oxygen-delivery system is based on a patient's need for oxygen support, the severity of the hypoxia/hypoxemia, and the disease process. Consider other factors such as the patient's age and developmental level, level of health and orientation, presence of an artificial airway, setting (home or hospital), type of home environment, and type of support and care needed after discharge.

Oxygen-delivery devices are classified into either high-flow or low-flow devices, depending on how much oxygen they deliver to the patient. Health care providers determine how much oxygen a device should deliver as well as the desired effects on the patient's respiratory pattern when choosing an oxygen-delivery device. High-flow devices include Venturi mask (Fig. 23.1), large-volume nebulizers, and blender masks and an HFNC (Fig. 23.2). Low-flow devices include nasal cannula (Fig. 23.3) and simple face mask (Fig. 23.4), and nonrebreather and partial rebreather masks (Fig. 23.5). These devices deliver set percentages of oxygen, and each one has advantages and disadvantages. You can estimate approximate FiO_2 by the flow rate (Table 23.1).

An oxygen flowmeter regulates the flow rate in liters per minute (Fig. 23.6). There are a variety of oxygen sources used in health care facilities, ranging from wall connections at the patient's bedside or cylinders or oxygen tanks. In addition, smaller, easily transported cylinders are available for home oxygen therapy. Patients using home oxygen commonly use concentrators, some of which are portable.

Several types of oxygen cannula are used to deliver oxygen to patients (see Table 23.1). A nasal cannula is a simple, effective,

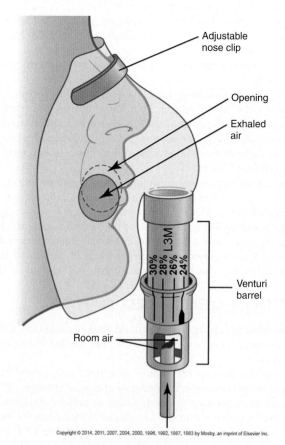

Copyright © 2014, 2011, 2007, 2004, 2000, 1996, 1992, 1987, 1983 by Mosby, an imprint of Elsevier Inc.

FIG. 23.1 Venturi mask.

and comfortable device for delivering oxygen (see Fig. 23.3). It allows a patient to breathe through the mouth or nose, is available for all age-groups, and is adequate for short- or long-term use. The two tips of the cannula, about 1.5 cm (½ inch) long, protrude from the center of a disposable tube and are inserted into the nostrils.

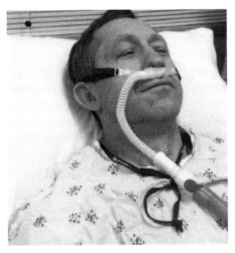

FIG. 23.2 High-flow nasal cannula. (*Courtesy Fisher & Paykel Healthcare.*)

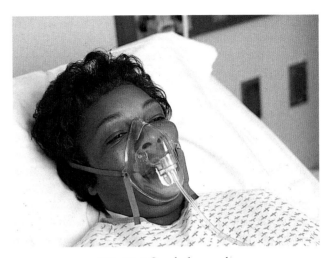

FIG. 23.4 Simple face mask.

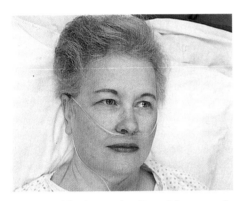

FIG. 23.3 Nasal cannula adjusted for proper fit.

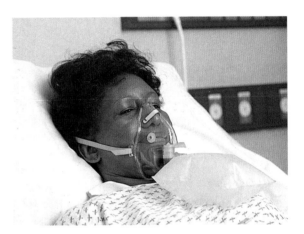

FIG. 23.5 Plastic face mask with reservoir bag.

TABLE 23.1

Oxygen-Delivery Systems

Delivery System	FiO$_2$ Delivered	Advantages	Disadvantages
Low-Flow Delivery Devices			
Nasal cannula	1–6 L/min: 24%–44%	Safe and simple Easily tolerated Effective for low concentrations Does not impede eating or talking Inexpensive, disposable	Unable to use with nasal obstruction Drying of mucous membranes Can dislodge easily May cause skin irritation or breakdown Patient's breathing pattern affects exact FiO$_2$
Oxygen-conserving cannula	8 L/min: up to 30%–60%	Indicated for long-term O$_2$ use in the home Allows increased O$_2$ concentration and lower flow	Cannula cannot be cleaned More expensive than standard cannula
Simple face mask	6–12 L/min: 35%–50%	Useful for short periods of time such as patient transportation	Contraindicated for patients who retain CO$_2$ May induce feelings of claustrophobia Therapy interrupted with eating or drinking Increased risk for aspiration
Partial nonrebreather (Bag should always remain partially inflated. Therefore flow rate must be high enough to prevent collapse of bag.)	10–15 L/min: 60%–90%	Useful for short periods Delivers increased FiO$_2$ Easily humidifies O$_2$ Does not dry mucous membranes	Hot and confining; may irritate skin; tight seal necessary Interferes with eating and talking Bag may twist or kink; should not totally deflate

Continued

TABLE 23.1

Oxygen-Delivery Systems—cont'd

Delivery System	FiO$_2$ Delivered	Advantages	Disadvantages
High-Flow Delivery Devices			
Venturi mask	24%–50%	Provides specific amount of O$_2$ with humidity added Administers low, constant O$_2$	Mask and humidity may irritate skin Interferes with eating, drinking, and talking
High-flow nasal cannula	Adjustable FiO$_2$ (0.21–1.0) with a modifiable flow (up to 60 L/min)	Wide range of FiO$_2$; can use on adults, children, and infants	FiO$_2$ dependent on patient respiratory pattern and input flow Risk for infection (Urden et al., 2024)

FiO$_2$, Fraction of inspired oxygen concentration.

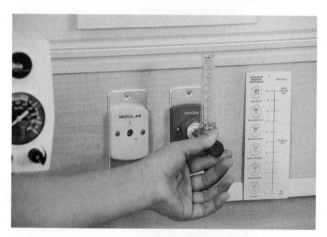

FIG. 23.6 Oxygen flowmeter.

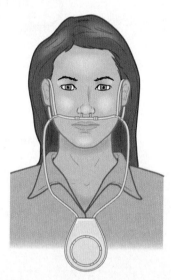

FIG. 23.7 Oxygen-reserving cannula. (*From Harding MM, Kwong J, Hagler D, Reinisch C: Lewis' medical-surgical nursing: assessment and management of clinical problems, ed 12, St Louis, 2023, Elsevier.*)

At flow rates greater than 4 L/min, humidification helps prevent drying of nasal and oral mucous membranes.

High-flow nasal cannula (HFNC) consists of an air-oxygen blender that has an adjustable FiO$_2$. It is used in patients in hypoxemic respiratory failure and in patients with respiratory failure and hypercapnia (Nishimura, 2019). For adults with COVID-19 and acute hypoxemic respiratory failure despite conventional oxygen therapy, HFNC oxygen is recommended over noninvasive positive pressure ventilation (NIPPV) (National Institutes of Health [NIH], 2023). This system can deliver a heated and humidified air/oxygen mixture at high flows, up to 50 to 60 L/min (Baird, 2023; Renda et al., 2018). The oxygen gas is then delivered to the patient via wide-bore nasal prongs. Heated high-flow nasal cannula (HHFNC) has been used in the neonatal population, and there is increasing evidence to support its use in adults with acute respiratory failure (Kim et al., 2018; Rochwerg et al., 2019).

An oxygen-conserving cannula is indicated for patients who require higher oxygen concentrations than what can be provided via traditional nasal cannula. The cannula possesses a built-in reservoir that allows for increasing oxygen concentration at a lower flow rate, which increases patient comfort (Fig. 23.7).

The simple oxygen face mask (see Fig. 23.4) is for short-term oxygen therapy. It fits loosely and delivers oxygen concentrations from 35% to 50% or 60%. A plastic face mask with a reservoir bag (see Fig. 23.5) and a Venturi mask (see Fig. 23.1) deliver higher concentrations of oxygen. When used as a nonrebreather, the plastic face mask with a reservoir bag delivers 60% to 90% oxygen when the flow rate setting is greater than 10 L/min. This oxygen mask maintains a high-concentration oxygen supply in the reservoir bag. The mask must have a tight seal on the face. Frequently inspect the bag to make sure that it is fully inflated. If it is *not* fully inflated, the patient may breathe in large amounts of exhaled carbon dioxide.

A Venturi mask is a cone-shaped high-flow device with entrainment ports of various sizes at the base of the mask, which delivers a more precise concentration of oxygen to a patient. The delivered FiO$_2$ remains constant despite patient respiratory rates or patterns. The concentration of oxygen delivered ranges from 24% to 40% and is based on the flow of the gas. The nurse or respiratory therapist adjusts the ports on the mask to permit regulation of FiO$_2$.

Delegation

Certain agencies allow the skill of applying a nasal cannula or oxygen mask be delegated to assistive personnel (AP) (check agency policy). The nurse is responsible for assessing the patient's respiratory system, response to oxygen therapy, and setup of oxygen therapy, including adjustment of oxygen flow rate. Instruct the AP:

• On how to safely adjust the device (e.g., loosening the strap on the oxygen cannula or mask) and clarifying its correct placement and positioning

• To inform the nurse immediately about any changes in vital signs; changes in pulse oximetry (SpO$_2$); changes in level of consciousness (LOC); skin irritation from the cannula, mask, or straps; or patient reports of pain or breathlessness

• To provide extra skin care around patient's ears and nose to prevent skin breakdown

Interprofessional Collaboration

- Health care providers such as pulmonary specialists or advanced practice nurses are responsible for prescribing the oxygen-delivery device, the flow rate, and the amount of oxygen to deliver.
- Respiratory therapists are usually responsible for the setup of the oxygen-delivery devices, especially HFNC. Communication includes patient assessment, patient vital signs (including trends in pulse oximetry values), tolerance of and response to interventions, and diagnostic lab results such as arterial blood gases (ABGs) or chest x-rays.

Equipment

- Oxygen-delivery device (as ordered)
- Oxygen tubing (consider extension tubing)

- Humidifier, if indicated
- Sterile water for humidifier
- Clean gloves and other personal protective equipment (PPE; e.g., gown or face mask) as patient condition warrants
- Oxygen source
- Oxygen flowmeter
- Appropriate "Oxygen in Use" signs (as required by health care agency)
- Pulse oximeter
- Stethoscope
- **NOTE:** If device is used in the home, the home care equipment vendor provides the equipment.

STEP	RATIONALE

ASSESSMENT

1. Identify patient using at least two identifiers (e.g., name and birthday or name and medical record number) according to agency policy.

   Ensures correct patient. Complies with The Joint Commission standards and improves patient safety (TJC, 2023).

2. Review patient's electronic health record (EHR), including health care provider's orders and nurses' notes. Include patient's vital signs, pulse oximetry values, baseline and trends in respiratory rate and effort of breathing, past medical history, past oxygen requirements, and most recent ABG results.

   Knowing the patient condition and past medical history helps to explain the amount of oxygen to deliver, patient's past responses to oxygen, and patient's trends in breathing rate and effort. Ensures safe and accurate oxygen administration. Safe oxygen delivery includes the seven rights of medication administration (see Chapter 20).

3. Review patient's EHR for health care provider's order for oxygen, noting delivery method, flow rate, duration of oxygen therapy, and parameters for titration of oxygen settings.

   Ensures safe and accurate oxygen administration. Safe oxygen delivery includes the seven rights of medication administration (see Chapter 20).

4. Assess patient's/family caregiver's health literacy.

   Determines degree to which individuals have the ability to find, understand, and use information and services to make informed health-related decisions and actions for themselves and others (Centers for Disease Control and Prevention [CDC], 2023a).

5. Perform hand hygiene and apply clean gloves.

   Reduces transmission of microorganisms.

6. Perform respiratory assessment, including symmetry of chest wall expansion, chest wall abnormalities (e.g., kyphosis), temporary conditions (e.g., pregnancy, trauma) affecting ventilation, respiratory rate and depth, sputum production, and lung sounds (see Chapter 6) and signs and symptoms associated with hypoxia (see Box 23.1).

   Changes in ventilation and gas exchange resulting in hypoxia require oxygen therapy.

7. Inspect condition of skin around nose and ears. Note if patient has history of impaired sensation, poor perfusion, altered tissue tolerance, poor nutrition, edema, and the tendency for moisture to develop under device—all known risk factors for medical adhesive–related skin injury (MARSI) and medical device–related pressure injury (MDRPI) (Barakat-Johnson et al., 2019; Jackson et al., 2019).

   Provides baseline for monitoring development of MARSI and MDRPI (Barakat-Johnson et al., 2019; Fumarola et al., 2020).

8. Observe for cognitive and behavioral changes (e.g., apprehension, anxiety, confusion, decreased ability to concentrate, decreased LOC, fatigue, and dizziness).

   Decreased levels of oxygen (hypoxia) or increased levels of carbon dioxide (hypercapnia) affect a person's cognitive abilities, interpersonal interactions, and mood (Harding et al., 2023).

Clinical Judgment *Patients with sudden changes in their vital signs, level of consciousness (LOC), or behavior may be experiencing profound hypoxia. Patients who demonstrate subtle changes over time may have worsening of a chronic or existing condition or a new medical condition (Harding et al., 2023).*

9. Assess airway patency and remove airway secretions by having patient cough and expectorate mucus or by suctioning (see Chapter 24). Auscultate lung sounds. Remove and dispose of gloves and perform hand hygiene. **NOTE:** Reapply gloves if further contact with mucus is likely.

   Secretions obstruct the airway, decreasing amount of oxygen that is available for gas exchange in lungs. Reduces transmission of microorganisms.

STEP	RATIONALE

Clinical Judgment *Excessive amounts of secretions, signs of respiratory distress (increased work of breathing, increased respiratory rate), presence of rhonchi on auscultation, excessive coughing, or decrease in patient pulse oximetry values can indicate need for suctioning.*

10. Assess patient's/family caregiver's knowledge and prior experience with oxygen administration and feelings about procedure.	Reveals need for patient/family caregiver instruction and/or support.

PLANNING

1. Expected outcomes following completion of procedure:	
• Patient's SpO$_2$ and/or ABGs return to or remain within normal limits or at baseline levels (usually SpO$_2$ greater than 95% or PaO$_2$ greater than 80 mm Hg).	Objective determinants of stable or improved oxygenation.
• Patient's vital signs remain stable or return to baseline.	When there is no underlying cardiovascular disease, patients adapt to decreased oxygen levels by increasing pulse and blood pressure (BP). This is a short-term adaptive response. Once signs of hypoxia are reduced or controlled, patient's vital signs usually return to normal.
• Patient's work of breathing decreases.	Pulmonary conditions such as pneumonia or asthma cause varying degrees of airway narrowing. With improved oxygenation, patient's airways are open, and work of breathing decreases.
• Patient experiences increased lung expansion.	Improved oxygenation helps to resolve collapsed and constricted airways, improves work of breathing, and thus improves lung expansion.
• Patient's LOC returns to baseline.	Improvement in oxygenation relieves hypoxia and improves patient's mental status.
• Patient verbalizes improved levels of comfort, and subjective sensations of anxiety, fatigue, and breathlessness decrease.	Increased oxygen levels in the blood reduce patient's anxiety, fatigue, and breathlessness.
• Patient displays no evidence of pressure injuries on ears or nares, and nasal mucosa remains intact.	Intact skin indicates no MDRPI to underlying skin and mucous membrane (Barakat-Johnson et al., 2019).
2. Provide privacy and explain procedure.	Protects patient's privacy; reduces anxiety. Promotes cooperation.
3. Organize and set up any equipment needed to perform procedure.	Ensures more efficiency when completing the procedure.
4. Instruct patient and/or family caregiver about need for oxygen. If the oxygen is for home use, this is a good time to begin education about oxygen safety in the home and the equipment that will be used.	Education decreases patient and family caregiver anxiety and reduces oxygen consumption. Proper education about the use of and need for the oxygen equipment will help to ensure the safe and proper use of the equipment.

IMPLEMENTATION

1. Perform hand hygiene. Apply face shield if risk of exposure to splashing mucus exists. Apply gloves if patient has oral or nasal secretions. Apply gown if agency protocol dictates the need for one or if there is a risk of splash or excessive secretions.	Reduces transmission of microorganisms.
2. Adjust bed to appropriate height and lower side rail on side nearest you. Position patient comfortably in semi-Fowler position.	Minimizes caregiver's muscle strain and prevents injury. Position promotes ventilation.
3. Attach oxygen-delivery device (e.g., cannula, mask) to oxygen tubing and attach end of tubing to humidified oxygen source (if needed) adjusted to prescribed flow rate (see Fig. 23.6). Check functioning.	Humidity prevents drying of nasal and oral mucous membranes and airway secretions. Flowmeters with smaller calibrations may be required for patients requiring low-dose oxygen such as pediatric patients or patients with COPD (Hockenberry et al., 2024; Walsh & Smallwood, 2017).
4. Apply oxygen device:	
a. *Nasal cannula:* Place tips of the nasal cannula into patient's nares. If tips are curved, they should point downward inside nostrils. Then loop cannula tubing up and over patient's ears. Adjust lanyard so cannula fits snugly but not too tightly, without pressure to patient nares and ears (see Fig. 23.3).	Tips of cannula direct flow of oxygen into patient's upper respiratory tract. Correct placement over ears reduces risk of MDRPI.

STEP	RATIONALE
b. *Mask:* Apply any type of oxygen mask by placing it over patient's mouth and nose. Then bring straps over patient's head and adjust to form a comfortable but tight seal (see Fig. 23.4).	A properly fitting device is one that does not create pressure on nares or ears and is comfortable. Thus patient is more likely to keep it in place and there is a reduced risk for MDRPI (Barakat-Johnson et al., 2019).
5. Maintain sufficient slack on oxygen tubing.	Allows patient to turn head and to have head of bed raised without causing mask to shift position or dislodge nasal cannula.
6. Observe for proper function of oxygen-delivery device:	Ensures patency of delivery device and accuracy of prescribed oxygen flow rate (see Table 23.1).
a. *Nasal cannula:* Cannula is positioned properly in nares; oxygen flows through tips (see Fig 23.3).	Provides prescribed oxygen rate and reduces pressure on tips of nares.
b. *Oxygen-conserving cannula:* Fit as for nasal cannula. Reservoir is located under patient's nose or worn as a pendant (see Fig. 23.7).	Delivers higher flow of oxygen with nasal cannula. Delivers 2:1 ratio (e.g., 6 L/min nasal cannula is approximately equivalent to 3.5 L/min with oxygen-conserving cannula device).
c. *Nonrebreather mask:* Apply as regular mask (see Fig. 23.5). Contains one-way valves with reservoir; exhaled air does not enter reservoir bag. Can be combined with nasal cannula to provide higher inspired oxygen concentration (FiO_2).	Device of choice for short-term high FiO_2 delivery. Valves on mask side ports permit exhalation but close during inhalation to prevent inhaling room air.
d. *Simple face mask:* Select appropriate flow rate (see Fig. 23.4).	Used for short-term oxygen therapy.
e. *Venturi mask* (see Fig. 23.1): Select appropriate flow rate (see Table 23.1).	Used when high-flow device is desired.
f. *HFNC* (see Fig. 23.2): Fit as for nasal cannula.	Provides adjustable O_2 delivery and flow rates that assist in reducing the work of breathing and increasing oxygen delivery (Drake, 2018).

Clinical Judgment *Changing of gloves and hand hygiene may need to be performed more often than indicated in these steps. If the gloves become contaminated with secretions while applying the delivery device, they should be changed prior to touching flowmeters or side rails in order to prevent transmission of organisms.*

STEP	RATIONALE
7. Verify setting on flowmeter and oxygen source for proper setup and prescribed flow rate.	Ensures delivery of prescribed oxygen therapy in conjunction with specific cannula/mask.
8. Check cannula/mask and humidity device (if used) every 8 hours or as agency policy indicates. Ensure that humidity container is filled at all times.	Ensures patency of cannula and oxygen flow. Oxygen is a dry gas; when it is administered via nasal cannula at 4 L/min or more, or administered to pediatric patients, you must add humidification to prevent thickening of secretions, minimize atelectasis, and prevent heat loss (Hockenberry et al., 2024; Walsh & Smallwood, 2017).
9. Post "Oxygen in Use" signs on wall behind bed and at entrance to room (check agency policy).	Alerts visitors and care providers that oxygen is in use.
10. Remove and dispose of gloves.	Reduces transmission of microorganisms.
11. Help patient to comfortable position.	Work of breathing is decreased when in a comfortable position. Some patients will need the head of the bed elevated in order to achieve that comfortable position. Ensures patient safety.
12. Raise side rails (as appropriate) and lower bed to lowest position, locking into position.	Ensures patient safety and prevents falls.
13. Place nurse call system in an accessible location within the patient's reach.	Ensures patient can call for assistance if needed.
14. Properly dispose of used equipment and perform hand hygiene.	Reduces transmission of microorganisms.

STEP	RATIONALE

EVALUATION

1. Monitor patient's response to changes in oxygen flow rate with SpO_2. **NOTE:** Monitor ABGs when ordered; however, obtaining ABG measurement is an invasive procedure, and ABGs are not measured frequently.

Continual monitoring with SpO_2 is required for patients on oxygen therapy. Base changes in supplemental oxygen on individual patient's oxygen saturation levels.

2. Perform respiratory assessment: auscultate lung sounds; palpate chest excursion; inspect color and condition of skin; and observe for decreased anxiety, improved LOC and cognitive abilities, decreased fatigue, and absence of dizziness. Obtain vital signs.

Evaluates patient's response to supplemental oxygen. As patient's oxygen level improves, physical signs and symptoms improve.

3. Assess adequacy of oxygen flow each shift or as agency policy dictates.

Ensures patency of oxygen-delivery device.

4. Observe patient's external ears, bridge of nose, nares, and nasal mucous membranes for evidence of skin breakdown.

Oxygen therapy sometimes causes drying of nasal mucosa. The oxygen-delivery device can cause MDRPI where device comes in contact with patient's face, neck, and ears (Barakat-Johnson et al., 2019).

5. **Use Teach-Back:** "I want to be sure I explained how oxygen will help you. Explain to me why oxygen is beneficial for you to use right now." Revise your instruction now or develop a plan for revised patient/family caregiver teaching if patient/family caregiver is not able to teach back correctly.

Teach-back is a technique for health care providers to ensure that they have explained medical information clearly so that patients and their families understand what is communicated to them (Agency for Healthcare Research and Quality [AHRQ], 2023).

Unexpected Outcomes	Related Interventions
1. Patient experiences skin irritation or breakdown (e.g., at ears, bridge of nose, nares, other pressure areas), sinus pain, or epistaxis.	• For sinus pain/epistaxis, increase humidification to oxygen-delivery system. • Provide appropriate skin/wound care (see Chapters 38 and 39). Do not use petroleum-based gel around oxygen because it is flammable. • Reposition device to alleviate pressure.
2. Patient experiences continued hypoxia.	• Notify health care provider. • Obtain health care provider's orders for follow-up SpO_2 monitoring or ABG determinations. • Consider measures to improve airway patency, including but not limited to coughing techniques and oropharyngeal or orotracheal suctioning.
3. Patient experiences nasal and upper airway mucosa drying.	• If oxygen flow rate is greater than 4 L/min, use humidification. At rates greater than 5 L/min, nasal mucous membranes dry, and pain in frontal sinuses may develop (American Lung Association, 2022; Harding et al., 2023). • Assess patient's fluid status and increase fluids if appropriate. • Provide frequent oral care.

Documentation

- Document the respiratory assessment findings, method of oxygen delivery, oxygen flow rate, patient's response to intervention, any adverse reactions or side effects; document patient's skin integrity.
- Document evaluation of patient and family caregiver learning.

Hand-Off Reporting

- Report patient status, including recent assessment findings, vital signs, SpO_2, and skin integrity before and after oxygen administration.
- Report the type of oxygen-delivery device initiated and used, the initial flow rates, and whether any adjustments to the flow rate were made during the shift. Include the patient response to the flow rate adjustments and what interventions were successful.
- Report any unexpected outcome to health care provider or nurse in charge.

Special Considerations

Patient Education

- Discuss signs of hypoxia and carbon dioxide retention (e.g., confusion, headache, decreased LOC, somnolence, carbon dioxide narcosis, respiratory arrest) that patient or family caregiver needs to report to the health care provider.
- Review oxygen safety guidelines if visitors fail to follow guidelines.

Pediatrics

- Some infants and small children are able to tolerate a nasal cannula. Secure the prongs of the cannula with transparent tape or strips of transparent dressing over the child's cheek.
- Inspect toys for safety and suitability when oxygen is in use. Any source of sparks (e.g., from mechanical or electrical toys) is a potential fire hazard (Hockenberry et al., 2024).
- Provide comfort and reassurance to a child. Make sure that the child is able to see someone nearby. Children may still be held by their parents while receiving oxygen (Hockenberry et al., 2024).

Older Adults

- Older adults have stiffer chest walls and weaker respiratory muscles, which increases their risk for having a disturbance in oxygenation that requires oxygen therapy (Touhy & Jett, 2022).
- Because of the fragility of older adults' skin and mucous membranes, offer oral hygiene and skin care more frequently.

Patients With Disabilities

- Initiation of oxygen may elicit different reactions in a person with a cognitive impairment or delirium. It is important to proceed slowly and observe patient for increased agitation. If agitation increases with the use of oxygen masks, try other methods such as high-flow oxygen cannula.

Home Care

- Teach patient and family caregiver the importance of and rationale for oxygen therapy, how to safely use the oxygen-delivery device, how to contact the supplier of medical equipment, and when to contact the health care provider (see Box 23.2 and Chapter 42).
- Obtain appropriate referrals to determine if patient meets the standards for third-party reimbursement (e.g., PaO_2 55 mm Hg or less or SaO_2 less than 88% while on room air at rest). Exceptions may apply when patients have pulmonary hypertension, cor pulmonale, erythrocytosis, edema, or impaired mental status.
- Oxygen tubing in the home setting is available in lengths of 15 m (50 feet), which allows patient to be ambulatory within the home and maintain oxygen use as ordered.
- Provide information about a reliable oxygen-therapy equipment vendor who can teach the patient and family caregiver how to use a home-fill system with an oxygen concentrator.
- Consider using oxygen-conserving devices that administer oxygen in a pulse-dosed flow during inhalation only. These reduce the use and cost of long-term oxygen therapy.

◆ SKILL 23.2   Administering Oxygen Therapy to a Patient With an Artificial Airway

Patients with artificial airways require constant humidification (see Chapter 24). An artificial airway bypasses the normal filtering and humidification process of the nose and mouth. The two devices that supply humidified gas to an artificial airway are a T tube and a tracheostomy collar.

The T tube, also called a *Briggs adapter*, is a T-shaped device with a 15-mm (1/3-inch) connector that attaches an oxygen source to an artificial airway such as an endotracheal (ET) tube or tracheostomy (Fig. 23.8). A tracheostomy mask is a curved device that fits over the tracheostomy opening and has an adjustable strap that fits around a patient's neck (Fig. 23.9).

Delegation

The skill of administering oxygen therapy to a patient with an artificial airway cannot be delegated to assistive personnel (AP). Instruct AP about:

- Patient-specific variations for application or adjustment of the T tube or tracheostomy collar (e.g., methods to avoid medical device–related pressure injury [MDRPI] or pulling on the artificial airway, methods for handling accumulated secretions in devices)
- Immediately reporting to the nurse increase in anxiety, changes in vital signs, and increase in airway secretions

Interprofessional Collaboration

- Respiratory therapists are usually responsible for the setup of the oxygen-delivery devices.
- Additional therapists, such as physical therapists, occupational therapists, or speech therapists, help with activities of daily living and mobility. Therapists need to be aware of the patient's most recent vital signs, pulmonary status, oxygen requirements, and activity tolerance.

Equipment

- T tube or tracheostomy collar
- Large-bore oxygen tubing
- Nebulizer
- Sterile water for nebulizer
- Oxygen or gas source
- Clean gloves
- Additional personal protective equipment (PPE), including mask, goggles, and/or barrier gown (if exposure to mucus or splash is likely or patient isolation orders dictate)
- Flowmeter
- Yankauer or tonsillar tip suction catheter
- Connecting tubing (at least 6 feet)
- Suction machine or wall suction device
- Pulse oximeter
- Stethoscope

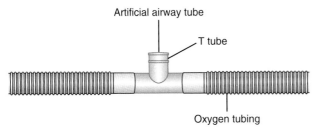

FIG. 23.8 T tube.

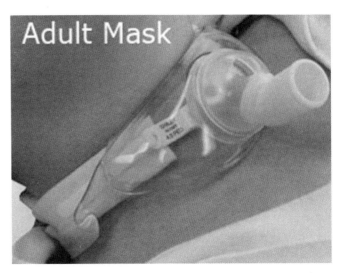

FIG. 23.9 Tracheostomy mask. (*Courtesy Marcpac Company.*)

STEP	RATIONALE

ASSESSMENT

1. Identify patient using at least two identifiers (e.g., name and birthday or name and medical record number) according to agency policy.

Ensures correct patient. Complies with the Joint Commission standards and improves patient safety (TJC, 2023).

2. Review patient's electronic health record (EHR), including health care provider's orders and nurses' notes. Note patient's normal and most recent pulse oximetry and $EtCO_2$ values, baseline and trends in respiratory rate and effort of breathing, past medical history, past oxygen requirements, and most recent arterial blood gas (ABG) results. Also review for medical order for oxygen, flow rate, and duration of oxygen therapy.

Knowing the patient's condition and past medical history helps to explain the amount of oxygen needed for delivery, patient's past responses to oxygen, and patient's trends in breathing rate and effort. Ensures safe and accurate oxygen administration. Safe oxygen delivery includes the seven rights of medication administration (see Chapter 20).

3. Assess patient's/family caregiver's health literacy.

Determines degree to which individuals have the ability to find, understand, and use information and services to make informed health-related decisions and actions for themselves and others (CDC, 2023a).

4. Perform hand hygiene Apply mask if there is risk of mucus splash. Assess patient's respiratory status, including symmetry of chest wall expansion, respiratory rate and depth, sputum production, and lung sounds (see Chapter 6); assess for signs and symptoms associated with hypoxia (see Box 23.1).

Changes in ventilation and gas exchange resulting in hypoxia require oxygen therapy.

5. Observe condition of tissues surrounding ET tube or tracheostomy tube (TT) for impaired skin integrity (e.g., blistering, abrasions, pressure injuries) on nares, lips, cheeks, corner of mouth, or neck; excess nasal or oral secretions; patient moving tube with tongue or biting tube or tongue; or foul-smelling mouth (see Chapter 24).

Provides baseline for monitoring for MDRPI. Increased risk for developing pressure injuries around ET tube or TT from impaired circulation as tube is pulled or pressed against oral mucosal tissues. Tube impairs ability of patient to swallow oral secretions.

6. Observe patency of airway: excess peristomal, intratracheal, or endotracheal secretions; diminished airflow; or signs and symptoms of airway obstruction (see Chapter 24).

Secretions plug airway, decreasing amount of oxygen available for gas exchange in lung. Secretions also occlude T tube or tracheostomy collar, impeding oxygen delivery to patient. Excess secretions in the artificial airways may indicate need for more frequent suctioning.

7. Observe for cognitive and behavioral changes (e.g., apprehension, anxiety, confusion, decreased ability to concentrate, decreased level of consciousness [LOC], fatigue, and dizziness).

Decreased levels of oxygen (hypoxia) or increased levels of carbon dioxide (hypercapnia) affect a person's cognitive abilities, interpersonal interactions, and mood (Harding et al., 2023).

Clinical Judgment *Patients with artificial airways who develop sudden changes in their vital signs, level of consciousness (LOC), or behavior may be experiencing hypoxia secondary to airway obstruction. The airway must be determined to be patent before oxygen is administered. If patients continue with signs of hypoxia once obstruction is removed or ruled out, oxygen should be applied.*

8. Monitor pulse oximetry (SpO_2) and, if available, note patient's most recent ABG results. Remove gloves and other PPE and perform hand hygiene.

Objectively documents patient's pH, arterial oxygen, arterial carbon dioxide, or arterial oxygen saturation. Reduces transmission of microorganisms.

9. Assess patient's/family caregiver's knowledge, prior experience with oxygen administration through an artificial airway, and feelings about procedure.

Reveals need for patient/family caregiver instruction and/or support.

PLANNING

1. Expected outcomes following completion of procedure:
   - Patient's signs of hypoxia are reduced or eliminated.

   Patient demonstrates improved oxygenation.

   - Patient's vital signs remain stable or return to baseline.

   When there is no underlying cardiovascular disease, patient adapts to decreased oxygen levels by increasing pulse and blood pressure. This is a short-term adaptive response. Once signs of hypoxia are reduced or controlled, patient's vital signs usually return to normal.

STEP	RATIONALE
• Patient's work of breathing decreases.	With improved oxygenation, tissue oxygen demand is met, and work of breathing decreases.
• Patient experiences increased lung expansion.	Improved oxygenation helps to resolve collapsed and constricted airways, improve work of breathing, and thus improve lung expansion.
• Patient's LOC returns to baseline.	Improvement in oxygenation relieves hypoxia and improves patient's mental status.
• ABG values or SpO$_2$ saturation returns to normal or baseline.	Documents physiological response to oxygen therapy.
• Tracheal stoma and peristomal area remain intact without irritation or pressure injury.	Stomal irritation and breakdown are common complications in patients with a tracheostomy (Karaca & Korkmaz, 2018; Urden et al., 2024).
2. Provide privacy and explain procedure.	Protects patient's privacy; reduces anxiety. Promotes cooperation.
3. Organize and set up any equipment needed to perform procedure.	Ensures more efficiency when completing the procedure.
4. Instruct patient and/or family caregiver about need for oxygen. If the oxygen is for home use, educate patient about oxygen safety in the home and the equipment that will be used.	Education decreases patient and family caregiver anxiety and reduces oxygen consumption. Proper education about the use of and need for the oxygen equipment will help to ensure the safe and proper use of the equipment.

IMPLEMENTATION

STEP	RATIONALE
1. Perform hand hygiene; apply clean gloves and PPE as needed (check agency policy).	Reduces transmission of microorganisms by preventing contact with pulmonary secretions. Patients with excessive secretions or forceful productive coughs place caregiver at risk for splash contact.
2. Adjust bed to appropriate height and lower side rail on side nearest you. Position patient comfortably in semi-Fowler position.	Minimizes caregiver's muscle strain and prevents injury. Position promotes ventilation.
3. Attach T tube or tracheostomy mask to large-bore oxygen tubing and to humidified room air or oxygen source as indicated. Ensure that humidity container is filled at all times.	Provides supplemental humidification to avoid drying of airway, which can lead to obstruction of the patient airway or the artificial airway (Billington & Luckett, 2019).
4. If health care provider orders oxygen, adjust flow rate to 10 L/min or as ordered. Adjust nebulizer to proper oxygen concentration (FiO$_2$) setting. Attach T tube to artificial airway. Place tracheostomy collar over TT and adjust straps so it fits snugly.	Nebulizer regulates FiO$_2$. Proper connection of devices ensures proper oxygen delivery to airway.
5. Observe that T tube does not pull on artificial airway or cause pressure on adjacent skin and tissue. Observe for secretions within T tube or tracheostomy collar, and suction as necessary (see Chapter 24).	Pulling effect on tube increases patient's discomfort and causes pressure to side of patient's mouth or tracheal stoma, which increases risk for MDRPI (Brophy et al., 2021).
6. Observe oxygen tubing frequently for accumulation of fluid caused by condensation. If fluid is present, drain tube away from patient, disconnect from collar or T tube, and discard fluid in proper receptacle.	Excess water is medium for bacterial growth. Draining contaminated water into proper receptacle prevents contamination of entire humidifying unit and decreases risk for infection (Sharma et al., 2023).
7. Set up suction equipment at patient's bedside.	Humidification increases airway secretions. Patients need a nonobstructed airway in order for oxygen to be effective, and suction equipment helps to clear the airway when needed (see Chapter 24).
8. Be sure patient remains in comfortable position.	Work of breathing is decreased when in a comfortable position. Some patients will need the head of the bed elevated in order to achieve that comfortable position.
9. Raise side rails (as appropriate) and lower bed to lowest position, locking into position.	Ensures patient safety and prevents falls.
10. Place nurse call system in an accessible location within the patient's reach.	Ensures that patient can call for assistance if needed.
11. Remove and dispose of PPE; perform hand hygiene.	Reduces transmission of microorganisms.

STEP	RATIONALE

EVALUATION

1. Monitor patient's vital signs and SpO_2.

Continuous monitoring of vital signs and SpO_2 allows for continual noninvasive, cost-effective trending of patient's vital signs and oxygen saturation.

2. Perform respiratory assessment and observe for any cognitive and behavioral changes indicative of hypoxia.

Monitors changes in patient's respiratory assessment and cognitive status in response to supplemental oxygen.

3. Observe position of oxygen-delivery device and condition of adjacent tissues to ensure that there is no pulling on artificial airway or pressure injuries.

Pulling on artificial airway or pressure on adjacent tissues results in complications such as tube displacement and MDRPI (Brophy et al., 2021; Urden et al., 2024).

4. Use Teach-Back: "I want to be sure I explained how oxygen will help your mother. Explain to me why oxygen is attached to your mother's tracheostomy tube." Revise your instruction now or develop a plan for revised patient/family caregiver teaching if patient/family caregiver is not able to teach back correctly.

Teach-back is a technique for health care providers to ensure that they have explained medical information clearly so that patients and their families understand what is communicated to them (AHRQ, 2023).

Unexpected Outcomes

1. Patient experiences tracheal stoma or lip irritation; thick, tenacious secretions; or pressure areas on neck or near stoma site.

2. Patient experiences continued hypoxia.

Related Interventions

- Implement measures to protect patient from MDRPI (see Chapter 39).
- Increase frequency of suctioning and airway care (see Chapter 24).
- Determine if cause of continued hypoxia is functioning of oxygen-delivery device, obstruction of airway, oxygen flow rate, or a new clinical problem.
- Notify health care provider of continued or worsening hypoxia.

Documentation

- Document the respiratory assessment findings; method of oxygen delivery; flow rate; condition of tracheal stoma, peristomal area, or lips; patient's response; and any adverse reactions.
- Document evaluation of patient and family caregiver learning.

Hand-Off Reporting

- Report patient status, including recent assessment findings, vital signs, and SpO_2 before and after oxygen administration.
- Report the type of oxygen-delivery device initiated and used, the initial flow rates, and whether any ordered adjustments to the flow rate were made during the shift. Include the patient response to the flow rate adjustments and what interventions were successful.

- Report any unexpected outcome to health care provider or nurse in charge.

Special Considerations

Patient Education

- See teaching considerations for Skill 23.1.

Home Care

- Some patients who are at home have both a permanent tracheostomy and a T tube or a tracheostomy collar. The patient and/ or family caregiver must be physically able to perform tracheostomy care and suctioning techniques, identify changes to stoma and peristomal skin, and understand how to manage oxygen (see Chapters 24 and 42).

◆ SKILL 23.3   Using Incentive Spirometry

Incentive spirometry encourages voluntary deep breathing by providing visual feedback to patients about inspiratory volume. It is a commonly used intervention that promotes deep breathing and is thought to prevent or treat atelectasis in the postoperative patient, especially patients who had thoracic surgery. Recent evidence suggests that the use of the incentive spirometer (IS) is not as effective at preventing postoperative pulmonary complications in all populations. However, there is an indication that IS can lead to a reduction in the incidence of postoperative pulmonary complications following thoracic surgery, including atelectasis, in patients with chronic pulmonary conditions, such as chronic obstructive pulmonary disease (COPD) (Kotta & Ali, 2021). A recent study noted that scheduled nurse-guided IS reduced the risk for pulmonary complications and length of hospital stay following thoracic surgery (Alwekhyan et al., 2022).

The use of an IS alone is not recommended to prevent postoperative pulmonary complications. It should be used in combination with other pulmonary maneuvers such as deep breathing and coughing, early mobilization of the patient, and directed coughing (Hanada et al., 2020; Urden et al., 2024).

There are two types of ISs. Flow-oriented ISs consist of one or more plastic chambers that contain freely moving colored balls. A patient inhales slowly and with an even flow to elevate the balls and keep them floating for as long as possible to ensure a maximally sustained inhalation (Fig. 23.10) Even if a very slow inspiration does not elevate the balls, this pattern helps a patient improve lung expansion (Eltorai et al., 2018a).

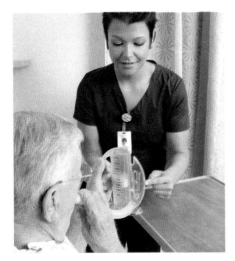

FIG. 23.10 Flow-oriented incentive spirometer.

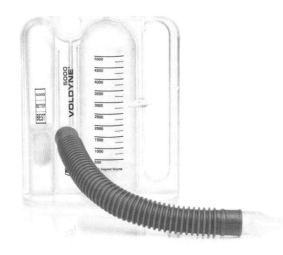

FIG. 23.11 Volume-oriented incentive spirometer.

Volume-oriented IS devices have a bellows that is raised to a predetermined volume by an inhaled breath (Fig. 23.11). The advantage of the volume-oriented IS is that a patient can achieve a known inspiratory volume and measure it with each breath. They are also associated with a decreased work of breathing (Kotta & Ali, 2021).

Delegation

The skill of helping a patient to use IS can be delegated to assistive personnel (AP). The nurse is responsible for assessing and monitoring the patient, evaluating the patient response, educating the patient about the proper use of the IS, and evaluating that education. Instruct the AP about:

- The patient's target goal for incentive spirometry

- Immediately notifying the nurse about any unexpected outcomes such as chest pain, excessive sputum production, and fever

Interprofessional Collaboration

- Respiratory therapists are often responsible for assessing the patient with potential disturbances in oxygenation.

Equipment

- Flow- or volume-oriented IS
- Stethoscope
- Pulse oximeter monitor
- Clean gloves

STEP	RATIONALE

ASSESSMENT

STEP	RATIONALE
1. Identify patient using at least two identifiers (e.g., name and birthday or name and medical record number) according to agency policy.	Ensures correct patient. Complies with the Joint Commission standards and improves patient safety (TJC, 2023).
2. Review patient's electronic health record (EHR), including health care provider's order and nurses' notes. Review if patients will benefit from IS use (e.g., patients who have undergone thoracic or abdominal surgery; surgical patients with a history of COPD; patients with asthma or preoperative chest infections) (Sweity et al., 2021).	Health care agencies often require a medical order for incentive spirometry to receive third-party reimbursement. Alerts health care personnel to patients at risk for respiratory complications during illness or after surgery.
3. Assess patient's/family caregiver's health literacy.	Determines degree to which individuals have the ability to find, understand, and use information and services to make informed health-related decisions and actions for themselves and others (CDC, 2023a).
4. Assess patient for confusion, cognitive impairments, ability to follow directions, age, developmental level, level of consciousness, and decrease in necessary motor skills.	Determines risks for difficulty with or ability to perform spirometry. Patients with some cognitive impairment benefit form nurse-guided incentive spirometry (Alwekhyan et al., 2022).

Clinical Judgment *Patients who are unable to follow directions or who are not developmentally or physically able to perform the actions associated with this skill are not candidates for this intervention. This assessment also enables the nurse to identify whether to use the flow-oriented or the volume-oriented IS.*

STEP	RATIONALE
5. Perform hand hygiene. Assess patient's respiratory status, including symmetry of chest wall expansion, respiratory rate and depth, sputum production, and lung sounds (see Chapter 6). Also obtain a pulse oximetry reading.	Reduces transmission of microorganisms. Decreased chest wall movement, crackles or decreased lung sounds, increased respiratory rate, or increased sputum production can indicate a need for incentive spirometry to improve lung expansion.
6. Assess character of patient's pain and rate acuity on a pain scale of 0 to 10.	Determines if comfort measures are effective.

Clinical Judgment *When the patient reports increased pain, administer prescribed analgesic prior to using the IS.*

| 7. Assess knowledge, prior experience of patient/family caregiver with use of the IS, and feelings about procedure. | Reveals need for patient/family caregiver instruction and/or support. |

PLANNING

1. Expected outcomes following completion of procedure:	
• Patient demonstrates correct use of IS.	Demonstrates learning.
• Patient achieves target volume and number of repetitions per hour.	Demonstrates increased lung expansion.
• Patient has improved breath sounds and increased pulse oximeter reading.	Incentive spirometry helps patient deep breathe and manage airway secretions.
2. Provide privacy and explain procedure.	Protects patient's privacy; reduces anxiety. Promotes cooperation.
3. Organize and set up any equipment needed to perform procedure.	Ensures more efficiency when completing the procedure.
4. Instruct patient about need for IS. Indicate to patient where target volume is on IS. **NOTE:** If possible, demonstrate to patient how to use IS.	Education decreases patient anxiety and will help to ensure the safe and proper use of the equipment. Encourages patients to "do better" with each breath and meet or exceed target volume. When patients have a visual target, they can gauge their improvement and have fewer hypoxic episodes (Alwekhyan et al., 2022).

IMPLEMENTATION

1. Perform hand hygiene. Apply clean gloves if there is risk of exposure to mucus.	Reduces transmission of microorganisms.
2. Adjust bed to appropriate height and lower side rail on side nearest you. Position patient in most erect position (e.g., high-Fowler if tolerated) in bed or chair.	Minimizes caregiver's muscle strain and prevents injury. Promotes optimal lung expansion during respiratory maneuver.
3. Instruct patient to hold IS upright, exhale normally and completely through mouth, and place lips tightly around mouthpiece (see illustration).	Allows for proper functioning of IS (Sweity et al., 2021). Showing patient how to correctly place mouthpiece is reliable technique for teaching psychomotor skill and enables patient to ask questions.

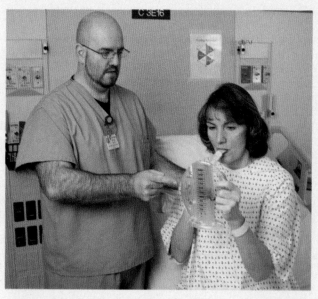

STEP 3 Proper placement of lips around incentive spirometer.

STEP	RATIONALE
4. Instruct patient to take a slow, deep breath and maintain constant flow, like pulling through a straw. The recommendation is 5 to 10 breaths per session every hour while awake (Cleveland Clinic, 2022). If flow-oriented IS, inhalation should raise the ball. If volume-oriented IS, inhalation should raise the piston. Remove mouthpiece at point of maximal inhalation; then have patient hold breath for 3 seconds and exhale normally.	Maintains maximal inspiration; reduces risk for progressive collapse of individual alveoli.

Clinical Judgment *Some patients are unable to hold their breath for 3 seconds. Encourage them to do their best and try to extend the duration of breath holding. Allow patients to rest between IS breaths to prevent hyperventilation and fatigue. Remind them it is more important to inhale slowly versus quickly.*

STEP	RATIONALE
5. Have patient repeat maneuver; encourage patient to reach prescribed goal.	Ensures correct use of IS and patient's understanding of use.
6. Encourage patient to independently use IS at prescribed frequency. An example of a frequently prescribed timing schedule includes 5 to 10 attempts every hour while awake (Cleveland Clinic, 2022).	Repeated use of IS improves lung expansion and promotes clearing of airways. Encouraging patients to perform independently gives them a sense of control over their care.
7. Encourage patient to cough after cycle of IS breaths.	Use IS in combination with other pulmonary measures, such as deep breathing and coughing. Early mobilization is recommended for patients who are at risk for atelectasis (Hanada et al., 2020). The effects of the IS are augmented when accompanied by coughing (Kotta & Ali, 2021; Eltorai et al., 2018b).
8. Help patient to comfortable position.	Work of breathing is decreased when in a comfortable position. Some patients will need the head of the bed elevated in order to achieve that comfortable position.
9. Raise side rails (as appropriate) and lower bed to lowest position, locking into position.	Ensures patient safety and prevents falls.
10. Place nurse call system in an accessible location within the patient's reach.	Ensures patient can call for assistance if needed.
11. Remove and properly dispose of gloves, if used, and perform hand hygiene.	Reduces transmission of microorganisms.

EVALUATION

1. Observe patient's ability to use incentive spirometry by return demonstration.	Determines patient's ability to perform breathing exercise correctly.
2. Assess if patient is able to achieve target volume or frequency.	Measures adherence to therapy and lung expansion.
3. Auscultate chest during respiratory cycle and obtain pulse oximeter reading.	Assesses lung expansion, identifies any abnormal lung sounds, and determines if airways are clear. Identifies improvement in pulse oximetry readings.
4. **Use Teach-Back:** "I want to be sure I explained how and when to use the IS. Show me how to use your IS and tell me how frequently you should use it." Revise your instruction now or develop a plan for revised patient teaching if patient is not able to teach back correctly.	Teach-back is a technique for health care providers to ensure that they have explained medical information clearly so that patients and their families understand what is communicated to them (AHRQ, 2023).

Unexpected Outcomes

1. Patient is unable to achieve IS target volume.

2. Patient has decreased lung expansion and/or abnormal breath sounds or decreased pulse oximetry readings.

3. Patient develops hyperventilation.

Related Interventions

- Encourage patient to attempt IS more frequently, followed by rest periods.
- Teach cough-control exercises.
- Teach patient how to splint and protect incision sites during deep breathing.
- Administer ordered analgesic if acute pain is inhibiting use of IS (Sweity et al., 2021).

- Teach patient cough-control exercises.
- Provide help with suctioning if patient cannot cough up secretions effectively.

- Encourage longer rest periods between breaths.

Documentation

- Document lung sounds, respiratory rate, and pulse oximetry readings before and after incentive spirometry; frequency of use; volumes achieved; and any adverse effects.
- Document evaluation of patient and/or family caregiver learning.

Hand-Off Reporting

- Report patient status, including recent lung sounds, vital signs, and SpO_2 before and after the use of the IS.
- Report the frequency of use of the IS, the desired volume/level the patient should reach, the actual volume/level attained, and patient tolerance of the procedure.
- Report the need for any analgesic medication prior to the use of the IS.
- Report any unexpected outcome to health care provider or nurse in charge.

Special Considerations

Patient Education

- Teach patient to examine sputum for consistency, amount, and color changes. Sputum should become clearer over time and decrease in volume.

- Teach patient that it should become easier to take deep breaths after the use of the IS.
- Teach patient that the use of the IS, in conjunction with ambulation and coughing and deep breathing, helps decrease the incidence of pulmonary complications in patients who have had surgery.

Pediatrics

- Incentive spirometry is used with school-age and older children. The pediatric patient needs the fine-motor skills and ability to follow instructions to use an IS effectively (Hockenberry et al., 2024).
- Allowing a child to play with and try out the IS helps to decrease anxiety and encourages participation in care.
- Use games or blowing bubbles and pinwheels to encourage small children to take deep breaths. These activities help achieve the same goals as incentive spirometry in some children.

Older Adults

- Weakened respiratory muscles and decreased elastic recoil properties of the lungs affect a patient's ability to cough and deep breathe. Therefore it takes an older adult longer to achieve the target volume (Touhy & Jett, 2022).

◆ SKILL 23.4 Care of a Patient Receiving Noninvasive Positive Pressure Ventilation

Noninvasive positive pressure ventilation (NIPPV or NPPV), or noninvasive ventilation (NIV), maintains positive airway pressure and improves alveolar ventilation without the need for an artificial airway. There are two types of NIPPV: continuous positive airway pressure (CPAP; Fig. 23.12) and bilevel positive airway pressure (BiPAP; Fig. 23.13). BiPAP and CPAP are usually applied via a mask covering the nose or both the mouth and the nose, but those who require home CPAP may wear nasal prongs instead (Hill et al., 2019; Urden et al., 2024).

NIPPV is used both in acute care settings and increasingly in home care settings to treat a variety of conditions, including obstructive sleep apnea (OSA), chronic obstructive pulmonary disease (COPD), cardiogenic pulmonary edema, hypoxic and/or hypercapnic respiratory failure, and neuromuscular disorders (e.g., amyotrophic lateral sclerosis [ALS]). It is commonly used in these conditions to reduce mortality and avoid the complications of invasive ventilation strategies, including pneumonia and aspiration (Enezi et al., 2018; Wu et al., 2022).

NIPPV should not be used in patients who cannot protect their airway or in patients with an inadequate respiratory drive or apnea.

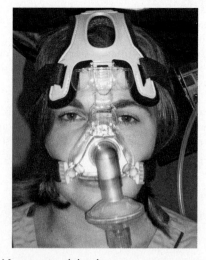

FIG. 23.13 Noninvasive bilevel positive airway pressure (BiPAP) ventilation. A mask is placed over the nose or nose and mouth. Positive pressure from a mechanical ventilator aids the patient's breathing efforts, decreasing the work of breathing. (*From Harding MM: Lewis's medical-surgical nursing: assessment and management of clinical problems, ed 12, St. Louis, 2023, Elsevier. Courtesy Richard Arbour, RN, MSN, CCRN, CNRN, CCNS, FAAN, and Anna Kirk, RN, MSN.*)

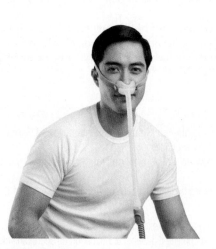

FIG. 23.12 Continuous positive airway pressure (CPAP) mask. ResMed's AirFit N30TM. (*Copyright © ResMed. All rights reserved.*)

TABLE 23.2

Problems Associated With Noninvasive Positive Pressure Ventilation (NIPPV)

Problem	Cause
Discomfort	Mask that fits over patient's nose is tight fitting.
	Oxygen flow rate causes dry mucous membranes.
Psychosocial	Relationship with sleep partner is difficult when NIPPV is used at home.
	There are possible sensations of claustrophobia.
Risks to skin integrity	Tight fit of mask causes diaphoresis, pressure, and increased risk for medical device–related pressure injury (MDRPI). Patients need to remove mask to relieve pressure.
	Exposure to medical adhesive to assist in securing mask increases risk for medical adhesive–related skin injury (MARSI).
Hypercapnia	Although CPAP improves alveolar function, which increases carbon dioxide clearance from the blood, it also causes air trapping. In some patients this causes a rise in carbon dioxide levels. Initially you need to monitor patient's ABG levels.
Gastric distention	CPAP and BiPAP force more air into the stomach, which causes distention and discomfort.
Noise	Some patients find the machines noisy, interfering with sleep and leisure activities such as watching television or listening to music.

ABG, Arterial blood gas; *BiPAP,* bilevel positive airway pressure; *CPAP,* continuous positive airway pressure.
Data from Miller K, et al: A multidisciplinary approach to reduction pressure injuries during noninvasive ventilation, *RT: The Journal for Respiratory Care Practitioners* 31(3):18–22, 2018; and Urden L, et al: *Priorities in critical care nursing,* ed 9, St. Louis, 2024, Elsevier.

It should be used with caution in patients with asthma, those with facial injuries, uncooperative patients, or hemodynamically unstable patients (Ghosh & Elliott, 2019; Hill et al., 2019).

The advantages of this type of ventilation versus invasive ventilation include an increased ability to communicate with caregivers and family, better ability to cough and clear secretions, and allowance for eating and drinking, if stable and not at risk for aspiration. There are disadvantages, problems, and concerns related to this type of ventilation (Table 23.2). The mask must fit tightly and have a good seal to prevent air from leaking. This pressure can cause feelings of claustrophobia and intolerance in patients, which can lead to issues with adherence to therapy. The tight-fitting mask can also lead to medical device–related pressure injuries (MDRPIs), particularly on the bridge of the nose (Hill et al., 2019; Jackson et al., 2019).

Delegation

The skill of caring for a patient receiving NIV cannot be delegated to assistive personnel (AP). However, the skills of patient positioning, therapeutic coughing, and CPAP/BiPAP mask application can be delegated to AP. Direct the AP to:
- Immediately report to the nurse any changes in patient's vital signs; oxygen saturation; mental status; skin color; or skin abrasions, bruising, or blistering around mask area.
- Immediately report to the nurse any ventilator or CPAP/BiPAP machine alarms or patient monitor alarms.
- Provide special care practices—for example, include how long the mask can be removed during oral care, any special skin care needs, and how to perform quick release of mask in case of vomiting.
- Immediately report to the nurse any changes in the patient's skin around the mask or securement devices. These include increased redness, blistering, and break in skin integrity.
- Immediately notify the nurse of any change in settings on the NIPPV or in patient comfort.

Interprofessional Collaboration
- Respiratory therapists are usually responsible for the setup of the NIPPV devices. Communication includes patient assessment, patient vital signs including trends in pulse oximetry values, tolerance and response to interventions, and diagnostic lab results such as arterial blood gases (ABGs) or chest x-rays.
- Other therapists, such as physical therapists, occupational therapists, or speech therapists need to be aware of patient's pulmonary status, oxygen requirements, NIPPV settings, and tolerance of activity in order to perform their prescribed activities accurately and safely.
- A wound, ostomy, continence nurse (WOCN) or skin expert/wound expert can individualize skin care to prevent and/or treat MDRPI (Barakat-Johnson et al., 2019; Fumarola et al., 2020).

Equipment
(**NOTE:** When device is used in the home, the home care equipment vendor provides the NIPPV equipment. In a health care agency, the respiratory therapy department will set up the NIPPV equipment.)
- Nasal mask/full face mask (with quick-release straps), or nasal pillows
- Oxygen source and tubing
- CPAP/BiPAP health care provider order
- Humidification source
- BiPAP and/or CPAP ventilator
- Delivery tubing
- Pulse oximetry
- Clean gloves
- Other personal protective equipment (PPE) as appropriate
- Stethoscope
- Suction equipment
- Self-inflating manual-resuscitation bag-valve mask device

STEP	RATIONALE

ASSESSMENT

1. Identify patient using at least two identifiers (e.g., name and birthday or name and medical record number) according to agency policy.

   Ensures correct patient. Complies with The Joint Commission standards and improves patient safety (TJC, 2023).

2. Review patient's electronic health record (EHR), including health care provider's order and nurses' notes, for patient's normal pulse oximetry values, baseline and trends in respiratory rate and effort of breathing, past medical history, past oxygen and NIPPV requirements, and most recent ABG results or SpO_2 value. Also review EHR for prescription for NIPPV, noting pressure settings, desired amount of oxygen, desired facial appliance, and duration of therapy.

   Knowing the patient condition and past medical history helps to explain the amount of oxygen to deliver, the amount of pressure to deliver, the patient's past responses to NIPPV, and patient's trends in breathing rate and effort. Ensures safe and accurate NIPPV. Safe oxygen delivery includes the seven rights of medication administration (see Chapter 20).

3. Assess patient's/family caregiver's health literacy.

   Determines degree to which individuals have the ability to find, understand, and use information and services to make informed health-related decisions and actions for themselves and others (CDC, 2023a).

4. Perform hand hygiene and apply clean gloves.

   Reduces transmission of microorganisms.

5. Assess patient's respiratory status, including symmetry of chest wall expansion, respiratory rate and depth, oxygen saturation, sputum production, and lung sounds (see Chapter 6). When possible, ask patient about dyspnea and observe for signs and symptoms associated with hypoxia (see Box 23.1).

   Decreased chest wall movement, crackles or decreased lung sounds, increased respiratory rate, increased sputum production, or signs of worsening hypoxia may make patient a candidate for NIPPV or changes in NIPPV settings.

6. Observe patient's skin over bridge of nose, around external ears, back of head.

   The mask places pressure on skin and increases risk for MDRPI.

7. Observe patient's ability to clear and remove airway secretions by coughing.

   Secretions plug the airway, decreasing amount of oxygen that is available for gas exchange in the lung.

8. Assess patient's level of consciousness, cognition and behaviors, and ability to maintain and protect airway.

   Patients who cannot maintain their own airway, who are uncooperative, or who need heavy sedation are not candidates for NIPPV (Urden et al., 2024).

Clinical Judgment *Noninvasive positive pressure ventilation (NIPPV) is contraindicated in patients with hemodynamic instability, arrhythmias, or apnea; patients who cannot cooperate or tolerate the mask; patients who have had recent upper airway or esophageal surgery; and patients who cannot maintain a patent airway, clear secretions, or properly fit the mask (Urden et al., 2024).*

9. Remove and discard gloves; perform hand hygiene.

   Reduces transmission of organisms.

10. Assess patient's/family caregiver's knowledge and prior experience of with NIPPV and feelings about procedure.

   Reveals need for patient/family caregiver instruction and/or support.

PLANNING

1. Expected outcomes following completion of procedure:
   - Patient has increased lung expansion.

     Patient experiences improved gas exchange when lungs are expanded from constant pressure of NIPPV.

   - Patient maintains ABG levels, and/or pulse oximetry (SpO_2) readings improve or remain normal.

     Improved gas exchange achieved with NIPPV delivered appropriately based on patient assessment data.

   - Patient experiences reduction in feelings of dyspnea and work of breathing.

     In patients with acute conditions, dyspnea usually improves. Patients with chronic pulmonary diseases often require nocturnal CPAP/BiPAP indefinitely to achieve long-term benefits.

   - Patient's vital signs and respiratory assessment parameters improve.

     Reduced pulse and respiratory rate, improved mental status, improved skin color, and decreased use of accessory and abdominal muscles occur because patient's work of breathing decreases as level of oxygenation improves.

Clinical Judgment *When first initiating CPAP/BiPAP, it is important to monitor gas exchange, lung sounds, and respiratory muscle effort. If there are any signs of respiratory distress, the health care provider should be notified and changes in ventilator settings should be anticipated. In the planning process, it is essential to be prepared to assess for patient tolerance to the NIPPV (Urden et al., 2024).*

STEP	RATIONALE
• Patient's skin around bridge of nose, ears, and back of head remains intact without signs of pressure injury.	Mask applied properly and monitored for MDRPI.
• Patient able to describe how to use NIPPV in the home setting, if required.	Demonstrates learning.
2. Provide privacy and explain procedure.	Protects patient's privacy; reduces anxiety. Promotes cooperation.
3. Collaborate with the respiratory therapist and gather and organize equipment or supplies to perform procedure at patient's bedside.	Ensures that you have necessary equipment to apply the NIPPV system. Ensures more efficiency when completing the procedure.
4. Instruct patient and/or family caregiver about need for NIPPV. If NIPPV is planned for home use, educate patient about oxygen safety, use of equipment, and appropriate vendor and community resources.	Education decreases patient and family caregiver anxiety. Proper education about NIPPV and use of equipment helps to ensure the safe and proper use of the equipment. Vendor and community resources will assist family in obtaining prompt assistance for equipment issues.

IMPLEMENTATION

1. Perform hand hygiene; apply clean gloves. Apply mask, gown, and goggles if secretions are projectile or if patient is in isolation.	Reduces transmission of microorganisms and exposure to pulmonary secretions.
2. Determine correct mask size. Use masking chart to determine correct size (S, M, L, XL). **NOTE:** It is imperative that masks have quick-release straps.	Mask should fit snugly over patient's nose (CPAP) or nose and/or mouth (BiPAP) to create a tight seal for delivering positive pressure. In case of emergency (e.g., vomiting, respiratory arrest), quick-release straps allow mask to be removed quickly. The patient should be able to remove the mask quickly as needed (Urden et al., 2024).

Clinical Judgment *A patient receiving NIPPV via a full-face mask should never be restrained. The patient must be able to remove the mask if patient begins to vomit, needs to remove excess secretions, or needs to reposition a mask that has moved. A shifted mask can force the patient's jaw inward, which can obstruct the patient's airway (Urden et al., 2024).*

3. Adjust bed to appropriate height and lower side rail on side nearest you. Check locks on bed wheels. Place patient in position of comfort with the head of the bed raised.	Minimizes caregiver's muscle strain and prevents injury. Prevents bed from moving. Proper patient position allows for optimal lung expansion and decreased work of breathing.
4. Connect CPAP/BiPAP device-delivery tubing to pressure generator.	Ensures that patient is receiving proper NIPPV as ordered.
5. Connect patient to pulse oximetry, if not already being monitored.	It is important to continually monitor patient's level of oxygenation when initiating NIPPV.
6. Set CPAP/BiPAP initial settings per health care provider order:	These settings allow health care team to determine initial patient response.
a. *CPAP*: Initially, pressure is typically set at 3 to 5 cm H_2O or less, and then changes are guided by ABG and patient tolerance (Oxford Medication Education [OME], 2023; Urden et al., 2024).	CPAP provides single positive pressure throughout breathing cycle, which helps to keep alveoli open at end expiration.
b. *BiPAP*: Inspiratory pressure is usually set at 5 to 15 cm H_2O initially and can be titrated up to 20 to 30 cm H_2O as patient condition dictates; expiratory pressure is usually set at 3 to 4 cm H_2O initially and can be titrated up as patient condition warrants (Ghosh & Elliott, 2019).	BiPAP supplies pressure at both inhalation and exhalation. The inhalation pressure (sometimes referred to as pressure support) is set according to health care provider's order and helps prevent airway closure. Expiratory pressure (sometimes referred to as positive end-expiratory pressure [PEEP]) is set according to health care provider's order and keeps alveoli open at end-expiration (OME, 2023; Urden et al., 2024).
7. Select FiO_2 level as indicated and per prescriber order.	Patients on NIPPV may also need supplemental oxygen to decrease signs and symptoms of hypoxia (Ghosh & Elliott, 2019).
8. Ensure that humidification and heating appliances are connected and on.	Humidification of gas is thought to improve comfort in patients receiving NIPPV (Elliott & Elliott, 2018; Restrepo & Walsh, 2022).
9. Ensure that mask is tight fitting, no air leak is present, and there are no excessive pressure points.	An ill-fitting mask leads to loss of pressure getting into airways or dyssynchrony with ventilator. It also can lead to air blowing into eyes, which can cause patient discomfort. Pressure points around mask area can cause MDRPI (Jackson et al., 2019).
10. If patient is to use CPAP at home, have patient or family caregiver demonstrate mask placement and adjustment of settings.	Return demonstration indicates learning.

STEP	RATIONALE
11. Return patient to comfortable position.	Restores comfort and sense of well-being.
12. Raise side rails (as appropriate) and lower bed to lowest position, locking into position.	Ensures patient safety and prevents falls.
13. Place nurse call system in an accessible location within patient's reach.	Ensures patient can call for assistance if needed.
14. Remove and dispose of gloves and other PPE, and perform hand hygiene.	Reduces transmission of microorganisms.
15. Continuous care of patient:	
a. Ensure that all ventilator alarms are on and active and that ventilator circuit is intact and properly functioning.	Ensures patient safety.
b. Ensure that emergency resuscitation equipment is at bedside.	Allows for quick resuscitation in case of worsening patient condition (Urden et al., 2024).
c. Investigate any and all alarms from ventilator/CPAP machine and/or patient monitor.	Alarms alert health care team to problems with patient or with circuit that adversely affects patient status.
d. Change patient's position every 2 hours or encourage patient to change position every 2 hours.	Reduces incidence of atelectasis or pneumonia secondary to stasis of secretions (Urden et al., 2024).

EVALUATION

1. Observe for decreased anxiety, improved level of consciousness and cognitive abilities, decreased fatigue, and absence of dizziness.	Determines patient's response to NIPPV. As hypoxia and hypercapnia are reduced or corrected, patient's behavioral assessment parameters improve.
2. Measure vital signs, perform respiratory assessment, and ask patient to describe sense of dyspnea.	Physical assessment parameters reveal oxygenation status.
3. Assess skin under mask every 1 to 2 hours for signs of skin breakdown/pressure injuries. Apply protective dressing/barrier if indicated.	Maintains vigilance for MDRPI due to pressure from the mask. The use of a protective barrier may help to prevent the development of skin breakdown or could prevent worsening of the breakdown (Fumarola et al., 2020; Jackson et al., 2019).
4. Monitor pulse oximetry. Obtain ABG values per health care provider.	Assesses patient's level of oxygenation and gas exchange.
5. If NIPPV is planned for use in the home, observe and monitor the patient's and family caregiver's ability to use the NIPPV ventilator and manipulate the mask to have a good fit.	Determines patient's and/or family caregiver's ability to perform self-care and adhere to the NIPPV plan.
6. Use Teach-Back: "I want to be sure I explained how NIPPV works and why you are receiving this therapy. Explain to me why this therapy is necessary." Revise your instruction now or develop a plan for revised patient/family caregiver teaching if patient/family caregiver is not able to teach back correctly.	Teach-back is a technique for health care providers to ensure that they have explained medical information clearly so that patients and their families understand what is communicated to them (AHRQ, 2023).

Unexpected Outcomes	Related Interventions
1. Patient experiences hypoxia, hypercapnia, or other signs of worsening respiratory function or barotrauma (pneumothorax).	• Notify health care provider immediately. • Reassess patient. • Determine correct settings and integrity of NIPPV. Consult with respiratory therapist.
2. Patient develops skin breakdown at mask sites or sites where mask straps are located such as bridge of nose, nasal septum, or ears.	• Notify health care provider. • Place protective synthetic coverings on nasal bridge or areas of irritation/possible irritation to protect skin (Fumarola et al., 2020). • Fit mask so it is tight enough to not cause air leak but loose enough to not cause skin breakdown. • Reassess patient (Jackson et al., 2019).
3. Patient states sense of smothering or claustrophobia.	• Explain system to patient again. • Demonstrate use of quick-release straps. • Have patient demonstrate use of quick-release straps.

Documentation

- Document type of NIPPV, including pressure settings, oxygen flow rates, assistance needed with positioning, coughing effectiveness, and respiratory assessment findings.
- Document patient tolerance of and adherence to NIPPV, mask fit, skin assessment findings, and patient subjective reports of comfort and daytime fatigue.
- Document evaluation of patient and family caregiver learning.

Hand-Off Reporting

- Report patient status, including recent assessment findings, vital signs, and SpO_2 before initiation of NIPPV.
- Report the type of NIPPV device initiated and used, the initial pressure settings and oxygen flow rates, and if any adjustments to the pressure settings and flow rate were made during the shift. Include the patient response to the flow rate adjustments and what interventions were successful.
- Report any unexpected outcome to health care provider or nurse in charge.

Special Considerations

Patient Education

- Teach patient and family caregiver the prescribed hours to use the machine. If not in use for 24 hours/day, work with the family caregiver to identify the ideal time for use (e.g., bedtime, watching television).
- Teach patient and family caregiver how to assess patient's skin under the mask, apply the mask, connect it to the machine, and add oxygen if ordered.
- Instruct family caregiver to bring the machine, along with a list of correct settings, to the hospital any time patient is admitted.

Pediatrics

- Children may not tolerate the NIPPV mask and may resist its use. Encourage the parents/family caregivers to assist the child in wearing the NIPPV device.

Patients With Disabilities

- Patients with a cognitive developmental delay may not tolerate the application of the full face mask for NIPPV use. Assess the patient's cognitive ability to understand the necessity for NIPPV and assess for signs of agitation or intolerance of the device.

Home Care

- The durable medical equipment provider, the home care nurse, and the primary care nurse develop a teaching plan to ensure that patient and family have working knowledge of the system before discharge.
- When patients require home NIPPV, instruct in complete care of the CPAP/BiPAP system. Skills include assembling the system, cleaning it, and maintaining the equipment daily.
- Teach patient and family caregiver what to do in case of respiratory distress or power failure.
- Notify appropriate power company so that in the event of a power outage, the home is on priority for restoring power.
- Follow the safety precautions for oxygen use (see Box 23.2).

PROCEDURAL GUIDELINE 23.1 *Use of a Peak Flowmeter*

For patients who have measurable changes in the flow of air through their airways, such as patients with asthma or reactive airway disease, peak expiratory flow rate (PEFR) measurements are useful. The PEFR is the maximum flow that a patient forces out during one quick, forced expiration and is measured in liters per minute. Use these measurements as an objective indicator of a patient's current status or the effectiveness of treatment. Decreased PEFR may indicate the need for further interventions such as increased doses of bronchodilators, antiinflammatory medications, or even seeking emergency medical attention. Normal PEFR values vary according to a person's age, gender, and size (American Lung Association [ALA], 2023).

Patients with asthma perform PEFR measures in the home to monitor the status of their airways. Health care providers usually recommend that patients measure and record their PEFR at the following times: same time every day (values are lowest in the morning and typically highest between noon and 5 p.m.), before taking asthma medicines, during asthma symptoms or an asthma attack, after taking medicine for an asthma attack, and at other times recommended by their health care provider (ALA, 2023).

Delegation

Initial assessment of the patient's condition is a nursing responsibility and cannot be delegated. The skills of follow-up PEFR measurements in a stable patient can be delegated to assistive personnel (AP). Instruct the AP to:

- Report immediately to the nurse patient's difficulty breathing or decrease in PEFR measurement

Interprofessional Collaboration

- Health care providers are responsible for prescribing any changes in medications that should be made based on PEFR measurements.
- Respiratory therapists are often responsible for administering any nebulized medications necessitated by PEFR measurements.

Equipment

Peak flowmeter (Fig. 23.14); patient diary/action plan (if appropriate); clean gloves (optional)

Steps

1. Identify patient using at least two identifiers (e.g., name and birthday or name and medical record number) according to agency policy (TJC, 2023).
2. Review electronic health record (EHR) for patient's baseline PEFR readings (if available).
3. Review the target set by patient's health care provider.
4. Assess patient's/family caregiver's health literacy (CDC, 2023a).
5. Perform hand hygiene and complete a respiratory assessment (lung sounds, respirations).
6. Assess if patient has the manual dexterity to correctly measure PEFR by having patient manipulate device.
7. Assess patient's/family caregiver's knowledge and prior experience with the peak flowmeter.
8. Assess patient's goals or preferences for how peak flow rate measurement should be performed.

Continued

PROCEDURAL GUIDELINE 23.1 *Use of a Peak Flowmeter—cont'd*

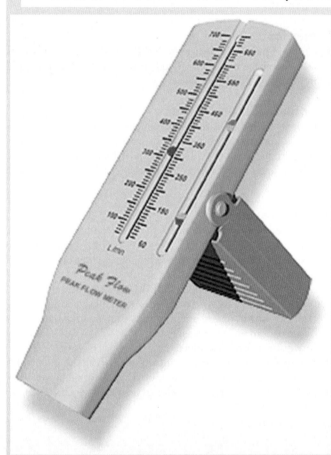

FIG. 23.14 Peak flowmeter. (*Courtesy Philips Respironics.*)

9. Gather peak flowmeter and diary at bedside.
10. Perform hand hygiene. Apply clean gloves if exposure to mucus is likely.
11. Close room door or curtains around bed.
12. Instruct the patient and/or family caregiver about the need for the peak flowmeter.
13. Help patient to stand or to assume a high-Fowler position or any other position that promotes optimum lung expansion. Remove any gum or food from mouth.
14. Slide the marker on the peak flowmeter to the bottom of the scale.
15. Slide clean mouthpiece into base of the numbered scale. Instruct patient on how to place mouthpiece in mouth and close lips, making a firm seal. Instruct patient to keep tongue away from mouthpiece.
16. Instruct patient to take a deep breath and blow out. Then have patient take another deep breath and hold. Have patient quickly place meter mouthpiece in mouth, close lips

firmly, and blow out as hard and fast as possible through mouth only. Note the number on scale and document on a piece of paper.
17. Repeat two more times or as ordered by health care provider.
18. Document the highest number.
19. Inform patient of the individualized acceptable range and mark on meter.
20. If patient is to record PEFR at home, have the patient or family caregiver demonstrate how to record it accurately on chart using "traffic light" pattern. A system of asthma zones—green, yellow, and red—is commonly used. Green indicates that the PEFR is 80% to 100% of patient's personal best value and means that patient should continue with the currently prescribed treatment regimen. Yellow indicates that the PEFR is 50% to 80% of the personal best and that the person should implement the health care provider's plan for yellow zone values. Interventions are typically to add the prescribed quick-relief medication to the treatment regimen and continue with the daily long-term control medications. Red indicates that the PEFR is less than 50% of the patient's personal best and that the person should take the prescribed quick-relief medication and contact health care provider immediately (ALA, 2023) (Fig. 23.15).
21. Instruct patient to measure peak flow rate every day, as close as possible to the same time every day.
22. Instruct patient to keep a chart or diary of daily peak flow values that can be shared with the health care provider.
23. Instruct patient to clean unit weekly, following manufacturer's instructions.
24. Help patient to comfortable position.
25. Raise side rails (as appropriate) and lower bed to lowest position, locking into position.
26. Place nurse call system in an accessible location within patient's reach.
27. Remove and dispose of gloves and other PPE (if used) and perform hand hygiene.
28. **Use Teach-Back:** "I want to make sure that I showed you how to correctly measure your PEFR. Show me how you would use this PEFR device." Revise your instruction now or develop a plan for revised patient/family caregiver teaching if patient/family caregiver is not able to teach back correctly.
29. Compare patient's PEFR with the patient's personal best.
30. Document PEFR measurement before and after therapy and patient's ability and effort to perform PEFR.
31. Report to health care provider if patient is in yellow or red zone.
32. Report to nurses/respiratory therapists the patient's PEFR values and tolerance of performance of peak flow measurements.

PROCEDURAL GUIDELINE 23.1 *Use of a Peak Flowmeter—cont'd*

Asthma Action Plan

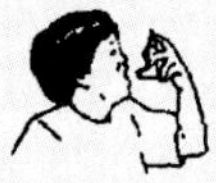

You can use the colors of a traffic light to help learn about your asthma medicines.

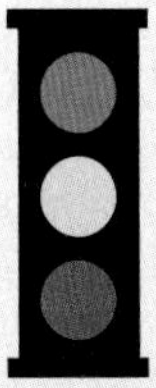

Name: _____

Doctor: _____ Date: _____

Phone for doctor or clinic: _____

Emergency contact phone and name: _____

1. **Green** means **Go.**
   Use preventive medicine.

2. **Yellow** means **Caution.**
   Use quick-relief medicine.

3. **Red** means **Stop.**
   Get help from a doctor.

1. Green — Go

- Breathing is good
- No cough or wheeze
- Can work and play

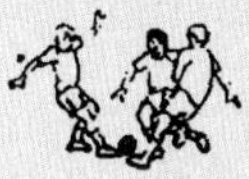

Peak flow number
_____ to _____

Personal best peak flow _____

Use preventive medicine.

Medicine	How much to take	When to take it

5 to 60 minutes before exercise, use this medicine:

_____

2. Yellow — Caution

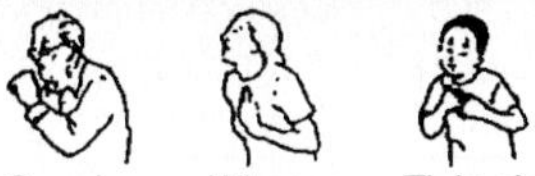

Cough Wheeze Tight chest

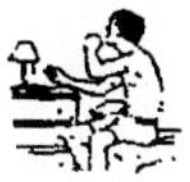

Wake up at night

Peak flow number
_____ to _____
(50% to 80% of my best peak flow)

Take quick-relief medicine to keep an asthma attack from getting bad

Medicine	How much to take	When to take it
(short-acting beta₂ agonist)		

If symptoms return to Green Zone after 1 hour of taking above quick-relief medication, take _____ (medicine) and _____ (medicine).

If symptoms **do not** return to Green Zone after 1 hour of taking the quick-relief medication, take _____ (medicine) and add _____ (medicine).
(short-acting beta₂ agonist)   (oral steroid)

Call your doctor if symptoms do not improve within ____ hours after taking the oral steroid or if your symptoms are in the Red Zone.

3. Red — Stop — Danger

- Medicine is not helping
- Breathing is hard and fast
- Nose opens wide
- Can't walk
- Ribs show
- Can't talk well

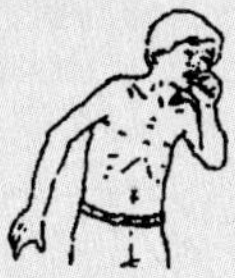

Peak flow number
_____ to _____
(50% or less of personal best)

Get help from a doctor now!
Take these medicines until you talk with the doctor.

Medicine	How much to take	When to take it
(short-acting beta₂ agonist)		
(oral steroid)		

Go to the emergency department immediately or call the ambulance if you cannot reach your doctor and you are still in the Red Zone after 15 minutes.

These signs signal **DANGER:**
- Difficulty walking or breathing
- Mental confusion
- Fingernails or lips are blue

Call the ambulance.

FIG. 23.15 Asthma action plan. (*From Hockenberry MJ, Duffy EA, Gibbs KD:* Wong's nursing care of infants and children, *ed 12, St Louis, 2024, Elsevier.*)

✦ SKILL 23.5   Care of a Patient on a Mechanical Ventilator

Mechanical ventilation, also referred to as positive pressure ventilation, is a life-saving therapy used for patients who have illnesses or conditions that can lead to respiratory failure. It controls or helps a patient's respirations when the patient is unable to maintain adequate gas exchange because of respiratory or ventilatory failure (Table 23.3). Clinical indications for invasive mechanical ventilation include cardiac or respiratory arrest, disorientation, failure to respond to bronchodilator therapy, and exhaustion (Urden et al., 2024). It can be used to either fully or partially replace spontaneous breathing, depending on the needs of the patient. Invasive mechanical ventilation also redistributes oxygen demand from working respiratory muscles to other vital organs.

The ventilator takes over the physical work of moving air into and out of the lungs, but it does not replace or alter the physiological function of the lung. It can be used for a short period of time or as a long-term means of support for those who cannot support their own respiratory effort, such as those with neuromuscular disorders (Harding et al., 2023; Urden et al., 2024). Patients receiving mechanical ventilation are most often in an intensive care unit but may be in skilled nursing facilities or home settings.

Positive pressure ventilation is the most common method of ventilation (Fig. 23.16). It delivers a positive pressure to inflate the lungs. An artificial airway such as an endotracheal (ET) tube or tracheostomy tube (TT) is necessary for positive pressure

TABLE 23.3

Modes of Mechanical Ventilation

Types	Description	Nursing Considerations
Continuous positive airway pressure (CPAP)	Applies positive pressure during entire respiratory cycle. Used to help open alveoli at end expiration, thereby improving oxygenation.	Used for patients who breathe spontaneously but have hypoxemic respiratory failure; useful during weaning. Patients with chronic obstructive pulmonary disease (COPD) may tire after long hours of CPAP and require increased pressure support. Is used in both invasive and noninvasive ventilation modes.
Pressure support ventilation (PSV)	Preset amount of positive pressure used to help augment patient's spontaneous inspiratory efforts. Patient controls rate, inspiratory flow, and tidal volume.	Spontaneous breathing mode. Helps overcome resistance of airway and ventilator tubing. Reduces patient work of breathing and improves ventilator-patient synchrony.
Assist-control (AC) or continuous mandatory ventilation (CMV)	Patient initiates breathing, but backup control delivers preset number of breaths at set volume.	Volume-controlled CMV used in patients with weak respiratory muscles that are spontaneously breathing. Watch for barotrauma. Pressure-controlled CMV used in patients with increased airway resistance or decreased lung compliance. Watch for hypercapnia. Sedation may be needed to control respiratory rate.
Synchronized intermittent mandatory ventilation (SIMV)	Ventilator delivers set number of breaths at specified volume. Some patients breathe spontaneously between SIMV breaths at volumes differing from those set on the machine.	Volume-controlled intermittent mandatory ventilation (IMV) is primary method of ventilation in many settings. Requires frequent monitoring during weaning from mechanical ventilation. May increase patient's work of breathing.
Pressure-regulated volume-control ventilation (PRVCV or PRVC)	Variation of CMV combining features of volume- and pressure-control settings. The ventilator delivers a preset tidal volume at the lowest possible airway pressure. That pressure will not exceed preset maximum pressure limit.	Used in patients with changing pulmonary mechanics and dynamics. Potential complications are limited when compared with AC or pressure controlled–intermittent mandatory ventilation (PC-IMV) modes.
Airway pressure release ventilation (APRV)	Two different levels of CPAP (inspiratory and expiratory) are applied for set periods of time, allowing for spontaneous breathing that can occur at both levels.	Spontaneous breathing mode that recruits alveoli with decreased risk of high peak pressures, decreasing risk of barotrauma. Patient should be monitored for hypercapnia.
High-Frequency		
High-frequency jet ventilation (HFJV)	Delivers gas rapidly under low pressure via special injector cannula. Delivers 100–600 cycles/min with lower-than-normal tidal volumes.	Patient on any mode of high-frequency ventilation requires continuous sedation and neuromuscular blocking agent administration. Not commonly used in adults; more commonly used in neonates. Requires intensive monitoring and care.
High-frequency oscillatory ventilation (HFOV)	Delivers 900–3000 cycles/min with very small tidal volumes. Airway pressure controlled.	Most common of high-frequency types maintains alveolar ventilation with low airway pressure; useful for treating esophageal or bronchopleural fistulas; helps avert barotraumas in high-risk patients if used early in treatment. Not commonly used in adults; more commonly used in infants and children. Requires use of continuous sedation and neuromuscular blocking agent. Requires intensive monitoring and care.

Data from Baird M: Manual of critical care nursing: Interprofessional collaborative management, ed 8, St. Louis, 2023, Elsevier and Urden L, et al: Priorities in critical care nursing, ed 9, St. Louis, 2024, Elsevier.

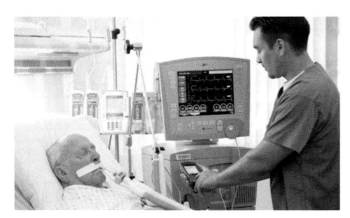

FIG. 23.16 Positive pressure ventilator. (*Courtesy and copyright © Becton, Dickinson and Company.*)

mechanical ventilation (see Chapter 24). Multiple complications are associated with positive pressure ventilation, including decreased cardiac output, aspiration, barotrauma, and ventilator-associated events (VAEs) such as ventilator-associated pneumonia (VAP) (see Chapter 24). Be alert for these adverse events by conducting cardiopulmonary assessment and evaluation (Elliott & Elliott, 2018; Urden et al., 2024).

It is important that patients remain on mechanical ventilation only as long as necessary because there is an increased mortality risk associated with positive pressure ventilation. In addition, as the length of time needed for mechanical ventilation increases, there is an increased risk of failure to wean from the ventilator (Urden et al., 2024).

Alarms and Settings

The mechanical ventilator has a number of settings to adjust the amount of oxygen delivered, the number of breaths per minute, the amount of tidal volume delivered, the time for inspiration and expiration, and the pressure at which each breath is delivered. The health care provider will prescribe the ventilator settings and the respiratory therapist (RT) will adjust the ventilator to the prescribed settings. The goal in adjusting settings is to use as little oxygen as possible (typically an FiO_2 can be set between 21% and 100% and is adjusted to maintain PaO_2 level >60 mm Hg or SpO_2 level >92%) with a tidal volume of 6 to 10 mL/kg order to help patients meet their SpO_2 and arterial blood gas (ABG) parameters (Elliott & Elliott, 2018; Urden et al., 2024). It is valuable for nurses to understand ventilator parameters and their significance so that appropriate assessments can be made along with timely communication with all health care providers (Table 23.4).

There are several alarms on the ventilator to ensure patient safety. Each ventilator is a little different; however, the basic alarms are similar. Alarms common to all ventilators include high-pressure, low-pressure, and low–exhaled volume alarms. Table 23.5 lists the common causes of ventilator alarms as well as the nursing interventions used to address the alarms. You need to know how to respond to the ventilator alarms and which nursing actions are required to preserve the patient's respiratory status (Elliott & Elliott, 2018; Urden et al., 2024).

The most frequently sounding alarms are the high-pressure and low-pressure alarms. The high-pressure alarm is usually set at 10 to 20 cm above peak inspiratory pressure (Urden et al., 2024). When this alarm sounds, it indicates that the ventilator has met resistance to delivering the tidal volume and requires more pressure to inflate the lungs. The low-pressure alarm sounds when the ventilator has no resistance to inflating the lung. All ventilator alarms

---

TABLE 23.4

Ventilator Parameters

Parameter	Definition	Ventilator Setting
Tidal volume (Vt)	Amount of air inspired and expired with each breath; can be set by ventilator or can measure patient's own spontaneous breaths	6–8 mL/kg of ideal body weight. Use lower volumes in patients with ARDS.
Respiratory rate (R or RR)	Number of breaths delivered by ventilator per minute	Usual rate is 10–16 breaths/min. However, the rate can be set 4–20 breaths/min, with lower rates used during ventilator weaning.
Fraction of inspired oxygen (FiO_2)	Amount of oxygen that patient receives	Ideally less than 40% to maintain PaO_2 >60 mm Hg and SpO_2 >90%.
Positive end-expiratory pressure (PEEP)	Positive pressure applied at end-expiration of ventilator breaths to open alveoli and improve oxygenation	5 cm H_2O may be used to approximate physiological PEEP. May require higher levels (10–20 cm H_2O) in respiratory failure (e.g., refractory hypoxemia). If patient has a PEEP greater than 10 cm H_2O, the circuit should not be interrupted.
Sensitivity	Determines patient's inspiratory effort required to trigger the ventilator	A breath can be triggered by a change in either flow or pressure. Pressure trigger is usually 0.5–1.5 cm below baseline. Flow trigger is usually 1–3 L/min below baseline.
I:E ratio	Comparison of inspiratory (I) to expiratory (E) time	Example: Inspiration 0.5 seconds, expiration 1 second, then I:E = 1:2. Usually set at 1:2 to 1:1.5 because expiration is typically longer than inspiration. Can use inverse ratios for certain disease states such as ARDS in attempt to open alveoli.
Exhaled minute ventilation (VE)	Measures exhaled minute ventilations in liters	Alarm set at 15% greater than patient's average VE.

ARDS, Acute respiratory distress syndrome.
Data from Baird M: *Manual of critical care nursing: Interprofessional collaborative management,* ed 8, St. Louis, 2023, Elsevier; and Urden L, et al: *Priorities in critical care nursing,* ed 9, St. Louis, 2024.

TABLE 23.5

Troubleshooting Mechanical Ventilation

Ventilator Alarm	Possible Causes	Nursing Interventions
Sudden increase in peak airway pressure (high-pressure alarm)	Coughing Airway plugging/excess secretions Changes in patient position Pneumothorax Incorrect endotracheal (ET) tube position Kinked ventilator circuit Excessive water in ventilator circuit Patient biting tube Patient not in synchrony with ventilator Ventilator malfunction	Clear secretions by suctioning. Reposition patient. Assess breath sounds and chest wall movement. Verify placement of ET tube. Verify centimeter level of ET tube. Check circuit; unkink tubing. Drain ventilator tubing. Insert bite block. Sedate patient. Notify respiratory therapist and health care provider if interventions do not fix the cause.
Gradual increase in peak airway pressure	Decreasing lung compliance Exacerbation of acute process	Evaluate breath sounds; suction. Check for reversible causes: airway plugging, bronchospasm. Notify respiratory therapist and health care provider if interventions do not fix the alarm.
Decrease in peak airway pressure (low-pressure alarm)	Patient disconnected from ventilator Leak in ventilator circuit ET tube displaced into pharynx Cuff not inflated properly Improved lung compliance Decrease in amount of secretions	Check for disconnection. Evaluate circuit connections; tighten loose connections. Assess cuff for appropriate pressure (see Skills 24.3 and 24.4). Notify respiratory therapist.
Change in minute ventilation or tidal volume	Leak in ET cuff Patient stops spontaneously breathing Other conditions that trigger low- or high-pressure alarms	Check cuff seal (see Skills 24.3 and 24.4). Notify respiratory therapist.
Increase in respiratory rate	Patient anxiety Increased metabolic demand Hypoxia	Reassure patient. Evaluate body temperature, heart rate and rhythm. Monitor pulse oximetry.
Apnea	Respiratory arrest Oversedation Incidental extubation	Reverse/discontinue sedating medications. Provide breaths via self-inflating resuscitation bag. Prepare for reintubation if tube dislodged and patient requires it. Institute emergency Rapid Response Team.
Ventilator inoperative or low battery	Equipment malfunction Machine not plugged in	Plug in machine. Notify respiratory therapist. Provide breaths via self-inflating resuscitation bag if necessary.

Data from Baird M: *Manual of critical care nursing: Interprofessional collaborative management,* ed 8, St. Louis, 2023, Elsevier; and Urden L, et al: *Priorities in critical care nursing,* ed 9, St Louis, 2024, Elsevier.

require immediate nursing intervention to prevent patient harm. When responding to a ventilator alarm, it is important to also assess the patient's vital signs, especially the pulse oximetry.

Ventilator-Associated Events

A VAE is a deterioration in patient condition after placement on mechanical ventilation, including sepsis, acute respiratory distress syndrome, and ventilator-associated pneumonia (VAP). There is a lengthy and complicated series of criteria that must be met in order for a patient to be diagnosed with VAE (CDC, 2023b). VAP and VAE are often used interchangeably in the literature, even though they are different. VAP is one of the most common hospital-acquired infections. It is simply defined as pneumonia in a patient who has been intubated and receiving mechanical ventilation for 48 to 72 hours (Urden et al., 2024). It can cost between $10,000 and $40,000 per patient, can increase patient length of stay, and is associated with increased morbidity and mortality rates (Alja'afreh et al., 2019; Darawad et al., 2018). To reduce rates of VAEs, health care facilities have implemented the use of practice bundles. The use of

evidence-based interventions targets efforts at decreasing the rates of VAEs (Box 23.3). Even though implementation of ventilator bundles is associated with reductions in VAP, a new surveillance model of VAEs has shifted the focus from VAP to objective, generalized signs of pulmonary decompensation not specific to VAP (CDC, 2023b; Kallet, 2019). The Institute for Healthcare Improvement (IHI) developed a widely used ventilator bundle that has been the basis for bundles used in medical centers today (IHI, 2019). This standard bundle is being revised as new studies support or refute specific therapies. Refer to your health care agency for ventilator bundle guidelines.

Delegation

The skill of caring for a patient on a mechanical ventilator cannot be delegated to assistive personnel (AP). Instruct the AP to:
- Report immediately to the nurse any change in the patient's respiratory status, vital signs, or oxygen saturation and if patient indicates breathlessness.
- Inform the nurse immediately if any of the ventilator alarms sound.

Interventions for Reducing Risk for Ventilator-Associated Pneumonia

- Good hand hygiene
- Internal endotracheal cuff pressure at 25–30 cm H_2O
- Head of bed (HOB) raised to at least 30 degrees unless contraindicated
- Prophylaxis for deep vein thrombosis (DVT)
- Daily interruptions of sedation to assess for readiness to extubate
- Oral care with chlorhexidine 0.12% every 6 hours and general oral care every 2 hours secondary to microbial colonization within the mouth (Alja'afreh et al., 2019; Urden et al., 2024)
- Complete subglottal suctioning to decrease risk of oral fluid aspiration (Letchford & Bench, 2018; Urden et al., 2024)
- Brushing the patient's teeth with a soft toothbrush and brushing the tongue and gums with a foam swab (Urden et al., 2024)
- Timely, not scheduled, ventilator circuit changes and removal of condensation
- Reduce risk of skin injury through turning and repositioning every 2 hours
- Use the prone position to improve oxygenation parameters (PaO_2; SaO_2) (Shelhamer et al., 2021)
- Reduce risk of cardiopulmonary deconditioning with early ambulation and mobility

NOTE: The use of probiotics has not been shown to have an effect on VAP rates (Mahmoodpoor et al., 2019). Their safety has not been established in critically ill patients (Virk & Wiersinga, 2019).

- Help in daily care such as bathing and repositioning the patient. Include special skin care needs and any positioning restrictions.

Interprofessional Collaboration

- RTs set up and maintain the ventilator and ventilator circuit. They are the staff members responsible for making the changes on the ventilator settings that have been ordered by the health care providers.
- A wound, ostomy, continence nurse (WOCN) or skin care specialist will assist in special skin care interventions to reduce

the risk of pressure injury, medical device–related pressure injury (MDRPI), and medical adhesive–related skin injury (MARSI) when needed.
- Physical and occupational therapists may be responsible for assisting with range-of-motion exercises or ambulation of the patient.

Equipment

- Artificial airway (ET tube or TT)
- Appropriate mechanical ventilator
- Heater and humidifier for circuit
- Oxygen source
- Pulse oximetry (SpO_2) probe and monitor
- Electrocardiogram (ECG) monitoring (if in intensive care unit or by institution policy)
- Capnography ($EtCO_2$) window and monitor (if available)
- Stethoscope
- 5- or 10-mL syringe
- Oral airway/bite block, as needed
- Manual self-inflating resuscitation bag (bag-valve mask) with oxygen connecting tubing and flowmeter and a positive end-expiratory pressure (PEEP) valve
- Appropriately sized resuscitation face mask
- Cuff pressure manometer
- Agency-approved sedation monitoring scale if patient receiving sedation
- Clean gloves, goggles (if splash risk exists); mask and gown if patient's isolation orders indicate
- Suction equipment at bedside (in-line/individual catheters)
- Suction equipment for subglottic and oral suctioning
- Chlorhexidine solution (0.12%), oral swab, and toothbrush for oral care
- Method for patient communication (e.g., letter/picture board, common word lists)
- Twill cloth tape, adhesive tape, or ETT/TT holder
- Ventilator flow sheet to document ventilator changes and settings (may be a paper flow sheet part of the electronic health record [EHR])

STEP	RATIONALE

ASSESSMENT

1. Identify patient using at least two identifiers (e.g., name and birthday or name and medical record number) according to agency policy.

Ensures correct patient. Complies with the Joint Commission standards and improves patient safety (TJC, 2023).

2. Review patient's EHR, including health care provider's order and nurses' notes. Note patient's normal pulse oximetry values, baseline and trends in respiratory rate and effort of breathing, past medical history, past oxygen and/or ventilatory requirements, and ABG results or SpO_2 values and $EtCO_2$ values.

Knowing the patient's baseline and ongoing condition and past medical history helps in understanding the amount of oxygen to deliver and the ventilator settings to be used.

3. Review the patient's EHR for prescription for oxygen requirements and ventilator settings, including ventilator rate, tidal volume, PEEP, and pressure to deliver. Note any titration parameters, such as for delivery of oxygen or changing of respiratory rate.

RT will make ventilator settings. Ensures safe and accurate oxygen delivery and ventilator settings.

4. Review EHR to determine patient's age and history of dehydration, malnutrition, exposure to radiation therapy, underlying chronic conditions (e.g., diabetes mellitus, immunosuppression), and edema of the skin.

Common risk factors for MARSI from adhesive (when used to secure ET tube) (Fumarola et al., 2020).

STEP	RATIONALE
5. Assess patient's/family caregiver's health literacy. Determine method for communication with patient. If possible, review previous communication techniques with patient and family. Use simple language to gather assessment.	Determines degree to which individuals have the ability to find, understand, and use information and services to make informed health-related decisions and actions for themselves and others (CDC, 2023a). Patients with an artificial airway and mechanical ventilation cannot communicate verbally, so communication aids need to be identified (Karlsen et al., 2019; Santiago et al., 2019).
6. Assess patient's level of consciousness (LOC) and ability to cooperate with mechanical ventilation and tolerate need for special positioning such as head of bed (HOB) at 30 degrees.	Determines patient's ability to cooperate and understand aspects of care. Anxious and combative patients may require sedation to tolerate mechanical ventilation.
7. Assess patient's need for sedation (check agency policy).	Sedation is often used in mechanically ventilated patients to reduce respiratory efforts, decrease oxygen demand, ensure patient synchrony with the ventilator, and improve ABG and oxygen saturation levels (Urden et al., 2024).

Clinical Judgment *When patients on mechanical ventilation become excessively anxious or combative or try to override the ventilator, sedation is often used. Be aware that heavy sedation is associated with increased length of time on the ventilator, increased risk of delirium, and increased mortality. Follow agency policy for the specific indications for sedation and the specific protocol for administering and monitoring sedation levels for these patients.*

8. Perform hand hygiene. Apply gloves and other personal protective equipment (PPE) as patient status indicates.	Reduces transmission of microorganisms.
9. Assess patient's respiratory status, including symmetry of chest wall expansion, respiratory rate and depth, sputum production, and lung sounds (see Chapter 6), and assess for signs and symptoms associated with hypoxia (see Box 23.1).	Decreased chest wall movement, crackles or decreased or absent lung sounds, increased respiratory rate, increased sputum production, or signs of worsening hypoxia indicate need for mechanical ventilation or changes in current ventilator settings to improve oxygenation and ventilation.
10. Assess patient's cardiovascular condition, including blood pressure, heart rate, regularity of heart rate, and quality of peripheral pulses (see Chapter 6).	Positive pressure mechanical ventilation can increase patient's intrathoracic pressure. This can cause a decrease in cardiac output and cardiovascular function (Urden et al., 2024).
11. Assess for signs and symptoms of inadvertent extubation (able to vocalize, low-pressure ventilator alarms, decreased or absent breath sounds, gastric distention, changes in ET tube depth according to markings, changes in $EtCO_2$ waveform and values, patient holding tube with hand).	Inadvertent extubation can lead to decrease in patient oxygenation and cardiopulmonary status.

Clinical Judgment *Sometimes patients tolerate inadvertent extubation. The nurse needs to carefully assess the patient and be prepared to apply a different type of oxygen-delivery device (nasal cannula, face mask, or noninvasive positive pressure ventilation [NIPPV]) or to reintubate the patient. The nurse may need to perform bag-valve-mask ventilation until a provider who can reintubate the patient arrives in the room.*

12. Check ventilator, $EtCO_2$ (if available), SpO_2, and cardiac alarms at beginning of each shift and periodically throughout care and compare with health care provider's orders.	Verifies that ventilator settings are as ordered by health care provider. Ensures patient safety.
13. Verify placement of artificial airway through auscultation of lung sounds, verification of distal tip marking on ET tube, and/or $EtCO_2$ value. Determine that tube is secure and stable (see Chapter 24).	Prevents migration of tube into right or left bronchus and accidental extubation.

Clinical Judgment *When patients have periodic chest x-ray examinations, use the x-ray images to verify placement of the artificial airway.*

a. Auscultate over trachea for presence of air leak. When air leak is present, you hear movement of air over trachea. Assess and compare inhaled and exhaled tidal volumes as measured by ventilator.	Cuff of artificial airway needs to be inflated to create a seal for positive pressure ventilation to occur.
b. Use cuff pressure monitoring device.	Cuff pressure of ET tube should be between 20 and 30 cm H_2O (Urden et al., 2024). Use 5- or 10-mL syringe to inflate or deflate cuff to achieve desired pressure.

Clinical Judgment *Endotracheal (ET) tube cuff pressures need to be monitored carefully. Pressures that are too low lead to microaspiration of oral and subglottic secretions, which increase the patient's risk of developing ventilator-associated pneumonia (VAP). If the cuff pressures are too high, the patient is at risk of developing tracheal mucosa damage. Hypopharyngeal suctioning should be performed before a cuff is deflated to decrease risk of aspiration of secretions (AACN, 2018; Turner et al., 2020).*

STEP	RATIONALE
14. Ensure that suctioning system is functioning properly.	It is important to know that the emergency equipment is functioning before it is needed.
15. Observe for patent airway and, if necessary, remove airway secretions by suctioning (see Chapter 24). Remove and dispose of gloves and perform hand hygiene.	Secretions plug airway, decreasing amount of oxygen that is available for gas exchange in lung. Secretions also occlude T tube or tracheostomy collar, impeding oxygen delivery to patient. Reduces transmission of microorganisms.
16. Reapply clean pair of gloves. Inspect integrity of patient's oral mucous membrane and skin around tube stabilization device or adhesives.	Provides baseline to recognize signs of MDRPI or MARSI on the surfaces around the artificial airway, stabilization, or any adhesive (Fumarola et al., 2020).
17. If available, note patient's most recent ABG results or SpO_2. Determine if any factors have changed during mechanical ventilation. Remove and dispose of gloves and perform hand hygiene.	Objectively determines if there is a recent change in patient's pH, arterial oxygen, arterial carbon dioxide, or arterial oxygen saturation. Reduces transmission of microorganisms.
18. Assess patient's/family caregiver's knowledge and prior experience with mechanical ventilation and feelings about procedure.	Reveals need for patient/family caregiver instruction and/or support.

PLANNING

1. Expected outcomes following completion of procedure: • Patient has improved lung expansion.	As patient's lungs and lung mechanics improve, lung expansion increases.
• Patient maintains or has improving PaO_2, $PaCO_2$, and pH levels, and oxygen saturation within normal range or at patient baseline.	Verifies that ventilator settings are effective in improving or maintaining patient's level of oxygenation and ventilation.
• Patient's vital signs and respiratory assessment parameters improve.	Reduced pulse and respiratory rate, improved mental status, improved skin color, and decreased use of accessory and abdominal muscles occur because patient's work of breathing decreases as level of oxygenation improves.
• Patient experiences reduction in feelings of dyspnea and work of breathing. **NOTE:** Dyspnea scales are available to provide more objective data.	Indicates effectiveness of therapy.
• Patient uses communication board, paper and pencil, or computer to state needs.	Appropriate communication system matches patient's abilities. Helps to express patient's needs and wishes.
2. Provide privacy and explain procedure.	Protects patient's privacy; reduces anxiety. Promotes cooperation.
3. Organize and set up any equipment needed to perform procedure.	Ensures more efficiency when completing the procedure.
4. Explain ventilator system to patient and family caregiver and be sure to include purpose of and reasons for initiation of mechanical ventilation.	Reinforces need for ventilation to improve patient condition. Education decreases patient and family caregiver anxiety.
5. Arrange for extra personnel to help as necessary.	Some patients are unable to assume positioning independently and require assistance.

IMPLEMENTATION

1. Perform hand hygiene; apply clean gloves. Apply PPE: mask, gown, and goggles if secretions are projectile or if isolation precautions secondary to infectious status are indicated.	Reduces transmission of microorganisms and exposure to pulmonary secretions.
2. Ensure that suction equipment is set up and functioning, including oral suctioning (see Chapter 24).	Suctioning of ET tube or TT as needed prevents plugging of airway and reduces risk for infection.
3. Ensure that subglottic suctioning equipment (if tube is equipped for such type of suction) is functioning appropriately.	The use of subglottic suctioning helps to prevent the development of VAE/VAP (Sanaie et al., 2022; Huang et al., 2018; Letchford & Bench, 2018).
4. Check need for airway suctioning, then position patient with HOB elevated 30 to 45 degrees (unless contraindicated).	Positioning patients with HOB elevated 30 to 45 degrees or higher significantly reduces gastric reflux, thereby decreasing risk for aspiration and VAP (IHI, 2019; Kallet, 2019).
5. Be sure there is proper connection of ET tube or TT to ventilator with mechanical ventilator functioning.	Artificial airway to ventilator must have a closed system, which enables ventilator to exert appropriate pressure or volume to meet patient's oxygen and ventilation demands.

STEP	RATIONALE

Clinical Judgment *The mechanical ventilator requires programming of accurate settings before attaching to the patient. This is the responsibility of the respiratory therapist (RT) as prescribed by the health care provider; however, it is usually a collaborative responsibility of the nurse to provide assessment information.*

6. Observe patient for synchronization with mechanical ventilation and response to therapy.	Ensures that patient is comfortable using ventilator and has not experienced any adverse hemodynamic effects.
7. Monitor heart rate, blood pressure, respiratory rate, temperature, and cardiac rhythm routinely during care (see agency policy).	Patient's condition can change quickly while on ventilator and during care. Implementation of mechanical ventilation results in decreased venous return and associated hemodynamic changes. The patient is also at increased risk for developing an infection; therefore temperature needs to be monitored.
8. Reassess and mark level of ET tube at the patient's teeth (see Chapter 24). Ensure that ET tube continues to be secured.	ET tube must be placed through vocal cords into trachea. Helps to ensure that tube is not malpositioned. ET tube may be secured with use of tape or commercial tube holder (see Chapter 24 and Skill 24.3).

Clinical Judgment *Marking the level of the endotracheal (ET) tube at the patient's teeth provides an accurate measure to compare with baseline for depth of ET tube placement. Using the lips as a baseline measure risks inaccurate subsequent tube placement, as the patient's lips may swell due to trauma, fluid imbalances, oral surgery, and so on.*

Clinical Judgment *Suction the oral cavity before any repositioning. Verify cuff pressures after repositioning.*

9. Reposition patient regularly (minimum of every 2 hours), maintaining HOB elevation of 30 to 45 degrees. In some instances, patient may even be placed in prone position. Monitor SpO₂ during and after positioning. Assess ET tube markings at teeth to ensure tube placement has not changed.	Elevated HOB positioning improves oxygenation and ventilation. It reduces stasis of secretions, which can lead to atelectasis or pneumonia. In addition, HOB elevation reduces risk for aspiration of stomach content secretions into patient's airway (AACN, 2018; Huang et al., 2018). SpO₂ drops during position change and recovers once patient is completely positioned. ET tube can be dislodged while turning the patient prone.

Clinical Judgment *Prone positioning is reserved for critically ill patients with severe illness and requires assistance of four or five staff members or a specialty bed (Shelhamer et al., 2021).*

10. Collaborate with health care provider frequently about status of patient, response to therapy, and ongoing monitoring.	Assesses oxygenation status and continued need for mechanical ventilation.
a. Monitor SpO₂ continuously.	Provides ability to continually assess oxygenation levels.
b. Monitor EtCO₂ continually (if available and indicated) to detect possible overventilation or inadequate alveolar ventilation.	Allows you to continuously monitor integrity of ventilator circuit and quickly evaluate response to therapy or changes to ventilator settings.
c. Obtain serial ABG levels with changes in patient's condition or ventilator changes per provider order.	Provides more accurate measure of oxygen saturation and partial pressures of oxygen and carbon dioxide.
11. Perform safety checks on patient and ventilator system:	Frequency of checks is dependent on agency policy but is usually every hour.
a. Place nurse call system in an accessible location within patient's reach.	Ensures patient can call for assistance if needed.
b. Check security of all ventilator connections; make sure that alarms are all turned on, including both high- and low-pressure alarms and volume alarms.	Ensures continuous safe and proper functioning of ventilator system. Enables you to identify and correct problems in a timely manner.
c. Collaborate with RT and verify that all ventilator settings are correct and correspond to health care provider's orders.	Maintains integrity of system and ensures that all settings are consistent with health care provider's orders.
d. Check and refill humidifier as needed. Check corrugated tubing for condensation; drain away from patient but not into humidifier and appropriately discard liquid.	Ensures continuous humidification. Condensation that returns to humidifier can cause possible bacterial contamination. Condensation that drains into patient can cause pneumonia or severe coughing episode that can lead to increased patient distress (Restrepo & Walsh, 2022).
e. When present, observe temperature gauges on panel of mechanical ventilator, making sure that gas is delivered at correct temperature. Desired temperature of inspired gas is 35°C to 37°C (95°F to 98.6°F). Confer with RT if settings need adjusting.	The temperature of inspired gas artificially alters patient's body temperature.

STEP	RATIONALE
12. Perform mouth care at least 4 times per 24 hours (see Chapter 18). Use 0.12% chlorhexidine to brush teeth, gums, and tongue with soft toothbrush at least twice a day. Apply water-based moisturizer every 2 to 4 hours.	VAEs are common and are associated with microaspiration of oropharyngeal secretions. Frequent oral care reduces patient's risk for VAP (CDC, 2023b; Urden et al., 2024).
13. Monitor for the development of oral or lip ulcers or facial skin tears.	The artificial airway, the oral suction catheter, or the tube stabilization device can cause skin breakdown (Landsperger et al., 2019).
14. Insert bite block if patient bites ET tube.	Prevents patient from occluding airway. Oral mucous membranes and tongue need to be monitored for any signs of breakdown.
15. Administer sedating drugs as indicated.	Sedating medications keep patient comfortable and allow patient to tolerate the work of the ventilator (Urden et al., 2024).
16. Perform daily interruption in sedation; assess readiness to extubate.	This step is part of the IHI ventilator bundle. Providing daily interruptions of sedation decreases length of time on mechanical ventilation (IHI, 2019; Urden et al., 2024).
17. Institute deep vein thrombosis (DVT) prophylaxis as ordered per the health care provider. This includes use of anticoagulants (if no contraindications such as bleeding are present) and sequential compression devices (see Chapter 12).	DVT prevention protocols reduce patient's risk of DVT (Urden et al., 2024).

Clinical Judgment *The use of probiotics has not been shown to have an effect on rates of ventilator-associated pneumonia (VAP) (Mahmoodpoor et al., 2019). Their safety has not been established in critically ill patients (Virk & Wiersinga, 2019).*

STEP	RATIONALE
18. Perform nursing activities to prevent hazards of immobility (e.g., help patient change position, perform joint range-of-motion exercise, and encourage independence and early mobility protocol as tolerated) (see Chapter 12).	Maintaining activity and promoting early mobility avoid deconditioning and other complications associated with decreased mobility such as pressure injuries, pneumonia, and DVT. Patients receiving mechanical ventilation need help with activity but can ambulate (Urden et al., 2024).
19. Ensure that communication method is in place for patient after administering care. This includes letter/picture boards, common word and phrase lists, writing utensil and paper, or a computer/tablet.	Patients report feeling frightened, anxious, and disconnected during their time of short-term mechanical ventilation. Communication strategies and aids, including lip reading, patient gestures, and message boards, help patient communicate needs and feelings, which helps to decrease anxiety and fear (Karlsen et al., 2019; Urden et al., 2024).
20. Keep patient and family informed about progress and plan for weaning from mechanical ventilator.	Apprehension and anxiety occur when patient and family are not properly informed about progress, changes in care, or changes in ventilator setting. Patients and families need information and emotional support to successfully tolerate and wean from mechanical ventilation (Urden et al., 2024).
21. Remove and dispose of PPE; perform hand hygiene.	Reduces transmission of microorganisms and exposure to pulmonary secretions.
22. Help patient to a comfortable position with HOB elevated 30 to 45 degrees.	Restores comfort and sense of well-being.
23. Raise side rails (as appropriate) and lower bed to lowest position, locking into position.	Ensures patient safety and prevents falls.
24. Place nurse call system in an accessible location within patient's reach.	Ensures patient can call for assistance if needed.
25. Perform hand hygiene.	Reduces transmission of microorganisms.

EVALUATION

1. Monitor and evaluate patient's response to mechanical ventilation every 1 to 4 hours.
  a. *Neurological assessment:* LOC, orientation, sleepiness, changes in anxiety, sedation levels
  b. *Pulmonary assessment:* Lung sounds, airway clearance, work of breathing, breathing pattern, rate of respirations, SpO$_2$, EtCO$_2$
  c. *Cardiovascular assessment:* Vital signs, heart rhythm, heart sounds, lower extremity edema, pulse quality
	Patients requiring mechanical ventilation have unstable physiological status. It is important to perform key focused evaluation measures frequently as patient's condition warrants.

2. Observe integrity of patient ventilator system.	Ensures adequate delivery of mechanical ventilation.

STEP	RATIONALE
3. Observe skin and oral mucosa around artificial airway and any securement devices every 2 hours.	Identifies early signs of skin injury related to pressure from the artificial airway or securement device or any medical adhesive material.

4. Observe and evaluate effectiveness of communication methods:
  a. Ask patient if needs and concerns are addressed.
  b. Observe for signs of frustration (e.g., patient shaking head in irritation, crying, withdrawal).
  c. Observe patient/family caregiver and health care personnel use communication methods.
	Communication, or lack of it, increases patient's frustration, sense of powerlessness, anxiety, and confusion during mechanical ventilation and weaning process.

5. **Use Teach-Back:** "I want to be sure I explained how the ventilator works and why we are using it to treat your husband. Explain to me why mechanical ventilation is necessary." Revise your instruction now or develop a plan for revised patient/family caregiver teaching if patient/family caregiver is not able to teach back correctly.	Teach-back is a technique for health care providers to ensure that they have explained medical information clearly so that patients and their families understand what is communicated to them (AHRQ, 2021).

Unexpected Outcomes	Related Interventions
1. Patient experiences a VAE.	• Notify health care provider. • Remain with patient. • Conduct complete cardiac and pulmonary assessment. • Be prepared for initiation of antibiotic therapy.
2. Patient's respiratory status does not improve or declines.	• Notify health care provider. • Reassess patient. • Assess integrity of ventilator system. • Expect ventilator change (increased PEEP levels, increase in respiratory rate or tidal volume).
3. Patient extubates artificial airway.	• Maintain patent airway by suctioning and inserting oral airway. • Provide oxygen. • Assess patient's respiratory status and level of oxygenation and ventilation. • Notify health care provider or rapid response team immediately. • Patient may need sedation and/or use of restraints to prevent this complication from occurring in the future (see Chapter 14).
4. Patient develops barotrauma such as tension pneumothorax (an emergency situation).	• Remain with patient, remove patient from ventilator, and ventilate with bag-valve mask (see Chapter 27). • Notify rapid response team, including respiratory therapist and health care provider. • Ask AP to obtain chest tube insertion kit. • Ask additional nursing personnel to obtain patient's vital signs.

Documentation

- Document the following: respiratory assessment findings, mode of mechanical ventilation, oxygen level, actual patient tidal volume, actual patient respiratory rate, peak inspiratory pressure, vital signs, size and level of the ET tube, ABG results (if performed as a point-of-care test), patient level of comfort, sedation level scores (if sedation is used), and degree of bed elevation.
- Document nursing interventions that are performed, including oral care, repositioning, range-of-motion exercises, medications that were administered, and suctioning.
- Document your evaluation of patient and family caregiver learning.

Hand-Off Reporting

- Report patient status, including recent assessment findings, vital signs, and SpO$_2$ before and after initiation of mechanical ventilation.

- Report the type of ventilator used and mode of ventilation. Include the patient response to any ventilator adjustments and what interventions were successful.
- Report patient tolerance to nursing interventions.
- Report any unexpected outcomes to health care provider or nurse in charge.

Special Considerations
Patient Education
- Teach patient and family caregiver about the rationale for mechanical ventilation and the alarms and what they mean.
- Teach patient and family caregiver alternative communication techniques to help reduce frustration and fear.
- Teach patient about rationale for all interventions, including oral care and frequent repositioning.

Pediatrics
- Increasing numbers of children are on home mechanical ventilation. For this reason, it is important to include the parent in

the child's care as appropriate. Parents also need to be prepared that, because of the chronic nature of the illness, when a readmission to a hospital occurs the child may not be readmitted to an intensive care unit but rather may remain in the general medical or surgical area (Hockenberry et al., 2024).

- Once the child is stable on the mechanical ventilator, promote normal or near-normal activities as the child's condition warrants (e.g., promote play, resume school activities, and encourage mobility).

Older Adults

- Presence of underlying chronic illnesses increases patient's risk for longer intensive care and hospital stays.
- Older adults are usually not able to tolerate the usual sedative or antianxiety medications ordered. The prescribed dose is based on patient's baseline kidney and liver functions (Touhy & Jett, 2022).

Home Care

- Planning for home ventilation is performed by an interprofessional team, including representatives of nursing, respiratory department, dietary service, and social services; the home care nurse; the home care durable medical equipment company; and the patient's insurance company/health care payer.
- Patients requiring home mechanical ventilation need to be assessed for acceptance of ventilator dependence and the ability to understand and demonstrate daily care of the artificial airway, ventilator, and ventilator circuit.
- Patients requiring home mechanical ventilation need their home environment, personal and monetary resources, and availability of home care nurses or staff assessed. Availability of community resources should also be assessed. The home electricity may need to be updated to support the equipment required to care for them.
- Evaluate the following areas during each visit: oxygen flow, alarm system, inspiratory pressure, high-pressure alarm, tidal volume setting, humidifier, respiratory rate, tubing, temperature, resuscitation bag, tracheostomy care, breath sounds, suctioning, and tubing changes.
- Teach patient and family caregiver what to do in case of respiratory distress or power failure. Check to determine availability of emergency batteries.
- Instruct family caregiver in use of the bag-valve mask (see Chapter 27).

✦ CLINICAL JUDGMENT AND NEXT-GENERATION NCLEX® EXAMINATION–STYLE QUESTIONS

A 59-year-old patient with a history of well-controlled COPD developed an upper respiratory tract infection 2 weeks ago and was treated with antibiotics. The patient completed the full course of antibiotics, but symptoms continued. The patient has a 4-day history of fever higher than 39.4°C (102.8°F), fatigue, productive cough with yellow sputum, worsening dyspnea, and decreased activity tolerance. The health care provider has ordered a chest x-ray examination and sputum culture. Preliminary chest x-ray results indicate right lower lobe pneumonia. The patient is admitted to a general medical floor. Vital signs on admission: T 39.4°C (102.8°F), HR 110 beats/min, RR 24 breaths/min, BP 140/90 mm Hg. Health care provider orders include intravenous (IV) antibiotics, supplemental oxygen at 2 L/min via nasal cannula, and pulmonary hygiene measures.

1. Which of the following interventions would the nurse delegate to assistive personnel (AP)? **Select all that apply.**
   1. Obtain vital signs every 4 hours.
   2. Assist with transfer from bed to chair.
   3. Auscultate lungs every 2 hours.
   4. Change position in bed every 2 hours.
   5. Teach cough and deep breathing exercises.
   6. Report pulse oximetry changes during ambulation.
   7. Evaluate skin for pressure caused by oxygen tubing.
   8. Perform nasotracheal suctioning.
   9. Assist with hygiene.
2. The nurse is performing an assessment during the morning shift. Which assessment finding indicates that the plan of care is ineffective at this time?
   1. Respiratory rate 20 breaths/minute
   2. Heart rate 90 beats/minute
   3. Oxygen saturation 88% on 2 L of oxygen
   4. Blood pressure 128/82 mm Hg

3. While the patient is receiving oxygen therapy, which assessment finding alerts the nurse to intervene?
   1. Decrease in the work of breathing
   2. Lung expansion increases
   3. Mild confusion
   4. SpO$_2$ 94%
4. The patient is discharged to home with a plan to use continuous oxygen. Which of the following patient statements indicate that teaching by the nurse has been effective? **Select all that apply.**
   1. "I will not use candles in my home."
   2. "I must have signs in my home showing where oxygen is used."
   3. "I can burn incense instead of using candles."
   4. "I am not going to let anyone smoke in my house."
   5. "I am going to use the microwave instead of cooking on my gas stove."
5. The patient's spouse becomes ill and is admitted to the hospital with COVID-19 and acute hypoxemic respiratory failure. Which method of oxygen delivery does the nurse anticipate will be prescribed?
   1. High-flow nasal cannula
   2. Simple oxygen face mask
   3. Noninvasive positive pressure ventilation
   4. Oxygen-conserving cannula

Visit the Evolve site for Answers to Clinical Judgment and Next-Generation NCLEX® Examination–Style Questions.

REFERENCES

Agency for Healthcare Research and Quality (AHRQ): *Teach-Back: intervention,* 2021. https://www.ahrq.gov/patient-safety/reports/engage/interventions/teach-back.html.

Alja'afreh M, et al: The effects of oral care protocol on the incidence of ventilator-associated pneumonia in selected intensive care units in Jordan, *Dimens Crit Care Nurs* 38(1):5, 2019.

Alwekhyan S, et al: Nurse-guided incentive spirometry use and postoperative pulmonary complications among cardiac surgery patients: a randomized controlled trial, *Int J Nurs Pract* 28(2):e13023, 2022.

American Association of Critical Care Nurses (AACN): *AACN practice alert: prevention of aspiration in adults*, 2018 update. https://www.aacn.org/clinical-resources/practice-alerts/prevention-of-aspiration. Accessed May 1, 2023.

American Lung Association (ALA): *Oxygen therapy: oxygen delivery devices and accessories*, 2022. https://www.lung.org/lung-health-diseases/lung-procedures-and-tests/oxygen-therapy/oxygen-delivery-devices. Accessed April 29, 2023.

American Lung Association (ALA): *Measuring your peak flow rate*, 2023. https://www.lung.org/lung-health-and-diseases/lung-disease-lookup/asthma/living-with-asthma/managing-asthma/measuring-your-peak-flow-rate.html. Accessed May 1, 2023.

American Thoracic Society (ATS): *Oxygen therapy*, 2019, updated 2020. https://www.thoracic.org/patients/patient-resources/resources/oxygen-therapy.pdf. Accessed May 1, 2023.

Baird M: *Manual of critical care nursing: interprofessional collaborative management*, ed 8, St. Louis, 2023, Elsevier.

Barakat-Johnson M, et al: The incidence and prevalence of medical device-related pressure ulcers in intensive care: a systematic review, *J Wound Care* 28(8):512–521, 2019.

Beran A, et al: High-flow nasal cannula oxygen versus non-invasive ventilation in subjects with COVID-19: a systematic review and meta-analysis of comparative studies, *Resp Care* 67(9):1177-1189, 2022.

Billington J, Luckett A: Care of the critically ill patient with a tracheostomy, *Nurs Stand* 34(2):59–64, 2019.

Brophy S, et al: What is the incidence of medical device-related pressure injuries in adults within the acute hospital setting? A systematic review, *J Tissue Viability* 30(4):489–498, 2021.

Centers for Disease Control and Prevention (CDC): *What is health literacy?* 2023a. https://www.cdc.gov/healthliteracy/learn/index.html.

Centers for Disease Control and Prevention (CDC): *National Healthcare Safety Network: ventilator-associated event*, 2023b. https://www.cdc.gov/nhsn/pdfs/pscmanual/10-vae_final.pdf. Accessed May 1, 2023.

Cleveland Clinic: *Incentive spirometer*, 2022. https://my.clevelandclinic.org/health/articles/4302-incentive-spirometer. Accessed May 1, 2023.

Darawad M, et al: Evidence-based guidelines for prevention of ventilator-associated pneumonia: evaluation of intensive care unit nurses' adherence, *Am J Infect Control* 46(6):711–713, 2018.

Drake MG: High-flow nasal cannula oxygen in adults: an evidence-based assessment, *Ann Am Thorac Soc* 15(2):145–155, 2018.

Elliott ZJ, Elliott SC: An overview of mechanical ventilation in the intensive care unit, *Nurs Stand* 32(28):41–49, 2018.

Eltorai A, et al: Clinical effectiveness of incentive spirometry for the prevention of postoperative pulmonary complications, *Respir Care* 63(3):347–352, 2018a.

Eltorai A, et al: Perspectives on incentive spirometry utility and patient protocols, *Respir Care* 63(5):519–531, 2018b.

Enezi F, et al: The effectiveness of non-invasive ventilation in neuromuscular patients in KAMC, *Electron J Gen Med* 15(5):75, 2018.

Fumarola S, et al: Overlooked and underestimated: medical adhesive-related skin injuries. Best practice consensus document on prevention, *J Wound Care* 29(Sup3c):S1-S24, 2020.

Ghosh D, Elliott M: Acute non-invasive ventilation—getting it right on the acute medical take, *Clin Med* 19(3):237–242, 2019.

Hanada M, et al: Aerobic and breathing exercises improve dyspnea, exercise capacity and quality of life in idiopathic pulmonary fibrosis patients: a systematic review and meta-analysis, *J Thorac Dis* 12(3):1041, 2020.

Harding MM, et al: *Lewis' medical-surgical nursing: assessment and management of clinical problems*, ed 12, St. Louis, 2023, Elsevier.

Hill N, et al: Noninvasive ventilatory support for acute hypercapneic respiratory failure, *Respir Care* 64(6):647–657, 2019.

Hockenberry M, et al: *Wong's nursing care of infants and children*, ed 12, St. Louis, 2024, Elsevier.

Huang X, et al: Influence of subglottic secretion drainage on the microorganisms of ventilator associated pneumonia, *Medicine (Baltimore)* 97(28):1–7, 2018.

Huether S, et al: *Understanding pathophysiology*, ed 7, St. Louis, 2020, Elsevier.

Institute for Healthcare Improvement (IHI): *How-to guide: prevent ventilator-associated pneumonia*, 2012 (Modified May 13, 2019). http://www.ihi.org/sites/search/pages/results.aspx?k=prevent+ventlatot+assciated+pneumonia#k=prevent%20ventilator%20associated%20pneumonia. Accessed May 1, 2023.

Jackson D, et al: Medical device-related pressure ulcers: a systematic review and meta-analysis, *Int J Nurs Stud* 92:109–120, 2019.

Kallet RH: Ventilator bundles in transition: from prevention of ventilator-associated pneumonia to prevention of ventilator-associated events, *Respir Care* 64(8):994–1006, 2019.

Karaca T, Korkmaz F: A quasi-experimental study to explore the effect of barrier cream on the peristomal skin of patients with a tracheostomy, *Ostomy Wound Manage* 3:32–39, 2018.

Karlsen M, et al: Communication with patients in intensive care units: a scoping review, *Nurs Crit Care* 24(3):115–131, 2019.

Kim E, et al: Effectiveness of high-flow nasal cannula oxygen therapy for acute respiratory failure with hypercapnia, *J Thorac Dis* 10(2):882–888, 2018.

Kotta PA, Ali JM: Incentive spirometry for prevention of postoperative pulmonary complications after thoracis surgery, *Respir Care* 66(2):327, 2021.

Landsperger J, et al: The effect of adhesive tape versus endotracheal tube fastener in critically ill adults: the endotracheal tube securement (ETTS) randomized controlled trial, *Crit Care* 23:161–167, 2019.

Letchford E, Bench S: Ventilator-associated pneumonia and suction: a review of the literature, *Br J Nurs* 27(1):13–18, 2018.

Lewarski J: Brief review of ATS CPG: *Home oxygen therapy for adults with chronic lung disease*, 2021, https://www.aarc.org/an21-brief-review-of-the-ats-cpg-home-oxygen-therapy-for-adults-with-chronic-lung-disease/. Accessed October 7, 2023.

Li J, et al: The effects of flow settings during high-flow nasal cannula support for adult subjects: a systematic review, *Crit Care* 27:78, 2023.

Mahmoodpoor A, et al: Effect of a probiotic preparation on ventilator-associated pneumonia in critically ill patients admitted to the intensive care unit: a prospective double-blind randomized controlled trial, *Nutr Clin Pract* 34(1):156–162, 2019.

National Institutes of Health (NIH): *Covid-19 treatment guidelines*: oxygenation and ventilation, 2023. https://www.covid19treatmentguidelines.nih.gov/critical-care/oxygenation-and-ventilation/. Accessed May 1, 2023.

Nishimura M: High-flow nasal cannula oxygen therapy devices, *Respir Care* 64(6):735–742, 2019.

Oxford Medication Education (OME): *Starting non-invasive ventilation*, 2023. https://oxfordmedicaleducation.com/clinical-skills/procedures/starting-niv/. Accessed May 1, 2023.

Renda T, et al: High-flow nasal oxygen therapy in intensive care and anaesthesia, *Br J Anaesth* 120(1):18–27, 2018.

Restrepo R, Walsh B: AARC clinical practice guideline—*Humidification during invasive and noninvasive mechanical ventilation*, 2022 update. https://www.guidelinecentral.com/guideline/10614/#section-anchor-328321. Accessed April 29, 2023.

Rochwerg B, et al: High flow nasal cannula compared with conventional oxygen therapy for acute hypoxemic respiratory failure: a systematic review and meta-analysis, *Intensive Care Med* 45(5):563–572, 2019. doi:10.1007/s00134-019-05590-5.

Sanaie S, et al: Comparison of subglottic vs. non-subglottic secretion drainage in prevention of ventilator associated pneumonia: a systematic review and meta-analysis, *Trends Anaesth Crit Care* 43:23–29, 2022.

Santiago C, et al: The use of tablet and communication app for patients with endotracheal or tracheostomy tubes in the medical surgical intensive care unit: a pilot, feasibility study, *Can J Crit Care Nurs* 30(1):17–23, 2019.

Sharma S, et al: *High flow nasal cannula*, Treasure Island, 2023, StatPearls.

Shelhamer MC, et al: Prone positioning in moderate to severe acute respiratory distress syndrome due to COVID-19: a cohort study and analysis of physiology, *J Intensive Care Med* 36(2):241, 2021.

Sweity E, et al: Preoperative incentive spirometry for preventing postoperative pulmonary complications in patients undergoing coronary artery bypass graft surgery: a prospective, randomized controlled trial, *J Cardiothorac Surg* 16:241, 2021.

The Joint Commission (TJC): *2023 National Patient Safety Goals*, Oakbrook Terrace, IL, 2023, The Joint Commission. https://www.jointcommission.org/standards/national-patient-safety-goals/.

Touhy T, Jett K: *Ebersole and Hess' gerontological nursing and healthy aging*, ed 6, St. Louis, 2022, Elsevier.

Turner M, et al: Improving endotracheal cuff inflation pressures: an evidence-based project in a military medical center, *AANA J*, 88(3):203–208, 2020

Urden L, et al: *Priorities in critical care nursing*, ed 9, St. Louis, 2024, Elsevier.

Virk H, Wiersinga J: Current place of probiotics for VAP, *Crit Care* 23:46, 2019.

Walsh B, Smallwood C: Pediatric oxygen therapy: a review and update, *Respir Care* 62(6):645–661, 2017.

Wu Z, et al: Baseline level and reduction in $OPaCO_2$ are associated with the treatment effect of long-term home noninvasive positive pressure ventilation in stable hypercapnic patients with COPD: a systematic review and meta-analysis of randomized controlled trials, *Int J Chron Obstruct Pulmon Dis* 22(17):719, 2022.

Xia J, et al: High-flow nasal cannula versus conventional oxygen therapy in acute COPD exacerbation with mild hypercapnia: a multicenter randomized controlled trial, *Crit Care*, 26:109, 2022.

Xia M, et al: A postoperative comparison of high-flow nasal cannula therapy and conventional oxygen therapy for esophageal cancer patients, *Ann Palliat Med* 10(3):2530, 2021.

Xu Z, et al: High-flow nasal cannula in adults with acute respiratory failure and after extubation: a systematic review and meta-analysis, *Respir Res* 19(1):202, 2018.

24 | Airway Management

SKILLS AND PROCEDURES

Skill 24.1 **Performing Oropharyngeal Suctioning, p. 755**

Skill 24.2 **Suctioning: Open for Nasotracheal/Pharyngeal and Artificial Airways, p. 759**

Procedural Guideline 24.1 **Closed (In-Line) Suction, p. 769**

Skill 24.3 **Performing Endotracheal Tube Care, p. 770**

Skill 24.4 **Performing Tracheostomy Care, p. 778**

OBJECTIVES

Mastery of content in this chapter will enable you to:

- Explain the safety guidelines for managing a patient's airway.
- Apply patient-centered approaches to airway management.
- Select nursing interventions for airway management.
- List measures to reduce the risk of medical device–related pressure injuries (MDRPIs) from artificial airways.

- Discuss the clinical judgment needed and the indications for airway suctioning.
- Discuss the indications for endotracheal or tracheostomy care.
- Demonstrate oropharyngeal, nasopharyngeal and nasotracheal, and tracheal suctioning; endotracheal tube care; and tracheostomy tube care.

MEDIA RESOURCES

- http://evolve.elsevier.com/Perry/skills
- Review Questions
- ▶ Video Clips
- Audio Glossary
- **NSO** Nursing Skills Online

- Answers to Clinical Judgment and Next-Generation NCLEX® Examination–Style Questions
- Animations
- Printable Key Points
- Skills Performance Checklists

PURPOSE

Safe and effective airway management involves interprofessional collaboration and nursing interventions designed to maintain the patency of a patient's upper, lower, or (in some cases) artificial airway. The primary goal of airway management is to protect the airway, which will help promote and maintain adequate tissue oxygenation.

PRACTICE STANDARDS

- American Association of Critical-Care Nurses (AACN) Practice Alert, 2018a: Prevention of Aspiration in Adults
- AACN Practice Alert, 2018b: Oral Care for Acutely and Critically Ill Patients
- AACN Practice Alert, 2017: Prevention of Ventilator-Associated Pneumonia in Adults—Suctioning and endotracheal (ET) care
- AARC Clinical Practice Guideline, 2010: Endotracheal Suctioning of Mechanically Ventilated Patients With Artificial Airways—Tracheal suctioning
- Martin-Loeches et al., 2018: New Guidelines for Hospital-Acquired Pneumonia/Ventilator-Associated Pneumonia: USA versus Europe—Prevention of ventilator pneumonia
- Mussa CC, et al., 2021: AARC Clinical Practice Guideline: Management of Adult Patients With Tracheostomy in the Acute Care Setting—Tracheostomy care

- The Joint Commission (TJC), 2023: National Patient Safety Goals—Patient identification

SUPPLEMENTAL STANDARDS

- AARC Clinical Practice Guideline, 2004: Nasotracheal Suctioning

PRINCIPLES FOR PRACTICE

- A patient's airway has the potential to become obstructed by mucus, mechanical obstruction (i.e., soft tissue in upper airway), or a foreign body. A nursing assessment will allow you to appropriately select and individualize the best airway management measures for maintenance of an open airway.
- Hydration, positioning, nutrition, chest physiotherapy techniques, deep breathing, coughing, humidity, incentive spirometry, and aerosol therapy are noninvasive techniques that keep airway secretions liquified and mobilized to maintain a patent airway and promote oxygenation.
- When patients are unable to protect their own airway or clear airway secretions with coughing, chest physiotherapy, or other noninvasive techniques, more invasive measures such as suctioning or inserting an artificial airway are needed.
- An artificial airway is a device (such as a tracheostomy or endotracheal tube) that is inserted into the upper respiratory tract to facilitate ventilation or the removal of secretions.

PERSON-CENTERED CARE

- Artificial airways alter a patient's ability to communicate, possibly causing feelings of fear, frustration, anxiety, and vulnerability (Santiago et al., 2019).
- Communication with patients with an altered airway can improve with the use of communication aids, such as pen and paper, message boards, picture boards, or eye tracking aids (Santiago et al., 2019).
- Thoroughly educate your patients and their families using plain language that is culturally appropriate, and then verify that they understand any equipment, procedures, or tests to be performed.
- Patients and families who have English as their second language or do not speak English require the use of an agency-approved translator any time there is communication between the patient and/or family and members of the health care team.
- Assess the functional skills of the patient. Ensure that functioning hearing aids are in place and working so that communication with a hearing-impaired patient is possible. Allow patients to wear their glasses.

EVIDENCE-BASED PRACTICE

Prevention of Ventilator-Associated Pneumonia (VAP)

Ventilator-associated pneumonia (VAP) is a common health care–associated infection (HAI) in intensive care units (ICUs). It is associated with increased hospital length of stay, increased mortality, and increased hospital costs of an estimated $40,000 per patient (Alja'afreh et al., 2019; Letchford & Bench, 2018). VAP is typically described as pneumonia that develops greater than 48 hours after insertion of an artificial airway or initiation of mechanical ventilation and is a type of ventilator-associated event (VAE) (Centers for Disease Control and Prevention [CDC], 2022; Ferrer & Torres, 2018). The primary cause of VAP is the migration of microorganisms into the lower respiratory tract (Alja'afreh et al., 2019; Mahmoodpoor et al., 2019). Implementation of ventilator bundles (evidence-based group of interventions) is associated with reductions in ventilator-associated pneumonia (VAP) (Kallet, 2019). However, new surveillance models of ventilator-associated events (VAEs) have shifted the focus from VAP to objective, generalized signs of pulmonary decompensation not specific to just VAP. Researchers are examining if bundled interventions for VAP have an impact on VAEs (Kallet, 2019). Ongoing research continues to identify the interventions that have the most impact on prevention. Kallet (2019) reported significant reductions in duration of intubation with early weaning, sedation, and head-of-bed elevation, as well as reduced mortality risk with weaning and a sedation bundle. While there is no single strategy, the use of care bundle interventions is effective (Martin-Loeches et al., 2018; Triamvisit, 2021). These bundled interventions include:

- Use proper hand hygiene measures before and after patient contact.
- Elevate the head of the bed to at least 30 degrees, unless contraindicated.
- Perform oral hygiene with chlorhexidine gluconate solution at least twice a day (AACN, 2018b; Alja'afreh et al., 2019).
- Institute peptic ulcer prophylaxis (Virk & Wiersinga, 2019).
- Institute venous thromboembolism prophylaxis (anticoagulants, venous sequential compression).

- Provide daily disruption of sedation.
- Encourage early mobilization (see Chapter 12).
- Initiate enteric feedings earlier rather than later.
- Provide subglottic secretion drainage, although it is not clear whether it should be continuous or intermittent manual suction (Huang et al., 2018; Letchford & Bench, 2018; Pozuelo-Carrascosa et al., 2020).
- Maintain artificial airway cuff pressure between 20 mm Hg and 30 mm Hg (AACN, 2017).
- Use silver-coated endotracheal tubes when possible (Lethongkam et al., 2020; Tokmaji et al., 2018).
- Have respiratory therapy change ventilator circuits only when dirty or contaminated and not on a routine basis (AACN, 2017).
- The use of probiotics has not been shown to have an effect on VAP rates (Mahmoodpoor et al., 2019). Their safety has not been established for use in critically ill patients (Virk & Wiersinga, 2019).
- The use of prophylactic antibiotics is controversial because their use may decrease rates of early-onset VAP, but they have no effect on late-onset VAP or mortality rates and they do increase the risk of antibiotic-resistant organism development (Mirtalaei et al., 2019).
- Closed suction systems have no clear advantage over open suction but may better prevent late-onset ventilator-associated pneumonia (Letchford & Bench, 2018)

SAFETY GUIDELINES

- Know a patient's baseline range of vital signs (VS) and oxygen saturation levels. Baseline physiological measures are important assessment data useful in determining the status of an illness and a patient's response to interventions.
- Know a patient's medical history. Smoking alters normal mucociliary clearance. Certain disorders such as chronic obstructive pulmonary disease, asthma, cystic fibrosis, pneumonia, thoracic surgery, chest trauma, and abdominal surgery place patients at increased risk for an obstructed airway.
- Identify conditions that increase a patient's risk for aspiration of gastric contents into the lung, resulting in airway obstruction or pneumonia. These include the presence of enteral feeding tubes or nasal and oral gastric tubes, a decreased level of consciousness, and a decreased swallowing ability (AACN, 2018a).
- Use caution when suctioning patients with head injuries. The suction procedure causes an elevation in intracranial pressure (ICP) (Harding et al., 2023; Urden et al., 2024). Reduce this risk by presuctioning hyperventilation, which results in hypocarbia. This in turn induces cranial vasoconstriction, thereby reducing the risk of elevated ICP.
- Determine if a patient has a history of nasal trauma, nasal polyps, deviated nasal septum, or chronic sinusitis. Allergy problems may cause mucosal swelling that narrows nasal passages, which affects the ability to easily pass a suction catheter.
- Review a patient's respiratory assessments from the past 12 or 24 hours. These are important assessment data that distinguish between gradual and acute changes in a patient's status. Ensure that you receive this information during the hand-off report.
- Before initiating an airway management intervention, perform a systematic pulmonary assessment of upper and lower airways, including identifying respiratory rate, respiratory pattern, accessory

muscle use, breath sounds, ability to cough effectively, integrity of the rib cage, and the characteristics of sputum production (Chapter 6).
- Identify and become familiar with the use of equipment available at the agency. Many types of artificial airways, suction catheters, and suction machines are available. Knowing how to operate the equipment before use promotes positive outcomes.
- Have adequate suctioning, airway, and oxygen supplies on hand at the bedside in case they are needed emergently.
- Test all equipment before use. Equipment must work properly to provide safe nursing care. Determine that the suction machine is generating adequate negative suction pressure and

that suction catheters and appropriate equipment are available at the bedside.
- Know the side effects of medications and other therapies. Some medications such as beta-adrenergic blockers have the side effect of bronchospasm. An adverse effect of opioids and sedatives is respiratory depression. Similarly, too much oxygen reduces the drive to breathe in patients with chronic hypercapnia (elevated arterial carbon dioxide levels). Some position changes affect a patient adversely. For example, in patients with impaired spinal cord innervations of the respiratory muscles, supine positions place the diaphragm at a mechanical disadvantage and increase the risk for aspiration.

✦ SKILL 24.1 Performing Oropharyngeal Suctioning

 Video Clip

A Yankauer, or tonsillar tip, suction device is used for oropharyngeal suctioning (i.e., the removal of pharyngeal secretions through the mouth) (Fig. 24.1). A Yankauer suction catheter is made of rigid, minimally flexible plastic. The tip of this suction catheter usually has one large and several small openings through which the mucus enters with application of negative pressure. The Yankauer suction catheter is angled to facilitate removal of secretions through a patient's mouth. Oropharyngeal suctioning only removes secretions from the mouth and back of the throat. Perform oral suctioning when a patient is able to cough effectively but is unable to clear secretions, such as for a patient with a neuromuscular injury who cannot manage oral secretions. Patients with artificial airways and impaired swallowing require use of the Yankauer suction device to provide oral hygiene.

Oropharyngeal suctioning does not replace subglottic suctioning for patients with tracheal or endotracheal tubes. Instead, use the special subglottic suction port on the tracheostomy tube (Skill 24.4) (Tracheostomy Education, 2020).

Delegation

The skill of performing oropharyngeal suctioning can be delegated to assistive personnel (AP). Do not delegate this skill for patients with oral or neck surgery in the immediate postoperative period.

The nurse is responsible for assessing the patient's respiratory status. Educate the AP about:
- Appropriate suction limits for oropharyngeal suctioning for a particular patient (e.g., appropriate suction pressure, expected frequency of suctioning, and expected color and volume of secretions).
- The risks of applying excessive or inadequate suction pressure.
- Avoiding mouth sutures, applying suction against sensitive tissues, and dislodging tubes in the patient's nose or mouth.
- How to avoid stimulation of the gag reflex.
- Immediately reporting to the nurse any change in VS, pulse oximetry (SpO_2), sputum (i.e., bloody), difficulty breathing, or discomfort during or after the procedure.

Interprofessional Collaboration

- Collaborate with health care providers, who need to be aware of the frequency of suctioning and the amount and characteristics of the secretions.
- Collaborate with respiratory therapists regarding the need for oropharyngeal suctioning, as well as the frequency of suctioning and the amount and characteristics of the secretions.
- Collaborate with physical therapists, occupational therapists, or speech therapists. Therapists need to be aware of patient pulmonary status and need for oropharyngeal suctioning before the implementation of their prescribed interventions.

Equipment

- Clean, nonsterile Yankauer or tonsillar tip suction catheter
- Clean gloves
- Other personal protective equipment (PPE): mask, goggles, or face shield; isolation gown if indicated
- Disposable cup or nonsterile basin
- Tap water or normal saline (about 100 mL)
- Suction machine or wall suction device with regulator
- Connecting tubing (6 feet)
- Oral airway (if indicated)
- Washcloth (if indicated)
- Towel, cloth, or disposable paper drape
- Pulse oximeter
- Stethoscope
- Manual self-inflating resuscitation bag (bag-valve mask) with oxygen connecting tubing

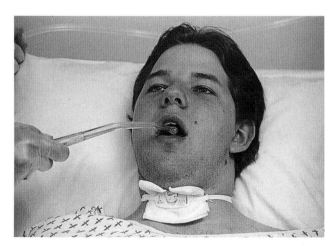

FIG. 24.1 Oropharyngeal suctioning.

STEP	RATIONALE

ASSESSMENT

1. Identify patient using at least two identifiers (e.g., name and birthday or name and medical record number) according to agency policy.

Ensures correct patient. Complies with The Joint Commission standards and improves patient safety (TJC, 2023).

2. Review patient's electronic health record (EHR), including health care provider's order and nurses' notes for patient's normal pulse oximeter values, baseline and trends in respiratory rate and effort of breathing, frequency of suctioning, and response to suctioning.

Knowing the patient condition helps to identify need for suctioning and predicts the patient response to interventions.

3. Review patient's medical history for risk factors for airway obstruction: impaired cough or gag reflex, weakened respiratory muscles, impaired swallowing, and decreased level of consciousness.

Risk factors prevent patient from protecting airway from aspiration or clearing secretions safely.

4. Review EHR for conditions including recent head and neck surgery or mouth trauma.

May contraindicate suctioning or require you to adapt oral suctioning approach.

5. Assess patient's/family caregiver's health literacy.

Determines degree to which individuals have the ability to find, understand, and use information and services to make informed health-related decisions and actions for themselves and others (CDC, 2023).

Clinical Judgment *If the presence of secretions is noted and/or upper airway obstruction is suspected, then immediate suctioning is warranted and should be performed before assessing patient or caregiver health literacy.*

6. Perform hand hygiene. Apply gloves and any other PPE equipment as patient condition dictates (e.g., risk of splashing).

Reduces transmission of microorganisms.

7. Assess patient's level of consciousness and obtain VS, noting signs and symptoms of hypoxia: anxiety, change in level of consciousness, recent change in VS (see Chapter 23, Box 23.1).

Clearing the oropharynx of secretions often assists in improving oxygenation.

8. Obtain patient's oxygen saturation level via SpO_2 (see Chapter 5). Do not remove the probe until after the oropharynx is suctioned.

Provides an objective baseline measure of oxygen saturation and an early indication of hypoxia. Aids in assessment of patient during and after oropharyngeal suctioning.

9. Assess for signs and symptoms of upper airway obstruction: gurgling on inspiration or expiration, restlessness, obvious excessive oral secretions, drooling, gastric secretions or vomitus in mouth, or coughing without clearing secretions from upper airway.

Secretions pool in upper airway, which can cause total airway obstruction and hypoxia. The risk for aspiration of gastric contents and airway obstruction is increased in patients with vomiting; delayed gastric emptying; impairment in esophageal sphincter control, cough, swallowing, or gag reflex; or those receiving enteral feedings.

10. Auscultate for presence of adventitious sounds (see Chapter 6).

Determines if lower airway secretions are present (indicating need for tracheal suction) and establishes baseline.

11. Assess patient's knowledge, prior experience with oropharyngeal suctioning, and feelings about procedure.

Reveals need for patient instruction and/or support.

PLANNING

1. Expected outcomes following completion of procedure:
   - No gurgling sounds are heard in patient's pharynx on inspiration and expiration.

Suctioning is effective. Secretions are removed from large upper airway.

   - Drooling is diminished or absent.

Excessive drooling indicates that patient is unable to handle oral secretions. Absence of secretions indicates that the suctioning was effective.

   - Vomitus or gastric secretions are absent from mouth.

Gastric secretions retained in oral cavity increase patient's risk for aspiration pneumonia. Absence of vomitus or secretions indicates that the suctioning was effective.

   - SpO_2 improves or remains at patient's normal baseline.

Removal of secretions helps to improve oxygen saturation level.

Clinical Judgment *In patients with chronic pulmonary disease, the SpO_2 value may remain the same after oropharyngeal suctioning. This baseline value may be lower than the typical normal values of greater than 95%.*

STEP	RATIONALE
2. Perform hand hygiene. Gather equipment/supplies at patient's bedside. Check the suction machine to ensure it is working properly.	Reduces transmission of microorganisms. Ensures that procedure is well organized and equipment is functioning appropriately.
3. Close the room door or curtain. Lower side rails and assist patient to comfortable position, typically semi-Fowler or high Fowler.	Provides privacy. Reduces stimulation of gag reflex, promotes patient comfort and secretion drainage, and prevents aspiration.
4. Explain to patient how procedure helps clear airway secretions and relieves some breathing problems. Explain that coughing, gagging, or (less commonly) sneezing is normal and lasts only a few seconds. Encourage patient to cough out secretions and show how to splint painful areas during procedure. Practice coughing if able.	Gagging or coughing occurs when posterior pharynx is suctioned or as a result of excess secretions. Coughing secretions out of lower airway or posterior pharynx decreases amount of suctioning required. Splinting reduces abdominal incision discomfort during coughing or gagging.

IMPLEMENTATION

1. Perform hand hygiene. Apply clean gloves. Apply mask or face shield if splashing is likely. Wear gown if isolation precautions are indicated.	Reduces transmission of microorganisms.

Clinical Judgment *If you do not leave the room between assessment and implementation, the isolation equipment can stay on, but hand hygiene should still be performed and a new pair of clean gloves should be worn.*

2. Place towel, cloth, or paper drape across patient's neck and chest. Place pulse oximeter on finger if not already in place.	Towel protects gown and bed linen from contamination by secretions. Pulse oximetry allows for continuous monitoring or patient's oxygenation level.
3. Fill cup or basin with approximately 100 mL of water or normal saline.	Helps to clean catheter after suctioning and assesses that equipment functions.
4. Connect one end of connecting tubing to suction machine and other to Yankauer suction catheter. Turn on suction machine; set vacuum regulator to appropriate suction, typically between 80 and 120 mm Hg (Hare & Seckel, 2024).	Prepares suction apparatus. Excessive pressures should be avoided because elevated pressure settings increase risk for hypoxemia, atelectasis, and airway trauma (Urden et al., 2024; Hare & Seckel, 2024).
5. Check that suction machine is functioning properly by placing tip of catheter in water or normal saline and suctioning small amount from cup or basin.	Ensures that equipment functions and lubricates catheter.
6. Remove patient's oxygen mask if present. Nasal cannula may remain in place. Keep oxygen mask near patient's face.	Allows access to mouth. Reduces chance of hypoxia.

Clinical Judgment *Be prepared to quickly reapply supplemental oxygen if SpO_2 value falls below 90% or respiratory distress develops during or at the end of oropharyngeal suctioning. Be prepared to use the bag-valve mask if patient has serious acute respiratory distress or decline in SpO_2.*

Clinical Judgment *If patients have been tracheally suctioned before oropharyngeal suctioning, they may require some recovery from the suctioning procedure before oropharyngeal suctioning is performed. Allow for that recovery to happen by reapplying the oxygen mask until just before oropharyngeal suctioning.*

7. Insert catheter into mouth along gum line to pharynx. Move catheter around mouth until secretions have cleared. Encourage patient to cough. Replace oxygen mask.	Movement of catheter prevents suction tip from invaginating oral mucosal surfaces and causing trauma. Coughing moves secretions from lower airway into mouth and upper airway.

Clinical Judgment *Use caution when using a Yankauer tip suction catheter with a patient who had recent oral or head/neck surgery. Aggressive suctioning and excessive coughing should not be used or encouraged in patients who have undergone throat surgery such as a tonsillectomy. These acts can aggravate the operative site, increasing the risk of infection or bleeding (Urden et al., 2024).*

8. Rinse catheter with water or normal saline in cup or basin until connecting tubing is cleared of secretions. Turn off suction. Place catheter in clean, dry area. Remove and dispose of gloves (and any other PPE). Perform hand hygiene.	Rinses catheter and reduces probability of transmission of microorganisms. Clean suction tubing enhances delivery of set suction pressure.
9. Observe respiratory status. Repeat procedure if indicated. May need to use standard suction catheter to reach into trachea if respiratory status not improved (see Skill 24.2).	Directs you to continue, cease intervention, or choose another intervention.

STEP	RATIONALE
10. Remove towel, cloth, or disposable drape and place in trash or laundry if soiled. Reposition patient comfortably; lateral recumbent or side-lying position encourages drainage and should be used if patient has decreased level of consciousness.	Reduces transmission of microorganisms. Facilitates drainage of oral secretions.
11. Discard remainder of water or normal saline into appropriate receptacle. Rinse basin in warm, soapy water and dry with paper towels or discard (check agency policy). Discard disposable cup into appropriate receptacle. Perform hand hygiene.	Reduces transmission of microorganisms. Moist environment encourages microorganism growth.

Clinical Judgment *Keep catheter in nonairtight container such as brown paper or plastic bag attached to bedrail or in suction canister. Do not store the catheter where it will come in contact with secretions or excretions, which promote bacterial growth.*

STEP	RATIONALE
12. Apply clean gloves to provide personal care, such as washing the patient's face or performing oral hygiene.	Promotes comfort.
13. Help patient to a comfortable position.	Restores comfort and sense of well-being.
14. Place nurse call system in an accessible location within the patient's reach.	Ensures patient can call for assistance if needed.
15. Raise side rails (as appropriate) and lower the bed to the lowest position, locking into position.	Ensures patient safety and prevents falls.
16. Remove and dispose of gloves. Perform hand hygiene.	Reduces transmission of microorganisms.

EVALUATION

1. Compare assessment findings before and after procedure.	Identifies physiological response to suction procedure.
2. Auscultate chest and airways for adventitious sounds.	Presence of lower airway adventitious sounds suggests need for lower airway suctioning.
3. Inspect mouth for any vomitus or remaining secretions.	A clear oral airway is necessary to prevent aspiration.
4. Obtain and document postsuction SpO₂ value. Compare with presuction level.	Provides objective measure of effectiveness of suction procedure (Urden et al., 2024).
5. **Use Teach-Back:** "I want to be sure I explained how to suction your mouth and why it should be done. Show me how you will use this suction catheter." Revise your instruction now or develop a plan for revised patient/family caregiver teaching if patient/family caregiver is not able to teach back correctly.	Teach-back is a technique for health care providers to ensure that they have explained medical information clearly so that patients and their families understand what is communicated to them (Agency for Healthcare Research and Quality [AHRQ], 2023).

Unexpected Outcomes	Related Interventions
1. Patient's respiratory distress increases.	• Suction further or implement nasal or tracheal suctioning (Skill 24.2). • Evaluate need for other means to protect airway (e.g., oral intubation, oral airway, positioning). • Provide supplemental oxygen. • Notify health care provider.
2. Bloody secretions are suctioned.	• Assess oral cavity for trauma or lesions. • Reduce amount of suction pressure used. • Observe catheter tip for nicks, which cause mucosal trauma. • Increase frequency of oral hygiene. • Notify the health care provider.

Documentation

- Document the amount, consistency, color, and odor of secretions; number of times suctioned; patient's response to suctioning; and presuction and postsuction cardiopulmonary assessment findings.
- Document your evaluation of patient learning.

Hand-Off Reporting

- Report any unresolved outcomes such as worsening respiratory distress to the health care provider.
- Report frequency of suctioning and patient response to suction, as well as presuction and postsuction assessments during hand-off.

Special Considerations

Patient Education

- Instruct patient and family caregiver not to allow suction catheter to fall to the floor. If this occurs, teach patient and caregiver to notify a member of the health care team.
- Provide information regarding signs and symptoms of worsening respiratory status.

Pediatrics

- Airways of infants and children are smaller than those of an adult. Even a small amount of mucus can cause airway obstruction. Smaller suction catheters may be necessary (Hockenberry et al., 2024).
- Bulb syringes may be used to suction the oral cavity in newborns and infants. To properly use a bulb syringe, compress the bulb before inserting into mouth to decrease the risk of forcing the secretions into lower airways. If the bulb syringe cannot remove the secretions, use appropriate-size mechanical suction equipment (Hockenberry et al., 2024).

- Use lower suction pressures with infants and children than with adults (Hockenberry et al., 2024).
- Position infants with breathing problems or excessive vomitus in side-lying position to decrease risk of aspiration. However, NEVER place an infant on a pillow (Hockenberry et al., 2024).

Older Adults

- Oral mucosa in older adults is fragile. Use a lower suction pressure if bleeding starts to occur.
- Older adults are prone to aspiration of oral secretions because of decreased cough and gag reflexes and increased incidence of dysphagia (Touhy & Jett, 2022).

Populations With Disabilities

- Patients with neuromuscular disabilities, such as muscular dystrophy or amyotrophic lateral sclerosis (ALS), have weak and ineffective swallowing and weak respiratory muscles and need oropharyngeal suctioning to assist in airway clearance (Hockenberry et al., 2024).
- Patients with dysphagia may benefit from oral suctioning before, during, and after meals.

Home Care

- Ensure that a family caregiver is present and explain the procedure, particularly if it is to be completed at home. The presence of a trusted caregiver may help to decrease a patient's anxiety during the procedure.
- Make sure that patient and family caregiver know how to clean and disinfect or change the secretion collection container every 24 hours according to home care protocol. Many agencies seal and dispose of the entire disposable secretion collection canister as biohazardous material.

◆ SKILL 24.2 Suctioning: Open for Nasotracheal/Pharyngeal and Artificial Airways

Suctioning of the airway is necessary when patients are unable to clear respiratory secretions. If the secretions are only in the nose and mouth, only the pharynx requires suctioning. You may suction secretions from the pharynx as often as needed using clean aseptic technique and oropharyngeal suctioning (see Skill 24.1). However, in many instances you will need to suction both the pharynx and trachea, requiring a more invasive procedure. Secretions that are not removed are more likely to be aspirated into the lungs, increasing the risk for infection, VAP, and respiratory failure. Retained lower airway secretions require nasotracheal suctioning.

Suctioning nasotracheally into the trachea and pharynx or directly into established artificial airways is more commonly performed using open suction. Open suctioning is performed with the suction catheter directly inserted through the nasotrachea or an artificial airway, or with the temporary disconnection of a patient from a ventilator and the introduction of the suction catheter into an artificial airway. Open suctioning is necessary with ventilated patients who have artificial airways and need to have sputum specimens obtained. Closed suctioning is described in Procedural Guideline 24.1.

Nasotracheal and artificial airway suctioning are sterile procedures. A suction catheter is extended into the lower airway (upper bronchus) to remove respiratory secretions and maintain optimum ventilation and oxygenation in patients who are unable to remove these secretions independently.

All forms of tracheal suctioning have many complications, including hypoxemia, cardiac dysrhythmias, changes in blood pressure

(can be either hypertensive or hypotensive), laryngeal or bronchospasm, pain, infection, or bradycardia. Bradycardia is associated with stimulation of the vagus nerve. Respiratory or cardiac arrest can even occur as a result of tracheal suctioning. Nasal trauma and bleeding can develop from a suction catheter being introduced nasotracheally (Urden et al., 2024).

Patient assessment guides the frequency of airway suctioning. Do not suction patients on the basis of an arbitrary or routine schedule. Suction on the basis of a patient's need for minimal excessive and unnecessary trauma. Patient assessment factors indicating the need for suctioning include oxygen saturation below 90%; visible secretions in the airway; patient's inability to produce an effective, productive cough; auscultation of coarse crackles over the trachea; and acute respiratory distress. If a patient has an artificial airway in place and/or is mechanically ventilated, other indications for suctioning include the presence of a saw-tooth pattern on the flow-volume loop on a ventilator monitor, increased peak inspiratory pressure or decreased tidal volumes noted on the ventilator monitor, abnormal capnography waveforms, or suspected aspiration (Urden et al., 2024; Hare & Seckel, 2024).

Artificial Airways

Endotracheal tubes (ETT) and tracheostomy tubes (TTs) are artificial airways inserted to maintain respiratory flow and prevent airway obstruction. They provide a route for mechanical ventilation, permit easy access for secretion removal, and protect the airway from gross aspiration in patients with impaired cough or gag reflexes.

Endotracheal Tubes

ET intubation is a procedure performed by the health care provider or other specially trained personnel (e.g., certified registered nurse anesthetist, respiratory therapist, rescue personnel). An ET is inserted through the nares (nasotracheal tube) or more commonly through the mouth (oral ET), past the epiglottis and vocal cords, and into the trachea (Fig. 24.2A–B). Adult (and some pediatric) sizes of ETs have a cuff molded onto the tube. When the cuff is inflated, it seals the airway around the tube to prevent the aspiration of oral secretions or gastric contents into the lung and/or to obstruct the escape of air from mechanical ventilator breaths through the upper airway. Some newer ETs also contain a port that can be connected for subglottal suctioning.

The length of time that an endotracheal tube (ETT) remains in place is controversial. Complications from long-term intubation include laryngeal and tracheal stenosis or a cricoid abscess (Urden et al., 2024). Sources differ on when a patient should be changed from an ETT to a tracheostomy tube (TT). The range of recommended length of time to be endotracheally intubated is 7 to 14 days (Urden et al., 2024; Wang et al., 2019). Collaborate with a health care provider if patients begin to show signs of complications from the airways themselves, such as erosion of the oral mucosa. Known benefits of having a TT versus an ETT include less need for sedation, shorter ventilator weaning time (time it takes to get a patient off a ventilator), and shorter ICU and hospital stay (Wang et al., 2019).

Tracheostomy Tubes

A TT can be temporary or permanent, depending on a patient's condition. It is inserted either surgically or percutaneously directly into the trachea through a small incision made in a patient's neck. Reasons for a TT include the need for prolonged mechanical ventilation, upper airway obstruction secondary to trauma or tumor, or difficulties with airway clearance that can occur in conditions such as spinal cord injury or neuromuscular disease (Urden et al., 2020). TTs are made of several different materials, including polyvinyl chloride or silicone-based plastics and, less commonly, stainless steel or metallic compounds. Metal TTs are thermal sensitive and must be protected from extreme heat and cold to prevent tissue injury in a patient. Most metal and plastic TTs contain an inner cannula that is withdrawn temporarily for cleaning airway-occluding mucus without removing the entire TT (see Skill 24.4) (Urden et al., 2024).

Delegation

The skill of open nasotracheal and artificial airway suctioning of newly inserted artificial airways cannot be delegated to nursing assistive personnel (AP). At some agencies, the AP may suction a patient with a well-established tracheostomy that the nurse has determined to be stable. Educate the AP about:
- Any modifications of the skill such as the need for supplemental oxygen or clean versus sterile technique.
- Appropriate suction limits for suctioning ETTs and TTs and risks of applying excessive or inadequate suction pressure.
- Reporting any changes in patient's respiratory status, level of consciousness, restlessness, secretion color and amount, and unresolved coughing or gagging.
- Reporting any change in patient's color, vital signs (VS), or complaints of pain.
- Reporting any signs of skin injury around the stoma and peristomal area.

Interprofessional Collaboration

- A respiratory therapist or health care provider can determine if there are any needed alterations to the suctioning procedure, such as not increasing oxygen before suctioning or not changing patient position.
- Respiratory therapists (RTs) in some agencies or settings are also responsible for suctioning patients. Communicate frequency of suctioning and patient response to suctioning.
- Collaborate with physical therapy, occupational therapy, or speech therapy staff, who may need to alert you to the need for suctioning. Their interventions may increase the need for you to suction the patient before and during therapies.

Equipment

- Stethoscope
- Pulse oximeter (*option* for artificial airway suction: end-tidal CO_2 monitor)
- Portable or wall suction machine
- Connecting tubing (4–6 feet)
- Bedside table
- Clean gloves, sterile gloves
- Mask, goggles, or face shield; gown if isolation procedures dictate
- Water-soluble lubricant
- Appropriate-size suction catheter. It should be the smallest diameter that will remove secretions effectively, preferably one

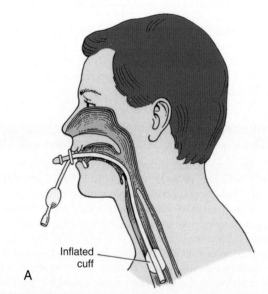
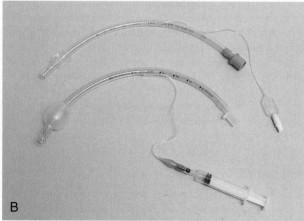

Inflated cuff

A

B

FIG. 24.2 (A) Endotracheal (ET) tube with inflated cuff. (B) ET tubes with uninflated and inflated cuffs and syringe for inflation.

that is no more than half of the internal diameter of the artificial airway to minimize the decrease in PaO_2 (Billington & Luckett, 2019).
- Clean towel or paper drape
- Small Y-adapter (if catheter does not have a suction control port)

- Sterile basin or solution container
- Sterile normal saline solution or sterile water, about 100 mL
- Manual self-inflating manual resuscitation bag-valve device with appropriate-size mask
- PEEP valve for resuscitation bag

STEP	RATIONALE

ASSESSMENT

1. Identify patient using at least two identifiers (e.g., name and birthday or name and medical record number) according to agency policy.

Ensures correct patient. Complies with The Joint Commission standards and improves patient safety (TJC, 2023).

2. Review patient's EHR for history of abnormal anatomy or head and neck surgery/trauma, tumors involving lower airway, pneumonia, chronic obstructive pulmonary disease, and neurological abnormalities.

Changes in neurological status and neuromuscular impairment increase likelihood that patient is unable to clear respiratory secretions. Abnormal anatomy or head and neck surgery/trauma and tumors in and around lower airway impair normal secretion clearance. Accumulating pulmonary secretions impede patient's ability to effectively clear airway through cough mechanism (Urden et al., 2024).

3. Review EHR for patient's normal pulse oximeter and end-tidal CO_2 values, VS, previous response and tolerance to suctioning procedure, and color and quantity of sputum.

Knowing the patient's recent condition and past response to suctioning helps predict or prevent unexpected outcomes.

4. Review sputum microbiology data in laboratory report.

Certain bacteria are easier to transmit or require isolation because of virulence or antibiotic resistance.

5. Assess patient's/family caregiver's health literacy.

Determines degree to which individuals have the ability to find, understand, and use information and services to make informed health-related decisions and actions for themselves and others (CDC, 2023).

6. Perform hand hygiene and apply clean gloves or other personal protective equipment (PPE) if risk of exposing self to secretions or if patient condition indicates.

Prevents transmission of microorganisms.

7. Auscultate lungs and assess for:

   a. Signs and symptoms of upper and lower airway obstruction requiring suctioning: abnormal respiratory rate, adventitious lung sounds, secretions in the airway, gurgling, drooling, restlessness, gastric secretions or vomitus in mouth, and coughing without clearing airway secretions and/or improving adventitious lung sounds.

Physical signs and symptoms result from secretions in upper and lower airways and decreased oxygen to the tissues. Presuction assessment provides baseline data to identify need for suctioning and measures the effectiveness of suction procedures (Urden et al., 2024).

   b. VS and oximetry signs and symptoms associated with respiratory distress or hypoxia and hypercapnia: decreased pulse oximetry (SpO_2), increased pulse and blood pressure, bradycardia, tachypnea, decreased breath sounds, apprehension, anxiety, lethargy, pallor, and cyanosis (a late sign of hypoxia). *Keep pulse oximeter on patient for continuous assessment of SpO_2.*

Physical signs and symptoms resulting from decreased tissue oxygenation. Provides presuction baseline to measure patient tolerance to suctioning and effectiveness of suctioning on SpO_2 levels.

8. Assess for risk factors for upper and lower airway obstruction, including chronic obstructive pulmonary disease, impaired mobility, decreased level of consciousness, nasal feeding tube, decreased cough or gag reflex, and decreased swallowing ability.

Risk factors can impair patient's ability to clear secretions from airway, increase risk for retaining secretions, and necessitate nasopharyngeal or nasotracheal suctioning (Urden et al., 2024).

9. Assess for excessive amounts of secretions visible in the artificial airway, signs of respiratory distress from obstructed airway (increased work of breathing, increased respiratory rate), presence of rhonchi on auscultation, excessive coughing, increased peak inspiratory pressures (if on mechanical ventilator), sawtooth pattern on ventilator monitor, or changes in capnography waveform (if patient on mechanical ventilator) or decrease in patient pulse oximeter (Hare & Seckel, 2024; Urden et al., 2024).

All factors indicate need for tracheal suctioning.

Clinical Judgment *Suctioning should only be performed after applying clinical judgment with patient assessment data to determine what patient's condition indicates and not suction in a scheduled fashion such as hourly (Urden et al., 2024; Harding et al., 2023).*

STEP	RATIONALE
10. Assess patency of ET with capnography/end-tidal carbon dioxide (CO_2) detector.	ET may become displaced or blocked by secretions. CO_2 detector is pH sensitive and can identify changes in CO_2 levels caused by retained secretions (Urden et al., 2024).
11. Assess factors that may affect volume and consistency of secretions.	Thickened or copious secretions increase risk for airway obstruction.
a. Fluid balance	Fluid overload increases amount of secretions. Dehydration can lead to thicker secretions.
b. Lack of humidity	Environment influences secretion formation and gas exchange. Airway suctioning is needed when patient cannot clear secretions effectively.
c. Infection (e.g., pneumonia)	Patients with respiratory infections are prone to increased secretions that are thicker and sometimes more difficult to expectorate.
12. For endotracheal suctioning, assess patient's peak inspiratory pressure when on volume-controlled ventilation or tidal volume during pressure-controlled ventilation.	Increased peak inspiratory pressure or decreased tidal volume may indicate airway obstruction (Urden et al., 2024; Hare & Seckel, 2024).

Clinical Judgment *The patient's VS, pulse oximetry, end-tidal CO_2, ventilator pressures and volumes (if receiving mechanical ventilation), and respiratory status are assessed before and continuously throughout suctioning (Hare & Seckel, 2024).*

STEP	RATIONALE
13. Identify contraindications to nasotracheal suctioning: occluded nasal passages; nasal bleeding; epiglottis or croup; acute head, facial, or neck injury or surgery; coagulopathy or bleeding disorder; irritable airway; laryngospasm or bronchospasm; gastric surgery with high anastomosis; myocardial infarction (Urden et al., 2024; American Association of Respiratory Care [AARC], 2004; Hare & Seckel, 2024).	These conditions are contraindicated because passage of suction catheter through nasal route causes trauma to existing facial trauma/surgery, increases nasal bleeding, or causes severe bleeding in presence of coagulopathy or bleeding disorders. In presence of epiglottitis or croup, laryngospasm, or irritable airway, passage of suction catheter through nose causes intractable coughing, hypoxemia, and severe bronchospasm, necessitating emergency intubation or tracheostomy. Hypoxemia could worsen cardiac damage in myocardial infarction (AARC, 2004).
14. Remove and dispose of gloves. Perform hand hygiene. (Other PPE may be kept on for actual suctioning.)	Reduces transmission of microorganisms.
15. Determine presence of apprehension, anxiety, decreased ability to concentrate, lethargy, decreased level of consciousness (especially acute), increased fatigue, dizziness, and/or behavioral changes (especially irritability).	These are signs and symptoms of hypoxia and/or hypercapnia, which can indicate need for suction. These signs can also help to identify patient's ability to cooperate with procedure.
16. Assess patient's knowledge, prior experience with suctioning procedure, and feelings about procedure.	Reveals need for patient instruction and/or support.

PLANNING

STEP	RATIONALE
1. Expected outcomes following completion of procedure:	
• Upper and lower airways demonstrate absent or diminished gurgles, crackles, rhonchi, and wheezes on inspiration and expiration.	Absent or diminished adventitious sounds indicate that airways are cleared of secretions and are patent.
• Heart rate, blood pressure, respiratory rate, and effort are within normal range for patient.	When airway secretions are removed and oxygenation improves, patient's VS and respiratory assessment findings improve.
• Patient's SpO_2 is at or above baseline, whereas end-tidal carbon dioxide concentration (E_tCO_2), if being monitored, is at or below baseline.	Demonstrates improvement in gas exchange (Urden et al., 2024).

Clinical Judgment *It is important to ensure that the patient's SpO_2 and E_tCO_2 values are back to their own personal normal baseline values. Patients with chronic pulmonary disease may have lower than normal SpO_2 or higher than normal E_tCO_2 values (Urden et al., 2024).*

STEP	RATIONALE
• Patient's peak inspiratory pressure decreases back to baseline, and exhaled tidal volume increases back to baseline.	Demonstrates removal of secretions.
2. Perform hand hygiene. Arrange supplies at patient's bedside. Close room door or curtain.	Enhances efficiency of procedure. Promotes privacy and patient comfort.
3. Explain to patient procedure and how it will help clear airway and relieve breathing difficulty. Explain that temporary coughing, sneezing, gagging, or shortness of breath is normal during procedure.	Encourages cooperation and minimizes risks, anxiety, and pain of procedure.

STEP	RATIONALE

IMPLEMENTATION

1. Perform hand hygiene and apply appropriate PPE, if not already applied during assessment (mask with face shield or goggles; gown if necessary).

   Reduces transmission of microorganisms.

2. If not already present, place pulse oximeter on patient's finger. Take reading and leave oximeter in place.

   Provides continuous SpO$_2$ value to determine patient's response to suctioning.

3. Adjust bed to appropriate height (if not already done) and lower side rail on side nearest you. Check locks on bed wheels. Assist patient to comfortable position, typically semi-Fowler or high Fowler.

   Minimizes caregiver's muscle strain and prevents injury. Prevents bed from moving. Positioning reduces stimulation of gag reflex, promotes patient comfort and secretion drainage, and prevents aspiration.

4. Connect one end of connecting tubing to suction device and place other end in convenient location near patient. Turn suction device on and set suction pressure to as low a level as possible and yet able to effectively clear secretions. This value is typically between 80 and 120 mm Hg (Mwakanyanga et al., 2018; Hare & Seckel, 2024). Occlude end of suction tubing to check pressure.

   Ensures equipment function. Excessive negative pressure damages tracheal mucosa and induces greater hypoxia (Hare & Seckel, 2024).

5. Prepare suction catheter for all types of open suctioning.

   a. Using aseptic technique, open suction kit or catheter package. If sterile drape is available, place it across patient's chest or on bedside table. Do not allow suction catheter to touch any nonsterile surfaces.

   Prepares catheter, maintains asepsis, and reduces transmission of microorganisms. Provides sterile surface on which to lay catheter between passes.

   b. Unwrap or open sterile basin and place on bedside table. Be careful not to touch inside of basin. Fill with about 100 mL sterile normal saline solution or water (see illustration).

   Saline or water is used to clean tubing after each suction pass.

   c. If performing nasotracheal suctioning, open packet of water-soluble lubricant and apply small amount to sterile field. **NOTE:** *Lubricant is not necessary for artificial airway suctioning.*

   Water-soluble lubricant helps avoid lipid aspiration pneumonia. Excessive amount of lubricant occludes catheter.

6. Apply sterile gloves to each hand or clean glove to nondominant hand and sterile glove to dominant hand.

   Reduces transmission of microorganisms and maintains sterility of suction catheter.

7. Pick up suction catheter with dominant hand without touching nonsterile surfaces. Pick up connecting tubing with nondominant hand. Secure catheter to tubing (see illustration).

   Maintains catheter sterility. Connects catheter to suction.

8. Place tip of catheter into sterile basin and suction small amount of normal saline solution from basin by occluding suction vent.

   Ensures equipment function. Lubricates internal catheter and tubing.

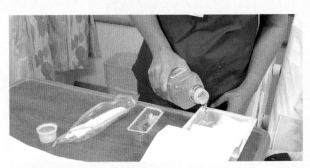

STEP 5b Pouring sterile saline into tray.

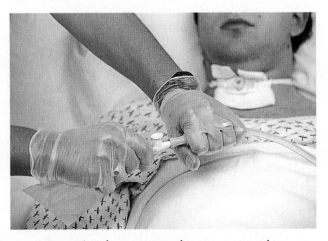

STEP 7 Attaching suction catheter to suction tubing.

STEP	RATIONALE
9. Suction airway.	
a. Nasotracheal and nasopharyngeal:	
(1) Ask patient to extend neck back slightly. Have patient take deep breaths, if able, or increase oxygen flow rate with delivery device through cannula or mask (if ordered).	Position opens access to airway.
(2) Lightly coat distal 6 to 8 cm (2−3 inches) of catheter with water-soluble lubricant.	Lubricates catheter for easier insertion.
(3) Remove oxygen-delivery device, if applicable, with nondominant hand.	May help to decrease risks of hypoxemia

Clinical Judgment *Be sure to insert catheter during patient inhalation, especially if inserting it into trachea, because epiglottis is open. Do not insert during swallowing or catheter will most likely enter esophagus. Never apply suction during insertion. Patient should cough. If patient gags or becomes nauseated, catheter is most likely in esophagus and you need to remove it (AARC, 2004; Urden et al., 2024).*

STEP	RATIONALE
(4) Introduce catheter and apply suction.	
(a) *Nasopharyngeal:* As patient takes deep breath, insert catheter (without applying suction) following natural course of naris; slightly slant catheter downward and advance to back of pharynx. Do not force through naris. In adults, insert catheter approximately 16 cm (6.5 inches); in older children, 8 to 12 cm (3–5 inches); in infants and young children, 4 to 7.5 cm (1.5–3 inches). Rule of thumb is to insert catheter distance from tip of nose (or mouth) to angle of mandible.	Ensures that catheter tip reaches pharynx for suctioning.

Clinical Judgment *If resistance is met during insertion, you may need to try the other naris. Do not force the catheter up the nares because this will cause mucosal damage.*

STEP	RATIONALE
(i) Apply intermittent suction for no more than 10 to 15 seconds by placing and releasing nondominant thumb over catheter vent. Slowly withdraw catheter while rotating it back and forth between thumb and forefinger.	Intermittent suction up to 10–15 seconds safely removes pharyngeal secretions. Suction time greater than 15 seconds increases risk for suction-induced hypoxemia (AARC, 2004; Urden et al., 2024).

Clinical Judgment *Do not advance catheter into trachea after suctioning nasopharyngeally. The mouth and pharynx contain more bacteria than trachea. You can introduce bacteria into airways and lungs causing serious infection.*

STEP	RATIONALE
(b) *Nasotracheal:* With head slighting extended, have patient takes deep breath, then advance catheter (without applying suction) following natural course of naris. Advance catheter slightly slanted and downward to just above larynx. Then as patient takes another deep breath, quickly insert catheter into larynx. Patient will begin to cough; then pull back catheter 1 to 2 cm (½ inch) before applying suction (see illustration).	Ensures that catheter tip reaches trachea for suctioning.

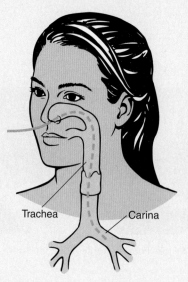

Trachea   Carina

STEP 9a(4)b Distance of insertion of nasotracheal catheter.

STEP	RATIONALE

Clinical Judgment *When there is difficulty passing the catheter, ask patient to cough or say "ahh" or try to advance the catheter during inspiration. Both measures help to open the glottis to permit passage of the catheter into the trachea.*

(i) *Positioning option:* In some instances, turning patient's head helps you suction more effectively. If you feel resistance after insertion of catheter, use caution; it has probably hit the carina of trachea. Pull catheter back 1 cm (0.4 inches) before applying suction (AARC, 2004; Hare & Seckel, 2024).	Turning patient's head to side elevates bronchial passage on opposite side. Turning head to right helps with suctioning of left main-stem bronchus; turning head to left helps you suction right main-stem bronchus. Suctioning too deeply may cause tracheal mucosa trauma.
(ii) Apply intermittent suction for no more than 10 to 15 seconds by placing and releasing nondominant thumb over catheter vent. Slowly withdraw catheter while rotating it back and forth between thumb and forefinger.	Suction time greater than 15 seconds increases risk for suction-induced hypoxemia (Urden et al., 2024; AARC, 2004). Intermittent suction and rotation of catheter prevents injury to tracheal mucosa. If catheter "grabs" mucosa, remove thumb to release suction.
(iii) If there are pharyngeal secretions present, suction just before removing catheter from naris. **Do not suction nasally again after suctioning mouth.**	Catheter is used for sterile airways first, then nonsterile pharyngeal cavity.

Clinical Judgment *Monitor patient's VS and SpO$_2$ throughout suctioning process. Stop suctioning if the patient becomes hemodynamically unstable (e.g., a 20 beats/min change [increase or decrease] in pulse rate) or SpO$_2$ falls below 90% or 5% from baseline.*

(5) Reapply oxygen-delivery device and encourage patient to take some deep breaths, if able.	Helps to decrease risk of hypoxia. Increases patient comfort.
(6) Rinse catheter and connecting tubing with normal saline or water until cleared.	Secretions that remain in suction catheter or connecting tubing decrease suctioning efficiency.
(7) Assess for need to repeat suctioning. Do not perform more than two passes with catheter. Allow patient to rest at least 1 minute (AARC, 2010). Ask patient to take deep breaths and cough.	Observe for alterations in cardiopulmonary status. Suctioning induces hypoxemia, irregular pulse, laryngospasm, and bronchospasm (AARC, 2010).

Clinical Judgment *Hyperoxygenation is based on patient assessment and should not be used routinely. Hyperoxygenation should be limited to those patients who desaturate during suctioning and those patients on high levels of oxygen or positive end-expiratory pressure (Urden et al., 2024; Hare & Seckel, 2024).*

b. Artificial airway:

(1) With assistance from respiratory therapy when patients have an artificial airway, hyperoxygenate, when appropriate, with 100% oxygen for at least 30 to 60 seconds before suctioning by (1) pressing suction hyperoxygenation button on ventilator, OR (2) increasing baseline fraction of inspired oxygen (FiO$_2$) level on mechanical ventilator, OR (3) disconnecting ventilator, attaching self-inflating resuscitation bag-valve device to tube with nondominant hand (or have assistant do this), and administering 5 to 6 breaths over 30 seconds (or have assistant do this). **NOTE:** Some mechanical ventilators have a button that, when pushed, delivers 100% oxygen for a few minutes and then resets to previous setting.	When hyperoxygenation is needed, it decreases the risk of decreased arterial oxygen levels while ventilation or oxygenation is interrupted and volume is lost during suctioning (Urden et al., 2024; AARC, 2010; Hare & Seckel, 2024).
(2) If patient is receiving mechanical ventilation, open swivel adapter or, if necessary, remove oxygen- or humidity-delivery device with nondominant hand.	Exposes artificial airway.

Clinical Judgment *Suctioning can cause elevations in intracranial pressure (ICP) in patients with head injuries. Reduce this risk by presuction hyperoxygenation, which results in hypocarbia and, in turn, induces vasoconstriction. Vasoconstriction reduces the potential for an increase in ICP (Urden et al., 2024).*

STEP	RATIONALE
(3) Advise patient that you are about to begin suctioning. Without applying suction, gently but quickly insert catheter into artificial airway using dominant thumb and forefinger (it is best to try to time catheter insertion into artificial airway with inspiration) (see illustration). Advance catheter until patient coughs, which is usually 0.5 to 1 cm below the level of the tube. Then pull back 1 cm (0.4 inch) before applying suction (Billington & Luckett, 2019).	Application of suction pressure while introducing catheter into artificial airway increases risk for damage to tracheal mucosa and increased hypoxia. Pulling back stimulates cough and removes catheter from mucosal wall so that catheter is not resting against tracheal mucosa during suctioning (Urden et al., 2024; AARC, 2010).

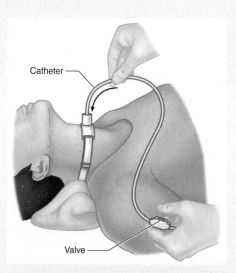

STEP 9b(3) Suctioning tracheostomy.

Clinical Judgment *If unable to insert catheter past the end of an ETT, the catheter is probably caught in the Murphy eye (i.e., side hole at the distal end of the ETT that allows for collateral airflow in the event of tracheal main-stem intubation). If this happens, pull the catheter back 1 cm (½ inch) and rotate the catheter to reposition it away from the Murphy eye, or withdraw it slightly and reinsert with the next inhalation. Usually the catheter meets resistance at the carina. One indication that the catheter is at the carina is acute onset of coughing because the carina contains many cough receptors (Urden et al., 2024; Billington & Luckett, 2019).*

STEP	RATIONALE
(4) Apply intermittent suction by placing and releasing nondominant thumb over valve of catheter. Apply suction for 10 seconds (Hare & Seckel, 2024; Urden et al., 2024). Slowly withdraw catheter while rotating it back and forth between dominant thumb and forefinger. Do not use suction for greater than 15 seconds. Encourage patient to cough. Watch for respiratory distress.	Suction time greater than 15 seconds increases risk for suction-induced hypoxemia (Urden et al., 2024; AARC, 2010; Hare & Seckel, 2024). Intermittent suction and rotation of catheter prevent injury to tracheal mucosa. If catheter "grabs" mucosa, remove thumb to release suction.

Clinical Judgment *If patient develops respiratory distress during the suction procedure, immediately withdraw catheter (without applying suction) and supply additional oxygen and breaths as needed. In an emergency, administer oxygen directly through the catheter. Disconnect suction and attach oxygen at prescribed flow rate through the catheter. If the patient does not tolerate the suctioning procedure, you may need to consider switching to closed (in-line) suctioning (Procedural Guideline 24.1) or allowing longer recovery times. Notify health care provider if patient develops significant cardiopulmonary compromise during suctioning (Urden et al., 2024).*

STEP	RATIONALE
(5) If patient is receiving mechanical ventilation, close swivel adapter or replace oxygen-delivery device. Hyperoxygenate patient for 30 to 60 seconds.	Reestablishes artificial airway. Helps to decrease risks of hypoxia.
(6) Rinse catheter and connecting tubing with normal saline until clear. Use continuous suction.	Removes catheter secretions. Secretions left in tubing decrease suctioning efficiency and provide environment for microorganism growth.
(7) Assess patient's VS, cardiopulmonary status, and ventilator measures for secretion clearance. Repeat Steps 9b(1) through 9b(6) once or twice more to clear secretions. Allow adequate time (at least 1 full minute) between suction passes.	Suctioning can induce dysrhythmias, hypoxia, and bronchospasm and impair cerebral circulation or adversely affect hemodynamic stability (Urden et al., 2024).

STEP	RATIONALE

Clinical Judgment *The number of suction passes should be based on patient assessment and presence of secretions. If secretions persist after two passes, hyperoxygenate and allow patient more time to rest and recover between suction catheter passes (Hare & Seckel, 2024).*

Clinical Judgment *The instillation of normal saline into the artificial airway to help remove secretions has not proven to be beneficial, and it may contribute to hypoxemia and lower airway microorganism colonization, resulting in ventilator-associated pneumonia (VAP) (Urden, 2024).*

STEP	RATIONALE
c. When trachea or artificial airways are sufficiently cleared of secretions, perform oropharyngeal suctioning (Skill 24.1) to clear mouth of secretions. Do not suction nose with catheter after suctioning mouth.	Removes upper airway secretions. Generally, more microorganisms are present in mouth. Upper airway is considered "clean," and lower airway is considered "sterile." You can use same catheter to suction from sterile to clean areas (e.g., tracheal suctioning to oropharyngeal suctioning) but not from clean (oropharynx) to sterile (trachea) areas.
10. When suctioning is complete, disconnect catheter from connecting tubing. Roll catheter around fingers of dominant hand. Pull glove off inside out so that catheter remains coiled in glove. Pull off other glove over first glove in same way. Discard in appropriate receptacle. Turn off suction device.	Seals contaminants in gloves. Reduces transmission of microorganisms.
11. Remove towel, place in laundry or appropriate receptacle, and reposition patient. (Apply clean gloves to continue personal care.)	Reduces transmission of microorganisms. Promotes comfort.
12. If oxygen level was changed during procedure, readjust oxygen to original ordered level because patient's blood oxygen level should have returned to baseline.	Prevents absorption atelectasis (i.e., tendency for airways to collapse if proximally obstructed by secretions). Prevents oxygen toxicity while allowing patient time to reoxygenate blood.
13. Discard remainder of normal saline. If basin is disposable, discard into appropriate receptacle. If basin is reusable, rinse it out and place it in soiled utility room.	Reduces transmission of microorganisms.
14. Help patient to comfortable position and provide oral hygiene as needed.	Restores comfort and sense of well-being. Work of breathing is decreased when in a comfortable position. Oral hygiene promotes comfort.
15. Remove and dispose of gloves and other PPE, if used, and perform hand hygiene.	Reduces transmission of microorganisms.
16. Place unopened suction kit on suction machine table or at head of bed.	Provides immediate access to suction catheter for next procedure.
17. Raise side rails (as appropriate) and lower bed to lowest position, locking into position.	Ensures patient safety and prevents falls.
18. Place nurse call system in an accessible location within the patient's reach.	Ensures patient can call for assistance if needed.

EVALUATION

1. Compare patient's VS, cardiopulmonary assessments, and E_tCO_2 and SpO_2 values before and after suctioning. If on ventilator, compare FiO_2 and tidal volumes and peak inspiratory pressures.	Identifies physiological effects of suction procedure to restore airway patency. Auscultation of lungs offers information about change in lung sounds.
2. Ask patient if breathing is easier and if congestion is decreased.	Provides subjective confirmation that suctioning procedure has relieved airway.
3. Observe character of airway secretions.	Provides data to document presence or absence of respiratory tract infection or thickened secretions.
4. **Use Teach-Back:** "I need to suction your father, and I want to be sure that I explained the suctioning procedure and when I need to do it. Please tell me in your own words why the suctioning is needed." Revise your instruction now or develop a plan for revised patient/family caregiver teaching if patient/family caregiver is not able to teach back correctly.	Teach-back is a technique for health care providers to ensure that they have explained medical information clearly so that patients and their families understand what is communicated to them (AHRQ, 2023).

STEP	RATIONALE
Unexpected Outcomes	**Related Interventions**
1. Patient has decrease in overall cardiopulmonary status as evidenced by decreased SpO_2, increased E_tCO_2, continued tachypnea, continued increased work of breathing, and cardiac dysrhythmias.	• Limit length of time for suctioning. • Determine need for more frequent suctioning, possibly of shorter duration. • Determine need for supplemental or increase in supplemental oxygen. Supply oxygen between suctioning passes. • Notify health care provider.
2. Bloody secretions are returned after suctioning.	• Determine amount of suction pressure used. May need to be decreased. • Ensure that suction is completed correctly using intermittent suction and catheter rotation. Do not apply suction until after catheter has been pulled back 1 cm (0.4 inches) to prevent applying suction while catheter is touching carina. • Evaluate suctioning frequency. • Provide more frequent oral hygiene. • Notify health care provider.
3. Patient has paroxysms of coughing or bronchospasm.	• Administer supplemental oxygen. • Allow patient to rest between passes of suction catheter. • Consult with health care provider regarding need for inhaled bronchodilators or topical anesthetics.
4. Inability to obtain secretions during suction procedure.	• Evaluate patient's fluid status and adequacy of humidification on oxygen-delivery device. • Assess for signs of infection. • Determine need for chest physiotherapy (refer to RT).

Documentation

- Document the amount, consistency, color, and odor of secretions; size of catheter; route of suctioning; and patient's response to suctioning.
- Document patient's presuctioning and postsuctioning VS, cardiopulmonary status, and ventilation measures.
- Document need for hyperoxygenation, type of hyperoxygenation, and FiO_2 used.
- Document your evaluation of patient and family learning.

Hand-Off Reporting

- Report patient's tolerance of and response to procedure, need for hyperoxygenation, frequency of suctioning, and the quantity and quality of the secretions.
- Report unexpected physiological changes to health care provider.

Special Considerations

Patient Education

- Instruct patient that coughing increases and that there will be some discomfort during the procedure.
- Explain why supplemental oxygen is given before and after suctioning if indicated.

Pediatrics

- Infants need less suction pressure than adults (AARC, 2010).
- Hyperoxygenate with 100% oxygen in pediatric patients and 10% increase of baseline in neonates before suctioning (Hockenberry et al., 2024).
- Thick secretions are more difficult to remove because of the small diameter of the suction catheter. Normal saline should not be instilled in the airway in an attempt to thin the secretions (AARC, 2010).
- Infant airways have less cartilage and may collapse easily, especially in premature infants or those with reactive airways.

Older Adults

- Capillaries of older adults are often fragile, predisposing patient to bleeding problems.

Populations With Disabilities

- Patients with intellectual disabilities may not understand the education that is provided. Ensure that a caregiver is present to help explain the procedure, particularly if it is to be completed at home.
- Patients with neuromuscular disabilities, such as muscular dystrophy or ALS, may have weak respiratory muscles and could have difficulties coughing and clearing their airways. Closely monitor their need for suctioning.

Home Care

- Most patients with airway clearance problems at home have a tracheostomy.
- Instruct patient and family caregiver to clean and disinfect or change the secretion collection container every 24 hours according to home care or agency protocol.
- In the home setting, stress the importance of brief intervals of applying suction pressure. Instruct those performing suctioning to hold their breath during the application of negative suction pressure to help them remember to not suction too long.

PROCEDURAL GUIDELINE 24.1 *Closed (In-Line) Suction*

The use of closed-system suction catheters for suctioning artificial airways has increased in recent years. When comparing closed versus open suctioning, the incidence of ventilator-associated pneumonia (VAP) is unchanged. However, there is a decreased risk of infection for a health care provider from exposure to patient secretions with a closed system (Letchford & Bench, 2018; Urden et al., 2024).

Closed-system catheter (in-line) suctioning allows quicker lower airway suctioning without applying sterile gloves or a mask and does not interrupt ventilation and oxygenation in critically ill patients. It involves the use of a multiuse suction catheter that is housed within a plastic sleeve and is attached to a patient's artificial airway (Fig. 24.3A–B). This method of suctioning is associated with decreased risk of hypoxia and cardiovascular complications when compared with open suctioning. It is also the recommended method of suctioning for patients who cannot tolerate loss of positive end-expiratory pressure (PEEP), such as those with severe respiratory disorders who require high amounts of PEEP or oxygen (Urden et al., 2024; Letchford & Bench, 2018; Hare & Seckel, 2024). With a closed-system method, the patient's artificial airway is not disconnected from the mechanical ventilator; therefore there is no loss of positive end-expiratory pressure (PEEP).

Delegation
The skill of airway suction with a closed (in-line) suction catheter is not delegated to assistive personnel (AP). In special situations, such as suctioning a well-established permanent tracheostomy, this procedure may be delegated to the AP (see agency policy). The nurse is responsible for cardiopulmonary assessment and evaluation of the patient. Direct the AP about:
- Individualized aspects of suctioning the patient (e.g., position, duration of suction, pressure settings).
- Expected quality, quantity, and color of secretions and to inform the nurse immediately if there are changes.
- Patient's anticipated response to suction and to immediately report to the nurse changes in vital signs, complaints of pain, shortness of breath, confusion, or increased restlessness.

Interprofessional Collaboration
- A respiratory therapist (RT) may also be responsible for suctioning the patient. Communicate frequency of suctioning and patient response to suctioning.
- Collaborate with physical, speech, or occupational therapists, who may need to alert you of need for suctioning. Their interventions may increase the need for you to suction the patient before and during therapies.

Equipment
Closed-system or in-line suction catheter, appropriately sized; 5- to 10-mL normal saline in syringe or vials; suction machine/source with regulator; connecting tubing 182.8 cm (6 feet); two clean gloves; oral suction kit/supplies for oropharyngeal suctioning (see Skill 24.1); mask, goggles, or face shield; gown if isolation precautions indicate; pulse oximeter; stethoscope; manual self-inflating resuscitation bag (bag-valve mask) with appropriate-size mask, while not necessary for the procedure, is safe to have on hand

Steps
1. Identify patient using at least two identifiers (e.g., name and birthday or name and medical record number) according to agency policy (TJC, 2023).
2. Perform respiratory and airway assessment as in Skill 24.2.
3. Perform hand hygiene. Gather equipment/supplies at bedside.
4. Close room door or curtains around bed.
5. Explain procedure to patient and caregiver and the importance of coughing during the suctioning procedure. Even when patients cannot speak, they need to have information regarding the procedure.
6. Perform hand hygiene; don personal protective equipment (PPE) as patient status indicates (e.g., gloves, mask, gown).
7. If not already placed during assessment, position pulse oximeter on patient's finger. Take reading and leave oximeter in place.
8. Adjust the bed to appropriate height and lower side rail on the side nearest you. Check locks on the bed.

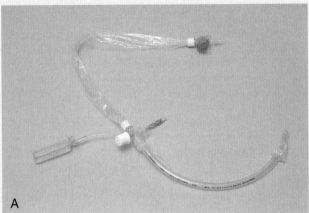

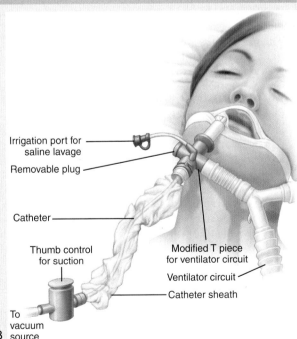

Irrigation port for saline lavage
Removable plug
Catheter
Thumb control for suction
To vacuum source
Modified T piece for ventilator circuit
Ventilator circuit
Catheter sheath

FIG. 24.3 (A) Closed-system suction catheter attached to endotracheal tube. (B) Closed suction system attached to an endotracheal tube. (*B from Blanchard B: Thoracic surgery. In Rothrock JC, McEwen DR, editors:* Alexander's care of the patient in surgery, *ed 14, St Louis, 2011, Mosby.*)

Continued

PROCEDURAL GUIDELINE 23.1 *Closed (In-Line) Suction—cont'd*

9. Help patient assume a position of comfort, usually semi- or high-Fowler position. Place towel across patient's chest.
10. Turn suction device on, set vacuum regulator to appropriate negative pressure (usually 80–120 mm Hg), and check pressure. Consult manufacturer guidelines for recommended pressure to use with the agency's brand of catheter.
11. Attach suction:
    a. In many agencies an RT attaches the catheter to the mechanical ventilator circuit. If catheter is not already in place, open suction catheter package using aseptic technique and attach closed-system suction catheter to ventilator circuit by removing swivel adapter and placing closed-system suction catheter apparatus on endotracheal tube (ET) or tracheostomy tube (TT). Connect Y on mechanical ventilator circuit to closed-system suction catheter with flex tubing.
    b. Connect one end of connecting tubing to suction machine; connect other end to the end of the closed-system or in-line suction catheter.
12. If ordered, hyperoxygenate patient (usually 100% oxygen) for at least 30 seconds by adjusting the fraction of inspired oxygen (FiO_2) setting on the ventilator or by using a temporary oxygen-enrichment program available on microprocessor ventilators according to agency policy or protocol. (Manual ventilation is not recommended.)

Clinical Judgment *Hyperoxygenation is based on patient assessment and should not be used routinely. Hyperoxygenation should be limited to those patients who desaturate during suctioning and those patients on high levels of oxygen or positive end expiratory pressure (Urden et al., 2024).*

13. Unlock suction control mechanism if required by manufacturer. Open saline port and attach saline syringe or vial.
14. Pick up suction catheter enclosed in plastic sleeve with dominant hand.
15. Suction patient:
    a. Wait until patient inhales to insert catheter. Then insert catheter using a repeating maneuver of pushing catheter and sliding plastic sleeve back between thumb and forefinger until resistance is felt or patient coughs.
    b. Pull back 1 cm (0.5 inches) before applying suction to avoid tissue damage to carina. **NOTE:** If patient has a history of bleeding during previous suction procedures, care should be taken to avoid hitting the carina with the suction catheter.
    c. Encourage patient to cough and apply suction by squeezing on suction control mechanism while withdrawing catheter. **NOTE:** It is difficult to apply

intermittent pulses of suction and nearly impossible to rotate the catheter compared with a standard catheter.
    d. Apply continuous suction for 10 to 15 seconds as you remove the suction catheter (Urden et al., 2024; AARC, 2010; Hare & Seckel, 2024). Be sure to withdraw the catheter completely into the plastic sheath and past the tip of the airway so that it does not obstruct airflow.
16. Reassess cardiopulmonary status, including pulse oximetry (SpO_2) and ventilator measures, to determine need for subsequent suctioning or complications. Repeat Steps 15a-d one more time to clear secretions if patient condition indicates. Allow adequate time (at least 1 full minute) between suction passes for ventilation and reoxygenation.
17. When airway is clear, withdraw catheter completely into sheath. Be sure that colored indicator line on catheter is visible in the sheath. Attach sterile solution lavage container or sterile saline or water syringe to side port of suction catheter. Squeeze vial or push syringe while applying suction to rinse inner lumen of catheter. **NOTE:** Do not let the saline go down the ETT or TT. Use at least 5 to 10 mL of saline to rinse the catheter until it is clear of retained secretions, which can cause bacterial growth and increase the risk for infection (AARC, 2010; Hare & Seckel, 2024). Lock suction mechanism if applicable and turn off suction.
18. Hyperoxygenate for at least 30 seconds (see Step 12).
19. If patient requires oral or nasal suctioning, perform Skill 24.1 or 24.2 with separate standard suction catheter.
20. Place the Yankauer catheter on a clean, dry area for reuse with suction turned off or within patient's reach with suction on if patient is capable of suctioning own mouth.
21. Help patient to a comfortable position.
22. Place nurse call system in an accessible location within patient's reach.
23. Raise side rails (as appropriate) and lower bed to lowest position, locking into position.
24. Compare patient's VS and SpO_2 before and after suctioning.
25. Auscultate lung fields and compare with baseline.
26. Observe airway secretions.
27. Ask patient if breathing is easier and congestion is decreased.
28. Remove gloves, face shield, and other PPE; discard into appropriate receptacle; and perform hand hygiene.
29. **Use Teach-Back:** "I want to be sure I explained this suctioning procedure correctly. Please squeeze my hand if you understand these steps. Each time I suction you, I will explain these steps again." Revise your instruction now or develop a plan for revised patient/family caregiver teaching if patient/family caregiver is not able to teach back correctly.

✦ SKILL 24.3 Performing Endotracheal Tube Care

Endotracheal tubes (ETTs) are flexible, plastic tubes placed in the mouth or through the nose and advanced down into the trachea to establish short-term artificial airways to administer mechanical ventilation, relieve upper airway obstruction, protect against aspiration, and clear secretions (see Fig. 24.2A–B). Routine care includes maintaining correct position of the tube, monitoring cuff

pressures, and preventing complications such as tracheal erosion, ventilator-associated events (VAEs), and medical device pressure injuries (MDRPIs).

After insertion of an ETT, the cuff is inflated and the tube is secured with a commercial holder device or tape. A cuff on an ETT prevents the escape of air between the tube and the walls of the trachea and reduces the risk of aspiration when a patient is receiving mechanical ventilation. The amount of cuff inflation is based on two factors: the size of the patient's trachea and the external diameter of the artificial airway. Cuff pressure should be between 20 and 25 mm Hg (Sanaie et al., 2019; Wen et al., 2018). When cuff pressures are too high, permanent damage to the tracheal mucosa occurs, leading to complications such as tracheomalacia; tracheoesophageal fistula; or erosion of the innominate artery, which is rare but almost always fatal (Turner et al., 2020; Urden et al., 2024). When cuff pressure is too low, mechanical ventilation is not effective and a patient has an increased risk of aspiration, which increases the risk of ventilator-associated pneumonia (VAP) (Sanaie et al., 2019; Urden et al., 2024).

Preventing tube-related complications is a critical component of care and depends on securing the tube and inflating the cuff properly. In many agencies these functions are the responsibility of respiratory therapists (RTs). However, nurses are responsible for assessing patients' respiratory status, ventilator settings and functioning, and integrity of the airway cuff.

Once a tube is inserted, confirmation of placement is achieved using a chest x-ray film and a disposable end-tidal CO_2 detector (Fig. 24.4) (Urden et al., 2024; Hare & Seckel, 2024). Capnography is the noninvasive measurement of the partial pressure of carbon dioxide (CO_2) in an exhaled breath expressed as the CO_2 concentration over time. The measure continuously monitors CO_2 once a patient is placed on mechanical ventilation. Continuous end-tidal CO_2 monitoring is a reliable indicator of proper tube placement and allows for detection of future tube dislodgement (Hare & Seckel, 2024). The CO_2 monitor measures CO_2 directly from the airway, with the sensor located on the airway adapter at the hub of the ETT.

Properly securing an ETT prevents inadvertent extubation from coughing, gagging, or accidental pulling on the tube. Tubes are secured with either commercial ETT holders/fasteners or tape. Use of tape increases the risk for medical adhesive–related skin injury (MARSI, Fumarola et al., 2020). Evidence suggests that the commercial fasteners are associated with fewer developments of lip ulcers or facial skin tears and decreased risk of tube dislodgments or excess movement (Landsperger et al., 2019). Commercial fasteners are easier to use and allow for quicker performance of ETT care, such as moving the ETT from one side of the mouth to the other (Landsperger et al., 2019). Proper securing of an ETT reduces the

risks of tracheal stenosis; tracheomalacia; barotrauma; erosion of the innominate artery; and tracheoesophageal fistula, particularly when the cuff is overinflated (Urden et al., 2024). In addition, properly securing the ETT and routine ETT care reduces the risk for MDRPIs, which develop due to pressure from the artificial airway on adjacent tissues (e.g., lips, oral mucosa) (Jackson et al., 2019).

After a tube is inserted and secured and the cuff is inflated, you need to maintain patency of the ETT and prevent a ventilator-associated event (VAE). Please refer to Chapter 23 for more information regarding VAE. In patients who cannot clear their secretions, periodic suctioning of the artificial airway achieves airway patency (Skill 24.2 and Procedural Guideline 24.1).

Delegation

The skill of performing ETT care cannot be delegated to assistive personnel (AP). AP may provide routine care for patients with an ETT and assist the nurse with ETT care. Direct the AP to:
- Immediately report any signs of respiratory problems or increased airway secretions.
- Immediately report if the ETT appears to have moved or becomes obstructed or dislodged.
- Immediately report changes in patient's mood, level of consciousness, irritability, VS, decreased pulse oximetry value, or changes in end-tidal CO_2 values.
- Immediately report any redness, irritation, or injury around the patient's mouth or lips.

Interprofessional Collaboration

- Collaborate with the RT in performing ETT care.
- Collaborate with other nurses and work together to perform tube care. Usually, this skill requires two people (either nurse and RT or two nurses) in order to be safely completed without risk for extubation.

Equipment

- Towel
- ET and oropharyngeal suction equipment (see Skills 24.1 and 24.2)
- Commercial ETT holder and mouth guard (follow manufacturer instructions for securing); for emergencies or when commercial devices not available, use 1.27-cm (½-inch) wide adhesive or waterproof tape (do not use paper or silk tape)
- Oral airway and bite block (both are optional and only used if patient is biting ETT)
- Clean gloves: mask, goggles, face shield (if indicated); gown if isolation procedures indicate
- Adhesive remover swab or acetone on cotton ball
- Oral hygiene supplies: soft toothbrush (or suction toothbrush); foam oral swab; cleaning solution: 0.12% to 0.20% chlorhexidine gluconate mouthwash, rinse, or gel
- Face hygiene equipment (e.g., wet washcloth, towel, soap, shaving supplies)
- Clean 2 × 2 gauze
- Normal saline solution
- Liquid adhesive or skin preparation pads
- Tongue blade (optional)
- Stethoscope
- Pulse oximeter, end-tidal CO_2 detector
- Another health care team member (need two people to perform some of the steps)
- Communication device (letter or picture board, tablet, paper, and pen)

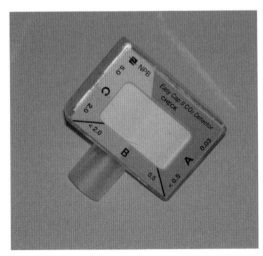

FIG. 24.4 End-tidal CO_2 detector. (*Used by permission from Nellcor Puritan Bennett, LLC, Boulder, CO, doing business as Covidien.*)

STEP	RATIONALE

ASSESSMENT

1. Identify patient using at least two identifiers (e.g., name and birthday or name and medical record number) according to agency policy.

Ensures correct patient. Complies with The Joint Commission standards and improves patient safety (TJC, 2023).

2. Review patient's EHR for depth of ETT insertion, previous ET cuff pressures, last time ETT was repositioned, and patient tolerance of care.

Knowing the patient information helps to guide planning of ETT care and improves patient safety.

3. Assess patient's/family caregiver's health literacy. Use communication board with patient.

Patient with ETT cannot speak. Determines degree to which individuals have the ability to find, understand, and use information and services to make informed health-related decisions and actions for themselves and others (CDC, 2023).

4. Identify if patient is at risk for medical adhesive–related skin injury (MARSI) from adhesive tape: age, dehydration, malnutrition, exposure to radiation therapy, underlying chronic conditions (e.g. diabetes, immunosuppression), and edema of skin

Common risk factors for MARSI (Fumarola et al., 2020). Factors raise your level of observation if patient has adhesive tape securing ETT.

5. Ask patient to describe history of allergies: known type of allergies and normal allergic reaction. Check patient's allergy wristband. Focus on adhesive or latex.

Reduces risk for exposing patient to allergens that can cause localized or systemic allergic reactions.

6. Perform hand hygiene, apply gloves and other personal protective equipment (PPE) as determined by patient condition and agency policy.

Reduces transmission of organisms.

7. Assess patient's cardiopulmonary status, including lung sounds, pulse oximetry, E_tCO_2, VS, and level of consciousness. *Keep pulse oximeter in place.*

Provides baseline measure of ventilation and oxygenation.

8. Observe for factors that increase risk for complications from ETT: type and size of tube, movement of tube up and down trachea, duration of tube placement, presence of facial trauma.

Tube rotating from side to side causes risk for MDRPI. Tube can become dislodged from lower airway (incidental extubation), or it can enter right main-stem bronchus. Longer duration of intubation is associated with increased risk for lower airway complications such as ventilator-associated pneumonia (VAP) (Urden et al., 2024; Wang et al; 2018).

9. Observe condition of tissues surrounding ETT for impaired skin integrity (e.g., blistering, abrasions, pressure injuries) on nares, lips, cheeks, or corner of mouth and for excess nasal or oral secretions. Note if patient moves tube with tongue, bites tube or tongue, and/or has foul-smelling mouth.

Presence of ETT impairs ability of patient to swallow oral secretions. Patient is at increased risk for developing MDRPI and MARSI from ETT as tube is positioned or pulled against lips and oral mucosal tissues (Fumarola et al., 2020; Jackson et al., 2019).

10. Observe patency of airway: excess secretions, diminished airflow, and signs and symptoms of airway obstruction.

Buildup of secretions in ETT impairs oxygen delivery and subsequent tissue oxygenation.

11. Observe for gurgling on expiration, decreased exhaled tidal volume (mechanically ventilated patient), signs and symptoms of inadequate ventilation (rising end-tidal carbon dioxide concentration [E_tCO_2], patient-ventilator dyssynchrony, or dyspnea), spasmodic coughing, tense test balloon on tube, flaccid test balloon on tube, and ability to speak or vocalize.

Cuff underinflation increases risk for aspiration, allows secretions to enter the trachea, and permits vocalization.

Cuff overinflation may cause ischemia or necrosis of tracheal tissue from obstruction of capillary bed, resulting in tracheomalacia or tracheoesophageal fistula (Sanaie et al., 2019; Turner et al., 2020; Urden et al., 2024). End-tidal carbon dioxide concentration (E_tCO_2) validates the correct placement of the ET (Urden et al., 2024; Hare & Seckel, 2024).

Clinical Judgment *When assessment indicates possible overinflation or underinflation of ET cuff (pressures less than 20 mm Hg or greater than 25 mm Hg), notify RT and follow agency policy for correcting cuff pressures (Sanaie, 2019; Hare & Seckel, 2024).*

12. Determine current ET depth as noted by centimeters at incisors or gum line. A line is marked on tube and documented in patient's EHR at time of intubation and every shift.

Ensures that tube is at proper depth to adequately ventilate both lungs and that it is not too high, which causes vocal cord damage, or too low, which results in right main-stem intubation, in which only the right lung is ventilated.

13. Remove and dispose of gloves. Perform hand hygiene. Remaining PPE may stay in place.

Reduces transmission of microorganisms.

14. Review EHR and determine when oral and airway care were last performed. Know the health care agency protocols and procedures, but be aware of patient-specific needs for more frequent care.

Oral care protocols help to reduce the incidence of ventilator-associated pneumonia (AACN, 2018b; Martin-Loeches et al., 2018).

STEP	RATIONALE
15. Assess patient's knowledge, prior experience with ETT care, and feelings about procedure. Use communication board.	Reveals need for patient instruction and/or support.

PLANNING

STEP	RATIONALE
1. Expected outcomes following completion of procedure:	
• ETT remains in correct position in patient's trachea, evidenced by depth of tube the same as when started or as ordered (same centimeter marking at gums or incisors); bilateral breath sounds are equal; E_tCO_2 values remain at patient baseline.	Maintaining ET position promotes adequate ventilation of lungs. Complications of lower airway and vocal cord trauma prevented.
• Patient's skin around mouth and oral mucous membranes remains intact without evidence of MARSI or MDRPI.	ET stabilized so as to not place undue pressure against corners of mouth. Patient is not able to bite inner cheeks or tongue. Commercial holder device avoids use of adhesive.
• Patient does not develop signs of tracheal damage.	Cuff pressure maintained at safe level.
2. Perform hand hygiene. Gather equipment/supplies and arrange at bedside.	Reduces transmission of microorganisms. Ensures efficiency in performing procedure.
3. Obtain assistance from available staff for this procedure.	Reduces risk for accidental extubation of ETT as tube is manipulated.
4. Close room door or curtains around bed.	Provides for patient privacy.
5. Explain procedure and patient's need to participate, including not biting or moving ETT with tongue, trying not to cough when tape/holder device is off ETT, keeping hands down, and not pulling on tubing.	Reduces anxiety, encourages cooperation, and reduces risk of accidental extubation.

Clinical Judgment *Patients with ETTs are not able to verbalize their wants, fears, anxieties, or needs easily. This impaired ability to communicate can lead to increased anxiety and apprehension. While patients can often understand what is being said to them, communication aids should be offered to patients to allow them to ask questions, confirm understanding, or communicate their concerns (Santiago et al., 2019).*

IMPLEMENTATION

STEP	RATIONALE
1. Perform hand hygiene. Apply clean gloves. Keep remaining PPE on. Have assistant apply PPE as well.	Reduces transmission of microorganisms.
2. Assist patient in assuming comfortable position. Elevate patient's head of bed at least 30 degrees, unless contraindicated.	Provides access to site and facilitates completion of procedure. Prepares patient for oropharyngeal suctioning and helps to decrease risk of aspiration (AACN, 2017).
3. Adjust bed to appropriate height and lower side rail on side nearest you. Check locks on bed wheel.	Minimizes caregiver's muscle strain and prevents injury. Prevents bed from moving.
4. Place clean towel across patient's chest.	Reduces soiling of bed clothes and linen.
5. Perform endotracheal or oropharyngeal suction if indicated (see Skills 24.1 and 24.2 and Procedural Guideline 24.1).	Removes secretions. Diminishes patient's need to cough during procedure.
6. Connect Yankauer suction catheter to suction source and have it ready to use. Ensure that suction source/machine for oral suctioning is on and functioning properly.	Need to have functioning equipment to perform oral care appropriately. Prepares suction apparatus.
7. Remove oral airway or bite block, if present, and place on towel.	Provides access to and complete observation of patient's oral cavity.

Clinical Judgment *If patient is biting the tube, do not remove bite block until absolutely necessary. The bite block prevents obstruction of the ETT and occlusion of the airway.*

STEP	RATIONALE
8. Brush teeth with soft toothbrush using toothpaste with fluoride (Hare & Seckel, 2024). Suction oropharyngeal secretions as needed.	There may be need for pediatric toothbrush depending on size of patient's oral cavity. It is recommended to brush teeth at least twice a day (AACN, 2018b; Hare & Seckel, 2024).
9. Use 0.12% chlorhexidine solution, 1.5% hydrogen peroxide, or 0.05% antiseptic solution and oral swabs to clean mouth (Hare & Seckel, 2024). Have your assistant suction oropharyngeal secretions as needed. Apply mouth moisturizer to oral mucosa and lips after each cleaning. Complete every 2 to 4 hours (check agency policy).	The use of chlorhexidine mouthwash or gel is effective in reducing VAP (AACN, 2018b; Alja'afreh et al., 2019).

Clinical Judgment *It is helpful to have the assistant on hand to frequently suction the oral cavity during the procedure. This helps to prevent the pooling and aspiration of oral secretions.*

STEP	RATIONALE

Clinical Judgment *Do not use lemon glycerin swabs due to irritation and drying of oral mucosa, which causes a worsening of xerostomia (Hare & Seckel, 2024).*

10. Secretions (subglottic) accumulate just above inflated cuff. Perform subglottic secretion drainage (SSD), if not continuously performed. **NOTE:** Many ventilators have an integrated subglottic secretion mechanism (see agency policy).	SSD allows for the suction of secretions above the cuff of the ETT. Its use, whether continuous or intermittent, helps to reduce the incidence of VAP (Letchford & Bench, 2018; Pozuelo-Carrascosa et al., 2020).

Clinical Judgment *The ability to perform SSD is not available on every ETT or at every institution. The provider must choose the tube that allows for SSD when intubating (Lacherade et al., 2018). Use SSD if a patient is intubated for more than 48 to 72 hours. Continuous SSD (available on some ventilators) has been associated with an increased risk of tracheal hemorrhage or necrosis, so those patients should be closely monitored (Huang et al., 2018).*

11. Prepare to secure the ETT.	
a. Open commercially available ETT holder package per manufacturer instructions. Set device aside with head guard in place and Velcro strips open.	Commercial devices are latex free, provide access to oral mucosa for cleansing, and are convenient and disposable.

Clinical Judgment *Commercially available ETT holders are recommended for ongoing use by patients. ETTs are usually stabilized for only short-term use with adhesive tape, such as during a surgical intubation when extubation is expected as the patient awakes from anesthesia or emergently in the emergency department (ED). However, the use of adhesive tape can lead to a MARSI. This injury occurs during removal of tape when the attachment between the skin and an adhesive is stronger than that between individual cells, causing either the epidermal layers to separate or the epidermis to detach completely from the dermis (mechanical trauma) (Fumarola et al., 2020). The procedure for taping an ETT can be found in Box 24.1.*

b. Remove Velcro strips from ETT and remove ETT holder from patient while assistant holds ETT securely in place.	Velcro strips hold ETT in place and provide marker to measure distance to patient's incisors or gums. These devices permit access to patient's mouth for ease in oropharyngeal suctioning, skin assessment, and oral hygiene.

Clinical Judgment *Clean exterior surface of ETT with soap and water as needed. If adhesive tape was initially used to secure ETT, DO NOT apply adhesive tape remover to the tube itself. This action will make it nearly impossible for the new commercial holder to appropriately stick to the ETT, which increases risk of tube dislodgement. Do not allow assistant to hold the tube away from the lips or nares. Doing so allows too much movement in the tube and increases the risk for tube movement and accidental extubation. Instruct assistant not to let go of the ETT because it could become dislodged.*

c. Remove excess secretions or adhesive from patient's face. Clean facial skin with mild soap and water and dry thoroughly.	The patient's face must be clean and dry in order for a new device to adhere properly if an adhesive product is used.

Clinical Judgment *If patient is actively biting, oral airway or bite block is not removed during hygiene. Wait until the new commercial device is partially or completely secured to ETT.*

d. Note level of ETT by looking at mark or noting centimeter value on tube itself. Move ETT to other side of mouth and ensure that tube marking at incisors or gum line is unchanged. Perform oral care as needed on side where tube was initially positioned. Clean oral airway or bite block (if patient is not biting) with warm soapy water and rinse well. Reinsert as needed.	The ETT should be repositioned at least daily. Changing sides of ETT redistributes pressure and decreases risk of tissue injury at corners of mouth and oral mucosa (Hare & Seckel, 2024).

Clinical Judgment *The cuff of the ETT may need to be deflated before changing its position. If this step is required, perform deep oral suctioning before deflation of the cuff and do not provide oral care until the cuff is properly reinflated.*

Clinical Judgment *The patient may cough excessively when the tube is being moved. The person who is holding the tube in place should be prepared for this and take extra caution while holding. The assistant needs to continue holding the ETT in place until oral care and, if necessary, shaving is completed and the commercial ETT holder is stabilized and secured. In some cases, the patient may need to be administered a dose of antianxiety or sedating medication.*

12. Secure tube. (**NOTE:** Assistant must continue to hold ETT in place.)	
a. Thread ET through opening in holder designed to secure it. Be sure that pilot balloon is accessible.	Commercially available holders have a slit in front of holder designed to secure ETT.
b. Place strips of ET holder under patient at occipital region of head.	

BOX 24.1

Steps for Securing an Endotracheal Tube With Tape

1. Prepare tape by cutting piece of tape long enough to go completely around patient's head from naris to naris plus 15 cm (6 inches). This is typically 30 to 60 cm (12–24 inches) in total length.
2. Lay tape adhesive side up on bedside table.

3. Cut and lay 8 to 15 cm (3–6 inches) of second piece of tape, adhesive sides together, in center of the long strip to prevent tape from sticking to hair. Smaller strip of tape should cover area between ears around back of head (see illustration A).

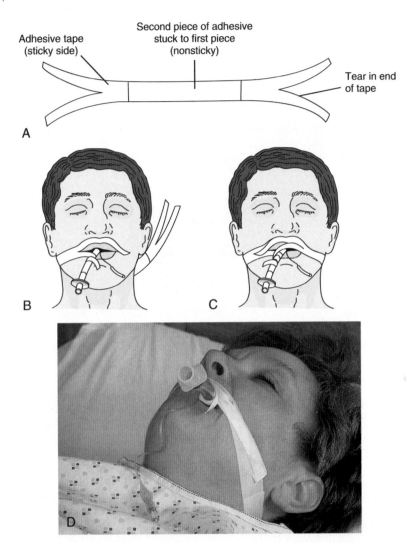

4. While one person is holding and stabilizing ET, the other person should remove old tape from patient's skin, using adhesive tape remover to remove sticky residue. The tape will also need to be removed from ET itself. **NOTE:** If the sticky adhesive residue is not removed, the new adhesive tape will not properly adhere to tube and/or patient's skin.
5. While one person continues to hold and stabilize ET, clean face and shave patient if needed. Apply tincture of benzoin as needed.
6. Slip prepared tape under patient's head and neck, adhesive side up. Take care not to twist tape or catch hair. Do not allow tape to stick to itself. Then slide tape under patient's neck. **NOTE:** In some situations, it may help to gently stick end of tape to tongue blade, which serves as guide.
7. Center tape so that double-faced tape extends around back of neck from ear to ear.

8. On one side of face, secure tape from ear to naris (nasal ET) or over lip to ET (oral ET).
9. Tear remaining tape in half lengthwise, forming two pieces that are 1 to 1.5 cm (0.4–0.6 inch) wide.
10. Secure top half of tape across upper lip (oral ET) or across top of nose (nasal ET) to opposite ear.
11. Wrap bottom half of tape around tube and up from bottom (see illustration B). Tape should encircle tube at least 2 times for security.
12. Gently pull other side of tape firmly to pick up slack and secure to opposite side of face and ET same as first piece (see illustrations C and D). **NOTE:** ET is secured.
13. Assistant can release hold.
14. Check depth mark at incisors or gum line.

Images A, B, C from Goodrich CA: Endotracheal intubation (Assist). In Johnson KL, editor: *AACN Procedural manual for progressive and critical care*, ed 8, St Louis, 2024, Elsevier.

STEP	RATIONALE
c. Verify that ET is at established depth using incisors or gum line marker as guide.	Ensures that ETT remains at correct depth as determined during assessment.
d. Attach Velcro strips at base of patient's head. Leave 1 cm (0.4 inch) slack in strips.	
e. Verify that tube is secure, it does not move forward from patient's mouth or backward down into patient's throat, and there are no pressure areas on oral mucosa or occipital region of head (see illustration).	Tube must be secure so that it remains at correct depth. It can be secured without being tight and causing pressure.

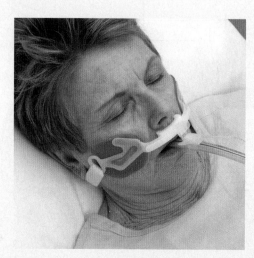

STEP 12e Commercial endotracheal tube holder. (*Modified from Sills JR: Entry-level respiratory therapist exam guide, St Louis, 2000, Mosby.*)

STEP	RATIONALE
13. For unconscious patient, reinsert oral airway without pushing tongue into oropharynx and secure with tape (see Skill 27.1).	Prevents patient from biting ET and allows access for oropharyngeal suctioning. An oral airway is not used in a conscious, cooperative patient because it causes excessive gagging and pressure areas to mouth and tongue (Goodrich, 2024).
14. Ensure proper cuff inflation by using the pressure manometer to keep the pressure between 20 and 25 mm Hg (Larrow & Klich-Heartt, 2016).	Underinflated cuffs lead to an increased risk of VAP while overinflated cuffs increase risk of tracheal ischemia or damage (Marjanovic et al., 2021).

Clinical Judgment *Other methods to check cuff pressure (minimal leak technique and minimal occluding volume) are used in agencies without access to manometers. These techniques have been found to be not as accurate and can lead to overinflation or underinflation of the cuff (Sanaie et al., 2019; Turner et al., 2020).*

STEP	RATIONALE
15. Clean rest of face and neck with soapy washcloth, rinse, and dry. Shave male patient as needed.	Moisture and beard growth cause irritation from holder straps.

Clinical Judgment *Be sure there is an assistant to hold the ETT in position while shaving. When shaving patients, take great care to keep the cuff inflation port away from the razor. The razor can inadvertently cut or nick the tubing, causing air loss from the cuff and the possible need for reintubation.*

STEP	RATIONALE
16. Remove gloves and mask, goggles, or face shield or gown; discard in receptacle; and perform hand hygiene. (Assistant performs same steps.) Place clean items (e.g., oral care solution, excess swabs) in place of storage in patient room.	Reduces transmission of microorganisms. Ensures that contaminated gloves and hands do not touch clean items.
17. Help patient to a comfortable position.	Restores comfort and sense of well-being.
18. Raise side rails (as appropriate) and lower bed to lowest position, locking into position.	Ensures patient safety and prevents falls.
19. Place nurse call system in an accessible location within patient's reach.	Ensures patient can call for assistance if needed.

EVALUATION

1. Compare respiratory assessments before and after ETT care.	Identifies any physiological changes, including presence and quality of breath sounds after procedure.

STEP	RATIONALE
2. Observe depth and position of ETT according to health care provider recommendation.	Position of ETT should not be altered.
3. Assess security of holder device or tape by *gently* tugging at tube.	Device or tape should remain secure. Patient may cough during tugging.
4. Assess skin around mouth and oral mucous membranes for intactness and MDRPI. Check for MARSI if using adhesive securement.	If using tape, it should not tear skin. MDRPI should be absent.
5. Compare E_tCO_2 and SpO_2 values from before and after ETT care.	Changes in E_tCO_2 and SpO_2 can help identify displacement or dislodgement of ETT.
6. Observe for excessive phonation, presence of gastric secretions in airway secretions, or tracheoesophageal fistula.	Occurs with inadequate or excessive cuff inflation.
7. Use Teach-Back: "I want to be sure I explained why this ETT care is necessary. I want you to nod yes or no as I explain each step." Revise your instruction now or develop a plan for patient/family caregiver teaching if patient/family caregiver is not able to teach back correctly.	Teach-back is a technique for health care providers to ensure that they have explained medical information clearly so that patients and their families understand what is communicated to them (AHRQ, 2023).

Unexpected Outcomes

1. Patient is extubated accidentally.

2. ET moves in airway and becomes malpositioned.

3. Patient has MDRPI in mouth or on lips and nares.

4. Cuff leak develops.

Related Interventions

- Remain with patient while calling for help. Notify health care provider.
- Ventilate with bag-valve mask as needed.
- Assess patient for airway patency, spontaneous breathing, and VS.
- Prepare for reintubation.
- Call for help and repeat securement or taping.
- Be prepared for chest x-ray film to confirm placement.
- Increase frequency of ETT care.
- Consult with skin care specialist regarding treatment per agency protocol.
- Align oxygen and humidity supply tubing so that they do not pull ETT, creating pressure injuries.
- Monitor for infection. If skin tear is present on cheeks or over nose or upper lip, consult with skin care specialist and apply protective barrier such as stoma adhesive patch or hydrocolloid dressing and apply tape to it.
- Notify health care provider.
- Verify position of tube, notify respiratory therapy, and follow agency policy.

Documentation

- Document time of care, respiratory assessments (including pulse oximetry and E_tCO_2) before and after care, cuff pressure after care, patient's tolerance of procedure, frequency and extent of ETT care, integrity of oral and nasal mucosa, and pressure injury care (if performed).
- Document your evaluation of patient/family caregiver learning.
- Document repositioning of ET, side on which it is placed, depth it is placed, and the securement technique used.

Hand-Off Reporting

- Report signs of infection immediately.
- Report unequal breath sounds, accidental extubation or displacement, cuff leak, or respiratory distress immediately to the health care provider.
- Report tolerance of procedure as well as assessment findings to the next shift nurse and the RT (if they did not assist during the procedure).

Special Considerations

Patient Education

- Instruct patient and family caregivers not to manipulate the ETT, tape, or ETT holder. If patient is complaining or appears uncomfortable, instruct caregiver to ask for the nurse.
- Instruct patient and family caregiver to inform the nurse if the tube causes gagging. Repositioning of the tube and/or sedation are options for reducing gagging.

Pediatrics

- Neonatal and pediatric procedures for securing ETTs and suctioning airways vary. Neonatal patients typically do not have cuffed tubes (Ahmed & Boyer, 2022). Refer to agency protocols for specific procedures (Hockenberry et al., 2024).
- Because of infants' delicate skin, it is more prone to tearing when removing tape. However, adhesive tape remover may be contraindicated in this population (Hockenberry et al., 2024).
- ETT holders are best used in this population as long as appropriate-size holders are available for the child.

Older Adults

- Older adult skin is more prone to tearing when removing tape or adhesive products (Touhy & Jett, 2022).
- Older adults with tendency toward inadequate nutrition are more prone to complications (e.g., infection, breakdown of oral mucosa).

◆ SKILL 24.4 *Performing Tracheostomy Care*

 Video Clip

A tracheostomy is a surgical or percutaneous creation of a stoma through the neck and into the trachea that allows for the insertion of an artificial airway, *tracheostomy tube (TT)*. TTs are placed in patients who require long-term airway management because of airway obstruction, airway clearance needs, and/or long-term need for mechanical ventilation (Bolsega & Sole, 2018). A TT offers advantages over long-term ETT placement such as decreased risk of laryngeal and tracheal injury, less sedation, shorter ventilator weaning time (time it takes to get a patient off a ventilator), and improved comfort for the patient. Some TTs even allow more patient freedom in the performance of activities of daily living such as feeding, speaking, and mobility (Wang et al., 2019).

TTs are composed of several components (Fig. 24.5A–B). The shaft is the main component of the TT and is what sits inside the trachea, keeping the airway open. Flanges rest against the patient's neck and prevent the TT from migrating into the trachea. The 15-mm connector is located on the shaft or inner cannula and is where the ventilator tubing or resuscitation bag attaches to the TT. The obturator is placed inside the TT and used during the TT insertion process. It is replaced with an inner cannula (if necessary) once inserted. The inner cannula is located inside the shaft of the TT and is a safety feature because it can be quickly removed and replaced if obstructed. TTs are curved and are commonly made of a synthetic material such as polyvinyl chloride (PVC), silicone, or polyurethane. The curved nature of the TT improves the ability of the tube to fit within the trachea. Metal tubes are rarely used because of their increased costs, rigidity, and lack of a cuff.

The pressure exerted by a TT against the neck creates the risk for medical device–related pressure injuries (MDRPIs). The AARC developed a tracheostomy bundle for preventing MDRPI

(Mussa et al., 2021). The bundle consists of four components: (1) placement of a hydrocolloid dressing underneath the tracheostomy flange in the postprocedure (trach creation) period, (2) removal of plate sutures within 7 days of the tracheostomy procedure, (3) placement of a polyurethane foam dressing after suture removal, and (4) neutral positioning of the head. The use of the bundle has shown a significant reduction in the rate of hospital-acquired tracheostomy-related pressure injuries (Mussa et al., 2021). In some settings the polyurethane dressing is applied postprocedure, as well as on an ongoing basis.

A TT is cuffed or uncuffed. A cuff on a TT serves the same purpose as the cuff on an ET. Cuffs are made of a balloon-like inflatable plastic typically inflated with air, although there are brands that are inflated with liquid such as water or saline. Uncuffed tubes allow patients the ability to clear the airway, but they provide no protection from aspiration. It is also more difficult to use positive-pressure ventilation in patients with uncuffed TTs (Przybyl, 2024). Monitoring and care of the cuff of the TT is similar to that of an ETT.

Speaking valves can be used with TTs. The patient must have a cuffless or fenestrated TT (see Fig. 24.5B) in place or be able to tolerate the cuff being deflated without risk of respiratory distress or aspiration. The openings in fenestrated tubes allow air to flow from the lungs over the vocal cords. However, these tubes must be used with caution and only in patients who can swallow without aspiration. This type of TT gives patients the ability to verbalize needs, and such communication often provides psychological benefits to the patient. Patients may not tolerate the speaking valves when first placed; therefore they will need to be carefully monitored for signs of intolerance or respiratory distress. Fenestrated

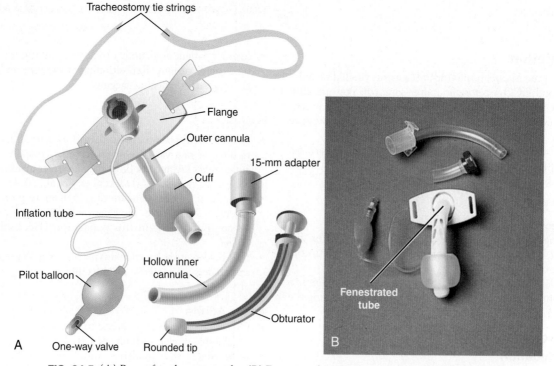

FIG. 24.5 (A) Parts of tracheostomy tube. (B) Fenestrated tracheostomy tube with cuff, inner cannula, decannulation plug, and pilot balloon. (*From Harding MM, et al: Medical-surgical nursing: assessment and management of clinical problems, ed 12, St Louis, 2023, Mosby.*)

BOX 24.2

Emergency Bedside Equipment for a Tracheostomy Patient

- Suction machine/equipment
- Suction tubing
- Suction catheters (Yankauer and tracheal)
- Sterile saline
- Additional tracheostomy tubes, one the same size as the current tube and another that is one size smaller
- Obturator
- Manual self-inflating resuscitation bag with appropriate-size mask
- 10-mL syringe

tubes are also associated with increased risk of granulation, which can lead to narrowing of the airway (Pandian et al., 2019).

Nurses also need to monitor for emergency events such as tube obstruction or dislodgement. Box 24.2 is a list of emergency bedside equipment for a patient who has a tracheostomy. Table 24.1 describes the signs of tracheal tube obstruction or dislodgement and interventions that should be performed.

Delegation

The skill of performing tracheostomy care is not routinely delegated to assistive personnel (AP). In some settings, patients who have permanent or well-established TTs may have the care delegated to AP (see agency policy). The nurse is responsible for assessing a patient and evaluating for proper artificial airway care, often in collaboration with a RT. The nurse is also responsible for educating the patient and caregivers regarding care of an established tracheostomy in the home. Direct the AP to:

- Immediately report any changes in patient's respiratory status, level of consciousness, confusion, restlessness or irritability, or level of comfort.

- Immediately report any dislodgement or excessive movement of the TT.
- Immediately report abnormal color of the tracheal stoma and drainage (e.g., yellow-green or bloody).

Interprofessional Collaboration

- Respiratory therapists (RTs) are often responsible for the care of the mechanical ventilator, as well as performing TT care.
- Collaborate with physical and occupational therapists. Therapists need to be aware of the signs of TT dislodgment that can occur during their prescribed exercises.
- Collaborate with speech therapists, who are often responsible for assessing the patient's ability to swallow and in assisting the patient in learning how to speak with the TT in place.

Equipment

- Bedside table
- Person to assist with changing the tracheostomy tie/holder
- Towel
- Artificial airway suction supplies (see Skill 24.2)
- Oropharyngeal suction supplies (see Skill 24.1)
- Sterile tracheostomy care kit, if available (be sure to collect supplies listed that are not available in kit)
- Three sterile 4 × 4–inch gauze pads
- Sterile cotton-tipped applicators
- Sterile hydrocolloid dressing or polyurethane foam dressing (if not available can use precut and sewn surgical gauze dressing)
- Sterile basin
- Sterile normal saline or water
- Small sterile brush (or disposable inner cannula)
- Commercial tracheostomy holder. Option: Roll of twill tape, tracheostomy ties
- Scissors
- Inner cannula that fits the patient's TT (may be disposable)
- Cuff pressure manometer

TABLE 24.1

Tracheostomy Emergencies

Emergency Type	Signs and Symptoms	Interventions
Tube dislodgement/ decannulation	• Inability to pass suction catheter past the length of the tube • Presence of subcutaneous emphysema near incision or stoma • Signs of respiratory distress • High-pressure alarm on ventilator • Flange of TT not flush with neck • Decreased SpO_2, increased E_tCO_2 • Decreased exhaled tidal volume • Patient able to speak around the TT	• Call for help • If stoma is less than 1 week old • Notify surgeon • Bag-mask ventilation • Prepare for intubation or surgical reinsertion of new TT • If stoma is well established (typically older than 1 week) • Replace with a new TT, inserting at a 90-degree angle into the trachea, then angling downward another 90 degrees
Tube obstruction	• Respiratory distress • Inability to pass suction catheter • Resistance felt when using the self-inflating resuscitation bag	• Ensure TT is in correct position • Call for help • Remove and inspect the inner cannula (if one present); clean or replace with a new one • Replace the TT (if changing inner cannula did not relieve the obstruction) • Patient may need more invasive intervention such as bronchoscopy • Prepare for possible oral endotracheal intubation, tracheostomy revision, or placement of a longer TT
Hemorrhage	• More than minimal bleeding at stoma site	• Notify health care provider • Provide oxygen, if not already in place

Data from Billington J, Luckett A: Care of the critically ill patient with a tracheostomy, *Nursing Standard* 34(2):59–65, 2019; Urden L, et al: *Priorities in critical care nursing*, ed 9, St Louis, 2024, Elsevier; Przybyl HL: Tracheostomy cuff and tube care, In Johnson KL, editor: *AACN procedure manual for high acuity, progressive, and critical care*, ed 8, St Louis, 2024, Elsevier.

- Pulse oximeter, end-tidal CO_2 detector
- Clean gloves (two pairs)
- Personal protective equipment (PPE): goggles, gown, or face shield if concern regarding contact with secretions
- Self-inflating manual resuscitation bag-valve device and appropriate-size mask
- One extra sterile tracheostomy kit
- Stethoscope
- Oxygen source

- 10 mL syringe
- Three-way stopcock
- Padded hemostats
- Tongue depressor
- Reintubation equipment (at the bedside in case of accidental TT dislodgment)
- Extra tracheostomy tubes (one same size as patient's current tube and one a size smaller, in case of accidental dislodgment)

STEP	RATIONALE

ASSESSMENT

1. Identify patient using at least two identifiers (e.g., name and birthday or name and medical record number) according to agency policy.	Ensures correct patient. Complies with The Joint Commission and improves patient safety (TJC, 2023).
2. Review the patient's EHR for time care was last performed; tolerance to procedure; type and size of TT and inner cannula, if present; any specific provider orders regarding the TT care; amount of air or fluid in TT cuff; and trends in patient VS and respiratory assessments.	Knowing the patient information guides the care delivery and ensures patient safety. Tracheostomy care is provided at least every 4 to 8 hours and more often if indicated (e.g., increased airway or stoma secretions, infection [airway or stoma]) (Urden et al., 2024).
3. Assess patient's/family caregiver's health literacy.	Determines degree to which individuals have the ability to find, understand, and use information and services to make informed health-related decisions and actions for themselves and others (CDC, 2023).
4. Perform hand hygiene and apply clean gloves and other PPE as patient condition dictates.	Reduces transmission of microorganisms.
5. Observe for signs and symptoms of tube dislodgement/ decannulation, and tube obstruction (see Table 24.1).	Addressing these findings promptly will reduce the negative effects of inadequate ventilation.
6. Observe for excess peristomal and intratracheal secretions, soiled or damp tracheostomy ties, soiled or damp tracheostomy dressing, diminished airflow through tracheostomy tube, or signs and symptoms of airway obstruction requiring suctioning (see Skill 24.2).	Indicate need for tracheostomy care caused by presence of secretions at stoma site or within tracheostomy tube. Irritation of mucosa caused by tube itself can also increase secretions (Przybyl, 2024). Assess for secretions and obstruction every 4 hours (Billington & Luckett, 2019).
7. Observe the tracheal stoma, skin around the stoma and under TT flange, and under tracheal ties (neck, face, back of neck) for pressure injury: blistering, erythema, drainage, or other discoloration.	Peristomal skin injuries are MDRPIs due to pressure from the tube, flange, or ties. These are one of the most common problems associated with tracheostomies, so patients should be closely monitored for this complication (Carroll et al., 2020). Sometimes, the patient's head position means that the tube will cause pressure areas on the skin of the neck or chest.
8. Assess patient's hydration status, humidity delivered to airway, status of any existing infection, patient's nutritional status, and ability to cough.	Determines factors that affect amount and consistency of secretions in tracheostomy and patient's ability to clear airway.
9. Assess patient's cardiopulmonary status, including pulse oximetry (SpO_2), E_tCO_2, VS, respiratory effort, lung sounds, and level of consciousness. Keep pulse oximeter in place.	Provides baseline to determine patient response to and tolerance of therapy.
10. Remove and dispose of gloves. Perform hand hygiene. Keep on remaining PPE.	Reduces transmission of microorganisms.
11. Assess patient's knowledge, prior experience with performing tracheostomy care, and feelings about procedure.	Reveals need for patient instruction and/or support.

Clinical Judgment *Patients who do not have or cannot tolerate speaking valves may not be able to verbalize their wants, fears, anxieties, or needs. This impaired ability to communicate can lead to increased anxiety and apprehension. Communication aids should be offered to patients to allow them to ask questions or communicate their concerns (Billington & Luckett, 2019).*

PLANNING

1. Expected outcomes following completion of procedure: • Inner and outer cannulas of TT are free of secretions; securement device is clean and secured snugly.	TT is patent and secure, optimizing amount of oxygen delivered to patient and limiting risk of infection from retained secretions.

STEP	RATIONALE
• Stoma site is pink; does not bleed; and is free of secretions, signs of infection, skin breakdown and pressure injuries, and signs of granuloma formation.	Indicates absence of infection at stoma site. Dry, intact tracheostomy stoma reduces risk for subsequent systemic infection.
• No evidence of skin injury or breakdown under tracheostomy ties or commercial tube holder.	Patients with excessive secretions or diaphoresis are at risk for skin breakdown under TT stabilizer.
• Cuff remains intact and cuff pressure remains at the desired level (usually between 20 and 30 Cm H_2O) (Urden et al., 2024; Przybyl, 2024).	Prevents aspiration, air leak, and tracheal damage.
2. Have another nurse or RT help in this procedure. Ensure that this employee performs hand hygiene, applies clean gloves, and dons appropriate PPE as patient condition dictates. All PPE should remain in place until end of procedures.	Assisting with procedure prevents accidental dislodgment of TT. Reduces transmission of infection.
3. Gather supplies and arrange at bedside. Close room door or curtain.	Ensures a well-organized procedure. Ensures patient privacy.
4. Raise head of bed at least 30 degrees, unless contraindicated. Be sure patient is comfortable. Adjust bed to appropriate height and lower side rail on side nearest you. Ensure bed is locked.	Provides access to site and facilitates completion of procedure. Prepares patient for any required suctioning. Positioning may decrease risk of aspiration (AACN, 2017, 2018a).
5. Explain procedure and patient's need to participate, including trying not to cough when tape or holder is off TT, keeping hands down, and not pulling on staff or tubing.	Encourages cooperation, minimizes risks or accidental dislodgment, and reduces anxiety.

Clinical Judgment *At some agencies it is standard practice to have an extra TT that is the same size as the patient's current TT and a TT one size smaller at the bedside at all times in case there is an emergent need to replace the TT because of obstruction or dislodgement (see Box 24.2) (Billington & Luckett, 2019).*

IMPLEMENTATION

1. Perform hand hygiene. Apply clean/sterile gloves for suctioning (see Skill 24.2) and other PPE if not already completed.	Reduces transmission of microorganisms.
2. Hyperoxygenate patient for 30 seconds or ask patient to take 5 to 6 deep breaths. Then suction tracheostomy (see Skill 24.2). Before removing gloves, remove soiled gauze or polyurethane foam tracheostomy dressing and discard in glove with coiled catheter. Hydrocolloid and polyurethane foam dressings may remain in place for a week depending on amount of tracheal secretions and manufacturer's directions.	Removes secretions to avoid occluding outer cannula while inner cannula is removed. Reduces need for patient to cough.

Clinical Judgment *Hyperoxygenation is based on patient assessment and should not be used routinely. Hyperoxygenation should be limited to those patients who desaturate during suctioning and those patients on high levels of oxygen or positive-end expiratory pressure (Urden et al., 2024).*

3. Perform hand hygiene. Prepare equipment on bedside table as follows:	Prepares equipment and allows for smooth, organized completion of tracheostomy care. Reduces transmission of microorganisms. Saline used for cleansing.
a. Open sterile tracheostomy kit. Open two 4 × 4–inch gauze packages using aseptic technique and pour normal saline on gauze in one package. Leave gauze in second package dry. Open two cotton-tipped swab packages and pour normal saline on swab tip in one package. Do not recap normal saline.	
b. Open sterile tracheostomy dressing package for hydrocolloid, polyurethane foam, or precut gauze.	
c. Unwrap sterile basin and pour about 0.5 to 2 cm (0.2 to 1 inch) of normal saline into it.	
d. Open small sterile brush package and place aseptically into sterile basin.	
e. Prepare TT fixation device.	
(1) If using commercially available TT holder, open package according to manufacturer directions.	
(2) If using twill tape: Prepare length of twill tape long enough to go around patient's neck 2 times, about 60 to 75 cm (24–30 inches) for an adult. Cut ends on diagonal. Lay aside in dry area.	Cutting ends of tie on diagonal aids in inserting tie through eyelet.

STEP	RATIONALE
f. Open inner cannula package (if new one is to be inserted, such as with disposable inner cannulas, or if patient does not tolerate being disconnected from oxygen source while cleaning reusable inner cannula).	
4. Apply sterile gloves. Keep dominant hand sterile throughout procedure.	Reduces transmission of microorganisms.
5. Remove oxygen source if present and if patient can tolerate.	Minimal time without oxygen reduces risk of hypoxia.

Clinical Judgment *It is important to stabilize TT at all times during tracheostomy care to prevent injury, unnecessary discomfort, or accidental extubation. Instruct assistant to stabilize the TT using gloved hands.*

6. Care of tracheostomy with reusable inner cannula:	
a. While touching only outer aspect of tube, unlock and remove inner cannula with nondominant hand following line of tracheostomy. Drop inner cannula into normal saline basin.	Should be cleaned either twice a day or every 8 hours, depending on agency policy (Billington & Luckett, 2019; Masood et al., 2018). Removes inner cannula for cleaning. Normal saline loosens secretions from inner cannula.

Clinical Judgment *If patient is on mechanical ventilation, instruct assistant to hold and stabilize TT and to remove the ventilator tube from the connection while you remove the inner cannula. This ensures that the TT itself is not removed accidentally if difficulties removing the ventilator from the TT or removing the inner cannula from the TT occur.*

b. Place tracheostomy collar, T tube, or ventilator oxygen source over outer cannula. (**NOTE:** May not be able to attach T tube and ventilator oxygen devices to all outer cannulas when inner cannula is removed.)	Maintains continuous supply of oxygen to patient as needed.

Clinical Judgment *If patient is unable to tolerate being disconnected from the ventilator, replace the inner cannula with a clean new one and reattach the ventilator to the tracheostomy. Then proceed with cleaning the original inner cannula as described in the next steps and store it in a sterile container until the next inner cannula change (Urden et al., 2024; Przybyl, 2024).*

c. To prevent oxygen desaturation in affected patients, quickly pick up inner cannula and use small brush to remove secretions inside and outside inner cannula (see illustration).	Tracheostomy brush provides mechanical force to remove thick or dried secretions.
d. Hold inner cannula over basin and rinse with sterile normal saline, using nondominant (clean) hand to pour normal saline.	Removes secretions and normal saline from inner cannula.
e. Remove oxygen source, replace inner cannula (see illustration), and secure "locking" mechanism. Reapply ventilator, tracheostomy collar, or T tube. Hyperoxygenate patient if needed.	Secures inner cannula and reestablishes oxygen supply.
7. Tracheostomy with disposable inner cannula:	
a. Remove new cannula from manufacturer packaging.	Prepares you for change of inner cannula. Should be changed twice a day (Masood et al., 2018).

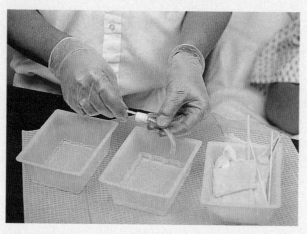

STEP 6c Cleaning tracheostomy inner cannula.

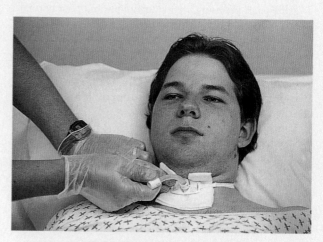

STEP 6e Reinserting inner cannula.

STEP	RATIONALE

b. While touching only outer aspect of tube, withdraw inner cannula and replace with new cannula. Lock into position.

Maintains a clean, sterile inner cannula for patient.

Clinical Judgment *If patient is on mechanical ventilation, instruct assistant to hold and stabilize TT and remove the ventilator tube from the connection while you remove the inner cannula. This ensures that the TT itself is not removed accidentally if difficulties removing the ventilator from the TT or removing the inner cannula from the TT occur.*

c. Dispose of contaminated cannula in appropriate receptacle and reconnect TT to ventilator or oxygen supply.

Prevents transmission of infection. Restores oxygen delivery.

8. Using normal saline-saturated cotton-tipped swabs and 4 × 4–inch gauze, clean exposed outer cannula surfaces and tracheal stoma under faceplate extending 5 to 10 cm (2−4 inches) in all directions from stoma (see illustration). Clean in circular motion from stoma site outward with dominant hand to handle sterile supplies. Do not go over previously cleaned area.

Aseptically removes secretions from stoma site. Moving in outward circle pulls mucus and other contaminants from stoma to periphery (Bolsega & Sole, 2018).

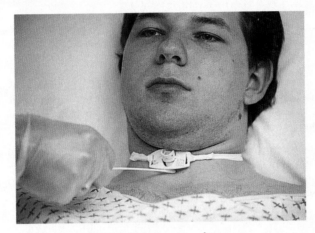

STEP 8 Cleaning around stoma.

9. Using dry 4 × 4–inch gauze, pat lightly at skin and exposed outer cannula surfaces. Inspect condition of skin under tracheostomy flange.

Dry surfaces prohibit formation of moist environment for microorganism growth and skin excoriation. Area under flange is common site for MDRPI (Urden et al., 2024).

10. Secure tracheostomy.

Clinical Judgment *Some agencies do not recommend changing the securement device for the first 72 hours after insertion of the TT because of risk of stoma closure if the tube were to become dislodged accidentally (Przybyl, 2024).*

a. Tracheostomy tube holder method:
  (1) Instruct assistant to continue holding TT in place. When an assistant is not available, leave old TT holder in place until new device is secure.

Ensures that tracheostomy stays in correct position.

  (2) Align strap under patient's neck. Be sure that Velcro attachments are on either side of TT.

Ensures proper fit and promotes patient comfort.

  (3) Place narrow end ties under and through faceplate eyelets. Pull ends even and secure with Velcro closures.

Ensures proper securement of TT.

  (4) Verify that there is space for only one loose or two snug finger widths to be inserted under neck strap.

Ensures proper securement of TT without securement device being too tight.

  (5) Insert new hydrocolloid, foam, or a 4 × 4–inch gauze precut tracheostomy dressing under clean neck plate (see illustration). *Option:* if using gauze dressing, apply barrier cream around stoma, if ordered.

Dressings absorb drainage and protect underlying skin. Dressing prevents pressure on clavicle heads (Bolsega & Sole, 2018). Gauze dressings may retain secretions and keep the area moist, leading to increased risk of skin breakdown. Barrier cream helps prevent skin breakdown around the stoma (Carroll et al., 2020). Hydrocolloid and foam dressing reduce risk of MDRPI (Mussa et al., 2021).

STEP	RATIONALE

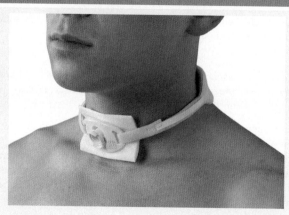

STEP 10a(5) Tracheostomy tube holder in place with foam dressing. (*Used with permission from TIDI Products, Inc.*)

b. Tracheostomy tie/twill tape method:

(1) Instruct assistant to continue to hold TT as you cut old tracheostomy ties. Ensure to not cut pilot balloon of cuff.

Secures TT to prevent incidental dislodgement. If pilot balloon is cut, there is no ability to inflate cuff (Urden et al., 2024).

Clinical Judgment *Assistant must not release hold on TT until new ties are firmly tied. If working without an assistant, do not cut old ties until new ties are in place and securely tied (Harding et al., 2023). When working with an assistant and the ties are removed, this is a good time to clean the back of the patient's neck and assess patient's skin under TT flange and under the ties or tube holder, making sure that skin is intact, free of pressure, and dry before applying securement device.*

(2) Take prepared twill tape, insert one end of tie through faceplate eyelet, and pull ends even (see illustration).

(3) Slide both ends of tie behind head and around neck to the other eyelet and insert one tie through second eyelet.

(4) Pull snugly.

(5) Tie ends securely in double square knot, allowing space for insertion of only one loose or two snug finger widths between tie and neck (see illustration).

(6) Insert new hydrocolloid, foam, or a 4 × 4–inch gauze precut tracheostomy dressing under clean neck plate. *Option:* If using gauze dressing, apply barrier cream around stoma, if ordered (see illustration).

Diagonal cuts ensure ease of threading end of tie through holes of eyelet (Przybyl, 2024).

Secures TT.

One finger width of slack prevents ties from being too tight when tracheostomy dressing is in place and also prevents movement of tracheostomy tube into lower airway (Przybyl, 2024).

Dressings absorb drainage and protect underlying skin. Dressing prevents pressure on clavicle heads (Bolsega & Sole, 2018). Gauze dressings may retain secretions and keep the area moist, leading to increased risk of skin breakdown. Barrier cream helps prevent skin breakdown around the stoma (Carroll et al., 2020). Hydrocolloid and foam dressing reduce risk of MDRPI (Mussa et al., 2021).

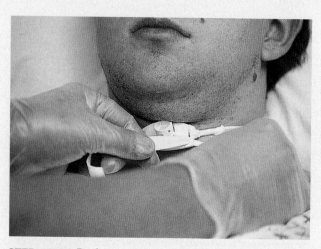

STEP 10b(2) Replacing tracheostomy ties. Do not remove old tracheostomy ties until new ones are secure.

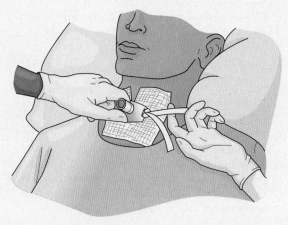

STEP 10b(5) Tracheostomy ties properly placed. (*From Sorrentino SA: Mosby's textbook for nursing assistants, ed 8, St Louis, 2013, Mosby.*)

STEP	RATIONALE

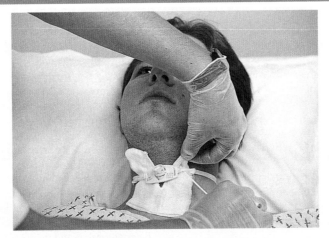

STEP 10b(6) Applying tracheostomy dressing.

> **Clinical Judgment** *Never cut a gauze pad to fit around TT. The cut fibers from the gauze pad may shed fibers that could be inhaled by patient and lead to pulmonary damage or infection. Use a manufactured pad for this purpose (Przybyl, 2024). Foam dressings have a keyhole opening to fit easily around stoma and are ideal in patients with excess secretions (Bolsega & Sole, 2018).*

STEP	RATIONALE
11. Ensure that the tracheostomy tube is midline and secure and no excess traction is applied. Assistant may release TT at this time.	Prevents the development of complications such as tracheal erosion or skin ulcerations (Urden et al., 2024).
12. Perform oral care with toothbrush or oral swabs and chlorhexidine rinse. Suction orally if needed. Perform subglottic suctioning if TT equipped with that capability.	Use of chlorhexidine may decrease patient risk of developing a ventilator-associated event (VAE)/ventilator-associated pneumonia (VAP) and promotes patient comfort (Urden et al., 2024; Pozuelo-Carrascosa et al., 2020).
13. Measure cuff pressure with the manometer; add or remove air/saline/water from cuff to maintain pressure between 20 and 25 mm Hg.	Complete at least once per shift or as often as every 2 to 4 hours (follow agency policy). Prevents aspiration of oral secretions and tracheal damage (Urden et al., 2024; Billington & Luckett, 2019).

> **Clinical Judgment** *If cuff is deflated during use of a speaking valve, then inflate cuff once the use of the valve is finished and measure cuff pressures. Perform oral and/or subglottic suctioning before a cuff is deflated (Pozuelo-Carrascosa et al., 2020).*

STEP	RATIONALE
14. Help patient to a comfortable position with head of bed remaining elevated at least 30 degrees (unless contraindicated) and assess respiratory status.	Restores comfort and sense of well-being. Some patients require post tracheostomy care suctioning. Keeping the head of the bed at 30 degrees minimizes risk of aspiration and reduces risk of VAP (Urden et al., 2024; Przybyl, 2024).
15. Be sure that oxygen- or humidification-delivery sources are in place and set at correct levels.	Humidification provides moisture for airway, makes it easier to suction secretions, and decreases risk of mucus plugs (Nakanishi et al., 2019).
16. Raise side rails (as appropriate) and lower bed to lowest position, locking into position.	Ensures patient safety and prevents falls.
17. Remove and properly dispose of gloves and other PPE, if used. Perform hand hygiene.	Reduces transmission of microorganisms.
18. Place nurse call system in an accessible location within the patient's reach.	Ensures patient can call for assistance if needed.
19. Replace cap on reusable normal saline bottles. Store reusable liquids, date container, and store unused supplies in appropriate place.	Once opened, normal saline is considered free of bacteria for 24 hours.

STEP	RATIONALE

EVALUATION

1. Compare respiratory assessments before and after tracheostomy care.
2. Assess fit of new tracheostomy securement device and ask patient if tube feels comfortable. Palpate tube for pulsation for air under the skin.

3. Inspect inner and outer cannulas for secretions.

4. Assess stoma, surrounding skin, and skin under ties for MDRPI: inflammation, edema, bleeding or discolored secretions.

5. Observe for excessive phonation, presence of gastric secretions in airway secretions, or tracheoesophageal fistula.
6. **Use Teach-Back:** "I want to be sure I explained how to clean your tracheostomy tube and place new ties. Let's take time now and show me how to clean the tubing and place new ties." Revise your instruction now or develop a plan for revised patient/family caregiver teaching if patient/family caregiver is not able to teach back correctly.

Determines effectiveness of tracheostomy care and patient's tolerance of procedure.

Tracheostomy ties are uncomfortable and place patient at risk for tissue injury when they are too loose or too tight. A pulsating feeling in TT can indicate early signs of innominate artery erosion. Air under skin suggests presence of subcutaneous emphysema.

Presence of secretions on cannulas indicates need for more frequent tracheostomy care.

Broken skin places patient at risk for infection. Stoma infection requires change in tracheostomy skin care plan.

Traction placed on the TT can lead to the rare complication of trachea-innominate artery fistula, which can lead to exsanguination and death (Przybyl, 2024).

Occurs with inadequate or excessive cuff inflation.

Teach-back is a technique for health care providers to ensure that they have explained medical information clearly so that patients and their families understand what is communicated to them (AHRQ, 2023).

Unexpected Outcomes	Related Interventions
1. Cuff leak develops.	• Verify position of tube. • Notify RT, and follow agency policy.
2. Inflammation of tracheostomy stoma or pressure area around TT.	• Increase frequency of tracheostomy care. • Apply topical antibacterial solution; apply bacterial barrier if ordered. • Apply hydrocolloid, foam, or transparent dressing around stoma to protect skin from breakdown. • Consult with skin care specialist.
3. Accidental decannulation/dislodgement.	• Call for help. • Notify health care provider and RT immediately. • Prepare for replacement of old TT with new tube. Some experienced nurses or RTs may be able to reinsert TT quickly. • Same-size ET can be inserted in stoma in an emergency. • Insert suction catheter to confirm that new tube is in trachea. • Be prepared to manually ventilate patients in whom respiratory distress develops with self-inflating resuscitation bag until tracheostomy is replaced.
4. Respiratory distress from mucus plugs in cannula.	• Remove inner cannula, if applicable, for cleaning or suction cannula. • Notify health care provider if TT requires replacement.

Documentation

- Document respiratory, stoma, and skin assessments before and after care; type and size of tracheostomy tube and inner cannula; frequency and extent of care, including inner cannula, dressing, and securement device changes; type, color, and amount of secretions; patient tolerance and understanding of procedure; and any interventions performed in event of unexpected outcomes.
- Document your evaluation of patient/family learning.

Hand-Off Reporting

- During hand-off, report patient status, frequency of care, tolerance and response to care, TT size and type of securement device, and last time care was performed.

- Report accidental decannulation, respiratory distress, or other unexpected outcomes to nurse in charge and health care provider.

Special Considerations

Patient Education

- Instruct caregivers not to lift up rigid faceplates/neck plates or they will dislodge tube.
- Some commercial TT holders require removal of excess tie material to fit properly.
- If you anticipate long-term placement of tracheostomy, plan to teach patient and caregiver tracheostomy care.
- Patients with new tracheostomy frequently have bloody secretions for 2 or 3 days after tube change (Przybyl, 2024).

Pediatrics

- Children generally have shorter necks, making the stoma more difficult to clean.
- Pediatric TTs (smaller than size 4) do not contain an inner cannula (Hockenberry et al., 2024).

Older Adults

- Some older adults may have more fragile skin and are more prone to skin breakdown from secretions or pressure (Touhy & Jett, 2022).
- Some older adults with impaired nutrition do not heal well after a surgical procedure. More frequent monitoring of the TT site may be necessary.

Populations With Disabilities

- Patients with intellectual or developmental disabilities may not understand the procedure, leading to increased anxiety and less cooperation. Try to perform the procedure at a time when a trusted caregiver is available and able to help calm and soothe the patient.

Home Care

- Coordinate with patient, family caregivers, and home care agencies to ensure ability to secure appropriate supplies for use at home.
- Coordinate with home care services to ensure that home has appropriate electricity to support the equipment, particularly if patient is receiving mechanical ventilation or requires suctioning.
- Coordinate with home care services and providers to ensure that patient and family caregivers are physically and emotionally able to perform the TT care at home, away from the hospital setting.
- Coordinate with home care services to provide support to family caregiver to prevent caregiver burden (Karaca et al., 2019).

✦ CLINICAL JUDGMENT AND NEXT GENERATION NCLEX® EXAMINATION–STYLE QUESTIONS

The nurse is caring for a 65-year-old patient who had a severe stroke 2 days ago and cannot communicate verbally. The health care team is monitoring the patient for the ability to control secretions and maintain an airway. Upon entering the room, the nurse notes that the patient is gasping for air, is tachypneic and dyspneic, and has a copious amount of oral secretions. The pulse oximeter reading is 78%.

1. Which action will the nurse take first?
   1. Apply oxygen via nasal cannula.
   2. Perform oropharyngeal suctioning.
   3. Call respiratory therapy.
   4. Prepare for insertion of an endotracheal tube.

2. The nurse uses oropharyngeal suctioning to clear the airway. Pulse oximetry improves to 82% after the initiation of oxygen at 10 L/min via nonrebreather mask. Which of the following assessments will the nurse perform at this time? **Select all that apply.**
   1. Gurgling upon inspiration or expiration
   2. Demonstration of restlessness
   3. Presence of drooling
   4. Chest wall motion
   5. Lung auscultation

3. The patient is stabilized and resting comfortably. One hour later, the nurse performs another assessment.
   Highlight the findings that require further nursing follow-up.

Body System	Findings
Neurological	PERRLA. Moves extremities equally yet weakly.
Pulmonary	Lungs clear to auscultation. Remains tachypneic.
Cardiovascular	Heart sounds regular without murmur. Capillary refill 4 seconds. All extremities cool to the touch. Pulses +1 in lower extremities.
Gastrointestinal	Abdomen round and soft to gentle touch. Bowel sounds present in all 4 quadrants.

4. The patient continues to have difficulty breathing easily. Which intervention will the nurse perform?
   1. Notify health care provider.
   2. Obtain sputum specimen for culture of microorganisms.
   3. Lower head of the bed while placing patient on unaffected side.
   4. Discontinue suctioning to facilitate easier breathing.

5. The health care provider decides to insert an endotracheal tube (ETT) to improve the patient's airway maintenance and oxygenation. The respiratory therapist sets up a mechanical ventilator to connect to the patient's ETT tube. What interventions will the nurse include in the plan of care for the patient's mechanical ventilation?
   1. Instill saline when suctioning the endotracheal tube.
   2. Use adhesive tape remover when cleaning the ETT.
   3. Ensure endotracheal tube cuff pressure is between 10 and 15 mm Hg.
   4. Brush the patient's teeth with a soft toothbrush at least twice a day.

Visit the Evolve site for Answers to Clinical Judgment and Next Generation NCLEX® Examination-Style Questions.

REFERENCES

Agency for Healthcare Research and Quality (AHRQ): *Teach-back: intervention,* 2023. https://www.ahrq.gov/patient-safety/reports/engage/interventions/teachback.html.

Ahmed RA, Boyer TJ: Endotracheal tube. In *Stat Pearls (Internet),* 2022, *National Institutes of Health.* https://www.ncbi.nlm.nih.gov/books/NBK539747/. Accessed October 9, 2023.

Alja'afreh M, et al: The effects of oral care protocol on the incidence of ventilator-associated pneumonia in selected intensive care units in Jordan, *Dimens Crit Care Nurs* 38(1):5–12, 2019.

American Association of Critical-Care Nurses (AACN): *AACN practice alert: Prevention of aspiration in adults,* 2018a. http://www.aacn.org/wd/practice/content/practicealerts/aspiration-practice-alert.pcms?menu=practice. Accessed June 2023.

American Association of Critical Care Nurses (AACN): AACN practice alert: oral care for acutely and critically ill patients, *Crit Care Nurse* 37(3):e19–e21, 2018b. https://aacnjournals.org/ccnonline/article-abstract/38/6/80/20842/Oral-Care-for-Acutely-and-Critically-Ill-Patients?redirectedFrom=fulltext. Accessed June 2023.

American Association of Critical Care Nurses (AACN): *AACN practice alert: prevention of ventilator-associated pneumonia in adults,* 2017. https://aacnjournals.org/ccnonline/article/37/3/e22/3571/Prevention-of-Ventilator-Associated-Pneumonia-in. Accessed June 2023.

American Association of Respiratory Care (AARC): *AARC clinical practice guideline: nasotracheal suctioning—2004 revision & update*, 2004. https://www.aarc.org/wp-content/uploads/2014/08/09.04.1080.pdf. Accessed October 9, 2023.

American Association of Respiratory Care (AARC): AARC clinical practice guidelines: endotracheal suctioning of mechanically ventilated patients with artificial airways, *Respir Care* 55(6):758, 2010.

Billington J, Luckett A: Care of the critically ill patient with a tracheostomy, *Nurs Stand* 34(2):59–65, 2019.

Bolsega T, Sole M: Tracheostomy care practices in a simulated setting: an exploratory study, *Clin Nurse Spec* 32(4):182–188, 2018.

Carroll D, et al: Implementation of an interdisciplinary tracheostomy care protocol to decrease rates of tracheostomy-related pressure ulcers and injuries, *Am J Otolaryngol* 41(4), 2020.

Centers for Disease Control and Prevention (CDC): *Ventilator-associated event (VAE)*, 2022. https://www.cdc.gov/nhsn/pdfs/pscmanual/10-vae_final.pdf. Accessed October 9, 2023.

Centers for Disease Control and Prevention (CDC): *What is health literacy?* 2023. https://www.cdc.gov/healthliteracy/learn/index.html.

Ferrer M, Torres A: Epidemiology of ICU-acquired pneumonia, *Curr Opin Crit Care* 24(5):325–331, 2018.

Fumarola S, et al: Overlooked and underestimated: medical adhesive-related skin injuries. Best practice consensus document on prevention, *J Wound Care* 29(Suppl 3c):S1–S24, 2020.

Goodrich CA: Endotracheal intubation (assist). In Johnson KL, editor: *AACN procedural manual for progressive and critical care*, ed 8, St. Louis, 2024, Elsevier.

Harding MM, et al: Medical surgical nursing: assessment and management of clinical problems, ed 12, St. Louis, 2023, Elsevier.

Hare E, Seckel MA: Suctioning: endotracheal or tracheostomy tube. In Johnson KL, editor: *AACN procedure manual of progressive and critical care*, ed 8, St. Louis, 2024, Elsevier.

Hockenberry M, et al: *Wong's nursing care of infants and children*, ed 12, St. Louis, 2024, Elsevier.

Huang X, et al: Influence of subglottic secretion drainage on the microorganisms of ventilator associated pneumonia, *Medicine* 97(28):1–7, 2018 https://www.ncbi.nlm.nih.gov/pmc/articles/PMC6076059/. Accessed October 9, 2023.

Jackson D, et al: Medical device-related pressure ulcers: a systematic review and meta-analysis, *Int J Nurs Stud* 92:109–120, 2019.

Kallet RH: Ventilator bundles in transition: from prevention of ventilator-associated pneumonia to prevention of ventilator-associated events, *Respir Care* 64(8):994–1006, 2019.

Karaca T, et al: Caring for patients with a tracheostomy at home: a descriptive, cross-sectional study to evaluate health care practices and caregiver burden, *Wound Manag Prev* 65(3):22–29, 2019.

Lacherade J, et al: Subglottic secretion drainage for ventilator-associated pneumonia prevention: an underused efficient measure, *Ann Transl Med* 6(21):422, 2018.

Landsperger J, et al: The effect of adhesive tape versus endotracheal tube fastener in critically ill adults: the endotracheal tube securement (ETTS) randomized controlled trial, *Crit Care* 23(161):1–7, 2019.

Larrow V, Klich-Heartt E: Prevention of ventilator-associated pneumonia in the intensive care unit: beyond the basics, *J Neurosci Nurs* 48(3):160 165, 2016.

Letchford E, Bench S: Ventilator-associated pneumonia and suction: a review of the literature, *Br J Nurs* 27(1):13–18, 2018.

Lethongkam S, et al: Prolonged inhibitory effects against planktonic growth, adherence, and biofilm formation of pathogens causing ventilator-associated pneumonia using a novel polyamide/silver nanoparticle composite-coated endotracheal tube, *Biofouling* 36(3):292-307, 2020.

Mahmoodpoor A, et al: Effect of a probiotic preparation on ventilator-associated pneumonia in critically ill patients admitted to the intensive care unit: a prospective double-blind randomized controlled trial, *Nutr Clin Pract* 34(1):156–162, 2019.

Marjanovic N, et al: Continuous pneumatic regulation of tracheal cuff pressure to decrease ventilator-associated pneumonia in trauma patients who were mechanically ventilated: the AGATE multicenter randomized controlled study, *Chest* 160(2):499–508, 2021.

Martin-Loeches I, et al: New guidelines for hospital-acquired pneumonia/ventilator-associated pneumonia: USA vs. Europe, *Curr Opin Crit Care* 24:347–352, 2018.

Masood M, et al: Association of standardized tracheostomy care protocol implementation and reinforcement with the prevention of life-threatening respiratory events, *JAMA Otolaryngeal Head Neck Surg* 144(6):527–532, 2018.

Mirtalaei N, et al: Efficacy of antibiotic prophylaxis against ventilator-associated pneumonia, *J Hosp Infect* 101:272–275, 2019.

Mussa CC, et al: AARC Clinical practice guideline: management of adult patients with tracheostomy in the acute care setting, *Respir Care* 66(1):156–169, 2021. https://rc.rcjournal.com/content/66/1/156. Accessed October 9, 2023.

Mwakanyanga ET, et al: Intensive care nurses' knowledge and practice on endotracheal suctioning of the intubated patient: a quantitative cross-sectional observational study, *PLoS One* 13(8):e0201743, 2018.

Nakanishi N, et al: Humidification performance of passive and active humidification devices within a spontaneously breathing tracheostomized cohort, *Respir Care* 64(2):130–135, 2019.

Pandian V, et al: Speech and safety in tracheostomy patient receiving mechanical ventilation: a systematic review, *Am J Crit Care* 28(6):441–450, 2019.

Pozuelo-Carrascosa DP, et al: Subglottic secretion drainage for preventing ventilator-associated pneumonia: an overview of systematic reviews and an updated meta-analysis, *Eur Respir Rev* 29(155):190107, 2020.

Przybyl HL: Tracheostomy cuff and tube care. In Johnson KL editor: *AACN procedural manual for progressive and critical care*, ed 8, St. Louis, 2024, Elsevier.

Sanaie S, et al: Comparison of tracheal tube cuff pressure with two techniques: fixed volume and minimal leak test techniques, *J Cardiovasc Thorac Res* 11(1):48–52, 2019.

Santiago C, et al: The use of tablet and communication app for patients with endotracheal or tracheostomy tubes in the medical surgical intensive care unit: a pilot, feasibility study, *Can J Crit Care Nurs* 30(1):17–23, 2019.

The Joint Commission (TJC): *2023 National Patient Safety Goals*, Oakbrook Terrace, IL, 2023, The Joint Commission. https://www.jointcommission.org/standards/national-patient-safety-goals/.

Tokmaji G, et al: Silver-coated endotracheal tubes for prevention of ventilator-associated pneumonia in critically ill patients (review), *Cochrane Database Syst Rev* 2015(8):1–39, 2018.

Touhy T, Jett K: *Ebersole and Hess' Gerontological Nursing & healthy aging*, ed 6, St. Louis, 2022, Elsevier.

Tracheostomy Education: *Subglottic Suctioning: Benefits, Covid-19 and Manual versus Automatic*, 2020. https://www.tracheostomyeducation.com/subglottic-suctioning-covid-19/. Accessed October 13, 2023.

Triamvisit S, et al: Effect of modified care bundle for prevention of ventilator-associated pneumonia in critically-ill neurosurgical patients, *Acute Crit Care* 36(4):294–299, 2021.

Turner M, et al: Improving endotracheal cuff inflation pressures: an evidence-based project in a military medical center, *AANA* 88(3):203–208, 2020.

Urden L, et al: *Priorities in critical care nursing*, ed 9, St. Louis, 2024, Elsevier.

Virk H, Wiersinga J: Current place of probiotics for VAP, *Crit Care* 23:46–48, 2019.

Wang R, et al: The impact of tracheotomy timing in critically ill patients undergoing mechanical ventilation: a meta-analysis of randomized controlled clinical trials with trial sequential analysis, *Heart Lung* 48(1):46–54, 2018.

Wen Z, et al: Is continuous better than intermittent control of tracheal cuff pressure? A meta-analysis, *Br Assoc Crit Care Nurses* 24(2):76–82, 2018.

25 | Cardiac Care

SKILLS AND PROCEDURES

Skill 25.1 **Obtaining a 12-Lead Electrocardiogram, p. 791**

Skill 25.2 **Applying a Cardiac Monitor, p. 794**

OBJECTIVES

Mastery of content in this chapter will enable you to:
- Identify the indications to obtain a 12-lead electrocardiogram (ECG) and cardiac monitor application.
- Determine correct electrode placement to obtain an accurate ECG tracing.
- Perform measures to reduce false cardiac monitor alarms.

MEDIA RESOURCES

- http://evolve.elsevier.com/Perry/skills
- Clinical Review Questions
- Audio Glossary
- Animations
- **NSO** Nursing Skills Online

- Answers to Clinical Judgment and Next-Generation NCLEX® Examination–Style Questions
- Skills Performance Checklists
- Printable Key Points

PURPOSE

The electrocardiogram (ECG) is the graphic representation of the electrical activities, or conduction system, of the heart used for diagnostic and treatment purposes. Accuracy of these waveforms depends on the correct placement and clean application of electrodes to the skin. Monitoring of the ECG can be done once or on a continuous basis.

PRACTICE STANDARDS

- Sandau K et al., 2017: Update to Practice Standards for Electrocardiographic Monitoring In Hospital Settings: A Scientific Statement From the American Heart Association—Cardiac monitoring
- The Joint Commission (TJC), 2023: National Patient Safety Goals—Patient identification

SUPPLEMENTAL STANDARDS

- Arnett D et al., 2019: ACC/ AHA Guideline on the Primary Prevention of Cardiovascular Disease

PRINCIPLES FOR PRACTICE

- A 12-lead ECG provides a snapshot of the electrical activity of the heart from multiple views. It is a diagnostic tool to determine cardiac rhythm, conduction system irregularities, and myocardial ischemia. In addition, an ECG can be used to monitor the heart's response to drug treatment and metabolic abnormalities. Accuracy and timeliness are the key principles of ECG acquisition (Rahimpour et al., 2021).
- Cardiac monitoring provides continuous ECG observation of the acutely ill patient. Proper placement of the ECG electrodes is essential to ensure real-time detection of arrhythmias (Jones, 2021) (Table 25.1).

PERSON-CENTERED CARE

- Placement of the electrodes requires exposure of a patient's chest. Measures to maintain the patient's modesty and privacy are essential.
- Placement of electrodes when there is breast tissue requires that the leads be placed as close to the chest wall as possible, avoiding the breast tissue (Jones, 2021).
- Patients and family caregivers, especially those with a need for modesty, may need detailed information about the procedure so that they do not misunderstand the intent and objective of cardiac monitoring.
- Always explain which type of physical interaction is involved to avoid misinterpretation of interventions.

EVIDENCE-BASED PRACTICE

Alarm Fatigue

Nurses can perceive alarms as burdensome and occurring too often and as interfering with patient care, resulting in distrust of alarms (Lewandowska et al., 2020). However, given the importance of these alarms, there has been an increase in quality improvement and research studies aimed at reducing alarm fatigue and improving alarm system safety. Efforts to reduce alarm fatigue led to a reduction in nuisance alarms; the reduction did not affect nurses' attitudes toward the alarm or reduce alarm fatigue. Nurses' ability to monitor navigation of the cardiac monitor is a complex cognitive

TABLE 25.1

Basic Cardiac Rhythms

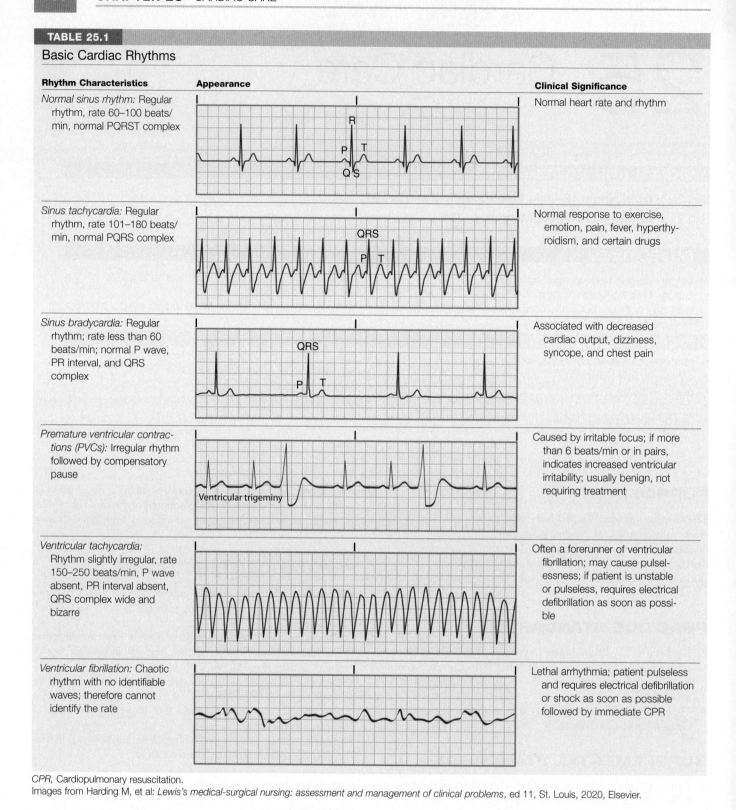

Rhythm Characteristics	Appearance	Clinical Significance
Normal sinus rhythm: Regular rhythm, rate 60–100 beats/min, normal PQRST complex		Normal heart rate and rhythm
Sinus tachycardia: Regular rhythm, rate 101–180 beats/min, normal PQRS complex		Normal response to exercise, emotion, pain, fever, hyperthyroidism, and certain drugs
Sinus bradycardia: Regular rhythm; rate less than 60 beats/min; normal P wave, PR interval, and QRS complex		Associated with decreased cardiac output, dizziness, syncope, and chest pain
Premature ventricular contractions (PVCs): Irregular rhythm followed by compensatory pause		Caused by irritable focus; if more than 6 beats/min or in pairs, indicates increased ventricular irritability; usually benign, not requiring treatment
Ventricular tachycardia: Rhythm slightly irregular, rate 150–250 beats/min, P wave absent, PR interval absent, QRS complex wide and bizarre		Often a forerunner of ventricular fibrillation; may cause pulselessness; if patient is unstable or pulseless, requires electrical defibrillation as soon as possible
Ventricular fibrillation: Chaotic rhythm with no identifiable waves; therefore cannot identify the rate		Lethal arrhythmia; patient pulseless and requires electrical defibrillation or shock as soon as possible followed by immediate CPR

CPR, Cardiopulmonary resuscitation.
Images from Harding M, et al: *Lewis's medical-surgical nursing: assessment and management of clinical problems,* ed 11, St. Louis, 2020, Elsevier.

process that requires specific policies and procedures, a monitor design that is usable, sufficient training on monitor capability, and the use of clinical judgment for appropriate monitoring parameters (Sowan et al., 2021). Current efforts should focus on maintaining safe patient care and reducing alarm fatigue. These include:

- Establishing guidelines for pulse oximetry and physiological monitors
- Customizing patient monitoring bundles and thresholds

- Individualizing the monitoring process
- Eliminating overmonitoring and undermonitoring
- Providing nursing education including monitor technology navigation (Gorisek et al., 2021)
- Adding bedside visual reminders
- Improving monitor screen visibility by increasing brightness
- Implementing an agency-specific alarm fatigue bundle based on identified alarm fatigue unit issues (Seifert et al., 2021)

SAFETY GUIDELINES

- Know the indications for the ordered 12-lead ECG. Patients with chest pain need to have their 12-lead ECG within 10 minutes of the assessment and onset of pain (Appold et al., 2021). A 12-lead ECG will determine the next step in the treatment plan.
- Know if the patient took any nitroglycerin prior to admission, as this may alter the ECG.
- Know a patient's current medications. Some medications—particularly beta blockers, some calcium channel blockers, and other antiarrhythmics—can cause dysrhythmias.
- The continued ECG monitoring of a patient creates the risk of a medical adhesive–related skin injury (MARSI) because the skin surface stays in contact with the adhesive around electrodes (Fumarola et al., 2020). Inspect the skin regularly for signs of redness, edema, blisters, or tearing.

◆ SKILL 25.1 Obtaining a 12-Lead Electrocardiogram

Electrical impulses of the heart are conducted to the surface of the body and are detected by electrodes placed on the skin of the limbs and torso. The electrodes carry these impulses to either a continuous monitor or a 12-lead electrocardiograph machine. The appearance of the electrocardiogram (ECG) pattern or wave form helps to diagnose whether there are any abnormalities in the electrical conduction through the heart. Each 12-lead ECG is a 10-second strip (see Table 25.1). The ECG strip is divided by large boxes and small boxes to help measure times and distances for electrical conduction. Each large box represents 0.20 seconds, and there are five small boxes in each large box; thus each small box is equivalent to 0.04 seconds. The 12-lead ECG provides a snapshot of the waveforms from 12 different angles or views of the heart. One electrode is placed on each of the four extremities, and six electrodes are placed at specific sites on the chest for a total of 10 electrodes on the patient's skin. They are bipolar limb leads I, II, and III; augmented limb leads aV_R, aV_L, aV_F; and precordial chest leads V_1 to V_6. The leads view a specific part of the surface of the heart and can help determine which part of the heart has sustained or is sustaining damage and the origin and flow of the impulse. A qualified health care professional evaluates the amplitudes of waves or complexes to determine abnormalities. Nurses must learn to recognize common ECG abnormalities to appropriately monitor patients at risk for cardiac problems.

Delegation

The skill of obtaining a 12-lead ECG can be delegated to assistive personnel (AP) who are specifically trained in obtaining the measurement. Direct the AP to:

- Immediately report to the nurse changes in the patient's cardiac status such as complaints of chest pain or heart rate
- Immediately deliver the completed 12-lead ECG recording to a health care provider for interpretation
- Use specific patient precautions related to disease, mobility status, or position restrictions

Interprofessional Collaboration

- The rapid response team or cardiac catheterization lab personnel are involved in possible emergency needs.

Equipment

- 12-lead electrocardiograph
- 10 ECG leads with alligator clip, suction cup, or snap-on attachments
- 10 ECG electrodes (disposable, self-adhesive)
- Clean, dry towel or sponge wipes
- Hair clippers (optional depending on hair at electrode sites)

STEP	RATIONALE

ASSESSMENT

1. Identify patient using at least two identifiers (e.g., name and birthday or name and medical record number) according to agency policy.

   Ensures correct patient. Complies with The Joint Commission standards and improves patient safety (TJC, 2023).

2. Review electronic health record (EHR) to determine indications for obtaining ECG. Assess patient's history and cardiopulmonary status (e.g., heart rate and rhythm, blood pressure, respirations).

   If 12-lead ECG is ordered for chest pain or other ischemic signs and symptoms, obtain ECG within 10 minutes of patient's pain report.

3. Review EHR to determine patient's age and history of dehydration, malnutrition, exposure to radiation therapy, underlying chronic conditions (e.g., diabetes mellitus, immunosuppression), and edema of the skin.

   Common risk factors for medical adhesive–related skin injury (MARSI) (Fumarola et al., 2020).

4. Assess patient's/family caregiver's health literacy.

   Determines degree to which individuals have the ability to find, understand, and use information and services to make informed health-related decisions and actions for themselves and others (Centers for Disease Control and Prevention [CDC], 2023).

5. Assess for chest pain; rate acuity on a pain scale of 0 to 10.

   Determines level of chest discomfort, which may be warning for cardiac ischemia.

Clinical Judgment *If chest pain is noted, notify health care provider immediately. Obtain ECG (per agency policy).*

6. Ask patient if there is a history of irritant contact dermatitis from use of adhesives.

   Dermatitis results from sensitivity to chemicals in adhesive. Actual adhesive allergy is less common.

STEP	RATIONALE
7. Assess patient's ability to follow directions and remain still in supine position.	Provides clear, accurate recording without artifact.
8. Assess patient's knowledge, prior experience with ECG, and feelings about procedure.	Reveals need for patient instruction and/or support.

PLANNING

1. Expected outcomes following completion of procedure: • Patient tolerates procedure without anxiety or discomfort. • Clear, accurate recording of ECG waveform is obtained.	Appropriate preparation and education decrease anxiety. ECG leads placed correctly, with patient remaining still.
2. Provide privacy and explain procedure to patient. Discuss the ECG and what the patient might experience.	Protects patient's privacy; reduces anxiety. Promotes cooperation.
3. Close room door and bedside curtain.	Provides patient privacy.
4. Obtain and organize equipment for ECG at bedside.	Ensures more efficiency when completing an assessment.

IMPLEMENTATION

1. Perform hand hygiene, apply clean gloves, and prepare patient for procedure:	Reduces transmission of microorganisms.
a. Remove or reposition patient's clothing to expose only patient's chest and arms. Keep abdomen and thighs covered.	Facilitates correct placement of cardiac leads and maintains patient's modesty. Improper lead placement produces artifact, which necessitates repeating test or causes interpretation errors.
b. Place patient in supine position with head of bed no higher than 30 degrees.	Electrodes must be placed on anterior chest for standard 12-lead ECG.
c. Instruct patient to lie still without talking and to not cross legs.	Body movement or talking produces artifact, which may necessitate repeating test.
2. Turn on machine; enter required demographic information.	Turning machine on first helps you identify electrode and lead issues on application.
3. Clean and prepare skin for isolated electrode placement with soap and water. Wipe area with rough washcloth or gauze or use edge of electrode to gently scrape skin. Clip excessive hair from electrode area. Where possible, avoid the use of products that dry the skin, such as alcohol-based skin preps (Fumarola et al., 2020).	Proper skin preparation before ECG electrodes are placed decreases skin impedance and signal noise, thereby producing clean, accurate recording. Do not use alcohol to clean area. It will dry out skin. Clipping hair in electrode area is preferred. Shaving leaves nicks that predispose to infection (Tanner & Melen, 2021).
4. Apply electrodes in correct positions. a. Chest (precordial) leads (Fig. 25.1) V_1—Fourth intercostal space (ICS) at right sternal border V_2—Fourth ICS at left sternal border V_3—Midway between V_2 and V_4 V_4—Fifth ICS at midclavicular line V_5—Left anterior axillary line at level of V_4 horizontally V_6—Left midaxillary line at level of V_4 horizontally b. Extremities: One lead on each extremity (Fig. 25.2); right wrist, left wrist, left ankle, right ankle	Proper placement of leads is very important for accurate interpretation of 12-lead ECG. Ensure that correct lead is in correct location. If any leads are misplaced, ECG reading will be inaccurate (Ajmal & Marcus, 2021).
5. Check 12-lead machine for messages to correct electrode or lead issues. If no messages occur, press button to obtain 12-lead ECG.	Establishes device readiness.
6. If you obtain ECG tracing without artifact, disconnect leads and gently remove from patient's skin.	Promotes comfort and hygiene.
7. If STAT, immediately deliver ECG tracing (if not computerized) to appropriate health care provider for interpretation.	If non-STAT 12-lead ECG, place in patient's chart or designated area.
8. Help patient to a comfortable position.	Restores comfort and sense of well-being.
9. Raise side rails (as appropriate) and lower bed to lowest position, locking into position.	Ensures patient safety and prevents falls.
10. Place nurse call system in an accessible location within patient's reach.	Ensures patient can call for assistance if needed.
11. Dispose of all contaminated supplies in appropriate receptacle, remove and dispose of gloves, and perform hand hygiene.	Reduces transmission of microorganisms.

STEP	RATIONALE

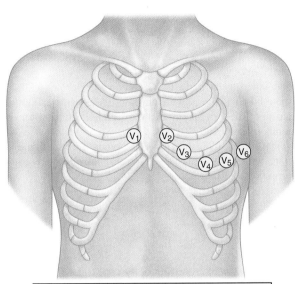

V₁ – 4th intercostal space (ICS) at right sternal border
V₂ – 4th ICS at left sternal border
V₃ – Midway between V₂ and V₄
V₄ – Fifth ICS at midclavicular line
V₅ – Left anterior axillary line at level of V₄ horizontally
V₆ – Left midaxillary line at level of V₄ horizontally

FIG. 25.1 Precordial (chest) lead placement for a standard 12-lead electrocardiogram (ECG).

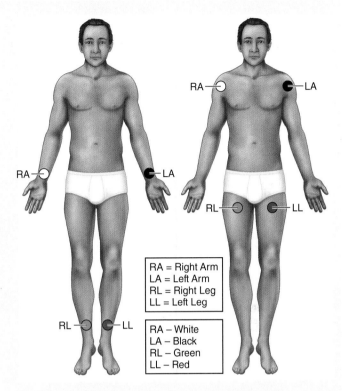

RA = Right Arm
LA = Left Arm
RL = Right Leg
LL = Left Leg

RA – White
LA – Black
RL – Green
LL – Red

FIG. 25.2 Limb lead placement for a standard 12-lead electrocardiogram (ECG).

EVALUATION

1. Note and document if patient is experiencing any chest discomfort during procedure.
2. Discuss findings and results of 12-lead ECG with health care provider to determine next steps in patient's treatment plan.

3. Inspect condition of skin after electrode removal for signs of MARSI (e.g., redness, blistering).
4. **Use Teach-Back:** "I want to be sure I explained why you need this ECG. Why are you receiving an ECG?" Revise your instruction now or develop a plan for revised patient/family caregiver teaching if patient/family caregiver is not able to teach back correctly.

Helps correlate ECG changes to symptoms of chest pain.

If myocardial infarction is identified, immediate steps will need to be taken to get patient to cardiac catheterization laboratory or consider use of thrombolytic medications.
MARSI can occur following placement or removal of an adhesive electrode (Fumarola et al., 2020).
Teach-back is a technique for health care providers to ensure that they have explained medical information clearly so that patients and their families understand what is communicated to them (Agency for Healthcare Research and Quality [AHRQ], 2023).

Unexpected Outcomes

1. ECG cannot be interpreted:
   - Absence of tracing on one or more leads
   - Presence of artifact in ECG tracings

Related Interventions

- Inspect electrodes for secure placement.
- Reposition any wires that move as a result of patient breathing or movement or vibrations in environment. Do not reposition electrodes if in correct position.
- Remind patient who is moving that lying still is necessary to obtain good tracing.
- If artifact looks like 60-cycle interference (very thick-lined waveform), unplug battery-operated equipment in room one item at a time to see if interference disappears. **NOTE:** 60-cycle interference is rare.
- Repeat tracing.

2. Patient has chest pain or anxiety.

- Continue to monitor patient.
- Reassess factors contributing to anxiety or distress.
- Follow specific orders related to findings.
- Notify health care provider.

Documentation

- Document date and time ECG was obtained, reason for obtaining ECG, and to whom ECG was given for interpretation.
- Document your evaluation of patient learning.

Hand-Off Reporting

- Report any chest pain or unexpected outcomes immediately.

Special Considerations

Patient Education

- Be aware that medications such as digitalis and amiodarone can affect ECG results.
- Ensure that electrodes are placed directly on the chest wall and not the breast tissue. The breast may need to be lifted to accommodate chest leads V_4, V_5, and V_6.

Pediatrics

- Most children with chest pain will be stable, but an ECG may be warranted if there are additional symptoms of cardiac disease.

- Keeping a child still while obtaining an ECG is challenging;, if appropriate, having the child held in parent's arms is helpful.

Older Adults

- First-degree heart block can be a normal finding in an older adult with no history of cardiac disease due to the fibrotic changes of aging (Ker & Outhoff, 2022).

Home Care

- There are now e-textile ECG systems used for rehabilitation of home-based patients with chronic diseases. The home-based nature of these programs means minimal disruption for the patient (Teferra et al., 2019).
- New wearable ECG systems are being used in the home for patients with arrhythmias; these systems allow for early intervention (Bouzid et al., 2022).

✦ SKILL 25.2   Applying a Cardiac Monitor

The use of continuous cardiac monitors is a common practice in health care agencies, clinics, and outpatient settings. The cardiac monitor can be a bedside, hard-wired monitor or a wireless transmitter used with telemetry systems. A continuous electrocardiogram (ECG) rhythm is obtained using three or five electrodes and leads on the patient. Cardiac monitors are attached to patients for immediate dysrhythmia detection, as some dysrhythmias can be life threatening. These devices can also monitor a decrease or increase in heart rate. Most cardiac monitor systems have dysrhythmia detection software and provide alarms when dysrhythmias appear or the identified heart rate limits are exceeded.

It is important to monitor only patients with clinical indications for cardiac monitoring. This can significantly decrease the number of false alarms (McGuffin & Ortiz, 2019). The American Heart Association (AHA) developed guidelines for ECG monitoring in hospitalized patients (Sandau et al., 2017) (Box 25.1).

Alarm fatigue develops when a person is exposed to an excessive number of alarms (McGuffin & Ortiz, 2019). This situation can result in sensory overload, which may cause the person to become desensitized to the alarms. Consequently, the response to alarms may be delayed or alarms may be missed altogether (McGuffin & Ortiz, 2019). Some patient deaths have been attributed to alarm fatigue; because of this, The Joint Commission (TJC, 2023) has made the reduction of alarm fatigue a National Patient Safety Goal. The American Association of Critical-Care Nurses (AACN) has provided a practice alert listing some strategies for alarm management to reduce alarm fatigue and improve patient safety (Box 25.2).

BOX 25.1

Indications for Continuous Cardiac Monitoring

- Postresuscitation patients
- Early phase of acute coronary syndromes (<24 hours)
- Emergency percutaneous coronary intervention (PCI) or nonurgent PCI with complications
- Adults and children undergoing cardiac surgery
- New implantable defibrillator and/or pacemaker placement
- Temporary or transcutaneous pacemaker
- Atrioventricular block
- Suspected or known accessory pathway conduction
- Long QT syndrome
- Heart failure/pulmonary edema
- Indication for intensive care admission
- Procedures requiring conscious sedation or anesthesia
- Diagnosis of dysrhythmia in children

Adapted from Sandau K, et al.: Update to practice standards for electrocardiographic monitoring in hospital settings: a scientific statement from the American Heart Association, *Circulation* 136(19):e273, 2017.

BOX 25.2

Reduction of Alarm Fatigue

Strategies for Nurses

- Ensure proper skin preparation for and placement of ECG electrodes.
- Use the appropriate oxygen saturation probes and site placement; change pulse oximeter probes as needed.
- Check alarm settings at the start of every shift, with any change in patient condition, and with any change in caregiver.
- Customize alarm parameter and default settings for individual patients according to unit or agency policy (Gorisek et al., 2021).

Strategies for Nursing Leaders

- Establish an interprofessional team to collect data and address issues related to ECG alarms.
- Develop unit-specific default monitor settings including alarm management policies.
- Provide initial and ongoing education on monitoring systems and alarm management (Gorisek et al., 2021).
- Develop policies and procedures for ECG monitoring in only those patients with clinical indications for monitoring.

ECG, Electrocardiogram.
Adapted from American Association of Critical-Care Nurses (AACN): *Practice alert on alarm management,* 2019. https://www.patientsafetysolutions.com/docs/April_16_2019_AACN_Practice_Alert_on_Alarm_Management.htm; Lewandowska K, et al: (2020). Impact of alarm fatigue on the work of nurses in an intensive care environment: a systematic review. *Int J Environ Res Public Health* 17(22):8409, 2020; Lewis CL, Oster CA: Research outcomes of implementing CEASE: an innovative, nurse-driven, evidence-based, patient-customized monitoring bundle to decrease alarm fatigue in the intensive care unit/stepdown unit. *Dimens Crit Care Nurs* 38(3):160–173, 2019.

Delegation

The skill of applying a cardiac monitor can be delegated to assistive personnel (AP) who are specifically trained. In some health care agencies, the responsible party for monitoring ECG rhythms and alarms may also be a specifically trained AP, such as a telemetry technician. Direct the AP to:

- Immediately report to the nurse monitor alarms or patient complaints of pain, shortness of breath, or hypotension

Interprofessional Collaboration

- The interprofessional team makes the decisions to ensure that continuous monitoring is clinically indicated.

Equipment

- Bedside cardiac monitor or telemetry transmitter
- Three or five ECG electrodes (disposable, self-adhesive)
- Three or five ECG leads with snap-on attachments
- Clean, dry towel, washcloth, or gauze
- Hair clippers (optional depending on hair at electrode sites)

STEP	RATIONALE

ASSESSMENT

1. Identify patient using at least two identifiers (e.g., name and birthday or name and medical record number) according to agency policy.

Ensures correct patient. Complies with The Joint Commission standards and improves patient safety (TJC, 2023).

2. Review electronic health record (EHR) to determine clinical indication for continuous cardiac monitoring: patient's history, cardiopulmonary status, and history of chest pain.

Knowing reason for monitoring allows for focused, improved response to an alarm.

3. Review EHR to determine patient's age and history of dehydration, malnutrition, exposure to radiation therapy, underlying chronic conditions (e.g., diabetes mellitus, immunosuppression), edema of the skin, and allergic dermatitis, erythema, blistering, or excoriation of the skin under or around monitor leads.

Common risk factors for medical adhesive–related skin injury (MARSI) (Fumarola et al., 2020). Continuous monitoring leads have an adhesive backing, and patients are at risk for developing symptoms associated with MARSI (Thayer et al., 2022).

4. Perform hand hygiene. Check skin for fragility, presence of oil or excess moisture, and local signs of irritation or damage at the site where the adhesive will be applied. If oil or moisture is present, wipe chest or limbs with clean, dry towel.

Clean, dry area without lesions should be chosen for electrode placement to avoid development of MARSI (Thayer et al., 2022). Provides clear, accurate recording without artifact.

5. Assess patient's/family caregiver's health literacy.

Determines degree to which individuals have the ability to find, understand, and use information and services to make informed health-related decisions and actions for themselves and others (CDC, 2023).

6. Assess patient's knowledge, prior experience with ECG monitoring, and feelings about procedure.

Reveals need for patient instruction and/or support.

PLANNING

1. Expected outcomes following completion of procedure:
   - Patient tolerates procedure without anxiety or discomfort.
   - Clear, accurate ongoing recording of ECG rhythm is obtained.

Appropriate preparation decreases anxiety.
ECG leads placed correctly.

2. Provide privacy and explain procedure to patient. Discuss need for ECG. If applicable, teach patient how to report chest pain.

Protects patient's privacy; reduces anxiety. Promotes cooperation.

3. Close room door and bedside curtain.

Provides patient privacy.

4. Obtain and organize equipment for ECG monitoring at bedside.

Ensures more efficient procedure.

IMPLEMENTATION

1. Perform hand hygiene, apply clean gloves, and prepare patient for procedure:

Reduces transmission of microorganisms.

   a. Remove or reposition patient's gown to expose only patient's chest. Keep abdomen and thighs covered.

Facilitates correct placement of cardiac leads and maintains patient's modesty.

   b. Place patient in supine position.

Electrodes must be placed on anterior chest.

2. Clean and prepare chest area for electrode placement with soap and water. Wipe area with rough washcloth or gauze or use edge of electrode to gently scrape area. Where possible, avoid the use of products that dry the skin, such as alcohol-based skin preps (Thayer et al., 2022; Fumarola et al., 2020). Clip excessive hair from electrode area rather than shaving.

Proper skin preparation before ECG electrodes are placed decreases skin impedance and signal noise, thereby producing a clean, accurate recording. Do not use alcohol to clean area. It will dry skin and predispose patient to a MARSI. Roughening skin helps remove epidermis outer layer to allow electrical signals to travel (Sandau et al., 2017). Clipping reduces risk for infection.

STEP	RATIONALE

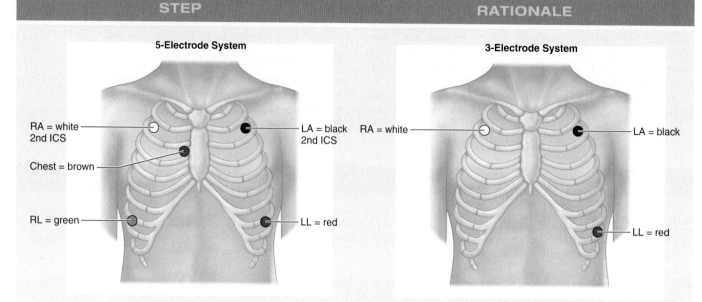

FIG. 25.3 Cardiac monitor lead placement: three- or five-electrode systems. *ICS*, Intercostal space; *LA*, left arm; *LL*, left leg; *RA*, right arm; *RL*, right leg.

3. Apply electrodes in correct positions for either a three- or a five-electrode system (Fig. 25.3).

Proper placement of leads is very important for accurate dysrhythmia interpretation.

   a. For females, the precordial leads (V_3–V_6) should be placed under the left breast.

Ensures that breast tissue does not interfere with ECG reading (Jones, 2021).

4. Attach monitor leads to electrodes. Colors of leads represent their polarity. White is negative. Black is positive. Red is ground or neutral. Two additional leads on five-lead system would include a green lead (positive or negative) and a brown lead (positive), which can be placed at a V lead location on precordial chest.

Coloring system allows for consistent application of leads.

5. Check bedside monitor or telemetry station for any messages indicating electrode or lead issues. Troubleshoot as needed.

Monitoring system itself may detect bad electrode contact with skin or loose connection.

6. Check that the ECG rhythm can be visualized on bedside monitor, central station, or remote viewing station.

If staff is watching monitor remotely, communicate with them before you leave the room so you can correct any issues while on the phone with viewers. This call can also serve as notification that monitoring has started.

7. Change ECG electrodes daily or more often if electrode contact to skin is loose. Inspect condition of skin for allergic dermatitis, erythema, blistering, or excoriation (Thayer et al., 2022).

Changing ECG electrodes decreases the number of false alarms (McGuffin & Ortiz, 2019). Monitors for development of MARSI.

8. Customize alarm limits within 1 hour of assuming care of patient and on condition changes. Changes made should be in accordance with agency policies and health care provider's orders.

Alarm settings need to be individualized, checked for accuracy, and detectable (McGuffin & Ortiz, 2019).

9. Help patient to a comfortable position.

Restores comfort and sense of well-being.

10. Place nurse call system in an accessible location within patient's reach.

Ensures patient can call for assistance if needed.

11. Raise side rails (as appropriate) and lower bed to lowest position, locking into position.

Ensures patient safety and prevents falls.

12. Dispose of all contaminated supplies in appropriate receptacle, remove and dispose of gloves, and perform hand hygiene.

Reduces transmission of microorganisms.

EVALUATION

1. Ensure that all appropriate alarms are ON.

Ensures accurate monitoring. Refer to agency policies.

2. Inspect condition of skin after electrode removal for signs of MARSI.

Continual electrode placement and removal can lead to development of MARSI.

STEP	RATIONALE
3. **Use Teach-Back:** "I want to be sure I explained why you needed this cardiac monitoring. Why is this monitoring important?" Revise your instruction now or develop a plan for revised patient/family caregiver teaching if patient/family caregiver is not able to teach back correctly.	Teach-back is a technique for health care providers to ensure that they have explained medical information clearly so that patients and their families understand what is communicated to them (AHRQ, 2023).

Unexpected Outcomes	**Related Interventions**
1. Monitor tracing cannot be interpreted: • Absence of tracing on one or more leads • Presence of artifact in ECG tracings	• Inspect electrodes for secure placement. Replace as needed and perform new skin preparation. • Reposition any wires that move as result of patient breathing or movement or vibrations in environment. Do not reposition electrodes if in correct position. • If artifact looks like 60-cycle interference (very thick-lined waveform), unplug battery-operated equipment in room one item at a time to see if interference disappears. **NOTE:** 60-cycle interference is rare. Consider electronic interference such as cell phone and personal computers that are too close to the remote monitor.
2. Signs of MARSI develop.	• Gently remove existing adhesive-backed electrode by supporting the skin at the adhesive/skin interface and apply adhesive remover to the skin (Thayer et al., 2022). • Cleanse skin with a non–alcohol-based cleaner or plain water. • Do not position new electrodes over irritated skin.

Documentation

- Document alarm trends and waveforms at least once a shift and on report of an alarm.
- Document at least one rhythm strip per shift per agency policy.
- Document your evaluation of patient and family caregiver learning.
- Document skin assessment.

Hand-Off Reporting

- Report any unexpected ECG patterns or waveforms immediately to the health care provider.

Special Considerations

Patient Education

- Educate patients on what information needs to be reported prior to an ECG (e.g., medications).

Pediatrics

- In general, the mechanisms of dysrhythmias are the same in children as they are in adults; however, the appearance of the dysrhythmias on the ECG may differ because of developmental issues such as heart size, baseline heart rate, sinus and atrioventricular (AV) node function, and autonomic innervation.
- Be aware that medications such as digitalis and antiarrhythmics can affect ECG rhythms.
- The position of the brown lead can be changed to mirror one of the precordial (chest) lead positions, V_1 to V_6. The standard placement is V_1 at fourth intercostal space (ICS), right sternal border.
- Strategies to provide continuous monitoring in a child may be required in order to prevent the removal of the electrodes.

Older Adults

- An ECG is not always indicated based on aging, but a baseline ECG can be part of a routine health visit.

Populations With Disabilities

- Performing an ECG in the home may be the safest route for patients with intellectual and developmental disabilities.

✦ CLINICAL JUDGMENT AND NEXT-GENERATION NCLEX® EXAMINATION–STYLE QUESTIONS

A 76-year-old patient is postoperative day 2 following a partial colectomy for colon cancer. The patient has a history of myocardial infarction (MI) 15 years ago with two stents. The patient reports nausea and vomiting, which began several moments ago. Vital signs: T 37.5°C (99.5°F); HR 120 beats/min; RR 28 breaths/min; BP 96/50 mm Hg; SpO_2 90% on RA. Lungs have crackles in the bases bilaterally. Apical pulse is very irregular. The patient reports pain at the surgical site of 4 on a 0-to-10 scale.

1. Which diagnostic test does the nurse anticipate the health care provider will order **initially**?
   1. ALT/AST
   2. Electrocardiogram
   3. CT scan of the abdomen
   4. Chest x-ray
2. Evaluation of which of the following conditions indicates to the nurse that an electrocardiogram is needed for a patient? **Select all that apply.**
   1. Suspected acute coronary syndromes
   2. Implanted defibrillators and pacemakers
   3. Syncope
   4. Metabolic disorders
   5. Effects and side effects of pharmacotherapeutics
3. The nurse is applying leads to the patient for an electrocardiogram. Where will the nurse place the precordial lead of V_1?
   1. Midway between V_2 and V_4
   2. Fifth intercostal space at the midclavicular line
   3. Left anterior axillary line at level of V_4 horizontally
   4. Fourth intercostal space at the right sternal border
4. The nurse determines the priority for the plan of care.
   Complete the following sentence by selecting from the list of word choices below.

   The *priorities* of care for the patient at this time are to **[Word Choice]** and **[Word Choice]**.

Word Choices
Treat pain at the surgical site
Determine origin of nausea and vomiting
Manage perfusion
Assess the surgical incision
Contact the family members

5. Cardiac monitoring via telemetry has begun, and an artifact continues to appear on the patient's ECG rhythm. Which of the following actions will the nurse perform to troubleshoot this finding? **Select all that apply.**
   1. Move electrodes to different locations on the chest.
   2. Wipe electrode skin areas with alcohol.
   3. Prepare skin by washing with soap and water and drying with a washcloth.
   4. Do not change electrodes for 2 days.
   5. Inspect electrodes for secure placement.

Visit the Evolve site for Answers to Clinical Judgment and Next-Generation NCLEX® Examination–Style Questions.

REFERENCES

Agency for Healthcare Research and Quality (AHRQ): *Teach-back: intervention.* Rockville, MD, November 2023, Agency for Healthcare Research and Quality. https://www.ahrq.gov/patient-safety/reports/engage/interventions/teachback.html.

Ajmal, M, Marcus F: Preoperative hair removal to reduce surgical site infection, *Cochrane Database Syst Rev* 8:CD004122, 2021.

Appold B, et al: Reining in unnecessary admission EKGs: a successful interdepartmental high-value care initiative, *Cureus* 13(9):e18351, 2021.

Arnett D, et al: *2019 ACC/AHA guideline on the primary prevention of cardiovascular disease,* 2019. https://www.ahajournals.org/doi/pdf/10.1161/CIR.0000000000000678.

Bouzid Z, et al: Remote and wearable ECG devices with diagnostic abilities in adults: a state-of-the-science scoping review, *Heart Rhythm* 19(7):1192-1201, 2022.

Centers for Disease Control and Prevention (CDC): *What is health literacy?* 2023. https://www.cdc.gov/healthliteracy/learn/index.html.

Fumarola S, et al: Overlooked and underestimated: medical adhesive-related skin injuries. Best practice consensus document on prevention, *J Wound Care* 29(Suppl 3c):S1–S24, 2020.

Gorisek R, et al: An evidence-based initiative to reduce alarm fatigue in a burn intensive care unit, *Crit Care Nurse* 41(4):29–37, 2021.

Jones S: ECG notes: *Interpretation and management guide,* ed 4, Philadelphia, 2021, FA Davis.

Ker J, Outhoff K: In a heartbeat: important cardiac arrhythmias in clinical practice, *S Afr Gen Pract J* 3(1):26–30, 2022.

Lewandowska K, et al: Impact of alarm fatigue on the work of nurses in an intensive care environment: a systematic review, *Int J Environ Res Public Health* 17(22):8409, 2020.

McGuffin S, Ortiz S: Daily electrocardiogram electrode change and the effect on frequency of nuisance alarms, *Dimens Crit Care Nurs* 38(4):187–191, 2019.

Rahimpour M, et al: Electrocardiogram interpretation competency among emergency nurses and emergency medical service (EMS) personnel: a cross-sectional and comparative descriptive study, *Nurs Open* 8:1712–1719, 2021.

Sandau K, et al: Update to practice standards for electrocardiographic monitoring in hospital settings: a scientific statement from the American Heart Association, *Circulation* 136(19):e273, 2017.

Seifert M, et al: Effect of bundle set interventions on physiologic alarms and alarm fatigue in an intensive care unit: a quality improvement project, *Intensive Crit Care Nurs* 67:103098, 2021.

Sowan A, et al: Improving the safety, effectiveness, and efficiency of clinical alarm systems: simulation-based usability testing of physiologic monitors, *JMIR Nurs* 4(1):e20584, 2021.

Tanner, J, Melen K: Standardization in performing and interpreting electrocardiograms, *Am J Med* 134(4):430–434, 2021.

Teferra M, et al: Electronic textile electrocardiogram monitoring in cardiac patients: a scoping review protocol, *JBI Database System Rev Implement Rep* 17(2):147–156, 2019.

Thayer D, et al: Prevention and management of moisture-associated skin damage (MASD), medical adhesive-related skin injury (MARSI), and skin tears. In McNichol LL, et al., editors: *WOCN Core Curriculum Wound Management,* ed 2, Philadelphia, 2022, Wolters Kluwer.

The Joint Commission (TJC): *2023 National Patient Safety Goals,* Oakbrook Terrace, IL, 2023, The Joint Commission. https://www.jointcommission.org/standards/national-patient-safety-goals/.

26 | Closed Chest Drainage Systems

SKILLS AND PROCEDURES

Skill 26.1 **Managing Closed Chest Drainage Systems, p. 803**

Skill 26.2 **Assisting With Removal of Chest Tubes, p. 813**

Skill 26.3 **Autotransfusion of Chest Tube Drainage, p. 817**

OBJECTIVES

Mastery of content in this chapter will enable you to:
- Explain the physiology of normal respiration.
- Identify three common sites for chest tube placement.
- Discuss three conditions requiring chest tube insertion.
- Explain closed chest drainage systems: water-seal systems, waterless systems, and flutter-valve systems.
- Explain principles and mechanisms of chest tube suction.
- Discuss measures to maintain patient safety during chest tube insertion, maintenance, and removal.
- Examine methods of troubleshooting chest tube systems.
- Discuss the nursing principles in caring for patients with chest tubes.
- Explain nursing principles for autotransfusion of chest tube drainage.

MEDIA RESOURCES

- http://evolve.elsevier.com/Perry/skills
- Review Questions
- Audio Glossary
- **NSO** Nursing Skills Online
- Answers to Clinical Judgment and Next-Generation NCLEX® Examination–Style Questions
- Skills Performance Checklists
- Printable Key Points

PURPOSE

Patients require chest tubes when air, blood, or fluid collects in the intrapleural space, disrupting the normal intrapleural and intrapulmonic pressures necessary for lung expansion. When air enters the pleural space, a pneumothorax occurs. When blood enters the pleural space, a hemothorax occurs. Pleural effusions occur when fluid enters the pleural space in response to infection, inflammation, or cancer. The management of chest tubes and drainage systems is a complex skill requiring knowledge of the cardiopulmonary system. Patients who require chest tubes are usually in the emergency department or intensive care settings (Basler & Englund, 2020).

The purpose of a closed chest drainage system, with or without suction, is to drain air and/or fluid from the pleural space. A chest tube is a catheter inserted through the rib cage into the pleural space to remove air, fluids, or blood; to prevent air or fluid from reentering the pleural space; and to reestablish normal intrapleural and intrapulmonic pressures after trauma or surgery (Chotai & Mosenifar, 2022; Porcel, 2018). Lung reexpansion occurs as the fluid and/or air is removed, and the patient's oxygenation improves (Mitsui et al., 2021).

PRACTICE STANDARDS

- Bauman H, Handley C, 2018: Best Practices: Chest Tube Management—Principles of chest tube management
- Sasa R, 2019: Evidence-Based Update on Chest Tube Management—Home care and best practices
- Slaughter C, 2024: Chest Tube Placement (Assist). In AACN Procedure Manual for Progressive and Critical Care (Johnson KL, editor)
- The Joint Commission (TJC), 2023: National Patient Safety Goals—Patient identification

SUPPLEMENTAL STANDARDS

- Hartjes T, 2023: AACN Core Curriculum for Progressive and Critical Care Nursing

PRINCIPLES FOR PRACTICE

- The chest cavity is a closed structure bound by muscle, bone, connective tissue, vascular structures, and the diaphragm. This cavity has three distinct sections, each sealed from the others: one section for each lung and a third section for the mediastinum, which surrounds structures such as the heart, esophagus, trachea, and great vessels.
- The lungs, except for the hilar region, are covered with a membrane called the *visceral pleura*. The interior chest wall is lined with a membrane called the *parietal pleura* (Fig. 26.1). The space between the visceral and parietal pleura is called the *pleural space* and is filled with just enough lubricating fluid to help the pleura slide during respiration (Patton et al., 2022). The pleural space normally functions with a negative pressure (subatmospheric pressure). Although it fluctuates during inspiration and expiration, intrapleural pressure remains approximately −4 mm Hg throughout the breathing cycle.

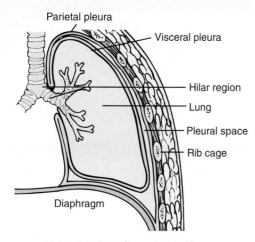

FIG. 26.1 Partial structures of lungs.

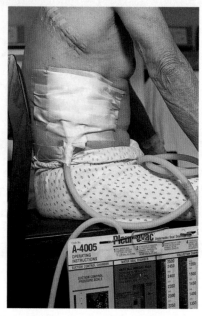

FIG. 26.2 Pleural chest tube in place following thoracic surgery.

- Trauma, disease, or surgery can result in air, blood, pus, or lymph fluid leaking into the intrapleural space, creating a positive pressure that collapses lung tissue (Chotai & Mosenifar, 2022). Small leaks (24% or less) are sometimes absorbed spontaneously and may not necessitate the use of a chest tube.

- Several clinical conditions such as cancer, infection, pancreatitis, connective tissue disease, autoimmune diseases, asbestos exposure, use of certain drugs, or collagen vascular diseases increase pleural fluid entry or decrease fluid exit from the lung. This is called a *pleural effusion*, and when it is present, a patient usually needs a diagnostic thoracentesis and pleural fluid analysis to determine the cause of the exudate (see Chapter 8) (Ignatavicius et al., 2022).

- A pneumothorax is a collection of air in the pleural space and is classified as either open (air entering through opening in chest wall) or closed (no external wound) (Harding et al., 2023). The loss of negative intrapleural pressure causes the lung to collapse. A traumatic pneumothorax develops as a result of penetrating chest trauma such as a stabbing (open) or the chest striking the steering wheel in an automobile accident (closed). One also can occur during an invasive procedure such as insertion of a subclavian intravenous (IV) line. A spontaneous or primary pneumothorax sometimes occurs from the rupture of a small bleb (air-filled sacs) on the surface of the lung (Harding et al., 2023). Secondary pneumothorax occurs because of underlying disease such as emphysema. A patient with a pneumothorax usually feels sharp chest pain that worsens on inspiration or coughing because atmospheric air irritates the parietal pleura (Banasik & Copstead, 2019).

- A tension pneumothorax, a life-threatening situation, occurs from a tear in the pleura causing a situation in which air has no way to escape from the pleural cavity. If left untreated, the lung on the affected side collapses, and the mediastinum shifts to the opposite (unaffected side), leading to tracheal deviation and pressure on the heart and great vessels with reduced venous return and subsequent decrease in cardiac output (Harding et al., 2023). Tracheal deviation is a late sign and may be absent in some cases (Huggins et al., 2023). Sudden chest pain, a fall in blood pressure, tachycardia, acute pleuritic pain, diaphoresis, dry cough, and cardiopulmonary arrest are signs and symptoms of the condition.

- A hemothorax is an accumulation of blood and fluid in the pleural space, usually as a result of trauma. It produces a counterpressure and prevents the lung from full expansion. A rupture of small blood vessels from inflammatory processes such as pneumonia or tuberculosis (TB) can cause a hemothorax, as

can trauma. In addition to pain and dyspnea, signs and symptoms of shock develop if blood loss is severe (Gomez & Tran, 2021; Ignatavicius et al., 2022).

- Chest tube insertion is the treatment for most types of effusions, pneumothorax, hemothorax, and postoperative chest surgery or trauma. A chest tube is a catheter inserted through the thorax to remove fluid (effusions), blood (hemothorax), and/or air (pneumothorax) (Fig. 26.2).

- If emergent treatment is required (e.g., with tension pneumothorax or with no availability of a chest tube), a needle thoracostomy is achieved with a large-gauge needle (14 or 16 gauge) inserted into the second to third intercostal space, midclavicular line. A "hissing" sound is noted, followed by a rapid stabilization of the patient's vital signs and respiratory status (Huggins et al., 2023). Another option in emergent situations is insertion of a small-gauge chest tube or catheter through the chest wall with a rubber, one-way "flutter" valve (e.g., a Heimlich valve) attached to the catheter (Fig. 26.3). As the patient exhales, the positive pressure generated by the air leaving the chest enters the tubing, causing the valve to open so air is released. During inspiration the tube collapses on itself, preventing air from re-entering the chest. This type of valve is not used when patients need fluid drained from a hemothorax or a pleural effusion (Harding et al., 2023).

- The location of a chest tube indicates the type of drainage expected. Apical (second or third intercostal space) and anterior chest tube placement promotes removal of air. Because air rises, these chest tubes are placed high, allowing evacuation of air from the intrapleural space and lung reexpansion (Fig. 26.4). The air is discharged into the atmosphere, and there is little or no drainage expected in the collection chamber.

- Chest tubes for removal of blood and fluid are placed low (usually in the fifth or sixth intercostal space) and posterior or lateral to drain fluid (see Fig. 26.4). Fluid in the intrapleural space is affected by gravity and localizes in the lower part of the lung cavity. Fluid drainage is expected after open-chest surgery, with pleural effusions, and with some chest trauma.

- A mediastinal chest tube is placed in the mediastinum, just below the sternum (Fig. 26.5), and is connected to a drainage

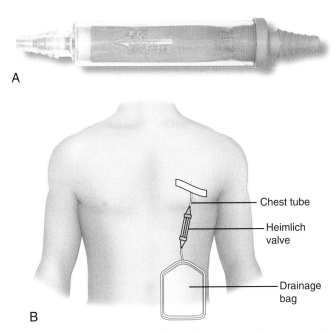

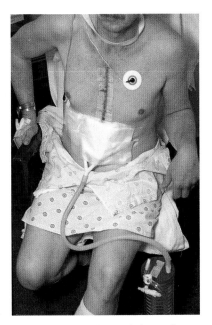

FIG. 26.5 Mediastinal chest tube.

FIG. 26.3 (A) Heimlich chest drain valve is a specially designed flutter valve that is used in place of a chest drainage unit for small uncomplicated pneumothorax with little or no drainage and no need for suction. The valve allows for escape of air but prevents reentry of air into the pleural space. (B) Placement of valve between chest tube and drainage bag, which can be worn under clothing. (*A courtesy and copyright © Becton, Dickinson and Company.*)

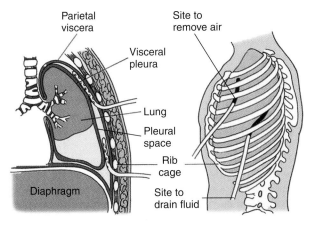

FIG. 26.4 Diagram of sites for chest tube placement.

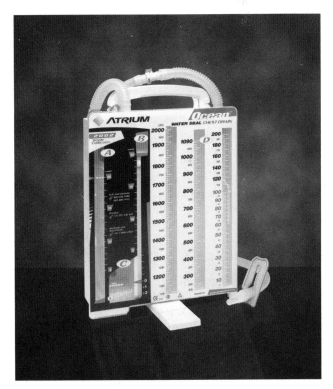

FIG. 26.6 Disposable water-seal chest drainage system with suction. (*Used with permission, Atrium Medical Corp.*)

system. This tube drains blood or fluid, preventing its accumulation around the heart. A mediastinal tube is commonly used after open-heart surgery.

- Small-bore "pigtail" chest tubes (SBCTs) have emerged as an effective and less traumatic alternative to traditional large-bore chest tubes for the removal of air or pleural fluid (Khan et al., 2021). These less invasive, smaller caliber tubes and their flexibility provide the patient the advantage of less pain during insertion. SBCTs are a reasonable first-line chest-tube alternative; however, they are not without complications, such as infection, catheter dislodgement, catheter malfunction, and pneumothorax (Broder et al., 2020). They can also be used for chronic pleural fluid or air removal and can be connected to small disposable systems (e.g., Atrium) for patients discharged to home.

- After a chest tube is inserted, it is attached to a drainage system. A traditional chest drainage unit (CDU) has three chambers for collection of drainage, water seal, and suction control. This unit can drain a large amount of both fluid and air. Disposable chest drainage systems, such as the Codman, Pleur-evac, or Atrium, allow for more mobility than previous bottle systems and are now more commonly used (see Skill 26.1 and Fig. 26.6). The disposable systems also allow for increased ability to maintain sterility of the system (Chotai & Mosenifar, 2022).

- A three-chamber system drains both a hemothorax and a pneumothorax effectively. A three-chamber system promotes the drainage of fluid and air with controlled suction. In both systems the first chamber provides a compartment for fluid or blood drainage and a second compartment for either a water seal or a one-way valve. In the three-chamber system, the third compartment is for suction control, which may or may not be used. Disposable units appear to be the system of choice because they are cost-effective, and some facilitate autotransfusion.
- Ongoing assessment is required to monitor for changes in the patient's baseline cardiopulmonary status. Signs and symptoms that may necessitate chest tube insertion or indicate malfunction of an existing chest tube include:
  - Vital sign changes: Tachypnea, decreased oxygen saturation, hypotension, tachycardia/bradycardia
  - Changes in respiratory assessment findings: Shortness of breath, dyspnea, decreased or absent breath sounds on affected side, asymmetrical chest expansion with respirations, subcutaneous emphysema, hyperresonance in the affected side, dullness to percussion in the affected side, tracheal deviation to the unaffected side
  - Changes in cardiovascular assessment findings: Tachycardia, neck vein distention, muffled heart sounds, cyanosis
  - Changes in neurological/behavioral assessment findings: Anxiety, restlessness, changes in level of consciousness
- Infections occur rarely with chest tubes. They can range from skin infections at the insertion site to empyema and even necrotizing infections (Chotai & Mosenifar, 2022).

PERSON-CENTERED CARE

- Following chest tube insertion, encourage deep-breathing exercises and early mobility, provide appropriate analgesia to promote activity, and provide patient education regarding these practices (Ignatavicius et al., 2022).
- Autotransfusion may pose a challenge for nurses owing to the religious beliefs of some patients. A patient may wish to discuss options with elders of the church before consenting to any blood transfusions.

EVIDENCE-BASED PRACTICE

Prevention of Occlusion

The clinical need for chest tube placement arises when there is a need to drain or remove air, blood, and other fluids from the pleural space. The purpose in removing the air and/or fluid from the thoracic cavity is so that a normal, negative intrathoracic pressure within the chest can be reestablished. This requires an open and functioning chest tube. Evidence exists for the proper methods to avoid occlusion.

- Clogging of the chest tube can occur when small chest tubes are used and become blocked by blood clots and fibrin. Large-bore catheters (such as 28 Fr) safely remove any fluid or drainage (Slaughter, 2024; Urden et al., 2024).
- Routine milking or stripping of the chest tubes is NOT recommended, as it can cause increased intrathoracic pressure and tissue damage. Chest drainage stripping or milking demonstrates no safety or efficacy benefits, slightly increases intrathoracic pressure, and risks tissue damage (Urden et al., 2024; Huggins et al., 2023; Sasa, 2019).
- Stripping or milking chest tubes to keep them patent is based on nursing assessment and, in some situations, may be necessary to remove clots in the tube (Urden et al., 2024; Abuejheisheh et al., 2021). Refer to agency policy.

- Careful management of chest tube drainage prevents chest tube occlusion (Abuejheisheh et al., 2021; Baird, 2023):
  - Avoid dependent loops of the drainage tube; or, when these loops cannot be avoided (such as when the patient is sitting), lift and clear the tube frequently.
  - Keep the chest drainage tubing and the collection system below the level of the patient's chest. Keep the tubing above the collection system and prevent dependent loops in order to allow drainage by gravity into the collection chamber.
- Hemothorax in children should be treated with a tube of an appropriate size to evacuate blood, monitor the rate of bleeding, and minimize risk of occlusion by clotting (Huggins et al., 2023).

SAFETY GUIDELINES

- Observe the water seal for intermittent bubbling and a rise and fall of the fluid in the water-seal chamber (tidaling) that is synchronous with respirations, which is expected (Baird, 2023; Ignatavicius et al., 2022). In a spontaneously breathing patient, the fluid level normally rises during inspiration and falls during expiration. When a patient is on a mechanical ventilator, the opposite occurs. If tidaling does not occur, suspect that the tubing is kinked or clamped or that a dependent tubing section has become filled with fluid (Bauman & Handley, 2018).
- Constant bubbling in the water seal or a sudden, unexpected stoppage of water-seal activity is considered abnormal and requires immediate attention (Slaughter, 2024; Baird, 2023; Sasa, 2019).
- After 2 or 3 days, tidaling or bubbling on expiration is expected to stop, indicating that the lung has reexpanded and that the chest tube can be removed (Baird, 2023; Sasa, 2019).
- Unexpected stoppage of chest tube activity may indicate a blockage. In these situations, immediate attention and correction are indicated. In a waterless system, look for a rise and fall of fluid in the diagnostic air-leak indicator synchronous with respirations. Constant left-to-right bubbling (when facing the indicator) or violent rocking are considered abnormal and indicate an air leak.
- Note the expected amount of chest tube drainage and monitor drainage on a regular basis (e.g., every hour initially and then every 4 hours). At the end of every shift, make a mark to indicate the fluid level with the date and time on the side of the drainage collection chamber.
- A sudden decrease in the amount of chest tube drainage needs to be reported to the surgeon or Rapid Response Team (Ignatavicius et al., 2022).
- Notify the health care provider when there is a sudden increase of more than 50 to 150 mL of drainage over 1 hour, or according to the health care provider order, which can indicate fresh bleeding (Good & Kirkwood, 2018; Sasa, 2019).
- Drainage from a pneumothorax is generally limited to fluid buildup from the trauma of chest tube insertion (Urden et al., 2024). However, when the drainage device becomes full of fluid, it must be changed.
- Be familiar with the expected color of chest drainage. Drainage from recent open-chest surgery initially is bright red and gradually becomes serous as the postoperative course continues. Blood-tinged fluid is expected from a malignancy, pulmonary infarction, or severe inflammation. Frank blood is expected from a hemothorax. Purulent drainage is expected when a chest tube is inserted for an empyema, which is a collection of pus in the pleural cavity (Urden et al., 2024; Williams et al., 2021).

- In a water-seal system, observe for constant, gentle bubbling in the suction-control chamber when it is connected to suction. In a waterless system, a designated amount of suction is maintained by setting the suction source and dialing the prescribed suction level in the float ball column.
- Assess both types of systems for air leaks. If an air leak exists, determine whether it is in the patient (patient-centered air leak such as at the tube insertion site or inside the chest cavity) or the chest tube system (system-centered air leak such as within the drain or tubing connections). The amount of bubbling in the water-seal chamber indicates the degree of the leak.
- To rule out an air leak, ask the patient to take deep breaths in and out. If there is no air leak, ask the patient to cough (Baird, 2023).
- If air is leaking from the patient's pleural space, intermittent bubbling is seen corresponding to respirations.
- Briefly occlude the chest tube at the dressing site (Baird, 2023). If bubbling in the water-seal chamber stops when the occlusion takes place, the air leak is inside the patient's chest or under the dressing. If this occurs, reinforce the dressing and notify the health care provider. If bubbling is continuous despite the previously mentioned skills, intermittently pinch the chest tube

tubing for a brief moment (i.e., less than a minute), beginning at the insertion site and progressing to the CDU (Baird, 2023).
- If the leak stops when the drainage tubing is occluded along its length, the air leak is likely between the occlusion and the patient's chest. This often is noted when air leaks occur at the point where the distal end of the chest tube connects to the drainage device tubing. Check this site to determine that it has not become loose and is tight. If bubbling continues with the occlusion, then replace the chest drainage device (Baird, 2023). With a significant leak occurring despite the aforementioned recommendations, it may be possible to palpate subcutaneous emphysema under the skin (Sasa, 2019). Document and report any changes in lung sounds, pulse oximetry, respiratory rate, or mentation.
- Be sure that the drainage system is stable and will not tip over. Most CDUs have attached adjustable hangers that allow the device to hang on the side or end of the patient's bed. Many have a swing-out floor stand to reduce the chance of accidentally knocking over the chest drainage system if it is placed on the floor. Some manufacturers make a reusable drain caddy that allows the chest drainage system to be connected to an IV pole to facilitate patient movement and eliminate a chance of knocking over the system.

◆ SKILL 26.1   Managing Closed Chest Drainage Systems

There are two types of commercial drainage systems: wet suction water-seal (see Fig. 26.6 and Table 26.1) and dry suction water-seal (Fig. 26.7) systems. It is important to note that patients in acute care agency settings have chest tubes with water seals. The water seal prevents backflow into the chest and can indicate if there is a leak in the system. The water in this location of the chest drainage device is typically located at the bottom of the collection system, and the water is dyed blue.

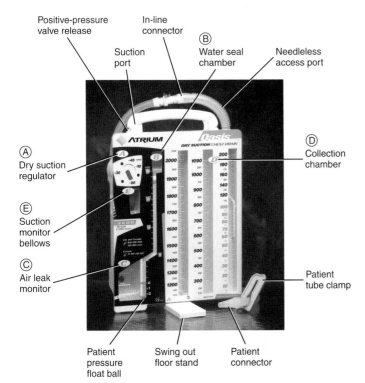

FIG. 26.7 Dry suction chest drainage system. (*Used with permission, Atrium Medical Corp.*)

Wet Suction Water-Seal Systems
Three-Chamber Water-Seal System
Wet suction water-seal systems have three chambers: the collection chamber, the water-seal chamber, and the suction chamber. If suction is used, the three-chamber water-seal system (see Fig. 26.6) is set up with sterile water added to the suction-control chamber to the water level that is marked as −20 cm H_2O. A prescribed amount of sterile fluid (e.g., 20 cm of water) is poured into the suction-control chamber, which is then attached to a suction source by tubing. The amount of sterile water added depends on the manufacturer's recommendations and the health care provider's order. The chamber is filled to the set volume for the prescribed amount of suction. It is the height of the water in the suction-control chamber that determines the amount of suction. Twenty centimeters of water suction is typically ordered for an adult; 10 to 20 cm of water suction may be ordered for pediatric patients; and 5 cm of water suction is commonly used for neonates. Sterile water is added as needed because of evaporation. As the fluid level decreases, the amount of suction also declines. Suction needs to be turned off momentarily in order to accurately assess the level of water in the chamber.

If the suction source is set too high, the force exerted will cause vigorous bubbling and will facilitate evaporation of the fluid added to the system. If this occurs, lower the suction source setting to reduce noise and evaporation of the fluid. The absence of bubbling indicates that no suction is being exerted into the system. Raise the suction setting to restore gentle bubbling.

The middle/bottom chamber is the water seal. The water seal allows air to exit from the pleural space on exhalation and prevents it from entering the pleural cavity or mediastinum on inhalation. Water in this chamber is typically dyed blue. When the appropriate amount of sterile water is added, a 2-cm water seal is established. To maintain an effective water seal, the chest drainage unit (CDU) must remain upright, and the water level in the water-seal chamber must be monitored to check for evaporation. It is normal to see intermittent bubbling in the water-seal chamber; this indicates that

TABLE 26.1

Comparison of Chest Tube Drainage Systems

Drainage System Type	Function	Advantage	Disadvantage
Wet suction water-seal system (see Fig. 26.6)	Three-chamber system provides a chamber to aid evacuation of chest drainage.	Easy setup and use Cost-effective	System must be kept upright to maintain water seal. Drainage chamber may fill up quickly if patient has large amount of drainage. Sterile water must be added as needed to maintain suction and water seal because of evaporation.
Dry suction system (see Fig. 26.7)	Provides two chambers; suction is controlled by an integrated valve.	Easy setup Quiet operation Can be used when higher levels of suction are required	Sterile water must be added to system to provide a water seal.

air is escaping the patient's pleural space appropriately. Continuous bubbling in the water-seal chamber indicates an air leak, and the source of the leak (physiological [within the patient] or mechanical [within the drainage system]) must be investigated, documented, and reported to the health care provider.

Dry Suction Water-Seal Systems

Two-Chamber Dry Suction Water-Seal System

Dry suction-control systems provide many advantages (see Fig. 26.7), including higher suction pressure levels if needed, easy setup, no water in the suction-control chamber (hence the name "dry"), and the absence of continuous bubbling, which provides for quiet operation. Note that there are only two chambers with this type of chest tube drainage device: the water-seal chamber and the collection chamber. A self-compensating regulator controls dry suction units. A dial is set to the prescribed suction-control setting. These units are preset to −20 cm of water pressure, but they are adjustable from −10 to −40 cm. However, the dry suction-control systems require or have presealed sterile water to use in the water-seal chamber (Baird, 2023; Ignatavicius et al., 2022).

When suction is ordered, attach the suction tubing to the port on the suction chamber and turn the suction regulator on; an orange plunger will bellow out. Set the suction indicator to the prescribed setting. If the orange plunger does not bellow out, increase the suction source setting until it does. The system is now functioning with suction.

Delegation

The skill of chest tube management cannot be delegated to assistive personnel (AP). Direct the AP about:
- Proper positioning of the patient with chest tubes to facilitate chest tube drainage and optimal functioning of the system
- Ambulating and transferring patient with a chest drainage system in place
- Reporting changes in vital signs, complaints of chest pain or sudden shortness of breath, or excessive bubbling in water-seal chamber to the nurse immediately
- Danger of any disconnection of the drainage system, change in type and amount of drainage, sudden bleeding, or sudden cessation of bubbling or tidaling

Interprofessional Collaboration

Insertion of chest tubes at the bedside requires interprofessional collaboration of all health care providers, including physicians, physician assistants, and advanced practice nurses who individualize care

practices based on patient assessment findings. These care practices include:
- Orders for patient transport: Orders are needed for when a patient requires transport from the room for any studies or procedures for which the provider approves suction being turned off (if it is on). **NOTE:** Chest tubes are not routinely clamped during patient transport unless clamping of the chest tube is specifically ordered by the health care provider.
- Observe and measure chest tube output after surgery. Patients typically have 50 to 150 mL of chest tube output per hour for the first several hours after surgery (Good & Kirkwood, 2018). Patients who require chest tube insertion following penetrating chest trauma may have different output limits; verify health care provider's order and monitor hourly output accordingly.
- Management of new or increasing air leaks in the chest or around the chest tube insertion site and signs and/or symptoms of increasing pneumothorax, cardiac tamponade, or hemothorax.
- Assisting in changing the chest drainage collection system as needed.

Equipment

- Water-seal system or waterless (dry) suction system: sterile water or normal saline (NS) per manufacturer's directions
- Suction source and setup
- Sterile skin preparation solution (chlorhexidine solution or povidone iodine)
- Clean gloves
- Sterile gauze sponges
- Local anesthetic, if not an emergent procedure
- Chest tube tray (all items are sterile): knife handle (1), knife blade No. 10 or disposable safety scalpel No. 10, chest tube clamp, small sponge forceps, needle holder, size 3-0 silk sutures, tray liner (sterile field), curved 8-inch Kelly clamps (2), 4 × 4–inch sponges (10), suture scissors, hand towels (3), sterile gloves
- Dressings: petrolatum or Xeroform gauze, split chest-tube dressings, several 4 × 4–inch gauze dressings, large gauze dressings (2), and 4-inch tape
- Personal protective equipment (PPE): head cover, face mask/face shield, sterile gloves
- Two rubber-tipped hemostats for each chest tube
- 2.5-cm (1-inch) waterproof adhesive tape or plastic zip ties for securing connections
- Stethoscope, sphygmomanometer, and pulse oximeter

STEP	RATIONALE

ASSESSMENT

1. Identify patient using at least two identifiers (e.g., name and birthday or name and medical record number) according to agency policy.

Ensures correct patient. Complies with The Joint Commission standards and improves patient safety (TJC, 2023).

2. Review patient's electronic health record (EHR), including health care provider's order and nurses' notes. Assess significant medical history, including recent trauma, chronic lung disease, spontaneous pneumothorax, pulmonary disease, therapeutic procedures, mechanism of injury, and hemoglobin and hematocrit levels (Urden et al., 2024; Baird, 2023).

Insertion of chest tube requires a health care provider order. History of medical condition or injury may provide the reason for the occurrence of the pneumothorax, hemothorax, empyema, and/or pleural effusion, providing a rationale for what to observe in chest tube system.

Hemoglobin and hematocrit reflect whether blood loss is occurring, which may affect oxygenation.

3. Verify that informed consent was obtained before administering any pain medication. See agency policy.

Federal regulations, many state laws, and accreditation agencies such as The Joint Commission require informed consent for procedure. Patients should provide informed consent prior to any procedure.

4. Review patient's medication record for anticoagulant therapy, including aspirin, warfarin, heparin, or platelet aggregation inhibitors such as ticlopidine or dipyridamole.

Anticoagulation therapy can increase procedure-related blood loss.

5. Assess patient for known allergies. Ask patient about any history of problems (such as skin sensitivity) with medications, latex, or anything applied to the skin. If allergy is identified, place allergy band on patient's wrist.

Chlorhexidine or povidone iodine are antiseptic solutions used to clean skin before tube insertion (Huggins et al., 2023). Lidocaine is a local anesthetic administered to reduce pain. The chest tube will be held in place with tape and sutures (Baird, 2023).

6. Review EHR to determine patient's age and history of dehydration, malnutrition, exposure to radiation therapy, underlying chronic conditions (e.g., diabetes mellitus, immunosuppression), and edema of the skin.

Common risk factors for medical adhesive–related skin injury (MARSI) (Fumarola et al., 2020).

7. If nonemergent, assess patient's/family caregiver's health literacy.

Determines degree to which individuals have the ability to find, understand, and use information and services to make informed health-related decisions and actions for themselves and others (Centers for Disease Control and Prevention [CDC], 2023).

8. Assess character of patient's pain and rate pain severity on a scale of 0 to 10.

Provides a baseline to compare after chest tube insertion.

Clinical Judgment *It may be necessary to administer prescribed analgesics or sedatives during the assessment phase. The medications reduce the patient's discomfort and anxiety and help to facilitate patient cooperation during assessment and the subsequent procedure (Huggins et al., 2023).*

9. Perform hand hygiene and inspect condition of skin around chest. If adhesive has been in place, note any redness, irritation, or blistering. Note if patient is diaphoretic or has history of impaired poor perfusion, altered tissue tolerance, poor nutrition, or edema.

Prevents transmission of microorganisms. Provides baseline for monitoring development of a medical device–related pressure injury (MDRPI) or MARSI (Fumarola et al., 2020).

10. Perform a complete respiratory assessment, baseline vital signs, and pulse oximetry (SpO_2).
    a. Assess for signs and symptoms of increased respiratory distress and hypoxia (e.g., decreased breath sounds over affected and unaffected lungs, marked cyanosis, asymmetrical chest movements, displaced trachea, shortness of breath, and confusion).
    b. Assess for sharp, stabbing chest pain or chest pain on inspiration, hypotension, and tachycardia. If possible, ask patient to again rate level of pain severity on a scale of 0 to 10.

Baseline assessment and vital signs are essential for any invasive procedure. Chest tube insertion often causes respiratory distress.

Signs and symptoms associated with respiratory distress are related to type and size of pneumothorax, hemothorax, or preexisting illness. Signs of hypoxia are related to inadequate oxygen to tissues. Provides baseline to later determine if tube insertion improves patient status.

Sharp stabbing chest pain with or without decreased blood pressure and increased heart rate may indicate tension pneumothorax. Presence of pneumothorax or hemothorax is painful, frequently causing sharp inspiratory pain. In addition, discomfort is associated with presence of a chest tube, not just with its insertion. As a result, patients tend to not cough or change position in an effort to minimize this pain (Chotai & Mosenifar, 2022).

11. For patients who have chest tubes in place:
    a. Perform hand hygiene and apply gloves. Inspect skin around chest tube dressing and site surrounding tube insertion. Keep a box of sterile 4 × 4–inch gauze pads and petroleum gauze at bedside.

Ensures that dressing is intact, that occlusive seal remains without air or fluid leaks, and that area surrounding insertion site is free of drainage or skin irritation (Chotai & Mosenifar, 2022).

The 4 × 4–inch gauze pads are used in the event of chest tube(s) dislodgment. Covering the site immediately and taping the dressing on three sides are essential.

STEP	RATIONALE
b. Inspect the amount and type of drainage by marking the drainage level on the outside of the drainage-collection chamber in hourly or shift increments, or in increments established by the health care provider or per the agency's policy.	Marking the container provides reference point for future measurements. Drainage should decrease gradually and change from bloody to pink to straw colored. Sudden flow of dark bloody drainage that occurs with position change is often old blood (Slaughter, 2024).
c. Observe tubing for kinks, dependent loops, or clots.	Maintains a patent, freely draining system, preventing fluid accumulation in chest cavity. When tubing is coiled, looped, or clotted, drainage is impeded and there is an increased risk for tension pneumothorax or surgical emphysema (Baird, 2023).
d. Verify position of chest drainage system. It should remain upright and below level of tube insertion. Remove gloves and perform hand hygiene.	An upright drainage system facilitates drainage and maintains water seal.
12. Assess patient's knowledge, prior experience with chest tubes, and feelings about procedure.	Reveals need for patient instruction and/or support.

PLANNING

1. Expected outcomes following completion of procedure:	
• Patient is oriented and less anxious.	Hypoxia is relieved.
• Vital signs are stable.	Decreased hypoxia improves vital sign measures.
• Patient reports reduced chest pain.	Reexpansion of lung reduces chest pain.
• Breath sounds are auscultated in all lobes. Lung expansion is symmetrical, SpO_2 is stable or improved, and respirations are unlabored.	Reexpansion of lung promotes normal respirations.
• Chest tube remains in place and free of kinks, and chest drainage system remains airtight.	Indicates correct placement and patency of chest tube drainage system.
• Gentle tidaling (fluctuations or rocking) is evident in water-seal or diagnostic indicator.	Indicates that system is functioning normally. Reflects changes in intrapleural pressure.
2. Provide privacy and explain procedure to patient. Discuss chest tube systems and the patient's role. If applicable, teach patient how to move with chest tube in place.	Protects patient's privacy; reduces anxiety. Promotes cooperation.
3. Organize and set up any equipment needed for chest tube management at bedside	Ensures more efficiency when completing the procedure.

IMPLEMENTATION

1. Confirm informed consent was obtained (if needed). Complete time-out procedure; verify procedure with patient.	Invasive medical procedures typically require informed consent. Time-out is part of Universal Protocol and is completed to determine right patient, procedure, and location of insertion or incision site (Dermenchyan, 2023; TJC, 2023).
2. Review health care provider's order for chest tube placement.	Insertion of the chest tube and setting up the closed drainage system is an interprofessional procedure. To maintain patient safety, each discipline must understand the procedure, expected outcomes, and how to observe for potential complications (Ghazali et al., 2021).
3. Perform hand hygiene. Don appropriate PPE.	Reduces transmission of microorganisms.
4. Set up water-seal or dry suction system; see manufacturer's guidelines.	The water-seal system contains two or three compartments or chambers. Fluid drains into the first chamber. The second chamber contains the water seal, which allows air to escape because of the force of expiration but not to reenter on inspiration. If suction is needed, a third chamber is used.
a. Prepare chest drainage system. Remove wrappers and prepare to set up two- or three-chamber system.	Maintains sterility of system for use under sterile operating room conditions.
b. While maintaining sterility of drainage tubing, stand system upright and add sterile water or NS to appropriate compartments.	Reduces possibility of contamination.
(1) *Two-chamber system (without suction):* Add sterile solution to water-seal chamber (second chamber), bringing fluid to required level as indicated or ordered by health care provider.	Water-seal chamber acts as one-way valve so air cannot enter pleural space (Sasa, 2019; Chotai & Mosenifar, 2022).

STEP	RATIONALE
(2) *Three-chamber system (with suction):* Add sterile solution to water-seal chamber (second chamber). Add amount of sterile solution prescribed by health care provider to suction-control chamber (third chamber), usually 20 cm H$_2$O pressure. Connect tubing from suction-control chamber to suction source. **NOTE:** Suction-control chamber vent must not be occluded when suction is used (see illustration).	Depth of fluid level dictates highest amount of negative pressure that can be present within system. For example, 20 cm of water is approximately 20 cm of water pressure. After chest tube is inserted, turn up the wall or portable suction device until water in suction-control bottle exhibits continuous, gentle bubbling.

Clinical Judgment *When increasing suction, remember that increased bubbling does not result in more suction to the chest cavity but serves only to evaporate the water more quickly. The suction pressure should not exceed −20 cm H$_2$O because lung tissue damage may occur (Chotai & Mosenifar, 2022).*

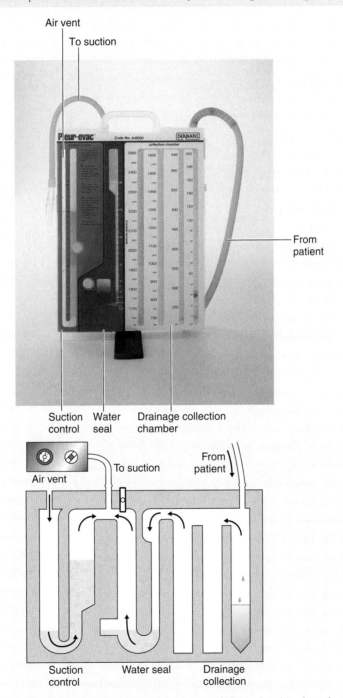

STEP 4b(2) *Top,* Pleur-evac drainage system, a commercial three-chamber chest drainage device. *Bottom,* Schematic of drainage device.

STEP	RATIONALE
(3) *Dry suction system:* Fill water-seal chamber with sterile solution. Adjust suction-control dial to prescribed level of suction; suction ranges from −10 to −40 cm of water pressure. Suction-control chamber vent is never occluded when suction is used. **NOTE:** On dry suction system, **DO NOT** obstruct positive pressure relief valve. This allows air to escape.	Automatic control valve on dry suction-control device adjusts to changes in patient air leaks and fluctuation in suction source and vacuum to deliver prescribed amount of suction.
5. Set up waterless system (see illustration) (see manufacturer's guidelines).	A waterless system is like a water-seal system except that sterile water is not required for suction. The suction-control chamber is replaced by a one-way valve located near the top of the system. The suction-control chamber contains a suction-control float ball that is set by a suction-control dial (Huggins et al., 2023).

6. Secure all system tubing connections with tape in double-spiral fashion using 2.5-cm (1-inch) adhesive tape or zip ties (Parham-Martin bands) with a clamp (Baird, 2023). Check system for patency by:
  a. Clamping drainage tubing that will connect to patient's chest tube.
  b. Connecting tubing from float ball chamber to suction source.
  c. Turning on suction to prescribed level.
	Prevents atmospheric air from leaking into system and patient's intrapleural space. Provides chance to ensure airtight system before connection to patient.

7. Turn off suction source and unclamp drainage tubing before connecting patient to system. Suction source is turned on again after patient is connected. Remove and dispose of gloves.	Having patient connected to suction when it is initiated could damage pleural tissues from sudden increase in negative pressure. Tubing that is coiled or looped may become clotted and cause tension pneumothorax (Baird, 2023).
8. If not already completed (see Assessment), administer premedication such as sedatives or analgesics as ordered.	Reduces patient anxiety and pain during procedure.

Clinical Judgment *During procedure, carefully monitor patient for changes in level of sedation.*

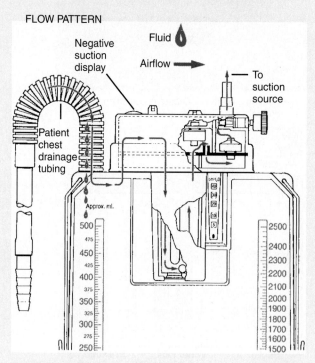

STEP 5 Disposable water-seal chest drainage system with suction.

STEP	RATIONALE
9. Provide psychological support to patient (Chapa & Akintade, 2023).	
a. Reinforce preprocedure explanation.	Reduces patient anxiety and helps complete procedure efficiently.
b. Coach and support patient throughout procedure.	
10. Perform hand hygiene and apply clean gloves. Position patient for tube insertion so side in which tube is to be inserted is accessible to health care provider.	Reduces transmission of microorganisms. For pneumothorax, place patient in lateral supine position. For hemothorax, place patient in semi-Fowler position (Chotai & Mosenifar, 2022). Ensures smooth insertion.
11. Assist health care provider with chest tube insertion by providing needed equipment and local analgesic. Health care provider anesthetizes skin over insertion site, makes small skin incision, inserts clamped tube, sutures it in place, and applies occlusive dressing.	
12. Help health care provider attach drainage tube to chest tube; remove any existing clamp. Turn on suction to prescribed level.	Connects drainage system and suction (if ordered) to chest tube.
13. Tape or zip-tie all connections between chest tube and drainage tube. (**NOTE:** Chest tube is usually taped by health care provider at time of tube placement; check agency policy.)	Secures chest tube to drainage system and reduces risk for air leak that causes breaks in airtight system (Chotai & Mosenifar, 2022).
14. Check systems for proper functioning. Health care provider orders chest x-ray film.	Verifies intrapleural placement of tube.
15. After tube placement, position patient:	Permits optimum drainage of fluid and/or air.
a. Semi-Fowler or high-Fowler position to evacuate air (pneumothorax) (Chotai & Mosenifar, 2022)	
b. High-Fowler position to drain fluid (hemothorax) (Chotai & Mosenifar, 2022)	
16. Check patency of air vents in system.	
a. Water-seal vent must have no occlusion.	Permits displaced air to pass into atmosphere.
b. Suction-control chamber vent is not occluded when suction is used.	Provides safety factor of releasing excess negative pressure into atmosphere.
c. Waterless systems have relief valves without caps.	Provides safety factor of releasing excess negative pressure.
17. Position excess tubing horizontally on mattress next to patient. Secure with clamp that attaches to bottom sheet so it does not obstruct tubing.	Prevents excess tubing from hanging over edge of mattress in dependent loop (Huggins et al., 2023).
18. Adjust tubing to hang in straight line from chest tube to drainage chamber.	Promotes drainage and prevents fluid or blood from accumulating in pleural cavity.

Clinical Judgment *Frequent gentle lifting of the drain allows gravity to help blood and other viscous material to move to the drainage bottle. Patients with recent chest surgery or trauma need to have the chest drain lifted on the basis of assessment of the amount of drainage; some patients might need chest tube drains lifted every 5 to 10 minutes until drainage volume decreases. However, when coiled or dependent looping of tubing is unavoidable, lift the tubing every 15 minutes at a minimum to promote drainage (Baird, 2023).*

STEP	RATIONALE
19. Place two rubber-tipped hemostats (for each chest tube) in easily accessible position (e.g., taped to top of patient's headboard). These should remain with patient when ambulating.	Chest tubes are clamped under specific circumstances: (1) to assess for air leak (Table 26.2), (2) to empty or quickly change disposable systems, (3) to assess whether patient is ready to have tube removed, or (4) if chest tube becomes accidentally disconnected from drainage system (Ignatavicius et al., 2022; Huggins et al., 2023).

Clinical Judgment *In the event of a chest tube disconnection and risk of contamination, submerge the tube 2 to 4 cm (1–2 inches) below the surface of a 250-mL bottle of sterile water or normal saline (NS) until a new chest tube unit can be set up (Harding et al., 2023).*

STEP	RATIONALE
20. Dispose of all contaminated supplies in appropriate receptacle, remove and dispose of gloves, and perform hand hygiene.	Reduces transmission of microorganisms.
21. Care of patient after chest tube insertion:	
a. Perform hand hygiene and apply clean gloves. Assess vital signs; oxygen saturation; pain; skin color; breath sounds; rate, depth, and ease of respirations; and insertion site every 15 minutes for first 2 hours and then at least every shift (see agency policy).	Provides immediate information about procedure-related complications such as respiratory distress and leakage.

STEP	RATIONALE

TABLE 26.2

Solving Problems Related to Chest Tubes

Assessment	Intervention
Air leak can occur at insertion site, at connection between tube and drainage device, or within drainage device itself. Determine when air leak occurs during respiratory cycle (e.g., inspiration or expiration). Continuous bubbling is noted in water-seal chamber that is attached to suction (Slaughter, 2024).	Check all connections between chest tube and drainage system to make sure they are tight. When in doubt, remove tape without disconnecting the tube to inspect connections. Inspect the chest drainage unit for cracks or breaks that can allow air into the system. Leaks are corrected when constant bubbling stops. If present on a chest drainage system such as the Sahara S 1100a Pleur-Evac, observe the air-leak meter to determine the size of the leak.
Assess for location of leak by squeezing the chest drainage tubing between your hands. If the bubbling stops, air leak is inside patient's thorax or at chest insertion site.	Release the pressure on the drainage tube, reinforce chest dressing, and notify health care provider immediately. Leaving chest tube clamped can cause collapse of lung, mediastinal shift, and eventual collapse of other lung from buildup of air pressure within the pleural cavity.
If bubbling continues, it indicates that leak is in the drainage system.	Change the drainage system.
Assess for tension pneumothorax: • Severe respiratory distress • Low oxygen saturation • Chest pain • Absence of breath sounds on affected side • Tracheal shift to unaffected side (seen on inspection or palpated) • Hypotension and signs of shock • Tachycardia	Make sure that chest tubes are patent: remove clamps, eliminate kinks, or eliminate occlusion. Notify health care provider immediately and prepare for another chest tube insertion. A one-way flutter (Heimlich) valve or large-gauge needle may be used for short-term emergency release of pressure in the intrapleural space. Have emergency equipment, oxygen, and code cart available because condition is life threatening.
Water-seal tube is no longer submerged in sterile fluid because of evaporation.	Add sterile water to water-seal chamber until distal tip is 2 cm under surface level. Most chest drainage units are marked at the 2-cm level to indicate the fill line.

   b. For severe pain, medicate with ordered analgesics and use complementary pain-relief methods as needed (e.g., repositioning).

   c. Monitor color, consistency, and amount of chest tube drainage every 15 minutes for first 2 hours. Indicate level of drainage fluid, date, and time on write-on surface of chamber.

    (1) From mediastinal tube, expect less than 100 mL/h immediately after surgery. Persistent excessive bleeding >500 mL/h or >300 mL for 2 to 3 hours indicates the need for further intervention (Good & Kirkwood, 2018).

    (2) From posterior chest tube, drainage is grossly bloody during first several hours after surgery and changes to serous (Harding et al., 2023).

    (3) Expect little or no output from anterior chest tube that is inserted for a pneumothorax (Baird, 2023).

Promotes patient's ability to breathe and fully expand lungs with less discomfort.

Provides baseline for continuous assessment of type and quantity of drainage. Ensures early detection of complications.

Sudden gush of drainage may result from coughing or changing patient's position (i.e., releasing pooled/collected blood rather than indicating active bleeding). Acute bleeding indicates hemorrhage. Notify health care provider if there is more than 500 mL (or per postoperative order) of bloody drainage in an hour (Harding et al., 2023; Good & Kirkwood, 2018).

Acute bleeding indicates hemorrhage. Health care provider should be notified if there is a sudden increase or more than 300 mL over 2 to 3 hours of bloody drainage in an hour (Harding et al., 2023; Good & Kirkwood, 2018).

Clinical Judgment *Routine stripping or milking of the chest tube is not a recommended practice. Doing so can result in increased pressure in the thoracic cavity, causing damage to the lungs or the pleural tissues. If there is a visible clot in the tubing, gentle milking of the tubing (manual squeezing and releasing of parts of the tubing) may be indicated, but only if the patient is at risk of further harm from the clot, such as the development of a tension pneumothorax (Abuejheisheh et al., 2021; Ignatavicius et al., 2022).*

   d. Observe chest dressing for drainage and determine whether it is still occlusive.

Drainage around tube may indicate blockage of the tube. Many health care agencies require the chest tube dressings to be occlusive in nature.

STEP	RATIONALE
e. Inspect condition of skin around adhesive tape for redness, blistering, and edema.	Inspection of skin determines if MARSI has developed (Fumarola et al., 2020).
f. Palpate around tube for swelling and crepitus (subcutaneous emphysema) as indicated by crackling.	Indicates presence of air trapping in subcutaneous tissues. Most occurrences of crepitus are minor, as small amounts are commonly absorbed. Large amounts are potentially dangerous, and the health care provider should be notified (Baird, 2023; Sasa, 2019).

Clinical Judgment *Some patients may develop subcutaneous emphysema (i.e., a collection of air under the skin after chest tube placement), which can occur if tubing is blocked or kinked. When this occurs, a crepitus (a crackling sensation) is felt on palpation of the skin where subcutaneous emphysema has occurred or spread.*

STEP	RATIONALE
g. Check tubing to ensure that it is free of kinks and dependent loops.	Promotes drainage and prevents the development of a tension pneumothorax.
h. Observe for fluctuation of drainage in tubing and water-seal chamber during inspiration and expiration. Observe for clots or debris in tubing.	If fluctuation or tidaling stops, it means that either the lung is fully expanded or the system is obstructed. In patient who is spontaneously breathing, fluid rises in water-seal or diagnostic indicator (waterless system) with inspiration and falls with expiration. The opposite occurs in patient who is mechanically ventilated. This indicates that system is functioning properly (Baird, 2023).
i. Keep drainage system upright and below level of patient's chest.	Promotes gravity drainage and prevents backflow of fluid and air into pleural space.
j. Check for air leaks by monitoring bubbling in water-seal chamber: Intermittent bubbling is normal during expiration when air is being evacuated from pleural cavity, but continuous bubbling during both inspiration and expiration indicates leak in system.	Absence of bubbling may indicate that lung is fully expanded in patient with pneumothorax. Check all connections and locate sources of air leak.
22. Instruct patient on how to regularly take deep breaths and to reposition as often as possible.	Maintains lung expansion.
23. Assist patient to semi- or high-Fowler position. Verify that patient is comfortable.	Facilitates lung expansion and chest tube drainage. Restores comfort and sense of well-being.
24. Raise side rails (as appropriate) and lower bed to lowest position, locking into position.	Ensures patient safety and prevents falls.
25. Place nurse call system in an accessible location within patient's reach.	Ensures patient can call for assistance if needed.
26. Dispose of all contaminated supplies in appropriate receptacle, remove and dispose of gloves, and perform hand hygiene.	Reduces transmission of microorganisms.

EVALUATION

1. Evaluate patient for decreased respiratory distress and chest pain. Auscultate patient's lungs and observe chest expansion.	Determines status of lung expansion.
2. Monitor vital signs and SpO$_2$.	Determines if level of oxygenation has improved.
3. Reassess patient's character of pain and level of severity on scale of 0 to 10, comparing level with comfort before chest tube insertion.	Indicates need for analgesia. Patient with chest tube discomfort hesitates to take deep breaths and as a result is at risk for pneumonia and atelectasis.
4. Evaluate patient's ability to use deep-breathing exercises while maintaining comfort.	Indicates patient's ability to promote lung expansion and prevent complications.
5. Monitor functioning of chest tube system (e.g., reduction in amount of drainage, resolution of air leak, and complete reexpansion of the lung).	Detects early signs of system complications or indicates possible need for removal of chest tube.
6. **Use Teach-Back:** "I want to be sure I explained why you have a chest tube. Tell me the reason why you have it." Revise your instruction now or develop a plan for revised patient/family caregiver teaching if patient/family caregiver is not able to teach back correctly.	Teach-back is a technique for health care providers to ensure that they have explained medical information clearly so that patients and their families understand what is communicated to them (Agency for Healthcare Research and Quality [AHRQ], 2023).

STEP	RATIONALE
Unexpected Outcomes	**Related Interventions**
1. Patient develops respiratory distress. Chest pain, decrease in breath sounds over affected and unaffected lungs, marked cyanosis, asymmetrical chest movements, presence of subcutaneous emphysema around tube insertion site or neck, hypotension, tachycardia, and/or mediastinal shift are critical and indicate severe change in patient status such as excessive blood loss or tension pneumothorax.	• Notify health care provider immediately. • Collect set of vital signs and SpO₂. • Prepare for chest x-ray examination. • Provide oxygen as ordered. • Be sure head of bed is elevated 45 degrees.
2. There is sudden, unexpected chest tube drainage.	• Observe for kink in chest drainage system. • Observe for possible clot in chest drainage system. • Observe for mediastinal shift or respiratory distress (medical emergency). • Notify health care provider.
3. Chest tube is dislodged.	• Immediately apply pressure over chest tube insertion site. • Have assistant obtain sterile petroleum gauze dressing. Apply as patient exhales. Secure dressing with tight seal. Dressing with tape over three of four sides may allow for escape of air if there is residual pneumothorax. • Notify health care provider.

Documentation

- Document respiratory assessment, type of chest tube and drainage device, amount of suction if used, amount and appearance of drainage in chamber, and presence or absence of an air leak.
- Document the integrity of the dressing, color and type of drainage, and condition of skin around tape for comparison between shifts.
- Document level of patient comfort and baseline vital signs, including oxygen saturation.
- Document patient teaching and validation of patient understanding.

Hand-Off Reporting

- Report patient tolerance of chest tube insertion, comfort level and any analgesia, and respiratory assessment before and after chest tube insertion.
- Report the quantity and quality of the chest tube drainage.

Special Considerations

Patient Education

- Instruct patient and family caregivers regarding proper functioning of chest tube and drainage system.
- Instruct patient to call for assistance before getting out of bed if the chest tube is attached to suction.
- Instruct patient to not lie on the tubing or allow it to get kinked to promote drainage).
- Instruct patient to immediately report any changes in chest comfort.
- Instruct patient to call immediately for help if the chest tube becomes dislodged.

Pediatrics

- If possible, using pictures and special dolls, familiarize child and family with equipment before inserting chest drainage system (Hockenberry et al., 2024).
- Chest tube drainage greater than 3 mL/kg/h for more than 3 consecutive hours is excessive and may indicate postoperative hemorrhage. Notify the health care provider immediately (Hockenberry et al., 2024).

Older Adults

- Fragility of the older adult's skin requires special care and planning for management of chest tube dressing. Frequently assess surrounding skin for signs of skin breakdown (Touhy & Jett, 2022).

Populations With Disabilities

- Patients with cognitive, mental, or physical impairments may have limited understanding and may not be able to tolerate their chest tube devices (Sullivan, 2018). Consider the need for use of soft restraints to ensure patient safety and prevention of patient removal of chest tube. Restraints will require health care provider order.
- Frequent nursing assessments should be done on these patients to assess for dyspnea and sputum retention due to ineffective cough (Porcel, 2018). Bronchoscopic suctioning may be required.

Home Care

- Patients with chronic conditions (e.g., uncomplicated pneumothorax, effusions, empyema) that require long-term chest tube placement may be discharged with smaller mobile drains (Sasa, 2019).
- Teach patient how to ambulate and remain active with a mobile chest tube drainage system.
- Instruct patient and family caregivers about when to contact health care provider or seek emergency medical care regarding changes in the drainage system (e.g., chest pain, breathlessness, change in color or amount of drainage, leakage on the dressing around the chest tube).
- Provide patient and family caregiver with information specific to the type of drain; when possible have patient demonstrate proper maintenance of the mobile drainage system. Most of these systems do not have a suction-control chamber and use a mechanical one-way valve instead of a water-seal chamber (Sasa, 2019).

✦ SKILL 26.2 Assisting With Removal of Chest Tubes

Removal of a chest tube is most often the function of a physician or health care provider such as a physician's assistant or advanced practice nurse (check agency policy). Prepare a patient for chest tube removal by assessing the need for pre-removal analgesia, obtaining the required medication orders, and instructing the patient about the process and what will be requested. There has been debate about the optimal timing of chest tube removal in relation to the respiratory cycle (Choi et al., 2021). The primary goal of chest tube removal is removal of the tubes without introducing air into the pleural space. Studies have shown that removal either at the end of inspiration or at the end of expiration does not affect the outcome (Huggins et al., 2023).

Make sure that the patient receives pain medication at least 30 minutes before removal. Some pain during chest tube removal is expected, and it is essential that patients practice how to exhale during removal so that they do not accidentally gasp during removal (Huggins et al., 2023). Instruct the patient to exhale while bearing down in a Valsalva maneuver (Patterson, 2022). An occlusive dressing is applied immediately after tube removal to maintain a tight seal.

An unplanned removal of the chest tube, such as the tube being accidentally removed while repositioning a patient, requires you to cover the site with a gloved hand and ask for help in retrieving supplies to cover the site. Petrolatum gauze, dry gauze, and tape will be needed to dress the site. If the chest tube becomes disconnected from the drainage system, clamp the tubing with a shodded hemostat or crimp the tubing with a gloved hand to prevent air from entering the pleural space. Ask for someone to get a new chest drainage system immediately and attach it to the chest tube in a sterile manner. **Do Not Keep Tube Clamped for an Extended Period.** Regardless of how the tube comes out, monitor the patient for signs of respiratory distress and auscultate lung sounds (Ignatavicius et al., 2022).

Delegation

The skill of assisting with removal of chest tubes cannot be delegated to assistive personnel (AP). Direct the AP to:
- Immediately report to the nurse any patient sensations of shortness of breath, increased chest pain, dizziness, or increased anxiety before and after procedure
- Report to the nurse any drainage on the dressing placed over the chest tube site

Interprofessional Collaboration

- The health care team, which includes physicians, physician assistants, and advanced practice nurses, determines chest tube removal based on individualized patient assessment.

Equipment

- Suture removal set
- Antiseptic swabs (chlorhexidine gluconate with alcohol)
- Sterile scissors
- Sterile forceps
- Clean gloves
- Sterile gloves
- Face mask/face shield
- Prepared sterile dressing: petrolatum-impregnated gauze, 4 × 4–inch gauze dressings, and large dressings (two to four)
- Rubber-tipped Kelly clamps
- 4-inch adhesive tape or elastic bandage (Elastoplast) cut into strips
- Stethoscope, sphygmomanometer, pulse oximeter
- Waterproof pad

STEP	RATIONALE
ASSESSMENT	
1. Identify patient using at least two identifiers (e.g., name and birthday or name and medical record number) according to agency policy.	Ensures correct patient. Complies with The Joint Commission standards and improves patient safety (TJC, 2023).
2. Review patient's electronic health record (EHR) regarding health care order, patient response to chest tube, and status of tube functioning.	Identifies any patient data relevant to preparation for chest tube removal.
3. Review EHR to determine patient's age and history of dehydration, malnutrition, exposure to radiation therapy, underlying chronic conditions (e.g., diabetes mellitus, immunosuppression), and edema of the skin.	Common risk factors for medical adhesive–related skin injury (MARSI) (Fumarola et al., 2020).
4. Assess patient's/family caregiver's health literacy.	Determines degree to which individuals have the ability to find, understand, and use information and services to make informed health-related decisions and actions for themselves and others (CDC, 2023).
5. Perform hand hygiene. Perform respiratory assessment and gather measures for indication of lung reexpansion.	Reduces transmission of microorganisms. Assesses for lung expansion.
a. Provide health care provider with results of most recent chest x-ray study.	Reveals position of lung tissue in chest cavity and whether sufficient lung reexpansion has occurred (Huggins et al., 2023).
b. Note trend in water-seal fluctuation over last 24 hours. Determine if bubbling is present.	Pleura of expanded lung seals the holes on internal tip of chest tube, halting fluctuation in water seal. Halt in fluctuation for 24 hours indicates that lung is expanded. When bubbling is present, it usually indicates that lung has not fully expanded (Huggins et al., 2023).

STEP	RATIONALE
c. Confirm that drainage has decreased to less than 50 to 100 mL/day (Patterson, 2022).	Pleural drainage was removed, allowing lung to reexpand.
d. Percuss lung for resonance (see Chapter 6).	Normal resonance occurs with reexpansion.
e. Auscultate lung sounds (see Chapter 6).	Normal breath sounds are heard bilaterally with reexpansion.

Clinical Judgment *If the following occur prior to the removal process, notify health care provider; removal of chest tube may be delayed:*
- *New or increasing air leaks in the chest or around the chest tube insertion site*
- *Any increase in excessive drainage (>100 mL/h)*
- *Signs and/or symptoms of increasing respiratory distress, pneumothorax, cardiac tamponade, or hemothorax*
- *Absence of or decline in reexpansion of lungs as shown on chest radiograph*

6. Assess patient's skin around and under chest tube insertion site for skin injury.	Medical adhesives are used to secure the chest tube dressing in place. These adhesives increase a patient's risk for MARS (Fumarola et al., 2020).
7. Assess patient's character of pain and rate severity on a scale of 0 to 10 and determine when last analgesic medication was given.	Chest tube removal is often painful; additional analgesia or breathing exercises are often necessary (Huggins et al., 2023).
8. Assess patient's knowledge, prior experience with chest tube removal, and feelings about procedure.	Reveals need for patient instruction and/or support.

PLANNING

1. Expected outcomes following completion of procedure:	
• Lung reexpansion is achieved.	Source of air or fluid loss is sealed or has healed.
• Patient does not experience discomfort.	Pain management is achieved.
• Spontaneous healing of chest tube insertion site occurs after removal of tube without infection or other complications.	Large, nonporous occlusive dressing at puncture site promotes uncomplicated healing.
2. Plan to administer prescribed medication for pain relief about 30 minutes before procedure.	Reduces discomfort and relaxes patient. Medication reaches peak effect at time of tube removal. Patients report sensations ranging from pain to pulling when chest tube is removed (Chotai & Mosenifar, 2022).
3. Provide privacy and explain procedure to patient.	Protects patient's privacy; reduces anxiety. Promotes cooperation.
4. Organize and set up equipment for chest tube removal at bedside.	Ensures more efficiency when completing the procedure.

IMPLEMENTATION

1. Perform hand hygiene and apply clean gloves and face shield and other personal protective equipment (PPE) as needed.	Reduces transmission of microorganisms.
2. Perform time-out procedure with health care provider to verify patient identification, planned procedure, and correct tube(s), and that chest tube is visible and patient position is correct.	The time-out step is intended to reliably identify patient as individual for whom procedure is intended and to match procedure to patient (TJC, 2023).
3. Help patient to sitting position on edge of bed, lying supine or on side without chest tubes. Place pad under chest tube site.	Health care provider prescribes patient's position to facilitate tube removal. Pad absorbs any drainage associated with tube removal.
4. Assist health care provider with preparation and procedure:	
a. Assist with discontinuing suction from chest-drainage system, and check for air leaks while patient coughs.	Bubbling in the air leak detector is associated with an air leak. When an air leak is present, removal of the chest tube may cause development of a pneumothorax.
b. Assist with gently removing existing tape, and clean area around tubes with antiseptic wipe.	Allows access to the chest tube at the skin level and prepares the sutures for removal.
c. Assist with clamping each tube to be removed with two Kelly clamps or clamp associated with chest-drainage setup.	Clamping chest tube before removal to assess patient's tolerance is controversial. This is based on preventing air from being introduced into the pleural space. Follow agency policy regarding clamping of chest tube at this time (Harding et al., 2023).

Clinical Judgment *Do not attempt to remove an adhesive medical device with one swift action. Fast, vertical pulling not only is more painful, but it also generates a higher peel force than slow removal. In addition, the adhesive product is likely to fold onto itself (Fumarola et al., 2020).*

STEP	RATIONALE
5. Assist health care provider in preparing an occlusive dressing of petrolatum-impregnated gauze on pressure dressing. Set it aside on sterile field while provider applies sterile gloves.	Essential to prepare in advance for quick application to wound on tube withdrawal.
6. Support patient physically and emotionally while health care provider removes dressing and clips sutures.	Patients state that when they know that the tube is being pulled, they can mentally prepare themselves for the procedure. Support from health care team reduces anxiety and promotes cooperation.
7. Health care provider asks patient to exhale completely and hold it while bearing down (Valsalva maneuver).	Prevents air from being sucked into chest as tube is removed (Huggins et al., 2023). A complication associated with removal of chest tubes is recurrent pneumothorax, which results from atmospheric air reentering pleural cavity. This occurs when patient inhales during tube removal.
8. Health care provider quickly pulls out chest tube. *Option:* may tighten and tie purse-string suture (if present), after which patient is instructed to breathe normally.	This forms an airtight seal and prevents entry of air through chest wound. Sutures aid in skin closure (Baird, 2023). Purse-string may not be used so that any blood near insertion site can drain out before dressing is applied.
9. Health care provider applies sterile occlusive dressing over wound and firmly secures it in position with wide tape. Assist as needed.	Keeps wound aseptic. Prevents entry of air into chest. Wound closure occurs spontaneously.
10. Health care provider inspects end of chest tube(s) before disposal to ensure entire removal.	On rare occasions, chest tube is damaged by instruments, surgical wires, or manipulation, which can lead to its breakage during removal. Inspection of end of chest tube helps to verify that all of tube was removed (Baird, 2023).
11. Help patient to upright position supported by pillows or in comfortable position.	Restores patient's comfort. Following chest tube removal, it is important that the patient be in a comfortable position and able to expand lungs with each breath. High- or semi-Fowler position is often preferred. Patients report that proper positioning following chest tube removal helps to relieve procedure-related sensations of pain and pulling (Chotai & Mosenifar, 2022).
12. Assess the patient's condition and level of comfort immediately after the procedure and compare with preprocedure findings.	Ensures stable respiratory status after the procedure.
13. Raise side rails (as appropriate) and lower bed to lowest position, locking into position.	Ensures patient safety and prevents falls.
14. Place nurse call system in an accessible location within patient's reach.	Ensures patient can call for assistance if needed.
15. Dispose of all contaminated supplies in appropriate receptacle, remove and dispose of gloves, and perform hand hygiene.	Reduces transmission of microorganisms.

EVALUATION

1. Auscultate lung sounds.	Helps to confirm that lung remains expanded.
2. Palpate skin over area where tube was inserted for subcutaneous emphysema and inspect for redness, inflammation, and blistering.	Subcutaneous emphysema results from entrance of air into subcutaneous space. It is painful, and as a result patient may not take full lung expansion (Baird, 2023). Skin irritation and damage are signs of MARSI (Fumarola et al., 2020).
3. Evaluate vital signs, oxygen saturation, and ventilatory movement to detect signs of respiratory distress after tube removal and during first few hours after removal.	Provides for early notification of health care provider if adverse symptoms or complications occur. Chest tubes may need reinsertion.

Clinical Judgment *If air is heard escaping from the chest tube site, reinforce the occlusive dressing and immediately notify health care provider.*

4. Evaluate patient's psychological status.	Determines level of patient's overall comfort or anxiety.
5. Review chest x-ray film, if ordered.	Evidence does not support routine postremoval x-rays in either adults or pediatric/neonatal patients (Huggins et al., 2023). If complications are noted, bedside ultrasound imaging or computed tomography (CT) scan, which is better at identifying the chest cavity, may be ordered.

STEP	RATIONALE
6. Evaluate character of patient's pain and level of severity on a scale of 0 to 10. Observe for nonverbal cues of pain.	Indicates that wound did not close well. Determines patient's tolerance of procedure.
7. Check chest dressing for drainage (see agency policy). When changing dressing, note wound for signs of healing.	Ensures occlusion and proper healing of chest wound. **NOTE:** Dressing is usually not changed initially for 1 to 2 days.
8. **Use Teach-Back:** "I want to be sure I explained what we are going to do as we remove your chest tube. Tell me in your own words what we plan to do and what you expect." Revise your instruction now or develop a plan for revised patient/family caregiver teaching if the patient/family caregiver is not able to teach back correctly.	Teach-back is a technique for health care providers to ensure that they have explained medical information clearly so that patients and their families understand what is communicated to them (AHRQ, 2023).

Unexpected Outcomes	Related Interventions
1. Dyspnea and labored respirations noted after chest tube removal; potential recurrence of pneumothorax, hemothorax, or effusion.	• Notify health care provider. • Obtain vital signs and oxygen saturation and administer supplemental oxygen as ordered. • Stay with patient.
2. Infection is noted at insertion site.	• Prepare for possible chest tube removal and possible reinsertion (Baird, 2023). • Assess patient's vital signs for elevated temperature, tachypnea, and tachycardia. Assess wound for drainage, odor, erythema, or increased pain. • Obtain wound culture.
3. MARSI results from adhesive exposure as evidenced by inflammation, edema, blistering, or skin tear.	• Provide good skin care by avoiding washing skin too often, hydrating skin, avoiding use of alcohol-based products, and handling the skin gently (Fumarola et al., 2020). • Refer to wound care specialist if blister or skin tear exists (see Chapter 38). • Provide pain management as needed (Fumarola et al., 2020).

Documentation

• Document removal of tube; amount and appearance of drainage in the collection bottle; appearance of wound, surrounding skin, and dressing; and patient's response/tolerance and understanding of the procedure.
• Document vital signs and respiratory assessment.
• Document the results of chest radiograph and any unexpected outcomes.
• Document patient learning.

Hand-Off Reporting

• Report patient tolerance of chest tube removal, comfort level and any analgesia, and respiratory assessment before and after chest tube removal.
• Report any persistent bleeding, crepitus, purulent drainage, tenderness, or warmth at the site.
• Report any continued or severe pain despite pain interventions.
• Report chest radiograph results.
• Report unexpected outcomes to nurse in charge or health care provider.

Special Considerations

Patient Education

• Instruct patient and family caregiver to immediately report signs of chest pain, shortness of breath, or sensations of chest discomfort.

Pediatrics

• Pediatric patients usually require analgesia before chest tube removal (Hockenberry et al., 2024).

• Eutectic mixture of local anesthetics (EMLA; locally applied lidocaine/prilocaine anesthetic patch) placed under an occlusive dressing at the chest tube insertion site 1 hour before tube removal reduces pain of procedure. However, child may still feel the "pulling" sensation (Hockenberry et al., 2024).

Older Adults

• Fragility of the older adult's skin requires special care and planning for management of chest tube dressing removal. Frequently assess surrounding skin for signs of MARSI.

Populations With Disabilities

• Patients with cognitive, mental, or physical impairments may have limited understanding and/or tolerance and may not be able to tolerate the chest tube removal process.
• Frequent nursing assessments should be done on these patients to assess for dyspnea and sputum retention due to ineffective cough (Porcel, 2018). Bronchoscopic suctioning may be required.

Home Care

• Teach patient the importance of ambulating and remaining active once the chest tube has been removed.
• Instruct patient and family caregivers about when to contact health care provider regarding changes to the patient's skin around the chest tube removal site (e.g., chest pain, breathlessness, change in color or amount of drainage, leakage on the dressing from the chest tube removal site).
• Provide patient and family caregiver information specific to the type of wound care needed; when possible, have patient demonstrate proper wound care (Sasa, 2019).

✦ SKILL 26.3 Autotransfusion of Chest Tube Drainage

Autotransfusion (AT) is when the patient's own blood is collected and transfused back; this is an established alternative to donor blood transfusion (Palmqvist et al., 2022). In autotransfusion, shed blood from the patient is collected, filtered, and reinfused. Shed blood is collected from the chest tube or the operative field and reinfused immediately (Baird, 2023). Autotransfusion is commonly used for trauma patients as well as patients undergoing cardiothoracic procedures. When bloody chest drainage from the mediastinal or pleural space is reinfused using special equipment made for that purpose, it is a relatively risk-free, inexpensive, and easy method of replacing blood. Benefits of autotransfusion include an immediate blood supply, little risk of transfusion reaction and disease transmission, and the ability to supply more oxygen to vital organs (McGinty, 2017). Patients must also have a patent intravenous (IV) line in place (see Chapter 28). Autotransfusion may be contraindicated in patients with coagulation disorders, infections, or cancer; however, the decision for autotransfusion in these patients is made on a case-by-case basis and includes the patient's current physiological status (Frank et al., 2020). It is also contraindicated with blood that has been in the collection system for longer than institutional standards allow, and in the presence of preexisting liver or kidney dysfunction. However, any of these contraindications can be overruled if the patient is exsanguinating and there is not an adequate supply of banked blood available (McGinty, 2017).

Delegation

The skill of autotransfusion of chest tube drainage cannot be delegated to assistive personnel (AP). Direct the AP to:
- Immediately inform nurse of changes in patient's vital signs or pulse oximetry (SpO_2) levels
- Immediately inform nurse about increased or decreased drainage from chest tube

Interprofessional Collaboration

- The health care team including physicians, physician assistants, and advanced practice nurses are responsible for determining when autotransfusion is used and assisting with setting up the equipment.

Equipment

- Adult/pediatric single-use chest drainage and agency autotransfusion (AT) system unit
- *Optional:* Continuous AT system with a blood-compatible infusion pump (check agency policy)
- Microaggregate blood filter (40-μm filter; see manufacturer's instructions)
- Nonvented blood-compatible IV administration set
- Normal saline
- Antiseptic swab
- Infusion pump (see manufacturer's instructions)
- PPE: Gown, clean gloves, face shield, and mask as needed

STEP	RATIONALE
ASSESSMENT	
1. Identify patient using at least two identifiers (e.g., name and birthday or name and medical record number) according to agency policy. Compare identifiers with information on patient's medication administration record (MAR) or electronic health record (EHR).	Ensures correct patient. Complies with The Joint Commission standards and improves patient safety (TJC, 2023).
2. Review patient's EHR regarding history of coagulation disorders, cancer, active infection, and kidney or liver disease, including health care provider's order and nurses' notes.	Conditions may contraindicate procedure. Verifies health care provider's order and identifies any pertinent patient data prior to procedure.

Clinical Judgment *Notify health care provider of any change in the patient's baseline condition/assessment findings, new onset of clots, sudden decrease or absence of drainage, or concern for infection or septicemia (Palmqvist et al., 2022; Frank et al., 2020).*

3. Assess patient's/family caregiver's health literacy.	Determines degree to which individuals have the ability to find, understand, and use information and services to make informed health-related decisions and actions for themselves and others (CDC, 2023).
4. See Assessment for Skill 26.1.	
5. Determine presence of active bleeding (at least 100 mL/h) through an existing chest tube or collection of more than 300 mL in a collection system (McGinty, 2017).	Indicates need for possible reinfusion of chest tube drainage.

Clinical Judgment *Reinfuse blood within 6 hours of collection and ensure that the transfusion is complete within 4 hours of starting it (McGinty, 2017). Check agency policy.*

6. Perform hand hygiene. Assess IV site (see Chapter 28). Note size of IV catheter; 18-gauge angiocatheter preferred.	Determines presence of adequate and patent IV site for administration of blood products.
7. Obtain baseline laboratory data (e.g., hemoglobin and hematocrit).	Provides data to measure effectiveness of reinfusion of chest drainage on patient's circulating blood volume.
8. Assess patient's knowledge, prior experience with autotransfusion, and feelings about procedure.	Reveals need for patient instruction and/or support.

STEP	RATIONALE

PLANNING

1. Expected outcomes following completion of procedure:
   - Vital signs, hematocrit, and hemoglobin stabilize.

   - Drainage system functions correctly and lung reexpands in 48 to 72 hours.
   - IV line remains patent.

2. Provide privacy and explain procedure to patient.
3. Organize and set up equipment for autotransfusion at bedside.

Reinfusion reduces significant blood loss associated with closed chest drainage.

Negative pressure is reestablished in intrapleural space.

Patent IV is necessary for reinfusion of cleansed mediastinal tube drainage.

Protects patient's privacy; reduces anxiety. Promotes cooperation.

Ensures more efficiency when completing the procedure.

IMPLEMENTATION

1. Perform hand hygiene and apply clean gloves and mask and/or face shield and other PPE as needed.

Reduces transmission of microorganisms.

2. Prepare AT System:
   a. Follow manufacturer's guidelines and agency policy.
   b. Make certain that all connections are tight and all clamps are open.
   c. A 200-μm double-sided mesh filter is located in AT bag to filter drainage (Palmqvist et al., 2022) (check manufacturer's instructions).

   d. The AT system collection bag has capacity of 1000 mL marked in increments of 25 mL and an area for marking times and amounts.

Ensure safe autotransfusion procedure.

Tight connections ensure airtight system, and open clamps allow chest drainage to enter AT system bag.

Filters should be used when transfusing salvaged blood. Filters remove extraneous materials and microemboli (Frank et al., 2020). In obstetric emergencies, a filter reduces the risk for amniotic emboli (Palmqvist et al., 2022; Frank et al., 2020).

Dark red drainage is expected only during immediate postoperative period. This drainage turns serous over time.

Clinical Judgment *Continuous autotransfusion may be prescribed following cardiac surgery. This is a closed system with a specific infusion pump and intravenous (IV) circuit. This system requires specific education and is used in selected situations. Check agency policy.*

3. Prepare chest drainage for reinfusion.
   a. Following manufacturer's directions, open replacement bag and close two white clamps.

   b. Use high-negativity relief valve to reduce excessive negativity.
   c. Bag transfer:
      (1) Close clamps on chest drainage tubing.

      (2) Close clamps on top of initial AT system collection bag.
      (3) Connect chest drainage tube to new AT system bag.
      (4) Make certain that all connections are tight.
      (5) Open all clamps on chest drainage tube and replacement bag.
   d. Connect connectors on top of initial collection bag and remove bag by lifting it from side hook and then from foot hook.
   e. Secure replacement bag by connecting foot hook, replacing metal frame into side hook of chest drainage unit (CDU), and pushing down to secure frame onto hook.
   f. Place thumbs on top of metal frame and push up with fingers to slide bag out; remove replacement bag.
4. Reinfuse chest drainage.
   a. Use new microaggregate filter to reinfuse each autotransfusion bag.
   b. Access bag by inverting it, wiping off port with antiseptic swab, and spiking through port with microaggregate filter by twisting.
   c. With bag upside down, gently squeeze it to remove air and prime filter with blood.

Contamination of unit provides ready source of contamination to patient. Closed clamps maintain closed system during replacement.

This eases removal of initial collection bag from metal support stand.

Prevents air from entering chest cavity through tube and collapsing lung.

Maintains closed system for reinfusion, preventing contamination of blood.

Establishes new autotransfusion.

Ensures airtight system.

Reestablishes autotransfusion.

Maintains closed system within bag and removes it for use in autotransfusion.

Provides safe attachment of replacement bag to CDU.

Prevents infusion of microemboli and provides maximal filtration for each bag.

Connects autotransfusion bag to transfusion tubing.

Gentle pressure is used to prevent hemolysis.

STEP	RATIONALE
d. Hang bag on IV pole and continue to prime tubing until all air is gone. Clamp tubing, attach it to patient's IV access, and adjust clamp to deliver reinfusion at appropriate rate.	Removes all air from transfusion tubing. Reinfusion is delivered by gravity, application of a blood cuff (not to exceed 150 mm Hg pressure), or blood-compatible IV pump (see Chapter 28).
e. If ordered, anticoagulants (sodium citrate, citrate-phosphate-dextrose-adenine [CPDA], heparin) are added to reinfusion through self-sealing port in autotransfusion connector (Palmqvist et al., 2022).	Prevents clotting in autotransfusion. Reversing heparin with protamine to preoperative levels or collection of nonheparinized blood following emergency chest trauma may require a citrate anticoagulant (Palmqvist et al., 2022).
f. Monitor patient's vital signs and SpO_2 according to patient condition and agency policy. For some patients this may be as frequently as every 15 minutes; for other patients it may be every hour.	Patients who require autotransfusion usually have complex physiological needs, and their vital signs change quite rapidly. Consistent, frequent monitoring allows for timely identification of changes and initiation of appropriate interventions to restore physiological stability.
5. Help patient to a comfortable position.	Restores comfort and sense of well-being.
6. Raise side rails (as appropriate) and lower bed to lowest position, locking into position.	Ensures patient safety and prevents falls.
7. Place nurse call system in an accessible location within patient's reach.	Ensures patient can call for assistance if needed.
8. Dispose of all contaminated supplies in appropriate receptacle, remove and dispose of gloves and other PPE, and perform hand hygiene.	Reduces transmission of microorganisms.

EVALUATION

1. Monitor vital signs every 15 minutes for the first hour and then according to agency policy, hematocrit, and hemoglobin.	Helps determine effects of treatment.
2. Monitor chest drainage system and patient's lung sounds.	Helps determine proper functioning of system and its effectiveness.
3. Evaluate IV infusion site for infiltration and phlebitis.	Patent IV infusion site is maintained.
4. Use Teach-Back: "I want to be sure I explained why you needed to receive this blood. Tell me why this was important." Revise your instruction now or develop a plan for revised patient/family caregiver teaching if patient/family caregiver is not able to teach back correctly.	Teach-back is a technique for health care providers to ensure that they have explained medical information clearly so that patients and their families understand what is communicated to them (AHRQ, 2023).

Unexpected Outcomes	Related Interventions
1. Chest tube is dislodged.	• Immediately apply pressure over chest tube insertion site. • Have assistant apply sterile petrolatum-impregnated occlusive dressing. • Notify health care provider.
2. Patient has dyspnea, chest pain, and labored respirations.	• Verify that chest tube is patent and draining. • Obtain vital signs. • Notify health care provider.
3. Patient has signs of infection, fever, and chills.	• Notify health care provider. • Obtain wound cultures as ordered. • Obtain vital signs. • Stop infusion. • Maintain a patent IV site.

Documentation

- Document drainage and reinfusion with times and amounts of each; include patient's response to reinfusion.
- Document condition of IV infusion site.
- Document patient teaching and validation of understanding.

Hand-Off Reporting

- Report to health care provider any drainage >200 mL/h, new-onset clots, absence of drainage, or any unexpected outcomes.

Special Considerations

Patient Education

- Prepare patient and family caregivers for the procedure so they will understand when the patient's blood is reinfused. Patients and their families may have had this instruction before surgery but need reinforcement.

Older Adults

- Pulmonary edema due to transfusion-associated circulatory or volume overload may occur, especially in patients with compromised cardiac function (Touhy & Jett, 2022).

◆ CLINICAL JUDGMENT AND NEXT-GENERATION NCLEX® EXAMINATION–STYLE QUESTIONS

The nurse in the intensive care unit is caring for a patient following surgery who has right pleural and mediastinal chest tubes to drainage. Vital signs: T 37.2°C (99.0°F) rectally; HR 90 beats/min; RR 16 breaths/min; BP 110/64 mm Hg. SpO_2 95% on 2 L of oxygen. The most recent hourly chest tube drainage was 75 mL from the pleural tube and 100 mL from the mediastinal tube. When the patient is transferred from the bed to a chair, the nurse notes drainage of 50 mL of dark red fluid, fluctuation of water in the water-seal chamber when the patient breathes in and out, and bubbling in the suction-control chamber.

1. Which action will the nurse take at this time?
   1. Contact the Rapid Response Team.
   2. Document the findings.
   3. Notify the surgeon of hemorrhage.
   4. Remove the chest tubes immediately.

2. The patient pushes the nurse call system to report something wrong with the chest tube. On arrival to the room, the nurse notices that the drainage system has fallen on its side and is leaking drainage onto the floor from a crack in the system. Which action will the nurse perform *first*?
   1. Notify the health care provider.
   2. Obtain a new drainage system.
   3. Disconnect the tubing from the drainage system.
   4. Insert the tubing 2.5 cm (1 inch) below the surface of a bottle of sterile water.

3. A new system for the patient has been obtained and implemented. When the patient is 12 hours postoperative, which assessment finding requires the nurse to intervene?
   1. Drainage from both chest tubes of 60 mL/h each
   2. Temporary increase in drainage when the patient coughs
   3. Small air leak within the first hour of insertion
   4. Sudden cessation of bleeding

4. The health care provider is preparing to remove the patient's chest tubes. Which of the following actions will the nurse perform when assisting? **Select all that apply.**
   1. Gather supplies needed for the procedure.
   2. Premedicate the patient with pain medicine prior to the tube removal as ordered.
   3. Place the patient in semi-Fowler position.
   4. Have the patient take a deep breath, exhale, and bear down during removal of the tube.
   5. Stay with the patient and provide emotional support during the procedure.
   6. Place a petroleum gauze over the site where the tube was removed.
   7. Clean with alcohol the site where the drain was located.

5. The patient follows up with the surgeon as an outpatient 1 week after discharge. Which finding indicates to the nurse that hospital nursing and collaborative interventions were effective?
   1. Clear breath sounds auscultated
   2. SpO_2 91% on room air
   3. Chest tube insertion site draining pus
   4. Respiratory rate 24 breaths/min

Visit the Evolve site for Answers to Clinical Judgment and Next-Generation NCLEX® Examination–Style Questions.

REFERENCES

Abuejheisheh A, et al: Chest drains: prevalence of insertion and ICU nurses' knowledge of care, *Heliyon* 7(8):e00719, 2021.

Agency for Healthcare Research and Quality (AHRQ): *Teach-back: intervention*, 2023. https://www.ahrq.gov/patient-safety/reports/engage/interventions/teachback.html.

Baird MS: *Manual of critical care nursing*, ed 8, St. Louis, 2023, Elsevier.

Banasik J, Copstead L: *Pathophysiology*, ed 6, St. Louis, 2019, Elsevier.

Basler J, Englund H: Chest tubes: importance of connecting the dots for students using simulation and theory, *Teach Learn Nursing* 15:201, 2020.

Broder JS, et al: Pigtail catheter insertion error: root cause analysis and recommendations for patient safety, *J Emerg Med* 58(3):464, 2020.

Centers for Disease Control and Prevention (CDC): *What is health literacy?* 2023. https://www.cdc.gov/healthliteracy/learn/index.html.

Chapa D, Akintade B: Psychosocial aspects of critical care. In Hartjes T, editors: *AACN core curriculum for progressive and critical care nursing*, ed 8, St. Louis, 2023, Elsevier.

Choi J, et al: Scoping review of traumatic hemothorax: evidence and knowledge gaps, from diagnosis to chest tube removal, *Surgery* 170(4):1260–1267, 2021.

Chotai P, Mosenifar Z. *Tube thoracostomy management*, 2022, Medscape. https://emedicine.medscape.com/article/1503275-overview?form=fpf. Accessed October 7, 2023.

Dermenchyan A: Professional caring and ethical practice. In Hartjes, T, editors: *AACN core curriculum for progressive and critical care nursing*, ed 8. St. Louis, 2023, Elsevier.

Frank SM, et al: Clinical utility of autologous salvaged blood: a review, *J Gastrointest Surg* 24:464, 2020.

Fumarola S: Overlooked and underestimated: medical adhesive–related skin injuries, Best practice consensus document on prevention, *J Wound Care* 29(Suppl 3c):S1–S24, 2020.

Ghazali D, et al: Interdisciplinary teamwork for chest tube insertion and management: an integrative review, *Anaesthesiol Intensive Ther* 53(5):456, 2021.

Good VS, Kirkwood PL: *Advanced critical care nursing*, ed 2, St. Louis, 2018, Elsevier.

Gomez LP, Tran V: *Hemothorax*, 2021, StatPearls. https://www.ncbi.nlm.nih.gov/books/NBK538219/. Accessed October 6, 2023.

Harding M, et al: *Lewis's medical-surgical nursing: assessment and management of clinical problems*, ed 12, St. Louis, 2023, Elsevier.

Hartjes T: *AACN core curriculum for progressive and critical care nursing*, ed 8, St. Louis, 2023, Elsevier.

Hockenberry MJ, et al: *Wong's nursing care of infants and children*, ed 12, St. Louis, 2024, Elsevier.

Huggins J, et al: *Thoracostomy tubes and catheters: indications and tube selection in adults and children*, UpToDate, 2023. https://www.uptodate.com/contents/thoracostomy-tubes-and-catheters-indications-and-tube-selection-in-adults-and-children. Accessed June 15, 2023.

Ignatavicius D, et al: *Medical-surgical nursing: concepts for interprofessional collaborative care*, ed 10, St. Louis, 2022. Elsevier.

Khan A, et al: All over the map: identifying best practices for chest tube management in pneumothorax, *Chest* 2021, Annual meeting 2021.

McGinty K: Autotransfusion. In Weigand D, editor: *AACN procedure manual for critical care*, ed 7, St. Louis, 2017, Elsevier.

Mitsui S, et al: Low suction on digital drainage devices promptly improves postoperative air leaks following lung resection operations: a retrospective study, *J Cardiothorac Surg* 16:105, 2021.

Palmqvist M, et al: Autotransfusion in low-resource settings: a scoping review, *BMJ Open* 12:e056018, 2022. doi:10.1136/bmjopen-2021-056018.

Patterson M: Several important issues in the diagnosis and treatment of chest trauma, *J Contemp Med Pract* 4(3):146–153, 2022.

Patton K, et al: *Anatomy & physiology*, ed 11, St. Louis. 2022. Elsevier.

Porcel JM: Chest tube drainage of the pleural space: a concise review for pulmonologists, *Tuberc Respir Dis (Seoul)* 81(2):106–115, 2018.

Ritchie M, et al: Chest tubes: indications, sizing, placement, and management, *Clin Pulm Med* 24(1):37–53, 2017.

Slaughter C: Chest tube placement (assist). In Johnson KL, editor: *AACN procedure manual for progressive and critical care*, ed 8, St. Louis, 2024, Elsevier.

Sullivan WF, et al: Primary care of adults with intellectual and developmental disabilities: 2018 Canadian consensus guidelines, *Can Fam Physician* 64:254, 2018.

The Joint Commission (TJC): *2023 National Patient Safety Goals*, Oakbrook Terrace, IL, 2023, The Joint Commission. https://www.jointcommission.org/standards/national-patient-safety-goals/.

Touhy TA, Jett K: *Ebersole & Hess' gerontological nursing & healthy aging*, ed 6, St. Louis, 2022, Elsevier.

Urden LD, et al: *Priorities in critical care nursing*, ed 9, St. Louis, 2024, Elsevier.

Williams E, et al: Study protocol for DICE trial: Video-assisted thoracoscopic surgery decortication versus interventional radiology guided chest tube insertion for the management of empyema, *Contemp Clin Trials Commun* 22:100777, 2021.

27 | Emergency Measures for Life Support

SKILLS AND PROCEDURES

Skill 27.1 **Inserting an Oropharyngeal Airway, p. 824**

Skill 27.2 **Using an Automated External Defibrillator, p. 827**

Skill 27.3 **Resuscitation Management, p. 830**

OBJECTIVES

Mastery of content in this chapter will enable you to:
- Discuss indications for an oral airway insertion.
- Identify a patient's need for automated external defibrillator (AED) application and indications for use.
- Examine the indications for cardiopulmonary resuscitation (CPR).
- Identify three key nursing roles during a cardiac arrest.

MEDIA RESOURCES

- http://evolve.elsevier.com/Perry/skills
- Review Questions
- Audio Glossary
- **NSO** Nursing Skills Online
- Answers to Clinical Judgment and Next-Generation NCLEX® Examination–Style Questions in Media Resources
- Skills Performance Checklists Printable
- Key Points

PURPOSE

Cardiopulmonary arrests are emergencies that can occur at any time. Nurses are expected to follow current resuscitation guidelines from the American Heart Association (AHA) in a systematic and organized manner. The goal is to provide resuscitation in a timely manner to restore cardiopulmonary function and avoid poor neurological outcomes. All nurses and nursing students are required to maintain certification in basic life support (BLS). Table 27.3 summarizes CPR skills for the adult, child, and infant techniques.

PRACTICE STANDARDS

- Merchant RM, et al., 2020: Executive Summary: American Heart Association Guidelines for Cardiopulmonary Resuscitation and Emergency Cardiovascular Care

SUPPLEMENTAL STANDARDS

- Atkins D, et al., 2022: Interim Guidance to Health Care Providers for Basic and Advanced Cardiac Life Support in Adults, Children, and Neonates With Suspected or Confirmed COVID-19
- Panchal AR, et al., 2020: Adult Basic and Advanced Life Support: Part 3: 2020 American Heart Association Guidelines for Adult Cardiopulmonary Resuscitation and Emergency Cardiovascular Care

PRINCIPLES FOR PRACTICE

- Early Defibrillation: In some cardiac arrests, circulating blood flow is lost due to an erratic heart rhythm known as a dysrhythmia. The cause of the dysrhythmia may include acute coronary syndrome, electrolyte disturbances, and certain prescribed or recreational medications. Two of the lethal dysrhythmias, ventricular tachycardia (VT) and ventricular fibrillation (VF), require a medically delivered electrical shock for treatment. Early defibrillation or shock may quickly return the heart to normal without further deterioration of a patient's status (Table 27.1).
- Early Warning Signs of Cardiac Arrest: Frequently, cardiac arrest is preceded with signs and symptoms of deterioration, which may include tachycardia, hypotension, tachypnea, decreasing oxygen saturation below 90% despite provision of supplemental oxygen, and a decreasing urine output of less than 50 mL in 4 hours. Early intervention can be provided by a Rapid Response Team—a group of clinicians designated to provide a rapid response to hospital patients who are showing objective or subjective signs of clinical deterioration. These teams have shown evidence of reducing mortality and length of stay when used appropriately (AHRQ, 2019).
- Initiating a Code Blue: Each health care agency has a specific code or signal to summon immediate assistance in the event of a cardiac and/or respiratory arrest; the arrest situation may be referred to as a "code" (e.g., "code blue," "Dr. Heart"). The team that responds is referred to as the code, code blue, or resuscitation team.

PERSON-CENTERED CARE

- Some research shows that family presence during resuscitation (FPDR) helps people meet their emotional needs and promotes the grieving process (Vardanjani et al., 2021). Know your agency's policy and procedure if witnessed resuscitation is allowed.
- Whenever a patient requires resuscitation, the family is also a prime nursing concern. Using resources like pastoral care and/or social work can provide support to the family during this trying event.

TABLE 27.1

Common Cardiac Dysrhythmias*

Rhythm Characteristics and Etiology	Clinical Significance and Management

Sinus Tachycardia

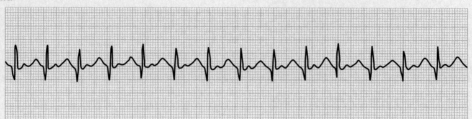

Regular rhythm, rate 100–180 beats/min (higher in infants), normal P wave, normal QRS complex.

Some patients with heart disease are unable to increase their heart rate to meet increased oxygen demands.

Rate increase is often a normal response to exercise; emotion; or stressors such as pain, fever, pump failure, hyperthyroidism, and certain drugs (e.g., caffeine, nitrates, epinephrine, nicotine).

Correct underlying factors; discontinue drugs producing the side effect.

Sinus Bradycardia

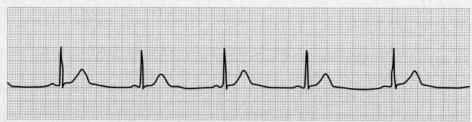

Regular rhythm, rate less than 60 beats/min, normal P wave, normal PR interval, normal QRS complex.

No clinical significance unless associated with signs and symptoms of reduced cardiac output, such as dizziness, syncope, change in mental status, dyspnea, or presence of chest pain.

Rate decrease is a normal response to sleep or in a well-conditioned athlete; diminished blood flow to SA node, vagal stimulation, hypothyroidism, increased intracranial pressure, or pharmacological agents (e.g., digoxin, propranolol, quinidine, procainamide) sometimes cause abnormal drops in rate.

Bradycardia with hypotension and decreased cardiac output is treated with atropine; pacemaker is sometimes necessary.

Atrial Fibrillation (A-fib)

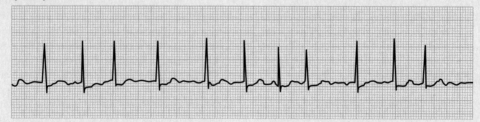

Chaotic, irregular atrial activity resulting in an irregular ventricular response. No identifiable P waves. Irregular ventricular response resulting in an irregular cardiac rate and rhythm. The conduction of the multiple atrial impulses across the atrioventricular (AV) node determines the rate.
Caused by aging, calcification of the sinoatrial (SA) node, or changes in myocardial blood supply.

There is loss of the atrial kick (part of the cardiac output squeezed in the ventricles with a coordinated atrial contraction), pooling of blood in the atria, and development of microemboli. The patient often complains of fatigue, a fluttering in the chest, or shortness of breath if the ventricular response is rapid. Dysrhythmia occurs commonly in the aging and older adult.

Ventricular Tachycardia

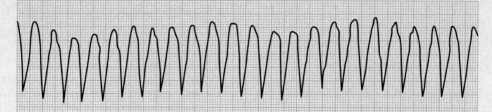

Common Cardiac Dysrhythmias—cont'd

Rhythm Characteristics and Etiology	Clinical Significance and Management
Rhythm slightly irregular, rate 100–200 beats/min, P wave absent, PR interval absent, QRS complex wide and bizarre, >0.12 second.	Results in decreased cardiac output caused by decreased ventricular filling time; often leads to severe hypotension and loss of pulse and consciousness.
Caused by changes in the normal pacemaker of the heart, such as decrease in blood flow, ischemia, or embolus.	Acute loss of pulse and respiration. Immediate chest compressions and defibrillation are required.

Ventricular Fibrillation

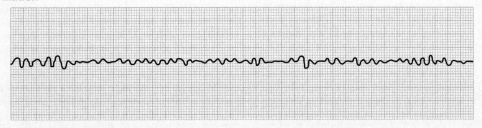

Uncoordinated electrical activity. No identifiable P, QRS, or T wave. Causes include sudden cardiac death, electrical shock, acute myocardial infarction, drowning, or trauma.	Acute loss of pulse and respiration. Immediate chest compressions and defibrillation are required. Availability of automated external defibrillator (AED) is recommended in public and/or private places where large numbers of people gather or where people who are at high risk for heart attack live.

Modified from Merchant RM, et al: Part 1: executive summary: 2020 American Heart Association Guidelines for cardiopulmonary resuscitation and emergency cardiovascular care, *Circulation* 142(16 suppl 2):S337–S357, 2020.

- Cardiac arrest often occurs without warning. When caring for patients from diverse cultures and religions, consider an individual's meaning and interpretation of life support and resuscitation when possible. Although individuals may be part of a specific cultural or religious group, an individual may not follow all aspects of that culture or religion. It is essential that you consider the individual's interpretation and wishes to ensure the right of self-determination.
- When necessary, use a professional language interpreter to explain the patient's status to the family and/or the patient. In addition, use cultural and religious support personnel to facilitate understanding of the events.
- Be prepared to handle large numbers of visitors who may remain at the bedside to provide support for the family. Collaborate with the family decision maker and leader to plan rotating visits at the bedside.
- Advance directives offer valuable information concerning a patient's choice for having resuscitation and individual patient decisions regarding resuscitation efforts. Although advance directives are often addressed before or during a patient's hospitalization, nurses play an important role in encouraging patients to complete their plan of care.

EVIDENCE-BASED PRACTICE

Cardiopulmonary Resuscitation (CPR)

The American Heart Association's Committee on Emergency Cardiac Care (Merchant et al., 2020) reviews and conducts research on cardiac arrest treatment and outcomes and has created evidence-based guidelines for both initial care (BLS) and ongoing measures (advanced cardiovascular life support [ACLS]). These guidelines emphasize the importance of high-quality cardiopulmonary resuscitation (CPR) to improve chances of patients' survival from a cardiac arrest.
- Strategies to improve survival after cardiopulmonary arrest include (Merchant et al., 2020):
  - Immediate recognition and activation of emergency medical response

- Early CPR and rapid defibrillation that emphasize high-quality chest compressions
- Effective advanced cardiac life support
- High-quality CPR improves survival from cardiac arrest and includes:
  - Ensuring chest compressions of adequate rate and depth
  - Allowing full chest recoil between compressions
  - Avoiding excessive ventilation
  - Minimizing interruptions in chest compressions
- Strategies to improve CPR techniques include real-time feedback to the health care providers who are chest compressors via audiovisual indicators for compression depth, rate, and recoil.
- Health care provider who is providing compression can adjust the speed, depth, and release on the basis of feedback. Feedback devices are available as stand-alone devices or incorporated into the AED or manual defibrillator or available as a smartphone app.
- Special tasks and guidelines exist for providing resuscitation to patients with COVID-19 (Atkins et al., 2022), including:
  - Don personal protective equipment (PPE) according to local guidelines and availability before beginning CPR.
  - Minimize the number of clinicians performing resuscitation, use a negative-pressure room whenever possible, and keep the door to the resuscitation room closed if possible.
  - May use a mechanical device, if resources and expertise are available, to perform chest compressions on adults and on adolescents who meet minimum height and weight requirements.
  - Use a high-efficiency particulate air (HEPA) filter for bag-mask ventilation (BMV) and mechanical ventilation.
- Postarrest care is encouraged to be delivered in a structured pathway approach to include targeted temperature management to preserve neurological function, early coronary angiography and intervention (if indicated), keeping mean arterial pressure above 65 mm Hg pressure, keeping end-tidal carbon dioxide levels within normal levels, pulse oximetry above 95%, and avoidance of fever and glucose control (Storm et al., 2019).

- Allowing family members to remain in a patient's room during resuscitative efforts requires support personnel to focus on the family and their needs (LaRocco & Toronto, 2019). It also involves an assessment of the individuals to screen for anyone who might become an obstacle in the room and interrupt care.

SAFETY GUIDELINES

- Know your patient's baseline vital signs, cardiac history, and current health problems. Conditions that place a patient at risk for dysrhythmias include coronary artery disease, myocardial infarction, open-heart surgeries, acid-base imbalances, and toxicities.

- Know your patient's most recent serum electrolyte values. Electrolyte imbalances (e.g., potassium, magnesium, calcium) can precipitate cardiopulmonary arrest.
- When a patient has been exposed to a chemical or drug, attempt to determine the type and amount of the substance involved. Certain chemicals (e.g., ethanol, tranquilizers, opioids) depress the respiratory center and can result in a respiratory arrest, which can lead to full cardiac arrest if not treated. Oversedation involving the use of patient-controlled analgesia (PCA) pumps or intermittent IV, epidural, or oral opioid administration can also contribute to respiratory depression.
- Clear communication to all others in the room is essential at the time of defibrillation so that everyone is aware and does not touch the patient or bed at the time of shock.

✦ SKILL 27.1 Inserting an Oropharyngeal Airway

An oropharyngeal airway (OPA) is a semicircular, rigid piece of plastic (Fig. 27.1) shaped to follow the curvature of the tongue. When inserted, it extends from just outside the lip, over the tongue, and toward the pharynx (Fig. 27.2). An OPA allows for the passage of a suction catheter or a fiberoptic scope through the channel of the airway. It will maintain airway patency in an unconscious patient by displacing the tongue forward and toward the oral cavity floor. The correct size of an OPA is based on width and length of the mouth for the patient's age. The size is correct when the flange is held parallel to the front teeth and the end of the OPA reaches the angle of the jaw (Table 27.2). Upper airway obstruction is common in the unconscious patient, especially during a cardiac arrest. An OPA is indicated if the patient cannot be ventilated using maneuvers like head tilt–chin lift or jaw thrust to open the airway. If the patient requires bag-mask ventilation, the airway may be accidently obstructed due to pressure placed on the face to seal the mask. It is common practice to use an OPA along with bag-mask ventilation. Due to the length of an OPA, it should only be used in the unconscious patient to avoid gagging and vomiting.

Delegation

The skill of inserting an OPA cannot be delegated to assistive personnel (AP). Direct the AP to:
- Immediately report to the nurse any signs of airway distress, vomiting, or change in level of consciousness.

Interprofessional Collaboration

- Respiratory therapists and anesthesia providers should be involved to troubleshoot OPA placement.

Equipment

- Appropriate-size OPA (see Table 27.2)
- Clean gloves
- Gown and mask/face shield if indicated
- Tissues or washcloths
- Suction equipment
- Nonallergenic tape
- Tongue blade
- Stethoscope
- Pulse oximeter

FIG. 27.1 Oropharyngeal airways.

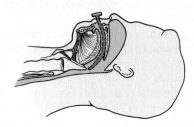

FIG. 27.2 Placement of oropharyngeal airway.

TABLE 27.2

Oral Airway Guidelines for Size* by Age

Size	Age
30 mm or size 000	Premature neonates
45 mm or size 00	Newborn
55 mm or size 0	Newborn to 1 year
60 mm or size 1	1–2 years
70 mm or size 2	2–6 years
80 mm or size 3	6–18 years
90 mm or size 4	Adult medium
100 mm or size 5	Adult large
110 mm or size 6	Adult extra large

*Measure from the corner of the mouth to the angle of the jaw just below the ear for size estimation (see Skill 27.1, Assessment, Step 4).
From Castro D, Freeman LA: *Oropharyngeal airway*, Bethesda, Maryland, 2022, National Library of Medicine, Treasure Island, StatPearls.

STEP	RATIONALE

ASSESSMENT

1. Identify need to insert an oropharyngeal airway (OPA). Signs and symptoms include the following in an unconscious patient: upper airway gurgling with breathing, absent cough or gag reflex, decline in PaO_2, increased oral secretions, excessive drooling, absent or labored respirations.

   These conditions place patient at risk for obstruction of the upper airway. Use an OPA only in unconscious patients. They may stimulate vomiting or gagging if inserted in a semiconscious or conscious patient.

2. Assess for factors that may contribute to upper airway obstruction, such as age (children have a proportionally larger tongue), altered mental status, seizures, sedation, and foreign objects (e.g., food, kinking of nasogastric drainage tube). **NOTE**: *This can be an urgent procedure. Once it is established that airway obstruction is developing, proceed immediately to implementation.*

   Allows you to accurately assess need for OPA placement.

3. Perform hand hygiene.

   Reduces transmission of microorganisms.

Clinical Judgment *Never insert an oral airway in a conscious patient or a patient with recent oral/facial trauma, oral surgery, or loose teeth. Never force an airway into place.*

4. Measure the OPA size for the patient (see illustration). Hold the flange of the OPA parallel to the front teeth. The end of the OPA should reach the angle of the jaw (Castro, 2022).

   Inserting an appropriate-size OPA will help to avoid damage to the soft palate or other oral structures. If the OPA is too large for the patient, it will further obstruct the airway.

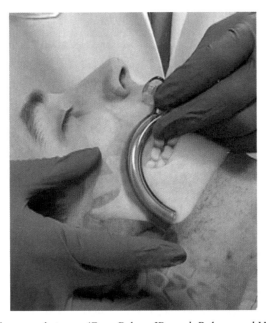

STEP 4 Measuring for an oral airway. (*From Roberts JR, et al: Roberts and Hedges' clinical procedures in emergency medicine and acute care, ed 7, Philadelphia, 2019, Elsevier.*)

PLANNING

1. Expected outcomes following completion of procedure:
   - Patient's respiratory status improves, as evidenced by ease of manual ventilations, pulse oximeter monitoring values improving, and easier removal of secretions.

     Airway should be suctioned before placement of OPA.

   - Patient is not able to grind teeth or bite tubes.

     Oral airway prevents tooth contact with other teeth or with tubes.

   - Patient's tongue does not obstruct airway.

     Oral airway keeps tongue in correct position to maintain patent airway.

2. Close room door and bedside curtain.

   Provides patient privacy.

3. Obtain and organize equipment for airway insertion at bedside.

   Ensures efficiency when completing a procedure.

4. Position unconscious patient in semi-Fowler position if possible.

   Provides easy access to oral cavity.

STEP	RATIONALE

IMPLEMENTATION

1. Perform hand hygiene and apply clean gloves and face shield (when possible).

Reduces transmission of microorganisms.

2. Ensure that patient does not have dentures in place before attempting an OPA insertion. Remove dentures that are in place.

OPA insertion can dislodge dentures and cause worsening airway obstruction.

3. If difficult to open mouth, use a padded tongue blade or use thumb and forefinger of nondominant hand to open jaws and teeth.

Provides access to oral cavity. To avoid a bite, **do not insert your fingers into patient's mouth.** Use extreme caution if manually opening patient's jaw and teeth.

4. Suction out the oral cavity to rid it of excess secretions (see Skill 24.1).

Cleaning out the oral cavity may prevent aspiration of secretions.

5. Insert oropharyngeal airway.

When inserting airway, take care not to push patient's tongue into pharynx.

   a. Hold oral airway with curved end toward the hard palate. As you are inserting the oropharyngeal airway and it approaches the posterior pharynx, rotate the oropharyngeal airway 180 degrees into the correct position. *Option:* Hold airway sideways, insert halfway, and rotate 90 degrees while gliding it over natural curvature of tongue. Make sure that outer flange is just outside patient's lips.

Proper insertion of airway prevents displacement of patient's tongue into posterior oropharynx. DO NOT insert the oropharyngeal airway in with the curve tip down. This will push the tongue posterior and further obstruct the airway.

Clinical Judgment *In a pediatric patient, DO NOT rotate the oral airway on insertion because the airway tip will damage the soft palate.*

6. Suction secretions as needed.

Removes secretions; maintains patent airway.

7. Reassess patient's respiratory status: auscultate lungs, check ease of manual ventilation and improvement of pulse oximetry values.

Verifies respiratory status and patent airway.

8. Clean patient's face with soft tissue or washcloth.

Promotes hygiene.

9. Help patient to comfortable position, preferably in side-lying position.

Promotes patient comfort, reduces risk of aspiration, and eases breathing.

10. Once airway is established, determine family caregiver's health literacy and knowledge of purpose of airway. Explain how airway functions and reasons patient requires one.

Determines degree to which individuals have the ability to find, understand, and use information and services to make informed health-related decisions and actions for themselves and others (CDC, 2023).
Reveals need for family caregiver instruction and support.

11. Place nurse call system in an accessible location within patient's reach so that it can be used if the patient regains consciousness.

Ensures patient or family caregiver can call for assistance if needed.

12. Raise side rails (as appropriate) and lower bed to lowest position, locking into position.

Ensures patient safety and prevents falls.

13. Dispose of all contaminated supplies in appropriate receptacle, remove and dispose of gloves and face mask, and perform hand hygiene.

Reduces transmission of microorganisms.

14. Administer mouth care frequently.

Increases patient comfort and removes debris. It also provides moisture to oral mucosal tissues.

Clinical Judgment *An oropharyngeal airway will need to be removed, cleaned, or discarded and replaced in patients with excessive oral secretions. Frequent suctioning of the oral cavity may be required. Oropharyngeal airways are not a long-term solution. They can create pressure on underlying tissue and cause significant lip and tongue erosion, which can result in a medical device–related pressure injury (TJC, 2022).*

EVALUATION

1. Observe patient's respiratory status and compare respiratory assessments before and after insertion of oropharyngeal airway.

Identifies patient's response to insertion of airway.

2. Evaluate that airway is patent and that patient's tongue does not obstruct it.

Ensures route for oxygen delivery to patient.

3. Observe adjacent and underlying tissue for signs of redness, abrasion, or bruising.

Identifies early signs of medical device.

4. Observe the patient for signs of improved mental status: pushing airway out with tongue or coughing may indicate the return of the patient's ability to protect their own airway.

Patient's ability to clear their own airway may have returned. Indicates need to remove the oropharyngeal airway.

STEP	RATIONALE
5. Use Teach-Back: "I want to be sure I explained why your loved one needs this oral airway. Tell me why it is important." Revise your instruction now or develop a plan for revised patient/family caregiver teaching if patient/family caregiver is not able to teach back correctly.	Teach-back is a technique for health care providers to ensure that they have explained medical information clearly so that patients and their families understand what is communicated to them (Agency for Healthcare Research and Quality [AHRQ], 2023).

Unexpected Outcomes	Related Interventions
1. Patient continually coughs and gags when oropharyngeal airway (OPA) is inserted.	• Do not continue inserting airway if patient begins to gag. Stimulation of gag reflex can cause vomiting and aspiration. • Remove OPA and position patient on the side.
2. Airway obstruction not relieved.	• Obtain immediate assistance. • Reinsert airway or determine if another form of airway is needed. • Assess for other causes of obstruction.
3. Patient pushes airway out of place or out of mouth.	• Reassess patient's need for OPA. • Do not reinsert if patient is awake or can protect their own airway.
4. Unable to insert oral airway; patient is combative, or you are unable to open the mouth.	• Get help. • Do not continue efforts to place OPA.

Documentation

- Document assessment findings; patient's status before and after airway insertion; size of oropharyngeal airway; other interventions performed at same time, especially positioning and suctioning; and patient's response to procedure.
- Document your evaluation of patient and family caregiver learning.

Hand-Off Reporting

- Report any airway obstruction, changes in secretions, or changes in patient's tolerance of airway (e.g., pushing airway out). Remember: If patient begins to push out the OPA, do not reinsert. Patient must be completely unconscious to safely tolerate an OPA.

Special Considerations
Pediatrics

- Oropharyngeal airways are seldom used in treatment of airway obstruction in infants and children. Because the airway is narrow, it is often more occlusive than beneficial (Hockenberry et al., 2022). A nasopharyngeal airway may be tolerated by children better than an oropharyngeal one (Ralston et al., 2022).
- For infants and small children, sliding the oropharyngeal airway along the side of the mouth rather than with the tip up is recommended because the soft palate is easily injured.

✦ SKILL 27.2   Using an Automated External Defibrillator

Defibrillation is the administration of an electrical shock to a patient's chest in an attempt to terminate a lethal cardiac arrhythmia. An automated external defibrillator (AED) is a device that allows a BLS provider to defibrillate. The device is attached to a patient's chest via two adhesive pads. Most AEDs have a simple three-step function (Fig. 27.3) with verbal prompts to guide the responder. All AEDs offer automated rhythm analysis, whereby the rhythm is compared with thousands of other rhythms stored in the AED computer software. AEDs recommend a shock based on the automated analysis and prompt the responder to press the shock button.

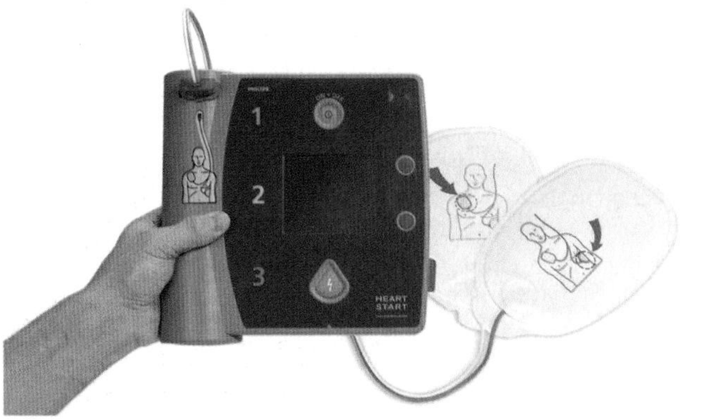

Delegation

BLS certification provides hands-on training with an AED for laypeople, assistive personnel (AP), and licensed health care professionals. Most agencies using AEDs have given the authority to use it to all BLS or CPR-certified personnel, including APs. Refer to specific agency policies for use of the AED.

Interprofessional Collaboration

- The code blue team members are present to resuscitate the patient (see Skill 27.3).

Equipment

- AED
- Pair of AED adhesive pads
- Barrier device or mouth-to-mask device or bag-valve mask device
- Gloves and other personal protective equipment

FIG. 27.3 Automated external defibrillator device. (*Courtesy Philips Medical Systems.*)

STEP	RATIONALE

ASSESSMENT

1. Establish person's unresponsiveness and call for help. (In community settings have someone call 9-1-1.)

This information helps to determine if individual is unresponsive rather than asleep, intoxicated, hearing impaired, or postictal. Rapid response by qualified professionals ensures ongoing resuscitation support.

2. Establish absence of respirations and lack of circulation within 10 seconds: no pulse, no respirations, no movement.

Indicates need for emergency measures, including AED.

Clinical Judgment *An AED should be applied only to a patient who is unconscious, not breathing, and pulseless. Children older than age 8 can be treated with a standard AED. For children ages 1–8, the AHA recommends pediatric pads. In infants <1 year of age, a manual defibrillator is preferred (Merchant et al., 2020).*

PLANNING

1. Expected outcomes following completion of procedure:
   - Patient's cardiac rhythm is converted back to stable rhythm.
   - Patient regains pulse and respirations.

Defibrillation provides electrical shock to convert a lethal dysrhythmia.

CPR and defibrillation were successful.

IMPLEMENTATION

1. Assess patient for unresponsiveness, not breathing and pulselessness, and no movement within 10 seconds.

These are indicators of cardiopulmonary arrest.

2. Activate code team in accordance with agency policy and procedure.

First available person brings resuscitation cart and AED.

Clinical Judgment *The AHA's COVID-19 guidelines recommend both EMS personnel and health care workers don personal protective equipment (PPE) to guard against contact with both airborne and droplet particles before entering a patient room or scene of a cardiac arrest. Only essential personnel should be allowed in the room or on the scene (Atkins, 2022).*

3. Start chest compressions and continue until AED is attached to patient and verbal prompt of device advises you, "Do not touch the patient."

To minimize interruption time of chest compressions, continue CPR while AED is being applied and turned on.

4. Place AED next to patient near chest or head.

Ensures easy access to device.

Clinical Judgment *If the AED is immediately available, attach it to patient as soon as possible. The faster defibrillation is delivered, the better the survival rate (Merchant et al., 2020).*

5. Turn on power (see illustration).

Turning on power begins verbal prompts to guide you through the next steps.

6. Attach device. Place first AED pad on upper right sternal border directly below clavicle. Place second AED pad lateral to left nipple with top of pad a few inches below axilla (see illustration). Ensure that cables are connected to AED.

Alternative pad placement of AED pads is not recommended. AEDs analyze most heart rhythms using lead II.

Clinical Judgment *Wet surfaces, implanted defibrillators, and medication patches reduce the effectiveness of the defibrillation attempt and result in complications.*

7. Do NOT touch patient when AED prompts you. Direct rescuers and bystanders to avoid touching patient by announcing "Clear!" Allow AED to analyze the rhythm. Some devices require that an analysis button be pressed. The AED takes approximately 5 to 15 seconds to analyze the rhythm.

Not touching patient when directed prevents artifact errors, avoids all movement during analysis (Panchal et al., 2020), and prevents shock from being delivered to bystanders.

8. Before pressing the shock button, announce loudly to clear the victim and perform a visual check to ensure that no one is in contact with the patient.

Clearing patient ensures safety for those involved in rescue efforts.

9. Immediately begin chest compression after the shock and continue for 2 minutes with a ratio of 30:2 (30 compressions and 2 breaths). Do NOT remove pads.

Continues cardiac perfusion.

STEP	RATIONALE

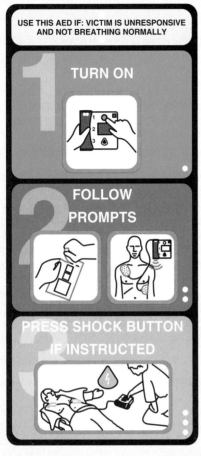

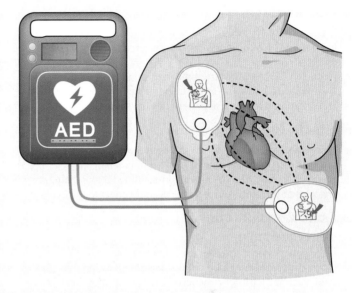

STEP 5 Power panel with automated external defibrillator prompts. (*Courtesy Philips Medical Systems.*)

STEP 6 Placement of automated external defibrillator pads with device next to patient.

10. Deliver two breaths using mouth-to-mouth with barrier device, mouth-to-mask device, or bag-valve mask device. Watch for chest rise and fall.
    If second rescuer is available, deliver 10 to 12 breaths/min or 1 breath every 5 to 6 seconds while continuing chest compressions.

In an agency setting where protected methods of artificial ventilation are available, mouth-to-mouth without a barrier device is not recommended because of risk for microbial contamination.

11. After 2 minutes of CPR, AED will prompt you not to touch patient and will resume analysis of patient's rhythm. This cycle will continue until patient regains a pulse or health care provider determines death.

Determines patient status.

12. Remove and dispose of gloves and other PPE. Perform hand hygiene.

Reduces transmission of microorganisms.

EVALUATION

1. Inspect pad adhesion to chest wall. If pads are not in good contact with chest wall, remove them and apply a new set.

Poor pad-skin contact reduces effectiveness of the shock, causes skin burns, or increases chance of shocking those involved in the rescue efforts. Always apply a new set of pads.

2. Check for palpable pulse and responsiveness. Continue resuscitative efforts until patient regains pulse or health care provider determines death.

Evaluates circulatory status.

3. Provide updates to family on patient's status.

Use resources to keep family informed, including providers, chaplain, and social workers. Screen family for possibly allowing family presence in the room (LaRocco & Toronto, 2019).

STEP	RATIONALE
Unexpected Outcomes	**Related Interventions**
1. Patient's heart rhythm does not convert into stable rhythm with pulse after defibrillation.	• Assess pad contact on patient's chest wall. • Do not touch patient during AED rhythm analysis. • Avoid placing AED pads over medication patches, pacemaker, or implantable defibrillator generators.
2. Patient's skin has burns under AED pads.	• Assess AED pad contact on chest. • Ensure that chest is dry before applying pads to chest. • Apply skin care as indicated if patient is resuscitated successfully.

Documentation

• Cardiopulmonary arrest requires immediate and accurate documentation. Most agencies use a form designed specifically for in-agency arrests.
• Document onset of arrest, time and number of AED shocks (you will not know the exact energy level used by the AED), and additional resuscitation activities (see Skill 27.3).

Hand-Off Reporting

• Immediately report arrest via the agency-wide communication system indicating exact location of victim.
• Share all information documented regarding patient status pre-arrest and postarrest to the to the postarrest team.

Special Considerations

Patient Education

• If the patient is at risk for repeat cardiopulmonary arrest, instruct the family caregiver in CPR or encourage certification through an American Red Cross or American Heart Association instructor.

• It is extremely helpful if the family caregiver maintains a list of the patient's current medications and a description of the medication's purpose at all times.

Pediatrics

• Most AEDs are specifically designed for adult use only and are therefore not recommended for use in children younger than 8 years old (Merchant et al., 2020). Adult pads can be used if child pads are not available; be sure not to overlap pads. Manual defibrillation performed by health care personnel using lower-energy settings (2 to 4 joules/kg) is the most common method of pediatric defibrillation.

Home Care

• Patient and family should keep emergency numbers readily available or consider programming them into a speed dial function on both home and mobile phones. Stress the use of 9-1-1.
• AEDs are available for use in the community and home setting.

◆ SKILL 27.3   Resuscitation Management

Initially a cardiac arrest is managed by first responders performing the basic skills of cardiopulmonary resuscitation (CPR). Basic CPR includes the primary survey (assessing the patient and then performing the appropriate action) of C (circulation), A (airway), B (breathing), and D (early defibrillation, as soon as available). These interventions continue until the resuscitation team arrives. The initial process also includes notification of the resuscitation or code team. Most of the code team members have been trained in the advanced cardiac life support (ACLS) guidelines and the performance of the secondary survey: C (rhythm analysis of cardiac rhythm), A (airway intubation), B (confirmation of airway and ventilation), and D (differential diagnosis of the cause). Both surveys must be reassessed continually and managed as appropriate throughout the code situation.

The code or resuscitation team usually includes a physician, intensive care nurse, respiratory therapist, anesthesia, and possibly pharmacy, radiology, and laboratory personnel. Clinical nurses on site will also participate as needed. A pastoral care representative is often available to be with the family.

The ability of a first-responder nurse to initiate basic resuscitative efforts such as CPR and defibrillation via an AED can prevent lethal dysrhythmias such as ventricular fibrillation from deteriorating to asystole (absence of cardiac electrical activity) and provide a chance for the heart to return to its normal rhythm (see Skill 27.2). Early CPR and defibrillation delivered within the primary

survey time period will help to preserve heart and brain function, leading to improved survivability. During the secondary survey, the code team will determine the patient's cardiac rhythm and provide the appropriate treatment for that rhythm. Table 27.2 summarizes basic cardiac arrhythmias. Equipment (stored in a resuscitation or crash cart) should be readily available to provide the emergency treatments at the bedside. It is the nurse's responsibility to know how to use this equipment and to know the location within the cart so that hand-offs of equipment/medications to members of the code team can be made quickly.

Delegation

Most skills involved with resuscitation management cannot be delegated to assistive personnel (AP). However, AP who are certified in BLS techniques can perform the basic skills of CPR, including AED use if deemed appropriate by the agency's policy. Most agencies reserve the skill of manual defibrillation for licensed personnel who are ACLS certified or have received competency validation to perform manual defibrillation. All other skills in the code situation are directed by the code team leader and performed by nurses, respiratory therapists, and other health care professionals.

Interprofessional Collaboration

Teamwork and clear, closed-loop communication during a cardiac arrest are essential. All the various tasks to be performed are directed by the code team leader. It is also essential that all team members in the room generally affirm their roles in the code, know their limitations, understand what interventions should be done, and predict what comes next. For example, all pulseless patients will receive the medication epinephrine. Knowing this will prompt the crash cart nurse to prepare epinephrine off the crash cart. The crash cart nurse, in turn, will notify the code team leader that epinephrine is ready to give and then hand off the epinephrine to the bedside nurse to administer. The bedside nurse announces to the room that epinephrine has just been administered. Hearing this, the recording nurse then documents the administration of epinephrine and notifies the code team leader when the next epinephrine dose is due in 2 minutes. All actions require calm and confident teamwork and an awareness of what everyone is doing in the room.

Equipment

Crash cart (Fig. 27.4)—Most adult carts have the following equipment:

- Clean and sterile gloves, gown, mask, protective eyewear
- Oxygen source
- Bag-valve mask device or resuscitation bag
- Oral pharyngeal airways (OPAs)
- Laryngoscope, handle, and laryngoscope straight and curved blades
- Endotracheal (ET) tubes, various sizes (5 to 9 mm for adults; 0 to 4 mm for pediatrics)
- Carbon dioxide detector to confirm ET tube placement
- Tape or commercial ET tube holder
- Backboard
- AED and/or manual defibrillator with AED/defibrillator pads
- Intravenous (IV) needles (sizes for adults and pediatrics)
- Central vascular access kit or intraosseous kit

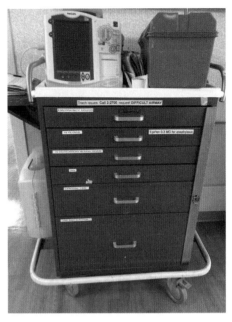

FIG. 27.4 Emergency resuscitation cart.

- IV tubing and fluids (normal saline [NS] and 5% dextrose in water [D$_5$W])
- Syringes
- Laboratory specimen tubes
- Arterial blood gas kit
- Emergency medications
- ACLS guidelines or algorithms
- Suction source and suction equipment if not with crash cart

STEP	RATIONALE

ASSESSMENT

1. Determine if patient is unconscious by shaking them and shouting, "Are you OK?" Assess patient unresponsiveness.	Confirms that patient is unresponsive rather than intoxicated, sleeping, or hearing impaired. Substance abuse, hypoglycemia, drug toxicities, seizures, trauma, ketoacidosis, and shock also can cause unconsciousness.

Clinical Judgment *If an unresponsive person has adequate respirations and pulse, remain until further help is present. Place victim in a modified lateral recovery position (see illustration). Continue to assess for the presence of respirations and pulse because a recurrent arrest may develop.*

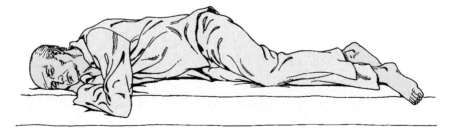

STEP 1 Recovery position.

PLANNING

1. Expected outcomes following completion of procedure:
  • Patient regains pulse and respirations.
  • Patient receives postresuscitation care.
  • Patient transported to intensive care unit (ICU) for ongoing care.
	CPR is successful.
	Ongoing treatment and support needed.
	Resuscitation will hopefully result in immediate survival.

STEP	RATIONALE
2. Immediately activate the agency's code team or emergency medical services (EMS). Tell co-workers to bring AED (if available) and crash cart to bedside.	Timely application of defibrillation, CPR, and ACLS to arrest victim will help to improve chances of survival.

IMPLEMENTATION

Primary Survey: *C* (Circulation) and *D* (Defibrillation, as soon as available)

STEP	RATIONALE
1. Apply clean gloves and face shield, if needed.	Reduces transmission of microorganisms.

Clinical Judgment *Following the COVID-19 pandemic, the AHA recommends the following (Atkins et al., 2022): Health care workers should don personal protective equipment (PPE) to guard against contact with both airborne and droplet particles before entering the scene of a cardiac arrest. Only essential personnel should be allowed on the scene. Intubation involves a high risk of aerosolization, but a closed-loop ventilation system has a lower risk of aerosolization than other ventilation methods. Health care workers should use a bag mask with a tight seal and an attached high-efficiency particulate air (HEPA) filter before intubation or if intubation must be delayed.*

STEP	RATIONALE
2. Check carotid pulse on adult or child; use brachial or femoral pulse in infant. Palpate for no more than 10 seconds (Merchant et al., 2020).	Carotid pulse is the easiest to locate in adults and children. Femoral pulse may also be palpated in child or infant.
3. If pulse is absent and an AED is unavailable, immediately initiate chest compressions.	
a. Place victim on hard surface, such as floor, ground, or backboard. Victim must be flat. Logroll victim to flat, supine position using spine precautions if trauma is suspected.	External compression of heart is facilitated on a hard surface. Heart is compressed between sternum and spinal vertebrae, which must be on hard and firm surface. Do *NOT* delay the start of CPR. Positioning patient on hard surface may take more than one or two rescuers. You may need to wait to safely move the patient. Place on backboard or position patient as soon as appropriate help is present.
b. Assume correct hand position and compression ratio for patient (30:2 adult compressions: breath ratio) (see Table 27.3; see illustrations).	Specific hand position, compression depth, and ratio are different for adults, children, and infants to avoid injury to heart, lung, or liver.

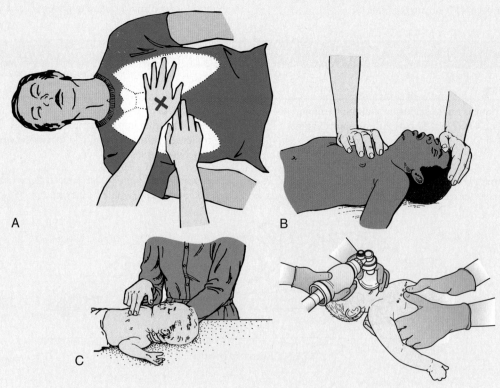

STEP 3b (A) Proper hand position—adult. (B) Proper hand position—child. (C) Proper hand position—infant. (D) Two thumb encircling hands method. (*D from Sorrentino SA, Remmert LN: Mosby's textbook for nursing assistants, ed 10, St Louis, 2021, Elsevier.*)

STEP	RATIONALE

TABLE 27.3

Adult, Child, and Infant Cardiopulmonary Resuscitation Techniques (Health Care Providers)

Technique	Adult	Child (1–8 Years Old)	Infant (Younger Than 1 Year) Does Not Include Newborns
Chest compressions: Push hard and fast to allow complete recoil of sternum	Begin compressions if no pulse Lower half of sternum Heel of 1 hand, other hand on top. Depth of 5–6 cm (2–2.4 inches) 1 to 2 rescuers: rate of 100–120/min and ratio of 30 compressions to 2 breaths (30:2) Continue until AED is available and ready to analyze rhythm	Begin compressions if no pulse or pulse <60/min Lower half of sternum, between nipples Heel of 1 hand or as for adults At least ⅓ depth of chest 1 rescuer: 30 compressions, 2 breaths (30:2) 2 rescuers: 15 compressions, 2 breaths (15:2)	Begin compressions if no pulse or pulse <60/min Just below nipple line (lower half of sternum) 2 fingers or 2 thumbs (encircling hands) 1 rescuer: 30 compressions, 2 breaths (30:2) 2 rescuers: 15 compressions, 2 breaths (15:2)
Defibrillation using AED	Use adult pads AED should be applied and turned on as soon as available, and shock as soon as advised Resume compressions immediately after shock	Use child pads whenever possible If none, use adult pads but do not overlap them Apply AED as soon as available, and shock as soon as advised	If there is a shockable rhythm, manual defibrillation is used
Airway	Head tilt–chin lift (HCP: Suspected trauma, use jaw thrust)	Head tilt–chin lift (HCP: Suspected trauma, use jaw thrust)	Head tilt–chin lift (HCP: Suspected trauma, use jaw thrust)
HCP: Rescue breathing mouth-to-mask or bag-valve mask without chest compressions	10–12 breaths/min (approximately 1 breath every 5–6 seconds)	12–20 breaths/min (approximately 1 breath every 3 seconds)	12–20 breaths/min (approximately 1 breath every 3 seconds)
HCP: Rescue breaths for CPR with advanced airway (endotracheal tube/tracheotomy)	8–10 breaths/min (approximately 1 breath every 6–8 seconds)	8–10 breaths/min (approximately 1 breath every 6–8 seconds)	8–10 breaths/min (approximately 1 breath every 6–8 seconds)

Modified from Merchant RM, et al: Part 1: executive summary: 2020 American Heart Association guidelines for cardiopulmonary resuscitation and emergency cardiovascular care, *Circulation* 142(16 suppl 2):S337–S357, 2020.
AED, Automated external defibrillator; *CPR*, cardiopulmonary resuscitation; *HCP*, health care provider.

4. If pulse is absent and AED is available, apply AED immediately as appropriate.

   a. After one shock, resume CPR for 5 cycles (30:2, adult compressions: breath ratio) and begin rhythm analysis and shock sequence again (Table 27.3).

Most successful defibrillation rates occur when AED is applied and used within 3 minutes following collapse. Survival rates decline the more defibrillation is delayed.
One shock followed by chest compressions for 5 cycles of 30:2 ratio provides sufficient blood flow and perfusion before another set of shocks is delivered (Panchal et al., 2020).

Primary Survey: A (Airway):
Performed after first 2 minutes of chest compression and AED use.
5. Open airway.
   a. Head tilt–chin lift (no trauma) (see illustration) *or*

   b. Jaw thrust (use if cervical trauma is suspected) (see illustration)

Tongue is most common cause of blocked airway in unresponsive patient.
Suspect spinal cord injury in patients with trauma. Jaw-thrust maneuver prevents head extension and neck movement and further paralysis or spinal cord injury. Apply rigid cervical collar and immobilize patient as soon as possible to reduce cervical spine motion.

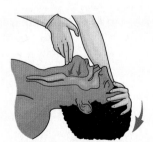

STEP 5a Head tilt–chin lift. (*From Kostelnick C:* Mosby's textbook for long-term care nursing assistants, *ed 8, St Louis, 2020, Elsevier.*)

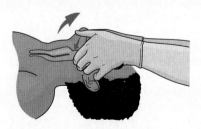

STEP 5b Jaw thrust without head tilt.

STEP	RATIONALE
6. Determine if patient has spontaneous respirations.	Determines level of resuscitation required.

Primary Survey: *B* (Breathing)

STEP	RATIONALE
7. Attempt to ventilate patient with slow breaths using one of these methods.	Slow breaths deliver air at low pressure to reduce risk of gastric distention.
a. Mouth-to-mouth using barrier device	Forms airtight seal to prevent air from escaping through nose.
b. Mouth-to-mask using pocket mask (see illustration)	Provides secure seal and permits use of supplemental oxygen.
c. Bag-mask device (see illustrations) **NOTE**: This is the method recommended if COVID-19 precautions are still in effect (Atkins et al., 2022).	Gives breaths with enough force to make chest rise.

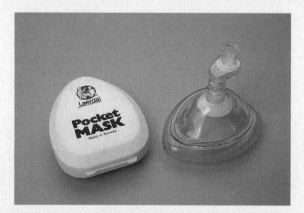

STEP 7b Pocket mask.

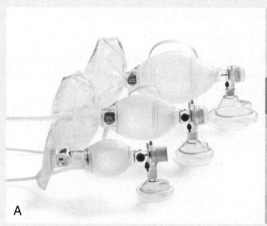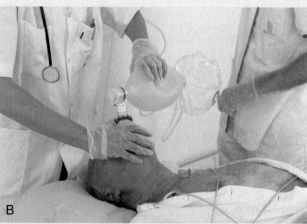

STEP 7c (A) Bag-valve mask devices. (B) Two-rescuer breathing with bag-valve mask device. (*Courtesy Ambu USA.*)

STEP	RATIONALE
8. If ventilation is difficult, insert an oral airway (see Skill 27.1).	Maintains tongue on anterior floor of mouth and prevents obstruction of posterior airway by tongue.
9. Suction secretions if necessary or turn victim's head to one side unless trauma is suspected.	Suctioning prevents airway obstruction. Turning patient's head to one side allows gravity to drain any secretions, decreasing risk of aspiration.

Secondary Survey: Implementation

STEP	RATIONALE
1. Give code leader brief verbal report on events performed before code team's arrival. Report immediate prearrest events, medical diagnosis, and any prearrival code intervention.	This information is critical in selection of appropriate treatment for patient.

STEP	RATIONALE

2. On arrival of sufficient personnel, delegate tasks as appropriate while the primary group continues with resuscitation efforts.

Delegation of duties and confirmation of these duties by each team member is essential to meet critical needs of the patient and family in a timely matter.

  a. Help victim's roommate and visitors away from code scene. Assign pastoral care or other nurses to communicate with patient's family. Consider allowing family to witness resuscitation (see agency policy).

Family members who were allowed to witness resuscitation efforts have been found to have a significant reduction in posttraumatic stress and self-reports of a greater sense of resolution and fulfillment (LaRocco & Toronto, 2019).

  b. Delegate someone to remove excess furniture or equipment from room.

Provides room for emergency equipment and responders.

  c. Have someone bring patient's chart to bedside or have access to patient's electronic health record (EHR).

Clarifies patient's medical condition, code status, and presence of any allergies.

  d. Assign nurses to one of three major roles:

Provides more direct care to the patient as directed.

    (1) Bedside Nurse: Gives medications, checks pulse, obtains vital signs, assists with direct patient tasks

    (2) Crash Cart Nurse: Retrieves medications and supplies from the crash cart to hand off to bedside nurse on code team, sets up manual defibrillator for use.

Provides code personnel with appropriate medication and equipment in timely fashion.

    (3) Recorder Nurse: Records/documents code events as they occur using a designated paper or electronic CPR worksheet

Ensures accurate documentation of events of code, medications, and treatments administered.

Secondary Survey: *C* (Analysis of Cardiac Rhythm)

3. Attach manual defibrillator/monitor to patient or switch over from the AED to the manual defibrillator using "hands-off" defibrillation electrode to visualize cardiac rhythm (see illustration).

A manual defibrillation/monitor provides immediate rhythm display for analysis. This device can also provide multiple leads to view the ECG and other functions like synchronized cardioversion and external pacemaker and continuous end-tidal CO_2 monitoring, if available.

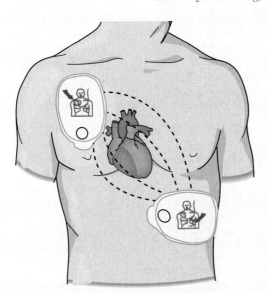

STEP 3 Pad placement for defibrillation.

4. If cardiac rhythm is "shockable," continue CPR and help code team with manual defibrillation.

Manual defibrillation is performed by ACLS-certified personnel.

  a. Turn on defibrillator and select proper energy level following agency policy and equipment directions.

Energy is delivered in prescribed doses. Manual biphasic devices deliver shocks at a lower level (200 joules), but some can deliver up to 360 joules; monophasic waveforms use 360 joules.

  b. Apply conductive gel or gel pads to patient's chest where defibrillator paddles will be placed. Most defibrillators use "hands-off pads" that are applied to patient's chest and directly connect to manual defibrillator.

Good skin-to-paddle/pad contact ensures appropriate discharge of current and decreases chance of skin burns (Panchal et al., 2020).

STEP	RATIONALE
c. Place paddles or pads on patient's chest wall. (See paddle placement, Skill 27.2.)	Ensures appropriate discharge of current.
d. Verify that no one is in physical contact with patient, bed, or any item contacting patient during defibrillation. A warning must be called out before initiating charge.	Prevents accidental delivery of shock or injury to personnel.
5. Establish IV access (see Chapter 28) with large-bore IV needle (14- to 22-gauge) and begin infusion of 0.9% NS or lactated Ringer solution.	Provides a route for rapid drug administration and access for blood samples and fluid administration. Physiological saline is isotonic. Rapid fluid infusion facilitates dispersal of medication throughout cardiovascular system.
a. If you cannot obtain peripheral IV access, health care provider may pursue central venous or intraosseous (IO) access.	Administration of emergency medications is dependent on vascular or IO access.
6. Help with procedures as needed.	Most equipment needed for special procedures during code is on the crash cart. Knowledge of crash cart contents is helpful in the code to provide personnel with appropriate equipment.
7. Continue CPR until relieved (i.e., until victim regains spontaneous pulse and respiration, rescuer is exhausted and unable to perform CPR effectively, or health care provider discontinues CPR). Rotate chest compressors every 2 minutes to maintain high-quality CPR.	Interruptions in chest compressions should be minimized and should never exceed 10 seconds (Panchal et al., 2020). CPR can be continued through the following actions: endotracheal intubation, defibrillator pad placement, brief interruption during chest compressor rotation, and only checking for pulse every 2 minutes during chest compressor rotation.

Secondary Survey: *A* (Intubate Airway)

STEP	RATIONALE
8. If respirations are absent, help code team with endotracheal intubation.	Intubation provides a patent airway and helps to protect patient against aspiration. Laryngeal mask airway (LMA) or esophageal-tracheal (Combi-tube) can also be used to provide advanced airway support.
a. Have available laryngoscope handle, laryngoscope blades, curved and straight blades, ET tubes, stylet, suction, and tape or ET tube holder. Ensure that light source on laryngoscope is functional. **NOTE:** During the COVID-19 pandemic, the AHA recommended using video laryngoscopy to reduce exposure to aerosolized particles during intubation (Atkins et al., 2022).	Light is necessary on laryngoscope to visualize vocal cords and intubate trachea. Batteries may need to be changed. All supplies should be readily available on the crash cart or in a designated airway box.

Secondary Survey: *B* (Confirmation of Airway and Ventilation)

STEP	RATIONALE
9. Help in confirmation of ET tube placement or advanced airway support by auscultating lungs for bilateral breath sounds and monitoring the carbon dioxide (CO_2) detector to confirm correct airway placement (Panchal et al., 2020).	Auscultation of lungs and monitoring of exhaled CO_2 or esophageal detector device further verify correct airway placement and adequacy of ventilation and gas exchange. Chest x-ray film is usually obtained after patient has been stabilized to confirm placement of ET tube and central venous catheters.
10. Ventilate using bag device on intubation. **Avoid hyperventilation.**	Increased intrathoracic pressure caused by incomplete exhalation results in reduced cardiac output (Panchal et al., 2020).

Secondary Survey: *D* (Differential Diagnosis)

STEP	RATIONALE
11. Obtain ordered laboratory and diagnostic studies.	Aids in determination of cause of arrest.

EVALUATION

1. Reassess primary and secondary surveys throughout code event.	Keeps process organized and addresses immediate needs of patient.
2. Palpate carotid or femoral pulse at 5 cycles or 2 minutes of CPR.	Documents adequacy of external cardiac compressions.
3. Observe for spontaneous return of respirations or heart rate every 2 minutes usually performed during chest compressors rotation. This should be performed in less than 10 seconds.	Assessment of pulse, respiration, heart rate, and cardiac rhythm can occur after chest compressions and ventilation have been interrupted briefly every 2 minutes.
4. Ensure that interruptions in CPR are minimized.	Interruptions are associated with reduced coronary artery perfusion pressure and lower mean coronary perfusion pressure (Merchant et al., 2020.)

STEP	RATIONALE
5. Use Teach-Back with Family Caregiver: "I want to be sure I clearly explained what has happened to your loved one and why we performed cardiopulmonary resuscitation, known as CPR. In your own words, tell me why we had to perform CPR." Revise your instruction now or develop a plan for revised family caregiver teaching if family caregiver is not able to teach back correctly.	Teach-back is a technique for health care providers to ensure that they have explained medical information clearly so that patients and their families understand what is communicated to them (Agency for Healthcare Research and Quality [AHRQ], 2023).

Unexpected Outcomes

1. Patient develops skeletal injury, such as fractured ribs or sternum or internal organ injury including lacerated lung or liver as result of chest compressions.

2. Patient's CPR is unsuccessful.

Related Interventions

- Obtain appropriate diagnostic tests to document injuries.
- Assess patient's postarrest breathing for symmetry and pain.
- Assess for intrathoracic or intraabdominal bleeding (hematomas, increasing abdominal girth).
- Contact chaplain services.
- Contact social worker.
- Complete postmortem care on patient (see Chapter 17).
- Notify coroner and organ procurement agency in accordance with local agency or state law.
- Provide for privacy for patient's family to grieve and mourn loss of loved one.

Documentation

- Document the onset of arrest, time and number of AED shocks (you will not know the exact energy level used by the AED), time and energy level of manual defibrillations, medications given (including time), procedures performed (e.g., intubation, specimens), cardiac rhythm, use of CPR, patient's response, education, and support provided to family.

Hand-Off Reporting

- Immediately report arrest, indicating exact location of victim. In agency setting, follow agency policy. In community setting, activate the emergency response system.
- Use the CPR worksheet as reference during a hand-off to accepting nurse. Report the prearrest assessment and major interventions during the arrest.

Special Considerations

Patient Education

- See Skill 27.2 for teaching considerations.

Pediatrics

- All people involved in administering CPR must understand different breathing/compression ratios, hand (fingers) placement, and depth of compression in children and infants compared with adults (see Table 27.3).

- Infants and children experience respiratory arrest much more frequently than full cardiopulmonary arrest.
- Quick reference, color-coded guides are frequently used in pediatric codes to quickly determine appropriate drug doses and equipment sizes based on the patient's length.

Older Adults

- In older adults, compressions often result in rib or cartilage fractures.
- Remove loose-fitting dentures to avoid obstructing the airway. If dentures fit securely, leave them in to provide a tight seal when providing ventilations.

Home Care

- In community and long-term care settings, patients may have implanted cardioverter defibrillators (ICDs) and/or pacemakers. For these patients, families need to know how to administer CPR and the specific capabilities of the patient's ICD/pacemaker. Placement of defibrillator or AED pads/paddles may need to be altered to avoid placement directly on top of an ICD or pacemaker generator. Remove medication patches from chest.
- Soft surfaces such as a mattress or car seat decrease efficiency of external cardiac compressions.

✦ CLINICAL JUDGMENT AND NEXT GENERATION NCLEX® EXAMINATION–STYLE QUESTIONS

This nurse is caring for a patient with acute kidney injury (AKI). During rounds, the nurse finds the patient lying on the floor of the bathroom. The patient is unresponsive when shaken and called by name. An automated external defibrillator (AED) is available down the hall.

1. Which action will the nurse take **first**?
   1. Apply automated external defibrillator (AED).
   2. Call for help.
   3. Check for a pulse.
   4. Open airway and provide two breaths.
2. Which of the following techniques would the nurse use to deliver high-quality cardiopulmonary resuscitation (CPR)? **Select all that apply.**
   1. Minimizing interruption in chest compressions
   2. Avoiding full chest recoil
   3. Providing more ventilations than recommended
   4. Assuring adequate depth and rate of compression
   5. Pausing chest compressions during defibrillation preparation
3. Another nurse arrives to the room with the automated external defibrillator (AED). The primary nurse is providing chest compressions. Which step will the primary nurse take **next**?
   1. Check for onset of a pulse.
   2. Clear the area to initiate the AED.
   3. Instruct the other nurse to apply the AED.
   4. Provide ongoing chest compressions.
4. The Rapid Response Team (RRT) arrives to continue resuscitation attempts. Which information will the nurse communicate to the arriving RRT? **Select all that apply.**
   1. Found patient on the floor
   2. How long cardiopulmonary resuscitation (CPR) has been administered
   3. Number of shocks delivered by the automated external defibrillator (AED)
   4. Reason patient is hospitalized
   5. Initial assessment data
5. The patient is stabilized and resting in bed. For each body system, select the potential nursing interventions that would be appropriate for the care of the patient. Each body system may support more than one potential nursing intervention.

System	Potential Nursing Interventions
Cardiovascular	• Document blood pressure • Apply cardiac monitor • Discuss cardiac rehabilitation with the patient
Respiratory	• Explain the cause of infection • Assess lung sounds every 2 hours • Monitor continuous pulse oximetry
Neurological	• Assess for changes in cognition • Ask to count backwards from 100 by 7s • Tell three words to the patient; ask patient to repeat the words 5 minutes later

Visit the Evolve site for Answers to Clinical Judgment and Next Generation NCLEX® Examination2Style Questions.

REFERENCES

Agency for Healthcare Research and Quality (AHRQ): *Teach-back: intervention*, 2023. https://www.ahrq.gov/patient-safety/reports/engage/interventions/teachback.html.

Agency for Healthcare Research and Quality (AHRQ): *Patient safety primer: rapid response systems*, January 2019. https://psnet.ahrq.gov/primers/primer/4/rapid-response-systems. Accessed November 16, 2023.

Atkins D, et al: 2022 Interim guidance to health care providers for basic and advanced cardiac life support in adults, children, and neonates with suspected or confirmed COVID-19: From the Emergency Cardiovascular Care Committee and Get With The Guidelines-Resuscitation Adult and Pediatric Task Forces of the American Heart Association in Collaboration With the American Academy of Pediatrics, American Association for Respiratory Care, the Society of Critical Care Anesthesiologists, and American Society of Anesthesiologists, *Circ Cardiovasc Qual Outcomes* 15(4):e008900, 2022.

Castro D, Freeman LA: *Oropharyngeal airway*, Treasure Island, 2022, StatPearls, National Library of Medicine.

Centers for Disease Control and Prevention (CDC): *What is health literacy?* 2023. https://www.cdc.gov/healthliteracy/learn/index.html.

Hockenberry MJ, et al: *Wong's essentials of pediatric nursing*, ed 11, St. Louis, 2022, Elsevier.

Merchant RM, et al: Part 1: executive summary: 2020 American Heart Association guidelines for cardiopulmonary resuscitation and emergency cardiovascular care, *Circulation* 142(16 Suppl 2):S337–S357, 2020.

LaRocco SA, Toronto CE: Clinical practice guidelines and family presence during cardiopulmonary arrest, *West J Nurs Res* 41(9):1219–1221, 2019.

Panchal AR, et al. Part 3: adult basic and advanced life support: 2020 American Heart Association Guidelines for Cardiopulmonary Resuscitation and Emergency Cardiovascular Care, *Circulation* 142(16 Suppl 2):S366–S468, 2020.

Ralston M, et al: *Basic airway management in children*, 2022, UpToDate. https://www.uptodate.com/contents/basic-airway-management-in-children. Accessed November 16, 2023.

Storm C, et al: Impact of structural pathways for postcardiac arrest care: a systemic review and meta-analysis, *Crit Care Med* 47(8):e710–e716, 2019.

The Joint Commission: Managing medical device-related pressure injuries, *Quick Safety* Issue 25, 2022. https://www.jointcommission.org/resources/news-and-multimedia/newsletters/newsletters/quick-safety/quick-safety-issue-25-preventing-pressure-injuries/#.YszpTnbMI2w.

Vardanjani A, et al: The effect of family presence during resuscitation and invasive procedures on patients and families: an umbrella review, *J Emerg Nurs* 47(5):752–760, 2021.

UNIT 9
Oxygenation: Next-Generation NCLEX® (NGN)–Style Unfolding Case Study

PHASE 1

QUESTION 1.
A client has been brought to the emergency department by their roommate. The triage nurse conducts an initial assessment.

Highlight the client findings that require **immediate** follow-up by the nurse.

History and Physical	Nurses' Notes	Vital Signs	Laboratory Results

2234: Client brought to the emergency department by roommate. The roommate states, "We live across the street from the hospital, and I made her come here. We were at a party and ate some cookies, and then she broke out in this weird rash." Medical history in the electronic health record (EHR) reveals a history of depression, which is controlled with sertraline by mouth daily, and anxiety, which is treated as needed with hydroxyzine by mouth PRN. Assessment reveals lung sounds with mild stridor and mildly decreased breath sounds, facial swelling, and urticaria on the neck and chest. Client reports, "I feel as if I am swallowing over something, but nothing is in my throat, and my heart feels as if it is going to beat out of my chest. I'm really scared!" S_1S_2 present without murmur. Bowel sounds present × 4 quadrants; strength equal in all extremities. Vital signs: T 37.6°C (99.6°F); HR 120 beats/min; RR 26 breaths/min; BP 168/100 mm Hg; SpO_2 89% on RA.

QUESTION 2.
The nursing assessment noted that the client has broken out in a rash.

Complete the following sentence by selecting from the lists of options below.

The nurse anticipates that the client is most likely experiencing 1 [Select] due to 2 [Select].

Options for 1	Options for 2
Cardiac arrest	Cardiac ischemia
Anaphylaxis	Sertraline
Asthma attack	Food allergy
Myocardial infarction	Hydroxyzine

PHASE 2

QUESTION 3.
The nursing assessment noted that the client had broken out in a rash.

Complete the following sentence by selecting from the list of word choices below.

The nurse will **first** address the client's [Word Choice].

Word Choice
Heart rate
Urticaria
Oxygen saturation
Fear
Consumption of cookies

QUESTION 4.
The nurse must identify interventions that would improve the client's status.

Complete the following sentence by selecting from the list of options below.

The nurse will prepare for the following interventions: 1 [Select] and 2 [Select].

Options for 1	Options for 2
Avoid airway collapse	Manage sertraline allergy
Prevent venous thromboembolism	Prevent respiratory arrest
Administer diphenhydramine	Increase the heart rate

PHASE 3

QUESTION 5.

The emergency team is present.

Which action does the nurse implement at this time? **Select all that apply.**

- ○ Apply wrist restraints.
- ○ Prepare for intubation.
- ○ Administer epinephrine.
- ○ Contact the client's family.
- ○ Place in Trendelenburg position.
- ○ Inform the roommate of what is happening.
- ○ Initiate rapid bolus infusion of 1000 mL normal saline.

QUESTION 6.

The client is intubated and stabilized in the emergency department and transferred to intensive care.

Highlight the findings that indicate that the client is progressing favorably.

History and Physical	Nurses' Notes	Vital Signs	Laboratory Results

0422: Client in ICU following stabilization after anaphylaxis in the emergency department. Resting comfortably. Cardiac monitor shows sinus rhythm at 72 beats/min. Other vital signs: T 37.2°C (99.0°F); RR 18 breaths/min; BP 128/88 mm Hg; SpO$_2$ 97%. Opens eyes to stimuli; PERRLA. Lung sounds clear bilaterally. S$_1$S$_2$ present without murmur.

UNIT 10
Fluid Balance

The skills used to support a patient's fluid balance apply principles of surgical asepsis and infection control, safe medication practices, patient safety and comfort, and protection of skin integrity. Patients who develop fluid balance problems are frequently in need of intravenous therapy. Sound clinical judgment for how to manage these patients safely requires application of knowledge about normal fluid and electrolyte balance and the impact of pathological conditions on a patient's fluid balance. Your knowledge base and experience in applying these principles aid in directing your patient assessments, identifying patient problems, and making decisions about applying the skills correctly.

Administration of intravenous and vascular access therapy is a complex, time-sensitive, and time-pressured nursing action. For safe therapy, remove any distractions as you apply all of the principles of safe medication practices, following the seven rights of medication administration, and know the action, purpose, side effects, and nursing implication of each fluid or additive medication.

Apply knowledge about a patient's clinical condition or physical risks, in the event that there are factors that might affect the rate of an intravenous infusion. Safe administration of intravenous therapy requires a careful check of a health care provider's order and accurate calculation and double checking of the prescribed infusion rate.

Inserting an intravenous catheter is an invasive procedure. Use your knowledge about infection control, surgical asepsis, and anatomical location of large peripheral veins and arteries when you select an insertion site. The preparation of the site requires measures to reduce the risk of central line–associated bloodstream infection (CLABSI). Apply the Infusion Nurses Society's infusion therapy standards and Standard Precautions for infection control. Your experience in vein selection is invaluable in being able to choose a site that is less likely to be compromised by patient positioning or physical care activities.

A thorough patient assessment is necessary when initiating, regulating, or maintaining any fluid therapy. Use clinical judgment in assessing for signs and symptoms of dehydration or fluid overload, signs of catheter site inflammation or CLABSI, any signs associated with medical device–related pressure injury (MDRPI) under catheter tubing or catheter-stabilization devices, and any signs of medical adhesive–related skin injury (MARSI) from adhesives used to secure intravenous catheters. Your assessment can identify cues that indicate fluid overload or deficit, infection, or early pressure or skin injury. If these problems arise, you may need to contact the health care provider to change a fluid order. Also, you can take preventive steps to minimize intravascular complications. For example, when a catheter insertion site shows early signs of infection, remove the catheter and select a new site for reinsertion. If a patient has an MDRPI forming around a catheter insertion site, you will provide appropriate skin and wound care to the pressure injury site. If the patient has signs of MARSI, you will change the type of adhesive to use for catheter securement, reposition any adhesive, and perform special periwound skin care.

Central vascular access devices (CVADs) are implanted devices inserted by a health care provider. The location of the device in the central circulation creates significant patient risks, particularly infection, thrombus, and dislodgement, among others. Thorough ongoing patient assessments are necessary to detect any complications early. Site care is particularly important in preventing CLABSI; follow current practice standards rigorously.

A patient who requires a CVAD has serious health problems that require ongoing fluid therapy, frequent blood sampling, and long-term intravenous medications, such as chemotherapy, intravenous antibiotics, or cardiac support medications. The safe use of a CVAD and administration of any fluid or medication requires critical thinking when you assess the integrity and function of the vascular access device and patient tolerance of the device and prescribed therapies, including medications and blood products.

28 | Intravenous and Vascular Access Therapy

SKILLS AND PROCEDURES

Skill 28.1 **Insertion of a Peripheral Intravenous Device, p. 846**

Skill 28.2 **Regulating Intravenous Flow Rates, p. 861**

Skill 28.3 **Changing Intravenous Solutions, p. 867**

Skill 28.4 **Changing Infusion Tubing, p. 871**

Skill 28.5 **Changing a Peripheral Intravenous Dressing, p. 874**

Procedural Guideline 28.1 **Discontinuing a Peripheral Intravenous Device, p. 878**

Skill 28.6 **Managing Central Vascular Access Devices, p. 879**

OBJECTIVES

Mastery of content in this chapter will you to:

- Discuss current evidence-based practices for intravenous (IV) therapy.
- Discuss patient conditions requiring IV therapy.
- Identify safety guidelines for IV fluid administration.
- Explain how to prepare a patient to receive IV therapy.
- Discuss nursing measures for preventing complications of IV therapy.
- Identify individualized outcomes for patients requiring IV therapy.
- Identify the educational needs of patients receiving IV therapy.
- Explain techniques for preventing transmission of infection for a patient receiving IV therapy.
- Demonstrate initiating IV therapy, regulating IV flow rate, changing IV solutions, changing IV tubing, changing IV dressings, and discontinuing a peripheral IV device.
- Identify common types of central vascular access devices (CVADs) and describe their care and maintenance.
- Identify the educational needs of patients with CVADs.

MEDIA RESOURCES

- http://evolve.elsevier.com/Perry/skills
- Review Questions
- ▶ Video Clips
- Audio Glossary
- **NSO** Nursing Skills Online
- Answers to Clinical Judgment and Next-Generation NCLEX® Examination–Style Questions
- Printable Key Points
- Skills Performance Checklists

PURPOSE

Intravenous (IV) therapy is used to provide parenteral nutrition, transfuse blood products, provide a route for hemodynamic monitoring and diagnostic testing, and administer fluids and medications. These functions offer the ability to change blood concentration levels of fluids, nutrients, and medications rapidly and accurately by either continuous, intermittent, or IV push method. Assessment of a patient's anatomy and physiology of the circulatory system, fluid and electrolyte balance, disease pathophysiology, type and duration of prescribed therapy, allergies, and the patient's response to illness plays a key role in clinical judgment and clinical decision making to ensure safe delivery of infusion solutions or medications.

Successful IV therapy depends on patient preparation, site selection, catheter selection, and catheter insertion. The goal of IV therapy is to maintain and prevent fluid and electrolyte imbalances, administer continuous or intermittent medications (e.g., antibiotics and analgesics), and replenish blood volume (Gorski, 2023). The use of IV therapy for a patient is common in nursing practice and thus requires skill competency.

PRACTICE STANDARDS

- Gorski L, et al., 2021: Infusion Therapy Standards of Practice
- Fumarola S, et al., 2020: Overlooked and Underestimated: Medical Adhesive–Related Skin Injuries (MARSI). Best Practice Consensus Document on Prevention—Assessment and prevention
- The Joint Commission (TJC), 2023:National Patient Safety Goals—Patient identification

SUPPLEMENTAL STANDARDS

- Centers for Disease Control and Prevention (CDC) National Health Safety Network (NHSN), 2022: Bloodstream Infection Event (Central Line–Associated Bloodstream Infection and Non–Central Line–Associated Bloodstream Infection)

- Occupational Safety and Health Administration (OSHA), n.d.: Bloodborne Pathogens Standard—Occupational safe exposure to bloodborne pathogens

PRINCIPLES FOR PRACTICE

- Evidence-based practices guide the safe, efficient, and high-quality care necessary to provide IV therapy.
- Safe IV therapy requires conscientious use of infection control practices.
- Indications and protocols for vascular access device (VAD) selection and placement; management; prevention, assessment, and management of complications; and infusion therapy administration are established in agency policies, procedures, and/or practice guidelines and according to manufacturer directions for use (Gorski et al., 2021).
- Follow the seven rights of medication administration when administering parenteral solutions or medications: *Right* patient, *Right* drug or solution, *Right* dose and concentration, *Right* route, *Right* date and time, *Right* documentation, and *Right* indication (Gorski, 2023).
- The seven rights of medication administration also include applying knowledge of the solution or medication and its purpose, knowing how to initiate and regulate an infusion, operating and maintaining infusion equipment, identifying and correcting any infusion-related complications, and discontinuing an infusion.

Vascular Access Devices

- For administration of IV solutions and medications, a VAD is inserted into a vein. VADs can be peripheral devices (i.e., peripheral, midline) or central vascular access devices (CVADs) (i.e., tunneled, nontunneled, peripherally inserted central catheter [PICC], implanted port). The choice depends on where the tip of the device needs to reside. For example, fluids of high concentration need to be infused into large blood vessels accessed with a CVAD.
- When selecting the appropriate VAD, consider a patient's prescribed therapy; length of treatment; duration the device remains in place; vascular characteristics; and patient's age, height, weight, co-morbidities, history of infusion therapy, preference for VAD location, and resources available to care for the device (Gorski et al., 2021).
- When continuous infusion of solutions or medications is not necessary, a peripheral IV line can stay in place but be locked with preservative-free 0.9% sodium chloride (normal saline [NS]) in adults (Gorski et al., 2021). Then the device can be reaccessed without needing to start a new IV. To maintain a saline lock, use commercially available prefilled syringes for flushing the device to reduce the risk of catheter-related bloodstream infection (CRBSI). Use a minimum volume equal to twice the internal volume of the catheter system (see agency policy) (Gorski et al., 2021).
- In the case of CVADs, fill a lock with either heparin 10 units per milliliter or preservative-free 0.9% NS according to the directions for use of the VAD and agency policy (Gorski et al., 2021).

Intravenous Solutions

- There are many prepared IV solutions available for use (Table 28.1).
- IV solutions fall into several categories based on fluid osmolality: isotonic, hypotonic, and hypertonic. Isotonic solutions have the same osmolality as body fluids.

TABLE 28.1

Intravenous Solutions

Solution	Concentration in IV Container and at Tip of VAD	Effective Concentration in Body	Comments
Dextrose (Glucose) in Water Solutions			
Dextrose 5% in water (D5W)	Isotonic	Hypotonic	Isotonic when first enters vein; dextrose enters cells rapidly, leaving free water, which dilutes ECF; most of the water then enters cells by osmosis.
Dextrose 10% in water (D10W)	Hypertonic	Hypotonic	Hypertonic when first enters vein; dextrose enters cells rapidly, leaving free water, which dilutes ECF; most of the water then enters cells by osmosis.
Saline (Sodium Chloride [NaCl] in Water) Solutions			
0.225% NaCl (¼ NS)	Hypotonic	Hypotonic	Expands ECV (vascular and interstitial) and rehydrates cells.
0.45% NaCl (½ NS)	Hypotonic	Hypotonic	Expands ECV (vascular and interstitial) and rehydrates cells.
0.9% NaCl (NS)	Isotonic	Isotonic	Expands ECV (vascular and interstitial); does not enter cells.
3% or 5% NaCl (hypertonic saline; 3% or 5% NaCl)	Hypertonic	Hypertonic	Draws water from cells into ECF by osmosis.
Dextrose in Saline Solutions			
Dextrose 5% in 0.45% NaCl (½ NS; D50.45% NaCl)	Hypertonic	Hypotonic	Dextrose enters cells rapidly, leaving 0.45% NaCl.
Dextrose 5% in 0.9% NaCl (D5NS; D50.9% NaCl)	Hypertonic	Isotonic	Dextrose enters cells rapidly, leaving 0.9% NaCl.
Multiple Electrolyte Solutions			
Lactated Ringer (LR) solution	Isotonic	Isotonic	LR contains Na$^+$, K$^+$, Ca^{2+}, Cl$^-$, and lactate, which liver metabolizes to HCO$_3^-$; expands ECV (vascular and interstitial); does not enter cells.
Dextrose 5% in LR (D5LR)	Hypertonic	Isotonic	Dextrose enters cells rapidly, leaving LR.

ECF, Extracellular fluid; *ECV,* extracellular volume; *IV,* intravenous; *NS,* normal saline; *VAD,* vascular access device.

- Administer IV solutions carefully; isotonic solutions can cause increased risk for fluid overload in patients with renal or cardiac disease; hypotonic solutions can exacerbate a hypotensive state; and hypertonic solutions are irritating to the vein and can cause increased risk of heart failure and pulmonary edema.
- To prevent infusion-related complications, solutions and medications with an osmolarity greater than 900 mOsm/L are infused through a CVAD. Peripheral catheters should not be used for continuous vesicant therapy, parenteral nutrition, or infusates with an osmolarity greater than 900 mOsm/L (Gorski et al., 2021). In addition, solution or medication characteristics (e.g., irritant, vesicant, osmolarity), along with anticipated duration of infusion therapy, should be considered when agents are administered with a peripheral or midline catheter, as they have the potential to cause infusion-related complications such as phlebitis (Gorski, 2023).
- Premixed solutions contain medications or electrolytes added by the manufacturer. However, the risk for medication errors increases because they come in varying dosages.
- A patient's specific fluid and electrolyte imbalance and serum electrolyte values guide health care providers in the selection of the appropriate IV fluid (Gorski, 2023).

PERSON-CENTERED CARE

- Communication, comfort, and education are essential components of patient-centered care when delivering IV therapy.
- Consider patient and family caregiver cultural and linguistic needs when educating about the prescribed IV therapy and goals and expected outcomes of therapy.
- Encourage patient participation in creating the plan of care, including the patient's preferences regarding the degree of active involvement. Although the skills in this chapter are performed by a registered nurse (RN), engaging patients in the decision-making process can give them a sense of control.
- Patient education includes clear and concise terms for all aspects of IV therapy and individualized training that includes patient-centered self-care practices.
- Patient teaching should also include the care of the VAD, infection prevention, and potential VAD complications and signs and symptoms to report (Gorski et al., 2021).
- Reduce anxiety and fear during the insertion of a VAD by preparing the patient before insertion of a peripheral IV catheter. Place patient in a comfortable position, speak directly to the patient, and answer questions as honestly as possible. Ask patients if they have had IV therapy in the past. Know their concerns and expectations.
- When preparing for an IV catheter insertion, use techniques that minimize discomfort. Consider using local anesthetic agents (see agency policy) based on patient condition, needs, risks, benefits, and anticipated discomfort of the procedure (Gorski et al., 2021).
- Allow a patient to have a family caregiver present and provide privacy during the procedure if possible.
- Pain is also expressed differently in different cultures, and you may see some cultures that encourage expressiveness and others that encourage stoicism; this is important to keep in mind when performing skills that may elicit a response to the pain of inserting or removing the tape and dressing from a VAD.
- Consider patients' religious beliefs, especially when using heparin in a saline lock for a VAD. Heparin is derived from animal products (e.g., porcine, bovine) and may be in conflict with a patient's religious beliefs (Gorski et al., 2021).

EVIDENCE-BASED PRACTICE

Reducing Complications in Infusion Therapy

Infusion therapy is practiced in health care settings spanning from the health care agency to home care. It is expected that the nurse providing infusion therapy understands and implements evidence-based practice and complies with laws, rules, regulations, standards, and policies to keep up with role changes, understand new products and technology, and prevent complications (Gorski, 2023; Gorski et al., 2021).

- Quality improvement includes surveillance, reporting and analysis of infection rates, infection prevention practices, and infusion-related patient quality indicators, such as occurrence of central line–associated bloodstream infection (CLABSI) and number of attempts for VAD insertion. Implementation of quality indicators and benchmarks develops a culture of accountability (Buetti et al., 2022; Gorski et al., 2021).
- Remove VADs when there is an unresolved complication, such as phlebitis or discontinuation of infusion therapy, or when the VAD is no longer necessary for the plan of care (Buetti et al., 2022; Gorski et al., 2021).
- Passive disinfection caps contain a sponge saturated with a disinfecting agent (usually isopropyl alcohol). A cap is often placed on an access port on infusion tubing. In addition, a cap is placed on the end of a needleless connector between intermittent infusions (such as a piggyback) when an infusion is not being used. It protects the end of a connector from the entrance of microorganisms, and therefore less disinfection time or no disinfection is needed before the IV infusion is reaccessed (Barton, 2019; Buetti et al., 2022; Gorski et al., 2021). These caps have been shown to reduce contamination within the lumen of an infusion tube and significantly reduce the rates of CLABSI (Buetti et al., 2022; Gorski et al., 2021).
- Primary and secondary continuous administration sets used to administer solutions other than lipid, blood, or blood products should be changed not more often than every 96 hours but at least every 7 days (Buetti et al., 2022; Gorski et al., 2021).
- Compared with all other dressing types, the use of chlorhexidine gluconate (CHG)–impregnated dressings, in a patch or in a transparent dressing, is more effective in reducing the incidence of bloodstream infections in CVADs (Buetti et al., 2022; Gorski et al., 2021).
- Randomized controlled trials have shown similar outcomes with heparin and sodium chloride lock solutions for keeping multiple-lumen nontunneled CVADs, PICCs, and implanted ports patent while accessed and when the access needle is removed. There is insufficient evidence to recommend one solution over the other (Gorski et al., 2021).

SAFETY GUIDELINES

- Clinician competence is required for the use, placement, and management of VADs; the ability to recognize signs and symptoms of VAD-related complications; the use of infusion equipment; and knowledge of all aspects of administering infusion therapy (Gorski et al., 2021).
- Conduct a complete history and physical assessment, including vital signs, and review laboratory findings before initiating any solutions.
- Know the indications for prescribed therapy before initiating IV therapy. Obtain and review the health care provider's order to ensure appropriateness of the prescribed solution for the

patient's age, health status, medical diagnosis, allergy status, and acuity (Gorski et al., 2021).

- Before initiating an IV infusion, assess the patency and functioning of the VAD for aspiration of a blood return using Aseptic Non-Touch Technique (ANTT), absence of resistance, patient complaints of pain or discomfort when flushing, and all VAD complications (Gorski et al., 2021). ANTT is achieved by integrating Standard Precautions, including hand hygiene, use of personal protective equipment (PPE) with appropriate aseptic field management, non-touch technique, and sterilized supplies (Box 28.1) (Gorski et al., 2021).

- Reduce risk for administration set misconnections by tracing the path between the IV fluid container and patient, labeling administration sets near patient connection and solution container, and routing tubing used for different purposes in different directions. In general, disconnections are not recommended.
- Maintain sterility of a patent IV system using Infusion Nurses Society (INS) standards (see Box 28.1).
- Know and implement the Standard Precautions for infection control and the Occupational Safety and Health Administration (OSHA) standards for occupational exposure to bloodborne pathogens (Box 28.2).

BOX 28.1

Infusion Nurses Society (INS) Standards to Decrease Intravascular Infection Related to Intravenous Therapy

- Aseptic Non-Touch Technique (ANTT) is designed for use in the placement, management, and infusion administration of vascular access devices (VADs). ANTT integrates Standard Precautions including hand hygiene, use of personal protective equipment (PPE) with appropriate aseptic field management, non-touch technique, and sterilized supplies. In the event of Key-Parts or Key-Sites (see below) requiring direct touch, then sterile gloves must be used.
- The five terms for using ANTT:
  - *Key Site:* Any portal of entry into the patient (e.g., VAD site, injection site).
  - *Key Part:* The part of the equipment that, if contaminated, is likely to contaminate the patient (e.g., syringe tip, male Luer end or spike of administration set, injection needle).
  - *General Aseptic Field:* A decontaminated and disinfected procedure tray or single-use procedure kit or barrier.
  - *Critical Aseptic Field:* A sterile drape or barrier that is used to ensure asepsis; all procedure equipment is placed upon the drape.
  - *Micro Critical Aseptic Field:* A small protective sterile surface or housing (e.g., sterile caps, covers, and the inside of recently opened sterile equipment packaging) that protects Key Parts individually.
- Perform hand hygiene, following ANTT, before placing and providing any VAD-associated interventions.
- Assess the VAD catheter-skin junction site and surrounding area for redness, tenderness, swelling, and drainage by visual inspection and palpation through the intact dressing and through patient report of symptoms of a complication.
- Assess central vascular access devices (CVADs) and midline catheters at least daily.
- Assess peripheral catheters minimally at least every 4 hours or more if clinically indicated.

- Assess VADs daily for outpatient or home care patients. For a continuous infusion via a peripheral catheter in the home, assess every 4 hours while patient is awake.
- Perform routine dressing changes at a frequency based on the type of catheter and dressing.
- Change a dressing on any VAD or peripheral IV site immediately to assess, clean, and disinfect the site in the event of drainage, tenderness, or other signs of infection, or if dressing becomes loose, visibly soiled, or dislodged.
- Change gauze dressings every 2 days.
- Change transparent semipermeable membrane (TSM) dressings every 5 to 7 days.
- Use approved antiseptic agents before venipuncture and when performing skin antisepsis. The preferred skin antiseptic is greater than 0.5% chlorhexidine gluconate (CHG) in alcohol solution. Tincture of iodine, an iodophor (povidone-iodine), or 70% alcohol may be used if CHG solution is contraindicated.
- Allow skin antiseptic to dry fully before dressing placement: alcoholic CHG for at least 20 seconds, and iodophors for up to 6 minutes.
- Use catheter stabilization device that allows visual inspection of access site.
- Use vigorous mechanical scrubbing methods when disinfecting needleless connectors before each access using 70% isopropyl alcohol, iodophors, or 0.5% CHG alcoholic solution. Disinfect before each access when multiple accesses are required.
- Change needleless connectors, using ANTT, every 96 hours or with the primary administration set changes.
- Use passive disinfection caps (e.g., isopropyl alcohol).
- Change administration sets based on solution administered and frequency of the infusion and immediately on suspected contamination or when integrity has been compromised.

Modified from Gorski L, et al: *Infusion therapy standards of practice*, ed 8, Norwood, MA, 2021, Infusion Nurses Society (INS).

BOX 28.2

Standards for Reducing Occupational Exposure to Bloodborne Pathogens

1. Gloves are required when there is a reasonable expectation that the employee may contact blood (e.g., during vascular access procedures or while changing intravenous [IV] administration sets).
2. Immediately place contaminated needles, needleless devices, and other sharps in puncture-resistant, leak-proof containers properly labeled as a biohazard; when the containers are full, seal and dispose of them properly.
3. Do not bend, shear, recap, or remove contaminated needles from the syringe after use.
4. Occupational Safety and Health Administration (OSHA) requires reports of needlestick injuries, and the health care agency must provide medical evaluation and follow-up.

5. Hepatitis B vaccinations should be made available to all employees who have occupational exposure to blood.
6. Training and education about exposure prevention and use of protective equipment must be offered to high-risk workers who initiate IV therapy.
7. Each agency must have an infection control plan, including methods to reduce health care workers' exposure to biohazardous wastes.
8. Agencies must have engineering and work practice controls to eliminate or minimize employee exposure. Controls may include sharps disposal containers and self-sheathing needles.

Modified from Occupational Safety and Health Administration (OSHA): *Bloodborne pathogens and needlestick prevention.* https://www.osha.gov/bloodborne-pathogens/general.

◆ SKILL 28.1 Insertion of a Peripheral Intravenous Device

 Video Clip

An intravenous (IV) device provides access to the venous system. Peripheral venous access is categorized into use of three types of peripheral IV catheters (Gorski et al., 2021): short peripheral (in superficial veins), long peripheral (superficial or deep peripheral veins), and midline (peripheral vein of the upper arm via the basilic, cephalic, or brachial vein with the terminal tip located at the level of the axilla). Reliable venous access for infusion therapy administration is essential. Several vascular access devices (VADs) are available. Fig. 28.1 shows the parts of two peripheral IV devices. Table 28.2 outlines the VAD options for peripheral administration. Commonly used devices include (1) an over-the-needle catheter (ONC) made of silicone, polyurethane, polyvinyl chloride, or polytetrafluoroethylene (Teflon) that threads into a vein and remains there for the infusion of fluid; and (2) a metal stylet to pierce the skin. Table 28.3 indicates appropriate uses for the more common peripheral catheter sizes.

Delegation

The skill of inserting a peripheral IV access device cannot be delegated to assistive personnel (AP). Delegation to licensed practical nurses (LPNs) varies by state nurse practice act. Direct the AP to:
- Notify the nurse if the patient complains of any IV site–related complications such as redness, pain, tenderness, swelling, bleeding, drainage, or leaking from under dressing
- Notify the nurse if the patient's IV dressing becomes wet

- Notify the nurse if the level of fluid in the IV bag is low or the electronic infusion device (EID) is alarming

Interprofessional Collaboration
- The health care provider and pharmacy services are involved in the management of VADs.

Equipment
- Peripheral IV start kit supplies (available in some agencies): single-use tourniquet, tape, dressing (integrated securement device, transparent semipermeable membrane [TSM] dressing or sterile gauze), sterile tape, antiseptic wipes (chlorhexidine

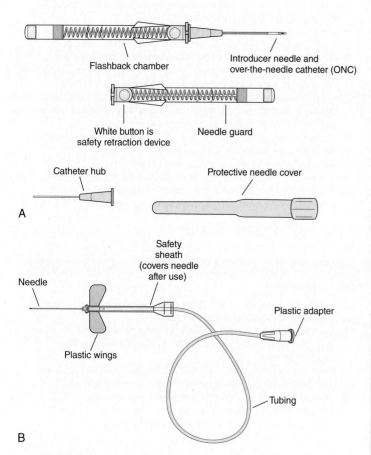

FIG. 28.1 Intravenous access device options. (A) Over-the-needle catheter device. (B) Steel butterfly needle.

TABLE 28.2

Peripheral Vascular Access Device Options

Type	Use	Types of Infusions
Short, over-the-needle catheter (ONC), placed in superficial veins	Continuous infusion, intermittent infusion, short-term duration (Gorski et al., 2021)	Solutions or medications with an osmolarity less than 900 mOsm/L (Gorski et al., 2021)
Long peripheral, placed in superficial or deep peripheral veins when a short peripheral cannot cannulate the vein	Continuous infusion, intermittent infusion, short-term duration (Gorski et al., 2021)	Solutions or medications with an osmolarity less than 900 mOsm/L (Gorski et al., 2021)
Midline peripheral catheters, placed in peripheral vein of the upper arm via the basilic, cephalic, or brachial vein with the terminal tip located at the level of the axilla	Continuous infusion and intermittent infusion (5–14 days) (Gorski et al., 2021)	Solutions or medications with an osmolarity less than 900 mOsm/L (Gorski et al., 2021)

TABLE 28.3

Recommendations for Peripheral Catheter Selection

Catheter Size (Gauge)	Clinical Indication
18	Trauma, surgery, rapid blood transfusions, and rapid fluid replacement
20	Continuous or intermittent infusions in adults; administration of blood transfusions in adults
22	Continuous or intermittent infusions in adults, children, neonates, and the elderly; administration of blood or blood product in adults, children, neonates, and older adults
24–26	Continuous or intermittent infusions in adults, children, neonates, and the elderly; administration of blood or blood product in adults, children, neonates, and older adults

Modified from Gorski LA, et al: Infusion therapy standards of practice. *J Infus Nurs* 44(suppl 1):S1-S224, 2021. doi:10.1097/NAN.0000000000000396.

gluconate [CHG] solution preferred, povidone-iodine, or 70% alcohol), 2 × 2–inch gauze pads, and label. **NOTE:** Plastic tape is preferred to prevent medical adhesive–related skin injury (MARSI) (Fumarola et al., 2020).
- If kit is not available, gather all items separately.
- Appropriate peripheral IV ONC or metal stylet needle. ONC has safety mechanism for venipuncture (see Table 28.3) (Gorski et al., 2021)
- Clean gloves (latex free for patients with latex allergy); sterile gloves are needed if key parts or key sites are touched (see Box 28.1) (Gorski et al., 2021)
- Single-use hair clippers or scissors for hair removal if indicated
- Short extension tubing with fused needleless connector or separate needleless connector (also called *injection cap, saline lock, heparin lock, IV plug,* or *PRN adapter*)
- 5-mL prefilled syringe with preservative-free 0.9% sodium chloride (normal saline [NS]) (Gorski et al., 2021)
- Antiseptic swabs

- Skin barrier: film, cream, or wipe
- Manufactured catheter stabilization device (if available)
- Prescribed IV solution or medication (see Chapter 22)
- IV infusion set (IV tubing), either macrodrip or microdrip, depending on prescribed rate; if using EID, appropriate administration set
- 0.2-micron filter for nonlipid (fat emulsion) solutions (may be incorporated into the infusion set)
- Personal protective equipment (PPE): goggles, face shield, and mask (based on agency policy)
- Electronic infusion device (EID) and IV pole
- Vein visualization device (optional based on agency policy)
- Stethoscope
- Watch with second hand to calculate drip rate
- Special patient gown with snaps at shoulder seams if available (makes removal with IV tubing easier)
- Needle disposal container (sharps container or biohazard container)

STEP	RATIONALE

ASSESSMENT

1. Review patient's electronic health record (EHR) for accuracy of health care provider's order: date and time, IV solution, route of administration, volume, rate, duration, and signature of ordering health care provider (Gorski, 2023). Follow the seven rights of medication administration (see Chapter 20) (Gorski, 2023).

   a. Use approved online database or drug reference book or consult pharmacist for information about IV solution composition, purpose, potential incompatibilities, adverse reactions, and side effects.

2. Assess patient's/family caregiver's health literacy.

3. Perform hand hygiene following Aseptic Non-Touch Technique (ANTT). Obtain data from patient's EHR for clinical factors and conditions that will respond to or be affected by administration of IV solutions, or perform physical examination of the following:

   a. Body weight

   b. Clinical markers of vascular volume:
     (1) Urine output (decreased, dark yellow)

     (2) Vital signs: blood pressure, respirations, pulse, temperature

     (3) Distended neck veins (Normally veins are full when person is supine and flat when person is upright.)

     (4) Auscultation of lungs

     (5) Capillary refill

   c. Clinical markers of interstitial volume:
     (1) Skin turgor (pinch skin over sternum or inside of forearm). Also assess skin temperature, color, moisture level, fragility, and overall integrity, including presence of irritation around potential IV site.

Before initiating IV therapy, an order from a health care provider is needed (Gorski et al., 2021).
Verification that order is complete prevents medication errors.

Ensures safe and correct administration of IV therapy and appropriate selection of VAD.

Determines degree to which individuals have the ability to find, understand, and use information and services to make informed health-related decisions and actions for themselves and others (CDC, 2023).
Reduces transmission of microorganisms. Provides baseline to determine effectiveness of prescribed therapy. A systems approach is recommended to assess for fluid and electrolyte imbalances (Gorski, 2023).

Changes in body weight can be an indication of fluid loss or gain (Gorski, 2023).

Kidneys respond to extracellular volume (ECV) deficit by reducing urine production and concentrating urine. Kidney disease can also cause oliguria.
Changes in blood pressure may be associated with fluid volume status (fluid volume deficit [FVD]) seen in postural hypotension.
Respirations can be altered in presence of acid-base imbalances.
Body temperature elevations of 38.3°C (101°F) to 39.4°C (103°F) increase need for fluid replacement (Gorski, 2023).
Indicator of fluid volume status: flat or collapsing with inhalation when supine with ECV deficit; full when upright or semi-upright with ECV excess.
Crackles or rhonchi in dependent parts of lung may signal fluid buildup caused by ECV excess.
Indirect measure of tissue perfusion (sluggish with ECV deficit).

Failure of skin to return to normal position after several seconds indicates FVD (Gorski, 2023). Skin characteristics can indicate risk for MARSI (Fumarola et al., 2020).

STEP	RATIONALE
(2) Dependent edema (pitting or nonpitting) (see Chapter 6).	Edema is not usually apparent until 2 to 4 kg (4.4–8.8 lb) of fluid is retained. A weight gain of 1 kg (2.2 lb) is equivalent to the retention of 1 L of body water (Gorski, 2023).
(3) Oral mucous membrane between cheek and gum (see Chapter 6).	More reliable indicator than dry lips or skin. Dry area between cheek and gums indicates ECV deficit.
d. Thirst	Occurs with hypernatremia and severe ECV deficit. Not a reliable indicator in older adults (Gorski, 2023).
e. Behavior and level of consciousness:	
(1) Restlessness and mild confusion	Occurs with FVD or acid-base imbalance. Occurs with severe ECV deficit.
(2) Decreased level of consciousness (lethargy, confusion, coma)	May occur with osmolality, fluid and electrolyte, and acid-base imbalances.
4. After completing any physical examination, perform hand hygiene.	Reduces transmission of microorganisms.
5. Review EHR to determine patient's risk for developing a MARSI with use of adhesive devices or tape: age, dehydration, malnutrition, exposure to radiation therapy, underlying chronic conditions (e.g., diabetes mellitus, immunosuppression, edema).	Common risk factors for MARSI (Fumarola et al., 2020).
6. Review EHR and ask patient about allergy to iodine, adhesive, latex, or chlorhexidine (CHG). If allergy identified, apply allergy ID band to patient's wrist.	Medications, solutions used during catheter insertion, and use of gloves and tape can cause serious allergic reactions. Latex allergy will require caregiver use of latex-free gloves.
7. Determine whether patient is to undergo any planned surgeries or procedures.	Allows anticipation and placement of appropriate VAD for infusion and avoids placement in an area that will interfere with medical procedures (Gorski et al., 2021).
8. Assess available laboratory data (e.g., hematocrit, serum electrolytes, arterial blood gases, and kidney functions [blood urea nitrogen, urine specific gravity, and urine osmolality]).	Helps determine priority assessments and establishes baseline for determining if therapy is effective. Laboratory values are an assessment of hydration status (Gorski, 2023).
9. Assess patient's knowledge, prior experience with infusion therapy, and feelings about procedure.	Reveals need for patient instruction and/or support.

PLANNING

1. Expected outcomes following completion of procedure:	
• Patient's VAD remains patent, and site is free from signs and symptoms of IV-related complications.	Ensures that patient receives prescribed infusion therapy and VAD without complications (Gorski et al., 2021).
• Vital signs are stable and within normal limits for patient.	Demonstrates response of body systems to fluid and electrolyte replacement (Gorski, 2023).
• Fluid and electrolyte balance return to normal.	Proper solution is infused at proper rate and monitored, resolving fluid and electrolyte imbalance (Gorski, 2023).
• Patient can explain purpose and risks of IV therapy.	Demonstrates learning.
2. Provide privacy and explain the rationale for infusion, including solution and medications ordered, procedure for initiating an IV line, and signs and symptoms of complications (e.g., redness, pain, tenderness, swelling, bleeding, drainage, or leaking from under dressing).	Protects patient's privacy; reduces anxiety. Promotes cooperation.
3. Collect and organize equipment on clean, clutter-free bedside stand or overbed table. Be sure you have the correct infusion set for the EID that is to be used. Select integrated securement device or proper adhesive tape to reduce risk of MARSI. *Option:* Have vein visualization device at hand.	Ensures more efficiency when completing a procedure. Reduces risk of microbial contamination and cross-contamination of equipment (Gorski et al., 2021). Easy access to equipment improves efficiency. Ensures patient safety. To reduce risk of MARSI, consider plastic tape for short-term wear (Fumarola et al., 2020).
4. Help patient to comfortable sitting or supine position. Change patient's gown to one more easily removed with snaps at shoulder if available. Provide adequate lighting.	Promotes comfort and relaxation of patient. Use of this gown decreases risk of inadvertently dislodging VAD or administration set when changing gown. Aids in successful vein location.

IMPLEMENTATION

1. Identify patient using at least two identifiers (e.g., name and birthday or name and medical record number) according to agency policy. Compare identifiers with information on patient's medication administration record (MAR) or EHR.	Ensures patient safety. Complies with The Joint Commission standards and improves patient safety (TJC, 2023).

STEP	RATIONALE

2. Perform hand hygiene following ANTT. Select appropriate-size catheter based on assessment; open and prepare sterile packages using sterile aseptic technique (see Chapter 9).

Reduces transmission of microorganisms. Use smallest-gauge peripheral catheter that will accommodate prescribed therapy and patient need (Gorski et al., 2021).

3. *Option:* Prepare a short extension tubing with fused needleless connector or separate needleless connector (injection cap) to be used to attach to catheter hub.

Needleless connectors protect health care workers by eliminating needles and potential for needlestick injuries when accessing VAD (Gorski et al., 2021).

  a. Remove protective cap from needleless connector and attach syringe with 1 to 3 mL 0.9% sodium chloride (NS), maintaining sterility. Slowly inject enough saline to prime (fill) short extension tubing and connector, removing all air. Leave syringe attached to end of tubing (see illustration).

Replaces air with NS, preventing air from entering patient's vein later during VAD insertion.

  b. Maintain sterility of end of connector by reapplying end caps, and set aside for attaching to catheter hub after successful venipuncture.

Prevents touch contamination, which allows microorganisms to enter infusion equipment and bloodstream.

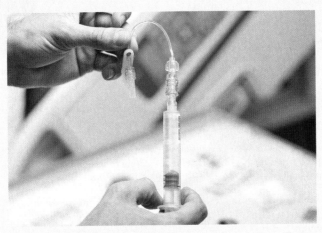

STEP 3a Prime short extension tubing and connector and leave syringe attached to tubing.

Clinical Judgment *Short extension sets may be used on peripheral catheters. Reduces catheter manipulation. Many agencies use short extension tubing for continuous infusions and standalone saline locks (capped catheters). For patient safety, all connections should be of Luer-Lok type (Gorski et al., 2021).*

4. Prepare IV infusion tubing and solution for continuous infusion.

  a. Check IV solution using seven rights of medication administration (see Chapter 20) (Gorski, 2023; Gorski et al., 2021) and review label for name and concentration of solution, type and concentration of any additives, volume, beyond-use and expiration dates, and sterility state. If using bar-code system, scan code on patient's wristband and then on IV fluid container. Be sure that prescribed additives such as potassium and vitamins have been added. Check solution for color and clarity. Check bag for leaks.

Reviewing label for accuracy reduces risk for medication errors (Gorski et al., 2021). Bar-code system reduces human error (Gorski et al., 2021).

Risk for medication errors can be reduced with safe medication practices, including (Gorski et al., 2021):
- Do not add medications to infusing containers of IV solutions (Gorski et al., 2021).
- Do not use IV solutions that are discolored, contain precipitates, or are expired.
- Risk for transmission of infection can be reduced by not using leaking bags because integrity has been compromised.

  b. Open IV infusion set, maintaining sterility. **NOTE:** EIDs sometimes have a dedicated administration set; follow manufacturer's instructions.

Prevents touch contamination, which allows microorganisms to enter infusion equipment and bloodstream.

  c. Place roller clamp (see illustration A) about 2 to 5 cm (1–2 inches) below drip chamber and move roller clamp to "off" position (see illustration B).

Close proximity of roller clamp to drip chamber allows more accurate regulation of flow rate. Moving clamp to "off" prevents accidental spillage of IV solution during priming.

  d. Remove protective sheath over IV tubing port on plastic IV solution bag (see illustration) or top of IV solution bottle while maintaining sterility.

Provides access for insertion of IV tubing spike into solution using sterile technique.

STEP	RATIONALE

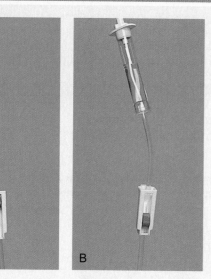

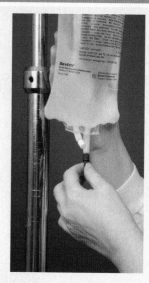

STEP 4c (A) Roller clamp in open position. (B) Roller clamp in closed position.

STEP 4d Removing protective sheath from IV tubing port.

   e. Insert spike into port of IV bag using a twisting motion (see illustration).

Flat surface on top of bottled solution may contain contaminants, whereas opening to plastic bag is recessed.

Clinical Judgment *If solution container is glass bottle, clean rubber stopper on glass-bottled solution with antiseptic swab and insert spike into rubber stopper of IV bottle. Bottles require vented tubing. Rationale: Prevents contamination of bottled solution during insertion of spike. If sterility of spike is compromised, discard IV tubing and obtain new tubing.*

   f. Compress drip chamber and release, allowing it to fill one-third to one-half full (see illustration).

   g. Prime air out of IV tubing by filling with IV solution: Remove protective cover on end of IV tubing (some tubing can be primed without removing protective cover) and slowly open roller clamp to allow fluid to flow from drip chamber to distal end of IV tubing. Return roller clamp to "off" position after priming tubing (filled with IV fluid). Replace protective cover on distal end of tubing. Label IV tubing with date according to agency policy and procedure.

   h. Be certain that IV tubing is clear of air and air bubbles. To remove small air bubbles, firmly tap tubing where bubbles are located (see illustration). Check entire length of tubing to ensure that all air bubbles are removed.

   i. If using optional long extension tubing (not short tubing mentioned in Step 3), remove protective cover and attach it to distal end of IV tubing, maintaining sterility. Then prime long extension tubing. Insert tubing into EID with power off.

5. Perform hand hygiene and apply clean gloves following ANTT.

6. Apply tourniquet around upper arm about 10 to 15 cm (4–6 inches) above proposed insertion site (see illustration). Do not apply tourniquet too tightly. Check for presence of pulse distal to tourniquet.

   (*Option A:* Apply tourniquet on top of thin layer of clothing such as gown sleeve to protect fragile or hairy skin.)

   (*Option B:* Blood pressure cuff may be used in place of tourniquet: activate cuff and hold at approximately 50 mm Hg. Avoid performing venipuncture too close to the blood pressure cuff.)

   (*Option C:* Instead of applying a tourniquet, use a vein visualization device) (see illustration).

Creates suction effect; fluid enters drip chamber to prevent air from entering tubing.

Priming ensures that IV tubing is clear of air and filled with IV solution before connecting to VAD. Slowly filling tubing decreases turbulence and chance of bubble formation.

Closing clamp prevents accidental loss of fluid.

Maintains sterility.

Labeling IV tubing allows for recognition of length of time that tubing has been in use and when to change it.

Large air bubbles may act as emboli (Gorski, 2023).

Priming removes air from long extension tubing so that it does not enter patient's vascular system.

Facilitates starting infusion as soon as IV site is ready.

Decreases transmission of microorganisms.

Tourniquet should be tight enough to impede venous flow while maintaining arterial circulation (Gorski et al., 2021).

If patient has fragile veins or bruises easily, tourniquet should be applied loosely or not at all to prevent damage to veins and bruising.

Reduces trauma to skin. Excessive back pressure may be seen if venipuncture is performed too close to the blood pressure cuff (Gorski, 2023).

Near-infrared (NIR) technology enables visualization of the superficial vasculature without a tourniquet in order to identify veins for optimal peripheral venous access.

STEP	RATIONALE

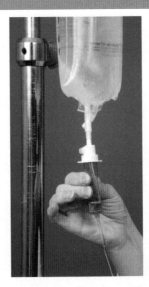
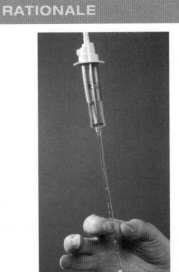

STEP 4e Inserting spike into IV bag. **STEP 4f** Squeezing drip chamber to fill with fluid. **STEP 4h** Removing air bubbles from tubing.

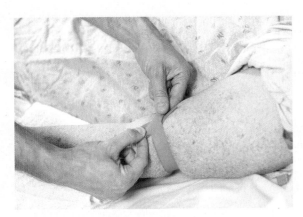

STEP 6 Tourniquet placed on arm for initial vein selection.

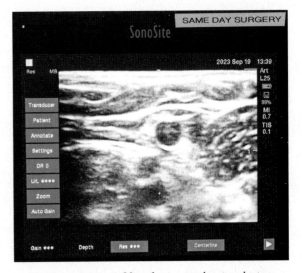

STEP 6, option C Use of vein visualization device.

7. Select vein for VAD insertion (see illustration). Veins on dorsal and ventral surfaces of arms (e.g., metacarpal, cephalic, basilic, or median) are preferred in adults.
   a. Use most distal site in nondominant arm if possible.

   b. Following ANTT, with your fingertip, palpate vein at intended insertion site by pressing downward. Note resilient, soft, bouncy feeling while releasing pressure (see illustration).
   c. Select well-dilated vein.

   d. Methods to improve vascular distention:
      (1) Position extremity lower than heart, have patient open and close fist slowly, and lightly stroke vein downward.
      (2) Use controlled warming (e.g., warm compress) to extremity for several minutes.

Ensures adequate vein that is easy to puncture and less likely to rupture. Better hemodilution is obtained in the larger veins of the forearms (Gorski, 2023).

Patients with VAD placement in their dominant hand have decreased ability to perform self-care.

Fingertip is more sensitive and better for assessing vein location and condition.

Increased volume of blood in vein at venipuncture site makes vein more visible.

Use of gravity promotes vascular distention (Gorski et al., 2021).

Controlled warming has been found to increase successful peripheral catheter insertion (Gorski et al., 2021).

Clinical Judgment *Avoid multiple tapping of a vein, especially in older adults with fragile veins, as it can cause damage to the vein (Gorski, 2023).*

STEP	RATIONALE

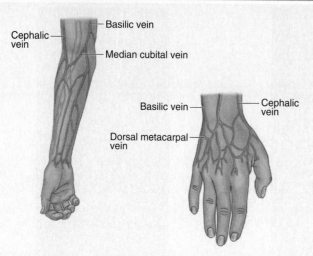

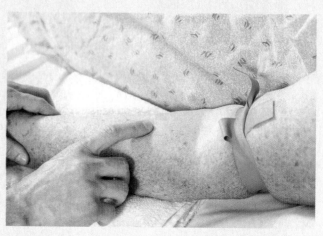

STEP 7 Cephalic, basilic, and median cubital veins are best for IV placement in adults.

STEP 7b Palpate vein.

8. When selecting a vein, avoid selection in:
   a. Dominant hand. Choose site that will not interfere with patient's activities of daily living (ADLs), use of assistive devices, or planned procedures.

   Patient will move dominant hand more often and freely. Preferred site is the nondominant side for insertion (Gorski et al., 2021).

   b. Areas with pain on palpation, compromised areas, sites distal to compromised areas (e.g., open wounds, bruising, infection, infiltration, or extravasation) (Gorski et al., 2021).

   It would be difficult to assess for any signs or symptoms of complications if an IV device were inserted in an area already compromised. Phlebitis has been associated with bruised insertion sites (Marsh et al., 2018).

   c. Upper extremity on side of breast surgery with axillary node dissection or lymphedema or after radiation; arteriovenous (AV) fistulas/grafts; or affected extremity from cerebrovascular accident (CVA) (Gorski et al., 2021).

   Increases risk for complications, such as infection, lymphedema, or vessel damage.

   d. Site distal to previous venipuncture site, sclerosed or hardened veins, previous infiltrations or extravasations, areas of venous valves, or phlebitic vessels.

   Such sites cause infiltration around newly placed VAD site and vessel damage.

   e. Fragile dorsal hand veins in older adults. Veins of lower extremities should not be used for routine IV therapy in adults because of risk of tissue damage and thrombophlebitis (Gorski et al., 2021).

   Veins have increased risk for infiltration.

   f. Areas of flexion such as wrist or antecubital area (Gorski et al., 2021).

   Veins have increased risk for infiltration, phlebitis, or dislodgement.

   g. Ventral surface of wrist (10–12.5 cm [4–5 inches]).

   Venipuncture in ventral surface of wrist is painful and has potential for nerve damage (Gorski et al., 2021).

9. Release tourniquet temporarily. Remove gloves and dispose of in appropriate container.

   Restores blood flow and prevents venospasm when preparing for venipuncture.

Clinical Judgment *If hair removal is needed, do not shave area with a razor. Shaving may increase risk of infection (Gorski et al., 2021). Clip hair with scissors or hair clippers to prepare area for application of transparent semipermeable membrane (TSM) dressing if necessary (explain to patient).*

Clinical Judgment *Local anesthetic reduces discomfort associated with placement of a vascular access device (VAD). Both topical and injectable drugs can be used to reduce pain and require a health care provider's order. Apply topical local anesthetic to intended IV site before insertion. Follow manufacturer's recommendations, and monitor for allergic reaction (Gorski, 2023; Gorski et al., 2021).*

10. Perform hand hygiene and apply clean gloves following ANTT. Wear eye protection and mask (see agency policy) if splash or spray of blood is possible.

    Decreases potential risk of microbial contamination and cross-contamination (Gorski et al., 2021).

11. Place adapter end of short extension set (prepared in Step 3) or needleless connector (injection cap) for saline lock nearby in the sterile package.

    Permits smooth, quick connection of infusion to peripheral catheter once vein is accessed.

STEP	RATIONALE

12. If area of insertion is visibly soiled, clean site with antiseptic soap and water first and dry. Perform skin antisepsis with alcoholic CHG solution in back-and-forth motion (see illustration) and allow to dry completely (follow manufacturer's recommendations). If using alcohol or povidone-iodine, clean in concentric circle, moving from insertion site outward with swab. Allow drying time between agents if agents are used in combination (alcohol and povidone-iodine).

Allow any skin antiseptic agent to fully dry for complete antisepsis; alcoholic CHG solutions take at least 20 seconds; iodophors may take up to 6 minutes for adequate antisepsis (Gorski, 2023).

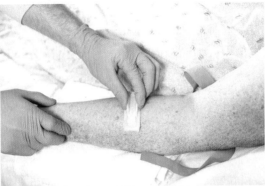

STEP 12 Clean site with 0.5% chlorhexidine alcoholic solution.

Clinical Judgment *If vein palpation is necessary after performing skin antisepsis, use sterile gloves for palpation or perform skin antisepsis again because touching cleaned area introduces microorganisms from your finger to site (Gorski et al., 2021).*

13. Use visualization device or reapply tourniquet 10 to 15 cm (4–6 inches) above anticipated insertion site. Check for presence of pulse distal to tourniquet.

Pressure of tourniquet promotes vein distention. Diminished arterial flow prevents venous filling.

14. Perform venipuncture. Anchor vein below anticipated insertion site by placing thumb over vein 4 to 5 cm (1½ to 2 inches) distal to site and gently stretching skin against direction of insertion. Instruct patient to relax hand.

Stabilizes vein for needle insertion; prevents vein from rolling; and stretches skin taut, decreasing drag during insertion. Some devices require loosening needle (stylet) from catheter before venipuncture. Follow manufacturer directions for use.

    a. Warn patient of a sharp stick. Hold ONC or metal stylet with needle bevel up. Align catheter on top of vein at 10- to 30-degree angle (see illustration A). Puncture skin and anterior vein wall (see illustration B).

Accessing vein at an angle reduces risk of puncturing posterior vein wall. Superficial veins require smaller angle. Deeper veins require greater angle.

Clinical Judgment *Use each over-the-needle catheter (ONC) only once for each insertion attempt.*

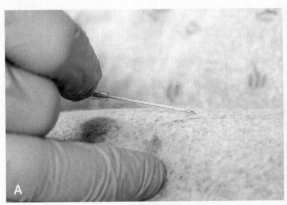
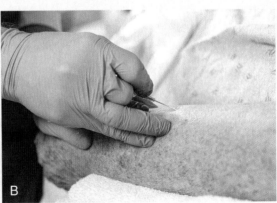

STEP 14 (A) Align catheter on top of vein at 10- to 30-degree angle. (B) Puncture skin and anterior vein wall.

STEP	RATIONALE
15. Observe for blood return in catheter or flashback chamber of catheter, indicating that bevel of needle has entered vein (see illustration A). Advance ONC approximately 0.6 cm (¼ inch) into vein and loosen stylet (needle) of ONC. Continue to hold skin taut while stabilizing ONC and, with index finger on push-off tab of ONC, advance catheter off needle into vein until hub rests at venipuncture site (see illustration B). *Do not reinsert stylet into catheter once catheter has been advanced into vein.* Advance catheter while safety device automatically retracts stylet (techniques for retracting stylet vary with different VADs). Place stylet directly into sharps container.	Increased venous pressure from tourniquet causes backflow of blood into catheter and/or flashback chamber. Some ONCs have a notch in the stylet, allowing flash of blood into catheter. Stabilizing ONC allows for placement of catheter into vein and advancement of catheter off stylet. Advancing entire stylet into vein may penetrate wall of vein, resulting in hematoma. Advancing catheter with finger on open hub causes contamination (Gorski et al., 2021). Reinsertion of stylet can cause catheter to shear off and embolize into vein. Proper sharps disposal prevents needlestick injury (OSHA, n.d.).

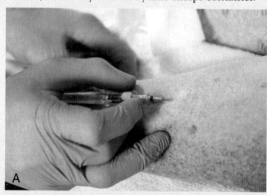 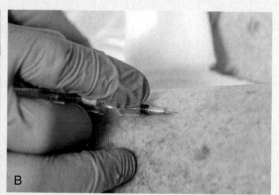

STEP 15 (A) Observe for blood return in catheter and/or flashback chamber. (B) Advance catheter into vein until hub rests at venipuncture site.

Clinical Judgment *A single clinician should not make more than two attempts at initiating IV access and should limit total attempts by all health care providers to no more than four (Gorski et al., 2021).*

STEP	RATIONALE
16. Stabilize ONC with nondominant hand and release tourniquet or blood pressure cuff with other. Apply gentle but firm pressure with middle finger of nondominant hand 3 cm (1¼ inches) above insertion site. Keep catheter stable with index finger.	Permits venous flow and reduces backflow of blood. Digital pressure minimizes blood loss and allows attachment of extension set needleless connector.
17. Quickly connect Luer-Lok end of short extension tubing with needleless connector to the end of catheter hub (see illustration). Secure connection. Avoid touching sterile connection ends. *Option:* Main IV tubing can be attached directly to catheter hub in place of short extension tubing with needleless connector.	Prompt connection maintains patency of vein, minimizes blood loss, and prevents risk of exposure to blood. Maintains sterility.

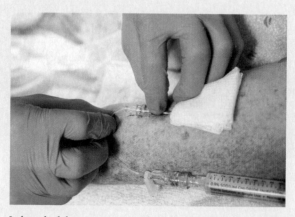

STEP 17 Connect Luer-Lok end of short extension tubing with needleless connector to end of catheter hub.

STEP	RATIONALE
18. Take the prefilled flush syringe of 0.9% sodium chloride already attached to short extension set and aspirate to assess blood return. (Do not reinject any air.) After blood return, slowly inject NS from prefilled syringe into ONC. Remove syringe and discard.	Blood return that is color and consistency of whole blood confirms placement of catheter in vein (Gorski et al., 2021). Flushing prevents reflux of blood into catheter and occlusion (Gorski et al., 2021). Initiates flow of fluid through IV catheter, preventing clotting of device. Swelling indicates infiltration, and catheter would need to be removed.
Option: To begin primary infusion, swab needleless connector of short extension set with antiseptic swab and attach Luer-Lok end of IV tubing. Open roller clamp of IV tubing, turn on EID, and program it. Begin infusion at correct rate. If using gravity flow instead of EID, begin infusion by slowly opening roller clamp to regulate rate.	Initiates flow of fluid through IV catheter, preventing clotting of VAD.

Clinical Judgment *Needleless connectors protect health care workers and decrease risk for needlestick injuries. They have different internal mechanisms for fluid displacement and vary in the flush-clamp-disconnect sequence to prevent reflux of blood into catheter on disconnection (Gorski et al., 2021). The sequence depends on the type of internal mechanism (Gorski, 2023). A typical ONC connected with short extension tubing and needleless connector maintains a positive pressure in saline locked line.*

19. Observe insertion site for swelling.	Swelling indicates infiltration, which necessitates immediate catheter removal.
20. Apply protective skin barrier: film, cream, or wipe over area around IV site insertion. Allow to dry completely.	Skin should be protected with a barrier product before an adhesive medical device (including tape) is applied, and this should be considered a standard part of the skin care protocol to prevent MARSI (Fumarola et al., 2020). Forms a mechanical barrier over the skin; the barrier is thin and nonmessy, and dressings can still adhere to the skin (Fumarola et al., 2020).
21. Apply sterile dressing over site. **a.** Integrated securement device, such as 3M Tegaderm:	Device combines a sterile dressing with securement functions; includes transparent, semipermeable window and a bordered fabric collar that secures to skin (Gorski et al., 2021). Protects insertion site and accidental dislodgment of catheter.
(1) Continue to secure catheter with nondominant hand. Take first securement strip and place over catheter hub; secure to skin (see illustration).	
(2) Peel paper liner from paper framed dressing. Use dressing handles and, using ANTT technique, place dressing over catheter so that transparent film covers insertion site (see illustration).	Ensures aseptic technique. Allows for visualization of insertion site.
(3) Remove paper border and press down on dressing edges (see illustration).	Secures dressing under catheter hub.
(4) Smooth over the soft cloth sections under the catheter hub (see illustration).	Improves adhesion to skin.
(5) Use second securement strip and place under catheter hub and across soft cloth section of dressing (see illustration).	Provides added securement.

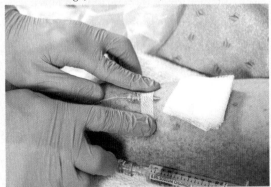

STEP 21a(1) Take first securement strip and place over catheter hub.

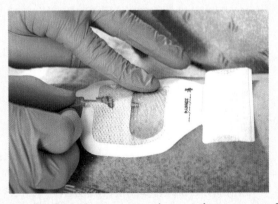

STEP 21a(2) Place dressing over catheter so the transparent film covers the insertion site.

STEP	RATIONALE

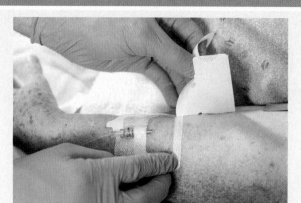

STEP 21a(3) Remove paper border and press down on dressing edges.

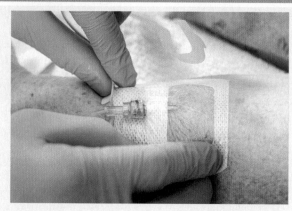

STEP 21a(4) Smooth over the soft cloth sections under the catheter hub.

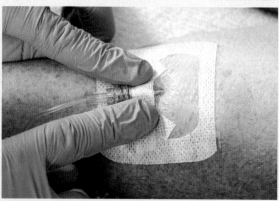

STEP 21a(5) Use second securement strip and place under catheter hub and across soft cloth section of dressing.

b. TSM dressing:
  (1) Continue to secure catheter with nondominant hand. Remove adherent backing of dressing. Apply one edge of dressing and gently smooth over IV insertion site. Do not apply with tension or stretching. Leave the Luer-Lok connection between tubing and catheter hub uncovered. Apply in the correct orientation to allow for stretching of body part if movement or swelling is anticipated. Smooth into place without gaps or wrinkles. Remove outer covering and smooth dressing gently over site (see illustration).

Protects catheter insertion site and minimizes risk for infection (Gorski, 2023). Allows visualization of insertion site and surrounding area for complications (Gorski et al., 2021). Access to Luer-Lok connection between tubing and catheter hub facilitates changing tubing if necessary. Steps of application follow evidence-based guidelines (Fumarola et al., 2020).

  (2) Place 2.5 cm (2-inch) piece of tape over Luer-Lok connector (see illustration). Do not cover connection between connector and catheter hub. Do not apply tape on top of TSM dressing.

Removal of tape from TSM dressing can tear dressing and cause catheter dislodgement.
Tape on top of TSM dressing prevents moisture from being carried away from skin.

c. Sterile gauze dressing:
  (1) Be sure skin is dry, and then place 5-cm (2-inch) piece of sterile tape over catheter hub (see illustration). **NOTE:** Plastic tape is preferred over other types of tape for short-term wear to prevent MARSI (Fumarola et al., 2020).

Used less frequently.
Moisture reduces effectiveness of adhesion (Fumarola et al., 2020). Stabilizes catheter under gauze dressing.

  (2) Place 2 × 2–inch gauze pad over insertion site and edge of catheter hub. Secure all edges with tape. Do not place tape over insertion site. Do not cover connection between IV tubing and catheter hub (see illustration).

Use gauze dressings for site drainage, excessive perspiration, or sensitivity/allergic reactions to TSM dressings (Gorski, 2023; Gorski et al., 2021).

  (3) Fold 2 × 2–inch gauze in half and cover with 2.5-cm-wide (1 inch) tape so that about 1 inch will extend on each side of dressing. Place under Luer-Lok connector.

Tape on top of gauze makes it easier to access hub/tubing junction. Gauze pad elevates hub off skin to prevent pressure area.

STEP	RATIONALE

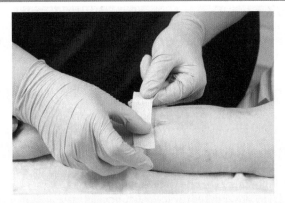

STEP 21b(1) Apply transparent semipermeable membrane dressing.

STEP 21b(2) Place tape over administration set tubing.

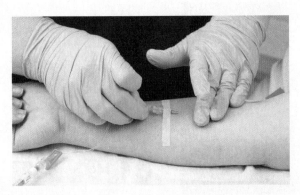

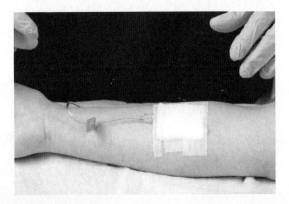

STEP 21c(1) Place sterile tape over catheter hub.

STEP 21c(2) Place 2 × 2–inch gauze over insertion site and catheter hub.

22. Secure Luer-Lok connector and tubing.
   a. Secure using engineered stabilization device (follow manufacturer directions and agency policy).

    (1) Apply skin protectant to area of skin where stabilization device is to be placed. Allow to dry completely.
    (2) Align anchoring pads with directional arrow pointing to insertion site. Press device retainer over top of Luer-Lok connection while supporting underneath connection (see illustration).
    (3) Stabilize catheter and peel off one side of liner and press to adhere to skin. Repeat on other side.

Reduces pulling on IV catheter

Use of engineered stabilization devices can reduce risk of ONC complications (i.e., phlebitis, occlusion/infiltration, dislodgment, and infection) and unintentional loss of access (Gorski et al., 2021).

Helps minimize risk for MARSI, which is increased as result of age, joint movement, and edema; use of skin protectant can decrease risk (Gorski et al., 2021).

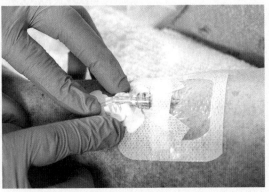

STEP 22a(2) Catheter stabilization device in place.

STEP	RATIONALE
b. Secure using tape. Apply 2.5-cm (1-inch) piece of tape over the folded gauze that is placed under Luer-Lok connector. Avoid applying tape or gauze around arm. Do not use rolled bandages with or without elastic to secure ONC. Taping Luer-Lok connection can be eliminated if engineered stabilization device is to be used.	Prevents back-and-forth motion of catheter. Rolled bandages do not secure ONC adequately, can impair circulation or flow of infusion, and obscure visualization for complications (Gorski et al., 2021).
23. *Option:* Apply site protection device (Fig 28.2).	Reduces risk of VAD dislodgement (Gorski et al., 2021).
24. Loop extension or IV tubing alongside dressing on arm and secure with second piece of tape directly over tubing.	Securing tubing reduces risk for dislodging catheter if IV tubing is pulled (i.e., loop comes apart before catheter dislodges).
25. For continuous infusion, verify ordered rate of infusion and be sure EID is programmed correctly. If infusing by gravity drip, adjust flow rate to correct drops per minute.	Prevents fluid overload.
26. Label dressing per agency policy. Include date and time of IV insertion, VAD gauge size and length, and your initials (see illustration).	Allows for recognition of type of device and length of time that device has been in place.

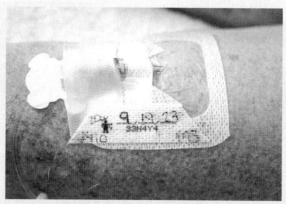

STEP 26 Label IV dressing.

27. Dispose of all contaminated supplies in appropriate receptacle; remove and dispose of gloves and any other PPE.	Reduces transmission of microorganisms. Use appropriate disposal receptacle if patient is on hazardous drugs (Oncology Nursing Society [ONS], 2018).
28. Assist patient to a comfortable position and instruct on how to move and turn without dislodging VAD.	Restores comfort and sense of well-being. Prevents accidental dislodgement of catheter and minimizes risk for falls.
29. Raise bed rails (as appropriate) and lower bed to lowest position, locking into position.	Ensures patient safety and prevents falls.
30. Place nurse call system in an accessible location within patient's reach. Instruct patient in its use.	Ensures patient can call for assistance if needed.
31. Perform hand hygiene.	Reduces transmission of microorganisms.

EVALUATION

1. Observe patient every 1 to 2 hours or at established intervals per agency policy and procedure for function, intactness, and patency of IV system and for correct infusion rate and accurate type/amount of IV solution infused by observing level in IV container.	Ensures delivery of prescribed volume over prescribed time and decreases risk for fluid and electrolyte imbalance.

STEP	RATIONALE
2. Evaluate patient to determine response to therapy (e.g., laboratory values, input and output [I&O], weights, vital signs, postprocedural assessments).	Early recognition of complications leads to prompt treatment.
3. Evaluate patient at established intervals per agency policy and procedure for signs and symptoms of phlebitis and infiltration by inspecting and gently palpating skin around and above IV site over the dressing.	Identifies complications that compromise integrity of VAD or cause inaccurate IV solution flow rate.
4. Monitor IV dressing site for MARSI: look for mechanical trauma (skin stripping, blistering, skin tears), dermatitis (irritation in response to adhesive), and maceration and folliculitis.	*Medical adhesive–related skin injury* (MARSI) refers to any skin damage related to the use of medical adhesive products or devices, such as tape.

Clinical Judgment *If IV is positional, fluid will run slowly or stop, depending on position of patient's arm; if this continues, you may have to restart IV line.*

STEP	RATIONALE
5. **Use Teach-Back:** "I want to make sure that I explained the problems that can happen with your IV. Tell me the signs or symptoms that you should tell me or the other nurses about." Revise your instruction now or develop a plan for revised patient/family caregiver teaching if patient/family caregiver is not able to teach back correctly.	Teach-back is a technique for health care providers to ensure that they have explained medical information clearly so that patients and their families understand what is communicated to them (Agency for Healthcare Research and Quality [AHRQ], 2023).

Unexpected Outcomes

1. Fluid and electrolyte imbalances:
   a. FVD: decreased urine output, dry mucous membranes, decreased capillary refill, disparity in central and peripheral pulses, tachycardia, hypotension, and shock.
   b. Fluid volume excess (FVE): dyspnea, crackles in lung, edema, and/or increased urine output.
   c. Electrolyte imbalances: abnormal serum electrolyte levels, changes in mental status, alterations in neuromuscular function, cardiac arrhythmias, and changes in vital signs.

2. IV-related complications
   a. Infiltration: pain, swelling, coolness to touch, or presence of blanching (white, shiny appearance at or above IV site) or redness (Gorski et al., 2021).

   b. Catheter occlusion can occur from bent catheter, positional catheter (catheter resting against vein wall), kink or knot in infusion tubing, clot formation, or precipitate formation from administration of incompatible medications or solutions.
   c. Phlebitis (i.e., vein inflammation): pain, redness, warmth, swelling, induration, or presence of palpable cord along course of vein (Table 28.4) (Gorski et al., 2021). Rate of infusion may be altered.

   d. Catheter-related infection can present as redness, swelling around or above IV site, pain, purulent drainage at insertion site, and body temperature elevations (Gorski et al., 2021).

Related Interventions

- Notify health care provider.
- Requires readjusting infusion rate per health care provider order.
- Requires adjusting additives in IV line or type of IV fluid per health care provider order.

- Stop infusion and remove IV catheter at first sign of infiltration (see Procedural Guideline 28.1).
- Elevate affected extremity.
- Avoid applying pressure, which can force solution into contact with more tissue, causing tissue damage.
- Determine cause and consider catheter removal.
- Positional catheters can be repositioned to improve IV flow.
- Remove occluded IV catheter. Occluded catheters should not be flushed (Gorski, 2023).
- Notify health care provider.
- Determine cause (i.e., chemical, mechanical, bacterial) and consider removal or replacement of VAD.
- *Chemical phlebitis:* Apply heat, elevate limb, and consider slowing infusion rate (Gorski et al., 2021).
- *Mechanical phlebitis:* Apply heat, elevate limb, monitor for 24 hours, consider catheter removal if signs and symptoms persist (Gorski et al., 2021).
- *Bacterial phlebitis:* Remove IV catheter, obtain wound culture from site, and monitor for signs of systemic infection (Gorski et al., 2021).
- Evidence does not allow for recommendation of use of topical agents/interventions in the prevention or treatment of IV-related phlebitis (Goulart et al., 2020).
- Document phlebitis using a standardized scale, including nursing interventions per agency policy and procedure (see Tables 28.4 and 28.5).
- Notify health care provider. Obtain order to culture drainage (Gorski et al., 2021).
- Remove IV catheter and culture purulent drainage from around IV site (see Chapter 7) (Gorski et al., 2021).

STEP	RATIONALE
e. Hematoma is bleeding under skin caused by trauma to vessel wall. It can occur during peripheral IV insertion if needle punctures either adjacent vessels or posterior vein wall or can be seen with multiple venipuncture attempts (Gorski, 2023).	• Remove IV catheter and apply pressure and dry, sterile dressing. • Apply ice and monitor for additional bleeding. • Elevate extremity and monitor for circulatory, neurological, or motor dysfunction (Gorski, 2023).
f. Nerve injuries during peripheral IV insertion can occur. Be alert for patient complaints of paresthesia, including shocklike pain, tingling or pins and needles, burning, or numbness on insertion.	• Notify health care provider of any signs and symptoms of nerve injury (Gorski et al., 2021). • Immediately stop VAD insertion and remove device if patient complains of symptoms of paresthesia (Gorski et al., 2021). • Continue to monitor neurovascular status (Gorski et al., 2021).
3. MARSI develops under adhesive covering IV site dressing.	• If IV site is to remain or if decision is made to remove IV ONC and insert a new one, protect skin with a skin barrier product. An alcohol-free product will not irritate skin if skin is broken (Fumarola et al., 2020). • Treat affected skin with appropriate emollient.

TABLE 28.4

Visual Infusion Phlebitis Scale

Score	Observation
1	IV site appears healthy
2	The following is evident: • Slight pain near IV site *or* slight redness near IV site
3	Two of the following are evident: • Pain at IV site • Erythema • Swelling
4	Both of the following signs are evident: • Pain along path of cannula • Induration
5	All of the following signs are evident and extensive: • Pain along path of cannula • Erythema • Induration • Palpable venous cord
6	All of the following signs are evident and extensive: • Pain along path of cannula • Erythema • Induration • Palpable venous cord • Pyrexia

IV, Intravenous.
Modified from Gorski LA, et al: Infusion therapy standards of practice. *J Infus Nurs* 44(suppl 1):S1–S224, 2021. doi:10.1097/NAN.0000000000000396.

TABLE 28.5

Phlebitis Scale

Grade	Clinical Criteria
0	No symptoms
1	Erythema at access site with or without pain
2	Pain at access site with erythema and/or edema
3	Pain at access site with erythema Streak formation Palpable venous cord
4	Pain at access site with erythema Streak formation Palpable venous cord >1 inch in length Purulent drainage

Modified from Gorski LA, et al: Infusion therapy standards of practice. *J Infus Nurs* 44(suppl 1):S1–S224, 2021. doi:10.1097/NAN.0000000000000396.

Hand-Off Reporting

• Report placement of ONC with reason for insertion with signs or symptoms of observed or patient-reported IV site–related complications, type of fluid, flow rate, status of ONC, amount of fluid remaining in present solution, expected time to hang subsequent IV container, and patient condition.

• Report to health care provider any adverse events occurring with ONC placement (e.g., persistent pain or suspected nerve damage, hematoma formation, arterial puncture).

Special Considerations

Patient Education

• Instruct patient and family caregiver to notify nurse or AP if any signs or symptoms of IV complications are noted (e.g., redness, pain, tenderness, swelling, bleeding, drainage, or leaking under dressing), if flow rate slows or stops, or if patient sees blood in the IV tubing or on the dressing.

• Teach patient how to ambulate with IV pole and protect IV when performing hygiene activities.

Pediatrics

• Perform venipuncture in a neutral space to allow the child's room to be a safe place.

• In addition to the usual venipuncture sites, the scalp veins may be used in infants younger than 18 months and, in toddlers, if not walking, the veins of the foot (Gorski, 2023).

Documentation

• Document number of attempts at insertion, both successful and unsuccessful; precise description of insertion site by location and vessel (if possible), brand, length, and gauge of IV device (e.g., cephalic vein on dorsal surface of right lower arm, 2.5 cm [1 inch] above wrist); type of solution and additives infusing; rate and method of infusion (e.g., gravity or name of EID); and patient's response to insertion (e.g., what patient reports).

• Document patient's status, purpose of infusion, when infusion was started, IV fluid, amount infused, and integrity and patency of system according to agency policy. Use an infusion therapy flow sheet when available.

• If using an EID, document type and rate of infusion and device identification number.

• Document patient's and family caregiver's level of understanding following instruction.

- Needle selection is based on age: 26- to 22-gauge for neonates and pediatric patients (Gorski et al., 2021).
- Use local anesthetics and distraction strategies to minimize distress associated with venipuncture (Gorski, 2023; Gorski et al., 2021).
- Apply latex-free tubing or use a blood pressure cuff inflated to just below diastolic blood pressure.
- Allow older children to select IV site to increase cooperation so that they believe they have some control over their treatment.
- To maintain safety in positioning, have extra help when starting an IV line on a child. Use therapeutic hugging, usually in a sitting position, to provide close contact (Hockenberry et al., 2022). AP can help with positioning.
- Choose age-appropriate activities compatible with the maintenance of the IV infusion to maintain normal growth and development.

Older Adults

- Veins of the older population are fragile; perform venipuncture gently and evaluate the need for a tourniquet (Gorski, 2023).
- Avoid sites that are easily moved or bumped, as well as the dorsal metacarpal veins, where hematoma formation may occur (Gorski, 2023). Use a commercial protective device to protect the site and reduce manipulation (Fig. 28.2).
- In older adults the use of a 26- to 22-gauge catheter is appropriate for most therapies (Gorski et al., 2021). Smaller-gauge catheters are less traumatizing to the vein but still allow blood flow to provide increased hemodilution of the IV solutions or medications (Gorski, 2023).
- As older adults lose subcutaneous tissue, the veins lose stability and roll away from the needle. To stabilize the vein, pull the skin taut and toward you with your nondominant hand and anchor the vein with your thumb.

Patients With Disabilities

- Ensure adequate stabilization of the venous access device to prevent dislodgement. Patients with cognitive disabilities may try to handle or manipulate site.
- Avoid the dominant arm for venipuncture because use of these sites interferes with patient independence.

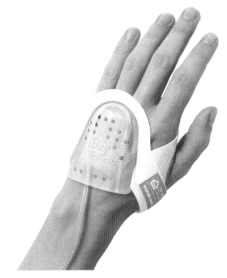

FIG. 28.2 I.V. House Protective Device. (*Courtesy I.V. House.*)

Home Care

- Determine if patient or family caregiver has the manual dexterity and cognitive ability to manage the infusion or seek assistance in an emergency for equipment malfunction while providing IV therapy care at home.
- Ensure that all sharps and equipment contaminated by blood are disposed of appropriately based on their community's standards. Some suppliers provide sharps containers for needle disposal. Teach patient and family caregiver appropriate sharps disposal (see Chapter 42).
- Instruct patient and family caregiver about procedures of IV therapy, including hand hygiene and aseptic technique while handling and proper disposal of syringes and other supplies. Observe patient and family caregiver performing tasks.
- Ensure availability of 24-hour assistance with provider of home infusion therapy pharmaceuticals and equipment.
- Teach patient about activity restrictions (e.g., avoiding strenuous exercise of the arm with the IV line, protecting site while bathing/showering).

◆ SKILL 28.2   Regulating Intravenous Flow Rates

 Video Clip

Accurate infusion rates in intravenous (IV) therapy are essential in the safe delivery of solutions and medications (see Chapter 22). Appropriate regulation of infusion rates can reduce complications (e.g., phlebitis, infiltration, fluid overload, or clotting of the vascular access device [VAD]) associated with IV therapy and allows patients to achieve therapeutic outcomes (Gorski, 2023).

Various methods for regulating infusion rates exist. Electronic infusion devices (EIDs) maintain correct flow rates and catheter patency and prevent an unexpected bolus of IV infusion for patient safety (Gorski et al., 2021). Many EIDs provide a record of the volume of fluid infused over a period of time while delivering a measured amount of fluid over a period of time (e.g., 100 mL/h) using positive pressure. An electronic sensor signals an alarm if the pressure in the system changes and the desired flow rate alters. The use of an EID does not absolve a nurse from regularly checking to ensure that a pump is functioning and infusing at the prescribed rate or to detect infiltration or extravasation at an IV site (Gorski et al., 2021).

Manual flow-control devices include flow regulators (i.e., dial or barrel-shaped) and mechanical infusion devices without a power source (i.e., elastomeric devices, piston-driven pumps). These may be used when flow rate is not critical (Gorski, 2023). They are not recommended for use in infants and children because accuracy cannot be guaranteed (Gorski, 2023).

Flow regulators such as volume-control devices deliver small volumes with the aid of gravity. Mechanical factors (e.g., height of the IV container, IV tubing size, or fluid viscosity) affect an IV gravity controller. One example of a volume-control device is a calibrated chamber placed between the IV container and the insertion spike and drip chamber of an administration set (see Chapter 22). A small volume of IV solution (usually limited to 2 hours of ordered solution) is placed in the chamber and regulated for administration. The advantage of this system is that if the rate of the IV infusion is inadvertently increased, only a limited amount of solution will infuse. With either type of device, consistent moni-

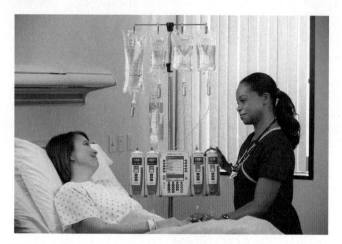

FIG. 28.3 Smart pump. (*Courtesy and copyright © Becton, Dickinson and Company.*)

toring is necessary to verify the accurate infusion of the IV solution and detect and prevent complications.

Dose-error reduction systems (DERSs) or "smart pumps" have an embedded computer system with a drug library and are associated with reduced risk for infusion-related medication errors (Gorski, 2023). The built-in software is programmed from health care pharmacy databases with unit-specific profiles (Fig. 28.3). The pump has an audible and visual alert when its setting does not match the preselected dose or volume limits, helping to prevent infusion errors. The use of a smart pump with the potential reduction in serious medication errors and improved patient outcomes is becoming the standard of care across all settings (Gorski, 2023). Know and follow your agency's and manufacturer's recommendations for selection and use of EIDs, alarm settings, pump controls, and features. Diligence is necessary on your part to assess and monitor patients because use of any EID or controller is not without risk of malfunction, placing a patient at risk for harm or injury.

Electronic infusion pumps are not foolproof. A systematic review of smart pump infusions found five error categories: (1) undocumented errors, (2) drug library errors, (3) programming errors, (4) administration errors, and (5) ancillary equipment errors (Kirkendall et al., 2020). The researchers found that some errors (e.g., drug library errors) are introduced by the implementation of smart pump technology, and some may be the result of workarounds. In workarounds, nurses find ways to circumvent work systems they perceive to be flawed (e.g., the procedure for programming and monitoring an EID) to provide more efficient or better care. Such workarounds involving IV therapy are dangerous. Follow policy and procedure guidelines judiciously when preparing and administering IV fluids.

Patients in alternative care settings (e.g., home care, long-term care) can receive infusion therapy with ambulatory pumps, which promote independence and improved quality of life. Most pumps weigh less than 2.7 kg (6 lb) and range from palm size to fitting in a backpack. Programming capabilities range from rate adjustments, remote site adjustments, and therapy-specific settings.

Delegation

The skill of regulating IV flow rates cannot be delegated to assistive personnel (AP). Delegation to licensed practical nurses (LPNs) varies by state nurse practice act. Direct the AP to:

- Inform the nurse when the EID alarm signals
- Inform the nurse when the fluid container or volume control device is near completion
- Report any patient complaints of discomfort related to infusion, such as pain, burning, bleeding, or swelling

Equipment

- Watch with second hand
- Calculator, paper, and pencil
- Tape
- Label
- IV solution bag and appropriate administration set
- IV administration set: EID (optional)
- Clean gloves

STEP	RATIONALE

ASSESSMENT

1. Review patient's electronic health record (EHR), including accuracy and completeness of health care provider's order for patient name, type and volume of IV fluid, additives, infusion rate, and duration of IV therapy. Follow seven rights of medication administration (see Chapter 20) (Gorski, 2023; Gorski et al., 2021).

Ensures delivery of correct IV solution and prescribed volume over prescribed time.

2. Review EHR to identify patient's risk for fluid and electrolyte imbalance given type of IV solution ordered (e.g., neonate, older adult, history of cardiac or renal disease).

Helps prioritize assessments. Volume control needs to be strict. Guides choice of infusion device.

3. Perform hand hygiene and apply clean gloves following Aseptic Non-Touch Technique (ANTT).

Reduces transmission of microorganisms.

4. Check infusion system from solution container down to VAD insertion site for integrity.

Identifies complications that can compromise integrity of VAD and patient safety.

   a. Assess IV container for discoloration, cloudiness, leakage, and expiration date.

Incompatibility of solutions or medications compromises integrity of VAD and patient safety (Gorski, 2023).

   b. Assess IV tubing for puncture, contamination, or occlusion.

Compromised tubing results in fluid leakage and bacterial contamination.

STEP	RATIONALE
5. Assess the integrity, patency, and functioning of the existing VAD. Assess the VAD catheter–skin junction site and surrounding area by visually inspecting and palpating through the intact dressing for redness, tenderness, swelling, and drainage.	Identifies complications that compromise integrity of VAD and may necessitate replacement of VAD. Reduces transmission of infection.
6. Remove and dispose of gloves and perform hand hygiene.	Reduces transmission of microorganisms.
7. Assess patient's/family caregiver's health literacy regarding positioning of IV site.	Determines degree to which individuals have the ability to find, understand, and use information and services to make informed health-related decisions and actions for themselves and others (CDC, 2023).
8. Assess patient's knowledge, prior experience with IV flow rates, and feelings about procedure.	Reveals need for patient instruction and/or support.

PLANNING

1. Expected outcomes following completion of procedure:	
• Fluid and electrolyte levels remain within normal limits.	IV solution helps to maintain fluid and electrolyte levels.
• Patient receives prescribed volume of solution over prescribed time interval.	IV rate maintained to achieve therapeutic outcomes.
• Patient's VAD remains patent.	IV infuses so that patient receives prescribed infusion therapy without occlusion complications (Gorski et al., 2021).
• Patient can explain how positioning of IV site affects rate and describe complications related to inaccurate flow rate.	Demonstrates learning.
2. Prepare and organize equipment at patient's bedside.	Ensures more efficiency when completing a procedure.
a. Have paper and pencil or calculator to calculate flow rate.	Calculating hourly flow rates ensures that the prescribed amount of fluid to be infused over the prescribed time frame is correct.
b. Check order to see how long each liter of fluid should infuse. If hourly rate (mL/h) is not provided in health care provider order, calculate it by dividing total volume in infusion container by hours of infusion. For example:	Basis of calculation to ensure infusion of solution over prescribed hourly rate.

$$mL/h = \frac{\text{Total infusion (mL)}}{\text{Hours of infusion}}$$
$$1000 \text{ mL/8 h} = 125 \text{ mL/h}$$

Or if 3 L is ordered for 24 hours:

$$3000 \text{ mL/24 hr} = 125 \text{ mL/hr}$$

Clinical Judgment *It is common for health care providers to write an abbreviated IV order such as "D5W with 20 mEq KCl 125 mL/h continuous." This order implies that the IV should be maintained at this rate until an order has been written for the IV to be discontinued or changed to another order.*

c. If a keep-vein-open (KVO) rate is ordered, check agency policy regarding flow rate of KVO. Rates may vary from 0.5 mL/h to 30 mL/h on the basis of the type of VAD, patient specific therapy, and method of infusion (gravity or EID).	Prevents catheter clotting, thus preserving venous access while infusing a minimal amount of fluid. An order for KVO rate must specify an infusion rate as required by the seven rights of medication administration (Gorski, 2023; Gorski et al., 2021).
d. Use hourly rate to program EID or, if gravity-flow infusion, use the hourly rate to calculate the minute flow rate (gtt/mL).	EID automatically delivers correct minute flow rate. Gravity infusion requires calculation of gtt/mL.
e. Know calibration (drop factor), in drops per milliliter (gtt/mL), of infusion set used by agency:	
(1) Microdrip: 60 gtt/mL. Used to deliver rates less than 100 mL/h.	Microdrip tubing universally delivers 60 gtt/mL. Used when small or very precise volumes are to be infused.
(2) Macrodrip: 10 to 15 gtt/mL (depending on manufacturer). Used to deliver rates greater than 100 mL/h.	There are different commercial parenteral administration sets for macrodrip tubing. Used when large volumes or fast rates are necessary. Know drip factor for tubing being used.

STEP	RATIONALE
f. Select one of the following formulas to calculate the minute flow rate (drops per minute) based on drop factor of infusion set: $$mL/h/60 \ min = mL/min$$ $$Drop \ factor \times mL/min = Drops/min$$ or $$mL/h \times Drop \ factor/60 \ min = Drops/min$$	Once you determine hourly rate, these formulas compute the correct flow rate.
Example: Calculate minute flow rate for a bag 1000 mL with 20 mEq KCl at 125 mL/h. Microdrip: $$125 \ mL/h \times 60 \ gtt/mL = 7500 \ gtt/h$$ $$7500 \ gtt \div 60 \ min = 125 \ gtt/min$$	When using microdrip, the milliliters per hour (mL/h) value always equals drops per minute (gtt/min).
Macrodrip: $$125 \ mL/h \times 15 \ gtt/mL = 1875 \ gtt/h$$ $$1875 \ gtt \div 60 \ min = 31 - 32 \ gtt/min$$	Multiply volume by drop factor and divide product by time (in minutes).
3. Provide privacy and explain procedure, its purpose, and what is expected of patient.	Protects patient's privacy; reduces anxiety. Promotes cooperation.

IMPLEMENTATION

1. Identify patient using at least two identifiers (e.g., name and birthday or name and medical record number) according to agency policy. Compare identifiers with information on patient's medication administration record (MAR) or EHR.	Ensures patient safety. Complies with The Joint Commission standards and improves patient safety (TJC, 2023).
2. Regulate gravity infusion. **a.** Ensure that IV container is at least 76.2 cm (30 inches) above IV site for adults, and increase height for more viscous fluids.	Pressure caused by gravity is necessary to overcome venous pressure and resistance from tubing and catheter.
b. Slowly open roller clamp on tubing until you can see drops in drip chamber. Hold a watch with second hand at same level as drip chamber and count drip rate for 1 minute (see illustration). Adjust roller clamp to increase or decrease rate of infusion.	Regulates flow to prescribed rate.
c. Monitor drip rate at least hourly.	Many factors influence drip rate; frequent monitoring ensures IV fluid administration as prescribed.

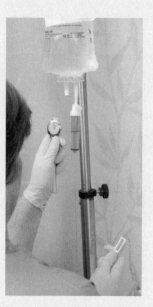

STEP 2b Nurse counting drip rate on gravity infusion.

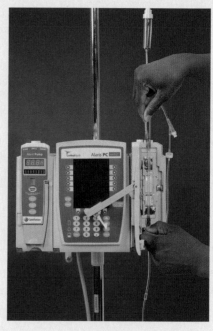

STEP 3b Insert IV tubing into chamber of control mechanism.

STEP	RATIONALE

3. **Regulate EID (infusion pump or smart pump):** Follow manufacturer guidelines for setup of EID. Be sure you are using infusion tubing compatible with EID.

Smart pumps with medication safety software are designed for administration of IV fluids that contain medications.

   a. Close roller clamp on primed IV infusion tubing.

Prevents fluid leakage.

   b. Insert infusion tubing into chamber of control mechanism (see manufacturer's directions) (see illustration). Roller clamp on IV tubing goes between EID and patient.

Most EIDs use positive pressure to infuse. Infusion pumps propel fluid through tubing by compressing and milking IV tubing.

   c. Secure part of IV tubing through "air in line" alarm system. Close door (see illustration A) and turn on power button, select required drops per minute or volume per hour, close door to control chamber, and press start button (see illustration B). If infusing medication, access the EID library of medications and set appropriate rate and dose limits. If smart pump alarms immediately and shuts down, your settings were outside unit parameters.

Ensures safe administration of ordered flow rate or medication dose. Smart pumps require additional information such as patient unit and medication. Computer will match the pump setting against a drug database (Wolf & Hughes, 2019).

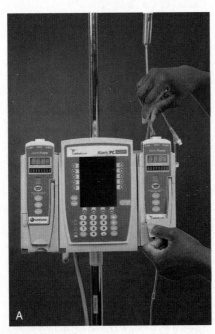 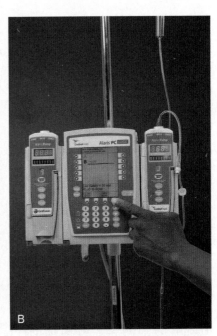

STEP 3c (A) Close door of control mechanism. (B) Select rate and volume to be infused and press start button.

Clinical Judgment *An anti–free-flow safeguard (preventing bolus infusion in the event of machine malfunction or when tubing is removed from machine) is an important element of an EID and is required. Always check and follow manufacturer's recommendations for specific device features.*

   d. Open infusion tubing drip regulator completely while EID is in use.

Ensures that pump freely regulates infusion rate.

   e. Monitor infusion rate and IV site for complications according to agency policy. Use watch to verify rate of infusion, even when using EID.

Flow controllers and pumps do not replace frequent, accurate nursing evaluation. EIDs can continue to infuse IV solutions after a complication has developed (Gorski et al., 2021).

   f. Assess IV system from container to VAD insertion site when alarm signals.

Alarm indicates situation that requires attention. Empty solution container, tubing kinks, closed clamp, infiltration, clotted catheter, air in tubing, and/or low battery can trigger EID alarm.

4. Attach label to IV solution container with date and time container changed (check agency policy).

Provides reference to determine next time for container change, especially with KVO rate that contains a specific infusion rate as ordered by health care provider.

5. Teach patient to avoid touching control clamp, lying on tubing, or raising hand or arm in a way that affects flow rate. If infusion therapy is delivered by EID, explain purpose of alarms and teach patient to avoid trying to adjust settings.

Information allows patient to protect IV site and informs patient about rationale for not altering control rate.

STEP	RATIONALE
6. Dispose of all contaminated supplies in appropriate receptacle.	Reduces transmission of microorganisms.
7. Assist patient to a comfortable position and instruct how to move and turn without dislodging VAD.	Restores comfort and sense of well-being. Prevents accidental dislodgement of catheter and minimizes risk for falls.
8. Raise bed rails (as appropriate) and lower bed to lowest position, locking into position.	Ensures patient safety and prevents falls.
9. Place nurse call system in an accessible location within patient's reach. Instruct patient in its use.	Ensures patient can call for assistance if needed.
10. Perform hand hygiene.	Reduces transmission of microorganisms.

EVALUATION

1. Observe patient every 1 to 2 hours (see agency policy), noting volume of IV fluid infused and rate of infusion.	Ensures delivery of prescribed volume over prescribed time and decreases risk for fluid and electrolyte imbalance.
2. Evaluate patient's response to therapy (e.g., laboratory values, intake and output [I&O], weights, vital signs, postprocedural assessments).	Provides ongoing evaluation of patient's fluid status, including monitoring for fluid volume excess (FVE) or fluid volume deficit (FVD). Early recognition of complications leads to prompt treatment.
3. Evaluate condition of IV site at established intervals per agency policy and procedure for signs and symptoms of IV site–related complications.	Prevents complications that compromise integrity of VAD or cause inaccurate IV solution flow rate.
4. **Use Teach-Back:** "I want to be sure that I explained the importance of your IV fluids running on time at the rate ordered. Tell me what you think may cause the pump to alarm and what you would do." Revise your instruction now or develop a plan for revised patient/family caregiver teaching if patient/family caregiver is not able to teach back correctly.	Teach-back is a technique for health care providers to ensure that they have explained medical information clearly so that patients and their families understand what is communicated to them (AHRQ, 2023).

Unexpected Outcomes

1. Solution does not infuse at prescribed rate.
   a. Sudden infusion of large volume of solution occurs; patient develops dyspnea, crackles in lung, dependent edema (edema in legs), and increased urine output, indicating FVE.

   b. IV solution runs slower than ordered.

2. IV patency is lost subsequent to IV solution container running empty.

Related Interventions

- Slow infusion rate: KVO rates must have specific rate ordered by health care provider.
- Notify health care provider immediately.
- Place patient in high-Fowler position.
- Anticipate new IV orders.
- Anticipate administration of oxygen per order.
- Administer diuretics if ordered.
- Check for positional change that affects rate, height of IV container, kinking of tubing, or obstruction.
- Check VAD site for complications.
- Consult health care provider for new order to provide necessary fluid volume.
- Discontinue present IV infusion and restart new peripheral catheter in new site.

Documentation

- Document IV solution and volume in container, rate of infusion in drops per minute (gtt/min) or milliliters per hour (mL/h), and integrity and patency of system.
- If using an EID, document type and rate of infusion and device identification number.
- Document patient response (e.g., laboratory values, I&O, weights, vital signs, postprocedural assessments) to therapy and unexpected outcomes (e.g., signs and symptoms of FVE, FVD, or IV site–related complications).
- Document patient's and family caregiver's level of understanding following instruction.

Hand-Off Reporting

- Report rate of infusing and remaining volume.
- Report to health care provider any infusion-related complications, interventions, and response to treatment.

Special Considerations
Patient Education

- Instruct patient to notify nurse if any signs or symptoms of IV complications are noted (e.g., redness, pain, tenderness, swelling, bleeding, drainage, leaking from under dressing).
- Patient using an EID should know the significance of alarms and when to notify nursing.
- Teach patient about factors affecting flow rate, to protect IV site, and about importance of not altering rate control.

Pediatrics

- The use of metered volume chamber sets filled with 1 to 2 hours of prescribed infusion fluid may be used for safe medication delivery if an EID or syringe pump is not used. Always use tamper-resistant volume-controlled EIDs to ensure accurate fluid delivery (Hockenberry et al., 2022).

Older Adults

- Use an EID and microdrip tubing to administer IV solutions. Monitor vital signs, electrolyte levels, blood urea nitrogen (BUN), creatinine, urine output, and body weight (Gorski, 2023).

Home Care

- Ensure that patient is able and willing to operate an EID and administer IV therapy. If patient is unable to provide self-care, be sure that a reliable family caregiver is available in the home.
- Discuss proper EID function with patient. Consider use of an ambulatory-type device. Observe patient or family caregiver operating EID and administering IV therapy.
- Teach patient and family caregiver what EID alarms mean, methods to troubleshoot them, and how to disconnect the IV tubing from the EID pump and then reregulate rate by gravity in the event of a pump failure.
- Ensure that patient's electrical outlets are properly grounded.
- Provide patient with a contact phone number to access 24 hours a day for problems.

✦ SKILL 28.3 Changing Intravenous Solutions

Patients receiving intravenous (IV) therapy periodically require changes of IV solutions: at the end of an infusion, at a time to avoid exceeding hang time of an existing solution, or in the middle of an infusion when orders for the type of solution change (Gorski, 2023). IV containers include plastic bags and glass bottles. You change a container when there is an order for a new solution or based on agency policy hang times (Gorski, 2023). It becomes clinically appropriate to change the type of solution, depending on a patient's fluid and electrolyte balance, response to therapy (e.g., therapeutic drug monitoring), and goals of therapy. The maximum hang time for routine replacement of IV containers is established by agency policy and procedure (Gorski, 2023). Maximum hang time is based on factors such as the use of strict aseptic technique, whether the system remains closed without injection ports or add-on tubing, stability of the solution or medication being infused, and how long the solution in the IV container will last (Gorski, 2023). Organizational and clinical judgment skills are necessary to manage changing IV containers or solutions in a manner that decreases the risk of infusion-related complications, such as an infusion container becoming empty or clotting of a vascular access device (VAD).

Delegation

The skill of changing an IV solution cannot be delegated to assistive personnel (AP). Delegation to licensed practical nurses (LPNs) varies by state nurse practice act. Direct the AP to:
- Inform the nurse when an IV container is near completion
- Report any cloudiness or precipitate in the IV solution
- Report alarm sounding on electronic infusion device (EID)
- Report any patient complaints of discomfort related to infusion, such as pain, burning, bleeding, or swelling

Equipment

- Clean gloves
- IV solution as ordered by health care provider
- Label

STEP	RATIONALE

ASSESSMENT

1. Review patient's electronic health record (EHR), including accuracy and completeness of health care provider's order for patient name and correct solution: type, volume, additives, infusion rate, and duration of IV therapy. Follow the seven rights of medication administration (see Chapter 20) (Gorski, 2023; Gorski et al., 2021).	Ensures delivery of correct IV solution and prescribed volume over prescribed time (Gorski et al., 2021).
2. Note date and time when IV tubing and solution were last changed.	Ensures correct timing of tubing changes.
3. Assess patient's/family caregiver's health literacy.	Determines degree to which individuals have the ability to find, understand, and use information and services to make informed health-related decisions and actions for themselves and others (CDC, 2023).

STEP	RATIONALE
4. Perform hand hygiene and apply clean gloves, following Aseptic Non-Touch Technique (ANTT); inspect and gently palpate skin around and above IV site over dressing. Assess VAD for patency and signs and symptoms of IV site–related complications (e.g., infiltration, occlusion of VAD, phlebitis, infection, patient complaints of pain, or leaking under dressing).	Identifies complications that compromise integrity of VAD and necessitate replacement of VAD.
5. Check infusion system from solution container down to VAD insertion site for integrity, including but not limited to discoloration, cloudiness, leakage, and expiration date. Determine compatibility of all IV solutions and additives by consulting approved online database, drug reference, or pharmacist. Remove and dispose of gloves and perform hand hygiene.	A break in integrity of solution container necessitates a container change (Gorski, 2023). May indicate need for IV tubing change. Incompatibilities cause physical, chemical, and therapeutic changes with adverse patient outcomes (Gorski, 2023). Reduces transmission of microorganisms.
6. Check pertinent laboratory data such as potassium level.	Compare data with baseline to determine ongoing response to IV solution administration.
7. Assess patient's/family caregiver's knowledge and understanding of need for continued IV therapy and feelings about procedure.	Reveals need for patient instruction and/or support.

PLANNING

STEP	RATIONALE
1. Expected outcomes following completion of procedure: • IV solution is correct. • Patient's VAD remains patent, and site is free from signs and symptoms of complications. • Patient and family caregiver can explain purpose of IV solution change.	Patient receives solution ordered for treatment of diagnosis. Ensures IV access for delivery of prescribed IV therapy (Gorski et al., 2021). Demonstrates learning.
2. Provide privacy and explain procedure, its purpose, and what is expected of patient.	Protects patient's privacy; reduces anxiety. Promotes cooperation.
3. Organize and set up any equipment needed to perform procedure.	Ensures more efficiency when completing a procedure.
4. Perform hand hygiene following ANTT. Collect equipment. Have next solution prepared at least 1 hour before needed. If solution is prepared in pharmacy, ensure that it has been delivered to patient care unit. Allow solution to warm to room temperature if it has been refrigerated. Check that solution is correct and properly labeled. Check solution expiration date. Ensure that any light sensitivity restrictions are followed.	Reduces transmission of microorganisms. Proper handling of solutions prevents IV-related complications, such as occlusion. Checking that solution is correct prevents medication error.

IMPLEMENTATION

STEP	RATIONALE
1. Identify patient using at least two identifiers (e.g., name and birthday or name and medical record number) according to agency policy. Compare identifiers with information on patient's medication administration record (MAR) or EHR.	Ensures patient safety. Complies with The Joint Commission standards and improves patient safety (TJC, 2023).
2. Change solution when fluid remains only in neck of container (about 50 mL), when new type of solution has been ordered, or when existing solution hang time has expired.	Prevents waste of solution. Prevents exposure to contaminated solution.
3. Prepare new solution for changing. If using plastic bag, hang on IV pole and remove protective cover from IV tubing port. If using glass bottle, remove metal cap and metal and rubber disks.	Permits quick, smooth, organized change from old to new container.
4. Apply clean gloves. Close roller clamp on existing solution to stop flow rate. Remove IV tubing from EID (if used). Then remove old IV solution container from IV pole. Hold container with tubing port pointing upward.	Prevents solution remaining in drip chamber from emptying while changing solutions. Prevents solution in bag from spilling.
5. Quickly remove spike from old solution container and, without touching tip, insert spike into new container (see illustrations).	Reduces risk for solution in drip chamber becoming empty and maintains sterility.

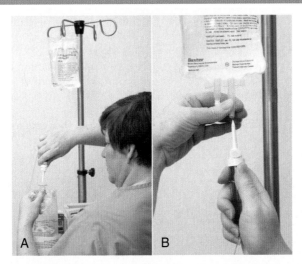

STEP 5 (A) Quickly remove spike from old solution container. (B) Without touching tip, insert spike into new container.

Clinical Judgment *If spike becomes contaminated by touching an unsterile object, you will need a new IV tubing set.*

6. Hang new container of solution on IV pole.
7. Check for air in IV tubing. If air bubbles have formed, remove them by closing roller clamp, stretching tubing downward, and tapping tubing with finger (bubbles rise in fluid to drip chamber) (see illustration).
8. Make sure that drip chamber is one-third to one-half full. If drip chamber is too full, level can be decreased by removing bag from IV pole, pinching off IV tubing below drip chamber, inverting container, squeezing drip chamber (see illustration), releasing, turning solution container upright, and releasing pinch on tubing.

Gravity helps with delivery of fluid into drip chamber.
Reduces risk of air entering tubing. Use of an air-eliminating filter also reduces risk.

Reduces risk for air entering IV tubing. If chamber is completely filled, you cannot observe or regulate drip rate.

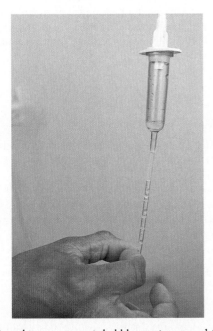

STEP 7 Tap tubing to cause air bubbles to rise up to drip chamber.

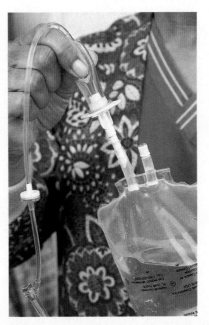

STEP 8 Squeeze drip chamber to fill with fluid. Be sure to leave chamber one-third to one-half full.

STEP	RATIONALE
9. Regulate flow to ordered rate by opening and adjusting roller clamp on IV tubing or by opening roller clamp and programming and turning on EID.	Maintains measures to restore fluid balance and deliver IV solution as ordered.
10. Place time label on side of container and label with time hung, time of completion, and appropriate hourly intervals. If using plastic bags, mark only on label and **not container**.	Provides visual comparison of volume infused compared with prescribed rate of infusion.
11. Instruct patient on purpose of new IV solution, additives, flow rate, potential side effects, how to avoid occluding tubing, and what to report.	Informs patient about purpose for continued IV therapy and what to report and protects VAD patency.
12. Dispose of all contaminated supplies in appropriate receptacle; remove and dispose of gloves.	Reduces transmission of microorganisms. Use appropriate disposal receptacle if patient is on hazardous drugs (ONS, 2018).
13. Assist patient to a comfortable position and instruct how to move and turn without dislodging VAD.	Restores comfort and sense of well-being. Prevents accidental dislodgement of catheter and minimizes risk for falls.
14. Raise bed rails (as appropriate) and lower bed to lowest position, locking into position.	Ensures patient safety and prevents falls.
15. Place nurse call system in an accessible location within patient's reach. Instruct patient in its use.	Ensures patient can call for assistance if needed.
16. Perform hand hygiene.	Reduces transmission of microorganisms.

EVALUATION

1. Observe patient every 1 to 2 hours or at established intervals per agency policy and procedure for function, intactness, and patency of IV system; correct infusion rate; and type and amount of IV solution infused.	Ensures delivery of prescribed volume over prescribed time and decreases risk for fluid and electrolyte imbalance.
2. Evaluate patient to determine response to therapy (e.g., laboratory values, intake and output [I&O], weights, vital signs, and postprocedural assessments).	Provides ongoing evaluation of patient's fluid status.
a. Monitor patient for signs of fluid volume excess (FVE), fluid volume deficit (FVD), or signs and symptoms of electrolyte imbalances.	Early recognition of complications leads to prompt treatment.
3. Evaluate IV site at established intervals per agency policy and procedure for signs and symptoms of phlebitis or infiltration.	Prevents complications that compromise integrity of VAD or cause inaccurate IV solution flow rate.
4. **Use Teach-Back:** "We talked about the importance of your IV solutions running continuously on time. I want to be sure I explained this clearly. Tell me in your own words what you should do if you notice that the IV is not dripping." Revise your instruction now or develop a plan for revised patient/family caregiver teaching if patient/family caregiver is not able to teach back correctly.	Teach-back is a technique for health care providers to ensure that they have explained medical information clearly so that patients and their families understand what is communicated to them (AHRQ, 2023).

Unexpected Outcomes	Related Interventions
1. Flow rate is incorrect; patient receives too little or too much solution.	• Notify health care provider if patient's anticipated infusion is 100 to 200 mL less than or greater than anticipated (per agency policy and procedure). • Evaluate patient for signs and symptoms of adverse effects of infusion (e.g., FVD or FVE). Notify health care provider if patient is symptomatic. • Determine and correct cause of incorrect flow rate (e.g., change in position, tubing kink, loss of IV patency or intactness). • Use EID when accurate flow rate is critical.
2. Fluid and/or electrolyte imbalances	• Notify health care provider. • Anticipate orders for changes in IV solution or additives.

Documentation

- Document solution changes, type of infusion solution including any additives, volume of container, time of change, rate of infusion, and integrity and patency of system.
- Document use of any EID or control device and identification number on that device.
- Document patient response to therapy and unexpected outcomes (e.g., causes of flow rate inaccuracy).

Hand-Off Reporting

- Report time and reason for IV solution change, new solution, rate of and volume left in infusion, and any significant information about IV site or system.

Special Considerations

Patient Education

- Inform patient of new solution, additives, and potential side effects, including those to report to the nurse.

- Instruct patient to notify nurse or AP if flow rate slows or IV container is empty.

Home Care

- Ensure that patient and family caregiver are willing and able to perform an IV solution change.
- Teach patient and family caregiver how to perform an IV solution change. Observe them performing procedure.

✦ SKILL 28.4   Changing Infusion Tubing

An important component of intravenous (IV) therapy is maintaining the integrity of the IV system through the conscientious use of infection-prevention principles during tubing changes. Administration sets are the primary method of delivering IV solutions to patients. In addition, patients may have add-on devices (e.g., filters, extension sets), which you connect to the primary administration set as indicated by the prescribed therapy. Secondary sets may be used as a method to administer medications in conjunction with the primary infusion (e.g., antibiotics). Any time a new IV infusion tubing or add-on device is added, Luer-Lok connections must be used to prevent accidental tubing disconnection (Gorski et al., 2021). When a peripheral IV site is rotated to a different site or a new CVAD is placed, the administration set should be changed (Gorski et al., 2021). Follow agency policy and procedures for specific requirements (Table 28.6). Administration sets used for parenteral nutrition (see Chapter 32) and blood or blood products (see Chapter 29) have specific criteria for tubing changes (see agency policy).

Whenever possible, schedule IV tubing changes when it is time to hang a new IV container (see Skill 28.3). To prevent entry of bacteria into the bloodstream, maintain sterility during tubing and solution changes. If the tubing and/or IV bag becomes damaged, is leaking, or becomes contaminated, it must be changed, regardless of the tubing change schedule.

Delegation

The skill of changing IV tubing cannot be delegated to assistive personnel (AP). Delegation to licensed practical nurses (LPNs) varies by state nurse practice act. Direct the AP to:
- Report any leakage from or around the IV tubing
- Report if tubing has become contaminated (e.g., is lying on the floor)

Equipment

- Clean gloves
- Antiseptic swabs (chlorhexidine gluconate [CHG] solution preferred, povidone-iodine, or 70% alcohol)
- Tubing label

Continuous IV Infusion

- Microdrip or macrodrip administration set of IV tubing as appropriate
- Add-on device as needed (e.g., filters, extension set, needleless connector)

Intermittent Extension Set

- 3- to 5-mL syringe filled with preservative-free 0.9% sodium chloride (normal saline [NS])
- Short extension tubing (if necessary), injection cap

STEP	RATIONALE

ASSESSMENT

1. Note date and time when IV tubing was last changed (see Table 28.6 for recommendations on administration set changes).	Decreases risk of infection.

TABLE 28.6

Intravenous Administration Set Changes

Primary and Secondary Continuous Infusions	Primary Intermittent Infusions	Use of Add-On Devices
Change no more frequently than every 96 hours for solutions *other than* lipid, blood, or blood products. In addition to routine changes, change the administration set whenever the peripheral IV site is changed or a new CVAD is placed. If the secondary set is removed from the primary set, the secondary set is now an intermittent set and should be changed every 24 hours.	Should be changed every 24 hours because of increased risk of infection with repeatedly disconnecting and reconnecting administration set. Aseptically attach a new, sterile covering device to the Luer end of the administration set after each intermittent use. *Avoid* attaching the exposed end of the administration set to port on the same set (e.g., looping).	Should be minimized because each is a potential source of contamination and disconnection. Use of administration sets with devices as part of the set is preferred. Aseptically change with insertion of new VAD or with each administration set replacement. Change if the integrity of the product is compromised or suspected of being compromised.

CVAD, Central vascular access device; *IV*, intravenous; *VAD*, vascular access device.
Modified from Gorski LA, et al: Infusion therapy standards of practice. *J Infus Nurs* 44(suppl 1):S1-S224, 2021. doi:10.1097/NAN.0000000000000396.

STEP	RATIONALE
2. Perform hand hygiene, following Aseptic Non-Touch Technique (ANTT). Assess IV tubing for puncture, contamination, or occlusion that requires immediate change.	Compromised tubing results in fluid leakage and bacterial contamination.
3. Assess patient's or family caregiver's health literacy.	Determines degree to which individuals have the ability to find, understand, and use information and services to make informed health-related decisions and actions for themselves and others (CDC, 2023).
4. Assess patient's knowledge, prior experience with need for IV tubing change, and feelings about procedure.	Reveals need for patient instruction and/or support.

PLANNING

1. Expected outcomes following completion of procedure:	
• Patient experiences no leakage of solution from or around IV tubing.	Intact system decreases risk for microbial contamination.
• Patient's IV tubing is patent, and patient receives prescribed IV therapy as ordered.	Brief interruption of IV infusion does not result in occlusion of vascular access device (VAD).
• Patient's VAD remains patent, and site is free from signs and symptoms of IV site–related complications.	Adherence to administration set changes decreases risk of complications.
• Patient and family caregiver can explain purpose of tubing change and how patient can avoid occluding tubing.	Demonstrates learning.
2. Provide privacy and explain procedure, its purpose, and what is expected of them.	Protects patient's privacy; reduces anxiety. Promotes cooperation.
3. Coordinate IV tubing changes with solution changes when possible.	Decreases number of times system is open.
4. Obtain and organize equipment for tubing change at bedside.	Ensures more efficiency when completing a procedure.
5. Assist patient to comfortable position with easy access to IV site.	Improves patient comfort and efficiency of procedure.

IMPLEMENTATION

1. Identify patient using at least two identifiers (e.g., name and birthday or name and medical record number) according to agency policy. Compare identifiers with information on patient's medication administration record (MAR) or electronic health record (EHR).	Ensures patient safety. Complies with The Joint Commission standards and improves patient safety (TJC, 2023).
2. Perform hand hygiene following ANTT. Open new infusion set and connect add-on pieces (e.g., filters, extension tubing) using aseptic technique. Keep protective coverings over infusion spike and distal adapter. Place roller clamp about 2 to 2.5 cm (1–2 inches) below drip chamber and move roller clamp to "off" position. Secure all connections.	Close proximity of roller clamp to drip chamber allows more accurate regulation of flow rate. Securing connections reduces later risk of air emboli and infection. Protective covers reduce entrance of microorganisms. All connections should be of Luer-Lok type (Gorski et al., 2021).
3. Apply clean gloves. If patient's IV cannula hub is not visible, remove IV dressing (see Skill 28.5). Do not remove tape or securement device securing cannula to skin.	Cannula hub must be visible to provide smooth transition when removing old and inserting new tubing.
4. Prepare IV tubing with new IV container. (See Skill 28.1, Step 4.)	
5. Prepare IV tubing with existing continuous IV infusion bag.	
a. Be sure roller clamp on new IV tubing is still in the "off" position.	Prevents fluid spillage.
b. Slow rate of infusion through old tubing to keep-vein-open (KVO) rate using electronic infusion device (EID) or roller clamp.	Prevents occlusion of VAD.
c. Compress and fill drip chamber of old tubing.	Ensures that drip chamber remains full until new tubing is changed.
d. Invert container and remove old tubing. Dispose of container. Old tubing may be held upright or hung on IV pole until end of change is over. Keep spike of tubing sterile and upright.	Solution in drip chamber will continue to run and maintain catheter patency.
e. Insert spike of new infusion tubing into solution container. Hang solution bag on IV pole, compress drip chamber on new tubing, and release, allowing it to fill one-third to one-half full.	Permits drip chamber to fill and promotes rapid, smooth flow of solution through tubing.

STEP	RATIONALE

f. Prime air out of IV tubing by filling with IV solution: Remove protective cover on end of tubing and slowly open roller clamp to allow solution to flow from drip chamber to distal end of IV tubing. Return roller clamp to "off" position after priming tubing (filled with IV solution). Replace protective cover on end of IV tubing. Place end of adapter near patient's IV site.

Priming ensures that IV tubing is clear of air before connection with VAD and filled with IV solution. Slow fill of tubing decreases turbulence and chance of bubble formation. Closing clamp prevents accidental loss of fluid.
Maintains sterility. Equipment is positioned for quick connection of new tubing.

g. Stop EID or turn roller clamp on old tubing to "off" position.

Prevents fluid spillage.

6. Prepare tubing with extension set or saline lock.

a. If short extension tubing is needed, use sterile technique to connect new injection cap to new extension set or IV tubing.

Prepares extension set for connecting with IV.

b. Scrub injection cap with antiseptic swab for at least 15 seconds and allow to dry completely. Attach syringe with 3 to 5 mL of NS flush solution and inject through injection cap into extension set.

Ensures effective disinfection (Gorski, 2023). Maintains patency of catheter.

7. Reestablish infusion.

a. Gently disconnect old tubing from extension tubing (or from IV catheter hub). Quickly insert Luer-Lok end of new tubing or saline lock into extension tubing connection (or IV catheter hub) (see illustrations for example of connecting tubing to short extension set).

Allows smooth transition from old to new tubing, minimizing time system is open.

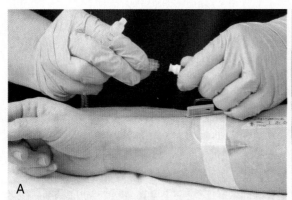 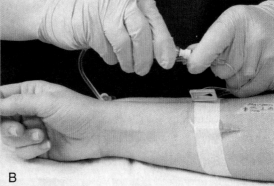

STEP 7a (A) Disconnect old tubing. (B) Insert adapter of new tubing.

b. For continuous infusion, open roller clamp on new tubing and regulate drip rate using roller clamp, or insert tubing into EID, program to desired rate, and push "on."

Ensures catheter patency and prevents occlusion.

c. Attach piece of tape or preprinted label with date and time of IV tubing change onto tubing below drip chamber.

Provides reference to determine next time for tubing change.

d. Form loop of tubing and secure it to patient's arm with strip of tape.

Avoids accidental pulling against site and stabilizes catheter.

8. Remove and discard old IV tubing. If necessary, apply new dressing (see Skill 28.5).

Reduces transmission of microorganisms.

9. Teach patient how to move and turn properly with IV tubing.

Prevents accidental occlusion or disconnection and contamination of IV tubing.

10. Dispose of all contaminated supplies in appropriate receptacle; remove and dispose of gloves.

Reduces transmission of microorganisms. Use appropriate disposal receptacle if patient is on hazardous drugs (ONS, 2018).

11. Assist patient to a comfortable position.

Restores comfort and sense of well-being.

12. Raise bed rails (as appropriate) and lower bed to lowest position, locking into position.

Ensures patient safety and prevents falls.

13. Place nurse call system in an accessible location within patient's reach. Instruct patient in its use.

Ensures patient can call for assistance if needed.

14. Perform hand hygiene.

Reduces transmission of microorganisms.

STEP	RATIONALE

EVALUATION

1. Observe patient every 1 to 2 hours or at established intervals per agency policy and procedure for function, intactness, and patency of IV system and leaking at connection sites.

Ensures that IV system is functioning appropriately and minimizes risk of infection caused by breach in system integrity.

2. Evaluate patient at established intervals per agency policy and procedure for signs and symptoms of IV site–related complications.

Prevents complications that compromise integrity of VAD or cause inaccurate IV solution flow rate.

3. **Use Teach-Back:** "Let's go over what we talked about earlier regarding the problems that can occur with your IV line. Tell me how you can prevent the tubing from being pinched off and which problems you would report to me or another nurse." Revise your instruction now or develop a plan for revised patient/family caregiver teaching if patient/family caregiver is not able to teach back correctly.

Teach-back is a technique for health care providers to ensure that they have explained medical information clearly so that patients and their families understand what is communicated to them (AHRQ, 2023).

Unexpected Outcomes

1. IV solution infuses more slowly than ordered.

Related Interventions

- Check for positional change that affects rate, height of IV container, kinking of tubing, or obstruction.
- Check for patency by opening roller clamp.
- Check VAD site for complications.
- Prepare for insertion of new VAD if existing one is occluded.

Documentation

- Document tubing change, type of solution, volume, and rate of infusion. Use an infusion therapy flow sheet for parenteral solutions per agency policy.
- If using an EID, document type and rate of infusion and device identification number.
- Document patient's and family caregiver's level of understanding following instruction, including what problems to report.

Hand Off-Reporting

- Report any significant information about IV site or system and time IV tubing was changed.

Special Considerations

Patient Education

- Instruct patient to notify nurse if fluid leaks from or around IV site or tubing or if tubing separates from catheter.

Home Care

- Ensure that patient or family caregiver is able and willing to perform IV tubing change and maintain IV access site or that there is a reliable person at home to provide this IV therapy care.
- Instruct patient or family caregiver in procedure for performing a sterile tubing change. Observe them performing procedure.

◆ SKILL 28.5   Changing a Peripheral Intravenous Dressing

Administration of solutions via the parenteral route is not without complications, which can be either systemic or local (Gorski, 2023). Systemic complications occur within the vascular system and are usually remote to the infusion site (e.g., septicemia, circulatory overload, embolism). Local complications result from trauma to the inner layer of the vein (tunica intima) as a direct result of many factors, such as poor insertion technique, inappropriate size of peripheral device (see Table 28.3), inadequate catheter stabilization, osmolarity of IV solution not within suggested ranges (see Table 28.2), and poor assessment and incorrect technique or frequency for peripheral catheter dressing change.

Another complication directly related to an intravenous (IV) site dressing is medical adhesive–related skin injury (MARSI). Such injuries can occur from any adhesive (e.g., tape, device adhesive) that results in mechanical injury (skin stripping, blistering, skin tears), dermatitis (irritation in response to the adhesive), and other complications (maceration and folliculitis) (Fumarola et al., 2020). Use of skin barriers during application of any adhesive device and the use of sterile adhesive removers is recommended for the prevention of MARSI (Fumarola et al., 2020).

Peripheral IV catheters require strict adherence to infection-prevention measures to avoid systemic and local complications. The skin insertion site is the most common source of colonization and catheter-related infections (Gorski, 2023). Peripheral catheter transparent semipermeable membrane (TSM) dressings (including integrated securement device dressings) should be changed at least every 7 days, and gauze dressing changes every 2 days (Gorski et al., 2021). If a gauze dressing is underneath a TSM, it should be changed every 2 days (Gorski et al., 2021). Apply IV catheter dressings securely and change any dressing immediately when it becomes wet, soiled, or loosened or if the integrity is compromised (Gorski et al., 2021). Stabilization of peripheral catheters decreases risk of catheter-related complications and premature loss of access. Preferred options for stabilization include an adhesive engineered stabilization device used with a standard peripheral IV catheter or an integrated feature on the IV catheter with use of a bordered polyurethane dressing (Gorski et al., 2021). Although sterile tape or surgical strips can be used, they are not as effective as an engineered stabilization device (Gorski, 2023).

Delegation

The skill of changing a peripheral IV dressing cannot be delegated to assistive personnel (AP). Direct the AP to:
- Report if a patient complains of moistness or loosening of an IV dressing
- Protect the IV dressing during hygiene and activities of daily living (ADLs)

Equipment

- Antiseptic swabs (chlorhexidine gluconate [CHG] solution preferred, povidone-iodine, or 70% alcohol)
- Sterile adhesive remover
- Skin barrier protectant (film, cream, swab, or wipe)
- Clean gloves
- Engineered stabilization device or precut strips sterile tape
- Commercially available IV site protection device (optional) (see Fig. 28.2)
- Sterile TSM dressing, integrated securement device, or sterile 2 × 2– or 4 × 4–inch gauze pad

STEP	RATIONALE
ASSESSMENT	
1. Refer to electronic health record (EHR) to determine when dressing was last changed. Dressing should also be labeled to include date and time last applied and size and type of vascular access device (VAD) with insertion date.	Provides information regarding length of time that present dressing has been in place and allows planning for dressing change.
2. Review EHR to determine patient's risk for developing a MARSI with use of adhesive devices or tape: age, dehydration, malnutrition, exposure to radiation therapy, underlying chronic conditions (e.g., diabetes, immunosuppression), and edema of extremity.	Common risk factors for MARSI (Fumarola et al., 2020).
3. Assess patient's/family caregiver's health literacy.	Determines degree to which individuals have the ability to find, understand, and use information and services to make informed health-related decisions and actions for themselves and others (CDC, 2023).
4. Perform hand hygiene and apply clean gloves, following Aseptic Non-Touch Technique (ANTT). Observe present dressing for moisture and intactness. Determine if moisture is from site leakage or external source.	Nonadhering dressing increases risk for insertion site infection or dislodgement of VAD. Moisture causes skin maceration.
5. Inspect and gently palpate skin around and above IV site over dressing, and ask if patient feels tenderness or discomfort. Is area swollen?	Detects possible phlebitis or infiltration.
a. Assess VAD for patency and check site for signs and symptoms of IV site–related complications (e.g., infiltration, occlusion of VAD, phlebitis, infection, or leaking under dressing).	Identifies complications that compromise integrity of VAD and may necessitate its replacement.
b. Assess skin around dressing: temperature, color, moisture level, turgor, fragility, and integrity. Observe for local signs of irritation or skin damage at the site where any adhesive has been or will be applied.	Signs and symptoms of MARSI (Fumarola et al., 2020).
6. Remove and dispose of gloves in appropriate receptacle and perform hand hygiene.	Reduces transmission of microorganisms.
7. Assess patient for allergy to iodine, adhesive, latex, or chlorhexidine (CHG). If you identify allergy, place allergy band on patient's wrist.	Medications, solutions used during catheter insertion, and use of latex gloves and tape can cause serious allergic reactions.
8. Assess patient's knowledge, prior experience with the need for IV dressing change, and feelings about procedure.	Reveals need for patient instruction and/or support.
PLANNING	
1. Expected outcomes following completion of procedure:	
• Patient's VAD remains patent, and site is free from signs and symptoms of IV site–related complications and MARSI.	Proper care maintains IV site. Diligent skin care prevents MARSI.
• Patient and family caregiver can explain procedure and purpose of VAD dressing change.	Demonstrates learning.
2. Provide privacy and explain procedure and purpose to patient and family caregiver. Explain that patient will need to hold affected extremity still. Explain how long procedure will take.	Protects patient's privacy; reduces anxiety. Promotes cooperation.
3. Assist patient to comfortable position with IV site easily accessible.	Promotes patient comfort.

STEP	RATIONALE
4. Collect equipment and organize on clean, clutter-free bedside stand or overbed table.	Ensures more efficiency when completing a procedure.

IMPLEMENTATION

STEP	RATIONALE
1. Identify patient using at least two identifiers (e.g., name and birthday or name and medical record number) according to agency policy. Compare identifiers with information on patient's electronic health record (EHR).	Ensures patient safety. Complies with The Joint Commission standards and improves patient safety (TJC, 2023).
2. Perform hand hygiene, following ANTT, and apply clean gloves. Remove existing dressing:	Reduces transmission of microorganisms. Technique minimizes discomfort during removal. Use sterile adhesive remover on integrated securement device/TSM dressing next to patient's skin to loosen dressing.
a. For integrated securement device/TSM dressing:	
(1) Stabilize catheter with nondominant hand (see illustration).	Guidelines for MARSI prevention (Fumarola et al., 2020).
(2) Loosen the edges of the dressing with the fingers of the nondominant hand by pushing the skin down and away from the integrated securement device/TSM dressing. (For integrated securement device, gently lift edges of two strips of tape covering dressing.)	

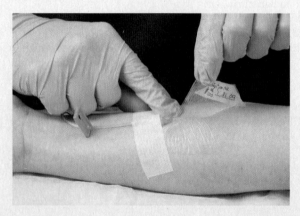

STEP 2a(1) Remove transparent semipermeable membrane dressing by pulling side laterally.

STEP	RATIONALE
(3) With fingers of the dominant hand, loosen a corner of the dressing and stretch it horizontally in the opposite direction of the wound (stretch-and-relax technique). Walk your fingers under the dressing to continue stretching it. One hand should continuously support the skin adhered to the dressing.	
(4) This process can be repeated around the dressing. Use medical adhesive remover if needed to loosen the adhesive bond. Follow the manufacturer's instructions for use.	
b. For gauze dressing:	Guidelines for MARSI prevention (Fumarola et al., 2020).
(1) Stabilize catheter hub.	
(2) Remove tape strips by slowly lifting and removing each side toward the center of dressing. When both sides are completely loosened, lift the strip up from the center of the dressing.	
(3) Remove old dressing one layer at a time by pulling toward insertion site. Be cautious if tubing becomes tangled between two layers of dressing. Use medical adhesive remover if needed to loosen the adhesive bond of tape.	

STEP	RATIONALE
3. Assess VAD insertion site for signs and symptoms of IV site–related complications. If complication exists, determine if VAD requires removal. Remove catheter if ordered by health care provider (see Procedural Guideline 28.1).	Presence of complication may necessitate VAD removal.
4. If catheter is to remain in place, assess integrity of engineered stabilization device. Continue to stabilize catheter and remove as recommended by manufacturer's directions for use. Inspect for signs of MARSI from adhesive-based engineered stabilization devices.	Removing stabilization device allows for appropriate skin antisepsis before applying dressing and new stabilization device (Gorski et al., 2021). Stabilization prevents accidental dislodgement of VAD. Guidelines for MARSI prevention (Fumarola et al., 2020).
5. **NOTE:** Some stabilization devices are designed to remain in place for length of time VAD is in, as long as adequate stabilization is evident.	

Clinical Judgment *Always keep one finger over catheter until dressing secures catheter hub. If patient is restless or uncooperative, it is helpful to have another nurse or AP help with procedure.*

STEP	RATIONALE
6. While stabilizing IV line, perform skin antisepsis to insertion site with CHG solution using friction in back-and-forth motion following manufacturer's guidelines. If using alcohol or povidone-iodine, clean in concentric circle, moving from insertion site outward with the swab. Allow any antiseptic solution to dry completely.	Reduces incidence of catheter-related infections (Gorski, 2023). Drying of antiseptic agent is necessary for complete antisepsis (Gorski et al., 2021).
7. *Optional:* Apply skin barrier protectant to area where you will reapply tape, dressing, or engineered stabilization device (Fumarola et al., 2020). Allow to dry.	Coats skin with protective solution to maintain skin integrity, prevents irritation from adhesive, and promotes adhesion of dressing.
8. While stabilizing catheter, apply sterile dressing over site (procedures differ; follow agency policy). Be sure skin surface is dry.	Moisture reduces effectiveness of adhesion.
a. *Integrated securement device/TSM dressing:* Apply dressings as directed in Skill 28.1, Step 21a, 21b.	Protects catheter insertion site and minimizes risk for infection (Gorski, 2023). The dressings allow visualization of insertion site and surrounding area for complications (Gorski et al., 2021).
b. *Sterile gauze dressing:* Apply sterile gauze dressing as directed in Skill 28.1, Step 21c.	Only use sterile tape (plastic preferred for short-term use) under sterile dressing to prevent site contamination. Gauze dressing obscures observation of insertion site and is changed every 2 days (Gorski et al., 2021).
9. *Option:* Secure with new engineered catheter stabilization device. Apply device as directed in Skill 28.1, Step 22.	Use of engineered stabilization devices can reduce risk for VAD complications (i.e., phlebitis, infection, migration) and unintentional loss of access (Gorski et al., 2021).

Clinical Judgment *Because Band-Aids are not occlusive and because nonsterile tape increases the risk for insertion site infection, do not use either over catheter insertion points.*

STEP	RATIONALE
10. *Optional:* Apply site protection device.	Reduces risk of VAD dislodgement (Gorski et al., 2021).
11. Anchor extension tubing or IV tubing alongside dressing on arm and secure with tape directly over tubing. When using integrated securement device/TSM dressing, avoid placing tape over dressing.	Prevents accidental dislodgement of VAD tubing.
12. Label dressing per agency policy. Information on label includes date and time of IV insertion, VAD gauge size and length, and your initials.	Communicates type of device and time interval for dressing change and site rotation.
13. Dispose of all contaminated supplies in appropriate receptacle. Remove and dispose of gloves.	Prevents transmission of microorganisms.
14. Assist patient to a comfortable position and instruct how to move and turn without dislodging VAD.	Restores comfort and sense of well-being. Prevents accidental dislodgement of catheter and minimizes risk for falls.
15. Raise bed rails (as appropriate) and lower bed to lowest position, locking into position.	Ensures patient safety and prevents falls.
16. Place nurse call system in an accessible location within patient's reach. Instruct patient in its use.	Ensures patient can call for assistance if needed.
17. Perform hand hygiene.	Prevents transmission of microorganisms.

STEP	RATIONALE

EVALUATION

1. Evaluate function, patency of IV system, and flow rate after changing dressing.

2. Evaluate patient at established intervals per agency policy and procedure for signs and symptoms of IV site–related complications.

3. **Use Teach-Back:** "I want to be sure that I explained reasons for why we changed the IV dressing. Tell me in your own words the problems that you would report that would require us to change the dressing." Revise your instruction now or develop a plan for revised patient/family caregiver teaching if patient/family caregiver is not able to teach back correctly.

Validates that IV line is patent and functioning correctly. Manipulation of catheter and tubing will affect rate of infusion.

Identifies complications that compromise integrity of VAD or cause inaccurate IV solution flow rate.

Teach-back is a technique for health care providers to ensure that they have explained medical information clearly so that patients and their families understand what is communicated to them (AHRQ, 2023).

Unexpected Outcomes

1. IV catheter is removed or dislodged accidentally.

Related Interventions

- Restart new peripheral IV line in other extremity or above previous insertion site if continued therapy is necessary.

Documentation

- Document the time peripheral dressing was changed, reason for change, type of dressing material used, patency of system, description of VAD site, and any complications, interventions, and response to treatment.
- Document patient's and family caregiver's understanding of what IV problems to report.

Hand-Off Reporting

- Report dressing was changed and any significant information about integrity of system.
- Report to health care provider any IV-related complications, interventions, and response to treatment.

Special Considerations

Patient Education

- Instruct patient to notify nurse or AP if the dressing is wet, soiled, or loosened.

Pediatrics

- Pediatric patients are not always able to understand explanations fully. Presence of parent or security toy during procedure helps to decrease fear and increase cooperation. Perform procedure on patient's toy or doll first.
- Help is necessary to keep patient still and protect IV catheter from dislodgement.

- Use commercially available IV site protectors to cover and protect the IV site in young, active children.
- Use CHG with care in preterm or low-birth-weight infants due to the risks of skin irritation and chemical burns (Gorski et al., 2021).
- Remove antiseptics after procedure with sodium chloride or sterile water for preterm or low-birth-weight infants (Gorski et al., 2021).

Older Adults

- Some older adults have fragile skin; therefore prevent skin tears by minimizing the use of tape or an engineered stabilization device directly on the skin and applying skin protectant before applying tape.
- Infiltration may go unnoticed because of the decreased elasticity of skin and loose skinfolds. Because of decreased tactile sensation, a large amount of fluid may infiltrate before pain occurs.

Home Care

- Instruct patient and family caregiver about the signs and symptoms of IV-related complications.
- Have patient or family caregiver demonstrate hand hygiene.
- Teach patient to protect IV site during bath or shower by wrapping in plastic bag and taping occlusively to keep dry.
- Teach patient and family caregiver what to do if dressing becomes compromised or catheter comes out. If catheter comes out, apply gauze pressure dressing at site and notify home health agency nurse.

PROCEDURAL GUIDELINE 28.1 *Discontinuing a Peripheral Intravenous Device*

A peripheral intravenous (IV) catheter is discontinued when the prescribed length of therapy is completed or a complication occurs (e.g., phlebitis, infiltration, or catheter occlusion). The technique for discontinuing a peripheral IV catheter follows infection-prevention guidelines to minimize the chance of the patient acquiring an infection. Care must also be taken because the risk of catheter emboli may occur if the catheter breaks off during removal.

Delegation

The skill of discontinuing a peripheral IV line cannot be delegated to assistive personnel (AP). Delegation to licensed practical nurses (LPNs) varies by state nurse practice act. Direct the AP to:

- Report any bleeding at the site after the catheter has been removed.

PROCEDURAL GUIDELINE 28.1 *Discontinuing a Peripheral Intravenous Device—cont'd*

- Report any complaints of pain or observation of redness at the site by the patient.

Equipment

Clean gloves; sterile 2 × 2–inch or 4 × 4–inch gauze sponge; antiseptic swabs (chlorhexidine gluconate [CHG] solution preferred, povidone-iodine, or 70% alcohol); tape

Steps

1. Review accuracy and completeness of health care provider's order for discontinuation of vascular access device (VAD).
2. Perform hand hygiene, following Aseptic Non-Touch Technique (ANTT), and collect equipment.
3. Identify patient using at least two identifiers (e.g., name and birthday or name and medical record number) according to agency policy. Compare identifiers with information on patient's electronic health record (EHR).
4. Apply clean gloves. Observe existing IV site for signs and symptoms of IV-related complications (redness, pain, tenderness, swelling, bleeding, drainage, or leaking from under dressing). Palpate catheter site through intact dressing.
5. Assess if patient is receiving an anticoagulant or has a history of a coagulopathy. These factors can increase bleeding at IV site once catheter is removed.
6. Assess patient's/family caregiver's health literacy and understanding of the reason for IV infusion to be discontinued.
7. Provide privacy and explain procedure to patient before you remove catheter. Explain that patient needs to hold affected extremity still.
8. Turn IV tubing roller clamp to "off" position or turn electronic infusion device (EID) off and roller clamp to "off" position.
9. Carefully remove VAD dressing, tape, and engineered stabilization device (follow guidelines in Skill 28.5 for preventing medical adhesive–related skin injury [MARSI]).
10. Stabilize IV catheter hub with middle finger of nondominant hand.

Clinical Judgment *Never use scissors to remove the tape or dressing because you may accidentally cut the catheter.*

11. Place clean sterile gauze above insertion site and, using dominant hand, withdraw catheter using a slow, steady motion and keeping the hub parallel to skin (see illustration).

Clinical Judgment *Do not raise or lift catheter before it is completely out of the vein to avoid trauma or hematoma formation.*

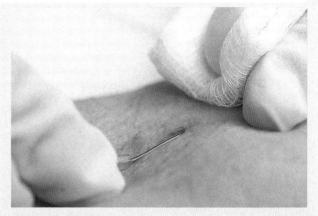

STEP 11 IV catheter is removed slowly, keeping catheter parallel to vein.

12. Apply pressure to site for a minimum of 30 seconds until bleeding has stopped. **NOTE:** Apply pressure for at least 5 to 10 minutes if patient is on anticoagulants.
13. Inspect catheter for intactness after removal; note tip integrity and length.
14. Observe IV site for evidence of redness, pain, tenderness, swelling, bleeding, or drainage. Monitor for 24 to 48 hours after removal for postinfusion phlebitis.
15. Apply clean, folded gauze dressing over insertion site and secure firmly with plastic tape.
16. Dispose of used supplies, remove and dispose of gloves, and perform hand hygiene.
17. Use **Teach-Back:** "I want to be sure that I explained to you why we are taking your IV out. In your own words, tell me why we are removing the IV and what problems we will watch for afterwards." Revise your instruction now or develop a plan for revised patient/family caregiver teaching if patient/family caregiver is not able to teach back correctly. Teach-back is a technique for health care providers to ensure that they have explained medical information clearly so that patients and their families understand what is communicated to them (AHRQ, 2023).
18. Document removal of peripheral IV device and patient's tolerance of procedure.
19. Provide hand-off reporting to oncoming nursing staff: time and reason for removal of peripheral IV device. Report to health care provider and document any complications.

✦ SKILL 28.6 Managing Central Vascular Access Devices

The need for safe and convenient intravenous (IV) therapy in seriously ill patients has led to the development of vascular access devices (VADs) designed for long-term access to the venous or arterial systems. A health care provider or specialty trained nurse places these devices into the central vascular system. A central vascular access device (CVAD) differs from a peripheral or midline catheter because the farthest tip of the catheter ends in a large blood vessel. This is necessary for the infusion of concentrated IV solutions such as total parenteral nutrition. The tip of a CVAD should be placed in the upper body in the lower segment of the superior or inferior vena cava at or near the cavoatrial junction (Fig. 28.4). Those placed in the lower body should end in the inferior vena cava above the level of the diaphragm (Gorski et al., 2021).

Factors considered when determining placement of a CVAD include type and expected duration of infusion therapy (greater than 5 days), patient's disease status, vascular characteristics, patient's age, co-morbidities, history of infusion therapy, and preference for VAD

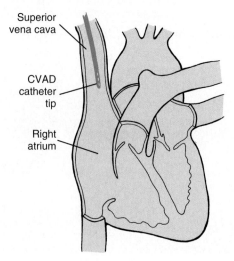

Superior vena cava

CVAD catheter tip

Right atrium

FIG. 28.4 Catheter tip from central vascular access device (CVAD) lies in superior vena cava.

location (Gorski et al., 2021). Also considered are osmolarity of the solution or medication to be administered. Your role is to anticipate a patient's need for a CVAD, assist the health care provider in placing a CVAD, care for and maintain the device, administer solutions or medications, and assess for signs and symptoms of IV-related complications.

Be aware of the similarities and differences between devices (Table 28.7). Characteristics of the devices and the type of patient education affect care and maintenance of each type of CVAD. These devices are composed of silicone or polyurethane and can be coated with antibiotics, silver, minocycline/rifampin, or chlorhexidine (Gorski, 2023).

Catheter tip configuration can be either open ended or valve ended. Open-ended devices (e.g., Hickman, Broviac) have a catheter tip that is open, like a straw. Valve-ended catheters (e.g., Groshong) have a rounded catheter tip with a three-way pressure-activated valve that prevents reflux of blood into the catheter to reduce the risk of hemorrhage, air embolism, and occlusion. This technology can also be located in the catheter hub (e.g., PASV, SOLO2). Manufacturers of valved catheters state that heparin is not needed to maintain patency and recommend flushing with only 0.9% sodium chloride (normal saline [NS]) (Gorski, 2023).

CVADs have single or multiple lumens (see Fig. 28.5). The choice of the number of lumens depends on a patient's condition and prescribed therapy. Critically ill patients requiring numerous infusions and blood samplings may have a device placed with more than one lumen, allowing simultaneous administration of solutions and medications. In addition, multiple lumens allow for administration of incompatible solutions or medications at the same time. You access a CVAD through the hub of the device located on the end of each external lumen.

An implanted venous port is a CVAD that has a reservoir placed in a pocket under the skin with the catheter inserted into a major vessel (e.g., subclavian). The CVAD has no external lumen or hub. Instead, you access an implanted venous port by inserting a special 90-degree–angle noncoring needle through the skin into the self-sealing injection port in the septum of the reservoir. It is common for a port not to be used for extended periods (i.e., weeks) between infusions, and it is not necessary that the port remain accessed during these periods. To maintain the patency of a port, it is necessary to flush every 4 to 12 weeks with heparin solution or 0.9% sodium chloride in accordance with agency policies and procedures and manufacturer's directions for use (Gorski et al., 2021).

Complications associated with CVADs can include local or systemic infection. A local infection can develop around the catheter insertion site. A more serious infection of the bloodstream may be caused by contamination of the catheter from the skin of the patient or poor infection-prevention practices during insertion, care, and maintenance (Gorski, 2023). The implementation of the central line–associated bloodstream infection care bundle to prevent infection includes (Gupta et al., 2021):

- Perform hand hygiene before catheter insertion; before and after palpating catheter insertion site; and before and after manipulating the catheter dressing, following Surgical Aseptic Non Touch Technique (ANTT), protecting key sites and key parts collectively using a sterile drape(s) and barrier precautions (Gorski et al., 2021).

TABLE 28.7

Central Vascular Access Devices

Short-Term Devices	Long-Term Devices
Nontunneled Percutaneous	**External Tunneled (Hickman, Broviac, Groshong)**
• Length of dwell: Days to several weeks	• Length of dwell: Considered permanent until therapy ends
• Insertion sites: Subclavian, external or internal jugular, and femoral veins	• Insertion sites: Chest region through subclavian or jugular vein
• Insertion technique: Not surgically placed; can be done at bedside; direct puncture into intended vein without passing through subcutaneous tissue	• Insertion technique: Surgery required; tunneling of proximal end subcutaneously from insertion site and bringing it out through skin at an exit site (Fig. 28.6)
• Held in place with sutures or engineered securement device	• Held in place by a Dacron cuff coated in antimicrobial solution; in approximately 2–3 weeks, scar tissue forms around cuff, fixing catheter in place
Peripherally Inserted Central Catheters (PICCs) (Fig. 28.5)	**Implanted Venous Ports**
• Length of dwell: As long as they function properly with no evidence of IV-related complications	• Length of dwell: Considered permanent until therapy ends
• Insertion sites: Antecubital fossa or upper arm (basilic or cephalic vein) and advanced until catheter tip reaches superior vena cava	• Insertion sites: Chest, abdomen, or inner aspect of forearm
• Insertion technique: Not surgically placed; can be done at bedside, in home setting, or in radiology setting	• Insertion techniques: Requires surgery; catheter placed via subclavian or jugular vein and attached to reservoir located within a surgically created subcutaneous pocket (Fig. 28.7)
• Held in place with sutures or engineered securement device	• Sutured in place within surgically created pocket and accessed using a noncoring needle through the skin (Fig. 28.8)

IV, Intravenous.

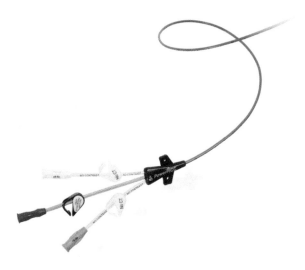

FIG. 28.5 Peripherally inserted central catheter. *(Courtesy and copyright © Bard Access Systems.)*

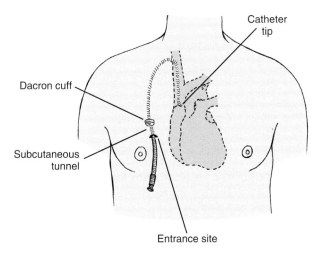

FIG. 28.6 Tunneled catheter is in place, threaded into superior vena cava.

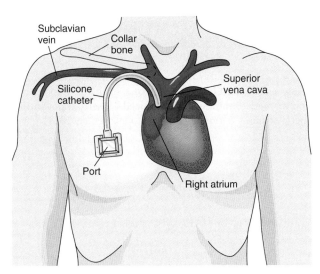

FIG. 28.7 Implanted port and catheter.

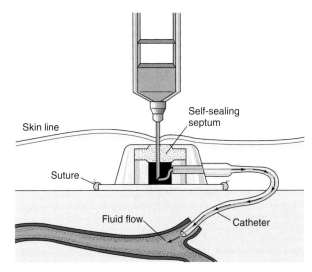

FIG. 28.8 Cross-section of implanted port showing access of port with noncoring needle.

- Maximal sterile barrier precautions with insertion. (Inserter wears a cap, mask, and sterile gloves and gown, and a large sterile drape is placed over patient during insertion.)
- Chlorhexidine gluconate (CHG) 0.5% skin antisepsis.
- Optimal catheter site selection, with avoidance of the femoral vein for central venous access in adult patients.
- Necessity of daily review of the condition of the line and insertion site with prompt removal of unnecessary lines.

Care of CVADs requires knowledge of the purpose and function of the devices and prevention of complications. Patients with CVADs require health education and teaching about infection-prevention practices and skin care.

Delegation

The skill of managing a CVAD cannot be delegated to assistive personnel (AP). Direct the AP to:
- Report immediately: bleeding or swelling around CVAD insertion site; shortness of breath; loosened or soiled dressing; or if the patient has a fever or complains of pain at the site or catheter becomes dislodged
- Inform nurse if the electronic infusion device (EID) alarm signals or if the fluid level in container is low or empty
- Help with positioning patient during insertion and care

Interprofessional Collaboration

- The health care provider and central supply and pharmacy services are involved in the management of CVADs.

Equipment

Insertion and Dressing Care
- Hair clippers
- CVAD insertion tray to include appropriate-length catheter and introducer needle, sterile gauze, sterile drapes, disposable tape measure
- Maximum barrier supplies, including head covering, sterile gowns, masks, sterile gloves (powder free), protective eyewear, large full-body sterile drape with fenestration for accessing IV insertion site
- Antiseptic solution (alcoholic chlorhexidine solution is preferred; 70% isopropyl alcohol and povidone-iodine for chlorhexidine sensitivities)

- Clean gloves
- Gauze pads
- Disinfecting caps for CVAD lumens
- Surgical towels
- 1% lidocaine for use as local anesthetic as ordered by health care provider
- 3-mL syringe and small-gauge needle for anesthetic administration
- 10-mL syringe
- Transparent semipermeable membrane (TSM) or 4 × 4–gauze dressing for catheter insertion site
- Engineered stabilization device
- Needleless connector for each lumen (if not provided)
- Polymer-based skin protectant spray, wipe, or swab (optional)
- Sterile tape: paper/cloth tape recommended for long-time wear (Fumarola et al., 2020)
- Electronic infusion device (EID)
- Ultrasound device (if available) with sterile wand cover and sterile transducer gel

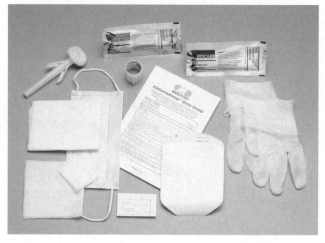

FIG. 28.9 Central vascular access device dressing change kit.

Site Care and Dressing Change
- CVAD dressing change kit (Fig. 28.9), which includes sterile gloves, mask, antiseptic swabs for skin disinfection (chlorhexidine 0.5% solution preferred, povidone-iodine, or 70% alcohol), TSM dressing, 4 × 4–inch gauze pads, tape measure, sterile tape, and label
- Engineered stabilization device (if not sutured) for peripherally inserted central catheter (PICC) or nontunneled catheters
- Adhesive remover
- Polymer-based skin protectant spray, wipe, or swab (optional)
- Clean gloves
- Needleless injection cap(s) for each lumen(s)

Blood Sampling
- Clean gloves
- Antiseptic swabs (CHG 0.5% solution, povidone-iodine, or 70% alcohol)
- 5-mL Luer-Lok syringes
- 10-mL Luer-Lok syringes
- Vacuum system or blood transfer device (see agency policy)
- Blood tubes, including waste tubes, labels
- Needleless injection cap
- Syringe (5 mL or 10 mL; see agency policy) for discarded blood

- 10-mL syringe with 5 to 10 mL preservative-free 0.9% sodium chloride (NS)
- 10-mL syringe with heparin flush solution
- Sterile cap to maintain sterility of distal end of IV tubing

Changing the Injection Cap
- Clean gloves
- Antiseptic swabs (CHG 0.5% solution, povidone-iodine, or 70% alcohol)
- Needleless injection cap(s)
- 10-mL syringe with 10 mL preservative-free 0.9% sodium chloride (NS)
- 10-mL syringe with heparin flush solution

Discontinuation of a Nontunneled Catheter
- Personal protective equipment (PPE) as indicated (goggles, gown, mask, and clean gloves)
- CVAD dressing change kit (see Fig. 28.9), which includes sterile gloves, mask, antiseptic swabs for skin disinfection, TSM dressing, 4 × 4–inch gauze pads, tape measure, sterile tape, label
- Petroleum-based ointment or petroleum-based gauze, sterile
- Suture removal kit (if sutures are in place)
- Stethoscope

STEP	RATIONALE

ASSESSMENT

1. Review patient's electronic health record (EHR), including accuracy and completeness of health care provider's order for insertion of CVAD for size and type. Assess treatment schedule: times for administration of IV solutions, medications, and blood sampling. Follow seven rights of medication administration (see Chapter 20) (Gorski, 2023; Gorski et al., 2021).
   Confirm that informed consent has been obtained and witnessed by health care provider who will perform procedure.

   Identifies patient's need for vascular access, evaluates response to therapy, and determines education needs. Insertion of central catheter requires informed consent (Gorski et al., 2021).

2. Review EHR to determine patient's risk for developing a medical adhesive–related skin injury (MARSI) with use of adhesive devices or tape: age, dehydration, malnutrition, exposure to radiation therapy, underlying chronic conditions (e.g., diabetes, immunosuppression), and edema of skin.

   Common risk factors for MARSI (Fumarola et al., 2020).

STEP	RATIONALE
3. Assess patient's/family caregiver's health literacy.	Determines degree to which individuals have the ability to find, understand, and use information and services to make informed health-related decisions and actions for themselves and others (CDC, 2023).
4. Perform hand hygiene, following ANTT. Apply gloves if risk of contacting blood. Assess patient's hydration status: skin turgor, dryness of mouth, skin texture, and fluid intake and output (I&O).	Reduces transmission of infection. Provides baseline to determine response to fluid therapy. In addition, dehydration makes insertion of CVAD more difficult.
5. Prior to a new insertion, assess patient for any surgical procedures of upper chest or anatomical irregularities of proposed insertion site.	Previous surgical procedures or central vascular catheterizations indicate that you should not use a site. Spinal deformities and contractions make positioning difficult.
6. Assess existing or potential CVAD placement site for skin integrity (open lesions) and signs of infection (i.e., redness, pain, tenderness, swelling, bleeding, or drainage). Also assess skin temperature, color, moisture level, fragility, and overall integrity, including presence of irritation around potential IV site. Apply gloves if drainage is present.	Compromised skin integrity contraindicates catheter insertion and can lead to secondary complications. Condition of skin creates risk for MARSI (Fumarola et al., 2020).
7. Assess patient for allergy to iodine, lidocaine, adhesive, latex, or chlorhexidine (CHG). If you identify allergy, place allergy band on patient's wrist.	Medications, solutions used during catheter insertion, and use of latex gloves and tape can cause serious allergic reactions.
8. Assess type of CVAD intended for placement. Review manufacturer's directions concerning catheter and maintenance.	Care and management depend on type and size of catheter or port, number of lumens, and purpose of therapy.
9. Assess for proper function of existing CVAD *before therapy*: integrity of catheter, ability to flush or infuse solution, and ability to aspirate blood. Remove and dispose of gloves (if worn). Perform hand hygiene.	Blood return should be obtained and patency confirmed before infusion of solutions or medications (Gorski et al., 2021). Reduces transmission of microorganisms.
10. Assess if any existing catheter lumens require flushing or if CVAD site needs dressing change by referring to EHR, nurses' notes, agency policies, and manufacturer-recommended guidelines for use.	Provides guidelines for maintaining catheter patency and preventing infection.
11. Assess patient's knowledge and prior experience with CVAD, including purpose, care, and maintenance, and feelings about procedure. For long-term use, ask patient or family caregiver to discuss steps in care and perform procedure (e.g., catheter site cleaning or dressing change).	Reveals need for patient instruction and/or support.

PLANNING

1. Expected outcomes following completion of procedure: • Insertion occurs without complication.	Placement of nontunneled CVAD carries risks such as pneumothorax, hematoma, air embolism, thrombosis, and infection.
• Catheter tip placement is appropriate at or near the cavoatrial junction as confirmed by electrocardiogram (ECG), fluoroscopy, x-ray, or ultrasound (preferred method).	Appropriate tip placement decreases risk of thrombotic complications or arrhythmias. Confirmation of tip location is required before use of CVAD (Gorski et al., 2021).
• CVAD site remains intact, with no evidence of signs or symptoms of postinsertion complications (e.g., catheter migration, redness, swelling, aching or pain).	Catheter is patent, properly placed, and without evidence of complications.
• Prescribed solutions and medications infuse without difficulty.	Catheter remains patent.
• Patient's CVAD is maintained routinely and remains patent; site is free from signs and symptoms of IV site–related complications.	Care and maintenance of CVAD includes assessment, site care, dressing changes, injection cap changes, and flushing with aseptic technique.
• Blood specimens are obtained, and CVAD patency is maintained.	Catheter remains patent after blood draws.
• Patient and family caregiver are able to explain purpose of CVAD and IV line therapy, care, and maintenance.	Demonstrates that patient and family caregiver have understanding and competency in caring for CVAD.

STEP	RATIONALE
2. Provide privacy and explain procedure and purpose to patient and family caregiver. Explain to patient that patient must not move during procedure. Offer opportunity at this time to toilet and offer pain medication (if needed).	Protects patient's privacy; reduces anxiety. Promotes cooperation.
3. Perform hand hygiene. Collect and organize equipment on clean, clutter-free bedside stand or overbed table.	Reduces transmission of microorganisms. Ensures more efficiency when completing a procedure.

IMPLEMENTATION

1. Identify patient using at least two identifiers (e.g., name and birthday or name and medical record number) according to agency policy. Compare identifiers with information on medication administration record (MAR) or EHR.	Ensures patient safety. Complies with The Joint Commission standards and improves patient safety (TJC, 2023).
2. **Catheter insertion:** nontunneled device:	Ultrasound-guided venous access is recommended when internal jugular vein is going to be used and equipment and clinical expertise are available to improve success of insertion and reduce the risk of procedure-related complications (La Greca et al., 2021). Ultrasound is also used to place PICCs using brachial or basilic vein in children and adults (La Greca et al., 2021).
a. Health care provider, with help from nurse, positions patient in Trendelenburg or supine position for placement of CVAD in vessels above heart, unless contraindicated.	Opens angle between clavicle and first rib; dilates veins to facilitate eventual catheter insertion.

Clinical Judgment *Trendelenburg position is contraindicated in patients with head injuries, increased intracranial pressure, certain respiratory conditions, and spinal cord injuries.*

(1) Nurse places rolled towel or bath blanket between patient's shoulder blades, rotating them slightly to 10-degree angle. Turn patient's head away from intended insertion site.	Head down, below heart, promotes maximum filling and distention with increase in diameter of subclavicular vein (Gorski, 2023); 10-degree tilt effectively achieves increase in diameter of vein.
b. If necessary, use scissors or electric clippers to remove any hair around insertion site. Explain rationale to patient.	Transient microorganisms reside in body hair. Shaving can cause increased risk for infection (Gorski et al., 2021).
c. Perform hand hygiene, following Surgical ANTT techniques.	Handwashing technique removes transient and resident bacteria from skin.
d. Health care provider and nurse apply cap, mask, eyewear, surgical gown, and powder-free sterile gloves. Patient applies mask.	Maximum barrier precautions using Surgical ANTT precautions are needed when inserting central vascular catheter (Gorski et al., 2021).
e. Nurse or health care provider opens central vascular access kit. Nurse adds additional needed sterile equipment to kit for use during insertion (see Chapter 10).	Maintains sterile field.
f. Site preparation:	Reduces incidence of catheter-related infections (Gorski, 2023; Gorski et al., 2021).
(1) Perform skin antisepsis over proposed insertion site with CHG solution, using friction in back-and-forth motion according to manufacturer's directions; allow to dry completely.	Allow any skin antiseptic agent to fully dry for complete antisepsis (Gorski et al., 2021).
g. After cleaning site, health care provider and nurse remove and dispose of gloves. Health care provider changes into second pair of sterile gloves, and nurse performs hand hygiene. (Check agency policy because some agencies require strict precautions.)	Gloves become contaminated from surface bacteria picked up in solution. Nurse functions as nonsterile circulator whose primary function is to ensure sterility of insertion field.
h. Health care provider uses large sterile drape and sterile towels to create sterile field. Health care provider finds anatomical landmarks and places sterile fenestrated drape appropriately over proposed insertion site.	Provides sterile workspace for catheter insertion (Gorski et al., 2021).
i. Health care provider arranges equipment in kit in preparation for catheter insertion.	Ensures smooth, orderly procedure.
j. Nurse sets up IV bag, primes and fills tubing, and covers end of tubing with sterile cap (see Skill 28.1).	IV tubing is ready to be connected to IV catheter.

STEP	RATIONALE
k. Nurse scrubs top of 1% lidocaine bottle with antiseptic swab, allowing to dry completely, and holds bottle upside down if not in insertion kit. *Optional:* Topical local anesthetic agents can be applied before insertion with health care provider's order.	Removes surface bacteria; allows health care provider to withdraw lidocaine while maintaining asepsis. Lidocaine has potential for creating allergic reaction and tissue damage.
l. Health care provider injects needle into bottle and withdraws approximately 3 to 4 mL lidocaine. Health care provider injects needle into site for internal jugular puncture and anesthetizes venipuncture site, waiting 1 to 2 minutes for effect to take place.	Use of anesthetic minimizes discomfort patient feels during venipuncture. Site has been documented to be safer for bedside insertion and ability to use ultrasound-guided insertion (Gorski et al., 2021).

Clinical Judgment *Just before time of catheter insertion, ask patient to hold breath and strain. This is a Valsalva maneuver, which increases central venous pressure to prevent entry of air into the catheter. The Valsalva maneuver is the preferred method, although breath holding and humming may be a necessary option in uncooperative patients. In addition, if patient is unable to perform maneuvers, compress patient's abdomen gently.*

STEP	RATIONALE
m. Health care provider uses ultrasound imaging with an introducer needle, micropuncture needle, or angiocath cannula to insert CVAD into internal jugular vein. Once vein is entered, health care provider removes needle from cannula, threading wire into cannula and vein, removing cannula over wire, advancing central vein catheter over wire to appropriate location, and removing the guidewire (Seldinger technique) (Gorski et al., 2021).	Large vein is selected because it will be less irritated by hypertonic solutions or medications.
n. Health care provider determines patency of line by withdrawing blood with 5-mL syringe, flushing with 0.9% sodium chloride, and placing needleless connectors on hub of each lumen. *Option:* VAD may be flushed with heparin based on type of catheter and agency policy and procedure.	Determines patency of device. Use of heparin, flush volume, and concentration vary by agency and type of catheter. Valved catheters are flushed with 0.9% sodium chloride only and do not require heparin.
o. Cover insertion site with integrated securement device/TSM dressing (see Skill 28.1). Health care provider applies catheter securement device (e.g., engineered stabilization device, sterile tape, or surgical Steri-Strips) to secure central vascular catheter in place. **NOTE:** Sutures are not recommended.	Catheter securement devices are noninvasive and preferred for preventing catheter dislodgement (Gorski et al., 2021). Suturing catheter to skin at insertion site increases risk for infection.
p. Health care provider removes sterile drapes and completes procedure. Patient can remove mask once dressing is applied. External catheter length is measured and documented by nurse.	Measurement allows for comparison if dislodgement of CVAD is suspected (Gorski et al., 2021).
q. Nurse initiates and regulates IV infusion to prescribed rate and connects to EID after receiving confirmation of appropriate tip placement. Although chest x-ray is still used for determining tip placement, the use of ECG methods, fluoroscopy, and ultrasound used during the insertion procedure are preferred due to greater accuracy, more rapid initiation of infusion therapy, and reduced cost (La Greca et al., 2021; Gorski et al., 2021).	Maintains patency of VAD. Confirmation of tip placement prevents complications.
3. Insertion site care and dressing change:	
a. Position patient in comfortable position with head slightly elevated. Have arm extended for PICC or midline device.	Provides access to patient.
b. Prepare dressing materials. • Integrated securement device/TSM dressing: Change at least every 7 days. • *Gauze dressing:* Change at least every 2 days. • *Gauze under TSM:* Change at least every 2 days (not recommended).	Integrated securement and TSM dressings have advantage of allowing visualization of IV site. Gauze dressings and TSM are associated with a lower rate of catheter tip infection (Gorski et al., 2021).
c. Perform hand hygiene and apply mask, following ANTT. Instruct patient to apply mask and turn head away from site during dressing change.	Reduces transfer of microorganisms; prevents spread of airborne microorganisms over CVAD insertion site.
d. Apply clean gloves. Carefully remove old dressing (See Skill 28.5).	Prevents unintentional catheter removal. Allows visualization of insertion site.

STEP	RATIONALE
e. Remove catheter stabilization device if used and requires changing. Must use adhesive remover to remove adhesive stabilization devices.	Allows greater visualization of insertion site and allows for appropriate skin antisepsis (Gorski et al., 2021). Use of adhesive remover minimizes risk for MARSI (Gorski et al., 2021).

Clinical Judgment *If sutures are used for initial catheter stabilization and become loosened or are no longer intact, alternative stabilization measures should be used. An engineered stabilization device is recommended because sutures are associated with increased risk of infection (Gorski, 2023; Gorski et al., 2021).*

STEP	RATIONALE
f. Inspect catheter, insertion site, and surrounding skin. Measure external CVAD length and compare to measurement from insertion if dislodgement is suspected. For PICC and midlines, measure upper-arm circumference 10 cm above antecubital fossa if clinically indicated and compare with baseline.	Insertion sites require regular inspection for early detection of signs and symptoms of IV-related complications and MARSI (Gorski et al., 2021; Fumarola et al., 2020). Measurement of external catheter length provides comparison to determine dislodgement; arm measurement with a 3-cm increase can indicate thrombosis (Gorski et al., 2021).
g. Remove and dispose of clean gloves; perform hand hygiene. Open CVAD dressing kit using sterile technique and *apply sterile gloves*, following surgical ANTT. Area to be cleaned should be same size as dressing.	Sterile technique is required to apply new dressing. Reduces transmission of microorganisms.
h. Clean site:	Reduces incidence of catheter-related infections.
(1) Perform skin antisepsis with CHG solution using friction in back-and-forth motion according to manufacturer's directions, and allow to dry completely.	Allow any skin antiseptic agent to dry fully for complete antisepsis (Gorski et al., 2021).
(2) Povidone-iodine and alcohol may be used in some settings or if patient is sensitive to CHG (see agency policy). Clean in concentric circle, moving from insertion site outward with swab. Allow to dry completely.	
i. Apply polymer-based skin protectant to area and allow to dry completely so that skin is not tacky. Skin protectant must be used if adhesive stabilization device will be used.	Protects irritated or fragile skin from dressing and stabilization device, if used, and minimizes risk for MARSI (Fumarola et al., 2020).
j. *Option:* Use CHG-impregnated dressing for short-term CVADs.	CHG-impregnated dressings can reduce risk of infection (Gorski et al., 2021). Use with caution in premature neonates and patients with fragile skin and/or complicated skin pathologies (Gorski et al., 2021).
k. Apply sterile integrated securement device/TSM dressing over insertion site (see Skill 28.1, Steps 21a and b).	Protects catheter insertion site and minimizes risk for infection (Gorski, 2023). Allows for clear visualization of catheter site between dressing changes (Gorski et al., 2021).
l. Apply new catheter stabilization device according to manufacturer directions for use (see Skill 28.1, Step 22). Apply new injection caps to lumens of CVAD every 72 hours (see agency policy) (see Step 6 below). Then apply disinfecting cap to end of injection caps of catheter.	Use of engineered stabilization devices that allow visual inspection of insertion site can reduce risk for VAD complications (i.e., phlebitis, infection, migration) and unintentional loss of access (Gorski et al., 2021). Injection caps provide non–Luer-Lok device for access to CVAD. Disinfecting caps reduce transmission of infection.
m. Apply label to dressing with date, time, and your initials.	Provides information about next dressing change.
n. Have patient remove mask. Dispose of all contaminated supplies in appropriate receptacle; remove and dispose of gloves, and perform hand hygiene.	Reduces transmission of microorganisms. Use appropriate disposal receptacle if patient is on hazardous drugs (ONS, 2018).
4. Blood sampling:	
a. Perform hand hygiene. Apply clean gloves and face mask using Surgical ANTT.	Reduces transmission of microorganisms.
b. Put the EID on hold for at least 1 to 5 minutes before drawing blood. **NOTE:** If you cannot stop infusion, draw blood from peripheral vein.	Prevents dilution of sample. Use of peripheral vein prevents interruption of critical IV therapy.
c. Use a dedicated lumen for blood sampling from a multilumen CVAD (Gorski et al., 2021). When drawing through staggered multilumen catheters, draw from the lumen exiting at the point farthest away from the heart (or one recommended by manufacturer).	Distal lumen is typically largest-gauge lumen (Gorski, 2023).

STEP	RATIONALE
d. Clamp the CVAD lumen using the small slide clamp (see illustration on next page). **Exception:** Valved catheter does not require clamping.	Prevents spillage. Valved catheters do not require clamping because clamp opens valve and allows reflux of blood into catheter.
e. Syringe method:	
(1) Remove disinfection cap from CVAD lumen. Scrub catheter injection cap hub with antiseptic swab for at least 15 seconds and allow to dry completely.	Reduces risk of infection. Drying is necessary for antimicrobial action to be effective.
(2) Attach syringe containing 5 to 10 mL of NS (see agency policy for volume) to end of hub. Unclamp CVAD (if necessary). Flush CVAD slowly with NS. Reclamp CVAD.	Ensures patency of CVAD lumen. Clamping prevents spillage.
(3) Clean catheter hub with antiseptic swab and allow to dry completely. Attach empty 5-mL syringe to hub and unclamp catheter (if necessary). To withdraw blood, first aspirate gently, pulling back 1 to 2 mL. Pause and hold pressure to allow valve to open. Then continue pulling plunger slowly, staying just ahead of the blood flow, until you obtain 2 to 25 mL of blood for discard sample depending on the internal volume of the CVAD (see agency policy) (Gorski et al., 2021).	Reduces transmission of infection. A discard sample reduces risk of drug concentrations or diluted specimen (Gorski, 2023).
(4) Reclamp catheter (if necessary); remove syringe with blood and discard in appropriate biohazard container.	Valved catheters do not require clamping because clamp opens valve and allows reflux of blood into catheter. Prevents spillage. Prevents transmission of infection.
(5) Scrub catheter hub with another antiseptic swab for 15 seconds and allow to dry completely.	Reduces transmission of infection.
(6) Attach syringe(s) to obtain required volume of blood needed for specimen(s) ordered.	Multiple syringes may be required, depending on specimens required and number of blood tubes needed.

Clinical Judgment *If multiple blood tests are ordered, anticipate timing so that accessing the CVAD is necessary only one time. Consult with laboratory about number of milliliters needed for any one sample (Gorski et al., 2021). This uses blood conservation strategy.*

STEP	RATIONALE
(7) Unclamp catheter (if necessary) to withdraw blood. Obtain necessary blood volume for specimens.	Minimum amount of blood is needed to perform any one blood test analysis.
(8) Once specimens are obtained, clamp catheter (if necessary) and remove syringe.	Prevents spillage.
(9) Scrub catheter hub with antiseptic swab for 15 seconds and allow to dry completely.	Reduces transmission of infection.
(10) Attach prefilled syringe with 10-mL 0.9% sodium chloride (NS). Unclamp catheter (if necessary). Flush catheter using the appropriate flush-clamp-disconnect sequence based on the type of needleless connector (e.g., neutral, negative, or positive pressure displacement). Ensure that clamp is engaged (if available).	Flush with 10 to 20 mL 0.9% sodium chloride (NS) (Gorski et al., 2021). Refer to agency policy and procedure for flush volume requirements. Reduces risk for catheter clotting after procedure.

Clinical Judgment *Always use a 10-mL syringe or syringe designed to generate lower injection pressure (i.e., 10 mL–diameter syringe barrel) on central lines in adults to minimize pressure during injection (Gorski et al., 2021).*

STEP	RATIONALE
(11) Remove syringe and discard into appropriate biohazard container.	Reduces transmission of microorganisms.
(12) Transfer blood from syringe into blood tubes using transfer vacuum device (see illustration).	Reduces risk of blood exposure.
(13) *Option:* Flush catheter with heparin flush based on type of catheter and agency policy and procedure using appropriate flush-clamp-disconnect sequence. Ensure that clamp is engaged (if available).	Prevents clot formation. Heparin flush volume and concentration vary by agency and type of catheter. Valved catheters are flushed with 0.9% sodium chloride (NS) only and do not require heparin.

STEP	RATIONALE

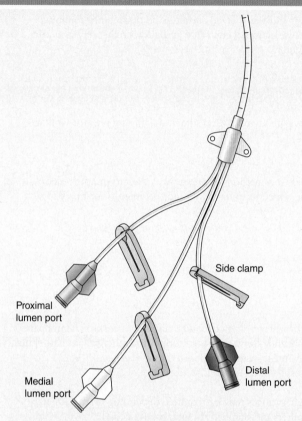

STEP 4d Slide clamps used to clamp CVAD.

Proximal lumen port

Medial lumen port

Side clamp

Distal lumen port

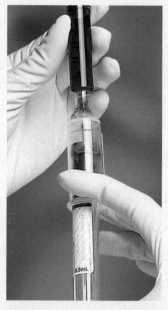

STEP 4e(12) Blood specimen transfer device. (*Courtesy and copyright © Becton, Dickinson and Company.*)

(14) Scrub exposed hub or CVAD with antiseptic swab for 15 seconds and allow to dry. Attach new injection cap (see Step 6 below) to accessed lumen. Apply disinfection cap to injection cap. Resume infusion as ordered.

Decreases risk of contamination.

f. NOTE: Check agency policy for use of vacuum tube method for blood sampling with CVADs.

Use vacuum tubes in the correct sequence (Gorski et al., 2021).

g. Dispose of all contaminated supplies in appropriate receptacle; remove and dispose of gloves and mask, and perform hand hygiene.

Reduces transmission of microorganisms. Use appropriate disposal receptacle if patient is on hazardous drugs (ONS, 2018).

5. Changing needleless injection cap:

a. Determine if injection caps should be changed.

Injection caps should be changed no more frequently than 72-hour intervals or when administration set is changed, if there is residual blood or debris in it, if it becomes contaminated, or according to agency policies and procedures (Gorski et al., 2021).

b. Prepare new injection cap(s):

Understanding of types of injection caps ensures appropriate flush-clamp-disconnect sequence based on type of device (e.g., positive, negative, or neutral displacement valves) (Gorski et al., 2021).

(1) Perform hand hygiene. Apply clean gloves and mask, following Surgical ANTT. (Have patient apply mask.) Remove cap from package. Do not contaminate sterile injection port.

Reduces transfer of microorganisms. Maintains sterility.

(2) Keep protective cover on tip of injection cap.

Maintains sterility.

(3) Attach prefilled syringe to end of injection cap by pushing in and then turning clockwise. Prime injection cap by flushing with preservative-free 0.9% sodium chloride (NS) through cap until fluid escapes from tip of cap. Keep syringe attached to cap and keep connection sterile.

Removes air from system, preventing it from being introduced into vein.

STEP	RATIONALE
c. Based on catheter type, clamp catheter lumen by using slide or squeeze clamp.	Prevents air from entering system when opened (Gorski, 2023).
d. Remove old injection cap by turning counterclockwise. Dispose of old injection cap using aseptic technique. Continue holding catheter lumen.	Reduces transmission of microorganisms.
e. Scrub exposed catheter hub with antiseptic swab, twisting back and forth vigorously for 15 seconds, and allow to dry completely. Take the new injection cap and attached syringe, remove the protective cover from tip, and connect new injection cap(s) on catheter hub, turning clockwise just until resistance is felt. Remove and dispose of syringe. *Option:* Place disinfecting cap on end of injection cap.	Drying allows time for maximum antimicrobial activity of agents. Turning cap on too tightly makes it difficult to remove for subsequent cap change.
f. Repeat procedure for additional CVAD lumens.	
g. Dispose of all contaminated supplies in appropriate receptacle, remove and dispose of gloves and mask, remove patient's mask (if worn), and perform hand hygiene.	Reduces transmission of microorganisms. Use appropriate disposal receptacle if patient is on hazardous drugs (ONS, 2018).
6. Discontinuing nontunneled catheters:	
a. Verify health care provider's order to discontinue line. Check agency policy because most require health care providers to discontinue CVAD. In some settings advanced practice nurses or specially credentialed nurses can remove devices.	Verifies appropriateness of procedure. Only specially trained health care professional can remove CVAD.
b. If IV solutions or medications are to continue, arrange placement of a peripheral or midline before CVAD discontinuation.	
c. **NOTE:** Be aware of osmolarity of solution or medication for appropriateness of conversion to peripheral or midline catheter.	Prevents interruption of IV therapy.
d. Position patient in supine flat or 10-degree Trendelenburg position unless contraindicated.	Position promotes venous filling and prevents air embolus during catheter removal.
e. Perform hand hygiene, following Surgical ANTT.	Prevents transmission of microorganisms.
f. Turn off IV solutions infusing through central line and convert to alternate VAD.	Prevents fluid loss during CVAD removal.
g. Place moisture-proof pad under central line site.	Minimizes soiling of bed linen. Provides clean environment.
h. Apply gown, clean gloves, mask, and goggles.	Prevents transmission of microorganisms and exposure to bloodborne pathogens.
i. Gently remove CVAD dressing by stabilizing catheter with nondominant hand, pulling up one corner, and gently pulling straight out and parallel to skin. Repeat on all sides until dressing has been removed.	Prevents skin tears. Allows inspection of CVAD insertion site before removal.
j. If catheter securement device is present, carefully remove catheter from device and remove device with adhesive remover.	Aids in removal of securement device without causing skin tear.
k. Remove and dispose of gloves and perform hand hygiene; open CVAD dressing change kit. Add items to sterile field. Apply sterile gloves.	Prevents transfer of organisms on soiled dressing to catheter insertion site using Surgical ANTT.
l. Perform skin antisepsis of insertion site with CHG solution using friction in back-and-forth motion according to manufacturer's guidelines and allow to dry completely.	Reduces risk of migration of microbes into catheter tract.

Clinical Judgment *All central vascular access devices (CVADs) require measurements of total length and external catheter on insertion. Peripherally inserted central catheter (PICC) lines also require measurement of upper-arm circumference.*

m. Using nondominant hand, apply sterile 4 × 4–inch gauze to site. Instruct patient to take deep breath and perform Valsalva maneuver as catheter is withdrawn.	Valsalva maneuver reduces risk for air embolus by decreasing negative pressure in respiratory system. Use Trendelenburg or left lateral decubitus position if Valsalva is contraindicated (Gorski et al., 2021).

STEP	RATIONALE
n. With dominant hand, slowly remove catheter in smooth, continuous motion an inch at a time. Keeping fingers near insertion site, immediately apply digital pressure to site and continue until bleeding stops. Stop removal procedure if resistance is met while removing catheter (Gorski et al., 2021).	Gentle removal of catheter prevents stretching and breaking it. Damaged catheter may break off and leave piece in patient's arm. Direct pressure reduces risk for bleeding and hematoma formation.

Clinical Judgment *It is often necessary to apply pressure longer if patient is receiving anticoagulation therapy or has prolonged clotting times.*

STEP	RATIONALE
o. Apply gauze to exit site. Apply sterile occlusive dressing, such as TSM dressing or sterile gauze, to site. Change dressing every 24 hours until healed.	Reduces chance of air embolism and seals skin-to-vein tract (Gorski, 2023). Allows for inspection of site for bleeding infection until it is healed.
p. Label dressing with date, time, and your initials.	Identifies date of catheter removal and need for dressing change.
q. Inspect catheter integrity for intactness, especially along tip; check that length is appropriate for device. Discard in appropriate biohazard container.	If catheter tip is broken or compromised, place in container, label for possible follow-up, and notify health care provider.
r. NOTE: Catheter cultures should be performed when catheter is removed for suspected catheter-related bloodstream infection (CRBSI). Catheter cultures should not be obtained routinely (Gorski et al., 2021).	
s. Position patient in a supine position for 30 minutes after nontunneled CVAD removal. Be sure that peripheral IV line or midline is infusing at correct rate.	Reduces chance of air embolism. Maintains prescribed IV solution therapy.
t. Dispose of all contaminated supplies in appropriate receptacle; remove and dispose of gloves and other PPE.	Reduces transmission of microorganisms. Use appropriate disposal receptacle if patient is on hazardous drugs (ONS, 2018).
7. Assist patient to a comfortable position and instruct how to move and turn without dislodging VAD.	Restores comfort and sense of well-being. Prevents accidental dislodgement of catheter and minimizes risk for falls.
8. Raise bed rails (as appropriate) and lower bed to lowest position, locking into position.	Ensures patient safety and prevents falls.
9. Place nurse call system in an accessible location within patient's reach. Instruct patient in its use.	Ensures patient can call for assistance if needed.
10. Perform hand hygiene.	Reduces transmission of microorganisms.

EVALUATION

1. Consult ECG, fluoroscopy, x-ray film, or ultrasound reports for catheter placement.	Ultrasound is the gold standard to confirm position of catheter tip and presence of pneumothorax. However, other technologies are proving reliable.
2. Determine daily, in consultation with health care provider, the continued need for the CVAD.	Daily review of need for line is a necessity. Prompt removal of unnecessary lines is a practice recommended in the central line–associated bloodstream infection (CLABSI) bundle (La Greca et al., 2021).
3. Evaluate for postinsertion complications:	Complications after insertion can include pneumothorax, cardiac arrhythmias, and nerve injury (Gorski, 2023). Prompt identification can allow for treatment, repositioning of catheter, or removal if necessary.
a. Auscultate breath sounds and evaluate for shortness of breath, chest pain, and absent breath sounds.	Signs and symptoms of pneumothorax (see Chapter 27) develop if CVAD pierces intrathoracic space.
b. Monitor vital signs, including heart rate and rhythm.	Evaluates for signs of cardiac arrhythmias.
c. Monitor patient complaints of pain, numbness, tingling, or weakness.	Signs of nerve injury from catheter insertion.
4. Evaluate patient to determine response to infusion therapy (e.g., laboratory values, I&O, weights, vital signs, postprocedural assessments).	IV solutions and additives maintain or restore fluid and electrolyte balance. Early recognition of complications leads to prompt treatment.
5. Evaluate patient at established intervals for signs and symptoms of CVAD-related complications (Table 28.8) according to agency policy and procedure.	Prevents complications that compromise integrity of CVAD or cause inaccurate IV solution flow rate and allows for prompt intervention.
6. Observe all connection points, being sure that they are secure as directed by agency policy and procedure.	An intact system prevents accidental blood loss or entrance of air or microbes into the vasculature.

TABLE 28.8

Complications of Vascular Access Devices

Complication	Assessment	Prevention	Intervention
Catheter damage, breakage	Every shift observe for pinholes, leaks, tears. Assess for drainage from site after flushing.	Follow proper clamping procedure. Avoid sharp objects near catheter. Use needleless system device. A 10-mL syringe is preferred for flushing CVADs to avoid excessive pressure and potential catheter damage. Never flush against resistance.	Clamp catheter near insertion site and place sterile gauze over break or hole until repaired. Use only repair kit that is recommended by manufacturer. Remove catheter with order.
Occlusion: thrombus, fibrin sheath, fibrin tail, precipitation, malposition	Assess insertion site and sutures. Assess for blood return. Assess for ability to infuse fluid. Assess equipment. If port is in place, reassess and verify noncoring needle placement. Assess with syringe directly on catheter. Assess for discomfort or pain in shoulder, neck, ear, or arm at insertion site. Assess for neck or shoulder edema.	Follow routine flushing with positive pressure and/or use positive-pressure valve injection cap. Secure with catheter stabilization device to prevent tension on CVAD. A 10-mL syringe is preferred for flushing CVADs to avoid excessive pressure and potential catheter damage. Do not flush against resistance. Flush between medications. Flush vigorously after viscous solutions. Avoid mixing incompatible drugs. Avoid kinking catheter.	Reposition patient. Have patient cough and deep breathe. Raise patient's arm overhead. Obtain venogram if ordered. Administer thrombolytics if ordered. Remove catheter (CVAD requires order). Obtain x-ray film as ordered. Do not use a 1-mL syringe to instill saline because pressure exceeds 200 psi.
Infection and sepsis: catheter-skin junction, tunnel, thrombus, port pocket, CLABSI	Assess catheter-skin junction for redness, drainage, edema, or tenderness. Assess for signs of systemic infection. Monitor laboratory findings.	Use aseptic technique. Prevent contamination of catheter hub. Adhere to dressing change technique. Apply TSM dressing over catheter-skin junction.	Obtain blood culture specimens from peripheral VAD and CVAD if ordered. Remove catheter (CVAD requires order). Replace catheter.
Dislodgement	Assess length of catheter daily. Inform patient of possible catheter dislodgement. Identify edema at catheter-skin junction or drainage. Palpate catheter-skin junction and tunnel for coiling (catheter can feel cord-like underneath the skin). Assess for distended neck veins.	Loop and tape catheter securely. Use catheter stabilization device and TSM dressing. Avoid pulling on CVAD. Avoid manipulating catheter by hand.	Insert new catheter. Secure with catheter stabilization device. Teach patient not to manipulate catheter.
Catheter migration (e.g., length of catheter moved from original position), pinch-off syndrome (e.g., compression of catheter between clavicle and first rib), port separation or catheter fracture (e.g., internal fracture or separation of catheter)	Assess for patient complaints of gurgling sounds. Assess for change in patency of catheter by evaluating change in flow rate, local irritation, swelling, occlusion, tenderness, pain, and inability to aspirate fluid and/or blood. Pain at site when flushed or symptoms of embolus. Obtain x-ray film examination. Assess edema of arm and hand on side of insertion. Assess for distended neck veins. Assess for inability to infuse solutions. Assess length of catheter daily.	Avoid trauma. Avoid placement near site of local infection, scarring, or skin disorder.	Reposition under fluoroscopy as ordered. Remove catheter as ordered. Stop all fluid administration.
Skin erosion (e.g., mechanical loss of skin tissue), hematomas (e.g., local collection of blood), cuff extrusion (e.g., tissue at edges of insertion site separate), scar tissue formation over port	Assess for loss of viable tissue over septum site. Assess for separation of exit site edges. Assess for drainage at catheter skin junction. Assess for redness. Assess for edema and contusions. Note if tunneled catheter is exposed (Dacron cuff is visible).	Maintain nutritional status. Avoid pressure or trauma. Rotate with each port access. Do not reinsert a noncoring needle in the same "hole" of a previous insertion. This creates a permanent hole in the septum. Do not use standard needle to access port.	Remove CVAD as ordered. Improve nutrition. Provide appropriate skin care.

Continued

TABLE 28.8

Complications of Vascular Access Devices—cont'd

Complication	Assessment	Prevention	Intervention
Infiltration, extravasation	Assess for erythema. Assess for edema. Assess for spongy feeling. Assess for swelling around IV site and at termination of catheter tip. Assess for labored breathing. Assess for aspiration of fluid and/or blood. Assess for complaints of pain with infusion of solutions or medications (e.g., burning). Assess for no free-flow IV drip.	Immediately stop vesicant administration. Administer antidote or therapeutic medications to maintain tissue integrity according to protocol.	Apply cold/warm compresses according to specific vesicant protocol. Provide emotional support. Obtain x-ray film if ordered. Use antidotes per protocol. Discontinue IV solutions.
Pneumothorax, hemothorax, air emboli, hydrothorax	Assess for subcutaneous emphysema by inspecting and palpating skin around insertion site and along arm. Inspection may reveal edema where air is located, and air may travel if skin is loose. Palpation reveals a crackling sensation such as popping plastic bubble wrap. Assess for chest pain. Assess for dyspnea, apnea, hypoxia, tachycardia, hypotension, nausea, and confusion.	Use injection cap on distal end when not in use. Do not leave catheter hub open to air. If appropriate for device, be sure that clamps are engaged.	Administer oxygen as ordered. Elevate feet. Aspirate air and fluid. If air emboli suspected, place patient on left side with head down. Remove catheter as ordered. Help with insertion of chest tubes as ordered.
Incorrect placement	Assess for cardiac dysrhythmias. Assess for hypotension. Assess for neck distention. Assess for narrow pulse pressure. Assess for inadequate blood withdrawal. Assess for retrograde flow of blood (flow of blood back into tubing usually caused by decreased pressure gradient between venous system and access device unit [e.g., IV infusion, heparin lock]).	Obtain ultrasound, echocardiogram, fluoroscopy, or x-ray film examination after placement. Reposition catheter as warranted.	Stop all fluid administration until placement is confirmed. Discontinue catheter (requires order). Obtain ultrasound, x-ray film, and/or electrocardiogram (for PICC and CVAD). Administer support medications as ordered.

CLABSI, Central line–associated bloodstream infection; *CVAD,* central vascular access device; *IV,* intravenous; *PICC,* peripherally inserted central catheter; *TSM,* transparent semipermeable membrane.

STEP	RATIONALE
7. **Use Teach-Back:** "I want to be sure that I explained the purpose and care of your intravenous catheter. This catheter is placed in a large vein in your body, and the problems we talked about can occur. Tell me in your own words the problems that might develop with your catheter and the signs and symptoms you would report to me or another nurse." Revise your instruction now or develop a plan for revised patient/family caregiver teaching if patient/family caregiver is not able to teach back correctly.	Teach-back is a technique for health care providers to ensure that they have explained medical information clearly so that patients and their families understand what is communicated to them (AHRQ, 2023).

Unexpected Outcomes	Related Interventions
1. For catheter complications, see Table 28.8.	• See Table 28.8.
2. Patient or family caregiver is unable to explain or perform CVAD care.	• Indicates need for home care referral or additional instruction.

Documentation

- Document catheter site insertion/care, including catheter location; size of catheter; number of lumens; condition of catheter insertion site or port site; skin integrity; external catheter length; mid-arm circumference for PICC; condition and type of securement device; date and time of dressing change; change of injection caps; patency of catheter, including presence or absence of blood return or resistance; and patient's tolerance of the procedure.
- Document catheter flushes to include solution, volume, and concentration.
- Document catheter removal: patient position, appearance of site, length of catheter removed, integrity of catheter after removal, dressing applied, patient's tolerance of procedure, presence or

absence of bleeding from site, and any problems with removal.

- Document blood draw: date, time, sample drawn and tests ordered, waste volume, and flushes used.
- Document unexpected outcomes and CVAD complications, interventions, and patient response to treatment.
- Document patient's and family caregiver's ability to explain instructions.

Hand-Off Reporting

- Report placement of CVAD with reason for insertion, signs or symptoms of observed or patient-reported IV-related complications, status of VAD, and patient condition.
- Report to health care provider any CVAD-related complications, interventions, and response to treatment.

Special Considerations
Patient Education

- Instruct patient to report discomfort around the site; discomfort in arms, shoulders, or side of the neck; or any shortness of breath.
- Provide written instruction for dressing changes, inspection of insertion site, flushing, and tubing changes.
- Arrange for instruction and return demonstration of skills by patient or family caregiver.
- Have patient or family caregiver maintain a list of caregivers and telephone numbers (e.g., health care provider, nurse, social worker, pharmacist, registered dietitian nutritionist).

Pediatrics

- Central vein catheters that are of a smaller diameter and shorter length are available for children and infants.
- Take care to secure infant catheters in a manner that does not allow them to twist. Small-diameter catheters are fragile, and twisting them causes them to tear.
- Amount and dosage of flush solution (heparin/sodium chloride) vary with age, size, and catheter diameter and length.
- Document volume of blood draws on I&O record.

Older Adults

- Some older adults have difficulty lying flat in bed, and a modification of the totally supine position during CVAD insertion is often necessary.
- PICC insertion may provide an alternative route of administration and reduce the risk of complications associated with subclavian or jugular insertion.

Home Care

- Initiate early referral for discharge planning to social service, counselor, or home care coordinator for assessment of resources.
- Assess home environment and determine suitable area for dressing changes, avoiding areas where contaminants are potential hazards.
- Discuss and provide written emergency measures and telephone numbers of health care personnel to be used in case of catheter damage, dislodgement, swelling, redness, or leakage at insertion site; occlusion of catheter; temperature above 38°C (100.4°F) (see agency policy); and shaking chills.
- Provide patient with comprehensive list of providers for supplies and equipment.
- Provide patient with Kelly clamp *without* teeth (bulldog clamp) that can be used in the event of catheter rupture to prevent air embolism, and instruct patient on use.
- Instruct patient or family caregivers in flushing technique, site care, and dressing change, and observe them performing procedures.
- Instruct patient and family caregivers in adaptations of agency procedures that they can make at home (e.g., good hand hygiene instead of sterile gloves).
- Provide education to the patient and family caregivers about how to recognize signs and symptoms of IV-related complications, actions to take, how to report, and methods for preservation of CVADs.
- Provide appropriate information about home disposal of soiled dressings and equipment (see Chapter 41).

✦ CLINICAL JUDGMENT AND NEXT-GENERATION NCLEX® EXAMINATION–STYLE QUESTIONS

An 88-year-old patient with a history of heart failure and stomach cancer was admitted to the health care agency 24 hours ago for dehydration with mild confusion, decreased urine output, postural hypotension, and poor oral intake after receiving chemotherapy. The patient has been receiving D5W at 100 mL/h through a peripheral intravenous (IV) line since admission. Today the family caregivers tell the nurse that the patient seems to be having difficulty breathing and is asking for another pillow for the bed.

1. Which of the following assessments would the nurse perform at this time to determine if the patient has fluid volume excess (FVE)? **Select all that apply.**
   1. Weight
   2. Urine output
   3. Neck veins
   4. Lung sounds
   5. Presence of edema

2. The health care provider determines that the patient is experiencing anxiety rather than fluid volume excess (FVE). Changes are made to the IV solution orders. Based on the patient's signs and symptoms, which type of solution would the nurse anticipate will be ordered?
   1. 0.45% saline
   2. D10W
   3. 0.9% saline
   4. 5% dextrose in lactated Ringer solution

3. During hospitalization, the health care provider places a tunneled central vascular access device (CVAD). Which action would the nurse take **next** when performing catheter care after first performing hand hygiene, donning gloves and mask, removing the old dressing, and cleaning the catheter site?
   1. Flush catheter
   2. Disinfect catheter hub
   3. Apply new injection cap
   4. Apply sterile labeled dressing

4. After the tunneled CVAD is removed later, a peripheral IV line needs to be inserted. Which of the following actions would the nurse take to insert a line? **Select all that apply.**

1. Apply tourniquet to arm 10 to 15 cm (4–6 inches) above the intended insertion site.
2. Clean skin using an approved antiseptic agent such as chlorhexidine or 70% isopropyl alcohol and allow to dry thoroughly.
3. Stabilize the vein by placing the thumb proximal to the insertion site, stretching the skin in the direction of insertion.
4. Use the smallest-gauge, shortest catheter available and insert with the bevel up at a 10- to 15-degree angle.
5. Observe for blood in the flashback chamber of the catheter, advance the catheter off the needle into the vein, and release the tourniquet.

5. The nurse has successfully inserted the new peripheral IV line. Select two assessment findings that would require the nurse to intervene.

1. Warm distal extremity
2. Increasing pain at the insertion site
3. Blood pressure 110/78 mm Hg
4. Capillary refill 2 sec
5. Redness at IV site
6. Ability to feel sensation on the hand

Visit the Evolve site for Answers to Clinical Judgment and Next-Generation NCLEX® Examination–Style Questions.

REFERENCES

Agency for Healthcare Research and Quality (AHRQ): *Teach-back: intervention*, Rockville, MD, 2023, Agency for Healthcare Research and Quality. https://www.ahrq.gov/patient-safety/reports/engage/interventions/teachback.html.

Barton A: The case for using a disinfecting cap for needlefree connectors, *Br J Nurs* 28(14):S22–S27, 2019.

Buetti N, et al: Strategies to prevent central line-associated bloodstream infections in acute-care hospitals: 2022 update, *Infect Control Hosp Epidemiol* 43(5): 553–569, 2022.

Centers for Disease Control and Prevention (CDC): *What is health literacy?* 2023. https://www.cdc.gov/healthliteracy/learn/index.html.

Centers for Disease Control and Prevention, National Health Safety Network (NHSN): *Bloodstream infection event (central line–associated bloodstream infection and non–central line–associated bloodstream infection)*, 2022. https://www.cdc.gov/nhsn/pdfs/pscmanual/4psc_clabscurrent.pdf.

Fumarola S, et al: Overlooked and underestimated: medical adhesive-related skin injuries. Best practice consensus document on prevention, *J Wound Care* 29(Suppl 3c):S1–S24, 2020.

Gorski L, et al: *Infusion therapy standards of practice*, ed 8, Norwood, Mass, 2021, Infusion Nurses Society (INS).

Gorski L: *Phillips's Manual of I.V. therapeutics: evidenced-based infusion therapy*, ed 8, Philadelphia, 2023, FA Davis.

Goulart CB, et al: Effectiveness of topical interventions to prevent or treat intravenous therapy-related phlebitis: a systematic review, *J Clin Nurs* 29(13–14): 2138–2149, 2020.

Gupta P, et al: Bundle approach used to achieve zero central line-associated bloodstream infections in an adult coronary intensive care unit, *BMJ Open Quality* 2021;10:e001200.

Hockenberry MJ, et al: *Wong's essentials of pediatric nursing*, ed 11, St. Louis, 2022, Elsevier.

Kirkendall ES, et al: Human-based errors involving smart infusion pumps: a catalog of error types and prevention strategies, *Drug Saf* 43:1073–1087, 2020. https://psnet.ahrq.gov/issue/human-based-errors-involving-smart-infusion-pumps-catalog-error-types-and-prevention. Accessed October 20, 2023.

La Greca A, et al: ECHOTIP: A structured protocol for ultrasound-based tip navigation and tip location during placement of central venous access devices in adult patients. *J Vasc Access* 24(4):535–544, 2023.

Marsh N, et al: Observational study of peripheral intravenous catheter outcomes in adult hospitalized patients: a multivariable analysis of peripheral intravenous catheter failure, *J Hosp Med* 3(2):83–89, 2018.

Occupational Safety and Health Administration (OSHA): *Bloodborne pathogens standard*, n.d., United States Department of Labor. https://www.osha.gov/pls/oshaweb/owadisp.show_document?p_table=STANDARDS&p_id=10051. Accessed October 31, 2023.

Oncology Nurses Society (ONS): *Toolkit for safe handling of hazardous drugs for nurses in oncology*, 2018. https://www.ons.org/sites/default/files/2018-06/ONS_Safe_Handling_Toolkit_0.pdf.

The Joint Commission (TJC): *2023 National Patient Safety Goals*, Oakbrook Terrace, IL, 2023, The Joint Commission. https://www.jointcommission.org/standards/national-patient-safety-goals/. Accessed July 15, 2023.

Wolf Z, Hughes R: Best practices to decrease infusion-associated medication errors, *J Infus Nurs* 42(4):183, 2019.

29 | Blood Therapy

SKILLS AND PROCEDURES

Skill 29.1 **Initiating Blood Therapy, p. 900**

Skill 29.2 **Monitoring for Adverse Transfusion Reactions, p. 908**

OBJECTIVES

Mastery of content in this chapter will enable you to:
- Discuss indications for blood therapy.
- Demonstrate the following skills on selected patients: initiating blood therapy, implementing autotransfusion, and monitoring for adverse reactions to transfusion.

- Discuss nursing implications for ensuring safe initiation of a blood transfusion.
- Compare various transfusion reactions.
- Explain rationale for the techniques used to manage symptoms of adverse transfusion reactions.

MEDIA RESOURCES

- http://evolve.elsevier.com/Perry/skills
- Review Questions
- Audio Glossary
- ▶ Video Clips
- Animations

- **NSO** Nursing Skills Online
- Answers to Clinical Judgment and Next-Generation NCLEX® Examination–Style Questions
- Skills Performance Checklists
- Printable Key Points

PURPOSE

Transfusion therapy or blood replacement is the intravenous (IV) administration of whole blood (Fig. 29.1), its components, (Fig. 29.2A–B) (e.g., packed red blood cells [PRBCs], cryoprecipitate, platelets), or a plasma-derived product for therapeutic purposes (Shaz et al., 2019). Transfusion therapy restores intravascular volume with whole blood or albumin; restores the oxygen-carrying capacity of blood with red blood cells (RBCs); provides clotting factors and/or platelets for patients with hematological disorders, cancer, or injury and during surgical intervention; and provides treatment for diseases related to coagulation deficiencies (AABB, 2022). The blood product can be allogeneic (blood donated from someone else) or autologous (a patient's own blood, which has been collected and is reinfused for intravascular volume replacement) (AABB, 2022).

Blood safety involves keeping the U.S. blood supply free of contaminants or infectious agents (National Heart, Lung, and Blood Institute [NHLBI], n.d.). Blood banks and transfusion centers follow protocols to ensure that blood is free of pathogens (Box 29.1). The rates of transfusion-transmitted viral infections such as the human immunodeficiency virus (HIV) and hepatitis have fallen over the last few decades due to the highly sensitive technique of viral nucleic acid testing (Wu et al., 2022). Recently there have been advances in technologies for identifying the genetic makeup of cells and microorganisms and creating diagnostic platforms that incorporate these technologies to allow for very rapid detection of several different pathogens simultaneously in donated blood (Duncan, 2022). There is a national public health surveillance system to monitor adverse events among patients who receive blood transfusions. It is designed to capture adverse reactions and process incidents related to blood transfusion (Centers for Disease Control and Prevention [CDC], 2022). Nurses have the responsibility to educate patients about blood safety and to use clinical judgment when identifying patients and blood products and following strict procedures for blood and blood product administration.

There are three primary blood-typing systems: ABO, Rh, and human leukocyte antigen (HLA). These systems are used during the cross-matching procedures. A competent nurse must know not only the complexities of the ABO and Rh systems, but also the numerous components of blood that can be transfused and the serious negative outcomes that can occur if not managed and monitored correctly. Never view the transfusion of blood products as routine; overlooking a minor detail is dangerous and can be life threatening to a patient (AABB, 2022; Gorski, 2023).

PRACTICE STANDARDS

- AABB (formerly American Association of Blood Banks), 2022: Standards for Blood Banks and Transfusion Services
- AABB (formerly American Association of Blood Banks), 2018: AABB Primer of Blood Administration
- Infusion Nurses Society (INS), 2021: Infusion Therapy Standards of Practice—Blood administration
- The Joint Commission (TJC), 2023: National Patient Safety Goals—Patient identification

SUPPLEMENTAL STANDARDS

- AABB (formerly American Association of Blood Banks), 2023: Technical Manual for Transfusing Blood and Blood Products

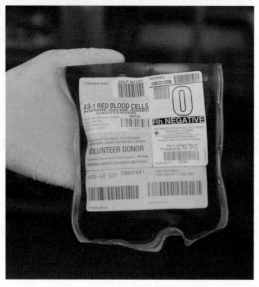

FIG. 29.1 Unit of blood. (*Image courtesy American Red Cross.*)

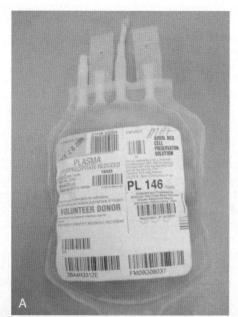

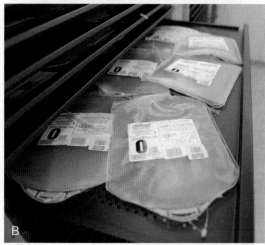

FIG. 29.2 (A) Bag of cryoprecipitate (Cryo). (B) Bags of platelets. (*Images courtesy American Red Cross.*)

BOX 29.1

Common Infectious Disease Pathogens Screened for During Blood Donation

Hepatitis B virus (HBV)
Hepatitis C virus (HCV)
Human immunodeficiency virus (HIV) types 1 and 2
Human T-lymphotropic virus (HTLV) types 1 and 2
Treponema pallidum (syphilis)
West Nile virus (WNV)
Bacterial contamination
Babesia (screening performed in endemic regions of the world)
Trypanosoma cruzi (Chagas disease)
Cytomegalovirus (CMV)

Adapted from Centers for Disease Control and Prevention (CDC): *Blood safety basics*, 2023.
https://www.cdc.gov/bloodsafety/basics.html. Accessed May 4. 2023.

PRINCIPLES FOR PRACTICE

- The most common method of blood transfusion is allogeneic blood (blood donated from someone else).
- Autologous transfusion, or autotransfusion, is a method in which a patient's own blood is collected and reinfused for the purpose of IV volume replacement (Gorski, 2023). Patients who have a concern about transfusion-related reactions or transmission of disease find advantages to autologous transfusion. It is ideal for preoperative blood donation, intraoperative cell salvage, and postoperative blood salvage. Preoperative blood donation is the most commonly used type of autologous donation. In this process, patients can donate several units of their own blood approximately 4 to 6 weeks before surgery via phlebotomy, which is performed weekly. The last donation must occur more than 72 hours before surgery.
- To decrease transfusion-related adverse events, blood and its components are treated and stored in controlled environments. Blood is a living tissue, and once obtained via the donor it must remain healthy before transfusion (Gorski, 2023).
- Caution is needed when infusing multiple units of blood or a unit of blood nearing its expiration. When blood is stored, RBCs are destroyed continually, which releases potassium (K) from the cells into the plasma. Often a laboratory test of a patient's potassium (K) level is ordered before a unit of blood is administered (Shaz et al., 2019).
- Your role during a blood transfusion is to carry out the health care provider's order by safely administering the blood or blood products; assessing the patient before, during, and after the transfusion; and promptly identifying and reporting any transfusion reactions.

ABO System

- The ABO, Rh, and HLA blood-typing systems ensure a close match between transfused products and a recipient's blood. The ABO system uses the presence or absence of specific antigens on the surface of RBCs to identify blood groups. When the type A antigen is present, the blood group is type A. When the type B antigen is present, the blood group is type B. When both A and B antigens are present, the blood group is type AB; when neither A nor B antigens are present, the blood group is type O (Gorski, 2023) (Table 29.1).
- Antibodies that react against the A and B antigens are naturally present in the plasma of people whose RBCs do not carry the antigen. These antibodies (agglutinins) react against foreign antigens (agglutinogens). Incompatible RBCs agglutinate

TABLE 29.1

ABO System

Patient Blood Type (Rh Factor)	Red Blood Cell Antigen	Transfuse With Type A	Transfuse With Type B	Transfuse With Type AB	Transfuse With Type O	Transfusion Options
A (+)	A	Yes	No	No	Yes	A+, A− O+, O−
A (−)	A	Yes	No	No	Yes	A−, O−
B (+)	B	No	Yes	No	Yes	B+, B− O+, O−
B (−)	B	No	Yes	No	Yes	B−, O−
AB (+)	AB	Yes	Yes	Yes	Yes	A+, A− B+, B− O+, O− Universal recipient
AB (−)	AB	Yes	Yes	Yes	Yes	A− B− O−
O (+)	None	No	No	No	Yes	O+, O−
O (−)	None	No	No	No	Yes	O− Universal donor

Data from Gorski L: Phillips's manual of IV therapeutics: evidence-based practice for infusion therapy, ed 8, Philadelphia, 2023, FA Davis.

(clump together) and result in a life-threatening acute hemolytic transfusion reaction (AHTR). People with type A blood have anti-B antibodies; people with type B blood have anti-A antibodies. People with type AB blood have neither antibody and can receive all blood types. People with type O blood have both A and B antibodies and can receive only type O blood (Gorski, 2023).

Rh System

- The Rh factor is considered when matching blood components for transfusion. The Rh factor is another antigen in RBC membranes. Although nearly 50 types of Rh antigen may be present on the surface of RBCs, the type D antigen is widely prevalent and is most likely to elicit an immune response. It is the presence or absence of the D antigen that determines a person's Rh type. A person with the D antigen is Rh positive, and a person without the D antigen is Rh negative (Gorski, 2023). Unlike the ABO antigens, naturally occurring antibodies to the Rh(D) antigen do not occur. A person with Rh-negative blood must first be exposed to Rh-positive blood before any Rh antibodies are formed.
- An Rh-negative mother previously exposed to Rh antigen can transfer Rh antibodies across the placenta to an Rh-positive fetus. This can result in severe fetal hemolysis (i.e., the breakdown of RBCs, with resultant anemia and jaundice) and is often fatal to the infant. To prevent current or future fetal hemolysis, Rh(D) immunoglobulin (RhoGAM) is given by intramuscular injection to the mother. RhoGAM can suppress or destroy the fetal Rh-positive blood cells that have passed from the fetal to the maternal circulation.

Human Leukocyte Antigen System

Although most commonly linked to transplant rejection, HLAs are highly immunogenic antigens that can cause serious transfusion complications. HLA antibodies are located on the cell surface of leukocytes but can be found on all cells of the body (Gorski, 2023). HLA complications most commonly seen include febrile nonhemolytic reaction, transfusion-related acute lung injury (TRALI), and transfusion-associated graft-versus-host disease (TA-GVHD).

PERSON-CENTERED CARE

- When administering blood products, consider patients' values, culture, and religious beliefs about blood therapy. Patients' perceptions of their disease or health condition affect how receptive they are to receiving blood. Blood transfusion is often equated to severity of illness.
- When possible, it is helpful to consult a religious leader when caring for patients in need of blood therapy. Be familiar with agency policies and procedures to follow when patients refuse blood transfusions, and inform the health care provider of a patient's decision.
- By law, parents are obligated to care for and make decisions about their minor children. However, the legal principle of *parens patriae* says that the state has an overriding interest in the health and welfare of its citizens. The parents' refusal can be interpreted as neglect. A nurse's role is to advocate for the patient and family. This may include seeking different forms of treatment or, if necessary, coordinating with officials to petition juvenile or family court for temporary guardianship of the child.

EVIDENCE-BASED PRACTICE

Prevention of Transfusion Reactions

Compliance with standards and policies and ongoing education are essential to maintain patient safety and reduce potential transfusion errors. Safety and risk management are key factors in transfusion therapy. ABO incompatibilities are one of the most serious errors associated with transfusions and can have fatal outcomes

(Gorski, 2023). Pretransfusion requirements to decrease transfusion-related errors include (Teruya, 2022; Uhl, 2022):

- Use proper labeling of the cross-and-match blood sample immediately on collection. Laboratories and transfusion departments usually require two separate specimens for blood-type verification to avoid transfusion errors.
- The blood sample label identifies the patient's blood type and antibodies present in the plasma at the time transfusion is administered. If the patient has been pregnant in the past 3 months, this specimen must be less than 3 days old.
- Compatibility testing is performed on plasma. Most laboratories use tubes with ethylenediaminetetraacetic acid (EDTA) (pink or lavender top), but tubes with acid citrate dextrose (ACD) (yellow top) or without anticoagulant (red top) are also acceptable if they have been validated by the laboratory (Fang & Pham, 2021). Serum from a clotted sample can be used, but plasma is preferred.
- Pretransfusion testing routinely includes ABO and Rh(D) typing including antibody screening. RBC genotyping may be used for patients with confusing serological results—for example, patients with sickle cell anemia or thalassemia (Teruya, 2022; Fang & Pham, 2021).

- For infants younger than 4 months, pretransfusion testing is difficult owing to their immature immune system and the presence of maternal antibodies (Teruya, 2022).
- Knowledge of the patient's prior transfusion history is needed to identify potential transfusion reaction areas, such as a history of transfusion antibodies.

SAFETY GUIDELINES

- The blood delivery pathway is a standard for ensuring delivery of the right blood product to the right patient (Gorski, 2023):
  - Identify the patient with two unique identifiers.
  - Connect the patient identifiers to all prepared lab samples, tests, and blood products by checking labels.
  - Deliver the right blood product to the right patient at the right time, confirming patient identification again.
- Administration of blood and blood components requires meticulous attention to detail (e.g., preparation, administration, and monitoring) to prevent life-threatening transfusion reactions (Table 29.2).
- Review agency policy and procedure regarding administration of blood or blood products.

TABLE 29.2

Transfusion Reactions

Reaction	Etiology	Onset	Signs and Symptoms	Prevention	Nursing Intervention
Acute Immediate (<24 Hours)					
Febrile, nonhemolytic	Most common type of transfusion reaction; caused by WBC antigen-antibody reaction	May begin early in transfusion or as long as several hours after completion	Temperature increase of >1°C (2°F) or more above baseline, chills, headache, vomiting	Premedicate as ordered with antipyretics if prior history of reaction. Use leukocyte-reduced blood products.	**Stop the transfusion.** Change administration set and administer 0.9% sodium chloride at rate to maintain patent IV access. Institute transfusion reaction protocol. Administer antipyretics as ordered to treat fever. Document clinical symptoms, when transfusion was stopped, notification of health care provider and blood bank, nursing interventions and response to interventions, and patient teaching.
Acute hemolytic transfusion reaction (AHTR)	Transfusion of ABO-incompatible RBCs; usually caused by misidentification or improper labeling	Within minutes of transfusion initiation	Fever with or without chills; tachycardia; hypotension; abdominal, chest, back, and flank pain; dyspnea; red/dark urine; shock	Use extreme care during the entire patient identification process; proper labeling of blood sample; meticulous verification of ABO/Rh compatibility between donor and recipient before administration; start transfusion slowly and monitor carefully for the first 15 minutes.	**Stop the transfusion.** Get help immediately. Change administration set and administer 0.9% sodium chloride at rate to maintain patent IV access. Notify health care provider and blood bank. Treat shock. Maintain blood pressure and renal perfusion. Insert Foley catheter. Monitor intake and output hourly. Dialysis may be required. Obtain blood and urine samples and send to laboratory with unused part of unit of blood. Document reaction according to agency policy.
Allergic reaction (mild to moderate)	Caused by recipient sensitivity allergens in the blood components	Within minutes of transfusion initiation	Urticaria, pruritus, facial flushing, mild wheezing	May administer antihistamines 30 minutes before transfusion if prescribed.	**Stop the transfusion.** Change administration set and administer 0.9% sodium chloride at rate to maintain patent IV access. Notify health care provider and blood bank. Administer antihistamines as ordered. Monitor and document vital signs every 15 minutes. Transfusion may be restarted if fever, dyspnea, and wheezing are not present.

TABLE 29.2

Transfusion Reactions—cont'd

Reaction	Etiology	Onset	Signs and Symptoms	Prevention	Nursing Intervention
Severe allergic reaction (anaphylaxis)	Caused by recipient allergy to a donor antigen (usually IgA) Agglutination of RBCs obstructing capillaries and blocking blood flow, causing symptoms in all major organ systems	Within minutes of transfusion initiation	Hypotension, tachycardia, urticaria, bronchospasm, anxiety, shock, nausea, vomiting, diarrhea, abdominal pain	Use autologous blood or blood from donors who are IgA deficient. Transfusion of saline-washed or leukocyte-depleted RBCs.	**Stop the transfusion.** Change administration set and administer 0.9% sodium chloride at rate to maintain patent IV access. Notify health care provider and blood bank. Administer antihistamines, corticosteroids, epinephrine, and antipyretics as ordered. Monitor and document vital signs until stable. Initiate cardiopulmonary resuscitation if necessary.
Transfusion-related acute lung injury (TRALI)	Presence of WBC antibodies from donor who has a WBC-activating agent in blood Leading cause of transfusion-related death	During or within 6 hours of transfusion	Fever, respiratory failure, hypoxemia, hypotension, pulmonary edema	Currently there is no method to identify patients at risk.	**Stop the transfusion.** Provide respiratory support; administer oxygen; frequently necessitates mechanical ventilation; administer vasopressor agents.
Transfusion-associated circulatory overload (TACO)	Related to volume overload; patients older than 70 years and infants are at highest risk	Usually occurs during or within 6 hours of transfusion	Dyspnea, orthopnea, cyanosis, tachycardia, jugular vein distention (JVD), hypertension, cough	Frequent patient monitoring required for those at high risk, including slowing infusion rate.	**Stop the transfusion.** Place patient in high-Fowler position; notify health care provider; administer oxygen and diuretics.
Delayed Transfusion Reactions					
Transfusion-associated graft-versus-host disease (TA-GVHD)	Usually rare but fatal Donor lymphocytes destroyed by recipient's immune system In immunocompromised patients the donor lymphocytes are identified as foreign; however, patient's immune system is not capable of destroying, and in turn patient's lymphocytes are destroyed	8–10 days after transfusion	Maculopapular rash, watery diarrhea, fever, jaundice caused by liver dysfunction, bone marrow suppression (pancytopenia)	Administration of irradiated blood and leukocyte-depleted RBC products as prescribed.	No effective therapy. Treatment of symptoms.
Iron overload	Iron from donated blood binds to protein and is not eliminated	Usually occurs when multiple units (>100 units of PRBCs) are transfused	Cardiac dysfunction, organ failure, arrhythmias, heart failure symptoms, increased serum transferrin, increased liver enzymes, jaundice	Iron chelation, phlebotomy, monitoring of serum iron levels.	No effective therapy. Iron chelation therapy. Monitor patient for heart failure, cardiac disorder, liver disorder, and serum transferrin.
Infection-Related Complications					
Bacterial contamination	Microorganism contamination of infused product during donation or in preparing component for infusion Highest risk when administering platelets	Occurs at time of donation; symptoms may appear during transfusion or within 4 hours of completion	High fever, severe chills, hypotension, flushed skin, shock, hemoglobinuria, renal failure, DIC	Use good skin antisepsis prior to venipuncture. Inspect blood unit carefully and do not administer if clots, bubbles, bag leaks, or discoloration of unit noted.	**Stop the transfusion.** Treat shock and administer ordered steroids and antibiotics. Culture patient's blood, blood components, and all intravenous solutions.

DIC, Disseminated intravascular coagulation; *IgA,* immunoglobulin A; *IV,* intravenous; *PRBCs,* packed red blood cells; *RBC,* red blood cell; *WBC,* white blood cell.
Data adapted from AABB (formerly American Association of Blood Banks): *Technical manual for transfusing blood and blood products,* ed 20, Bethesda, MD, 2023, AABB; and Gorski L: *Phillips's manual of IV therapeutics: evidence-based practice for infusion therapy,* ed 8, Philadelphia, 2023, FA Davis.

- Two nurses verify blood unit label for accuracy and correct patient at the patient's bedside before administration.
- Despite precautions, transfusion therapy carries risks. Compatibility of the patient and donor is essential. Human-related errors (e.g., improper labeling, poor hand-off between nurses and the person transporting blood, or the method used to complete

a blood requisition) that may lead to the administration of incompatible transfusions can occur at every step of the process. Complications resulting from immunological response to blood or blood products can be reduced by modifications such as use of washed or irradiated RBCs or leukocyte-reduced blood (Shaz et al., 2019).

✦ SKILL 29.1 Initiating Blood Therapy

 Video Clip

Blood is administered for different clinical indications (Table 29.3). A patient's medical condition determines when and which blood component is indicated. A health care provider's order is required for the administration of a blood product. As a nurse, you will be

responsible for understanding which components are appropriate in various situations. Always ensure that a blood sample for typing and compatibility screening has been collected and sent to the laboratory within 72 hours. The blood sample collector follows standards

---

TABLE 29.3

Blood and Blood Component Products[a]

Blood Product and Source	Volume and Infusion Time	Able to Transmit HIV/HBV	ABO/Rh Testing Needed	Actions/Uses
Whole blood—Single donor: allogeneic or autologous	300–550 mL Within 4 h	Yes	Yes—Must be ABO identical Rh—Yes	Replaces red cell mass and plasma volume; expected to raise Hgb 1 g/100 mL and Hct by 3% in nonhemorrhaging adult.
Red blood cells (RBCs)— Single donor: allogeneic or autologous	225–350 mL Within 4 h	Yes	Yes/Yes	Preferred method of replacing RBC mass; expected to raise Hgb/Hct level same as whole blood.
Leukocyte-poor RBCs— Single donor: allogeneic or directed	200–250 mL Within 4 h	Yes	Yes/Yes	Replaces RBCs while preventing febrile, nonhemolytic transfusion reactions; reduces risk for CMV transmission.
Irradiated RBCs—Single donor: allogeneic or directed	250–350 mL Within 4 h	Yes	Yes/Yes	Replaces RBCs while preventing transfusion-associated graft-versus-host disease TA-GVHD); used in immunodeficient patients (any blood component can be irradiated).
Fresh frozen plasma (FFP)—Single donor	200–250 mL Within 24 h of thawing Within 4 h	Yes	Yes/No	Replaces plasma without RBCs or platelets; contains most coagulation factors and complement; used in control of bleeding when replacement of coagulation factors is needed (e.g., DIC, TTP).
Cryoprecipitate—Multiple donors, pooled	5–20 mL/unit; 1 unit/10 kg body weight 1–2 mL/min Infuse within 6 h of thawing or 4 h of pooling	Yes	No/No	Replaces factors VIII, XIII, von Willebrand factor, and fibrinogen.
Platelets—Multiple/random donor, pooled	40–70 mL/unit; 1 unit/10 kg body weight Within 6 h of pooling	Yes	Yes/Yes	Used in patients with thrombocytopenia. Certain microaggregate filters are not to be used with platelets—check manufacturer's instructions.
Platelets—Single donor	200–500 mL Within 4 h	Yes	Yes/Yes	Single-donor platelets are most useful in immunologically refractory patients when given as HLA matched with recipient. Each unit expected to raise platelet count by 5000–10,000/mL in a 70-kg patient.
Colloid components— Albumin 5% pooled	250–500 mL 1–10 mL/min	No	No/No	Oncotically equivalent to plasma; used to treat hypoproteinemia in burns and hypoalbuminemia in shock and ARDs; used to support blood pressure in dialysis and acute liver failure.
Colloid components—Albumin 25% pooled	50–100 mL 0.2–0.4 mL/min	No	No/No	Increases circulating blood volume by increasing intravascular oncotic pressure.

ARD, Acute respiratory disease; *CMV,* cytomegalovirus; *DIC,* disseminated intravascular coagulation; *HBV,* hepatitis B virus; *Hct,* hematocrit; *Hgb,* hemoglobin; *HIV,* human immunodeficiency virus; *HLA,* human leukocyte antigen; *TTP,* thrombotic thrombocytopenic purpura.
[a]Other, less commonly used blood components include factors VIII and IX concentrates, granulocytes, immunoglobulin, and saline-washed RBCs.
Data modified from AABB (formerly American Association of Blood Banks): *Technical manual for transfusing blood and blood products,* ed 20, Bethesda, MD, 2023, AABB; and Gorski L: *Phillips's manual of IV therapeutics: evidence-based practice for infusion therapy,* ed 7, Philadelphia, 2023, FA Davis.

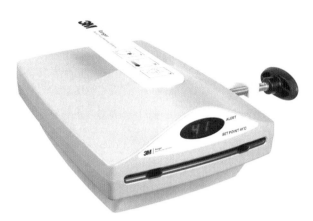

FIG. 29.3 3M™ Ranger™ Blood/Fluid Warming Unit, model 24500. *(Image courtesy 3M, St. Paul, MN.)*

when labeling the blood tube and ensures that the label includes the patient's name and identification information based on agency policy (Gorski, 2023; TJC, 2023).

Blood is stored in a refrigerated environment. The refrigeration unit is regulated by the blood bank; blood should not be stored in refrigerators on the patient care unit. In emergency situations, rapid transfusion of cold blood may lead to dysrhythmias and a reduction of core temperature. Sometimes a blood-warmer device is used for rapid transfusions (Fig. 29.3). *Do not heat blood products in a microwave or with hot water because this is dangerous and may destroy blood cells and result in hemolysis and severe reactions* (Gorski, 2023).

Delegation

The skill of initiating transfusion therapy cannot be delegated to assistive personnel (AP). The skill of initiating transfusion therapy by a licensed practical nurse (LPN) varies by state practice acts. After a transfusion has been started and a patient is stable, monitoring of a patient by the AP does not relieve a registered

nurse (RN) of the responsibility to continue to assess the patient during the transfusion. Instruct the AP about:

- Frequency of vital sign monitoring needed
- What to observe, such as complaints of shortness of breath, hives, and/or chills, and reporting this information to the nurse
- Obtaining blood components from the blood bank (check agency policy)

Interprofessional Collaboration

- Contact blood bank personnel as per agency policy for any guidelines related to blood administration.

Equipment

- Y-type blood administration set (in-line filter) (**NOTE:** Depending on blood product, special tubing and filter are necessary.)
- Prescribed blood product
- 250-mL bag 0.9% sodium chloride (normal saline [NS]) intravenous
- 5- to 10-mL prefilled syringe with preservative-free 0.9% sodium chloride (NS)
- Antiseptic swabs (chlorhexidine solution preferred, povidone-iodine, or 70% alcohol)
- Clean gloves
- Tape
- Vital sign equipment: thermometer, blood pressure cuff, stethoscope, and pulse oximeter
- Electronic infusion pump designated for transfusion of whole blood and blood products
- Signed transfusion consent form

Optional Equipment

- Rapid infusion pump
- *Option:* Leukocyte-depleting filter (**NOTE:** Agency may irradiate blood products within the blood bank.)
- Blood warmer (used mainly when rapid transfusion is needed)
- Pressure bag (used for rapid infusion in acute blood loss)
- Cardiac monitor for emergencies

STEP	RATIONALE

ASSESSMENT

1. Identify patient using at least two identifiers (e.g., name and birthday or name and medical record number) according to agency policy. Compare identifiers with information on patient's medical administration record (MAR) or electronic health record (EHR).	Ensures correct patient. Complies with The Joint Commission standards and improves patient safety (TJC, 2023).
2. Verify health care provider's order for specific blood or blood product with appropriate date, time to begin transfusion, special instructions (e.g., irradiated, leukocyte depleted), duration, and any pretransfusion or posttransfusion medications to administer.	A health care provider's order must be present before a blood product is transfused. Verifying order helps to ensure that appropriate blood component will be administered (Gorski, 2023; Infusion Nurses Society [INS], 2021). Premedication such as an antihistamine or antipyretic may be ordered if patient demonstrated previous transfusion sensitivity.

Clinical Judgment *A health care provider's order must be present before a blood product can be transfused. When more than one blood product is to be given, the sequence or order of transfusion should be specified. Any additional medications such as an antihistamine (given when the history shows previous allergic response), antipyretics (given when the history shows previous febrile nonhemolytic response), diuretics (given when the history shows potential for heart failure), or other special treatment of the components should also be included in a written transfusion order.*

3. Verify that any pretransfusion laboratory studies are completed and in patient's EHR. Review current laboratory values: hematocrit (Hct), coagulation values, platelet count, and potassium (K).	Provides baseline for later evaluation of patient response to transfusion (INS, 2021). When blood is stored, there is continual destruction of red blood cells, which releases potassium (K) from the cells into the plasma.

STEP	RATIONALE
4. Obtain patient's transfusion history; note known allergies and previous transfusion reactions. Verify that type and crossmatch have been completed within 72 hours of transfusion.	Identifies patient's prior response(s) to transfusion of blood components. If patient has experienced reaction in the past, anticipate similar reaction and be prepared to rapidly intervene.
5. Assess patient's/family caregiver's health literacy.	Determines degree to which individuals have the ability to find, understand, and use information and services to make informed health-related decisions and actions for themselves and others (CDC, 2023).
6. Perform hand hygiene and apply clean gloves. Verify that intravenous (IV) cannula is patent and without complications such as infiltration or phlebitis (see Chapter 28).	Reduces transmission of microorganisms. Presence of a patent and appropriate VAD is needed for a transfusion (INS, 2021).
• Assess the vascular access device (VAD) catheter-skin junction site and surrounding area for catheter-related complications by visually inspecting and palpating through the intact dressing for redness, tenderness, swelling, and drainage.	
• Assess the patency of the VAD by aspiration of a blood return, absence of resistance when flushing, and complaints of patient pain or discomfort when flushing.	
• If necessary, place a VAD for transfusion purposes:	
a. Administer blood or blood components to an adult through short peripheral catheter (an 18- to 20-gauge catheter is appropriate for the general population) (Gorski, 2023; INS, 2021).	The gauge of the IV cannula should be appropriate for accommodating the infusion of blood and/or blood components (INS, 2021).
b. Transfuse an adult patient using proper gauge catheter (INS, 2021): *Adults:* Use a 20- to 24-gauge device. For rapid transfusion, use an 18- to 20- gauge device. *Infants/children:* Use umbilical vein for neonates; 22- to 24-gauge device for other children.	Use of smaller cannula gauges such as 24 gauge often requires the blood bank to divide the unit so each half can be infused within allotted time or with pressure-assisted devices.
c. Central vascular access devices (CVADs) may be used for a transfusion (INS, 2021).	Use for blood administration depends on catheter gauge and manufacturer recommendations for use.
7. Remove and dispose of gloves. Perform hand hygiene.	Reduces transmission of microorganisms.
8. Check that patient has completed and signed transfusion consent form properly before retrieving blood. Determine if patient has any remaining questions.	Informed consent is required before transfusion and includes risks, benefits, and treatment alternatives; right to accept or refuse transfusion; and opportunity to ask questions (AABB, 2018; INS, 2021). Administration of albumin does not require informed consent.
9. Review EHR to confirm indications or reasons for transfusion (e.g., packed red blood cells [PRBCs] for patient with low Hct level from gastrointestinal bleeding or surgery blood loss).	Allows you to anticipate patient's response to therapy.
10. Obtain and document pretransfusion baseline vital signs (temperature, pulse, respirations, and blood pressure) within 30 minutes prior to transfusion (INS, 2021). If patient is febrile (temperature greater than 37.8°C [100°F]), notify health care provider before initiating transfusion.	Change from baseline vital signs during infusion alerts nurse to potential transfusion reaction or adverse effect of therapy (Gorski, 2023).

Clinical Judgment *A fever may be a cause for delaying a transfusion (INS, 2021).*

11. Assess patient's need for IV fluids or medications to be given while transfusion is infusing. Administer blood or blood components only with 0.9% sodium chloride (NS) (INS, 2021).	If IV medications need to be administered during transfusion, a second IV site is necessary. Do not add or infuse any other solutions or medications through same IV administration set with blood or blood components, including piggyback (INS, 2021).
12. Assess patient's knowledge of a prior experience with a blood transfusion and feelings about procedure. Allow patient to express religious/cultural beliefs about transfusion (INS, 2021).	Reveals need for patient instruction and/or support.

STEP	RATIONALE

PLANNING

1. Expected outcomes following completion of the procedure:
   - Patient verbalizes understanding of rationale for therapy.

   - Mucous membranes are pink, and patient has brisk capillary refill.
   - Patient's cardiac output returns to baseline.
   - Patient's systolic blood pressure improves from baseline, and urine output is 0.5 to 1 mL/kg/h.
   - Patient's laboratory values improve in targeted areas.

2. Close room doors and prepare environment.
3. Ask patient to void. If patient is unable to void, apply clean gloves and empty urine drainage collection container.

4. Perform hand hygiene. Collect equipment and organize on clean, clutter-free bedside stand or over-bed table.
5. Explain procedure to patient and family caregiver: Review compatibility testing and vascular access. Explains signs and symptoms associated with complications of transfusion (e.g., chills, uneasy feeling, flushing or fever, nausea) (INS, 2021).

Indicates patient's understanding and ability to make informed decision for consent.
Tissue perfusion is improved.

Intravascular volume is restored.
Parameters reflect optimal fluid status and adequate renal blood flow.
Indicates that patient responds appropriately to blood or blood component infusion.
Promotes patient comfort and efficiency of procedure.
Provides baseline urine specimen. If transfusion reaction occurs, urine specimen containing urine produced after initiation of transfusion will be obtained and sent to laboratory for comparison.
Reduces transmission of infection and contamination of equipment.

Decreases anxiety, promotes cooperation, and gives patient knowledge to recognize problems.

IMPLEMENTATION

1. Preadministration protocol:
   a. Obtain blood component from blood bank, following agency protocol (see illustration). Check patient and blood product identification.
   b. Observe and check blood bag for any signs of contamination at the time it is released from blood bank. Do not use if container not intact or if abnormal color, clots, excessive air/bubbles, or unusual odor is present (INS, 2021).
   c. At bedside, identify patient using at least two identifiers (e.g., name and birthday or name and medical record number) according to agency policy. Compare identifiers with information on patient's medication administration record (MAR) or electronic health record (EHR).

Timely acquisition ensures that product is safe to administer. Agency protocol usually encompasses safeguards to ensure quality control throughout transfusion process.
Blood should not be infused if integrity is compromised. Blood is a medium for bacterial growth. Air bubbles, clumping, clots, and discoloration can indicate bacterial contamination or inadequate anticoagulation of stored component. Findings contraindicate transfusion of that product (Gorski, 2023).
Ensures correct patient. Complies with The Joint Commission standards and improves patient safety (TJC, 2023). Two independent identifiers are required for transfusion (INS, 2021).

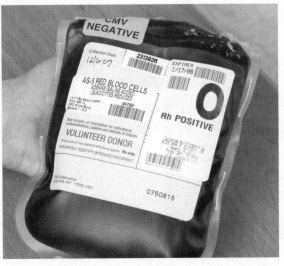

STEP 1a Unit of blood with label.

STEP	RATIONALE
d. With another RN at patient's bedside, verify information on blood unit and in EHR (see illustration): • Check that transfusion record number and patient's identification number match • Check that patient's name is correct on all documents • Check unit number on blood bag with blood bank form to ensure they match • Check that blood type matches on transfusion record and blood bag. Verify that component received from blood bank is same component that health care provider ordered (e.g., PRBCs, platelets). • Check that patient's blood type and Rh type are compatible with donor blood type and Rh type (e.g., Patient A+: Donor A+ or O+). • Check special transfusion requirements • Check expiration date/time on blood unit and date/time released from blood bank	Standards for ensuring right blood is administered to right patient (INS, 2021). Independent double check by two adults in presence of patient is required (INS, 2021). Verifies accurate blood donor type and compatibility with patient. Never infuse expired blood. Blood components deteriorate.

Clinical Judgment *If you notice a discrepancy during the verification procedure, do not administer the product. Notify blood bank and appropriate personnel as indicated by agency policy. The product should be returned to the blood bank until the discrepancy has been resolved (Gorski, 2023; INS, 2021).*

STEP	RATIONALE
e. Just before initiating transfusion, check patient identification information one more time with blood unit label information (see illustration). Be sure patient's name is on label. Do not administer blood to patient without identification bracelet or blood identification bracelet (see agency policy). Check one more time that patient's blood type and Rh type are compatible with donor blood type and Rh type.	Serves as last point of patient and blood confirmation (Gorski, 2023). Verifies accurate donor blood type and compatibility (INS, 2021).
f. Both nurses verify patient and unit identification record process as directed by agency policy.	Documentation is legal medical record.
g. Review purpose of transfusion and ask patient to report any changes noticed during the transfusion.	Signs and symptoms of transfusion reactions include chills, low back pain, shortness of breath, rash, hives, or itching (Gorski, 2023). Prompt notification aids in early intervention.

Clinical Judgment *Blood transfusion should be initiated within 30 minutes from time of release from blood bank. If this cannot be completed because of factors such as an elevated temperature, immediately return the blood to the blood bank and retrieve it when you can administer it (Gorski, 2023). Repeat preadministration process. It is important that the blood bag not be spiked until you ensure that no factors exist preventing transfusion.*

2. Administration:

STEP	RATIONALE
a. Perform hand hygiene. Apply clean gloves. Reinspect blood product for signs of leakage or unusual appearance.	Using Standard Precautions reduces risk for transmission of microorganisms. Provides ongoing verification of blood product.

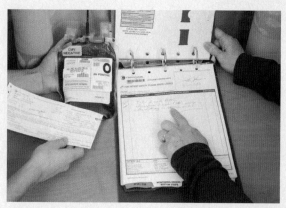

STEP 1d Two clinicians verifying blood type with health care provider order.

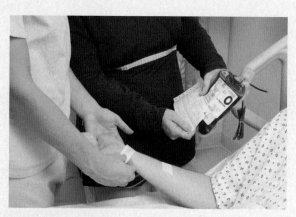

STEP 1e Two clinicians verifying identification of patient and blood product.

STEP	RATIONALE

b. Open standard Y-tubing blood administration set with filter, for single unit. Use multiset if multiple units are to be transfused.

Y-tubing facilitates maintenance of IV line access with NS in case patient will need more than 1 unit of blood.

c. Set all clamp(s) to "off" position.

Setting clamps to "off" position prevents accidentally spilling and wasting product.

d. Use aseptic technique and spike 0.9% sodium chloride (NS) IV bag with one of Y-tubing spikes (INS, 2021). Hang bag on IV pole and prime tubing. Open upper clamp on NS side of tubing and squeeze drip chamber until fluid covers filter and one-third to one-half of drip chamber.

Primes tubing with fluid to eliminate air in Y-tubing. Closing clamp prevents spillage and waste of fluid.

e. Maintain clamp on blood product side of Y-tubing in "off" position. Open common tubing clamp to finish priming tubing to distal end of tubing connector with NS. Close tubing clamp when tubing is filled with saline. All three tubing clamps should now be closed. Maintain protective sterile cap on tubing connector.

This will completely prime tubing with saline, and IV line is ready to be connected to patient's VAD.

f. Prepare blood component for administration. Gently invert bag 2 or 3 times, turning back and forth. Remove protective covering from access port. Spike blood component unit with the other Y-connector. Close the NS clamp above filter. Open clamp above filter to blood unit, and prime tubing with blood. Blood will flow into drip chamber (see illustration). Tap filter chamber to remove residual air. Close clamp when tubing is filled. Apply cap to end of tubing.

Gentle agitation suspends red blood cells in anticoagulant. Protective barrier drape may be used to catch any potential blood spillage. Tubing is primed with blood unit and ready for transfusion into patient.

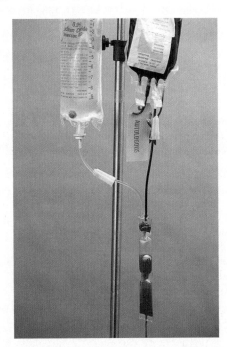

STEP 2f Unit of blood connected to Y-tubing setup.

Clinical Judgment *Normal saline (NS; 0.9% sodium chloride) is compatible with blood products, unlike solutions that contain dextrose, which cause blood coagulation. Use only 0.9% NS to administer blood. No other solutions are to be administered with blood (piggybacked) (Gorski, 2023; INS, 2021).*

g. *Option:* Infuse with electronic infusion device (EID). Maintaining asepsis, insert infusion tubing into chamber of control mechanism of EID. Be sure you are using EID indicated for blood administration (follow manufacturer's directions) (INS, 2021). Roller clamp on IV tubing goes between EID and patient. Secure tubing through "air in line" alarm system. Close door and turn on power button. Select required administration rate.

Reduces transmission of microorganisms from catheter hub. Establishes infusion line. Avoid use of needleless connectors for rapid flow rates for red blood cell infusion, which can greatly reduce blood flow (INS, 2021). EIDs that have a labeled indication for blood transfusion should be used. EIDs can be used to deliver blood or blood components without significant risk of hemolysis of RBCs or platelet damage (INS, 2021).

STEP	RATIONALE
h. Remove cap and attach primed tubing to patient's VAD by first cleansing the catheter hub with an antiseptic swab. Then connect NS-primed blood administration tubing directly to patient's VAD.	Establishes sterile intact system.
i. Open common tubing clamp and the clamp to blood bag. Regulate blood infusion to allow only 2 mL/min to infuse in initial 15 minutes. Remain with patient during first 15 minutes of transfusion (INS, 2021). Initial flow rate during this time should be 1–2 mL/min or 10–20 gtt/min (using macrodrip of 10 gtt/mL).	Many transfusion reactions occur within first 15 minutes of transfusion (Gorski, 2023). Infusing small amount of blood component initially minimizes volume of blood to which patient is exposed, thereby minimizing severity of reaction (Gorski, 2023).
j. Monitor patient's vital signs within 15 minutes of initiating transfusion, upon completion of transfusion, and 1 hour after transfusion completed or more often if patient condition is warranted (INS, 2021; Gorski, 2023).	Frequently monitoring patient helps to quickly alert you to transfusion reaction. The three most common causes of transfusion-related mortality are transfusion-related acute lung injury (TRALI), acute hemolytic transfusion reaction (AHTR), and transfusion-associated circulatory overload (TACO) (AABB, 2022).
k. Assess the patient for any adverse reactions at least every 30 minutes during transfusion (INS, 2021).	Ensures early identification of transfusion complication.

Clinical Judgment *If signs of a transfusion reaction occur (see Table 29.2),* **stop the transfusion,** *start 0.9% sodium chloride (normal saline [NS]) with a new primed tubing attached directly to the vascular access device (VAD) hub, and notify the health care provider immediately (see Skill 29.2). Do not discard the blood product or tubing because they need to be returned to the blood bank. Do not infuse saline through existing tubing because it will cause blood in tubing to enter patient.*

l. If there is no transfusion reaction, regulate rate of transfusion according to health care provider's orders based on drop factor for blood administration tubing (see Chapter 28).	Maintaining prescribed rate of flow decreases risk for fluid volume excess while restoring vascular volume. Drop factor for most blood tubing is 10 gtt/mL.

Clinical Judgment *Administer and complete each unit of blood or blood component within 4 hours. Administer platelets over 1 to 2 hours. Administer plasma as quickly as tolerated by patient or over 15 to 60 minutes (INS, 2021). When a longer transfusion time is indicated clinically, the unit may be divided by the blood bank, and the part not being transfused can be properly refrigerated. Administration sets should be changed in conjunction with manufacturer's directions (INS, 2021).*

Clinical Judgment *Do not infuse medications and solutions into the same intravenous (IV) line with a blood component because of the possibility of incompatibility unless the drug or solution has been approved by the U.S. Food and Drug Administration (FDA) for use with blood administration. Maintain a separate IV access if patient requires IV solutions or medications (Gorski, 2023).*

m. After blood has infused, turn off EID and turn off clamp to blood bag. Remove tubing from EID. Clear IV line with 0.9% sodium chloride (NS) by opening clamp to NS bag and infusing slowly. Once tubing is clear, regulate IV (using EID to ordered rate). Discard blood bag according to agency policy. When consecutive units are ordered, maintain line patency with 0.9% sodium chloride (NS) at a keep vein open (KVO) rate as ordered by health care provider and retrieve subsequent unit for administration.	Infusing IV NS allows remainder of blood in IV tubing to infuse and keeps IV line patent for supportive measures in case of transfusion reaction (Gorski, 2023). KVO rate must specify infusion rate as required by the seven rights of medication administration.
3. Help patient to a comfortable position.	Restores comfort and sense of well-being.
4. Place nurse call system in an accessible location within patient's reach.	Ensures patient can call for assistance if needed.
5. Raise side rails (as appropriate) and lower bed to lowest position, locking into position.	Ensures patient safety and prevents falls.
6. Dispose of all contaminated supplies in appropriate receptacle, remove and dispose of gloves, and perform hand hygiene.	Reduces transmission of microorganisms. Use appropriate disposal receptacle if patient is on hazardous drugs (Nyhus, 2022).

STEP	RATIONALE

EVALUATION

1. Observe IV site and status of infusion each time vital signs are taken.

Detects presence of IV-related complications (e.g., infiltration, occlusion, phlebitis) and verifies continuous and safe infusion of blood product.

2. Observe for any signs of transfusion reactions (see Table 29.2) for at least 4 to 6 hours to detect febrile or pulmonary reactions (INS, 2021).

Compare presenting signs and symptoms to baseline assessment of patient before transfusion.

3. Observe patient and assess laboratory values to determine response to administration of blood component.

Determines whether goals of therapy have been reached or if further blood component therapy will be required. Laboratory results may not reflect transfusion reaction for several hours.

4. Monitor urine output.

Reflects adequate renal blood flow.

5. Use Teach-Back: "I want to be sure that I explained the reason for your blood transfusion, including the risks and benefits. How can this transfusion help you?" Revise your instruction now or develop a plan for revised patient/family caregiver teaching if patient/family caregiver is not able to teach back correctly.

Teach-back is a technique for health care providers to ensure that they have explained medical information clearly so that patients and their families understand what is communicated to them (Agency for Healthcare Research and Quality [AHRQ], 2023).

Unexpected Outcomes

Related Interventions

1. Patient displays signs and symptoms of transfusion reaction (see Table 29.2). The most common side effects include fever, chills, urticaria, and itching (Suddock & Crookston, 2022).

- Stop transfusion immediately.
- See Table 29.2 for interventions.
- Do not administer emergency medications through the blood administration set; prime a new administration set with 0.9% sodium chloride for infusion through the VAD (INS, 2021).

2. Patient develops infiltration or phlebitis at venipuncture site.

- Stop transfusion at first sign of infiltration, and remove IV line (see Procedural Guideline 28.1).
- Insert new VAD in area above previous location or opposite arm.
- Restart product if remainder can be infused within 4 hours of initiation of transfusion.
- Institute nursing measures to reduce discomfort at infiltrated or phlebitic area.

3. Fluid volume overload occurs, and/or patient exhibits difficulty breathing or has crackles on auscultation of lungs.

- Slow or stop transfusion, elevate head of bed, and inform health care provider of physical findings.
- Administer diuretics, morphine, and/or oxygen as ordered by health care provider.
- Continue frequent assessments and closely monitor vital signs and intake and output.

Documentation

- Before transfusion, document pretransfusion medications, vital signs, location and condition of IV site, and patient/family caregiver education.
- Document the type and volume of blood component, blood unit/donor/recipient identification, compatibility, and expiration date according to agency policy, along with patient's response to therapy.
- Document volume of NS and blood component infused.
- Document amount of blood received by autotransfusion and patient's response to therapy.
- Document vital signs 15 minutes after initiating transfusion, on completion of transfusion, and 1 hour after completion.
- Document your evaluation of patient and family caregiver learning.

Hand-Off Reporting

- Report signs and symptoms of a transfusion reaction immediately to the health care provider.

- Report to health care provider any intratransfusion or post-transfusion deterioration in cardiac, pulmonary, and/or renal status.

Special Considerations

Patient Education

- Instruct patient and family caregiver about rationale for transfusion, anticipated amount of time for completion of transfusion, and possible signs and symptoms of complications.
- Discuss with patient and family caregiver the rationale for patient monitoring throughout transfusion.
- Instruct patient and family caregiver to notify nurse if patient experiences itching, swelling, dizziness, fever, dyspnea, low back pain, and/or chest pain (indicators of a transfusion reaction).
- Instruct patient and family caregiver to inform nurse if redness, pain, tenderness, swelling, bleeding, drainage, or leaking from under dressing occurs at IV site.

Pediatrics

- Infuse the first 50 mL or 20% of volume (whichever is smaller) of a blood transfusion very slowly in a pediatric patient. Stay with the child during this time (Hockenberry et al., 2024).

Older Adults

- Some older adults have decreased cardiac function and therefore require a slower infusion time. Half units may be obtained if a patient is unable to tolerate the volume in a whole unit of blood or blood component.
- In older adults at risk for circulatory overload, regulate flow rate at 1 mL/kg/h.

Home Care

- Blood administration within the home setting is not routine. However, it is available to increase the accessibility and convenience of care to chronically ill patients (Fridey, 2022). The Infusion Nurses Society (INS, 2021) recommends the following for home transfusions:
  - Documentation showing no identified adverse events during previous transfusions
  - Immediate access to the health care provider by phone during the transfusion
  - Presence of another competent adult in the home who is available to assist with patient identification and call for medical assistance if needed
  - Ability to transport blood product in appropriate containers
  - Ability to appropriately dispose of medical waste
- Have family caregiver return the waste container, empty blood unit bags, and tubing to the home care agency after completion of the transfusion.

✦ SKILL 29.2 Monitoring for Adverse Transfusion Reactions

Adverse transfusion reactions may occur at any time during a transfusion of blood products. Life-threatening reactions usually occur within the first 15 minutes of transfusion; however, the Infusion Nurses Society (INS, 2021) recommends monitoring patients for reactions for at least 4 to 6 hours after a transfusion. Several types of adverse reactions may result from a blood transfusion (see Table 29.2). An acute hemolytic transfusion reaction (AHTR) is a systemic response to the administration of a blood product that is incompatible with the recipient. The product contains allergens to which the recipient is sensitive or allergic, or it is contaminated with pathogens. Some patients who have a history of frequent transfusion may receive premedication with diphenhydramine to combat acquired sensitivities.

Before a transfusion, each blood unit undergoes extensive serological testing to reduce the risk that patients will acquire a blood-borne disease. Symptoms that indicate an adverse reaction range from fever, chills, and skin rash to hypotension and cardiac arrest. Some patients also experience a delayed transfusion reaction, which sometimes does not occur for days or weeks after the transfusion (Gorski, 2023). Other possible adverse outcomes that result from transfusion therapy include transmission of diseases, circulatory overload, and transfusion-related acute lung injury (TRALI), characterized by noncardiogenic pulmonary edema with an onset within 6 hours of transfusion. The greatest risk for transfusion-associated death is the erroneous transfusion of ABO-incompatible allogeneic units (Gorski, 2023).

Microchimerism is the presence of cells from one person in another genetically different individual, usually the result of pregnancy. Transfusion-associated microchimerism (TA-MC) has been identified as one of the complications of blood transfusion. Microchimerism from non-leukoreduced blood products has been found to persist for months to years after the transfusion. This most commonly occurs from a transfusion-related reaction as the result of an antigen-antibody reaction (Shrivastava et al., 2019).

Delegation

The skill of monitoring for blood transfusion reactions cannot be delegated to assistive personnel (AP). The skill of monitoring for adverse blood transfusion reactions by a licensed practical nurse (LPN) varies by state nurse practice acts. After a transfusion has been started and the patient is stable, monitoring of a patient by AP does not relieve a registered nurse (RN) of the responsibility to continue to assess the patient during the transfusion. Instruct the AP about:

- Frequency of vital sign monitoring needed
- The signs and symptoms of a transfusion reaction that patient may exhibit and to immediately report these to the nurse

Interprofessional Collaboration

- Contact blood bank personnel as per agency policy if a reaction occurs.
- Collaborate with the respiratory therapist and other critical care health care providers as needed to manage patients with blood transfusion reactions.

Equipment

- Vital sign equipment (stethoscope, sphygmomanometer, thermometer, pulse oximeter)

STEP	RATIONALE

ASSESSMENT

1. Identify patient using at least two identifiers (e.g., name and birthday or name and medical record number) according to agency policy.	Ensures correct patient. Complies with The Joint Commission standards and improves patient safety (TJC, 2023).
2. Assess patient's/family caregiver's health literacy.	Determines degree to which individuals have the ability to find, understand, and use information and services to make informed health-related decisions and actions for themselves and others (CDC, 2023).

STEP	RATIONALE
3. Perform hand hygiene and apply clean gloves (as needed). Monitor vital signs and pulse oximetry continuously every 15 minutes or per agency policy. Specifically note the following:	
a. With initiation of a transfusion, observe patient for fever with or without chills.	Fever indicates onset of AHTR, febrile nonhemolytic reaction, or bacterial sepsis.
b. Assess patient for tachycardia and/or tachypnea and dyspnea.	Indicates AHTR or circulatory overload. In case of circulatory overload, cough may accompany these symptoms.
c. Assess patient for drop in blood pressure.	Hypotension indicates infectious disease transmission, AHTR, and anaphylaxis.
d. Auscultate lungs before and during procedure and observe patient for wheezing, chest pain, and possible cardiac arrest.	These are all indications of anaphylactic reaction.
4. Observe patient for urticaria or skin rash and itching, including assessment of trunk and back.	These are early indications of an allergic reaction, anaphylaxis, or graft-versus-host disease, which occurs after transfusion.
5. Observe patient for flushing.	Early indication of AHTR or febrile nonhemolytic reaction. Sometimes localized flushing presents with an allergic reaction.
6. Observe patient for gastrointestinal symptoms (e.g., nausea and vomiting).	Present in AHTR, anaphylactic reactions, or infectious disease transmission.
7. Be alert to patient complaints of headache or muscle pain in presence of fever.	Both indicate febrile nonhemolytic reaction.
8. Monitor patient for disseminated intravascular coagulation (DIC), renal failure, anemia, and hemoglobinemia/hemoglobinuria by reviewing laboratory test results (complete blood count [CBC] with differential, hemoglobin [Hgb], hematocrit [Hct]).	All are late signs of AHTR.
9. Monitor pulse oximetry and central venous pressure (CVP) if possible.	Crackles in bases of lungs and rising CVP are indications of circulatory overload. Oxygen saturation improves with red blood cell (RBC) transfusion.
10. Observe patient for jaundice and laboratory values for increased liver enzyme levels, indicating liver damage; and for decreased RBCs, white blood cells (WBCs), and platelets, indicating bone marrow suppression.	These indicate graft-versus-host disease and would occur following transfusion.
11. In patients receiving massive transfusions, observe for mild hypothermia, cardiac dysrhythmias, hypotension, hypocalcemia, and hemochromatosis (iron overload).	Cold blood products affect cardiac conduction system, resulting in ventricular dysrhythmias. Other cardiac dysrhythmias, hypotension, and tingling indicate hypocalcemia, which occurs when citrate (used as a preservative for some blood products) combines with patient's calcium. Iron overload may occur after 10 transfusions (see Table 29.2). It usually occurs in patients who require chronic transfusions.
12. Be sure patient is understanding what is occurring during your response.	Promotes patient cooperation with aim of reducing anxiety.
13. Assess patient's knowledge of and prior experience with transfusion reaction and feelings about outcome.	Reveals need for patient instruction and/or support.

PLANNING

1. Expected outcomes following completion of procedure:	
• Patient's cardiac parameters (heart rate, blood pressure, SpO$_2$, CVP) return to baseline.	Intravascular volume is restored, reaction reversed.
• Patient maintains core body temperature of 36°C to 37.2°C (97°F to 99°F).	Helps to confirm absence of transfusion reaction, infection, and sepsis.
• Patient has urine output of 0.5 to 1 mL/kg/h.	Reflects optimal fluid status.
• Patient maintains oxygen saturation greater than 95%.	Improved tissue perfusion.
• Patient is comfortable.	Absence of transfusion reaction. Appropriate nursing measures keep patient at ease.
2. Explain need for monitoring to patient. Discuss signs and symptoms of transfusion reaction.	Reduces anxiety and promotes cooperation.
3. Close room door and bedside curtain. Perform hand hygiene.	Provides patient privacy. Reduces transmission of microorganisms.

STEP	RATIONALE

IMPLEMENTATION

1. If you suspect transfusion reaction:

    a. Immediately stop transfusion.

    Severity of reaction is related to amount of blood component infused and cause of reaction. It is critical to prevent any more blood from infusing into patient.

    b. Remove blood component and tubing containing blood product. Replace them with new bag of 0.9% sodium chloride (normal saline [NS]) and tubing (see Chapter 28) (INS, 2021). Connect tubing directly to hub of vascular access device (VAD).

    Prevents additional blood in tubing from being infused.

        Exception: If patient symptoms suggest mild allergic reaction, stop transfusion, administer antihistamine, and later restart or discontinue transfusion per health care provider's order.

    c. Maintain patent VAD by opening 0.9% sodium chloride (NS) infusion and regulate at a keep vein open (KVO) rate until you contact health care provider for order.

    NS keeps patent IV and provides route for emergency medications and fluids.

    d. Notify health care provider.

    Transfusion reactions require immediate medical intervention. Follow protocol for emergency interventions for anaphylactic reactions.

    e. Notify blood bank.

    Blood bank has procedure to follow when notified of transfusion reaction.

    f. Remain with patient for continuous monitoring and assessment. *Do not leave patient alone.*

    Patient's response will dictate treatment ordered.

    g. Obtain blood samples (if needed) from extremity opposite extremity receiving transfusion. Check agency policy regarding number and type of tubes to be used.

    Typically, one tube of blood will be cross-matched to pretransfusion sample to ensure that correct blood was given to recipient. Blood will be checked for antibodies to determine type of reaction. Second sample will be checked for free Hgb in serum, indicating hemolysis, and bilirubin level should be obtained.

    h. Return remainder of blood component and attached blood tubing to blood bank according to agency policy.

    Sample of this blood will be cross-matched to patient's pretransfusion and posttransfusion samples to determine if error in cross-matching occurred.

    i. Administer prescribed medications according to type and severity of transfusion reaction.

    Follow medical protocol or health care provider's orders.

        (1) Epinephrine

        Stimulates sympathetic nervous system to relieve respiratory distress and combat vasodilation in anaphylaxis.

        (2) Antihistamine

        Diminishes allergic response by blocking histamine receptors.

Clinical Judgment *Antihistamines have been linked to patient falls (Cho, 2018). Carefully monitor patients who attempt to ambulate.*

        (3) Antibiotics

        Administered when bacterial contamination/sepsis is suspected.

        (4) Antipyretics/analgesics

        Administered to relieve fever and discomfort in reactions and bacterial sepsis.

        (5) Diuretics/morphine

        Treats circulatory overload by reducing intravascular volume (diuresis) and decreasing vascular tone (opioid effect).

        (6) Corticosteroids

        Stabilizes cell membranes, decreasing histamine release. Administered in severe allergic reactions.

        (7) Intravenous (IV) fluids

        Rapid administration of IV fluids counteracts some symptoms of anaphylactic shock.

    j. In the event of cardiac arrest, initiate cardiopulmonary resuscitation (see Chapter 27).

    Anaphylaxis can quickly lead to cardiopulmonary arrest. Prompt resuscitation may prevent further complications.

    k. Obtain first voided urine sample following reaction and send to laboratory. You may need to insert Foley catheter to obtain urine (see Chapter 33).

    Hemoglobinuria occurs with AHTR. Degree of damage to kidneys is influenced by pH of urine and rate of urinary excretion. Attempts will be made to initiate diuresis and alkalinize urine. If kidney damage is severe, dialysis may be required.

2. Help patient to a comfortable position.

Restores comfort and sense of well-being.

3. Place nurse call system in an accessible location within patient's reach.

Ensures patient can call for assistance if needed.

STEP	RATIONALE
4. Raise side rails (as appropriate) and lower bed to lowest position, locking into position.	Ensures patient safety and prevents falls.
5. Dispose of all contaminated supplies in appropriate receptacle, remove and dispose of gloves, and perform hand hygiene.	Reduces transmission of microorganisms.

EVALUATION

1. Continue monitoring patient for signs and symptoms of transfusion reactions.	Continued monitoring of patient's cardiopulmonary status and physiological response will indicate if reaction has been reversed.
2. **Use Teach-Back:** "I want to be sure that I explained the reactions that developed as you were getting your blood transfusion. What signs and symptoms told us you were having a reaction?" Revise your instruction now or develop a plan for revised patient/family caregiver teaching if patient/family caregiver is not able to teach back correctly.	Teach-back is a technique for health care providers to ensure that they have explained medical information clearly so that patients and their families understand what is communicated to them (AHRQ, 2023).

Unexpected Outcomes

1. Patient's physiological status worsens.

Related Interventions

- Appropriate interventions depend on type of transfusion reaction. Table 29.2 provides general guidelines.

Documentation

- Document the exact time transfusion reaction was first noted, all vital signs and other physiological assessments, treatments instituted, and patient response. Complete transfusion reaction report (see agency policy).
- Document your evaluation of patient and family caregiver learning.

Hand-Off Reporting

- Immediately report presence of transfusion reaction and patient's physical assessment findings to nurse in charge and health care provider.

Special Considerations

Patient Education

- Teach patient and family caregiver signs and symptoms of transfusion reactions and steps to take if they occur.

Pediatrics

- Irradiated RBCs and platelets are preferable in children younger than 6 years because of their immature immune systems and to avoid graft-versus-host disease.

Older Adults

- Administer blood components cautiously to older adults, considering both rate and amount of infusion, because they are at risk for developing circulatory overload.

Home Care

- Certain adverse outcomes (development of hepatitis) or transfusion reactions (delayed hemolysis) occur days to weeks after patient has received transfusion and may become evident in the home setting. It is important that patient, family caregiver, and home care workers be aware of signs and symptoms of adverse occurrences and steps to be taken should they occur.

A 72-year-old patient was to have a hip replacement a month ago and donated 1 unit of autologous blood in case a transfusion was needed. Three weeks ago the patient developed bleeding colon polyps, which were surgically repaired yesterday. Today the patient reports feeling very tired and has passed blood with several bowel movements during the night and earlier this morning. The nurse assesses the patient to be pale, with skin that is cool to the touch. The blood pressure has changed from 130/80 mm Hg to 110/72 mm Hg. The heart rate is 82 beats/min, and the respiratory rate is 14 breaths/min. The patient had blood drawn this morning; the hematocrit (Hct) has dropped from 36% to 32%. Blood glucose is 92 mg/dL. The patient asks the nurse, "If I need a transfusion, can you use the blood I donated before surgery?"

1. The nurse will address the patient's **1 [Select]** and **2 [Select]** as the priorities of care.

Options for 1	Options for 2
Heart rate	Hematocrit
Blood in stool	Blood glucose
Blood pressure	Fatigue
Respiratory rate	Question about autologous blood donation

2. The health care provider orders a blood transfusion, and a unit of packed red blood cells (PRBCs) is sent to the unit. Prior to arrival of the PRBCs, the patient is taken for a CT scan of the abdomen and is not expected to return for over an hour. Which action will the nurse take?
   1. Place the PRBCs in a refrigerator on the unit.
   2. Return the PRBCs to the blood bank.
   3. Go to the imaging location to administer the PRBCs.
   4. Leave the PRBCs in the patient's room to administer upon return.

3. When the patient returns to the unit, the blood bank sends up PRBCs again. Which of the following items must be verified at the patient's bedside to ensure that the correct blood component is transfused to the correct patient? **Select all that apply.**
   1. Identify the patient's identity verbally using two approved patient identifiers.
   2. Confirm that the transfusion record number matches the patient's identification number.
   3. Check that the blood unit expiration date is not passed.
   4. Verify that the blood component and type to be infused match the patient's.
   5. Have two qualified individuals perform verifications before initiation of transfusion.

4. The nurse has set up supplies to administer the transfusion. Which of the following actions would the nurse take to administer the PRBCs? **Select all that apply.**
   1. Verify the health care provider's order for PRBCs, number of units, date and time to give, duration, and pretransfusion medications.
   2. Ensure that the patient has a patent, working VAD, then obtain PRBCs from blood bank.
   3. Verify that the correct product was obtained and patient's ABO and Rh types are compatible, and match product obtained with another qualified person (e.g., nurse).
   4. Administer PRBCs over 2 hours; take vital signs before transfusion, 15 minutes after beginning transfusion, and at completion of transfusion.
   5. Prior to initiating transfusion, check product expiration date and verify that patient identification number matches transfusion number and that PRBC unit number matches blood bank form with another qualified person (e.g., nurse).

5. During the infusion, the patient begins to exhibit shortness of breath. Which action will the nurse take first?
   1. Obtain vital signs.
   2. Stop the infusion of PRBCs.
   3. Contact the blood bank.
   4. Notify the health care provider.

Visit the Evolve site for Answers to the Clinical Judgment and Next-Generation NCLEX® Examination–Style Questions.

REFERENCES

Agency for Healthcare Research and Quality (AHRQ): *Teach-back: intervention*, 2023. https://www.ahrq.gov/patient-safety/reports/engage/interventions/teach-back.html.

AABB (formerly American Association of Blood Banks): *Technical manual for transfusing blood and blood products*, ed 20, Bethesda, MD, 2023, AABB.

AABB (formerly American Association of Blood Banks): *Standards for blood banks and transfusion services*, ed 33, Bethesda, MD, 2022, AABB.

AABB (formerly American Association of Blood Banks): *AABB primer of blood administration*, Bethesda, MD, 2018, AABB.

Centers for Disease Control and Prevention (CDC): *Monitoring blood safety*, 2022. https://www.cdc.gov/bloodsafety/monitoring/blood_safety.html. Accessed May 4, 2023.

Centers for Disease Control and Prevention (CDC): *What is health literacy?* 2023. https://www.cdc.gov/healthliteracy/learn/index.html.

Cho H, et al: Antihistamine use and the risk of injurious falls or fracture in elderly patients: a systematic review and meta-analysis, *Osteoporos Int* 29(10):2163–2170, 2018.

Duncan R: *Food and drug administration (FDA): advanced technology for reducing the risk of transmission by transfusion*, 2022. https://www.fda.gov/vaccines-blood-biologics/biologics-research-projects/advanced-technology-reducing-risk-transmission-transfusion.

Fang DC, Pham HP: *Transfusion medicine: blood bank testing, pretransfusion testing*, Pathology Outlines.com, 2021. https://www.pathologyoutlines.com/topic/transfusionmedpretransfusiontesting.html. Accessed October 23, 2023.

Fridey JL: *General principles of home blood transfusion*, 2022, Up-To-Date. https://www.uptodate.com/contents/general-principles-of-home-blood-transfusion#!. Accessed May 4, 2023.

Gorski L: *Phillips's manual of IV therapeutics: evidence-based practice for infusion therapy*, ed 8, Philadelphia, 2023, FA Davis.

Hockenberry MJ, et al: *Wong's nursing care of infants and children*, ed 12, St. Louis, 2024, Elsevier.

Infusion Nurses Society (INS): Infusion therapy standards of practice, 8 edition, *J Intraven Nurs* 44(1S):S1-S224, 2021.

National Heart, Lung, and Blood Institute (NHLBI): *Blood disorders and blood safety*, n.d. https://www.nhlbi.nih.gov/science/blood-disorders-and-blood-safety. Accessed May 4, 2023.

Nyhus J: *Handling hazardous drugs in healthcare*, 2022, American Nurse. https://www.myamericannurse.com/handling-hazardous-drugs-in-healthcare/. Accessed May 3, 2023.

Shaz B, et al: *Transfusion medicine and hemostasis: clinical and laboratory aspects*, ed 3, St. Louis, 2019, Elsevier: Science Direct.

Shrivastava S, et al: Microchimerism: a new concept, *J Oral Maxillofac Pathol* 23(2):311, 2019.

Suddock JT, Crookston KP: Transfusion reactions. In *StatPearls* [Internet], NIH, National Library of Medicine, 2022. https://www.ncbi.nlm.nih.gov/books/NBK482202/. Accessed May 4, 2023.

Teruya J: *Red blood cell transfusion in infants and children: selection of blood products*, 2022, UpToDate. https://www.uptodate.com/contents/red-blood-cell-transfusion-in-infants-and-children-selection-of-blood-products.

The Joint Commission (TJC): *2023 National Patient Safety Goals*, Oakbrook Terrace, IL, 2023, The Joint Commission. https://www.jointcommission.org/standards/national-patient-safety-goals/. Accessed May 4, 2023.

Uhl L: *Pretransfusion testing for red blood cell transfusion*, 2022, UpToDate. https://www.uptodate.com/contents/pretransfusion-testing-for-red-blood-cell-transfusion. Accessed May 4, 2023.

Wu D, et al: The impact of nucleic acid testing to detect human immunodeficiency virus, hepatitis C virus, and hepatitis B virus yields from a single blood center in China with 10-years review, *BMC Infect Dis* 22:279, 2022.

UNIT 10
Fluid Balance: Next-Generation NCLEX® (NGN)–Style Unfolding Case Study

PHASE 1

QUESTION 1.
The nurse is reviewing notes for a client who is to receive a simple transfusion.

Highlight the findings that indicate to the nurse why the client may be here for a transfusion.

History and Physical	Nurses' Notes	Vital Signs	Laboratory Results

0902 52-year-old client here for transfusion today. History of seasonal allergies to pollens. Was recently seen at urgent care after twisting their ankle while walking. Client is scheduled in several weeks for elective rhinoplasty surgery to reduce the size of their nose. Has a history of hemophilia. Preoperative hemoglobin is 7 g/dL and hematocrit is 32%. Vital signs: T 37.2°C (99°F); HR 72 beats/min at rest; RR 18 breaths/min; BP 132/78 mm Hg.

QUESTION 2.
The nurse is reviewing options for the transfusion.

Complete the following sentence by selecting from the list of word choices below.

The nurse anticipates that the client is most likely to be prescribed an infusion of [Word Choice] and [Word Choice].

Word Choices
Colloid components–albumin 5% pooled
Red blood cells
Whole blood
Clotting factor concentrates
Cryoprecipitate

PHASE 2

QUESTION 3.
The nurse is preparing the client for the transfusion.

Complete the following sentence by selecting from the list of word choices below.

Prior to administering RBCs, the nurse will *first* [Word Choice].

Word Choices
Review pretransfusion laboratory studies
Verify the health care provider's order for transfusion
Select an 18-gauge catheter
Assure that informed consent was signed by the client

QUESTION 4.
The nurse is preparing for the transfusion.

Complete the following sentence by selecting from the lists of options below.

Once the blood arrives, the nurse plans to *initially* **1 [Select]** and **2 [Select]**.

Options for 1	Options for 2
Set tubing clamps to "off" position	Open Y-tubing blood administration set for a single unit
Inspect the bag for any signs of contamination	Spike 0.9% sodium chloride (NS) IV bag
Review the purpose of the transfusion with the client	Compare the blood product with the client's identifiers with another nurse

PHASE 3

QUESTION 5.

The nurse starts the transfusion. Within the first 5 minutes, the client reports feeling flushed and developing itching. Vital signs: BP 140/82 mm Hg; HR 88 beats/min; RR 24 breaths/min; T 37.4°C (99.3°F).

Which actions does the nurse implement at this time? **Select all that apply.**

- ○ Stop the infusion.
- ○ Offer sips of water.
- ○ Restart the infusion at a faster rate.
- ○ Set the infusion to deliver more slowly.
- ○ Provide reassurance that this is a normal feeling.
- ○ Delegate monitoring of vital signs to assistive personnel.
- ○ Give the client a magazine to read to provide distraction.

QUESTION 6.

It is determined the client experienced a mild allergic reaction to the RBC infusion. Soon, the client's symptoms resolve after the nurse follows all appropriate policies regarding, a transfusion reaction. The unit of packed cells is restarted, and the patient receives a prescribed dose of diphenhydramine (Benadryl).

Highlight the findings that indicate that the client is progressing favorably.

History and Physical	Nurses' Notes	Vital Signs	Laboratory Results

1355: Client resting comfortably in chair as RBCs infuse. Vital signs include 37.0°C (98.6°F); RR 16 breaths/min; HR 76 beats/min; BP 118/72 mm Hg; SpO$_2$ 99%. Alert and oriented × 4. Lung sounds clear bilaterally. S$_1$S$_2$ present without murmur.

Providing patients with adequate nutrition requires application of knowledge about normal nutritional needs, the nutritional deficiencies caused by various health conditions, and patients' physical ability to take in nutrients. In addition, knowledge is needed regarding patients' risk for nutritional deficiencies and patients' values and cultural beliefs about food and eating habits. Because there are patients who are unable to swallow easily or who require nutritional elements to be delivered by routes other than oral intake, knowledge of the risks involved must be considered in order to prevent complications such as aspiration and infection. Nutritional standards such as the national *Dietary Guidelines for Americans* provide direction for determining a patient's dietary requirements so that you can compare what is recommended with a patient's actual dietary deficits.

A thorough patient assessment allows you to make dietary recommendations and educate patients and families about nutrition and the role it plays in maintaining health. In outpatient and home health settings, nurses are in an ideal position to better understand a patient's food preferences, meal patterns, and eating habits so that any recommendations are more individualized and likely to be accepted. In acute care, nurses often must focus on assessing whether patients are physically able to self-feed or swallow safely. Patient-centered nutritional care requires patients to partner with you in making decisions about ways to improve their nutritional intake. These decisions also affect how you can support patients in need of assistance with self-feeding.

A patient who is on aspiration precautions is at risk for aspirating mucous secretions or food from the oral cavity into the tracheobronchial tree. Aspiration often leads to pneumonia, a serious complication. Your knowledge of patient conditions that pose risks for dysphagia (e.g., stroke, Parkinson disease, head and neck surgery), the signs of dysphagia, and the presence of cognitive changes allows you to critically anticipate the need for precautions to take during oral feeding. You apply the same knowledge along with therapeutic communication skills and teaching principles to educate family caregivers who assist patients with feeding. Often, the resource of a speech-language pathologist is needed to ensure that foods of the right consistency are offered to patients with dysphagia.

A patient who requires enteral nutrition has serious health problems preventing oral intake of nutrients. The safe administration of enteral nutrition requires clinical judgment in your assessment of the integrity and function of a feeding tube and whether the patient has risks for tube displacement and aspiration. Standards for enteral nutrition practices offer the framework for how to identify patient risks, maintain function of a feeding tube, and prevent complications. For example, while preparing to administer a tube feeding, you check the pH of an aspirate taken from the tube and find it to be highly alkaline, above what is normally expected. You apply critical thinking to problem solve and determine if the abnormal pH is due to medications the patient is receiving or possible tube displacement. Similarly, once you have administered a feeding, you critically apply appropriate assessment skills to judge if the patient is tolerating the feeding. You also apply clinical judgment to make adaptations to administering a tube feeding when needed. For example, a standard exists for keeping the head of the bed elevated during administration of a tube feeding to prevent aspiration. But what if a patient has a stage 4 pressure injury? Is an upright position safe? Assessment of the patient's condition and priority needs along with collaboration with dietitians and health care providers guides you in the best action to take.

Parenteral nutrition poses significant risks to patients because it is delivered intravenously at a high nutrient concentration. A patient's database must include continuous measurements of intake and output, serum blood tests, vital signs, and body weight. You use these data for ongoing monitoring to detect complications as early as possible. The high concentration of glucose in parenteral solutions predisposes patients to infection both at the site of intravenous insertion and systemically. You apply knowledge of the infectious process to anticipate clinical signs. Also, you apply standards of the Infusion Nurses Society (INS) in providing meticulous site care and sterile aseptic dressing changes. You also apply INS standards to correctly monitor parenteral solution infusion rates and know when to act if metabolic or electrolyte imbalances develop.

30 | Oral Nutrition

SKILLS AND PROCEDURES

Skill 30.1 **Performing a Nutrition Screening, p. 919**

Skill 30.2 **Assisting an Adult Patient With Oral Nutrition, p. 925**

Skill 30.3 **Aspiration Precautions, p. 931**

OBJECTIVES

Mastery of content in this chapter will enable you to:
- Create an accurate nutrition screening.
- Summarize the nutritional components of a healthy diet.
- Identify the need and collaborate with a registered dietitian nutritionist (RDN) for a patient's nutrition assessment.
- Assess a patient's ability to swallow.
- Identify risk factors for aspiration.
- Evaluate a patient's tolerance of oral nutrition.
- Develop a nursing care plan to prevent a patient from aspirating.
- Demonstrate how to properly feed a patient who cannot self-feed.

MEDIA RESOURCES

- http://evolve.elsevier.com/Perry/skills
- Review Questions
- ▶ Video Clips
- Audio Glossary
- Answers to Clinical Judgment and Next-Generation NCLEX® Examination–Style Questions
- Printable Key Points
- Skills Performance Checklists

PURPOSE

Nutrition is a basic component of health and is essential for normal growth and development, tissue maintenance and repair, cellular metabolism, and organ function. The quality of individuals' nutritional intake affects their rate of recovery from short-term and chronic illness, surgery, and injury. The nutrition and weight status goal of *Healthy People 2030* is to promote health and reduce chronic disease risk through the consumption of healthful diets and achievement and maintenance of healthy body weights (Office of Disease Prevention and Health Promotion [ODPHP], n.d.). As a nurse, you play a role in counseling and educating patients about diverse types of nutrition problems, such as digestive disorders, swallowing problems, and metabolic alterations. A consistent theme in promoting the nutrition of these patients is promoting healthy diets and good eating habits. The *Healthy People 2030* initiative provides these guidelines for Americans for a healthful diet (ODPHP, n.d.):
- Consume a variety of nutrient-dense foods within and across the food groups, especially whole grains, fruits, vegetables, low-fat or fat-free milk or milk products, and lean meats and other protein sources.
- Limit the intake of saturated and *trans* fats, cholesterol, added sugars, sodium (salt), and alcohol.
- Limit caloric intake to meet caloric needs.

All Americans should avoid unhealthy weight gain, and those whose weight is too high may also need to lose weight.

Malnutrition among hospitalized patients and those in long-term care agencies is a serious issue that has been underdiagnosed and undertreated for decades. Malnutrition is a syndrome that occurs when there is a deficiency of intake or utilization of vital nutrients needed for tissue maintenance and repair that negatively affects growth, physical health, mood, behavior, and other functions of the body (Jensen et al., 2019). The malnutrition Healthcare Cost and Utilization Project (HCUP) found that individuals affected most by malnutrition during hospitalization include adults aged 65 and older, those already underweight, those of Black race/ethnicity, and adults with a lower socioeconomic status (Agency for Healthcare Research and Quality [AHRQ], 2022). Malnutrition is a major health concern, particularly for older adults and patients with limited financial resources. Research shows that one in two older adults is either malnourished or at risk of becoming malnourished—typically persons over 60 years of age (Haines et al., 2020; Richardson, 2019). Malnourishment in older adults leads to loss of strength and function, increased risk of falls, depression, lethargy, immune dysfunction, increased risk of infection, delayed recovery from illness, pressure injuries, poor wound healing, and an increase in hospitalizations resulting in increased health care costs (Brennan, 2023; Haines et al., 2020; Richardson, 2019). The Joint Commission (TJC, 2022) requires routine identification of malnutrition with screening of patients in health care settings. As a nurse you will provide nutrition screening and collaborate with registered dietitian nutritionists (RDNs) and health care providers to determine the safest and best approaches for supporting patients' nutritional health.

PRACTICE STANDARDS

- International Dysphagia Diet Standardisation Initiative (IDDSI), 2019—Types of dysphagia diets
- The Joint Commission (TJC), 2022: Nutritional and functional screening

- The Joint Commission (TJC), 2023: National Patient Safety Goals—Patient identification
- Office of Disease Prevention and Health Promotion (ODPHP), n.d.: *Healthy People 2030*—Nutrition and healthy eating
- U.S. Department of Agriculture and U.S. Department of Health and Human Services (USDA/USDHHS), 2020: Dietary Guidelines for Americans, 2020–2025
- U.S. Department of Agriculture (USDA), n.d.a: MyPlate— MyPlate guidelines
- U.S. Department of Agriculture (USDA), n.d.b: MyPlate— Older adults

SUPPLEMENTAL STANDARDS

- Compher C, et al., 2022: Guidelines for the Provision of Nutrition Support Therapy in the Adult Critically Ill Patient— American Society for Parenteral and Enteral Nutrition (ASPEN) clinical guidelines

PRINCIPLES FOR PRACTICE

- A nutrition screening must be completed within 24 hours of a patient's admission to a hospital, within 14 days of admission to a long-term care agency, or within an agency-defined period of time in ambulatory and home care settings (Grodner et al., 2020; TJC, 2022).
- When performing a nutrition screening, one aim is to identify common risk factors for nutrition problems (Box 30.1).
- A thorough nutrition assessment is performed by an RDN. Recommendations for improving nutritional status such as change in diet, alternative feeding methods, or further medical assessment and intervention stem from nutrition assessments.

BOX 30.1

Risk Factors for Potential Nutrition Problems

- Age
- Frailty in institutionalized persons
- Excessive polypharmacy
- General health decline including physical function
- Parkinson disease
- Constipation
- Poor or moderate self-reported health status
- Cognitive decline, dementia
- Eating dependencies; difficulty feeding self
- Loss of interest in life
- Poor appetite
- Basal oral dysphagia
- Signs of impaired efficacy of swallowing
- Institutionalization
- Clear- or full-liquid diets for more than 3 days without nutrient supplementation or with inappropriate or insufficient nutrient supplementation
- Intravenous feeding (dextrose and saline or saline) or nothing by mouth (NPO) status for more than 3 days without nutrient supplementation
- Low intake of prescribed diet or tube feedings
- Pregnancy weight gain deviating from normal patterns
- Remaining NPO

Adapted from Haines J, et al: *Malnutrition in the elderly: underrecognized and increasing in prevalence,* 2020. https://www.clinicaladvisor.com/home/topics/geriatrics-information-center/malnutrition-in-the-elderly-underrecognized-and-increasing-in-prevalence/3/. Accessed October 27, 2023; and O'Keeffe M, et al.: Potentially modifiable determinants of malnutrition in older adults: a systematic review. *Clin Nutr* 38(6):2477–2498, 2019.

- In an acute care setting, high-quality nutrition care requires you to document weight, appetite loss, and reduced self-feeding ability and to collaborate with health care providers to make dietary referrals (Compher et al., 2022; Ukleja et al., 2018).
- Hospitalizations in adults with a diagnosis of malnutrition involve longer lengths of stay, higher costs, more co-morbidities, and increased mortality rates compared with hospital stays in adults without malnutrition (Abugroun et al., 2021; AHRQ, 2021).
- Nurses are responsible for preparing patients who are on oral diets by offering the type of assistance needed to help them successfully eat an adequate amount of food at a safe and comfortable pace.
- The updated *Dietary Guidelines for Americans, 2020–2025* (USDA/USDHHS, 2020) acknowledge that the nutritional quality of foods has improved dramatically over the past century. However, rates of chronic diseases—many of which are related to poor-quality diet and physical inactivity—have increased. About half of all American adults have one or more preventable, diet-related chronic diseases, including cardiovascular disease (CVD), type 2 diabetes, and overweight and obesity. Scientific evidence incorporated in the guidelines shows that healthy eating patterns and regular physical activity can help people achieve and maintain good health and reduce the risk of chronic disease throughout all stages of the life span. The *Dietary Guidelines for Americans* are reflected in the user-friendly MyPlate guidelines (USDA, n.d.a; USDA, n.d.b).

PERSON-CENTERED CARE

- Social and cultural norms influence values held about nutrition and physical activity, including patients' preferences for certain types of foods, acceptable ranges of body weight, and values placed on physical activity and healthy food. The Social-Ecological Model (Fig. 30.1) shows that implementing multiple changes at various levels of the model can be effective in improving an individual's eating behavior (USDA/USDHHS, 2015).
- Having access to healthy, safe, and affordable food choices is crucial for an individual to achieve a healthy eating pattern. This includes having proximity to food retail outlets (e.g., distance to a store or the number of stores in an area), individual resources (e.g., income or personal transportation), and neighborhood-level resources (e.g., average income of the neighborhood and availability of public transportation) (USDA/USDHHS, 2020).
- Collaborate with RDNs in considering a patient's knowledge and attitudes about food and health, skills in being able to feed self and properly store and prepare food, social support, and access to and use of food assistance programs, as well as the economic price system affecting the patient (ODPHP, n.d.).
- Some cultures believe in the hot-and-cold theory of health and illness. Foods are classified as cold or hot on the basis of their characteristics, independent of the temperature at which they are served. There is no universal agreement across cultures about which foods are hot and which foods are cold (Giger & Haddad, 2021).
- MyPlate (Fig. 30.2) offers ideas and tips to help people create a healthier eating style that meets their individual needs and improves their health (USDA, n.d.a; USDA, n.d.b). A nurse's role is to match patient food preferences with healthier food choices when possible.

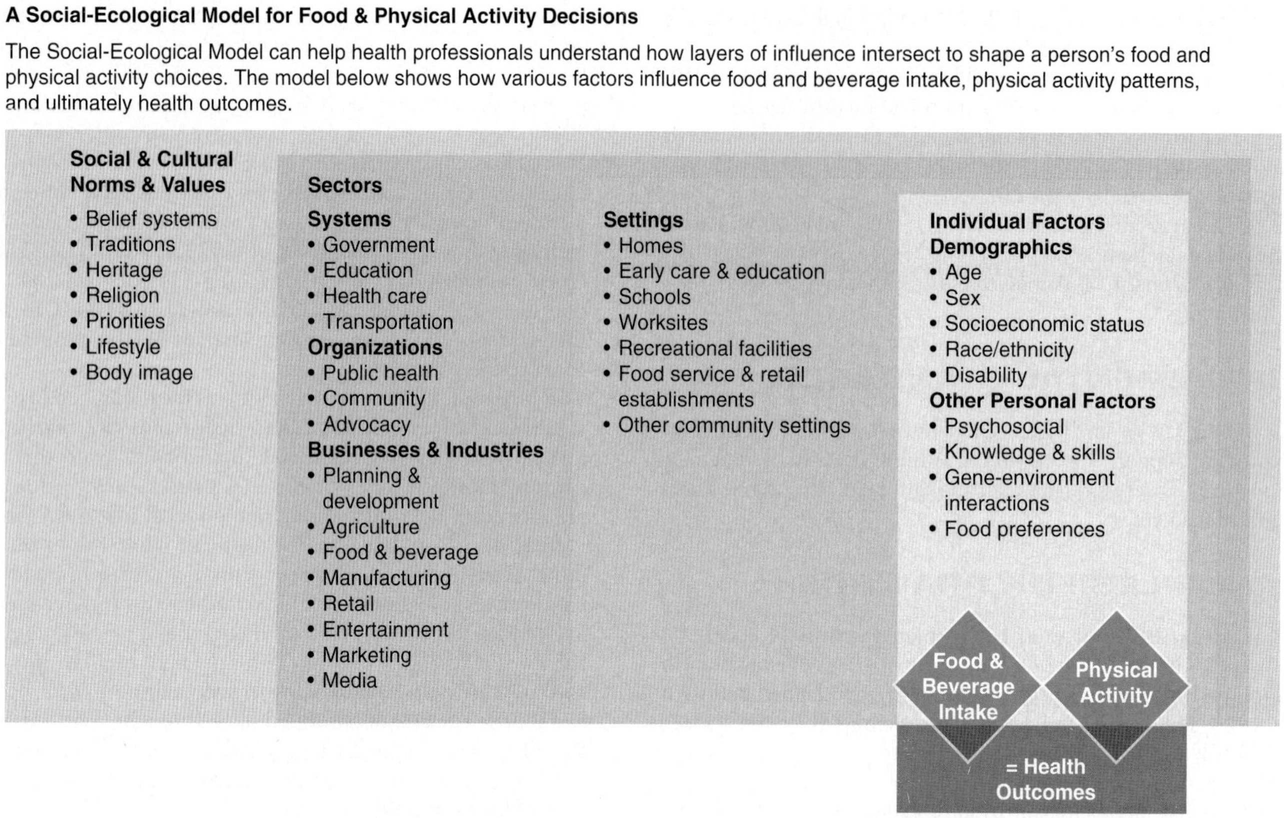

A Social-Ecological Model for Food & Physical Activity Decisions

The Social-Ecological Model can help health professionals understand how layers of influence intersect to shape a person's food and physical activity choices. The model below shows how various factors influence food and beverage intake, physical activity patterns, and ultimately health outcomes.

Social & Cultural Norms & Values
- Belief systems
- Traditions
- Heritage
- Religion
- Priorities
- Lifestyle
- Body image

Sectors

Systems
- Government
- Education
- Health care
- Transportation

Organizations
- Public health
- Community
- Advocacy

Businesses & Industries
- Planning & development
- Agriculture
- Food & beverage
- Manufacturing
- Retail
- Entertainment
- Marketing
- Media

Settings
- Homes
- Early care & education
- Schools
- Worksites
- Recreational facilities
- Food service & retail establishments
- Other community settings

Individual Factors
Demographics
- Age
- Sex
- Socioeconomic status
- Race/ethnicity
- Disability

Other Personal Factors
- Psychosocial
- Knowledge & skills
- Gene-environment interactions
- Food preferences

Food & Beverage Intake   Physical Activity

= Health Outcomes

FIG. 30.1 The Social-Ecological Model for Food and Physical Activity Decisions. *(From U.S. Department of Agriculture and U.S. Department of Health and Human Services [USDA/USDHHS]: Dietary Guidelines for Americans, 2015–2020, 2015. https://www.researchgate.net/figure/Social-ecological-framework-for-nutrition-and-physical-activity-decisions-Source_fig1_276060761. Accessed October 27, 2023.)*

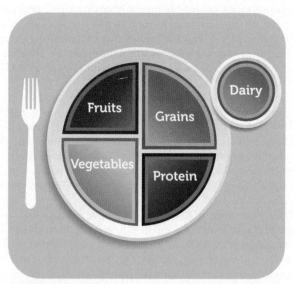

FIG. 30.2 MyPlate showing the five essential food groups. *(From the U.S. Department of Agriculture [USDA]: What is MyPlate? n.d. https://www.myplate.gov/eat-healthy/what-is-myplate. Accessed October 27, 2023.)*

- Food insecurity, common among vulnerable populations, occurs when access to nutritionally adequate and safe food is limited or uncertain. Help patients with food insecurity to find resources for the delivery of food and other resources to reach people who are in need and when community services are scarce (USDA/USDHHS, 2020).

EVIDENCE-BASED PRACTICE

Improving Oral Intake of Older Adults

Numerous factors affect the oral intake of older adults. Several age-related physiological changes, including more rapid and longer satiation, dental and chewing problems, being less hungry and thirsty, and impairments in smell and taste, can change eating behavior (Linnell et al., 2021). Older adults may eat more slowly, consume smaller meals, and snack less, leading to lower food consumption and ultimately to weight loss (Lutz et al., 2019; Norman et al., 2021). Age-related and behavior changes in eating can be compounded by the effects of co-morbidities and medication that causes anorexia (Rashid et al., 2020). Evidence shows that the following approaches can improve dietary intake among older adults:

- During mealtime, incorporate activities in which there is social support and social interaction (National Council on Aging, 2021). Meal sharing provides an opportunity to develop social relationships and can lead to better diet quality (Alne et al., 2021).
- When caring for community-dwelling older adults, the provision of meals (e.g., Meals on Wheels), meal enhancements, and, for those who need them, nutritional supplements can improve diet quality (Fleury et al., 2021).
- Hospitalized older adults require early nutrition screening and may benefit from the lifting of dietary restrictions, encouragement of frequent nutrient-dense meals, and use of oral nutritional supplements (ONSs) to increase caloric or nutrition consumption.
- Hospital nutrition care plans should result from interprofessional teamwork and involve both patient and family caregivers (Haines et al., 2020; Ukleja et al., 2018).
- Dietary modifications in hospitals aim to optimize the provision of essential nutrients to the body. They include adjustments

Food Safety Tips

Clean: Wash your hands and food preparation surfaces often.
- Germs that cause food poisoning can survive in many places and spread around a kitchen. Wash hands for 20 seconds with soap and water before, during, and after preparing food and before eating.
- Wash utensils, cutting boards, and countertops with hot, soapy water.
- Rinse fresh fruits and vegetables under running water.

Separate meats from vegetables; do not cross-contaminate.
- Raw meat, poultry, seafood, and eggs can spread germs to ready-to-eat foods unless you keep them separated. Use separate cutting boards and plates for raw meat, poultry, and seafood.
- When grocery shopping, keep raw meat, poultry, seafood, and their juices away from other foods.
- Keep raw meat, poultry, seafood, and eggs separate from all other foods in the refrigerator.

Cook to the right temperature.
- The only way to tell if food is safely cooked is to use a food thermometer. You cannot tell if food is safely cooked by checking its color and texture.

- Use a food thermometer to ensure that foods are cooked to a safe internal temperature:
  - 145°F for whole cuts of beef, pork, veal, and lamb (then allow the meat to rest for 3 minutes before carving or eating)
  - 160°F for ground meats, such as beef and pork
  - 165°F for all poultry, including ground chicken and turkey
  - 165°F for leftovers and casseroles
  - 145°F for fresh ham (raw)
  - 145°F for finned fish, or cook until flesh is opaque

Refrigerate food promptly to avoid food poisoning.
- Bacteria can multiply rapidly if left at room temperature or in the "danger zone" between 40°F and 140°F. Never leave perishable food out for more than 2 hours (or 1 hour if it is hotter than 90°F outside).
- Keep the refrigerator below 40°F and know when to throw food out.
- Refrigerate perishable food within 2 hours. (If outdoor temperature is above 90°F, refrigerate within 1 hour.)
- Thaw frozen food safely in the refrigerator, in cold water, or in the microwave. Never thaw foods on the counter because bacteria multiply quickly in the parts of the food that reach room temperature.

Adapted from Centers for Disease Control and Prevention (CDC): *Four steps to food safety,* 2023. https://www.cdc.gov/foodsafety/keep-food-safe.html. Accessed October 27, 2023.

regarding consistency; presentation; energy value; nutrient content; protein, fat, and carbohydrate content; and number of meals (Lutz et al., 2019).

SAFETY GUIDELINES

- Each year, one in six Americans becomes ill from eating contaminated food (USDHHS, 2020). There are four principles for food safety in the home (Centers for Disease Control and Prevention [CDC], 2023a): Wash the hands and food preparation surfaces thoroughly, separate different types of food (poultry, eggs, raw meat, seafood) during preparation, cook to the right temperature, and refrigerate promptly (Box 30.2).
- Identify patients at risk for dysphagia and collaborate with other members of the health care team, especially a speech-language pathologist (SLP), to minimize complications such as aspiration

pneumonia. The role of SLPs is to identify signs and symptoms of dysphagia, to identify indications and contraindications specific to each patient for assessment procedures, to identify signs of potential swallowing disorders and work collaboratively with medical professionals to provide safe and effective treatment, and to evaluate the stages of the swallow and make recommendations to physicians, nurses, dietitians, and family members (American Speech-Language-Hearing Association [ASHA], 2023b).
- Ensure that patients receive the correct therapeutic diets. TJC and the Centers for Medicare and Medicaid Services (CMS) report that common dietary errors include wrong diet, delivery of meals meant for other patients, and delivery of meals to patients who are to receive nothing by mouth (NPO).
- Assess a patient's level of consciousness and ability to swallow before attempting any oral feeding.

SKILL 30.1 Performing a Nutrition Screening

Nurses screen for patients' actual and potential nutritional alterations on an ongoing basis by focusing on the effects of an illness, disease, or lifestyle on a patient's nutritional status, such as recent weight loss and decreased oral intake. A nutrition risk screening is a rapid and simple set of questions that have been validated to predict if a patient is malnourished or at risk for malnutrition, helping to determine if a detailed nutrition assessment is indicated (Box 30.3). Although there are multiple easy-to-use, reliable, and valid nutrition screening tools available, the Academy of Nutrition and Dietetics recommends use of the Malnutrition Screening Tool (MST) in adults (Academy of Nutrition and Dietetics, 2023a, 2023b). Completion of a nutrition screening is mandated by TJC (2022) within 24 hours of a patient's admission to an acute health care agency. In long-term care facilities, screening and assessments must be completed on all residents within 14 days of admission (Grodner et al., 2020). TJC also requires behavioral health care programs to screen all individuals served in order to identify those in whom a more detailed nutrition assessment is indicated. Behavioral health care organizations provide a wide range of community-based services (e.g., mental health, eating disorders, addiction programs) within a variety of settings across the continuum of care.

At a minimum, the screening includes questions about the following (Barrins & Associates, 2018; Dodd, 2020):
- Food allergies
- Weight loss or gain of 4.5 kg (10 lb) or more in the past 3 months
- Decrease in food intake and/or appetite
- Dental problems
- Eating habits or behaviors that may be indicators of an eating disorder, such as bingeing or induced vomiting

If a nutrition screening indicates that a patient is at risk for malnutrition, a more comprehensive assessment must be conducted, usually by a registered clinical dietitian or, in some settings, an advanced practice nurse (Ukleja et al., 2018). In addition, assessment findings can lead to a medical referral to a speech-language pathologist (SLP) if the patient has swallowing difficulties. High-quality and accurate nutrition assessments rely on the integration of data from multiple sources, including a review of systems (medical, nutrition, and psychosocial histories); physical examination; anthropometric data (height, weight, body mass index [BMI], and ratio of lean body tissue to body fat); functional outcomes; and examination of the intake of energy and nutrients. As reported by the National Association of Clinical Nurse Specialists (NACNS, 2017), the

Examples of Nutrition Screening Tools

- The Malnutrition Screening Tool (MST) is a simple, three-question tool assessing recent weight and appetite loss; the MST has been validated for use in general medical, surgical, and oncology patients. It was designed for use by non–nutrition-trained staff and uses a scoring system to identify patients at high nutrition risk, which can then provide a basis for dietetic referrals and intervention. In an analysis of screening tools, the MST was the only tool shown to be both valid and reliable for identifying undernutrition in the acute care and hospital-based ambulatory care settings (Academy of Nutrition and Dietetics, 2020).
- The Malnutrition Universal Screening Tool (MUST) was designed to detect both undernutrition and obesity in adults. It can be used in multiple settings, including hospitals and nursing homes. Body mass index (BMI), unplanned weight loss, and the presence or absence of serious disease allow a score to be derived to indicate whether nutrition intervention is necessary. It is not valid for children or renal failure patients.
- Nutrition Risk Screening (NRS-2002) uses recent weight loss, decreased BMI, and reduced dietary intake, combined with a subjective assessment of disease severity (based on increased nutrition requirements and/or metabolic stress), to generate a nutrition risk score. The NRS tool has been recommended for use in hospitalized patients and may be useful for prompting the initiation of nutrition support.
- The Subjective Global Assessment (SGA) is one of the most commonly used nutrition assessment tools. It requires completion of a questionnaire, which includes data on weight change, dietary intake change, gastrointestinal symptoms, changes in functional capacity in relation to malnutrition, and assessment of fat and muscle stores and the presence of edema and ascites. This tool allows for malnutrition diagnosis and classifies patients as A, well-nourished; B, mildly/moderately malnourished; or C, severely malnourished.

Modified from Academy of Nutrition and Dietetics: *Nutrition screening adults: tool descriptions (2018),* 2023. https://www.andeal.org/topic.cfm?menu=5382. Accessed November 16, 2023; Dodd K: *Which malnutrition tool is best?* 2020. https://thegeriatricdietitian.com/malnutrition-screening-tool/. Accessed October 27, 2023; and National Association of Clinical Nurse Specialists(NACNS): *Malnutrition in hospitalized adult patients: the role of the clinical nurse specialist,* 2017. https://nacns.org/wp-content/uploads/2017/01/Malnutrition-Report.pdf. Accessed November 16, 2023.

Physical Signs of Nutritional Status Alteration

Body Area	Indicators of Malnutrition
General appearance	Listless, apathetic, cachectic
Posture	Sagging shoulders, sunken chest, humped back
Hair	Stringy, dull, brittle, dry, thin and sparse, depigmented, easily plucked
Face and neck	Greasy, discolored, scaly, swollen, dark skin over cheeks and under eyes, lumpiness or flakiness of skin around nose and mouth
Skin	Rough, dry, scaly, pale, pigmented, irritated; bruises and petechiae
Lips	Dry, scaly, swollen, redness and swelling (cheilosis), angular lesions at corner of mouth or fissures or scars
Mouth, oral mucous membranes	Swollen, deep red or magenta mucous membranes, oral lesions
Gums	Spongy, bleed easily, marginal redness, inflamed, receding
Tongue	Swelling, scarlet and raw, magenta color, beefy (glossitis), hyperemic and hypertrophic or atrophic papillae
Teeth	Missing, broken teeth
Eyes	Conjunctivae pale, redness of conjunctivae, dryness or infection, redness and fissuring of eyelid corners (angular palpebritis), Bitot spots
Neck (glands)	Thyroid or lymph nodes enlarged
Nails	Spoon shaped (koilonychias), brittle, ridged
Legs and feet	Edema, tender calf, tingling, weakness, lesions
Muscles	Flaccid, poor tone, undeveloped, tender, impaired ability to walk
Nerve conduction and mental status	Inattentive, irritable, confused, burning and tingling of hands and feet, loss of position and vibratory sense

Adapted from Nix S: *Williams' basic nutrition and diet therapy,* ed 16, St. Louis, 2022, Elsevier.

presence of two or more of the following six characteristics identifies the presence of malnutrition:

- Insufficient energy intake as measured by nutrients consumed and/or administered compared with estimated body energy requirements
- Weight loss as measured by a percentage of weight loss from baseline
- Loss of muscle mass as measured by wasting seen at temples, clavicles, shoulders, interosseous muscles, scapula, and thigh and calf muscles using a scale ranging from mild to severe
- Loss of subcutaneous fat as measured by loss, especially from orbital and triceps areas, and/or fat overlying the ribs using a scale ranging from mild to severe
- Localized or generalized fluid accumulation in extremities or vulva or scrotum, and/or ascites that can mask weight loss
- Diminished functional status as measured by handgrip

Registered nurses working in clinical areas can be invaluable in screening patients for nutritional risks and recognizing signs of alterations. During any physical examination or while administering direct care, learn to recognize the physical signs that indicate a nutritional alteration (Table 30.1). Also, routinely review the patient's laboratory results (e.g., albumin, prealbumin, ferritin, total iron binding capacity, vitamin B_{12}) and the dietary information from a nursing admission history. These data provide helpful information that will allow you to identify the adequacy of a patient's current diet, appetite changes, type of assistance a patient will need to eat, and food preferences.

Registered dietitian nutritionists (RDNs) are qualified to assess patients' nutritional treatment plans and design and implement nutritional treatment plans in consultation with the care team (Grodner et al., 2020). When you make referrals to RDNs, it is important to know their role. RDNs use a problem-solving method, the Nutrition Care Process (NCP), to think critically and make decisions regarding nutrition therapy. It provides a framework for the RDN to individualize care, considering the patient's needs and values and using the best evidence available to make decisions (Academy of Nutrition and Dietetics, 2023a).

Delegation

The skill of performing and interpreting a nutrition screening and physical examination cannot be delegated to assistive personnel (AP). However, measurement of a patient's height and weight can be delegated. Direct the AP to:

- Measure the patient's weight after voiding, at the same time of day and with the patient wearing the same clothing
- Use an internal bed scale (if available) according to agency guidelines (if applicable)
- Report inability to measure height if the patient is not ambulatory

Interprofessional Collaboration

- Following an initial nutrition screening, collaborate with the health care provider for a referral to an RDN or consult with an agency advanced practice nurse.

Equipment

- Scale (beam, electronic, bed with scale, wheelchair/chair)
- Nutrition screening form (data sheet and pen or computerized assessment form)
- Tongue blade, clean gloves, penlight for physical examination

STEP	RATIONALE

ASSESSMENT

1. Identify patient using at least two identifiers (e.g., name and birthday or name and medical record number) according to agency policy.

Ensures correct patient. Complies with The Joint Commission standards and improves patient safety (TJC, 2023).

2. Assess patient's/family caregiver's health literacy.

Determines degree to which individuals have the ability to find, understand, and use information and services to make informed health-related decisions and actions for themselves and others (CDC, 2023b).

3. Ask patient to report usual body weight (UBW), noting recent changes in weight. Ask if weight loss was intentional or unintentional.

In adults, weight is usually stable. A weight loss of more than 5% within 1 month is an indicator for further assessment, especially in an adult older than 65 years (Table 30.2).

4. Perform hand hygiene. Measure actual body weight (ABW).

Reduces transmission of infection.

   a. Have patient void. Be sure that patient is wearing underwear or hospital gown. Weigh with patient barefoot or with same shoes. Weigh at same time of day (e.g., before breakfast).

Improves accuracy of ABW for comparison over time (Nix, 2022).

   b. Make sure that beam scale has been calibrated. If ambulatory, have the patient stand as straight as possible, without shoes or a hat (Nix, 2022). Be sure weight is evenly distributed on both feet with heels together.

Accurate measurement requires regularly calibrated and maintained scales. Standing still with equal weight distribution helps to obtain accurate weight (Grodner et al., 2020).

   c. If patient is unable to stand, use wheelchair or bed scale.

Decreases risk of falling.

   d. Document weight to nearest 0.1 kg (¼ lb).

Provides precise measurement of weight.

5. Measure actual height.

On average, when asked, people report being slightly taller than they are, and the extent of overstating increases as people age (Grodner et al., 2020).

   a. Help patient to a standing position, standing erect with weight equally distributed on both feet and heels together.

Ensures accurate height, which is needed for calculation of protein and energy requirements (Grodner et al., 2020).

   b. Instruct patient to let arms hang freely at sides with palms facing thighs.

Prevents movement of shoulders, which would result in inaccurate measurement.

   c. Have patient look straight ahead, take a deep breath, and hold position while you bring horizontal bar firmly on top of head. Measure to nearest 0.1 cm (⅛ inch). Make sure that your eyes are level with bar to read measurement.

Steady position ensures accurate measurement. Provides precise measurement of height.

6. Know the formula for calculating ideal body weight (IBW).

This is usually calculated by RDN or advanced practice nurse.

   a. Calculate via standard height and weight chart. IBW range for normal is 10% above and 10% below IBW.

Use IBW to compare with patient's actual weight to determine if at risk for nutritional alteration.

   b. Use the following formulas:
     Male: 48.1 kg (106 lb) for first 5 ft; add 2.7 kg (6 lb) per additional 2.5 cm (inch).
     Female: 45.4 kg (100 lb) for first 5 ft; add 2.25 kg (5 lb) per additional 2.5 cm (inch).

7. Calculate BMI (see illustration):

$$BMI = \frac{Actual\ body\ weight\ (kg)}{Height^2\ (m^2)}$$

Usually calculated by RDN or advanced practice nurse. BMI is a measure of body fat based on height and weight that applies to adults (National Heart, Lung, and Blood Institute [NHLBI], n.d.). Use this link for an automatic calculation: http://www.nhlbi.nih.gov/health/educational/lose_wt/BMI/bmicalc.htm (NHLBI, n.d.)

   a. Divide ABW in pounds by 2.2.

Converts pounds into kilograms.

   b. Convert height to inches. Multiply inches by 2.54.

Converts height in inches to centimeters.

   c. Divide height in centimeters by 100.

Converts height to meters.

   d. Divide weight in kilograms by the square of height in meters (m^2).

Computes BMI (Box 30.4).

   e. Optional formula for BMI:
     Weight (lb)/[Height (inches)]^2 × 703

TABLE 30.2

Weight Change as an Indicator of Nutrition Status

Weight Change (%)	Time Period	Nutrition Status
1–2	1 week	Moderate weight loss
Greater than 2	1 week	Severe weight loss
5	1 month	Moderate weight loss
Greater than 5	1 month	Severe weight loss

From Grodner M, et al: Nutritional foundations and clinical applications: a nursing approach, ed 7, St. Louis, 2020, Elsevier; and American Dietetic Association (ADA): ADA/A.S.P.E.N: Clinical characteristics that the RD can obtain and document to support a diagnosis of malnutrition, n.d. http://www.cmcgc.com/media/handouts/320121/t21_jane_white.pdf. Accessed October 28, 2023.

BOX 30.4

Classification of Body Mass Index in Adults

Degree of Adiposity	Body Mass Index
Underweight	Less than 18.5 kg/m^2
Normal or healthy weight	18.5–24.9 kg/m^2
Overweight	25–29.9 kg/m^2
Obesity	30 kg/m^2 and above
Obesity (class 2)	35–39.9 kg/m^2
Extreme obesity (class 3)	Greater than or equal to 40 kg/m^2

From Centers for Disease Control and Prevention (CDC): *About adult BMI,* 2022. https://www.cdc.gov/healthyweight/assessing/bmi/adult_bmi/index.html. Accessed July 12, 2023.

To use the table, find the appropriate height in the left-hand column labeled Height. Move across to a given weight (in pounds). The number at the top of the column is the BMI at that height and weight. Pounds have been rounded off.

BMI	19	20	21	22	23	24	25	26	27	28	29	30	31	32	33	34	35
Height (inches)							Body Weight (pounds)										
58	91	96	100	105	110	115	119	124	129	134	138	143	148	153	158	162	167
59	94	99	104	109	114	119	124	128	133	138	143	148	153	158	163	168	173
60	97	102	107	112	118	123	128	133	138	143	148	153	158	163	168	174	179
61	100	106	111	116	122	127	132	137	143	148	153	158	164	169	174	180	185
62	104	109	115	120	126	131	136	142	147	153	158	164	169	175	180	186	191
63	107	113	118	124	130	135	141	146	152	158	163	169	175	180	186	191	197
64	110	116	122	128	134	140	145	151	157	163	169	174	180	186	192	197	204
65	114	120	126	132	138	144	150	156	162	168	174	180	186	192	198	204	210
66	118	124	130	136	142	148	155	161	167	173	179	186	192	198	204	210	216
67	121	127	134	140	146	153	159	166	172	178	185	191	198	204	211	217	223
68	125	131	138	144	151	158	164	171	177	184	190	197	203	210	216	223	230
69	128	135	142	149	155	162	169	176	182	189	196	203	209	216	223	230	236
70	132	139	146	153	160	167	174	181	188	195	202	209	216	222	229	236	243
71	136	143	150	157	165	172	179	186	193	200	208	215	222	229	236	243	250
72	140	147	154	162	169	177	184	191	199	206	213	221	228	235	242	250	258
73	144	151	159	166	174	182	189	197	204	212	219	227	235	242	250	257	265
74	148	155	163	171	179	186	194	202	210	218	225	233	241	249	256	264	272
75	152	160	168	176	184	192	200	208	216	224	232	240	248	256	264	272	279
76	156	164	172	180	189	197	205	213	221	230	238	246	254	263	271	279	287

Key

Obese (30+)
Overweight (25-29)
Normal (19-24)

STEP 7 Body mass index (BMI) 35 and lower. (*Data from National Heart, Lung, and Blood Institute [NHLBI]: Body mass index table 1: calculate your body mass index, n.d. http://www.nhlbi.nih.gov/health/educational/lose_wt/BMI/bmicalc.htm. Accessed October 28, 2023.*)

8. Assess patient's knowledge, prior experience with nutrition screening and physical examination, and feelings about procedure.

Reveals need for patient instruction and/or support.

PLANNING

1. Expected outcomes following completion of procedure:
   • Patient receives individualized therapeutic diet plan following assessment.

A comprehensive nutrition assessment determines the presence of malnutrition and offers guideline for types of nutritional interventions (NACNS, 2017).

STEP	RATIONALE
2. Explain to patient and/or family caregiver intent of assessment and how the information will allow the health care team to develop a diet plan.	Allows patient/family opportunity to collaborate and time to ask questions.
3. Close room door and bedside curtain.	Provides patient privacy.

IMPLEMENTATION

STEP	RATIONALE
1. Review the dietary information that you collected from the nursing history (see Chapter 6):	
a. Assess patient's dietary history, including current diet, food choices and preferences, appetite, food allergies, and food intolerances. **NOTE:** In outpatient settings, have patient bring 7-day food diary report.	Assesses factors affecting diet adequacy and appetite based on 24-hour diet recall (Grodner et al., 2020).
b. Assess for any cultural, social, and religious preferences and/or restrictions in diet.	Knowing patient preferences will improve ability to plan diet that patient will accept. As a resource, the Food and Agriculture Organization of the United Nations (FAO) provides guidelines on food, food groups, and dietary patterns for more than 100 countries in line with current evidence (FAO, 2023). Guidelines are adapted to each country's nutrition situation, food availability, culinary cultures, and eating habits.
c. Determine medications and other dietary/herbal supplements that patient is taking (over the counter and prescribed). Be aware of common drug-drug and drug-nutrient interactions (consult pharmacist).	Certain medications inhibit or increase action of other medications. Some nutrients interact with medications. For example, vitamin K–rich foods (green leafy vegetables) interfere with action of warfarin (anticoagulant). Medications such as mineral oil laxatives impair nutrient use.
2. Synthesize information gathered during physical assessment (see Chapter 6) (see Table 30.1), including fluid assessment, functional status, wound status, physical changes reflecting nutritional deficiencies, patient's level of consciousness, responsiveness, and ability to swallow.	The most obvious signs of malnutrition on physical examination are apparent in the skin, mouth, muscles, and central nervous system. Difficulty swallowing predisposes patient to aspiration when eating. Functional alterations impair self-feeding ability.
3. Review results of relevant laboratory tests (e.g., albumin, prealbumin, hemoglobin, immune factors [zinc, vitamin A], vitamin D). Compare with known standards.	Test data provide clues about nutritional status. No single test is available for evaluating short-term response to nutrition therapy. Serial testing will give more accurate information but usually is not practical in acute care setting (Grodner et al., 2020).
4. During first meal, determine patient's ability to manipulate eating utensils and self-feed.	Difficulty in self-feeding creates significant risk for malnutrition (Rashid et al., 2020).
5. Complete a nutrition screening tool within 24 hours of patient admission (see Box 30.3) (see agency policy).	Valid tools include key elements for detecting patient's nutritional risk.
6. While critically analyzing findings, conduct education sessions with patient and family caregiver about the *Dietary Guidelines for Americans, 2020–2025* and healthy food choices. Use MyPlate as a guide. Adapt to patient's food preferences when possible.	Equips patient and family caregiver with knowledge needed to plan and execute a healthy daily meal plan.
7. Provide patient help with feeding based on assessment findings (see Skill 30.2).	Level of assistance required depends on patient's motor skills, ability to attend, and ability to swallow and chew normally.
8. Institute aspiration precautions (see Skill 30.3) if needed.	Precautions lessen chance of patient aspirating food or liquid into tracheobronchial tree.
9. Help patient to a comfortable position.	Restores comfort and sense of well-being.
10. Raise side rails (as appropriate) and lower bed to lowest position, locking into position.	Ensures patient safety and prevents falls.
11. Place nurse call system in an accessible location within patient's reach.	Ensures patient can call for assistance if needed.

EVALUATION

STEP	RATIONALE
1. Review history and physical findings. Note abnormal findings or areas of concern.	Permits prompt identification of risk for malnutrition and need for nutritional interventions.
2. Compare patient's actual weight for height with IBW. Compare BMI with recommended BMI for height and weight.	Determines if weight status is a nutritional risk factor.

STEP	RATIONALE
3. Compare normal laboratory test levels (e.g., plasma proteins, liver enzymes, hemoglobin, electrolytes) with patient's levels.	When considered with other nutritional parameters, abnormal values can indicate malnutrition (Nix, 2022).
4. Compute and review score on nutrition screening tool.	Valid tools use scoring system to identify patients at high nutritional risk.
5. **Use Teach-Back:** "I want to be sure I explained how the results of your nutrition screening will help us create a diet plan. Tell me what foods to include in your diet plan. Show me a meal plan for a day." Revise your instruction now or develop a plan for revised patient/family caregiver teaching if patient/family caregiver is not able to teach back correctly.	Teach-back is a technique for health care providers to ensure that they have explained medical information clearly so that patients and their families understand what is communicated to them (AHRQ, 2023).

Unexpected Outcomes	Related Interventions
1. Patient is overweight if BMI is greater than 25 kg/m^2 in an adult. Patient is obese if BMI is greater than 30 kg/m^2.	• Ensure that patient is receiving correct caloric diet. • Check that patient is being weighed on same scale, with same type of clothing and shoes, and at same time of day. • Consult with RDN or health care provider so that RDN can calculate patient's caloric and protein intake and route of nutrition (enteral versus parenteral) (see Chapters 31 and 32).
2. Patient is underweight, taking in insufficient intake.	• Consult with RDN to determine needed calorie and protein intake and proper route of nutrition. • Implement measures to improve patient's appetite: appearance of served food, comfort of room, providing comfort measures before meal. • Include patient and family caregiver in developing a meal plan.
3. Nutrition screening tool score reflects high nutritional risk.	• Refer patient to RDN.

Documentation

- Document assessment results.
- Document your evaluation of patient and family caregiver learning.

Hand-Off Reporting

- Notify health care provider and RDN of abnormal findings.

Special Considerations

Patient Education

- To increase the awareness of healthy nutrition, educate patient and family caregiver about the *Dietary Guidelines for Americans, 2020–2025* (USDA/USDHHS, 2020) with a healthy eating pattern at the 2000-calorie level, and use teaching resources such as the MyPlate Plan (USDA, n.d.a) (Box 30.5).
- Introduce technological nutrition tools, such as nutrition smartphone applications and websites, to encourage patient engagement with diet plan.
- Educate patients and family caregivers about the benefits of healthy meal services for improving diet quality (Howley, 2020).

Pediatrics

- Anthropometric data include length, weight, and head circumference in children. Compare these measurements with standard growth charts to determine percentiles.
- The most commonly used growth charts are from the National Center for Health Statistics (Hockenberry et al., 2024). These charts now include BMI for age and weight for stature percentiles.

Older Adults

- Older adults, ages 65 years and older, who are overweight or obese are encouraged to prevent additional weight gain. Among

---

BOX 30.5

Building a Healthy Eating Style

Following the USDA (n.d.a) MyPlate guidelines will result in a healthier eating style:

- When selecting foods and beverages, focus on variety, amount, and nutrients. Include all five food groups—fruits, vegetables, grains, protein foods, and dairy—to get the nutrients you need.
- Eat the right number of calories for you based on your age, sex, height, weight, and physical activity level.
- Choose an eating style low in saturated fat, sodium, and added sugars.
- Use nutrition fact labels and ingredient lists to find the amounts of saturated fat, sodium, and added sugars in the foods and beverages you choose. Make food choices that follow guidelines.
- Look for food and drink choices that are lower in saturated fat, sodium, and added sugar. Eating fewer calories from foods high in saturated fat and added sugars can help you manage your calories and prevent overweight and obesity. Most people eat too many foods that are high in saturated fat and added sugar.
- Eating foods with less sodium can reduce your risk of high blood pressure.
- Make small changes to create a healthier eating style. Think of each change as a personal "win" on your path to living healthier. Each win is a change you make to build your healthy eating style. Find little victories that fit into your lifestyle, and celebrate each one.
- Start with a few of these small changes: Make half your plate fruits and vegetables, focus on whole fruits, vary your veggies, make half your grains whole grains, move to low-fat or fat-free milk or yogurt, and vary your protein routine.
- Create settings where healthy choices are available and affordable to you and others in your community.
- Professionals, policy makers, partners, industries, families, and individuals can help others in their journey to make healthy eating a part of their lives.

See more at https://www.myplate.gov/eat-healthy/what-is-myplate. Accessed October 27, 2023.

older adults who are obese, particularly those with cardiovascular disease (CVD) risk factors, intentional weight loss can be beneficial and result in improved quality of life and reduced risk of chronic diseases and associated disabilities (USDA, n.d.b; USDA/USDHHS, 2020).

- Food insecurity is the limited or uncertain availability of nutritionally adequate and safe foods or limited or uncertain ability to acquire acceptable foods in socially acceptable ways (Feeding America, 2022a, 2022b; USDA, 2023). Food insecurity remains a concern for many older adults; their rate of household food insecurity has been estimated at 6.8% or 1 in 15 older adults (Feeding America, 2022b). For adults aged 50 to 59 years, the rate of food insecurity was 10.4% or 1 in 10 adults in this age-group (Feeding America, 2022b).
- Older adults often benefit from sharing meals with others or socializing with others during mealtimes, particularly at local senior centers (Alne et al., 2021; National Council on Aging, 2021).

Populations With Disabilities

- To promote healthy outcomes in disabled children, a nutrition assessment and measurements of height, weight, and BMI will more accurately estimate intake (Pelizzo et al., 2019).
- Infants and young children who are malnourished as defined by underweight (low weight for age) and stunting (low height for age) are also more likely to screen positive for disability. Macronutrient and micronutrient deficiencies are risk factors for physical, sensory, and cognitive impairment (Feng et al., 2022).
- Nutrition and disability are linked in pediatric patients. Those with neurophysical impairment may have inappropriate dietary energy intake, oral motor dysfunction, increased loss of nutrients, and increased basal metabolic rate (Pelizzo et al., 2019).

Home Care

- Instruct patient and family caregiver about strategies for safe handling, preparation, and storage of food in the home.
- Assess home environment to determine if patient or family caregiver can prepare a meal safely.

◆ SKILL 30.2 Assisting an Adult Patient With Oral Nutrition

Some patients are unable to feed themselves adequately because of the severity of their illness, fatigue, pain, or debilitation from their condition. For example, a patient who loses fine-motor skills from a neuromuscular disease will have difficulty getting food from the plate into the mouth. Helping adults with feeding requires time, patience, knowledge of their physical limitations and nutritional needs, and understanding of their preferences for foods and how to eat a meal. You can improve patients' nutritional intake by helping with feedings directly or teaching family caregivers how to do so safely. It is also important to maintain patients' dignity during feeding and to actively involve them in eating. Encourage patients to make decisions about food choices and times for eating, and help them remain independent by encouraging them to use assistive devices correctly (when needed) or offering finger foods.

Hospitalized patients often receive therapeutic oral diets based on their ability to chew, swallow, and digest food and liquids. However, hospitalized patients who receive prescribed therapeutic diets (particularly fluid-only diets) have been found to be at risk for malnutrition (Range & Samra, 2022). A patient's health condition will often require temporary therapeutic diets (Table 30.3), but there are also patients who need to follow disease-specific therapeutic diets (e.g., low salt, diabetic, gluten free) on a long-term basis. As a nurse, collaborate closely with registered dietitian nutritionists (RDNs) to find the best nutritive foods that can be incorporated into these diets. There are two ways to modify a regular diet: quantitatively or qualitatively (Grodner et al., 2020). Quantitative diets include modifications in number or size of meals served or amounts of specific nutrients, such as six small feedings or a specific number of kilocalories. Qualitative diets include modifications in consistency, texture, or nutrients, such as clear or full liquid. You can supplement any diet with oral nutritional supplements. In a health care setting, you will often receive an order for a calorie count, which requires you to document the percentage of each food that a patient eats next to the food choice directly on the meal menu. The RDN collects the menus to calculate caloric intake and determine the need for nutritional supplements or dietary change.

Altered dentition, improperly fitted dentures, oral lesions or infections, or diseases causing impaired digestion limit the types and consistencies of foods tolerated. Hemiplegia, a fractured arm, quadriplegia, debilitating illness, or generalized weakness limits self-feeding ability and appetite. The presence of intravenous (IV) catheters or tubing, dressings, and bandages also limits mobility needed for self-feeding. Collaborate with an occupational therapist (OT) who can assess a patient's ability to self-feed and make recommendations for adaptive equipment and supplies for self-feeding. An adult who needs help to eat needs compassion and understanding.

Delegation

The skill of assisting a patient with oral nutrition can be delegated to assistive personnel (AP). However, the nurse is responsible for assessing whether a patient can receive or tolerate oral nutrition. Direct the AP by:

- Explaining any specific swallowing strategies or techniques unique to the patient (see Skill 30.3)
- Reviewing when to stop feeding and report immediately to the nurse incidences of coughing, gagging, pocketing of food in the mouth, or difficulty swallowing
- Cautioning to not rush the patient during eating

Interprofessional Collaboration

- Consult with an RDN on the amount, frequency, and quality of feedings.
- Consult with an OT if self-feeding assistive devices are needed.

Equipment

- Stethoscope
- Washcloths and towels
- Tongue blade
- Adaptive utensils as needed for self-feeding
- Straw
- Oral hygiene supplies; *Option:* solution for stomatitis care
- Clean gloves

TABLE 30.3

Progressive and Therapeutic Diets

Diet	Description
Clear liquid	Foods that are clear and liquid at room or body temperature (e.g., water, coffee, tea, clear fruit juices, gelatin, popsicles), that leave little residue, and that are easily absorbed. Commonly ordered for short-term use (24–48 hours) after surgery, before diagnostic tests, and after episodes of diarrhea and vomiting.
Full liquid	Includes foods on clear-liquid diet plus addition of smooth-textured dairy products (e.g., milk, yogurt drinks, ice cream), strained soups and custard, refined cooked cereals, vegetable juice, pureed vegetables, and all fruit juices. Commonly ordered before or after surgery or for patients who cannot chew or tolerate solid foods; must verify that patients are able to tolerate lactose before providing dairy products.
Pureed	Includes foods on clear- and full-liquid diet plus easily swallowed foods that do not require chewing (e.g., scrambled eggs, pureed meats, vegetables, fruits, mashed potatoes). Ordered for patients with swallowing difficulties. Can be modified for low sodium, fat, or calorie count.
Mechanical or dental, soft	Consists of all previous diets plus addition of lightly seasoned ground or finely diced meats, flaked fish, cottage cheese, cheese, rice, potatoes, pancakes, light breads, cooked vegetables, cooked or canned fruit, bananas, and peanut butter; avoid tough meats, nuts, bacon, and fruits with tough skins or membranes. Ordered for patients who have chewing problems or mild GI problems; used as a transition diet from liquids to regular.
Soft/low residue	Addition of low-fiber, easily digested foods such as pastas, casseroles, moist tender meats, and canned cooked fruits and vegetables; includes foods that are easy to chew and simply cooked; does not permit fatty, rich, and fried foods; sometimes referred to as *low-fiber diet*.
High fiber	Addition of fresh uncooked fruits, steamed vegetables, bran, oatmeal, and dried fruits; includes sufficient amounts of indigestible carbohydrates to relieve constipation, increase GI motility, and increase stool weight.
Regular or diet as tolerated	No restrictions; permits patient preferences and allows for postoperative diet progression.
Sample Therapeutic Diets	
Restricted fluids	Required in severe heart failure or kidney failure.
Sodium restricted	Low levels of sodium: may include a 4-g (no added salt), 2-g (moderate), 1-g (strict), or 500-mg (very strict) diet. May be ordered for patients with heart failure, renal failure, cirrhosis, or hypertension.
Fat modified	Low total and saturated fat and low cholesterol intake limited to less than 300 mg daily, and fat intake 30% to 35%; eliminates or reduces fatty foods for hypercholesterolemia, malabsorption disorders, and diarrhea.
Diabetic	Essential treatment for patients with diabetes mellitus; provide patient with a diet recommended by the American Diabetes Association, which allows patients to select set amount of food from basic food groups.

GI, Gastrointestinal.
Adapted from Grodner M, et al: Nutritional foundations and clinical applications: a nursing approach, ed 7, St. Louis, 2020, Elsevier.

STEP	RATIONALE

ASSESSMENT

1. Identify patient using at least two identifiers (e.g., name and birthday or name and medical record number) according to agency policy.

Ensures correct patient. Complies with The Joint Commission standards and improves patient safety (TJC, 2023).

2. Review electronic health record (EHR) for patient's most recent weight and laboratory values.

Provides ongoing monitoring of patient's nutritional status.

3. Review EHR for history of conditions that might impair patient's ability to eat normally (e.g., cerebrovascular accident, dementia, laryngectomy, neuromuscular disease, blindness).

The most common diseases leading to feeding difficulty are characterized by perceptual deficits, cognitive impairment, or a lack of motor control required to (1) recognize food and eating utensils, (2) effectively use utensils to get the food into the mouth, or (3) effectively control chewing and swallowing food.

4. Assess patient's/family caregiver's health literacy.

Determines degree to which individuals have the ability to find, understand, and use information and services to make informed health-related decisions and actions for themselves and others (CDC, 2023b).

5. Perform hand hygiene. Assess presence and condition of teeth. (Apply clean gloves if there is risk of exposure to saliva.) Determine if dentures are poorly fitted. If patient has mouth discomfort, measure pain severity on a pain scale of 0 to 10.

Reduces transmission of microorganisms. Absence of teeth and ill-fitting dentures inhibit normal chewing and influence preparation of food for safe swallowing (see Skill 30.3). Pain can reduce patient's appetite and ability to chew or swallow. These factors increase risk for dysphagia.

STEP	RATIONALE
6. Have patient speak and swallow. Watch for laryngeal movement. Ask patient to say "Ah" while using tongue blade and penlight. Check for midline uvula and symmetrical rise of uvula and soft palate. Use tongue blade to elicit gag reflex (see Chapter 6).	Patients with chronic neurological disease may experience cranial nerve damage, resulting in impaired swallowing (cranial nerve IX) or loss of gag reflex, hoarseness, and nasal voice (cranial nerve X).
7. Assess physical motor skills (e.g., hand motor control [ability to move utensil to mouth] and strength of grasp [ability to grasp utensils, hold cup]).	Determines to what extent patient can self-feed. Patients with any level of independence should be encouraged to feed self as much as possible. Thorough understanding of patient's physical limitations alerts you to type of assistance patient needs.
8. Assess patient's cognitive status, level of consciousness, and ability to attend to feeding.	Patients with cognitive limitations may experience difficulty in recognizing food, handling food on a plate, attending to the task of eating, transporting food to the mouth, manipulating food in the mouth, and swallowing.
9. Assess patient's visual acuity and peripheral vision (Chapter 6).	Reduced visual acuity and peripheral vision make it difficult for patients to see food and utensils (particularly when there is little color contrast between the table, plate, and food).
10. Assess patient's appetite, recent food and fluid intake, cultural and religious preferences for participating in mealtime, and food likes and dislikes.	Determines patient's interest in eating and the type of foods and size of meals that can potentially improve oral intake.
11. Assess for presence of generalized fatigue, pain, or shortness of breath.	Symptoms affect appetite and ability to participate in feeding. Patients eat better when rested.
12. Ask if patient feels nauseated. Also assess recent bowel pattern. Is patient passing flatus? Auscultate for bowel sounds.	Determines baseline assessment of gastrointestinal function.
13. Assess need for toileting, handwashing, and oral care (including dentures) before feeding.	Reduces interruptions and improves patient's appetite.
14. Assess patient's/family caregiver's knowledge, prior experience regarding eating limitations, and need for assistance with nutritional intake.	Reveals need for patient/family caregiver instruction and/or support.

PLANNING

1. Expected outcomes following completion of procedure:	
• Patient's weight is maintained or trends toward desired level.	Nutritional intake meets daily needs.
• Patient's nutrition-related laboratory values trend toward normal.	Biochemical markers along with nutrition assessment indicate nutritional status.
• Patient demonstrates increased ability to self-feed or open items on tray as appropriate.	Indicates increased strength, improved mental status, and increased well-being.
• Patient coughs appropriately with no indication of respiratory compromise.	Feeding method did not compromise respiratory status to cause aspiration.
• Patient completes meal.	Indicates improved nutritional intake.
• Patient able to describe foods allowed within prescribed diet.	Demonstrates learning.
2. After assessment, allow patient to rest 30 minutes before mealtime.	Assessment activities can be tiring. Short rest improves patient's energy level and ability to participate in feeding.
3. Administer ordered analgesic 30 minutes before meal if patient has discomfort.	Analgesic will reach peak effect during meal, improving patient's ability to self-feed.
4. Explain to patient how you plan to set up and help with meal. Allow time for questions.	Minimizes any anxiety and engages patient in mealtime.
5. Prepare patient's room for mealtime.	
a. Perform hand hygiene. Clear over-bed table and arrange any needed supplies.	Reduces transmission of microorganisms and prepares room for food tray.
b. Help patient with elimination needs and hand hygiene.	Increases patient's comfort and enjoyment of meal, which helps increase patient's nutritional intake.
c. Help patient to comfortable sitting position in chair or place bed in high-Fowler position. If patient is unable to sit, turn on side with head of bed elevated and chin in downward position.	Upright position facilitates swallowing, reducing aspiration risk. Conditions such as pressure injury, traction, or spinal surgery prevent positioning with head elevated.

STEP	RATIONALE

IMPLEMENTATION

1. Prepare patient for meal.

   a. Apply clean gloves and offer oral hygiene. If patient has dentures, remove and rinse thoroughly and reinsert. Remove and dispose of gloves and perform hand hygiene.

   Moist, clean oral mucosa and teeth improve taste and appetite. Reduces transmission of microorganisms.

   b. Patients with oral mucositis (inflammation of mucous membranes) benefit from rinsing with solutions such as 0.9% saline, 0.9% saline plus sodium bicarbonate mouthwash, sodium bicarbonate solution, and topical anesthetics or from using mucosal coating agents (National Cancer Institute [NCI], 2022). Consult with health care provider to determine best therapy.

   Pain of mucositis causes patients to avoid eating. Dry mouth makes swallowing difficult.

   c. Help patient put on eyeglasses or insert contact lenses if used.

   Enhances patient's ability to self-feed and makes meal more visually appealing.

2. Check environment for distractions. Reduce noise level from care activities if possible. *Option:* If patient enjoys music, play a soothing, low-volume selection.

   Pleasant environment enhances mealtime experience. Dining music in some settings (e.g., long-term care) has increased food intake, possibly by reducing agitation.

3. Obtain special assistive devices as needed and instruct on use. For example:

   Devices facilitate self-feeding by improving ability to grasp, pick up foods with utensils, and drink liquids.

   • Nonskid mats

   Hold dishes in place when patient has functional use of only one hand or arm (Swiech et al., 2020).

   • Nosey cup or glass

   Useful for patients with reduced neck motion and inability to tip head or neck back (Dodd, 2022).

   • Two-handled cup with wide or weighted base and spout in lid

   Easier to drink and hold or lift a cup. Avoids spills. Wide base prevents tipping over (Swiech et al., 2020).

   • Plate with plate guard (see illustration) and nonskid bottom

   Helps person with limited flexibility of hands or poor motor coordination or who uses only one hand (Dodd, 2022).

   • Knife, fork, and spoon with large handles and options of being bendable, curved, and coated (see illustration)

   Improves ability to place food on utensil (Dodd, 2022).

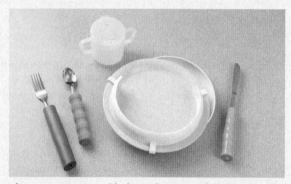

STEP 3 Mealtime adaptive equipment. *Clockwise from upper left:* Two-handled cup with lid, plate with plate guard, utensils with splints, and utensils with enlarged handles.

4. Assess meal tray for completeness and correct diet. Use this time (and during actual feeding) to instruct patient about diet, rationale for diet, food options, and dysphagia risks. Focus on principles (e.g., safe swallowing, nutritional value, comfort) that are easily applied at home.

   Prevents intake of incomplete or incorrect diet. Instruction is more meaningful when applied during real-time activity.

5. Begin feeding. Ask in which order patient would like to eat the meal. Help to set up meal tray if patient unable to do so: open packages, cut up food, apply seasonings or condiments, place napkin.

   Allows patient more independence and control. Small pieces are easier to chew and minimize risk for aspiration.

6. Watch patient successfully swallow first bites of food and drink. If patient is able to eat independently, stop here. Reinforce positive results. Return after 15 or 20 minutes or stay at side for communication and additional teaching.

   Aim is to make patient as self-sufficient as possible. Providing positive feedback to the learner reinforces competency (Reynolds et al., 2020).

STEP	RATIONALE

7. Help patient who cannot eat independently.

   a. Assume comfortable position.

      Being comfortable prevents you from rushing patient through meal.

   b. If patient is visually impaired, identify food location on plate as if it were a clock (e.g., vegetables at 9 o'clock, meat at 3 o'clock) (see illustration).

      Helps patient locate food items; patient may be able to feed self if given adequate information about food placement on tray.

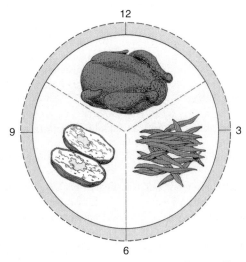

STEP 7b Clock setup to prepare food on a plate for the visually impaired patient.

   c. Ask in what order the patient prefers to eat, and cut food into bite-size pieces.

      Gives patient more independence and control. Small bites reduce risk of aspiration (see Skill 30.3).

   d. Provide fluids as requested. Discourage patient from drinking all fluids at beginning of meal.

      Promotes swallowing. Prevents patient from filling up on fluids.

   e. Pace feeding to avoid patient fatigue. Interact with patient during mealtime. Verbally encourage self-feeding attempts.

      Social interaction may improve appetite. Providing positive feedback reinforces competency (Reynolds et al., 2020).

   f. Use mealtime as opportunity to communicate with and educate patient about nutrition topics and discharge plan.

      Offers extended time for teaching.

   g. Feed patient in manner that facilitates chewing and swallowing. Position patient's chin down and place food in stronger side of the mouth.

      Chin-down position may help to reduce aspiration risk (see Skill 30.3).

8. Use appropriate feeding techniques for patients with special needs:

   a. *Older adult:* Feed small amounts at a time, observing biting, chewing, ability to manipulate tongue to form bolus of food, swallowing, and fatigue between bites. Be sure that patient has swallowed food. Offer variety of foods and frequent rest periods.

      Decreased saliva production in older adults impairs swallowing. Dementia progressively leads to dysphagia. Aspiration results from decreased or absent gag reflex.

   b. *Neurologically impaired patient:* Feed small amounts at a time and observe ability to chew, manipulate tongue to form bolus, and swallow. Have patient open mouth, and check for food left inside cheeks (pocketing). Give small amount of thin liquid between bites.

      Some patients with limited tongue strength and control are unable to move food to back of mouth for swallowing. Checking for pocketed food in mouth prevents aspiration.

   c. *Patients with cancer:* Check for food aversions before and during meal. Monitor for fatigue.

      Strong, abnormal sense of taste and smell are side effects of chemotherapy. Cancer patients can tire easily.

9. Help patient with hand hygiene and mouth care after meal is completed. (Apply gloves as needed.)

      Maintains comfort.

STEP	RATIONALE
10. Help patient to comfortable resting position; leave head of bed elevated at least 45 degrees for 30 to 60 minutes after meal.	Reduces risk of aspiration from regurgitation.
11. Place nurse call system in an accessible location within patient's reach.	Ensures patient can call for assistance if needed.
12. Raise side rails (as appropriate) and lower bed to lowest position, locking into position.	Ensures patient safety and prevents falls.
13. Return patient's tray to appropriate place, remove and dispose of gloves and perform hand hygiene.	Reduces transmission of microorganisms.

EVALUATION

1. Monitor body weight daily or weekly.	Determines ongoing nutritional status.
2. Monitor laboratory values as indicated.	Biochemical markers such as albumin and prealbumin help to identify changes in nutritional status over time.
3. Monitor intake and output (I&O) (see Chapter 6) and complete intake measurement (e.g., observed intake, calorie count).	Monitors fluid intake and fluid balance.
4. Observe patient's ability to self-feed, including ability to feed certain items, part or all of meal.	Helps to determine what assistance patient needs with feeding.
5. Observe patient for choking, coughing, gagging, or food left in mouth during eating.	Indicates dysphagia and possible aspiration.
6. **Use Teach-Back:** "We discussed ways you can help feed your husband that make it easier for swallowing. Tell me two ways to help with feeding and why it is important." Revise your instruction now or develop a plan for revised family caregiver teaching if family caregiver is not able to teach back correctly.	Teach-back is a technique for health care providers to ensure that they have explained medical information clearly so that patients and their families understand what is communicated to them (AHRQ, 2023).

Unexpected Outcomes	Related Interventions
1. Patient is unable to eat entire meal or refuses to eat.	• Determine if patient has other food preferences and cultural factors or religious restrictions.
	• Ask what is affecting patient's ability to eat.
	• Determine if patient's ability or desire to eat is better at other times of the day.
	• Determine if patient is in pain or nauseated. Does patient have constipation? Implement appropriate interventions (e.g., administering analgesic, antiemetic, or cathartic; offering food or liquid at temperature patient prefers; offering small frequent meals).
	• Provide more frequent oral care.
	• If inability to eat meal is a repeated problem, collaborate with health care provider and RDN.
2. Patient chokes on food.	• Stop feeding immediately; place on side with head forward and pointing down; suction food and secretions from mouth and airway.
	• Contact health care provider if choking occurs repeatedly.
	• Suggest appropriate referrals (e.g., speech-language pathologist, RDN) (see Skill 30.3).

Documentation

• Document the patient's type of diet, amount of feeding assistance needed, tolerance of diet, amount or percentage of the meal eaten (e.g., 25% of food consumed at breakfast), and calorie count (if ordered).
• If measuring I&O, document fluid intake (see Chapter 6).
• If patient is receiving oral nutritional supplements (e.g., Ensure, Boost), document the amount taken and patient's tolerance (absence of nausea or feeling full) and likes and dislikes in EHR or chart.
• Document evaluation of patient/family caregiver learning.

Hand-Off Reporting

• Report any swallowing difficulties, food dislikes or intolerance, or refusal to eat to health care provider and RDN.
• Report to registered nurse (RN) on upcoming shift any new approaches needed that promote patient's ability to eat.

Special Considerations

Patient Education

• Family caregivers report increased fear and anxiety related to their responsibilities when feeding patients with dementia, including worry about the patient's nutritional status and risk for choking (Namasivayam-MacDonald & Shune, 2018). Provide frequent education sessions and have family caregivers demonstrate feeding techniques.

- Suggest to family caregivers these strategies when feeding patients with dementia (Alzheimer's Society, 2022; Cleveland Clinic, 2019):
  - Avoid "food fights." Make mealtime as pleasant as possible. Encourage someone to eat, but do not demand, cajole, or threaten.
  - Someone with dementia may not be able to express what food choices are desired. If giving choices, give only two things to choose between. Even if a choice is made, the person may not want it when it is presented. Do not take it personally.
  - If you know a patient's favorite foods, have them available for backup. Favorite foods might change.
  - People often crave sweet things, so make them available, in limited quantities, unless medically not recommended (e.g., diabetes). Fruit can often fulfill this need.
  - People will often not eat a large meal or the traditional three meals a day. Try offering smaller, more frequent meals. Always have water or other liquids available and offer them often so that the person does not get dehydrated.
  - Use small plates, as large ones can be overwhelming. Use color contrast of plate and food for the person to distinguish the food more easily.

Pediatrics

- Human milk is the most desirable complete diet for infants during the first 6 months. Infants who are breastfed or bottle-fed do not require additional fluids, especially water or juice, during the first 4 months of life. Excessive intake of water causes water intoxication, failure to thrive, and hyponatremia.
- Typically infants do not consume solid foods until 6 months of age. Iron-fortified infant cereal is usually the first solid food to offer. A common sequence for introducing solid food is one new food every 5 to 7 days; it is recommended that strained fruits be introduced first, followed by vegetables, and finally meats (Hockenberry et al., 2024).
- Do not mix solid foods in a bottle and feed through a nipple with a larger hole (Hockenberry et al., 2024).

Older Adults

- The U.S. Department of Agriculture (USDA) MyPlate (USDA, n.d.b) recommendations for older adults encourage making small adjustments to help individuals enjoy the foods and beverages they eat and drink by:
  - Adding flavor to foods with spices and herbs instead of salt and looking for low-sodium packaged foods.
  - Adding sliced fruits and vegetables to meals and snacks. Look for presliced fruits and vegetables on sale if slicing and chopping are a challenge.
  - Asking the doctor to suggest other options if the medications taken affect appetite or change the desire to eat.
  - Drinking 3 cups of fat-free or low-fat milk throughout the day. If milk is not tolerated, small amounts of yogurt, buttermilk, hard cheese, or lactose-free foods can be tried. Drink water instead of sugary drinks.
  - Consuming foods fortified with vitamin B_{12}, such as fortified cereals.
- Being physically active can help individuals stay strong and independent as they grow older. If a patient is overweight or obese, weight loss can improve quality of life and reduce the risk of disease and disability.
- Older adults may refuse to eat certain foods because of the way they look and smell or because the food conflicts with their culture or personal history, even if they can feed themselves. Be culturally sensitive in food selection.

Populations With Disabilities

- For patients with intellectual disabilities, assess for risk factors for malnutrition, such as abuse (Sullivan et al., 2018).

Home Care

- Assess financial resources of patient and family caregiver to determine if they can purchase nutritionally complete foods for patient.
- Help patient and family caregiver identify ways to make meals in the home pleasant and enjoyable.

✦ SKILL 30.3 Aspiration Precautions

 Video Clip

Dysphagia, or difficulty swallowing, refers to a sensation of food or liquid being delayed or hindered in its passage from the mouth to the stomach (Audag et al., 2019). It is classified anatomically as either oropharyngeal or esophageal. Dysphagia occurs in patients with multiple diseases and conditions (Box 30.6). Patients with dysphagia are at risk for aspiration. Conditions that suppress the cough reflex (such as sedation) further increase the risk for aspiration (Metheny, 2018). Aspiration is the misdirection of oropharyngeal secretions or gastric contents into the larynx and lower respiratory tract (Chen et al., 2021; Metheny, 2018). It occurs when secretions in the oral pharynx enter the trachea, or it may occur as a result of reflux of gastric content that enters the throat and then goes down the trachea. The prevalence of aspiration ranges from 43% to 51% in patients with dysphagia (Chen et al., 2021). Harmful results of dysphagia include aspiration pneumonia, malnutrition, and dehydration, which can lead to increased hospital length of stay, hospital readmission, or death (Chen et al., 2021). Emotional responses to dysphagia may include altered body image, embarrassment, social isolation, and depression.

The inability to coordinate the complex, sequential swallowing mechanism slows eating, results in food being left in the mouth, and may lead to aspiration (Audag et al., 2019). Gastric material and secretions in the mouth and pharynx and pathogenic bacteria enter the trachea and lungs. Aspiration pneumonia can be a fatal complication of dysphagia, especially in older adults. However, aspiration pneumonia develops only if the material aspirated is pathogenic to the lungs and the patient's natural resistance to the material is compromised (Makhnevich et al., 2019).

A nurse's role when feeding patients or supervising them during eating is to recognize dysphagia to prevent aspiration. Reliable and valid screening tools are available to use to detect dysphagia (Audag et al., 2019). Symptoms of dysphagia vary, depending on the swallowing alteration. You should suspect dysphagia if a patient has coughing during or right after eating or drinking, a wet or gurgling sounding voice during or after eating or drinking, extra effort

BOX 30.6

Causes of Dysphagia

Neurogenic
- Stroke
- Cerebral palsy
- Guillain-Barré syndrome
- Multiple sclerosis
- Amyotrophic lateral sclerosis (Lou Gehrig disease)
- Diabetic neuropathy
- Parkinson disease

Myogenic
- Myasthenia gravis
- Aging
- Muscular dystrophy
- Polymyositis

Obstructive
- Benign peptic stricture
- Lower esophageal ring
- Candidiasis
- Head and neck cancer
- Inflammatory masses
- Trauma/surgical resection
- Anterior mediastinal masses
- Cervical spondylosis

Other
- Gastrointestinal or esophageal resection
- Rheumatological disorders
- Connective tissue disorders
- Vagotomy

BOX 30.7

Criteria for Dysphagia Referral

Before referral:
If the answer is yes to either of the following two questions, referral at this time is not appropriate.
- Is patient unconscious or drowsy?
- Is patient unable to sit in an upright position for a reasonable length of time?

Also consider the next two questions before making a referral:
- Is the patient near the end of life?
- Does the patient have an esophageal problem that will require surgical intervention?

When observing a patient or giving mouth care, look for the following:
- Open mouth (weak lip closure)
- Drooling liquids or solids
- Facial or tongue weakness
- Difficulty moving or swallowing secretions in the mouth
- Slurred, indistinct speech
- Hoarseness
- Poor posture or head control
- Weak, involuntary cough
- Delayed cough (up to 2 minutes after swallow)
- General frailty, confusion, or dementia
- No spontaneous swallowing movements

If any of the above is present, the patient may have swallowing problems and need referral to a speech-language pathologist.

---

or time needed to chew or swallow, food or liquid leaking from the mouth or getting stuck in the mouth after multiple attempts to swallow, recurring chest congestion after eating, and weight loss or dehydration from not being able to eat enough (National Foundation of Swallowing Disorders, 2023). The clinical symptoms of resultant aspiration are tachypnea (an early symptom of respirations above 26), cough, dyspnea (trouble breathing), decreased breath sounds, and abnormal breath sounds such as wheezing, rales, and rhonchi (see Chapter 6).

Small-volume aspirations that produce no overt symptoms are common and are often not discovered until the condition progresses to aspiration pneumonia (Metheny, 2018). Silent or asymptomatic aspiration refers to passage of food or liquid into the trachea and lungs without producing a productive cough or other signs consistent with aspiration. As patients with dysphagia age, their perception of the urge to cough decreases, which further increases the risk for silent aspiration. The condition often results from sensory damage to the pharynx and muscle weakness in the throat and mouth that produces a lack of a protective cough reflex (Chen et al., 2021). Lack of outward signs such as coughing reduces awareness by the patient, family caregiver, and health team members that aspiration is occurring. This can result in longer periods of ingestion of food and liquid into the lungs. The more subtle signs associated with silent aspiration are easy to miss and include lack of speech, depressed alertness, wet quality to voice, drooling, difficulty controlling secretions, and absence of gag reflex.

As a nurse you are in a key position to identify patients' swallowing difficulties and make referrals to appropriate health care professionals. Early screening and intervention are crucial to preventing aspiration and pneumonia. Conduct your initial nutrition

screening (see Skill 30.1) to determine the potential for both aspiration and safe oral intake. When you detect risk factors, consult the speech-language pathologist (SLP) for a more comprehensive examination (Box 30.7). The single most important measure to prevent aspiration is to place the patient on nothing-by-mouth (NPO) status until a dysphagia evaluation by a certified SLP can be performed, and then a safe diet can resume.

Dysphagia Management

The primary approaches to managing dysphagia and preventing aspiration during oral intake include texture modification of food and liquids and positional swallowing maneuvers, such as chin-tuck or head rotation (Chen et al., 2021; Kollmeier & Keenaghan, 2022). Dietary modification by altering the consistency of food and liquids is most effective when implemented using an interprofessional approach recommended by the SLP (McGinnis et al., 2019). The SLP and registered dietitian nutritionist (RDN) are central to dysphagia management. Appropriate food choices and consistency of liquids are individualized and based on which phase of swallowing is dysfunctional (IDDSI, 2019).

In October 2002 the American Dietetic Association published the National Dysphagia Diet Task Force national dysphagia diet. In 2019, the International Dysphagia Diet Standardisation Initiative (IDDSI, 2019) published standardization of the terminology for food textures and liquid consistencies for use around the world. The diet standards provide guidelines and standard terminology for food and texture modifications. The diet comprises eight levels (Table 30.4) (IDDSI, 2019).

Delegation

The skill of following aspiration precautions while feeding a patient can be delegated to assistive personnel (AP). However, the nurse is responsible for the ongoing assessment of a patient's risk for

TABLE 30.4

International Dysphagia Diet Framework

Level and Description	Characteristics	Examples
0: Thin liquid	Flows like water, can be drunk easily through a straw *Rationale:* Functional ability to safely manage liquids of all types	Coffee, tea, lemonade, juice, water
1: Slightly thick liquid	Thicker than water, requires more effort to drink, still flows through a straw or nipple *Rationale:* Primarily used for the pediatric population to reduce speed of flow	Commercially available oral supplements similar in viscosity to an infant "antiregurgitation" formula, nectar-thick juices
2: Mildly thick liquid	Flows off a spoon, effort required to drink through a straw *Rationale:* Suitable if tongue control is slightly reduced	Milkshake
3: Liquidized, moderately thick	Can be drunk from a cup, some effort to suck through a straw, cannot be eaten with a fork, will drip between prongs, no oral processing or chewing required, smooth texture with no lumps *Rationale:* Allows more time for oral control, needs some tongue propulsion effort	Runny rice cereal, runny pureed fruit, sauces and gravies, honey-thickened beverages
4: Pureed, extremely thick	Cannot be drunk from a cup, usually eaten with a spoon, cannot be sucked through a straw, does not require chewing, can be molded, no lumps, not sticky *Rationale:* If tongue control is significantly reduced, requires less propulsion, no biting or chewing is required; used in patients with missing teeth or poorly fitting dentures	Pureed meat, vegetables, fruits, and thick cereals
5: Minced and moist	Can be eaten with a fork or spoon, soft and moist with no separate thin liquid, small lumps that are easy to squash with tongue *Rationale:* Biting is not required, minimal chewing, tongue force alone can be used to break soft small particles; used in patients with some missing teeth	Finely minced or ground tender meats served in extremely thick, smooth, nonpouring sauce or gravy; mashed potatoes; mashed fruits; very thick cereals Fluid or milk should *not* separate from items, pre-gelled soaked breads
6: Soft and bite-sized	Can be eaten with a fork or spoon; can be mashed/broken down with pressure from utensils; knife is not required to cut; chewing is required before swallowing; soft, tender, and moist throughout *Rationale:* Tongue force and control are required to move the food for chewing and to keep it within the mouth during chewing; tongue force is required to move the bolus for swallowing	Soft cooked meat cut in small pieces, flakey fish, casseroles, stews, soft-cooked vegetables in bite-sized pieces, mashed fruits
7: Regular	Normal, everyday foods of various textures *Rationale:* Ability to bite hard or soft foods, chew all textures without tiring	No restrictions

Adapted from the International Dysphagia Diet Standardisation Initiative (IDDSI): *The International Dysphagia Diet Standardisation Initiative 2019: complete IDDSI framework detailed definitions 2.0*, 2019. https://iddsi.org/IDDSI/media/images/Complete_IDDSI_Framework_Final_31July2019.pdf. Accessed October 28, 2023.

aspiration and determination of positioning and any special feeding techniques. Direct the AP to:
- Position patient upright (90 degrees preferred) or in highest position allowed by patient's medical condition, during and after feeding
- Use aspiration precautions while feeding patients who need help and explain feeding techniques that are successful for specific patients
- Immediately report any onset of coughing, gagging, a wet voice, or pocketing of food to the nurse

Interprofessional Collaboration

- When you suspect a patient has dysphagia, refer to an SLP and RDN.
- An SLP specializes in swallowing disorders and makes treatment recommendations for food and liquid texture modifications.

- The RDN ensures that recommendations are balanced with the nutritional and caloric needs of patients.

Equipment

- Chair or bed that allows patient to sit upright
- Thickening agents as designated by SLP (rice, cereal, yogurt, gelatin, commercial thickener)
- Tongue blade
- Penlight
- Oral hygiene supplies (see Chapter 18)
- Suction equipment (see Chapter 24)
- Clean gloves
- *Option:* Pulse oximeter

STEP	RATIONALE

ASSESSMENT

1. Identify patient using at least two identifiers (e.g., name and birthday or name and medical record number) according to agency policy.	Ensures correct patient. Complies with The Joint Commission standards and improves patient safety (TJC, 2023).
2. Review patient's medical history, nutritional risks, and results of nutrition screening in electronic health record (EHR). Assess for presence of conditions that cause dysphagia (see Box 30.7). Note patient's weight.	Reveals patient risk patterns for altered nutrition and dysphagia. Weight provides baseline for determining change in nutritional status.
3. Assess patient's current medications for use of sedatives, hypnotics, or other agents that may impair cough or swallowing reflex and for any medications that dry oral secretions (e.g., calcium channel blockers, diuretics) (O'Brien, 2020).	Medication side effects may increase risk of developing dysphagia.
4. Assess patient's/family caregiver's health literacy.	Determines degree to which individuals have the ability to find, understand, and use information and services to make informed health-related decisions and actions for themselves and others (CDC, 2023b).
5. Perform hand hygiene. Assess patient for signs and symptoms of dysphagia. Use a screening tool if recommended by agency.	Patient symptoms aid in determining if further swallow evaluation is needed and approach to feeding.

Clinical Judgment *If screening is positive for dysphagia, consult with speech-language pathologist (SLP).*

6. Assess patient's mental status: alertness, orientation, and ability to follow simple commands (e.g., open your mouth; stick out your tongue).	Disorientation and inability to follow commands present higher risk for dysphagia. Patients with progressive dementia develop dysphagia.
7. Apply gloves. Assess patient's oral cavity, level of dental hygiene, missing teeth, or poorly fitting dentures. Remove and dispose of gloves and perform hand hygiene.	Poorly fitting dentures and absence of teeth can cause chewing and swallowing difficulties, increasing aspiration risk. Poor oral hygiene and periodontal disease can result in growth of bacteria in oropharynx, which, if aspirated, can lead to pneumonia (Thomas et al., 2019; O'Brien, 2020). Findings indicate level of oral hygiene needed and food consistency needed. Reduces transmission of microorganisms.
8. *Option:* Obtain baseline assessment oxygen saturation. A decline in SpO_2 of 2% or more has been regarded as a possible marker of aspiration (Marian et al., 2017). Perform hand hygiene. (Keep oximeter in place if preparing for mealtime.)	Despite the clinical use of oximetry, research findings question whether it can reliably be used to detect aspiration (ASHA, 2023a; Marian et al., 2017; Britton et al., 2018).
9. Indicate in patient's health record that dysphagia/aspiration risk is present. *Option:* Some agencies use different-colored meal trays to signify patients at risk for aspiration.	Identifying patient as dysphagic reduces risk of receiving improperly prepared oral nutrition without supervision.
10. Assess patient's/family caregiver's knowledge of and experience with dysphagia risk and diet options.	Reveals need for patient/family caregiver instruction and/or support.

PLANNING

1. Expected outcomes following completion of procedure: • Patient does not exhibit signs or symptoms of aspiration. • Patient maintains stable weight.	Interventions for preventing aspiration are successful. Patient is able to maintain adequate oral nutrition.
2. Provide patient 30 minutes of rest.	Fatigue increases risk of aspiration.
3. Explain why you are observing patient during eating.	Signs or symptoms associated with aspiration that develop during eating indicate need for further swallowing evaluation
4. Explain to patient and family caregiver about aspiration precautions and specifically what you are going to do and why.	Increases patient cooperation and prepares family caregiver for being able to help.
5. Close room door and bedside curtain.	Provides patient privacy.
6. Obtain and organize equipment for aspiration precautions at bedside.	Ensures more efficient procedure.

IMPLEMENTATION

1. Perform hand hygiene and have patient or family caregiver (if going to help with feeding) perform hand hygiene.	Prevents transmission of microorganisms. Educates patient and family caregiver about need to maintain infection control practices.

STEP	RATIONALE
2. Apply clean gloves. Provide thorough oral hygiene, including brushing tongue, before meal.	Risk for aspiration pneumonia has been associated with poor oral hygiene (Thomas et al., 2019).
3. Position patient upright (90 degrees) in chair or elevate head of patient's bed to a 90-degree angle or highest position allowed by medical condition during meal.	Position facilitates safe swallowing and enhances esophageal motility (Metheny, 2018; Thomas et al., 2019). Side-lying position is an option if patient cannot have head elevated.
4. *Option:* If not previously applied, place pulse oximeter on patient's finger; monitor during feeding.	Pulse oximetry continues to be used in many agencies to predict aspiration, but research has raised questions about its efficacy (Britton et al., 2018; Marian et al., 2017).
5. Using penlight and tongue blade, gently inspect mouth for pockets of food.	Pockets of food found inside cheeks occur when patient has difficulty moving food from mouth into pharynx; may lead to aspiration (Nova Scotia Health Authority, 2020; Chen et al., 2021). Patient is usually unaware of pocketing left after prior feeding.
6. Provide appropriate thickness of liquids per SLP and type of liquids per RDN (IDDSI, 2019) (see Table 30.4). Encourage patient to feed self.	Thin liquids are difficult to control in mouth and pharynx and are more easily aspirated.
7. Have patient assume chin-down position. Remind patient to not tilt head backward when eating or while drinking. *Option:* Have patient assume head-turn-plus-chin-down position.	Chin-down position may help reduce aspiration (Metheny, 2018). One study has suggested that a head-turn-plus-chin-down maneuver may be more successful (Chen et al., 2021).
8. Adjust the rate of feeding and size of bites to match the patient's tolerance. If patient unable to feed self, place ½ to 1 teaspoon of food in unaffected side of mouth, allowing utensil to touch mouth or tongue.	Small bites help patient swallow (Grodner et al., 2020; Metheny, 2018). Provides tactile cue to food being eaten; avoids pocketing of food on weaker side.
9. Observe patient during eating for signs of dysphagia. Observe patient attempt to feed self; note type of food consistencies and liquids able to swallow. Note during and at end of meal if patient tires.	Detects abnormal eating patterns such as frequent clearing of throat or prolonged eating time. Chewing and sitting up for feeding bring on onset of fatigue (Meiner & Yeager, 2019). Provides data for future planning of meal assistance.
10. Provide verbal coaching: remind patient to chew and think about swallowing. • Open your mouth. • Feel the food in your mouth. • Chew and taste the food. • Raise your tongue to the roof of your mouth. • Think about swallowing. • Close your mouth and swallow. • Swallow again. • Cough to clear your airway.	Verbal cueing keeps patient focused on normal swallowing (Metheny, 2018). Positive reinforcement enhances patient's confidence in ability to swallow.
11. Avoid mixing food of different textures in same mouthful. Alternate liquids and bites of food (Metheny, 2018). Refer to SLP for next meal if patient has difficulty with a particular consistency.	Gradual increase in types and textures combined with constant monitoring helps patient to eat more safely. Single textures are easier to swallow than multiple textures. Alternating solids with liquids removes food residue in mouth.
12. During the meal, explain to patient and family caregiver the techniques being used to promote swallowing. Allow family caregiver to coach patient.	Enhances patient and family caregiver's ability to use techniques in the home. Optimizes teaching time during patient contact.
13. Monitor swallowing and observe for any respiratory difficulty. Observe for throat clearing, coughing, choking, gagging, and drooling of food; suction airway as needed (see Chapter 24).	These are indications that suggest dysphagia and thus pose risk for aspiration.
14. Minimize distractions, do not talk (except for explanations being provided), and do not rush patient. Allow time for adequate chewing and swallowing. Provide rest periods as needed during meal.	Environmental distractions and conversations during mealtime increase risk for aspiration. Avoiding fatigue reduces aspiration risk.

Clinical Judgment *If patient remains stable without difficulty, this is a good time to delegate continued feeding to AP so that you can attend to other patients and assigned priorities.*

15. Use sauces, condiments, and gravies (if part of dysphagia diet) to facilitate cohesive food bolus formation.	Cohesive food bolus helps to prevent pocketing or small food particles from entering the airway.

STEP	RATIONALE
16. Ask patient to remain sitting upright for at least 30 to 60 minutes after a meal. Provide access to nurse call system to patient and instruct patient to use if needed.	Remaining upright after meals or snacks reduces chance of aspiration by allowing food particles remaining in pharynx to clear (Metheny, 2018). Promotes patient safety. Ensures patient can call for assistance if needed.
17. Apply clean gloves. Provide thorough oral hygiene after meal (see Chapter 18).	Rigorous oral hygiene reduces plaque and secretions containing bacteria, with studies showing reduction in incidence of pneumonia (Chen et al., 2021; Thomas et al., 2019).
18. Be sure patient is comfortable in upright position.	Promotes patient comfort and safety.
19. Place nurse call system in an accessible location within patient's reach.	Ensures patient can call for assistance if needed.
20. Return patient's tray to appropriate place. Remove and dispose of gloves, if worn.	Reduces spread of microorganisms.
21. Raise side rails (as appropriate) and lower bed to lowest position, locking into position. Perform hand hygiene.	Ensures patient safety and prevents falls. Reduces transmission of microorganisms.

EVALUATION

1. Observe patient's ability to swallow food and fluids of various textures and thickness without choking.

   Indicates if there is ease with swallowing and absence of signs related to aspiration.

2. Monitor pulse oximetry readings (if ordered) for high-risk patients during eating.

   Deteriorating oxygen saturation levels may indicate aspiration, but research has raised questions about predictive ability (Britton et al., 2018; Marian et al., 2017).

3. Monitor patient's intake and output (I&O), calorie count, and food intake.

   Helps to detect malnutrition and dehydration resulting from dysphagia.

4. Weigh patient daily or weekly.

   Determines if weight is stable and reflects nutritional status.

5. Observe patient's oral cavity after meal.

   Determines presence of food pockets after meal that has included foods of various textures.

6. **Use Teach-Back:** "We talked about why your husband is at risk to aspirate food. Tell me the things to observe for that will tell you whether your husband is having trouble swallowing. What should you do if these things happen during a meal?" Revise your instruction now or develop a plan for revised family caregiver teaching if family caregiver is not able to teach back correctly.

   Teach-back is a technique for health care providers to ensure that they have explained medical information clearly so that patients and their families understand what is communicated to them (AHRQ, 2023).

Unexpected Outcomes

1. Patient coughs, gags, complains of food "stuck in throat," and has wet quality to voice when eating.

2. Patient experiences weight loss over next several days/weeks.

Related Interventions

- Stop feeding immediately and place patient on NPO.
- Notify health care provider and suction as needed (Chapter 24).
- Anticipate further consultation with SLP for swallowing exercises and techniques to improve swallowing.
- Discuss findings with health care provider and RDN. Determine if increasing frequency or quality of foods is needed.
- Nutritional supplements may be needed.

Documentation

- Document positioning for eating, assessment findings, type of patient's diet, tolerance of liquids and food textures, amount of assistance required, response to instruction, absence or presence of any symptoms of dysphagia, fluid intake, and amount of food eaten.
- Document your evaluation of patient/family caregiver learning.

Hand-Off Reporting

- Describe patient's tolerance to diet and degree of assistance required during hand-off reporting.
- Report any coughing, gagging, choking, or other swallowing difficulties to health care provider.

Special Considerations
Patient Education
- In any situation when a patient has difficulty eating, educate patient and family caregiver about aspiration precautions, particularly the techniques most effective for the patient, to prevent pneumonia.
- Recommend to patients and family caregivers appropriate websites for how to prepare pureed foods. An example is from the University Health Network, available at https://www.uhn.ca/PatientsFamilies/Health_Information/Health_Topics/Documents/Pureed_Foods_for_people_with_Dysphagia.pdf.

Pediatrics
- Long-term effects for a child diagnosed with pediatric dysphagia include poor weight gain velocity and/or undernutrition (failure to thrive), aspiration pneumonia and/or compromised pulmonary status, food aversion, oral aversion, dehydration, and ongoing need for enteral or parenteral nutrition (ASHA, 2023c).
- The primary goals of feeding and swallowing interventions for children are to safely support adequate nutrition and hydration, determine the optimum feeding methods/technique to maximize swallowing safety and feeding efficiency, collaborate with family caregiver to incorporate dietary preferences, attain age-appropriate eating skills in the most normal setting and manner possible, minimize the risk of pulmonary complications, and maximize the quality of life (ASHA, 2023c).

Older Adults
- People with dementia often have eating difficulties before hospitalization, but they are likely to worsen in the hospital because people with dementia often become more confused in an unfamiliar place. Different mealtime routines and foods add to the problem.
- Patients with dementia may not be able to tell anyone that they are hungry or that they need help eating or more time to chew and swallow.
- Minimize the use of sedatives and hypnotics because these agents may impair the cough reflex and swallowing (Metheny, 2018).

Populations With Disabilities
- Assess patients with intellectual disabilities for overt or silent aspiration because they may be at increased risk for aspiration pneumonia (Sullivan et al., 2018).

Home Care
- Warn family caregiver that older adults with pneumonia often complain of significantly fewer symptoms than their younger counterparts; for this reason, aspiration pneumonia is underdiagnosed in this group. Delirium may be the only manifestation of pneumonia in elderly people.
- Dysphagia is best managed with an interprofessional approach that includes patient, family caregiver, health care provider, nurse occupational therapist, and SLP (Kollmeier & Keenaghan, 2022; Thomas et al., 2019).

◆ CLINICAL JUDGMENT AND NEXT-GENERATION NCLEX® EXAMINATION–STYLE QUESTIONS

A 66-year-old patient with amyotrophic lateral sclerosis (ALS) has been admitted to the hospital with bilateral pneumonia for antibiotic therapy. On physical examination, the nurse notes a diminished gag reflex, clear oral cavity, and reduced strength in the hands and arms bilaterally. The nurse also notes that the patient has bilateral decreased lung sounds in the bases. Pulse oximetry is 92% on room air. The nurse observes during mealtime and notes that the patient chews and swallows very slowly and frequently coughs when swallowing and that food and liquids leak from the corners of the mouth while eating.

1. The nurse analyzes the findings to determine the patient's condition.
   Choose the *most likely* options for the information missing from the statement below by selecting from the lists of options provided.
   The patient is at highest risk for **1 [Select]** as evidenced by **2 [Select]**.

Options for 1	Options for 2
Dehydration	Reduced strength in hands
Malnutrition	Diminished gag reflex
Sepsis	Decreased lung sounds
Aspiration	Pulse oximetry 92%

2. While caring for the patient, which of the following activities can the nurse delegate to an AP? **Select all that apply.**
   1. Taking the medication history
   2. Patient height and weight
   3. Completing nutrition screening tool
   4. Assisting patient to the bathroom
   5. Assisting the patient to order meals for the next day

3. The nurse assess that the patient consistently eats only about 25% of each meal. Which of the following interventions would the nurse implement to improve the patient's food intake? **Select all that apply.**
   1. Provide meals at scheduled times established by the hospital.
   2. Remind that the patient must eat to heal.
   3. Determine if the patient is experiencing pain.
   4. Offer larger servings of food more often.
   5. Provide between-meal snacks.

4. The patient is soon discharged back to the residence at an assisted-living facility. Two weeks later the nurse is in a team conference discussing that the patient is losing weight. Which of the following factors place the patient at risk for malnutrition? **Select all that apply.**
   1. Difficulty feeding self
   2. Poor appetite
   3. Residence in assisted-living facility
   4. BMI of 21
   5. Family members who take the patient out to eat

5. The nurse collaborates with the registered dietitian nutritionist (RDN) to enhance the patient's nutritional status with a minced and moist diet. Which of the following foods would the nurse provide to the patient? **Select all that apply.**
   1. Pureed fruit
   2. Ground beef in gravy
   3. Flakey fish
   4. Thick cereal
   5. Stew

Visit the Evolve site for Clinical Judgment and Next-Generation NCLEX® Examination–Style Questions.

REFERENCES

Abugroun A, et al: Impact of malnutrition on hospitalization outcomes for older adults admitted for sepsis, *Am J Med* 134(2):221–226, 2021.

Academy of Nutrition and Dietetics: Position of the Academy of Nutrition and Dietetics: malnutrition (undernutrition) screening tools for all adults, *J Acad Nutr Diet* 120(4):709–713, 2020.

Academy of Nutrition and Dietetics: *Eat Right Pro—Nutrition Care Process*, 2023a. https://www.eatrightpro.org/practice/nutrition-care-process. Accessed October 30, 2023.

Academy of Nutrition and Dietetics: *Nutrition screening adults*, 2023b. https://www.andeal.org/topic.cfm?menu=5382. Accessed October 28, 2023.

Agency for Healthcare Research and Quality (AHRQ): *Healthcare cost and utilization project (HCUP)*, 2022. https://www.ahrq.gov/data/hcup/index.html. Accessed November 16, 2023.

Agency for Healthcare Research and Quality (AHRQ): *Malnutrition in hospitalized adults*, 2021, Comparative Effectiveness Review No. 249: Malnutrition in Hospitalized Adults: a Systematic Review (ahrq.gov). https://effectivehealthcare.ahrq.gov/sites/default/files/related_files/cer-249-malnutrition-hospitalized-adults-evidence-summary_0.pdf. Accessed October 27, 2023.

Agency for Healthcare Research and Quality (AHRQ): *Teach-Back: Intervention*, 2023. https://www.ahrq.gov/patient-safety/reports/engage/interventions/teach-back.html. Accessed October 28, 2023.

Alne EKF, et al: Sharing meals: promising nutritional interventions for primary health care including nursing students and elderly people, *BMC Nutr* 7(8):1–11, 2021.

Alzheimer's Society: *Improving the eating experience*, 2022. https://www.alzheimers.org.uk/get-support/daily-living/improving-eating-experience-dementia#content-start. Accessed October 28, 2023.

American Speech-Language-Hearing Association (ASHA): *Adult dysphagia*, 2023a. https://www.asha.org/practice-portal/clinical-topics/adult-dysphagia/. Accessed October 28, 2023.

American Speech-Language-Hearing Association (ASHA): *Pediatric feeding and swallowing*, 2023b. https://www.asha.org/practice-portal/clinical-topics/pediatric-feeding-and-swallowing/#collapse_3. Accessed October 23, 2023.

American Speech-Language-Hearing Association (ASHA): *Speech-language pathologists: about speech-language pathology*, 2023c. https://www.asha.org/students/speech-language-pathologists/#:~:text=Speech%2Dlanguage%20pathologists%20(SLPs),disorders%20in%20children%20and%20adults. Accessed October 28, 2023.

Audag N, et al: Screening and evaluation tools of dysphagia in adults with neuro-muscular diseases: a systematic review, *Ther Adv Chronic Dis* 10:1–15, 2019.

Barrins and Associates: *Joint Commission nutrition screening requirements for behavioral healthcare programs*, 2018. https://barrins-assoc.com/tjc-cms-blog/behavioral-health/joint-commission-nutrition-screening-requirements-for-behavioral-healthcare-programs/. Accessed October 28, 2023.

Brennan D: *What to know about malnutrition in older adults*, 2023. https://www.webmd.com/healthy-aging/what-to-know-about-malnutrition-in-older-adults. Accessed November 21, 2023.

Britton D, et al: Utility of pulse oximetry to detect aspiration: an evidence-based systematic review, *Dysphagia* 33(3):282–292, 2018.

Centers for Disease Control and Prevention (CDC): *Four steps to food safety: clean, separate, cook, chill*, 2023a. https://www.cdc.gov/foodsafety/keep-food-safe.html. Accessed October 30, 2023.

Centers for Disease Control and Prevention (CDC): *What is health literacy?* 2023b. https://www.cdc.gov/healthliteracy/learn/index.html.

Chen S, et al: Interventions to prevent aspiration in older adults with dysphagia living in nursing homes: a scoping review, *BMC Geriatr* 21:429, 2021.

Cleveland Clinic: *Eating and nutritional challenges in patients with Alzheimer's Disease: tips for caregivers*, 2019. https://my.clevelandclinic.org/health/articles/9597-eating-and-nutritional-challenges-in-patients-with-alzheimers-disease-tips-for-caregivers. Accesseed October 28, 2023.

Compher C, et al: Guidelines for the provision of nutrition support therapy in the adult critically ill patient: the American Society for Parenteral and Enteral Nutrition, *JPEN* 46(1):12–41, 2022.

Dodd K: *Which malnutrition tool is best?* 2020. https://thegeriatricdietitian.com/malnutrition-screening-tool/. Accessed October 28, 2023.

Dodd K: *Adaptive equipment for eating: what, when, why*, 2022. https://thegeriatricdietitian.com/adaptive-equipment-for-eating/. Accessed October 28, 2023.

Feeding America: *Hunger and food insecurities*, 2022a. https://www.feedingamerica.org/hunger-in-america/food-insecurity. Accessed October 27, 2023.

Feeding America: *Senior food insecurities studies: the state of senior hunger in America*, 2022b. https://www.feedingamerica.org/research/senior-hunger-research/senior. Accessed October 27, 2023.

Feng L, et al: Malnutrition is positively associated with cognitive decline in centenarians and oldest-old adults: a crosssectional study, *EClinicalMedicine* 47:101336, 2022.

Fleury S, et al: The nutritional issue of older people receiving home-delivered meals: a systematic review, *Front Nutr* 8:Article 629580, 2021.

Food and Agriculture Organization of the United Nations (FAO): *Food-based dietary guidelines*, 2023. http://www.fao.org/nutrition/education/food-dietary-guidelines/home/en/. Accessed October 30, 2023.

Giger JN, Haddad LG: *Transcultural nursing: assessment and intervention*, ed 8, St. Louis, 2021, Elsevier.

Grodner M, et al: *Nutritional foundations and clinical applications: a nursing approach*, ed 7, St. Louis, 2020, Elsevier.

Haines J, et al: *Malnutrition in the elderly: underrecognized and increasing in prevalence*, 2020. https://www.clinicaladvisor.com/home/topics/geriatrics-information-center/malnutrition-in-the-elderly-underrecognized-and-increasing-in-prevalence/. Accessed October 30, 2023.

Howley EK: *Senior meal delivery services*, 2020. https://health.usnews.com/wellness/delivery-kits/articles/senior-meal-delivery-services. Accessed October 23, 2023.

Hockenberry MJ, et al: *Wong's nursing care of infants and children*, ed 12, St. Louis, 2024, Elsevier.

International Dysphagia Diet Standardisation Initiative (IDDSI): *The International Dysphagia Diet Standardisation Initiative 2019: complete IDDSI Framework Detailed definitions 2.0*, 2019. https://iddsi.org/IDDSI/media/images/Complete_IDDSI_Framework_Final_31July2019.pdf. Accessed October 30, 2023.

Jensen GL, et al: GLIM Criteria for the diagnosis of malnutrition: a consensus report from the global clinical nutrition community, *JPEN* 43(1):32–40, 2019.

Kollmeier BR, Keenaghan M: *Aspiration risk*, 2022, StatPearls [Internet]. https://www.ncbi.nlm.nih.gov/books/NBK470169/. Accessed October 30, 2023.

Linnell D, et al: *Nutrition for older adults: preventing malnutrition as the body ages*, 2021. https://extension.oregonstate.edu/sites/default/files/catalog/auto/PNW767.pdf. Accessed May October 30, 2023.

Lutz M, et al: Considerations for the development of innovative foods to improve nutrition in older adults, *Nutrients* 11:1275, 2019.

Makhnevich A, et al: Aspiration pneumonia in older adults, *J Hosp Med* 14:429–435, 2019.

Marian T, et al: Measurement of oxygen desaturation is not useful for the detection of aspiration in dysphagic stroke patients, *Cerebrovasc Dis Extra* 7(1):44, 2017.

McGinnis CM, et al: Dysphagia: interprofessional management, impact, and patient-centered care, *Nutr Clin Pract* 34(1):80–95, 2019.

Meiner S, Yeager J: *Gerontologic nursing*, ed 6, St. Louis, 2019, Elsevier.

Metheny N: Preventing aspiration in older adults with dysphagia. *Try This: Best Practices in Nursing Care to Older Adults*, Issue No. 20, 2018. https://consultgeri.org/try-this/general-assessment/issue-20.pdf. Accessed October 30, 2023.

Namasivayam-MacDonald AM, Shune SE: The burden of dysphagia on family caregivers of the elderly: a systematic review, *Geriatrics (Basel)* 3(2):30, 2018.

National Association of Clinical Nurse Specialists (NACNS): *Malnutrition in hospitalized adult patients: the role of the clinical nurse specialist*, 2017. https://nacns.org/wp-content/uploads/2017/01/Malnutrition-Report.pdf. Accessed November 21, 2023.

National Cancer Institute (NCI): *Oral complications of chemotherapy and head/neck radiation—for health professionals (PDQ®): oral mucositis*, 2022. http://www.cancer.gov/about-cancer/treatment/side-effects/mouth-throat/oral-complications-hp-pdq#section/_337. Accessed October 30, 2023.

National Council on Aging: *Facts and benefits about senior centers you probably didn't know*, 2021. https://www.ncoa.org/article/facts-and-benefits-about-senior-centers-you-probably-didnt-know. Accessed October 30, 2023.

National Foundation of Swallowing Disorders: *Swallowing disorder basics*, 2023. https://swallowingdisorderfoundation.com/about/swallowing-disorder-basics/. Accessed October 30, 2023.

National Heart, Lung, and Blood Institute (NHLBI): *Calculate your body mass index*, n.d. http://www.nhlbi.nih.gov/health/educational/lose_wt/BMI/bmicalc.htm. Accessed October 30, 2023.

Nix S: *Williams' basic nutrition and diet therapy*, ed 16, St. Louis, MO, 2022, Elsevier.

Norman K, et al: Malnutrition in older adults—recent advances and remaining challenges, *Nutrients* 13:2764, 2021.

Nova Scotia Health Authority: *Patient and family guide: foods that may increase the risk of aspiration*, Nova Scotia, 2020, Nova Scotia Health Authority.

O'Brien S: *Making oral health a priority for NPO patients*, 2020. https://dietitian-sondemand.com/making-oral-health-a-priority-for-npo-patients/. Accessed October 30, 2023.

Office of Disease Prevention and Health Promotion (ODPHP): Nutrition and healthy eating. *Healthy People 2030*, n.d., US Department of Health and Human Services. https://health.gov/healthypeople/objectives-and-data/browse-objectives/nutrition-and-healthy-eating. October 30, 2023.

Pelizzo G, et al: Malnutrition and associated risk factors among disabled children. Special considerations in pediatric surgical "fragile" patients, *Front Pediatr* 7(86):2, 2019.

Range TL, Samra NS. *Full liquid diet*, 2022, StatPearls [Internet]. https://www.ncbi.nlm.nih.gov/books/NBK554389/. Accessed October 30, 2023.

Rashid I, et al: Malnutrition among elderly a multifactorial condition to flourish: evidence from a cross-sectional study, *Clin Epidemiol Glob Health* 8:91–95, 2020.

Reynolds L, et al: Nurses as educators: creating teachable moments in practice, *Nurs Times* 116(2):25–28, 2020.

Richardson B: *Preventing and managing malnutrition in older adults: heightened focus in health care*, 2019. https://www.anfponline.org/docs/default-source/legacy-docs/docs/ce-articles/nc082019.pdf. Accessed October 27, 2023.

Sullivan W, et al: Primary care of adults with intellectual and developmental disabilities: clinical practice guidelines, *Can Fam Physician* 64:254, 2018.

Swiech PC, et al: *Self-feeding with the adult population: back to basics*, 2020, American Occupational Therapy Association.

The Joint Commission (TJC): *2023 National Patient Safety Goals*, Oakbrook Terrace, IL, 2023, The Joint Commission. https://www.jointcommission.org/standards/national-patient-safety-goals/. Accessed October 27, 2023.

The Joint Commission (TJC): *Nutritional and functional screening—requirement*, 2022. https://www.jointcommission.org/standards/standard-faqs/critical-access-hospital/provision-of-care-treatment-and-services-pc/000001652/. Accessed October 28, 2023.

Thomas L, et al: Aspiration prevention: a matter of life and breath, *Nursing* 49(3):64, 2019.

Ukleja A, et al: Standards for nutrition support: adult hospitalized patients, *Nutr Clin Pract* 33(6):906–920, 2018.

U.S. Department of Agriculture (USDA): *MyPlate*, n.d.a. https://www.myplate.gov/. Accessed October 30, 2023.

U.S. Department of Agriculture (USDA): *MyPlate: older adults*, n.d.b. https://www.myplate.gov/life-stages/older-adults. Accessed October 30, 2023.

U.S. Department of Agriculture (USDA) Economic Research Service: *Food security in the United States: overview*, 2023. https://www.ers.usda.gov/topics/food-nutrition-assistance/food-security-in-the-us/. Accessed October 30, 2023.

U.S. Department of Agriculture (USDA) and U.S. Department of Health and Human Services (USDHHS): *Dietary guidelines for Americans, 2015–2020*, 2015. https://health.gov/dietaryguidelines/2015/resources/2015-2020_Dietary_Guidelines.pdf. Accessed October 30, 2023.

U.S. Department of Agriculture (USDA) and U.S. Department of Health and Human Services (USDHHS): *Dietary guidelines for Americans, 2020–2025*, ed 9, 2020. https://www.dietaryguidelines.gov/sites/default/files/2021-03/Dietary_Guidelines_for_Americans-2020-2025.pdf. Accessed October 30, 2023.

U.S. Department of Health and Human Services (USDHHS): *Food poisoning*, 2020. https://www.foodsafety.gov/food-poisoning#:~:text=While%20the%20American%20food%20supply,128%2C000%20hospitalizations%20and%203%2C000%20deaths. Accessed October 30, 2023.

31 | Enteral Nutrition

SKILLS AND PROCEDURES

Skill 31.1 **Insertion and Removal of a Small-Bore Feeding Tube, p. 942**

Skill 31.2 **Verifying Placement of a Feeding Tube, p. 949**

Skill 31.3 **Irrigating a Feeding Tube, p. 953**

Skill 31.4 **Administering Enteral Nutrition: Nasogastric, Nasointestinal, Gastrostomy, or Jejunostomy Tube, p. 955**

Procedural Guideline 31.1 **Care of a Gastrostomy or Jejunostomy Tube, p. 962**

OBJECTIVES

Mastery of content in this chapter will enable you to:
- Assess patients who are to have enteral tubes inserted.
- Assess patients who are to receive enteral tube feedings.
- Apply practice standards to properly insert a nasogastric/small-bore feeding tube.
- Identify the rationale for methods used to determine nasogastric or nasoenteric feeding tube placement.
- Discuss the reasons for risks of pulmonary complications during the insertion and maintenance of a feeding tube.
- Make use of appropriate technique for irrigating a feeding tube.
- Apply three appropriate techniques for administering enteral formulas.
- Evaluate a patient's tolerance of enteral feeding.

MEDIA RESOURCES

- http://evolve.elsevier.com/Perry/skills
- Review Questions
- Audio Glossary
- **NSO** Nursing Skills Online
- Answers to Clinical Judgment and Next-Generation NCLEX® Examination–Style Questions
- Skills Performance Checklists
- Printable Key Points

PURPOSE

Enteral nutrition (EN) refers to the delivery of nutritional formulas through a tube that has been inserted into the gastrointestinal (GI) tract. Nasogastric (NG) feedings are delivered through a feeding tube introduced through the nose into the stomach. Nasointestinal (NI) feedings are delivered through a feeding tube introduced through the nose into the small intestine. Tubes are sometimes placed orally if a patient has trauma to the nose, cranial injury or surgery, or facial surgery. Surgically or endoscopically placed tubes into the stomach or intestine are preferred for long-term feeding (more than 6 weeks). Candidates for EN are patients with a functioning GI tract who have adequate digestion and absorption but are unable to ingest, chew, or swallow food safely or in adequate amounts.

PRACTICE STANDARDS

- Boullata et al., 2017: American Society for Parenteral and Enteral Nutrition (ASPEN) Safe Practices for Enteral Nutrition Therapy—Enteral tube insertion and maintenance, enteral feeding guidelines
- Institute for Safe Medication Practices (ISMP), 2022: 2022–2023 Targeted Medication Safety Best Practices for Hospitals—Liquid medication administration and EnFit connectors
- The Joint Commission (TJC), 2023: 2023 National patient safety goals—Patient identification

SUPPLEMENTAL STANDARD

- Bischoff et al., 2022: European Society for Clinical Nutrition and Metabolism (ESPEN) Practical Guideline: Home Enteral Nutrition

PRINCIPLES FOR PRACTICE

- The selection of an enteral feeding tube and placement method depends on the anticipated duration of feeding and other patient-related factors such as gastric emptying, GI anatomy, and risk for gastric reflux.
- The reflux of tube-feeding formula into the oropharynx can lead to aspiration into the lung.
- The Institute for Safe Medication Practices (ISMP) strongly recommends that liquid medication for patients with feeding tubes be prepared and dispensed in exact doses by the pharmacy (ISMP, 2022).
- Radiographic verification is recommended to confirm correct placement of any blindly inserted enteral tube before its initial use for feedings or medication administration (Anderson, 2019; Boullata et al., 2017; Duan et al., 2020; Sigmon & An, 2022).

- Marking and documenting the exit site of an enteral tube at the time of radiographic confirmation of correct placement will be helpful in subsequent monitoring of the location of the tube during its use for feedings (Anderson, 2019; Boullata et al., 2017; Gardner & Wallace, 2021).

PERSON-CENTERED CARE

- The insertion and use of a feeding tube often raise emotional and psychological concerns. A patient and family caregiver need reassurance and encouragement throughout the insertion procedure and once the tube feeding is in progress.
- Nursing interventions such as oral hygiene and care of the nasal passage or tube insertion site promote patient comfort during tube feeding and can reduce complications.
- Although tube feedings offer life-sustaining treatment, artificial nutrition can never replace the social and symbolic benefits of sharing meals. Social, religious, and cultural events involve food; patients requiring long-term tube feeding may feel a sense of loss regarding their ability to participate in life activities.
- An interprofessional team approach can help patients and family caregivers use nutritional strategies to preserve or enhance quality of life. A speech language pathologist can be involved to evaluate the ability of a patient to swallow safely.
- Encourage patients who require long-term tube feedings to use resources available to them such as the Oley Foundation (https://oley.org), which can provide them with education, outreach, and networking.
- Patients with living wills or other forms of advance directives may refuse the use of artificial feeding via a feeding tube. An interprofessional approach that considers cultural, spiritual, and psychological dimensions of this issue should be considered based on the patient's treatment goals.

EVIDENCE-BASED PRACTICE

Enteral Feeding Tube Placement and Maintenance

Evidence-based guidelines ensure correct technique for placing enteral feeding tubes, initiating and maintaining EN, and reducing risks for feeding tube complications.

- Obtain radiographic confirmation of correct placement of any blindly inserted tube before its initial use for feeding or medication administration (Anderson, 2019; Boullata et al., 2017; Metheny et al., 2019). The most common complication of blindly inserted feeding tubes is improper placement in the esophagus or pulmonary system (Boullata et al., 2017; Gardener & Wallace, 2021; Metheny et al., 2019).
- Critically ill patients experiencing acute respiratory distress syndrome (ARDS) are often managed in the prone position to improve respiratory status, especially during COVID-19. The frequent change in position necessitates checks for NG tube placement at each position change. Ultrasonography was found to be an effective method to verify NG tube placement after position change (Mak & Tam, 2020; Tsolaki et al., 2022). Enteral feedings have been well tolerated in patients in the prone position (Allen & Hoffman, 2019). Elevating the head of the bed 10 degrees while the patient is prone is often beneficial to tolerance of feedings (Allen & Hoffman, 2019).
- NI feeding tubes are positioned into the small bowel to reduce the incidence of pulmonary aspiration of stomach contents and allow the enteral feeding to be initiated sooner and improve nutritional patient outcomes (Metheny et al., 2019; Wang et al., 2021). Research has not consistently demonstrated this benefit, but newer techniques for detecting aspiration pro-

vide some evidence that small-intestine feeding reduces the incidence of pulmonary aspiration (Boullata et al., 2017; Clore et al., 2019; Irving et al., 2018; Metheny et al., 2019).
- The testing of gastric pH is useful in distinguishing between gastric and small-bowel tube positions. This method is of minimal benefit during continuous feedings because enteral formula buffers the gastric pH (Anderson, 2019; Boullata et al., 2017; Glen et al., 2021).
- Capnography and carbon dioxide (CO_2) detectors have been used to assess the position of small-bore feeding tubes and can reveal a tube placed in the airway by measuring CO_2 in expired air, which directly reveals CO_2 being eliminated from the lungs. However, capnography does not verify proper position of the tube in the GI tract; final tube placement should therefore be verified with an x-ray (Gardner & Wallace, 2021; Metheny et al., 2019).
- Maintaining and monitoring tube location during enteral feeding and, when the patient is in a supine or lateral position, keeping the head-of-bed elevation at a minimum of 30 degrees (preferably 45 degrees) effectively reduce aspiration and subsequent pneumonia (Boullata et al., 2017; Metheny et al., 2019; Koontalay et al., 2020).
- Gastric residual volumes (GRVs) are measured routinely during tube feeding to identify risk for regurgitation and pulmonary aspiration of gastric contents. This technique involves withdrawing and measuring stomach contents at regular intervals during tube feeding. Feeding is stopped when GRVs exceed a specified level; however, studies have failed to demonstrate a consistent relationship between GRV and risk of pulmonary aspiration, regurgitation, or pneumonia (Boullata et al., 2017; Koontalay et al., 2020; Yasuda et al., 2019). Recommendations for stopping tube feeding for elevated GRVs range from 250 to 500 mL, but automatic cessation of feeding should not occur for GRVs less than 500 mL in the absence of other signs of intolerance (Boullata et al., 2017; Koontalay et al., 2020; Yasuda et al., 2019).

SAFETY GUIDELINES

- Be aware of factors that increase a patient's risk for complications related to feeding tube insertion: altered level of consciousness, abnormal clotting, or impaired gag or cough reflex.
- Nasal tubes are associated with sinusitis, otitis, vocal cord paralysis, and medical device–related pressure injuries (MDRPIs) to the nose.
- Know the purpose of the feeding and the intended location of the tip of the feeding tube.
- Take precautions to prevent microbial contamination of enteral formulas including using within 2 hours of removal from refrigerator, using clean technique when handling formula, and minimizing handling during preparation.
- Be aware of safety measures to prevent pulmonary aspiration of gastric contents and accidental tube displacement by patients.
- Consult with a pharmacist regarding a patient's medications and their route of delivery to determine if administration via feeding tube is appropriate.
- Use ENFit connector for all EN sets, syringes, and feeding tubes to improve patient safety. The ENFit connector is not compatible with Luer-Lok connections or any other small-bore medical connectors and thus prevents misadministration of an enteral feeding or medication by the wrong route (Glanz, 2022; ISMP, 2022; Stay Connected, 2023).
- An MDRPI is a localized injury to the skin or underlying tissue that forms as a result of sustained pressure from a device. Choose the correct size of medical device(s) to fit the individual, and cushion and protect the skin with dressings in high-risk areas (e.g., nares, nasal bridge). Remove adhesive or tube fixation device daily to assess skin around the tube. When possible, move the device daily (Galetto et al., 2019; Seong et al., 2021).

✦ SKILL 31.1 Insertion and Removal of a Small-Bore Feeding Tube

Small-bore feeding tubes placed by means of either the nasal (via the nose) or the oral (via the mouth) route may be used to deliver enteral nutrition (EN) directly into the stomach (nasogastric [NG] tube) or small intestine (nasointestinal [NI] tube). These feeding tubes are soft and flexible and therefore may require a removable guidewire or stylet to provide stiffness during insertion. Some evidence suggests that postpyloric feeding (tip of the tube placed past the pyloric sphincter) may reduce the risk of aspiration and allow for greater delivery of prescribed nutrition (Wang et al., 2021). Placement of a small-bore tube into the intestine can be technically difficult, and assistive devices (electromagnetic tracing, capnography) provide improved safety and rate of successful bedside placement, although they should be used in conjunction with other methods of placement verification (Gardner & Wallace, 2021; Powers et al., 2021). However, radiographic confirmation remains the gold standard in confirming tube placement (Anderson, 2019; Boullata et al., 2017; Powers et al., 2021). In some cases, the health care provider may order a prokinetic agent such as metoclopramide to assist with advancement of a tube beyond the pylorus. Confirmation of the correct position of a newly inserted tube is mandatory before any feeding or medication is administered (see Skill 31.2).

Placement of a feeding tube requires a health care provider's order. All candidates for NG or NI tube placement require an assessment of their coagulation status. Anticoagulation and bleeding disorders pose a risk for epistaxis during nasal tube placement; the health care provider may order platelet transfusion or other corrective measures before tube insertion.

Delegation

The skill of feeding tube insertion cannot be delegated to assistive personnel (AP). However, the AP may help with patient positioning and comfort measures during tube insertion.

Interprofessional Collaboration

- The skill of inserting a nasoenteric feeding tube with a stylet is done by collaborating with an advanced practice nurse (APN) or other certified health care provider. Check agency policy to determine if you need to collaborate with other medical personnel.

Equipment
Insertion
- Small-bore feeding tube with or without stylet (select the smallest diameter possible to enhance patient comfort) (Fig. 31.1)

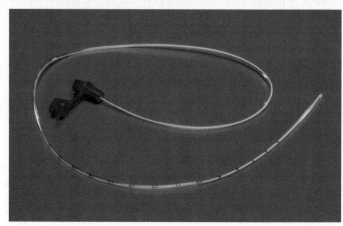

FIG. 31.1 Small-bore feeding tube. (*Courtesy Kendall Brands, Mansfield, MA.*)

- 60-mL ENFit syringe
- Stethoscope, pulse oximeter, capnograph (optional)
- Hypoallergenic tape, semipermeable (transparent) dressing, or tube fixation device
- Tincture of benzoin or other skin barrier protectant
- pH indicator strip (scale 0–11.0)
- Cup of water and straw or ice chips (for patients able to swallow)
- Water-soluble lubricant
- Emesis basin
- Towel or disposable pad
- Facial tissues
- Clean gloves
- Suction equipment in case of aspiration
- Penlight to check placement in nasopharynx
- Tongue blade
- Oral hygiene supplies

Removal
- Disposable pad
- Tissues
- Clean gloves
- Disposable plastic bag
- Towel

STEP	RATIONALE

ASSESSMENT

STEP	RATIONALE
1. Identify patient using at least two identifiers (e.g., name and birthday or name and medical record number) according to agency policy.	Ensures patient safety. Complies with The Joint Commission standards and improves patient safety (TJC, 2023).
2. Verify health care provider's order for type of tube and enteric feeding schedule. Also check order to determine if health care provider wants prokinetic agent (e.g., metoclopramide) given before tube placement.	Health care provider's order is needed to insert feeding tube. Prokinetic agent given before tube placement may help advance tube into intestine.
3. Review patient's electronic health record (EHR) medical history (e.g., for basilar skull fracture, nasal problems, nosebleeds, facial trauma, nasal-facial surgery, deviated septum, anticoagulant therapy, coagulopathy).	History of these problems may require you to consult with health care provider to change route of nutritional support. Passage of tube intracranially can cause neurological injury.

Clinical Judgment *If a patient is at risk for intracranial passage of the tube, avoid the nasal route. Oral placement or placement under medical supervision using fluoroscopic direct visualization is preferable. Insertion of a gastrostomy or jejunostomy tube is another alternative.*

STEP	RATIONALE
4. Review EHR to determine patient's risk for developing a medical adhesive–related skin injury (MARSI) with use of adhesive devices or tape: age, dehydration, malnutrition, exposure to radiation therapy, underlying chronic conditions (e.g., diabetes, immunosuppression), and edema of extremity.	These are common risk factors for MARSI. If medical adhesive is used to anchor enteral tube to nose, patient is at risk for MARSI (Fumarola et al., 2020).
5. Assess patient's height, weight, hydration status, electrolyte balance, caloric needs, and intake and output (I&O).	Provides baseline information to measure nutritional improvement after enteral feedings.
6. Ask patient to describe history of allergies; know type of allergies and normal allergic reaction. Focus on foods and adhesives. Check patient's allergy wristband.	Communication of patient allergies is essential for safe patient care.
7. Perform hand hygiene. Have patient close each nostril alternately and breathe. Examine each naris for patency and skin breakdown (apply clean gloves if drainage present).	Reduces transmission of microorganisms. Sometimes nares are obstructed or irritated, or septal defect or facial fractures are present. Place tube in more patent naris.
8. Assess patient's/family caregiver's health literacy.	Determines degree to which individuals have the ability to find, understand, and use information and services to make informed health-related decisions and actions for themselves and others (Centers for Disease Control and Prevention [CDC], 2023).
9. Assess patient's mental status (ability to cooperate with procedure, sedation), presence of cough and gag reflex, ability to swallow, critical illness, and presence of artificial airway.	These are risk factors for inadvertent tube placement into tracheobronchial tree (Boullata et al., 2017; Metheny, 2018; Vadivelu et al., 2023).

Clinical Judgment *Recognize situations in which blind placement of a feeding tube poses an unacceptable risk for placement. Devices designed to detect pulmonary intubation, such as CO_2 sensors or electromagnetic tracking devices, enhance patient safety. Alternatively, to avoid insertion complications from blind placement in high-risk situations, clinicians trained in the use of visualization or imaging techniques should place tubes (Boullata et al., 2017; Powers et al., 2021; Metheny et al., 2019).*

10. Perform physical assessment of abdomen (see Chapter 6). Remove and dispose of gloves (if worn). Perform hand hygiene.	Absence of bowel sounds or the presence of abdominal pain, tenderness, or distention may indicate medical problem contraindicating feedings.
11. Assess patient's knowledge of and prior experience with small-bore feeding tube insertion and feelings about procedure.	Reveals need for patient instruction and/or support.

PLANNING

1. Expected outcomes following completion of procedure: • Tube is successfully placed in stomach or small intestine. • Feeding tube remains patent. • Patient has no respiratory distress (e.g., increased respiratory rate, coughing, poor color) or signs of discomfort or nasal trauma.	Proper position is essential before initiating feeding tube. Proper irrigation clears tube of formula residue (Boullata et al., 2017). Correctly placed tube causes no interference with airway.
2. Explain procedure to patient, including sensations (e.g., burning in nasal passages) that will be felt during insertion.	Increases patient's cooperation with intubation procedure and helps lessen anxiety.
3. Provide privacy and explain to patient how to communicate during intubation by raising index finger to indicate gagging or discomfort.	Protects patient's privacy; reduces anxiety. Promotes cooperation. Patient must have a way of communicating to alleviate stress and enhance cooperation.
4. Organize and set up equipment for small-bore feeding tube insertion at bedside.	Ensures more efficiency when completing the procedure.

IMPLEMENTATION

1. Perform hand hygiene. Stand on same side of bed as naris chosen for insertion, and position patient upright in high-Fowler position (unless contraindicated). If patient is comatose, raise head of bed as tolerated in semi-Fowler position with head tipped forward, using a pillow chin to chest. If necessary, have the AP help with positioning of confused or comatose patients. If patient is forced to lie supine, place in reverse Trendelenburg position.	Reduces transmission of microorganisms. Allows for easier manipulation of tube. Fowler position reduces risk of aspiration and promotes effective swallowing. Forward head position helps with closure of airway and passage of tube into esophagus.
2. Apply pulse oximeter/capnograph and measure vital signs. Maintain oximetry or capnography continuously.	Provides baseline for objective assessment of respiratory status during tube insertion and throughout time a tube is in place. Lowered oxygen saturation or increased end-tidal CO_2 can indicate tube misplacement into the lungs or movement out of the stomach and into the lungs (Heidarzadi et al., 2020).

STEP	RATIONALE

Clinical Judgment *If patient has increase in end-tidal CO_2 or decrease in oxygen saturation, tube should not be inserted until you determine patient stability.*

3. Place bath towel over patient's chest. Keep facial tissues within reach.

Prevents soiling of gown. Insertion of tube frequently produces tearing.

4. Determine length of tube to be inserted and mark location with tape or indelible ink.

Ensures organized procedure and estimation of the proper length of tube for insertion.

   a. *Option, Adult:* Measure distance from tip of nose to earlobe to xiphoid process (NEX) of sternum (see illustration). Mark this distance on tube with tape.

Most traditional method. Length approximates distance from nose to stomach. Research has shown that this method may be least effective compared with others, although additional research is needed (Torsy et al., 2020; Vadivelu et al., 2023).

   b. *Option, Adult:* Measure distance from tip of nose to earlobe to mid-umbilicus (NEMU) to estimate appropriate NG tube placement.

Promotes placement of the tube end holes in or closer to the gastric fluid pool (Gardner & Wallace, 2021).

   c. *Option, Adult:* Measure distance from xiphoid process to earlobe to nose (XEN) + 4 inches (10 cm).

Provides best estimate of NG insertion length (Monica et al., 2019; Torsy et al., 2020).

   d. *Option, Child:* Use the NEMU option.

Estimates the proper length of tube insertion for pediatric patient.

   e. Add 8 to 12 inches (20–30 cm) for postpyloric tubes.

Length approximates distance from nose to jejunum.

Clinical Judgment *Tip of prepyloric tubes must reach stomach to avoid the risk for pulmonary aspiration, which occurs when tubes terminate in the esophagus. Research findings are mixed regarding the best technique for estimating tube length (Monica et al., 2019; Torsy et al., 2020). Confirmation of placement via x-ray immediately after completed insertion is still needed.*

5. Prepare tube for intubation. **NOTE:** Do not ice tubes.

Iced tube becomes stiff and inflexible, causing trauma to nasal mucosa.

   a. Obtain order for stylet tube and check agency policy for trained clinician to insert tube.

   b. If tube has guidewire or stylet, inject 10 mL of water from ENFit syringe into tube.

Aids in guidewire or stylet removal. Activates lubrication of tube for easier passage and ensures that tube is patent. ENFit devices will not be compatible with Luer-Lok connection or any other type of small-bore medical connector, thus preventing misadministration of an enteral feeding (Boullata et al., 2017; ISMP, 2022).

   c. If using stylet, make certain that it is positioned securely within tube. Inject 10 mL of water from ENFit syringe into tube.

Promotes smooth passage of tube into gastrointestinal (GI) tract. Improperly positioned stylet can cause tube to kink or injure patient. Ensures that tube is patent and aids in stylet removal. Once tube insertion is confirmed, have trained clinician remove stylet.

6. Prepare tube fixation materials. Cut hypoallergenic tape 4 inches (10 cm) long or prepare membrane dressing or other tube fixation device (e.g., bridle).

Used to secure tubing after insertion. Fixation devices allow tube to float free of nares, thus reducing pressure on nares, preventing medical device–related pressure injury (MDRPI) (see illustration).

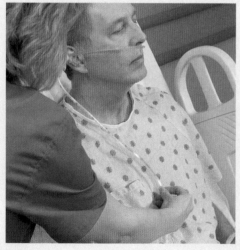

STEP 4a Measure to determine length of tube to insert.

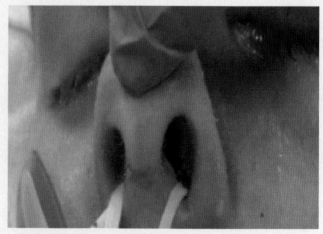

STEP 6 Medical device–related pressure injury under nose.

STEP	RATIONALE
7. Perform hand hygiene and apply clean gloves.	Reduces transmission of microorganisms.
8. *Option:* Dip tube with surface lubricant into glass of room-temperature water or apply water-soluble lubricant (see manufacturer's directions).	Activates lubricant to facilitate passage of tube into naris and GI tract.
9. Offer alert patient a cup of water with straw (if able to safely swallow).	Patient is asked to swallow water to facilitate tube passage.
10. Explain next steps and gently insert tube through nostril to back of throat (posterior nasopharynx). This may cause patient to gag. Aim back and down toward ear (see illustration).	Natural contours facilitate passage of tube into GI tract.
11. Have patient take deep breath, relax, and flex head toward chest after tube has passed through nasopharynx.	Closes off glottis and reduces risk for tube entering trachea.
12. Encourage patient to swallow small sips of water. Advance tube as patient swallows. Rotate tube gently 180 degrees while inserting.	Swallowing facilitates passage of tube past oropharynx. Distinct tug may be felt as patient swallows, indicating that tube is following expected path.
13. Emphasize need to mouth breathe and swallow during insertion.	Helps facilitate passage of tube and alleviates patient's fears during procedure.
14. Do not advance tube during inspiration or coughing because it is more likely to enter respiratory tract. Monitor oximetry and capnography at this time.	Can cause tube to inadvertently enter patient's airway, which will be reflected in changes in oxygen saturation and/or capnography.
15. Advance tube each time patient swallows until desired length has been reached (see illustration).	Reduces discomfort and trauma to patient. Helps facilitate tube passage.

Clinical Judgment *Do not force the tube or push against resistance. If patient starts to cough, experiences a drop in oxygen saturation, or shows other signs of respiratory distress, withdraw the tube into the posterior nasopharynx until normal breathing resumes.*

16. Check for position of tube in back of throat using penlight and tongue blade.	Tube may be coiled, kinked, or entering trachea.
17. Temporarily anchor tube to nose with small piece of tape.	Movement of tube stimulates gagging. Temporary anchoring of tube allows for assessment of general tube position before anchoring tube more securely.
18. Keep tube secure and check its placement by aspirating stomach contents to measure gastric pH (see Skill 31.2). Also measure amount, color, and quality of return.	Proper tube position is essential before initiating feeding.

Clinical Judgment *Insufflation of air into tube while auscultating abdomen is not a reliable means to determine position of feeding tube tip (Boullata et al., 2017; Heidarzadi et al., 2020; Kisting et al., 2019; Metheny et al., 2019).*

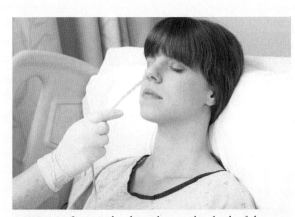

STEP 10 Insert tube through nostril to back of throat.

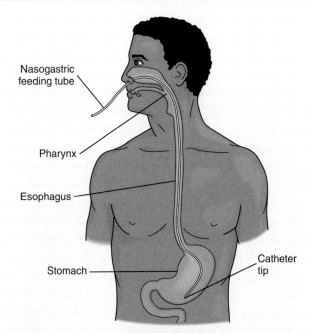

STEP 15 Nasogastric tube inserted through nasopharynx and esophagus into stomach.

STEP	RATIONALE
19. Anchor tube to patient's nose, avoiding pressure on nares. Mark exit site on tube with indelible ink. Make sure skin over nose is clean and dry. Apply liquid barrier spray or wipe on bridge of patient's nose and allow it to dry completely. Select one of the following options for anchoring:	Marking tube can alert nurses to possible displacement of tube. Properly secured tube allows patient more mobility and prevents trauma to nasal mucosa (Powers et al., 2021). Skin should be protected with a barrier product before an adhesive medical device is applied (Fumarola et al., 2020).
a. Apply membrane dressing or tube fixation device:	Permits longer securement without need to change dressing.
(1) Membrane dressing:	Allows membrane to adhere to skin.
(a) Apply tincture of benzoin or other skin protector to patient's cheek and area of tube to be secured.	Reduces risk of MARSI (Fumarola et al., 2020).
(b) Place tube against patient's cheek and secure tube with membrane dressing, out of patient's line of vision.	Eliminates application of tape around naris. Decreases risk for patient's inadvertent extubation.
(2) Tube fixation device:	Secures tube and reduces friction on naris.
(a) Apply wide end of patch to bridge of nose (see illustration).	Use of fixation devices on the bridge of a patient's nose reduces inadvertent nasal feeding tube dislodgement (Powers et al., 2021).
(b) Slip connector around feeding tube as it exits nose (see illustration).	

Clinical Judgment *Adhesive fixation materials create high risk for medical adhesive–related skin injury (MARSI) (Fumarola et al., 2020). If possible, use product with least adhesive content.*

b. Apply tape:	Prevents pulling of tube. May require frequent change if tape becomes soiled.
(1) Apply tincture of benzoin or other skin adhesive on tip of patient's nose and allow it to become "tacky."	Helps tape adhere better. Protects skin.
(2) Remove gloves and tear two horizontal slits on each side of tape at one-third and two-thirds length. Do not split tape. Fold middle sections forward.	Creates a gap in tape that will allow tube to float and exert less pressure on naris.
(3) Tear vertical strip at bottom of tape. Print date and time on nasal part of tape.	Secures tube firmly and provides date of insertion and subsequent adhesive tape changes.
(4) Place intact end of tape over bridge of patient's nose. Wrap each strip around tube as it exits (see illustration).	Tube is free floating in the naris with this taping method, resulting in movement of tube in pharynx. Securing tape to naris in this method reduces pressure on naris and risk for MDRPI (Powers et al., 2021).
20. Fasten end of tube to patient's gown using clip (see illustration) or piece of tape. Do not use safety pins to secure tube to gown.	Reduces traction on naris if tube moves, which can cause MDRPI. Safety pins can become unfastened and cause injury to patients.
21. Help patient to comfortable position but keep head of the bed elevated at least 30 degrees (preferably 45 degrees) unless contraindicated (Metheny et al., 2019). For intestinal tube placement, place patient on right side when possible until radiographic confirmation of correct placement is made.	Promotes patient comfort and lowers risk of aspiration should patient receive tube feeding. Placing patient on right side promotes passage of NI tube into small intestine.
22. Remove and dispose of gloves and perform hand hygiene.	Reduces transmission of microorganisms.

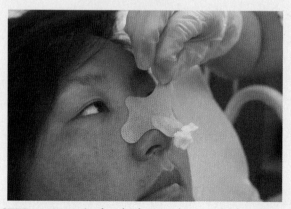

STEP 19a(2)(a) Apply tube fixation device to bridge of nose.

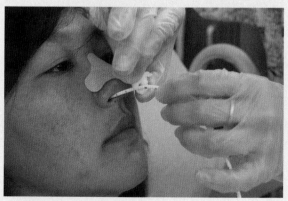

STEP 19a(2)(b) Slip connector around feeding tube.

STEP	RATIONALE

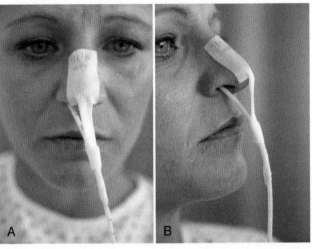

STEP 19b(4) (A) Applying tape to anchor nasoenteral tube. (B) Naris is free of pressure from tape and tube.

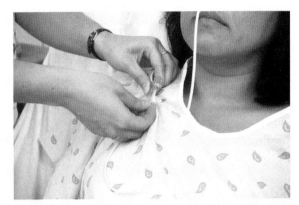

STEP 20 Fasten feeding tube to patient's gown.

Clinical Judgment *Leave stylet in place until correct position is verified by x-ray film. Never try to reinsert a partially or fully removed stylet while feeding tube is in place. This can cause perforation of tube and injure patient.*

23. Contact radiology department to obtain x-ray film of chest/abdomen.

Radiographic examination is most accurate method to determine feeding-tube placement (Boullata et al., 2017; Metheny et al., 2019; Powers et al., 2021; Vadivelu et al., 2023).

24. Perform hand hygiene and apply clean gloves. Administer oral hygiene (see Chapter 18). Clean tubing at nostril with washcloth dampened in mild soap and water.

Promotes patient comfort and integrity of oral mucous membranes. Reduces transmission of microorganisms.

25. Place nurse call system in an accessible location within patient's reach.

Ensures patient can call for assistance if needed.

26. Raise side rails (as appropriate) and lower bed to lowest position, locking into position.

Ensures patient safety and prevents falls.

27. Dispose of all contaminated supplies in appropriate receptacle, remove and dispose of gloves, and perform hand hygiene.

Reduces transmission of microorganisms. Use appropriate disposal receptacle if patient is on hazardous drugs (Elsevier, 2020; Nyhus, 2022).

28. Tube removal:
    a. Verify health care provider's order for tube removal.
    b. Gather equipment.
    c. Provide privacy and explain procedure to patient and that patient will be instructed to take a deep breath and hold it.

Health care provider's order is needed to remove feeding tube.
Ensures organized procedure.
Encourages cooperation, reduces anxiety, and minimizes risks. Specifies what patient needs to do during the procedure and identifies teaching needs.

    d. Perform hand hygiene. Apply clean gloves.
    e. Position patient in high-Fowler position unless contraindicated.

Reduces transmission of microorganisms.
Reduces risk for pulmonary aspiration in event patient should vomit.

    f. Place disposable pad or towel over patient's chest.

Prevents mucus and gastric secretions from soiling patient's clothing.

    g. Disconnect tube from feeding administration set (if present) and clamp or cap end.

Prevents formula from spilling from tube as it is removed.

    h. Remove tape or tube fixation device from patient's nose. Unclip tube from patient's gown.

Allows tube to be removed easily.

    i. Instruct patient to take deep breath and hold it. Then, as you kink end of tube securely (folding it over on itself), completely withdraw it by pulling it out steadily and smoothly onto towel or disposable bag. Dispose of it into appropriate receptacle.

Prevents inadvertent aspiration of gastric contents while tube is removed. Kinking prevents leakage of fluid from tube. Promotes patient comfort. Reduces transmission of microorganisms.

    j. Offer tissues to patient to blow nose.
    k. Provide oral hygiene.
    l. Help patient to a comfortable position.

Clears nasal passages of remaining secretions.
Promotes patient comfort.
Restores comfort and sense of well-being.

STEP	RATIONALE
m. Place nurse call system in an accessible location within the patient's reach.	Ensures patient can call for assistance if needed.
n. Raise side rails (as appropriate) and lower bed to lowest position, locking into position.	Ensures patient safety and prevents falls.
o. Dispose of all contaminated supplies in appropriate receptacle, remove and dispose of gloves, and perform hand hygiene.	Reduces transmission of microorganisms. Use appropriate disposal receptacle if patient is receiving hazardous medications (Elsevier, 2020; Nyhus, 2022).

EVALUATION

1. Observe patient's response to tube placement. Assess lung sounds; have patient speak; check vital signs; note any coughing, dyspnea, cyanosis, or decrease in oxygen saturation or increase in end-tidal CO_2.	Symptoms may indicate placement in respiratory tract. Auscultation of crackles, wheezes, dyspnea, or fever may be delayed response to aspiration. Lowered oxygen saturation or increased end-tidal CO_2 may reveal tip of tube in trachea or lung.
2. Confirm radiographic film results with health care provider.	Verifies position of tube before initiating enteral feeding.
3. Remove stylet after radiographic film verification of correct placement. Review agency policy regarding requirement of trained clinician for insertion.	If placement needs adjustment, stylet is still in place.
4. Routinely observe condition of nares, location of external exit site marking on tube, and color and pH of fluid aspirated from tube.	Routine evaluation helps to prevent MDRPI and verifies correct placement of tube.
5. After removal, assess patient's level of comfort.	Provides for continued comfort of patient.
6. **Use Teach-Back:** "I want to be sure that I explained to you what you can do during insertion of the NG tube so you can communicate with me. Tell me how you are going to communicate with me during tube insertion." Revise your instruction now or develop a plan for revised patient/family caregiver teaching if patient/family caregiver is not able to teach back correctly.	Teach-back is a technique for health care providers to ensure that they have explained medical information clearly so that patients and their families understand what is communicated to them (Agency for Healthcare Research and Quality [AHRQ], 2023).

Unexpected Outcomes	Related Interventions
1. Aspiration of stomach contents into respiratory tract (delayed response or small-volume aspiration), evidenced by auscultation of crackles or wheezes, dyspnea, or fever.	• Report a change in patient condition to health care provider; if there has not been a recent chest x-ray, suggest ordering one. • Position patient on side to protect airway. • Suction nasotracheal and orotracheally. • Prepare for possible initiation of antibiotics.
2. Displacement of feeding tube to another site (e.g., from duodenum to stomach) possibly occurs when patient coughs or vomits.	• Aspirate GI contents and measure pH. • Remove displaced tube and insert and verify placement of new tube. • If there is question of aspiration, obtain chest x-ray film.

Documentation

• Document type and size of tube placed, location of distal tip of tube, patient's tolerance of procedure, condition of naris, and confirmation of tube position by radiographic film examination.
• Document removal of tube, condition of naris, and patient's tolerance.
• Document your evaluation of patient learning.

Hand-Off Reporting

• Report any type of unexpected outcome and the interventions performed to the health care provider.
• During hand-off, report tube placement, when confirmation of placement was received, and condition of nares.

Special Considerations

Patient Education

• Instruct patient or family caregiver to offer oral hygiene frequently and keep patient's lips lubricated.
• Teach patient or family caregiver to report tension on feeding tube or displacement of tape or tube fixation device;

instruct patient or caregiver to stabilize the tube and call for help.

Pediatrics

• The distance from nose to ear to mid-umbilicus better predicts insertion length for gastric tube placement in neonates and children than traditional distance from nose to ear to xiphoid (Hockenberry et al., 2024; Kisting et al., 2019).
• Radiographic film confirmation is the most accurate assessment of proper tube placement. The best bedside assessment of tube placement is to aspirate gastric contents for color and pH (Hockenberry et al., 2024; Kisting et al., 2019). When inserting a feeding tube in an infant, the heart rate and blood pressure may change in response to vagal stimulation.

Older Adults

• Ensure adequate lubrication of tube to decrease discomfort for the older adult because of the potential for decreased oral or nasopharyngeal secretions.

Populations With Disabilities

- Aspiration is a common cause of death for individuals with intellectual and developmental disabilities. Assess for signs of difficulty swallowing and silent aspiration (Landes et al., 2021).

Home Care

- Assess patient's or family caregiver's ability to maintain a tube for a feeding program.

- Prior to discharge from a health care agency, patients at risk of malnutrition should be considered for home EN (Bischoff et al., 2022).
- Assess the environmental safety and sanitation of patient's home to determine potential for infection or injury.
- Teach patient or family caregiver how to assess tube placement (see Skill 31.2).
- Teach family caregiver correct method for securing a feeding tube and the routine care necessary to reduce pressure injuries.

✦ SKILL 31.2 Verifying Placement of a Feeding Tube

Once a feeding tube is inserted (see Skill 31.1), it is essential to routinely check its location and patency. It is possible for the tip of a feeding tube to move or migrate into a different location (e.g., from the stomach into the intestine or esophagus, from the intestine into the stomach). Although all tubes should be marked to document correct position, tube dislocation can sometimes occur without any external evidence that the tube has moved. The risk of aspiration of regurgitated gastric contents into the respiratory tract increases when the tip of the tube accidentally dislocates upward into the esophagus.

Following initial radiographic film verification of correct feeding tube position, you must monitor the tube to ensure that the tube tip remains in the intended site. Based on a patient's clinical condition and agency policies, assess feeding tube position at regular intervals (often every 4–6 hours) and before administering formula or medications through the tube. Radiographic film verification is impractical every 4 to 6 hours and costly, but the reports of routine chest and abdominal films should be monitored for reference to the feeding tube location. No single bedside method of monitoring tube position during feeding is completely reliable;

there are several techniques to use in combination to detect feeding tube dislocation:

- Monitor the external length of the tube and observe the appearance, volume, and pH of fluid aspirated through it. The color of the fluid can help differentiate gastric from intestinal placement. Because most intestinal aspirates are stained by bile to a distinct yellow color and most gastric aspirates are not, the difference in color can often be used to distinguish the sites (Fig. 31.2).
- Testing the pH of an aspirate at the bedside using pH paper offers some information regarding the position of a feeding tube. However, the pH test has no value if a patient is receiving acid-suppression medication. Results are also less reliable during continuous feeding and should be used in combination with other indicators with careful assessment of a patient in the clinical setting (Boullata et al., 2017; Clore et al., 2019; Metheny et al., 2019).
- To ensure a high confirmation rate for a correctly placed prepyloric or gastric tube, the pH or gastric aspirate should be less than or equal to 5 (Boullata et al., 2017; Gardner & Wallace,

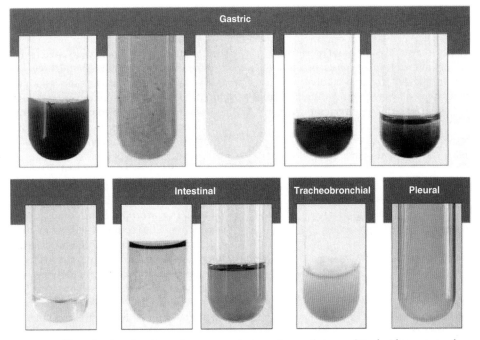

FIG. 31.2 Typical color of aspirates from stomach, intestine, and airway. (*Used with permission from Metheny NA, et al: pH, color, and feeding tubes, RN 61:25, 1998.*)

2021). If pH levels are greater than 5, additional confirmation techniques are needed.

- Observe for presence of bubbling; biochemical markers such as pepsin, capnography, ultrasound, electromagnetic tracing, and manometer techniques have all been used and studied and have advantages and disadvantages (Metheny et al., 2019; Powers et al., 2021).
- Consult with health care provider to obtain repeat radiographic verification of tube placement if bedside methods create any doubt regarding feeding tube location.

Delegation

The skill of verifying tube placement cannot be delegated to assistive personnel (AP). Direct the AP to:
- Immediately inform the nurse if patient's respirations change or patient complains of shortness of breath, coughing, or choking
- Immediately inform the nurse if the patient vomits or the AP notices vomitus in patient's mouth during oral hygiene
- Immediately inform the nurse if nasal skin irritation or excoriation is present

- Immediately inform the nurse if a change in the external length of the tube occurs, which could indicate displacement of the tube.

Interprofessional Collaboration

- Confirm radiographic film verification with radiology report and health care provider prior to initiating feeding or medications.

Equipment

- 60-mL ENFit syringe
- Stethoscope
- Clean gloves
- pH indicator strip (scale of 0–11.0)
- Small medication cup
- Water (tap water or sterile [see agency policy], in a dated and initialed container at patient's bedside)
- Towel
- Pulse oximeter

STEP	RATIONALE

ASSESSMENT

1. Identify patient using at least two identifiers (e.g., name and birthday or name and medical record number) according to agency policy.

   Ensures correct patient. Complies with The Joint Commission standards and improves patient safety (TJC, 2023).

2. Review agency policy and procedures for frequency and method of checking tube placement. **Do not insufflate air into tube to check placement.**

   Following agency standards maintains quality of patient care. Insufflation of air is not a reliable way to determine tube placement.

3. Review patient's medication record for orders for enteral feeding, a gastric acid inhibitor (e.g., cimetidine, ranitidine, famotidine, nizatidine), or a proton pump inhibitor (e.g., omeprazole).

   The presence of enteral formula in aspirated secretions diminishes usefulness of pH measurements by buffering pH of stomach. Similarly, H_2 receptor antagonists reduce acid content of secretions, also raising pH value (Boullata et al., 2017; Clore et al., 2019; Metheny et al., 2019).

4. Review patient's electronic health record (EHR) for history of prior tube displacement.

   Patients with such a history are at increased risk for repeated tube displacement.

5. Identify conditions that increase risk for spontaneous tube migration or dislocation: altered level of consciousness, agitation, retching, vomiting, nasotracheal suction.

   Feeding tubes may become dislocated by increases in intraabdominal pressure or coughing, but most frequently they are displaced when patient moves or pulls on tube.

6. Observe for signs and symptoms of respiratory distress during feeding: coughing, choking, or reduced oxygen saturation.

   Once a tube has been correctly placed into the gastrointestinal (GI) tract, movement into the pulmonary system is unlikely. However, a tube that has been pulled back into the esophagus can lead to regurgitation and aspiration of feeding.

7. Perform hand hygiene. Assess bowel sounds and abdomen.

   Determines presence of peristalsis. Bowel sounds are not needed to begin feeding; however, high-pitched or hyperactive sounds may indicate bowel changes or obstruction.

8. Observe external part of tube for movement of ink or tape mark away from mouth or naris (see Skill 31.1).

   Increased external length of tube indicates that distal tip is no longer in correct position.

9. Obtain baseline pulse oximetry reading.

   Baseline is used to compare with oximetry changes in determining if tube has been misplaced into trachea.

10. Assess patient's/family caregiver's health literacy.

    Determines degree to which individuals have the ability to find, understand, and use information and services to make informed health-related decisions and actions for themselves and others (CDC, 2023).

11. Assess patient's knowledge of and prior experience with tube placement verification and feelings about procedure.

    Reveals need for patient instruction and/or support.

STEP	RATIONALE

PLANNING

1. Expected outcomes following completion of procedure:
- Color, pH, and appearance of gastric aspirate are consistent with findings at initial tube placement.

Indicates that tube has likely remained in correct location, initially confirmed by x-ray film (Boullata et al., 2017; Clore et al., 2019; Metheny et al., 2019).

2. Explain procedure to patient. Discuss need for procedure prior to tube feeding. If applicable, teach patient or family caregiver how to check tube placement.

Reduces anxiety and promotes cooperation.
Self-care supports patient's sense of autonomy.

3. Close room door and bedside curtain.

Provides patient privacy.

4. Obtain and organize equipment for tube feeding at bedside.

Ensures more efficient procedure.

IMPLEMENTATION

1. Perform hand hygiene and apply clean gloves. Ensure pulse oximeter is in place.

Reduces transmission of microorganisms.
Used to monitor change in oxygen saturation.

2. Verify tube placement at the following times.

Clinical Judgment *Listening to insufflated air instilled through tube to check tube tip position is unreliable (Boullata et al., 2017; Metheny et al., 2019; Vadivelu et al., 2023).*

a. For intermittent tube feedings, test placement immediately before each feeding (usually a period of at least 4 hours will have elapsed since previous feeding) and before medications.

Each administration of feeding/medication can lead to pulmonary aspiration if tube is displaced. More frequent checking has been associated with increased clogging of small-bore tubes.

b. For continuous tube feedings, follow agency policy to test placement of the tube. Feedings may need to be held for up to 30 minutes to improve accuracy of pH testing (Powers et al., 2021).

Feedings should not be stopped only for purpose of pH testing. pH testing may be helpful when feedings are interrupted for procedures or diagnostic studies (Boullata et al., 2017; Clore et al., 2019; Metheny et al., 2019).

c. Wait to verify placement at least 1 hour after medication administration by tube or mouth.

Premature withdrawal of contents will remove unabsorbed medication, reducing dose delivered to patient.

3. To access the gastric or small-bore feeding tube to verify placement when tube feeding is infusing, first turn off or place tube feeding on hold. Then clamp or kink feeding tube and disconnect from end of infusion bag tubing. For intermittent feedings, remove plug at end of feeding tube.

4. Draw up 30 mL of air into a 60-mL ENFit syringe. Place tip of syringe into end of gastric or small-bore tube and flush with air before attempting to aspirate fluid. Repositioning patient from side to side is helpful. In some cases, more than one bolus of air is necessary.

Burst of air helps to aspirate fluid more easily. Smaller syringes generate unnecessarily high pressures inside tube.
It is often difficult to aspirate fluid from the small intestine or from a smaller tube (Chauhan et al., 2021; Metheny et al., 2019).

5. Draw back on syringe slowly and obtain 5 to 10 mL of gastric aspirate. Observe appearance of aspirate. Aspirates from gastric tubes of continuously tube-fed patients often look like curdled enteral formula. Gastric aspirates from intermittently tube-fed patients typically are not bile stained (unless intestinal fluid has refluxed into stomach) (Metheny et al., 2019).

Drawing back quickly or using smaller syringe may cause tube to collapse.
Quantity is sufficient for pH testing.
Appearance of aspirate helps to assess position of tube.

6. Gently mix aspirate in syringe. Expel a few drops into clean medicine cup. Note color of aspirate. Measure pH of aspirated GI contents by dipping pH strip into fluid or applying a few drops of fluid to strip. Compare color of strip with color on chart (see illustration) provided by manufacturer.

Mixing ensures equal distribution of contents for testing.
Most-accurate readings of gastric pH levels are provided by pH paper covering minimal range of 0 to 11.0.

a. Gastric fluid from patient who has fasted for at least 4 hours usually has pH range of 5.0 or less.

A pH value of 5.5 or below will exclude 100% of pulmonary placements and more than 93.9% of placements in small intestine (Metheny et al., 2019).

b. Fluid from tube in small intestine of fasting patient usually has pH greater than 6.0 (Zhang et al., 2023).

Intestinal contents are more basic than stomach contents. A pH greater than 6.0 indicates intestinal or pulmonary placement (Metheny et al., 2019).

c. The pH of pleural fluid from the tracheobronchial tree is generally greater than 6.

pH values of pleural contents are more alkaline and usually greater than 6.0 (Metheny et al., 2019).

STEP	RATIONALE

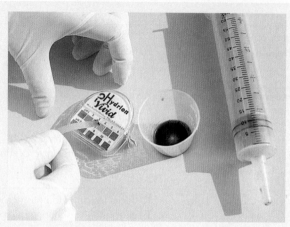

STEP 6 Compare color on test strip with color on pH chart.

7. If after repeated attempts it is not possible to aspirate fluid from tube that was confirmed by x-ray film to be in desired position and if (1) there are no risk factors for tube dislocation, (2) tube has remained in original taped position, and (3) patient is not in respiratory distress, assume that tube is correctly placed. Continue with irrigation (Boullata et al., 2017; Metheny et al., 2019).

Reports of routine chest or abdominal radiographic films can be used to monitor tube location. Repeat radiographic confirmation of tube position is indicated if external length of tube changes, tape holding tube comes loose, or patient coughs forcefully or vomits (Boullata et al., 2017; Metheny et al., 2019; Powers et al., 2021).

8. Irrigate tube (see Skill 31.3).

Keeps tube patent.

9. Help patient to a comfortable position.

Restores comfort and sense of well-being.

10. Place nurse call system in an accessible location within patient's reach.

Ensures patient can call for assistance if needed.

11. Raise side rails (as appropriate) and lower bed to lowest position, locking into position.

Ensures patient safety and prevents falls.

12. Dispose of all contaminated supplies in appropriate receptacle, remove and dispose of gloves, and perform hand hygiene.

Reduces transmission of microorganisms. Use appropriate disposal receptacle if patient is receiving hazardous medications (Elsevier, 2020; Nyhus, 2022).

EVALUATION

1. Observe patient for respiratory distress: persistent gagging, paroxysms of coughing, drop in oxygen (O_2) saturation, or respiratory patterns (e.g., rate and depth) that are inconsistent with baseline measures.

Indicates that tube may be displaced in respiratory tract.

2. Verify that external length of tube, pH, and appearance of aspirate are consistent with initial tube placement.

Indicates that tip of tube is likely to be positioned in same place as it was following x-ray film confirmation.

3. **Use Teach-Back:** "I want to go over what I explained earlier. Tell me why it is important for me to test gastric pH and the color of the gastric secretions before feedings." Revise your instruction now or develop a plan for revised patient/family caregiver teaching if patient/family caregiver is not able to teach back correctly.

Teach-back is a technique for health care providers to ensure that they have explained medical information clearly so that patients and their families understand what is communicated to them (AHRQ, 2023).

Unexpected Outcomes	Related Interventions
1. Red or brown coloring (coffee grounds appearance) of fluid aspirated from feeding tube indicates new or old blood, respectively, in GI tract.	• If color is not related to medications recently administered, notify health care provider.
2. Patient develops severe respiratory distress (e.g., dyspnea, decreased oxygen saturation, increased pulse rate) as a result of aspiration or tube displacement into lung.	• Stop any enteral feedings. • Notify health care provider. • Obtain radiographic film as ordered.
3. Tube cannot be irrigated after testing.	• Reattempt to irrigate tube. Do not force fluid. If unsuccessful, notify health care provider.

Documentation
- Document pH, appearance of aspirate, and any irrigation.
- Document your evaluation of patient and family caregiver learning.

Hand-Off Reporting
- Report to health care provider if tubing is clogged or there are indications of tube displacement.
- During hand-off report, note most current gastric pH and status of feeding.

Special Considerations
Patient Education
- Have family caregiver or patient demonstrate how to check tube placement while still in health care setting.
- Instruct patient to not pull or alter position of enteral tube.

Pediatrics
- Decrease the amount of air insufflated according to patient's size (e.g., an infant may need only 1 mL of air; a small child, 5 mL) before withdrawal of gastric secretions.
- pH testing and abdominal x-ray examination are the best practices for verifying the location of gastric enteral tubes (Northington et al., 2022).

- Calorimetric carbon dioxide detectors can detect tube displacement inserted in the lungs of children at the bedside (Hockenberry et al., 2024).

Older Adults
- Some older adults have delayed gastric emptying, and formula remains in the stomach longer than in younger patients. This population may benefit from intestinal feedings.

Home Care
- Instruct the patient or family caregiver on the following topics:
  - How to administer feedings and monitor for symptoms of discomfort, diarrhea, and aspiration (see Skill 31.4)
  - How to monitor intake and output (I&O) with household devices and what target intake should be
  - How to provide skin care to nares or around gastrostomy or jejunostomy tube
  - How to resecure a feeding tube and check for tube placement
  - Signs and symptoms of complications to report to the health care provider
- Instruct patient or family caregiver not to proceed with feedings or medication administration via the tube if there is any doubt as to its proper placement.

✦ SKILL 31.3 Irrigating a Feeding Tube

Feeding tubes must remain patent to ensure that liquid nutritional formulas can pass through easily. All types of feeding tubes require routine irrigation to keep a tube patent. Inability to instill air or fluid suggests that a tube is occluded. Curdled enteral formula and improperly crushed medications are the most common causes of feeding tube occlusion.

Delegation
The skill of irrigating a feeding tube cannot be delegated to assistive personnel (AP). Direct the AP to:
- Report when a continuous tube feeding stops infusing

Interprofessional Collaboration
- Report any difficulty irrigating feeding tube to the health care provider.

Equipment
- 60-mL ENFit syringe
- Water (tap water or sterile [see agency policy], dated and initialed container at patient's bedside)
- Towel
- Clean gloves
- Stethoscope

STEP	RATIONALE
ASSESSMENT	
1. Identify patient using at least two identifiers (e.g., name and birthday or name and medical record number) according to agency policy.	Ensures correct patient. Complies with The Joint Commission standards and improves patient safety (TJC, 2023).
2. Perform hand hygiene and apply clean gloves. Inspect volume, color, and character of previous gastric aspirates (if obtainable) (see Skill 31.2).	Excess volume of secretions (more than 250 mL) may indicate delayed gastric emptying.
3. Auscultate for bowel sounds.	Determines if peristalsis is present. Removal of tube will be delayed if peristalsis is not present. **NOTE:** Bowel sounds should be present when a patient is receiving enteral feedings.
4. Note ease with which tube feeding infuses through tubing.	Failure of formula to infuse as desired may indicate developing obstruction and the need for irrigation.
5. Monitor volume of continuous enteral formula administered during shift and compare with ordered amount.	Indicates whether sufficient volume of feeding is infusing. Serves as baseline to determine tube patency.
6. Refer to agency policies regarding routine irrigation or health care provider's order.	Determines frequency of irrigations.
7. Assess patient's/family caregiver's health literacy.	Determines degree to which individuals have the ability to find, understand, and use information and services to make informed health-related decisions and actions for themselves and others (CDC, 2023).

STEP	RATIONALE
8. Assess patient's knowledge of and prior experience with feeding tube irrigation and feelings about procedure.	Reveals need for patient instruction and/or support.

PLANNING

STEP	RATIONALE
1. Expected outcomes following completion of procedure: • Feeding tube remains patent.	Irrigation fluid clears inner lumen of feeding tube of solids and secretions.
2. Explain procedure to patient. Discuss need for and procedure related to feeding tube irrigation. If applicable, teach patient or family caregiver how to perform feeding tube irrigation.	Reduces anxiety and promotes cooperation. Self-care supports patient's sense of autonomy.
3. Provide privacy and explain procedure to patient	Protects patient's privacy; reduces anxiety. Promotes cooperation.
4. Obtain and organize equipment for feeding tube irrigation at bedside.	Ensures more efficiency when completing the procedure.
5. Position patient in high-Fowler (if tolerated) or semi-Fowler position.	Reduces reflux and risk for pulmonary aspiration during irrigation.

IMPLEMENTATION

STEP	RATIONALE
1. Perform hand hygiene and apply clean gloves.	Reduces transmission of microorganisms.
2. Verify tube placement (see Skill 31.2) if fluid can be aspirated for pH testing.	With tip of tube correctly placed in stomach or intestine, irrigation will not increase risk for pulmonary aspiration.
3. Irrigate routinely before, between, and after final medication (before feedings are reinstituted), and before an intermittent feeding is administered.	Certain formulas have properties that predispose to tube clogging. Irrigation prevents mixing of medications in tube, which may cause clogging.
4. Draw up 30 mL of water in ENFit syringe. Do not use irrigation fluids from bottles that are used on other patients. Patient should have individual bottle of solution.	This amount of solution will flush length of tube. Water is most effective agent for preventing tube clogging.
5. Change irrigation bottle every 24 hours. Irrigation trays, which hold both irrigation fluid and syringe, are considered open systems and may be more easily contaminated than sterile water bottles. **NOTE:** Be sure that syringe in tray has ENFit adaptor.	Ensures sterile solution. Sterile water is required for neonates and patients who are immunosuppressed or critically ill (Hockenberry et al., 2024; Kisting et al., 2019).
6. Stop continuous or intermittent feeding. Kink feeding tube while disconnecting it from administration tubing or while removing plug at end of tube.	Prevents leakage of gastric secretions.
7. Insert tip of ENFit syringe into end of feeding tube. Release kink and slowly instill irrigation solution.	Infusion of fluid clears tubing.
8. If unable to instill fluid, reposition patient on left side and try again.	Tip of tube may be against stomach wall. Changing patient's position may move tip away from stomach wall.
9. When water has been instilled, remove syringe. Reinstitute tube feeding or administer medication as ordered. Flush each medication completely through tube.	Tubing is clear and patent. Ensures that full dose reaches stomach and medications do not mix with formula.
10. Help patient to a comfortable position.	Restores comfort and sense of well-being.
11. Place nurse call system in an accessible location within patient's reach.	Ensures patient can call for assistance if needed.
12. Raise side rails (as appropriate) and lower bed to lowest position, locking into position.	Ensures patient safety and prevents falls.
13. Dispose of all contaminated supplies in appropriate receptacle, remove and dispose of gloves, and perform hand hygiene.	Reduces transmission of microorganisms. Use appropriate disposal receptacle if patient is receiving hazardous medications (Elsevier, 2020; Nyhus, 2022).

EVALUATION

STEP	RATIONALE
1. Observe ease with which tube feeding instills through tubing.	Successfully irrigated tube is patent, allowing for free flow of solution.
2. **Use Teach-Back:** "I want to be sure that I explained to you and your wife why you need to flush your tube when you return home. Tell me why it is important to flush your tube." Revise your instruction now or develop a plan for revised patient/family caregiver teaching if patient/family caregiver is not able to teach back correctly.	Teach-back is a technique for health care providers to ensure that they have explained medical information clearly so that patients and their families understand what is communicated to them (AHRQ, 2023).

STEP	RATIONALE

Unexpected Outcomes

1. Tube cannot be irrigated and remains obstructed.

2. Fluid and electrolyte imbalances occur. Insufficient irrigation can cause water deficiency; excessive irrigations can cause fluid volume excess.

Related Interventions

- Repeat irrigation; if unsuccessful, notify health care provider.
- Tube may need to be removed and a new tube placed.
- Notify health care provider of abnormal electrolyte levels or imbalanced intake and output (I&O).

Documentation

- Document time of irrigation and amount and type of fluid instilled.
- Document your evaluation of patient and family caregiver learning.

Hand-Off Reporting

- Report to health care provider if tubing has become clogged.

Special Considerations

Pediatrics

- Irrigation of a tube requires a smaller volume of solution in children: 1 to 2 mL for smaller tubes and 5 to 15 mL for larger tubes (Hockenberry et al., 2024; Kisting et al., 2019).

◆ SKILL 31.4 Administering Enteral Nutrition: Nasogastric, Nasointestinal, Gastrostomy, or Jejunostomy Tube

Enteral nutrition (EN), or tube feeding, is a method for providing nutrients to patients who are not able to meet their nutritional requirements orally. As a rule, candidates for EN must have a sufficiently functional gastrointestinal (GI) tract to digest and absorb nutrients. Examples of indications for enteral feeding include the following:

- Situations in which normal eating is unsafe because of high risk for aspiration: altered mental status, swallowing disorders, impaired gag reflex, dependence on mechanical ventilation, esophageal conditions (e.g., strictures or dysmotility), and delayed gastric emptying.
- Clinical conditions that interfere with normal ingestion or absorption of nutrients or create hypermetabolic states: surgical resection of oropharynx, proximal intestinal obstruction or fistula, pancreatitis, burns, and severe pressure injuries.
- Conditions in which disease- or treatment-related symptoms reduce oral intake: anorexia, nausea, pain, fatigue, shortness of breath, or depression.

Gastric feedings are the most common type of EN, allowing tube-feeding formulas to enter the stomach and then pass gradually through the intestinal tract to ensure absorption. In contrast, small-bowel feeding occurs beyond the pyloric sphincter of the stomach, which theoretically reduces the risk for pulmonary aspiration, provided that feedings do not reflux back into the stomach (Metheny et al., 2019; Powers et al., 2021). To avoid bloating, cramping, and diarrhea, use of an enteral infusion pump controls the administration rate of small-bowel feedings and many continuous gastric feedings. Inadequate delivery of nutrients, potentially leading to caloric deficit or electrolyte disturbances, sometimes occurs because of frequent interruptions in feeding.

Nasally or orally placed feeding tubes are used for short-term feeding (less than 4–6 weeks) and are inserted with tips located in the stomach (nasogastric [NG] tube) or small bowel (nasointestinal [NI] tube). For long-term feeding (more than 4–6 weeks), feeding tubes may be inserted directly through a patient's abdominal wall into the stomach (gastrostomy, jejunostomy). The majority of patients will tolerate feeding into the stomach. Conversion to intestinal feeding should be done only when gastric feeding is poorly tolerated owing to ileus (decreased or absent peristalsis of the stomach but not the intestine), gastroparesis (delayed gastric emptying), high risk for aspiration, or mechanical issues (gastric resection) (Tatsumi, 2019). Feeding tubes that end in the stomach are used for gravity bolus or continuous infusion feedings by infusion pumps. The small intestine does not have the storage capacity of the stomach, and therefore a tube feeding administered into the small intestine is delivered more slowly and continuously with an infusion pump.

Delegation

The skill of administration of nasoenteric tube feeding can be delegated to assistive personnel (AP) (refer to agency policy). A registered nurse (RN) or licensed practical nurse (LPN) must first verify tube placement and patency. Direct the AP to:

- Elevate head of bed to 30 to 45 degrees or sit patient up in bed or a chair unless contraindicated
- Not adjust feeding rate; infuse feeding as ordered
- Report any difficulty infusing the feeding or any discomfort voiced by the patient
- Report any gagging, paroxysms of coughing, or choking
- Provide frequent oral hygiene

Interprofessional Collaboration

- Collaborate with registered dietitian nutritionist (RDN) and health care provider for determination of patient's caloric and protein requirements. Then set goal for delivery of EN.

Equipment

- Disposable feeding bag, tubing, or ready-to-hang system
- 60-mL or larger ENFit syringe
- Stethoscope
- Enteral infusion pump for continuous feedings
- pH indicator strip (scale 0–11.0)
- Water for flushing tube; purified or sterile as indicated
- Prescribed enteral formula (standard polymetric, high protein, or disease specific) (Allen & Hoffman, 2019; Ukleja et al., 2018)
- Clean gloves
- ENFit connector

STEP	RATIONALE

ASSESSMENT

1. Identify patient using at least two identifiers (e.g., name and birthday or name and medical record number) according to agency policy.

Ensures correct patient. Complies with The Joint Commission standards and improves patient safety (TJC, 2023).

2. Verify health care provider's order for type of formula, rate, route, and frequency.

Ensures that correct formula will be administered in appropriate volume. Enteral formulas are not interchangeable.

3. Assess patient's/family caregiver's health literacy.

Determines degree to which individuals have the ability to find, understand, and use information and services to make informed health-related decisions and actions for themselves and others (CDC, 2023).

4. Assess patient for food allergies. If allergy present, apply allergy wrist band.

Prevents patient from developing localized or systemic allergic responses to feeding.

5. Assess patient for factors that increase risk for aspiration: sedation, mechanical ventilation, nasotracheal suctioning, neurological compromise, lying flat, and sepsis (Kollmeier & Keenaghan, 2023; Makhnevich et al., 2019).

Identifies patients at high risk so that nurse can take steps to minimize aspiration risk.

6. Perform hand hygiene. Perform physical assessment of abdomen, including auscultation for bowel sounds, before feeding (see Chapter 6).

Objective measures for assessing tolerance include changes in bowel sounds, expanding girth, tenderness, firmness on palpation, increasing NG output, and vomiting (Tatsumi, 2019). Report findings to health care provider to determine if tube feeding can proceed safely (Harding et al., 2023).

7. Obtain baseline weight and review serum electrolytes and blood glucose measurement. Assess patient for fluid volume excess or deficit, electrolyte abnormalities, and metabolic abnormalities (e.g., hyperglycemia).

Enteral feedings should restore or maintain patient's nutritional status. Measures provide objective data and baseline to determine selection of formula and measure effectiveness of feedings.

8. Collaborate with RDN to determine patient's caloric and protein requirements. Then set goal for delivery of EN (Ukleja et al., 2018).

Sets objective measure for determining percent of prescribed calories and protein to be delivered.

9. Assess patient's knowledge of and prior experience with enteral feedings and feelings about procedure.

Reveals need for patient instruction and/or support.

PLANNING

1. Expected outcomes following completion of procedure:
- Patient achieves established target for body weight over time.

Indicates that patient's nutritional status is maintained or improved.

- Patient has no sign of respiratory distress.

Feeding tube does not enter airway, and patient does not aspirate feeding.

- Patient achieves established target for calories and protein.

Scheduled feedings are administered as ordered.

- Patient is free of abdominal cramping, distention, pain, nausea, vomiting, or diarrhea.

Feeding administered without abdominal distention demonstrates tolerance of tube feeding (Tatsumi, 2019).

2. Provide privacy and explain procedure to patient. Discuss need for and procedure related to EN. If applicable, teach patient or family caregiver how to perform enteral feeding.

Reduces anxiety and promotes cooperation.
Self-care supports patient's sense of autonomy.

3. Obtain and organize equipment for enteral feeding at bedside.

Ensures more efficiency when completing the procedure.

IMPLEMENTATION

1. Perform hand hygiene. Apply clean gloves.

Reduces transmission of microorganisms and potential contamination of enteral formula.

2. Reverify correct formula and check expiration date; note integrity of container and appearance of formula.

Ensures that correct therapy is to be administered and checks integrity of formula.

3. Prepare formula for administration, following manufacturer guidelines.

Clinical Judgment *Discard unused reconstituted and refrigerated formula within 24 hours of preparation (Boullata et al., 2017).*

a. Have formula at room temperature.

Cold formula causes gastric cramping and discomfort because liquid is not warmed by mouth and esophagus.

b. Use aseptic technique to connect tubing to container as needed. Use proper ENFit connector and avoid handling feeding system or touching can tops, container openings, spike, and spike port.

Bag, connections, and tubing must be free of contamination to prevent bacterial growth. The use of a closed system lowers the risk of infections due to bacterial contaminants (Boullata et al., 2017).

STEP	RATIONALE

c. Shake formula container well. Clean top of canned formula with alcohol swab before opening it.

Ensures integrity of formula; prevents transmission of microorganisms.

d. Connect administration tubing to formula bag. If using open system, pour formula from brick pack or can into administration bag (see illustration).

Formulas are available in closed-system containers that contain a 24- to 48-hour supply of formula or in an open system, in which formula must be transferred from brick packs or cans to a bag before administration.

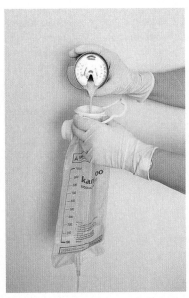

STEP 3d Pour formula into open feeding container.

4. Open roller clamp and allow administration tubing to fill. Clamp off tubing with roller clamp. Hang container on intravenous (IV) pole.

Prevents introduction of air into stomach once feeding begins.

5. Keep patient in high-Fowler position or elevate head of bed at least 30 degrees (45 degrees is recommended). For patient forced to remain supine, place in reverse Trendelenburg position, which raises head.

Elevated head helps prevent pulmonary aspiration (ASPEN, 2023; Boullata et al., 2017). Researchers recommend head-of-bed elevation of 45 degrees for patients receiving mechanical ventilation or who are heavily sedated, but lowering the head of bed to 30 degrees might be done periodically for patient comfort and in patients at risk for developing pressure injuries (Kim & Shin, 2021; Metheny et al., 2019).

6. Verify tube placement using EnFit 60 mL syringe (see Skill 31.2). Observe appearance of aspirate and note pH. When checking a jejunostomy tube, check pH if significant amounts are returned that resemble gastric secretions.

A pH value of 5.5 or below will exclude 100% of pulmonary placements and more than 93.9% of placements in small intestine (Metheny et al., 2019).

Intestinal contents are more alkaline than stomach contents. A pH greater than 6.0 indicates intestinal or pulmonary placement (Metheny et al., 2019).

pH values of pleural contents are more alkaline and are usually greater than 6.0 (Metheny et al., 2019).

7. Check gastric residual volume (GRV) per agency policy. Routine use is no longer recommended (Boullata et al., 2017; Jordan & Moore, 2020), and GRV should not be used as a single measure of tolerance.

GRV has poor correlation with pneumonia, regurgitation, and aspiration. Frequent checking may delay feeding. However, if other signs (e.g., abdominal distention or pain) of intolerance are present, GRV of 250 to 500 mL may indicate the need to take measures to prevent aspiration or hold feeding completely (Boullata et al., 2017). Intestinal residual volume is usually small. If residual volume is greater than 10 mL, displacement of intestinal tube into stomach may have occurred. Determines if gastric emptying is delayed.

STEP	RATIONALE

Clinical Judgment *Limit gastric residual checks to recommended standard intervals because acidic gastric contents may cause protein in enteral feeding to precipitate within the lumen of the tube, causing risk for obstruction. Frequent gastric residual volume (GRV) measurements lead to an increased risk of tube occlusion and decreased amount of enteral nutrition delivered to the patient (Boullata et al., 2017).*

a. Draw up 10 to 30 mL of air into ENFit syringe and connect to end of feeding tube. Inject air slowly into tube. Pull back slowly and aspirate total amount of gastric contents you can aspirate.

b. Return aspirated contents to stomach slowly. Refer to agency policy for any cutoff to hold aspirated contents (Boullata et al., 2017; Clore et al., 2019).

c. GRVs in range of 200 to 500 mL should raise concern and lead to implementation of measures to reduce risk of aspiration. Automatic cessation of feeding should not occur for GRV less than 500 mL in absence of other signs of intolerance (Jordan & Moore, 2020; Metheny et al., 2019).

d. Flush feeding tube with 30 mL of water (see Skill 31.3).

GRV may not be easy to obtain from small-bore feeding tube owing to smaller tube diameter, which can result in gastric tube collapse (Harding et al., 2023). A 60-mL syringe prevents gastric tube collapse.

Prevents loss of nutrients and electrolytes in discarded fluid. Some questions exist regarding safety of returning high volumes of fluid into stomach.

Raising cutoff value for GRV from lower number to higher number does not increase risk for regurgitation, aspiration, or pneumonia. Elevated GRV should raise concern and lead to measures to reduce risk of aspiration (Boullata et al., 2017; Metheny et al., 2019).

Prevents clogging of tubing and ensures that complete feeding is administered.

Clinical Judgment *Minimize the use of sedatives in patients receiving continuous feeding because airway clearance is reduced in patients when they are sedated (Boullata et al., 2017).*

8. Intermittent feeding (administered at certain times during the day):

a. Pinch proximal end of feeding tube and remove cap. Attach distal end of administration set tubing to ENFit connection system on feeding tube and release tubing (see illustration).

Prevents excessive air from entering patient's stomach and leakage of gastric contents during connection. ENFit devices are not compatible with Luer-Lok connections. The use of these devices ensures that feeding will be administered into the correct tubing and prevents administration of enteral feeding or medication by the wrong route, such as IV tubing (ISMP, 2022).

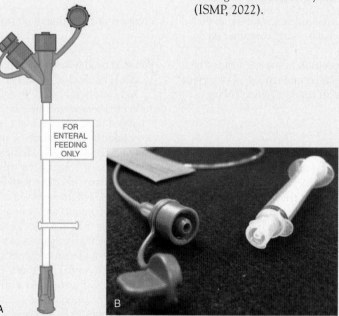

STEP 8a (A) ENFit connection system. (B). Enteral connector.

STEP	RATIONALE

Clinical Judgment *Use pumps designated for tube feeding, not intravenous (IV) fluids.*

b. Set rate by adjusting roller clamp on tubing (see illustration) or attach tubing to feeding pump (see Step 9 below). Allow bag to empty gradually over 30 to 45 minutes (length of time of a comfortable meal). Label bag with patient identifiers, formula type, enteral delivery site (route and access), administration method, and volume and frequency of water flushes (Boullata et al., 2017; Ukleja et al., 2018). Also include label with date, time, and initials when hanging a feeding.

Gradual emptying of tube feeding reduces risk for abdominal discomfort, vomiting, or diarrhea induced by bolus or too-rapid infusion of tube feedings. Critical elements for an EN order should be on EN label (Boullata et al., 2017; Ukleja et al., 2018). Labeling provides means to determine when to change administration set and confirms that right patient is receiving feeding.

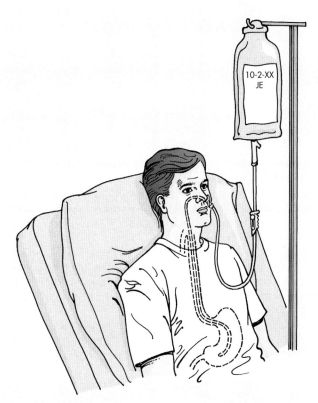

STEP 8b Administer intermittent feeding.

c. Immediately follow feeding with prescribed amount of water (per health care provider's orders or agency policy). Cover end of feeding tube with cap when not in use. Keep bag as clean as possible. Change administration set every 24 hours.

Prevents tube from clogging. Prevents air from entering stomach between feedings and limits microbial contamination of system.

9. Continuous infusion method:

Method delivers prescribed hourly rate of feeding and reduces risk for abdominal discomfort.

a. Remove cap on tubing and connect distal end of administration set tubing to feeding tube using ENFit connector as in Step 8a.

Prevents excess air from entering patient's stomach and leakage of gastric contents.

b. Thread tubing through feeding pump; set rate on pump and turn on (see illustrations).

Delivers continuous feeding at steady rate and pressure. Feeding pump alarms for increased resistance.

c. Advance rate of tube feeding (and concentration of feeding) gradually, as ordered.

Tube feeding can usually begin with full-strength formula. Conservative initiation and advancement of EN depend on factors such as patient's age, medical condition, nutritional status, and expected patient tolerance (Boullata et al., 2017; Grodner et al., 2021).

Clinical Judgment *Limit infusion time for open enteral nutrition (EN) feeding systems to 4 to 8 hours maximum (12 hours in the home setting) (Boullata et al., 2017). Follow the manufacturer's recommendations for duration of infusion through an intact closed delivery system (Boullata et al., 2017).*

STEP	RATIONALE

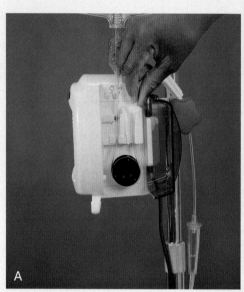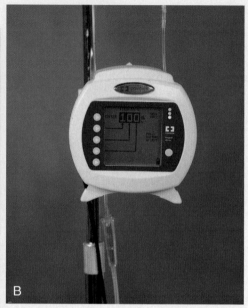

STEP 9b (A) Nurse threads tube through infusion pump. (B) Set pump as ordered.

10. After feeding, flush tubing with 30 mL water every 4 hours during continuous feeding (see agency policy) or before and after an intermittent feeding. Have RDN recommend total free-water requirement per day and obtain health care provider's order (see Skill 31.3).

Provides patient with source of water to help maintain fluid and electrolyte balance. Clears tubing of formula.

11. Rinse bag and tubing with warm water whenever feedings are interrupted. Use new administration set every 24 hours.

Rinsing bag and tubing with warm water clears old tube feedings and reduces bacterial growth.

12. Help patient to assume and remain in comfortable position with head of bed elevated 30 to 45 degrees.

Promotes patient comfort and reduces risk for aspiration of EN.

13. Place nurse call system in an accessible location within patient's reach.

Ensures patient can call for assistance if needed.

14. Raise side rails (as appropriate) and lower bed to lowest position, locking into position.

Ensures patient safety and prevents falls.

15. Dispose of all contaminated supplies in appropriate receptacle, remove and dispose of gloves, and perform hand hygiene.

Reduces transmission of microorganisms. Use appropriate disposal receptacle if patient is on hazardous drugs (Elsevier, 2020; Nyhus, 2022).

EVALUATION

1. Monitor patient's tolerance to feeding by evaluating for abdominal distention, firmness, feeling of fullness, or nausea (Boullata et al., 2017). Measure GRV per agency policy but should be limited.

GI tolerance of tube feedings must be monitored closely to avoid complications.

2. Monitor intake and output (I&O) at least every 8 hours and calculate daily totals every 24 hours.

I&O is an indication of fluid balance, which can indicate fluid volume excess or deficit.

3. Weigh patient daily until maximum administration rate is reached and maintained for 24 hours; then weigh patient 3 times per week.

Slow weight gain is indicator of improved nutritional status; however, sudden gain of more than 0.9 kg (2 lb) in 24 hours usually indicates fluid retention.

4. Monitor patient for appropriate tube feeding placement at least every 4 hours or per agency policy. Monitor visible length of tubing or marking at tube exit site and check placement when deviation is noted (Boullata et al., 2017).

Accidental displacement of tip of tube could lead to aspiration.

5. Monitor laboratory values as ordered by health care provider.

Determines correct administration of formula rate and strength.

6. Observe patient's respiratory status for coughing, dyspnea, tachypnea, change in oxygen saturation, hoarseness, or crackles in lungs.

Change in respiratory status may indicate aspiration of tube feeding into respiratory tract.

STEP	RATIONALE
7. For gastrostomy and jejunostomy tubes, inspect site for signs of impaired skin integrity and symptoms of infection, injury, or tightness of tube (see Procedural Guideline 31.1).	Enteral tubes often cause pressure and excoriation at insertion site. Feeding tube fixation devices use medical adhesives, and some patients may react to the adhesive and develop medical adhesive–related skin injury (MARSI).
8. Observe nasoenteral tube insertion site at least daily (see agency policy). Note skin integrity and look for edema under device, excoriation, or presence of injury.	Allows for early detection of excoriation, which can progress to a medical device–related pressure injury (MDRPI).
9. **Use Teach-Back:** "I want to be sure that I explained to you what you need to look for that may tell us you are not tolerating your tube feeding. Tell me two things that may tell us that you are not tolerating your tube feeding." Revise your instruction now or develop a plan for revised patient/family caregiver teaching if patient/family caregiver is not able to teach back correctly.	Teach-back is a technique for health care providers to ensure that they have explained medical information clearly so that patients and their families understand what is communicated to them (AHRQ, 2023).

Unexpected Outcomes	Related Interventions
1. Feeding tube becomes clogged.	• Attempt to flush tube with water. • Special products are available for unclogging feeding tubes; **do not** use carbonated beverages and juices. • Hold feeding and notify health care provider. • Maintain patient in semi-Fowler position. • Contact pharmacist to change medications to liquid form and flush before and after intermittent feedings and medications (Boullata et al., 2017).
2. Patient develops large amount of diarrhea (more than three loose stools in 24 hours).	• Notify health care provider. • Consult registered dietitian nutritionist (RDN) about need to change formula to prevent malabsorption. • Identify and treat underlying medical/surgical issues and infections. • Provide perianal skin care after each stool. • Determine other causes of diarrhea (e.g., *Clostridium difficile* infection, contaminated tube feeding, medication containing sorbitol).
3. Patient aspirates formula (auscultation of crackles or wheezes, dyspnea, or fever).	• Immediately report change in condition to health care provider. • Immediately position patient on side. • Suction nasotracheally or orotracheally.

Documentation

- Document amount and type of feeding, infusion rate (continuous feeding) or time of infusion (bolus method), GRV measurements, position of feeding tube, patient's response to tube feeding, patency of tube, and condition of skin at tube site.
- Document your evaluation of patient and family caregiver learning.
- Document volume of formula and any additional water.

Hand-Off Reporting

- Report adverse outcomes to the health care provider.
- During hand-off, report the type of feeding, infusion rate, and patient's tolerance, and trace the administration set tubing to the enteral tube connection point to ensure feeding is being infused enterally (Boullata et al., 2017).

Special Considerations

Patient Education

- Instruct patients and family caregivers not to reconnect lines that have separated but to seek clinical assistance.
- Teach patient and family caregiver that, if tolerated, patient should remain upright for 1 hour after feedings.

- Instruct patient or family caregiver that patient may express feelings of fullness, increased gas, belching, or diarrhea.
- Teach patient or family caregiver how to determine correct placement of feeding tube (see Skill 31.2).

Pediatrics

- Preterm infants who are at risk for necrotizing enterocolitis frequently receive minimal enteral feeding (MEF) to limit stress on the GI tract. Breast milk is the preferred "formula" in this situation. MEF is usually administered slowly with a pump and supplemented with IV nutrition (Bozkurt et al., 2020).

Older Adults

- Some older adults have decreased gastric emptying; therefore, formula remains in the stomach longer than in younger patients. GRV checks are especially important in patients with impaired cognition to decrease the risk for pulmonary aspiration.

Home Care

- Instruct patient or family caregiver on technique for administering feedings in the home and proper storage and refrigeration of supplies.

- Instruct patient or family caregiver about any symptoms or discomfort that may occur during enteral feedings. Reinforce instruction to contact health care provider if symptoms of discomfort occur.
- Teach patient or family caregiver how to perform skin care around the gastrostomy or jejunostomy tube and signs

and symptoms of infection at insertion site (see Procedural Guideline 31.1).
- Provide support for the patient and family caregiver as they are coping with the feeding tube and the change in lifestyle and social life the feeding tube creates.

PROCEDURAL GUIDELINE 31.1 *Care of a Gastrostomy or Jejunostomy Tube*

Feeding tubes can be placed directly into the gastrointestinal (GI) tract through the abdominal wall in patients who cannot tolerate nasoenteric feeding tubes or who require long-term enteral nutrition (EN). The stomach (gastrostomy tube) and jejunum (jejunostomy tube) are the most common sites for long-term feeding tubes. Long-term tubes require endoscopic, radiological, or surgical placement. The insertion method used to place tubes may call for specific nursing interventions in the postinsertion period, but otherwise these tubes are used in a similar way as other feeding tubes. Feedings delivered via a gastrostomy tube are relatively safe to administer, provided the patient has normal gastric emptying. Gastrostomy tubes are often called G *tubes*, but they are also commonly referred to as *percutaneous endoscopic gastrostomy (PEG) tubes*, a term used to describe tubes placed endoscopically. Gastrostomy tubes range in size from 16 Fr to 28 Fr and exit through an incision in the upper left quadrant of the abdomen, where an internal bumper or balloon and an external bumper or disk hold the tube in place (Fig. 31.3).

Jejunostomy tubes are indicated when the risk of regurgitation and aspiration is especially high, as in cases of severely delayed gastric emptying or conditions such as pancreatitis that limit the use of the stomach for feeding. They can be placed directly into the small intestine in a surgical procedure or threaded through the stomach into the jejunum under fluoroscopy. Some jejunal tubes inserted with this transgastric approach are dual-channel devices that have openings in both the stomach and the small-intestine part of the tube. These *combination tubes*, as they are called, allow simultaneous gastric decompression and intestinal feeding for patients with impaired gastric emptying or upper GI

cancers. Each lumen of a combination tube is clearly labeled to distinguish between the gastric and the jejunal ports (Fig. 31.4).

Sometimes a jejunostomy tube is placed through an existing PEG tube. The percutaneous endoscopic jejunostomy (PEJ) tube is passed through the PEG tube and advanced into the jejunum (Fig. 31.5). The PEJ tube occupies the lumen of the PEG tube; this tube-through-a-tube design does not allow drainage of the stomach during small-intestine feeding. In the case of both combination tubes and PEJ tubes, you must know whether the intended site for formula delivery is gastric or jejunal to ensure safe and effective nutritional care.

Delegation
Care of a new PEG or PEJ tube cannot be delegated to assistive personnel (AP). However, there may be some exceptions (refer to nurse practice acts and agency policy). Direct the AP to:
- Inform the nurse of any patient complaints of discomfort at the insertion site
- Inform the nurse of any drainage on the insertion site dressing

Interprofessional Collaboration
- Collaborate with registered dietitian nutritionist and health care provider for determination of patient's caloric and protein requirements. Then set goal for delivery of EN.

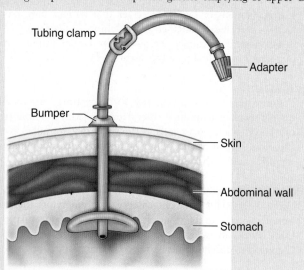

FIG. 31.3 Placement of percutaneous endoscopic gastrostomy (PEG) tube into stomach.

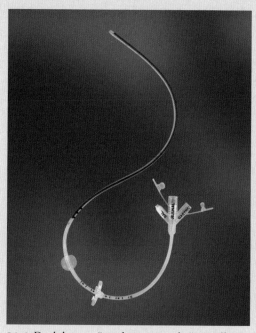

FIG. 31.4 Dual lumen "combination tube" to allow jejunal feeding and gastric decompression. (*Image used with permission from Kimberly-Clark Health Care. All rights reserved.*)

PROCEDURAL GUIDELINE 31.1 *Care of a Gastrostomy or Jejunostomy Tube—cont'd*

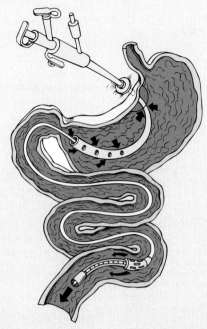

FIG. 31.5 Endoscopic insertion of jejunostomy tube.

Equipment

Normal saline, dated and initialed container at patient's bedside; 4 × 4–inch gauze; prepared drain-gauze dressing; paper tape; clean gloves; warm soapy water (see agency policy); protective skin barrier (if indicated)

Steps

1. Identify patient using at least two identifiers (e.g., name and birthday or name and medical record number) according to agency policy.
2. Determine whether exit site is left open to air or if a dressing is indicated. Check health care provider's order or verify agency policy. If dressing is indicated, obtain and organize dressing supplies.
3. Provide privacy and explain procedure to patient. Arrange equipment for care of tube at bedside. Perform hand hygiene.
4. Position patient in comfortable position lying supine or supine with head of bed slightly elevated.
5. Assess patient's/family caregiver's health literacy. Explain procedure to patient.
6. Assess patient's knowledge of and prior experience with PEG or PEJ tube care and feelings about procedure.
7. Perform hand hygiene and apply clean gloves. Remove old dressing. Fold dressing with drainage contained inside; remove gloves inside out over dressing. Discard in appropriate container. Perform hand hygiene.
8. Assess exit site for evidence of tenderness, leakage, swelling, excoriation, infection, bleeding, or excessive movement (more than 6 mm [¼ inch]) of the tube in or out of the stomach.
9. Apply clean gloves. Clean skin around stoma site with warm water and mild soap or saline (according to agency policy) with 4 × 4–inch gauze. Clean starting next to the stoma site and work outward using circular strokes.
10. Rinse and dry site completely.
11. Apply thin layer of protective skin barrier to exit site if indicated (e.g., site excoriated).
12. If dressing is ordered, place a drain-gauze dressing over external bar or disk. **NOTE:** Do not place dressing under external bar; this can cause gastric tissue erosion or internal abdominal wall pressure.
13. Secure dressing with tape.
14. Place date, time, and initials on new dressing.
15. Remove gloves and dispose of supplies in appropriate receptacle. Perform hand hygiene.
16. Help patient to comfortable position. Place nurse call system in an accessible location within patient's reach. Raise side rails (as appropriate) and lower bed to lowest position, locking into position.
17. Evaluate condition of site routinely (see agency policy).
18. **Use Teach-Back:** "I want to be sure I explained clearly how to care for your G tube. Tell me what steps you take to clear your G tube site." Revise your instruction now or develop a plan for revised patient/family caregiver teaching if patient/family caregiver is not able to teach back correctly.
19. Document appearance of exit site, drainage noted, and dressing application.
20. Report to health care provider any exit site complications.
21. Provide hand-off report to health care provider of any changes or abnormal findings.

◆ CLINICAL JUDGMENT AND NEXT-GENERATION NCLEX® EXAMINATION–STYLE QUESTIONS

The nurse is caring for a 72-year-old patient admitted to the acute stroke unit following a cerebral hemorrhage. Currently there is left-sided paralysis. The patient recognizes family members and at times has spoken a few words. Nothing by mouth (NPO) status has been maintained since admission. The nutrition support team has recommended that a small-bore NG feeding tube be inserted for nutritional support, and a continuous tube feeding of Isosource HN has been ordered to run at 55 mL/h.

1. Which of the following methods is the most reliable to verify the location of the small-bore feeding tube prior to beginning the ordered feeding?
   1. pH testing of fluid withdrawn through the tube
   2. Auscultating over the epigastrium while instilling air through the tube
   3. Observing the color and appearance of fluid aspirated through the tube
   4. Obtaining x-ray confirmation of tube placement
2. The nurse aspirates a gastric residual volume (GRV) of 150 mL after the enteral feeding has been infusing via enteral pump for 4 hours. The patient has bowel sounds; a soft, nondistended nontender abdomen; and no reports of nausea. Which of the following actions would the nurse take at this time? **Select all that apply.**
   1. Consult the registered dietitian nutritionist (RDN).
   2. Stop the feeding immediately.
   3. Continue tube feeding as ordered.
   4. Refeed the gastric aspirate withdrawn through the tube.
   5. Continue to assess feeding tolerance.
3. The patient continues to receive the enteral feeding at 55 mL/h as ordered. Which intervention will the nurse include in the patient's ongoing plan of care?
   1. Ensure that formula is kept refrigerated to prevent bacterial growth.
   2. Elevate the head of the bed to at least 20 degrees.
   3. Asses the capillary blood glucose level prior to the infusion.
   4. Flush the tube with water every 4 hours during the continuous feeding.
4. The nurse notes that the patient still has difficulty moving the left arm and leg. Vital signs: temperature = 37.2°C (99.0°F); heart rate (HR) = 82 beats/min; respirations = 12 breaths/min; blood pressure (BP) = 142/86 mm Hg. SpO₂ 91% on RA. Auscultation of the lungs showed crackles in bilateral upper and lower lobes. The GRV was 275 mL. The nurse notes that the patient's abdomen is hard and distended, without bowel sounds.

   Complete the following sentence by selecting from the list of word choices below.

   The assessment findings that require immediate follow-up include **[Word Choice]**, **[Word Choice]**, and **[Word Choice]**.

Word Choices
Left-sided paralysis
BP 142/86 mm Hg
Pulse oximetry 91% on RA
Hard, distended abdomen
GRV 275 mL
Crackles in lungs
Respirations 12 breaths/min

5. The nurse has just inserted a nasogastric (NG) tube in the patient's left naris. How will the nurse document this procedure?
   1. 18 Fr NG tube inserted into the left naris, patient tolerated well.
   2. 18 Fr NG tube inserted as ordered, radiographic film obtained, and tip is positioned in stomach; both nares are in good condition and intact.
   3. 18 Fr NG tube inserted in left naris; patient tolerated procedure with minimal discomfort; the left naris is intact with no skin breakdown or redness noted; x-ray called and confirmed that the tip of the tube is in the stomach.
   4. 18 Fr NG tube inserted for the first time by the nurse; patient tolerated procedure; gastric pH was noted to be 5.0.

Visit the Evolve site for Answers to Clinical Judgment and Next-Generation NCLEX® Examination–Style Questions.

REFERENCES

Agency for Healthcare Research and Quality (AHRQ): *Teach-Back: intervention*, 2023. https://www.ahrq.gov/health-literacy/quality-resources/tools/literacy-toolkit/healthlittoolkit2-tool5.html. Accessed May 5, 2023.

Allen K, Hoffman L: Enteral nutrition in the mechanically ventilated patient, *Nutr Clin Pract* 34(4):540-557, 2019.

Anderson L: Enteral feeding tubes: an overview of nursing care, *Br J Nurs* 28(12):748754, 2019. doi:10.12968/bjon.2019.28.12.748.

American Society for Parenteral and Enteral Nutrition (ASPEN): *Standards*, 2023. https://www.nutritioncare.org/Guidelines_and_Clinical_Resources/Clinical_Practice_Library/Standards/. Accessed May 5, 2023.

Bischoff SC, et al: ESPEN practical guideline: home enteral nutrition, *Clin Nutr* 41:468–488, 2022.

Boullata JI, et al: ASPEN safe practices for enteral nutrition therapy, *JPEN J Parenter Enteral Nutr* 41(1):15, 2017.

Bozkurt O, et al: Prolonged minimal enteral nutrition versus early feeding advancements in preterm infants with birth weight ≤1250g: a prospective randomized trial, *J Matern Fetal Neonatal Med* 35(2):341–347, 2020.

Centers for Disease Control and Prevention (CDC): *What is health literacy?* 2023. https://www.cdc.gov/healthliteracy/learn/index.html.

Chauhan D, et al: Nasogastric tube feeding in older patients: a review of current practice and challenges faced, *Curr Gerontol Geriatr Res* 2021:Article 6650675, 2021.

Clore A, et al: Early feeding tube placement in burn patients and the impact on nutritional outcomes, *J Burn Care Res* 40:S176, 2019.

Duan M, et al: A review of location methods of nasogastric tube in critically ill patients, *Open J Nurs* 10(10):Online, 2020. https://www.scirp.org/journal/paperinformation.aspx?paperid=103507. Accessed May 5, 2023.

Elsevier: *Clinical skills: safe handling of hazardous medications*, 2020. https://www.elsevier.com/__data/assets/pdf_file/0015/1002318/Safe-Handling-of-Hazardous-Medications-Skill-COVID-19-toolkit_140420.pdf. Accessed May 5, 2023.

Fumarola S, et al: Overlooked and underestimated: medical adhesive-related skin injuries: best practice consensus document on prevention, *J Wound Care* 29(Suppl 3c):S1–S24, 2020.

Galetto SGS, et al: Medical device-related pressure injuries: an integrative literature review, *Rev Bras Enferm* 72(2):505–512, 2019.

Gardner LE, Wallace S: Nasogastric tube placement: a cross-comparison of verification methods used in Pennsylvania hospitals and how they align with guidelines, *Patient Saf* 3(3):37–45, 2021.

Glanz S: *ENFit®: Your "hook-up" on the new tube feeding connectors*, 2022. https://dietitiansondemand.com/enfit-your-hook-up-on-the-new-tube-feeding-connectors/. Accessed May 5, 2023.

Glen K, et al: Ongoing pH testing to confirm nasogastric tube position before feeding to reduce the risk of adverse outcomes in adult and paediatric patients: a systematic literature review, *Clin Nutr ESPEN* 45:9–18, 2021.

Grodner M, et al: *Nutritional foundations and clinical applications: a nursing approach*, ed 8, St. Louis, 2021, Elsevier.

Harding M, et al: *Lewis's medical-surgical nursing: assessment and management of clinical problems*, ed 12, St. Louis, 2023, Elsevier.

Heidarzadi E, et al: The comparison of capnography and epigastric auscultation to assess the accuracy of nasogastric tube placement in intensive care unit patients, *BMC Gastroenterol* 20(Article 196):1–6, 2020. https://www.ncbi.nlm.nih.gov/pmc/articles/PMC7306926/pdf/12876_2020_Article_1353.pdf. Accessed May 5, 2023.

Hockenberry MJ, et al: *Wong's nursing care of infants and children*, ed 12, St. Louis, 2024, Elsevier.

Institute for Safe Medication Practices (ISMP): *Three new best practices in the 2022-2023 targeted medication safety best practices for hospitals*, 2022. https://www.ismp.org/resources/three-new-best-practices-2022-2023-targeted-medication-safety-best-practices-hospitals. Accessed May 5, 2023.

Irving SY, et al: Pediatric nasogastric tube placement and verification: best practice recommendations from the NOVEL project, *Nutr Clin Pract* 33(6):921–927, 2018. doi:10.1002/ncp.10189.

Jordan EA, Moore SC: Enteral nutrition in critically ill adults: literature review of protocols, *Nurs Crit Care* 25:24–30, 2020.

Kim SY, Shin YS: A comparative study of 2-hour interface pressure in different angles of laterally inclined, supine, and Fowler's position, *Int J Environ Res Public Health* 18(Article 9992):1–14, 2021.

Kisting MA, et al: Lose the whoosh: an evidence-based project to improve NG tube placement verification in infants and children in the hospital setting, *J Pediatr Nurs* 46:1–5, 2019. doi:10.1016/j.pedn.2019.01.011.

Kollmeier BR, Keenaghan M: *Aspiration risk*, 2023, StatPearls [Internet], https://www.ncbi.nlm.nih.gov/books/NBK470169/. Accessed May 5, 2023.

Koontalay A, et al: Effect of a clinical nursing practice guideline of enteral nutrition care on the duration of mechanical ventilator for critically ill patients, *Asian Nurs Res (Korean Soc Nurs Sci)* 14:17–23, 2020.

Landes SD, et al: Cause of death in adults with intellectual disability in the United States, *J Intellect Disabil Res* 65(1):47-59, 2021.

Makhnevich A, et al: Aspiration pneumonia in older adults, *J Hosp Med* 14:429–435, 2019.

Mak MY, Tam G: Ultrasonography for nasogastric tube placement verification: an additional reference, *Brit J Comm Nurs* 25(7):Online, 2020, https://doi.org/10.12968/bjcn.2020.25.7.328. Accessed May 5, 2023.

Metheny N, et al: A review of guidelines to distinguish between gastric and pulmonary placement of nasogastric tubes, *Heart Lung* 48:226–235, 2019.

Metheny N: *Preventing aspiration in older adults with dysphagia*, 2018, Try This: Best Pract Nurs Care Older Adults (20), 2018. https://hign.org/sites/default/files/2020-06/Try_This_General_Assessment_20.pdf. Accessed May 5, 2023.

Monica FJP, et al: Adequacy of different measurement methods in determining nasogastric tube insertion lengths: an observational study, *Int J Nurs Stud* 92:73, 2019.

Northington L, et al: Evaluation of methods used to verify nasogastric feeding tube placement in hospitalized infants and children: a follow-up study, *J Pediatr Nurs* 6:72–77, 2022.

Nyhus J: *Handling hazardous drugs in healthcare*, 2022, https://www.myamericannurse.com/handling-hazardous-drugs-in-healthcare/. Accessed October 16, 2023.

Powers J, et al: Development of a competency model for placement and verification of nasogastric and nasoenteric feeding tubes for adult hospitalized patients, *Nutr Clin Pract* 36:517–533, 2021.

Seong Y, et al: Development and testing of an algorithm to prevent medical device–related pressure injuries, *Inquiry* 58:1–11, 2021.

Sigmon DF, An J. Nasogastric tube. In *StatPearls* [Internet], Treasure Island, FL, 2022, StatPearls Publishing. https://www.ncbi.nlm.nih.gov/books/NBK556063/. Accessed May 5, 2023.

Stay Connected: *EnFit pharmacy resource guide*, 2023. https://stayconnected.org/pharmaguide/. Accessed May 5, 2023.

Tatsumi H: Enteral tolerance in critically ill patients, *J Intensive Care* 7(30):1–10, 2019.

The Joint Commission (TJC): *2023 National Patient Safety Goals*, Oakbrook Terrace, IL, 2023, https://www.jointcommission.org/standards/national-patient-safety-goals/.

Torsy T, et al: Accuracy of the corrected nose-earlobe-xiphoid distance formula for determining nasogastric feeding tube insertion length in intensive care unit patients: a prospective observational study, *Int J Nurs Stud* 110 (Article 103614):1–7, 2020.

Tsolaki V, et al: Ultrasonographic confirmation of nasogastric tube placement in the COVID-19 Era, *J Pers Med* 12:337, 2022.

Ukleja A, et al: Standards for nutrition support: adult hospitalized patients, *JPEN J Parenter Enteral Nutr* 33(6):906, 2018.

Vadivelu N, et al: Evolving therapeutic roles of nasogastric tubes: current concepts in clinical Practice, *Adv Ther* 40:828–843, 2023.

Wang Q, et al: Blind placement of postpyloric feeding tubes at the bedside in intensive care, *Crit Care* 25(Article 168):1–3, 2021. https://ccforum.biomedcentral.com/track/pdf/10.1186/s13054-021-03587-5.pdf. Accessed May 5, 2023.

Yasuda H, et al: Monitoring of gastric residual volume during enteral nutrition, *Cochrane Database Syst Rev* 5:CD013335, 2019. https://www.ncbi.nlm.nih.gov/pmc/articles/PMC6514529/. Accessed May 5, 2023.

Zhang G, et al: Programmed pH-responsive core-shell nanoparticles for precisely targeted therapy of ulcerative colitis, *Nanoscale* 15(4):1937–1946, 2023.

SKILLS AND PROCEDURES

Skill 32.1 **Administering Central Parenteral Nutrition, p. 970**

Skill 32.2 **Administering Peripheral Parenteral Nutrition With Lipid (Fat) Emulsion, p. 975**

OBJECTIVES

Mastery of content in this chapter will enable you to:

- Discuss the purpose and components of parenteral nutrition (PN).
- Explain the factors that make patients candidates for PN.
- Explore the safety and infection risks associated with PN.

- List the monitoring procedures used for patients receiving PN.
- Explain nursing measures used to prevent complications of PN.
- Demonstrate appropriate nursing care and use of safe precautions when caring for a patient receiving PN.

MEDIA RESOURCES

- http://evolve.elsevier.com/Perry/skills
- Review Questions
- Audio Glossary

- Answers to Clinical Judgment and Next-Generation NCLEX® Examination–Style Questions
- Skills Performance Checklists
- Printable Key Points

PURPOSE

Parenteral nutrition (PN), which includes central parenteral nutrition (CPN) and peripheral parenteral nutrition (PPN), is a specialized form of nutrition support that is delivered intravenously through a venous access device (e.g., a central line) (see Chapter 28), a peripherally inserted central catheter [PICC], or a venous port) by an infusion pump to patients who have significant gastrointestinal (GI) dysfunction. Use of the enteral route (see Chapter 31) is preferred over the parenteral route for nutrition support whenever feasible (Gorski et al., 2021). A PN infusion through a central line or port meets long-term nutrition needs in infusions administered in the home if GI dysfunction is expected to be long-term (months to years) (Box 32.1). A basic PN formula is a combination of crystalline amino acids, hypertonic dextrose, electrolytes, vitamins, and trace elements. The hypertonicity of a central PN infusion is why venous access into a large vein is indicated.

PRACTICE STANDARDS

- Compher C et al., 2022: Guidelines for the Provision of Nutrition Support Therapy in the Adult Critically Ill Patient: The American Society for Parenteral and Enteral Nutrition—Central parenteral nutrition (CPN) infusion rate
- Guenter P et al., 2018: Standardized Competencies for Parenteral Nutrition Administration: The ASPEN Model—Fat emulsions
- Gorski et al., 2021: Infusion Therapy Standards of Practice—Parenteral nutrition infusion
- The Joint Commission (TJC), 2023: National Patient Safety Goals—Patient identification

- Ukleja A et al., 2018: Standards for Nutrition Support: Adult Hospitalized Patients, American Society for Parenteral and Enteral Nutrition—Total parenteral nutrition (TPN) and CPN administration

SUPPLEMENTAL STANDARDS

- American Society for Parenteral and Enteral Nutrition (ASPEN), 2019: Appropriate Dosing for Parenteral Nutrition: ASPEN Recommendations
- American Society for Parenteral and Enteral Nutrition (ASPEN), 2023: Parenteral Nutrition Resources

PRINCIPLES FOR PRACTICE

- PN is used when the GI tract is not sufficiently functional. The solution is delivered through a catheter placed in a central venous line in a vein in the arm, neck, or chest. Total parenteral nutrition (TPN) means that all daily nutritional requirements are received via the intravenous (IV) route. Typically, about 2 L of fluid with added nutrients are given, with the nutrient combination varying according to the patient's specific health condition, disorders, and age (Thomas, 2022).
- TPN through a central venous access device (CVAD) involves administration of solutions or emulsions containing concentrations that result in an osmolarity greater than 900 mOsm/L. In contrast, PPN solutions should not exceed an osmolarity of 900 mOsm/L (Gorski et al., 2021).
- The type of catheter to use for administration of PN depends on patient factors and the expected length of PN therapy. The

Indications for Parenteral Nutrition

- Chronic intestinal obstruction as in colon cancer
- Bowel pseudo-obstruction with food intolerance
- Resting the bowel in cases of gastrointestinal (GI) fistulas with high flow
- When an infant's GI system is immature or the infant has a congenital GI malformation
- When there is a postoperative bowel anastomosis leak

- When a patient is unable to maintain nutritional status due to severe diarrhea or vomiting
- Small bowel obstruction
- Hypercatabolic states due to sepsis, polytrauma, and major fractures
- An anticipated period of nothing by mouth (NPO) status greater than 7 days, as in patients with inflammatory bowel disease exacerbations and critically ill patients

Adapted from Hamdan M, Puckett Y: *Total parenteral nutrition,* National Library of Medicine, StatPearls (Internet), 2022. https://www.ncbi.nlm.nih.gov/books/NBK559036/. Accessed September 13, 2023.

location of the catheter is defined on the basis of where the distal tip of the catheter lies. Concentrated PN solutions are diluted quickly when infused into a large-diameter central vein such as the subclavian (Fig. 32.1).

- PPN is delivered through a vein via a PICC line (see Chapter 28) (Fig. 32.2). The tip of the PICC line extends to the superior vena cava. The veins used are the cephalic, basilica, median antecubital, and median antebrachial in the arm. The use of peripheral veins creates a greater risk for phlebitis and is used when a central line or port is not available or when the anticipated need is no more than 14 days (Gorski et al., 2021).
- Patients who self-administer their PN solutions at home will require a central catheter, which may be an implanted subcutaneous port or a tunneled central access device (Fig. 32.3; see Chapter 28).
- Patients who require PN infusions usually have medical or surgical conditions that are often associated with GI fluid losses (e.g., obstruction, diarrhea, fistula) and organ dysfunction; therefore electrolyte monitoring is paramount. A routine laboratory panel relative to PN infusions would include a baseline assessment of electrolytes, serum proteins, complete blood count, triglyceride level, and liver function tests (Box 32.2).
- The components of the PN solution are amino acids, glucose, and lipids as energy sources, with the addition of electrolytes, minerals, trace elements, vitamins, and water. The addition of lipid emulsion to the PN solution results in a preparation called a *3:1, 3-in-1,* or *total nutrition admixture (TNA).*

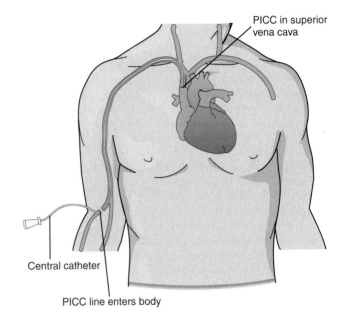

FIG. 32.2 Peripherally inserted central catheter *(PICC).*

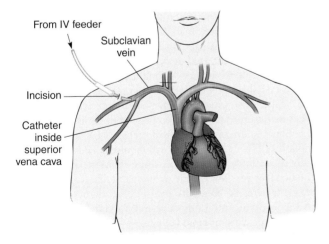

FIG. 32.1 Placement of central venous catheter inserted into subclavian vein. IV, Intravenous. *(Courtesy Rolin Graphics.)*

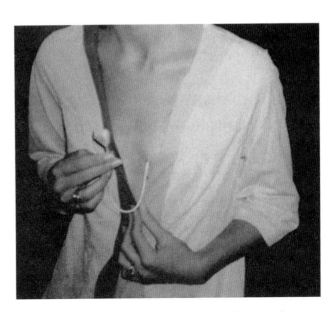

FIG. 32.3 Tunneled catheter used for home central parenteral nutrition. *(From Morgan SL, Weinsier RL: Fundamentals of clinical nutrition, ed 2, St. Louis, 1998, Mosby.)*

Typical Monitoring and Laboratory Orders for Patients With Parenteral Nutrition (PN)

Monitor
- Fluid intake, urine, and gastrointestinal output every 8 hours
- Vital signs every 4 hours
- Body weight at least 3 times weekly

Initial and Repeated Weekly
- Complete metabolic panel with sodium (Na), potassium (K), chloride (Cl), carbon dioxide (CO_2), glucose, calcium (Ca), phosphate (PO_4), magnesium (Mg), triglycerides, transaminases, liver function
- Complete blood count (CBC) with hemoglobin, hematocrit, white blood cell (WBC) count, red blood cell (RBC) count, lymphocyte count
- Serum proteins, often including albumin, transferrin, C-reactive protein, and/or prealbumin

Daily Until Stable
- Electrolyte panel daily until stable; then weekly
- Blood glucose every 6 hours until within normal limits for 48 hours; then daily
- Blood glucose in preparation for cyclic home parenteral nutrition (HPN); monitor 2 hours after PN begins and 2 hours after PN ends; adjust insulin per orders

Monthly or Biannually
- Trace elements such as zinc, copper, manganese, and selenium (depending on underlying condition such as gastrointestinal malabsorption) for long-term HPN patients
- Selected vitamins for long-term HPN patients

- Because hyperglycemia has been linked to increased infection rates, monitoring blood glucose levels during a PN infusion is an important procedure.
- When the goal is to prepare a patient for a cyclic home infusion of PN, it is very important to monitor glucose levels approximately 2 hours after an infusion begins (peak level) and 2 hours after it ends (trough level) to evaluate the need for adding regular human insulin to the infusion bag.
- Because PN solution is typically provided in response to GI dysfunction and to support nutrition needs, it is important for you to monitor data that describe patient progress (see Box 32.2). Measurement of intake and output is very important in order to document when a patient's GI function is changing and to provide information regarding the adequacy of fluid intake from the PN solution.

PERSON-CENTERED CARE

- Include patient and family caregiver in decisions to maintain patient control of self-care, activity level, personal decision making, and socialization with friends and family.
- PN may pose concerns for those with beliefs that include dietary restrictions. The components of PN are largely synthetic and do not contain pork. The lipid emulsion contains egg phospholipid, a product that may be objectionable to vegan patients.

EVIDENCE-BASED PRACTICE

Critically Ill Patients

Key evidence-based practice guidelines for management of critically ill patients in intensive care units (ICUs) include the following (Guenter et al., 2018; Hamdan & Puckett, 2022).
- If the patient was healthy before a critical illness with no evidence of protein calorie malnutrition, use of PN should be reserved and initiated only after the first 7 to 10 days of hospitalization when enteral nutrition is not available.
- PN should be initiated only if the duration is anticipated to be greater than or equal to 7 days.
- An interprofessional team including nutritionists and pharmacists should assess probable drug-nutrient interactions on a daily basis.
- Because the main adverse effects of PN include metabolic abnormalities, infection risk, or venous access complications, monitoring of laboratory values and careful inspection of venous

access sites and infusion line functioning is critical. Unstable and critically ill patients should be monitored daily until stable.
- In patients stabilized on PN, efforts should be made to reintroduce oral or enteral nutrition.
- PN should not be terminated until greater than or equal to 60% of energy and protein requirements are met by means of the oral or enteral route.
- The introduction of vascular access devices for PN will increase the risk for catheter-associated bloodstream infection. The INS (Gorski et al., 2021) recommends these steps to reduce infection risk:
  - Avoid blood sampling via a CVAD used for PN.
  - Consider dedication of a single lumen to PN administration when a multilumen CVAD has been placed. (**NOTE:** More research needed in this area.)
  - Avoid attaching administration sets until the time of infusion.

SAFETY GUIDELINES

- The most frequent complication with PN is central line–associated bloodstream infection (CLABSI), a risk that is found in both hospitalized patients and those with PN at home (Table 32.1). It is critically important that appropriate care of the vascular access device, dressing, and site be instituted to minimize CLABSI (see Chapter 28).
- Use Aseptic Non-Touch Technique (ANTT®) during manipulation of catheter and infusion tubing, site care, and dressing changes (Gorski, 2023; Gorski et al., 2021). When key parts (e.g., tubing and catheter connection) or key sites (e.g., CVAD insertion site) require direct touch, use sterile gloves (Surgical ANTT®) (Gorski, 2023; Gorski et al., 2021).
- CPN using concentrated dextrose solutions should not be infused into a peripheral IV or midline catheter because of the increased risk for phlebitis. If only peripheral lines are available, the health care provider's orders should clearly state that the administration route should be via a peripheral IV line so that the compounding pharmacy will prepare PPN with a lower osmolarity (Table 32.2), which will require added fluid volume.
- PPN is used only for very short-term situations or when there is the need for very low caloric requirements. It is difficult to meet total nutrient requirements with PPN owing to the limitation of dextrose concentration peripherally and the inability to meet caloric goals without large volumes.
- Many health care agencies use PICCs, termed *PICC lines* (see Fig. 32.2), which are placed by radiologists or by nurses who have been specially trained.

TABLE 32.1

Complications of Parenteral Nutrition

Problem	Cause	Symptoms	Immediate Action	Prevention
Pneumothorax	Tip of catheter enters pleural space during insertion, causing lung to collapse.	Sudden chest pain, difficulty breathing, decreased breath sounds, cessation of normal chest movement on affected side, tachycardia	Per health care provider's order, the properly trained health care provider may remove the central catheter. Nurse administers oxygen via nasal cannula. Health care provider inserts chest tube to remove air under water-seal drainage or dry one-way valve system.	Medical personnel should be properly trained to insert central catheters. Evidence recommends use of ultrasonography when placing CVCs (Gorski, 2023; Gorski et al., 2021). Catheter should be secured properly to prevent migration and movement.
Air embolism	IV tubing disconnected; part of catheter system open or removed without being clamped.	Sudden onset of dyspnea, gasping, continued coughing, breathlessness, chest pain, hypotension, tachyarrhythmias, wheezing, tachypnea, altered mental status and speech, change in facial appearance, numbness or paralysis (Gorski et al., 2021)	Immediately close, fold, clamp, or cover the existing catheter or cover the puncture site with an air-occlusive dressing or pad if the catheter has been removed (Gorski et al., 2021). Immediately place the patient on the left side in the Trendelenburg position or in the left lateral decubitus position if not contraindicated (Gorski et al., 2021). Call code team, notify health care provider, and administer 100% oxygen if available (Gorski et al., 2021).	Make sure that all catheter connections are secure; clamp catheter when not in use. Never use a stopcock with a CVC. Unless contraindicated, instruct patient in Valsalva maneuver during venipuncture procedure to reduce the risk of air embolism (Gorski, 2023).
Localized infection (exit site or tunnel)	Poor aseptic technique in removal of skin flora during site preparation and dressing care.	*Exit site:* Erythema, tenderness, induration, or purulence within 2 cm (0.8 inches) of skin at exit site *Tunnel:* Same as above but extends beyond 2 cm from exit site	Call health care provider. *Exit:* Apply warm compress, daily care of site, oral antibiotics. *Infection:* Collaborate with health care provider regarding removal of catheter (Gorski, 2023). *Tunnel:* Remove catheter.	Use Aseptic Non-Touch Technique (ANTT) during site care and dressing changes (Gorski, 2023; Gorski et al., 2021). If key parts or key sites require direct touch, use sterile gloves (Gorski et al., 2021; Gorski, 2023). Implement a postinsertion care bundle (cleaning site, applying new stabilization device, and applying sterile dressing per guideline) during daily care and management (Gorski et al., 2021). Assess VAD site and surrounding area by palpation and inspection, including catheter pathway, for integrity of skin, dressing, and securement device. Change transparent dressings at least every 7 days and gauze dressings at least every 2 days. Change dressing if damp, loosened, or soiled or when inspection of site is necessary (Gorski, 2023; Gorski et al., 2021). Use chlorhexidine wipes to cleanse site. For adults, consider the use of chlorhexidine-impregnated dressings (Gorski, 2023; Gorski et al., 2021).
Catheter-related sepsis or bacteremia	Catheter hub contamination; contamination of infusate; spread of bacteria through bloodstream from distant site.	*Systemic:* Isolation of same microorganism from blood culture and catheter segment, with patient showing fever, chills, malaise, elevated white blood cell count	*Systemic:* Do not exceed hang time of 24 hours for PN that contains dextrose and amino acids either alone or with fat emulsion added as a 3-in-1 formulation (Gorski, 2023). Administer antibiotics intravenously; catheter removal by proper professional (CRNP, PA-C, or physician).	Use full sterile-barrier precautions during catheter insertion and dressing change. Consider the use of antibiotic-impregnated catheters (Gorski, 2023). Do not disconnect tubing unnecessarily. Replace IV tubing and filter every 24 hours. In some situations it is necessary to change administration sets with each new PN container (Gorski, 2023).
Hyperglycemia	Possible blood-draw error; confirm with bedside glucose device. Patient receiving too little insulin in PN solution. Patient receiving steroids. New-onset infection.	Excessive thirst, urination, blood glucose greater than 160 mg/100 dL, confusion	Call health care provider; may need to slow infusion rate (health care provider order).	Review medical history for blood drawn through central line with PN infusing (repeat peripheral blood draw or obtain fingerstick), glucose intolerance or diabetes, new infection, new medication such as steroids; keep rate as ordered; never increase PN to "catch up." Maintain blood glucose in range ordered by health care provider. Use aseptic technique and routine blood glucose monitoring.

Continued

TABLE 32.1

Complications of Parenteral Nutrition—cont'd

Problem	Cause	Symptoms	Immediate Action	Prevention
Hypoglycemia	PN abruptly discontinued; too much insulin	Patient shaky, dizzy, nervous, anxious, hungry; blood glucose level <80 mg/100 dL	Call health care provider; if PN discontinued abruptly, may need to restart D10W at previous PN rate. If patient has oral intake, give ½ cup fruit juice. Perform blood glucose monitoring; retest in 15 to 30 min.	Decrease PN, "tapering" gradually until discontinued; blood glucose monitoring is used to ensure adequate insulin.

CRNP, Certified registered nurse practitioner; *CVC,* central venous catheter; *IV,* intravenous; *PA-C,* physician's assistant, certified; *PN,* parenteral nutrition; *VAD,* venous access device.

TABLE 32.2

Comparison of Central Versus Peripheral Parenteral Nutrition Orders

	Central Parenteral Nutrition	**Peripheral Parenteral Nutrition**
Osmolality	>900 mOsm	<900 mOsm
Route of administration	Central venous catheter	Small peripheral vein
Usual daily caloric intake	20–35 kcal/kg/day	5–10 kcal/kg/day
Usual daily volume (mL)	1000–2000	2000–3000
Fat emulsion	Minor caloric source	Major caloric source

Data from Ukleja A, et al: Standards for nutrition support: adult hospitalized patients, American Society for Parenteral and Enteral Nutrition, *Nutr in Clin Prac* 33(6), 2018; and Gorski, et al: Infusion therapy standards of practice, ed 8, *J Intraven Nurs* 44(15):S1-S224, 2021.

- Following central venous catheter insertion, do not initiate PN until placement of the venous catheter tip is confirmed by a radiograph or through the use of electrocardiograph-based tip verification technology (Gorski, 2023).
- Appropriate aseptic technique is needed when handling the central line, dressings, tubing, and needleless end cap PN port (see Skill 28.6).
- PN without lipids can be infused using tubing with a 1.2 μm filter, including lipid-containing emulsions (3-in-1) (Gorski, 2023). A filter is necessary because it prevents particulate matter or large droplets of lipid from reaching a patient, which could potentially result in a pulmonary embolism. The filter should be placed as close to the patient as possible to reduce the potential for patient harm due to particulates, microparticulates, microorganisms, and air emboli (Guenter et al., 2018).
- In very malnourished patients, during a process termed *refeeding syndrome,* some electrolytes (e.g., potassium [K], magnesium [Mg], and phosphorus [P]) may shift intracellularly with glucose provided in the PN, potentially resulting in low serum levels with risk for arrhythmias and muscle weakness. Adequate electrolyte replacement should occur before the initiation of PN. There is an increased risk of pulmonary edema and heart failure when initiating feeding in malnourished patients who are at greater risk of refeeding syndrome.
- Because there is a risk of bloodstream infection in patients with catheters, regular monitoring of vital signs is important.

♦ SKILL 32.1 **Administering Central Parenteral Nutrition**

Infusion of total parenteral nutrition (TPN) via a central line is described as central parenteral nutrition (CPN). It involves placement of an intravenous (IV) catheter tip into a large, high–blood flow vein, such as the superior vena cava. A central venous catheter terminates in the superior vena cava or the right atrium and is used to administer nutrition, medication, chemotherapy, and other therapies. Venous access is established through a peripherally inserted central catheter (PICC), a central venous catheter, or an implanted port (Hamdan & Puckett, 2022).

The procedure requires the use of standard Aseptic Non-Touch Technique (Gorski, 2023; Gorski et al., 2021) and application of critical thinking to make accurate clinical judgments regarding a patient's response to the infusion and anticipation of possible complications. Because of the composition of PN fluids, patients can experience metabolic and fluid balance changes quickly. In addition, the clinical condition of patients receiving PN may be poor, especially when they have alterations in host defenses, severe underlying illnesses, and extremes of age. Anticipate changes (e.g., infection, fluid imbalance, pulmonary complications) in a patient's condition and maintain the IV system to ensure that it is functioning properly.

Delegation

The skill of administering CPN to a hospitalized patient cannot be delegated to assistive personnel (AP). Direct the AP to:
- Report when the pump alarms or if the patient develops shortness of breath, headaches, weakness, shaky feeling, or discomfort or bleeding at IV site
- Perform fingerstick blood glucose monitoring as directed and report any abnormal results to the nurse
- Report to nurse any vital signs (VS) that are out of normal range
- Measure urinary output and weigh patient per agency protocol

Interprofessional Collaboration

- CPN is administered often without the oversight of a dedicated, knowledgeable nutrition support team. To minimize the risk to patients receiving this therapy and to promote the clinical benefits of CPN, the following health care team is recommended: nurses, physicians, registered dietitians, and pharmacists. The team is responsible for (Ukleja et al., 2018):
  - Recognizing clinical indications for CPN as well as situations in which the therapy is not likely to be beneficial
  - Developing a CPN prescription that meets individual requirements
  - Monitoring the response to therapy
  - Adjusting the therapeutic plan as indicated
  - Promoting a seamless transition in nutritional care when CPN is no longer required
  - Encouraging a collaborative approach across professional and departmental boundaries

Equipment

- CPN solution (IV)
- Electronic infusion device (EID) with anti–free-flow protection and alarms for occlusion. Consider the use of electronic infusion pumps with dose error reduction software (DERS) (i.e., smart pumps), as they are associated with reduced risk for infusion-related medication errors (Gorski et al., 2021).
- 1.2-μm filter for parenteral nutrition (PN) solution infusion, including lipid injectable emulsions (Gorski, 2023; Gorski et al., 2021)
- IV infusion tubing with Luer-Lok tip
- 5- to 10-mL syringe with sterile saline flush
- Bedside glucose monitoring kit
- Adhesive tape or tubing label
- Aqueous and alcohol-based chlorhexidine antiseptic swab
- Clean gloves (sterile gloves if a key part or site requires direct touch) (Gorski, 2023; Gorski et al., 2021)
- Stethoscope
- Medication administration record (MAR) or computer printout

STEP	RATIONALE

ASSESSMENT

1. Identify patient using at least two identifiers (e.g., name and birthday or name and medical record number) according to agency policy.

Ensures correct patient. Complies with The Joint Commission standards and improves patient safety (TJC, 2023).

2. Review electronic health record (EHR) for lab test measurement of levels of electrolytes, serum albumin, total protein, transferrin, prealbumin, and triglycerides.

Document baseline nutrition parameters that may influence the prescription and administration of nutrition support (Ukleja et al., 2018).

3. Assess patient's medical history for factors influenced by CPN administration: electrolyte levels; renal, cardiac, and hepatic function. Assess for history of allergies, including egg allergy with lipids.

Some patients require CPN solution to be adapted by composition or volume (requires health care provider order) based on medical history. CPN includes constituents (e.g., medications) to which patient may be allergic.

4. Review EHR to determine patient's age and history of dehydration, malnutrition, exposure to radiation therapy, underlying chronic conditions (e.g., diabetes mellitus, immunosuppression), and edema of the skin.

Common risk factors for medical adhesive–related skin injury (MARSI). Erythema, blistering, and excoriation are signs of MARSI and are related to the skin's reaction to an adhesive (Hitchcock et al., 2021; Thayer et al., 2022)

5. Assess patient's/family caregiver's health literacy.

Determines degree to which individuals have the ability to find, understand, and use information and services to make informed health-related decisions and actions for themselves and others (Centers for Disease Control and Prevention [CDC], 2023).

6. Assess indications of and risks for protein/calorie malnutrition: weight loss from baseline or ideal, muscle atrophy/weakness, edema, lethargy, failure to wean from ventilatory support, chronic illness, and nothing by mouth for more than 7 days. Confer with nutrition support team.

Identifies nutrition risk factors and specific nutrition deficits to determine individual nutrition needs and identify medical factors that may influence prescription and administration of CPN (Ukleja et al., 2018).

7. Perform hand hygiene and apply clean gloves. Check blood glucose level by fingerstick (see Chapter 7). Remove and dispose of gloves and perform hand hygiene.

Reduces transmission of microorganisms. Serum glucose determines patient's baseline and tolerance to high levels of glucose in CPN solution.

8. Apply new pair of clean gloves. Inspect condition of central vein access site for presence of inflammation, edema, and tenderness. Inspect tubing of access device for patency and kinking. **NOTE:** If necessary to touch site or connections, apply sterile gloves (Gorski et al., 2021; Gorski, 2023).

Reduces transmission of infection. Inspection identifies early signs of infection, infiltration, or disruption in system integrity. Development of complication contraindicates infusion of fluids and indicates need to establish new IV site.

9. Assess VS, auscultate patient's lung sounds, inspect for edema of extremities, and measure weight. Remove and dispose of gloves and perform hand hygiene.

Provides baseline for monitoring patient's response to fluid infusion and nutrients. Crackles in lungs are early indication of fluid volume excess. Reduces transmission of microorganisms.

10. Consult with members of nutrition support team on calculation of calorie, protein, and fluid requirements for patient.

Provides multidisciplinary plan for patient's nutrition support.

11. Verify order for nutrients, minerals, vitamins, trace elements, electrolytes, added medications, and flow rate. Check for compatibility of added medications.

CPN is often ordered daily in hospital setting after review of laboratory values. In home setting, orders may be obtained less frequently (e.g., weekly). Pharmacies that prepare parenteral solutions will check medication compatibility.

STEP	RATIONALE

Clinical Judgment *Medications are not added to or co-infused with a parenteral nutrition (PN) solution before or during infusion without consultation with a pharmacist regarding compatibility and stability (Gorski et al., 2021).*

12. Assess patient's knowledge, prior experience with CPN, and feelings about procedure.	Reveals need for patient instruction and/or support.

PLANNING

1. Expected outcomes following completion of procedure:	
• Patient's ideal weight gain is between 0.5 and 1.5 kg (1 and 3 lb) per week.	Weight is indicator of patient's nutritional status and determines fluid volume. Weight gain greater than 0.5 kg (1 lb) per day indicates fluid retention.
• Blood glucose levels are maintained per health care provider's order for desired glucose range.	Diabetes self-management education and support should be person centered. Glucose levels differ based on the degree of illness, so a specific health care provider order is needed (American Diabetes Association [ADA], 2019).
• Central venous access device (CVAD) is patent and site is free of pain, swelling, redness, or inflammation.	Ensures that CPN is infusing into vein rather than into surrounding tissues and that there are no signs of an access device extravasation or inflammation.
• Patient is afebrile.	Absence of systemic infection.
• Patient and family caregiver are able to discuss purpose and steps for care associated with PN.	Proper instruction informs patient and family caregiver and prepares for home care if needed.
2. Explain purpose of CPN to patient and family caregiver.	Promotes understanding and reduces anxiety.
3. If CPN solution is refrigerated, remove from refrigeration 1 hour before infusion.	Ensures solution will be administered at room temperature.
4. Perform hand hygiene. Assemble necessary equipment and supplies at bedside.	Reduces transmission of infection. Promotes efficiency of procedure.

IMPLEMENTATION

1. Perform hand hygiene.	Reduces transmission of microorganisms.
2. In medication room, check label on CPN bag with health care provider's order on MAR or computer printout and patient's name. Also check any additives and note solution expiration date.	Prevents medication error. *This is the first check for accuracy.*
3. Inspect 2:1 CPN solution for particulate matter.	Presence of particulate matter requires that solution be discarded. *This is the second check for accuracy.*
4. Before leaving medication room, check IV solution a second time using seven rights of medication administration (see Chapter 20). Check label of CPN bag against MAR or computer printout.	
5. Take new CPN solution to patient before the existing PN infusion solution empties. Compare names of solution and additives with MAR at bedside.	*This is the third check for accuracy.*
6. Identify patient again using at least two identifiers (e.g., name and birthday or name and medical record number) according to agency policy. Compare identifiers with information on patient's MAR or EHR.	Ensures correct patient. Complies with The Joint Commission standards and improves patient safety (TJC, 2023).
7. Close room doors and/or bedside curtain.	Provides patient privacy.
8. Position patient comfortably, either sitting or lying supine with head of bed elevated.	Promotes patient comfort.
9. Perform hand hygiene. Apply clean gloves. Prepare IV tubing for CPN solution:	Maintains sterility of solution. Air introduced into central circulation could result in air embolus, a fatal IV complication.
a. Attach 1.2-μm filter to IV tubing.	
b. Position filter to be as close to patient as possible (Gorski, 2023; Gorski et al., 2021).	
c. Prime tubing with CPN solution, making sure that no air bubbles remain, and turn off flow with roller clamp (see Chapter 28). Some infusion pumps and IV tubing require that priming be done by pump rather than by gravity. Add sterile-capped needle or place sterile cap on end of tubing.	

STEP	RATIONALE
10. Scrub end port of the CVAD with chlorhexidine antiseptic swab, allow to dry, attach syringe of 0.9% normal saline (NS) solution to needleless port, aspirate for blood return, and flush saline per agency policy (see illustration).	Scrubbing hub decreases microorganisms (Gorski, 2023). Determines patency of IV device before CPN is infused.
11. Remove syringe. Remove sterile cap and connect sterile Luer-Lok end of CPN IV tubing to dedicated end port of CVAD; for multilumen lines, label the tubing used for CPN.	Ensures that tubing is securely connected to IV line. Dedicated line should be used for CPN when a multilumen device is in place. Labeling of high-risk catheters prevents connection with inappropriate tube or catheter.

Clinical Judgment *An independent double-check verification should be performed by a second clinician prior to beginning a parenteral nutrition infusion (Ukleja et al., 2018).*

12. Place IV tubing in EID. Open roller clamp. Set and regulate flow rate as ordered (see illustration).	CPN flow rates are ordered to meet patient's metabolic and electrolyte needs. Maintaining rates prevents electrolyte imbalances.
a. *Continuous infusion:* Flow rate is immediately set at ordered rate and given over 24-hour period.	Ensures that blood glucose levels are maintained to prevent hypoglycemia or hyperglycemia (Guenter et al., 2018).
b. *Cycle infusion:* Flow rate is initiated at about 40 to 60 mL/h, and the rate is gradually increased until patient's nutrition needs are met. Before completion of infusion, rate is decreased at about the same rate in milliliters per hour until the CPN is completed. The infusion is usually given over a shorter time frame (12–18 hours).	Infusion rates are usually increased and decreased to prevent hypoglycemia or hyperglycemia (Guenter et al., 2018).

Clinical Judgment *Infuse all intravenous (IV) medications or blood through alternative IV site or different lumen of multilumen device. Do not obtain blood samples or central venous pressure readings through same lumen used for central parenteral nutrition (CPN). Prevents drug incompatibility and IV device occlusion (Gorski et al., 2021).*

13. Do not interrupt CPN infusion (e.g., during showers, transport to procedure, blood transfusion), and be sure that rate does not exceed ordered rate.	Prevents development of catheter-related bacteremia (Gorski, 2023).
14. A 3-in-1 CPN solution containing the three macronutrients (dextrose, amino acids, lipid emulsions) should have a hang time not to exceed 24 hours. Fat emulsions alone should have a hang time not to exceed 12 hours (see Skill 32.2).	Prevents bacterial infection and deterioration of emulsion (Guenter et al., 2018).

Clinical Judgment *American Society for Parenteral and Enteral Nutrition (ASPEN) guidelines suggest parenteral nutrition (PN) feeding between 12 and 25 kcal/kg/day in the first 7 to 10 days of an intensive care unit stay (Compher et al., 2022).*

15. Change IV administration sets with each new CPN solution container, which is usually every 24 hours and immediately on suspected contamination.	Reduces transmission of infection.

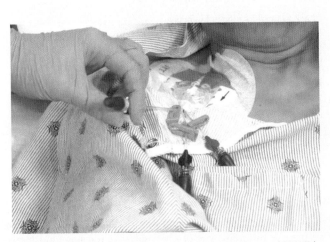

STEP 10 End port of central vascular access device (CVAD). *(From Elsevier: Clinical Skills: Essentials Collection, St. Louis, 2021, Mosby. Elsevier Education Portal.)*

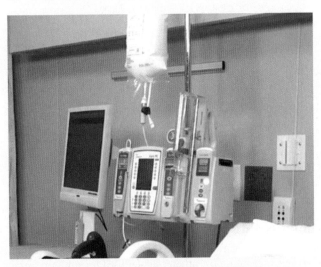

STEP 12 Parenteral nutrition solution infusing via infusion pump. *(From Elsevier: Clinical Skills: Essentials Collection, St. Louis, 2021, Mosby. Elsevier Education Portal.)*

STEP	RATIONALE
16. Remove and dispose of supplies and gloves. Perform hand hygiene.	Reduces transmission of microorganisms. Use appropriate disposal receptacle if patient is on hazardous drugs (Kennedy et al., 2023).
17. Help patient to a comfortable position.	Restores comfort and sense of well-being.
18. Place nurse call system in an accessible location within patient's reach.	Ensures patient can call for assistance if needed.
19. Raise side rails (as appropriate) and lower bed to lowest position, locking into position.	Ensures patient safety and prevents falls.

EVALUATION

1. Monitor flow rate according to agency policy and procedure. If infusion is not running on time, do not attempt to catch up.
   - Too-rapid or too-slow infusion could result in metabolic disturbances such as hyperglycemia and fluid overload.
2. Monitor fluid intake and urine and gastrointestinal (GI) fluid output every 8 hours.
   - Prevents fluid imbalance from too-slow or too-rapid infusion.
3. Measure VS every 4 hours.
   - Monitors for fluid overload response.
4. Obtain initial weight and then weigh at least 3 times weekly.
   - Routine measurement of weights will reflect a gain or loss resulting from either caloric intake or fluid retention. Gradual weight gain, if weight gain is the goal, indicates adequate tolerance.
5. Evaluate for fluid retention; palpate skin of extremities; auscultate lung sounds.
   - Weight gain in excess of 0.5 kg (1 lb) per day, dependent edema, lung crackles, and intake greater than output per each 24-hour period indicate fluid retention.
6. Monitor patient's glucose levels daily or as ordered and other laboratory parameters daily or as ordered.
   - Maintenance of normal electrolyte levels, satisfactory fluid balance, acceptable serum glucose levels, and improvement in serum proteins indicate adequate tolerance to PN.
7. Inspect central venous access site for signs and symptom of swelling, inflammation, drainage, redness, warmth, tenderness, or edema.
   - Determines IV patency and absence of infection, infiltration, or phlebitis.
8. Monitor for temperature, elevated white blood cell count, and malaise.
   - Signs of systemic infection.
9. **Use Teach-Back:** "I want to be sure I explained what can happen with your central parenteral nutrition. What signs and symptoms should you report to the nurse or doctor?" Revise your instruction now or develop a plan for revised patient/family caregiver teaching if patient/family caregiver is not able to teach back correctly.
   - Teach-back is a technique for health care providers to ensure that they have explained medical information clearly so that patients and their families understand what is communicated to them (Agency for Healthcare Research and Quality [AHRQ], 2023).

Unexpected Outcomes	Related Interventions
1. There is redness, swelling, and tenderness around central venous access site, indicating possible exit site infection.	• Notify health care provider. • Apply warm compress and initiate daily site care as ordered. • Systemic antibiotic therapy may be ordered.
2. Patient develops fever, malaise, and chills, indicating systemic infection.	• Check exit site for signs of infection. • Notify health care provider and consult about need to obtain cultures of exit site or blood. • Systemic antibiotic therapy may be ordered.
3. Serum glucose level is greater than 150 mg/dL or target set by health care provider. Indicates intolerance to glucose load in solution or may indicate new-onset infection.	• Notify health care provider. • Verify that blood was not drawn with PN infusing and that proper procedure to interrupt PN and discard first blood draw was followed. • Possible need for addition of insulin to CPN, modification of CPN solution, or sliding-scale insulin coverage.

Documentation

- Document condition of CVAD site, function of CVAD, rate and type of infusion, catheter lumen used for infusion, intake and output (I&O), blood glucose levels, VS, and weights.
- Document any adverse reactions.
- Document your evaluation of patient and family caregiver learning.

Hand-Off Reporting

- In a hand-off report, communicate condition of CVAD site, status of infusion, type of CPN solution infusing, and patient response.
- If signs of infection, occlusion, fluid retention, or infiltration occur, notify the health care provider.

Special Considerations

Patient Education

- Educate patient and family caregiver about purpose of nutrition support therapy, goals, and expectations. Incorporate the wishes of the patient and/or caregiver. Describe the route of administration, estimated duration of therapy, and criteria for discontinuation of therapy (Ukleja et al., 2018).
- As a home health nurse, you will likely provide several instructional sessions.
- Inform patient of signs of central line infection to report to the nurse.

Pediatrics

- Consider children's developmental needs when they are on long-term CPN. Perform regular assessments of development to determine child's progress. Implement interventions to encourage expected milestones.

Older Adults

- Some older adults have impaired ability to tolerate higher fluid volumes because of cardiac or renal impairment.
- When comparing older patients with younger patients receiving home parenteral nutrition (HPN), older adults had fewer catheter-related bloodstream infections (CRBSIs) but higher 2-year mortality (Daoud et al., 2022).

Home Care

- ASPEN has resources for patients and caregivers about parenteral nutrition at http://www.nutritioncare.org/About_Clinical_Nutrition/What_is_Parenteral_Nutrition/.

- Patient teaching for home CPN administration will be given by home infusion nurses after discharge or may be initiated in the hospital and continued at home.
- Patients requiring long-term CPN benefit from a referral to a home nutrition therapy team.
- Patients should have a home safety and physical, nutritional, and psychological needs assessment (Gorski, 2023).
- Patients receiving home CPN may have a PICC line or a tunneled or implanted catheter to reduce the possibility of infection. Patients or family caregivers need to learn to perform catheter site care, dressing changes, techniques for connecting and disconnecting PN solutions, and infusion pump management.
- Some patients receive home CPN at night during sleep (cyclic CPN) to allow the freedom to leave home during the day. Some patients may also take an oral diet as tolerated, although their impaired GI function limits nutrient absorption. Encourage food and fluid intake for pleasure, but monitor for diarrhea or increased output if eating in order to assess for dehydration.
- Teach patient and family caregiver to monitor patient's temperature, weight, I&O, and serum glucose level and recognize signs and symptoms of PN-related complications.
- Teach patient and family caregiver about actions to take in case of emergency or unexpected outcomes such as telephoning the health care provider or home infusion provider or going to the hospital, depending on the circumstances.
- If home CPN patients require insulin in their CPN, they will need a home glucose monitoring device and instruction in its use.
- Telehealth support groups may be available to improve maintenance and access for home parenteral nutrition (HPN) patients.

◆ SKILL 32.2 Administering Peripheral Parenteral Nutrition With Lipid (Fat) Emulsion

The administration of peripheral parenteral nutrition (PPN) requires a lower dextrose content (lower osmolarity) and is more appropriate for short-term use until central access can be achieved or the patient can be fed orally or enterally (see Table 32.2). Patients with elevated nutritional requirements from hypermetabolic illnesses or conditions and patients with fluid restrictions are not suitable candidates (Worthington et al., 2017). This therapy is for short-term use (no more than 14 days), in part because of increased risk for phlebitis (Gorski et al., 2021). Adding lipid emulsion provides a source of calories with minimal impact on the osmolality. A lipid emulsion must be administered through vented intravenous (IV) tubing as a primary IV infusion or a piggyback.

This skill describes a piggyback administration of PPN. You replace administration sets used for lipid emulsion with each new infusion; hang time for lipid emulsion should not exceed 12 hours (Gorski et al., 2021). The administration set must have a Luer-Lok design. Indications for PPN include the following:

- *Adequate peripheral access:* Despite its lower osmolality, PPN tends to cause phlebitis and often requires frequent changes in the access location. The use of midline catheters for PPN has not been studied; the location of midline catheters in a deeper vein may mask early signs of phlebitis (Gorski et al., 2021).
- *Ability to tolerate larger volumes of fluid:* Because of the lower concentration of dextrose in PPN, a larger volume of fluid is required to attain adequate calories. Some patients with impaired renal or cardiac function do not tolerate PPN.

- *Ability to tolerate lipid emulsions:* Lipid is the most calorically dense nutrient. A 1-L amount of 10% dextrose without lipid provides only 340 kcal. A 250-mL amount of 20% lipid solution provides 500 kcal.

Delegation

The skill of administering PPN cannot be delegated to assistive personnel (AP). Direct the AP to:

- Report patient complaint of burning, pain, or redness at peripheral IV site; moist IV site dressing; and any infusion pump alarms
- Report to nurse any patient complaints of shortness of breath and change in vital signs (VS)

Interprofessional Collaboration

- PPN is administered at times without the oversight of a dedicated, knowledgeable nutrition support team. To minimize the risk to patients receiving this therapy and to promote the clinical benefits of PPN, the following health care team is recommended: nurses, physicians, registered dietitians, and pharmacists. See Skill 32.1 for team responsibilities.

Equipment

- PPN solution or lipid emulsion (prepared by pharmacy)
- IV tubing with a 1.2-μm filter for amino acid/dextrose solution (PPN) and fat emulsion (Gorski, 2023)

- Bedside glucose monitoring kit
- Aqueous and alcohol-based chlorhexidine antiseptic
- Electronic infusion device (EID) with anti–free-flow control and alarms (Gorski, 2023)

- Clean gloves (**NOTE:** Use sterile gloves if necessary to touch site or connections.)
- Medication administration record (MAR) or computer printout
- Stethoscope

STEP	RATIONALE

ASSESSMENT

1. Identify patient using at least two identifiers (e.g., name and birthday or name and medical record number) according to agency policy.	Ensures correct patient. Complies with The Joint Commission standards and improves patient safety (TJC, 2023).
2. Review electronic health record (EHR) for history of patient having hypertriglyceridemia. Consult with health care provider and obtain orders for serum triglyceride level before initiation of PPN and weekly.	Determines patient's ability to metabolize lipid.
3. Assess patient's/family caregiver's health literacy.	Determines degree to which individuals have the ability to find, understand, and use information and services to make informed health-related decisions and actions for themselves and others (CDC, 2023).
4. Assess for history of allergies, including egg allergy with lipids.	PPN contains elements to which patient may be allergic.
5. Obtain patient's weight and VS.	Provides baseline information to determine effectiveness and tolerance of PPN solution.
6. Perform hand hygiene, and apply clean gloves using ANTT®. **NOTE:** *If necessary to touch site or connections, apply sterile gloves (Gorski et al., 2021; Gorski, 2023).* Select or initiate appropriate functional IV site to administer PPN and lipid emulsion. Assess its patency and function (see Chapter 28).	PPN may cause phlebitis; appropriate vein selection is important.
7. Obtain blood glucose level by fingerstick (see Chapter 7). Remove and dispose of gloves and perform hand hygiene.	Provides baseline to determine tolerance to glucose infusion. Reduces transmission of microorganisms.
8. Assess patient for edema in extremities, lung sounds, or fluid intake greater than fluid output.	Determines patient's fluid balance. Fluid intake that is given with PPN may cause fluid overload in elderly patients or those who have impaired renal or cardiac function.
9. Assess patient's knowledge, prior experience with PPN, and feelings about procedure.	Reveals need for patient instruction and/or support.

PLANNING

1. Expected outcomes following completion of procedure:	
• Triglyceride level is at targeted range per health care provider.	Indicates adequate clearance of lipid.
• Blood glucose levels are maintained per health care provider's order for desired glucose range.	Diabetes self-management education and support should be patient centered. Glucose levels differ based on the degree of illness, so a specific health care provider order is needed (ADA, 2019).
• Venipuncture site is free of phlebitis, pain, swelling, redness, and inflammation.	Ensures proper administration and monitoring of PPN with lipids.
• Patient does not show signs of systemic infection (e.g., elevated temperature).	VS are indication of possible systemic infection related to PPN.
• Patient does not show signs of allergy to lipids.	Monitoring infusion requires observation for allergic response to infusion.
• Patient and family caregiver are able to explain purpose of PPN and complications to observe for.	Proper instruction informs patient and family caregiver.
2. Explain purposes of PPN and fat emulsion.	Promotes understanding and reduces anxiety.
3. If PPN solution is refrigerated, remove from refrigeration 1 hour before infusion.	Solution should be removed from refrigeration before administration (Gorski, 2023).
4. Place patient in comfortable position for IV line insertion or initiation of infusion.	When patients are comfortable, they tolerate procedures more readily.

STEP	RATIONALE

IMPLEMENTATION

1. Perform hand hygiene.
2. Check health care provider's order against MAR for volume of fat emulsion, PPN solution, and administration time for PPN solution/fat emulsion. Then check name of solution on label with MAR.

3. Read label of fat emulsion solution.

4. Compare label of PPN bag/lipid emulsion bottle with MAR or computer printout; check for correct additives and solution expiration date. Also check patient's name.
5. Examine lipid solution for separation of emulsion into layers or fat globules or presence of froth.
6. Identify patient again at bedside using at least two identifiers (e.g., name and birthday or name and medical record number) according to agency policy. Compare identifiers with information on patient's MAR or EHR.
7. Compare identifiers with information on solution bag label and patient's MAR or EHR at the bedside.

8. Take new PPN solution to patient before the existing PPN infusion solution empties.
9. Close room doors and/or bedside curtain.
10. Position patient comfortably, either sitting or lying supine with head of bed elevated.
11. Perform hand hygiene. Apply clean gloves (surgical gloves if touching key connecting parts).
12. Prepare IV tubing and administer PPN solution:
    a. Apply 1.2-μm filter to PPN solution tubing using ANTT (Gorski, 2023).
    b. Position filters to be as close to patient as possible (Gorski et al., 2021).
    c. Run solution through PPN tubing to remove excess air. Turn roller clamp to "off" position. Some infusion pumps and tubing require priming through the infusion pump. Add sterile-capped needle or place sterile cap on end of tubing.
    d. Wipe end port of PPN IV infusion tubing with antimicrobial swab and allow to dry. Remove cap and prepare to connect needleless connector at end of PPN tubing to end port of patient's functional peripheral IV line. Gently disconnect old PPN tubing from IV site and insert adapter of new PPN infusion tubing. Open roller clamp on new tubing. Allow solution to run to ensure that tubing is patent; regulate IV drip rate using EID.

Reduces transmission of microorganisms.

Health care provider must order fat emulsions and PPN. Fat emulsions may cause adverse symptoms if infused too rapidly as separate infusion. Infusion time is normally at least 8 hours. Fat emulsions should hang no longer than 12 hours as separate infusion from original container (Gorski et al., 2021). *This is the first check for accuracy.*

Lipid emulsions are white and opaque; be sure to avoid confusing enteral tube feeding formula with parenteral lipids.

Prevents medication error. *This is the second check for accuracy..*

Do not administer if these elements appear.

Ensures correct patient. Complies with The Joint Commission standards and improves patient safety (TJC, 2023).

Ensures patient receives correct infusion. *This is the third check for accuracy.*

Provides patient privacy.

Promotes patient comfort.

To prevent air from entering vascular system, clear all tubing.

Reduces transmission of infection.

Prevents disruption of existing IV infusion and ensures patent infusion. Pump will deliver PPN infusion at prescribed rate.

Clinical Judgment *An independent double-check verification should be performed by a second clinician prior to beginning a parenteral nutrition (PN) infusion (Ukleja et al., 2018).*

13. Prepare IV tubing and administer lipid emulsion:
    a. Apply the 1.2-μm filter for lipid infusion to infusion tubing using ANTT (Gorski, 2023).
    b. Position filter to as close to patient as possible.
    c. Run lipid solution through tubing to remove excess air. Turn roller clamp to "off" position. Some infusion pumps and tubing require priming through the infusion pump. Add sterile-capped needle or place sterile cap on end of tubing.
    d. Clean needleless peripheral IV line tubing injection cap with antimicrobial swab and allow to dry.

Removes surface organisms at injection site and prevents organisms from entering blood system.

STEP	RATIONALE
e. Attach end of fat emulsion infusion tubing to injection cap of PPN IV line. Label tubing.	Labeling high-risk catheters prevents connection with an inappropriate tube or catheter (TJC, 2023).
f. Open roller clamp completely on fat emulsion infusion and check flow rate on infusion pump.	Initial slow infusion allows you to observe for allergic response.

g. Infuse lipids as follows (Harvard University, 2022):
    (1) Infuse at 0.1 mL/min for the first 10 to 15 minutes (i.e., 1.5 mL dose over 15 minutes, which would run at a rate of 6 mL/h).
    (2) If no allergic reaction, then increase to the ordered hourly rate of IV lipid emulsion (e.g., infuse at 1 mL/min for adults and 0.1 mL/min for child for first 15 to 30 minutes; then increase rate as ordered).
	Up to 2 to 2.5 g of fat per kilogram of body weight per day may be infused (Harvard University, 2022), but current practice is generally to give <1 g of fat per kilogram of body weight per day in adults.
	
	Lower concentration of dextrose allows most patients to tolerate full administration rate without difficulty.

Clinical Judgment *Not more than 500 mL of intralipid 10% (10% intravenous fat emulsion) should be infused into adults on the first day of therapy. If the patient has no untoward reactions, the dose can be increased on the following day (Drugs.com, 2022).*

14. Remove and dispose of gloves and used supplies. Perform hand hygiene.	Reduces transmission of microorganisms. Use appropriate disposal receptacle if patient is on hazardous drugs (Kennedy et al., 2023).
15. Help patient to a comfortable position.	Restores comfort and sense of well-being.
16. Place nurse call system in an accessible location within patient's reach.	Ensures patient can call for assistance if needed.
17. Raise side rails (as appropriate) and lower bed to lowest position, locking into position.	Ensures patient safety and prevents falls.

EVALUATION

1. Monitor flow rate routinely on an hourly basis or more frequently if necessary (see agency policy).	Too-rapid or too-slow infusion could result in metabolic disturbances such as hyperglycemia.
2. Measure VS and patient's general comfort level every 10 minutes for first 30 minutes, then VS every 4 hours.	Monitors patient for lipid allergic response.
3. Monitor patient's laboratory values (e.g., triglycerides, liver function test results) daily and perform blood glucose monitoring as ordered. Measure serum lipids 4 hours after discontinuing infusion.	Provides objective data to measure response to therapy (e.g., ability of liver to metabolize lipids). Measurement of lipids too soon after infusion will yield incorrect blood values.
4. Monitor temperature every 4 hours, and regularly inspect venipuncture site for signs of phlebitis or infiltration.	Determines onset of fever, a complication of intolerance to fat emulsion or sepsis. Determines integrity of IV system.
5. Evaluate patient's weight, intake and output (I&O), condition of peripheral extremities (for edema), and breath sounds.	Weight gain, I&O imbalance, peripheral edema, and crackles in lungs indicate fluid retention.
6. Use Teach-Back: "I want to be sure I explained to you what to look out for when you are on your peripheral parenteral nutrition. Tell me what to report to your nurse when you receive this type of nutrition." Revise your instruction now or develop a plan for revised patient/family caregiver teaching if patient/family caregiver is not able to teach back correctly.	Teach-back is a technique for health care providers to ensure that they have explained medical information clearly so that patients and their families understand what is communicated to them (AHRQ, 2023).

Unexpected Outcomes	Related Interventions
1. There is intolerance to fat emulsion, as evidenced by increased triglyceride levels (>200 mg/dL), increased temperature (3°F–4°F), chills, flushing, headache, nausea and vomiting, diaphoresis, muscle ache, chest and back pain, dyspnea, pressure over eyes, or vertigo (Harvard University, 2022).	• Turn off lipid infusion immediately. Maintain regular peripheral IV line if established. • Notify health care provider. • Hold lipids for 4 hours. • If triglycerides remain elevated, consider decreasing IV lipid emulsion rate. • Prepare to treat anaphylactic reaction according to health care provider's orders. • Document lipid allergy. Apply allergy arm band.

2. See Unexpected Outcomes and Related Interventions for Skill 32.1.

Documentation

- Document location and condition of IV site, type of solutions, rate and status of infusion, catheter lumen size used for infusion, I&O, blood glucose levels, VS, weights, and other assessment findings.
- Document any adverse reactions.
- Document your evaluation of patient and family caregiver learning.

Hand-Off Reporting

- During hand-off, report type of infusion, rate and status of IV access site, patient's response, and any abnormal assessment findings.
- If signs of fat intolerance, infection, occlusion, fluid retention, or infiltration occur, notify the health care provider.

Special Considerations

Patient Education

- While a patient is hospitalized, provide an overview of PPN, the reason patient requires the therapy, risks, and what to expect (e.g., insertion of venous access device, care and maintenance of infusion, frequency of PPN with lipids).

Pediatrics

- See Skill 32.1.

Older Adults

- Some older adults may have fragile peripheral veins or poor fluid tolerance because of cardiac or renal dysfunction, making PPN undesirable.

Home Care

- A PPN feeding cycle is usually adjusted so that it infuses overnight, freeing patients and family caregivers from the pump during the day.
- See Skill 32.1.

✦ CLINICAL JUDGMENT AND NEXT-GENERATION NCLEX® EXAMINATION–STYLE QUESTIONS

A 43-year-old patient is admitted to the hospital with a severe exacerbation of Crohn disease and a history of asthma. The patient lost 4.5 kg (10 lb) in the last 3 weeks and reports recurrent abdominal pain, cramping, and loose stools. The patient is unable to tolerate food orally, becoming easily nauseated. The patient is to receive bowel rest and nutrition support with central parenteral nutrition (CPN) via a central line inserted by the health care provider.

1. The nurse is preparing to perform a baseline assessment for comparison with future assessments. Which of the following physical parameters can change quickly when a patient first receives CPN? **Select all that apply.**
   1. Vital signs
   2. Level of consciousness
   3. Weight
   4. Lung sounds
   5. Blood glucose level

2. Which action will the nurse take **next** to administer CPN after applying clean gloves?
   1. Scrub end port of CVAD with alcohol swab.
   2. Connect Luer-Lok end of CPN IV tubing to end port of CVAD and place IV tubing in EID.
   3. Attach appropriate filter to IV tubing, and prime tubing with CPN solution.
   4. Attach syringe of 0.9% NS solution to needleless port and flush saline.

3. On the third day after central line insertion and bowel rest, the patient develops a fever and malaise, preferring to stay in bed.
   Complete the following sentence by selecting from the lists of options below.

   The patient is at risk for having **[Condition]** due to **[Patient Finding]**.

Conditions	Patient Findings
Dehydration	Dietary deficiency
Chronic fatigue syndrome	Newly inserted central line
Kidney failure	Exacerbation of Crohn disease
Central line–associated blood-stream infection (CLABSI)	History of asthma
Ileus	Loss of 4.5 kg (10 lb) recently

4. Which of the following parameters will the nurse monitor when the patient is suspected of having a central line–associated blood stream infection (CLABSI)? **Select all that apply.**
   1. Temperature
   2. Lung Sounds
   3. Catheter insertion site
   4. Pulse rate
   5. Signs of chills
   6. Weight

5. Two days after beginning CPN infusion, the patient experiences a 2.3-kg (5-lb) weight gain and comments, "I'm glad to be gaining back some of the weight I lost." Which of the following elements will the nurse include in an assessment? **Select all that apply.**
   1. Reflex responses
   2. Palpation of lower extremities
   3. Serum protein levels
   4. Auscultation of lungs
   5. Intake and output

Visit the Evolve site for Answers to Clinical Judgment and Next-Generation NCLEX® Examination–Style Questions.

REFERENCES

Agency for Healthcare Research and Quality (AHRQ): *Teach-Back: Intervention*, 2023. https://www.ahrq.gov/patient-safety/reports/engage/interventions/teach-back.html. Accessed July 21, 2023.

American Diabetes Association (ADA): Lifestyle management: standards of medical care in diabetes, *Diabetes Care* 42(Suppl 1):S46–S60, 2019. https://care.diabetesjournals.org/content/42/Supplement_1/S46. Accessed July 20, 2023.

American Society for Parenteral and Enteral Nutrition: *Parenteral nutrition resources*, 2023, https://www.nutritioncare.org/PNResources/. Accessed November 26, 2023.

American Society for Parenteral and Enteral Nutrition (ASPEN): *Appropriate dosing for parenteral nutrition: ASPEN Recommendations*, January 2020. http://www.nutritioncare.org/PNDosing. Accessed July 20, 2023.

Centers for Disease Control and Prevention (CDC): *What is health literacy?* 2023. https://www.cdc.gov/healthliteracy/learn/index.html. Accessed July 20, 2023.

Compher C, et al: Guidelines for the provision of nutrition support therapy in the adult critically ill patient: the American Society for Parenteral and Enteral Nutrition, *JPEN J Parenter Enteral Nutr* 46(1):12–41, 2022.

Daoud DC, et al: Home parenteral nutrition in older vs younger patients: clinical characteristics and outcomes, *JPEN J Parenter Enteral Nutr* 46(2):348–356, 2022.

Drugs.com: *Intralipid dosage*, 2022. Accessed July 21 2023.

Gorski L: *Phillips's manual of IV therapeutics: evidence-based practice for infusion therapy*, ed 8, Philadelphia, 2023, Davis.

Gorski LA, et al: Infusion therapy standards of practice, ed 8, *J Infus Nurs* 44(Suppl 1):S1–S224, 2021.

Guenter P, et al: Standardized competencies for parenteral nutrition administration: the ASPEN Model, *Nutr Clin Pract* 33(2):295–304, 2018.

Hamdan M, Puckett Y: Total *parenteral nutrition*. In *Stat Pearls*, 2022, National Library of Medicine. https://www.ncbi.nlm.nih.gov/books/NBK559036/.

Harvard University: *Intravenous lipid emulsions*, 2022, Harvard University. https://hpn.hms.harvard.edu/lipids. Accessed July 21, 2023.

Hitchcock J, et al: Preventing medical adhesive-related skin injury (MARSI), *Br J Nurs* 30(15):S48, 2021.

Kennedy K, et al: Safe handling of hazardous drugs, *J Oncol Pharm Practice* 29(2):401–412, 2023.

Thayer DM, et al: Top down injuries: prevention and management of moisture-associated skin damage, medical adhesive–related skin injury, and skin tears. In McNichol LM, et al., editors: *Core curriculum: wound management*, ed 2, Philadelphia, 2022, Wolters Kluwer.

The Joint Commission (TJC): *2023 National Patient Safety Goals*, Oakbrook Terrace, IL, 2023, The Joint Commission. https://www.jointcommission.org/standards/national-patient-safety-goals/.

Thomas DR: *Total parenteral nutrition (TPN)*, April 2022, Merck Manual Professional Version. https://www.merckmanuals.com/professional/nutritional-disorders/nutritional-support/total-parenteral-nutrition-tpn?query=TPN. Accessed July 20, 2023.

Ukleja A, et al: Standards for nutrition support: adult hospitalized patients, American Society for Parenteral and Enteral Nutrition, *Nutr Clin Pract* 33(6):906–920, 2018. https://aspenjournals.onlinelibrary.wiley.com/doi/10.1002/ncp.10204#:~:text=ASPEN%27s%20mission%20is%20to%20improve%20patient%20care%20by,without%20a%20formal%20nutrition%20support%20service%20%28or%20team%29. Accessed July 20, 2023.

Worthington P, et al: When is parenteral nutrition appropriate? *JPEN J Parenter Enteral Nutr* 41(3):324–377, 2017.

Nutrition: Next-Generation NCLEX® (NGN)–Style Unfolding Case Study

PHASE 1

QUESTION 1.

The nurse has documented an intake assessment for a client admitted from a long-term care agency with weakness and failure to thrive.

Highlight the findings that indicate to the nurse that the client may be malnourished.

History and Physical	Nurses' Notes	Vital Signs	Laboratory Results
1442: 91-year-old client admitted from long-term care agency with weakness and failure to thrive. Client has reportedly lost 5 kg (11 lb) in the past 3 months. Assessment reveals a cachectic individual with brittle hair, dry skin, red mucous membranes, lungs clear to auscultation, heart rate regular at 64 beats/min, and lower extremities with poor tone. Height 177.8 cm (70 inches), weight 56.2 kg (124 lb). BMI 17.8.			

QUESTION 2.

The nurse contacts the long-term care agency and learns that the client often refuses meals or portions of meals and does not drink much water.

Complete the following sentence by selecting from the list of word choices below.

The nurse anticipates that the client is at highest risk for [Word Choice].

Word Choices
Fluid retention
Dehydration
Dysphagia
Reflux

PHASE 2

QUESTION 3.

The nurse must identify interventions that would improve and correct the client's fluid balance.

Complete the following sentence by selecting from the list of word choices below.

The nurse *prioritizes* facilitating the client's intake of [Word Choice].

Word Choices
Fats
Protein
Fluids
Carbohydrates

QUESTION 4.

After 2 days, the client refuses to eat and has difficulty drinking. The client becomes too weak to make medical decisions. The son, the client's power of attorney, consents to having a feeding tube placed. A small-bore feeding tube placed through the nose is ordered by the health care provider.

In addition to the small-bore feeding tube, which supplies will the nurse plan to gather to prepare to insert the tube? **Select all that apply.**

- 60-mL ENFit syringe
- Skin barrier protectant
- Water-soluble lubricant
- Emesis basin
- Tongue blade
- Sterile gloves
- Hypoallergenic tape

PHASE 3

QUESTION 5.

The small-bore feeding tube is inserted.

Which **4** actions will the nurse take at this time?

- ○ Maintain head-of-bed elevation at 20 degrees.
- ○ Document how the client tolerated the procedure.
- ○ Print the date and time on the nasal portion of the tape.
- ○ Immediately begin feeding through the newly placed tube.
- ○ Fasten the end of the tube to the client's gown using a clip or tape.
- ○ Clean tubing at the nostril with a cotton pad dipped in alcohol.
- ○ Ensure that an order for an x-ray of the chest/abdomen has been placed.

QUESTION 6.

The client has been receiving enteral nutrition for several weeks after being returned to the long-term care agency.

Highlight the findings recorded by the long-term care agency nurse that indicate that the client's nutritional status is improving.

History and Physical	Nurses' Notes	Vital Signs	Laboratory Results

0808: Client sitting up in bed taking sips of water. Client reports being tired but "feeling better." Mucous membranes pink and moist. Lung sounds clear; S_1S_2 present without murmur; bowel sounds present × 4 quadrants. No skin breakdown noted. Vital signs: 36.9°C (98.4°F); HR 70 beats/min; RR 14 breaths/min; BP 108/68 mm Hg; SpO_2 99% on RA. Height 177.8 cm (70 inches), weight 59.0 kg (130 lb). BMI 18.7.

UNIT 12
Elimination

The skills used in support of normal urinary elimination apply principles of infection control, patient comfort, protection of skin integrity, and maintenance of patient dignity and privacy. Your knowledge base regarding these principles will direct your assessments, identification of patient problems, and decisions about administering the skills correctly. For example, when offering a bedpan to a female patient who is overweight, you consider the patient's weight and how to more comfortably position the bedpan. To avoid skin breakdown, you make sure the perineal and anal areas within skinfolds are cleansed thoroughly afterward. Your attention to perineal cleansing may be less stringent for a patient of normal weight. Any skill involving urinary elimination means that a patient needs assistance with a basic need. Thus your clinical judgment must include consideration of the patient's feelings and perceptions about being unable to provide self-hygiene.

When it is necessary to perform invasive procedures such as urinary catheter insertion or suprapubic catheter care, you rely on your knowledge base about the principles of surgical and medical asepsis to ensure that infectious microorganisms are not transmitted to patients. Infection control measures based on clinical guidelines for preventing catheter-associated urinary tract infection (CAUTI) are required to prevent microorganisms from entering an existing catheter. Clinical judgment is key when making assessments and planning care to decide when an indwelling catheter can be removed safely and in a timely manner.

Delivering skills to support normal bowel elimination also involves application of principles to promote patient comfort, protect skin integrity, and maintain patient dignity and privacy. The administration of an enema is uncomfortable and embarrassing and makes a patient feel helpless. Monitoring a patient's response to your approach and slowly instilling the enema solution reduces cramping, makes it easier for the patient to relax, and allows you to instill more solution for better results. Critical thinking comes into play when you have to adapt a skill such as enema administration—for example, adjusting the position of a patient who cannot turn to the left side.

The insertion, maintenance, and removal of nasogastric tubes used for gastric decompression require you to apply knowledge regarding the nature of a patient's gastrointestinal disease or condition. This knowledge guides what you monitor (e.g., type and amount of drainage and condition of abdomen) to determine patient response. The procedure for nasogastric tube insertion is uncomfortable. You assess how much a patient either knows or desires to know so that you can effectively partner and make certain that each step causes the least amount of discomfort possible. For example, knowing what is involved in nasogastric tube insertion, a patient can prepare for swallowing and head positioning to assist in making insertion easier. A nasogastric tube creates a high risk for skin irritation on the patient's nares and development of a medical device–related pressure injury (MDRPI). You are responsible for conducting ongoing assessments of the condition of a patient's nares and applying clinical judgment and critical thinking regarding frequency of assessment, especially if the patient has other problems contributing to skin breakdown such as diaphoresis or malnutrition.

Surgically placed ostomies for urinary or fecal drainage pose potential problems requiring you to apply knowledge of pathologic conditions, normal elimination, and how ostomies are designed to function. The existence of an ostomy creates a risk for skin breakdown, medical adhesive–related skin injury (MARSI), resultant pain, and difficulty in ostomy pouch placement if skin breakdown is severe. Ostomy care can be complicated, requiring you to rely on an important assessment data resource: a wound, ostomy, and continence (WOC) nurse specialist. Collaboratively, you can identify the best strategies for managing patients' ostomies and supporting the patient. The psychological impact of an ostomy can never go unnoticed. Apply principles of therapeutic communication, cultural sensitivity, and grief and loss to better understand the meaning an ostomy has for a patient and the person-centered approaches to best educate and support the patient.

33 | Urinary Elimination

SKILLS AND PROCEDURES

Procedural Guideline 33.1 **Assisting With Use of a Urinal, p. 986**

Skill 33.1 **Insertion of a Straight or an Indwelling Urinary Catheter, p. 987**

Skill 33.2 **Care and Removal of an Indwelling Catheter, p. 998**

Procedural Guideline 33.2 **Bladder Scan, p. 1003**

Skill 33.3 **Performing Catheter Irrigation, p. 1004**

Skill 33.4 **Applying an Incontinence Device, p. 1008**

Skill 33.5 **Suprapubic Catheter Care, p. 1013**

OBJECTIVES

Mastery of content in this chapter will enable you to:
- Explain approaches for delivering patient-centered care to patients with urinary elimination problems.
- Identify appropriate assessments needed for patients requiring urinary elimination interventions.
- Develop nursing interventions that promote normal micturition when toilet access is compromised or after a catheter is removed.
- Compare the relationship between fluid balance and urinary elimination.
- Identify factors that increase risk for catheter-associated urinary tract infection (CAUTI).
- Demonstrate the following skills: place and remove urinal, insert urinary catheter, care for an indwelling urinary catheter, measure postvoid residual (PVR) with catheterization and bladder scan, irrigate a catheter, remove an indwelling catheter, apply a condom catheter, and care for a suprapubic catheter.

MEDIA RESOURCES

- http://evolve.elsevier.com/Perry/skills
- Review Questions
- ▶ Video Clips
- Case Studies
- Audio Glossary

- **NSO** Nursing Skills Online
- Skills Performance Checklists
- Printable Key Points
- Answers to Clinical Judgment and Next-Generation NCLEX® Examination–Style Questions

PURPOSE

A basic human function is urinary elimination, which can be compromised by a wide variety of illnesses and conditions. A nurse's role is to identify a patient's elimination problems and then implement care measures to support normal bladder emptying with privacy and dignity by assisting patients as needed in toileting. During acute illness, a patient may require urinary catheterization for close monitoring of urine output or to facilitate bladder emptying when bladder function is compromised. Some patients require long-term indwelling catheters, urethral or suprapubic, when the bladder fails to empty effectively. When invasive therapies are used to promote bladder emptying, nurses implement meticulous measures to minimize risk for infection and promote urinary emptying. To avoid catheterization in female patients, consider using a low-pressure wall suction such as the PureWick female external catheter system. It functions by wicking the urine away from the patient and into a collection device.

PRACTICE STANDARDS

- Lawrence et al., 2019: The CAUTI Prevention Toolkit: A Professional Practice and Collaborative Project of the Wound, Ostomy, and Continence Nurses Society
- The Joint Commission (TJC), 2023: National Patient Safety Goals—Patient identification

SUPPLEMENTAL STANDARDS

- Gould et al., 2019: Guideline for Prevention of Catheter Associated Urinary Tract Infections
- Oncology Nurses Society (ONS), 2018: Toolkit for Safe Handling of Hazardous Drugs for Nurses in Oncology

PRINCIPLES FOR PRACTICE

- Adequate oral intake is essential for bladder health, especially if a patient has an indwelling urinary catheter. Some patients with urinary problems limit fluid intake in fear of incontinence and/or increased urinary frequency. Explain to the patient the importance of fluid intake in maintaining urinary health.

- Hormone changes can occur in the genitalia secondary to gender hormone transitioning therapy, especially for trans men. Changes to the lower urinary tract can cause urgency, frequency, dysuria, and recurrent urinary tract infections (UTIs). One way to improve the health of the lower urinary tract is hydration with water (Fosnight, 2023).
- Evaluate urinary output.
  - Know the average output range for a patient. Adult urinary output averages 2200 to 2700 mL in 24 hours. An hourly output of less than 30 mL/h for 2 hours identifies the need for further evaluation.
  - Know the signs of dehydration and fluid overload. Start measurement of intake and output (I&O) when there is an actual or anticipated change in fluid balance.
- Assess a patient's most recent serum electrolyte measurements. Abnormal values reflect alterations in fluid balance that can lead to deterioration in patients' health.
- Weigh a patient to determine fluid status. Ask the patient to empty the bladder. Weigh with the same scale; at the same time of day; and with comparable articles of clothing, including bed linen if bed weights are necessary.

PERSON-CENTERED CARE

- The personal level of touch required when you assist patients with problems in urinary elimination requires you to understand values and preferences.
- Determine how patients feel about having to undergo procedures such as catheterization. Try to adapt procedures to minimize the invasive nature of catheterization and maintain a patient's dignity and respect.
- When caring for patients from different cultures, it is important to incorporate into the plan of care sensitivity and awareness of factors that may impact how you deal with urinary elimination problems.
- Provide for a same-gender caregiver when a patient's culture emphasizes modesty and prohibits nonrelated individuals from touching.
- Variations within a cultural group are common. Assess and care for each patient as an individual. Many cultures have specific beliefs and practices related to elimination, privacy, and gender-specific care. For example:
  - Some cultures emphasize interdependence over independence; thus, family presence at the bedside for important decision making is common.
  - Drape a patient carefully when privacy is a value of their culture.

EVIDENCE-BASED PRACTICE

Prevention of Catheter-Associated Urinary Tract Infection

Major recommendations incorporated into evidence-based guidelines to reduce catheter-related problems and infection include reducing inappropriate catheter use and removing catheters as soon as possible (Lawrence et al., 2019; Shadle et al., 2021; Siregar et al., 2021; TJC, 2022). Evidence-based interventions for the prevention of catheter-associated urinary tract infection (CAUTI) include:

- Use aseptic catheter insertion technique using sterile equipment (Shadle et al., 2021).

- Use prevention checklists and evaluation of catheter indications (Siregar et al., 2021).
- Use smallest catheter possible individualized to the patient (Siregar et al., 2021).
- Remove catheter as soon as possible (Siregar et al., 2021).
- Secure indwelling catheters to prevent movement and pulling on the catheter.
- Maintain a sterile, closed urinary drainage system (Siregar et al., 2021).
- Maintain an unobstructed flow of urine through the catheter, drainage tubing, and drainage bag.
- Always keep the urinary drainage bag below the level of the bladder.
- When emptying the urinary drainage bag, use a separate measuring receptacle for each patient. Do not let the drainage spigot touch the receptacle.
- Perform routine perineal hygiene daily and after soiling (Shadle et al., 2021).
- Quality improvement/surveillance programs should be in place to alert providers that a catheter is in place and should include regular educational programming about catheter care.

SAFETY GUIDELINES

- Patients requiring assistance with urinary elimination often have a limitation in mobility (due to illness or medical treatment), requiring nurses to employ safe handling and transfer techniques (Chapter 11).
- The risk of exposing the sterile urinary tract requires nurses to use aseptic techniques and know an individual patient's risk for infection.
- Assess patients' mobility and functional status to determine the ability to safely stand and/or transfer to a toilet or commode and to ambulate safely when an indwelling catheter is in place.
- Assess a patient's normal pattern of urination. Patients taking diuretic medications should have a toilet, commode, and/or urinal close to the bed or chair. Respond to any request for toileting assistance promptly.
- Patients who need assistance with toileting should have a nurse call light within easy reach and the offer for help at regular intervals, especially in the morning after awakening, after meals, and before bedtime.
- Maintain aseptic technique when catheterizing patients and performing irrigation.
- Maintain personal safety in handling bodily wastes for patients receiving hazardous drugs (Box 33.1).

BOX 33.1

Disposal, Cleaning, Spills, and Exposure to Bodily Wastes of Patients Receiving Hazardous Drugs in Oncology

- Double chemotherapy gloves
- Protective chemotherapy gown
- Eye/face protection
- If liquid could splash
- Always use for spills
- Respiratory protection
- If inhalation potential
- Always use for spills

Data from Oncology Nurses Society (ONS): *Toolkit for safe handling of hazardous drugs for nurses in oncology*, 2018. https://www.ons.org/sites/default/files/2018-06/ONS_Safe_Handling_Toolkit_0.pdf. Accessed July 28, 2023.

PROCEDURAL GUIDELINE 33.1 *Assisting With Use of a Urinal*

 Video Clip

Patients who are limited in being able to stand and ambulate (e.g., lower extremity weakness, severe dyspnea) or who are restricted from being able to get out of bed because of a medical condition or treatment restriction are forced to use a urinal to micturate. A urinal is a container that collects and holds urine when access to a toilet is restricted. In some instances, a male patient may be able to stand at the bedside and use a urinal. Most urinals are used by men, but there are specially designed urinals for women (Fig. 33.1). The female urinal has a larger opening at the top with a defined rim, which helps position the urinal closely against the genitalia.

Delegation

The skill of assisting a patient with a urinal can be delegated to assistive personnel (AP). Direct the AP to:

- Help the patient with special needs or adaptations such as a need to hold a urinal for a patient.
- Provide personal hygiene as needed after urination.
- Report immediately any changes in urine color, clarity, and odor; development of incontinence (involuntary loss of urine); patient-reported dysuria, which could indicate an infection; and any changes in the frequency and amount of urine.

Interprofessional Collaboration

- Occupational therapy may be required for patients requiring use of a urinal at home so that appropriate adaptive devices can be identified.

Equipment

Urinal; clean gloves; graduated cylinder (used for measuring volume if on intake and output [I&O]); supplies for diagnostic urine tests and specimen collection (see Chapter 7); wash basin, washcloths, towels, and soap for perineal hygiene; toilet tissue

Steps

1. In determining need for a urinal, assess patient's electronic health record (EHR) for conditions that may place them at risk for falling during ambulation to bathroom: arthritis, benign prostatic hyperplasia (BPH), or overactive bladder (OAB).

Clinical Judgment *These conditions do not prohibit ambulation. Your role is to promote patient independence. But if patient is not to ambulate without assistance and experiences a sudden urge to urinate without a caregiver present, a urinal can be a helpful option for toileting.*

2. Assess patient's normal urinary elimination habits, including normal frequency and any episodes of incontinence.
3. Determine how much help is needed to place and remove the urinal. (Ask the patient or observe previous use.)
4. Review EHR for health care provider orders to determine if a urine specimen is to be collected.
5. Assess patient's/family caregiver's health literacy.
6. Provide privacy and explain procedure to patient.
7. Perform hand hygiene and apply clean gloves.
8. Assess for a distended bladder by inspecting the lower one-third of the abdomen or palpating gently above symphysis pubis.

Clinical Judgment *Always consider need for specific personal protective equipment (PPE) based on patient assessment and whether patient is receiving any hazardous drugs (ONS, 2018).*

9. Help patient into appropriate position:
   - Male patient on side, back, sitting with head of bed elevated, or in standing position
   - Female patient lying supine
10. If needed, place an absorbent pad under patient's buttocks to protect bed linens from accidental spills.

Clinical Judgment *Before having a patient stand to void, assess lower-extremity strength and mobility and assess blood pressure for orthostatic hypotension (Chapter 5), especially if there has been a period of prolonged bed rest.*

11. If possible, a patient of male gender should hold urinal and position penis in urinal. If needed, help patient by positioning penis completely in urinal and holding urinal in place or by helping to hold urinal. Ensure that the urinal is placed dependent of the flow of urine.
12. Help a patient of female gender by positioning the urinal against the genitalia and stabilizing it to keep it in position

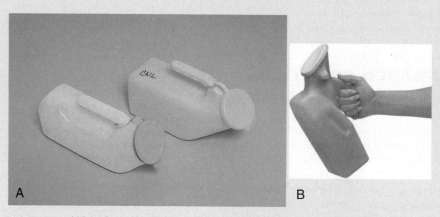

A   B

FIG. 33.1 (A) Male urinals. (B) Female urinal. (*B courtesy Briggs Medical Service Co.*)

PROCEDURAL GUIDELINE 33.1 *Assisting With Use of a Urinal—Cont'd*

and dependent of urine flow. *Option:* If the female urinal does not fit, have patient void into a bedpan.

13. Cover patient with bed linens and place nurse call system within reach. If possible, give patient further privacy by leaving the bedside after ensuring that they are in a safe and comfortable position. Remove and dispose of gloves and perform hand hygiene.

14. After patient has finished voiding, apply gloves and remove urinal and assess characteristics of the urine for color, clarity, odor, and amount. Help patient wash and dry genitalia.

15. Empty and clean urinal. Return urinal to patient for future use. Remove and dispose of gloves.

Clinical Judgment *Dispose of urine in appropriate receptacle based on special consideration if the patient is receiving any hazardous drugs (ONS, 2018).*

16. Help patient perform hand hygiene as needed.
17. Perform hand hygiene.
18. Help patient to a comfortable position.
19. Place nurse call system in an accessible location within patient's reach.

20. Raise side rails (as appropriate) and lower bed to lowest position, locking into position.

21. **Use Teach-Back:** "I want to be sure I explained clearly how to use a urinal. Tell me in your own words the steps for using this urinal." Revise your instruction now or develop a plan for revised patient/family caregiver teaching if patient/family caregiver is not able to teach back correctly.

22. Document amount and character of urine on I&O form.

23. Provide hand-off report to health care provider of any changes or abnormal findings.

Urinary catheterization (straight and indwelling) is the placement of a hollow flexible tube into the bladder to remove urine. It is an invasive procedure that requires the order of a health care provider and use of strict sterile technique. The use of an indwelling urinary catheter is associated with numerous complications, particularly catheter-associated urinary tract infection (CAUTI). This results in patient discomfort, increased hospital stays (by as much as 2–5 additional days), increased costs, and mortality (from sepsis). Urinary tract infections (UTIs) are the fourth most common type of health care–associated infection (HAI), with an estimated 62,700 UTIs in acute care hospitals in 2015 (Centers for Disease Control and Prevention [CDC], 2023a).

Because of the risk of CAUTI, there are recommendations for the appropriate and inappropriate use of an indwelling catheter (Box 33.2). Indwelling urinary catheterization may be short term (≤2 weeks) or long term (>14 days). Intermittent urinary catheterization is the insertion of a flexible single-use catheter for urinary retention and specimen collection. After urine has been drained, the catheter is removed. The steps for inserting an indwelling and an intermittent single-use straight catheter are the same. The difference lies in the inflation of a balloon to keep the indwelling catheter in place and the presence of a closed drainage system.

Urinary catheters are made with one to three lumens (Fig. 33.2). Single-lumen catheters (see Fig. 33.2A) are used for intermittent catheterization. Double-lumen catheters, designed for indwelling catheters, provide one lumen for urinary drainage and a second lumen for balloon inflation to keep the catheter in place (see Fig. 33.2B). Double- and triple-lumen catheters (see Fig. 33.2C) are used for continuous bladder irrigation (CBI) or to

---

BOX 33.2

Indications for Indwelling Urethral Catheter Use

Appropriate Use

- Patient has acute urinary retention or bladder outlet obstruction.
- Need for accurate measurements of urinary output in critically ill patients.
- Perioperative use for selected surgical procedures:
  - Patients undergoing urologic surgery or other surgery on contiguous structures of the genitourinary tract
  - Anticipated prolonged duration of surgery (catheters inserted for this reason should be removed in Post-Anesthesia Care Unit [PACU])
  - Patients anticipated to receive large-volume infusions or diuretics during surgery
  - Need for intraoperative monitoring of urinary output
- To assist in healing of open sacral or perineal wounds in incontinent patients.
- Patient requires prolonged immobilization (e.g., potentially unstable thoracic or lumbar spine, multiple traumatic injuries, such as pelvic fractures).
- To improve comfort for end-of-life care if needed.

Inappropriate Use

- As a substitute for nursing care of the patient or resident with incontinence.
- As a means of obtaining urine for culture or other diagnostic tests when the patient can voluntarily void.
- For prolonged postoperative duration without appropriate indications (e.g., structural repair of urethra or contiguous structures, prolonged effect of epidural anesthesia).

From Gould CV, et al: *Guideline for prevention of catheter-associated urinary tract infections 2019 update, Healthcare Infection Control Practices Advisory Committee*, Update June 2019. https://www.cdc.gov/infectioncontrol/pdf/guidelines/cauti-guidelines-H.pdf. Accessed September 29, 2023.

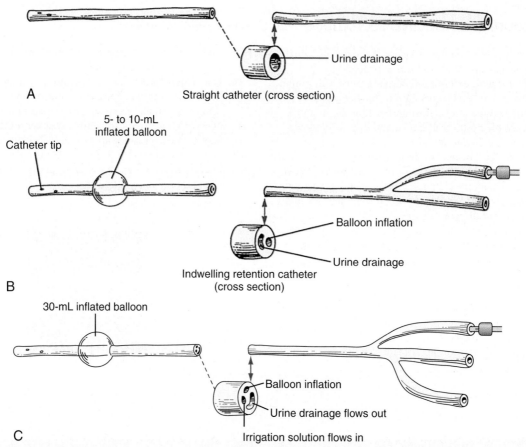

A

Straight catheter (cross section)

B

Indwelling retention catheter
(cross section)

C

FIG. 33.2 (A) Single-lumen or straight catheter (cross section). (B) Double-lumen or indwelling retention catheter (cross section). (C) Triple-lumen catheter for continuous closed irrigation (cross section).

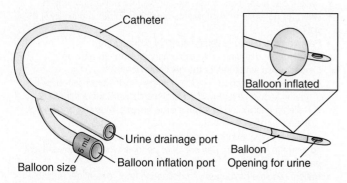

FIG. 33.3 Size of catheter and balloon printed on catheter inflation valve. *(From Wilk MJ, Sorrentino SA, Remmert LN:* Sorrentino's Canadian textbook for the support worker, *ed 5, St. Louis, 2022, Elsevier.)*

instill medications into the bladder. One lumen drains the bladder, a second lumen is used to inflate the balloon, and a third lumen delivers fluid from an irrigation bag into the bladder. Indwelling catheters come in a variety of balloon sizes. The size of the balloon is usually printed on the catheter port (Fig. 33.3). A nurse is responsible for maintaining the sterility of the urinary tract during catheter insertions and in the ongoing care and maintenance of indwelling catheters.

Delegation

The skill of inserting a straight or indwelling urinary catheter cannot be delegated to assistive personnel (AP). Direct the AP to:
- Assist the nurse with patient positioning, focus lighting for the procedure, maintain privacy, empty urine from collection bag, and help with perineal care.
- Report postprocedure patient discomfort or fever to the nurse.
- Report abnormal color, odor, amount of urine in drainage bag, and if the catheter is leaking or causes pain.

Interprofessional Collaboration

- Involve the health care provider and rehabilitation services in the management of long-term indwelling catheters.
- Wound ostomy services can assist in patient care if a catheter is being used for incontinence.

Equipment

- Catheter kit containing sterile items (**NOTE:** Catheter kits vary)
- Straight catheterization kit: Single-lumen catheter (12–14 Fr), drapes (one fenestrated—has an opening in the center), sterile gloves, lubricant, cleansing solution incorporated in an applicator or to be added to cotton balls, and specimen container and label
- Indwelling catheterization kit (Fig. 33.4): Double-lumen catheter, drapes (one fenestrated—has an opening in the center),

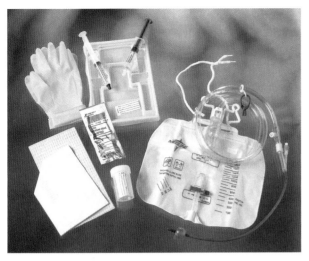

FIG. 33.4 Indwelling catheterization kit. *(Image used with permission Medline Industries. All rights reserved.)*

sterile gloves, lubricant, antiseptic cleansing solution incorporated in an applicator or to be added to cotton balls, specimen container and label, and a prefilled syringe with sterile water (to inflate balloon) (**NOTE:** Some kits contain a catheter with attached drainage bag; others contain only a catheter; others have no catheter.)
- Sterile drainage tubing and bag (if not included in indwelling catheter insertion kit)
- Device to secure catheter (catheter strap or other device)
- Extra sterile gloves and catheter (optional)
- Clean gloves
- Basin with warm water, washcloth, towel, and soap for perineal care (*Option*: chlorhexidine cloths, which can be used for perineal and catheter care)
- Flashlight or other additional light source
- Bath blanket, waterproof absorbent pad
- Measuring container for urine

STEP	RATIONALE

ASSESSMENT

1. Identify patient using at least two identifiers (e.g., name and birthday or name and medical record number) according to agency policy.

   Ensures correct patient. Complies with The Joint Commission standards and improves patient safety (TJC, 2023).

2. Review patient's EHR for previous catheterization, including catheter size, response of patient, and time of catheterization.

   Identifies purpose of inserting catheter (such as for measurement of PVR, preparation for surgery, or specimen collection) and potential difficulty with catheter insertion.

3. Review EHR for any pathological or anatomical conditions that may impair passage of catheter (e.g., enlarged prostate gland in men, urethral strictures).

   Obstruction of urethra may prevent passage of catheter into bladder. Urethral strictures are a common complication after genital gender-affirming surgery (GGAS) in transmasculine patients (Waterschoot et al., 2021).

4. Review EHR to determine patient's age and history of dehydration, malnutrition, exposure to radiation therapy, underlying chronic conditions (e.g., diabetes mellitus, immunosuppression), and edema of the skin.

   Common risk factors for medical adhesive–related skin injury (MARSI) (Fumarola et al., 2020). Adhesive product may be used to stabilize indwelling catheter.

5. Assess patient's gender. For example: Simply inquire, "I want to be respectful, so what name and pronouns would you like us to use?" (CDC, 2020).

   Respects patient's identity and assists with selection of catheter size.

6. Assess patient's/family caregiver's health literacy.

   Determines degree to which individuals have the ability to find, understand, and use information and services to make informed health-related decisions and actions for themselves and others (CDC, 2023b).

7. Ask patient and check EHR for history of allergies. Check allergy bracelet.

   Catheter made of different material is needed if patient has latex allergy.

8. Perform hand hygiene. Assess patient's weight, level of consciousness, developmental level, ability to cooperate, and mobility.

   Determines positioning to use for catheterization; indicates how much help is needed to properly position patient, ability of patient to cooperate during procedure, and level of explanation needed.

9. Assess for pain and bladder fullness. Palpate bladder over symphysis pubis or use bladder scanner (if available) (see Procedural Guideline 33.2).

   Palpation of full bladder causes pain and/or urge to void, indicating full or overfull bladder.

10. Apply clean gloves. Inspect perineal region, observing for perineal anatomical landmarks, erythema, drainage or discharge, and odor. Remove and dispose of gloves and perform hand hygiene.

    Assessment of perineum (especially female perineal landmarks) improves accuracy and speed of catheter insertion. Reduces transmission of microorganisms.

11. Assess patient's knowledge, prior experience with catheterization, and feelings about procedure.

    Reveals need for patient instruction and/or support.

STEP	RATIONALE

PLANNING

1. Expected outcomes following completion of procedure:
   - Patient's bladder is not palpable.
   - Patient verbalizes absence of abdominal discomfort or bladder pressure/fullness.
   - Patient has urine output of at least 30 mL/h as measured in urinary drainage bag.
   - Patient verbalizes purpose and expectations about procedure.
2. Provide privacy and explain procedure to patient.
3. Organize and set up equipment needed to perform procedure at bedside.
4. Arrange for extra personnel to help as needed.

Rationale:

Bladder successfully emptied.
Catheterization and free flow of urine through catheter relieve bladder distention and discomfort.
Verifies presence of catheter in bladder, catheter patency, and adequate kidney function.
Reflects patient understanding of procedure.
Protects patient's privacy; reduces anxiety. Promotes cooperation.
Ensures more efficiency when completing a procedure.

Some patients are unable to assume positioning independently for procedure.

IMPLEMENTATION

1. Check patient's plan of care for size and type of catheter (if this is a reinsertion). Use smallest-size catheter possible. Size 14 Fr to 16 Fr is most common for adults, and for older adults (12–14 Fr). Larger sizes (20–22 Fr) are needed in special circumstances, such as after urological surgery or in the presence of gross hematuria.

   Rationale: Ensures that patient receives correct size and type of catheter. Larger catheter diameters increase the risk for urethral trauma. Small catheter allows for adequate drainage of periurethral glands.

Clinical Judgment *If a transgender patient has undergone gender-confirming surgery involving the urethra, such as a vaginoplasty, or phalloplasty with urethral lengthening, placement of a urinary catheter may necessitate using a smaller catheter. In some circumstances, a urologist or other practitioner experienced with transgender anatomy may need to be consulted (Tollinche et al., 2018).*

2. Perform hand hygiene.

   Rationale: Reduces transmission of microorganisms.

3. Raise bed to appropriate working height. If side rails are in use, raise side rail on opposite side of bed and lower side rail on working side.

   Rationale: Promotes good body mechanics. Use of side rails in this manner promotes patient safety.

4. Have patient log roll or bend knees and raise hips to place a waterproof pad underneath.

   Rationale: Prevents soiling bed linen.

Clinical Judgment *Obtain help to position and support patients who have mobility restrictions or who are weak, frail, obese, or confused.*

5. Position patient:
   a. **Female patient:**
      (1) Help to dorsal recumbent position (on back with knees flexed). Ask patient to relax thighs so that you can rotate hips.

      Rationale: Exposes perineum and allows hip joints to be externally rotated.

      (2) Alternate female position: Position side-lying position with upper leg flexed at knee and hip. Support patient with pillows, if necessary, to maintain position.

      Rationale: Alternate position is more comfortable if patient cannot abduct leg at hip joint (e.g., patient has arthritic joints or contractures).

   b. **Male patient:**
      (1) Position supine with legs extended and thighs slightly abducted.

      Rationale: Comfortable position for patient aids in visualization of penis.

6. Drape patient:

   Rationale: Protects patient dignity and privacy by avoiding unnecessary exposure of body parts.

   a. **Female patient:**
      (1) Drape with bath blanket. Place blanket diamond fashion over patient, with one corner at patient's midsection, side corners over each thigh and abdomen, and last corner over perineum (see illustration).
   b. **Male patient:**
      (1) Drape patient by covering upper part of body with small sheet or towel; drape with separate sheet or bath blanket so that only perineum is exposed (see illustration).

7. Position portable light to illuminate genitals or have assistant available to hold light.

   Rationale: Adequate visualization of urinary meatus assists with accuracy of catheter insertion.

8. Apply clean gloves. Clean perineal area with soap and water, rinse, and dry. Use fingers to retract tissues for examining chapter and identify urinary meatus. Remove and dispose of gloves. Perform hand hygiene.

   Rationale: Hygiene before initiating aseptic catheter insertion removes secretions, urine, and feces that could be inserted into urethral canal and increase risk for catheter-associated urinary tract infection (CAUTI). Perform hand hygiene immediately before catheter insertion (Siregar et al., 2021). Reduces transmission of microorganisms.

STEP	RATIONALE

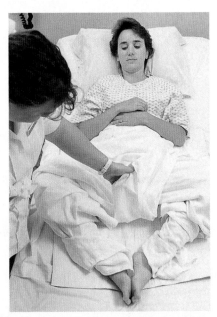

STEP 6a(1) Female patient draped and in dorsal recumbent position.

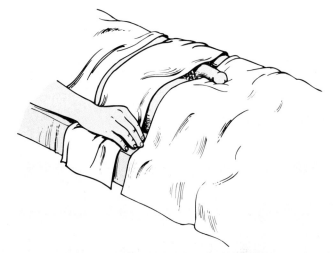

STEP 6b(1) Drape male patient with blankets.

9. Open outer wrapping of catheterization kit. Place inner wrapped catheter kit tray on clean, accessible surface such as bedside table or, if possible, between patient's open legs. Patient size and positioning dictate exact placement.

10. Remove the cover of the tray by taking the edge of the outer cover, peeling it away to open the tray, and ensuring hand does not extend over the sterile contents (see Chapter 10).
   a. Indwelling catheterization open system: Open separate package containing drainage bag, check to make sure that clamp on drainage port is closed, and place drainage bag and tubing in easily accessible location. Open outer package of sterile catheter, maintaining sterility of inner wrapper (see Chapter 10).
   b. Indwelling catheterization closed system: All supplies are in sterile tray and arranged in sequence of use.
   c. Straight catheterization: All needed supplies are in sterile tray that contains supplies and can be used for urine collection.

11. Apply sterile gloves. **NOTE:** Special gloves or double gloving may be needed if patient is receiving hazardous drugs.

12. *Option:* Apply sterile drape with ungloved hands when drape is packed as first item. Touch only 2.5 cm (1-inch) edges of drape. Then apply sterile gloves.

13. Drape perineum, keeping gloves and working surface of drape sterile (see Chapter 10).
   a. **Drape female:**
      (1) Pick up square sterile drape touching only edges (2.5 cm [1 inch]).
      (2) Allow drape to unfold without touching unsterile surfaces. Allow top edge of drape (2.5–5 cm [1 to 2 inches]) to form cuff over both gloved hands.
      (3) Place drape with shiny side down on bed between patient's thighs. Slip cuffed edge just under buttocks as you ask patient to lift hips. Take care not to touch contaminated surfaces or patient's thighs with sterile gloves. If gloves are contaminated, remove and apply new pair.

Provides easy access to supplies during catheter insertion. Tray provides a sterile field.

Sequence prevents you from reaching over sterile field.

Open drainage bag systems have separate sterile packaging for sterile catheter, drainage bag and tubing, and insertion kit.

Closed drainage bag systems have catheter preattached to drainage tubing and bag.

Maintains surgical asepsis. If patient is receiving chemotherapy, then double gloving is needed (ONS, 2018).
Maintains surgical asepsis.

Sterile drapes provide sterile field over which you will work during catheterization.

When creating cuff over sterile gloved hands, sterility of gloves and workspace is maintained.

STEP	RATIONALE

(4) Pick up fenestrated sterile drape out of tray. Allow drape to unfold without touching unsterile surfaces. Allow top edge of drape to form cuff over both gloved hands. Apply drape over perineum so that opening is over exposed labia (see illustration).

Opening in drape creates sterile field around labia.

b. Drape male:

(1) Use of square drape is optional; you may apply fenestrated drape instead.

(2) Pick up edges of square drape and allow to unfold without touching unsterile surfaces. Place over thighs, with shiny side down, just below penis. Take care not to touch contaminated surfaces with sterile gloves.

(3) Place fenestrated drape with opening centered over penis (see illustration).

14. Place sterile tray with cleaning solution (premoistened swab sticks or cotton balls, forceps, and solution), lubricant, catheter, and prefilled syringe for inflating balloon (indwelling catheterization only) on sterile drape close to patient. Arrange any remaining sterile supplies on sterile field, maintaining sterility of gloves.

Provides easy access to supplies during catheter insertion and helps to maintain aseptic technique. Appropriate placement is determined by size of patient and position during catheterization.

a. If kit contains sterile cotton balls, open package of sterile antiseptic solution and pour over cotton balls. Some kits contain package of premoistened swab sticks. Open end of package for easy access (see illustration).

Use of sterile supplies and antiseptic solution reduces risk of CAUTI (Siregar et al., 2021).

b. Open sterile specimen container if specimen is to be obtained (see Chapter 7).

Makes container accessible to receive urine from catheter if specimen is needed.

c. For indwelling catheterization, open sterile inner wrapper of catheter and leave catheter on sterile field or in tray. If part of closed system kit, remove tray with catheter and preattached drainage bag and place on sterile drape. Make sure that clamp on drainage port of bag is closed. If needed and if part of sterile tray, attach catheter to drainage tubing.

Indwelling catheterization trays vary. Some have preattached catheters; others need to be attached but are part of the sterile tray; others do not have catheter or drainage system as part of tray.

d. Open packet of lubricant and squeeze out on sterile field. Lubricate catheter tip by dipping it into water-soluble gel 2.5 to 5 cm (1–2 inches) for women and 12.5 to 17.5 cm (5–7 inches) for men (see illustration).

Lubrication minimizes trauma to urethra and discomfort during catheter insertion.
Male catheter needs enough lubricant to cover length of catheter inserted.

Clinical Judgment *Pretesting a balloon on an indwelling catheter by injecting fluid from the prefilled sterile normal saline syringe into the balloon port is not recommended. Testing the balloon may distort and stretch it and lead to damage, causing increased trauma on insertion.*

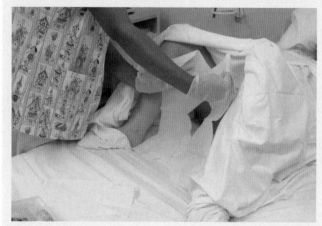

STEP 13a(4) Place sterile fenestrated drape (with opening in center) over female's perineum.

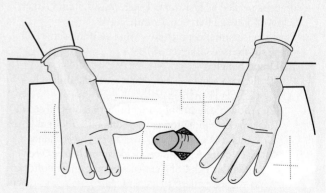

STEP 13b(3) Drape male with fenestrated drape.

STEP	RATIONALE

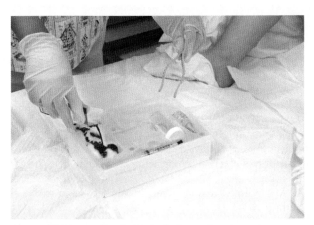

STEP 14a Sterile kit includes antiseptic swabs.

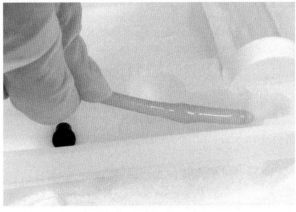

STEP 14d Lubricate catheter.

15. Clean urethral meatus:
   a. **Female patient:**
      (1) Separate labia with fingers of nondominant hand (now contaminated) to fully expose urethral meatus.
      (2) Maintain position of nondominant hand throughout procedure.

      (3) While maintaining sterility, pick up one moistened cotton ball with forceps or pick up one swab stick at a time. Clean labia and urinary meatus from clitoris toward anus. Use new cotton ball or swab for each area that you clean. Clean by wiping far labial fold, near labial fold, and last, directly over center of urethral meatus (see illustration).
   b. **Male patient:**
      (1) With nondominant hand (now contaminated), retract foreskin (if uncircumcised) and gently grasp penis at shaft just below glans. Hold shaft of penis at right angle to body. This hand remains in position for remainder of procedure.
      (2) Using dominant hand and maintaining sterility, clean meatus with cotton balls and forceps/swab sticks using circular strokes, beginning at meatus and working outward in spiral motion.
      (3) Repeat cleaning 3 times using clean cotton ball/swab stick each time (see illustration).

Optimal visualization of urethral meatus is possible.

Closure of labia during cleaning means that area is contaminated and requires cleaning procedure to be repeated.
Front-to-back cleaning moves from area of least contamination toward highly contaminated area. Follows principles of medical asepsis (see Chapter 9). Dominant gloved hand remains sterile.

When grasping shaft of penis, avoid pressure on dorsal surface to prevent compression of urethra.
Losing grasp during cleaning means that area is contaminated and requires cleaning procedure to be repeated.

Circular cleaning pattern follows principles of medical asepsis (see Chapter 9).

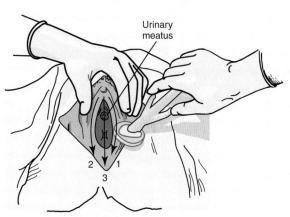

STEP 15a(3) Clean female perineum.

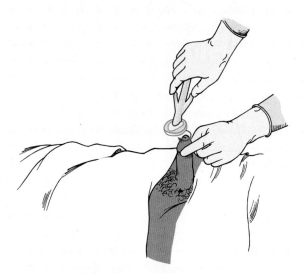

STEP 15b(3) Clean male urinary meatus.

STEP	RATIONALE

16. Pick up and hold catheter 7.5 to 10 cm (3 to 4 inches) from catheter tip with catheter loosely coiled in palm of hand. If catheter is not attached to drainage bag, make sure to position urine tray so that end of catheter can be placed there once insertion begins.

Holding catheter near tip allows for its easier manipulation during insertion. Coiling catheter in palm prevents distal end from striking nonsterile surface.

17. Insert catheter. Explain to patient that feeling of discomfort or pressure may be experienced as catheter is inserted into urethra. This sensation is normal and will go away quickly.

Helps to minimize patient anxiety.

  a. Female patient:

  (1) Ask patient to bear down gently and slowly insert catheter through urethral meatus (see illustration).

Bearing down may help visualize urinary meatus and promotes relaxation of external urinary sphincter, aiding in catheter insertion.

  (2) Advance catheter total of 5 to 7.5 cm (2–3 inches) or until urine flows out of catheter. Stop advancing with straight catheter. When urine appears, advance catheter another 2.5 to 5 cm (1–2 inches) for indwelling catheter. Do not use force to insert catheter.

Urine flow indicates that catheter tip is in bladder or lower urethra.

  (3) Release labia and hold catheter securely with nondominant hand.

Prevents accidental expulsion of catheter from the patient's bladder.

  b. Male patient:

  (1) Lift penis to position perpendicular (90 degrees) to patient's body and apply gentle upward traction (see illustration).

Straightens urethra to ease catheter insertion.

  (2) Ask patient to bear down as if to void and slowly insert catheter through urethral meatus.

Relaxation of external sphincter aids in insertion of catheter.

  (3) Advance catheter 17 to 22.5 cm (7–9 inches) or until urine flows out end of catheter. Do not use force to advance catheter.

Length of male urethra varies. Flow of urine indicates that tip of catheter is in bladder or urethra but not necessarily that balloon part of indwelling catheter is in bladder.

  (4) Stop advancing with straight catheter. When urine appears in indwelling catheter, advance it to bifurcation (inflation and deflation ports exposed) (see illustration).

Further advancement of catheter to bifurcation of drainage and balloon inflation port ensures that balloon part of catheter is not still in prostatic urethra.

  (5) Lower penis and hold catheter securely in nondominant hand.

Prevents accidental expulsion of catheter from the patient's bladder.

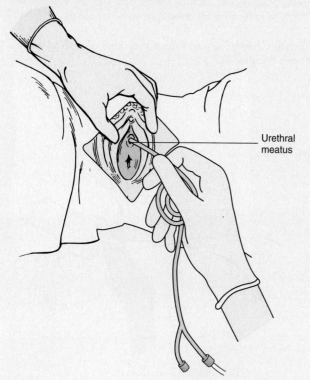

Urethral meatus

STEP 17a(1) Insert catheter into female urinary meatus.

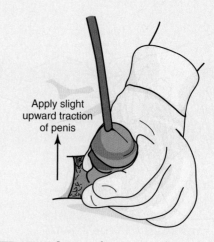

Apply slight upward traction of penis

STEP 17b(1) Insert catheter into male urinary meatus.

STEP	RATIONALE

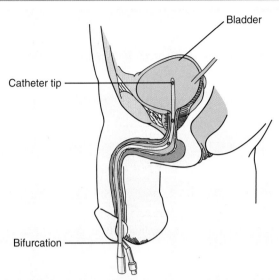

STEP 17b(4) Male anatomy with correct catheter insertion to bifurcation.

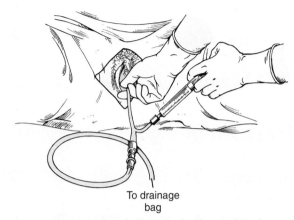

STEP 21c Inflate balloon (indwelling catheter).

18. Allow bladder to empty fully unless agency policy restricts maximum volume of urine drained (see agency policy).

There is no definitive evidence regarding whether there is benefit in limiting maximal volume drained.

19. Collect urine specimen as needed (see Chapter 7). Fill specimen container to 20 to 30 mL by holding end of catheter over the cup. Set container aside. Keep end of catheter sterile.

Sterile specimen for culture analysis can be obtained.

20. Option for straight catheterization: When urine stops flowing, withdraw catheter slowly and smoothly with dominant hand until removed.

Minimizes trauma to urethra.

21. For indwelling catheter: Inflate catheter balloon with amount of fluid designated by manufacturer.

Indwelling catheter balloon should not be underinflated. Underinflation causes balloon distortion and potential bladder damage.

　a. Continue to hold catheter with nondominant hand.

Holding on to catheter before inflating balloon prevents expulsion of catheter from urethra.

　b. With free dominant hand, connect prefilled syringe to injection port at end of catheter.

Tight connection needed to instill solution.

　c. Slowly inject total amount of solution (see illustration).

Full amount of solution needed to inflate balloon properly.

Clinical Judgment *If patient reports sudden pain during inflation of a catheter balloon or when resistance is felt when inflating the balloon, stop inflation, allow the fluid from the balloon to flow back into the syringe, advance catheter farther, and reinflate balloon. The balloon may have been inflating in the urethra. If pain continues, remove catheter and notify the health care provider.*

　d. After inflating catheter balloon, release catheter from nondominant hand. *Gently* pull catheter until resistance is felt. Then advance catheter slightly.

By moving catheter slightly back into bladder, pressure on bladder neck is avoided.

　e. Connect drainage tubing to catheter if it is not already preconnected.

22. Secure indwelling catheter with catheter strap or another securement device. Attach securement device at tubing just above catheter bifurcation.

Securing catheter reduces risk of movement, urethral erosion, CAUTI, or accidental catheter removal (Siregar et al., 2021). Attachment of securement device above catheter bifurcation prevents occlusion of catheter.

　a. **Female patient:**
　　(1) Secure catheter tubing to inner thigh, allowing enough slack to allow leg movement and prevent tension (see illustration).

　b. **Male patient:**
　　(1) Secure catheter tubing to upper thigh (see illustration) or lower abdomen (with penis directed toward chest). Allow slack in catheter so that movement does not create tension on catheter.

Anchoring catheter reduces traction on urethra and minimizes urethral injury.

　　(2) If retracted, replace foreskin over glans penis.

Leaving foreskin retracted can cause discomfort and dangerous penile edema.

STEP	RATIONALE

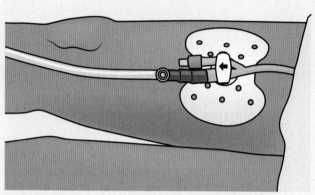

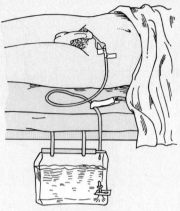

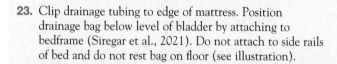

STEP 22a(1) Secure indwelling catheter on female with adhesive securement device.

STEP 22b(1) Secure indwelling catheter on male with tape.

23. Clip drainage tubing to edge of mattress. Position drainage bag below level of bladder by attaching to bedframe (Siregar et al., 2021). Do not attach to side rails of bed and do not rest bag on floor (see illustration).

24. Check to ensure that there is no obstruction to urine flow. Coil excess tubing on bed and fasten to bottom sheet with clip or another securement device.

25. Provide perineal hygiene as needed. Help patient to a comfortable position.

26. Label and bag specimen according to agency policy. Label specimen in front of patient. Have specimen sent to laboratory as soon as possible.

27. Measure urine and document.

28. Dispose of supplies in appropriate receptacles.

29. Remove and dispose of gloves.

30. Raise side rails (as appropriate) and lower bed to lowest position, locking into position.

31. Place nurse call system in an accessible location within patient's reach.

32. Perform hand hygiene.

Keeping the collection bag below the level of the bladder at all times prevents backflow into bladder, which can cause risk for CAUTI (Siregar et al., 2021). Bags attached to movable objects such as side rail increase risk for urethral trauma because of pulling or accidental dislodgement.

Keeping the catheter and collecting tube free from kinking may reduce risk of CAUTI.

Promotes patient comfort.

Fresh urine specimen ensures more accurate findings. Labeling ensures that diagnostic results will be connected to correct patient.

Provides baseline for urine output.

Reduces transmission of microorganisms.

Reduces transmission of microorganisms.

Ensures patient safety and prevents falls.

Ensures patient can call for assistance if needed.

Reduces transmission of infection.

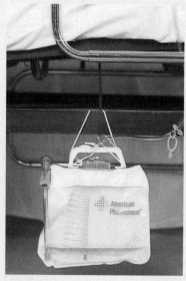

STEP 23 Drainage bag below level of bladder.

STEP	RATIONALE

EVALUATION

1. Palpate bladder for distention or use bladder scan (see Procedural Guideline 33.2) as per agency protocol.

2. Ask patient to describe level of comfort and if sensation of bladder fullness was relieved.

3. Indwelling catheter: Observe character and amount of urine in drainage system.

4. Indwelling catheter: Determine that there is no urine leaking from catheter or tubing connections.

5. **Use Teach-Back:** "I want to be sure I explained clearly about your urinary catheter and some things you can do to ensure the urine flows out of the catheter. Tell me what you can do to keep the urine flowing." Revise your instruction now or develop a plan for revised patient/family caregiver teaching if patient/family caregiver is not able to teach back correctly.

Determines if distention is relieved.

Determines if patient's sensation of discomfort or fullness has been relieved.

Determines if urine is flowing adequately and whether changes develop (e.g., color) that might indicate CAUTI.

Prevents injury to patient's skin and ensures closed sterile system.

Teach-back is a technique for health care providers to ensure that they have explained medical information clearly so that patients and their families understand what is communicated to them (Agency for Healthcare Research and Quality [AHRQ], 2023).

Unexpected Outcomes

1. Catheter goes into vagina.

2. Sterility is broken during catheterization by nurse or patient.

3. Patient complains of bladder discomfort, and catheter is patent as evidenced by adequate urine flow.

Related Interventions

- Leave catheter in vagina.
- Clean urinary meatus again. Using another catheter kit, reinsert sterile catheter into meatus (check agency policy). **NOTE:** If gloves become contaminated, start procedure again.
- Remove catheter in vagina after successful insertion of second catheter.

- Replace gloves if contaminated and start over.
- If patient touches sterile field but equipment and supplies remain sterile, avoid touching that part of sterile field.
- If equipment and/or supplies become contaminated, replace with sterile items or start over with new sterile kit.

- Check catheter to ensure that there is no traction on it.
- Notify health care provider. Patient may be experiencing bladder spasms or symptoms of urinary tract infection (UTI).
- Monitor catheter output for color, clarity, odor, and amount.

Documentation

- Document reason for catheterization, type and size of catheter inserted, amount of fluid used to inflate balloon, specimen collection (if applicable), characteristics and amount of urine, patient's response to procedure, and evaluation of patient learning.
- Document I&O.

Hand-Off Reporting

- Report reason for catheterization, type and size of catheter inserted, amount of fluid used to inflate balloon, and specimen collection and verify it was sent to the lab (if applicable), characteristics and amount of urine, patient's response to procedure, and any education.
- Report to health care provider persistent catheter-related pain and discomfort.

Special Considerations
Patient Education

- Teach patients and family caregivers signs and symptoms of UTI, how to prevent UTI, signs of MARSI/skin irritation, and how to manage these conditions.

- Educate patients and family caregivers about the problems to report to a health care provider immediately.
- If a patient or family caregiver must handle or empty a urine drainage bag, instruct on proper way to empty and importance of hand hygiene.

Pediatrics

- Catheterization in infants and children may be more comfortable with the use of an adequate amount of lubricant containing 2% lidocaine (Xylocaine) (Hockenberry et al., 2024).

Older Adults

- The urethral meatus of an older woman may be difficult to identify because of urogenital atrophy.
- Older adults may exhibit atypical signs and symptoms of UTI such as a change in mental status, which is wrongly attributed to delirium (Ignatavicius et al., 2021). A change in mental status may include confusion, agitation, or lethargy.
- Older adults have an increased risk for UTI related to increased prevalence of chronic disease, such as diabetes, prostatic hypertrophy in men, and a higher prevalence of incontinence (Ignatavicius et al., 2021).

Populations With Disabilities

- Insertion of an indwelling catheter may elicit different reactions for a person with a developmental or intellectual disability (ID). It is important to carefully consider the needs of the individual and provide care in a sensitive and respectful manner (Tremayne & Pawlyn, 2019).

Home Care

- In the nonacute care setting, clean (i.e., nonsterile) technique for intermittent catheterization is an acceptable and more practical alternative to sterile technique for patients requiring chronic intermittent catheterization.

✦ SKILL 33.2   **Care and Removal of an Indwelling Catheter**

 Video Clip

If an indwelling catheter is in place, ongoing monitoring for signs of a UTI and proper cleansing of the external portion of the catheter and the patient's perineum are necessary to reduce risk of infection. The maintenance of a closed drainage system is also essential to reduce entrance of microorganisms into the urinary tract. Timely removal of indwelling catheters has been shown to reduce the risk of CAUTI (Siregar et al., 2021). When removing a catheter, always be sure that the catheter balloon is fully deflated to minimize trauma to the urethra. Evidence is unclear that the practice of clamping a catheter to achieve bladder fullness for several minutes before removal actually improves bladder function after removal.

All patients should have their voiding monitored after catheter removal for at least 24 to 48 hours by using a voiding record or bladder diary to document the time and amount of each voiding, including any incontinence. A bladder scanner can be used to monitor bladder functioning by measuring PVR (see Procedural Guideline 33.2). Abdominal pain and distention, a sensation of incomplete emptying, incontinence, constant dribbling of urine, and voiding in small amounts can indicate inadequate bladder emptying that requires intervention. Symptoms of infection can develop 2 or more days after catheter removal. Always inform patients about the risk for infection, prevention measures, and signs and symptoms that need to be reported right away to the health care provider.

Delegation

The skill of performing routine catheter care can be delegated to assistive personnel (AP). The skill of removing an indwelling catheter can be delegated to AP (see agency policy); however, the nurse must first assess a patient's status and verify the order. Direct the AP to:

- Report characteristics of the urine (color, clarity, odor, and amount) before and after removal.
- Report the condition of the patient's genital area (e.g., color, rashes, open areas, odor, soiling from fecal incontinence, trauma

to tissues around urinary meatus) and skin around securement device (redness, swelling, blistering).

- Check size of balloon and syringe needed to deflate balloon and report if balloon does not deflate and if there is bleeding after removal.
- Report time and amount of first voiding after catheter is removed.
- Report patient complaints of fever, chills, burning, flank pain, back pain, and blood in the urine, which may indicate an upper UTI (e.g., kidney infection).
- Report patient complaints of dysuria, hematuria, urgency, frequency, lower abdominal pain, change in mental status, and lethargy, which may indicate a lower UTI (e.g., bladder infection).

Interprofessional Collaboration

- The wound/ostomy nurse is involved in patient care for specific skin care measures if there is perineal skin irritation from the catheter, from adhesive of catheter stabilization device, or from drainage around catheter insertion.

Equipment

Catheter Care

- Clean gloves
- Waterproof pad
- Bath blanket
- Soap, washcloth, towel, and basin filled with warm water (*Option:* Chlorhexidine 2% cloth)

Removing a Catheter

- 10-mL or larger syringe without needle (information on balloon size [mL] is printed directly on balloon inflation valve [see Fig. 33.3])
- Graduated cylinder to measure urine
- Toilet, bedside commode, urine "hat," urinal, or bedpan
- Bladder scanner (if indicated)
- Clean gloves

STEP	RATIONALE

ASSESSMENT

1. Identify patient using at least two identifiers (e.g., name and birthday or name and medical record number) according to agency policy.

Ensures correct patient. Complies with The Joint Commission standards and improves patient safety (TJC, 2023).

2. Assess patient's/family caregiver's health literacy.

Determines degree to which individuals have the ability to find, understand, and use information and services to make informed health-related decisions and actions for themselves and others (CDC, 2023b).

STEP	RATIONALE
3. Perform hand hygiene	Reduces transmission of microorganisms.
4. **Assess need for catheter care:**	
a. Observe urinary output and urine characteristics.	Sudden decrease in urine output may indicate occlusion of catheter. Cloudy, foul-smelling urine associated with other systemic symptoms may indicate CAUTI.
b. Assess for recent history or presence of bowel incontinence.	Most common bacteria to cause CAUTI are *Escherichia coli*, a major colonizer of the bowel; thus, fecal incontinence increases risk for CAUTI (Gould et al., 2019).
c. Apply clean gloves. Position patient and retract labial or foreskin to observe for any discharge, redness, bleeding, or presence of tissue trauma around urethral meatus (this may be deferred until catheter care).	Indicates inflammatory process, possible infection, or erosion of catheter through urethra.
d. Remove and dispose of gloves and perform hand hygiene.	Reduces transmission of microorganisms.
5. **Assess need for catheter removal:**	
a. Review patient's EHR for length of time catheter has been in place.	Catheters in place for more than a few days cause higher risk for catheter encrustation and UTI.
b. Assess urine color, clarity, odor, and amount. Note any urethral discharge, irritation of genital region, or trauma to urinary meatus (this may be deferred until just before removal).	May be indicator of inflammation or UTI and source of discomfort during catheter removal.
c. Assess patient for history of dehydration, malnutrition, exposure to radiation therapy, underlying chronic conditions (e.g., diabetes mellitus, immunosuppression), and edema of the skin.	Common risk factors for medical adhesive–related skin injury (MARSI) (Fumarola et al., 2020). Adhesive product may be used to stabilize indwelling catheter.
d. Determine size of catheter inflation balloon by looking at balloon inflation valve.	Determines size of syringe needed to deflate balloon and amount of fluid expected in syringe after deflation.
e. Assess patient's knowledge, prior experience with catheter care and/or catheter removal, and feelings about procedure.	Reveals need for patient instruction and/or support.

PLANNING

1. Expected outcomes following catheter care:	
• Genital area is free of secretions, fecal matter, and irritation.	Basic hygiene, especially perineal care, reduces risk for CAUTI (Siregar et al., 2021).
• Skin under and around securement device is free of MARSI.	Patient shows no sensitivity to adhesive.
• Patient verbalizes feeling of comfort around catheter exit site.	Cleaning relieves local discomfort from irritation of catheter.
2. Expected outcomes after catheter removal:	
• Patient voids at least 150 mL with each voiding no more than 6 to 8 hours after removal.	Indicates return of voluntary bladder function without urinary retention.
• Patient verbalizes feeling of complete bladder emptying and absence of discomfort.	
• Patient identifies signs and symptoms of UTI.	Indicates patient learning.
3. Provide privacy and explain procedure to patient. Discuss signs and symptoms of UTI and MARSI. If patient is to be discharged with a catheter, teach patient or family caregiver how to perform catheter hygiene.	Protects patient's privacy; reduces anxiety. Promotes cooperation.
4. Obtain and organize equipment at bedside.	Ensures more efficiency when completing a procedure.

IMPLEMENTATION

1. Perform hand hygiene.	Reduces transmission of microorganisms.
2. Raise bed to appropriate working height. If side rails are raised, lower side rail on working side.	Promotes use of proper body mechanics.
3. Position patient with waterproof pad under buttocks and cover with bath blanket, exposing only genital area and catheter (see Skill 33.1).	Shows respect for patient dignity by only exposing genital area and catheter.
a. Female in dorsal recumbent position.	
b. Male in supine position.	
4. Apply clean gloves.	Reduces transmission of microorganisms.
5. Remove catheter securement device while maintaining connection with drainage tubing.	Provides ability to easily clean around catheter and to remove it.

STEP	RATIONALE

6. Catheter care:

a. *Female:* Use nondominant hand to gently separate labia to fully expose urethral meatus and catheter. Maintain position of hand throughout procedure.

Provides full visualization of urethral meatus. Full separation of labia prevents contamination of meatus during cleaning.

b. *Male:* Use nondominant hand to retract foreskin if not circumcised and hold penis at shaft just below glans. Maintain hand position throughout procedure.

Retraction of foreskin provides full visualization of urethral meatus.

c. Grasp catheter with two fingers of nondominant hand to stabilize it.

Prevents unnecessary traction on catheter.
Pulling on catheter causes discomfort for patient and can damage urethra and bladder neck.

d. If not performed earlier, assess urethral meatus and surrounding tissues for inflammation, swelling, discharge, or tissue trauma and ask patient if burning or discomfort is present.

Determines frequency and type of ongoing care required. Indicates possibility of CAUTI or catheter erosion through urethra.

e. Provide perineal hygiene using mild soap and warm water (see Chapter 18). *Option:* Use chlorhexidine gluconate (CHG) 2% cloth.

Antiseptic cleaners have not been shown to definitively decrease CAUTI; mild soap and water is appropriate (Gould et al., 2019; Siregar et al., 2021). Although chlorhexidine 2% cloth can be used, there is no clear scientific evidence for use of antiseptics versus nonantiseptics to reduce rates of CAUTI (Gould et al., 2019; Rea et al., 2018).

f. Using clean washcloth or CHG cloth, clean along length of catheter.

Removes residue containing microorganisms that can ascend catheter.

(1) Starting close to urinary meatus, clean catheter in circular motion along its length for about 10 cm (4 inches), moving away from body (see illustration). Remove all traces of soap. *For male patients:* Reduce or reposition foreskin after care.

Moves from an area with potentially more microorganisms to an area of fewer microorganisms.

g. Reapply catheter securement device. Allow slack in catheter so that movement does not create tension on it.

Securing indwelling catheter reduces risk of urethral trauma, urethral erosion, CAUTI, or accidental removal (Gould et al., 2019; Lawrence et al., 2019; Siregar et al., 2021).

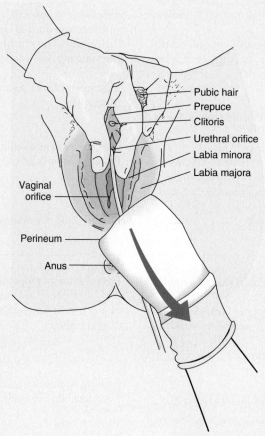

STEP 6f(1) Clean catheter starting at meatus and moving downward while holding it securely.

STEP	RATIONALE
7. Routinely check drainage tubing and bag.	
a. Catheter is secured to upper thigh.	Maintains unobstructed flow of urine out of bladder (Gould et al., 2019).
b. Tubing is positioned without loops and secured onto bed linen.	Assists in the prevention of CAUTI (Siregar et al., 2021).
c. Tubing is not kinked or clamped.	
d. Drainage bag is positioned below level of bladder with urine flowing freely into bag.	Assists in the prevention of CAUTI (Siregar et al., 2021).
e. Drainage bag is not overfull. Empty drainage bag when half full.	Overfull drainage bag creates tension and pulls on catheter, resulting in trauma to urethra and/or urinary meatus. Facilitates unobstructed flow of urine (Gould et al., 2019).
8. **Catheter removal:** (Perform catheter care [Step 6] before catheter removal.)	
a. With clean gloves still on, move syringe plunger up and down to loosen and then pull it back to 0.5 mL. Insert hub of syringe into inflation valve (balloon port). Allow balloon fluid to drain into syringe by gravity. Syringe should fill. Make sure that entire amount of fluid is removed by comparing removed amount with volume needed for inflation.	Partially inflated balloon can traumatize urethral wall during removal. Passive drainage of catheter balloon prevents formation of ridges in balloon. These ridges can cause discomfort or trauma during removal.
b. Pull catheter out smoothly and slowly. Examine it to ensure that it is whole. Catheter should slide out easily. Do not use force. If you note any resistance, repeat Step 8a to remove remaining water.	Non–whole catheter means that pieces of catheter may still be in bladder. Notify health care provider immediately.
c. Wrap contaminated catheter in waterproof pad. Unhook collection bag and drainage tubing from bed.	Promotes patient comfort and safety.
d. Empty, measure, and document urine present in drainage bag (see Chapter 6). Ensure proper gloving if patient on hazardous drugs.	Documents urinary output. Double gloving is needed along with appropriate disposal if patient is on hazardous drugs (ONS, 2018).
e. Encourage patient to maintain or increase fluid intake (unless contraindicated).	Maintains normal urine output.
f. Initiate voiding record or bladder diary. Instruct patient to tell you when need to empty bladder occurs and that all urine needs to be measured. Make sure that patient understands how to use collection container.	Evaluates bladder function.
g. Explain that many patients experience mild burning, discomfort, or small-volume voiding with first voiding, which soon subsides.	Burning results from urethral irritation.
h. Measure PVR volume (if ordered) (Procedure Guideline 33.2) within 5 to 15 minutes after helping the patient to void.	Provides the most reliable PVR reading. A PVR volume less than 50 mL is normal (Rogers, 2023).
i. Inform patient to report any signs of UTI.	
j. Ensure easy access to toilet, commode, bedpan, or urinal. Place urine "hat" on toilet seat if patient is using toilet.	Reduces incidence of falls during toileting. Urine hat collects first voided urine.
9. Provide patient personal hygiene as needed.	Promotes patient comfort and safety.
10. Help patient to a comfortable position.	Restores comfort and sense of well-being.
11. Place nurse call system in an accessible location within patient's reach.	Ensures patient can call for assistance if needed.
12. Raise side rails (as appropriate) and lower bed to lowest position, locking into position.	Ensures patient safety and prevents falls.
13. Dispose of all contaminated supplies in appropriate receptacle, remove and dispose of gloves, and perform hand hygiene.	Reduces transmission of microorganisms. Use appropriate disposal receptacle if patient on hazardous drugs (ONS, 2018).

STEP	RATIONALE

EVALUATION

1. Inspect catheter, securement area, and genital area for soiling, irritation, signs of MARSI, and skin breakdown. Ask patient about discomfort.

Determines if area is cleaned properly and/or if patient has any irritation.

2. Observe time and measure amount of first voiding after catheter removal.

Indicates return of bladder function after catheter removal.

3. Evaluate patient for signs and symptoms of UTI.

Any patient who has a catheter or has had a catheter removed recently is at risk for UTI.

4. Use Teach-Back: "I want to be sure I clearly explained the signs of a urinary tract infection and some things you should do to prevent infection. In your own words, tell me ways you can prevent a urinary tract infection." Revise your instruction now or develop plan for revised patient/family caregiver teaching if patient/family caregiver is not able to teach back correctly.

Teach-back is a technique for health care providers to ensure that they have explained medical information clearly so that patients and their families understand what is communicated to them (Agency for Healthcare Research and Quality [AHRQ], 2023).

Unexpected Outcomes

1. Normal saline equivalent to amount used for balloon inflation does not return into syringe.

Related Interventions

- Reposition patient; ensure that catheter is not pinched or kinked.
- Remove syringe. Attach new syringe and allow enough time for passive emptying.
- Attempt to empty balloon by gently pulling back on syringe plunger.
- If catheter balloon does not deflate, *do not* cut balloon inflation valve to drain water. Notify health care provider.

2. Patient has cloudy urine, foul urine odor, fever, chills, dysuria, flank pain, back pain, hematuria, urgency, frequency, lower abdominal pain, change in mental status, and lethargy.

- Assess for bladder distention and tenderness.
- Monitor vital signs and urine output.
- Report findings to health care provider; signs and symptoms may indicate UTI.
- Consult with health care provider for order to remove catheter.

3. Patient is unable to void within 6 to 8 hours after catheter removal, has sensation of not emptying, strains to void, or experiences small voiding amounts with increasing frequency.

- Assess for bladder distention.
- Help to normal position for voiding and provide privacy.
- Perform bladder ultrasound or scan (see Procedural Guideline 33.2) to assess for excessive urine volume in bladder.
- If patient is unable to void within 6 to 8 hours of catheter removal and/or experiences abdominal pain, notify health care provider.

Documentation

- Document time catheter was removed; teaching related to increasing fluid intake and signs and symptoms of UTI; and time, amount, and characteristics of first voiding.
- Document intake and voiding times and amounts.
- Document patient symptoms experienced upon and after catheter removal.
- Document your evaluation of patient learning.

Hand-Off Reporting

- Report time catheter was removed; teaching provided to patient; and time, amount, and characteristics of first voiding.
- Report hematuria, dysuria, inability or difficulty voiding, and any new incontinence after a catheter is removed to health care provider.

Special Considerations

Patient Education

- Unless contraindicated, patients with a catheter should drink at least 2200 mL of fluid per day to promote continuous flushing of the bladder and prevent sediment from collecting in the catheter tubing.

- Instruct patient to hold collection bag below the level of the bladder when ambulating.
- Instruct patient not to disconnect the catheter from the collection tubing and bag.

Pediatrics

- During catheter removal, do not force catheter out of bladder if you meet resistance. When excessive tubing has been inserted in bladder, there have been occurrences of knotting of the tube (Hockenberry et al., 2024).

Older Adults

- Older adults may exhibit atypical signs and symptoms of CAUTI, such as a change in mental status attributed to delirium. A change in mental status may include confusion, agitation, and/or lethargy.
- In contrast to UTI, asymptomatic bacteriuria (ASB) is more common in older adults than in younger adults (Touhy & Jett, 2022). Nursing home residents often experience significant cognitive deficits, impairing their ability to communicate, and chronic genitourinary symptoms (e.g., incontinence, urgency, frequency), which makes the diagnosis of symptomatic UTI in this group particularly challenging. Furthermore, when infected, nursing home residents are more likely to present with

nonspecific symptoms of UTI, such as anorexia, confusion, and a decline in functional status; fever may be absent or diminished.

Populations With Disabilities

- Poststroke patients are at increased risk for the development of a UTI, requiring you to assess for signs and symptoms more often (Elnady et al., 2018).
- There is high risk for a lack of continuity in care for patients with dementia and psychiatric disorders including the risk for UTIs (Jorgensen et al., 2018).

Home Care

- Urinary retention and urinary incontinence are the two main indications for long-term catheters. Before considering a long-term catheter, explore alternatives such as pads, sheaths, collection devices, and intermittent catheters (Murphy et al., 2018).
- Assess patient and family caregiver for ability and motivation to participate in routine catheter care.
- Collaborate with patients to adapt the home so that those with urinary frequency, urgency, nocturia, and urinary incontinence can reach toileting facilities quickly and safely. Conduct a safety review of the bedroom and bath (see Chapter 41).

PROCEDURAL GUIDELINE 33.2 *Bladder Scan*

Purpose

A bladder scanner (Fig. 33.5) is a noninvasive portable three-dimensional device that creates an ultrasound image of the bladder for measuring the volume of urine in the bladder. The device makes calculations to report accurate urine volumes, especially lower volumes. Use a bladder scanner to assess bladder volume whenever inadequate bladder emptying is suspected, such as following surgery (general anesthetic and spinal) and after the removal of indwelling urinary catheters. Nurses are able to assess the presence of urinary retention, monitor the volume and the excessive relaxation of the bladder, and avoid unnecessary catheterizations. The most common use for the bladder scan is to measure postvoid residual (PVR) (i.e., the volume of urine in the bladder after a normal voiding). To obtain the most reliable reading, measure PVR within 5 to 15 minutes of voiding (Rogers, 2023). A volume less than 50 mL is considered normal. Two or more PVR measurements greater than 100 mL require further investigation. If a bladder scanner is not available, obtain a PVR by measuring urine emptied from the bladder after a straight catheterization (see Skill 33.1).

Delegation

The skill of measuring bladder volume by bladder scan can be delegated to assistive personnel (AP). The nurse first determines the timing and frequency of the bladder scan measurement and interprets the measurements obtained. The nurse also assesses the patient's ability to toilet before measuring PVR and the abdomen for distention if urinary retention is suspected. Direct the AP to:

- Follow manufacturer recommendations for the use of the device.
- Measure PVR volumes within 5 to 15 minutes after helping the patient to void.
- Report and document bladder scan volumes.

Equipment

Bladder scanner (follow manufacturer instructions for use); ultrasound gel; cleaning agent for scanner head such as an alcohol pad; urethral catheterization tray with single-use catheter for straight/intermittent catheterization (see Skill 33.1); paper towel or washcloth

Steps

1. Identify patient using at least two identifiers (e.g., name and birthday or name and medical record number) according to agency policy (TJC, 2023).
2. Assess intake and output (I&O) record to determine urine output trends and check the plan of care to verify correct timing of the bladder scan measurement.
3. Assess patient's/family caregiver's health literacy.
4. Assess patient for inadequate bladder emptying including abdominal pain and distention, a sensation of incomplete emptying, incontinence, constant dribbling of urine, and voiding in small amounts.
5. Provide privacy and explain procedure to patient.
6. Perform hand hygiene and apply clean gloves.
7. Raise bed to appropriate working height. If side rails are raised, lower side rail on working side.
8. If measurement is for PVR, ask patient to void and measure voided urine volume. Measurement should be within 5 to 15 minutes of voiding.
9. Measure PVR with the bladder scan.
   a. Help patient to supine position with head slightly elevated.
   b. Expose patient's lower abdomen.
   c. Turn on scanner per manufacturer guidelines.
   d. Set gender designation per manufacturer guidelines. Women who have had a hysterectomy should be designated as male.

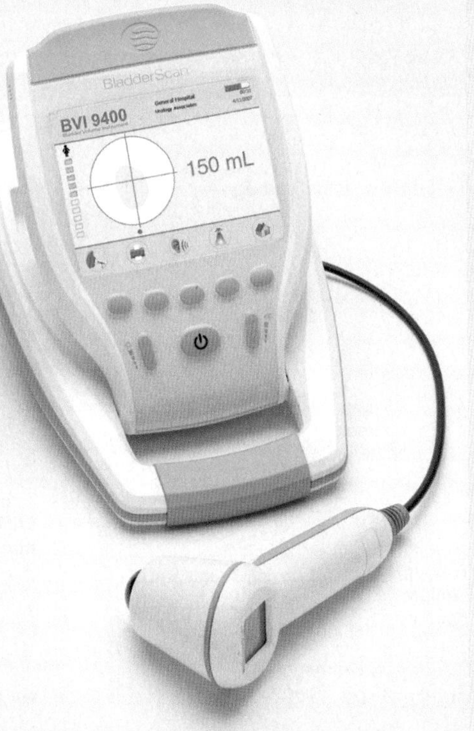

FIG. 33.5 Bladder scanner with image.

Continued

PROCEDURAL GUIDELINE 33.2 *Bladder Scan—cont'd*

e. Wipe scanner head with alcohol pad or other cleaner and allow to air dry.

f. Palpate patient's symphysis pubis (pubic bone). Apply generous amount of ultrasound gel (or if available a bladder scan gel pad) to midline abdomen 2.5 to 4 cm (1–1.5 inches) above symphysis pubis.

g. Place scanner head on gel, ensuring that scanner head is oriented per manufacturer guidelines.

h. Apply light pressure, keep scanner head steady, and point it slightly downward toward bladder. Press and release the scan button (see illustration).

i. Verify accurate aim (refer to manufacturer guidelines). Complete scan and print image (if needed).

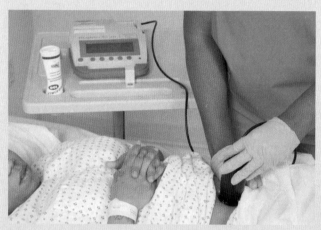

STEP 9h Placement of bladder scan head.

10. Remove ultrasound gel from patient's abdomen with paper towel or moist cloth.

11. Remove ultrasound gel from scanner head and wipe with alcohol pad or other cleaner; allow to air-dry.

12. Help patient to a comfortable position.

13. Place nurse call system in an accessible location within patient's reach.

14. Raise side rails (as appropriate) and lower bed to lowest position, locking into position.

15. Measure PVR after voiding or after using straight/intermittent catheterization (see Skill 33.1). Compare results with prevoiding scan; urine volume should be less. For patients with expected urinary retention, determine if results reveal residual urine in bladder.

16. Dispose of all contaminated supplies in appropriate receptacle and remove and dispose of gloves.

17. Perform hand hygiene.

18. **Use Teach-Back:** "I want to be sure I explained clearly why you need to have your bladder scanned and why there might be a need to catheterize you for residual urine. In your own words, tell me why the bladder scan is needed." Revise your instruction now or develop a plan for revised patient/family caregiver teaching if patient/family caregiver is not able to teach back correctly.

19. Review health care provider's order to determine how often to assess residual urine.

20. Review I&O record to determine urine output trends.

21. Document findings of scan, PVR, and patient tolerance of procedure.

22. Report to health care provider outcome of bladder scan and need to catheterize for residual volume.

◆ SKILL 33.3 | Performing Catheter Irrigation

Following surgery on the bladder and other GU structures, it is common to have hematuria for several days. Intermittent or continuous urinary catheter irrigations maintain catheter patency by keeping the bladder clear and free of blood clots or sediment. However, irrigation poses a risk for causing a UTI and thus must be done maintaining a closed urinary drainage system. Closed catheter irrigations do not disrupt the sterile connection between the catheter and the drainage system (Fig. 33.6). Continuous bladder irrigation (CBI) is an example of a continuous infusion of a sterile solution into the bladder, usually using a three-way irrigation closed system with a triple-lumen catheter.

Delegation

The skill of a closed catheter irrigation cannot be delegated to assistive personnel (AP). Direct the AP to:

• Report if the patient complains of pain, discomfort, or leakage of fluid around the catheter.

• Monitor and document intake and output (I&O); report immediately any decrease in urine output.

• Report any change in the color of the urine, especially the presence of blood clots.

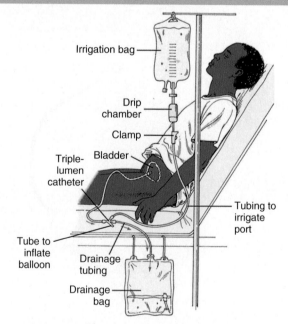

FIG. 33.6 Closed continuous bladder irrigation.

Interprofessional Collaboration

- The urologist or surgeon is included in the support of patients with bladder irrigation needs (e.g., volume to administer, signs and symptoms to report).

Equipment

- Sterile irrigation solution at room temperature (as prescribed)
- Intravenous (IV) pole (closed continuous or intermittent)
- Antiseptic swabs
- Clean gloves

Closed Intermittent Irrigation

- Sterile 50 mL syringe to access system: Luer-Lok syringe for needleless access port (per manufacturer's instructions)
- Screw clamp or rubber band (used to occlude catheter temporarily as irrigant is instilled)

Closed Continuous Irrigation

- Irrigation tubing with clamp to regulate irrigation flow rate
- Y connector (optional) to connect irrigation tubing to triple-lumen catheter

STEP	RATIONALE

ASSESSMENT

1. Identify patient using at least two identifiers (e.g., name and birthday or name and medical record number) according to agency policy.

   Ensures correct patient. Complies with The Joint Commission standards and improves patient safety (TJC, 2023).

2. Verify in EHR:
   a. Order for irrigation method (continuous or intermittent), type (sterile saline or medicated solution), and amount of irrigant.

   Health care provider's order is required to initiate therapy. Frequency and volume of solution used for irrigation may be in the order or standardized as part of agency policy.

   b. Type of catheter in place (see Fig. 33.2).

   Triple-lumen catheters are used for both intermittent and continuous closed irrigation.

3. Assess patient's/family caregiver's health literacy.

   Determines degree to which individuals have the ability to find, understand, and use information and services to make informed health-related decisions and actions for themselves and others (CDC, 2023b).

4. Perform hand hygiene. Palpate bladder for distention and tenderness or use bladder scan (see Procedural Guidelines 33.2).

   Reduces transmission of microorganisms. Bladder distention indicates that flow of urine may be blocked from draining.

5. Assess patient for abdominal pain or spasms, sensation of bladder fullness, or leaking around catheter. Wear clean gloves if risk of contacting urine.

   May indicate overdistention of bladder caused by catheter blockage. Offers baseline to determine if therapy is successful.

6. Observe urine for color, amount, clarity, and presence of mucus; clots; or sediment.

   Indicates if patient is bleeding or sloughing tissue, which would require increased irrigation rate or frequency of catheter irrigation.

7. Monitor I&O. If CBI is being used, amount of fluid draining from bladder should exceed amount of fluid infused into bladder.

   If output does not exceed irrigant infused, catheter obstruction (i.e., blood clots, kinked tubing) should be suspected, irrigation stopped, and prescriber notified (Ignatavicius et al., 2021).

8. Assess patient's knowledge, prior experience with catheter irrigation, and feelings about procedure.

   Reveals need for patient instruction and/or support.

PLANNING

1. Expected outcomes following completion of this procedure:
   - With CBI: Urine output is greater than volume of irrigating solution instilled.

     Indicates patency of drainage system, allowing for drainage of urine and irrigating solution.

   - Patient reports relief of bladder pain or spasms.

     Indicates bladder emptying.

   - Urine output has increased and/or there is an absence of blood clots and sediment. (**NOTE:** Urine will be bloody following bladder/urethral surgery, gradually becoming lighter and blood tinged in 2 to 3 days.)

     Indicates that catheter is at decreased risk for occlusion with blood clots.

   - Absence of fever, lower abdominal pain, and cloudy and/or foul-smelling urine.

     Signs of UTI are not present.

   - Patient or family caregiver can explain purpose of procedure and what to expect.

     Demonstrates learning.

2. Provide privacy and explain procedure to patient. Discuss what is involved in catheter irrigation and what the patient may expect to experience.

   Protects patient's privacy; reduces anxiety. Promotes cooperation.

3. Obtain and organize equipment at bedside.

   Ensures more efficiency when completing a procedure.

STEP	RATIONALE

IMPLEMENTATION

1. Perform hand hygiene. Raise bed to appropriate working height. If side rails are raised, lower side rail on working side.

Reduces transmission of microorganisms.
Promotes use of good body mechanics. Position provides access to catheter.

2. Position patient supine and expose catheter junctions (catheter and drainage tubing).

Position provides access to catheter and promotes patient dignity as much as possible.

3. Remove catheter securement device.

Eases access to catheter parts.

4. Closed continuous irrigation:

   a. Close clamp on new irrigation tubing and hang bag of irrigating solution on IV pole. Insert (spike) tip of sterile irrigation tubing into designated port of irrigation solution bag using aseptic technique (see illustration).

Prevents air from entering tubing. Air can cause bladder spasms. Technique prevents transmission of microorganisms.

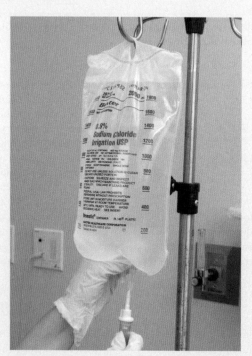

STEP 4a Spiking bag of sterile irrigation solution for continuous bladder irrigation.

   b. Fill drip chamber half full by squeezing chamber. Remove cap at end of tubing, and then open clamp and allow solution to flow (prime) through tubing, keeping end of tubing sterile. Once fluid has filled tubing, close clamp and recap end of tubing.

Priming tubing with fluid prevents introduction of air into bladder. Recapping keeps end of tubing sterile.

   c. Using aseptic technique, cleanse port on catheter with antiseptic swab, remove cap on tubing, and connect end of tubing securely to port for infusing irrigation fluid into double/triple-lumen catheter.

Reduces transmission of microorganisms.

   d. Adjust clamp on irrigation tubing to begin flow of solution into bladder. If a set volume rate is ordered, calculate drip rate and adjust rate at roller clamp. If urine is bright red or has clots, increase irrigation rate until drainage appears pink (according to ordered rate or agency protocol).

Continuous drainage is expected. It helps to prevent clotting in presence of active bleeding in bladder and flushes clots out of bladder.

   e. Observe for outflow of fluid into drainage bag. Empty catheter drainage bag as needed.

Discomfort, bladder distention, and possible injury can occur from overdistention of bladder when bladder irrigant cannot adequately flow from bladder. Bag will fill rapidly and may need to be emptied every 1 to 2 hours.

STEP	RATIONALE
5. Closed intermittent irrigation:	Fluid is instilled through catheter in a bolus, flushing system. Fluid drains out after irrigation is complete.
a. Pour prescribed sterile irrigation solution into sterile container.	
b. Draw prescribed volume of irrigant (usually 30–50 mL) into sterile syringe using aseptic technique. Place sterile cap on tip of needleless syringe.	Ensures sterility of irrigating fluid.
c. Clamp catheter tubing below soft injection port with screw clamp (or fold catheter tubing onto itself and secure with rubber band).	Occluding catheter tubing below point of injection will allow irrigating solution to enter catheter and flow into bladder.
d. Using circular motion, clean catheter port (specimen port) with antiseptic swab.	Reduces transmission of microorganisms.
e. Insert tip of needleless syringe into port using twisting motion.	Ensures that catheter tip enters lumen of catheter.
f. Inject solution using slow, even pressure.	Gentle instillation of solution minimizes trauma to bladder mucosa.
g. Remove syringe and clamp (or rubber band), allowing solution to drain into urinary drainage bag.	Allows drainage to flow out by gravity. Medications must be instilled long enough to be absorbed by lining of bladder. Clamped drainage tubing and bag should not be left unattended.

Clinical Judgment *Some medicated irrigants may need to dwell in the bladder for a prescribed period, requiring the catheter to be clamped temporarily before being allowed to drain.*

STEP	RATIONALE
6. Anchor catheter with catheter securement device (see Skill 33.1).	Prevents trauma to urethral tissue caused by pulling catheter.
7. Help patient to a comfortable position.	Restores comfort and sense of well-being.
8. Place nurse call system in an accessible location within patient's reach.	Ensures patient can call for assistance if needed.
9. Raise side rails (as appropriate) and lower bed to lowest position, locking into position.	Ensures patient safety and prevents falls.
10. Dispose of all contaminated supplies in appropriate receptacle, remove and dispose of gloves, and perform hand hygiene.	Reduces transmission of microorganisms. Use appropriate disposal receptacle if patient on hazardous drugs (ONS, 2018).

EVALUATION

STEP	RATIONALE
1. Measure actual urine output by subtracting total amount of irrigation fluid infused from total volume drained into basin.	Determines accurate urinary output.
2. Review I&O flow sheet to verify that hourly output into drainage bag is in appropriate proportion to irrigating solution entering bladder. Expect more output than fluid instilled because of urine production.	Determines urinary output in relation to irrigation.
3. Inspect urine for blood clots and sediment and be sure that tubing is not kinked or occluded.	Decrease in blood clots means that therapy is successful in maintaining catheter patency. System is patent.
4. Evaluate patient's comfort level.	Indicates catheter patency by absence of symptoms of bladder distention.
5. Monitor for signs and symptoms of infection.	Patients with indwelling catheters remain at risk for infection.
6. **Use Teach-Back:** "I want to be sure I explained clearly about the irrigation of your catheter. Tell me in your own words the reason we are doing the irrigation." Revise your instruction now or develop a plan for revised patient/family caregiver teaching if patient/family caregiver is not able to teach back correctly.	Teach-back is a technique for health care providers to ensure that they have explained medical information clearly so that patients and their families understand what is communicated to them (AHRQ, 2023).

Unexpected Outcomes	Related Interventions
1. Irrigating solution does not return (closed intermittent irrigation) or is not flowing at prescribed rate (CBI).	• Examine drainage tubing for clots, sediment, and kinks. • Notify health care provider if irrigant does not flow freely from bladder, patient complains of pain, or bladder distention occurs. • Inspect urine for presence of or increase in blood clots and sediment. • Evaluate patient for pain and distended bladder. • Notify health care provider.

STEP	RATIONALE
2. Bright-red bleeding with the irrigation (CBI) infusion wide open.	• Assess for hypovolemic shock (vital signs, skin color and moisture, anxiety level). • Leave irrigation infusion wide open, ensuring catheter is draining, and notify health care provider.
3. Patient experiences pain with irrigation.	• Examine drainage tubing for clots, sediment, or kinks. • Evaluate urine for presence of or increase in blood clots and sediment. • Evaluate for distended bladder. • Notify health care provider.

Documentation

- Document irrigation method, amount of and type of irrigation solution, amount returned as drainage, characteristics of output, and urine output.
- Document I&O.
- Document your evaluation of patient learning.

Hand-Off Reporting

- Report status of urine output, catheter occlusion, sudden bleeding, infection, or increased pain.

Special Considerations

Patient Education

- Instruct patient and family caregiver to observe urine daily for changes in color, presence of mucus or blood, and odor.

- Inform patients that bleeding is common after many urologic procedures and to expect bright red–tinged urine during the first 48 hours after surgery, followed by a change in urine ranging from pink-tinged to clear.
- Instruct patient to maintain adequate oral intake of 2 L/day (unless contraindicated).

Home Care

- Patients and family caregivers can be taught to perform catheter irrigations with adequate support, demonstration/return demonstration, and written instructions.
- Teach patients and family caregivers to observe urine color, clarity, odor, and amount.
- Arrange for home delivery and storage of catheter/irrigation supplies.
- Teach patients and family caregivers signs of catheter obstruction or UTI.

✦ SKILL 33.4 Applying an Incontinence Device

A male incontinence device, also called a *condom catheter,* penile sheath, or Texas catheter, is a soft, pliable condom-like sheath that fits over the penis, providing a safe and noninvasive way to contain urine for men who have complete and spontaneous bladder emptying. Most external catheters are made of soft silicone that reduces friction. They are clear to allow for easy visualization of skin under the catheter. Latex catheters are still available, so it is important to verify that a patient does not have a latex allergy before applying this type of catheter.

Condom-type external catheters are held in place by an adhesive coating on the internal lining of the sheath, a double-sided self-adhesive strip, brush-on adhesive applied to the penile shaft, or an external strap. **Never use tape to secure a condom catheter.** A catheter may be attached to a small-volume (leg) urinary drainage bag or a large-volume (bedside) drainage bag, both of which need to be kept lower than the level of the bladder. Various styles and sizes are available, so it is important to refer to the manufacturer's guidelines for fitting and correct application. For men who cannot be fitted for a condom-type external catheter, other externally applied catheters are available.

An option to the condom catheter is an incontinence device made of a 100% latex-free, hydrocolloid material. The device fits onto the tip of the penis and not over the penile shaft. It reduces occurrence of soiling of skin by urine. This device is helpful for patients with retracted anatomy or a small penile tip, causing a traditional condom catheter to dislodge.

In the acute care setting, the use of a female external collection device (Fig. 33.7) has effectively collected urine and prevented external tissue damage. The PureWick female external catheter system is a tube that lies between the labia near the urethral opening and extends in between the buttocks. The tube is secured in the

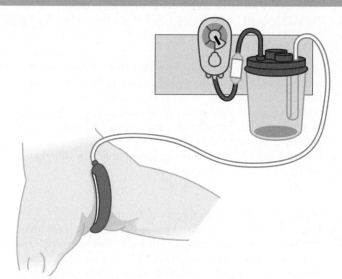

FIG. 33.7 External female catheter attached to wall suction. (*Courtesy and © Becton, Dickinson and Company.*)

suprapubic area and attached to a low and continuous suction system. The goal is for the system to wick the urine away as it leaks from the urethral opening (Ignatavicius et al., 2021). This type of device is useful for patients who are either in sitting or lying positions.

Delegation

Assessment of the skin of a patient's genitalia and penile shaft and determination of a latex allergy are done by a nurse before catheter application. The skill of applying an incontinence device can be delegated to assistive personnel (AP), depending on agency policy. Direct the AP to:

- Follow manufacturer directions for applying the incontinence device and securing device.
- Monitor urine intake and output (I&O) and document if applicable.
- Immediately report any redness, swelling, or skin irritation or breakdown of the genitalia, glans penis, or penile shaft.

Interprofessional Collaboration

- The health care provider and wound ostomy continence (WOC) nurse may be involved in the care of patients who may need an alternative to a traditional condom catheter.

Equipment

- Male incontinence device catheter kit—condom sheath of appropriate size, securing device (internal adhesive, strap), skin preparation solution (per manufacturer's recommendations)
  - *Option:* hydrocolloid incontinence device
  - Urinary collection bag with drainage tubing or leg bag and straps
- PureWick female external catheter system—collection cannister with lid, pump tubing, collector tubing with port, external catheter
- Basin with warm water and soap
- Towels, washcloth, bath blanket
- Clean gloves
- Scissors, hair guard, or paper towel

STEP	RATIONALE
ASSESSMENT	
1. Identify patient using at least two identifiers (e.g., name and birthday or name and medical record number) according to agency policy.	Ensures correct patient. Complies with The Joint Commission standards and improves patient safety (TJC, 2023).
2. Review electronic health record (EHR) and assess urinary pattern, ability to empty bladder effectively, and degree of urinary continence.	Incontinent patients are at risk for skin breakdown and thus candidates for condom catheter.
3. Review EHR for history of allergy to rubber or latex. Check patient's allergy wristband and confirm with patient.	Condoms are made of latex and can cause serious skin reaction.
4. Review EHR to determine patient's age and history of dehydration, malnutrition, exposure to radiation therapy, underlying chronic conditions (e.g., diabetes mellitus, immunosuppression), and edema of the skin.	Common risk factors for medical adhesive–related skin injury (MARSI) (Fumarola et al., 2020).
5. Assess patient's/family caregiver's health literacy.	Determines degree to which individuals have the ability to find, understand, and use information and services to make informed health-related decisions and actions for themselves and others (CDC, 2023b).
6. Perform hand hygiene and apply clean gloves. Assess skin of penis or genitalia for rashes, erythema, and/or open areas. (This may be deferred until just before device application.)	Reduces transmission of microorganisms. Provides baseline to compare changes in condition of skin after application of incontinence device.

Clinical Judgment *Apply an incontinence device only when the skin on the penile surface or around genitalia is intact and without erythema.*

7. Verify patient's size and type of male incontinence device from plan of care or use manufacturer measuring guide to measure length and diameter of penis in flaccid state (apply gloves for measurement). Remove and dispose of gloves and perform hand hygiene.	Identifies proper size of device needed. To measure the penile circumference, begin from the penile base where the diameter is the largest. To choose the right size of device if it is between two sizes, choose the smallest size (Sinha et al., 2018). Reduces transmission of microorganisms.
8. Assess patient's knowledge and prior experience with and feelings about an incontinence device.	Reveals need for patient instruction and/or support.

PLANNING

1. Expected outcomes following completion of procedure:	
• Patient's skin is free from urine wetness.	Device is applied correctly.
• Genitalia, glans, and penile shaft are free of skin irritation, erythema, MARSI, or breakdown.	Device is secure and not too tight. Patient free of MARSI.
• Patient explains purpose of procedure and what to expect.	Helps to minimize anxiety and promotes cooperation.
2. Provide privacy and explain procedure to patient. Discuss the type of device, why it is being placed, and how to manage the device.	Protects patient's privacy; reduces anxiety. Promotes cooperation.
3. Obtain and organize equipment at bedside.	Ensures more efficiency when completing a procedure.

IMPLEMENTATION

1. Perform hand hygiene.	Reduces transmission of microorganisms.
2. Raise bed to appropriate working height. Lower side rail on working side.	Promotes use of good body mechanics and easy access to perineum.
3. **Condom catheter**. Prepare urinary drainage collection bag and tubing (large-volume drainage bag or leg bag). Clamp off drainage bag port. Place nearby, ready to attach to condom after applied.	Provides easy access to drainage equipment after applying condom catheter.

STEP	RATIONALE
4. Help patient to supine or sitting position. Place bath blanket over upper torso. Fold sheets so that only penis is exposed.	Respects patient dignity; draping prevents unnecessary exposure of body parts.
5. Apply clean gloves. Provide perineal care (see Chapter 18). Dry thoroughly before applying device. In uncircumcised male, ensure that foreskin has been replaced to normal position before applying condom catheter. Do not apply barrier cream.	Prevents skin breakdown from exposure to secretions. Removes any residual adhesives. Perineal care minimizes skin irritation and promotes adhesion of new external catheter. Barrier creams prevent sheath from adhering to penile shaft.
6. Remove and dispose of gloves. Perform hand hygiene. Reapply clean gloves.	Reduces transmission of microorganisms.
7. Clip hair at base of penis as needed before application of condom sheath.	Hair adheres to condom and is pulled during condom removal or may get caught in adhesive as external catheter is applied.

Clinical Judgment *The pubic area should not be shaved because any microabrasions in skin increase risk for skin irritation and infection.*

8. Apply incontinence device.	
a. **Condom catheter.** With nondominant hand, grasp penis along shaft. With dominant hand, hold rolled condom sheath at tip of penis with head of penis in cone. Smoothly roll sheath onto penis. Allow 2.5 to 5 cm (1–2 inches) of space between tip of glans penis and end of condom catheter (see illustration).	Excessive wrinkles or creases in external catheter sheath after application may mean that patient needs smaller size.
b. **Hydrocolloid device.** Place the device onto the tip of the penis, not the shaft (see manufacturer's directions).	Hydrocolloid material makes device less irritating to the skin and is suitable for patients with latex allergy. Allows the skin to breathe and the urine to be directed away from the body, making urination as natural as possible.

Clinical Judgment *Some manufacturers provide a hair guard that is placed over penis before applying the device. Remove the hair guard after applying the catheter. An alternative to a hair guard is to tear a hole in a paper towel, place it over the penis, and remove it after application of the device.*

9. Apply appropriate securement device as indicated in manufacturer guidelines.	Condom must be secured firmly so that it is snug and stays on but not tight enough to cause constriction of blood flow.
a. Self-adhesive condom catheters: After application, apply gentle pressure on penile shaft for 10 to 15 seconds.	Ensures adherence of adhesive with penile skin. Secures catheter in place.
b. Outer securing strip-type condom catheters: Spiral wrap penile shaft with strip of supplied elastic adhesive. Strip should not overlap itself. Elastic strip should be snug, not tight (see illustration).	Using spiral wrap technique allows supplied elastic adhesive to expand so that blood flow to penis is not compromised.
c. Hydrocolloid incontinence device: Remove release papers from adhesive on faceplate of device. Center faceplate over opening of urinary meatus. Smooth hydrocolloid adhesive backing strips onto tip of penis. Then cover with hydrocolloid seal (see illustration).	Follow manufacturer's directions to ensure device covers tip of penis only.

Clinical Judgment *Never use regular adhesive tape to secure a condom catheter. Constriction from tape can reduce blood flow to the penile tissues.*

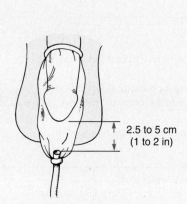

2.5 to 5 cm
(1 to 2 in)

STEP 8a Condom catheter.

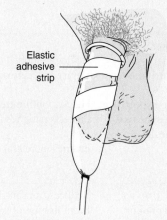

Elastic adhesive strip

STEP 9b Spiral application of adhesive strip.

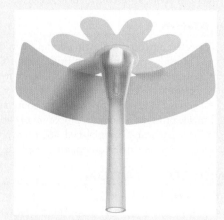

STEP 9c Men's Liberty Acute Male Incontinence Device. (*Courtesy BioDerm, Inc. Largo, Florida.*)

STEP	RATIONALE
10. Remove hair guard if used. Connect drainage tubing to end of condom catheter. Be sure that condom is not twisted. If using large drainage bag, place excess tubing on bed and secure to bottom sheet.	Allows urine to be collected and measured. Keeps patient dry. Twisted condom obstructs urine flow, causing urine pooling, skin irritation, and weakening and deterioration of adhesive, causing catheter to come off.
11. Prepare PureWick Urine Collection System:	
a. Plug the power cord into device outlet and into an A/C power outlet. **NOTE:** Be sure the power switch is in the OFF position.	
b. Insert the collection canister into the base of device and press the lid down firmly, ensuring the lid is sealed.	Prevents leakage.
c. Attach the short pump tubing to the PureWick Urine Collection System connector port and to the connector port on canister lid.	
d. Attach the elbow connector to the long collector tubing, then attach other end of the elbow connector to the connector port on canister lid.	
e. Connect the PureWick Female External Catheter to the PureWick Urine Collection canister:	
(1) Perform hand hygiene and apply clean gloves. Perform perineal care and assess skin integrity.	Reduces transmission of microorganisms.
(2) Separate the patient's legs, gluteus muscles, and labia.	Provides visual access for accurate application.
(3) With the soft gauze side of the device facing the patient, align the distal end of the PureWick Female External Catheter at the gluteal cleft.	
(4) Gently tuck the soft gauze side between the gluteus and labia. Ensure that the top of the gauze is aligned to the pubic bone.	
(5) Slowly place the legs back together once the PureWick Female External Catheter is positioned.	
12. Help patient to a comfortable position.	Restores comfort and sense of well-being.
13. Place nurse call system in an accessible location within patient's reach.	Ensures patient can call for assistance if needed.
14. Raise side rails (as appropriate) and lower bed to lowest position, locking into position.	Ensures patient safety and prevents falls.
15. Dispose of all contaminated supplies in appropriate receptacle, remove and dispose of gloves, and perform hand hygiene.	Reduces transmission of microorganisms. Use appropriate disposal receptacle if patient on hazardous drugs (ONS, 2018).
16. Remove and reapply condom catheter daily following Steps 8 to 10 unless an extended-wear device is used. To remove condom, wash penis with warm, soapy water and gently roll sheath and adhesive off penile shaft.	Prevents trauma and irritation to penile sheath.
17. Remove and replace PureWick Female External Catheter every 8 to 12 hours or if soiled with feces or blood. Perform perineal care before replacement of system.	To avoid injury to tissues, gently pull the system outward when removing and ensure that suction is maintained during removal.

EVALUATION

1. Observe urinary drainage.	Twisted condom prevents urine from draining into collection bag.
2. Inspect penis with condom catheter in place within 15 to 30 minutes after application. Assess for swelling and discoloration and ask patient if there is any discomfort.	Determines if condom is applied too tightly, impeding circulation to penis.
3. Inspect skin on penile shaft or genitalia for signs of erythema, irritation, or skin breakdown at least daily, when performing hygiene, and before reapplying condom or PureWick Female External Catheter.	Changing external catheter decreases chance of infection. Exposure to adhesive may cause MARSI.

STEP	RATIONALE
4. Use Teach-Back: "I want to be sure I explained clearly about your incontinence device and some things you can do to prevent it from falling off. Tell me how you can help keep the device on without it slipping off." Revise your instruction now or develop a plan for revised patient/family caregiver teaching if patient/family caregiver is not able to teach back correctly.	Teach-back is a technique for health care providers to ensure that they have explained medical information clearly so that patients and their families understand what is communicated to them (AHRQ, 2023).

Unexpected Outcomes	Related Interventions
1. Skin around penis is erythematous, ulcerated, has blistering, or is denuded.	• Check for latex allergy, allergy to skin preparation or adhesive device, or MARSI. • Remove condom and notify health care provider. • Do not reapply until penis and surrounding tissue are free from irritation. • Ensure that condom is not twisted and urine flow is unobstructed after application.
2. Penile swelling or discoloration occurs.	• Remove external catheter. • Notify health care provider. • Reassess current condom size. See manufacturer size chart.
3. Incontinence device does not stay on.	• Ensure that catheter tubing is anchored and patient understands to not pull or tug on catheter. • Reassess incontinence device size. Refer to manufacturer guidelines for sizing. • Observe whether incontinence device outlet is kinked and urine is pooling at tip of condom, bathing penis in urine; reapply as needed and avoid catheter obstruction. • Consult with WOC nurse. • Assess need for another brand of incontinence device (i.e., one that is self-adhesive).

Documentation

• Document condom/device application; condition of genitalia or penis, skin, and scrotum; urinary output and voiding pattern; patient response to external catheter application; and patient learning.

Hand-Off Reporting

• During hand-off reporting, communicate condition of skin and incontinence device.
• Report erythema, rashes, or skin breakdown to health care provider.

Special Considerations

Patient Education

• Teach patient and family caregiver about signs of skin breakdown or trauma.
• Teach patient and family caregiver to keep catheter kink free and positioned below level of bladder.
• Teach patient with leg bag to assess leg straps periodically for tightness and loosen as needed.

Pediatrics

• Use of condom catheters is uncommon in children. When used in adolescents, take precautions to minimize embarrassment.

Older Adults

• Evaluate patients with neuropathy carefully before applying a condom catheter. Patient may not feel sensation of pressure

from condom device. Assess penile skin at more frequent intervals, at least twice daily.
• Condom catheters are not recommended in patients with prostatic obstruction.

Populations With Disabilities

• Use of male incontinence devices in patients with paraplegia need routine special assessments, as patient may not be able to identify pain from improper placement. Improper placement can cause pressure and result in a medical device–related pressure injury (MDRPI) (see Chapter 39).

Home Care

• Teach patient and family caregivers appropriate assessments, such as signs and symptoms of UTI, signs of pressure injury, skin irritation and blistering, or poor-fitting catheter sheath.
• Loose-fitting clothing may be needed to accommodate the catheter and drainage system.
• Ensure that patient and family caregiver understand correct steps in applying the condom catheter. Manufacturers often supply patient educational materials.
• Teach patient or family caregiver to empty drainage bag frequently when half full to avoid unnecessary tension on the catheter, which can lead to problems keeping the catheter intact.
• Consult with health care provider or home care nurse regarding approach to use to clean urinary drainage bag. Typical options include vinegar and water or chlorine bleach and water. Have an extra bag available when cleaning.

✦ SKILL 33.5 Suprapubic Catheter Care

A suprapubic catheter is a urinary drainage tube inserted surgically through a small incision in the abdominal wall above the symphysis pubis into the bladder (Fig. 33.8). The catheter may be sutured to the skin, secured with an adhesive material, or retained in the bladder with a fluid-filled balloon like an indwelling catheter. Suprapubic catheters are placed when there is blockage of the urethra (e.g., enlarged prostate, urethral stricture, after urological surgery) and in situations when a long-term urethral catheter causes irritation or discomfort or interferes with sexual functioning.

Delegation

The skill of caring for a newly established suprapubic catheter cannot be delegated to assistive personnel (AP); however, care of an established suprapubic catheter may be delegated (refer to agency policy). Direct the AP to:

- Report patient's discomfort (bladder fullness, abdominal pain, skin irritation) related to the suprapubic catheter.
- Empty drainage bag and document urinary output on intake and output (I&O) record.
- Report any change in the amount and character of the urine.
- Report any signs of redness, foul odor, or drainage around catheter insertion site.

Interprofessional Collaboration

- The surgeon and WOC nurse are involved in the management of the suprapubic catheter and possible need for bladder training after removal.

Equipment

- Clean gloves (sterile may be necessary in some cases, see agency policy)
- Cleaning agent (sterile normal saline solution)
- Sterile cotton-tipped applicators
- Sterile surgical drainage gauze (split gauze)
- Sterile gauze dressing
- Washcloth, towel, soap, and water
- Tape
- Hook-and-loop fastener tube holder or tube stabilizer (optional)
- Thermometer

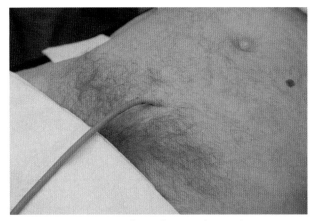

FIG. 33.8 Suprapubic catheter without a dressing.

STEP	RATIONALE

ASSESSMENT

1. Identify patient using at least two identifiers (e.g., name and birthday or name and medical record number) according to agency policy.

Ensures correct patient. Complies with The Joint Commission standards and improves patient safety (TJC, 2023).

2. Review electronic health record (EHR) for history of allergies.

Determines supplies used for catheter care. Identifies known patient allergies.

3. Review EHR to determine patient's age and history of dehydration, malnutrition, exposure to radiation therapy, underlying chronic conditions (e.g., diabetes mellitus, immunosuppression), and edema of the skin.

Common risk factors for medical adhesive–related skin injury (MARSI) (Fumarola et al., 2020).

4. Assess patient's/ family caregiver's health literacy.

Determines degree to which individuals have the ability to find, understand, and use information and services to make informed health-related decisions and actions for themselves and others (CDC, 2023b).

5. Assess urine in drainage bag for amount, clarity, color, odor, and sediment.

Abnormal findings indicate potential complications, such as UTI, decreased urinary output, and catheter occlusion.

6. Perform hand hygiene and apply clean gloves. Observe dressing around catheter insertion site for drainage and intactness.

Reduces transmission of infection. Drainage indicates potential complication, such as infection. Dressing may become nonocclusive because of tape choice or drainage.

7. Remove outer dressing and dispose in proper receptacle. Assess catheter insertion site (may be deferred until you clean site) for signs of inflammation (i.e., pain, erythema, edema, and drainage) and for growth of overgranulation tissue. Ask patient if there is any pain at site; if so, have patient rate on scale of 0 to 10. Remove and dispose of gloves and perform hand hygiene.

If insertion is new, slight inflammation may be expected as part of normal wound healing but can also indicate infection. Overgranulation tissue can develop at insertion site as reaction to catheter. In some instances, intervention may be necessary. Reduces transmission of microorganisms.

STEP	RATIONALE
8. Assess for elevated temperature and chills.	Increased temperature may indicate UTI or skin site infection.
9. Assess patient's knowledge and prior experience with and feelings about management of a suprapubic catheter.	Reveals need for patient instruction and/or support.

PLANNING

1. Expected outcomes following completion of procedure:	
• Patient verbalizes no pain or discomfort at insertion site and over bladder.	Patent catheter system keeps bladder empty and patient comfortable.
• Urine output is 30 mL or greater per hour.	Indicates that catheter is patent.
• Urine remains clear without foul odor, and patient is afebrile.	Indicates that patient is free of catheter-associated urinary tract infection (CAUTI).
• Catheter exit site is free of infection (i.e., erythema, edema, drainage, tenderness) or MARSI (redness, skin irritation, blistering).	Indicates absence of infection and irritation of skin.
• Patient and/or family caregiver can explain purpose of and methods for suprapubic catheter care.	Evaluates learning.
2. Provide privacy and explain procedure to patient. Discuss signs and symptoms of UTI and MARSI. If applicable, teach patient and family caregiver how to perform suprapubic catheter hygiene.	Protects patient's privacy; reduces anxiety. Promotes cooperation.
3. Obtain and organize equipment at bedside.	Ensures more efficiency when completing a procedure.

IMPLEMENTATION

1. Perform hand hygiene.	Reduces transmission of infection.
2. Raise bed to appropriate working height. If side rails are raised, lower side rail on working side.	Promotes use of good body mechanics and access to catheter site.
3. Prepare supplies and open gauze packets in same manner as for applying dry dressing (see Chapter 40).	Keeps dressing sterile until application.
4. Apply clean gloves. Loosen tape and remove existing dressing. Note type and presence of drainage. Remove and dispose of gloves and perform hand hygiene.	Provides baseline for condition of suprapubic wound. Reduces transmission of infection from dressing.
5. Clean insertion site using sterile aseptic technique for newly established catheter: *Option:* Review agency policy or consider individual patient need. In some agencies, clean gloves are appropriate.	Catheter site is made surgically and therefore is treated similarly to other incisions as designated by agency policy. Confirm if using either medical aseptic or sterile technique is recommended.
a. Apply sterile gloves (see agency policy).	
b. Without creating tension, hold catheter up with nondominant hand while cleaning. Use sterile gauze moistened in saline and clean skin around insertion site in circular motion, starting near insertion site and continuing in outward widening circle. Use new sterile gauze for each circular swipe out to approximately 5 cm (2 inches) (see illustration).	Moves from area of least contamination to area of most contamination. Tension on catheter may cause discomfort or damage to wall of bladder or catheter to slip out of place.
c. With fresh, moistened gauze, gently clean base of catheter, moving up and away from site of insertion (proximal to distal).	Removes microorganisms that reside on any drainage that adheres to tubing.
d. Once insertion site is dry, use sterile gloved hand to apply drain dressing (split gauze) around catheter (see illustration). Tape in place.	Moist skin can cause maceration and breakdown. Dressing collects drainage that develops around catheter insertion site.

STEP	RATIONALE

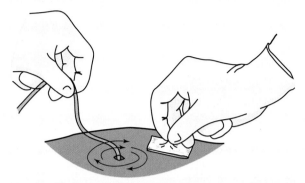

STEP 5b Clean around suprapubic catheter in circular pattern.

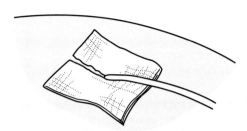

STEP 5d Split drain dressing for suprapubic catheter.

6. Clean insertion site using medical aseptic technique for long-term/established catheter:
   a. Apply clean gloves.
   b. Without creating tension, hold catheter erect with nondominant hand while cleaning. Clean with soap and water in circular motion, starting near catheter insertion site and continuing in outward widening circles for approximately 5 cm (2 inches).
   c. With a fresh washcloth or gauze, gently clean base of catheter, moving up and away from site of insertion (proximal to distal).
   d. *Option:* Apply drain dressing (split gauze) around catheter and tape in place.
7. Secure catheter to lateral abdomen with tape or hook-and-loop fastener multipurpose tube holder.
8. Coil excess tubing on bed. Keep drainage bag below level of bladder at all times.
9. Help patient to a comfortable position.
10. Place nurse call system in an accessible location within patient's reach.
11. Raise side rails (as appropriate) and lower bed to lowest position, locking into position.
12. Dispose of all contaminated supplies in appropriate receptacle, remove and dispose of gloves, and perform hand hygiene.

Rationale column:

Cleaning and drying suprapubic insertion site require general hygienic measures; dressing is an option if drainage is not present.

Removes microorganisms that reside in any drainage that adheres to tubing.

Secures catheter and reduces risk of excessive tension on suture and/or catheter.
Maintains free flow of urine, thus decreasing risk for CAUTI (Siregar et al., 2021).
Restores comfort and sense of well-being.
Ensures patient can call for assistance if needed.

Ensures patient safety and prevents falls.

Reduces transmission of microorganisms. Use appropriate disposal receptacle if patient on hazardous drugs (ONS, 2018).

EVALUATION

1. Ask patient to describe discomfort from suprapubic catheter and rate severity on scale of 0 to 10.
2. Monitor for signs of infection (e.g., fever, elevated white blood count) and observe urine for clarity, sediment, unusual color, or odor.
3. Observe catheter insertion site for erythema, edema, discharge, or tenderness. Check dressing at minimum of every 8 hours.
4. If catheter secured with adhesive device, evaluate for presence of MARSI.
5. **Use Teach-Back:** "I want to be sure I explained clearly about the care of your suprapubic catheter. Tell me about some of the things you need to do to care for it at home." Revise your instruction now or develop a plan for revised patient/family caregiver teaching if patient/family caregiver is not able to teach back correctly.

Rationale column:

Determines if bladder is draining and patient is free of infection.

Suprapubic catheters increase risk for UTI.

Indicators of an insertion site infection.

Determines if patient has sensitivity to adhesive.

Teach-back is a technique for health care providers to ensure that they have explained medical information clearly so that patients and their families understand what is communicated to them (AHRQ, 2023).

STEP	RATIONALE
Unexpected Outcomes	**Related Interventions**
1. Patient develops symptoms of UTI or catheter site infection.	• Increase fluid intake to at least 2200 mL in 24 hours (unless contraindicated). • Monitor vital signs and I&O; observe amount, color, consistency of urine; assess site. • Notify health care provider.
2. Suprapubic catheter becomes dislodged.	• Cover site with sterile dressing. • Notify health care provider. If newly established catheter, it will need to be reinserted immediately.
3. Skin surrounding catheter exit site or adhesive securement device becomes red or irritated and/or develops blisters or open areas.	• Notify health care provider. • Change dressing (if used) more frequently to keep site dry. • Consult with wound care nurse.

Documentation

- Document condition of insertion site, character of urine, type of dressing change, and patient's comfort level with the catheter and dressing change.
- Document urine output on I&O. In a situation in which there is both a suprapubic and a urethral catheter, document outputs from each catheter separately.
- Document your evaluation of patient learning.

Hand-Off Reporting

- Report condition of insertion site, character of urine, type of dressing change, and patient's comfort level with the catheter and dressing change.
- Report any complications with catheter to health care provider.

Special Considerations

Patient Education

- If not contraindicated, encourage patients to consume a minimum of 2200 mL of fluids daily.
- Teach patient to keep the drainage bag lower than the bladder and to keep tubing free of kinks.
- Patients who have suprapubic catheters may shower. Caution against use of creams, powders, or sprays near the catheter insertion site.

Home Care

- Teach patients and/or family caregivers how to clean and apply a dressing (if applicable) using clean technique.
- Caution patients and family caregivers about avoiding the use of powders or creams around the catheter unless specifically instructed to do so.
- Patient or family caregiver will learn how to change a suprapubic catheter every 4 to 6 weeks using sterile technique. Patients with suprapubic catheters should drink 8 to 12 glasses of water every day for a few days after changing a catheter and avoid physical activity for a week or two (Medline Plus, 2021).
- Teach patients and family caregivers how to properly position the drainage bag; empty the urinary drainage bag; and observe urine color, clarity, odor, and amount.
- Arrange for home delivery of catheter supplies, always ensuring that there is at least one extra catheter and drainage bag in the home.
- Teach patient and family caregiver signs of catheter obstruction, UTI, wound infection, and MARSI.
- Consult with health care provider regarding approach to use to clean urinary drainage bag. Typical options include vinegar and water or chlorine bleach and water. Have an extra bag available when cleaning.

✦ CLINICAL JUDGMENT AND NEXT-GENERATION NCLEX® EXAMINATION–STYLE QUESTIONS

A 78-year-old patient is in the preoperative unit preparing for abdominal surgery for a colon tumor. The patient needs to have an indwelling urinary catheter placed. She has an IV line in her right forearm, which is patent and infusing at 80 mL per hour on an intravenous pump. The patient is awake, oriented, and asking questions.

1. Which action will the nurse take **next** to insert the indwelling catheter into the patient after performing hand hygiene and donning gloves?
   1. Lubricate the catheter
   2. Cleanse the urinary meatus
   3. Prepare the sterile field
   4. Place a drape over the patient

2. After surgery, the patient is returned to the medical surgical floor. Indicate whether each nursing action below is indicated or not indicated when attempting to prevent a catheter-associated urinary tract infection (CAUTI) until the catheter is removed.

Nursing Action	Indicated	Not Indicated
Cleanse the urinary meatus with alcohol daily		
Hang the urinary drainage bag above the level of the bladder		
Change the urinary drainage bag daily		
Irrigate the catheter daily with normal saline		
Eliminate any kinking in urinary drainage tubing		
Use sterile technique each time emptying the drainage bag		

3. When assessing the patient one day after surgery, which finding associated with CAUTI will the nurse report to the health care provider? **Select all that apply.**
   1. Temperature 38.9°C (102°F)
   2. Report of dysuria
   3. Hematuria in the urinary drainage bag
   4. Lower abdominal pain
   5. Change in mental status

4. The nurse has delegated specific aspects of care to the assistive personnel (AP). When supervising, which AP action requires the nurse to intervene?
   1. Provides privacy when helping with perineal care
   2. Reports the patient is passing urine that is red in color to the nurse
   3. Applies petroleum jelly to lubricate the catheter tubing for comfort
   4. Obtains the assistance of another AP to help with patient positioning

5. The nurse has completed discharge teaching to the patient who will be returning home with the indwelling catheter in place. Which patient statement requires further nursing teaching?
   1. "I will call my health care provider if I develop a fever."
   2. "Bladder spasms are to be expected while I have this catheter."
   3. "It is important to be sure there is no traction on the tubing."
   4. "Periodically I will need to empty the catheter bag so it does not overfill."

Visit the Evolve site for Answers to Clinical Judgment and Next Generation NCLEX® Examination–Style Questions.

REFERENCES

Agency for Healthcare Research and Quality (AHRQ): *Teach-back: intervention*, Rockville, MD, November 2023, Agency for Healthcare Research and Quality. https://www.ahrq.gov/patient-safety/reports/engage/interventions/teachback.html. Accessed July 29, 2023.

Centers for Disease Control and Prevention (CDC): *Taking a sexual history*, 2020. https://www.cdc.gov/hiv/clinicians/transforming-health/health-care-providers/sexual-history.html. Accessed July 29, 2023.

Centers for Disease Control and Prevention (CDC): *Urinary tract infection (catheter-associated urinary tract infection [CAUTI] and non-catheter-associated urinary tract infection [UTI]) and other urinary system infection [UTI] events*, 2023a. https://www.cdc.gov/nhsn/pdfs/pscManual/7pscCAUTIcurrent.pdf. Accessed July 29, 2023.

Centers for Disease Control and Prevention (CDC): *What is health literacy?*, 2023b. https://www.cdc.gov/healthliteracy/learn/index.html. Accessed July 29, 2023.

Elnady H, et al: Stroke severity is the major player in post-stroke urinary tract infection in patients with first-ever ischemic stroke, *Neurosci Med* 9(2):99, 2018.

Fosnight A: *Urinary health concerns in the trans community*, 2023. https://uqora.info/blogs/learning-center/urinary-health-and-transgender-community. Accessed July 29, 2023.

Fumarola S, et al: Overlooked and underestimated: medical adhesive-related skin injuries. Best practice consensus document on prevention, *J Wound Care* 29(Suppl 3c):S1–S24, 2020.

Gould CV, et al: *Guideline for prevention of catheter-associated urinary tract infections 2019 update*, Healthcare Infection Control Practices Advisory Committee, Update June 2019. https://www.cdc.gov/infectioncontrol/pdf/guidelines/cauti-guidelines-H.pdf. September 29, 2023.

Hockenberry MJ, et al: *Wong's nursing care of infants and children*, ed 12, St. Louis, 2024, Elsevier Health Sciences.

Ignatavicius D, et al. *Medical-surgical nursing: concepts for interprofessional collaborative care*, ed 10, St. Louis, 2021, Elsevier.

Jorgensen S, et al: Risk factors for early return visits to the emergency department in patients with urinary tract infections, *Am J Emerg Med* 36(1):12, 2018.

Lawrence K, et al: The CAUTI prevention tool kit: a professional and collaborative project of the Wound, Ostomy and Continence Nurses Society, *J Wound Ostomy Continence Nurs* 46(2):154, 2019.

Medline Plus: *Suprapubic catheter care*, US National Library of Medicine, 2021. https://medlineplus.gov/ency/patientinstructions/000145.htm. Accessed July 29, 2023.

Murphy C, et al: Managing long term indwelling urinary catheters, *BMJ* 363:k3711, 2018.

Oncology Nurses Society (ONS): *Toolkit for safe handling of hazardous drugs for nurses in oncology*, 2018. https://www.ons.org/sites/default/files/2018-06/ONS_Safe_Handling_Toolkit_0.pdf. Accessed July 29, 2023.

Rea K, et al: A technology intervention for nurses engaged in preventing catheter-associated urinary tract infection, *Comput Inform Nurs* 36(6):305, 2018.

Rogers JL: *McCance & Huether's Pathophysiology. The biologic basis for disease in adults and children*, ed 9, St. Louis, 2023, Elsevier.

Shadle H, et al: A bundle-based approach to prevent catheter-associated urinary tract infections in the Intensive Care Unit, *Crit Care Nurse* 41(2):62–71, 2021.

Sinha A, et al: Condom catheter induced penile erosion, *J Surg Case Rep* 10:275, 2018.

Siregar S, et al: Strategies for preventing catheter-associated urinary tract infection in pediatric: a systematic review, *Int Med J* 28(4):411–416, 2021.

Tollinche LE, et al: Perioperative care of the transgender patient, *Anesth Analg* 127(2):359–366, 2018.

Touhy TA, Jett KF: *Ebersole and Hess' gerontological nursing and healthy aging*, ed 6, St. Louis, 2022, Elsevier.

Tremayne P, Pawlyn J: Care and management of indwelling urinary catheters, *Learn Disabil Pract* (In Press), 2019.

The Joint Commission (TJC): *2023 National patient safety goals*, Oakbrook Terrace, IL, 2023, The Joint Commission. https://www.jointcommission.org/standards/national-patient-safety-goals/Accessed July 29, 2023.

Waterschoot M, et al: Treatment of Urethral Strictures in Transmasculine Patients, *J Clin Med* 10(17):3912, 2021.

SKILLS AND PROCEDURES

Procedural Guideline 34.1 **Providing and Positioning a Bedpan, p. 1020**

Procedural Guideline 34.2 **Removing Fecal Impaction Digitally, p. 1022**

Skill 34.1 **Administering an Enema, p. 1024**

Skill 34.2 **Insertion, Maintenance, and Removal of a Nasogastric Tube for Gastric Decompression, p. 1029**

OBJECTIVES

Mastery of content in this chapter will enable you to:

- Compare factors that promote and impede normal bowel elimination.
- Discuss methods to relieve constipation or impaction.
- Identify precautions to follow when administering an enema.

- Analyze approaches for managing a patient's comfort during nasogastric (NG) tube insertion.
- Apply clinical judgment to perform the following skills: helping a patient use a bedpan, removing a fecal impaction, administering an enema, and inserting and removing an NG tube.

MEDIA RESOURCES

- http://evolve.elsevier.com/Perry/skills
- Review Questions
- Audio Glossary
- ▶ Video Clips
- NSO Nursing Skills Online

- Case Studies
- Answers to Clinical Judgment and Next-Generation NCLEX® Examination–Style Questions
- Skills Performance Checklists
- Printable Key Points

PURPOSE

Regular elimination of bowel waste products is essential for normal body functioning. Alterations in bowel elimination often indicate early signs, symptoms, or problems in the gastrointestinal (GI) system or other body systems (National Institutes of Health [NIH] National Institute of Diabetes and Digestive Kidney Diseases [NIDDK], 2018). A patient's lifestyle patterns, food and fluid intake, medications, functional status, and chronic conditions influence bowel function. To manage a patient's bowel elimination problems, you need to understand factors that promote, impede, or alter normal bowel elimination.

Patients may require your help to meet bowel elimination needs such as toileting or using a bedpan. Privacy needs related to bowel elimination must be considered, and patients may have culturally sensitive needs that must be respected. If a patient is constipated, you may instruct the patient in increasing fluid intake or adding fiber to the diet or administer medications or enemas. If a fecal impaction is present, it may be necessary to digitally remove impacted stool. If severe or chronic diarrhea exists, medications, containment products, and close attention to skin protection are needed. After abdominal surgery, an alteration in peristalsis or movement of fluid through the GI tract may cause a condition called an ileus, which in turn causes abdominal distention, nausea, and vomiting. The stomach does not empty properly, and a nasogastric (NG) tube may need to be inserted. Other conditions such as obstruction in the intestinal tract may also necessitate NG tube insertion.

PRACTICE STANDARDS

- Fumarola S, et al., 2020: Overlooked and Underestimated: Medical Adhesive-Related Skin Injuries—Prevention of medical adhesive–related skin injuries
- National Institutes of Health (NIH) National Institute of Diabetes and Digestive and Kidney Diseases (NIDDK), 2018: Constipation
- Ermer-Seltun J, Engberg S, 2022: Wound, Ostomy and Continence Nurses Society (WOCN) Core Curriculum: Continence Management—Continence management
- The Joint Commission (TJC), 2023—National Patient Safety Goals—Patient identification

PRINCIPLES OF PRACTICE

- Constipation is a functional GI symptom and not a disease. It is defined as infrequent or fewer than three bowel movements per week of hard lumpy stool. It is seen in all age-groups and is frequently encountered in clinical practice (Box 34.1). Approximately 30% of people encounter constipation during their lifetime; older adults are most affected (NIDDK, 2018). Constipation is often seen in patients with neurological illnesses, impaired mobility, and sensory deficits.

Common Causes of Constipation

- Irregular bowel habits and ignoring the urge to defecate
- Chronic illnesses (e.g., Parkinson disease, multiple sclerosis, rheumatoid arthritis, chronic bowel diseases, depression, eating disorders)
- Low-fiber diet high in animal fats (e.g., meats and carbohydrates); low fluid intake
- Stress (e.g., illness of a family member, death of a loved one, divorce)
- Physical inactivity
- Medications, especially use of opiates
- Changes in life or routine such as pregnancy, aging, and travel
- Neurological conditions that block nerve impulses to the colon (e.g., stroke, spinal cord injury, tumor)
- Chronic bowel dysfunction (e.g., colonic inertia, irritable bowel)

- Constipation occurs frequently in patients taking opioid medications. Opioids stimulate μ opioid receptors, which induce analgesia. However, activation of these receptors reduces gastric emptying; increases pyloric, anal, and biliary sphincter tone; reduces biliary track secretions; and increases water absorption from the bowel. All of these factors greatly increase the risk of constipation (Viscusi, 2019).
- Patients with diarrhea need frequent observation of their perineal and perianal skin. Skin barrier creams may be needed to protect from the enzymatic quality of liquid stools.
- There are also fecal-management systems available for short-term use with high-volume diarrhea. They are intended for use primarily in acute care settings. The devices have an intra-anal soft silicone catheter with a retention balloon, much like a Foley catheter, for insertion into the rectal vault to divert liquid stool away from the skin in immobilized patients. The catheter is connected to a drainage bag for collection of liquid fecal effluent. Strict adherence to manufacturer's instructions and application by competent health care providers are essential when using these devices (Ermer-Seltun & Enberg, 2022).
- Postoperative ileus or obstruction in the intestinal tract, with or without nausea and/or vomiting, may necessitate NG tube insertion to empty the stomach. This relieves abdominal distention but may cause patient discomfort, increased recovery time, and increased length of stay.

PERSON-CENTERED CARE

- Show respect for a patient's privacy, provide necessary comfort and hygiene measures, and attend to the patient's emotional needs when performing required skills.
- Determine patient's normal pattern of bowel elimination and accommodate that pattern while the patient is in a health care setting. Determine the time a patient normally has a bowel movement and the amount of help needed.
- There may be cultural considerations related to bowel elimination. Encourage the patient to express these concerns and make any accommodation that is possible in the health care setting.
- Design and follow individualized bowel management protocols to reduce patient's risk for constipation and diarrhea secondary to the illness process, medications, and/or lack of activity.
- Consider developmental changes that affect bowel functioning throughout the life span. For example, an older adult who becomes less active and has decreased muscle tone and changes in eating patterns is at higher risk for experiencing constipation

(Huether & McCance, 2020). Constipation in children may be due to anorectal malformation or to neurological lesions such as in spina bifida, or it may be classified as functional. Ninety-five percent of children with constipation have the latter; the causes may be developmental, behavioral, or psychological (Ermer-Seltun & Engberg, 2022). Careful evaluation must be done to determine a treatment plan.

EVIDENCE-BASED PRACTICE

Nasogastric Tube Placement

NG tubes continue to be an essential intervention in the care of patients who have undergone surgery or those with GI conditions that affect peristalsis. Research studies continue to investigate methods to correctly verify NG tube placement. This is crucial to avoid tube position complications, and nurses must be aware of best practices to ensure the effectiveness of placement and patient safety. The following placement considerations can be used to assess NG placement:

- Radiographic verification of placement of the tube immediately following insertion is the gold standard and provides for a clear and measurable placement of the tube (Nihal & Dilek, 2022; Judd, 2020; Powers et al., 2021).
- Aspiration of gastric contents and measured pH of 5 or lower are likewise used in subsequent verifications of tube placement (Judd, 2020).
- Researchers have found that gastric pH usually falls within a range from 1 to 5, whereas intestinal or respiratory pH is usually 6 or higher. Therefore, aspirates with pH of 5 or lower would likely indicate a gastric placement (Judd, 2020).
- Auscultation to determine tube placement has been proved to be unreliable in multiple studies (Gardner & Wallace, 2021; Judd, 2020).

SAFETY GUIDELINES

- Promote comfort when a patient uses a bedpan. Encourage patient to use the bathroom when able.
- Answer the nurse call system promptly to prevent a patient from attempting to get out of bed without help. This is a common factor related to patient falls. If a patient is at high risk for falls, especially if cognitively impaired, the bedside commode should not be left within reach so the patient will be less likely to attempt to try to get on the commode without assistance.
- Patients with cognitive, sensory, and/or motor deficits are prone to constipation. Place them on an individualized bowel training schedule and offer help with toileting at recommended intervals (Ermer-Seltun & Engberg, 2022).
- When digital removal of impacted fecal material is ordered, obtain patient baseline vital signs and periodically monitor heart rate during the procedure. Digital removal of fecal impaction stimulates the vagus nerve, which can cause a decrease in heart rate (Ermer-Seltun & Engberg, 2022).
- Follow agency policies to verify correct placement of NG tubes, which include radiographic verification after insertion and subsequent pH verification (pH ≤5).
- When a patient with an NG tube complains of nausea or vomits, assess both placement and patency of tube. Reposition and irrigate tube as needed.
- Check suction on an NG tube to be sure it is set on intermittent at the beginning of each shift and whenever the patient returns to the room and is reconnected to suction if the tube has been clamped for ambulation or transportation to another part of the

hospital for a procedure. Intermittent suction should be maintained, as continuous suction could damage the tissue that lines the stomach or small intestine (Judd, 2020).

- Pressure from an NG tube applied to the mucous membranes lining the nares can cause medical device–related pressure injuries (MDRPIs) (Fumarola et al., 2020). Tube fixation

methods that remove pressure from the nares help to reduce the risk for MDRPI. Conduct routine and ongoing assessment of nares and secondary pressure sites underlying medical devices, and implement skin-care practices such a taping method to reduce risk for MDRPI (Seong et al., 2021; Stellar et al., 2020).

PROCEDURAL GUIDELINE 34.1 *Providing and Positioning a Bedpan*

A patient restricted to bed must use a bedpan for bowel elimination. Two types of bedpans are available (Fig. 34.1). The regular and most commonly used bedpan has a curved, smooth upper end and a tapered lower end. The upper end (wide end) of the regular pan fits under a patient's buttocks toward the sacrum, with the lower end (tapered end) fitting just under the upper thighs toward the foot of the bed. A fracture pan, designed for patients with body or leg casts or those who are restricted from raising their hips (e.g., following total hip joint replacement), slips easily under a patient. The shallow upper end of the pan with a flat, wide rim fits under a patient's buttocks toward the sacrum, with the deep and lower open end toward the foot of the bed.

Delegation
The skill of providing a bedpan can be delegated to assistive personnel (AP). Instruct the AP to:

- Correctly position patients with mobility restrictions or those who have therapeutic equipment such as wound drains, intravenous (IV) catheters, or traction
- Provide perineal and hand hygiene for patient as necessary after use of a bedpan
- Report to the nurse stool color and characteristics, perianal skin integrity, and patient tolerance

Equipment
Clean gloves; bedpan (regular or fracture); bedpan cover; toilet tissue or premoisturized perineal wipes; specimen container (if necessary); plastic bag clearly labeled with date, patient's name, and identification number; basin; washcloths; towels; soap; waterproof absorbent pads (if necessary)

Steps
1. Assess patient's normal bowel elimination habits: routine pattern, character of stool, effect of certain foods or fluids and eating habits on bowel elimination, effect of stress and level of activity on normal bowel elimination patterns, current medications, and normal fluid intake.
2. Determine need for stool specimen prior to bedpan use.
3. Perform hand hygiene.
4. Assess patient to determine level of mobility, including ability to sit upright and lift hips or turn.

5. Assess patient's level of comfort. Ask about presence of rectal or abdominal pain, presence of hemorrhoids, or irritation of skin surrounding anus.
6. Provide privacy by closing curtains around bed or door of room.
7. Apply clean gloves. Inspect condition of perianal and perineal skin. Remove gloves and perform hand hygiene.

Clinical Judgment *Use a fracture pan if the patient had a total hip replacement. An abduction pillow must be placed between the legs when turning patient to prevent dislocation of new joint.*

8. For patient comfort, prepare metal bedpan by running warm water over it for a few minutes.
9. Apply clean gloves.
10. Raise side rail on opposite side of bed.
11. Raise bed horizontally according to your height.
12. Assist patient to the supine position.
13. Place patient who can assist on bedpan.
    a. Raise head of patient's bed 30 to 60 degrees.
    b. Remove upper bed linens so they are out of the way, but do not expose patient.
    c. Have patient flex knees and lift hips upward.
    d. Place hand closest to patient's head palm up under patient's sacrum to help lift. Ask patient to bend knees and raise hips. As patient raises hips, use other hand to slip bedpan under the patient (see illustration). Be sure that open rim of bedpan is facing toward foot of bed. Do not force bedpan under patient's knees (see illustration).

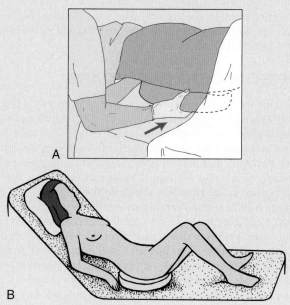

STEP 13d (A) Placing bedpan under patient's hips. (B) Correct positioning for placing mobile patient on bedpan.

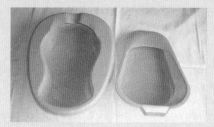

FIG. 34.1 Types of bedpans. *Left,* Regular bedpan. *Right,* Fracture bedpan.

PROCEDURAL GUIDELINE 34.1 *Providing and Positioning a Bedpan—cont'd*

    e. *Optional:* If using fracture pan, slip it under patient as hips are raised (see illustration). Be sure that deep, open, lower end of bedpan is facing toward foot of bed.

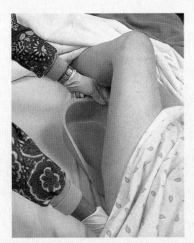

STEP 13e Patient lifts hips as fracture pan is positioned.

14. Place patient who is immobile or has mobility restrictions on bedpan.
    a. Lower head of bed flat or raise head slightly (if tolerated by medical condition).
    b. Remove top linens as necessary to turn patient while minimizing exposure.
    c. Assist patient to roll onto side with back toward you. Place bedpan firmly against patient's buttocks and down into mattress. Be sure that open rim of bedpan is facing toward foot of bed (see illustrations).
    d. Keep one hand against bedpan; place other hand around far hip of patient. Help patient to roll back onto bedpan, flat in bed. Do not force pan under patient.
    e. Raise patient's head 30 degrees or to a comfortable level (unless contraindicated).
    f. Have patient bend knees (unless contraindicated).
15. Maintain patient's comfort, privacy, and safety. Cover patient for warmth. Place small pillow or rolled towel under lumbar curve of back.
16. Place nurse call system in an accessible location within patient's reach. Ensure toilet tissue is within reach for patient.
17. Raise side rails (as appropriate) and lower bed to lowest position, locking into position.
18. Remove and dispose of supplies and gloves and perform hand hygiene.
19. Leave the room. Allow patient to be alone but monitor status and respond promptly.
20. Remove bedpan:
    a. Perform hand hygiene and apply clean gloves.
    b. Maintain privacy; determine if patient is able to wipe own perineal area. If you clean perineal area, use clean gloves and several layers of toilet tissue or disposable washcloths. For female patients, clean from mons pubis toward rectal area.

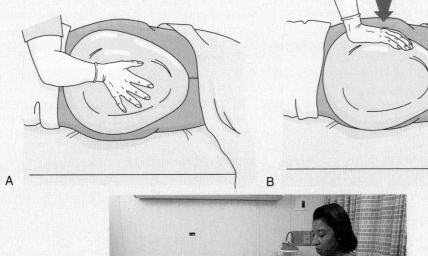

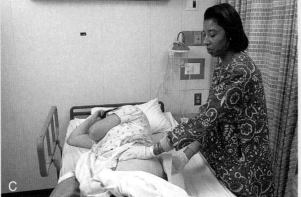

STEP 14c (A) Position patient on one side and place bedpan firmly against buttocks. (B) Push down on bedpan and toward patient. (C) Nurse places bedpan in position. (*A and B from Sorrentino SA: Mosby's textbook for nursing assistants, ed 7, St Louis, 2009, Mosby.*)

Continued

PROCEDURAL GUIDELINE 34.1 *Providing and Positioning a Bedpan—cont'd*

c. Deposit contaminated tissue in bedpan if no specimen or intake and output (I&O) is needed.

d. **For mobile patient:** Ask patient to flex knees, placing body weight on lower legs, feet, and upper torso; lift buttocks up from bedpan. At same time, place hand farther from patient on side of bedpan to support it (prevent spillage), and place other hand (closer to patient) under sacrum to help lift. Have patient lift and remove bedpan.

e. **For immobile patient:** Lower head of bed. Help patient roll onto side away from you and off bedpan. Hold bedpan flat and steady while patient is rolling off; otherwise, spillage will occur. Place bedpan on draped bedside chair, and cover.

f. Assist patient with hand and perineal hygiene as needed.

g. Change soiled linens, remove and dispose of gloves, perform hand hygiene, and return patient to comfortable position.

h. Raise side rails (as appropriate) and lower bed to lowest position, locking into position.

i. Place nurse call system in an accessible location within patient's reach.

j. Place drinking water and desired personal items within easy access.

21. *Option:* Obtain stool specimen as ordered. Wear clean gloves when emptying contents of bedpan into toilet or in special receptacle in utility room. Use spray faucet attached to most institution toilets to rinse bedpan thoroughly. Use disinfectant if required by agency; store pan. Remove and dispose of gloves. Perform hand hygiene.

22. **Use Teach-Back:** "Since your leg is immobilized, I want to make sure you're comfortable getting off and on the bedpan by using the trapeze to pull your torso off the bed. Show me how you use the trapeze to move your torso." Revise your instruction now or develop a plan for revised patient/family caregiver teaching if patient/family caregiver is not able to teach back correctly. Teach-back is a technique for health care providers to ensure that they have explained medical information clearly so that patients and their families understand what is communicated to them (Agency for Healthcare Research and Quality [AHRQ], 2023).

23. Assess and document characteristics of stool. Note color, odor, consistency, frequency, amount, shape, and constituents.

24. Include hand-off report if patient voided in bedpan. Report any skin irritation, discoloration, or break in skin integrity noted when cleansing patient.

PROCEDURAL GUIDELINE 34.2 *Removing Fecal Impaction Digitally*

Fecal impaction is the inability to pass a collection of hard stool. This condition occurs in all age-groups. Physically and mentally incapacitated individuals and institutionalized older adults are at greatest risk. Patients with acute stroke and spinal cord injuries are also at greater risk for fecal impaction.

Functional constipation includes a group of disorders associated with persistent, difficult, infrequent, or seemingly incomplete defecation without evidence of a structural or biochemical explanation (Sood, 2023). Ask patients to describe the characteristics of the stools; whether the quality is normally watery or formed, soft or hard; and the typical color. Ask the patient to describe the shape of a normal stool and the number of stools per day. Use a scale such as the Bristol Stool Form Scale to get an objective measure of stool characteristics (Fig. 34.2).

Symptoms of fecal impaction include constipation, rectal discomfort, anorexia, nausea, vomiting, abdominal pain, abdominal bloating, small liquid stools (leaking around the impacted stool), and urinary frequency. Prevention is the key to managing fecal impaction. With newer bowel management techniques such as safe long-term use of osmotic laxatives, which pull fluid into the stool and soften it, or transanal irrigation for patients with a neurogenic motility impairment, the need for regular digital removal of fecal material has been reduced. However, once impaction has occurred, digital removal of stool is the only alternative (Ermer-Seltun & Engberg, 2022).

Intra-anal catheters may be inserted in an adult patient with a large volume of liquid stool to contain the output and protect the perianal skin. These devices are used in hospitalized patients and should be inserted with strict adherence to the manufacturer's instructions. The insertion should be done by an experienced caregiver trained in use of the device; in some patients this device is contraindicated (Ermer-Seltun & Engberg, 2022) (Box 34.2).

Delegation

The skill of removing a fecal impaction digitally cannot be delegated to assistive personnel (AP). Instruct the AP to:
- Assist in positioning a patient for the procedure, and monitor heart rate as nurse removes impaction
- Provide perineal care following each bowel movement

Interprofessional Collaboration
- Include health care team members in planning bowel management program to avoid further fecal impactions.

Equipment
Bedpan, waterproof pad, water-soluble lubricant, washcloths, towels, soap, and clean gloves

Steps
1. Identify patient using at least two identifiers (e.g., name and birthday or name and medical record number) according to agency policy (TJC, 2023).
2. Assess patient's/family caregiver's health literacy (Centers for Disease Control and Prevention [CDC], 2023).
3. Perform hand hygiene, pull curtains around bed, obtain patient's baseline vital signs and assess level of comfort, and palpate for abdominal distention before the procedure.
4. Explain the procedure and help patient lie on left side in the lateral position with knees flexed and back toward you.

PROCEDURAL GUIDELINE 34.2 *Removing Fecal Impaction Digitally—cont'd*

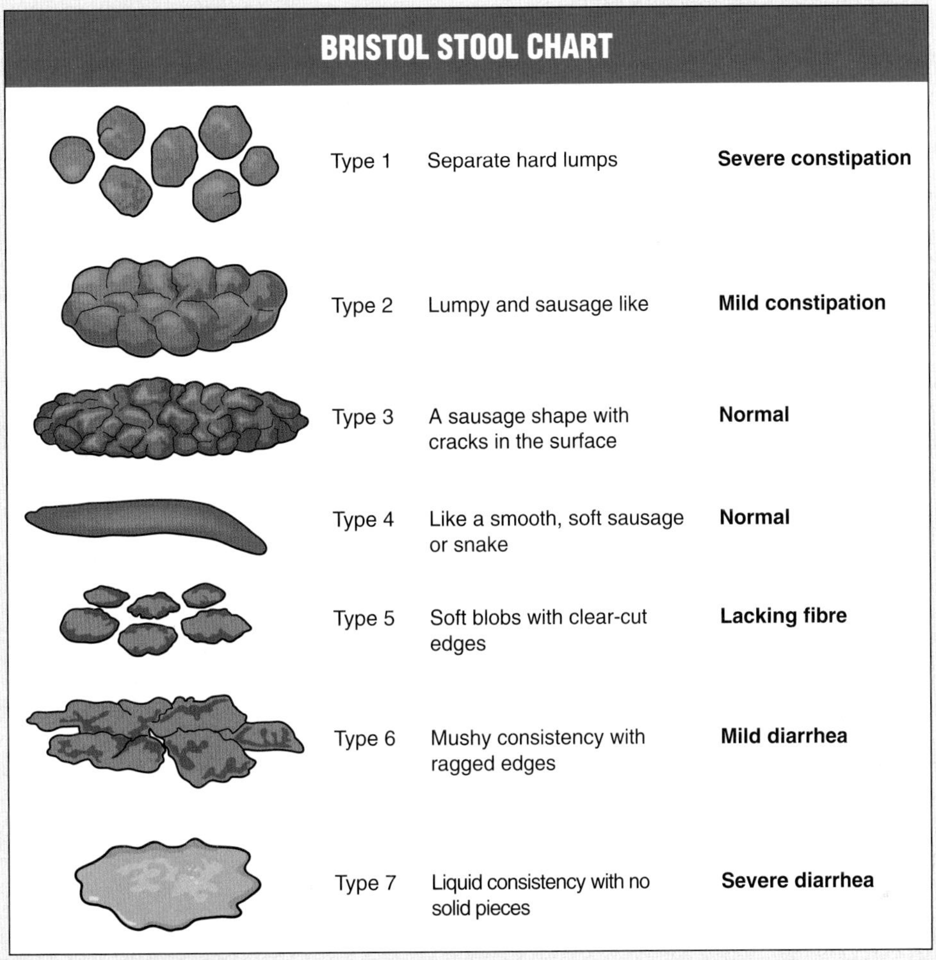

BRISTOL STOOL CHART

	Type 1	Separate hard lumps	**Severe constipation**
	Type 2	Lumpy and sausage like	**Mild constipation**
	Type 3	A sausage shape with cracks in the surface	**Normal**
	Type 4	Like a smooth, soft sausage or snake	**Normal**
	Type 5	Soft blobs with clear-cut edges	**Lacking fibre**
	Type 6	Mushy consistency with ragged edges	**Mild diarrhea**
	Type 7	Liquid consistency with no solid pieces	**Severe diarrhea**

FIG. 34.2 Bristol Stool Form Scale. *(From Scheibel P, et al:* Diagnosis in primary care, *ed 6, St. Louis, 2020, Elsevier.)*

BOX 34.2

Contraindications for Use of Internal Bowel Management Systems

- Known sensitivity or allergy to any of the components of the device
- Clotting disorders
- History of rectal or anal surgery in the last year
- Rectal or anal injury, incompetent sphincter, severe hemorrhoids, fecal impaction, rectal tumor, severe stricture or stenosis
- Rectal mucosal impairment, severe proctitis, ischemic proctitis, active inflammatory bowel disease

Clinical Judgment *Many older adults are especially prone to dysrhythmias and other problems related to vagal stimulation; monitor heart rate and rhythm closely (Ball et al., 2023).*

5. Apply clean gloves. Drape trunk and lower extremities with a bath blanket and place a waterproof pad under buttocks. Keep a bedpan next to patient.
6. Lubricate index finger of dominant hand with water-soluble lubricant.

7. Instruct patient to take slow, deep breaths. Gradually and gently insert index finger into the rectum and advance the finger slowly along the rectal wall.
8. Gently loosen the fecal mass by massaging around it. Work the finger into the hardened mass.
9. Work the feces downward toward the end of the rectum. Remove small pieces one at a time and discard into bedpan.
10. Periodically reassess patient's pulse and look for signs of fatigue. Stop the procedure if pulse rate drops significantly (check agency policy) or rhythm changes.
11. Continue to clear rectum of feces and allow patient to rest at intervals.
12. After completion, wash and dry buttocks and anal area.
13. Remove bedpan; inspect feces for color and consistency. Dispose of feces. Remove gloves by turning them inside out and then discard.
14. Help patient to toilet or onto a bedpan if urge to defecate develops (return to bedside to remove bedpan or return to assist patient back to bed).
15. Perform hand hygiene.
16. Follow procedure with enemas or cathartics as ordered by health care provider.

Continued

PROCEDURAL GUIDELINE 34.2 *Removing Fecal Impaction Digitally—cont'd*

17. Help patient to a comfortable position. Reassess patient's vital signs and level of comfort and observe status of abdominal distention.
18. Place nurse call system in an accessible location within patient's reach.
19. Raise side rails (as appropriate) and lower bed to lowest position, locking into position.
20. **Use Teach-Back:** "I want to make sure you include the high-fiber foods and fluids we recommended for your diet to help increase the passage of stool. Tell me which foods you will add to your diet." Revise your instruction now or

develop a plan for revised patient/family caregiver teaching if patient/family caregiver is not able to teach back correctly. Teach-back is a technique for health care providers to ensure that they have explained medical information clearly so that patients and their families understand what is communicated to them (AHRQ, 2023).
21. Document patient's tolerance of procedure, fecal characteristics, amount of stool removed, vital signs, and adverse effects.
22. Report any changes in vital signs and adverse effects to health care provider.

◆ SKILL 34.1   Administering an Enema

 Video Clip

An enema is the instillation of a solution into the rectum and sigmoid colon to promote defecation by stimulating peristalsis. Although first-line recommendations include dietary changes, bulk-forming laxatives, and non–bulk-forming laxatives to treat constipation, an enema may be prescribed for immediate relief. Other reasons to give an enema may be to prepare a patient for surgery or diagnostic procedures (Caffrey & Pensa, 2019). Table 34.1 describes common types of enemas. They act by stimulating peristalsis through infusion of large volumes of solution. Oil-retention enemas act by lubricating the rectum and colon, allowing feces to absorb oil and become softer and easier to pass.

Medicated enemas contain pharmacological therapeutic agents. Some are prescribed to reduce dangerously high serum potassium levels (e.g., sodium polystyrene sulfonate enema) or to reduce bacteria in the colon before bowel surgery (e.g., neomycin enema).

Delegation

The skill of administering an enema can be delegated to assistive personnel (AP) in some agencies. Check policy before delegating. **NOTE:** If a medicated enema is ordered, then it must be administered by a nurse. Instruct the AP to:
- Properly position patients who have mobility restrictions or therapeutic equipment such as drains, intravenous (IV) catheters, or traction
- Inform the nurse immediately about patient's new abdominal pain (*Exception:* a patient reports cramping) or rectal bleeding
- Inform the nurse immediately about the presence of blood in the stool or around the rectal area or any change in vital signs

Equipment

- Clean gloves
- Water-soluble local anesthetic lubricant (**NOTE:** Some agencies require use of water-soluble lubricant without anesthetic when nurse performs procedure.)

TABLE 34.1

Types of Enemas

Type of Enema	Description and Implications
Tap-water (hypotonic) enema	Large volume stimulates peristalsis. Do not repeat after first instillation because water toxicity or circulatory overload can develop.
Physiological normal saline	Safest enema to administer. Infants and children can tolerate only this type because of their predisposition to fluid imbalance.
Hypertonic solution	Useful for patients who cannot tolerate large volumes of fluid.
Harris flush enema	A return-flow enema that helps to expel intestinal gas. Administer small amount (100–200 mL) of enema solution into patient's rectum and colon. Lower the enema container to allow the total volume of solution to flow back. The repeated back-and-forth administration and return of the fluid reduces flatus and promotes return of peristalsis.
Soapsuds enema (SSE)	Pure castile soap added to either tap water or normal saline. Use only pure castile soap. Recommended ratio of pure soap to solution is 5 mL (1 teaspoon) to 1000 mL (1 quart) warm water or saline. Add soap to enema bag after water is in place to reduce excessive suds.
Oil-retention enema	Oil-based solution. The colon absorbs a small volume, which softens stool for easier evacuation.
Other enemas—follow health care provider order and agency policy in giving these	Carminative—relieves gaseous distention. Example: MGW solution, which contains 30 mL of magnesium, 60 mL of glycerin, and 90 mL of water Milk and molasses Medication administration as prescribed by health care provider, such as sodium polystyrene sulfate to lower serum potassium level

- Waterproof, absorbent pads
- Bedpan
- Bedpan cover (optional if available)
- Bath blanket
- Washbasin, washcloths, towels, and soap

Enema Bag Administration

- Enema container
- IV pole
- Tubing and clamp (if not already attached to container)
- Appropriate-size rectal tube (adult, 22–30 Fr; child, 12–18 Fr)
- Correct volume of warmed (tepid) solution (adult, 750–1000 mL; 11 years, 480–720 mL; 4–10 years, 360–480 mL; 2–4 years, 240–360 mL; infant, 120–240 mL) (Hockenberry et al., 2024)

Prepackaged Enema

- Prepackaged enema container with lubricated rectal tip (Fig. 34.3)

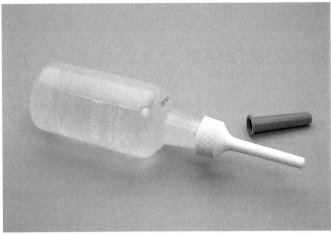

FIG. 34.3 Prepackaged enema container with rectal tip and cap.

STEP	RATIONALE

ASSESSMENT

1. Identify patient using at least two identifiers (e.g., name and birthday or name and medical record number) according to agency policy.

Ensures correct patient. Complies with The Joint Commission standards and improves patient safety (TJC, 2023).

2. Review health care provider's order for enema and clarify reason for administration.

Order by health care provider is usually required for hospitalized patient. Order states the number and type of enema patient will receive.

3. Assess patient's/family caregiver's health literacy.

Determines degree to which individuals have the ability to find, understand, and use information and services to make informed health-related decisions and actions for themselves and others (CDC, 2023).

4. Check electronic health record (EHR) to assess last bowel movement, normal versus most recent bowel pattern, presence of hemorrhoids, and presence of abdominal pain or cramping.

Determines need for enema and type of enema used. Also establishes baseline for bowel function. Hemorrhoids may obscure rectal opening and cause discomfort or bleeding during evacuation.

5. Assess patient's mobility and ability to turn and position on side.

Determines if assistance is needed for positioning patient.

6. Assess patient for allergy to any active ingredients of prepackaged enema.

Reduces risk for allergic reaction.

7. Perform hand hygiene.

Reduces transmission of microorganisms.

8. Inspect and palpate abdomen for presence of distention.

Establishes assessment baseline prior to enema administration.

9. Assess patient's knowledge, prior experience with enemas, and feelings about procedure.

Reveals need for patient instruction and/or support.

Clinical Judgment *When "enemas until clear" is ordered, the water expelled may be tinted but should not contain solid fecal material. It is essential to observe contents of solution passed. Check agency policy, but a patient should receive only three consecutive enemas to prevent fluid and electrolyte imbalance.*

PLANNING

1. Expected outcomes following completion of procedure:
   - Stool is evacuated.
   - Enema return is clear.
   - Abdomen is flat and nontender, with no distention.

Solution clears rectum and lower colon of stool.
Indicates all solid fecal material in colon has passed.

2. Explain enema administration procedure to patient and/or caregiver. Provide privacy and perform hand hygiene.

Decreases patient anxiety and promotes patient cooperation. Reduces transmission of microorganisms.

3. Arrange supplies at bedside. Place bedpan or bedside commode in easily accessible position. If patient will be expelling contents in toilet, ensure that toilet is available and place patient's nonskid slippers and bathrobe in easily accessible position.

Bedpan is used if patient is unable to get out of bed. Nonskid slippers help prevent falls.

STEP	RATIONALE

IMPLEMENTATION

1. Check accuracy and completeness of each medication administration record (MAR) with health care provider's written order. Check patient's name, type of enema, and time for administration. Compare MAR with label of enema solution.

The health care provider's order is most reliable source and only legal record of drugs or procedure that patient is to receive. Ensures that patient receives correct enema.

2. Perform hand hygiene. Apply clean gloves.

Reduces transmission of microorganisms.

3. With side rail raised on patient's right side and bed raised to appropriate working height, help patient turn onto left side-lying position with right knee flexed. Determine that patient is comfortable and encourage patient to remain in position until procedure is complete. **NOTE:** Place a child in the dorsal recumbent position.

Allows enema solution to flow downward by gravity along natural curve of sigmoid colon and rectum, thus improving retention of solution.

Clinical Judgment *Patients with poor sphincter control require placement of a bedpan under the buttocks. Administering enema with patient sitting on toilet is unsafe because curved rectal tubing can abrade rectal wall.*

4. Place waterproof pad, absorbent side up, under hips and buttocks. Cover patient with bath blanket, exposing only rectal area, clearly visualizing anus.

Pad prevents soiling of linen. Blanket provides warmth, reduces exposure of body parts, and allows patient to feel more relaxed and comfortable.

5. Separate buttocks and examine perianal region for abnormalities, including hemorrhoids, anal fissure, and rectal prolapse.

Findings influence approach for inserting enema tip. Prolapse contraindicates enema.

6. Administer enema. Verbalize to the patient when you will be touching their buttocks and inserting the enema tubing.
   a. Administer prepackaged disposable enema:
      (1) Remove plastic cap from tip of container. Tip may already be lubricated. Apply more water-soluble lubricant as needed (see Fig. 34.3).

Lubrication provides for smooth insertion of rectal tube without causing rectal irritation or trauma. With presence of hemorrhoids, extra lubricant provides added comfort.

      (2) Gently separate buttocks and locate anus. Instruct patient to relax by breathing out slowly through mouth. Inform patient when tip is to be inserted.

Breathing out promotes relaxation of external rectal sphincter.

      (3) Hold container upright and expel any air from enema container.

Introducing air into colon causes further distention and discomfort.

      (4) Insert lubricated tip of container gently into anal canal toward umbilicus (see illustration).
      Adult: 7.5–10 cm (3–4 inches)
      Adolescent: 7.5 cm–10 cm (3–4 inches)
      Child: 5–7.5 cm (2–3 inches)
      Infant: 2.5–3.75 cm (1–1½ inches)

Gentle insertion prevents trauma to rectal mucosa.

Clinical Judgment *If pain occurs or you feel resistance at any time during procedure, stop and discuss with health care provider. Do not force insertion.*

      (5) Squeeze and roll plastic bottle from bottom to tip until all of solution has entered rectum and colon. Instruct patient to retain solution until urge to defecate occurs, usually in 2 to 5 minutes.

Prevents instillation of air into colon and ensures that all content enters rectum. Hypertonic solutions require only small volumes to stimulate defecation.

   b. Administer enema in standard enema bag:
      (1) Add warmed prescribed type of solution and amount to enema bag. Warm tap water as it flows from faucet. Place saline container in basin of warm water before adding saline to enema bag. Check temperature of solution by pouring small amount of solution over inner wrist.

Hot water burns intestinal mucosa. Cold water causes abdominal cramping and is difficult to retain.

      (2) If soapsuds enema (SSE) is ordered, add castile soap after water.

Reduces suds in enema bag.

      (3) Raise container, release clamp, and allow solution to flow long enough to fill tubing.

Removes air from tubing.

      (4) Reclamp tubing.

Prevents further loss of solution.

      (5) Lubricate 6–8 cm (2½–3 inches) of tip of rectal tube with lubricant.

Allows smooth insertion of rectal tube without risk for irritation or trauma to mucosa.

STEP	RATIONALE

(6) Gently separate buttocks and locate anus. Verbalize when enema tip will be inserted. Instruct patient to relax by breathing out slowly through mouth. Touch patient's skin next to anus with tip of rectal tube.

Breathing out and touching of skin with tube promote relaxation of external anal sphincter.

(7) Insert tip of rectal tube slowly by pointing it in direction of patient's umbilicus. Length of insertion varies (see Step 6a[4]).

Careful insertion prevents trauma to rectal mucosa from accidental lodging of tube against rectal wall. Insertion beyond proper limit can cause bowel perforation.

Clinical Judgment *If tube does not pass easily, do not force. Consider allowing a small amount of fluid to infuse, and then try to reinsert the tube slowly. The instillation of fluid relaxes the sphincter and provides additional lubrication. If fecal impaction is present, remove it before administering the enema.*

(8) Hold tubing in rectum constantly until end of fluid instillation.

Prevents expulsion of rectal tube during bowel contractions.

(9) Open regulating clamp and allow solution to enter slowly with container at patient's hip level.

Rapid infusion stimulates evacuation of tubing and can cause cramping.

(10) Raise height of enema container slowly to appropriate level above anus: 30–45 cm (12–18 inches) for high enema; 30 cm (12 inches) for regular enema (see illustration); 7.5 cm (3 inches) for low enema. Instillation time varies with volume of solution administered (e.g., 1 L may take 10 minutes). You may use an IV pole to hold an enema bag once you have established a slow flow of fluid.

Allows for continuous, slow instillation of solution. Raising container too high causes rapid instillation and possible painful distention of colon. High pressure can result in bowel rupture.

Clinical Judgment *Temporary cessation of infusion minimizes cramping and promotes ability to retain solution. Lower container or clamp tubing if patient complains of cramping or if fluid escapes around rectal tube.*

(11) Instill all solution, and clamp tubing. Tell patient that procedure is completed and that you will remove tubing.

Prevents entrance of air into rectum. Patients may misinterpret sensation of removing tube as loss of control.

7. Place layers of toilet tissue around tube at anus and gently withdraw rectal tube and tip.

Provides for patient's comfort and cleanliness.

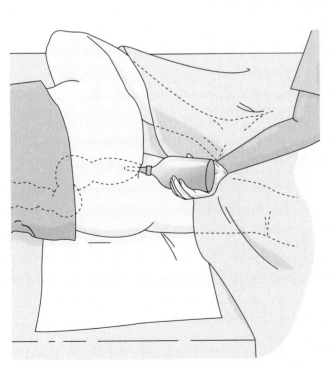

STEP 6a(4) With patient in left lateral position, insert tip of commercial enema into rectum. (*From Sorrentino SA: Mosby's textbook for nursing assistants, ed 7, St Louis, 2009, Mosby.*)

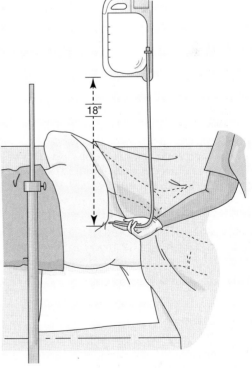

STEP 6b(10) Intravenous (IV) pole is positioned so bottom of enema bag is 45 cm (18 inches) above anus. (*From Sorrentino SA: Mosby's textbook for nursing assistants, ed 7, St Louis, 2009, Mosby.*)

Continued

STEP	RATIONALE
8. Explain to patient that some distention and abdominal cramping are normal. Ask the patient to retain solution as long as possible until urge to defecate occurs. This usually takes a few minutes. Stay at bedside. Have patient lie quietly in bed if possible. (For infant or young child, gently hold buttocks together for a few minutes.)	Solution distends bowel. Length of retention varies with type of enema and patient's ability to contract rectal sphincter. Longer retention promotes stimulation of peristalsis and defecation.
9. Discard enema container or disposable bag and tubing in proper receptacle. Remove and discard gloves and perform hand hygiene.	Reduces transmission and growth of microorganisms.
10. Help patient to bathroom or commode if possible. If using bedpan, apply clean gloves and help patient to as near a normal position for evacuation as possible (see Procedural Guideline 34.1).	Normal squatting position promotes defecation.
11. Observe character of stool and solution (instruct patient not to flush toilet before inspection).	Determines if enema was effective.
12. Help patient as needed to wash anal area with warm soap and water (use gloves for perineal care).	Fecal contents irritate skin. Hygiene promotes patient's comfort.
13. Remove and dispose of gloves and perform hand hygiene.	Reduces transmission of microorganisms.
14. Help patient to a comfortable position.	Restores comfort and sense of well-being.
15. Place nurse call system in an accessible location within patient's reach.	Ensures patient can call for assistance if needed.
16. Raise side rails (as appropriate) and lower bed to lowest position, locking into position.	Ensures patient safety and prevents falls.

EVALUATION

1. Inspect color, consistency, and amount of stool; odor; and fluid passed.
2. Palpate for abdominal distention.
3. **Use Teach-Back:** "I want to be sure I explained the proper diet to follow to reduce your constipation. Tell me the foods and liquids you can take to lessen the chance of constipation." Revise your instruction now or develop a plan for revised patient/family caregiver teaching if patient/family caregiver is not able to teach back correctly.

Determines if stool is evacuated or fluid is retained. Note abnormalities such as presence of blood or mucus.
Determines if distention is relieved.
Teach-back is a technique for health care providers to ensure that they have explained medical information clearly so that patients and their families understand what is communicated to them (AHRQ, 2023).

Unexpected Outcomes

1. Severe abdominal cramping, bleeding, or sudden abdominal pain develops and is unrelieved by temporarily stopping or slowing flow of solution.

2. Patient is unable to hold enema solution.

Related Interventions

- Stop enema.
- Notify health care provider.
- Obtain vital signs.

- If this occurs during instillation, slow rate of infusion.

Documentation

- Document the time, type, and volume of enema administered; patient's signs and symptoms; response to enema; and results, including color, amount, and appearance of stool.

Hand-Off Reporting

- Report to health care provider failure of patient to defecate or any adverse reactions.

Special Considerations
Pediatrics

- Increased fiber and fluid in the diet is the initial recommended treatment of constipation in children. If these measures are not effective, polyethylene glycol is commonly used as a softener/laxative for children (Hockenberry et al., 2024).
- Children and infants usually do not receive prepackaged hypertonic enemas because hypertonic solutions cause rapid fluid shift (Hockenberry et al., 2024).

Older Adults

- Caution is necessary when enemas are ordered "until clear" in older adults. Some older adults become tired, are at risk for fluid and electrolyte imbalances, and experience changes in vital signs.
- Sodium phosphate enemas should be used with caution in older adults because they may lead to severe metabolic disorders associated with high mortality and morbidity (Touhy & Jett, 2022). Any adult with renal disease should not receive sodium phosphate enemas.

- Some older adults may have difficulty retaining fluid. You may gently hold buttocks together to help with retention of fluid.

Populations With Disabilities

- For patients with mobility and sensory challenges, enemas may provide an effective method of bowel cleansing.
- Assess patient's and family caregiver's ability and motivation to administer enema, and provide instruction as needed.

◆ SKILL 34.2 **Insertion, Maintenance, and Removal of a Nasogastric Tube for Gastric Decompression**

There are times following major surgery or with conditions affecting the gastrointestinal (GI) tract when normal peristalsis is altered temporarily. Because peristalsis is slowed or absent, a patient cannot eat or drink fluids without developing abdominal distention. The temporary insertion of a nasogastric (NG) tube into the stomach serves to decompress the stomach, keeping it empty until normal peristalsis returns.

An NG tube is a hollow, pliable tube inserted through a patient's nasopharynx into the stomach. It allows for the removal of gastric secretions and the introduction of solutions into the stomach. Sometimes an NG tube is used for enteral feedings, but a softer small-bore feeding tube is preferred for feeding purposes (see Chapter 31). The Levin and Salem sump tubes are the most common for stomach decompression. The Levin tube is a single-lumen tube with holes near the tip (Fig. 34.4). It is connected to a drainage bag or an intermittent suction device to drain stomach secretions.

The Salem sump tube is preferable for stomach decompression. The tube has two lumens: one for removal of gastric contents and one to provide an air vent, which prevents suctioning of gastric mucosa into eyelets at the distal tip of a tube. A blue "pigtail" is the air vent that connects with the second lumen (Fig. 34.5). When the main lumen of the sump tube is connected to suction, the air vent permits free, continuous drainage of secretions. **Never clamp off the air vent, connect to suction, or use for irrigation.**

Delegation

The skill of inserting and maintaining an NG tube cannot be delegated to assistive personnel (AP). Direct the AP to:
- Measure and document the drainage from an NG tube
- Provide oral and nasal hygiene measures

- Perform selected comfort measures such as positioning or offering ice chips if allowed
- Anchor the tube to patient's gown during routine care to prevent accidental displacement
- Immediately report to the nurse any signs or patient complaints of burning or signs of redness or irritation to nares

Equipment

- 14 Fr or 16 Fr NG tube (catheters with a smaller lumen are not used for decompression in adults because the tube must be able to remove thick secretions)
- Water-soluble lubricating jelly
- pH test strips 1.0 to 11.0 or higher (measure gastric aspirate acidity)
- Tongue blade
- Clean gloves
- Flashlight
- Emesis basin
- Asepto bulb or catheter-tipped syringe
- Commercial fixation device or 2.5-cm (1-inch)–wide hypoallergenic tape (*Option:* bridle nasal tube system)
- Rubber band and plastic clip to attach tube to gown
- Clamp, drainage bag, or suction machine or pressure gauge if wall suction is to be used
- Towel
- Glass of water with straw
- Facial tissues
- Normal saline
- Tincture of benzoin (optional)
- Gastric suction equipment
- Stethoscope
- Pulse oximeter

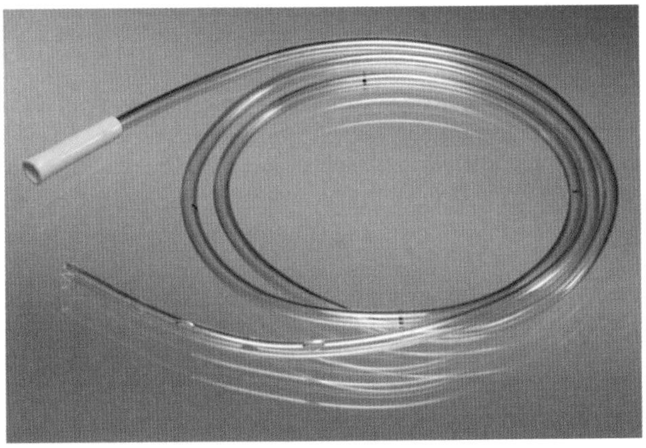

FIG. 34.4 Levin tube. (*Courtesy and copyright © Becton, Dickinson and Company.*)

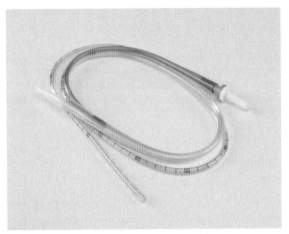

FIG. 34.5 Salem sump tube. (*Courtesy Covidien, Mansfield, MA.*)

STEP	RATIONALE

ASSESSMENT

STEP	RATIONALE
1. Identify patient using at least two identifiers (e.g., name and birthday or name and medical record number) according to agency policy.	Ensures correct patient. Complies with The Joint Commission standards and improves patient safety (TJC, 2023).
2. Verify health care provider order for type of NG tube to be placed and whether tube is to be attached to suction or drainage bag.	Requires order from health care provider. Adequate decompression depends on NG suction.
3. Assess patient's level of consciousness and ability to follow instructions.	Determines patient's ability to help in procedure.
4. Assess patient's/family caregiver's health literacy.	Determines degree to which individuals have the ability to find, understand, and use information and services to make informed health-related decisions and actions for themselves and others (CDC, 2023).
5. Ask patient or family caregiver about history of allergies and type of allergic reaction.	Avoid use of adhesive tape to anchor NG tube. Adhesive can cause medical adhesive–related skin injury (MARSI) (Fumarola et al., 2020).
6. Perform hand hygiene and apply gloves. Inspect condition of skin integrity around patient's nares and nasal and oral cavity.	Provides baseline data on the condition of the patient's skin prior to NG tube insertion. All patients with any medical device are at risk for pressure injury (Seong et al., 2021). If adhesive tape is used for anchoring, there is a risk for MARSI (Fumarola et al., 2020).
7. Ask if patient has history of nasal surgery or congestion and note if deviated nasal septum is present.	Poses risk for potential obstruction. Insert tube into uninvolved nasal passage. Procedure may be contraindicated if surgery is recent.
8. Auscultate for bowel sounds. Palpate patient's abdomen for distention, pain, and rigidity. Remove and dispose of gloves and perform hand hygiene.	In presence of diminished or absent bowel sounds, auscultate abdomen in all four quadrants (Ball et al., 2023). Documents baseline for any abdominal distention, GI ileus, and general GI function, which later serves as comparison once tube is inserted.

Clinical Judgment *If patient is confused, disoriented, or unable to follow commands, get help from another staff member to insert the tube.*

STEP	RATIONALE
9. Determine if patient had previous NG tube and, if so, which naris was used.	Patient's previous experience complements any explanations and prepares patient for NG tube placement.
10. Assess patient's knowledge, prior experience with NG tubes, and feelings about procedure.	Reveals need for patient instruction and/or support.
11. Assess patient's goals or preferences for how skill is to be performed or what patient expects.	Allows care to be individualized to patient.

PLANNING

STEP	RATIONALE
1. Expected outcomes following completion of procedure: • Abdomen is soft, nontender, and without distention.	Correctly positioned NG tube remains patent, drains gastric secretions, and relieves gastric distention.
• Nares, nasal mucosa, and skin around nares remain intact, clear, and without abrasions, skin tears, or excoriation.	Ensures absence of irritation, pressure injury, or MARSI formation from NG tube.
• Patient's level of comfort improves or remains the same.	Correctly inserted NG tube prevents abdominal discomfort from progressing.
2. Explain procedure. Inform patient that procedure may make them gag and that there will be a burning sensation in nasopharynx as tube is passed. Develop hand signal with patient.	Increases patient's cooperation and ability to anticipate nurse's action. If patient is unable to tolerate procedure, use of hand signal will alert nurse.
3. Provide privacy. Organize and set up any equipment needed to perform procedure.	Protects patient's privacy; reduces anxiety. Ensures more efficiency when completing an assessment.

IMPLEMENTATION

STEP	RATIONALE
1. Perform hand hygiene and apply gloves. Raise the bed to working height. Position patient upright in high-Fowler position unless contraindicated. If patient is comatose, raise head of bed as tolerated, with patient in semi-Fowler position and head tipped forward, chin to chest.	Promotes patient's ability to swallow during procedure. Good body mechanics prevent injury to you or patient.
2. Place bath towel over patient's chest; give facial tissues to patient. Allow to blow nose if necessary. Place emesis basin within reach.	Prevents soiling of patient's gown. Tube insertion through nasal passages may cause tearing and coughing with increased salivation.

STEP	RATIONALE

3. Wash bridge of nose with soap and water or alcohol swab. Dry thoroughly.

Removes oils from nose to allow fixation devices to adhere completely.

Clinical Judgment *Adhesives used in regular tape and fixation devices can cause medical adhesive–related skin injury (MARSI) if not applied correctly or if removed repeatedly. In patients at risk for MARSI (e.g., older age, dehydration, immunosuppression, dermatological conditions), avoid use of alcohol-based skin preps that dry the skin (Fumarola et al., 2020).*

4. Stand on patient's right side if right-handed, left side if left-handed. Lower side rail.

Allows easiest manipulation of tubing.

5. Instruct patient to relax and breathe normally while occluding one naris. Then repeat this action for other naris. Select nostril with greater airflow.

Tube passes more easily through naris that is more patent.

Clinical Judgment *Insertion of an NG tube is a painful procedure. Research provides evidence that in some instances, topical lidocaine, either as a gel or a spray, significantly reduces pain (Judd, 2020).*

6. Determine length of tube to be inserted and mark location with tape or indelible ink.

Ensures organized procedure and estimation of the proper length of tube to insert into patient.

   a. *Option, Adult:* Measure distance from tip of nose to earlobe to xiphoid process (NEX) of sternum (see illustration). Mark this distance on tube with tape.

Most traditional method. Length approximates distance from nose to stomach. Research has shown that this method may be least effective compared with others, although additional research is needed (Torsy et al., 2020; Vadivelu et al., 2023).

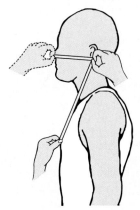

STEP 6a Determine length of tube to be inserted.

   b. *Option for Adult:* Measure distance from tip of nose to earlobe to mid-umbilicus (NEMU) to estimate appropriate NG tube placement.

Promotes placement of the tube end holes in or closer to the gastric fluid pool (Gardner & Wallace, 2021).

   c. *Option for Adult:* Measure distance from xiphoid process to earlobe to nose (XEN) + 10 cm (4 inches).

Provides best estimate to insert nasogastric tube (Torsy et al., 2020).

   d. *Option for Child:* Use the NEMU method.

Estimates proper length of tube insertion for the pediatric patient.

   e. Add 20 to 30 cm (8–12 inches) for postpyloric tubes.

Length approximates distance from nose to jejunum.

Clinical Judgment *Tip of prepyloric tube must reach stomach to avoid the risk for pulmonary aspiration, which occurs when tubes terminate in the esophagus. Research has mixed findings with regard to the best technique for estimating tube length (Fan et al., 2019; Torsy et al., 2020). Confirmation of placement via x-ray immediately after completed insertion is still needed.*

7. With small piece of tape placed around tube, mark length that will be inserted.

Indicates length of tube you will insert.

8. Prepare materials for tube fixation. Tear off a 7.5- to 10-cm (3- to 4-inch) length of hypoallergenic tape, or open membrane dressing or another fixation device (see Step 22a[2]).

Fixation devices allow tube to float free of nares, thus reducing pressure on nares and preventing medical device–related pressure injuries (MDRPIs). However, adhesive of fixation device can cause MARSI (Fumarola et al., 2020).

9. Remove and dispose of gloves. Perform hand hygiene and apply clean gloves.

Reduces transmission of infection.

10. Apply pulse oximetry/capnography device and measure vital signs. Monitor oximetry/capnography during insertion.

Provides objective assessment of respiratory status before and during tube insertion.

11. *Option:* Dip tube with surface lubricant into glass of room temperature water or lubricate 7.5 to 10 cm (3–4 inches) of end of tube with water-soluble lubricant (see manufacturer directions).

Water activates lubricant, minimizes friction against nasal mucosa, and aids in insertion of tube. Water-soluble lubricant is less toxic than oil-based lubricant if aspirated.

STEP	RATIONALE
12. Hand an alert patient a cup of water if able to hold cup and swallow. Explain that you are about to insert tube.	Swallowing water facilitates tube passage. Explanation decreases patient anxiety and increases patient cooperation.
13. Explain next steps. Insert tube gently and slowly through naris to back of throat (posterior nasopharynx). Aim back and down toward patient's ear.	Natural contour facilitates passage of tube into GI tract and reduces gagging.
14. Have patient relax and flex head toward chest after tube is passed through nasopharynx.	Closes off glottis and reduces risk of tube entering trachea.
15. Encourage patient to swallow by taking small sips of water when possible. Advance tube as patient swallows. Rotate tube gently 180 degrees while inserting.	Swallowing facilitates passage of tube past oropharynx. A tug may be felt as patient swallows, indicating that tube is following desired path.
16. Emphasize need to mouth breathe during procedure.	Helps facilitate passage of tube and alleviates patient's anxiety and fear during procedure.
17. Do not advance tube during inspiration or coughing because it will likely enter respiratory tract. Monitor oximetry/capnography.	When tube inadvertently enters airway, changes in oxygen saturation or end-tidal CO_2 (capnography) may occur.
18. Advance tube each time patient swallows until you reach desired length.	Reduces discomfort and trauma to patient.

Clinical Judgment *Do not force NG tube. If patient starts to cough or has a drop in O_2 saturation or an increased CO_2 level, withdraw tube into the posterior nasopharynx until normal breathing resumes.*

19. Using penlight and tongue blade, check to be sure that tube is not positioned in back of throat.	Tube could become coiled or kinked or could enter trachea.
20. Temporarily anchor tube to nose with small piece of tape.	Securing tube prevents movement of tube and subsequent gagging.
21. Verify tube placement. Check agency policy for recommended methods of checking tube placement.	It is important that the tube be in the stomach and not in the esophagus or respiratory tract.
a. Follow order for bedside x-ray study and notify radiology department for examination of chest and abdomen.	Radiography remains the gold standard for verification of initial placement of tube (Nihal & Dilek, 2022; Judd, 2020; Powers et al., 2021). This must be done before any medication or liquid is administered.
b. While waiting for x-ray film, follow these procedures: Attach Asepto or catheter-tipped syringe to end of tube. Aspirate gently back on syringe to obtain gastric contents, observing amount, color, and quality of return (see illustration).	Observation of gastric contents is useful to determine initial tube placement. Gastric contents are usually green but are sometimes off-white, tan, bloody, or brown. Other common aspirate colors include yellow or bile stained (duodenal placement) or possibly saliva-like (esophagus).
c. Use pH test paper to measure aspirate for pH with color-coded pH paper. Be sure that paper range of pH is at least 1.0 to 11.0 (see illustration).	Evidence supports pH test to be used as an indicator for placement (Judd, 2020), but radiographic confirmation is the most accurate way to be sure that the tube is in the stomach. (Nihal & Dilek, 2022).

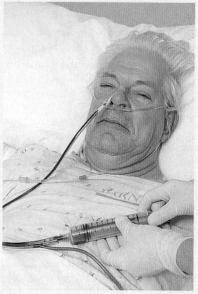

STEP 21b Aspiration of gastric contents.

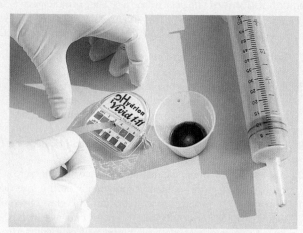

STEP 21c Checking pH of gastric aspirate.

STEP	RATIONALE

22. After tube is properly inserted and positioned, either clamp end or connect it to drainage bag or suction source. Anchor tube with a fixation device, avoiding pressure on the nares. Select one of the following fixation methods.

    a. Apply tape.

      (1) Be sure skin on bridge of nose is dry, not oily.

      (2) Remove gloves. Tear two small horizontal slits at one-third and two-thirds length of tape without splitting tape (see illustration). Fold middle sections toward each other to form a closed strip.

      (3) Tear vertical strip at bottom of tape. Print date and time on tape and place top end of tape over bridge of patient's nose.

      (4) Place intact end of tape over bridge of patient's nose. Wrap bottom end of tape around tube as it exits nose (see illustrations).

Drainage bag is used for gravity drainage. Intermittent low suction is most effective for decompression. Proper anchoring and marking of tube helps prevent migration of tube and pressure injury formation.

Improves adhesive adherence. Use of agents such as benzoin could affect risk for MARSI (Fumarola et al., 2020).

The strip holds tubing to lessen rubbing against soft palate and naris.

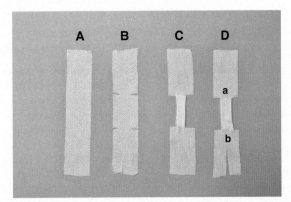

STEP 22a(2) Taping method. (A) Start with piece of tape. (B) Make two slits on both sides of tape. (C) Fold middle section inward. (D) Tear a new slit in bottom of tape. Top part *(a)* should attach to patient's nose; bottom part *(b)* should be wrapped around tube.

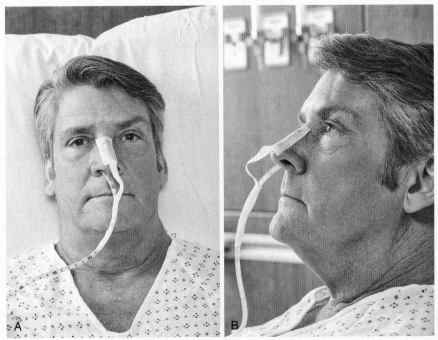

STEP 22a(4) (A) Tape applied to anchor nasogastric tube. (B) Nares are free of pressure from tape and tube.

STEP	RATIONALE

b. Apply tube fixation device, using shaped adhesive patch (see manufacturer's directions). *Option:* Place small strip of skin barrier directly on nose; apply patch over it.
  (1) Apply wide end of patch to bridge of nose (see illustration)
  (2) Slip connector around tube as it exits nose (see illustration).
	Secures tube, reduces friction on nares, and decreases risk for MDRPI. Skin barrier reduces risk of MARSI (Fumarola et al., 2020).

Clinical Judgment *Assess at least twice daily the condition of the naris and mucosa and skin around adhesive for inflammation, blistering, excoriation, or any type of skin or tissue injury. Injury can develop for many reasons: rigidity of device rubbing against mucosa, difficulty in securing or adjusting the device to the body, increased moisture surrounding the tubing, tight securement of the device, and poor positioning or fixation of the device (Seong et al., 2021). Irritation and blistering can occur from reaction to adhesive, causing MARSI (Fumarola et al., 2020).*

23. Fasten end of NG tube to patient's gown using clip (see illustration) or piece of tape. Do not use safety pins to fasten tube to gown.	Anchors tubing to prevent pulling on nose.
24. Keep head of bed elevated 30 to 45 degrees (preferably 45 degrees) unless contraindicated (Colwell & Goldberg, 2021).	Patients receiving NG tube feedings have an increased risk for aspiration. Head-of-bed elevation reduces risk for aspiration of stomach contents.

Clinical Judgment *If inserting a Salem sump tube, keep the blue "pigtail" of the tube above level of the stomach. This prevents a siphoning action that clogs the tube. The blue pigtail is the air vent that connects with the second lumen. When the main lumen of the sump tube is connected to suction, the air vent permits free, continuous drainage of secretions.* **Never clamp off the air vent, connect to suction, or use for irrigation.**

25. Assist radiology staff as needed in obtaining ordered x-ray film of chest and abdomen.	X-ray verification is the gold standard for NG tube verification (Judd, 2020; Nihal & Dilek, 2022).
26. Remove and dispose of gloves, perform hand hygiene, and help patient to comfortable position. Clean tubing at nostril with washcloth dampened in mild soap and water. Administer oral hygiene.	Reduces transmission of microorganisms. Restores comfort and sense of well-being.
27. Once placement is confirmed, measure amount of tube that is external and mark exit of tube at nares with indelible marker as guide for any tube displacement. Document this information in electronic health record (EHR).	The mark alerts nurses and other health care providers to possible tube displacement, which will require confirmation of tube placement.

Clinical Judgment *Never reposition an NG tube of a gastric surgical patient, because positioning can rupture the suture line.*

28. Attach NG tube to suction as ordered. Suction settings should be confirmed any time the patient is disconnected or at the beginning of each nurse's shift.	Suction setting is usually ordered at low intermittent setting, which decreases gastric irritation from NG tube.

Clinical Judgment *If lumen of tube is narrow and secretions are thick, NG tube will not drain as desired. Irrigate tube (see Step 29). Consult with health care provider for higher suction setting if unable to irrigate tube because of thick secretions.*

29. NG tube irrigation:
  a. Perform hand hygiene and apply clean gloves.
  b. Verify tube placement in stomach by disconnecting NG tube, connecting irrigating syringe, and aspirating contents (see Step 21b). Temporarily clamp NG tube or reconnect to connecting tube and remove syringe.
  c. Empty syringe of aspirate and use it to draw up 30 mL of normal saline.
	Reduces transmission of microorganisms.
	pH of gastric aspirate must measure between 1.0 and 5.0 to ensure that NG tube is in the stomach (Judd, 2020). Prevents accidental entrance of irrigating solution into lungs.
	
	Use of saline minimizes loss of electrolytes from stomach fluids.

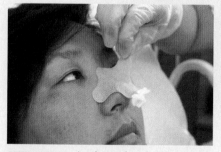

STEP 22b(1) Apply patch to bridge of nose.

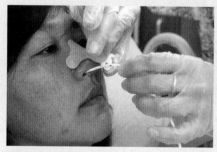

STEP 22b(2) Slip connector around naso-gastric tube.

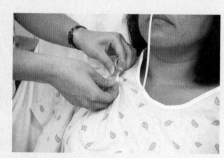

STEP 23 Fasten nasogastric tube to patient gown.

STEP	RATIONALE
d. Disconnect NG from connecting tubing and lay end of connection tubing on towel.	Reduces soiling of patient's gown and bed linen.
e. Insert tip of irrigating syringe into end of NG tube. Remove clamp. Hold syringe with tip pointed at floor and inject saline slowly and evenly. Do not force solution.	Position of syringe prevents introduction of air into vent tubing, which causes gastric distention. Solution introduced under pressure causes gastric trauma.

Clinical Judgment *Do not introduce saline through blue "pigtail" air vent of Salem sump tube.*

STEP	RATIONALE
f. If resistance occurs, check for kinks in tubing. Turn patient onto left side. Repeated resistance should be reported to health care provider.	Tip of tube may lie against stomach lining. Repositioning on left side may dislodge tube away from stomach lining. Buildup of secretions causes distention.
g. After instilling saline, immediately aspirate or pull back slowly on syringe to withdraw fluid. If amount aspirated is greater than amount instilled, document difference as output. If amount aspirated is less than amount instilled, document difference as intake.	Irrigation clears tubing, so stomach should remain empty. Measure and document amount of irrigant fluid inserted in tube as intake.
h. Use an Asepto syringe to place 10 mL of air into blue pigtail.	Ensures patency of air vent.
i. Reconnect NG tube to drainage or suction. (Repeat irrigation if solution does not return.)	Reestablishes drainage collection; may repeat irrigation or repositioning of tube until NG tube drains properly.
30. Removal of NG tube:	
a. Verify health care provider order to remove NG tube.	A health care provider order is required for procedure.
b. Per agency policy, stop suction briefly to auscultate abdomen for presence of bowel sounds or clamp the tube for a short period of time, assessing for nausea or discomfort.	Verifies return of peristalsis.
c. Provide privacy and explain procedure to patient and that patient will be instructed to take a deep breath and hold it.	Minimizes anxiety and increases cooperation. Tube passes out smoothly.
d. Perform hand hygiene and apply clean gloves.	Reduces transmission of microorganisms.
e. Position patient in high-Fowler position unless contraindicated.	Reduces risk for pulmonary aspiration in event patient should vomit.
f. Turn off suction and disconnect NG tube from drainage bag or suction. With irrigating syringe, insert 20 mL of air into lumen of NG tube. Gently remove tape or fixation device from bridge of nose and patient's gown.	Have tube free of connections before removal. Clears gastric fluids from tube to prevent aspiration of contents or soiling of clothing and bedding. Gentle adhesive removal reduces the risk of MARSI (Fumarola et al., 2020).
g. Hand patient facial tissue; place disposable towel across chest. Instruct patient to take and hold breath as tube is removed.	Some patients wish to blow nose after tube is removed. Towel keeps gown from soiling. Temporary airway obstruction occurs during tube removal.
h. Clamp or kink tubing securely and pull tube out steadily and smoothly into towel held in other hand while patient holds breath.	Clamping prevents tube contents from draining into oropharynx. Reduces trauma to mucosa and minimizes patient's discomfort. Towel covers tube, which is an unpleasant sight. Holding breath helps to prevent aspiration.
i. Inspect intactness of tube.	
j. Measure amount of drainage and note character of content. Dispose of tube and drainage equipment into proper container.	Provides accurate measure of fluid output. Reduces transfer of microorganisms.
k. Clean nares and provide oral hygiene.	Promotes comfort.
l. Position patient comfortably and explain procedure for drinking fluids if not contraindicated. Instruct patient to notify you if nausea occurs.	Sometimes patients are not allowed anything by mouth (NPO) for up to 24 hours. When fluids are allowed, orders usually begin with small amount of ice chips each hour and increase as patient is able to tolerate more.
31. For all procedures, clean equipment and return to proper place. Place soiled linen in utility room or proper receptacle.	Proper disposal of equipment prevents spread of microorganisms and ensures proper exchange procedures.
32. Remove and dispose of gloves and perform hand hygiene.	Reduces transmission of microorganisms.
33. Help patient to a comfortable position.	Restores comfort and sense of well-being.
34. Place nurse call system in an accessible location within patient's reach.	Ensures patient can call for assistance if needed.
34. Raise side rails (as appropriate) and lower bed to lowest position, locking into position.	Ensures patient safety and prevents falls.

STEP	RATIONALE

EVALUATION

1. Observe amount and character of contents draining from NG tube. Ask if patient feels nauseated.

Determines if tube is decompressing stomach of contents.

2. Auscultate for presence of bowel sounds. Turn off suction while auscultating. Assess for nausea and patient discomfort if tube is clamped for short trial period.

Sound of suction apparatus is sometimes misinterpreted as bowel sounds. Nausea and discomfort will occur if peristalsis is not returned.

3. Palpate patient's abdomen periodically. Note any distention, pain, and rigidity.

Determines success of abdominal decompression and return of peristalsis.

4. Inspect condition of nares, nose, and all skin and tissue around NG tubing as per agency policy.

Evaluates onset of skin and tissue irritation.

5. Observe position of tubing.

Prevents tension applied to nasal structures.

6. Explain that it is normal if patient feels sore throat or irritation in pharynx.

Result of tube irritation.

7. **Use Teach-Back:** "I need to be sure I explained the importance of letting me know if you are nauseated. Tell me why it is important for me to know if you feel nauseated." Revise your instruction now or develop a plan for revised patient/family caregiver teaching if patient/family caregiver is not able to teach back correctly.

Teach-back is a technique for health care providers to ensure that they have explained medical information clearly so that patients and their families understand what is communicated to them (AHRQ, 2023).

Unexpected Outcomes	Related Interventions
1. Patient complains of nausea, or patient's abdomen is distended and painful.	• Assess patency of tube. NG tube may be occluded or no longer in stomach. Verify placement. • Irrigate tube. • Verify that suction is on as ordered. • Notify health care provider if distention is unrelieved.
2. Patient develops irritation or erosion of skin around naris.	• Provide frequent skin care to area, keeping it dry. • Use taping method designed to reduce MDRPI (see taping methods [Step 22]). • Consider switching tube to other naris. • Try alternative tape or use of skin barrier to reduce MARSI (Fumarola et al., 2020).
3. Patient develops signs and symptoms of pulmonary aspiration: fever, shortness of breath, or pulmonary congestion.	• Perform complete respiratory assessment. • Notify health care provider. • Obtain chest x-ray examination as ordered.

Documentation

- Document length, size, and type of gastric tube inserted and naris in which tube was introduced. Also document patient's tolerance of procedure, confirmation of tube placement, character and pH of gastric contents, results of x-ray film, whether the tube is clamped or connected to drainage bag or to suction, and amount of suction supplied.
- When irrigating NG tube, document difference between amount of normal saline instilled and amount of gastric aspirate removed. Document amount and character of contents draining from NG tube every shift.
- Document removal of tube "intact," patient's tolerance of procedure, and final amount and character of drainage.

Hand-Off Reporting

- Set up a schedule to remove the tape and assess the skin and mucosa to avoid MDRPI and MARSI.
- Report occurrence of abdominal distention, unexpected increase or sudden stoppage in gastric drainage, and patient complaint of gastric distress to health care provider.

Special Considerations

Pediatrics

- Children usually have an NG tube for feeding, and often the tube is removed between feedings and reinserted as needed. If a tube is to be left in place for a young child, the child will need some type of hand restraint to keep the child from pulling the tube out (Hockenberry et al., 2024).

Older Adults

- In an older patient, it is important to assess cognitive status so that measures can be taken to keep the patient from pulling out the tube if the patient cannot understand why it has been placed.
- Skin and tissue integrity becomes more fragile in older patients, so extra care must be taken to avoid MDRPI in the nares or MARSI on the skin on the nose (Touhy & Jett, 2022).

Populations With Disabilities

- If the disability involves a developmental delay, careful watching will be required to ensure that the patient does not remove the tube.

◆ CLINICAL JUDGMENT AND NEXT-GENERATION NCLEX® EXAMINATION–STYLE QUESTIONS

An older adult with mild dementia was admitted to the hospital with a fractured hip 3 days ago. Surgical repair of the hip was done, and the patient took opioid medication for pain for 2 days after surgery. A stool softener was also ordered once a day. In reviewing the patient's health record, the nurse finds that the patient had two small liquid incontinent bowel movements last evening. The patient reports "pressure in my bottom." The family caregiver recalls that the patient reported constipation several days prior to surgery.

1. The health care provider orders a regular soapsuds enema (SSE) to be instilled. Determine whether each nursing action below is indicated or not indicated when administering the SSE.

Nursing Action	Indicated	Not Indicated
Use castile soap to prepare the SSE.		
Use cold water to mix with soap to prepare the SSE.		
Assist patient to a side-lying position.		
Prime tubing so it is filled with solution before administering SSE.		
Insert tip of rectal tube 10–12.7 cm (4–5 inches) into rectum.		
Raise enema container to approximately 12 inches above the anus to be instilled.		

2. When the nurse unclamps the tubing to begin to administer the enema, the fluid does not flow into the patient. When the second and third attempt at administration fail, which factor does the nurse anticipate **most likely** has caused this problem?
   1. Faulty tubing
   2. Broken clamp
   3. Fecal impaction
   4. Patient clenching

3. The nurse contacts the health care provider to report the issue with administration of the enema. Which order will the nurse request as the **priority**?
   1. Stool softener to be included in the medication regimen
   2. Digital removal of the stool mass present in the rectum
   3. Changes to the diet to increase fiber and fluids
   4. Reduction in opioid drug with transition to nonopioid pain medication

4. Later in the evening, the patient develops nausea and vomiting, and the health care provider orders an NG tube to be inserted. After verifying the order, performing hand hygiene and donning gloves, and confirming the patient's identity, which action will the nurse take **next**?
   1. Tape the tubing to the nose for stability.
   2. Pass the tube along the floor of nasal passage, then just past the nasopharynx.
   3. Instruct patient to flex head forward and swallow while the tube is advanced.
   4. Measure and mark tube to determine the correct tubing length.

5. The patient has recovered enough to be discharged home. Which of the following teachings will the nurse provide about management of chronic constipation? **Select all that apply.**
   1. Increase intake of fiber and fluids.
   2. Use a low-volume enema daily.
   3. Avoid gluten in the diet.
   4. Take laxatives twice a day.
   5. Incorporate movement into the daily routine.

Visit the Evolve site for Answers to Clinical Judgment and Next-Generation NCLEX® Examination–Style Questions.

REFERENCES

Agency for Healthcare Research and Quality (AHRQ): *Teach-Back: intervention,* 2023. https://www.ahrq.gov/patient-safety/reports/engage/interventions/teachback.html.
Ball J, et al: *Seidel's guide to physical examination,* ed 10, St. Louis, 2023, Mosby.
Caffrey J, Pensa G: Who gets constipation? What are the causes? What is an evidence-based approach management? In Graham A, Carlberg D, editors: *Gastrointestinal emergencies,* New York, 2019, Springer.
Centers for Disease Control and Prevention (CDC): *What is health literacy?* 2023. https://www.cdc.gov/healthliteracy/learn/index.html.
Colwell J, Goldberg M: *Wound, Ostomy, and Continence Nurses Society (WOCN) core curriculum: ostomy management,* ed 2, Philadelphia, 2021, Wolters Kluwer.
Ermer-Seltun J, Engberg S: *Wound, Ostomy, and Continence Nurses Society (WOCN) Core curriculum: continence management,* ed 2, Philadelphia, 2022, Wolters Kluwer.
Fan P, et al: Adequacy of different measurement methods in determining nasogastric tube insertion lengths: an observational study, *Int J Nurs Stud* 92:73–78, 2019.
Fumarola S, et al: Overlooked and underestimated: medical adhesive-related skin injuries. Best practice consensus document on prevention, *J Wound Care* 29(Suppl 3c):S1–S24, 2020.
Gardner LE, Wallace S: Nasogastric tube placement: a cross-comparison of verification methods used in Pennsylvania hospitals and how they align with guidelines, *Patient Safety* 3(3):37–45, 2021.
Hockenberry MJ, et al: *Wong's nursing care of infants and children,* ed 12, St. Louis, 2024, Elsevier.
Huether S, McCance K: *Understanding pathophysiology,* ed 7, St. Louis, 2020, Mosby.
Judd M: Confirming nasogastric tube placement in adults, *Nursing 2020* 50(4):43–46, 2020.
National Institutes of Health (NIH): National Institute of Diabetes and Digestive Kidney Diseases (NIDDK): *Constipation,* 2018. https://www.niddk.nih.gov/health-information/digestive-diseases/constipation/eating-diet-nutrition. Accessed June 2, 2023.
Nihal T, Dilek S: The effectiveness of auscultatory, colorimetric capnometry and pH measurement methods to confirm placement of nasogastric tubes: a methodological study, *Int J Nurs Pract* 28(2):e13049, 2022.
Powers J, et al: Development of a competency model for placement and verification of nasogastric and nasoenteric feeding tubes for adult hospitalized patients, *Nutr Clin Pract* 36:517–533, 2021.
Seong Y, et al: Development and testing of an algorithm to prevent medical device–related pressure injuries, *Inquiry* 58:469580211050219, 2021.
Sood M: *Chronic functional constipation and fecal incontinence in infants, children, and adolescents: Treatment,* 2023. https://www.uptodate.com/contents/chronic-functional-constipation-and-fecal-incontinence-in-infants-children-and-adolescents-treatment. Accessed June 2, 2023.
Stellar J, et al: Medical device–related pressure injuries in infants and children, *J Wound Ostomy Continence Nurs* 47(5):459–469, 2020.
The Joint Commission (TJC): *2023 National patient safety goals,* Oakbrook Terrace, IL, 2023, The Joint Commission. https://www.jointcommission.org/standards/national-patient-safety-goals/.
Torsy T, et al: Accuracy of the corrected nose-earlobe-xiphoid distance formula for determining nasogastric feeding tube insertion length in intensive care unit patients: a prospective observational study, *Int J Nurs Studies* 110:103614, 2020.
Touhy TA, Jett KJ: *Ebersole and Hess' gerontological nursing & healthy aging,* ed 6, St. Louis, 2022, Elsevier.
Vadivelu N, et al: Evolving therapeutic roles of nasogastric tubes: Current concepts in clinical Practice, *Adv Ther* 40:828–843, 2023.
Viscusi ER: Clinical overview and considerations for the management of opioid-induced constipation in patients with chronic noncancer pain, *Clin J Pain* 34(2):174–188, 2019.

35 | Ostomy Care

SKILLS AND PROCEDURES

Skill 35.1 **Pouching a Colostomy or an Ileostomy, p. 1040**

Skill 35.2 **Pouching a Urostomy, p. 1046**

Skill 35.3 **Catheterizing a Urinary Diversion, p. 1050**

OBJECTIVES

Mastery of content in this chapter will enable you to:
- Discuss the similarities and differences in the types of fecal and urinary diversions.
- Recall the differences in consistency of effluent based on the type of ostomy.
- Apply clinical decision making to perform an ostomy pouch change.
- Explain methods used to maintain integrity of the peristomal skin.
- Apply clinical decision making to catheterize a urinary diversion.

MEDIA RESOURCES

- http://evolve.elsevier.com/Perry/skills
- Review Questions
- Audio Glossary
- ▶ Video Clips
- **NSO** Nursing Skills Online
- Answers to Clinical Judgment and Next-Generation NCLEX® Examination–Style Questions
- Skills Performance Checklists
- Printable Key Points

PURPOSE

With certain diseases (e.g., cancer, inflammatory bowel disease) or conditions (e.g., neurogenic bowel or bladder, damage from radiation), a surgically created opening in the abdominal wall, called a *stoma*, is necessary to allow for the passage of urine or fecal matter. It is essential that a pouch be placed over a stoma correctly so that the output from the stoma is contained, the skin around the stoma is protected, and a patient is free from odor or leakage.

PRACTICE STANDARDS

- Colwell J, Goldberg M, 2021: Wound, Ostomy and Continence Nurses Society (WOCN) Core Curriculum: Ostomy Management—Ostomy site care and pouching
- Burgess-Stocks J, et al., 2022: Ostomy and Continent Diversion Patient Bill of Rights: Research Validation of Standards of Care—Body image changes
- The Joint Commission (TJC), 2023: National Patient Safety Goals—Patient identification

SUPPLEMENTAL STANDARDS

- World Council of Enterostomal Therapists (WCET), 2020: WCET International Ostomy Guideline—Cultural implications

PRINCIPLES FOR PRACTICE

- An ostomy is an artificial opening in an organ of the body created during a surgical procedure. For example, a colostomy is a surgical operation in which a section of the colon is diverted to an artificial opening in the abdominal wall so as to bypass a damaged or surgically removed part of the colon (Fig. 35.1). A colostomy is usually placed in the descending colon and results in a stool similar to that normally passed through the rectum.
- An ileostomy is a stoma placed in the ileum or lower portion of the small intestine. It drains fecal effluent that is watery-to-thick liquid and contains some digestive enzymes (Fig. 35.2).
- The character of the output of an intestinal stoma (called *effluent*) is influenced by a patient's medications, hydration status, and the foods eaten. Diet and fluid therapy are important therapies in managing ostomy effluent.
- If removal of the urinary bladder is necessary, a section of the ileum or small intestine is resected and the ureters are inserted into it, creating an ileal conduit or a urostomy (Fig. 35.3) from which urine exits the body through the stoma.
- A patient with a colostomy, ileostomy, or ileal conduit has no sensation or control over the time or frequency of the output and must wear a pouch to collect effluent.
- There are surgical procedures that create continent internal fecal or urinary pouches, eliminating the need to wear an external pouch. An ileal pouch is an internal reservoir formed from a segment of the ileum that is then connected to the anal canal above the anal sphincter (Fig. 35.4). A continent urinary diversion (Fig. 35.5) is a reservoir created from the intestine. A small stoma on the abdominal wall allows access via a catheter inserted to empty urine from the pouch. These surgeries are less common than the ileostomy or urostomy.

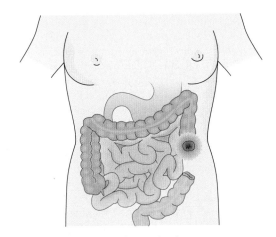

FIG. 35.1 Sigmoid colostomy.

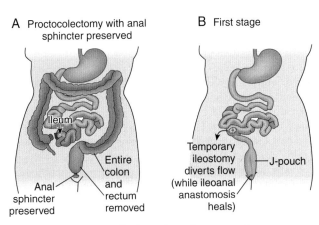

A Proctocolectomy with anal sphincter preserved

B First stage

Ileum

Anal sphincter preserved

Entire colon and rectum removed

Temporary ileostomy diverts flow (while ileoanal anastomosis heals)

J-pouch

FIG. 35.4 Ileal pouch anal anastomosis.

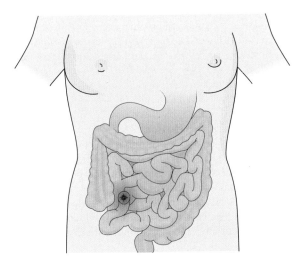

FIG. 35.2 Ileostomy.

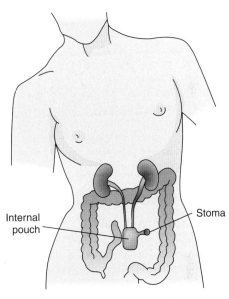

Internal pouch

Stoma

FIG. 35.5 Continent urinary diversion.

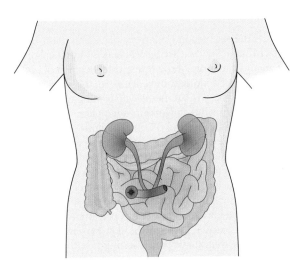

FIG. 35.3 Urostomy (ileal conduit).

PERSON-CENTERED CARE

- Persons with newly created stomas for the elimination of urine or fecal matter from the body need to be taught to care for their ostomy to regain autonomy in self-care for basic elimination.
- Some patients accept their stoma with minimal emotional difficulty; some may never completely adjust to it. Individualize care according to each patient's situation and circumstances (Goldberg et al., 2018).
- With any ostomy requiring a pouching system, a secure seal to the skin to prevent leakage of the effluent and protect the skin around the stoma (peristomal skin) is vital to helping patients resume normal activities and accept the changes in their bodies as a result of surgery (Burgess-Stocks et al., 2022).
- In addition to the stress of illness and surgical recovery, patients with ostomies face body image changes, fear of social rejection, concern about sexual function and intimacy, and the need for help with personal care (Colwell & Goldberg, 2021).
- Patients from some ethnic backgrounds and religious practices may find monitoring urinary or intestinal output from their

stomas to be more invasive and embarrassing than patients from cultures that are more open about bodily functions (World Council of Enterostomal Therapists [WCET], 2020). Discuss with patients their preferences.

- Consider the impact that caring for a person with an ostomy has on a family caregiver's quality of life (Goldberg et al., 2018).
- When you communicate with a patient during ostomy care, be sensitive and avoid communicating anything that the patient may interpret as disrespect or disgust. As always, prepare adequately for the procedure; seek necessary help; and maintain a calm, professional demeanor. Do not act offended by the odor or appearance of the effluent in the pouch or the appearance of the stoma. A negative reaction (e.g., a frowning facial expression) from caregivers only reinforces patients' feelings that the alteration in bodily function makes them personally and socially unacceptable.
- When patients come to a health care agency with an ostomy, encourage them to resume self-care as soon as possible. Respect a patient's routine of care even if it differs from usual care in the health care agency. Offer educational materials to support the patient's adaptation to the new ostomy (American Cancer Society [ACS], 2019a; ACS, 2019b; ACS, 2019c).
- Ostomy support groups and home health care nurses can offer ongoing community support. Research has shown that participation in an ostomy support group allows individuals with ostomies to function at more advanced levels than before participation in the support group (Byfield, 2020). In the same study, the patients' lived experiences were characterized by hope, willingness to live fully again, participating in different activities, and making new friends.

EVIDENCE-BASED PRACTICE

Peristomal Skin Breakdown

Evidence-based studies have shown a direct relationship between peristomal skin health and health-related quality of life (HRQOL), which is a multidimensional concept that includes domains related to physical, mental, emotional, and social functioning (Office of Disease Prevention and Health Promotion [ODPHP], n.d.). It is estimated that more than 80% of persons with ostomies will at

some point develop peristomal skin breakdown, and this may occur at any time after stoma creation (Zelga et al., 2021). More than 60% of this skin breakdown is from irritant dermatitis or exposure of the skin to fecal effluent, which occurs from a poorly placed stoma or an ill-fitting or inappropriate pouch (Fellows, 2021). Irritation of the skin, including blistering, skin stripping, and dermatitis, can also occur from exposure to adhesive, causing medical adhesive–related skin injury (MARSI) (Fumarola et al., 2020). The result of peristomal skin breakdown is pain and suffering, lack of confidence in providing care for an ostomy, social isolation due to leakage of the pouching system, and poor HRQOL (Fellows, 2021). As a result of these studies, patients having ostomy surgery should have access to:

- An ostomy nurse with specialized training (wound, ostomy, continence [WOC] nurse)
- Preoperative education and stoma site marking
- Instruction in proper care of the ostomy after surgery
- An appropriate pouching system
- Follow-up care as an outpatient (Burgess-Stocks et al., 2022)

SAFETY GUIDELINES

- Empty ostomy pouches when they are one-third to one-half full to avoid leakage. Leakage on the skin, especially from an ileostomy, can cause irritant dermatitis and peristomal skin breakdown.
- Know the signs of a healthy stoma and surrounding skin:
  - *Color/moisture:* Stoma should be red or pink and moist. Report a gray, purple, black, or very dry stoma to the charge nurse or health care provider.
  - *Size:* In the 4 to 6 weeks after surgery, the stoma will likely decrease in size as postoperative edema and abdominal distention decrease. Measure with each pouch change and adjust the size of the opening cut in the wafer.
  - *Peristomal skin:* It normally is intact with some reddening after the adhesive wafer is removed. Presence of blisters, a rash, or excoriated skin is abnormal and can indicate MARSI (Fumarola et al., 2020).
- Wear clean gloves during pouch and stoma care to avoid contact with body fluids.

◆ SKILL 35.1 | **Pouching a Colostomy or an Ileostomy**

 Video Clip

Immediately after a fecal surgical diversion, it is necessary to place a pouch over a newly created stoma to contain effluent when the stoma begins to function. The pouch keeps a patient clean and dry, protects the skin from damage, and provides a barrier against odor. A cut-to-fit, transparent pouching system is preferred because it protects the peristomal skin, allows the stoma to be visualized, and adapts to changes in stoma size as swelling decreases after surgery.

Recognize the difference between a budded stoma (Fig. 35.6) and a flush or retracted stoma (Fig. 35.7). Immediately after surgery, a stoma may be edematous, and the abdomen distended. These symptoms will resolve over a 4- to 6-week period after surgery, but during this time it will be necessary to revise the pouching system to meet the changing size of the stoma and the changes in body contours (Colwell & Goldberg, 2021).

There are many types of pouching systems. All have a protective adhesive layer that adheres to the skin, called a *skin barrier* or *wafer*, and a pouch. The wafer is a solid skin barrier that creates the seal

and protects the skin around the stoma. It is important to select a skin barrier that achieves a secure seal and is individualized to the size, shape, and curvature of the stoma (McNichol et al., 2021).

There are several unique ingredients in the skin barrier that make for a sticky backing. A one-piece pouching system (Fig. 35.8) has the two parts integrated together. A two-piece system (Fig. 35.9) has a separate skin barrier and pouch. The flush or retracted stoma may require a convex wafer (Fig. 35.10) for successful placement of a pouch. This type of skin barrier provides gentle pressure on the peristomal skin to push the stoma through the opening in the wafer. You apply the pouch to the skin barrier by attaching it to a flange (a plastic ring) on the wafer. You must use the skin barrier with a flange that fits the corresponding size pouch from the same manufacturer to avoid leakage between the skin barrier and the pouch. Some pouching systems have precut openings in the barrier for the stoma, whereas others need to be custom cut to size for a patient's stoma measurement. It is important to understand how to use each

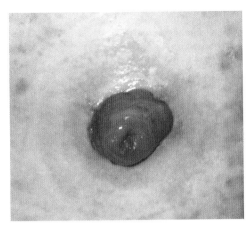

FIG. 35.6 Budded stoma. (*Courtesy Jane Fellows.*)

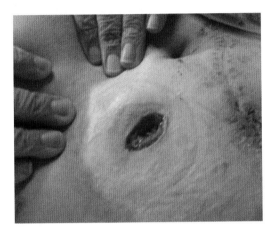

FIG. 35.7 Retracted stoma. (*Courtesy Jane Fellows.*)

of these different pouching systems before applying them on patients (Colwell & Goldberg, 2021). The websites for the companies that make ostomy supplies have both patient and health care provider instructions that are helpful in understanding how to use the pouching systems (e.g., http://www.convatec.com; http://www.us.coloplast.com; and http://www.hollister.com). The risk of medical adhesive–related skin injury (MARSI) is low when ostomy pouches are applied and removed correctly. The companies that make ostomy products strive for a wafer that does not require an additional skin barrier. The best pouching system is one that is applied to clean, dry skin without other products. When skin is not intact, added products may need to be used to absorb moisture.

Delegation

The skill of pouching a new ostomy should not be delegated to assistive personnel (AP). In some agencies, care of an established

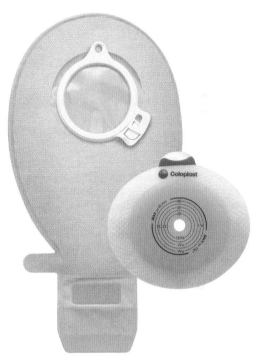

FIG. 35.9 Two-piece pouching system with separate skin barrier and attachable pouch. (*Courtesy Coloplast, Minneapolis, MN.*)

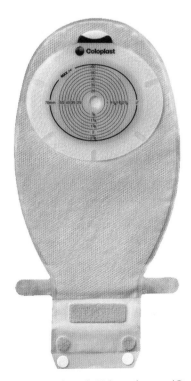

FIG. 35.8 One-piece pouch with Velcro closure. (*Courtesy Coloplast, Minneapolis, MN.*)

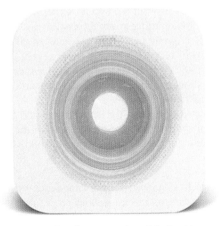

FIG. 35.10 Convex skin barrier wafer. (*Used with permission from Convatec, Inc. All rights reserved.*)

ostomy (2–3 weeks or more after surgery) can be delegated to AP. Instruct the AP about:

- The expected amount, color, and consistency of drainage from an ostomy
- The expected appearance of the stoma
- Special equipment needed to complete the procedure
- The changes in a patient's stoma and surrounding skin integrity that should be reported

Interprofessional Collaboration

- Refer to a WOC nurse, when available, for postsurgical assessment, selection of proper barrier and pouch, and patient education on self-care.

Equipment

- Wafer (skin barrier)/pouch—clear, drainable one-piece or two-piece, cut to fit or precut size
- Ostomy measuring guide
- Adhesive releaser
- Clean gloves
- Washcloth
- Towel or disposable waterproof barrier
- Basin with warm tap water
- Scissors
- Waterproof bag for disposal of pouch
- *Optional:* Gown or goggles if there is any risk of splashing when emptying pouch

STEP	RATIONALE

ASSESSMENT

1. Identify patient using at least two identifiers (e.g., name and birthday or name and medical record number) according to agency policy.	Ensures patient safety. Complies with The Joint Commission standards and improves patient safety (TJC, 2023).
2. Assess patient's/family caregiver's health literacy.	Determines degree to which individuals have the ability to find, understand, and use information and services to make informed health-related decisions and actions for themselves and others (Centers for Disease Control and Prevention [CDC], 2023).
3. Review electronic health record (EHR) and assess if patient is at risk for MARSI: age, dehydration, malnutrition, exposure to radiation therapy, underlying chronic conditions (e.g., diabetes mellitus, immunosuppression), and edema of skin.	Common risk factors for MARSI (Fumarola et al., 2020). Factors raise your level of observation if patient has a stoma product containing adhesive tape.
4. Perform hand hygiene and apply clean gloves.	Reduces transmission of microorganisms.
5. Have patient assume semi-reclining or supine position. Observe existing skin barrier and pouch for leakage and check EHR for length of time in place. Pouch should be changed every 3 to 7 days, not daily (Colwell & Goldberg, 2021). If an opaque pouch is being used, remove it (see Step 7) to fully observe stoma. Empty and measure effluent and dispose of pouch in proper receptacle.	Provides access to view stoma. Assesses effectiveness of pouching system and detects potential for problems. To minimize skin irritation, avoid unnecessary changing of entire pouching system. When pouch leaks, skin damage from effluent causes more skin trauma than early removal of wafer (Colwell & Goldberg, 2021).

Clinical Judgment *Repeated leaking may indicate need for different type of pouch or addition of products such as stoma paste or seal. If the pouch is leaking, change it. Taping or patching it to contain effluent leaves the skin exposed to chemical or enzymatic irritation.*

6. Observe amount of effluent in pouch and empty it when it is one-third to one-half full (WOCN, 2018) by opening the pouch and draining it into a container for measurement of output. Note consistency of effluent, and document output.	Weight of pouch may disrupt seal of adhesive on skin. Monitors fluid balance and bowel function after surgery. Normal colostomy effluent is soft or formed stool; normal ileostomy effluent is liquid.
7. Observe stoma (if pouch is transparent) for type, location, color, swelling, presence of sutures, trauma, and healing or irritation of peristomal skin.	Stoma characteristics influence selection of an appropriate pouching system. Convexity in skin barrier is often necessary with a flush or retracted stoma (Colwell et al., 2022).
8. Inspect area for placement of stoma in relation to abdominal contours and presence of scars or incisions. Remove and dispose of gloves; perform hand hygiene.	Determines if current pouching system is effective or if new selection is needed. Abdominal contours, scars, or incisions affect type of system and adhesion to skin surface. Reduces transmission of microorganisms (McNichol et al., 2021; Colwell & Goldberg, 2021).
9. Assess patient's knowledge, prior experience with stoma and ostomy care, and feelings about procedure.	Reveals need for patient instruction and/or support.
10. Discuss interest in learning self-care. Identify others who will be helping patient after leaving agency.	Assesses patient's body image. Facilitates teaching plan and timing of care to coincide with availability of family caregivers (Goldberg et al., 2018).

STEP	RATIONALE

PLANNING

1. Expected outcomes following completion of procedure:

- Stoma is red and moist; peristomal skin is intact and free of irritation; sutures are intact.
- Stoma drains moderate amount of liquid or soft stool (small amount of blood normal immediately after surgery), and flatus is in pouch, which can be seen with bulging of pouch. (Flatus may not be observable if pouch has gas filter.)
- Patient and/or family caregiver observes stoma and steps of procedure.
- Patient asks questions about procedure and attempts to help with pouch change.

2. Explain procedure to patient; encourage patient's interaction and questions.

3. Perform hand hygiene. Assemble equipment at bedside and close room curtains or door.

Normal findings in patient with postoperative ostomy that is healing.

Stoma is functioning normally. Snug seal around stoma has been attained. Flatus indicates return of peristalsis after surgery.

Reveals acceptance of alteration in body image and interest in self-care.

Indicates readiness to learn and begin self-care.

Lessens patient's anxiety and promotes patient's participation.

Reduces transmission of microorganisms. Ensures efficient procedure; provides privacy.

IMPLEMENTATION

1. Make patient comfortable, continuing to assume semi-reclining or supine position. (**NOTE:** Some patients with established ostomies prefer to stand.) If possible, provide patient with mirror for observation.

2. Perform hand hygiene and apply clean gloves.

3. Place towel or disposable waterproof barrier under patient and across patient's lower abdomen.

4. If not done during assessment, remove used pouch and skin barrier gently by pushing skin away from barrier in direction hair grows (WOCN, 2018). Loosen and lift the edge with one hand and press down on the skin near the sticky backing with the other hand. You may find it helpful to start at the top and work down to the bottom so you can see what you are doing. This will also allow the pouch to catch any urine or stool the stoma produces (Colwell & Goldberg, 2021). Use adhesive releaser to facilitate removal of skin barrier. Empty pouch and dispose of it in an appropriate receptacle. Measure output if needed. **NOTE:** There may be no output at time of first pouch change.

5. Clean peristomal skin gently with warm tap water using washcloth; do not scrub skin. If you touch stoma, minor bleeding is normal. Pat skin dry. Have washcloth handy for additional cleaning if there is output from the stoma while preparing pouch.

6. Measure stoma (see illustration). Expect size of stoma to change for first 4 to 6 weeks after surgery.

7. Trace pattern of stoma measurement on pouch backing or skin barrier (see illustration).

8. Cut opening on backing or skin barrier wafer (see illustration). If using a moldable or a shape-to-fit barrier, use fingers to mold shape-to-fit stoma.

When patient is semi-reclining, there are fewer skinfolds, which allows for ease of application of pouching system.

Reduces transmission of microorganisms.

Protects bed linen; maintains patient's dignity.

Reduces skin trauma. Improper removal of pouch and barrier can cause peristomal skin irritation or breakdown. Use of adhesive releaser reduces risk of MARSI (Fumarola et al., 2020).

Soap leaves residue on skin, which may irritate skin. Pouch does not adhere to wet skin. Ileostomies have frequent output, especially after eating.

Allows for proper fit of pouch that will protect peristomal skin. Swelling related to normal postoperative response.

Prepares for cutting opening in pouch.

Customizes pouch to provide appropriate fit over stoma.

Clinical Judgment *Instruct patients to remeasure stomas occasionally if they notice that the stoma has changed shape or size (Colwell & Goldberg, 2021).*

9. Remove protective backing from adhesive backing or wafer (see illustration).

10. Apply pouch over stoma (see illustration). Press firmly into place around stoma and outside edges. Have patient hold hand over pouch to apply heat to secure seal.

Prepares skin barrier for application to skin over stoma.

Pouch adhesives are heat and pressure sensitive and hold more securely at body temperature.

STEP	RATIONALE

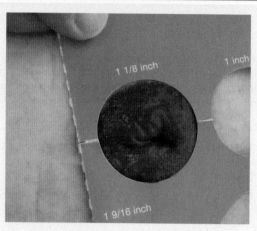

STEP 6 Measure stoma. *(Courtesy Coloplast, Minneapolis, MN.)*

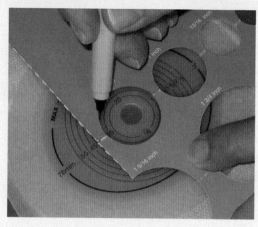

STEP 7 Trace measurement on skin barrier. *(Courtesy Coloplast, Minneapolis, MN.)*

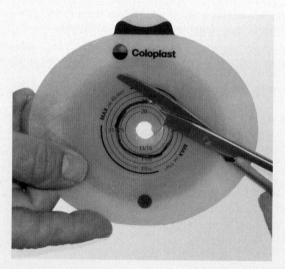

STEP 8 Cut opening in wafer. *(Courtesy Coloplast, Minneapolis, MN.)*

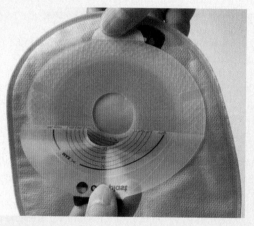

STEP 9 Remove protective backing. *(Courtesy Coloplast, Minneapolis, MN.)*

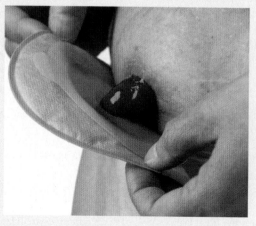

STEP 10 Apply pouch over stoma. *(Courtesy Coloplast, Minneapolis, MN.)*

STEP	RATIONALE
11. Close end of pouch with clip or integrated closure. Remove drape from patient. Help patient to assume comfortable position.	Ensures that pouch is secure. Contains effluent. Promotes patient comfort.
12. Place disposables in the trash. Remove and dispose of gloves. Perform hand hygiene.	Reduces transmission of microorganisms.
13. Raise side rails (as appropriate) and lower bed to lowest position, locking into position.	Ensures patient safety and prevents falls.
14. Place nurse call system in an accessible location within patient's reach.	Ensures patient can call for assistance if needed.

EVALUATION

1. Observe condition of skin barrier and adherence of pouch to abdominal surface.	Determines presence of leaks.
2. During pouch change, observe appearance of stoma, peristomal skin, abdominal contours, and suture line.	Determines condition of stoma and peristomal skin and progress of wound healing.
3. Note if there is presence of any flatus during pouch change.	Determines if peristalsis is returning.
4. Observe patient's and family caregiver's willingness to view stoma and ask questions about procedure.	Determines level of adjustment and understanding of stoma care and pouch application. Allows planning for future education needs and progress toward acceptance of altered body image (Colwell & Goldberg, 2021).
5. Use Teach-Back: "I want to be sure you understand how often you should change your ostomy pouch and why. Tell me what you should do to prevent your skin from becoming irritated and the frequency with which you should empty your pouch." Revise your instruction now or develop a plan for revised patient/family caregiver teaching if patient/family caregiver is not able to teach back correctly.	Teach-back is a technique for health care providers to ensure that they have explained medical information clearly so that patients and their families understand what is communicated to them (Agency for Healthcare Research and Quality [AHRQ], 2023).

Unexpected Outcomes

1. Skin around stoma is irritated, blistered, or bleeding or a rash is noted. May be caused by undermining of pouch seal by fecal contents, causing irritant dermatitis, or by adhesive exposure and removal, causing skin stripping or fungal or other skin eruption.

2. Necrotic stoma manifesting with purple or black color, dry instead of moist texture, failure to bleed when washed gently, or tissue sloughing.

3. Patient refuses to view stoma or participate in care.

Related Interventions

- Remove pouch more carefully.
- Change pouch more frequently or use different type of pouching system.
- Use only water to cleanse skin.
- Consult wound, ostomy, continence [WOC] nurse.
- Avoid use of alcohol or acetone-based products (Colwell & Goldberg, 2021).
- Pat skin dry after washing; do not rub the skin.

- Report to nurse in charge or health care provider.
- Document appearance.

- Obtain referral for ostomy care nurse.
- Allow patient to express feelings.
- Encourage family support.

Documentation

- Document type of pouch and skin barrier applied; time of procedure; amount and appearance of effluent in pouch; location, size, and appearance of stoma; and condition of peristomal skin.
- Document patient's and family caregiver's level of participation, teaching that was done, and response to teaching.

Hand-Off Reporting

- Report any of the following to nurse and/or health care provider: abnormal appearance of stoma, suture line, peristomal skin, or character of output.

Special Considerations

Patient Education

- Teach whenever you are doing a pouch change, even if patient does not appear interested. Do not insist that patient look at stoma; allow time for adjustment.
- Teach a family caregiver how to provide ostomy care when the patient is not self-managing elimination before surgery. Consult with a WOC nurse to provide instruction to patient/caregiver if available.
- Instruct patients to contact their WOC nurse or health care provider if (WOCN, 2018):
  - They are changing pouching systems more often than expected.
  - They are suddenly changing more often than normal wear time.
  - Their skin is red or sore.
- Give patient plain-language teaching materials that clearly state each step for a pouch change. Audiotaped or videotaped instructions are also available. Consider using materials that have illustrations for each step. For patients who do not speak English, provide a professional interpreter.
- Give patients a list of equipment and name, address, and phone number of a supplier.

Pediatrics

- Select pediatric pouches are designed especially for neonates, infants, and children. The pouches are smaller and have a more skin-sensitive adhesive on the barrier.
- Because most ostomy surgery done on neonates is for emergencies, often no time is available for preoperative selection of stoma site. The surgery is usually done because the neonate has necrotizing enterocolitis (NEC), Hirschsprung disease, or a congenital disorder (Colwell & Goldberg, 2021,). The stomas frequently are temporary, with closure of the ostomy performed when the surgical repair has healed and the neonate is medically ready for surgery. Children and adolescents may have ostomy surgery for conditions such as cancer, inflammatory bowel disease, and trauma.
- Neonates may have multiple stomas on their tiny abdomens after corrective bowel surgeries. Select a cut-to-fit pouch that allows multiple stoma openings in the skin barrier yet still fits on neonate's abdomen (Colwell & Goldberg, 2021).

- Because infants swallow air while sucking, it is normal to expect flatus. Make sure that the pouch can accommodate an increased amount of flatus after feeding or be prepared to release flatus frequently by opening the end of the pouch and releasing accumulated gas (Colwell & Goldberg, 2021).
- The skin of a preterm infant is not fully developed and is more absorbent than that of a full-term infant. Use skin sealants and adhesive releasers according to agency policy for preterm infant care (Colwell & Goldberg, 2021).
- As an infant grows in size, so does the stoma. Measure the stoma frequently and make appropriate adjustments in pouching and skin barrier size. Skin barriers for preterm infants must have flexibility to cover the infant's rounded abdominal contour (Colwell & Goldberg, 2021).
- Adolescents requiring an ostomy benefit from presurgical contact with other adolescents who have an ostomy (Colwell & Goldberg, 2021).

Older Adults

- Evaluate an older adult's cognitive status for understanding ostomy self-care instructions. Include a family caregiver in the care plan (if appropriate).
- Adapt care approaches for older patients who have impaired manual dexterity or limited vision. If a patient is unable to custom cut the size of the skin barrier, consider having barriers precut by an ostomy equipment supplier or using a precut pouching system.
- Costs of ostomy supplies and reimbursement are an issue for patients on a fixed income if not covered by insurance.

Populations With Disabilities

- Evaluate home toileting facilities and patients' ability to position to empty pouch directly into a toilet.
- Assess family caregiver ability and availability to aid with pouch emptying several times a day and pouch changes twice a week and as needed.
- Consider pouching systems that will allow for the greatest self-care success given the person's disability.

Home Care

- Evaluate home toileting facilities and patients' ability to position to empty pouch directly into a toilet.
- A patient may shower without covering a pouch or may take the pouch off in the shower to clean the peristomal skin if the patient wishes to do so and if cleared by health care provider.
- When patients are away from home, instruct them to carry plastic bags in a pocket or purse to throw away used pouching systems. If they use washable items such as a washcloth to clean the skin, they may be washed with household laundry (WOCN, 2018).
- If a pouching system has a clamp to close the pouch, have patients carry an extra clamp with them in case one breaks or gets lost.
- Patients should avoid storing pouches in extremely hot or cold locations. Temperature affects barrier and adhesive materials.

♦ SKILL 35.2   Pouching a Urostomy

Because urine flows more frequently from a urinary diversion, placement of a pouch is more challenging than with a fecal diversion. It can be difficult to keep the skin dry as you prepare a pouch application. In the immediate postoperative period, urinary stents extend out from a stoma (Fig. 35.11). A surgeon places the stents to prevent stenosis of the ureters at the site where the ureters are attached to the conduit. The stents are removed during the hospital stay or at the first postoperative visit with the surgeon.

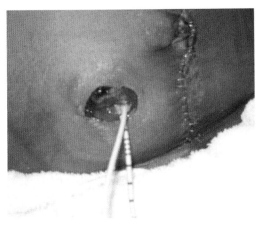

FIG. 35.11 Urostomy stoma with stents in place. (*Courtesy Jane Fellows.*)

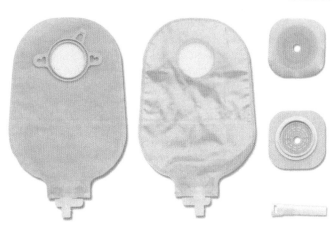

FIG. 35.12 Urostomy pouching system with adapter to connect pouch to bedside drainage bag. (*Courtesy Hollister Inc, Libertyville, IL.*)

The stoma is normally red and moist. It is made from part of the intestinal tract, usually the ileum. A normal stoma protrudes above the skin. An ileal conduit is usually located in the right lower quadrant of a patient's abdomen. While the patient is in bed, the pouch may be connected to a bedside drainage bag to decrease the need for frequent emptying. When the patient goes home, a bedside drainage bag may be used at night to avoid having to get up to empty the pouch. Each type of urostomy pouch comes with a connector for the bedside drainage bag (Fig. 35.12). A patient must understand the importance of draining the pouch frequently and using clean technique during stomal and skin care. As in the case of a colostomy or ileostomy pouching (see Skill 35.1), patients are at risk for medical adhesive–related skin injury (MARSI) unless proper skin barrier and pouch application are performed.

Delegation

The skill of pouching a new incontinent urinary diversion cannot be delegated to assistive personnel (AP). In some agencies care of an established urostomy (4–6 weeks or more after surgery) can be delegated to AP. Instruct the AP about:
- Expected appearance of the stoma
- Expected amount and character of the output and when to report changes
- Change in patient's stoma and surrounding skin integrity that should be reported
- Special equipment needed to complete procedure

Interprofessional Collaboration

- Refer to a wound, ostomy, continence (WOC) nurse, when available, for postsurgical assessment, pouch selection, and patient education.

Equipment

- Wafer (skin barrier) and clear urinary pouch, one-piece or two-piece, cut to fit or precut size
- Appropriate adapter for connection to bedside drainage bag
- Measuring guide
- Bedside urinary drainage bag
- Clean gloves
- Washcloth
- Towel or disposable waterproof barrier
- Basin with warm tap water
- Scissors
- Adhesive releaser
- Absorbent wick made from gauze rolled tightly in the shape of a tampon (optional)
- Waterproof bag for disposal of pouch
- Mirror for patient to observe ostomy
- *Optional:* Gown and goggles if there is any risk of splashing when emptying pouch

STEP	RATIONALE

ASSESSMENT

1. Identify patient using at least two identifiers (e.g., name and birthday or name and medical record number) according to agency policy.	Ensures patient safety. Complies with The Joint Commission standards and improves patient safety (TJC, 2023).
2. Assess patient's/family caregiver's health literacy.	Determines degree to which individuals have the ability to find, understand, and use information and services to make informed health-related decisions and actions for themselves and others (CDC, 2023).
3. Review electronic health record (EHR) and assess if patient is at risk for MARSI: age, dehydration, malnutrition, exposure to radiation therapy, underlying chronic conditions (e.g., diabetes, immunosuppression), and edema of skin.	Common risk factors for MARSI (Fumarola et al., 2020). Factors raise your level of observation if patient has a stoma product containing adhesive tape.
4. Perform hand hygiene and apply clean gloves.	Reduces transmission of microorganisms.

STEP	RATIONALE
5. Have patient assume semi-reclining or supine position. Observe existing skin barrier and pouch for leakage and length of time in place. Pouch should be changed every 3 to 7 days, not daily. If urine is leaking under wafer, change pouch.	Provides access to view stoma. Assesses effectiveness of pouching system and allows for early detection of potential problems. To minimize skin irritation, avoid changing entire pouching system unnecessarily. Repeated leakage may indicate need for different type of pouch to provide reliable seal (Colwell & Goldberg, 2021).
6. Observe characteristics of urine in pouch or bedside drainage bag. Empty pouch before it is one-third to one-half full by opening valve and draining it into container for measurement.	There may be blood or large amounts of mucus in urine after surgery, but this should resolve in the first 1 to 2 weeks after surgery. Weight of pouch can disrupt seal. Urine from ileal conduit will contain mucus because of flow through intestinal segment.
7. Observe stoma for color, swelling, presence of sutures, trauma, and healing of peristomal skin. Assess type of stoma. Remove and dispose of gloves. Perform hand hygiene.	Consider stoma characteristics in selecting appropriate pouching system. Convexity in skin barrier is often necessary with a flush or retracted stoma. Reduces transmission of microorganisms.
8. Assess patient's knowledge, prior experience with urostomy pouching, and feelings about procedure.	Reveals need for patient instruction and/or support.
9. Explore patient's perceptions, acceptance of change in function, and interest in learning self-care. Identify others who will be helping patient after leaving hospital.	Assesses patient's body image. Facilitates teaching plan and timing of care to coincide with availability of family caregivers (Goldberg et al., 2018).

PLANNING

1. Expected outcomes following completion of procedure:	
• Stoma is red and moist with stents protruding from it. Peristomal skin is free of irritation and intact. Sutures are intact.	Normal findings for postoperative urinary diversion (Colwell & Goldberg, 2021).
• Urine drains freely from stents or stoma.	These are normal findings after surgery.
• Urine is yellow with mucous shreds and is without foul odor. Urine may be pink or contain small blood clots after surgery.	Mucous shreds are normal when urine flows through intestinal segment.
• Volume of output is within acceptable limits (≥30 mL/h).	Normal output reveals ureters draining without obstruction.
• Patient and family caregiver observe stoma and procedural steps.	Shows adjustment to body image change and willingness to learn self-care.
• Patient asks questions about procedure and may help with pouch change.	Indicates readiness to learn and begin self-care.
2. Explain procedure to patient; encourage questions and interaction.	Lessens patient's anxiety and promotes participation.
3. Perform hand hygiene. Assemble equipment at bedside and close room curtains or door.	Reduces transmission of microorganisms. Ensures efficient procedure; provides privacy.

IMPLEMENTATION

1. Make patient comfortable, continuing to assume semi-reclining or supine position. If possible, provide patient with mirror for observation.	When patient is semi-reclining versus sitting, there are fewer skin wrinkles, which allows for ease of pouch application.
2. Perform hand hygiene and apply clean gloves.	Reduces transmission of microorganisms.
3. Place towel or disposable waterproof barrier under patient and across patient's lower abdomen.	Protects bed linen; maintains patient's dignity.
4. If not done during assessment, remove used pouch and skin barrier gently by pushing skin away from barrier, away from direction of hair growth (WOCN, 2018). Loosen and lift the edge with one hand and press down on the skin near the sticky backing with the other hand (WOCN, 2018). If stents are present, pull pouch gently around them and lay towel underneath. Empty pouch and measure output. Dispose of pouch in appropriate receptacle.	Reduces risk for trauma to skin and for dislodging stents. Keeps urine from leaking onto skin. Urine output provides information about renal status and whether volume is within acceptable limits (≥30 mL/h).
5. If stoma is draining continuously, may use rolled gauze placed at stoma opening. Encourage patient or family caregiver to hold gauze at stoma opening continuously during pouch measurement and change.	Using wick at stoma opening prevents peristomal skin from becoming wet with urine during pouch change. Allows patient/family caregiver participation during procedure.
6. While keeping rolled gauze in contact with stoma, clean peristomal skin gently with warm tap water and washcloth; do not scrub skin. If you touch stoma, minor bleeding is normal. Pat skin completely dry.	Avoid soap. It leaves residue on skin, which can irritate it. Pouch does not adhere to wet skin.

STEP	RATIONALE
7. Measure stoma (see Skill 35.1, Step 6). Expect size of stoma to change for first 4 to 6 weeks after surgery.	Allows for proper fit of pouch that will protect peristomal skin. Normal postoperative swelling.
8. Trace pattern on pouch backing or skin barrier (see Skill 35.1, Step 7).	Prepares for cutting opening in pouch.
9. Cut opening in pouch (see Skill 35.1, Step 8). If using a moldable or a shape-to-fit barrier, use fingers to mold shape-to-fit stoma.	Customizes pouch to provide appropriate fit over stoma.

Clinical Judgment *Instruct patients to remeasure stomas occasionally if they notice that the stoma has changed shape or size (Colwell & Goldberg, 2021; Goldberg et al., 2018).*

STEP	RATIONALE
10. Remove protective backing from adhesive backing or wafer surface (see Skill 35.1, Step 9). Remove rolled gauze from stoma.	Removing backing prepares skin barrier for application to skin over stoma.
11. Apply pouch (see Skill 35.1, Step 10). Press adhesive barrier firmly into place around stoma and outside edges. Have patient hold hand over pouch for 1 to 2 minutes to secure seal.	Pouch adhesives are heat and pressure sensitive and will hold more securely at body temperature.
12. Use adapter provided with pouches to connect pouch to bedside urinary bag. Keep tubing below level of bag.	Allows patient to rest without frequent emptying of pouch. Tubing position allows for collection and measurement of urine and prevents backflow of urine into pouch.
13. Remove drape from patient. Help patient to assume comfortable position.	Promotes patient comfort.
14. Place disposables in the trash. Remove and dispose of gloves. Perform hand hygiene.	Reduces transmission of microorganisms. Use appropriate disposal receptacle if patient is on hazardous drugs (Kennedy et al., 2023).
15. Raise side rails (as appropriate) and lower bed to lowest position, locking into position.	Ensures patient safety and prevents falls.
16. Place nurse call system in an accessible location within patient's reach.	Ensures patient can call for assistance if needed.

EVALUATION

1. Observe appearance of stoma, peristomal skin, and suture line during pouch change.	Determines condition of stoma and peristomal skin and progress of wound healing.
2. Evaluate character and volume of urinary drainage.	Determines if stoma and/or stents are patent. Character of urine reveals degree of concentration and whether there is possible urinary tract infection (Colwell & Goldberg, 2021).
3. Observe patient's and family caregiver's willingness to view stoma and ask questions about procedure.	Determines level of adjustment and understanding of stoma care and pouch application.
4. **Use Teach-Back:** "I want to be sure you know how to change your urostomy pouch. Let's review what we discussed. Tell me how often you should empty your pouch and how often you should change it." Revise your instruction now or develop a plan for revised patient/family caregiver teaching if patient/family caregiver is not able to teach back correctly.	Teach-back is a technique for health care providers to ensure that they have explained medical information clearly so that patients and their families understand what is communicated to them (AHRQ, 2023).

Unexpected Outcomes	Related Interventions
1. Skin around stoma is irritated, blistered, or bleeding; or maceration is noted as result of chronic exposure to urine.	• Check stoma size and opening in skin barrier. • Resize skin barrier opening if necessary. • Remove pouch more carefully. • Consult WOC nurse. • Pat skin dry after washing with water; do not rub the skin
2. No urine output for several hours, or output is less than 30 mL/h. Urine has foul odor.	• Increase fluid intake (if allowed). • Notify health care provider. • Obtain urine specimen for culture and sensitivity if ordered. (See Procedure 35.3.)
3. Patient and family caregiver are unable to observe stoma, ask questions, or participate in care.	• Consult WOC nurse. • Allow patient to express feelings. • Encourage family support.

Documentation

- Document type of pouch, time of change, condition and appearance of stoma/stents and peristomal skin, and character of urine.
- Document urinary output.
- Document patient's and family caregiver's reaction to stoma and level of participation. Document your evaluation of patient and family caregiver learning.

Hand-Off Reporting

- Report abnormalities in stoma or peristomal skin and absence of urinary output to nurse in charge or health care provider.

Special Considerations
Patient Education

- Follow patient education considerations in Skill 35.1.
- Teach patients the significance and importance of drinking 2 L (2 quarts) of fluid daily to prevent urinary tract infections (UTIs) (Colwell & Goldberg, 2021). Explain that some mucus in urine is expected but that patients should report any blood in their urine, excessively cloudy urine, chills, fever (38.3°C [101°F] or higher), and back (flank) pain to their health care provider.

Pediatrics

- In neonates, urinary diversions are less common than fecal ostomies.

- Select pediatric pouches designed especially for neonates, infants, and children; these pouches are smaller and have a more skin-sensitive adhesive on the barrier.

Older Adults

- Follow considerations for gerontological patients in Skill 35.1.
- Older patients have decreased thirst and may not normally consume adequate fluids. Explain importance of fluid intake to promote healthy renal function and decrease risk for UTIs.

Populations With Disabilities

- Follow considerations for disabled patients in Skill 35.1.
- If disabled patient cannot empty pouch as needed, use of urinary drainage bag connected to pouch during the day as well as at night may be considered. A smaller leg bag is available for daytime use.

Home Care

- Follow home care considerations in Skill 35.1.
- Instruct patient that pouch can be connected to straight drainage at night. Make sure patient understands that adapter will be needed to connect pouch to the bedside drainage bag (see Fig. 35.12).
- Urinary drainage bag should be rinsed with tap water after use.

◆ SKILL 35.3 Catheterizing a Urinary Diversion

Catheterization of a urinary diversion is the best method to obtain an accurate culture and sensitivity specimen to screen a patient with a urostomy for infection. When it is necessary to obtain a urine specimen from a urinary diversion, you insert a sterile catheter into a stoma. Obtaining a specimen of urine in a pouch does not provide an accurate finding because of the likely risk for contamination by microorganisms growing in the stagnant urine. With the use of aseptic technique, catheterization is relatively safe and easy. If a patient uses a two-piece system, remove the pouch from the skin barrier and replace it after catheterization without disturbing the skin barrier. If a patient uses a one-piece system, you must remove the pouch to obtain the specimen and replace it with a new pouch after the procedure. To prevent trauma to the tissues, understand how the stoma and implanted ureters are constructed for a patient (see Fig. 35.11).

Delegation

The skill of catheterizing a urinary diversion cannot be delegated to assistive personnel (AP). Instruct the AP to:
- Inform nurse if patient complains of peristomal or flank pain (sign of kidney infection)

- Inform nurse if there is a change in color, odor, or amount of urine or if there is blood in the urine

Equipment

- Urinary catheterization supplies (contained in prepackaged sterile catheter kit or may need to be gathered separately):
  - 14- to 16-Fr sterile catheter
  - Water-soluble lubricant
  - Antiseptic swabs (e.g., povidone-iodine or chlorhexidine)
  - Sterile gloves
  - Sterile specimen container
  - Absorbent gauze wick
- Bed protection barrier
- Towels
- Urinary pouch if needed
- Clean gloves

STEP	RATIONALE

ASSESSMENT

1. Identify patient using at least two identifiers (e.g., name and birthday or name and medical record number) according to agency policy. | Ensures patient safety. Complies with The Joint Commission standards and improves patient safety (TJC, 2023). |

2. Review electronic health record (EHR) and observe for signs and symptoms of urinary tract infection (UTI): elevated temperature, chills, foul-smelling urine, and elevated white blood cell (WBC) count. | Determines the indications for performing a catheterization to obtain sterile specimen from urinary diversion. Having urinary diversion poses risk for reflux of urine back to kidneys, resulting in infection (Colwell & Goldberg, 2021). |

STEP	RATIONALE
3. Obtain health care provider's order for catheterization.	Invasive and diagnostic procedure requires health care provider's order.
4. Assess patient's/family caregiver's health literacy.	Determines degree to which individuals have the ability to find, understand, and use information and services to make informed health-related decisions and actions for themselves and others (CDC, 2023).
5. Assess patient's understanding of need for procedure and how it is done.	Determines willingness to cooperate and reduces patient's anxiety.
6. Assess patient's knowledge, experience with urinary diversion catheterization, and feelings about procedure.	Reveals need for patient instruction and/or support.
7. Assess for allergies to antiseptics and substitute chlorhexidine for another antiseptic if patient has shown a skin reaction or allergic reaction to this solution. Have patient describe typical allergic response when allergy identified.	This is important for patient safety and to prevent an untoward effect from this topical application to the stoma.

PLANNING

1. Expected outcomes following completion of procedure:	
• Urine specimen is not contaminated with bacteria during procedure.	Urine was obtained correctly. Laboratory results are accurate.
• Patient describes risks for infection and techniques to prevent infection.	Demonstrates patient's learning.
2. Perform hand hygiene. Assemble equipment at bedside and close room curtain or door.	Reduces transmission of microorganisms. Ensures efficient procedure; provides privacy.
3. Explain procedure to patient, including sensations that will be felt. If possible, obtain specimen when patient is due to change pouch (see Skill 35.2) if using one-piece system.	Lessens anxiety and promotes patient's cooperation. Cleaning stoma and surrounding skin may cause cool sensation. Insertion of catheter may cause sensation of mild pressure, or it may not be felt at all. Changing pouch too frequently could result in skin trauma.

IMPLEMENTATION

1. If possible, position patient sitting and drape towel across lower abdomen.	Gravity facilitates flow of urine. Maintains patient's dignity. Towel absorbs urine.
2. Perform hand hygiene and apply clean gloves.	Reduces transmission of microorganisms.
3. Remove pouch (see Skill 35.2). If patient uses two-piece system, remove pouch but leave skin barrier attached to skin.	Allows access to stoma.
4. Remove and dispose of gloves and perform hand hygiene.	Avoids contamination.
5. Open sterile catheterization set according to instructions or open needed equipment and place on sterile barrier using aseptic technique (see Chapter 9). If not using catheterization kit, place gauze pad on sterile field and squeeze small amount of lubricant onto gauze. Apply sterile gloves.	Prepares sterile work field.
6. If needed, have patient hold absorbent gauze wick on stoma while you prepare catheterization supplies.	Prevents leakage of urine on peristomal skin, linens, and clothing.
7. Clean surface of stoma with antiseptic swabs using circular motion from center outward. Use new swab each time; repeat twice. Allow chlorhexidine antiseptic to dry completely or, if another antiseptic is used, wipe off excess antiseptic with dry sterile gauze or cotton ball.	Removes surface bacteria. Chlorhexidine must dry to achieve antibacterial effect.
8. Remove lid from sterile specimen container.	Sterile container collects small volume of urine.

Clinical Judgment *If patient has stents in place, use antiseptic swab to clean the ends of the stents and place the stents in the sterile cup. Allow urine to drip into the cup until you obtain an adequate amount for a specimen. Then go directly to Step 13.*

9. Lubricate tip of catheter with water-soluble lubricant, keeping catheter sterile.	Facilitates passage of catheter through stoma.
10. With dominant hand, gently insert catheter tip into stoma. Do not force catheter; redirect course as needed. Place distal end of catheter into specimen container. Have patient cough; massage abdomen near stoma or turn patient on the side.	Use care to avoid trauma to conduit. Movement and coughing may facilitate flow of urine from conduit (Colwell & Goldberg, 2021).

STEP	RATIONALE
11. Hold container below level of stoma. If needed, wait several minutes to get adequate amount of urine.	Culture and sensitivity studies require only 3 to 5 mL of urine (check agency policy).
12. Withdraw catheter slowly; place absorbent pad over stoma.	Keeps skin dry.
13. Apply lid to specimen container.	Prevents accidental spillage.
14. Reapply new pouch or reattach pouch if patient uses two-piece system (see Skill 35.2).	Pouch is necessary to contain urine.
15. Dispose of used pouch and equipment properly.	Avoids unpleasant odor in room. Reduces transmission of microorganisms. Use appropriate disposal receptacle if patient is on hazardous drugs (Kennedy et al., 2023).
16. Remove and dispose of gloves; perform hand hygiene. Label specimen in presence of patient (TJC, 2023), place in biohazard bag, and send to laboratory at once.	Reduces transmission of microorganisms. Ensures that laboratory results are assigned to correct patient. Labeling ensures acceptance and processing of specimen by laboratory. Urine that sits for long periods at room temperature will adversely affect laboratory results.
17. Help patient to a comfortable position.	Restores comfort and sense of well-being.
18. Place nurse call system in an accessible location within patient's reach.	Ensures patient can call for assistance if needed.
19. Raise side rails if appropriate and lower bed to lowest position, locking into position.	Ensures patient safety and prevents falls.

EVALUATION

1. Compare results of culture and sensitivity with expected findings. Mucus is normal finding if patient has ileal conduit.

2. **Use Teach-Back:** "I want to be sure you understand the reason we needed to collect the urine. Tell me in your own words why we did this procedure to get urine from your stoma. What are the signs of a urinary tract infection when you have a urostomy?" Revise your instruction now or develop a plan for revised patient/family caregiver teaching if patient/family caregiver is not able to teach back correctly.

Determines presence of infection. If contamination appears likely, second specimen will be needed.

Teach-back is a technique for health care providers to ensure that they have explained medical information clearly so that patients and their families understand what is communicated to them (AHRQ, 2023).

Unexpected Outcomes	Related Interventions
1. Unable to obtain urine specimen.	• Reposition patient. • If there is still no urine, have patient drink more fluids or consult with health care provider regarding increasing rate of intravenous fluids and try again later. • Inform health care provider if unable to obtain specimen on second attempt.
2. Skin or stoma reveals complications.	• Notify nurse and/or health care provider. • Consult with wound, ostomy, continence (WOC) nurse about pouching system or skin barrier to use.

Documentation
• Document time specimen collected; patient's tolerance of procedure; and appearance of urine, skin, and stoma.
• Document your evaluation of patient and family caregiver learning.

Hand-Off Reporting
• Report results of laboratory test to nurse in charge or health care provider.

Special Considerations
Patient Education
• Explain common symptoms of UTI to patient and family caregiver: flank pain; dark, cloudy, or bloody urine; foul-smelling urine; fever (38.3°C [101°F] or higher); confusion.
• Encourage patient to notify health care provider if symptoms of infection develop.
• Reinforce importance of fluid intake (2 L/day).

✦ CLINICAL JUDGMENT AND NEXT-GENERATION NCLEX® EXAMINATION–STYLE QUESTIONS

The nurse is caring for a 24-year-old patient who had surgery this week. The patient now has an ileostomy and urostomy and is having trouble coping with the change in body image. When the nurse attempts to provide education on self-care, the patient tearfully says, "I really don't think I can do any of that."

1. With which member of the interprofessional team will the nurse **most** closely collaborate to address the patient's fear?
   1. Surgeon who performed the procedure
   2. Wound, ostomy, continence nurse
   3. Registered dietitian nutritionist
   4. Patient's primary care provider

2. When initially caring for the patient's urostomy, which of the following assessments will the nurse conduct that could indicate the presence of a urinary tract infection (UTI)? **Select all that apply.**
   1. Urine appearance
   2. Intake of solid food
   3. Temperature
   4. Patient's report of lower abdominal discomfort
   5. Peristomal skin condition

3. The nurse provides health teaching about ostomy pouch emptying and pouch changing for the patient and family caregiver in preparation for discharge. Indicate whether each teaching by the nurse would be indicated or not indicated before the patient's discharge tomorrow.

Health Teaching	Indicated	Not Indicated
"Empty the ostomy pouch when it is one-third to one-half full to avoid leakage."		
"Only change the pouch if you notice leakage from under the wafer."		
"The stoma will normally be red and moist."		
"The skin around the stoma is normally intact with some reddening after the adhesive wafer is removed."		
"If you notice blisters on the skin around your stoma, scrub them well to make sure the skin is clean."		
"Pouches should be changed every 3 to 7 days."		
"Use alcohol- or acetone-based products to clean stoma thoroughly."		

4. The nurse is assisting the patient in learning how to change the ostomy pouch. After hand hygiene, donning gloves, and removing the old pouch, which action will the nurse tell the patient to take next?
   1. Measure the stoma.
   2. Cut a hole in the wafer.
   3. Observe the stoma and the skin around it.
   4. Cleanse and dry the peristomal skin.

5. The patient has been discharged to home. The home health care nurse notes that there is a raw, weeping, tender area of skin surrounding the stoma. The patient says, "The pouch overfilled a few times before I changed it." Which of the following actions will the nurse take? **Select all that apply.**
   1. Clean the area with alcohol to help dry the raw skin.
   2. Consult a wound, ostomy, continence nurse.
   3. Review the importance of emptying the pouch before it is half full.
   4. Cut the opening in the skin barrier larger than the last one.
   5. Measure the stoma again to see if it may have changed size since surgery.

Visit the Evolve site for Answers to Clinical Judgment and Next-Generation NCLEX® Examination–Style Questions.

REFERENCES

Agency for Healthcare Research and Quality (AHRQ): *Teach-Back: intervention*, 2023. https://www.ahrq.gov/patient-safety/reports/engage/interventions/teach-back.html. Accessed August 2, 2023.

American Cancer Society (ACS): *Colostomy guide*, Atlanta, GA, 2019a, ACS. https://www.cancer.org/cancer/managing-cancer/treatment-types/surgery/ostomies/colostomy.html. Accessed August 2, 2023.

American Cancer Society (ACS): *Caring for an Ileostomy*, Atlanta, GA, 2019b, ACS. https://www.cancer.org/cancer/managing-cancer/treatment-types/surgery/ostomies/ileostomy/management.html. Accessed August 2, 2023.

American Cancer Society (ACS): *Caring for a Urostomy*, Atlanta, GA, 2019c, ACS. https://www.cancer.org/cancer/managing-cancer/treatment-types/surgery/ostomies/urostomy/management.html. Accessed August 2, 2023.

Burgess-Stocks J, et al: Ostomy and continent diversion patient bill of rights: research validation of standards of care, *J Wound Ostomy Continence Nurs* 2022;49(3):251–260.

Byfield D: The lived experiences of persons with ostomies attending a support group: a qualitative study, *J Wound Ostomy Continence Nurs* 47(5):489–495, 2020. doi:10.1097/WON.0000000000000696.

Centers for Disease Control and Prevention (CDC): *What is health literacy?* 2023. https://www.cdc.gov/healthliteracy/learn/index.html. Accessed August 2, 2023.

Colwell JC, et al: Use of a convex pouching system in the postoperative period: a national consensus, *J Wound Ostomy Continence Nurs* 49(3):240–246, 2022.

Colwell J, Goldberg M: *Wound, Ostomy, and Continence Nurses Society (WOCN) Core Curriculum: Ostomy Management*, ed 2, Philadelphia, 2021, Wolters Kluwer.

Fellows J, et al: Multinational survey on living with an ostomy: prevalence and impact of peristomal skin complications, *Br J Nurs* 30(16):S22–S30, 2021.

Fumarola S, et al: Overlooked and underestimated: medical adhesive-related skin injuries. Best practice consensus document on prevention, *J Wound Care* 29(Suppl 3c):S1–S24, 2020.

Goldberg M, et al: Management of the adult patient with a fecal or urinary ostomy—an executive summary, *J WOCN* 45(1):50–58, 2018.

Kennedy K, et al: Safe handling of hazardous drugs. *J Oncol Pharm Practice* 29(2):401–412, 2023.

Office of Disease Prevention and Health Promotion (ODPHP): *Health-related quality of life and well-being*, n.d. https://health.gov/healthypeople/priority-areas/social-determinants-health. Accessed August 2, 2023.

The Joint Commission (TJC): *2023 National patient safety goals*, Oakbrook Terrace, IL, 2023, The Joint Commission. https://www.jointcommission.org/standards/national-patient-safety-goals/. Accessed August 2, 2023.

McNichol L, et al: Characteristics of convex skin barriers and clinical application, *J Wound Ostomy Continence Nurs* 48(6):524, 2021.

World Council of Enterostomal Therapists (WCET): *WCET international ostomy guideline*. Chabal L, Prentice J, Ayello E editors: Perth Australia, 2020, WCET.

Wound, Ostomy, and Continence Nurses Society (WOCN): *Basic ostomy skin care: a guide for patients and healthcare providers*, Mount Laurel, NJ, 2018. https://www.ostomy.org/wp-content/uploads/2018/11/wocn_basic_ostomy_skin_care_2018.pdf. Accessed August 2, 2023.

Zelga P, et al: Patient-related factors associated with stoma and peristomal complications following fecal ostomy surgery: a scoping review, *J Wound Ostomy Continence Nurs* 48(5):415–430, 2021.

UNIT 12
Elimination: Next-Generation NCLEX®
(NGN)–Style Unfolding Case Study

PHASE 1

QUESTION 1.
The nurse has documented an assessment for a client admitted to the hospital from a long-term care agency.

Highlight the findings that require **immediate** further assessment by the nurse.

History and Physical	Nurses' Notes	Vital Signs	Laboratory Results

1300: 88-year-old client of female gender identity with a history of dementia admitted from long-term care agency. Long-term care agency nurse states that the client began to decline this morning and has experienced intermittent hallucinations after developing a fever of 40°C (104.0°F). Other vital signs include HR 90 beats/min; RR 20 breaths/min; BP 150/92 mm Hg; SpO$_2$ 98% on RA. Assessment reveals a well-nourished individual with PERRLA, lungs clear to auscultation, regular heart rate with no murmurs, and a soft, nontender abdomen. Not oriented to person, time, location, or situation. The client has an indwelling urinary catheter present; urine is cloudy and dark colored. The long-term care nurse reports the catheter has been in place for 10 days.

QUESTION 2.
The nurse reviews the documentation to determine the need for additional information about the client.

Complete the following sentence by selecting from the list of word choices below.

The nurse will contact the long-term care agency nurse to inquire about the client's [**Word Choice**] and [**Word Choice**].

Word Choices
Current weight
Psychiatric history
Amount and type of usual fluid intake
Food preferences
Client's ability to feed self

PHASE 2

QUESTION 3.
The nurse prepares to talk with the health care provider about assessment findings and impressions.

Complete the following sentence by selecting from the list of word choices below.

The nurse will **prioritize** communicating to the health care provider about the client's **Word Choice** and **Word Choice**.

Word Choices
Disorientation to person, place, time, and situation
Temperature of 40°C (104.0°F)
History of dementia
Blood pressure of 150/92 mm Hg
Indwelling urinary catheter with dark cloudy urine

QUESTION 4.
The client is admitted to a medical unit for monitoring. Assessment reveals the client to be very weak and confused. The health care provider orders a urine culture to be obtained, removal of the existing catheter, and insertion of a new indwelling urinary catheter.

In addition to the new actual indwelling catheter, which supplies will the nurse plan to gather to prepare for insertion? **Select all that apply.**
o Soap
o Washcloth
o Clean gloves
o Sterile gloves
o Drainage bag
o Waterproof absorbent pad
o Syringe prefilled with sterile water

PHASE 3

QUESTION 5.

The nurse prepares the woman for catheterization.
   Which actions will the nurse take during the insertion process?

o Separate labia with nondominant hand.
o Don sterile gloves and cleanse perineum.
o Place sterile drape under client with shiny side up.
o Lubricate catheter tip before insertion with petroleum jelly.
o Cleanse labia and urinary meatus from anus toward clitoris.
o Inflate catheter balloon by using syringe prefilled with sterile water.

QUESTION 6.

The nurse has completed insertion of the indwelling urinary catheter.
   Select **2** findings that indicate that the task was completed accurately.

o The meatus is chafed.
o The client is restless.
o A bladder scan reveals no urine in the bladder.
o Bladder palpation reveals distention.
o Urine leaks around the tubing connection.
o The bag is noted to have 80 mL of urine collected.

UNIT 13
Care of the Surgical Patient

The care of a surgical patient involves a number of routine skills: patient education about perioperative preparation, physical preparation of the patient for surgery, monitoring during surgical recovery, and the comprehensive approach to support a patient through recovery and discharge. However, the manner in which you perform these skills is highly individualized. Patient education in particular must be patient-centered to ensure that a patient is properly informed and prepared to participate in the surgical experience and to then follow necessary postoperative guidelines. For example, a young adult with limited health literacy and visual limitations will require you to adapt instruction much differently compared with an older adult with no known health problems. Because surgery invokes anxiety and fear, your application of therapeutic communication techniques and knowledge of the stress response is key in identifying potential problems and then adapting teaching strategies accordingly. Also, critical assessment of a patient's resources in the home or community care setting allows you to anticipate how to adjust routine explanations so that recommended guidelines fit the patient's home environment.

Use clinical judgment when you conduct a preoperative assessment. A comprehensive patient database includes the patient's current health status, physical risks for undergoing surgery, and knowledge of the impending procedure. Include the family caregiver or close friend who will assist with postoperative care after discharge. You will apply critical thinking attitudes and intellectual standards to ensure the data you collect are thorough and relevant to the patient. Each category of preoperative assessment will trigger various questions leading to clarity and relevance. For example, consider assessing a patient for chronic disease; if one exists, you must explore the effects the condition has on the physical systems most affected by surgery and if the patient poses unique risks. If a patient has a history of bronchitis, knowing the impact on lung function, you will assess if the patient is able to cough effectively, the amount of mucous production normally expressed, and the status of lung sounds. Such information guides you to the interventions to deliver (e.g., coughing, incentive spirometry, hydration for mucous clearing) and provides a database for evaluating the patient response after interventions are performed.

The physical preparation of a patient for surgery is usually standardized, but there are variations on the basis of the type of scheduled surgery. For example, a patient undergoing surgery involving the intestines will have to follow a preoperative bowel preparation protocol. A patient undergoing a hip replacement may be required to exercise more physically and even visit a physical therapist before entering the health care agency. Many patients require chlorhexidine baths or scrubs the night before and/or the morning of surgery. As a nurse, you are responsible for anticipating the standard and individualized forms of preparation required and educating patients about the rationale for the therapies. Standard physical preparation just before surgery involves inserting an intravenous line for fluid administration, verifying allergies and blood type, and gathering a patient's personal items. During this process, the ongoing provision of psychological support and educational instruction informs the patient and potentially minimizes anxiety.

Knowledge of the anticipated effects of surgery, a patient's preoperative health status, and the standard postoperative assessments of airway, breathing, and circulation place you in a position to critically judge how a patient initially recovers from surgery. Always be alert. Let the patient's ongoing responses guide you in choosing the frequency and type of assessments needed. Then allow those assessments to direct your interventions. For example, when working in a recovery room, if a patient seems slow to awaken from anesthesia, focus on monitoring vital signs and level of consciousness, and if breathing is shallow, turn the patient to one side with the head elevated. If a patient awakens quickly with stable vital signs, focus on pain management and preventive therapies such as coughing and incentive spirometry.

As a patient recovers from the initial postoperative phase of recovery, your assessment and scope of interventions broaden to include all body systems. Airway, breathing, and circulation remain priorities. Pain becomes a priority as well because if it is left uncontrolled, patient recovery will be slowed. For example, acute pain will limit the ability of a patient to be mobile and initiate self-care. Postoperative assessment and corresponding supportive care include all body systems most likely to be affected by a particular surgery. Skin integrity will apply to all surgeries, requiring you to conduct a precise and accurate description of a surgical wound to monitor healing. Patients forced to be more immobile after surgery, such as knee or hip replacement and spinal surgery, require close examination of circulatory status to monitor for risk of deep vein thrombosis. Patients placed on early ambulation protocols will require monitoring of tolerance to exercise and the effects of ambulation on comfort.

Clinical judgment during postoperative recovery of a patient requires knowledge of surgical conditions, use of evidence-based knowledge for prevention of complications, and application of what you assess about each patient to make patient-centered adaptations needed for recovery.

36 | Preoperative and Postoperative Care

SKILLS AND PROCEDURES

Skill 36.1 **Preoperative Assessment, p. 1061**

Skill 36.2 **Preoperative Teaching, p. 1065**

Skill 36.3 **Patient Preparation for Surgery, p. 1075**

Skill 36.4 **Providing Immediate Anesthesia Recovery in the Postanesthesia Care Unit, p. 1079**

Skill 36.5 **Providing Early Postoperative (Phase II) and Convalescent Phase (Phase III) Recovery, p. 1087**

OBJECTIVES

Mastery of content in this chapter will enable you to:

- Apply principles of patient-centered care into preoperative and postoperative care.
- Discuss the patient preparations needed for a patient having surgery.
- Identify risk factors that can potentially affect a patient's clinical outcomes postoperatively.
- Discuss cultural differences that might affect the implementation of preoperative and postoperative procedures.
- Identify the benefits of structured preoperative teaching.
- Develop a rationale for each of the postoperative exercises.
- Formulate a plan to teach a patient to perform postoperative exercises.
- Discuss the differences in nursing assessment during the immediate postoperative period and the convalescent phase of recovery.
- Demonstrate an assessment of a postoperative patient.

MEDIA RESOURCES

- http://evolve.elsevier.com/Perry/nursinginterventions
- Audio Glossary
- Checklists
- Case Studies
- Review Questions
- ▶ Video Clips

- Answers to Clinical Judgment and Next-Generation NCLEX® Examination–Style Questions
- Skills Performance Checklists
- Printable Key Points

PURPOSE

Surgical care of patients has been impacted by advancements in technology that result in less invasive surgery and shortened inpatient lengths of stay. Surgery takes place in a variety of settings, including hospitals, ambulatory surgery centers, health care providers' offices, and even mobile units. The principles of caring for perioperative patients are basically the same, regardless of the setting, except for the timing and extent of therapy.

During preoperative preparation, a nurse focuses on physical, psychological, sociocultural, and spiritual preparation; assessment and validation of existing clinical information; reinforcement of teaching that applies to the perioperative period; and provision of nursing care to complete preparation for the surgical experience (American Society of PeriAnesthesia Nurses [ASPAN], 2022). Postoperative care involves stabilizing a patient's physical condition, educating a patient and family caregiver, and preparing for effective management of the condition during recovery. The care of postoperative patients returning from the operating room (OR) requires a nurse to complete a thorough assessment, provide ongoing monitoring, and educate both the patient and family caregiver.

PRACTICE STANDARDS

- American Society of PeriAnesthesia Nurses (ASPAN), 2022: 2021–2022 Perianesthesia Nursing Standards, Practice Recommendations, and Interpretive Statements—Paranesthesia nursing standards of practice during recovery
- Association of periOperative Registered Nurses (AORN), 2022: Perioperative Standards and Recommended Practices—Guidelines for perioperative practice
- Berrios-Torres et al., 2017: Centers for Disease Control and Prevention Guideline for the Prevention of Surgical Site Infection (SSI)—Steps to prevent SSI
- The Joint Commission, 2023: National Patient Safety Goals—Patient identification, universal protocol

SUPPLEMENTAL STANDARDS

- National Healthcare Safety Network (NHSN), 2023: Surgical Site Infection Event (SSI)

PRINCIPLES FOR PRACTICE

- Various diagnostic tests are coordinated before surgery to ensure that the surgeon and anesthesia care providers have the information needed to determine a patient's risks during surgery and the postoperative period.
- The American Society of PeriAnesthesia Nurses (ASPAN, 2022; Schick & Windle, 2021) identifies levels of care provided to the surgical/procedural patient that focus on stabilizing the patient so that the nurse may focus efforts on returning the patient to a functional level of wellness as soon as possible within the limitations created by surgery.
- The speed of a patient's recovery depends on how effectively you anticipate potential complications, initiate necessary supportive and preventive therapies, and actively involve the patient and family caregiver in the recovery process.
- Preoperative and postoperative patient education improves outcomes after surgery. Because most patients undergo surgery in an ambulatory setting, it is essential that they receive adequate information to ensure that postoperative care activities can be managed in the home setting.
- American Society of PeriAnesthesia Nurses (ASPAN, 2022) advocates for an ethical culture of accountability and safety with a systems analysis approach when exploring errors and unsafe practice. In addition, the society encourages reviewing errors/unsafe practices in a nonpunitive manner.

PERSON-CENTERED CARE

- Engaging and involving patients and their family caregivers in their care results in safer and more patient-centered care.
- To provide culturally sensitive care to a surgical patient, begin by assessing the family to determine not only who should be involved in the care of the patient but also who is legally responsible for making decisions and giving consent for surgery if the patient is unable.
- To better understand the culture and religious needs of a patient, you may be required to request specific information from the patient, family caregiver, or religious leader.
- When providing preoperative teaching, include family caregivers. The use of professional interpreters for patients who do not speak English is beneficial and required in providing competent informed patient care.
- Identify cultural and religious beliefs and practices that may affect patients' and/or family caregivers' reactions to the surgical experience, such as diet, pain, blood transfusions, and disposal of body parts, including hair.
- Before surgery it is important to accommodate a patient's religious and cultural needs and adapt the patient's care to encompass these practices and beliefs whenever possible.
- Explore patient's fears regarding surgery in both preoperative and postoperative assessments (Ralph & Norris, 2018).
- Both before and after surgery it will be helpful to assess patient preferences for pain medication. Explain the value and importance of pain medication after surgery, as many patients believe that pain medication leads to addiction and will attempt to endure the pain without medication.
- Some religions and/or cultures may request to wear articles such as jewelry, medallions, or undergarments. Allow such articles (e.g., medals, underclothing) to be worn until just before surgery. If articles are removed, ensure that they are returned promptly after surgery.

EVIDENCE-BASED PRACTICE

Surgical Site Infections

Among surgical patients, surgical site infections (SSIs) account for 20% of hospital-acquired infections (NHSN, 2023). The Centers for Disease Control and Prevention (CDC), the Institute for Healthcare Improvement (IHI), and current research suggest interventions for reducing the incidence of SSIs (Calegaril et al., 2021; Kushner et al., 2022) including:

- Preoperative measures:
  - Bath with antimicrobial or nonantimicrobial soap
  - No hair removal or, if necessary, removal only with an electric trimmer (Calegaril et al., 2021; Kushner et al., 2022)
  - Glycemic control <200 mg/dL
  - Normothermia (Calegaril et al., 2021; Kushner et al., 2022)
  - Cleaning and disinfection of environmental surfaces in operating room
  - Surgical antisepsis of the OR team
  - Administration of antibiotic prophylaxis 60 minutes before incision (Calegaril et al., 2021; Kushner et al., 2022)
- Postoperative measures:
  - Maintenance of oxygen therapy after extubation
  - Glycemic control <200 mg/dL
  - Maintain normothermia
  - Protection of closed incisions with sterile dressing for 24–48 hours after the surgery (Calegaril et al., 2021)
  - Enhanced recovery protocols (Kushner et al., 2022)

SAFETY GUIDELINES

Preparing patients to undergo surgery and anesthesia involves essential skills and a thorough preoperative assessment. Regardless of the setting, the preoperative assessment forms the basis for a plan of care that will follow a patient during and after surgery. Safety guidelines include the following:

- Follow safety measures such as verifying correct patient, correct procedure, and correct surgical site; obtaining signed consent and recording thorough documentation (e.g., history and physical examination, nursing assessment, and preanesthesia assessment); and ensuring the availability of required blood products, implants, devices, or special equipment for the procedure (TJC, 2023).
- Timing and duration of antibiotic administration and proper surgical site preparation are essential to prevent SSIs.
- The surgical site must be marked before surgery by the licensed independent practitioner who is ultimately accountable for the procedure (and who will be present during surgery) to allow staff to clearly identify the intended site for the procedure (TJC, 2023).
- A time-out must be performed immediately before beginning the procedure to ensure right surgery, patient, and site (TJC, 2023).
- Patient assessment in the immediate postoperative recovery phase emphasizes the ABCs—A, airway; B, breathing; and C, circulation. Postoperative patients are still under sedation and can become hypoxic. Nurses routinely monitor oxygen saturation levels and provide supplemental oxygen (when ordered) for as long as needed.
- During the postoperative period, assess the wound size, location, and depth, all of which influence the type and amount of drainage. It is important to know what type of drainage to anticipate from the dressing, tubes, and catheters to differentiate what is expected from what is abnormal.

- Implement prophylactic venous thromboembolism measures as ordered.
- Remove wound drains as clinically indicated and ordered to prevent SSI.
- Patients who are smokers, overweight, or obese have increased risk of postoperative complications such as obstructive sleep apnea (OSA), which predisposes them to airway management problems in the postanesthesia care unit (PACU) and possible postoperative pulmonary complications. Longer lengths of stay and unanticipated postoperative intensive care admission may be required for these patients.
- A patient having surgery performed in an ambulatory surgery center must be accompanied by a family member or friend to allow for discharge after the procedure.

✦ SKILL 36.1   Preoperative Assessment

A thorough preoperative assessment provides a baseline for intraoperative and postoperative care. Many health care agencies have a designated department devoted to completing thorough preoperative screening and testing before a patient is admitted for surgery. Laboratory tests, electrocardiograms (ECGs), chest x-ray films, and other tests are often obtained in these facilities 1 to 2 weeks in advance of the scheduled procedure so that abnormalities can be addressed before surgery. During this screening, a private location free of interruption is ideal to encourage open communication. It is not unusual for a patient to remember and report facts that may not have previously been reported to the surgeon. A nurse will again assess patients 1 to 2 hours before the actual surgical procedure to ensure that there are no medical changes. A preprocedure verification process should be followed (TJC, 2023).

Typically, the surgeon, anesthetist, or nurse completes an assessment, and the patient signs a consent form. Current test results and notices of any special considerations during the procedure, such as a need for blood products or special equipment, should be available.

Delegation
The skill of preoperative assessment cannot be delegated to assistive personnel (AP). Direct the AP to:
- Obtain vital signs and weight and height measurements.

Interprofessional Collaboration
- All designated departments are included to ensure all preoperative diagnostic tests are completed and results are available.

Equipment
- Stethoscope
- Blood pressure monitoring equipment
- Pulse oximetry
- Thermometer
- Watch or clock with a second hand
- Method to measure height and weight
- Access to laboratory, ECG, x-ray films, and other diagnostic equipment as needed
- Preprocedure checklist
- Preoperative assessment form

STEP	RATIONALE

ASSESSMENT

1. Identify patient using at least two identifiers (e.g., name and birthday or name and medical record number) according to agency policy.

Ensures correct patient. Complies with The Joint Commission standards and improves patient safety (TJC, 2023).

2. Perform hand hygiene. Prepare equipment and room for assessment.

Reduces transmission of infection. Makes assessment more efficient.

3. Assess patient's/family caregiver's health literacy.

Determines degree to which individuals have the ability to find, understand, and use information and services to make informed health-related decisions and actions for themselves and others (CDC, 2023).

4. Determine if patient has any communication impairment (e.g., blindness, hearing loss), can read and understand English, and is mentally competent. For example, give patient an informational brochure and have them explain part of the contents. Obtain a professional interpreter if needed.

Patient may not fully comprehend a diagnosis, understand proposed treatment, or effectively consider alternatives that are presented without effective communication. Relying on a family member as an interpreter cannot guarantee the accuracy of explanations.

5. Assess patient's understanding of the intended surgery and anesthesia. Ask patient to offer a description rather than asking a simple yes or no question (e.g., "Tell me in your own words what your surgery will involve"). Ask about patient's and family caregiver's expectations of surgery and care. Include questions concerning fears, cultural practices, and religious beliefs if applicable.

Patients may have misconceptions and incomplete knowledge. Asking about fears, cultural practices, and religious beliefs allows you to anticipate priorities of patient and family caregiver and adapt your plan so that you can give appropriate instruction and support.

6. Ask about advance directives (see Chapter 17).

Advance directives protect patient's rights by communicating patient's treatment preferences if they are unable to communicate.

7. Collect nursing history and identify surgical risk factors, including:

Allows for anticipation of possible complications and planning for interventions to reduce patient risks.

STEP	RATIONALE

Clinical Judgment *If patient is having emergency surgery, focus on assessment of primary body system affected.*

a. Condition requiring surgery.

b. Chronic illnesses and associated risks (e.g., hypertension—bleeding, and stroke; postoperative respiratory depression and arrest; asthma—impaired ventilation; hiatal hernia—aspiration; diabetes mellitus—poor wound healing; methicillin-resistant *Staphylococcus aureus*—impaired wound healing and sepsis).

Allows you to anticipate postoperative needs and possible complications.

Some chronic conditions increase risk of complications from surgery and anesthesia.

c. Determine if patient has obstructive sleep apnea (OSA). Many agencies use the STOP-BANG assessment tool (**any question answered *Yes* is a risk factor**):

STOP
- Do you SNORE loudly (louder than talking or loud enough to be heard through closed doors)?
- Do you often feel TIRED, fatigued, or sleepy during the daytime?
- Has anyone OBSERVED you stop breathing during your sleep?
- Do you have or are you being treated for high blood PRESSURE?

BANG
- BMI greater than 35 kg/m^2
- AGE older than 50 years old
- NECK circumference 40 cm (16 inches)
- GENDER: Male

In the surgical population, a STOP-BANG score greater than 5 identifies patients with high probability of moderate/severe obstructive sleep apnea (OSA). The STOP-BANG score helps the health care team to stratify patients for unrecognized OSA, practice perioperative precautions, or triage patients for diagnosis and treatment (Kawada, 2019; Nurgul, 2021).

Patients with OSA will require special anesthesia precautions. Patients with OSA are often sensitive to sedative medications, especially if the OSA is untreated. Even minimal sedation can cause airway obstruction and ventilatory arrest, thus requiring close monitoring postoperatively (Deslate et al., 2021; Nurgul, 2021).

d. Last menstrual period (for patients in childbearing years).

e. Previous hospitalizations.

f. Full medication history, including prescription, over-the-counter (OTC), and herbal remedies and date and time of last doses.

Anesthetic agents and other medications could injure fetus.

Determines if patient is familiar with agency procedures.

Patient may not report OTC medications and herbal remedies unless specifically asked. All may interact with anesthetic agents or other medications given during surgery. Patient may be instructed to take any routine blood pressure, cardiac, or seizure medications preoperatively. Changes in dosages of oral diabetic agents or insulin may be ordered.

g. Previous experience with surgery and anesthesia; have patient clarify if any undesirable outcomes occurred, such as postoperative nausea and vomiting.

h. Family history of complications from surgery or anesthesia.

Information helps to prevent recurrent problems with planned surgery.

Family history of reactions to anesthetic agents may indicate familial condition such as malignant hyperthermia, which is life threatening.

i. Patient history of chronic pain disorders and treatments used at home.

Preoperative assessment is essential to identify signs and symptoms of opioid abuse and later, postoperatively, opioid withdrawal, which can complicate patient pain management postoperatively.

j. Allergies to medications, food, topical solutions or adhesive, and natural rubber latex. Ask patients about any problem with medication or anything placed on their skin. If you identify an allergy, place allergy band on patient's wrist.

Allergies to medications or latex can be life threatening. Prevention of latex allergy in sensitized patients requires specific precautions. Often patients with latex allergies are scheduled as first case of the day. In addition, many patients do not understand that rubber and latex are the same. Using both words helps obtain accurate information.

k. Physical impairment (e.g., paralysis, reduced range of motion of extremity).

Physical impairments may cause limited mobility and situations that could lead to problems with positioning and risk for pressure injury (PI) formation. Communicate this information to the operating room (OR) nurse because these patients may need special positioning or OR bed surfaces.

l. Prostheses and implants (e.g., implantable medication-delivery pump, dentures, hearing aid, pacemaker, internal defibrillator, hip prosthesis).

These devices could become damaged or malfunction from electrical equipment used during surgery. Report this information to the OR nurse.

STEP	RATIONALE
m. Smoking, alcohol, and illicit drug use.	Preoperative alcohol consumption is associated with delayed postoperative recovery (Myoga et al., 2021). Preoperative use of illicit drugs can lead to pulmonary complications, poor pain control, and withdrawal symptoms. Smoking can lead to cardiopulmonary complications.
n. Occupation.	Anticipates how postoperative restrictions will affect patient's return to work.
8. Obtain patient's weight, height, and vital signs (see Chapters 5 and 6).	Height and weight are used to calculate drug dosages. Vital signs provide a baseline for postoperative comparison.

Clinical Judgment *Many patients with OSA are morbidly obese, placing them at increased risk for aspiration of acidic gastric fluid at the time of induction of anesthesia (Kohno et al., 2022). For this reason, many of these patients receive medications to suppress gastric acid production, neutralize the acid, or stimulate emptying of the stomach. Consult with health care provider regarding order for acid-suppressing medication.*

STEP	RATIONALE
9. Assess patient's respiratory status, including auscultation of lungs to detect adventitious sounds, assessment of character and rate of respirations, oxygen saturation, ability to breathe lying flat, use of oxygen or continuous positive airway pressure (CPAP) at home, and chest x-ray film report.	Poor respiratory condition can affect patient's response to general anesthesia. Use of CPAP may indicate that patient has OSA, a condition that poses risks after surgery.
10. Auscultate heart sounds and assess patient's circulatory status, including apical pulse, ECG report, peripheral pulses, and capillary refill (see Chapters 5 and 6).	Screens for possible cardiac problems that may contraindicate surgery. Circulation may be a factor in positioning patient on OR table.
11. Assess for patient's risk for postoperative thrombus formation (e.g., older adults, immobilized patients, patients with personal or family history of blood clots, use of birth control pills, hormones). Ask patient about any leg pain. Observe calves for swelling, warmth, and redness; observe calves for symmetry; and palpate pedal pulses.	Circulation slows after general anesthesia, increasing tendency for blood clot formation. Immobilization during surgical procedure promotes venous stasis. Manipulation and positioning can cause accidental trauma to leg veins.

Clinical Judgment *Do not routinely assess for Homans sign; stop patient's calf movement immediately if any pain is noted. If you suspect a VTE, notify the surgeon and refrain from manipulating the extremity any further. Surgery will usually need to be postponed. Antiembolism stockings or venous flexus foot pump (Fig. 36.1) may be ordered for patients at risk for thrombus formation (see Chapter 12).*

STEP	RATIONALE
12. Complete a gastrointestinal assessment; identify time of patient's last intake of food or drink (see Chapter 6).	With patient under general anesthesia, the esophageal sphincter relaxes and the stomach contents can be aspirated.
13. Complete neurological assessment; determine patient's neurological status, including level of consciousness (LOC), cognitive function, and sensation, and note neurological deficits (see Chapter 6).	Patient's neurological status affects attentiveness to instruction. Offers important baseline for postoperative evaluation.
14. Assess patient's musculoskeletal system, including range of motion (ROM) of joints (see Chapter 6).	If range of motion (ROM) is limited, extra care is needed to prevent injury related to positioning in surgery and during postoperative exercise.

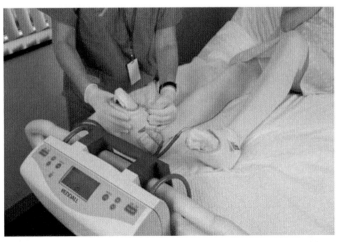

FIG. 36.1 Venous plexus foot pump with bedside controls. *(Courtesy Tyco Healthcare Group LP.)*

STEP	RATIONALE
15. Examine patient's skin; identify any breaks in skin integrity and determine level of hydration (see Chapter 6). Pay attention to area of body on which patient will be positioned.	If skin is thin, broken, or bruised, extra padding is needed in surgery. Hydration may affect skin integrity.
16. Determine patient's age and history of dehydration, malnutrition, exposure to radiation therapy, underlying chronic conditions (e.g., diabetes mellitus, immunosuppression), and edema of the skin.	Common risk factors for medical adhesive–related skin injury (MARSI) (Fumarola et al., 2020). Erythema, blistering, and excoriation are signs of MARSI and are related to the skin's reaction to an adhesive (Hitchcock et al., 2021; Thayer et al., 2022).
17. Assess patient's emotional status, including level of anxiety, coping ability, and family caregiver support. Consider using Hospital Anxiety and Depression Scale (HADS). Assess potential for abuse from a partner or family member.	If patient has high level of anxiety or fear, consultation with social worker, pastoral care, or advanced practice nurse might be useful.
18. Review results of laboratory tests, including complete blood count, electrolytes, urinalysis, and other diagnostic tests.	Laboratory work provides an assessment of major body systems.
19. Assess patient's knowledge, prior experience with preoperative assessment, and feelings about procedure.	Reveals need for patient instruction and/or support.

PLANNING

1. Expected outcomes following completion of procedure:	
• Patient understands the surgical rationale, preparation, and procedure.	Instruction successfully provides patient with knowledge about preoperative plan of care.
• Patient remains alert and appropriately responsive to assessment questions.	Identifies patient's readiness to learn.
• Patient's risks for postoperative complications are identified.	Thorough assessment reveals surgical risks.
• Patient does not incur positional or skin injury during preoperative preparation in OR.	Precautions taken as a result of assessment findings prevent positional and skin injury.
2. Provide privacy and explain assessment procedure to patient. Encourage patient to ask questions. If applicable, teach patient how to perform postoperative exercises (see Skill 36.2).	Protects patient's privacy; reduces anxiety. Promotes cooperation.
3. Obtain and organize equipment for preoperative assessment at bedside.	Ensures more efficiency when completing a procedure.

IMPLEMENTATION

1. Communicate to preoperative team risk factors that have the potential for making the patient vulnerable to intraoperative complications.	Limitations in mobility and sensation should affect how patient is positioned for surgery. Presence of OSA and any cardiopulmonary abnormalities can influence anesthesia approach.

Clinical Judgment *Even though the surgeon and anesthesia provider will conduct separate assessments, your findings may reveal surgical risk factors not identified previously.*

2. On the basis of the patient's cognitive status, experience, and nature of planned surgery, present preoperative instruction to patient and family caregiver (see Skill 36.2).	Assessment findings influence approach to instructions and topics to discuss.
3. Help patient to comfortable positions to enhance assessment process.	Promotes patient comfort and safety and ease in performing assessments.
4. At end of assessment, place nurse call system in an accessible location within patient's reach.	Ensures patient can call for assistance if needed.
5. Raise side rails (as appropriate) and lower bed to lowest position, locking into position.	Ensures patient safety and prevents falls.
6. Dispose of all contaminated supplies in appropriate receptacle, remove and dispose of gloves, and perform hand hygiene.	Reduces transmission of microorganisms.

EVALUATION

1. Review any available information in electronic health record (EHR) with your assessment findings to determine if patient information is complete so that plan of care can be established. Validate unclear information with family caregiver.	Provides valid preoperative baseline of assessment data.

STEP	RATIONALE
2. **Use Teach-Back:** "I want to be sure I explained what you need to know about your intended surgery and anesthesia. Tell me when your surgery is scheduled and the reason you are having surgery." Revise your instruction now or develop a plan for revised patient/family caregiver teaching if patient/family caregiver is not able to teach back correctly.	Teach-back is a technique for health care providers to ensure that they have explained medical information clearly so that patients and their families understand what is communicated to them (Agency for Healthcare Research and Quality [AHRQ], 2023).

Unexpected Outcomes

1. Patient does not understand what surgery will be performed.
2. Patient reports allergy to latex and/or adhesive.

Related Interventions

- Notify surgeon.
- Remove all supplies containing latex from patient's room.
- Post latex precautions sign on door or stretcher.
- Notify surgeon, anesthesia provider, and OR nurse.
- Avoid use of adhesive for attaching medical devices.

Documentation

- Document findings on the preoperative flow sheet or preoperative note in the EHR.
- Document your evaluation of patient and family caregiver learning.

Hand-Off Reporting

- Report abnormal laboratory values or other operative risks to the surgeon, anesthesiologist, and OR nurse. If patient has known history of opioid use for pain control or previous history of postoperative nausea and vomiting, communicate to health care provider.

Special Considerations

Patient Education

- During preoperative assessment, explain to patient the rationale for the type of data you collect, including any ordered lab or diagnostic tests. Offer opportunity for questions

Pediatrics

- When preparing a child for surgery, keep parent-child separation to a minimum.
- Consider a child's developmental level when performing preoperative assessment and preparation.

Older Adults

- Age-related changes may result in diminished short-term memory. Additional assessment and teaching may be necessary (Touhy & Jett, 2022).
- An older adult may have some limitation in ROM. If this limitation is significant, notify the OR nurse so that surgical position can be modified.

Populations With Disabilities

- Provide for education that is adapted to the needs of people with intellectual and developmental disabilities (IDDs) (Sullivan et al., 2018).

◆ SKILL 36.2 Preoperative Teaching

With shortened hospital lengths of stay and growth in ambulatory surgical procedures, there is a greater demand for early patient preparation and support. Patient education must go beyond simply providing information because patients and family caregivers must be prepared to assume more preoperative and postoperative responsibilities. Patients and family caregivers must also learn self-care skills. Comprehensive preoperative patient education has traditionally been provided to patients with the intent of improving patients' knowledge, health behaviors, and health outcomes. The content of preoperative education varies across settings but frequently includes discussion of presurgical procedures; the actual steps in a surgical procedure; postoperative care (e.g., monitoring, positioning, exercises); potential stressful scenarios associated with surgery; potential surgical and nonsurgical complications; postoperative pain management and physical movements to avoid after surgery; and how to eliminate high-risk behaviors (Association of PeriOperative Registered Nurses [AORN], 2022; Rothrock, 2019).

Tailor teaching based on the preoperative assessment. For example, a patient with a history of lung disease will need to focus on postoperative breathing; a patient with a history of diabetes mellitus must learn short- and long-term signs of wound infection. Select the best learning method for a patient, which may include videotape or streaming videos and written materials. Involve the

family caregivers whenever possible. Plan to have the patient demonstrate expected postoperative skills to allow for practice and to facilitate understanding.

To decrease anxiety, teach about expected perioperative sensations and set postoperative expectations about pain management and average length of surgery so that the patient knows what to expect during the postoperative recovery phase.

Delegation

The skills of preoperative teaching cannot be delegated to assistive personnel (AP). AP can reinforce and help patients perform postoperative exercises. If patient is hospitalized, direct the AP about:

- Any precautions or safety issues unique to the patient (e.g., fall precautions, mobility limitations, bleeding precautions, weight-bearing issues, dietary concerns).
- Informing the nurse of any identified concerns (e.g., patient is unable to perform the exercises correctly).

Interprofessional Collaboration

- Physical therapy and/or respiratory therapy may be included if needed for patient support of postoperative exercise education.

Equipment

- *Option:* Clean gloves
- Pillow
- Incentive spirometer

- Preoperative education flow sheet
- Positive expiratory pressure (PEP) device
- Stethoscope

STEP	RATIONALE

ASSESSMENT

1. Identify patient using at least two identifiers (e.g., name and birthday or name and medical record number) according to agency policy.

Ensures correct patient. Complies with The Joint Commission standards and improves patient safety (TJC, 2023).

2. Assess patient's electronic health record (EHR) for type of surgery and approach.

The surgical procedure itself may require patients to limit activities postoperatively. Anticipating any limitations that might affect how patient can perform postoperative exercises allows you to adapt your instruction preoperatively.

3. Assess patient's/family caregiver's health literacy.

Determines degree to which individuals have the ability to find, understand, and use information and services to make informed health-related decisions and actions for themselves and others (CDC, 2023).

4. Ask about patient's previous experiences with surgery and anesthesia.

This allows you to individualize teaching and address specific patient concerns.

5. Assess patient's level of alertness and orientation and identify primary language and culture. If patient does not speak English, have a professional interpreter to assist you.

These factors may alter patient's ability to understand meaning of surgery and can affect postoperative recovery if there are mixed messages or misunderstandings.

6. Assess patient's risk for postoperative respiratory complications (see Skill 36.1). Check nursing history for patient's height and age.

General anesthesia predisposes patient to respiratory problems (see Chapters 23 and 24). Presence of underlying respiratory conditions or patient's inability to perform postoperative respiratory exercises increases patient's risk for pulmonary complications. Height and age are used to set incentive spirometer parameters.

7. Assess patient's anxiety related to surgery.

Directs you to provide additional emotional support and indicates patient's readiness to learn.

8. Assess family caregiver's willingness to learn and support patient following surgery.

Family caregiver's presence after surgery can be potential motivating factor for patient recovery. In addition, caregiver can coach patient through postoperative exercise and observe for any postoperative problems.

9. Assess patient's understanding of the intended surgery and anesthesia. Ask patient to offer a description rather than asking a simple yes-or-no question (e.g., "Tell me what your surgery will involve"). Ask about patient's and family caregiver's expectations of surgery and care. Include questions concerning time frame for surgery and recovery, fears, cultural practices, and religious or spiritual beliefs.

Patients may have misconceptions and incomplete knowledge. Asking about fears, cultural practices, and religious or spiritual beliefs allows you to anticipate priorities of care and adapt teaching and support accordingly.

10. Assess patient's knowledge, prior experience with preoperative teaching, and feelings about procedure.

Reveals need for patient instruction and/or support.

PLANNING

1. Expected outcomes following completion of procedure:
- Patient demonstrates eye contact and asks and answers questions appropriately.

Identifies patient's readiness to learn.

- Patient correctly performs splinting, turning and sitting, breathing exercises, and leg exercises.

Patient will be prepared to participate in postoperative exercises following surgery.

- Family caregiver identifies location of waiting room and time frame when to expect status on family member.

Family caregiver anxiety may be reduced with preoperative expectations clearly provided.

- Family caregiver verbalizes ability to help prepare patient at home before surgery.

Family caregiver can assist patient with necessary preparations before surgery at home.

- Family caregiver provides emotional support for patient before surgery.

Both patient and family caregiver have support for surgery.

2. Provide privacy and explain importance of patient participation in performing postoperative exercises. Discuss surgical procedure and expected postoperative experiences and exercises.

Protects patient's privacy; reduces anxiety. Promotes cooperation.

3. Obtain and organize equipment for preoperative teaching at bedside.

Ensures more efficiency when completing a procedure.

STEP	RATIONALE

IMPLEMENTATION

1. Perform hand hygiene. Inform patient and family caregiver of date, time, and location of surgery; anticipated length of surgery; additional time in postanesthesia recovery area; and where to wait.

2. Encourage and answer questions patient and family caregiver ask.

3. Instruct patient about preoperative bowel or skin preparations as needed. Check medical orders and agency policy regarding number of preoperative showers and agent to be used for each shower (2% or 4% chlorhexidine gluconate is used most often). Following each preoperative shower, instruct patient to rinse the skin thoroughly and dry with a fresh, clean, dry towel. Patient should don clean clothing.

4. Instruct patient about extent and purpose of food and fluid restrictions for period specified before surgery (e.g., no clear liquids at least 2 hours before surgery, no light meal [e.g., toast and a clear liquid] 6 hours or more before surgery, no meat or fried foods 8 hours before surgery, unless otherwise specified by surgeon or anesthesiologist) (American Society of Anesthesiologists [ASA], 2017; Rothrock, 2019).

5. Describe perioperative routines applicable to patient (e.g., time-out, site marking, intravenous [IV] therapy, urinary catheterization, enema, hair clipping or removal, laboratory tests, transport to operating room [OR]).

6. Describe planned effect of preoperative medications.

7. Review which routine medications patient needs to discontinue before surgery and when.

8. Describe perioperative sensations to expect (e.g., blood pressure cuff tightening, electrocardiogram [ECG] leads, cool room, beep of monitor).

9. Describe pain-control methods to be used after surgery. Many patients have a patient-controlled analgesia (PCA) pump (see Chapter 16).

10. Describe what patient will experience after surgery (e.g., where patient will be on awakening, frequent vital signs, catheters, drains, tubes, alternating pressure from sequential compression device, postoperative exercises).

11. Teach Turning:
    a. Instruct patient on turning and sitting up (especially suited for abdominal and thoracic surgery):
       (1) Turn onto right side: Have patient assume supine position and move to side of bed (in this case, left side) if permitted by surgery. Have patient move by bending knees and pressing heels against mattress to raise and move buttocks (see illustration) to the side (left). Top side rails on both sides of bed should be in up position.
       (2) Have patient splint incision with right hand or with right hand with small pillow over incisional area; keep right leg straight and flex left knee up (see illustration); grab right side rail with left hand, pull toward right, and roll onto right side. Reverse process to turn to left side.

Reduces transmission of infection. Accurate information helps reduce stress associated with surgery.

Responding to patient and family caregiver questions helps to decrease anxiety and demonstrates your concern for them.

Proper skin preparation is critical element in preventing surgical site infections (SSIs). Rinsing skin removes residual antiseptic preparation that may cause skin irritation. After use, towels contain microorganisms that can grow in presence of moisture. Using fresh towel after each shower and donning clean clothing minimizes risk of reintroducing microorganisms to clean skin (Ammanuel et al., 2021; Berrios-Torres et al., 2017).

During general anesthesia, muscles relax and gastric contents can reflux into esophagus, leading to aspiration. Anesthetic eliminates patient's ability to gag.

Allows patient to anticipate and recognize routine procedures, reducing anxiety.

Provides information about what to expect, decreasing anxiety.

Some medications are discontinued several days before surgery or the morning of surgery to minimize effects that can cause surgical risks. For example, anticoagulants may increase bleeding and are usually discontinued 5 or more days before surgery. Insulin dosages are usually adjusted because of reduced intake of food before surgery.

Misconceptions and concerns about anesthesia have been ranked high among preoperative patients.

Patients are fearful of postoperative pain. Explaining pain-management techniques reduces this fear. Establishes what pain is acceptable, knowing that they will not be pain free, but their pain will be managed.

Provides concrete description of what patient can expect after surgery so that patient is prepared.

Promotes circulation and ventilation.

Positioning begins on side of bed so that turning to other side does not cause patient to roll toward edge of bed. Buttocks lift prevents shearing force against sheets. If patient's bed has a turn-assist feature, use it to help with positioning.

Supports incision and decreases discomfort while turning.

STEP	RATIONALE

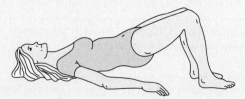

STEP 11a(1) Buttocks lift for moving to side of bed.

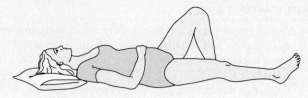

STEP 11a(2) Leg position when turning to right.

(3) Instruct patient to turn every 2 hours from side to side while awake. Often patient requires assistance with turning after surgery.	Reduces risk of vascular, pulmonary, and pressure injury (PI) complications.

Clinical Judgment *Some patients, such as those who have had back or hip surgery or vascular repair, are restricted from flexing their legs after surgery. Some patients are restricted from turning or may need help for positioning (see Chapter 11).*

(4) Sit up on right side of bed. Elevate head of bed and have patient turn onto right side. While lying on right side, patient pushes on mattress with left arm and swings feet over edge of bed with nurse's help. To sit up on left side of bed, reverse this process. Monitor for signs of orthostatic hypotension when patient performs maneuver (Skill 11.1).	Sitting position lowers diaphragm to permit fuller lung expansion. Sudden positional change can lower blood pressure.

Clinical Judgment *Caution patient to always ask for assistance, particularly first time sitting up on side of bed, to reduce risk of a fall.*

12. Teach coughing and deep breathing (especially suited for abdominal and thoracic surgery):	Patient may be unable or reluctant to deep breathe because of weakness or pain, resulting in secretions remaining in base of lungs. Collection of secretions increases risk of pulmonary atelectasis and pneumonia.
a. Assist patient to high-Fowler position in bed with knees flexed, or have patient sit on side of bed or chair in upright position.	Sitting position facilitates diaphragmatic expansion.
b. Instruct patient to place palms of hands across from one another lightly along lower border of rib cage or upper abdomen (see illustration).	This allows patient to feel rise and fall of abdomen during deep breathing.
c. Have patient take slow, deep breaths, inhaling through nose. Explain that patient will feel normal downward movement of diaphragm during inspiration. Demonstrate as needed.	Helps to prevent hyperventilation or panting. Slow, deep breath allows for more complete lung expansion.
d. Have patient avoid using chest and shoulder muscles while inhaling.	Increases unnecessary energy expenditure and does not promote full lung expansion.
e. Have patient take slow, deep breath; hold for count of 3 seconds; and slowly exhale through mouth as if blowing out candle (pursed lips).	Resistance during exhalation helps to prevent alveolar collapse.

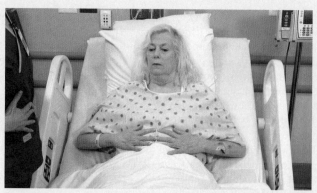

STEP 12b Deep-breathing exercise—placement of hands on upper abdomen during inhalation.

STEP	RATIONALE
f. Have patient repeat breathing exercise 3 to 5 times.	Repetition reinforces learning.
g. Have patient take two slow, deep breaths, inhaling through nose and exhaling through pursed lips.	Deep breaths expand lungs fully so that air moves behind mucus to facilitate coughing.
h. Have patient inhale deeply a third time and hold breath to count of 3. Cough fully for two to three consecutive coughs without inhaling between coughs.	Deep breathing moves up secretions in respiratory tract to stimulate cough reflex without voluntary effort on part of patient (Harding et al., 2020).
i. Caution patient against just clearing throat.	Clearing throat does not remove mucus from deeper airways.
j. Have patient practice several times. Instruct patient to perform turning, coughing, and deep breathing every 2 hours. Have family caregiver coach patient to exercise.	Ensures mastery of technique. Frequent pulmonary exercises and movement decrease risk of postoperative pneumonia (Harding et al., 2020).
13. Teach use of an incentive spirometer (see also Skill 23.3):	Provides visual aid of respiratory effort. Encourages deep breathing to loosen secretions in lung bases.
a. Position patient in sitting position in chair or in reclining position with head of bed elevated at least 45 degrees in bed.	Facilitates diaphragm lowering and lung expansion.
b. Set targeted tidal volume on the incentive spirometer according to manufacturer directions. Explain that this is the volume level to be reached with each breath.	Establishes goal of volume level necessary for adequate lung expansion. Manufacturers determine target on basis of patient height and age.
c. Explain to patient how to place mouthpiece of incentive spirometer so that lips completely cover mouthpiece (see illustration). Have patient demonstrate until position is correct.	Validates patient's understanding of instructions, evaluates psychomotor skills, and lets patient ask questions.
d. Instruct patient to exhale completely, and then position mouthpiece so that lips completely cover it. Inhale slowly, maintaining constant flow through unit until reaching goal volume (see illustration).	Promotes complete inflation of lungs and minimizes atelectasis.
e. Once maximum inspiration is reached, have patient hold breath for 2 to 3 seconds and exhale slowly.	Promotes alveolar inflation.
f. Instruct patient to breathe normally for short period between each of the 10 breaths taken on incentive spirometer. Repeat every hour while awake.	Prevents hyperventilation and fatigue.
14. Teach positive expiratory pressure (PEP) therapy and "huff" coughing (especially suited for any patient with lung disease or recent history of smoking):	
a. Set PEP device for setting ordered.	Higher settings require more effort.
b. Instruct patient to assume semi-Fowler or high-Fowler position in bed or to sit in a chair and place nose clip on patient's nose (see illustration).	Promotes optimum lung expansion and expectoration of mucus.

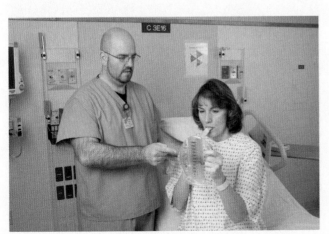

STEP 13c Patient demonstrates incentive spirometry.

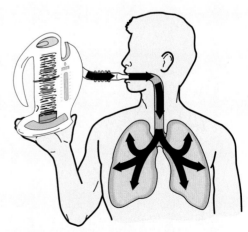

STEP 13d Diagram of use of incentive spirometer.

STEP	RATIONALE
c. Have patient place lips around mouthpiece. Instruct patient to take full breath and exhale 2 or 3 times longer than inhalation. Repeat pattern for 10 to 20 breaths.	Ensures that patient does all breathing through mouth. Ensures that patient uses device properly. Monitor patient for hyperventilation.
d. Remove device from mouth and have patient take slow, deep breath and hold for 3 seconds.	Promotes lung expansion before coughing.
e. Instruct patient to exhale in quick, short, forced "huffs." Repeat exercise every 2 hours while awake.	"Huff" coughing, or forced expiratory technique, promotes bronchial hygiene by increasing expectoration of secretions.
15. Teach controlled coughing (especially suited for any patient with lung disease, recent history of smoking, or abdominal or thoracic surgery):	Deep breaths expand lungs fully so that air moves behind mucus and facilitates effective coughing.
a. Apply clean gloves if you expect patient to cough and expectorate mucus. Explain importance of maintaining upright position.	Position facilitates diaphragm excursion and enhances thorax and abdominal expansion.
b. Demonstrate coughing. Take two slow, deep breaths, inhaling through nose and exhaling through (pursed lips) mouth.	Consecutive coughs help remove mucus more effectively and completely than one forceful cough.
c. To exhale, have patient lean forward, pressing arms against their abdomen. Cough 2 to 3 times without inhaling between coughs. Cough through a slightly open mouth. Coughs should be short and sharp (see illustration). (Tell patient to push all air out of lungs.)	Clearing throat does not remove mucus from deeper airways. Full, forceful cough is most effective in removing mucus.
d. Caution patient against just clearing throat instead of coughing deeply.	Clearing throat does not remove mucus from deeper airways.
e. If surgical incision is either thoracic or abdominal, teach patient to place either hands or pillow over incisional area and place hands over pillow to splint incision (see illustration). During breathing and coughing exercises, press gently against incisional area for splinting and support.	Surgical incision cuts through muscles, tissues, and nerve endings. Deep-breathing and coughing exercises place additional stress on suture line and cause discomfort. Splinting incision with hands or pillow provides firm support and reduces incisional pulling and pain.
f. Instruct patient to practice coughing exercises, splinting imaginary incision (see illustrations). Instruct patient to cough 2 to 3 times every 2 hours while awake.	Deep coughing with splinting effectively expectorates mucus with minimal discomfort.
g. Instruct patient to examine sputum for consistency, odor, amount, and color changes and notify a nurse if any changes are noted.	Sputum consistency, odor, amount, and color changes indicate presence of pulmonary complication such as pneumonia.

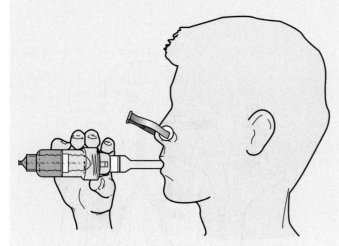

STEP 14b Diagram of use of positive expiratory pressure device.

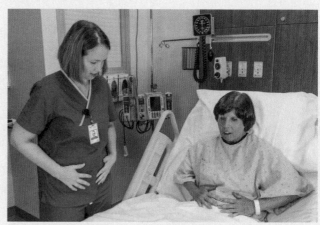

STEP 15c Controlled coughing with placement of hands on upper abdomen.

STEP	RATIONALE

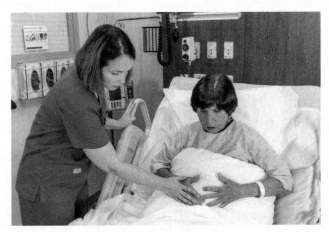

STEP 15e Patient splinting abdomen with pillow.

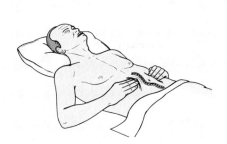 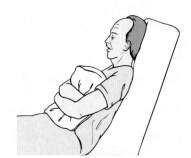 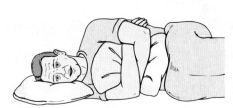

STEP 15f Techniques for splinting incisions.

16. Teach leg exercises (especially suited for any patient at risk for thromboembolic disease):

   a. Instruct and encourage patient in leg exercises to be performed every 1 to 2 hours while awake: ankle rotation, dorsiflexion and plantar flexion, leg extension and flexion, and straight leg raises (see illustration).

       Leg exercises facilitate venous return from lower extremities and reduce risk of circulatory complications such as venous thrombus.

Clinical Judgment *Leg exercises are recommended for patients who have been immobile or restricted to bed or during times when patients are ambulatory but resting in bed or in a chair. The ideal exercise to promote venous return and improve lung vital capacity is early mobility (see Chapter 12).*

   b. Position patient supine.

   c. Instruct patient to rotate each ankle in complete circle and draw imaginary circles with big toe 5 times.

       Promotes joint mobility.

   d. Alternate dorsiflexion and plantar flexion while instructing patient to feel calf muscles tighten and relax. Repeat 5 times.

       Helps maintain joint mobility and promote venous return to prevent thrombus formation.

   e. Perform quadriceps setting by tightening thigh and bringing knee down toward mattress and relaxing. Repeat 5 times.

       Quadriceps-setting exercises contract muscles of upper legs, maintain knee mobility, and improve venous return to heart.

   f. Instruct patient to alternate raising knee and leg straight up from bed surface. Leg should be kept straight and then knee drawn up. Repeat 5 times.

       Causes quadriceps muscle contraction and relaxation, which help promote venous return.

17. Have patient continue to practice exercises before surgery at least every 2 hours while awake. Teach patient to coordinate turning and leg exercises with diaphragmatic breathing and use of incentive spirometer.

       Leg exercises stimulate circulation, which prevents venous stasis to help prevent formation of deep vein thrombosis (DVT).

18. Verify that patient's expectations of surgery are realistic. Correct expectations as needed.

       Can prevent postoperative anxiety or anger.

STEP	RATIONALE

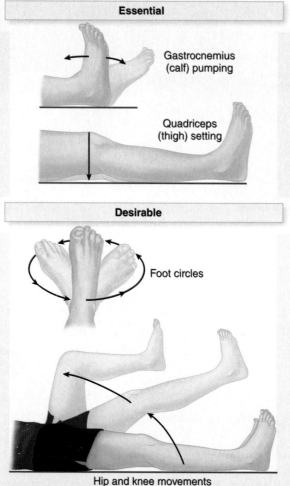

STEP 16a Postoperative leg exercises. (*From Silvestri LA, Silvestri A:* Saunders comprehensive review for the NCLEX-RN® Examination, *ed 8, St. Louis, 2022, Elsevier.*)

STEP	RATIONALE
19. Reinforce therapeutic coping strategies. If ineffective, encourage alternatives.	Therapeutic coping strategies promote postoperative adherence and recovery.
20. Help patient to a comfortable position.	Restores comfort and sense of well-being.
21. Place nurse call system in an accessible location within patient's reach.	Ensures patient can call for assistance if needed.
22. Raise side rails (as appropriate) and lower bed to lowest position, locking into position.	Ensures patient safety and prevents falls.
23. Dispose of all contaminated supplies in appropriate receptacle, remove and dispose of gloves (if worn), and perform hand hygiene.	Reduces transmission of microorganisms.

EVALUATION

1. Observe patient demonstrating splinting, turning and sitting, deep breathing, use of incentive spirometer, PEP therapy, and leg exercises.	Validates patient's ability to perform postoperative exercises and use devices.
2. Ask family caregiver to identify location of waiting room and validate if correct.	Establishes family caregiver's knowledge of where they can wait for patient information.
3. Ask family caregiver to explain how to help prepare patient at home before surgery.	Establishes that family caregiver can coach patient on exercises both before and after surgery.
4. Observe level of emotional support family caregiver provides patient.	Identifies preoperative emotional support for patient.

STEP	RATIONALE
5. **Use Teach-Back:** "I want to be sure I explained what you need to know about getting ready for surgery. Tell me which medications you should not take before surgery." Revise your instruction now or develop a plan for revised patient/family caregiver teaching if patient/family caregiver is not able to teach back correctly.	Teach-back is a technique for health care providers to ensure that they have explained medical information clearly so that patients and their families understand what is communicated to them (AHRQ, 2023).

Unexpected Outcomes

1. Patient identifies incorrect procedure, site, date, or time of surgery.

2. Patient incorrectly performs one of the postoperative exercises.

Related Interventions

- Provide correct information verbally and in writing for patient and family caregiver.
- Explain and demonstrate correct exercise technique.
- Explain importance of the postoperative exercise as it pertains to patient recovery.
- Instruct patient to repeat demonstration.

Documentation

- Document all preoperative patient and family caregiver teaching and their response to teaching.

Hand-Off Reporting

- Report patient's inability to identify procedure and site of surgery, as well as understanding of postoperative exercise(s) and teaching to health care provider.

Special Considerations

Patient Education

- Whenever you provide printed educational materials about a patient's surgery or recovery process, be sure the materials are age appropriate and at the patient's literacy level.
- It is important that any preoperative educational strategy focuses on improving a patient's sense of empowerment.
- Present information written at a sixth grade reading level.
- Nurses are responsible for ensuring that patient education material is clear, concise, in plain language, patient centered, and based on the patients' needs and abilities. In addition, the nurse must evaluate the effectiveness of the teaching (Box 36.1) (Schick & Windle, 2020).

Pediatrics

- Preoperative education involving use of videos, multifaceted programs, and interactive games to reduce preoperative anxiety in children undergoing elective surgery has been found most effective, whereas music therapy and Internet programs are less effective (Hockenberry et al., 2022).
- Use an age-appropriate level of communication and provide simple explanations using familiar terms.
- The use of pictures, models, equipment, and play rather than verbal explanations increases learning in preschool and school-age children.

Older Adults

- Physiological changes that occur with aging may require admission to health care agency before surgery for additional diagnostic tests and stabilization of condition (Table 36.1).
- Age-related changes in the central nervous system may diminish short-term memory. Additional time and reinforcement may be necessary for older adults to learn and comprehend information. The greater the number of different exposures to new material, the higher the probability that the material will be learned.

BOX 36.1

The Joint Commission Patient and Family Education Standards

Education provided is appropriate to the patient's needs. Assessment of learning needs addresses cultural and religious beliefs, emotional barriers, desire to learn, physical or cognitive limitations, and barriers to communication as appropriate. When called for by the age of the patient and the length of stay, the hospital assesses and provides for patient's education needs. Patients are educated about:

- The plan for care, treatment, and services (i.e., postoperative monitoring).
- Basic health practices and safety (i.e., out of bed [OOB] only with help).
- Safe and effective use of medication (i.e., the patient is only one allowed to self-administer patient-controlled analgesia [PCA]).

- Nutrition interventions, modified diets, or oral health (i.e., progression of diet after surgery).
- Safe and effective use of medical equipment or supplies when provided by the hospital (i.e., incentive spirometer).
- Pain—Understanding pain, the risk for pain, the importance of effective pain management, the pain-assessment process, and methods for pain management (i.e., reporting pain, frequency of medications, nonpharmacological pain-relief techniques).
- Habilitation or rehabilitation techniques to help the patient reach the maximum independence possible (i.e., early ambulation).

Modified from The Joint Commission (TJC): *Comprehensive accreditation manual for hospitals*, Oakbrook, IL, 2022, The Joint Commission; and Schick L, Windle P: *PeriAnesthesia nursing core curriculum: preprocedure, phase I and phase II PACU nursing*, ed 4, St Louis, 2020, Saunders.

TABLE 36.1

Physiological Factors That Place Older-Adult Patients at Risk for Surgery

Alterations	Surgery Risks	Nursing Implications
Cardiovascular		
Degenerative change in myocardium and valves	Reduced cardiac reserve	Assess baseline vital signs.
Rigidity of arterial walls and reduction in sympathetic and parasympathetic innervation to heart	Predisposes patient to postoperative hemorrhage and rise in systolic and diastolic blood pressure	Maintain adequate fluid balance to minimize stress to heart. Ensure that blood pressure is adequate to meet circulatory demands.
Increase in calcium and cholesterol deposits within small arteries; arterial walls thickened	Predisposes patient to clot formation in lower extremities	Teach patient techniques for performing leg exercises and proper turning. Apply bilateral antiembolism stockings, sequential compression devices (SCDs) (see Chapter 12).
Integumentary System		
Decreased subcutaneous tissue and increased fragility of skin	Prone to PIs and skin tears	Assess skin every 4 hours; pad all bony prominences during surgery. Turn or reposition.
Pulmonary		
Rib cage stiffens and enlarges	Reduced vital capacity	Teach patient proper technique for coughing and deep-breathing exercises and use of incentive spirometer.
Reduced diaphragm excursion	Greater residual capacity or volume of air left in lung after normal breath increases, reducing amount of new air brought into lungs with each inspiration	Encourage deep breathing. Use incentive spirometer to enhance exhalation.
Lung tissue less distensible; alveoli enlarged	Reduced blood oxygenation	Assess oxygen saturation via oximetry (SpO_2).
Renal		
Reduced blood flow to kidneys	Blood loss that causes decrease in circulation to the kidney	Monitor urinary output and laboratory data (i.e., blood urea nitrogen [BUN], creatinine).
Reduced glomerular filtration rate and excretory times	Limits ability to remove drugs or toxic substances	Assess for adverse effects of medications.
Reduced bladder capacity	Increase in voiding frequency; larger amount of urine stays in the bladder after voiding	Instruct patient to notify nurse immediately when sensation of bladder fullness develops.
	Sensation of need to void may not occur until bladder is filled	Keep call light or bedpan within easy reach.
Neurological		
Sensory losses, including reduced tactile sense, increased pain tolerance	Patient less able to respond to early warning signs of surgical complications	Inspect bony prominences for signs of pressure.
Decreased reaction time	Patient becomes confused easily after anesthesia	Orient patient to surrounding environment. Observe for nonverbal signs of pain. Maintain safe environment. Institute fall precautions.
Metabolic		
Lower basal metabolic rate	Reduced total oxygen consumption and nutritional needs	Ensure adequate nutritional intake once diet is resumed.
Reduced number of red blood cells and hemoglobin levels	Reduces ability to carry adequate oxygen to tissues	Administer necessary blood products. Assess for adequacy of oxygenation, fatigue, and infection.
Change in total amounts of body potassium and water volume	Greater risk for fluid or electrolyte imbalance	Monitor electrolyte levels.

- Reinforce teaching with verbal explanations, audiovisual resources, pamphlets, and demonstrations. Consider sight and hearing deficits when providing both written and verbal instructions.

Populations With Disabilities
- Patients with physical disabilities may require perioperative accommodations, such as an alternative position or equipment. In addition, patients with limited mobility are at increased risk

for venous thromboembolism. Preoperative surgical planning should include discussions with the patient, family caregivers, and OR staff about these physical limitations.

Home Care
- Review coughing, deep breathing, abdominal splinting, relaxation, leg exercises, and ambulation before admission to hospital or surgical clinic and after discharge.

✦ SKILL 36.3 Patient Preparation for Surgery

 Video Clip

Preparation of a patient for surgery involves confirming key assessment findings, providing ordered preoperative procedures, verifying patient understanding of surgery, verifying that required procedures and tests have been performed and any abnormal results reported, and documenting care in the patient's record. Preparation begins when the patient is admitted to the surgical center and continues to the transfer to the operating room. The physical care procedures depend on the type of surgery being performed and the risks involved. For example, compression stockings, intermittent sequential compression devices (ISCDs), and the venous foot pump (see Fig. 36.1) are frequently used for adult patients undergoing surgery that will last several hours and require a long period of immobilization afterward. Because many patients are admitted on the day of surgery, much of the preoperative preparation is often the responsibility of the patient or the family caregiver the day before. Regardless of the type of surgery, the goal of surgical preparation is to ensure the patient is in the best condition possible to minimize the risks of the planned surgery and achieve subsequent best outcomes.

The Association of periOperative Registered Nurses (AORN) offers a Comprehensive Surgical Checklist (AORN, 2019 [see Chapter 37]) that ensures effective communication and safe practices during three perioperative periods: before administration of anesthesia, before skin incision, and before the patient leaves the operative area. Hospitals and surgical outpatient centers can modify or add to the checklist on the basis of their practice guidelines.

The Joint Commission National Patient Safety Goals (NPSGs) implement the Universal Protocol for Preventing Wrong Site, Wrong Procedure, Wrong Person surgery (TJC, 2023). This protocol offers an added safety measure to ensure that the correct person, procedure, and surgical site are verified at the time of scheduling the procedure, on admission or entry into the agency, and

each time the responsibility for care of the patient is transferred to another health care provider. A final verification check involving the entire surgical team occurs immediately before the start of the procedure.

Delegation
The skill of coordinating the patient's preparation for surgery cannot be delegated to assistive personnel (AP). Direct the AP about:
- Observing and using precautions if the patient has an intravenous (IV) catheter or other invasive devices in place.
- Obtaining vital signs in stable patients, applying antiembolism stockings, and helping patients remove clothing, jewelry, and prostheses.

Interprofessional Collaboration
- Collaboration may be needed with the admission department, agency pharmacist, laboratory department, and diagnostics to ensure all preoperative patient needs have been met.

Equipment
NOTE: Equipment varies by procedure.
- Vital sign equipment: stethoscope, blood pressure (BP) cuff, thermometer, pulse oximeter
- Hospital gown
- IV solution and administration set (see Chapter 28)
- Skin-cleaning solution
- Compression (antiembolism) stockings (see Chapter 12)
- Intermittent sequential compression devices (ISCDs)
- Venous foot pump
- Urinary catheterization kit (see Chapter 33)
- Preoperative checklist
- Medications (e.g., sedative)
- Clean gloves

STEP	RATIONALE

ASSESSMENT

1. Identify patient using at least two identifiers (e.g., name and birthday or name and medical record number) according to agency policy.

Ensures correct patient. Complies with The Joint Commission standards and improves patient safety (TJC, 2023).

2. Perform hand hygiene. Complete preoperative assessment, including patient health literacy (see Skill 36.1).

Assessment provides baseline for monitoring patient's intraoperative course. Determines degree to which individuals have the ability to find, understand, and use information and services to make informed health-related decisions and actions for themselves and others (CDC, 2022).

STEP	RATIONALE

3. Assess and document patient's heart rate, blood pressure, respiratory rate, oxygen saturation, and temperature. *Option:* Keep oximeter attached to patient (Palese et al., 2019).

Provides baseline for patient's preoperative status. Continuous oximetry monitoring will occur during surgery.

4. If patient is same-day admit or ambulatory patient, validate that admission preparations (e.g., enema, shower with antiseptic, withholding medications) were completed at home as ordered. Ensure that patient has followed appropriate fluid and food restrictions per surgeon or anesthesiologist order (see Skill 36.2).

Failure to complete preparation could lead to perioperative or postoperative complications and may necessitate postponement or cancellation of surgery.

5. Ask if patient has an advance directive. If so, be certain a copy is in the electronic health record (EHR).

Document conveys patient's wishes if life support measures are necessary.

6. Assess patient's knowledge, prior experience with surgical preparation, and feelings about procedure.

Reveals need for patient instruction and/or support.

PLANNING

1. Expected outcomes following completion of procedure:
   • Patient can state which surgical procedure is being performed and risks and benefits of surgery.
   • Patient states that anxiety is decreased.

Identifies readiness to sign informed consent (Table 36.2).

Decreased anxiety increases participation.

2. Provide privacy and explain preoperative preparations to patient.

Protects patient's privacy; reduces anxiety. Promotes cooperation.

3. Plan preparation of any preoperative medications to avoid interruptions. Create a quiet environment. Do not take phone calls or talk with others. Follow agency "No Interruption Zone" policy.

Interruptions contribute to medication errors (Palese et al., 2019; Wang et al., 2021).

4. Obtain and organize equipment for preparing patient at bedside.

Ensures more efficiency when completing a procedure.

IMPLEMENTATION

1. Perform hand hygiene. Help patient put on hospital gown and remove personal items. Patients are often anxious before surgery. Before any procedure, decrease anxiety by explaining how equipment or preparation will feel (e.g., cold, tight) before touching patient.

Reduces transmission of infection. Orients patient to surroundings and understanding of presurgical procedures.

2. Instruct patient to remove makeup, nail polish, hairpins, and jewelry (see agency policy). (**NOTE:** This is usually instructed before admission to surgical center.)

Hair appliances and jewelry anywhere on body may become dislodged and cause injury during positioning and intubation. Rings decrease circulation in fingers. Makeup, nail polish, and false nails impede assessment of skin and oxygenation. In addition, acrylic nails harbor pathogenic organisms (Dogan et al., 2021).

TABLE 36.2

Information Needed for Informed Consent

Parameters	Examples
Name of procedure/surgery	Abdominal hysterectomy under general anesthesia
Description of procedure/surgery	Removal of uterus only through an incision in the abdominal wall at the top of the pubic hairline; done while unconscious
Person performing procedure/surgery	Dr. Richard Jones assisted by Dr. William Smith
Benefits of procedure/surgery	To remove uterus with fibroids and stop excessive bleeding Abdominal route necessary because of anticipated adhesions from prior abdominal surgery
Potential risks and adverse effects of procedure/surgery	Risk of hemorrhage and infection from surgery; risk of excessive sedation and allergic reaction to drugs used with general anesthesia; accidental damage to bladder, intestines, and/or nerves controlling these organs
Approximate length of time for procedure/surgery	About 1 hour; 1 to 2 hours in postanesthesia care unit (PACU)
Approximate length of time needed for recovery	2 to 3 days on surgical unit; 4 to 6 weeks before resuming physically stressful work
Alternative treatments	Removal of uterus vaginally; radiation to shrink fibroids
Consequences of refusing treatment	Continuation of pain and vaginal bleeding, risk for developing anemia; after menopause, fibroids should regress

STEP	RATIONALE
3. Ensure that money and valuables have been locked up or given to a family caregiver (see agency policy).	Patient may not return to same location after surgery. Prevents valuables from being misplaced or lost.
4. Verify that patient has followed appropriate medication, fluid, and food restrictions per surgeon or anesthesiologist order (see Skill 36.2).	Extent and type of restriction vary by agency and health care provider. Under general anesthesia, sphincters in the stomach relax, and contents can reflux into esophagus and trachea.
5. Verify presence of allergies and ensure that allergy/sensitivity band is present.	Alerts surgeons and health care team to potential allergies.
6. Assess patient's fall risks; apply fall risk armband if appropriate.	Alerts all health care providers to patient's risk for falling.
7. Verify that bowel preparation (e.g., laxative, cathartic, enema) has been completed by patient or family caregiver at home if ordered.	Proper bowel evacuation needed for surgery to be performed.

Clinical Judgment *In some situations, additional enemas and/or cathartics are ordered. Emptying the bowel is necessary for bowel surgery to decrease the risk of infection and postoperative ileus. Enemas are also used when surgery is near the lower intestine (e.g., gynecological and urological surgeries).*

STEP	RATIONALE
8. Ensure that medical history and physical examination results are in the EHR.	Ensures that pertinent laboratory and diagnostic test results are available and that all preoperative preparations are completed.
9. Verify that surgical consent, anesthesia consent, and consent for blood transfusion are complete. The name of procedure; name of surgeon; date; name of person authorized to obtain surgical consent; signature of surgeon (or authorized person) obtaining consent, anesthesia provider delivering anesthesia, and witness (often the nurse); and patient's signature should all be present.	Ensures patient's agreement to undergo intended procedure. In most settings, surgeon obtains consent, and nurse verifies that it is complete and consistent with patient's understanding (refer to agency policy).
10. Ensure that necessary laboratory work, electrocardiogram (ECG), and chest x-ray film studies are completed and results are documented.	Diagnostic test results may indicate medical problem and provide data for postoperative comparison.
11. Verify that blood type and crossmatch are completed if ordered by surgeon and that blood transfusions are available as needed.	In many cases surgery cannot begin without availability of blood units.
12. Instruct patient to void.	Prevents risk of bladder distention or rupture during surgery.
13. Perform hand hygiene and apply clean gloves. Start IV line; refer to unit standards or surgeon's orders (see Chapter 28). Remove and dispose of gloves. Perform hand hygiene.	IV line provides access for fluids and medications to be administered when in operating room (OR). Reduces transmission of microorganisms.
14. Administer preoperative medications as ordered (e.g., antibiotics, prophylactic agents). Manage potential for postoperative nausea and vomiting (PONV): administer preoperative and intraoperative antiemetics, recommend modifying anesthetics, and use nonpharmacologic approaches.	Preoperative medications are used for various reasons and should be administered as ordered for maximum effectiveness. Management of PONV should include multimodal preventive measures (Moore et al., 2021).
15. *Option:* Apply compression stockings (see Chapter 12) (if ordered).	Compression stockings promote circulation during periods of immobilization, reducing risk of embolism.
16. *Option:* Apply intermittent sequential compression devices (ISCDs) if ordered. **NOTE:** Compression stockings may or may not be used in combination with ISCDs. Verify order.	ISCDs push blood from superficial veins into deep veins, decreasing venous stasis.

Clinical Judgment *ISCDs do not provide effective deep vein thrombosis (DVT) prophylaxis if the device is not applied correctly or if the patient does not wear the device continuously except during bathing, skin assessment, and ambulation. ISCDs are not to be worn when a patient has an active DVT because of risk of pulmonary embolism.*

STEP	RATIONALE
17. Apply clean gloves. Clean and prepare surgical site if ordered. Remove and dispose of gloves.	Cleaning with antimicrobial soap decreases bacterial flora on skin. Reduces transmission of microorganisms.
18. *Option:* Perform hand hygiene and apply sterile gloves. Insert urinary catheter if ordered (see Chapter 33). **NOTE:** There are times when urinary catheter is placed in OR. Remove and dispose of gloves and perform hand hygiene.	Maintains bladder decompression and provides for monitoring output during surgery. Reduces transmission of microorganisms.

STEP	RATIONALE
19. Allow patient to wear eyeglasses or hearing aid if possible before surgery so that patient can sign consents and read materials. Remove contact lenses, eyeglasses, hairpieces, and dentures just before surgery (see checklist completed before surgery, noting that all items are removed before proceeding to OR).	These aids facilitate patient cooperation by ensuring that patient has clear vision and maximal auditory perception throughout preoperative phase.
20. Place head cover over patient's head and hair.	Contains hair and minimizes OR contamination during surgery. **NOTE:** Plastic or reflective caps reduce heat loss during surgery.
21. Place patient on bed rest with nurse call system within reach and forbid getting out of bed without help. Allow family members to remain at bedside until patient is transferred to surgical area. Maintain quiet and relaxing environment.	There is increased chance of injury by trying to ambulate to void when patient is sedated and unattended.
22. Transfer patient via stretcher to OR. Raise side rails appropriately.	Facilitates transportation to OR suite. Provides patient safety. Some ambulatory surgery patients walk to OR.
23. Dispose of all contaminated supplies in appropriate receptacle, remove and dispose of gloves, and perform hand hygiene.	Reduces transmission of microorganisms.

EVALUATION

1. Have patient describe surgical procedure and its benefits and risks.	Confirms level of knowledge needed to sign informed consent (see Table 36.2).
2. Have patient repeat preoperative instructions.	Provides evidence that patient understands instructions.
3. Monitor patient for signs and symptoms of anxiety and ask how patient and family are feeling.	Increased heart rate and blood pressure, dilated pupils, dry mouth, increased sweating, and muscle rigidity or shaking are responses to stress and anxiety. Asking patient about feelings gives permission to express concerns, which can be further explored.
4. Confirm IV is infusing at a keep-open or ordered rate.	Patent and functional IV is needed when patient enters OR suite.
5. **Use Teach-Back:** "I want to be sure you are ready for surgery. Tell me what you expect to happen once you get to the recovery room." Revise your instruction now or develop a plan for revised patient/family caregiver teaching if patient/family caregiver is not able to teach back correctly.	Teach-back is a technique for health care providers to ensure that they have explained medical information clearly so that patients and their families understand what is communicated to them (AHRQ, 2023).

Unexpected Outcomes	Related Interventions
1. Patient is unable to give consent, and appropriate family member is unavailable.	• In emergency situations, obtain telephone consent from next of kin or designated executor. Two people must witness oral consent (according to agency policy).
	• Document explanation of situation and fact that oral consent was obtained and witnessed.
	• At earliest opportunity, person giving oral consent must sign written consent. Signed telegram or signed fax may also be considered oral consent. Follow agency policy.
2. Patient did not remain NPO, which may create risk for aspiration and may indicate that instructions were not understood or were forgotten.	• Notify surgeon and anesthesiologist. Surgery may be postponed or cancelled.
3. Informed consent has not been signed and witnessed. Surgeon and anesthesiologist did not provide information and/or ensure that consent forms were signed.	• Patient is not ready for surgery. Patient must sign consent before administration of preoperative medications or any medication that alters central nervous system. Notify surgeon and anesthesiologist.

Documentation

- Document preoperative physical preparation on preoperative checklist.
- Document that informed consent (see Table 36.2) has been completed.
- Document disposition of patient valuables/belongings (i.e., whether locked up according to agency policy or sent with family).
- Document your evaluation of patient and family caregiver learning.

Hand-Off Reporting

- Report lack of signed and witnessed consent form or failure of patient to maintain NPO status and action taken.
- Report to nursing staff receiving patient in OR that preoperative physical preparation has been successfully completed, any deviations from appropriate preparation, and that completed informed consent is available in the patient's record.

Special Considerations

Pediatrics

- Give the child as many choices related to procedures as possible.
- Keep parent-child separation to the minimum time possible. When a parent cannot be present, it is important to leave a favorite possession with the child.

Older Adults

- Because of cognitive, sensory, or physical impairments, it may take an older patient increased time to dress for surgery and complete needed physical preparation.

Populations With Disabilities

- Patients with physical disabilities in need of special operative accommodations need to be identified, and operative staff need to be informed.

✦ SKILL 36.4 Providing Immediate Anesthesia Recovery in the Postanesthesia Care Unit

The first phase of postoperative care takes place during the immediate recovery period. This phase extends from the time the patient leaves the operating room (OR) until stabilization in the postanesthesia care unit (PACU) and the patient meets discharge criteria. Then the patient is either discharged as an outpatient or transferred to a nursing unit.

The first 1 to 2 hours are the most critical for assessing the aftereffects of anesthesia, including airway clearance, cardiovascular complications, temperature control, and neurological function (Table 36.3). A patient's condition can change rapidly; assessments must be timely, knowledgeable, and accurate. You need to be aware of the common complications and problems associated with the specific types of anesthesia (Table 36.4). Clinical judgment regarding selection of the most appropriate interventions is essential. A patient is usually ready for discharge home or to a general patient care unit in a hospital when specific standardized criteria are met. The Postanesthetic Discharge Scoring System (PADSS) (Table 36.5) and the Aldrete scoring system are types of scoring systems for assessment. The Aldrete scoring system uses parameters of activity, respiration, circulation, consciousness, and oxygen saturation. A score of greater than 9 indicates the patient may be discharged from the PACU.

Recovery from ambulatory surgery requires the same assessments. However, the depth of general anesthesia may be less because the surgery is less involved and of shorter duration. Some patients have only intravenous (IV) conscious sedation, and intensive monitoring is required for a shorter time period. As soon as the patient is stable and alert, give instructions for home care to the patient and caregiver, including demonstrations and written instructions.

Delegation

The skill of initiating immediate anesthesia recovery of a patient cannot be delegated to assistive personnel (AP). The AP may provide basic comfort and hygiene measures. Direct the AP by:

- Explaining any restrictions for how to provide comfort measures (e.g., repositioning, turning, applying warming blanket).
- Offering instruction in providing needed supplies.

NOTE: AP may be allowed to do more in ambulatory surgery recovery such as provide initial PO liquids.

Interprofessional Collaboration

- For ambulatory surgery, collaborate with patient's primary health care provider, home care department, and agency pharmacy to ensure a transition to home postoperatively.
- A pain management specialist may be involved in the care of the patient if the patient has a known history of opioid dependence to design a postoperative pain management plan.

Equipment

- Blood pressure monitoring equipment
- Oxygen equipment such as mask, oxygen regulator and tubing, and positive-pressure delivery system
- Various types and sizes of artificial airways
- Constant and intermittent suction
- Pulse oximeter
- End-tidal carbon dioxide (CO_2) monitor
- Electrocardiogram (ECG) monitor
- Portable ultrasound to assess pulses
- Thermoregulation equipment, including thermometers, blanket warmers, and cooling devices
- Bladder scanner
- IV supplies (if ordered) (see Chapter 28)
- Adult and pediatric emergency cart with defibrillator
- Stock supplies (e.g., facial tissues, dressings, bedpans, urinals, emesis basin)
- Adjustable lighting
- Personal protective equipment
- Latex-free supplies and equipment

TABLE 36.3

Postanesthesia Monitoring and Management of Complications

Condition	Interventions
Airway	
Mechanical obstruction: Decreased LOC and muscle relaxants, resulting in flaccid muscles and tongue blocking airway	Hyperextend neck; pull mandible forward; use nasal or oral airway; encourage deep breathing.
Retained thick secretions: Irritation from anesthesia; anticholinergic medications; history of smoking	Suction; encourage coughing.
Laryngospasm: Stridor from excessive secretions or airway irritation	Encourage to relax and breathe through the mouth. If extreme, it may require positive-pressure ventilation with oxygen, small dose of muscle relaxant (ordered by anesthesiologist), and intubation.
Laryngeal edema: Allergic reaction, irritation from ET tube, fluid overload	Administer humidified oxygen, antihistamines, steroids, sedatives; in some cases, perform reintubation.
Bronchospasm: Preexisting asthma, anesthetic irritation (expiratory wheeze)	Administer bronchodilators as ordered.
Aspiration: Vomiting from hypotension, accumulated gastric secretions and delayed gastric emptying, pain, fear, position changes	Position on side; suction airway; administer antiemetic as ordered.
Breathing: Hypoventilation/Hypoxemia	
CNS depression: Anesthesia, analgesics, muscle relaxants (respiratory rate shallow)	Encourage to cough and deep breathe; use mechanical ventilator; administer narcotic antagonist and muscle-relaxant reversal agent.
Mechanical restriction: Obesity, pain, tight cast or dressings, abdominal distention	Reposition; give analgesic; loosen cast or dressings; implement measures to reduce gastric distention (e.g., NG intubation, NG suction).
Circulation	
Hypovolemia: Blood loss, dehydration	Administer IV fluids or blood replacement.
Hypotension: Anesthesia/drug effects, vasodilation (possibly from spinal anesthesia), narcotics	Elevate legs; give oxygen, IV fluids, or blood replacement; administer vasopressors; monitor I&O, stimulation, hemoglobin, and hematocrit.
Cardiac failure: Preexisting cardiac disease; circulatory overload; excessive/too-rapid fluid replacement	Provide digitalization and diuretics; monitor ECG.
Cardiac arrhythmias: Hypoxemia; MI; hypothermia; imbalance of potassium, calcium, magnesium	Provide IV fluid replacement; monitor ECG and urine output; identify and treat cause.
Hypertension: Pain, distended bladder, preexisting hypertension, vasopressor drugs	Compare with preoperative baseline; identify and determine cause.
Compartment syndrome: Pressure from edema causing enough compression to obstruct arterial and venous circulation resulting in ischemia, permanent numbness, loss of function; forearm and lower leg most common sites	Obtain compartment pressures to diagnose and elevate extremity no higher than heart level; remove or loosen bandage or cast to relieve compression; if left untreated, amputation may be required. Do not apply ice. Check status of any intravenous (IV) fluid administration for infiltration.

CNS, Central nervous system; *ECG,* electrocardiogram; *ET,* endotracheal; *I&O,* intake and output; *IV,* intravenous; *LOC,* level of consciousness; *MI,* myocardial infarction; *NG,* nasogastric.

TABLE 36.4

Focused Assessment of Patient Problems Related to Anesthesia Type

Anesthesia Type	Focused Assessment
General	Hypotension; changes in heart rate or rhythm; lowered body temperature; respiratory depression; postoperative nausea and vomiting; emergence delirium in the form of shivering, trembling, confusion, or hallucinations
Spinal	Headache, hypotension, decreased cardiac output, cyanosis, difficulty breathing
Neuromuscular blocking drugs (NMBDs)	Intraocular pressure, intracranial pressure
Local	Skin rash; allergic reaction with edema of the face, lips, mouth, or throat; restlessness; bradycardia; hypotension; ischemic necrosis at injection site
Moderate (conscious) sedation	Respiratory depression, bradycardia, hypotension, nausea and vomiting
Epidural	Cyanosis, breathing difficulties, decreased heart rate, irregular heart rate, pale skin color, nausea and vomiting

Data from Lilley L, et al: *Pharmacology and the nursing process,* ed 10, St Louis, 2022, Elsevier.

TABLE 36.5

Postanesthetic Discharge Scoring System (PADSS)

		Score
Vital signs	BP + pulse within 20% preop baseline	2
	BP + pulse within 20–40% preop baseline	1
	BP + pulse >40% preop baseline	0
Activity	Steady gait, no dizziness, or meets preop level	2
	Requires assistance	1
	Unable to ambulate	0
Nausea and vomiting	Minimal/treated with PO medication	2
	Moderate/treated with parenteral medication	1
	Severe/continues despite treatment	0
Pain	Controlled with oral analgesics and acceptable to patient: Yes	2
	Controlled with oral analgesics and acceptable to patient: No	1
Surgical bleeding	Minimal/no dressing changes	2
	Moderate/up to two dressing changes required	1
	Severe/more than three dressing changes required	0

From American Society of PeriAnesthesia Nurses (ASPAN): *2021-2022 Perianesthesia nursing standards, practice recommendations and interpretive statements*, Cherry Hill, NJ, 2022, ASPAN.
BP, Blood pressure; *PO*, by mouth.

STEP	RATIONALE

ASSESSMENT

1. Identify patient using at least two identifiers (e.g., name and birthday or name and medical record number) according to agency policy.

   Ensures correct patient. Complies with The Joint Commission standards and improves patient safety (TJC, 2023).

2. Receive hand-off report from circulating nurse and anesthesia provider, including procedure performed, range of vital signs, any complications, estimated blood loss (EBL), other fluid loss, fluid replacement during surgery, type of anesthesia, medications given, type of airway and size, extent of surgical wound, restrictions to movement of position during surgery, and any preoperative medical and/or nursing diagnoses.

   Determines patient's general status and allows you to anticipate type of ongoing assessment needed, the need for special equipment, potential treatment measures, and nursing care interventions in PACU.

3. On patient's arrival in PACU, review surgeon's orders.

   Allows you to focus on priority interventions; assists you in organizing your care.

4. Consider type of surgical procedure, restrictions to movement, and type of anesthesia used.

   Influences type of assessments necessary, type of complications for which to observe, and specific nursing interventions needed.

5. Perform hand hygiene. Apply clean gloves. Perform thorough patient assessment, including vital signs; pulse oximetry (ASPAN, 2022); pain; and assessment of body systems, including respiratory, cardiac, neurological, gastrointestinal (GI), genitourinary (GU), metabolic, and fluid status. Assess patient's surgical site and drains, skin integrity, safety, and anxiety level.

   Reduces transmission of infection. Provides baseline for ongoing postoperative evaluations. Identifies priority nursing interventions.

6. Discharge from phase I level of care is based on specific criteria, not a time limit. Criteria should include assessment of airway patency, oxygenation, hemodynamic stability, thermoregulation, neurological stability, intake and output, tube patency, dressings, pain and comfort management, and postanesthesia recovery score if used. Each agency defines frequency of assessment.

   Discharge instructions are developed in consultation with anesthesia department.

Clinical Judgment *Be sure to turn patient on side (when possible) to observe underlying skin and check for accumulation of blood or serous drainage not visible in dependent areas (e.g., leg or arm).*

STEP	RATIONALE

PLANNING

1. Expected outcomes following completion of procedure:
   - Patient's airway remains clear; respirations are deep, regular, and within normal limits by time of transfer or discharge. Oxygen saturation remains greater than 95%.
   - Patient's BP, pulse, and temperature remain within previous baseline or normal expected range by time of discharge or transfer.
   - Dressings are clean, dry, and intact by discharge from recovery.
   - Intake and output (I&O) is within expected parameters by transfer or discharge from recovery.
   - Patient reports relief of discomfort after analgesia or other pain-relief measures by time of discharge or transfer from immediate recovery area (usually 1 to 2 hours).
   - Patient's physical examination measurements are within expected normal postoperative parameters.
2. Provide privacy and explain PACU activities to patient and family caregiver (when allowed into recovery).
3. Remove and dispose of gloves. Perform hand hygiene and apply new pair of clean gloves. Organize and set up equipment for continued monitoring and care activities.

No occurrence of pulmonary changes except those expected from effects of anesthetic or analgesic.

No occurrence of cardiovascular, pulmonary, or thermoregulatory changes except those expected from effects of anesthetic or analgesic.

Indicates wound stabilization without signs of bleeding or infection.

Adequate urinary elimination maintained. Fluid intake (IV and/or by mouth [PO]) adequately maintained.

Pain-relief measures effectively alter patient's reception or perception of pain.

Patient stable and may be prepared for next phase of postoperative recovery.

Protects patient's privacy; reduces anxiety. Promotes cooperation.

Reduces transmission of infection and promotes readiness for next priorities of care.

IMPLEMENTATION

1. Recovery activities will vary by type of surgery and patient status. While receiving hand-off report as patient enters PACU on stretcher/bed, immediately attach oxygen tubing to regulator, hang IV fluids, and check IV flow rates. Connect any drainage tubes to gravity drainage or continuous or intermittent suction as ordered. Attach cardiac monitor. Ensure that indwelling catheter and bag are in drainage position and patent.

Maintaining oxygenation and circulation are two priorities. Inhaled oxygen improves percentage of oxygen delivered to alveoli. IV fluids maintain circulatory volume and provide route for emergency drugs. Drainage tubes must remain patent and in proper position to allow fluid to drain.

2. Continue ongoing assessment of all vital signs every 5 to 15 minutes until patient stabilizes or more frequently if clinically indicated (see agency protocol). Compare findings with patient's baseline. Provide warm blankets as needed for patient comfort.

Vital signs reveal onset of postoperative complications from surgery or anesthesia (e.g., respiratory depression, hypothermia, hyperthermia, pulse irregularity, hypotension). Acute blood loss may lead to hypovolemic shock with signs of reduced BP, elevated heart and respiratory rates, pale skin, and restlessness. General anesthetic may affect temperature-regulating center, and lower metabolic rate causes hypothermia. Malignant hyperthermia is rare inherited condition that develops after receiving an anesthetic and is medical emergency (Schick & Windle, 2020).

Clinical Judgment *If patient underwent a short procedure under procedural sedation, check agency policy for sedation recovery guidelines. The perianesthesia registered nurse (RN) monitoring a patient who receives procedural sedation/analgesia should have no other responsibilities that compromise continuous patient monitoring (AORN, 2022; ASPAN, 2022). Monitor oxygenation until patients are no longer at risk for hypoxemia. Monitor ventilation and circulation at regular intervals until patients are suitable for discharge.*

3. Maintain patent airway after general anesthesia:
   a. Position patient on side with head facing down and neck slightly extended (see illustration). Never position patient with hands over chest (reduces chest expansion).

Ensures appropriate oxygenation.

Extension prevents occlusion of airway at pharynx. Downward position of head moves tongue forward, and mucus or vomitus can drain out of mouth, preventing aspiration.

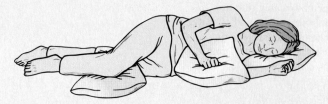

STEP 3a Position of patient during recovery from general anesthesia.

STEP	RATIONALE

Clinical Judgment *Always stay with a sedated patient until respirations are well established. Patients with an artificial airway may gag and vomit, become restless, or stop breathing. Closely monitor patients with a history of obstructive sleep apnea.*

b. Place small, folded towel or small pillow under patient's head. If patient is restricted to supine position, elevate head of bed approximately 10 to 15 degrees, extend neck, and turn head to side. Have emesis basin available if patient becomes nauseated.

Supports head in extended position. Prevents aspiration if patient should vomit.

Clinical Judgment *If patient is not able to extend neck, turn head to side if possible; suction oropharynx frequently (see Chapter 24).*

c. Encourage patient to cough and deep breathe on awakening and every 15 minutes.

Promotes lung expansion and expectoration of mucus secretions.

d. Suction artificial airway and oral cavity as secretions accumulate.

Clears airway of secretions.

e. Once gag reflex returns, have patient spit out oral airway (see illustration). Do not tape oral airway.

Indicates that patient can clear airway independently. If airway is taped, patient will gag and may obstruct airway.

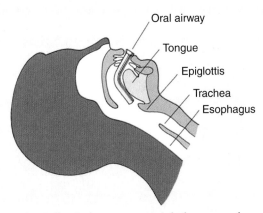

Oral airway
Tongue
Epiglottis
Trachea
Esophagus

STEP 3e Oral airway position before removal.

Clinical Judgment *Because of shorter half-life of drugs used today, many patients have oral airway removed before leaving the OR. PACU nurse must assess that respiratory effort is adequate; otherwise, airway may need to be replaced, and patient may need a ventilator.*

f. Avoid rapid position changes in patients who had spinal anesthesia, which can cause changes in patient's BP. Good body alignment is needed. Maintain IV infusion. Encourage fluid intake (only if patient can take fluids, such as with ambulatory surgery).

Rapid movements are avoided so as not to cause spinal headache from loss of cerebrospinal fluid. Increased IV or PO fluids help body replace cerebrospinal fluid.

4. Call patient by name in normal tone of voice. If there is no response, attempt to arouse patient by touching or gently moving a body part. Explain that surgery is over, and patient is in recovery area.

Determines patient's level of consciousness and ability to follow commands.

5. Assess circulatory perfusion by inspecting color of nail beds, mucous membranes, and skin. Palpate for skin temperature. Test for capillary refill (see Chapter 6).

Pink or normal color of skin, nail beds, and mucous membranes and brisk (3 seconds or less) capillary refill indicate adequate tissue perfusion. Warm extremities reveal adequate circulation.

6. Assess closely for any behavioral or clinical changes reflecting potential cardiovascular and pulmonary complications of general anesthesia (see Table 36.3). Monitor laboratory findings.

Postoperative patients who are sedated often become hypoxic. Any internal hemorrhage may be reflected in CBC.

7. When patients have general anesthesia: As patient arouses, introduce yourself and orient to surroundings.

Relieves patient anxiety.

8. For spinal or epidural anesthesia, monitor sensory, circulatory, pulmonary, and neurological responses:

Reflects return of spinal function.

  a. Monitor for hypotension, bradycardia, and nausea and vomiting.

Blockage of sympathetic nervous system results in vasodilation of major vessels and systemic hypotension.

  b. Maintain adequate IV infusion.

Maintains BP by increasing fluid volume and fills temporarily expanded vascular space.

STEP	RATIONALE
c. Keep patient supine or with head slightly elevated and maintain position.	Minimizes risk of postspinal anesthesia headache from leakage of spinal fluid at injection site, with increased pressures caused by elevation of upper body. Headache is more common with spinal than epidural anesthesia (Jabbari et al., 2021).
d. Assess respiratory status, level of spinal sensation, and mobility in lower extremities. Drowsiness will be apparent after IV sedation. Level of anesthesia depends on location of sensation change. Have patient close eyes and use alcohol wipe to test sensation along sensory dermatomes. Have patient identify if warm or cold. Remind patient that loss of extremity sensation and movement is normal and will return in several hours.	Spinal block is set within 20 minutes of onset. However, if level of anesthesia moves above sixth thoracic vertebra (T6), respiratory muscles are affected. Patients often feel short of breath and may require mechanical ventilation if respiratory muscles are severely affected.
e. Observe patients in PACU until they regain movement in extremities.	Patients fear permanent loss of function.
9. Monitor sources of intake and output:	
a. Observe dressing and drains for any evidence of bright red blood. Inspect surgical incision for swelling or discoloration. Note condition of surgical dressing, including amount, color, odor, and consistency of drainage. Mark dressing with circle around drainage using black pen. Place time of marking and check area every 10 to 15 minutes, marking any changes and noting vital signs.	Determines extent of fluid loss and condition of underlying wound. Size, location, and depth of wound influence amount of drainage.
b. Reinforce pressure dressing or change simple dressing if ordered (see Chapter 40). Continue to monitor condition of incision, surrounding tissue, and amount and color of any drainage if incision is exposed or covered with transparent dressing.	Pressure dressing should not be removed because it helps to maintain hemostasis (termination of bleeding) and absorb drainage. Changing dressings immediately after surgery can disrupt wound edges and aggravate drainage. First dressing changes most often occur 24 hours after surgery and are usually done by surgeon. Minor surgical wounds may not have dressings but simply skin closure, or wounds may be covered with transparent dressing, which allows for observation of incision and surrounding tissue.
c. Inform surgeon of unexpected bloody drainage and reinforce dressing as indicated. Apply direct pressure. Also look underneath patient for any pooling of bloody drainage. Monitor for decreased BP and increased pulse.	Progressive increase or changes in characteristics of drainage warrant call to surgeon because they could indicate hemorrhage (Harding et al., 2020; Schick & Windle, 2020). Hemorrhage from surgical wound is most likely within first few hours, indicating inadequate hemostasis during surgery. As dressing becomes saturated, blood often oozes down patient's side and collects underneath.
d. Inspect condition and contents of any drainage tubes and collecting devices. Note character and volume of drainage.	Determines patency of drainage tube and extent of wound drainage.
e. Observe amount, color, and appearance of urine from indwelling Foley catheter (if present).	Urine output of less than 30 mL/h is sign of decreased renal perfusion or altered renal function.
f. If nasogastric (NG) tube is present, assess drainage. If not draining, check placement and irrigate, if necessary, with normal saline (see Chapter 34).	Maintains patency of tube to ensure gastric decompression. Expected drainage is dark or pale, yellow or green, and 100 to 200 mL/h. Bloody drainage occurs after some surgeries.
g. Monitor and maintain IV fluid rates. Observe IV site for signs of infiltration (see Chapter 28).	Provides adequate hydration and circulatory function.
10. Promote comfort:	
a. Provide mouth care by placing moistened washcloth to lips, swabbing oral mucosa with dampened swab or soft toothbrush, or applying petrolatum to lips.	Mouth is dry from NPO status and preoperative anticholinergics.
b. Provide warm blanket or active warming device to promote warmth and minimize shivering.	General anesthesia impairs thermoregulation, OR environment is cold, and exposure of body cavity results in internal heat loss. Shivering increases oxygen consumption, predisposes patient to arrhythmias and hypertension, impairs platelet function, alters drug metabolism, impairs wound healing, and increases hospitalization costs. Skin surface warming such as forced-air is available postoperatively (Cho et al., 2021).

STEP	RATIONALE
c. Help with position changes and provide supportive pillows. Encourage leg exercises.	Improves ventilation and circulation.
11. Continue monitoring pain as patient awakens and until transfer to surgical unit or discharge, including quality, severity, and location (see Chapter 16). Do not assume that all postoperative pain is incisional pain.	Pain is often not directly related to surgical procedure (e.g., chest pain [myocardial infarction or pulmonary embolism] or muscle pain [trauma from positioning]). Referred pain (in shoulder) often occurs after laparoscopy. Pain control regimens should be individualized to the needs of the patient, considering age, medical and physical condition, level of fear/anxiety, personal preferences, type of surgical procedure, and individual patient response. An optimal plan for perioperative pain control should include a multimodal approach to minimize the need for opioids.
a. Provide pain medication as ordered and when vital signs have stabilized.	Promotes patient comfort.
12. Explain patient's condition to patient and inform of plans for transfer to nursing unit or discharge to alternate setting.	Decreases anxiety that can interfere with recovery process.
13. Appropriately dispose of supplies and equipment used in PACU setting. Remove and dispose of gloves. Perform hand hygiene.	Reduces transmission of infection.
14. When patient's condition stabilizes, contact anesthesiologist to approve transfer to nursing unit or release to home.	Surgeon is responsible for authorizing transfer or discharge.
15. Before discharge to home from ambulatory surgery unit, provide verbal and written instructions (Box 36.2).	Patients and home care providers must be aware of potential complications and follow-up care.
16. For patients transferring to the next point of care by stretcher, raise side rails and request transport team. Perform hand hygiene.	Ensures patient safety. Reduces transmission of microorganisms.

Clinical Judgment *If patient is to be discharged to home, ensure that someone is coming to drive the patient home and observe the patient for signs and symptoms of complications. Review with patient and driver reportable signs and symptoms and emergency care needed.*

EVALUATION

1. Compare all vital sign assessment measurements with patient's baseline and expected normal levels.	Evaluates patient's respiratory, cardiovascular, and thermoregulatory status throughout recovery.
2. Inspect surgical wound and dressings for drainage. Be sure to assess for wound drainage under patient.	Provides data to measure progress of wound healing.
3. Measure I&O. Urine output should be at least 30 to 50 mL/h.	Indicates onset of fluid imbalances.
4. Auscultate bowel sounds and ask if patient has passed flatus.	Allows you to evaluate return of peristalsis and diet tolerance.
5. Measure patient's perception of pain after implementing pain-relief measures.	Determines level of comfort achieved and effectiveness of pain-relief measures.
6. Complete system-specific physical assessments as appropriate according to patient's unique type of surgery (e.g., craniotomy—neurological assessment; neck surgery—airway status; vascular surgery—circulation and bleeding; orthopedic surgery—neurovascular status and immobility or positioning).	Evaluates course of recovery.

BOX 36.2

Postanesthesia and Ambulatory Surgery Discharge Criteria

Postanesthesia Discharge Criteria
- Patient is awake (or returns to baseline)
- Vital signs stable, within 20% of baseline
- Temperature ≥36°C and patient reports acceptable comfort level without symptoms of hypothermia or shivering
- No excess bleeding or drainage
- No respiratory depression
- Pain controlled
- Absence of bladder distention
- Hand-off report given

Ambulatory Surgery Discharge Criteria
- All postanesthesia care unit (PACU) discharge criteria met
- No intravenous (IV) opioids for past 30 minutes
- Minimal nausea and vomiting
- Pain controlled
- Voided (if appropriate to surgical procedure/orders)
- Able to ambulate if age appropriate and not contraindicated
- Responsible adult present to accompany patient
- Discharge instructions given and understood using teach-back

STEP	RATIONALE

7. Use Teach-Back: "I want to be sure you know what to expect when you go home. Tell me the signs and symptoms to expect if you were to get an infection." Revise your instruction now or develop a plan for revised patient/family caregiver teaching if patient/family caregiver is not able to teach back correctly.

Teach-back is a technique for health care providers to ensure that they have explained medical information clearly so that patients and their families understand what is communicated to them (AHRQ, 2023).

Unexpected Outcomes

1. Patient exhibits respiratory depression (pulse oximetry <95%, respiratory rate <10 breaths/min or shallow; see agency standards for range). Serious hypoxemic episode: oxygen saturation <90% for ≥1 hour. **NOTE:** A combination of "too much anesthesia" from excessive opioid use, inadequate reversal of neuromuscular blockade agents, or prolonged persistence of these agents in the system as a result of liver or renal disease is common for respiratory depression in the PACU.

2. Patient exhibits signs of hypovolemia related to internal or incisional hemorrhage.

3. Patient complains of severe incisional pain.

Related Interventions

- Promptly report assessment findings to surgeon.
- Administer oxygen as ordered by nasal cannula. Give patients with chronic obstructive pulmonary disease (COPD) 2 L/min or less of oxygen (as ordered) to prevent hypercapnia.
- Encourage deep breathing every 5 to 15 minutes.
- Position to promote chest expansion (on side or semi-Fowler).
- Administer prescribed medications (e.g., epinephrine, opioid reversal agent).

- Elevate patient's legs enough to maintain downward slope toward trunk of body. Do not lower head past flat position because this position increases respiratory effort and potentially decreases cerebral perfusion.
- Promptly report patient's present status to surgeon.
- Administer oxygen at 6 to 10 L/min by mask per order.
- Increase rate of IV fluid or administer blood products as ordered.
- Monitor BP and pulse every 5 to 15 minutes.
- Apply pressure dressings as follows per order:
  - *Abdominal dressing:* Cover bleeding area with several thicknesses of gauze compresses and place tape 7 to 10 cm (3 to 4 inches) beyond width of dressing with firm, even pressure on both sides close to bleeding source. Maintain pressure as you tape entire dressing to maximize pressure at source of bleeding.
  - *Dressing on extremity:* Apply rolled gauze, pressing gauze compress over bleeding site. Refrain from taping around entire extremity.
  - *Dressing in neck region:* Cover with several thicknesses of gauze and place tape 7 to 10 cm (3 to 4 inches) beyond width of dressing. Apply with pressure, but do not occlude carotid artery or airway. Assess every 5 to 15 minutes for carotid pulse and evidence of airway obstruction.
- Patient remains NPO because it is often necessary to return to surgery for control of bleeding.

- Administer analgesics; reassess and provide analgesia before pain is severe.
- Pain sometimes lowers BP; analgesia may restore vital signs to normal. Monitor vital signs carefully.
- For patients with patient-controlled analgesia (PCA), be sure that patient is using device correctly. Teach family caregiver not to manipulate PCA.
  - *Orthopedic surgery:* Earliest symptom of compartment syndrome in extremity is pain unrelieved by analgesics. Other symptoms include numbness, tingling, pallor, coolness, and absent peripheral pulses. Surgeon **must** be notified. Do not elevate extremity above level of heart because this increases venous pressure. Application of ice is contraindicated because vasoconstriction will occur (Harding et al., 2020).

Documentation

- Document patient's arrival time at PACU; include vital signs, I&O, and other physical parameters; level of consciousness (LOC); and pain location and severity. Also include condition of dressings and tubes, character of drainage, condition of IV infusion, and all nursing measures.

- Document your evaluation of patient and family caregiver learning.

Hand-Off Reporting

- Report any abnormal assessment findings and signs of complications to surgeon.

Special Considerations

Patient Education

- If patient had spinal or epidural anesthetic, remind family caregiver that loss of extremity movement is normal for several hours.
- Reinforce preoperative teaching regarding incentive spirometry, coughing, deep breathing, leg exercises, and information concerning ambulation and pain control.
- Provide the following instruction for ambulatory surgical patients:
  - Surgeon's office and surgery center telephone number (24-hour answer)
  - Follow-up appointment, date, time
  - Review of prescribed medications
  - Activity or diet restrictions related to specific surgery
  - Dressing and wound care
  - Pain control
  - Guidelines related to possible effects of anesthesia
  - Dietary restrictions
  - Activity restrictions
  - Signs and symptoms of complications

Pediatrics

- Maintenance of body temperature in infants and children after surgery is a priority because of their immature temperature-control mechanisms.
- Infants and children normally have higher metabolic rates and differences in physiological makeup than adults, resulting in greater oxygen, fluid, and calorie needs.

- Vomiting is a major concern in young children because of increased risk for fluid and electrolyte imbalances and risk for aspiration. Vomiting is also more likely because surgery in children is often necessitated by accidental injuries without benefit of NPO status.

Older Adults

- The ability of older adults to tolerate surgery depends on the extent of physiological changes that have occurred with aging, the presence of any chronic diseases, and the duration of the surgical procedure.
- When communicating with older adults, be aware of any auditory, visual, or cognitive impairment that may be present.

Populations With Disabilities

- Opioid-dependent patients may require postoperative pain control plans tailored to their needs. Opioid requirements for these patients may be unpredictable because of their individual opioid tolerance. A plan for postoperative pain management should be designed before surgery, including possible collaboration with a pain management specialist.

Home Care

- Teach ambulatory surgery patient and family caregiver about any postoperative exercises, home modifications, or activity limitations.
- If patient is discharged with dressing changes, suggest that bedroom or bathroom is usually ideal for procedure.
- Assess need for a home health care referral.

◆ SKILL 36.5 Providing Early Postoperative (Phase II) and Convalescent Phase (Phase III) Recovery

Early postoperative (phase II) anesthesia recovery focuses on preparing a patient for self-care, care by family caregivers, or care in an extended care environment (ASPAN, 2022). Convalescent (phase III) anesthesia recovery focuses on providing ongoing care for patients who require extended observation or intervention after transfer from phase I or phase II. Interventions are directed toward preparing the patient for self-care or care by family caregivers. Phases of recovery are not locations but levels of care (ASPAN, 2022).

Teaching is important to promote patient independence, inform the patient and family caregiver about limitations and restrictions, and provide resources needed to achieve an optimal state of wellness. Teaching begins preoperatively, continues during the early postoperative recovery period, and then extends from the time a patient is discharged from the PACU to the time of discharge or movement to the next point of care. Patients who have outpatient surgery undergo convalescence at home. Individualize your nursing care depending on the type of surgery, preexisting medical conditions, the risk for or development of complications, and the rate of recovery.

Many health care agencies have developed enhanced recovery after surgery (ERAS) protocols. The protocols are evidence based and designed to standardize care to minimize surgical stress and postoperative pain, reduce postoperative complications, improve patient outcomes, decrease length of stay, and promote early recovery (Sun & Qi, 2022). Elements of an ERAS protocol might include education, nutritional management, management of sleep and pain, maintenance of body temperature, IV fluid management, postoperative diet therapy, and early mobilization (Sun & Qi, 2022).

Delegation

The skill of providing early postoperative and convalescent phase recovery cannot be delegated to assistive personnel (AP). AP may obtain vital signs (if patient is stable), apply nasal cannula or oxygen mask (but not adjust oxygen flow), and provide hygiene or repositioning for comfort. Direct the AP by:
- Explaining how often to take vital signs.
- Reviewing specific safety concerns and what to observe and report back to the nurse.
- Explaining any precautions that affect how to provide basic hygiene and comfort measures.

Interprofessional Collaboration

- Transitional care health care team (e.g., long-term care) is included in care if patient will be discharged to these settings.

Equipment

- Postoperative bed (recliner for day surgery recovery)
- Stethoscope, sphygmomanometer, thermometer, pulse oximeter
- Intravenous (IV) fluid poles and infusion pumps as needed
- Emesis basin
- Washcloth and towel
- Waterproof pads
- Equipment for oral hygiene
- Pillows
- Facial tissue
- Oxygen equipment and bag-valve masks and emergency cart with defibrillator available for adult and children

- Suction equipment (to suction airway)
- Dressing supplies
- Intermittent suction (to connect to nasogastric [NG] or wound drainage tubes)
- Orthopedic appliances (if needed)

- Clean gloves
- Personal protective equipment as indicated
- Malignant hyperthermia cart (Schick & Windle, 2020)
- Latex-free supplies and equipment
- Transport equipment, including wheelchairs and carts

STEP	RATIONALE

ASSESSMENT

STEP	RATIONALE
1. Obtain phone report from postanesthesia care unit (PACU) nurse summarizing patient's current status (see Chapter 3).	Allows you to prepare hospital room with necessary supplies and equipment for patient's specific needs.
2. Perform hand hygiene and arrange equipment at bedside.	Reduces transmission of microorganisms. Arrangement of equipment facilitates safety and smooth transfer process.
3. Identify patient using at least two identifiers (e.g., name and birthday or name and medical record number) according to agency policy.	Ensures correct patient. Complies with The Joint Commission standards and improves patient safety (TJC, 2023).
4. If patient has been transported by stretcher, prepare for transfer with bed in high position (level with stretcher), with sheet folded to side and room for stretcher to be placed beside bed easily (see Chapter 11). Transfer patient to bed using safe patient handling.	Ensures safe patient transfer.
5. Collect more detailed hand-off report from nurse accompanying patient (if a nurse transferred the patient)	Detailed report helps you plan appropriate assessment and nursing care measures. Data provide baseline to detect any change in patient's condition.
6. Collect an initial set of vital signs.	Allows for comparison with patient's status in operating room (OR) and PACU.
7. Assess character and location of patient's surgical pain; rate severity on scale of 0 to 10.	Pain management is a postoperative priority. Data used for comparison during recovery process.
8. Review electronic health record (EHR) for information pertaining to type of surgery; postoperative complications; medications administered in PACU; preoperative medical risks; baseline vital signs, PACU vital signs, and other assessment findings; and patient's usual medications given/not given before surgery. Compare and validate with information from hand-off report.	Surgical review identifies intraoperative complications and presence of medical risks that dictate complications for which to observe. Vital signs provide way to detect postoperative changes. List of patient's usual medications may necessitate call to surgeon or hospitalist for orders concerning timing and dose of drugs not given before surgery.
9. Review postoperative medical orders.	Offers additional guidelines for type of care to provide.

Clinical Judgment *Postoperatively, the health care provider writes a set of new medication orders. It is common that the medications the patient was previously taking are not among the ordered medications. Patients must clarify with their regular health care provider after discharge if any previous medications need to be added or resumed for the daily regimen.*

STEP	RATIONALE

10. Assess patient's risk for postoperative urinary retention (POUR):
  a. Patient factors: older age, male, history of urinary retention, neurological disease
  b. Procedural factors: anorectal surgery, hernia repair, joint arthroplasty, incontinence surgery
  c. Anesthetic factors: excess fluid administration, select medications (e.g., anticholinergic, opioids), prolonged anesthesia, neuroaxial anesthesia
	Up to 14% of surgical patients may develop POUR, but it is usually transient (Lajiness, 2022).

11. Assess patient's risk for postoperative nausea and vomiting (PONV):
  a. Patient risk factors: preoperative nausea and vomiting, female, history of PONV or motion sickness, age younger than 50 years of age
  b. Anesthetic factors: general anesthesia, volatile anesthetics, nitrous oxide (N_2O), duration of anesthesia, use of opioids
  c. Surgical factors: type of surgery (e.g., cholecystectomy, gynecologic, laparoscopic)
	Postoperative nausea and vomiting (PONV) can occur in one of three patients based on individual, anesthetic, and surgical factors (Moore et al., 2021).

12. Refer to nurses' notes or, if necessary, reassess a patient's/family caregiver's health literacy.	Determines degree to which individuals have the ability to find, understand, and use information and services to make informed health-related decisions and actions for themselves and others (CDC, 2023).

STEP	RATIONALE
13. Ask patient or refer to nurses' notes regarding a patient's knowledge, prior experience with surgery, and feelings about procedure.	Reveals need for patient instruction and/or support.

PLANNING

STEP	RATIONALE
1. Expected outcomes following completion of procedure:	
• Patient's breath sounds remain clear bilaterally.	No occurrence of pulmonary changes except those expected from effects of anesthetic or analgesic.
• Patient's vital signs remain within normal limits consistent with preoperative baseline.	No occurrence of cardiovascular, pulmonary, or thermoregulatory changes except those expected from effects of anesthetic or analgesic.
• Incision wound edges are well approximated; no drainage is noted.	Indicates wound healing without signs of bleeding or infection.
• Fluid balance is evident by intake and output (I&O) records.	Adequate urinary elimination maintained. Fluid intake (IV and/or by mouth [PO]) adequately maintained.
• Patient describes character of pain and rates it at less than 4 on scale of 0 to 10 while engaged in moderate activity by discharge.	Pain-relief measures effectively alter patient's reception or perception of pain.
• Normal bowel sounds are present after bowel surgery or general anesthesia within 48 to 72 hours after surgery.	Indicates return of GI function.
• Patient does not experience nausea or vomiting.	Antiemetics administered for nausea are effective.
2. Provide privacy and explain all postoperative care measures to patient. Provide postoperative teaching during all care measures. If applicable, teach patient how to report complications or side effects from surgery.	Protects patient's privacy; reduces anxiety. Promotes cooperation.
3. Attach any existing oxygen tubing, hang IV fluids, verify IV flow-rate settings on infusion pump, and check drainage tubes (e.g., Foley catheter or wound drainage).	Provides continuity of therapies.

IMPLEMENTATION

STEP	RATIONALE
1. Perform hand hygiene. Apply clean gloves for any necessary procedures.	Reduces transmission of microorganisms.
2. **Early recovery initial postoperative care:**	
a. Maintain airway. If patient remains sleepy or lethargic, keep head extended and support in side-lying position.	Minimizes chances of aspiration and obstruction of airway with tongue.
b. Assess level of consciousness (LOC) and continue measuring vital signs per frequency of agency policy or health care provider order. Compare findings with vital signs taken in PACU and patient's baseline.	Patient's status may change during transfer. Movement of patient and pain level influence stability of vital signs. Change in vital signs may reveal onset of postoperative complications.
c. Encourage coughing, deep breathing, and use of incentive spirometry and positive expiratory pressure (PEP) device (see Skill 36.2) to prevent atelectasis.	Anesthesia, medications, and intubation irritate airways, resulting in secretions and atelectasis. Coughing and use of devices expand chest, aerate lungs, and mobilize secretions.
d. Assess for return of bowel sounds.	Indicates return of GI function.
(1) Manage postoperative nausea and vomiting (PONV): opioid-sparing pain management, use of postoperative antiemetics, and nonpharmacological techniques (e.g., relaxation).	Management for PONV should include multimodal preventive measures based on patient's identified risk and evidence-based interventions when PONV occurs (Moore et al., 2021).
(2) If NG tube is present, check placement and irrigate per policy (see Chapter 35). Connect to proper drainage device. Connect all other drainage tubes to appropriate suction or collection device. Secure to prevent tension on tubing.	Transfer and movement may dislodge tubes, which would interfere with drainage.
e. Inspect patient's surgical dressing for appearance, presence, and character of drainage. Unless contraindicated by surgeon, outline drainage along edges with pen and reassess in 1 hour for change. If no dressing is present, inspect condition of wound (see Chapter 38).	Wound can hemorrhage quickly during early postoperative period. Observations of wound and dressings provide data to measure progress of wound healing.

Clinical Judgment *If unable to change dressing, mark area of drainage and label with time, date, and initials. Document frequency of reinforcement. Never use felt-tip marker to mark dressing because ink can bleed into gauze, contaminating incision site.*

STEP	RATIONALE
f. Palpate abdomen for bladder distention or use bladder ultrasound when available. If Foley catheter is present, check placement. Ensure that it is draining freely and properly secured. Patient may have continuous bladder irrigations or suprapubic catheter (see Chapter 33).	Anesthesia often contributes to urinary retention. Urinary stasis increases risk for urinary tract infection.
(1) Manage postoperative urinary retention (POUR): Use bladder ultrasound for high-risk patients who have not voided within 4 hours; if greater than 600 mL of urine is present, consider a single-time catheterization.	Patients who are unable to void in the PACU may not complain of bladder fullness or lower abdominal discomfort, and physical examination does not detect bladder distention; patients should be reviewed for risk factors of POUR (Lajiness, 2022).
(2) If no urinary drainage system is present, explain that voiding within 8 hours after surgery is expected. Male patients may void successfully if allowed to stand.	Anesthetics and analgesics depress sensation of bladder fullness. Patient may still have no sensations below level of spinal or epidural anesthetic.
g. Measure all sources of fluid intake and output (I&O).	Altered fluid and electrolyte balance is potential complication of major surgery.
h. Describe purpose of equipment and frequent observations to patient and family caregivers.	Unfamiliar sights (e.g., equipment, patient's appearance) often provoke anxiety.
i. Provide pain management. Position patient for comfort, maintaining correct body alignment. Avoid tension on surgical wound site. Assess last time analgesic given.	Reduces stress on suture line. Helps patient relax and promotes comfort.
(1) Patient-controlled analgesia (PCA) may be used for pain control (see Chapter 16). Medicate patient as ordered either around the clock or prn as ordered during first 24 to 48 hours. Give PRN analgesic as soon as possible when patient reports increase in pain. Explain pain-management measures to patient. Know the symptoms of opioid use and withdrawal.	Determines level of discomfort. Adequate pain control is needed to permit patient to participate fully with recovery activities. Consider time of the last opioid dose; withdrawal symptoms will occur upon abrupt discontinuation of opioids or when opioid antagonists are administered (ASA, 2023).
j. Place nurse call system in an accessible location within patient's reach.	Ensures patient can call for assistance if needed.
k. Raise side rails (as appropriate) and lower bed to lowest position, locking into position.	Ensures patient safety and prevents falls.
l. Dispose of all contaminated supplies in appropriate receptacle, remove and dispose of gloves, and perform hand hygiene.	Reduces transmission of microorganisms. Use appropriate disposal receptacle for items soiled with urine or feces if patient is on hazardous drugs (ONS, 2018).
3. **Continued postoperative care:**	
a. Continue to assess vital signs at least every 4 hours or as ordered.	Temperature greater than 38°C (100.4°F) in first 48 hours may indicate atelectasis, the normal inflammatory response, or dehydration. Temperature greater than 37.8°C (100°F) on third day or after often indicates wound infection, pneumonia, or phlebitis (Harding et al., 2020). Altered blood pressure or pulse is associated with cardiovascular complications (see Table 36.3).
b. Closely monitor progress of wound healing and change dressings as needed or ordered.	Wound infection occurs most often within 3 to 6 days after surgery. Wound dehiscence occurs most often 3 to 11 days after surgery (see Chapter 38).
c. Monitor (see illustration A) and maintain wound drainage devices such as Jackson-Pratt, Hemovac, or Penrose drains. Jackson-Pratt and Hemovac drainage systems must be emptied when they are half full of drainage or air and recharged (compressed to discharge air) (see illustration B).	Wound drainage devices promote healing from inside to outside and relieve pressure on suture line. Compressing flexible closed container and then plugging drainage hole creates negative suction pressure.
d. Provide oral care at least every 2 hours as needed. If permitted, offer ice chips.	Medication such as anticholinergic given before surgery makes mouth dry. Oral care and ice chips promote comfort.
e. Encourage patient to turn, cough, deep breathe, and use incentive spirometer and PEP device at least every 2 hours (see Skill 36.2).	Promotes adequate ventilation and minimizes hypoventilation and atelectasis. Especially necessary for patients with a history of smoking, pneumonia, or chronic obstructive pulmonary disease (COPD) or patients who are confined to bed rest.

STEP	RATIONALE

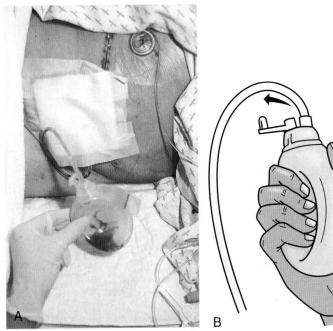

STEP 3c (A) Note color of drainage from Jackson-Pratt device. (B) Charging Jackson-Pratt drainage system.

f. Apply or monitor function of sequential compression devices or elastic stockings on lower extremities (see Chapter 12). Devices may be applied preoperatively. Explain to patient that compression device will inflate and deflate intermittently.

Compression devices and stockings increase venous return (Pai & Douketis, 2019). Explanation decreases anxiety and fosters cooperation.

Clinical Judgment *Remove sequential compression devices before patient ambulation. Exception: Mobile compression devices that allow for ambulation with assistance are available.*

g. Promote early ambulation and activity per agency protocol (see Chapter 12). Assess vital signs before and after activity to assess tolerance. Patients are often ambulating within first 12 hours of arrival to patient care unit. Set goals for patient to increase ambulation progressively.

Early ambulation is critical to prevent resultant postoperative complications (Sun & Qi, 2022). Mobility promotes circulation, lung expansion, and peristalsis. Postural hypotension is caused by sudden position changes.

h. Progress from clear liquids to regular diet as tolerated if nausea and vomiting do not occur.

Nausea and vomiting are associated with anesthesia and surgery. Implement PONV protocols if needed (Moore et al., 2021). IV fluids are usually discontinued when oral intake is tolerated. Some patients must be NPO for several days until flatus returns or bowel sounds are heard.

i. Include patient and family caregiver in decision making; answer questions as they arise.

Promotes patient's sense of control and independence and improves self-esteem.

j. Provide opportunity for patients who must adjust to change in body appearance or function to verbalize feelings.

Radical surgery, amputation, or inoperable cancer often results in anxiety and depression. Grief response to loss of body organ is common and should be expected.

4. Convalescent phase:

a. Assess patient's home environment for safety, cleanliness, and availability of community resources and help for patient. (**NOTE:** This may be done by a case manager and not a staff nurse.) Use the information to revise any teaching as needed.

Provides information about patient's environment after discharge and the possible need for home care. Verifies patient's and family caregiver's level of knowledge and any additional teaching needs for discharge. Helps to facilitate transition management and patient's independence and participation in care.

b. Provide instruction on care activities that patient or family caregiver will perform at home (e.g., dressing change, medication administration, exercises, IV therapy).

Enables patient to achieve self-care at home.

STEP	RATIONALE
c. Keep patient and family caregiver informed of progress made toward recovery. Explain time expected for discharge from health care agency. Provide answers to individual patient questions or concerns.	Decreases anxiety and helps patient know what to anticipate for discharge planning.
d. Following any procedure, remove and dispose of gloves; perform hand hygiene.	Reduces transmission of microorganisms.
e. Prepare patient for discharge home. Be sure patient and family caregiver have all necessary printed instructions. Provide a hand-off report if patient is being discharged to an agency such as a long-term care facility.	Ensures continuity of care and safe transitions of care.

EVALUATION

1. Auscultate breath sounds bilaterally.	Determines status of airways.
2. Monitor trends in vital signs.	Provides data to measure progress of postoperative status.
3. Evaluate I&O records. Assess time of patient's first postoperative urination.	Indicates onset of urination.
4. Auscultate bowel sounds and evaluate for presence of nausea.	Allows you to evaluate return of peristalsis and diet tolerance.
5. Ask patient to describe character of pain and rate acuity on a scale of 0 to 10 after moderate activity.	Determines level of comfort achieved and effectiveness of pain-relief measures.
6. Inspect incision (wound edges well approximated, no drainage noted).	Provides data to measure progress of wound healing.
7. Monitor progress of patient ambulation.	Progressive improvement reflects improved exercise tolerance.
8. Have patient or family caregiver describe incision care, dietary modifications or restrictions, activity restrictions, medication schedule, and plans for follow-up visit.	Identifies need for further teaching.
9. **Use Teach-Back:** "I want to be sure I explained what you need to know about your postoperative activity level. Explain for me how you will increase your activity level during the first week at home." Revise your instruction now or develop a plan for revised patient/family caregiver teaching if patient/family caregiver is not able to teach back correctly.	Teach-back is a technique for health care providers to ensure that they have explained medical information clearly so that patients and their families understand what is communicated to them (AHRQ, 2023).

Unexpected Outcomes	Related Interventions
1. Vital signs are above or below patient's baseline or expected range. Initially this could be related to anesthesia effects, pain, hypovolemic shock, airway obstruction, fluid and electrolyte imbalance, or hypothermia.	• Identify contributing factors. • Notify surgeon.
2. Patient complains of severe incisional pain.	• Report to surgeon; discuss alternative analgesic option. • Try nonpharmacological pain control measures (see Chapter 16).

Documentation

- Document patient's arrival at nursing unit; include vital signs, I&O, body system assessment findings, and all nursing measures initiated.
- Continue to document assessment measures every 4 hours or more frequently as patient's condition warrants.
- Document your evaluation of patient and family caregiver learning.

Hand-Off Reporting

- Report onset of any postoperative complications to surgeon or other health care provider immediately.
- During hand-off report, communicate patient's assessment findings pertinent to surgery, patient response, and progress with postoperative instruction.
- If transitioned to any other environment than home, report preoperative course and postoperative summary, as well as current status, to receiving nurse.

Special Considerations

Patient Education

- Instruct patient and family caregiver to identify signs and symptoms and appropriate actions to take for infection, respiratory, circulatory, or GI difficulties and wound disruptions.
- Provide important phone numbers to patient and family caregiver for use in emergency and follow-up care on discharge.
- Teach patient about appropriate wound care, diet recommendations, and activity restrictions.

Pediatrics

- Maintenance of body temperature in infants and children after surgery is a priority because of their immature temperature-control mechanisms (Hockenberry et al., 2022).
- Infants and children normally have higher metabolic rates and differences in physiological makeup compared with adults, resulting in greater oxygen, fluid, and calorie needs. Vomiting is

a concern because of increased risk for fluid and electrolyte imbalances and risk for aspiration.
- Use appropriate pain assessment tools to determine child's pain level.

Older Adults
- Older adults often experience a longer and more difficult postoperative recovery. Assess carefully for the development of postoperative complications.
- Assess for postoperative delirium and changes in mental status along with potential causes.

Populations With Disabilities
- Patients with preexisting heart failure or stroke are at increased risk for cardiac instability in the postoperative period.

Home Care
- Teach patient and family caregiver about postoperative exercises, home modifications, activity limitations, wound dressing care, medications, and nutritional needs.
- If patient is discharged with dressing changes, the bedroom or bathroom is usually ideal for the procedure. Have patient and family caregiver perform return demonstration of dressing change.
- Make referral to home health services if patient and family caregiver will have difficulty providing the expected level of care needed.
- Patients having surgery performed in ambulatory surgery centers must be accompanied by a family member or friend to allow for discharge after the procedure (see Box 36.2).

✦ CLINICAL JUDGMENT AND NEXT GENERATION NCLEX® EXAMINATION–STYLE QUESTIONS

The nurse is preparing to care for a 52-year-old female patient who is 5 feet tall and weighs 113.6 kg (250 lb). She will soon be admitted to the surgical unit from the PACU following an abdominal hysterectomy. Her previous medical history includes 30-year, 2-pack-per-day cigarette smoking and type 2 diabetes mellitus. She has been taking birth control pills for 30 years. She is on 2 L of oxygen via nasal cannula, has an abdominal dressing that has a small amount of serosanguineous fluid on it, and has both a Foley catheter draining pink-tinged urine and an IV of $D_5\frac{1}{2}$ normal saline (NS) infusing at 125 mL/h. She has a patient-controlled analgesia (PCA) device. She received cefazolin IV piggyback approximately 45 minutes before her incision was made and is to receive her second dose 8 hours later.

1. For each body system, select the tasks the nurse will delegate to the assistive personnel (AP). Each system may support more than one possible task to delegate to AP.

Body System	Possible Tasks to Delegate to Assistive Personnel (AP)
General	○ Assess for postoperative pain ○ Perform initial assessment upon arrival to unit ○ Provide repositioning every 2 hours
Integumentary	○ Monitor IV site for infiltration or signs of infection ○ Provide general hygiene and oral care AS and PM ○ Assess incision site twice per shift
Respiratory	○ Document pulse oximetry reading every 4 hours ○ Assess lung sounds every 2 hours ○ Teach how to cough and deep breathe
Renal	○ Empty Foley catheter bag ○ Provide perineal care twice daily ○ Assess kidney function for signs of infection

2. The next morning, the nurse notes that the patient can be woken but falls back to sleep easily. Current vital signs include blood pressure 104/68 mm Hg, pulse 68 beats/min, respirations 12 breaths/min, temperature 37.7°C (99.9°F), and oxygen saturation 98% on 2 L of oxygen. Which factor does the nurse anticipate is **most likely** the reason the patient has trouble staying awake?
   1. Fever
   2. Low blood pressure
   3. Opioid medication
   4. Fatigue after surgery

3. Which factor is the earliest indicator that gastrointestinal function has returned following the patient's surgery?
   1. First stool
   2. Passing of gas
   3. Normal bowel sounds
   4. Patient's report of abdominal growling

4. Which activities will the nurse teach the patient to enhance pulmonary status following surgery? **Select all that apply.**
   1. Cough and deep breathe.
   2. Get up to move regularly.
   3. Use incentive spirometer.
   4. Take an antihistamine if breathing is difficult.
   5. Splint the abdomen with a pillow when rising from bed.

5. On the day of discharge, the nurse performs an assessment. Which finding will the nurse report to the health care provider?
   1. No IV opioids have been taken today.
   2. Fluid intake is 950 mL in the last 8 hours.
   3. Abdominal binder is free from drainage.
   4. Temperature is 38°C (100.4°F).

Visit the Evolve site for Answers to Clinical Judgment and Next Generation NCLEX Examination–Style Questions.

REFERENCES

Agency for Healthcare Research and Quality (AHRQ): *Teach-back: intervention*, Rockville, MD, November 2023, Agency for Healthcare Research and Quality. https://www.ahrq.gov/patient-safety/reports/engage/interventions/teachback.html.
Ammanuel S, et al: Are preoperative chlorhexidine gluconate showers associated with a reduction in surgical site infection following craniotomy? A retrospective cohort analysis of 3126 surgical procedures, *J Neurosurg* 135:1889–1897, 2021.
American Society of PeriAnesthesia Nurses (ASPAN): *2021-2022 Perianesthesia nursing standards, practice recommendations and interpretive statements*, Cherry Hill, NJ, 2022, ASPAN.
Association of periOperative Registered Nurses (AORN): *AORN comprehensive surgical checklist*, Denver, CO, 2019, AORN.
Association of periOperative Registered Nurses (AORN): *Perioperative standards and recommended practices*, Denver, CO, 2022, AORN.
American Society of Anesthesiologists (ASA): Practice guidelines for preoperative fasting and the use of pharmacologic agents to reduce the risk of pulmonary aspiration: application to healthy patients undergoing elective procedures, *Anesthesiology* 126(3):376, 2017.
American Society of Anesthesiologists (ASA): *ASA-AAOS pain alleviation toolkit*. https://www.asahq.org/advocacy-and-asapac/advocacy-topics/pain-medicine-talking-points/the-pain-toolkit, 2023. Accessed November 6, 2023.

Berrios-Torres S, et al: Centers for Disease Control and Prevention guideline for the prevention of surgical site infection, *JAMA Surg* 152(8):784, 2017.

Calegaril I, et al: Adherence to measures to prevent surgical site infection in the perioperative period: a cohort study, *Rev enferm UERJ* 29:e62347, 2021.

Centers for Disease Control and Prevention (CDC): *What is health literacy?* 2023. https://www.cdc.gov/healthliteracy/learn/index.html.

Cho C, et al: Incidence of postoperative hypothermia and its risk factors in adults undergoing orthopedic surgery under brachial plexus block: a retrospective cohort study, *Int J Med Sci* 18(10):2197–2203, 2021.

Deslate S, et al: Assessment tool to predict intraprocedure airway maneuvers and adverse events in a gastrointestinal laboratory, *AANA J* 89(1):45–52, 2021.

Dogan S, et al: The effect of nail polish and henna on the measures of pulse oximeters in healthy persons, *J Perianesth Nurs* 36(5):532–535, 2021.

Fumarola S, et al: Overlooked and underestimated: medical adhesive-related skin injuries. Best practice consensus document on prevention, *J Wound Care* 29(Suppl 3c):S1–S24, 2020.

Harding M, et al: *Lewis's medical-surgical nursing: assessment and management of clinical problems*, ed 11, St. Louis, 2020, Elsevier.

Hitchcock J, et al: Preventing medical adhesive-related skin injury (MARSI), *Br J Nurs* 30(15):S48–S56, 2021.

Hockenberry MJ, et al: *Wong's essentials of pediatric nursing*, ed 11, St. Louis, 2022, Mosby.

Jabbari A, et al: A narrative review on prevention and treatment strategies of post spinal anesthesia headache, *Arch Anesth & Crit Care* 7(4):245–252, 2021.

Kawada T: Screening ability of STOP-BANG questionnaire for obstructive sleep apnea, *Anesth Analg* 128(3):e48, 2019.

Kohno A, et al: Swallowing and aspiration during sleep in patients with obstructive sleep apnea versus control individuals, *Sleep* 45(4):zsac036, 2022.

Kushner B, et al: Infection prevention plan to decrease surgical site infections in bariatric surgery patients, *Surg Endosc* 36:2582–2590, 2022.

Lajiness M: Non-urological postoperative urinary retention (POUR), *Urol Nurs* 42(1):25–33, 2022.

Moore C, et al: Preventing postoperative nausea and vomiting during an ondansetron shortage, *AANA J* 89(2):161–167, 2021.

Myoga Y, et al: The effects of preoperative alcohol, tobacco, and psychological stress on post operative complications: a prospective observational study, *BMC Anesthesiol* 21:245, 2021.

National Healthcare Safety Network (NHSN): *Surgical Site Infection Event (SSI)*, 2023. https://www.cdc.gov/nhsn/pdfs/pscmanual/9pscssicurrent.pdf. Accessed November 6, 2023.

Nurgul Y, et al: A simple and validated test for detecting patients with OSA: STOP-BANG questionnaire, *Ann Card Anaesth* 24(3):313–314, 2021.

Oncology Nurses Society (ONS): *Toolkit for safe handling of hazardous drugs for nurses in oncology*, 2018. https://www.ons.org/sites/default/files/2018-06/ONS_Safe_Handling_Toolkit_0.pdf.

Palese A, et al: "I am administering medication-please do not interrupt me": Red tabards preventing interruptions as perceived by surgical patients, *J Patient Saf* 15(1):30, 2019.

Ralph N, Norris P: Current opinion about surgery-related fear and anxiety, *J Perioper Nurs* 31(4):3–6, 2018.

Rothrock JC: *Alexander's care of the patient in surgery*, ed 16, St. Louis, 2019, Elsevier.

Schick L, Windle P: *PeriAnesthesia nursing core curriculum: preoperative, phase I and phase II PACU nursing*, ed 4, St. Louis, 2021, Saunders.

Sullivan W, et al: Primary care of adults with intellectual and developmental disabilities: clinical practice guidelines, *Can Fam Physician* 64:254, 2018.

Sun Z, Qi Y: Application of enhanced recovery after surgery care protocol in the perioperative care of patients undergoing lumbar fusion and internal fixation, *J Orthop Surg Res* 17:240, 2022.

Thayer DM, et al: Top down injuries: prevention and management of moisture-associated skin damage, medical adhesive–related skin injury and skin tears. In McNichol LM, et al., editors: *Core curriculum: wound management*, ed 2, Philadelphia, 2022, Wolters Kluwer.

The Joint Commission (TJC): *2023 National patient safety goals*, Oakbrook Terrace, IL, 2023, The Joint Commission. https://www.jointcommission.org/standards/national-patient-safety-goals/.

Touhy TA, Jett KF: *Ebersole and Hess' gerontological nursing and healthy aging*, ed 6, St. Louis, 2022, Elsevier.

Wang W, et al: Current status and influencing factors of nursing interruption events, *Am J Manag Care* 27(6):e188–e194, 2021.

SKILLS AND PROCEDURES

Skill 37.1 **Surgical Hand Antisepsis, p. 1098**

Skill 37.2 **Donning a Sterile Gown and Closed Gloving, p. 1102**

OBJECTIVES

Mastery of content in this chapter will enable you to:
- Discuss the meaning and implications of a sterile conscience.
- Explain the roles of a registered nurse in the operating room.
- Outline guidelines for use of sterile technique in the operating room.

- Examine actions to take when a break in sterile technique occurs in the operating room.
- Demonstrate surgical hand antisepsis correctly.
- Explain how to correctly don a sterile surgical gown.
- Apply sterile gloves using the closed technique.

MEDIA RESOURCES

- http://evolve.elsevier.com/Perry/skills
- Review Questions
- Audio Glossary

- Answers to Clinical Judgment and Next-Generation NCLEX® Examination–Style Questions
- Skills Performance Checklists
- Printable Key Points

PURPOSE

Nurses practicing in the operating room (OR) support patients' surgical experiences from the preoperative phase throughout the intraoperative period and into the various postoperative phases (see Chapter 36). Perioperative nurses exercise clinical judgment, critical thinking, and interpersonal communication skills while applying the nursing process to ensure that patients receive appropriate nursing care throughout their surgical experience (Association of periOperative Registered Nurses [AORN], 2023). Safety is a key principle in monitoring and managing intraoperative patients.

PRACTICE STANDARDS

- Association of periOperative Registered Nurses (AORN), 2023: Guidelines for Perioperative Practices
- The Joint Commission (TJC), 2023: Office-Based Surgery: 2023 National Patient Safety Goals
- World Health Organization (WHO), 2009: Surgical Safety Checklist

SUPPLEMENTAL STANDARDS

- American Society of PeriAnesthesia Nurses (ASPAN), 2023–2024: PeriAnesthesia Nursing Standards, Practice Recommendations and Interpretive Statements
- Association of Surgical Technologists (AST), 2019: Guidelines for Best Practices for Establishing the Sterile Field in the Operating Room

PRINCIPLES FOR PRACTICE

- The interprofessional surgical team includes the surgeon (doctor of medicine [MD] or doctor of osteopathy [DO]), physician's assistant (PA), registered nurse first assistant (RNFA), certified registered nurse anesthetist (CRNA) and/or physician anesthesiologist (MD or DO), circulating nurse (RN), and scrub nurse/technician (RN, licensed practical nurse [LPN] [Box 37.1], or certified surgical technologist [CST]).
- The responsibilities of the RNFA can vary depending on agency policies, settings, and patient populations. Some general responsibilities can include working preoperatively with other team members to perform a focused preoperative assessment, using instruments and providing hemostasis during the intraoperative period, and postoperatively assisting with patient discharge (AORN, 2022).
- The intraoperative phase begins when a patient enters the operating room (OR) or surgical suite and ends with admission to the post anesthesia care unit (PACU).
- A circulating nurse (Box 37.2) is an RN who both manages and collaborates closely with the interprofessional team while using the nursing process to guide the patient through the intraoperative phase (Rothrock, 2023). This "nonsterile" member of the surgical team assumes responsibility and accountability for maintaining patient safety and continuity of quality care. This includes supervising the conduct of the scrub technician and delegating tasks to assistive personnel (AP) as appropriate. The circulating nurse also assists the first assistant, scrub nurse/technician, and surgeon.
- It is a moral obligation for the perioperative nurse to develop a sterile conscience, always knowing the location of a sterile field and

BOX 37.1

Role of the Scrub Nurse

- Helps circulating nurse prepare the OR and open supplies
- Performs surgical hand antisepsis and dons sterile gown and gloves
- Prepares sterile field with procedure-appropriate supplies and instruments, verifying that all are in working order
- Participates in "time-out" procedure with other surgical team members (safety measure taken to ensure correct patient, correct procedure, correct site and side, correct patient position, and correct implants/equipment present) (TJC, 2023)
- Performs sponge, sharps, and instrument counts with circulating nurse before incision is made, at the beginning of wound closure, and at the end of the surgical procedure

- Labels all liquids and/or medications on sterile field with sterile marking pen when liquid or medication is out of the original container or package
- Gowns and gloves surgeons and assistants as they enter the OR
- Assists surgeons with sterile draping of patient
- Keeps sterile field orderly and monitors progress of procedure and any breaks in aseptic technique
- Passes sterile instruments and supplies to surgeons and assistants
- Handles surgical specimens per agency policy
- Constantly monitors location of all sponges and sharps in the sterile field

OR, Operating room.

BOX 37.2

Role of the Circulating Nurse

- Incorporates nursing process in plan of care
- Organizes and prepares OR before start of surgical procedure; checks to see that equipment works properly
- Gathers supplies for surgical procedure and opens sterile supplies for scrub nurse/technician
- Counts sponges, sharps, and instruments with scrub nurse/technician before incision is made, at the beginning of wound closure, and at the end of the surgical procedure
- Ensures that all liquids and/or medications on the sterile field are labeled with sterile marking pen when liquid or medication is out of the original container or package
- Sends for patient at appropriate time
- Conducts preoperative patient assessment, including the following:
  - Explaining role and identifying patient
  - Reviewing electronic health record (EHR) and verifying procedure and consents
  - Confirming dentures and prostheses removed
  - Confirming patient's allergies, NPO status, laboratory values, ECG, x-ray film studies, skin condition, and circulatory and pulmonary status
- Safely helps patient to operating table and positions patient according to surgeon preference and procedure type, using safety

precautions (e.g., safety belt, securing arms, padding bony prominences)
- Participates in "time-out" procedure with other surgical team members (safety measure taken to ensure correct patient, correct procedure, correct site and side, correct patient position, and correct implants/equipment present) (TJC, 2023)
- Applies conductive pad to patient if electrocautery used; may prepare patient's skin; may apply ECG electrodes
- Applies antiembolism stockings and sequential compression device per physician order
- Explains briefly to patient what circulating nurse and scrub nurse/technician are doing
- Assists surgical team by tying gowns and arranging equipment
- Assists anesthesia personnel during induction and extubation
- Continuously monitors procedure for any breaks in aseptic technique and anticipates needs of the team; opens additional sterile supplies for scrub nurse/technician
- Handles surgical specimens per agency policy
- Documents on perioperative nurses' notes
- Communicates to family and PACU personnel during the surgical procedure

ECG, Electrocardiogram; *NPO*, nothing by mouth; *OR*, operating room; *PACU*, post anesthesia care unit.

what items are sterile versus nonsterile and maintaining patient safety (Duff et al., 2022). A sterile conscience requires knowledge of the principles of aseptic technique; self-discipline; good communication skills to identify, address, and correct any breaks in sterile technique; and the maturity to overcome personal preferences.

- While a patient is in the OR and the OR team is gowned and gloved, it is recommended that a surgical safety checklist be completed (WHO 2009) (Fig. 37.1). The WHO checklist includes key safety checks and is designed for use in all types of facilities (e.g., hospital ORs, ambulatory surgery settings, physician offices).
- The checklist identifies three phases of an operation, each corresponding to a specific period in the normal flow of work: before induction of anesthesia, before skin incision, and before patient leaves the OR (WHO, 2009). In each phase a checklist coordinator must confirm that the surgery team has completed the listed tasks before it proceeds with the operation.
- The surgical checklist verifies the patient's identity, ascertains if the patient has any allergies, checks if the surgical site is marked and verifies the site marking, and asks the patient if there are any questions (TJC, 2023; WHO, 2009).
- A time-out is conducted immediately before starting any invasive procedure or making an incision (TJC, 2023). Time-outs are standardized by each agency, initiated by a designated

member of the team, and involve all the immediate members of the surgical/procedure team who will be participating in the procedure from the beginning. It is during the time-out that the team members agree at a minimum that the correct patient has been identified and the correct procedure is scheduled to be done and on the proper body part or area. The time-out is documented before the procedure begins (TJC, 2023).

PERSON-CENTERED CARE

- The patient may be unsure of what to expect and have concerns regarding pain, disfigurement, and length of recovery. It is a nurse's responsibility to provide this information and encourage questions.
- Care of the surgical patient requires specialized knowledge when the nurse is required to closely monitor a patient's intraoperative response to the experience (Duff et al., 2022).
- Patient needs vary on the basis of preoperative health, type of surgical procedure, and cultural and religious beliefs. Nurses obtain information regarding culture and religious preferences that may affect acceptance of education, blood administration, and surgical interventions.
- Information is communicated to the interprofessional team to ensure comprehensive intraoperative care.

Surgical Safety Checklist

Before induction of anaesthesia	Before skin incision	Before patient leaves operating room
(with at least nurse and anaesthetist)	(with nurse, anaesthetist and surgeon)	(with nurse, anaesthetist and surgeon)

Before induction of anaesthesia
(with at least nurse and anaesthetist)

Has the patient confirmed his/her identity, site, procedure, and consent?
☐ Yes

Is the site marked?
☐ Yes
☐ Not applicable

Is the anaesthesia machine and medication check complete?
☐ Yes

Is the pulse oximeter on the patient and functioning?
☐ Yes

Does the patient have a:

Known allergy?
☐ No
☐ Yes

Difficult airway or aspiration risk?
☐ No
☐ Yes, and equipment/assistance available

Risk of >500ml blood loss (7ml/kg in children)?
☐ No
☐ Yes, and two IVs/central access and fluids planned

Before skin incision
(with nurse, anaesthetist and surgeon)

☐ **Confirm all team members have introduced themselves by name and role.**

☐ **Confirm the patient's name, procedure, and where the incision will be made.**

Has antibiotic prophylaxis been given within the last 60 minutes?
☐ Yes
☐ Not applicable

Anticipated Critical Events

To Surgeon:
☐ What are the critical or non-routine steps?
☐ How long will the case take?
☐ What is the anticipated blood loss?

To Anaesthetist:
☐ Are there any patient-specific concerns?

To Nursing Team:
☐ Has sterility (including indicator results) been confirmed?
☐ Are there equipment issues or any concerns?

Is essential imaging displayed?
☐ Yes
☐ Not applicable

Before patient leaves operating room
(with nurse, anaesthetist and surgeon)

Nurse Verbally Confirms:
☐ The name of the procedure
☐ Completion of instrument, sponge and needle counts
☐ Specimen labelling (read specimen labels aloud, including patient name)
☐ Whether there are any equipment problems to be addressed

To Surgeon, Anaesthetist and Nurse:
☐ What are the key concerns for recovery and management of this patient?

This checklist is not intended to be comprehensive. Additions and modifications to fit local practice are encouraged.   Revised 1 / 2009   © WHO, 2009

FIG. 37.1 The World Health Organization surgical safety checklist. (*Used with permission, World Health Organization.*)

EVIDENCE-BASED PRACTICE

Surgical Conscience

Honesty and integrity are the cornerstones of surgical practice, with surgical conscience being seen as a vital and necessary element to provide safe, ethical, and competent surgical patient care (Farley, 2022). Surgical conscience has been compared to integrity and has been defined as what you do when no one is looking (Farley, 2022). It will impact workflow, operating room culture, and ultimately patient care and must be upheld to protect patients at one of their most vulnerable times.

- Optimal patient outcomes, including prevention of surgical site infections (SSIs), have been tied to surgical conscience as perioperative nurses are encouraged to listen to their "inner voice" in providing safe patient care and making critical clinical decisions (Farley, 2022).
- Aspects of teamwork tied to surgical conscience include working together, helping each other, shared responsibility, emphasizing and prioritizing patient safety, compassion for each patient, keeping high standards, and addressing any issue as soon as it is safe to do so, even after a case is finished (Farley, 2022).
- Qualities of selflessness and self-discipline will evolve surgical conscience in the nurse. Be a patient advocate and be accountable for nursing practice that supports safe patient care, achieves better outcomes, and prevents SSIs (Farley, 2022).
- Speak up for the patient, be an advocate, and uphold and defend surgical asepsis and patient safety by being vigilant for potential breaches in asepsis (Duff et al., 2022).

- Do not let fear or concerns of repercussions for speaking up stop you from doing what is right. Use moral reasoning, place the patient's well-being above everything else, and let your morals and values help guide you (Duff et al., 2022).
- Strategies to communicate effectively in a nonconfrontational manner are often lacking in perioperative education. Offer mentors to support new perioperative nurses and help socialize them into the unique culture and practice of the operating room, which will help develop surgical conscience (Duff et al., 2022).

SAFETY GUIDELINES

- Reduce intraoperative errors using a time-out, active communication, decreasing distractions, real-time documentation, and increasing staff education (TJC, 2023).
- All items used within a sterile field must be sterile. The sterile field must always be maintained. The presence of numerous personnel, complicated traffic patterns, unidirectional airflow, and use of multiple pieces of equipment may increase air contaminants in the room (Link, 2019).
- Sterile surgical gowns and gloves protect patients and the interprofessional team from transmission of pathogens. After donning, the front of a sterile gown is considered sterile from the chest to the level of the sterile field. Sleeves are considered sterile from 5 cm (2 inches) above the elbow to the cuff circumferentially.
- Surgical gowns should be an adequate size to wrap around and completely cover the scrubbed team member's body. Select the

surgical gown needed for the procedure according to the barrier performance class (e.g., reinforced gown) as per manufacturer recommendations and agency policy (Link, 2019).

- Scrubbed team members must keep their hands in view above waist level, in front of axillae and below neckline, to avoid contamination.
- When wearing a sterile gown, do not fold arms with hands tucked in the axillary region. This area is not considered sterile once you have donned the gown.
- Sterile-draped tables are sterile only at table level. Sides of the drape extending below table level are unsterile. The portion of the sterile drape that establishes the sterile field should not be moved after initial positioning (Link, 2019).

- All personnel moving around or within a sterile field must do so in a manner consistent with maintaining the sterility of that field. Scrubbed persons move from sterile areas to other sterile areas, contacting a sterile field only with sterile gowns and gloves. Unscrubbed team members always stay at least 30 cm (12 inches) away from the sterile field while keeping it in constant view; they touch only unsterile areas.
- Group all sterile supplies and equipment around the sterile-draped patient.
- Unsterile team members must avoid reaching over the sterile field.
- Scrubbed team members remain close to the sterile field. When changing position, turn face to face or back to back.

◆ SKILL 37.1 Surgical Hand Antisepsis

In the operating room (OR) setting it is imperative that you achieve surgical hand antisepsis through effective surgical scrub or antiseptic hand rub (AORN, 2023). To reduce patient risk for acquiring postoperative infections, use of an antimicrobial preparation for hand antisepsis is an integral part of the presurgical scrubbing procedure for OR personnel. Although the skin cannot be sterilized, you can reduce the number of microorganisms greatly by chemical, physical, and mechanical means.

Through the use of an antimicrobial agent and sterile sponges, the surgical hand scrub removes debris and transient microorganisms from the nails, hands, and forearms; reduces the resident microbial count to a minimum; and inhibits rapid/rebound growth of microorganisms (AORN, 2023). Evidence suggests that completing a brushless hand-rub technique using approved hand-hygiene products, with or without water, is an alternative to the traditional hand scrub with the same microbial efficacy (AORN, 2023). The AORN (2023) recommends a scrub for the length of time recommended by the manufacturer to allow adequate product contact with the skin. Both hand-antiseptic methods are currently used in OR settings.

Delegation

The skill of surgical hand antisepsis can be delegated to a surgical technologist or licensed practical nurse. Routinely observe surgical hand antisepsis for staff compliance.

Interprofessional Collaboration

An interprofessional team should develop a protocol and select hand hygiene/antisepsis products on the basis of an analysis of product effectiveness, user acceptance, and cost.

Equipment

- Deep sink with foot or knee controls for dispensing water and soap
- Antimicrobial agent approved by agency (dispenser with foot controls)
- Surgical scrub brush/sponge with plastic nail file
- Paper face mask, cap or hood, surgical shoe covers
- Protective eyewear/face shield
- Sterile towel
- Sterile pack containing sterile gown

STEP	RATIONALE

ASSESSMENT

1. Determine type and length of time for hand hygiene (see agency policy).
2. Remove bracelets, rings, and watches.

3. Inspect fingernails, which must be short (2 mm), clean, and healthy. Check with the agency policy to see if fingernail polish is permitted. Never wear artificial nails or extenders.

4. Inspect condition of cuticles, hands, and forearms for presence of abrasions, cuts, or open lesions.

Guidelines vary according to manufacturer's recommendations for surgical scrub.
Jewelry harbors and protects microorganisms from removal. Skin under rings has been shown to harbor more pathogens and should not be worn (AORN, 2023).
Long nails increase the risk of harboring potential pathogens, limit the effectiveness of hand hygiene, and can injure patients during patient handling (AORN, 2023). Long fingernails can also puncture gloves, causing contamination. Artificial nails harbor gram-negative microorganisms and fungus (AORN, 2023).
Cuts, abrasions, exudative lesions, fresh tattoos, or hangnails tend to ooze serum, which may contain pathogens. Individuals with these conditions should not have patient contact until conditions heal (AORN, 2023).

PLANNING

1. Expected outcome following completion of procedure:
   - Patient does not develop signs of surgical site infection.

Indicates that microorganisms are not transferred to patient and sterile field.

STEP	RATIONALE

IMPLEMENTATION

1. Don surgical shoe covers, cap or hood, face mask, and protective eyewear.

Protective eyewear prevents exposure to blood or body fluids splashing from sterile field, which causes risk for infection (e.g., human immunodeficiency virus [HIV], hepatitis B virus [HBV]).

Clinical Judgment *Laser surgery requires special protective eyewear to prevent eye damage from stray laser energy.*

2. Perform prescrub wash at beginning of work shift:

   Prevents contamination of hands after scrub.

   a. Turn water on using foot or knee control and adjust to comfortable temperature.
   b. Wet hands thoroughly with water. Follow manufacturer directions for application of soap.
   c. Rub hands, covering all surfaces with lather, including backs of hands, fingertips, inner webs, and palms, washing for at least 15 seconds.

   A short prescrub wash/rinse at least 15 seconds at beginning of work shift removes gross debris and superficial microorganisms (AORN, 2023).

   d. Rinse hands well. Dry hands thoroughly with disposable towel and discard towel.

   Rinsing removes all soap and remaining debris.

3. **Surgical hand scrub (with sponge):**

   a. Turn on water using foot or knee control. Clean under nails of both hands with disposable nail pick or cleaner (see illustration). Rinse hands and forearms under running water, keeping hands and forearms elevated and elbows down.

   Removes dirt and organic materials that harbor microorganisms.

   b. Dispense antimicrobial scrub agent according to manufacturer instructions. Apply agent to wet hands and forearms with soft, nonabrasive sponge.

   Scrub designed to remove resident microorganisms on all surfaces of hands and arms (AORN, 2023).

   c. Scrub for the length of time recommended by the manufacturer. Visualize each finger, hand, and arm as having four sides (see illustrations). Pay particular attention to cleansing of fingernails. Wash all four sides of fingers effectively, keeping hand elevated, elbow down. Repeat for other hand, fingers, and arm.

   Scrubbing all surfaces ensures removal of resident microorganisms on hands and arms (AORN, 2023). Keeping hands elevated and elbows down prevents microorganisms from flowing back onto hands. Fingernails have been found to have greater bacterial loads than skin on the fingertips (Vallejo et al., 2018).

   d. Avoid splashing surgical attire. Discard sponges in appropriate container.

   Splashing causes contamination and requires changing gown.

   e. Rinse hands and arms, running water from fingertips to elbows in one continuous motion, holding hands higher than elbows (see illustration).

   Hands remain cleanest part of upper extremities.

   f. Turn off water using foot or knee controls and back into OR holding hands higher than elbows and away from surgical attire.

   Water contaminates field.

   g. Approach sterile setup and grasp sterile towel, taking care not to drip water on sterile field (see illustration).

   Avoids sterile towel contacting unsterile scrub attire and transferring contamination to hands. Dries skin from cleanest (hands) to least clean (elbows).

   h. Keeping hands and arms above waist and outstretched, carefully grasp one end of sterile towel to dry one hand thoroughly, moving from fingers to elbow in rotating motion (see illustration).

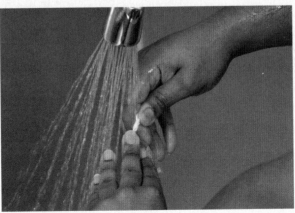

STEP 3a Clean under fingernails.

STEP	RATIONALE

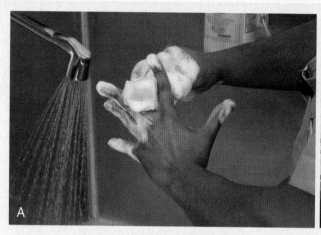 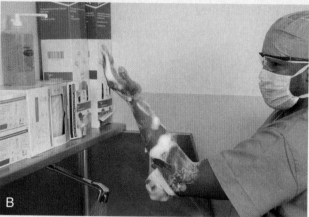

STEP 3c (A) Scrub sides of fingers. (B) Scrub forearms.

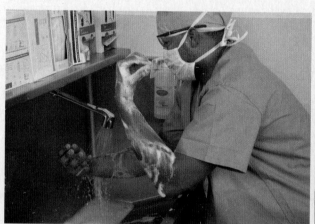

STEP 3e Rinse arms.

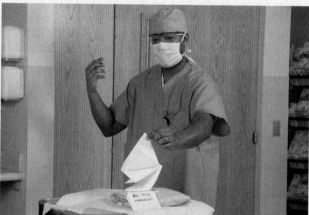

STEP 3g Grasp sterile towel.

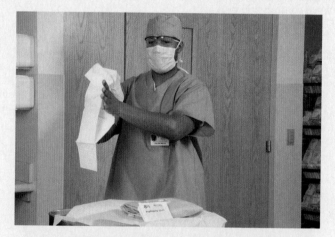

STEP 3h Dry hands thoroughly.

STEP	RATIONALE

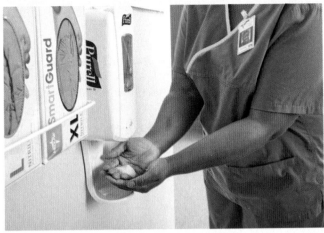

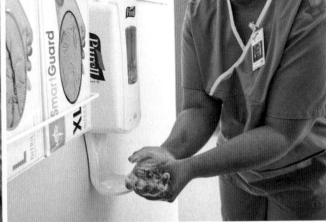

STEP 4b Dispense antimicrobial agent into hands.

STEP 4d Rub thoroughly until completely dry.

<table>
<tr><td>

i. Use opposite end of towel to dry other hand.

j. Drop towel into linen hamper or into circulating nurse's hand, making certain that hands do not fall below waist level.

</td><td>

Avoids transfer of microorganisms from elbow to opposite hand.

</td></tr>
<tr><td>

4. **Perform spongeless surgical hand scrub with alcohol-based hand-rub product:**

   a. After prescrub wash (Step 2), turn on water using foot or knee control. Clean under nails of both hands with disposable nail pick or cleaner and rinse hands and forearms under running water. Dry hands thoroughly with paper towel. Turn off water.

</td><td>

Prevents contamination of hands after wash.

</td></tr>
</table>

Clinical Judgment *Use approved brushless, alcohol-based surgical hand-rub products (with added emollients) that limit damage to the user's skin, improve adherence to hand antisepsis protocols, simplify application technique, and reduce material waste (i.e., water, brushes, and packaging) (Rothrock, 2023).*

<table>
<tr><td>

b. Dispense manufacturer-recommended amount of antimicrobial agent hand preparation (see illustration). Apply agent to hands and forearms according to manufacturer instructions for application, recommended volume, and specified time.

c. Repeat antimicrobial product application if indicated in manufacturer instructions.

d. Rub thoroughly until completely dry (see illustration). Proceed to OR to don gloves.

</td><td>

Promotes reduction in microorganisms on all surfaces of hands and arms (AORN, 2023).

Wet hands promote growth of microorganisms.

</td></tr>
</table>

EVALUATION

1. Monitor patient after surgery for signs of surgical site infection (usually occurs 2 to 3 days after surgery).	Signs of infection include redness, heat, swelling, pain, and purulent drainage at operative site.

Unexpected Outcomes

1. Redness, heat, swelling, pain, or purulent drainage may develop at surgical site, which often indicates wound infection.

Related Interventions

- Individualize interventions based on patient's situation (e.g., wound care, antibiotic therapy).

Documentation

- Documentation is not required for surgical hand antisepsis.
- Document area and description of surgical site after surgery to provide baseline for monitoring wound.

Hand-Off Reporting

- Report area and description of surgical site after surgery.

◆ SKILL 37.2   Donning a Sterile Gown and Closed Gloving

Immediately following surgical hand antisepsis, apply a sterile gown and then apply sterile gloves. All members of the surgical team must prepare in this manner before entering the sterile field. Once applied, the surgical gown is considered sterile in the front from chest to waist or table level. The sleeves are considered sterile from 5 cm (2 inches) above the elbow to fingertips. The back of the gown is not considered sterile when worn. Surgical gowns should cover all garments worn underneath. All sterile gowns that are free of tears, punctures, strain, and abrasion provide an effective barrier against microorganisms, particulates, and fluids passing between unsterile and sterile areas (AORN, 2023).

Use the closed-glove method to apply gloves when you enter the sterile field. If a glove becomes contaminated during the surgery, the circulating nurse, wearing protective unsterile gloves, grasps the outside of the glove and pulls it off inside out, leaving the stockinette cuff of the gown in place. Another sterile team member assists in regloving. The open method can be used when only one glove has been contaminated. In most settings the scrub nurse will wear two pairs of sterile gloves. If both of the scrub nurse/technician's gloves become contaminated, the gown is removed first, then the gloves are removed, and then the nurse regowns and regloves using the closed-glove method.

Delegation

The skills of donning a sterile gown and closed gloving can be delegated to a surgical technologist or licensed practical nurse. Routinely observe sterile gown application and closed gloving for staff compliance.

Interprofessional Collaboration

The surgeon and the interprofessional team members follow sterile practices to prevent infection and achieve optimal patient outcomes.

Equipment

- Package of proper-size sterile gloves (latex-free if sensitivity or allergy present)
- Sterile pack containing sterile gown
- Clean, flat, dry surface (table or Mayo stand) on which to open gown and gloves
- Paper face masks, cap or hood, surgical shoe covers
- Protective eyewear/face shield

STEP	RATIONALE
ASSESSMENT	
1. Select proper size and type of sterile gloves. Select latex-free gloves if you know that patient or any surgical personnel in room are latex sensitive.	Proper fit ensures ease of handling instruments and supplies. Prevents latex allergic response.
Clinical Judgment *Become familiar with your agency's policy since double gloving may be recommended and encouraged to reduce the risk for glove perforation during a surgical procedure (AORN, 2023; Link, 2019).*	
2. Select proper size and type of sterile surgical gown.	Ill-fitting gown impedes movement of extremities.
PLANNING	
1. Expected outcomes following completion of procedure: • Patient does not develop signs of surgical site infection.	Nurse maintains aseptic technique and does not contaminate gown or gloves.
IMPLEMENTATION	
1. **Donning sterile gown:** a. Open sterile gown and glove package on clean, dry, flat surface. Scrub nurse (before scrubbing hands) or circulating nurse can assist you, preferably on small table separate from sterile field containing sterile instruments and supplies.	Provides sterile area for gloving.
b. Perform surgical hand antisepsis (see Skill 37.1). Dry hands thoroughly.	
c. Pick up gown (folded inside out) from sterile package, grasping inside surface at collar.	Hands are not completely sterile. Inside surface of gown will contact surface of skin and thus is considered contaminated.
d. Lift folded gown directly upward and step back, away from table.	Prevents gown from touching unsterile object.
e. Locate neckband; with both hands grasp inside front of gown just below neckband.	Clean hands may touch inside of gown without contaminating outer surface.
f. Keeping gown at arm's length away from body, allow it to unfold with inside of gown toward body. Do not touch outside of gown or allow it to touch floor.	Outside of gown remains sterile.

STEP	RATIONALE

g. With hands at shoulder level, slip both arms into armholes simultaneously (see illustration). Do not allow hands to move through cuff opening. Have circulating nurse pull gown over shoulders by reaching inside arm seams. Pull gown on, leaving sleeves covering hands.

Careful application prevents contamination. Gown covers hands to prepare for closed gloving.

h. Have circulating nurse tie gown at neck and waist (see illustration). If gown is wraparound style, do not touch sterile front flap until scrub nurse/technician has gloved.

Secures gown without contaminating it.

2. Applying gloves using closed-glove method:

a. With hands covered by gown cuffs and sleeves, open inner sterile glove package (see illustration).

Sterile gown cuff touches sterile glove surface.

b. Grasp folded cuff of glove for dominant hand with nondominant hand.

Sterile gown touches sterile glove.

c. Extend covered dominant hand and forearm forward with palm up and place palm of glove against palm of dominant hand. Glove fingers point toward elbow.

Positions glove for application over cuffed hand, keeping glove sterile.

d. While holding glove cuff through gown with dominant hand on which it was placed, grasp back of glove cuff with nondominant hand and turn glove cuff over end of dominant hand and gown cuff (see illustration).

Positions glove over gown for hand insertion.

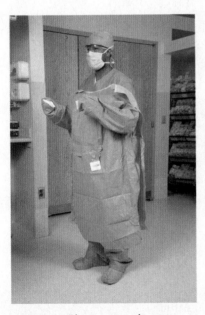

STEP 1g Place arms in sleeves.

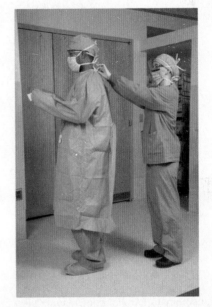

STEP 1h Circulating nurse ties scrub gown.

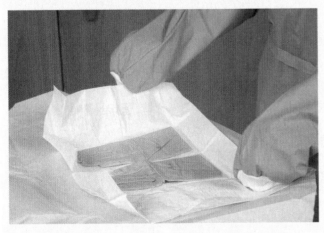

STEP 2a Scrub nurse opens glove package.

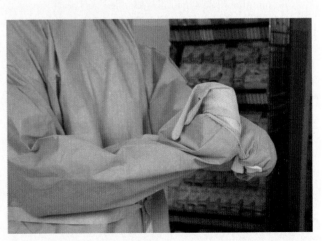

STEP 2d Glove applied as hands remain inside cuffs.

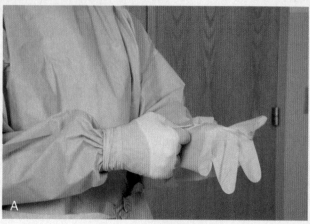 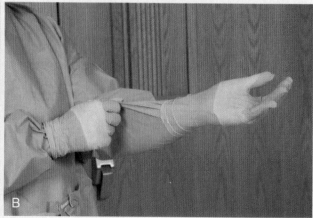

STEP 2f (A) Second glove applied. (B) Gloved fingers extended.

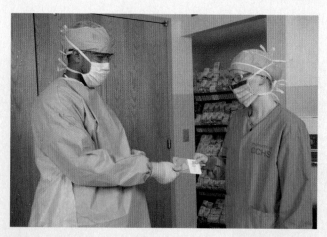

STEP 3b Paper tab on disposable gown is passed to circulating nurse.

e. Grasp top of glove and underlying gown sleeve with covered nondominant hand. Carefully extend fingers into glove, being sure that cuff of glove covers cuff of gown.	
f. Glove nondominant hand in same manner with gloved, dominant hand (Steps 2a-2e). Keep hand inside sleeve. Be sure that fingers are fully extended into both gloves (see illustrations).	Gloves remain sterile.
3. Donning wraparound gown:	
a. Grasp sterile front flap/paper tab with gloved hands and untie.	Front of gown is sterile.
b. Pass sterile paper tab to member of sterile surgical team or to nonsterile team member (e.g., circulating nurse) (see illustration). Keep gown tie in right hand. Circulating nurse stands still as scrub nurse/technician turns.	Nonsterile team member uses caution not to touch sterile tie when taking sterile paper tab while scrub nurse/technician turns.
c. Allowing margin of safety, turn to left one-half turn, covering back with extended gown flap. Retrieve sterile tie only from team member and secure both ties in place.	Maneuver covers entire body with gown. Nonsterile team member pulls off paper tab and discards.

STEP	RATIONALE

EVALUATION

1. Monitor patient after surgery for signs of surgical site infection (usually occurs 2 to 3 days after surgery).

Signs of infection include redness, heat, swelling, pain, and purulent drainage at operative site.

Unexpected Outcomes

1. Redness, heat, swelling, pain, or purulent drainage develops at surgical site, which often indicates wound infection.

Related Interventions

- Individualize interventions based on patient's situation (e.g., wound care, antibiotic therapy).

Documentation

- Documentation is not required for sterile gowning and gloving.
- Document area and description of surgical site after surgery to provide baseline for monitoring wound.

Hand-Off Reporting

- Report area and description of surgical site after surgery.

✦ CLINICAL JUDGMENT AND NEXT GENERATION NCLEX® EXAMINATION–STYLE QUESTIONS

The perioperative team is preparing to care for a 78-year-old patient who is scheduled for a total left knee replacement surgery.

1. Which information will the preoperative surgical nurse confirm with the patient during the preprocedure time?
1. Identity of patient
2. Procedure to be performed
3. Site that is to be operated on
4. Name of person who is driving the patient home in 48 hours
5. Previous reactions to any type of anesthesia

2. To perform surgical hand asepsis prior to the patient's surgery, which action will the nurse take first?
1. Inspect fingernails and cuticles.
2. Turn water on using foot or knee.
3. Wet hands thoroughly.
4. Dispense antimicrobial scrub agent.

3. In which circumstance will the nurse and other members of the perioperative team practice hand hygiene throughout intraoperative care? **Select all that apply.**
1. Before touching the patient
2. Before a procedure
3. After body fluid exposure
4. After touching the patient
5. After touching the environment

4. Complete the following sentence by selecting from the list of word choices below.

During the time-out right before surgery, the nurse and operative team will confirm **[Word Choice]** and the **[Word Choice]**.

Word Choices
Presence of advance directives in the health record
Patient identity
Unit the patient will be transferred to after PACU
Correct location of the surgery
Patient's next of kin
Insurance coverage for surgery

5. The circulating nurse is monitoring the sterile field to ensure sterile technique is maintained. Principles of sterile technique include: **Select all that apply.**
1. The back of a sterile gown is considered sterile from the neck to the level of the sterile field.
2. Unscrubbed team members always stay at least 15.2 cm (6 inches) away from the sterile field while keeping it in constant view.
3. Surgical gowns should be an adequate size to wrap around and completely cover the scrubbed team member's body.
4. Sterile-draped tables are sterile from table level to the floor.

Visit the Evolve site for Answers to Clinical Judgment and Next Generation NCLEX® Examination–Style Questions.

REFERENCES

American Society of PeriAnesthesia Nurses (ASPAN): *2023–2024 PeriAnesthesia nursing standards, practice recommendations and interpretive statements*, Cherry Hill, NJ, 2019, ASPAN.

Association of periOperative Registered Nurses (AORN): AORN Position Statement on RN First Assistants, *2022*. https://www.aorn.org/docs/default-source/guidelines-resources/position-statements/first-assisting/posstat-rnfa-0908.pdf?sfvrsn=7d9f3037_6. Accessed September 22. 2023.

Association of periOperative Registered Nurses (AORN): *Guidelines for perioperative practices*, Denver, 2023, AORN.

Association of Surgical Technologists (AST): *Guidelines for best practices for establishing the sterile field in the operating room*, 2019. https://www.ast.org/uploaded-Files/Main_Site/Content/About_Us/Guidelines%20Establishing%20the%20Sterile%20Field.pdf. Accessed September 22, 2023.

Duff J, et al: What does surgical conscience mean to perioperative nurses? An interpretive description, *Collegian* 29:147, 2022.

Farley M: Surgical conscience and its role in patient safety and care, *ORNAC J* 40:15, 2022.

Link T: Guideline implementation: sterile technique, *AORN J* 110(4):416, 2019.

Rothrock J: *Alexander's care of the patient in surgery*, ed 17, St. Louis, 2023, Elsevier.

The Joint Commission (TJC): *Office-based surgery: 2023 National patient safety goals*, 2023. https://www.jointcommission.org/standards/national-patient-safety-goals/office-based-surgery-national-patient-safety-goals/. Accessed August 21, 2023.

Vallejo RB, et al: Effectiveness of surgical hand antisepsis using chlorhexidine digluconate and parachlorometaxylenol hand scrub: Cross-over trial, *Medicine (Baltimore)* 97(42):e12831, 2018.

World Health Organization (WHO): *Surgical safety checklist*, 2009. https://www.who.int/teams/integrated-health-services/patient-safety/research/safe-surgery/tool-and-resources. Accessed March 13, 2023.

Care of the Surgical Patient: Next-Generation NCLEX® (NGN)– Style Unfolding Case Study

PHASE 1

QUESTION 1.

The nurse is performing a preoperative visit for a client who is scheduled to have surgery in 2 weeks for a knee replacement.

Highlight the findings that require follow-up by the nurse.

History and Physical	Nurses' Notes	Vital Signs	Laboratory Results

1030: 76-year-old client scheduled for knee replacement surgery in 2 weeks. Medical history includes type 2 diabetes mellitus, hypercholesterolemia, and hypertension. Medication history includes metformin 500 mg by mouth twice daily, lovastatin 20 mg by mouth every night, and amlodipine 5 mg by mouth at night. Has recently been on a prednisone oral dose pack when the client's jaw became very inflamed following a dental procedure. Family history positive for malignant hyperthermia. Vital signs: T 36.8°C (98.2°F); HR 74 beats/min; RR 16 breaths/min; BP 160/98 mm Hg; SpO$_2$ 98% on RA. Assessment reveals a well-nourished client. PERRLA, cranial nerves intact. Skin without lesions. Lungs clear to auscultation, heart regular rate and rhythm with no murmurs, and a soft, nontender abdomen. Alert and oriented × 4.

QUESTION 2.

The nurse must use the client's history to identify risks.

Complete the following sentence by selecting from the list of word choices below.

Based on the history, the nurse notes that the client is at high risk for developing **[Word Choice]**.

Word Choices
Malignant hyperthermia
Dehiscence
Evisceration
Hemorrhage

PHASE 2

QUESTION 3.

The nurse prioritizes client teaching points.

Complete the following sentence by selecting from the list of word choices below.

The nurse will provide *prioritized* teaching to the client about **[Word Choice]**.

Word Choices
Postoperative infection
Malignant hyperthermia
Activity restrictions
Preoperative laboratory testing

QUESTION 4.

After undergoing surgery, the client is transferred to the postsurgical unit from the postanesthesia care unit (PACU).

Which assessment will the nurse plan to perform? **Select all that apply.**

- Percuss liver.
- Auscultate lungs.
- Evaluate mental status.
- Palpate surgical knee.
- Observe cardiac monitor.
- Record output in urinary catheter bag.

PHASE 3

QUESTION 5.

Once the client awakens several hours later, he reports moderate pain. The family is at the bedside.

Which **3** actions will the nurse take at this time?

○ Ask the client to quantify the pain on a 0-to-10 scale.
○ Explain that pain medication must be reserved for severe pain.
○ Tell the spouse to push the patient-controlled anesthesia (PCA) button if the client is too tired to do so.
○ Prepare to administer the next dose of pain medication as ordered.
○ Provide teaching on how to use the PCA pump.
○ Teach that nonpharmacologic methods of pain control are preferable to opioids.

QUESTION 6.

The nurse has given pain medication as ordered. Thirty minutes later, the nurse checks on the client.

Highlight the assessment findings that indicate that pain was effectively managed.

History and Physical	Nurses' Notes	Vital Signs	Laboratory Results

1313: 76-year-old client returned 4 hours ago from right knee replacement surgery. Family at bedside. Vital signs: T 37.1°C (98.8°F); HR 72 beats/min; RR 18 breaths/min; BP 122/78 mm Hg. Client initially rated pain at 7 on 0-to-10 scale; now rates pain at 3. Skin flushed and red. Appears to be drifting off to sleep.

UNIT 14
Dressings and Wound Care

Implementing proper dressing and wound care is essential to patient comfort and safety. When patients have wounds from surgeries, trauma, or pressure injuries, the outermost layer of their skin is no longer intact, and that fact alone increases the patient's risks for further infection, tissue damage, and decreased mobility and dependence. It is important to use your clinical judgment to continually assess and evaluate your patient's skin integrity to determine if wound healing is occurring. Note the ongoing status of any wounds and the effectiveness of therapeutic measures, such as specific wound care therapies and irrigations, pressure injury prevention and care, and specialized dressings.

Excellent wound care requires application of the knowledge of wound healing and the nature of any condition causing the wound. Also consider a patient's risks for poor wound healing. Think critically about the specific assessment parameters you will use when observing your patient's wound. As you collect assessment data, identify cues and use clinical judgment to determine the specific wound care problem. For example, your postoperative patient shows signs of a wound infection and, as a result, the health care provider has opened the surgical incision, which now requires twice-a-day wound irrigations. You need to critically assess for changes in wound drainage and changes in the wound margin and review results of any wound cultures. Evaluate the patient's response to the wound irrigation and use clinical judgment to determine if the interventions are effective or if different therapies are needed.

Prevention of pressure injuries is one goal for safe patient care. Many patients are at risk for these injuries, which can begin as small, blistered areas on the skin that can rapidly progress. Frequent skin assessment of high-risk areas, such as the pressure points on skin underlying patients in bed or the skin under medical devices, is crucial. Use knowledge of your patient's current activity and mobility status, current and concurrent illnesses, and nutritional status when you perform physical assessment to identify skin and areas at risk. Your experience in caring for patients allows you to anticipate problems. For example, experience in caring for patients with feeding tubes prompts you to assess for early signs of a medical device–related pressure injury (MDRPI). As you collect the assessment data

and identify cues, use clinical judgment to plan and implement appropriate skin care and prevention interventions. Your initial assessments are a baseline to later clinically judge your patient's response to these interventions. Preventing pressure injuries from starting or progressing is a major nursing responsibility and starts immediately for all patients, especially those at high risk.

Dressings are applied to prevent some injuries to wounds, as well as being therapeutic in promoting wound healing. However, adhesives used to secure dressings pose risks to patients for medical adhesive–related skin injury (MARSI). Use clinical judgment when assessing your patient's skin around the wound (periwound) and the wound itself for early indications of tissue damage. Consider a patient's physical condition and care status to anticipate what to assess. For example, you have a male patient who is underweight and has limited mobility related to bilateral traction for leg fractures. Because of the immobility, you know to assess dependent areas of the skin and note that there is a reddened, intact, small blister on his sacrum. After consulting with a wound care specialist, you choose a transparent film dressing to protect the area while allowing for ongoing assessment of the wound status. In another example, you are caring for a patient with an open abdominal wound that requires irrigation followed by packing with fine mesh gauze. Because this wound needs frequent irrigation, wound packings, and dressing changes, you use Montgomery ties to secure the dressing and lessen the risk for MARSI for this patient. This choice of dressing promotes wound healing within the wound and reduces damage from medical adhesives to the periwound area.

In both examples, you will use clinical judgment to determine the effectiveness of the dressing with regard to wound healing. In the first example, you evaluate the response to the transparent dressing. Was it protective or did the wound progress? In the second example, you fully assess the wound bed and periwound area critically to analyze findings against wound healing criteria. Is the wound base showing signs of healing? Numerous factors affect the ongoing condition of any wound, including the patient's nutrition level, circulation, mobility, and hydration. Excellent wound care requires your vigilance and support of all factors that promote healing.

38 | Wound Care and Irrigation

SKILLS AND PROCEDURES

Procedural Guideline 38.1 **Performing a Wound Assessment, p. 1114**

Skill 38.1 **Performing a Wound Irrigation, p. 1117**

Skill 38.2 **Removing Sutures and Staples, p. 1122**

Skill 38.3 **Managing Wound Drainage Evacuation, p. 1128**

Skill 38.4 **Negative-Pressure Wound Therapy, p. 1133**

OBJECTIVES

Mastery of content in this chapter will enable you to:

- Discuss the response of the body during each stage of the wound-healing process.
- Compare and contrast the difference between primary, secondary, and tertiary intention wound healing.
- Explain factors that promote or impair normal wound healing.
- Explain the signs and symptoms of wound-healing complications.

- Apply clinical judgment and assess wounds correctly.
- Explain nursing interventions to take for impairment in wound healing.
- Demonstrate how to perform a wound irrigation.
- Demonstrate how to remove sutures or staples.
- Demonstrate care of a wound drainage system.
- Demonstrate care related to negative-pressure wound therapy (NPWT).

MEDIA RESOURCES

- http://evolve.elsevier.com/Perry/skills
- Review Questions
- ▶ Video Clips
- **NSO** Nursing Skills Online

- Answers to Clinical Judgment and Next-Generation NCLEX® Examination–Style Questions
- Skills Performance Checklists
- Printable Key Points

PURPOSE

Proper wound care is necessary to promote healing that restores an intact skin layer. Intact skin is the first line of defense of the body, a barrier protecting against invasion by infectious microorganisms. The skin defends the body in other ways by serving as a sensory organ for pain, touch, and temperature, and it has an acid pH, often called the *acid mantle*. It also plays a major role in thermoregulation, metabolism, immunity, and fluid balance regulation (Bryant & Nix 2024; Mufti et al., 2022). Use clinical judgment by applying scientific knowledge to correctly assess wound status and implement patient-centered nursing interventions.

PRACTICE STANDARDS

- European Pressure Ulcer Advisory Panel (EPUAP), National Pressure Injury Advisory Panel (NPIAP), and Pan Pacific Pressure Injury Alliance (PPPIA), 2019a: Treatment of Pressure Ulcers/Injuries: Clinical Practice Guideline. The International Guideline
- Wound, Ostomy, and Continence Nurses Society (WOCN), 2016: Guideline for Prevention and Management of Pressure Ulcers (Injuries)

SUPPLEMENTAL STANDARDS

- The Joint Commission (TJC), 2023: National Patient Safety Goals—Patient identification

PRINCIPLES FOR PRACTICE

- The skin is the largest external organ. It has two layers: the epidermis and the dermis (Fig. 38.1). The epidermis has five layers.
- Stratum corneum, the outermost layer, consists of flattened dead keratinized cells. Stratum corneum prevents dehydration of underlying cells and is a physical barrier to the entry of certain chemicals. This layer is like the shingles on a roof that provide protection from outside elements.
- The next layers of the epidermis are the stratum lucidum, stratum granulosum, and stratum spinosum.
- Stratum germinativum, the innermost layer, is sometimes called the *basal layer*. Important features of the stratum germinativum are the epidermal protrusions, or "peaks and valleys," that point downward into the dermis. These provide resiliency and integrity to the skin structure. Melanocytes, the cells that give the skin its color, are also in this layer.

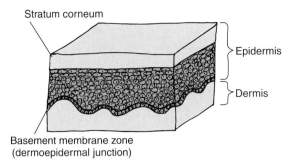

FIG. 38.1 Diagram of layers of skin and subcutaneous tissue.

- The area that separates the epidermis from the dermis is called the *dermoepidermal junction* or the *basement membrane zone*.
- Beneath the epidermis is the dermis. Collagen (a tough fibrous protein layer), blood vessels, and nerves compose the dermal layer. Collagen composes about 70% of the dermis and is extremely important in wound healing. The dermis restores the physical properties of the skin and its structural integrity. Restoration of both the epidermal and dermal layers is necessary to promote healing. Risk for local or systemic infection, impaired circulation, and breakdown of tissue directly impairs the wound-healing ability of the skin layers (Bohn & Bryant, 2024; Mufti et al., 2022).

- Wounds should be assessed on a scheduled basis to determine if they are moving toward healing. If the assessment reveals that the wound is not progressing as expected, the plan of care can be changed to facilitate wound healing (see Procedural Guideline 38.1).
- A thorough wound assessment includes identification of the type of wound healing (e.g., primary, secondary, or tertiary intention), type of tissue in the wound base, and condition of the wound; these parameters will be used to choose the proper wound intervention.
- A thorough head-to-toe skin assessment should be done on admission, daily, and if there is a change in the patient's condition (Bates-Jensen, 2022). All skin should be inspected closely, as a patient may not be aware of an issue with the skin because it is hidden under the clothes or on the back. The healing process proceeds in a series of events, generally described as *phases*. In a full-thickness wound, the phases are hemostasis, inflammation, proliferation, and remodeling (Box 38.1).
- During the proliferative stage, fibroblasts are at the site of injury. These fibroblasts increase synthesis of collagen, which forms the healing ridge that can be palpated under an intact healing incision by days 5 to 9 (Fig. 38.2) (Beitz, 2022).
- Wound healing occurs by primary, secondary, and tertiary intention (Fig. 38.3).
- Healing by primary intention occurs when the edges of a clean surgical incision remain close together. The wound heals

---

Phases of Wound Healing (Full-Thickness Wounds)

Hemostasis Phase
Blood vessels constrict; clotting factors activate coagulation pathways to stop bleeding. Clot formation seals the disrupted vessels so that blood loss is controlled and acts as a temporary bacterial barrier. Platelets release growth factors, which attract cells needed to begin the repair process.

Inflammatory Phase
Vasodilation occurs, allowing plasma and blood cells to leak into the wound, noted as edema, erythema, and exudate. Leukocytes (white blood cells) arrive in the wound to begin wound cleanup. Macrophages, a type of white blood cell, appear and begin to regulate the wound repair. The result of the inflammatory phase is a clean wound bed in a patient with a noncomplicated wound.

Proliferative Phase
Epithelialization (the construction of new epidermis) begins. At the same time, new granulation tissue is formed. New capillaries (angiogenesis) are created, restoring the delivery of oxygen and nutrients to the wound bed. Collagen is synthesized and begins to provide strength and structural integrity to the wound. Contraction, which occurs in open wounds, reduces the size of the wound.

Maturation (Remodeling) Phase
Collagen is remodeled to become stronger and provide tensile strength to the wound. Outer appearance in an uncomplicated wound will be that of a well-healed scar.

Wound Assessment: Anatomy of a Wound

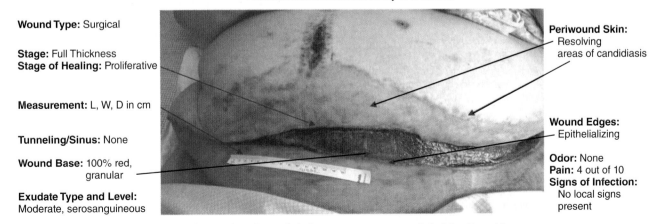

Wound Type: Surgical

Stage: Full Thickness
Stage of Healing: Proliferative

Measurement: L, W, D in cm

Tunneling/Sinus: None

Wound Base: 100% red, granular

Exudate Type and Level: Moderate, serosanguineous

Periwound Skin: Resolving areas of candidiasis

Wound Edges: Epithelializing

Odor: None
Pain: 4 out of 10
Signs of Infection: No local signs present

FIG. 38.2 Surgical wound with epithelialization occurring epithelial healing ridge apparent. (*Courtesy BS Rolstad.* Bryant RA, Nix DP, *editors:* Acute and chronic wounds: current management concepts, *ed 5, St Louis, 2016, Mosby.*)

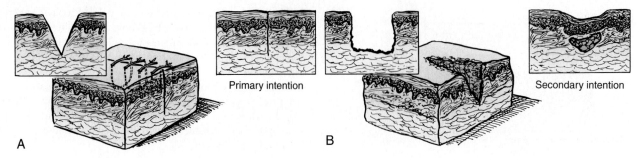

FIG. 38.3 Wound healing by primary intention such as with a surgical incision. (A) Wound edges are pulled together and approximated with sutures, staples, or adhesive tapes, and healing occurs by connective tissue deposition. (B) Wound healing by secondary intention. Wound edges are not approximated, and healing occurs by granulation tissue formation and contraction of the wound edges. (*From Bryant RA, Nix DP, editors:* Acute and chronic wounds: current management concepts, *ed 5, St Louis, 2016, Mosby.*)

quickly, and tissue loss is minimal or absent (Beitz, 2022). The skin cells regenerate quickly, and capillary walls stretch across under the suture line to form a smooth surface as they join.

- Wounds that are left open and allowed to heal by scar formation are classified as healing by secondary intention (Beitz, 2022). There is tissue loss and open wound edges. Granulation tissue gradually fills in the area of the defect (Fig. 38.4). This process is

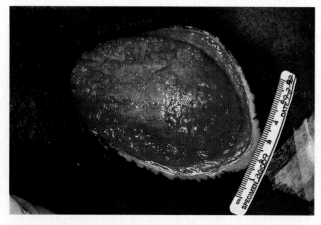

FIG. 38.4 Open wound with granulation tissue.

seen in a contaminated surgical wound such as a leak of a bowel anastomosis or massive surgical intervention with skin loss.

- In secondary intention there is a gap between the edges. Connective tissue develops, which supports new capillaries. This form of healing results in the formation of scar tissue to close the wound. The slowness of this process places a patient at greater risk for infection because there is no epidermal barrier until later in the healing process (Beitz, 2022).
- Healing by tertiary intention is sometimes called *delayed primary intention* or *closure*. It occurs when surgical wounds are not closed immediately but are left open for 3 to 5 days to allow edema or infection to diminish. Then the wound edges are sutured or stapled closed (Beitz, 2022).
- The percentage and type of tissue in the wound bed that is healing by secondary intention provide insight into the severity and duration of the wound, the extent to which it is progressing toward healing, and the effectiveness of current interventions (Nix, 2024). Viable tissue is normally red to pink in color and moist in appearance (Table 38.1). This type of tissue is called *granulation tissue* and indicates a wound moving toward healing. Black, brown, or tan tissue in the wound is slough or eschar and should be removed, or wound healing will be delayed.
- The location, severity, and extent of the injury and the tissue layer or layers involved all affect the wound-healing process

TABLE 38.1

Wound Color/Tissue

Color	Tissue Appearance
Black/brown wounds/eschar	Black or brown tissue is eschar, which represents full-thickness tissue destruction. Black is used to describe necrotic tissue or desiccated tissue such as tendon. It is also related to gangrenous lesions secondary to peripheral vascular disease.
	If the goal for a wound covered with eschar is debridement, sharp debridement is used to quickly remove the tissue, chemical debridement is used to soften the tissue for removal, or a moist dressing is also considered to loosen the tissue. The method of debridement depends on the overall goal for the patient.
Yellow wounds/ slough	Yellow tissue represents nonviable tissue and, in some cases, the presence of an infection. Slough tissue can be yellow; cream colored; or gray slough, which is usually accompanied by purulent drainage.
	For patients with a low infection risk, the use of moisture-retentive dressings enhances debridement of the yellow/slough tissue. Moisture-retentive dressings may include moist dressings, hydrocolloids, hydrogels, or alginates. If the wound is infected, antibiotics may be necessary.
Red wounds/ granulation	Red tissue represents the presence of granulation tissue. The red color is the result of an increasing amount of new blood vessels in the wound and is considered healthy.
	The goal in management of a red granulated wound is to select a dressing that maintains a clean and moist wound environment and minimizes damage to healing tissue.

Factors That Influence Wound Healing

- Hypovolemia, hypotension, vasoconstriction, edema, and hypoxia negatively affect wound healing because adequate perfusion and oxygenation are necessary for new vessel development, collagen synthesis, and development of tensile strength.
- An adequate nutritional status is critical for collagen synthesis, tensile strength, and immune function.
- Wound infection prolongs the inflammatory response, and the microorganisms use nutrients and oxygen needed for wound repair.
- A patient with diabetes mellitus or other peripheral vascular disease may have impaired wound healing because of abnormal and

prolonged inflammation, reduced collagen synthesis, impaired microcirculation, and impaired epithelial migration. Hyperglycemia is associated with compromised neutrophil function and impaired migration.
- Corticosteroid therapy or the use of other immunosuppressive agents such as chemotherapy increases the patient's susceptibility to infection.
- Advanced age can contribute to a diminished proliferation of cells critical to repair.

From Bohn G & Bryant RA: Wound healing physiology. In Bryant RA, Nix DP, editors: *Acute and chronic wounds: intraprofessionals from novice to expert*, ed 6, St Louis, 2024, Mosby.

(Bohn & Bryant, 2024). In addition, there are underlying factors that prevent the ability of cells and tissues to regenerate, return to normal structure, or resume normal functioning (Box 38.2).

- Partial-thickness wounds (loss of tissue limited to epidermis and possible partial loss of the dermis) heal by the process of regeneration.
- Full-thickness wounds (total loss of skin layers and some deeper tissues) heal by scar formation.

PERSON-CENTERED CARE

- Patient-centered care helps to improve a patient's wound care outcomes as it values the patient's perspectives, beliefs, and autonomy and considers the holistic needs of the patient When caring for patients from other cultures who have acute or chronic wounds, it is important to understand their cultural beliefs and practices and how these might impact wound care (Gethin et al., 2020). For example, in some cultures there is a belief that certain categories of people such as pregnant, lactating, or menstruating women should be prohibited from changing dressings (Koka et al., 2016).
- Using gender-congruent caregivers and having the family caregiver and a professional translator help with translation and care issues relieves some of the patient's and family caregiver's anxiety.
- In some cultures the meaning of blood and secretions is perceived as dirty; thus it would be advisable to promptly change stained bed linens and gowns.
- Be sure to recognize family caregivers when giving explanations about the nursing care regimen. In collectivist cultures the presence of family members at the bedside is customary. It is important to recognize that in some cultures, individuals may not be comfortable exposing body parts to a member of the opposite sex (Padela et al., 2019).
- Remind patients to tell health care providers about traditional home remedies and practices. In some cases these practices need to be avoided because they may increase the risk for delayed wound healing or infection in open wounds.

EVIDENCE-BASED PRACTICE

Wound Healing Process

Regardless of the etiology or extent of tissue loss, wounds heal by regeneration or scar formation. Regeneration is the preferred healing method, as the skin maintains its normal function and appearance (Beitz, 2022; Bryant & Nix, 2024). Wounds heal by

regeneration (cells replicate and move across the wound) if the wounds are confined to epidermal and superficial dermal layers. These wounds are classified as partial-thickness wounds. If wounds reach deeper dermal structures (e.g., hair follicles, sebaceous glands, sweat glands), subcutaneous tissue, muscle, tendons, ligaments, and bone, these structures are unable to regenerate and the wounds must heal by scar formation (Bryant & Nix, 2024). These wounds are classified as full-thickness wounds.

Newer research supports a moist wound environment. Moist wound healing is the practice of keeping a wound in an optimally moist environment (The Wound Source, 2016). Wound dressings can be used to establish and maintain a moist—not wet—wound environment and promote autolysis and epithelial migration (Bryant & Nix 2024). Examples of moist wound dressing that can be used are films, foams, hydrocolloids, hydrogels, and alginates (Nuutila & Eriksson, 2021). The benefits of providing a moist wound healing environment are increased cell migration and reepithelization, increased collagen synthesis, increased autolytic debridement, decreased necrosis, decreased pain, decreased inflammation, and decreased scarring (Nuutila & Eriksson, 2021).

- Nonviable tissue in a wound can delay wound healing and contribute to wound infection. Debridement of the wound or pressure injury of devitalized tissue—the removal of this tissue from the wound—is an essential objective of topical therapy and a critical component of optimal wound healing (EPUAP/NPIAP/PPPIA, 2019a, 2019b).
- Wound healing is also enhanced by various debridement techniques, including enzymatic, mechanical, and autolytic. The type of debridement chosen depends on the condition of the wound, the goal of wound treatment, and the patient's overall condition (EPUAP/NPIAP/PPPIA, 2019a).
- Enzymatic debridement is the topical application of enzymes such as collagenase over the necrotic tissue. Collagenase digests the necrotic tissue by dissolving the collagen in the dead tissue. When collagenase is used on a wound, the necrotic tissue is covered with the collagenase, and a moisture-retentive dressing can be used to soften the tissue (Manna et al., 2022; Bryant & Nix, 2024). Moisture is necessary to activate the collagenase enzyme (Manna et al., 2022).
- Antimicrobial-coated sutures have a significant benefit in reducing surgical site infection incidence in patients undergoing surgical procedures compared with noncoated sutures (Ahmed et al., 2019).
- Psychological distress impairs immune function and prolongs the inflammatory phase of healing, which results in impaired wound healing (Basu et al., 2022). Clinicians should consider psychological factors that may affect their patients when

treating the wounds, as these may increase the amount of time it takes to heal the wound. Other unhealthy behaviors that are linked to poor wound healing are decreased sleep, smoking, reduced exercise, and increased alcohol use (Gallagher & Barbe, 2022).

- Air fluidized therapy (AFT)/continuous low-pressure (CLP) pressure redistributing beds facilitate healing of advanced wounds in complex patients when part of a comprehensive wound care program (Arnold et al., 2020).

SAFETY GUIDELINES

- When changing wound dressings, follow proper aseptic technique. Keep a plastic bag within reach to discard dressing and prevent cross-contamination. Keep extra gloves within reach in case of contamination or additional wound assessment.
- Do not remove an initial surgical dressing for direct wound inspection until the health care provider writes an order for removal. Recommendation guidelines for surgical site infection prevention include leaving the sterile dressing that was applied in the operating room in place for 48 hours postoperatively (Brindle & Creehan, 2022).
- Provide analgesia 30 minutes before a dressing change when necessary.
- Healed skin from a prior injury is weaker than skin that has never had an injury and continues to be susceptible to tissue injury.
- Recognize the impact of aging on wound management. With aging, vascular changes occur, collagen tissue is less pliable, and scar tissue is tighter. Because the dermoepidermal junction becomes flatter in older adults, their skin may tear easily from mechanical trauma of tape removal (Thayer et al., 2022). Remove tape slowly using the push-pull technique and/or an adhesive remover or releaser (Hitchcock et al., 2021).
- Know a patient's nutritional status. Tissue repair and infection resistance are directly related to adequate nutrition, including proteins, carbohydrates, lipids, vitamins, and minerals.
- Understand the risks of obesity. Inadequate vascularization decreases delivery of nutrients and cellular elements required for

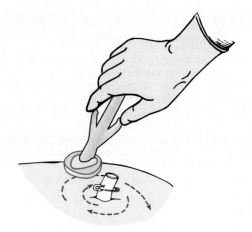

FIG. 38.5 Cleaning drain site.

healing. The patient is at greater risk for wound infection and dehiscence or evisceration (Bryant & Nix, 2024; Gallagher, 2022).

- When a drain is present, clean the drain site of infectious microorganisms using a circular stroke, starting with the area immediately next to the drain (Fig. 38.5). Using a new swab, clean immediately next to the drain and attempt to clean a little farther out from the drain.
- Identify factors that decrease oxygenation such as a decreased hemoglobin level, smoking, and underlying cardiopulmonary conditions. Adequate oxygenation at the tissue level is essential for new vessel development, promoting fibroblast proliferation, killing bacteria, collagen synthesis, and development of tensile strength (Bryant & Nix, 2024).
- Know the types of medications prescribed. Steroids reduce the inflammatory response and slow collagen synthesis. Cortisone depresses fibroblast activity and capillary growth. Chemotherapy depresses bone marrow production of white blood cells and impairs immune function.
- Identify the presence of chronic diseases or chronic trauma such as diabetes mellitus or radiation therapy. Decreased tissue perfusion and failure to release oxygen to tissues result from diabetes mellitus.

PROCEDURAL GUIDELINE 38.1 *Performing a Wound Assessment*

 Video Clip

An initial wound assessment provides the baseline for planning treatment options and the plan of care to promote the wound healing progress (Bates-Jensen, 2022). Normal wound healing occurs in an organized fashion, and repeated assessments of the wound status provides an ongoing evaluation of wound healing and helps to determine wound treatments. The frequency of wound assessment depends on the patient's overall condition, policy of the health care setting, type of dressings used, and overall patient goals. Acute care settings generally require wound assessment daily or with each dressing change. Long-term care facilities may require an initial admission wound assessment and weekly assessment for chronic wounds. Check agency policy for frequency of wound assessment and use of a specific wound assessment tool. Digital photography is a tool used for both assessment and documentation of wounds.

Wound assessment is necessary after every wound cleansing, and clinical judgment determines wound status (Bates-Jensen, 2022; Bryant & Nix, 2024). For example, is wound healing progressing as expected, or is it delayed? Is there new drainage (color and volume)? Wound size may increase in a wound with necrotic tissue. Removal of the necrotic tissue may result in a larger wound and is an expected finding. An increase in the amount and consistency of the drainage and new presence of odor may indicate a wound infection.

The following parameters are included in a wound assessment:
- *Location:* Note the anatomical position of the wound and periwound area.
- *Type of wound:* If possible, note the etiology of the wound (i.e., surgical, pressure, trauma).
- *Extent of tissue involvement:* Full-thickness wound involves both the dermis and epidermis. Partial-thickness wound

PROCEDURAL GUIDELINE 38.1 *Performing a Wound Assessment—cont'd*

involves only the epidermal layer. If the wound is a pressure injury, use the staging system of the European Pressure Ulcer Advisory Panel (EPUAP), National Pressure Injury Advisory Panel (NPIAP), and Pan Pacific Pressure Injury Alliance (PPPIA) (2019a) (see Chapter 39).

- *Type and percentage of tissue in wound base:* Describe the type of tissue (i.e., granulation, slough, eschar) and the approximate amount of each tissue present in wound bed.
- *Wound size:* Follow agency policy to measure wound dimensions, which include width, length, and depth. If a wound has undermining or tunneling, document that information as well.
- *Wound exudate:* Describe the amount, color, and consistency. Serous drainage is clear like plasma; sanguineous or bright red drainage indicates fresh bleeding; serosanguineous drainage is pink; and purulent drainage is thick and yellow, pale green, or white.
- *Presence of odor:* Note the presence or absence of odor, which may indicate infection.
- *Periwound area:* Assess the color, temperature, and integrity of the skin.
- *Pain:* Use a validated pain assessment scale to evaluate pain.

Delegation

The skill of wound assessment cannot be delegated to assistive personnel (AP). It is the nurse's responsibility to assess and document wound characteristics. Instruct the AP to:

- Report drainage from the wound that is present on sheets or as strikethrough from the dressing to the nurse for further assessment
- Report the presence of odor in the area of the wound
- Report any dressing that is no longer adherent

Interprofessional Collaboration

- Schedule the wound assessment by a wound care nurse specialist at a time when the nursing staff is present. This will reinforce correct wound healing assessment and reduce the number of times the patient will undergo a wound assessment in a single day.
- If the findings of the previous wound assessment were noted to be abnormal, include the primary medical or wound care surgical service to assess the wound together.

Equipment

Protective equipment: clean gloves, gown, and goggles if splash/spray risk exists; agency wound assessment tool to document assessment; measuring guide; cotton-tipped applicator; dressing supplies as ordered; disposable waterproof biohazard bag

Steps

1. Identify patient using at least two identifiers (e.g., name and birthday or name and medical record number) according to agency policy (TJC, 2023).
2. Examine the electronic health record (EHR) for findings from the last wound assessment to use as a comparison for this wound assessment. Review the record to determine the etiology of the wound.
3. Review EHR to determine patient's age and history of dehydration, malnutrition, exposure to radiation therapy, underlying chronic conditions (e.g., diabetes mellitus,

immunosuppression), and edema of the skin, which increase patient's risk for medical adhesive–related skin injury (MARSI) (Fumarola et al., 2020).

4. Determine agency-approved wound assessment tool and review the frequency of assessment. Examine the last wound assessment to use as comparison for this assessment.
5. Assess patient's/family caregiver's health literacy.
6. Assess patient's knowledge, prior experience with wound assessment, and feelings about procedure.
7. Assess character of patient's pain and rate acuity on a pain scale of 0 to 10. Offer pain medication 30 minutes before assessment as needed.
8. Perform hand hygiene. Close room door or bed curtains and position patient.
   a. Position comfortably to permit observation of wound in well-lit room.
   b. Expose only the area of the wound.
9. Explain procedure of wound assessment to patient.
10. Form a cuff on waterproof biohazard bag and place near bed.
11. Apply clean gloves and remove soiled dressings; remove gauze one layer at a time.
12. Examine dressings for quality of drainage (color, consistency), presence or absence of odor, and quantity of drainage (note if dressings were saturated, slightly moist, or had no drainage). Discard dressings in waterproof biohazard bag. Remove and discard gloves.
13. Perform hand hygiene and apply clean gloves.
14. Inspect wound and determine type of wound healing (e.g., primary or secondary intention).
15. Use agency-approved assessment tool and assess the following (Bates-Jensen, 2022):
    a. Wound healing by primary intention (surgical wound):
       (1) Assess anatomical location of wound on body.
       (2) Note if incisional wound margins are approximated or closed together. The wound edges should be together with no gaps.
       (3) Observe for presence of drainage. A closed incision should not have any drainage.
       (4) Look for evidence of infection (presence of erythema, odor, or wound drainage).
       (5) Lightly palpate along incision to feel a healing ridge (see Fig. 38.2). The ridge will appear as an accumulation of new tissue presenting as firmness beneath the skin, extending to about 1 cm ($\frac{1}{2}$ inch) on each side of the wound between 5 and 9 days after the incision was created. This is an expected positive sign (Bohn & Bryant, 2024).
    b. Wound healing by secondary intention (e.g., pressure injury or contaminated surgical or traumatic wound):
       (1) Assess anatomical location of wound.
       (2) Assess wound dimensions: Measure size of wound (including length, width, and depth) using a centimeter measuring guide. Measure length by placing the disposable measuring guide over wound at the point of greatest length (or head to foot). Measure width from side to side (Bates-Jensen, 2022) (see illustration).

Continued

PROCEDURAL GUIDELINE 38.1 *Performing a Wound Assessment—cont'd*

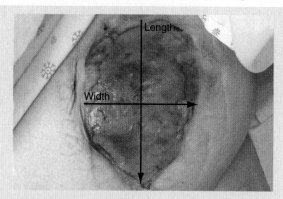

STEP 15b(2) Measuring wound length and width.

Measure depth by inserting cotton-tipped applicator in area of greatest depth and placing a mark on applicator at skin level; use measuring guide to determine depth. Discard measuring guide and cotton-tipped applicator in a biohazard bag.

(3) Assess for undermining: Use cotton-tipped applicator to gently probe wound edges. If undermining is present, measure depth and note location using the face of a clock as a guide. The 12 o'clock position (top of wound) would be the head of patient, and the 6-o'clock position would be the bottom of the wound toward patient's feet. Document the number of centimeters that area extends from wound edge underneath intact skin.

(4) Assess extent of tissue loss: If wound is a pressure injury, determine the deepest viable tissue layer in wound bed and determine stage. If necrotic tissue does not allow visualization of base of wound, the stage cannot be determined. If it is a pressure injury, use the staging system of the National Pressure Injury Advisory Panel (EPUAP/NPIAP/PPPIA, 2019b).

Clinical Judgment *If the wound is not a pressure injury, determine if there is partial-thickness loss (epidermis and part of the dermis) or full-thickness loss (loss of both the epidermis and the dermis).*

(5) Observe tissue type, including percentage of granulation, slough, and necrotic tissue.

(6) Note presence of exudate: amount, color, consistency, and odor. Indicate amount of exudate by using part of dressing saturated (completely or partially saturated or in terms of quantity—e.g., scant, moderate, or copious). Exposure to wound exudate places the periwound skin at risk for moisture-associated skin damage (MASD) such as erythema, dermatitis, maceration, or candidiasis (Earlam & Woods, 2022). Periwound maceration and prolonged contact with wound exudate can enlarge the wound and impede healing (Bryant & Nix, 2024).

(7) Determine if wound edges are rounded toward wound bed; this may be an indication of delayed wound healing. Describe presence of epithelialization at wound edges (if present) because this indicates movement toward healing.

Clinical Judgment *Compare the wound assessment to previous assessment and determine progress toward healing. If there is no movement toward healing or if you notice deterioration, consider a wound care consultation. Lack of wound healing is often related to infection. Notify health care provider and wound, ostomy, continence nurse (WOCN) or wound care team.*

16. Inspect the periwound skin, including color, texture, and temperature, and describe skin integrity (e.g., open macerated areas, blistering, excoriation). Periwound assessment provides clues about the effectiveness of wound treatment, possible wound extension, and any skin reactions to medical adhesive from the dressings (Hitchcock et al., 2021; Thayer et al., 2022).

17. Apply dressings per order. Place time, date, and initials on new dressing.

18. Reassess patient's pain and level of comfort, including pain at wound site, using a scale of 0 to 10 after dressing is applied.

19. Discard biohazard bag and soiled supplies per agency policy. Remove and dispose of gloves. Perform hand hygiene.

20. Help patient to a comfortable position.

21. Place nurse call system in an accessible location within patient's reach.

22. Raise side rails (as appropriate) and lower bed to lowest position, locking into position.

23. **Use Teach-Back:** "I want to be sure I explained clearly when it is important to frequently assess your wound. In your own words tell me why the nurses observe your wound." Revise your instruction now or develop a plan for revised patient/family caregiver teaching if patient/family caregiver is not able to teach back correctly.

24. Document wound assessment findings and compare assessment with previous wound assessments to monitor wound healing.

25. Provide hand-off report to health care provider regarding any serious complication such as new bleeding or signs of dehiscence.

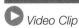

◆ SKILL 38.1   Performing a Wound Irrigation

▶ *Video Clip*

Irrigation is a common method of delivering a wound-cleansing solution to a wound. Wound irrigation cleans and debrides necrotic tissue with pressure that can remove debris from a wound bed without damaging healthy tissue (Ramundo, 2022). Typically, the irrigation of an open wound involves the use of clean technique with clean gloves.

Irrigation involves introducing a cleaning solution directly into the wound with a syringe, syringe and catheter, pulsed lavage device, or a handheld shower. A proper wound-cleaning solution is one that does not harm the tissue and uses an adequate force to agitate and wash away surface debris and devitalized tissue that contain bacteria (Table 38.2) (Jaszarowski & Murphree, 2022; Weir & Schultz, 2022).

Keep the tip of the syringe or catheter 2.5 cm (1 inch) above the wound. If a patient has a deep wound with a narrow opening, attach a soft catheter to the syringe to permit the fluid to enter the wound. Pulsed lavage delivers kinetic and mechanical energy and suction (a form of subatmospheric pressure). When pulsed lavage is used, normal saline may be delivered at between 4 and 15 psi (pressurized irrigation) through a mechanical apparatus (Bryant & Nix, 2024). Suction (subatmospheric pressure) may be used to aspirate wound debris and remove microorganisms. The use of mechanical energy through a pressurized spray also helps with the removal of wound debris. Ambulatory patients often benefit from the use of a handheld shower for wound cleaning, holding the shower spray approximately 30 cm (12 inches) from the wound. Another method to ensure an irrigation pressure within the correct range is to use a 19-gauge angiocatheter and a 35-mL syringe, which delivers saline to a wound bed between 4 and 15 psi (Fig. 38.6) (Bryant & Nix, 2024).

Delegation

The skill of wound irrigation cannot be delegated to assistive personnel (AP) unless it is an established chronic wound. It is the nurse's responsibility to assess and document wound characteristics. Instruct the AP to:
- Notify the nurse when the wound is exposed so that an assessment can be completed

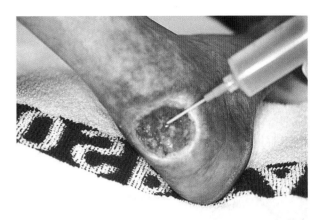

FIG. 38.6 Ensure irrigation pressure for cleaning wound.

- Report to the nurse patient's pain, presence of blood, and drainage

Interprofessional Collaboration

- Consider coordinating the wound irrigation with the primary health care provider if there are any questions about wound integrity. Coordination of the irrigation between disciplines helps in planning and organizing wound care interventions.
- Consult with a wound, ostomy, and continence nurse (WOCN) who can offer suggestions if there is a need for a change in dressing covering.

Equipment

- Personal protective equipment (PPE): clean gloves, sterile gloves, gown, face mask, and goggles if splash or spray risk exists (check agency policy)
- Irrigation/cleansing solution (type per order), volume 1.5 to 2 times the estimated wound volume
- Irrigation delivery system (per order), depending on amount of desired pressure: sterile irrigation 35-mL syringe with sterile soft

---

TABLE 38.2

Wound-Cleaning Considerations

	Mechanical Force	
	High Pressure	**Low Pressure**
Wound base characteristics	Presence of necrotic tissue (eschar, fibrin slough), debris, or other particulate matter Significant bacterial burden Moderate/large amount of exudate	Presence of granulation tissue or new epithelial cells No or minimum serous or serosanguineous exudate
Clinical outcome(s)	Loosen, soften, and remove devitalized tissue from wound Separate eschar from fibrotic tissue/fibrotic tissue from granulating base	Prevent trauma to viable wound tissue Remove wound care product residue
Solution	Normal saline Volume of solution depends on size of wound	Normal saline Volume of solution depends on size of wound
Delivery systems	35-mL syringe/19-gauge angiocatheter	Pouring saline directly from bottle Bulb syringe Piston syringe

TABLE 38.3

Common Wound Dressing Categories

Category	Description and Function	Indications	Side Effects	Contraindications
Hydrogel	Composed of water or glycerin-based polymers Provides moisture to wound bed Autolytic debridement	Partial- and full-thickness wounds Dry to light wound exudate Necrotic wounds	Potential for periwound maceration (MASD)	Contraindicated in third-degree burns
Alginate	Highly absorptive products that are retentive gel or fiber-gelling dressings	Partial or full thickness without depth or with depth (add fillers) Moderate to heavy exudate Not appropriate for dry wounds	May contribute to wound desiccation if wound exudate is minimal and gel dries	Contraindicated for narrow tunnels, third-degree burns, dry eschar, surgical implantation, or heavy bleeding
Foam	Absorption and protection Available in adhesive and no adhesive forms	Partial- or full-thickness without depth or with depth (add fillers) Absorption of moderate to heavy exudate Dressing should extend at least 1 inch larger than wound	May increase risk for wound dehydration	Contraindicated in ischemic wound with dry eschar and third-degree burns
Gauze	Available in woven or nonwoven, cotton or synthetic, sterile and nonsterile	Protection of surgical wounds Moist-to-dry dressings Wound-packing material	May adhere to healthy tissue and cause injury on removal	Traumatic wound debridement from dry gauze
Hydrocolloids	Adhesive dressings that contain a gel-forming agent, mold to body contours Autolytic debridement Maintain moist environment by forming a gelatinous mass	Partial- or full-thickness wound without depth Absorption of minimal to moderate exudate	Some products leave residue in wound on removal Potential for periwound maceration (MASD)	Contraindicated in third-degree burns Avoid acutely infected wound or eschar.

Data from Bryant, Nix DP: Principles of wound healing and topical management. In Bryant RA, Nix DP, editors: *Acute and chronic wounds: intraprofessionals from novice to expert*, ed 6, St Louis, 2024, Mosby.

angiocatheter or 19-gauge needle (Bryant & Nix, 2024; Jaszarowski & Murphree, 2022) or handheld shower
- Waterproof underpad if needed
- Dressing supplies (Table 38.3 and Table 40.1)
- Disposable waterproof biohazard bag
- Extra towels and padding (to protect bed)
- Wound assessment supplies (see Procedural Guideline 38.1)

STEP	RATIONALE

ASSESSMENT

1. Identify patient using at least two identifiers (e.g., name and birthday or name and medical record number) according to agency policy.

Ensures correct patient. Complies with The Joint Commission standards and improves patient safety (TJC, 2023).

2. Review patient's electronic health record (EHR), including health care provider's order and nurses' notes. Note previous status of wound and type of solution to be used.

Open-wound irrigation requires medical order, including type of solution(s) to use.

3. Review EHR for most current signs and symptoms related to patient's open wound.

   a. Extent of impairment of skin integrity, including size of wound

Provides ongoing data to indicate change in wound status (Bryant & Nix, 2024).

   b. Determine patient's age and history of dehydration, malnutrition, exposure to radiation therapy, underlying chronic conditions (e.g., diabetes mellitus, immunosuppression), and edema of the skin

Common risk factors for medical adhesive related skin injury (MARSI) (Fumarola et al., 2020). Erythema, blistering, and excoriation are signs of MARSI and are related to the skin's reaction to an adhesive (Hitchcock et al., 2021; Thayer et al., 2022).

   c. Number of drains present

Awareness of drain position facilitates safe dressing removal and determines need for special dressings.

   d. Drainage, including amount, color, consistency, and any odor noted

Ongoing data; drainage should decrease in healing wound. When drainage increases, it is often related to infection (Bohn & Bryant, 2024).

STEP	RATIONALE
e. Wound tissue color	Color represents balance between necrotic and new scar tissue. Proper selection of wound care products on basis of wound color facilitates removal of necrotic tissue and promotes new tissue growth (Bryant & Nix, 2024).
f. Culture reports	Culture reports identify type of bacteria and proper treatment.
4. Assess patient's/family caregiver's health literacy.	Determines degree to which individuals have the ability to find, understand, and use information and services to make informed health-related decisions and actions for themselves and others (CDC, 2023).
5. Assess character of patient's pain and rate acuity on a pain scale of 0 to 10.	Determines if comfort measures are effective. Provides baseline to determine tolerance to procedure and need to plan for analgesia prior to irrigation.
6. Assess patient for history of allergies to antiseptics, solutions, medications, tapes, latex, or dressing material. If allergy identified, apply allergy wrist band.	Known allergies suggest applying sample of prescribed wound treatment as skin test before flushing wound with large volume of solution or selecting different tape or dressing material. Latex allergies require the use of "latex-free" gloves and wound care products.
7. Assess if patient is taking an anticoagulant or has coagulopathy.	Caution must be used if patient has a bleeding tendency. Irrigation could cause bleeding.
8. Assess patient and family caregiver's understanding of need for irrigation and signs of wound infection.	Determines extent of instruction required.
9. Assess patient's knowledge, prior experience with wound irrigation, and feelings about procedure.	Reveals need for patient instruction and/or support.

PLANNING

1. Expected outcomes following completion of procedure:	
• Patient states acceptable level of comfort and rates a decreased severity of pain on a scale of 0 to 10 after wound irrigation.	Premedication, gently administered irrigation, application of clean dressing, and repositioning patient ensures comfort.
• Wound shows signs of healing; wound is free of excessive drainage, exudate, and inflammation.	Healing progresses in absence of debris.
• Skin integrity is maintained; no redness, edema, or inflammation noted in surrounding tissue.	No further skin and tissue damage has resulted from wound irrigation.
• Patient is able to describe signs of wound healing and infection.	Demonstrates learning.
2. Perform hand hygiene. Administer analgesic at least 30 minutes before starting wound irrigation procedure.	Promotes pain control and permits patient to move more easily and to be positioned to facilitate wound irrigation (Bryant & Nix, 2024; Oropallo & Quraishi, 2024).
3. Provide privacy and explain procedure to patient and family caregiver, instructing not to touch wound or sterile supplies.	Relieves anxiety and promotes understanding of healing process. Prevents contamination of sterile supplies.
4. Organize and set up any equipment needed and position patient properly to perform procedure.	Ensures more efficiency when completing the procedure.
a. Position comfortably to promote gravitational flow of irrigating solution over wound and into collection receptacle (see illustration).	Directing solution from top to bottom of wound and from clean to contaminated area prevents further infection.
b. Ensure that irrigant solution is at room temperature, and position patient so wound is vertical to collection basin.	Room temperature solution increases comfort and reduces vascular constriction response in tissues.
c. Place padding or extra towel on bed under area where irrigation will take place.	Protects bedding from becoming wet.

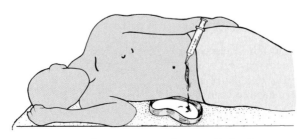

STEP 4a Patient position for wound irrigation.

STEP	RATIONALE

IMPLEMENTATION

1. Perform hand hygiene.

Reduces transmission of microorganisms.

2. Form cuff on waterproof biohazard bag and place near bed.

Cuffing helps to maintain large opening, thereby permitting placement of contaminated dressings without touching bag itself.

3. Apply PPE: gown, mask, and goggles as indicated; apply clean gloves and remove old dressing. Dispose of dressing in proper biohazard receptacle. Remove and discard gloves. Perform hand hygiene.

Reduces transmission of microorganisms. Protects nurse from splashes or sprays of blood and body fluids.

4. Apply clean or sterile gloves. Clean periwound either with normal saline or cleansing agent recommended by health care provider or wound care consultant. Remove and dispose of gloves. Perform hand hygiene.

While cleaning wound, use meticulous hand hygiene and proper infection control procedures before and after removing soiled dressings to limit risk for health care–acquired infection (Jaszarowski & Murphree, 2022).
Reduces transmission of microorganisms.

5. Apply clean or sterile gloves (check agency policy). Expose area near wound only, perform wound assessment, and examine recent documented assessment of patient's open wound (see Procedural Guideline 38.1).

Provides privacy and prevents chilling of patient. Provides ongoing wound-healing data. Use sterile precautions when sterile gloves are needed.

Clinical Judgment *Inspect periwound area for signs of MARSI and gently palpate wound edges for bogginess or patient report of increased pain.*

6. Irrigate wound:

The cleansing solution is introduced directly into the wound with a syringe, a syringe and catheter, or a pulsed lavage device.

  a. Fill 35-mL syringe with irrigation solution.

Irrigating wound uses mechanical force, which helps with separation and removal of necrotic debris and surface bacteria (Bryant & Nix, 2024; Jaszarowski & Murphree, 2022). Flushing wound helps remove debris and facilitates healing by secondary intention.

  b. Attach 19-gauge angiocatheter (see Fig. 38.6).

Catheter lumen delivers ideal pressure for cleaning and removing debris (Jaszarowski & Murphree, 2022; Ramundo, 2022). Mechanical debridement through use of 35-mL syringe with 19-gauge angiocatheter delivers irrigation pressures between 4 and 15 psi (Bryant & Nix, 2024).

Clinical Judgment *Pulsatile high-pressure lavage is an alternative to using the 35-mL syringe and the 19-gauge angiocatheter. A pulsatile lavage involves delivery of an irrigating solution under pressure with or without suction to loosen necrotic tissue and facilitate removal by other methods of debridement (Jaszarowski & Murphree, 2022; Ramundo, 2022).*

  c. Hold syringe tip 2.5 cm (1 inch) above upper end of wound and over area being cleaned.

Prevents syringe contamination. Careful placement of syringe prevents unsafe pressure of flowing solution.

  d. Using continuous pressure, flush wound; repeat until solution draining into basin is clear.

Flushing wound helps to remove debris; clear solution indicates removal of all debris.

7. Irrigate deep wound with very small opening:

  a. Attach soft catheter to filled irrigation syringe.

Catheter permits direct flow of irrigant into wound. Expect wound to take longer to empty when opening is small.

  b. Gently insert tip of catheter into opening about 1.3 cm (0.5 inch).

Prevents tip from touching fragile inner wall of wound.

Clinical Judgment *Do not force catheter into the wound because this will cause tissue damage.*

  c. Using slow, continuous pressure, flush wound.

Use of slow mechanical force of stream of solution loosens particulate matter on wound surface and promotes healing (Jaszarowski & Murphree, 2022).

Clinical Judgment *Pulsatile high-pressure lavage is often the irrigation of choice for necrotic wounds. Pressure settings should be set per provider order, usually between 4 and 15 psi, and should not be used on skin grafts, exposed blood vessels, muscle, tendon, or bone. Use with caution if patient has coagulation disorder or is taking anticoagulants (Jaszarowski & Murphree, 2022).*

  d. While keeping catheter in place, pinch it off just below syringe.

Avoids contamination of sterile solution.

  e. Remove and refill syringe. Reconnect to catheter and repeat irrigation until solution draining into basin is clear.

8. Clean wound with handheld shower:

STEP	RATIONALE

Clinical Judgment *When assisting patient into and out of shower, follow fall precautions (see Chapter 14).*

a. With patient seated comfortably in shower chair or standing if condition allows, adjust spray to gentle flow; make sure that water is warm.	Useful for patients able to shower with help or independently. May be accomplished at home.
b. Shower for 5 to 10 minutes with shower head 30 cm (12 inches) from wound.	Ensures that wound is cleaned thoroughly.
9. When indicated, obtain wound cultures (see Chapter 7) only after cleaning with nonbacteriostatic saline.	WOCN (2016) recommends using quantitative bacterial cultures (tissue biopsy or swab cultures). Most common methods for wound cultures are swab technique, aspirated wound fluid, or tissue biopsy (Hurlow & Kalan, 2024).

Clinical Judgment *Obtain an ordered wound culture, usually indicated by the presence of inflammation around the wound, purulent odor or drainage, new drainage, or a febrile patient.*

10. Dry wound edges with gauze; dry patient after shower.	Prevents maceration of surrounding tissue from excess moisture.
11. Remove and dispose of gloves. Perform hand hygiene. Apply clean or sterile gloves (see agency policy). Apply appropriate dressing and label with time, date, and your initials (see Chapter 40).	Reduces transmission of microorganisms. Maintains protective barrier and healing environment for wound.
12. Remove and dispose of gloves, mask, goggles, and gown.	Prevents transfer of microorganisms.
13. Dispose of equipment and soiled supplies. Perform hand hygiene.	Prevents transfer of microorganisms.
14. Help patient to a comfortable position.	Restores comfort and sense of well-being.
15. Raise side rails (as appropriate) and lower bed to lowest position, locking into position.	Ensures patient safety and prevents falls.
16. Place nurse call system in an accessible location within patient's reach.	Ensures patient can call for assistance if needed.

EVALUATION

1. Have patient describe pain and rate level of comfort on a scale of 0 to 10.	Patient's pain should not increase as result of wound irrigation.
2. Monitor type of tissue in wound bed.	Identifies wound-healing progress and determines type of wound cleaning and dressing needed.
3. Inspect dressing periodically (see agency policy).	Determines patient's response to wound irrigation and need to modify plan of care.
4. Inspect periwound skin integrity.	Determines if extension of wound has occurred or signs of infection are present (warm red periwound skin).
5. Observe for presence of retained irrigant.	Retained irrigant is medium for bacterial growth and subsequent infection.
6. **Use Teach-Back:** "I want to be sure that I explained why your wound was irrigated today. Tell me why it is important to irrigate your wound." Revise your instruction now or develop plan for revised patient/family caregiver teaching if patient/family caregiver is not able to teach back correctly.	Teach-back is a technique for health care providers to ensure that they have explained medical information clearly so that patients and their families understand what is communicated to them (AHRQ, 2023).

Unexpected Outcomes

Related Interventions

1. Bleeding or serosanguineous drainage appears. **NOTE:** Some bleeding may occur as necrotic tissue is removed and exposes new granulation tissue.	• Flush wound during next irrigation using less pressure. • Apply pressure with sterile gauze to wound to stop bleeding. • Notify health care provider of bleeding.
2. Increased pain or discomfort occurs.	• Decrease force of pressure during wound irrigation. • Assess patient for need for additional analgesia before wound care.
3. Suture line opening extends.	• Notify health care provider. • Reevaluate amount of pressure to use for next wound irrigation.

Documentation

- Document wound assessment before and after irrigation; appearance of wound before and after irrigation; amount, color, and odor of drainage on dressing removed; amount and type of solution used; irrigation device; patient's tolerance of the procedure; and type of dressing applied after irrigation.
- Document patient's and family caregiver's understanding through teach-back for reasons for wound irrigations.

Hand-Off Reporting

- Immediately report to the health care provider any evidence of fresh bleeding, sharp increase in pain, retention of irrigant, or signs of shock.

Special Considerations

Patient Education

- Instruct patient and family caregiver regarding wound care technique, observe them doing a return demonstration, and provide written instructions.
- Explain the need for specialized supplies such as irrigating solutions and dressings and the need to maintain asepsis when performing care.
- Teach patient and family caregiver signs of healing wound, improper wound healing, and wound infection.

Pediatrics

- Some pediatric patients are frightened. They might verbally and physically try to prevent you from cleaning the wound. Having the child take an active part in the procedure or working out feelings about wound irrigation with play therapy on a doll with a wound helps the child to be more cooperative (Hockenberry et al., 2024).

- The skin of premature and neonatal infants is easily damaged from pressure and wound care products. Check that products are approved for use with this population (Lund & Singh, 2022). Remember that in neonates, the skin readily absorbs products (Hockenberry et al., 2024).

Populations With Disabilities

- Be aware of patient's cognitive level of understanding when performing wound irrigation. If agitation worsens, stop procedure for a few moments and calmly explain steps to the patient (Mendes, 2018).

Home Care

- Assess patient's home environment to determine adequacy of resources for performing wound care; check especially for adequate lighting, running water, and storage of supplies.
- Solutions to use for irrigation in the home include potable tap water, distilled water, cooled boiled water, and normal saline (WOCN, 2016). Teach patient and family caregiver how to make normal saline by using 8 teaspoons of salt in 1 gallon of distilled water; can keep refrigerated for 1 month. The saline solution should be allowed to reach room temperature before use.
- Instruct the family caregiver on irrigation technique, and have the caregiver demonstrate.
- Be sure the patient and family caregiver know signs of infection and when to notify the health care provider.
- Provide support for patient and caregiver during the wound-healing process. Chronic wounds do not heal properly and do not close in a timely manner (Bohn & Bryant, 2024).

◆ SKILL 38.2 Removing Sutures and Staples

Sutures are threads of metal or other materials used to sew body tissues together. They come in different sizes and are absorbent or nonabsorbent. Most commonly, sutures are used to close surgical wounds, but they are also used to close clean cuts. Sutures are placed within tissue layers in deep wounds and superficially as the final means for wound closure. The choice of suture technique depends on the type of wound, depth, degree of tension, and desired cosmetic outcome (Fig. 38.7) (Azmat & Council, 2023). A patient's history of wound healing, site of wound, tissues involved, and the purpose of the sutures determine the suture material selected. For example, a patient with repeated abdominal surgeries might

require wire sutures for greater strength to promote wound closure. Sutures are available in a variety of materials, including silk, steel, cotton, linen, wire, nylon, and Dacron. Sutures of materials such as polydioxanone (PDS), Vicryl, and Monocryl can be absorbed. Those made of nylon, silk, and steel, are nonabsorbable and must be removed. Removal requires the use of sterile scissors.

Staples are stainless steel wires, are quick to use, and provide strength. The location of the incision sometimes restricts their use because there must be adequate distance between the skin and structures that lie below the skin, including bone and vascular structures. They are used for skin closure of abdominal incisions and orthopedic surgery when appearance of the incision is not critical. Removal requires a sterile staple extractor and aseptic technique.

There is an increase in the use of surgical glue (cyanoacrylate glue) to close certain wounds. This glue is a liquid tissue adhesive that forms a strong waterproof barrier across approximated wound edges, allowing normal healing to occur below. Its transparency makes the wound easier to inspect and reduces time associated with dressing changes. There is some clinical evidence that surgical glue has antimicrobial properties against gram-positive bacteria, which are common SSI pathogens (Machin et al., 2019). It can be used to replace small sutures for incisional repair. The wound edges are held (approximated) together until the solution dries, providing an adhesive closure.

Agency policy determines whether *only* a health care provider *or* nurse may remove sutures and staples. The health care provider

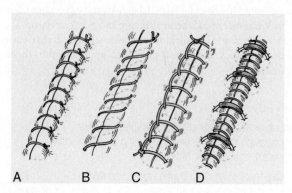

FIG. 38.7 Types of sutures. (A) Intermittent. (B and C) Continuous. (D) Blanket.

must determine and order removal of all sutures or staples at one time or removal of every other suture or staple as the first phase, with the remainder removed in the second phase.

Sutures should be removed within 2 weeks of their placement, depending on anatomic location (Oropallo, 2024). Staples generally are removed within 7 to 14 days after surgery if healing is adequate (deLemos, 2023). Retention sutures usually remain in place 14 to 21 days. Timing the removal of sutures and staples is important. They must remain in place long enough to ensure initial wound closure with enough strength to support internal tissues and organs. Sutures left in too long lead to suture marks, local tissue reaction, and scaring (Oropallo, 2024). The inflammatory process may cause the skin around staples to appear slightly red and edematous.

If there is any sign of suture line separation during the removal process, the remaining sutures or staples are left in place, and a description is documented and reported to the health care provider. In some cases these are removed several days to 1 week later. After removing sutures or staples, apply Steri-Strips over the incision to provide support. Steri-Strips are not removed and are allowed to fall off gradually.

Delegation

The skill of staple and/or suture removal cannot be delegated to assistive personnel (AP). Instruct the AP to:
- Report to the nurse drainage, bleeding, swelling at the incision site, or an elevation in patient's temperature
- Report to the nurse patient's complaints of pain
- Provide special hygiene practices following suture removal

Equipment
- Disposable waterproof biohazard bag
- Sterile suture removal set (forceps and scissors) or sterile staple extractor
- Sterile antiseptic swabs
- Gauze pads
- Steri-Strips or butterfly adhesive strips
- Clean gloves (sterile gloves optional)

STEP	RATIONALE
ASSESSMENT	
1. Identify patient using at least two identifiers (e.g., name and birthday or name and medical record number) according to agency policy.	Ensures correct patient. Complies with The Joint Commission standards and improves patient safety (TJC, 2023).
2. Review patient's electronic health record (EHR), including health care provider's order and nurses' notes for the following information:	Health care provider's order is required for removal of sutures.
a. Review specific directions related to suture or staple removal.	Indicates specifically which sutures are to be removed (e.g., every other suture).
b. Determine history of conditions that may pose risk for impaired wound healing: advanced age, cardiovascular disease, dehydration, diabetes, edema, immunosuppression, radiation, obesity, smoking, poor nutrition, and infection.	Preexisting health disorders affect speed of healing and sometimes result in dehiscence if sutures are removed too early. These are also common risk factors for medical adhesive–related skin injury (MARSI) (Fumarola et al., 2020).
3. Assess patient's/family caregiver's health literacy.	Determines degree to which individuals have the ability to find, understand, and use information and services to make informed health-related decisions and actions for themselves and others (CDC, 2023).
4. Assess patient for history of allergies. If allergy is identified, apply an allergy wrist band.	Determines if patient is sensitive to antiseptic or tape because Steri-Strips will be used.
5. Assess character of patient's pain and rate acuity on a pain scale of 0 to 10.	Provides baseline of patient's comfort level to determine response to therapy. Determines if comfort measures are effective.
6. Defer direct assessment of wound and periwound skin to implementation, just before suture removal.	Provides for more efficient procedure. Limits wound exposure when dressing is in place.
7. Assess patient's knowledge, prior experience with suture removal, and feelings about procedure.	Reveals need for patient instruction and/or support.
PLANNING	
1. Expected outcomes following completion of procedure:	
• All suture material or staples are removed.	Removes source of infection or irritation from retained sutures.
• Suture line is intact.	Wound is healing and does not require protective dressings.
• Patient states acceptable level of comfort and rates severity on a scale of 0 to 10 following removal of sutures or staples.	Analgesic effective in relieving pain.
• Patient or family caregiver is able to describe wound care following suture removal.	Demonstrates learning.
2. Provide privacy, and explain to patient how you will remove staples or sutures and that removal is usually not a painful procedure, but patient may feel pulling or tugging of skin.	Protects patient's privacy; reduces anxiety. Promotes cooperation.

STEP	RATIONALE
3. Administer prescribed analgesic, if needed, at least 30 minutes before procedure.	Promotes patient comfort to help minimize movement during suture removal.
4. Organize and set up any equipment and supplies needed to perform procedure.	Ensures more efficiency when completing the procedure.

IMPLEMENTATION

1. Perform hand hygiene and position patient comfortably while exposing suture line. Ensure that direct lighting is on suture line.	Reduces transmission of microorganisms. Aids visibility and correct placement of forceps or extractor during removal process, ultimately reducing soft tissue injury.
2. Place cuffed waterproof disposal bag within easy reach.	Provides for easy disposal of contaminated sutures and dressings (if present) and prevents passing items over sterile work area.
3. Open sterile packages of equipment needed for suture/staple removal:	Ensures an organized procedure.
a. Open sterile suture removal kit or staple extractor kit.	
b. Open sterile antiseptic swabs and place on inside surface of kit.	Avoids contamination of the antiseptic swabs.
c. Obtain gloves (sterile gloves if policy indicates).	
4. Perform hand hygiene. Apply clean gloves. Remove any gauze dressing covering wound. Dispose of soiled dressing in proper receptacle. Inspect incision for healing ridge and skin integrity of suture line for uniform closure of wound edges, normal color, and absence of drainage and inflammation (see illustration). Palpate around suture line gently, look for expression of drainage, and note any tenderness. Remove and dispose of gloves. Perform hand hygiene.	Indicates adequate wound healing for support of internal structures without continued need for sutures or staples (Oropallo, 2024). Reduces transmission of infection.

Clinical Judgment *If wound edges are separated or signs of infection are present, the wound has not healed properly. Notify the health care provider because sutures or staples may need to remain in place and/or other wound care may need to be initiated.*

5. Apply clean or sterile gloves as required by agency policy.	Reduces transmission of infection.
6. Clean sutures or staples and healed incision with antiseptic swabs. Start at sides next to incision and then wipe across suture line using new antiseptic swab for each swipe.	Removes surface bacteria from incision and sutures or staples.
7. **Remove staples:**	
a. Place lower tips of staple extractor under first staple. As you close handles, upper tip of extractor depresses center of staple, causing both ends of staple to be bent upward and simultaneously exit their insertion sites in dermal layer (see illustration).	Avoids excess pressure on suture line and secures smooth removal of each staple.
b. Carefully control staple extractor.	Avoids pressure on suture line and patient discomfort.
c. As soon as both ends of staple are visible, lift up and move it away from skin surface (see illustration) and continue until staple is over refuse bag. In some health care facilities, contaminated staples may be disposed of in a sharps container.	Prevents scratching tender skin surface with sharp pointed ends of staple for comfort and infection control.

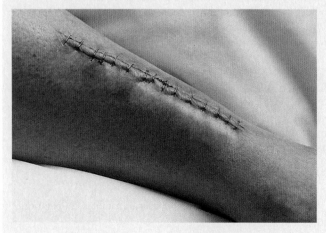

STEP 4 Suture line secured with staples.

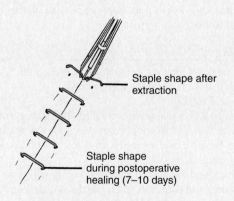

Staple shape after extraction

Staple shape during postoperative healing (7–10 days)

STEP 7a Staple extractor placed under staple.

STEP	RATIONALE
d. Release handles of staple extractor, allowing staple to drop into refuse bag.	Avoids contaminating sterile field with used staples.
e. Repeat Steps 7a through 7d until all staples have been removed.	
8. Remove interrupted sutures:	
a. Place gauze few inches from suture line. Hold scissors in dominant hand and forceps (clamp) in nondominant hand.	Gauze serves as receptacle for removed sutures. Placement of scissors and forceps allows for efficient suture removal.

Clinical Judgment *Placement of scissors and forceps is important. Avoid pinching the skin around the wound when lifting up the suture. Likewise, avoid cutting the skin around the wound by accident when snipping the suture.*

b. Grasp knot of suture with forceps and gently pull up knot while slipping tip of scissors under knot of suture near skin (see illustration).	Releases suture.
c. Snip suture as close to skin as possible at end distal to knot.	

Clinical Judgment *Never snip both ends of suture; there will be no way to remove the part of the suture situated below the surface.*

d. Grasp knotted end with forceps and, in one continuous smooth action, pull suture through from the other side (see illustration). Place removed suture on gauze.	Smoothly removes suture without additional tension on suture line.

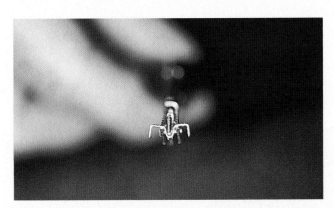

STEP 7c Metal staple removed by extractor.

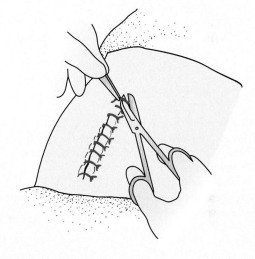

STEP 8b Removal of intermittent suture. Cut suture as close to skin as possible, away from knot.

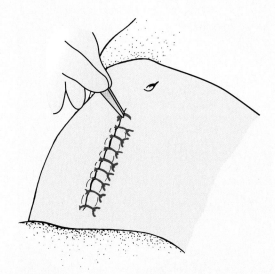

STEP 8d Remove suture and never pull contaminated stitch through tissues.

STEP	RATIONALE

Clinical Judgment *Never pull exposed surface of any suture into tissue below epidermis. The exposed surface of any suture is considered contaminated.*

    e. Repeat Steps 8a through 8d until you have removed every other suture.

    f. Observe healing level. On the basis of the observations of wound response to suture removal and the health care provider's original order, determine whether remaining sutures will be removed at this time. If so, repeat Steps 8a to 8d until you have removed all sutures. | Determines status of wound healing and if suture line will remain closed after all sutures have been removed.

    g. If any doubt, stop and notify health care provider.

  9. **Remove continuous and blanket stitch sutures:**

    a. Place sterile gauze a few inches from suture line. Grasp scissors in dominant hand and forceps in nondominant hand. | Gauze serves as receptacle for removed sutures. Placement of scissors and forceps allows for efficient suture removal.

    b. Snip first suture close to skin surface at end distal to knot. | Releases suture.

    c. Snip second suture on same side. | Releases interrupted sutures from knot.

    d. Grasp knotted end and gently pull with continuous smooth action, removing suture from beneath skin. Place suture on gauze. | Smoothly removes sutures without additional tension to suture line. Prevents pulling of contaminated part of suture through skin.

    e. Repeat Steps 9a to 9d in consecutive order until entire line is removed.

 10. Inspect incision to make sure that all sutures have been removed and identify any trouble areas. Gently wipe suture line with antiseptic swab to remove debris and clean incision. | Reduces risk for further incision line separation.

 11. To maintain contact between wound edges, apply Steri-Strips if *any* separation greater than two stitches or two staples in width is apparent. | Steri-Strips support wound by distributing tension across wound and eliminate scarring from closure techniques.

    a. Cut Steri-Strips to allow them to extend 4 to 5 cm (1½ to 2 inches) on each side of incision.

    b. Remove from backing and apply across incision (see illustration).

    c. Instruct patient to take showers rather than soak in bathtub according to health care provider's preference. | Steri-Strips are not removed; strips loosen over time (5–7 days) and are allowed to fall off gradually.

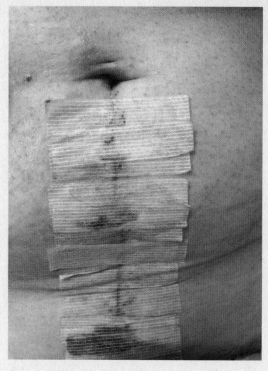

STEP 11b Steri-Strips over incision.

STEP	RATIONALE
12. Remove and discard gloves. Perform hand hygiene and apply new pair of gloves. Apply light dressing or expose to air if no clothing will come in contact with suture line. Instruct patient about applying own dressing if needed at home.	Reduces transmission of microorganisms. Healing by primary intention eliminates need for dressing.
13. Dispose of sharps (disposable staple extractor and/or scissors) in designated sharps disposal bin.	Prevents exposure to bloodborne organisms. Instruments are sharp and contaminated.
14. Remove and dispose of supplies; remove and dispose of gloves.	Reduces transmission of microorganisms.
15. Help patient to a comfortable position.	Restores comfort and a sense of well-being.
16. Raise side rails (as appropriate) and lower bed to lowest position, locking into position.	Ensures patient safety and prevents falls.
17. Place nurse call system in an accessible location within patient's reach.	Ensures patient can call for assistance as needed.
18. Perform hand hygiene.	Reduces transmission of microorganisms.

EVALUATION

1. Examine site where sutures or staples were removed; inspect condition of soft tissues, including skin. Look for any pieces of removed suture left behind.	Ensures that sources of infection have been removed.
2. Determine if patient has pain along incision and rate severity using pain rating scale.	Determines comfort level and can indicate if suture material remains in skin.
3. **Use Teach-Back:** "I want to be sure that I have adequately explained the signs of a wound or incision infection before you are discharged. Tell me the signs of infection and what you need to tell your health care provider if this happens." Revise your instruction now or develop a plan for revised patient/family caregiver teaching if patient/family caregiver is not able to teach back correctly.	Teach-back is a technique for health care providers to ensure that they have explained medical information clearly so that patients and their families understand what is communicated to them (AHRQ, 2023).

Unexpected Outcomes	Related Interventions
1. Retained suture is present.	• Notify health care provider. • Instruct patient to notify health care provider if signs of suture line infection develop following discharge from agency.
2. Patient experiences wound separation or drainage secondary to healing problems.	• Leave remaining sutures or staples in place. • Place Steri-Strip closures across suture line. • Notify health care provider.

Documentation

- Document the time the sutures or staples were removed and the number of sutures or staples removed; document the cleaning of the suture line, appearance of the wound, level of healing of the wound, and type of dressing applied; document patient's response to suture or staple removal.
- Document patient's and family caregiver's level of understanding following instruction.

Hand-Off Reporting

- Immediately report to the health care provider if suture line separation, dehiscence, evisceration, bleeding, or purulent drainage occurs.
- During hand-off, report the removal of the staples or sutures, integrity of the incision, use of a dressing (if indicated), and patient's response to removal of the staples or sutures.

Special Considerations

Patient Education

- Teach patient to observe for any sign of separation of wound edges before removing remaining sutures or staples and inspect incision for continued healing.

- Reinforce instruction about resuming bathing and showering activities, preventing abdominal strain during defecation, and providing adequate nutrition and ambulation.
- Teach patient not to put additional stress on suture line from such activities as lifting or bending. Patients with abdominal surgery or injury need to avoid lifting heavy packages or equipment for several weeks.
- Instruct patient that sometimes there is a small amount of drainage from wound immediately after suture removal.
- Skin glue is a clear gel or paste applied to the edges of clean small wounds to hold the edges of the wound together. Skin glue is not used over joints, the hand, or the groin area. It takes only a few minutes for the glue to set, and it usually peels off in 5 to 10 days (National Health Service [NHS], 2021). Patients will go home with the skin glue in place. Instruct patient to avoid touching the glue for 24 hours.
- Instruct patient to try to keep the wound dry for the first 5 days. Showers are preferable to baths to avoid soaking the wound; use a shower cap if the wound is on the head, and pat the wound dry if it gets wet. Do not rub the wound (NHS, 2021).

Pediatrics

- Help is sometimes necessary to keep infants from moving during the suture removal procedure.
- Virtual reality games and techniques are nonpharmacological and user-friendly interventions to reduce anxiety and pain during suture removal in school-aged children (LeMay et al., 2021).
- Topical anesthetic solutions (e.g., lidocaine, EMLA [eutectic mixture of local anesthetics]) applied to intact skin may provide

short-term (20 minutes) anesthesia (Hockenberry et al., 2024; Oropallo & Quraishi, 2024).

Older Adults

- Some older adults need reassurance about suture or staple removal procedure. Depending on their mental status, they may not understand the procedure.
- Wound healing is prolonged in older adults, and the risk for dehiscence after suture or staple removal increases (Richbourg, 2022).

✦ SKILL 38.3 Managing Wound Drainage Evacuation

When drainage accumulates in a wound bed, wound healing is delayed. Drains provide a means for fluid or blood that accumulates within a wound bed to drain out of the body. Drainage is facilitated when the surgeon inserts either a closed- or an open-drain system, even if the amount of drainage is small. The drain is inserted directly through a small stab wound near the suture line into the area of the wound.

An open-drain system (e.g., a Penrose drain, Fig. 38.8) removes drainage passively from the wound and deposits it onto the skin surface. A sterile safety pin is inserted through this drain, outside the skin, to prevent the tubing from moving into the wound. As the drainage decreases, the Penrose drain is gradually advanced to the surface of the wound and eventually removed. A split gauze dressing collects any drainage and helps to protect the patient's skin.

A closed-drain system such as the Jackson-Pratt (JP) drain (Fig. 38.9) or Hemovac drain is a convenient portable unit that connects to tubular drains lying within a wound bed and exerts a safe, constant low-pressure vacuum to remove and collect drainage. This provides active drainage. A JP drain collects fluid at a rate in the range of 100 to 200 mL/24 h. A Hemovac or ConstaVac drainage system is used for larger amounts of drainage (500 mL/24 h). The collection device is connected to a clear plastic drain with multiple perforations. Drainage collects in a closed reservoir or a suction bladder. When the drainage device is half full, empty the chamber and measure the drainage. After measurement, reestablish the vacuum and ensure that all drainage tubes are patent.

Delegation

The assessment of wound drainage and maintenance of drains and drainage systems cannot be delegated to AP. However, you may delegate to the AP emptying a closed drainage container or pouch, measuring the amount of drainage, and documenting the amount on the patient's intake and output (I&O) record. Instruct the AP by:

- Discussing any increase in frequency of emptying the drain other than once a shift

- Instructing to report to the nurse any a change in amount, color, or odor of drainage
- Reviewing the I&O procedure

Interprofessional Collaboration

- Contact wound care team if you note a change in the volume and/or consistency of the drainage, a presence of a strong odor in the drainage, and a change in wound-healing status.

Equipment

- Graduated measuring cylinder or specimen container
- Antiseptic wipes
- Gauze sponges, including split gauze sponges for drain site
- Sterile gauze dressings as needed
- Clean gloves
- Safety pin(s)
- Protective equipment: goggles, mask, and gown if risk of spray from drain is present
- Disposable drape or barrier
- *Optional:* Normal saline for cleaning insertion site

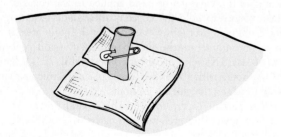

FIG. 38.8 Penrose drain with drain-split gauze.

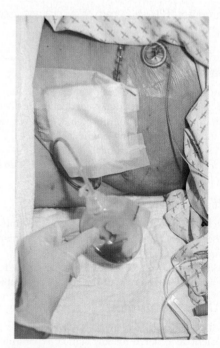

FIG. 38.9 Jackson-Pratt wound drainage system.

STEP	RATIONALE

ASSESSMENT

1. Identify patient using at least two identifiers (e.g., name and birthday or name and medical record number) according to agency policy.
2. Review patient's electronic health record (EHR), including health care provider's order and nurses' notes. Note presence, location, and purpose of closed wound drain and drainage system as patient returns from surgery.
3. Review EHR to determine patient's age and history of dehydration, malnutrition, exposure to radiation therapy, underlying chronic conditions (e.g., diabetes mellitus, immunosuppression), edema of the skin, and presence of erythema, blistering, or excoriation of skin under or adjacent to adhesive's securing dressing.
4. Assess patient's/family caregiver's health literacy.

5. Perform hand hygiene. Apply clean gloves. Assess drainage present on patient's dressing. Identify number of wound drain tubes and what each one is draining. Label each drain tube with a number or label.
6. Inspect drainage system to determine presence of one straight tube or Y-tube arrangement with two tube insertion sites.
7. Inspect active drainage system to ensure proper functioning, including insertion site, drainage moving through tubing in direction of reservoir, patency of drainage tubing, airtight connection sites, and presence of any leaks or kinks in system. Remove and dispose of gloves. Perform hand hygiene.
8. Determine if drain tube needs self-suction, wall suction, or no suction by checking health care provider's orders.
9. Identify type of drainage containers that patient has.
10. Assess patient's knowledge, experience with drainage system, and feelings about procedure.

Ensures patient safety. Complies with The Joint Commission standards and improves patient safety (TJC, 2023).

Identifies type and location of drainage system. Drainage tubing is usually placed near wound through small surgical incision.

Common risk factors for medical adhesive–related skin injury (MARSI) (Fumarola et al., 2020). Erythema, blistering, and excoriation are signs of MARSI and are related to the skin's reaction to an adhesive (Hitchcock et al., 2021; Thayer et al., 2022).

Determines degree to which individuals have the ability to find, understand, and use information and services to make informed health-related decisions and actions for themselves and others (CDC, 2023).

Assigning labeling system to each drain helps with consistent documentation when patient has multiple drainage tubes.

Allows you to plan skin care and identifies quantity of sterile dressing supplies needed.

Properly functioning system maintains suction until reservoir is filled or drainage is no longer being produced or accumulated. Tension on drainage tubing increases injury to skin and underlying muscle.

Some drain tubes such as Hemovac can be used with self-suction or wall suction.

Determines frequency for emptying drainage.

Reveals need for patient instruction and/or support.

PLANNING

1. Expected outcomes following completion of procedure:
   - Wound healing continues.
   - Vacuum is reestablished.
   - Tubing is patent.
   - Patient describes precautions to avoid drain removal.
2. Provide privacy and explain procedure to patient.
3. Organize and set up any equipment needed to perform procedure.

Patient is comfortable, and wound drainage is collected.

Suction system is intact.

Fluid is draining away from wound area.

Demonstrates learning.

Protects patient's privacy; reduces anxiety. Promotes cooperation.

Ensures more efficiency when completing the procedure.

IMPLEMENTATION

1. Perform hand hygiene and apply clean gloves.
2. Place open specimen container or measuring graduate container on bed between you and patient.
3. **Empty Hemovac or ConstaVac:**
   a. Maintain asepsis while opening plug on port indicated for emptying drainage reservoir.
      (1) Tilt suction container in direction of plug.
      (2) Slowly squeeze two flat surfaces together, tilting toward measuring container.

Reduces transmission of microorganisms.

Permits measuring and discarding of wound drainage.

Avoids entry of pathogens.

Vacuum will be broken, and reservoir will pull air in until chamber is fully expanded.

Drains fluid toward plug.

Prevents splashing of contaminated drainage. Squeezing empties reservoir of drainage.

STEP	RATIONALE
b. Drain all contents into measuring container (see illustration).	Contents counted as fluid output (see Chapter 6).
c. Hold open antiseptic swab in dominant hand. Place suction device on flat surface with open outlet facing upward; continue pressing downward until bottom and top are in contact (see illustration).	Cleaning plug reduces transmission of microorganisms into drainage evacuation.
d. Holding device flat with one hand and using antiseptic swab, quickly clean opening, plug with other hand, and immediately replace plug; secure suction device on patient's bed.	Compression of surface of Hemovac creates vacuum.
e. Check device for reestablishment of vacuum, patency of drainage tubing, and absence of stress on tubing.	Facilitates wound drainage and prevents tension on drainage tubing.
4. Empty Hemovac with wall suction:	Empties drainage and reestablishes suction to wound bed.
a. Turn off suction.	
b. Disconnect suction tubing from Hemovac port.	Allows port to be opened.
c. Empty Hemovac as described in Step 3.	
d. Use an antiseptic swab to clean port opening and the end of suction tubing. Reconnect tubing to port.	Cleaning plug reduces transmission of microorganisms.
e. Set suction level as prescribed or on low if health care provider does not specify suction level.	Reestablishes wound suction.
5. Empty JP suction drain:	
a. Open port on top of bulb-shaped reservoir (see illustration). **NOTE:** Open device away from you to prevent sprays to face.	Breaks vacuum for drain.
b. Tilt bulb in direction of port and drain toward opening. Empty drainage from device into measuring container (see illustration). Clean end of emptying port and plug with antiseptic wipe.	Reduces transmission of microorganisms.
c. Compress bulb over drainage container. While compressing bulb, replace plug immediately.	Reestablishes vacuum.
6. Place and secure drainage system below site with safety pin on patient's gown. Be sure that there is slack in tubing from reservoir to wound.	Pinning drainage tubing to patient's gown prevents tension or pulling on tubing and insertion site.
7. Note characteristics of drainage in measuring container; measure volume and discard by flushing in commode.	Contents count as output.

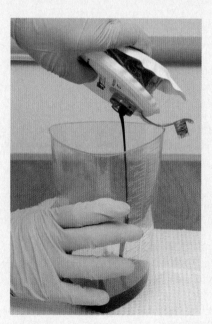

STEP 3b Hemovac contents drained into measuring container.

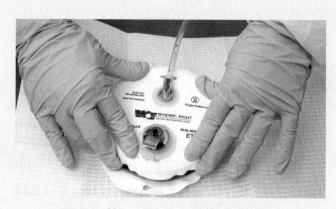

STEP 3c Hemovac compressed to create suction.

STEP	RATIONALE

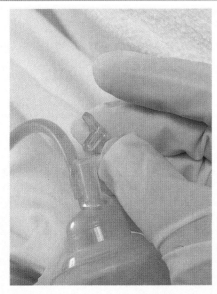

STEP 5a Opening port of Jackson-Pratt device.

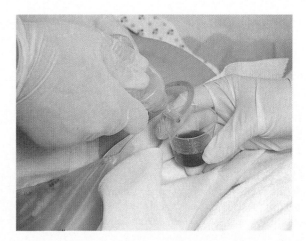

STEP 5b Emptying contents from Jackson-Pratt drainage device.

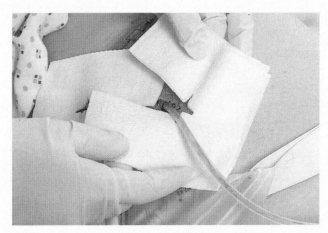

STEP 9 Applying split gauze dressing around Jackson-Pratt drain tube.

8. Discard soiled supplies and remove and dispose of gloves. Perform hand hygiene.

Reduces transmission of microorganisms.

9. Apply clean gloves. Proceed with dressing change (see Chapter 40) around drain site and inspection of drain insertion site and periwound skin. Split-drain sponge dressings are often used around drain tubes (see illustration) and taped in place.

Dressing reduces the risk for bacteria entering surgical wound and irritation to the periwound areas from drainage exudate. Periwound skin is at risk for MASD from wound exudate and MARSI due to potential skin reaction to the dressing adhesive (Bryant & Nix, 2024; Hitchcock et al., 2021; Thayer et al., 2022).

10. Remove and discard contaminated material and supplies, remove and dispose of gloves, and perform hand hygiene.

Reduces transmission of microorganisms.

11. Help patient to a comfortable position.

Restores comfort and a sense of well-being.

12. Raise side rails (as appropriate) and lower bed to lowest position, locking into position.

Ensures patient safety and prevents falls.

13. Place nurse call system in an accessible location within patient's reach.

Ensures patient can call for assistance if needed.

STEP	RATIONALE

EVALUATION

STEP	RATIONALE
1. Observe for drainage in suction device.	Indicates presence of vacuum, patency of tubing, and functioning of drainage suction device.

Clinical Judgment *Inspect for clots or cellular debris. Clots or large collections of debris may block drainage flow. The Y-site in the drainage tubing is especially prone to clogging.*

STEP	RATIONALE
2. Inspect wound for drainage or collection of drainage fluid under skin, which can cause a seroma.	Drainage should not be significant under suture line. May indicate inadequate functioning of drainage suction device.
3. Measure drainage from drainage system, and document on I&O form at least every 8 to 12 hours and as needed for large drainage volume (check agency policy).	Determines status of wound healing. Collect diagnostic specimen in presence of unexpected purulence or pungent odor, report findings to health care provider, and document in progress note.
4. Inspect periwound skin for any signs of irritation from wound exudate or dressing adhesive material.	Periwound tissue is fragile and at risk for injury from moisture or wound exudate and medical adhesives. These wounds can progress into severe skin injury (Bryant & Nix, 2024; Earlam & Woods, 2022).
5. Use **Teach-Back:** "I want to be sure I explained clearly why it is important not to pull on your drain. Tell me what can happen if you pull the drain out accidentally." Revise your instruction now or develop a plan for revised patient/family caregiver teaching if patient/family caregiver is not able to teach back correctly.	Teach-back is a technique for health care providers to ensure that they have explained medical information clearly so that patients and their families understand what is communicated to them (AHRQ, 2023).

Unexpected Outcomes	Related Interventions
1. Site where tube exits skin becomes infected: purulent drainage, odor, reddened site, increased white blood cell count, and temperature elevation.	• Notify health care provider about presence of signs of infection. • Use aseptic technique when changing dressings.
2. Bleeding appears in or around drainage collector.	• Determine amount of bleeding and notify health care provider if excessive. • Assess for tension on patient's drainage tubing. • Secure tubing to prevent pulling and pain.
3. Patient experiences pain at drain exit site.	• Medicate patient as ordered. • Stabilize drainage tubing to reduce tension and pulling against incision. • Notify health care provider if signs of wound infection are present.
4. Drainage suction device is not accumulating drainage.	• Assess drainage tubing for clots. • Assess drainage system for air leaks or kinks. • Notify health care provider.

Documentation

- Document emptying the drainage suction device; reestablishing vacuum in suction device; amount, color, odor of drainage; dressing change to drain site; and appearance of drain insertion site.
- Document amount of drainage.
- Document your evaluation of patient and family caregiver learning.

Hand-Off Reporting

- Immediately report a sudden change in amount of drainage, either output or absence of drainage flow, to the health care provider. Also report pungent odor of drainage or new evidence of purulence, severe pain, or dislodgment of the drainage tube to the health care provider.

Special Considerations

Patient Education

- Instruct patient about anticipated postoperative drainage, expected progress of wound healing and drainage volume, and estimated date of removal of drain as volume diminishes.
- Teach patient or family caregiver how to empty and document amount of drainage. If patient is going home with drainage

device, ask patient or family caregiver to document amount emptied and bring the documentation to the next outpatient visit.

Pediatrics

- Have parents help to prevent pediatric patients from dislodging drainage tubes. Placing mittens on infants and young children may help. Keep the tubing out of sight if possible.

Older Adults

- Be aware that older adults with large amounts of drainage will need additional fluid intake because they are more likely to become dehydrated.
- Take measures to prevent a confused patient from pulling out drain collector.

Home Care

- Provide written instructions in drain care. Include importance of measuring and documenting the amount of drainage. Patient should measure the volume of drainage on a daily basis and share with the health care provider at their next outpatient visit.

✦ SKILL 38.4   Negative-Pressure Wound Therapy

Negative-pressure wound therapy (NPWT) incorporates foam or gauze and subatmospheric (negative) pressure to a wound through suction to facilitate healing and collect wound fluid (Lund & Singh, 2022; Netsch & Nix, 2024; Nix & Bryant, 2022). NPWT (Figs. 38.10 and 38.11) stimulates the wound repair process by removal of edema and wound exudates and reduction of edema, macrodeformation and wound contraction, and microdeformation and mechanical stretch perfusion. Secondary effects include angiogenesis, granulation tissue formation, and reduction in bacterial bioburden (Netsch & Nix, 2024; Nix & Bryant, 2022). Some NPWT systems (iNPWT) allow the intermittent instillation of fluids into a wound and liquefy infectious material and wound debris, especially in wounds not responding to traditional NPWT (Fernandez et al., 2019). Research also supports the use of an instillation of wound-rinsing agents to facilitate healing in some chronic wounds (Matiasek et al., 2018). Instilled fluid lowers wound fluid viscosity, facilitating more effective removal of thick exudate. A clean wound environment may allow cellular resources to focus on cellular proliferation and matrix production rather than immune and inflammatory responses (Crumley, 2021).

Indications for NPWT include chronic, acute, traumatic, subacute, and dehisced wounds; closure of fistula tracts; partial-thickness burns; injuries (e.g., diabetic and pressure); flaps and grafts once nonviable tissue has been removed; and select high-risk postoperative surgical incisions (e.g., orthopedic, sternal). NPWT is also used in wounds with tunnels, undermining, or sinus tracts as long as the wound filler can fill the dead space and is easily retrieved. Mechanisms for wound healing include reduction in edema, with associated improvement in perfusion, and mechanical deformation of cells, which stimulates the wound repair process (Nix & Bryant, 2022).

Contraindications to NPWT include necrotic tissue with eschar present; untreated osteomyelitis; nonenteric and unexplored fistulas; malignancy in a wound; exposed vasculature; and exposed nerves, anastomotic site, or organs. Other safety precautions to consider are patients at high risk for bleeding or hemorrhage; patients taking anticoagulants; and patients requiring magnetic resonance imaging (MRI), hyperbaric chamber, or defibrillation (Netsch & Nix, 2024).

There are a number of different NPWT systems, some of which are gauze or foam based; some are designed for acute care settings or for outpatient care (Netsch & Nix, 2024). NPWT can be delivered intermittently or continuously. A review of evidence shows improved microvascular blood flow and granulation tissue formation with intermittent versus continuous therapy delivered at 125 mm Hg (WOCN, 2016). However, for patients with severe pain, lower levels of pressure (75–80 mm Hg) can be used to reduce pain and discomfort without compromising effectiveness (EPUAP/NPIAP/PPPIA, 2019a; EPUAP/NPIAP/PPPIA, 2019b; Netsch & Nix, 2024).

Delegation

The skill of NPWT cannot be delegated to assistive personnel (AP). Direct the AP to:
- Use caution in positioning or turning patient to avoid tubing displacement
- Report any change in dressing shape or integrity to the nurse
- Report any change in patient's temperature or comfort level to the nurse
- Report any wound fluid leakage around the edges of the adhesive drape
- Report any alarms on the NPWT system

Interprofessional Collaboration

- Collaborate with wound care specialists when needed if there is difficulty applying the NPWT dressing or in maintaining an airtight seal on larger or more complex wounds.

Equipment

- NPWT power unit (requires health care provider's order) (For this skill, the vacuum-assisted closure [V.A.C.] unit is used for illustration; several other systems are available, and their applications may differ; see manufacturer instructions.)
- NPWT dressing (gauze or foam, see manufacturer recommendations) and transparent dressing
- NPWT pad and connecting tubing
- NPWT drainage canister

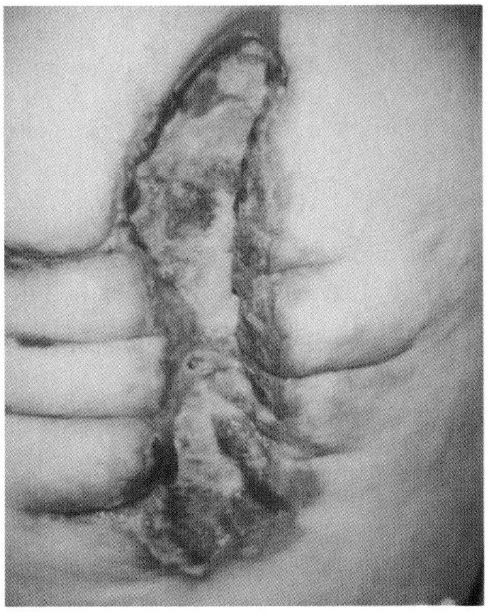

FIG. 38.10 Dehisced wound before negative-pressure wound therapy. *(Courtesy KCI Licensing, San Antonio, TX.)*

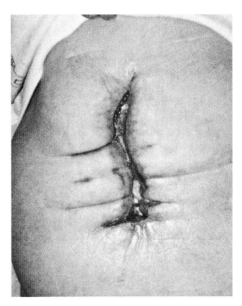

FIG. 38.11 Dehisced wound after negative-pressure wound therapy. *(Courtesy KCI Licensing, San Antonio, TX.)*

- Supplies for wound irrigation if needed (see Skill 38.1)
- Three pairs of gloves, clean and sterile (as needed)
- Scissors, sterile
- Skin preparation/skin barrier protectant/hydrocolloid dressing/skin barrier

- Adhesive remover (if needed)
- Personal protective equipment (PPE): gown, mask, goggles (used when splashing from wound is a risk)
- Waterproof biohazard bag for disposal

STEP	RATIONALE

ASSESSMENT

1. Identify patient using at least two identifiers (e.g., name and birthday or name and medical record number) according to agency policy.

Ensures correct patient. Complies with The Joint Commission standards and improves patient safety (TJC, 2023).

2. Review patient's electronic health record (EHR), including health care provider's order and nurses' notes, for frequency of dressing change, amount of negative pressure, type of foam or gauze to use, pressure cycle (intermittent or continuous), and appearance of wound at last dressing change.

Determines frequency of dressing change, negative-pressure setting, and special instructions. Health care provider's order is also necessary for reimbursement. Baseline appearance used to evaluate state of healing.

3. Review EHR to determine patient's age and history of dehydration, malnutrition, exposure to radiation therapy, underlying chronic conditions (e.g., diabetes mellitus, immunosuppression), edema of the skin, and the presence of erythema, blistering, or excoriation of skin under or adjacent to adhesive's securing dressing.

Provides baseline to compare findings with previous dressing change assessments and reflects wound-healing progress. Identifies common risk factors for medical adhesive related skin injury (MARSI) (Fumarola et al., 2020). Erythema, blistering, and appearance of wound at last dressing change and excoriation are signs of MARSI and are related to the skin's reaction to an adhesive (Hitchcock et al., 2021; Thayer et al., 2022).

4. Assess patient's/family caregiver's health literacy.

Determines degree to which individuals have the ability to find, understand, and use information and services to make informed health-related decisions and actions for themselves and others (CDC, 2023).

5. Assess character of patient's pain and rate acuity on a pain scale of 0 to 10.

Serves as baseline to measure patient's level of comfort during and after wound therapy. Determines if comfort measures are effective.

6. Perform hand hygiene. Apply clean gloves and appropriate PPE. Assess condition of skin around wound and status of NPWT dressing without disrupting NPWT (see Procedural Guideline 38.1). Remove and dispose of gloves. Perform hand hygiene.

Provides information regarding condition of skin around wound and existing dressing, presence of complications, and proper type of supplies and help needed.

Reduces transmission of microorganisms.

7. Assess patient's knowledge, prior experience with NPWT, and feelings about procedure.

Reveals need for patient instruction and/or support.

PLANNING

1. Expected outcomes following completion of procedure:
- Patient's wound shows evidence of healing as wound decreases in size with less drainage, redness, or swelling.
- Patient reports acceptable level of comfort and rates severity on a scale of 0 to 10 after dressing changes.
- Dressing remains intact with airtight seal and prescribed negative pressure.
- Patient or family caregiver demonstrates correct method of dressing changes.

Dressing is effective in promoting healing and preventing infection.

Analgesic and comfort measures effective in controlling pain.

Dressing is applied correctly and maintains negative pressure.

Indicates that patient and family caregiver learning has occurred.

2. Provide privacy and position the patient so that only the area currently being examined is exposed; use sheet to cover rest of the body.

Provides privacy and comfort.

3. Administer prescribed analgesic as needed 30 minutes before dressing change.

Comfortable patient will be less likely to move suddenly, causing wound or supply contamination.

4. Organize and set up supplies at patient's bedside.

Ensures more efficiency when completing the procedure.

5. Explain procedure to patient and family caregiver, instructing patient not to touch wound or sterile supplies.

Relieves anxiety and promotes understanding of healing process. Prevents contamination of sterile supplies.

IMPLEMENTATION

1. Cuff top of disposable waterproof biohazard bag and place within reach of work area.

Cuff prevents accidental contamination of top of outer bag.

2. Perform hand hygiene and apply clean gloves and appropriate PPE (if not previously applied) (e.g., if risk for spray exists, apply protective gown, goggles, and mask).

Reduces transmission of infectious organisms.

STEP	RATIONALE

3. Follow manufacturer directions for removal and replacement (units will vary). (Following are steps for Wound Vac by KCI). Turn off NPWT unit by pushing therapy on/off button.
  a. Close clamp on dressing tubing.
  b. Close clamp on pump tubing.
  c. Disconnect the tubes; allow any fluid in pump tubing to drain into collection device.
	Deactivates therapy and allows for proper drainage of fluid in drainage tubing.
	
	Prevents drainage from backflowing into wound when reconnected.

4. Remove transparent film by gently stretching, and slowly pull away from skin.	Prevents injury to wound tissue. Protects periwound skin breakdown from transparent adhesive.
5. Remove old foam one layer at a time and discard in bag. Be sure all pieces of foam are removed. Observe drainage on dressing. Use caution to avoid tension on any drains that are present near the wound or surrounding area. Remove and dispose of gloves.	Determines type and amount of dressings needed for replacement. Prevents accidental removal of drains.
6. Perform hand hygiene and conduct a wound healing assessment. Observe surface area and tissue type, color, odor, and drainage within wound. Measure length, width, and depth of wound as ordered (see Procedural Guideline 38.1).	Measurement of wound is necessary as a key assessment of wound-healing progression in addition to justification of continuation of NPWT with third-party payers (Netsch & Nix, 2024). Determines condition of wound and need for replacement of dressing.

Clinical Judgment *This is a time when a WOCN or health care provider might debride the wound. Debridement of eschar or slough, if present, should be performed for removal of devitalized tissue to prepare the wound bed (Netsch, 2022).*

STEP	RATIONALE
7. Remove and discard gloves in biohazard bag. Avoid having patient seeing old dressing because sight of wound drainage may be upsetting.	Reduces transmission of microorganisms. Lessens patient anxiety during procedure.

8. Clean wound per order or recommendations of WOCN or wound care specialist.
  a. Perform hand hygiene. Apply sterile or clean gloves, depending on agency policy and wound status.
  b. If ordered, irrigate wound with normal saline or other solution ordered by health care provider (see Skill 38.1). Gently blot periwound with gauze to dry thoroughly.
	Cleaning periwound is essential to remove wound surface debris and create an airtight seal.
	Reduces transmission of infectious organisms.
	
	Irrigation removes wound debris and cleans wound bed. Cleaning and removal of infectious material showed reduced infection and improved healing (EPUAP/NPIAP/PPPIA, 2019a; Fernandez et al., 2019).

Clinical Judgment *Health care providers may order wound cultures routinely. However, when drainage is more copious, looks purulent, or has a foul odor, obtain wound culture. This may be an indication that NPWT may need to be discontinued.*

Clinical Judgment *Health care providers may use normal saline instillation with large, complex wounds. NPWT with instillation in wounds that needed cleaning and removal of infectious material showed reduced infection and improved wound healing (Fernandez et al., 2019).*

STEP	RATIONALE
9. Apply skin protectant, barrier film, solid skin barrier sheet, or hydrocolloid dressing to periwound skin.	Maintains airtight seal needed for NPWT wound therapy (Netsch & Nix, 2024). Protects periwound skin from moisture-associated skin damage (MASD) (Bryant & Nix, 2024).
10. Fill any uneven skin surfaces (e.g., creases, scars, skinfolds) with skin-barrier product (e.g., paste, strip).	Creates a level wound surface, which further helps to maintain airtight seal (Netsch & Nix, 2024).
11. Remove and dispose of gloves. Perform hand hygiene.	Prevents transmission of microorganisms.
12. Depending on type of wound, apply sterile or new clean gloves (see agency policy).	Fresh sterile wounds require sterile gloves. Chronic wounds require clean technique (WOCN, 2016).

13. Apply NPWT dressing.
  a. Prepare NPWT filler dressing. Consult with wound care expert for appropriate type.
 	
    (1) Measure clean wound and select appropriate-size dressing.
	Filler dressing depends on NPWT used and can include foam or gauze dressings with or without antimicrobials such as silver. Type of dressing may be adjusted based on undermining, tunneling, or sinus tracts present (Netsch & Nix, 2024).
	Establishes baseline for wound size.
	Black polyurethane (PU) foam has larger pores and is most effective in stimulating granulation tissue and wound contraction. White soft foam is denser with smaller pores and used when growth of granulation tissue needs to be restricted (Amit et al., 2022; Netsch & Nix, 2024).

STEP	RATIONALE
(2) Using sterile scissors, cut filler dressing foam to wound size, making sure to fit exact size and shape of wound, including tunnels and undermined areas.	Proper size of foam dressing maintains negative pressure to entire wound (Netsch & Nix, 2024).

Clinical Judgment *In some instances an antimicrobial product such as silver-impregnated gauze or topical antibiotic is in order. These products help reduce the bioburden of the wound.*

STEP	RATIONALE
b. Place filler dressing in wound following manufacturer instructions. Be sure that filler dressing is in contact with entire wound base, margins, and tunneled and undermined areas. Count number of filler dressings and document in patient's chart.	Maintains negative pressure to entire wound. Edges of foam dressing must be in direct contact with patient's skin. Dressing count provides the number of filler dressings that should be removed at next dressing change.
c. Apply NPWT transparent dressing over foam wound dressing.	
(1) Trim dressing to cover wound and dressing so it will extend onto periwound skin approximately 2.5 to 5 cm (1–2 inches).	Prepares dressing of appropriate size for wound.
(2) Apply transparent dressing (see illustration).	
(a) Retain blue handling tab on portion of dressing used. Peel back one side of layer one. Then place adhesive side down over wound.	Dressing should be airtight with no wrinkles or tunnels to maintain a negative-pressure environment. A snug and tight application of the dressing must be applied to ensure an airtight seal (Box 38.3).
(b) Remove remaining side of layer one.	
(c) Remove green striped stabilization layer two. Remove blue handling tabs.	
(3) Apply connecting pad and tubing to dressing:	
(a) Identify site over dressing for pad application. Pinch transparent dressing and cut at least a 2 cm round hole.	Provides opening for wound drainage.

Clinical Judgment *Do not cut a slit or X as it may seal off the opening.*

STEP	RATIONALE
(b) Remove backing layers from pad. Place connecting tube opening of pad directly over hole in dressing.	Ensures free flow of drainage.
(c) Apply gentle pressure to secure. Remove any remaining stabilization layer and discard.	Prevents tubing from becoming dislocated.
(d) Connect pad tubing to canister tubing and open all clamps.	Creates open route for drainage.

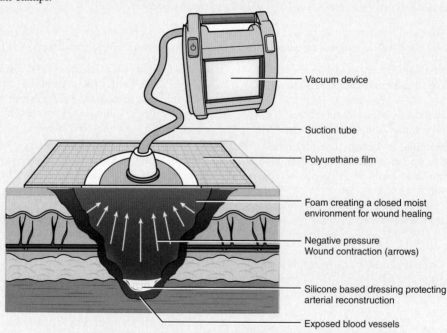

Vacuum device

Suction tube

Polyurethane film

Foam creating a closed moist environment for wound healing

Negative pressure
Wound contraction (arrows)

Silicone based dressing protecting arterial reconstruction

Exposed blood vessels

STEP 13d(2) Foam wound filler; transparent dressing over existing wound.

STEP	RATIONALE

BOX 38.3

Maintaining an Airtight Seal With Negative-Pressure Wound Therapy

To avoid loss of suction (negative pressure), the wound and dressing must stay sealed after therapy is initiated. Problem seal areas include wounds around joints; near skin creases and folds; and near moisture such as diaphoresis, wound drainage, and urine or stool. The following points may help to maintain an airtight seal:

- Clip hair on skin around wound (check agency policy).
- Fill uneven skin surfaces with a skin-barrier product such as paste or strips.
- Make sure that periwound skin surface is dry.
- Cut transparent film to extend 2.5 to 5 cm (1–2 inches) beyond wound perimeter.

- Frame periwound area with skin sealant, solid skin barrier, hydrocolloid, or transparent film dressing.
- Cut or mold transparent dressing to fit wound.
- Avoid wrinkles when applying transparent film.
- Identify any air leaks and repair them with a sealant dressing (e.g., transparent dressing). Use only one or two additional layers for large leaks. Multiple layers reduce moisture vapor transmission and cause maceration of wound.
- If an adhesive remover is used, be sure to cleanse periwound well because it leaves a residue that can hinder film adherence.

Data from Netsch DS: Refractory wounds. In Wound, Ostomy, and Continence Nurses Society (WOCN): *Core curriculum: wound management,* ed 2, Philadelphia, 2022, Wolters Kluwer; and Netsch DS and Nix DP: Negative pressure wound therapy. In Bryant RA, Nix DP, editors: *Acute and chronic wounds: intraprofessionals from novice to expert,* ed 6, St Louis, 2024, Mosby.

---

14. Turn on power to vac unit and set appropriate mode and pressure levels.

Negative pressure can be delivered intermittently or continuously, most often continuously. Review of evidence by national guidelines has concluded that there is improved microvascular blood flow and granulation tissue formation with intermittent therapy compared with continuous therapy delivered at 125 mm Hg (Netsch & Nix, 2024; WOCN, 2016).

15. Secure tubing several centimeters away from dressing, avoiding pressure points.

Drainage tubes over bony pressure prominences can cause medical device-related pressure injuries (Fu et al., 2022; TJC, 2022).

16. Remove and dispose of gloves. Perform hand hygiene.

Reduces transmission of microorganisms.

17. Inspect NPWT system.
    a. Verify that the system is on. **NOTE:** This is different for each type of NPWT unit. For example, on some units the display screen shows "Therapy On." Check agency policy and procedure for specific information.
    b. Verify that all clamps are open and all tubing is patent.
    c. Examine system to be sure that seal is intact and therapy is working.
    d. If a leak is present, use strips of transparent film to patch areas around edges of wound.

Negative pressure is achieved when a tight seal is present (Netsch & Nix, 2024).

18. Write initials, date, and time on new dressing.

Provides reference for next dressing change.

19. Dispose of sharps (scissors) in designated sharps disposal bin, and if gloves are not already removed, remove them and perform hand hygiene.

Reduces transmission of infection. Provides a safe environment because instruments are sharp and contaminated.

20. Help patient to a comfortable position. Patients may ambulate with NPWT.

Restores comfort and a sense of well-being.

21. Raise side rails (as appropriate) and lower bed to lowest position, locking into position.

Ensures patient safety and prevents falls.

22. Place nurse call system in an accessible location within patient's reach.

Ensures patient can call for assistance if needed.

EVALUATION

1. Inspect condition of wound, wound bed, and periwound area on an ongoing basis; note drainage and odor.

Determines status of wound healing and integrity of the periwound area (Bryant & Nix, 2024).

2. Ask patient to describe character of pain and rate severity using scale of 0 to 10.

Determines patient's level of comfort following procedure and while NPWT is in place.

3. Verify airtight dressing seal and correct negative-pressure setting.

Determines effective negative pressure being applied.

STEP	RATIONALE
4. Measure wound drainage output in canister on regular basis.	Monitors fluid balance and wound drainage.
5. **Use Teach-Back:** "I want to be sure I explained clearly what the function of NPWT is. Explain to me how NPWT helps your wound heal." Revise your instruction now or develop a plan for revised patient/family caregiver teaching if patient/family caregiver is not able to teach back correctly.	Teach-back is a technique for health care providers to ensure that they have explained medical information clearly so that patients and their families understand what is communicated to them (AHRQ, 2023).

Unexpected Outcomes	Related Interventions
1. Wound appears inflamed and tender, drainage has increased, and odor is present.	• Notify health care provider. • Obtain wound culture. • Increase frequency of dressing changes.
2. Patient reports increase in pain.	• Consult with health care provider about changing analgesia. • Instill normal saline to moisten foam and other filler dressings to allow them to loosen from granulation tissue. • Decrease pressure setting. • Change from intermittent to continuous cycling. • Change type of NPWT system.
3. Negative-pressure seal has broken.	• Take preventive measures (see Box 38.3).
4. Wound hemorrhages.	• Stop NPWT immediately and notify health care provider.
5. Patient or family caregiver is unable to perform dressing change.	• Provide additional teaching and support. • Obtain services of home care agency.

Documentation

- Document appearance of wound, characteristics of drainage, placement of NPWT (time and type of dressing, pressure mode and setting), and patient response to dressing change.
- Document whether the patient or caregiver is participating in changing the NPWT dressing.
- Document your evaluation of patient and family caregiver learning.

Hand-Off Reporting

- Report brisk, bright-red bleeding; evidence of poor wound healing; evisceration or dehiscence; and possible wound infection to health care provider immediately.

Special Considerations

Patient Education

- Successful NPWT relies on patient's and family caregiver's cooperation and participation with treatment, and the following things are important to know, especially if NPWT is continued at home:
  - Signs and symptoms that indicate development of an infection should be reported to health care provider immediately.
  - Expected wound appearance with use of NPWT. Instruct patient and caregiver in appearance of foam dressings.
  - When to call health care provider and specific phone numbers for medical equipment vendor or health care provider.
  - How to maintain negative-pressure seal.
  - Meaning of NPWT system alarms and when and how to call manufacturer for assistance.
  - The frequency of dressing changes.

- Patients and family caregivers need to learn how to administer analgesics appropriately. Patient tolerance of and adherence to NPWT are difficult if dressing changes are painful (Netsch & Nix, 2024).

Pediatrics

- NPWT can be used in some infants, and lower limits of pressure −50 to −75 mm Hg are recommended (Lund & Singh, 2022).
- Lower limits of −50 to −75 mm Hg are recommended in hemodynamically unstable children (Lund & Singh, 2022).
- Parents need to actively participate in NPWT treatment.

Older Adults

- Use skin-care practices to protect periwound tissue. Transparent film may be irritating to fragile skin. A skin protectant is one method to reduce the risk for tissue injury. When removing transparent film, consider using an adhesive releaser (Thayer et al., 2022).

Home Care (see Patient Education)

- The wound specialist will need to obtain information about the physical environment (e.g., stairways, electrical outlets) and the patient's ability to see the device controls and hear the alarms (Netsch & Nix, 2024).
- Be sure that patient and family caregiver understand the importance of maintaining a seal on the NPWT dressing and have been educated on how to seal the dressing. Explain whom to call if the alarm warns of a leak in the system and the patient or caregiver is unable to reestablish the seal.
- Review how to attach the device to a wall outlet to recharge the battery.

◆ CLINICAL JUDGMENT AND NEXT GENERATION NCLEX® EXAMINATION–STYLE QUESTIONS

A patient who is 8 days postoperative was readmitted because of excessive and odorous drainage from her midline abdominal incision and a high fever. A computed tomography (CT) scan revealed an anastomotic leak. The patient returned to surgery for a colon resection and the creation of a diverting colostomy. There was abdominal contamination related to leakage of stool into the abdominal cavity. At the time of surgery, a Jackson-Pratt (JP) drain was placed near the incision; because of the fecal contamination, the incision was left open to heal by secondary intention.

1. Which assessments will the nurse perform when the patient is returned to the medical surgical unit following PACU? **Select all that apply.**
   1. Percentage of viable tissue in wound bed
   2. Type of tissue visualized in wound bed
   3. Presence or absence of exudate
   4. Degree of pain experienced
   5. Periwound skin condition
   6. Size of wound
   7. Presence or absence of wound odor

2. Several days later, the nurse receives a hand-off report indicating that the wound has developed necrotic tissue. Which assessment findings does the oncoming nurse anticipate? **Select all that apply.**
   1. Elevated temperature and pulse
   2. Blood pressure within patient's baseline range
   3. Dressings with new thick yellow drainage
   4. Presence of foul odor from the wound
   5. Warmth and redness of the periwound skin

3. The nurse notes approximately 60 mL of bright red drainage in the JP drain 6 hours after surgery. Which intervention will the nurse take?
   1. Shake the bulb to thin the drainage.
   2. Call the surgeon to report the finding.
   3. Secure the drain above the level of the wound.
   4. Empty the drain immediately.

4. It has been 10 days after surgery, and wound irrigation has removed necrotic tissue. The wound bed now has granulation, and there is no further leakage of stool into the abdominal cavity. Which order does the nurse anticipate from the health care provider at this time?
   1. NPWT
   2. Leave wound open to air
   3. Return to surgery for suturing of the wound
   4. Begin course of antifungal medication

5. The nurse reviews the health care provider's order for NPWT pressure to be set on 200 mm Hg continuous. Which action will the nurse take?
   1. Apply the NPWT as ordered.
   2. Call the health care provider and verify the order.
   3. Fill the wound bed with white foam before application of black foam.
   4. Contact the manufacturer to determine the appropriate setting.

Visit the Evolve site for Answers to Clinical Judgment and Next Generation NCLEX® Examination–Style Questions.

REFERENCES

Ahmed I, Boulton AJ, Rizvi S, et al: The use of triclosan-coated sutures to prevent surgical site infections: a systematic review and meta-analysis of the literature, *BMJ Open* 9(9):e029727, 2019. https://doi.org/10.1136/bmjopen-2019-029727.

Agency for Healthcare Research and Quality (AHRQ): *Teach-back: intervention.* Agency for Rockville, MD, 2023, Healthcare Research and Quality. https://www.ahrq.gov/patient-safety/reports/engage/interventions/teachback.html. Accessed August 28, 2023.

Amit G, et al: Mechanical and contact characteristics of foam materials within wound dressings: theoretical and practical considerations in treatment, *Int Wound J* 20:1960–197, 2023.

Arnold M, et al: Wound Healing in the long-term acute care setting using fluidized therapy/continuous low-pressure therapeutic bed: a multiple case series, *J WOCN* 47(3):284, 2020.

Azmat CD, Council M: *Wound closure techniques,* StatPearls Publishing; In StatPearls.

Basu S, et al: Psychological stress on wound healing: a silent player in a complex background, *Int J Low Extrem Wounds* 15347346221077571, 2022.

Bates-Jensen BM: Wound assessment. In McNichol LL, et al., editors: *WOCN Core curriculum wound management,* ed 2, Philadelphia, 2022, Wolters Kluwer.

Beitz JM: Wound healing. In McNichol LL, et al., editors: *WOCN Core curriculum wound management,* ed 2, Philadelphia, 2022, Wolters Kluwer.

Bochert K: Pressure injury prevention and maintaining a successful plan and program. In McNichol LL, et al., editors: *WOCN Core curriculum wound management,* ed 2, Philadelphia, 2022, Wolters Kluwer.

Bohn G, Bryant RA: Wound-healing physiology and factors that affect the repair process. In Bryant RA, Nix DP, editors: *Acute and chronic wounds: intraprofessionals from novice to expert,* ed 6, St. Louis, 2024, Elsevier.

Brindle T, Creehan S: Management of surgical wounds: In McNichol LL, et al., editors: *WOCN wound curriculum wound management,* ed 2, Philadelphia, 2022, Wolters Kluwer.

Bryant RA, Nix DP: Principles of wound healing and topical management. In Bryant RA, Nix DP, editors: *Acute and chronic wounds: intraprofessionals from novice to expert,* ed 6, St. Louis, 2024, Mosby.

Centers for Disease Control and Prevention (CDC): *What is health literacy?* 2023. https://www.cdc.gov/healthliteracy/learn/index.html. Accessed August 28, 2023.

Crumley C: Negative pressure wound therapy devices with instillation/irrigation, *J Wound Ostomy Continence Nurs* 48(3):199, 2021.

deLemos D: *Skin laceration repair with sutures,* UpToDate, 2023. https://www.uptodate.com/contents/skin-laceration-repair-with-sutures. Accessed August 28, 2023.

Earlam AS, Woods L: Moisture-associated skin damage: the basics, *Am Nurse J* 17(10):6, 2022.

European Pressure Ulcer Advisory Panel (EPUAP), National Pressure Injury Advisory Panel (NPIAP), Pan Pacific Pressure Injury Alliance (PPPIA): Treatment of pressure ulcers/injuries: Clinical Practice Guideline. In Haesler E, editor: *The International Guideline,* 2019a, EPUAP/NPIAP/PPPIA.

European Pressure Ulcer Advisory Panel (EPUAP), National Pressure Injury Advisory Panel (NPIAP), Pan Pacific Pressure Injury Alliance (PPPIA): Treatment of pressure ulcers/injuries. In Haesler E, editor: *Quick Reference Guide,* 2019b, EPUAP/NPIAP/PPPIA.

Fernandez L, et al: Use of negative pressure wound therapy with instillation in the management of complex wounds in critically ill patients, *Wounds* 31(1):E1, 2019.

Fu F, et al: Knowledge of intensive care unit nurses about medical device-related pressure injury and analysis of influencing factors, *Int Wound J* 20:1219–1228, 2023.

Fumarola S, Allaway R, Callaghan R, et al: Overlooked and underestimated: medical adhesive-related skin injuries. Best practice consensus document on prevention, *J Wound Care* 29(Suppl 3c):S1–S24, 2020.

Gallagher S: Skin and wound care for the bariatric population. In McNichol LL, et al., editors: *WOCN Core curriculum wound management,* ed 2, Philadelphia, 2022, Wolters Kluwer.

Gallagher S, Barbe M: The impaired healing hypothesis: a mechanism by which psychosocial stress and personal characteristics increase MSD risk? *Ergonomics* 65(4):573–586, 2022.

Gethin D, et al: Evidence for person-centered care in chronic wound care: a systematic review and recommendations for practice, *J Wound Care* 29(Sup9b):S1–S22, 2020.

Hitchcock J, et al: Preventing medical adhesive-related sin injury (MARSI), *Br J Nurs* 30(15):S48–S56, 2021.

Hockenberry ML, et al: *Wong's nursing care of infants and children,* ed 12, St. Louis, 2024, Elsevier.

Hurlow J, Kalan L: Wound infection and bioburden: detection and management. In Bryant RA, Nix DP, editors: *Acute and chronic wounds: Intraprofessionals from novice to expert,* ed 6, St. Louis, 2024, Elsevier.

Jaszarowski KA, Murphree RW: Wound cleansing and dressing selection. In McNichol LL, et al., editors: Wound, Ostomy, and Continence Nurses Society (WOCN): *Core curriculum: wound management*, ed 2, Philadelphia, 2022, Wolters Kluwer.

Koka E, et al: Cultural understanding of wounds, buruli ulcers and their management at the Obon subdistrict of the Ga south municipality of the Greater Accra region of Ghana, *PLoS Negl Trop Dis* 10(7):1, 2016.

LeMay S, et al: Immersive virtual reality vs. non-immersive distraction for pain management of children during bone pins and suture removal: a randomized clinical trial protocol, *J Adv Nurs* 77(1):439, 2021.

Lund CL, Singh C: Skin and wound care for neonatal and pediatric population. In McNichol LL, et al., editors: *WOCN Core curriculum wound management*, ed 2, Philadelphia, 2022, Wolters Kluwer.

Machin M, et al: Systematic review of the use of cyanoacrylate glue in addition to standard wound closure in the prevention of surgical site infection, *Int Wound J* 16:387, 2019.

Manna B, Nahirniak P, Morrison CA. *Wound debridement*, In StatPearls, StatPearls Publishing, 2022. http://www.ncbi.nlm.nih.gov/books/NBK507882/.

Matiasek J, et al: Negative pressure wound therapy with instillation: effects on healing of category 4 pressure ulcers, *Plast Aesthet Res* 5(9):36, 2018.

Mendes A: Meeting the care needs of a person with dementia who is distressed, *Br J Nurs* 27(4):219, 2018.

Mufti A, et al: Anatomy and physiology of the skin. In McNichol LL, et al., editors: *WOCN core curriculum wound management*, ed 2, Philadelphia, 2022, Wolters Kluwer.

National Health Service (United Kingdom): *How do I care for a wound treated with skin glue?* 2021. https://www.nhs.uk/common-health-questions/accidents-first-aid-and-treatments/how-do-i-care-for-a-wound-treated-with-skin-glue/. Accessed August 28, 2023.

Netsch DS, Nix DP: Negative pressure wound therapy. In Bryant RA, Nix DP, editors: *Acute and chronic wounds: intraprofessionals from novice to expert*, ed 6, St. Louis, 2024, Mosby.

Netsch DS: Refractory wounds. In Wound, Ostomy, and Continence Nurses Society, editor: *Core curriculum: wound management*, ed 2, Philadelphia, 2022, Wolters Kluwer.

Nix DP: Skin and wound assessment. In Bryant RA, Nix DP, editors: *Acute and chronic wounds: intraprofessionals from novice to expert*, ed 6, St. Louis, 2024, Elsevier.

Nix D, Bryant RA: Fistula management. In McNichol LL, et al., editors: *WOCN Core curriculum wound management*, ed 2, Philadelphia, 2022, Wolters Kluwer.

Nuutila K, Eriksson E: Moist wound healing with commonly available dressings, *Adv Wound Care* 10(12):685–698, 2021. https://doi.org/10.1089/wound.2020.1232.

Oropallo A: Perfusion, oxygenation, and incision care. In Bryant RA, Nix DP, editors: *Acute and chronic wounds: intraprofessionals from novice to expert*, ed 6, St. Louis, 2024, Elsevier.

Oropallo A, Quraishi W: Wound Pain. In Bryant RA, Nix DP, editors: *Acute and chronic wounds: intraprofessionals from novice to expert*, ed 6, St. Louis, 2024, Elsevier.

Padela AI, et al: The development and validation of a modesty measure for diverse Muslim populations, *J Relig Health* 58(2):408, 2019.

Ramundo J: Principles and guidelines for wound debridement. In McNichol et al., editors: *Core curriculum: wound management*, ed 2, Philadelphia, PA, 2022, Wolters Kluwer.

Richbourg L: Skin and wound care for the geriatric population. In McNichol LL, et al., editors: *WOCN Core curriculum wound management*, ed 2, Philadelphia, 2022, Wolters Kluwer.

Thayer DM, et al: Top down injuries: prevention and management of moisture-associated skin damage, medical adhesive–related skin injury and skin tears. In McNichol LM, et al., editors: *Core curriculum: wound management*, ed 2, Philadelphia, PA, 2022, Wolters Kluwer.

The Joint Commission (TJC): *2023 National patient safety goals*, Oakbrook Terrace, IL, 2023, The Joint Commission. https://www.jointcommission.org/standards/national-patient-safety-goals/. Accessed August 28, 2023.

The Joint Commission (TJC): *Quick safety 25: preventing pressure injuries*, 2022. https://www.jointcommission.org/resources/news-and-multimedia/newsletters/newsletters/quick-safety/quick-safety-issue-25-preventing-pressure-injuries/preventing-pressure-injuries/. Accessed August 28, 2023.

Weir D, Schultz G: Assessment and Management of wound-related infections, In McNichol LL et al., editors: *WOCN Core curriculum wound management*, ed 2, Philadelphia, 2022, Wolters Kluwer.

Wound, Ostomy, and Continence Nurses Society (WOCN): *Guideline for prevention and management of pressure ulcers (injuries)*, Mount Laurel, NJ, 2016, WOCN.

Zabaglo M, Sharman T: Postoperative wound infection. In StatPearls, 2022, StatPearls Publishing. http://www.ncbi.nlm.nih.gov/books/NBK560533/.

39 | Pressure Injury Prevention and Care

SKILLS AND PROCEDURES

Skill 39.1 **Risk Assessment, Skin Assessment, and Prevention Strategies, p. 1146**

Skill 39.2 **Treatment of Pressure Injuries, p. 1154**

OBJECTIVES

Mastery of content in this chapter will enable you to:

- Explain the link between patient risk factors and development of pressure injuries.
- Analyze individual patient risk factors for pressure injury.
- Discuss how a nurse applies clinical judgment when using risk assessment tools during patient assessment of risk for pressure injury.
- Apply guidelines for prevention and treatment of pressure injuries.

- Use outcome criteria for patients at risk for pressure injuries or impaired skin integrity.
- Discuss indications for the use of topical agents in the treatment of pressure injuries.
- Explain teaching needs of patient and family caregiver regarding pressure injury prevention and treatment.

MEDIA RESOURCES

- http://evolve.elsevier.com/Perry/skills
- Review Questions
- ▶ Video Clips
- Case Studies
- Audio Glossary

- **NSO** Nursing Skills Online
- Answers to Clinical Judgment and Next-Generation NCLEX® Examination–Style Questions
- Skills Performance Checklists
- Printable Key Points

PURPOSE

A pressure injury prevention program (PIPP) is essential to safe patient care. A PIPP consists of a *best-practice bundle* and organizational *support* (Nix & Bryant, 2024). Comprehensive skin assessment identifies factors increasing a patient's risk for developing a pressure injury. Once a pressure injury has occurred, there are specific treatments to promote healing. A pressure injury is localized injury to the skin and/or underlying soft tissue, usually over a bony prominence, as a result of pressure or pressure in combination with shear (European Pressure Ulcer Advisory Panel [EPUAP], National Pressure Injury Advisory Panel [NPIAP], and Pan Pacific Pressure Injury Alliance [PPPIA], 2019a). In addition, tissue injury can result from pressure related to placement of a medical device. The injury occurs as a result of intense and/or prolonged pressure or pressure in combination with shear. The injury can present as intact nonblanchable skin or an open wound, which may be painful. The tolerance of soft tissue for pressure and shear may also be affected by microclimate, nutrition, perfusion, co-morbidities, and condition of the soft tissue. The term *pressure injury* replaces *pressure ulcer* in the National Pressure Ulcer Advisory Panel Pressure Injury Staging System as of April 2016 (EPUAP/NPIAP/PPPIA, 2019a). The change in terminology more accurately describes pressure injuries to both intact and ulcerated skin.

PRACTICE STANDARDS

- European Pressure Ulcer Advisory Panel (EPUAP), National Pressure Injury Advisory Panel (NPIAP), and Pan Pacific Pressure Injury Alliance (PPPIA), 2019a: Treatment of Pressure Ulcers/Injuries: Clinical Practice Guideline
- The Joint Commission (TJC), 2022: Preventing Pressure Injuries
- The Joint Commission (TJC), 2023: National Patient Safety Goals—Patient identification
- Wound, Ostomy, and Continence Nurses Society (WOCN), 2016: Guideline for Prevention and Management of Pressure Ulcers

SUPPLEMENTAL STANDARDS

- European Pressure Ulcer Advisory Panel (EPUAP), National Pressure Injury Advisory Panel (NPIAP), and Pan Pacific Pressure Injury Alliance (PPPIA), 2019b: Treatment of Pressure Ulcers/Injuries

PRINCIPLES FOR PRACTICE

- Pressure injuries occur from unrelieved, prolonged soft tissue compression, which interferes with blood flow to the tissue. When this compression continues for a prolonged period of time, the tissue dies from lack of blood flow, or tissue ischemia. Ischemia develops when pressure on the skin is greater than vascular pressure inside the vessels, causing the vessels to collapse and decreasing tissue perfusion.

- The most common sites for the development of pressure injuries are over bony prominences and can include the sacrum, coccyx, ischial tuberosities, greater trochanters, heels, scapula, iliac crests, and lateral and medial malleoli (Al Aboud & Manna, 2023). Fig. 39.1 shows pressure points over bony prominences where pressure injuries can develop in sitting or lying positions.
- Pressure injury can occur on any skin area subjected to pressure over nonbony locations from a poorly positioned or ill-fitting device or incorrect device use. These types of skin injuries are called *medical device–related pressure injuries* (MDRPIs). They have been defined as those that result from prolonged pressure or shear from a medical device on any location of the body, including mucosal cavities (Brophy et al., 2021).
- MDRPIs are pressure injuries that can cause pain, loss of function, increased length of stay, and increased health care costs. Timely assessment of risk for or actual MDPRI provides for prompt prevention or treatment (TJC, 2022).
- Factors such as incontinence and shear contribute to pressure injury formation. Chronic moisture from fecal and urinary incontinence compromises the protective barrier of the skin and may overhydrate it, making skin more susceptible to breakdown. Shear can damage the skin in one of two ways: shear stress, defined as the force per unit area exerted parallel to the plane of interest, and shear strain, defined as the distortion or deformation of tissue as a result of shear stress (EPUAP/NPIAP/PPPIA, 2019a; EPUAP/NPIAP/PPPIA, 2019b).
- Shear stress can result in skin tears (shearing of the epidermal layer from the dermal layer, such as inappropriate tape removal) or in deep damage, such as pressure injuries. Shear strain occurs when the subcutaneous tissue shears against the dermal layer

and blood flow becomes disrupted to the compressed area (e.g., when the patient slides down in bed, resulting in deep tissue injury) (Bohn & Bryant, 2024; Brophy et al., 2021).

- Medical adhesive–related skin injuries (MARSIs) result when erythema and/or other injuries such as erosions, tears, and bullae persist 30 minutes after removal of the adhesive (Bryant, 2024).
  - Types of MARSI include epidermal stripping, skin tears, tension blisters, maceration, irritant contact dermatitis, and allergic contact dermatitis (Bryant, 2024; Fumarola et al., 2020).
  - Factors related to tape trauma include product, user or caregiver technique, patient factors (e.g., age, co-morbidities), and anatomical site.
- Other risk factors that can contribute to the development of pressure injuries include immobility, loss of sensory perception, decrease in activity, and malnutrition (EPUAP/NPIAP/PPPIA, 2019a):
  - Immobility often restricts a patient's ability to change and control body position, thus increasing the pressure over bony prominences.
  - Loss of sensory perception, such as impairments caused by spinal cord injuries or cerebrovascular accidents, decreases the individual's ability to respond to increased, prolonged pressure in an area of the body and change positions accordingly.
  - Level of activity refers to the person's normal physical movement. A person who is bed bound is at greater risk for skin breakdown than a person who is fully or partially mobile.
  - Research indicates that malnutrition contributes to the development of pressure injuries (EPUAP/NPIAP/PPPIA, 2019a).
- Pressure injuries pose serious risks to a patient's health. A break in the skin, seen in stage 2 to 4 pressure injuries (Box 39.1), eliminates the first line of defense of the body against infection.

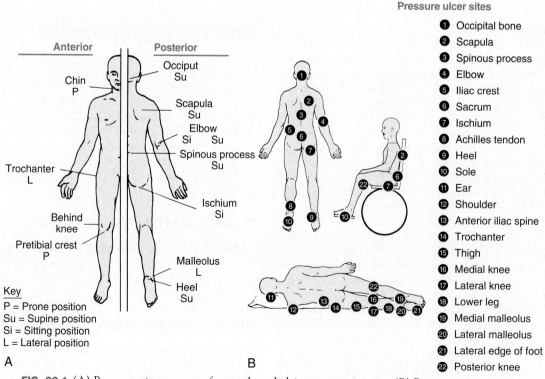

FIG. 39.1 (A) Bony prominences most frequently underlying pressure injuries. (B) Pressure injury sites. (From Trelease CC: Developing standards for wound care. *Ostomy Wound Manage* 26:50, 1988.)

BOX 39.1

Staging of Pressure Injuries

Stage 1

Pressure Injury: Nonblanchable Erythema of Intact Skin

Intact skin with a localized area of nonblanchable erythema, which may appear differently in darkly pigmented skin. Presence of blanchable erythema or changes in sensation, temperature, or firmness may precede visual changes. Color changes do not include purple or maroon discoloration; these may indicate deep tissue pressure injury (Bryant & Nix, 2024; EPUAP/NPIAP/PPPIA, 2019b).

Lightly Pigmented

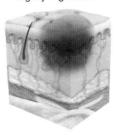 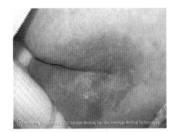

Darkly Pigmented

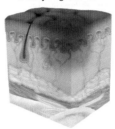

Stage 2

Pressure Injury: Partial-Thickness Skin Loss With Exposed Dermis

Partial-thickness loss of skin with exposed dermis. The wound bed is viable, pink or red, and moist and may also present as an intact or ruptured serum-filled blister. Adipose (fat) and deeper tissues are not visible. Granulation tissue, slough, and eschar are not present. These injuries commonly result from adverse microclimate and shear in the skin over the pelvis and shear in the heel. This stage should not be used to describe moisture-associated skin damage (MASD), including incontinence-associated dermatitis (IAD), intertriginous dermatitis (ITD), medical adhesive–related skin injury (MARSI), or traumatic wounds (skin tears, burns, abrasions) (Bryant & Nix, 2024; EPUAP/NPIAP/PPPIA, 2019b).

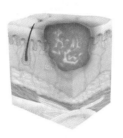 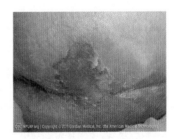

Stage 3

Pressure Injury: Full-Thickness Skin Loss

Full-thickness loss of skin, in which adipose (fat) is visible in the injury and granulation tissue and epibole (rolled wound edges) are often present. Slough and/or eschar may be visible. The depth of tissue damage varies by anatomical location; areas of significant adiposity can develop deep wounds. Undermining and tunneling may occur. Fascia, muscle, tendon, ligament, cartilage, and/or bone is not exposed. If slough or eschar obscures the extent of tissue loss, this is an unstageable pressure injury (Bryant & Nix, 2024; EPUAP/NPIAP/PPPIA, 2019b).

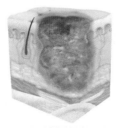 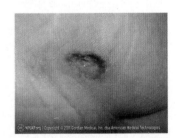

Stage 4

Pressure Injury: Full-Thickness Skin and Tissue Loss

Full-thickness skin and tissue loss with exposed or directly palpable fascia, muscle, tendon, ligament, cartilage, or bone in the injury. Slough and/or eschar may be visible. Epibole (rolled edges), undermining, and/or tunneling often occur. Depth varies by anatomical location. If slough or eschar obscures the extent of tissue loss, this is an unstageable pressure injury (Bryant & Nix, 2024; EPUAP/NPIAP/PPPIA, 2019b).

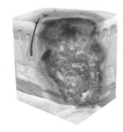 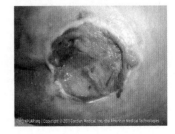

Continued

BOX 39.1

Staging of Pressure Injuries—cont'd

Suspected Deep Tissue Injury

Purple or maroon localized area of discolored, intact skin or blood-filled blister due to damage of underlying soft tissue from pressure and/or shear. The area may be preceded by tissue that is painful, firm, mushy, boggy, or warmer or cooler than adjacent tissue. Deep tissue injury may be difficult to detect in individuals with dark skin tones. Evolution may include a thin blister over a dark wound bed. The wound may further evolve and become covered by thin eschar. Evolution may be rapid, exposing additional layers of tissue even with treatment (EPUAP/NPIAP/PPPIA, 2019a).

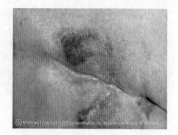

Unstageable Pressure Injury
Obscured Full-Thickness Skin and Tissue Loss

Full-thickness skin and tissue loss in which the extent of tissue damage within the ulcer cannot be confirmed because it is obscured by slough or eschar. If slough or eschar is removed, a stage 3 or stage 4 pressure injury will be revealed. Stable eschar (i.e., dry, adherent, intact without erythema or fluctuance) on the heel or ischemic limb should not be softened or removed (Bryant & Nix, 2024; EPUAP/NPIAP/PPPIA, 2019b).

Dark Eschar

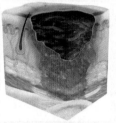

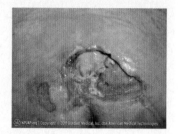

Slough Eschar

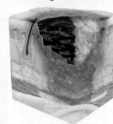

Deep Tissue Pressure Injury (DTPI)
Persistent Nonblanchable Deep Red, Maroon, or Purple Discoloration

Intact or nonintact skin with localized area of persistent nonblanchable deep red, maroon, or purple discoloration or epidermal separation revealing a dark wound bed or blood-filled blister. Pain and temperature change often precede skin color changes. Discoloration may appear differently in darkly pigmented skin. This injury results from intense and/or prolonged pressure and shear forces at the bone-muscle interface. The wound may evolve rapidly to reveal the actual extent of tissue injury or may resolve without tissue loss. If necrotic tissue, subcutaneous tissue, granulation tissue, fascia, muscle, or other underlying structures are visible, this indicates a full-thickness pressure injury (unstageable, stage 3, or stage 4). Do not use DTPI to describe vascular, traumatic, neuropathic, or dermatological conditions (Bryant & Nix, 2024; EPUAP/NPIAP/PPPIA, 2019b).

Additional Pressure Injury Definitions
Medical Device–Related Pressure Injury

Medical device–related pressure injuries result from the use of devices designed and applied for diagnostic or therapeutic purposes. The resultant pressure injury generally conforms to the pattern or shape of the device. The injury should be staged using the staging system (Bryant & Nix, 2024).

Mucosal Membrane Pressure Injury

Mucosal membrane pressure injuries are found on mucous membranes with a history of a medical device in use at the location of the injury. Due to the anatomy of the tissue, these ulcers cannot be staged (Bryant & Nix, 2024).

Data from European Pressure Ulcer Advisory Panel (EPUAP), National Pressure Injury Advisory Panel (NPIAP), Pan Pacific Pressure Injury Alliance: *Treatment of pressure ulcers/injuries: Clinical Practice Guideline. The International Guideline,* Emily Haesler (editor). 2019a, EPUAP/NPIAP/PPPIA; European Pressure Ulcer Advisory Panel (EPUAP), National Pressure Injury Advisory Panel (NPIAP), Pan Pacific Pressure Injury Alliance: *Treatment of pressure ulcers/injuries: Quick reference guide,* Emily Haesler (editor). 2019b, EPUAP/NPIAP/PPPIA; and Bryant RA, Nix DP: Principles of wound healing and topical management. In Bryan RA, Nix DP, editors: *Acute and chronic wounds: intraprofessionals from novice to expert,* ed 6, St. Louis 2024, Mosby.
Images used with permission of the European Pressure Ulcer Advisory Panel (EPUAP), National Pressure Injury Advisory Panel (NPIAP), Pan Pacific Pressure Injury Alliance: *Treatment of pressure ulcers/injuries: Quick reference guide,* Emily Haesler (editor). 2019, EPUAP/NPIAP/PPPIA.

- Reports vary as to the number of patients who are at risk for and develop pressure injuries, but the number of patients who develop them is significant. Patients are now older, with more co-morbidities and mobility impairments putting them at increased risk (Bohn & Bryant, 2024; Brophy et al., 2021). These changes contribute to an increased number of patients at risk for developing pressure injuries. Therefore it is critical to respond with an aggressive preventive approach. As a nurse you must identify the factors that place your patients at risk for the development of pressure injuries. Once you identify these factors, begin interventions to reduce or relieve the negative effects of each factor.
- When a pressure injury develops, explore the factors that contributed to skin breakdown, vigorously attempt to minimize the effects of these variables, and use current wound-healing principles in the management of injuries (see Chapters 38 and 40).

PERSON-CENTERED CARE

- Pressure injuries and the associated treatments affect patients' lives emotionally, mentally, physically, economically, and socially. Patients are aware of the amount and quality of care they receive, including levels of comfort during dressing changes and the timing of interventions. The presence of a pressure injury increases hospital stays, rates of readmissions, and health care costs (Nix & Bryant, 2024; WOCN, 2016). Given that it affects a patient's quality of life, providing culturally appropriate information about treatment and wound-healing expectations is an important aspect of care.
- When planning care for a patient, consider issues such as skin tones, patient and family caregiver education, and the social effects of a pressure injury. Skin assessment depends on skin color, and detection becomes a challenge in dark-toned patients (Nix & Bryant, 2024; EPUAP/NPIAP/PPPIA, 2019b). Palpation in patients with darker skin tones is particularly important for identification of erythema in darkly pigmented skin. Redness in dark-toned skin is difficult to determine without the use of palpation and a comparison with other, unaffected body parts (Box 39.2).

- When providing pressure injury care, remember that in some cultures hair has significance and should not be shaved. When shaving is absolutely necessary to prevent pain or trauma from taping hair around an injury, you may need the help of a patient's family or cultural elder.
- When you educate patients and family caregivers, consider their primary language and reading ability when using printed materials. Use pictures to determine if reading skills are adequate for printed educational materials.
- Consider how the presence of a pressure injury will affect the patient's social situation (e.g., if a wound would prevent a patient from socializing in the community). The presence of a pressure injury can also cause pain and resultant disability, which affect family dynamics.

EVIDENCE-BASED PRACTICE

Pressure Injury Risk Assessment

Risk assessment is a central component of clinical practice aimed at identifying individuals susceptible to pressure injuries to target appropriate preventative strategies (Borchert, 2022; EPUAP/NPIAP/PPPIA, 2019a; EPUAP/NPIAP/PPPIA, 2019b). Pressure injury risk assessment tools such as the Braden Scale aid in identifying those patients at greatest risk (Nix & Bryant, 2024; Huang et al., 2021). Nurses recognize the importance of this risk assessment for the following reasons:

- On admission to an agency or clinical division, a complete skin assessment is part of the risk assessment screening policy in place in all health care settings (Nix & Bryant, 2024: EPUAP/NPIAP/PPPIA, 2019a; Borchert, 2022; WOCN, 2016).
- Daily skin assessment is recommended to detect early signs of pressure injury (Nix & Bryant, 2024).
- Skin integrity bundles that identify key areas of assessment, skin-care measures, repositioning, and pressure-reducing strategies are effective in reducing frequency and severity of pressure injuries in critically ill patients (EPUAP/NPIAP/PPPIA, 2019a).
- Use validated risk assessment scores to further improve identification of at-risk patients, such as patients with incontinence, poor nutrition, advanced age, mobility issues, elevated body

---

BOX 39.2

Person-Centered Care for Skin Assessment of Pressure Injuries: Patients With Dark Skin Tone

There is evidence that standard visual inspection for erythema and stage 1 pressure injuries are unreliable in individuals with dark skin tones or darkly pigmented skin. Areas of redness are more difficult to assess with darker skin tones (Nix, 2024; EPUAP/NPIAP/PPPIA, 2019a). Patients with darkly pigmented skin cannot be assessed for pressure injury risk by examining only skin color (WOCN, 2016).

1. Use natural lighting, but note that visual inspection techniques to identify pressure injuries are unreliable in darkly pigmented skin.
2. Carefully inspect any discoloration over pressure areas and surrounding skin for temperature changes, edema (nonpitting swelling), change in tissue consistency, and pain/discomfort at site (Nix, 2024; EPUAP/NPIAP/PPPIA, 2019a). Assess localized skin color changes. Any of the following may appear:
   - Skin color may not change or balance when pressure is applied.
   - Color changes occur at site of pressure, which differ from patient's usual skin color.
   - If patient previously had a pressure injury, that area of skin may be lighter than original color.
   - Localized area of skin may be darker than the natural skin tone or purple/blue or violet instead of red (Nix, 2024). Purple or maroon discoloration may indicate deep tissue injury (WOCN, 2016).

3. Assessment of skin temperature changes: Circumscribed area of intact skin may be warm to touch. As tissue changes color, intact skin will feel cool to touch. **NOTE:** Gloves may decrease sensitivity to changes in skin temperature (EPUAP/NPIAP/PPPIA, 2019a; WOCN, 2016).
   - Localized heat (inflammation) is detected by making comparisons to surrounding skin. Localized area of warmth eventually will be replaced by area of coolness, which is a sign of tissue devitalization.
4. Edema (nonpitting) may occur with induration of more than 15 mm in diameter and may appear taut and shiny.
5. Palpate tissue consistency in surrounding tissues to identify any changes in tissue consistency between area of injury and normal tissue (EPUAP/NPIAP/PPPIA, 2019a).
6. Patient complains of discomfort at a site that is predisposed to pressure injury development (e.g., bony prominence, under medical devices).

temperature, and smoking (Nix & Bryant, 2024; Hotaling & Black, 2021; EPUAP/NPIAP/PPPIA, 2019a).

- The Braden Scale is very reliable. Braden Scale scores are grouped according to level of risk: not at risk (>18), mild risk (15–18), moderate risk (13–14), high risk (10–12), and very high risk (9 or lower); a cutoff score of 18 is useful in identifying risk (Nix & Bryant, 2024; Huang et al., 2021).
- A modified Norton Scale, the optimized Norton Scale (oNS), had high pressure injury prediction in critically ill patients. In the critical care setting the oNS was easier to administer, more specific to critical care, and more focused on the vulnerabilities of patients with critical illness (Sullivan et al., 2020).

- In individuals at risk of pressure injuries, conduct a comprehensive skin assessment as soon as possible after admission or transfer to the health care agency or nursing division (or at the first visit in community settings), as part of every risk assessment, in an ongoing manner based on the clinical setting and the individual's degree of risk, and before the individual's discharge (EPUAP/NPIAP/PPPIA, 2019a; EPUAP/NPIAP/PPPIA, 2019b).
- Individuals with pressure injuries or those at risk for pressure injuries should be placed on a support surface rather than a standard hospital mattress (EPUAP/NPIAP/PPPIA, 2019a; WOCN, 2016). A support surface must not be selected based *solely* on the patient's wound assessment findings but rather on the patient's individual needs (Nix & Milne, 2024).
- The use of dressings, such as a soft silicone multilayered foam dressing, as part of pressure injury prevention helps to reduce the incidence of pressure injuries in at-risk patients (EPUAP/NPIAP/PPPIA, 2019a; EPUAP/NPIAP/PPPIA, 2019b).
- Medical devices are commonly used in hospital settings and can create pressure injuries (MDRPIs). When placing a medical device, ensure that the device is the correct size and shape for the patient and is properly secured, and follow the manufacturer's instructions (EPUAP/NPIAP/PPPIA, 2019a; EPUAP/NPIAP/PPPIA, 2019b). Prompt and routine assessment of skin under the device helps to reduce the risk for pressure injury, identifies early stages of skin breakdown, and prompts interventions (EPUAP/NPIAP/PPPIA, 2019a; EPUAP/NPIAP/PPPIA, 2019b). Other ways to help decrease the risk of MDRPI are to regularly rotate or reposition the medical device, provide support for medical device to reduce pressure and shear, and remove the medical device as soon as medically possible (EPUAP/NPIAP/PPPIA, 2019a; EPUAP/NPIAP/PPPIA, 2019b).

SAFETY GUIDELINES

- Routinely and consistently assess patients for individual risks for development of pressure injuries. Select and use an appropriate agency risk assessment tool (Nix & Bryant, 2024; Hotaling & Black, 2021). For example, a separate risk assessment tool is often used in the operative setting when patient is immobile or positioned on a hard surface for a length of time

(EPUAP/NPIAP/PPPIA, 2019a). **NOTE:** Risk assessment tools incorporate many, but not all, relevant risk factors. Clinical judgment, which is based on up-to-date best evidence, is an essential component of any risk assessment (EPUAP/NPIAP/PPPIA, 2019a; WOCN, 2016).

- Perform pressure injury risk assessment on all patients who have one or more risk factors when admitted to an acute care agency, home care, hospice, or an extended care agency (EPUAP/NPIAP/PPPIA, 2019a; WOCN, 2016).
- Assess and inspect skin on a schedule that is based on patient acuity, as well as if there is a change in the patient's condition. Note all pressure points, and document relevant skin assessment findings (Nix & Bryant, 2024; WOCN, 2016).
- Position patients to redistribute the amount and duration of pressure to prevent ischemic tissue injury. The development of pressure injuries—especially stage 3 or 4 injuries and any unstageable ulcers—in a care setting is a serious reportable event. These events are called "never" events, and the U.S. Department of Health and Human Services (USDHHS), Centers for Medicare and Medicaid Services (CMS) will not financially reimburse acute care hospitals if a patient acquires one of these injuries during hospitalization (CMS, 2022).
- Turn and reposition a patient often to redistribute pressure from the superficial capillaries and allow tissues to compensate for temporary ischemia. Use safe patient-handling measures to turn and reposition patients every 1 to 2 hours as their condition allows. Proper positioning helps minimize formation of pressure injuries (see Chapter 11).
- Specialized beds, overlays, and mattresses (see Chapter 13) redistribute pressure over the entire body surface to prevent excess pressure over bony prominences. By distributing pressure evenly over a patient's body surface, these support surfaces enable less pressure to be applied at the skin level (Nix & Milne, 2024). Place patients at high risk for pressure injury formation on these devices as soon as possible. Consider the use of a chair cushion to redistribute pressure when a patient is seated.
- Clean patients who are incontinent of stool or urine as soon as possible. Prolonged skin moisture and wetness from urinary and fecal incontinence is a risk factor for skin breakdown (Borchert, 2022). Protect areas subjected to repeated episodes of incontinence with a barrier ointment or barrier paste. Fecal containment devices are available (see Chapter 34).
- Use approaches to minimize shear. When repositioning patients, use lift sheets to reduce rubbing skin against sheets. Raise the head of the bed no more than 30 degrees (unless medically contraindicated) to prevent sliding and shear injury (WOCN, 2016).
- Adequate nutrition helps to prevent and treat pressure injuries (WOCN, 2016). A diet high in protein with enough calories, vitamins, and minerals helps maintain normal tissue status and promotes healing. With tissue injury, the body needs more calories for healing; nutrient deficiencies may result in impaired or delayed healing. Make sure that monitoring the nutritional status is part of your total assessment (WOCN, 2016).

◆ **SKILL 39.1** **Risk Assessment, Skin Assessment, and Prevention Strategies**

The goal in preventing the development of pressure injuries is early identification of an at-risk patient and the implementation of prevention strategies. The *Prevention and Treatment of Pressure Ulcers/Injuries: Quick Reference Guide 2019* (EPUAP/NPIAP/PPPIA, 2019b) presents findings from an extensive literature review on the prevention and management of pressure injuries. The *Clinical*

Practice Guideline (EPUAP/NPIAP/PPPIA, 2019a) identifies the best available evidence in the prevention and management of pressure injuries. Overall management goals include the following:

- Identify individuals at risk for developing pressure injuries and initiate A Pressure Injury Prevention Program (Nix & Bryant, 2024).

TABLE 39.1

Guidelines for Pressure Injury Risk Assessment

Level of Care	Initial	Reassessment
Acute care	Within 8 hours of admission (EPUAP/NPIAP/PPPIA, 2019a; EPUAP/NPIAP/PPPIA, 2019b)	• On a defined schedule (e.g., every 24–48 hours) • Whenever major change in patient's condition occurs
Critical care	On admission	• Every 24 hours
Long-term care	On admission	• Weekly for first 4 weeks after admission • Routinely on quarterly basis • Whenever patient's condition changes or deteriorates
Home care	On admission	• Every registered nurse visit

- Implement appropriate strategies and plans to:
  - Attain and maintain intact skin.
  - Prevent complications.
  - Promptly identify or manage complications.
  - Involve patient and family caregiver in self-management.
  - Implement cost-effective strategies and plans that prevent and treat pressure injuries.

The Braden Scale is a reliable clinical tool to assess the etiological factors contributing to pressure injury development (Borchert, 2022). The scale includes six risk factors that contribute to pressure injury risk: sensory perception (ability to respond meaningfully to pressure-related discomfort), moisture (degree to which skin is exposed to moisture), activity (degree of physical activity), mobility (ability to change and control body position), nutrition (usual food intake pattern), and friction and shear (Borchert, 2022; Huang et al., 2021). The total score and each subscale score should be used to implement prevention strategies for every deficit that is identified (McNichol et al., 2022).

Inspect a patient's skin and bony prominences on admission, following any change in the patient's condition, on transfer to a different level of care, and at least daily; check agency policy (Table 39.1) (Borchert, 2022). Remove medical devices or tape securing these devices, shoes, socks, antiembolic stockings, and heel and elbow protectors to inspect the skin under all medical devices (EPUAP/NPIAP/PPPIA, 2019b; WOCN, 2016). Inspect all bony prominences, including back of head, shoulders, rib cage, elbows, hips, ischium, sacrum, coccyx, knees, ankles, and heels (see Fig. 39.1). Palpate any reddened or discolored areas with a gloved finger to determine if the erythema (redness of the skin caused by dilation and congestion of the capillaries) blanches (lightens in color). Blanching is normal. If you palpate an area that does not blanch (abnormal reactive hyperemia), this area is a site for potential skin breakdown and is considered a stage 1 pressure injury.

When a patient has adhesive dressings or an adhesive medical device, assess periwound or peristomal skin for skin injury. Medical adhesive–related skin injury (MARSI) results in skin tears; if these are not treated properly or if the area is exposed to pressure, the risk for localized pressure injury increases (Bryant, 2024; Thayer et al., 2022; Fumarola et al., 2020).

Delegation

The skill of pressure injury risk assessment cannot be delegated to assistive personnel (AP). Instruct the AP to:
- Frequently change a patient's position and the specific positions individualized for the patient
- Keep a patient's skin dry and provide hygiene following fecal or urinary incontinence and exposure of skin from wound drainage
- Report any changes in a patient's skin, such as redness or a break
- Report any redness and/or abrasion from medical devices

Interprofessional Collaboration

- When a patient's risk for pressure injuries increases, a wound, ostomy, continence nurse or skin care specialist can identify specific skin care and positioning interventions to reduce the patient's risk for developing pressure injuries and preventing worsening of existing injury.

Equipment

- Risk assessment tool (Use agency-approved tool; see agency policy.)
- Electronic health record (EHR)
- Pressure-redistribution mattress, bed, and/or chair cushion
- Positioning aids
- Clean gloves

STEP	RATIONALE

ASSESSMENT

1. Identify patient using at least two identifiers (e.g., name and birthday or name and medical record number), according to agency policy.

2. Review electronic health record (EHR) to determine patient's age and history of dehydration, malnutrition, exposure to radiation therapy, underlying chronic conditions (e.g., diabetes mellitus, immunosuppression), erythema, and edema of the skin.

Ensures correct patient. Complies with The Joint Commission standards and improves patient safety (TJC, 2023).

Common risk factors for MARSI (Bryant, 2024; Fumarola et al., 2020).

STEP	RATIONALE
3. Review patient's EHR, including health provider's orders and nurses' notes, to assess patient's risk for pressure injury formation:	Determines need to administer preventive care and identifies specific factors that place patient at risk (EPUAP/NPIAP/PPPIA, 2019a; EPUAP/NPIAP/PPPIA, 2019b).
a. Paralysis or immobilization caused by injury, such as spinal cord injury, or restrictive devices (Hotaling & Black, 2021)	Patient is unable to turn or reposition independently to relieve pressure.
b. Presence of medical device such as nasogastric (NG) tube, oxygen equipment, artificial airways, drainage tubing, or mechanical devices (Nix & Bryant, 2024; Doughty & McNichol, 2022)	Medical devices have potential to exert pressure on patient's skin near or adjacent to devices such as artificial airways and drainage tubes (Borchert, 2022; Hotaling & Black, 2021; TJC, 2022).

Clinical Judgment *Perform frequent assessment around and under medical devices (Nix & Bryant, 2024). If not medically contraindicated, remove medical device to observe tissues under and around each medical device. Pressure area assumes same configuration or shape as medical device (Brophy et al., 2021; WOCN, 2016).*

STEP	RATIONALE
c. Sensory loss (e.g., hemiplegia, spinal cord injury)	Patient is unable to feel discomfort from pressure and does not independently change position.
d. Circulatory disorders (e.g., critical illness, vasopressor use, peripheral vascular diseases, vascular changes from diabetes mellitus, neuropathy)	Reduced perfusion, circulation, and oxygenation of tissue increase risk for pressure injury (EPUAP/NPIAP/PPPIA, 2019b; Hotaling & Black, 2021).
e. Prone positioning	The prone position increases risk for pressure injury because there is little soft tissue padding on patient's forehead and upper chest area. Extra padding and more frequent skin assessments are needed (Hotaling & Black, 2021).
f. Fever	Increases metabolic demands of tissues. Accompanying diaphoresis leaves skin moist.
g. Anemia	Decreased hemoglobin level reduces oxygen-carrying capacity of blood and amount of oxygen available to tissues.
h. Malnutrition	Inadequate nutrition leads to weight loss, muscle atrophy, and reduced tissue mass. Nutrient deficiencies result in impaired or delayed healing (Brophy et al., 2021).
i. Fecal or urinary incontinence	Skin becomes exposed to moist environment, which alters skin flora. Excessive moisture macerates skin, which can lead to pressure injuries (Johansen et al., 2023).
j. Heavy sedation and anesthesia	Heavy sedation and prolonged anesthesia increase risk for pressure injury (Hotaling & Black, 2021). Patient is not mentally alert and does not turn or change position independently.
k. Age	Neonates and very young children are at high risk, with the head being the most common site of pressure injury occurrence (Hockenberry et al., 2024). There is loss of dermal thickness in older adults, impairing ability to distribute pressure (Rogers, 2023).
l. Dehydration	Results in decreased skin elasticity and turgor.
m. Edema	Edematous tissues are less tolerant of pressure, friction, and shear.
n. Existing pressure injuries or history of pressure injury	Specific information from a patient's history can help determine any potential risk factors for wound development and potential for nonhealing (Mondragon & Zito, 2022).
4. Select agency-approved risk assessment tool. Perform risk assessment when patient enters health care setting and repeat on regularly scheduled basis or when there is significant change in patient's condition (TJC, 2022).	Identifying risk factors that contribute to the potential for skin breakdown allows you to target specific interventions for decreasing risk for skin breakdown (Nix & Bryant, 2024).

Clinical Judgment *In acute care settings, perform initial assessment within 8 hours of admission and reassess every 24 hours or as patient condition changes; in critical care areas, perform assessment on admission and reassess every 24 hours or as patient condition changes; and in long-term and home care settings, perform assessment on admission. In long-term care settings, reassess weekly and then according to agency standards or when patient condition changes. In home care settings, reassess with every registered nurse visit.*

STEP	RATIONALE
5. Obtain risk score (see Table 39.1) and evaluate its meaning based on patient's condition and unique risk factors. When using the Braden Scale, there are risk scores identified for specific patient populations: intensive care patients, score less than 18 (Huang et al., 2021); older adults, score of 14 or lower (Alderden et al., 2017; Cox et al., 2022).	Risk cutoff score depends on instrument and patient's condition. Score involves identifying risk factors that contributed to it and minimizing these specific deficits (Hotaling & Black, 2021; EPUAP/NPIAP/PPPIA, 2019a).

STEP	RATIONALE
6. Assess patient's/family caregiver's health literacy.	Determines degree to which individuals have the ability to find, understand, and use information and services to make informed health-related decision and actions for themselves and others (Centers for Disease Control and Prevention [CDC], 2023).
7. Provide privacy and explain procedure.	Protects patient's privacy; reduces anxiety. Promotes cooperation.
8. Perform hand hygiene. Assess condition of patient's skin over regions of pressure (see Fig. 39.1). Apply clean gloves as needed with open and/or draining wounds.	Body weight against bony prominences places underlying skin at risk for breakdown.
a. Inspect for skin discoloration (see Box 39.2 for patients with darkly pigmented skin) and tissue consistency (firm or boggy feel) and/or palpate for abnormal sensations (Nix & Bryant, 2024; Pusey-Reid et al., 2023).	Indicates that tissue was under pressure; hyperemia is a normal physiological response to hypoxemia in tissues.
b. Palpate discolored area on skin and under and around medical devices, release your fingertip, and look for blanching. If on palpation an area of redness blanches (lightens in color), this indicates normal reactive hyperemia; tissue is not at risk for the development of an injury.	Blanchable erythema should resolve within 30 minutes of off-loading. If it persists, consider a support surface or change the repositioning schedule (Borchert, 2022). Tissue that does not blanch when palpated indicates abnormal reactive hyperemia; indication of possible stage 1 pressure injury.
c. Inspect for pallor and mottling.	Persistent hypoxia in tissues that were under pressure; an abnormal physiological response.
d. Inspect for absence of superficial skin layers.	Represents early pressure injury formation; usually a partial-thickness wound that may have resulted from shear.
e. Inspect for changes in skin temperature, edema, and tissue consistency, especially in individuals with darkly pigmented skin (EPAUP/NPIAP/PPPIA, 2019a; EPAUP/NPIAP/PPPIA, 2019b).	Localized heat, edema, and induration have been identified as warning signs for pressure injury development. Because it is not always possible to observe changes in skin color on darkly pigmented skin, these additional signs should be considered in assessment (EPUAP/NPIAP/PPPIA, 2019a; Pusey-Reid et al., 2023).
f. Inspect for wound drainage.	Wound drainage increases risk for skin breakdown because it is caustic to skin and underlying tissues.
	Tubing from drainage devices (e.g., Jackson-Pratt, Hemovac) causes pressure under device and on adjacent skin (Hotaling & Black, 2021; EPUAP/NPIAP/PPPIA, 2019a).
9. Assess skin and tissue around and beneath medical devices twice daily for areas of potential pressure injury resulting from medical devices (Nix & Bryant, 2024; Brophy et al., 2021; EPUAP/NPIAP/PPPIA, 2019a) (Table 39.2).	Patients at high risk need more frequent assessments and have multiple sites for pressure necrosis from medical devices in areas other than bony prominences (Chaboyer et al., 2017). Patients at higher risk of medical device–related pressure injuries (MDRPIs) are those who require mechanical ventilation or who are vulnerable to fluid shifts and/or edema (EPUAP/NPIAP/PPPIA, 2019a).
	Pressure points around medical devices (e.g., oxygen cannula and masks, drainage tubing) can cause pressure injury to underlying tissue and can become full-thickness pressure injuries (EPUAP/NPIAP/PPPIA, 2019a). Typically the MDRPI conforms to the same size and shape as the medical device that caused the injury (EPUAP/NPIAP/PPPIA, 2019a).
a. Nares: NG tube, oxygen cannula	Pressure to nares occurs from tape and other materials used to secure NG tube.
b. Ears: oxygen cannula, pillow	Oxygen equipment is a significant risk for pressure injuries (Duerst et al., 2022; Padula et al., 2017). Patients' ears and tips of nares are at risk for pressure from nasal cannula (Yiğitoğlu & Aydoğan, 2023).
c. Tongue and lips: oral airway, endotracheal (ET) tube	Mucosal tissues of the mouth are at increased risk for MDRPI as the devices placed to secure an artificial airway cause pressure on the mucosa, which causes the skin to become ischemic and leads to ulceration (EPUAP/NPIAP/PPPIA, 2019a).
d. Forehead: pulse oximetry device	May cause pressure injury to forehead or ears due to the securement device.
e. Drainage or other tubing	Stress and pressure against tissue can occur at exit site or from tubing lying under any part of patient's body.

STEP	RATIONALE
f. Indwelling urethral (Foley) catheter	The urinary meatus orifice is at risk for pressure injury when an indwelling urinary catheter is in place (Saleh & Ibrahim, 2023).
g. Orthopedic and positioning devices such as casts, neck collars, splints	Applied devices have potential to cause pressure to underlying and adjacent skin and tissue.
h. Compression stockings	Compression stockings have potential to cause pressure, especially if they fit poorly or are rolled down.

Clinical Judgment *Compression stockings must be completely removed for adequate assessment of the feet, heels, and legs.*

i. Immobilization device and restraints	If device is too tight or poorly placed or if patient strains, pressure points occur under it.
10. Remove and dispose of gloves and perform hand hygiene.	Reduces transmission of microorganisms.

TABLE 39.2

Strategies to Prevent Medical and Immobilization Device–Related Pressure Injuries

Device	Pressure Areas	Prevention Strategies[a]
Nasogastric tubes	Nares Skin on nasal bridge	Secure tube using pressure-relieving techniques, which direct the pressure from the tube away from the nares (see Chapters 32 and 35). Reposition tube.
Endotracheal tubes	Lips Tongue	Tubes should be moved laterally to relieve pressure over different portions of the lips and tongue (EPUAP/NPIAP/PPPIA, 2019a). Ensure that the depth of the endotracheal tube does not change when moving the tube laterally (EPUAP/NPIAP/PPPIA, 2019a).
Nasotracheal tube	Nose/nasal bridge Nares	Remove securing device daily and inspect for pressure injury (EPUAP/NPIAP/PPPIA, 2019a; Yiğitoğlu & Aydoğan, 2023). Reposition.
Tracheostomy tube	Front of neck and stoma site Back of neck	Remove securing device daily. Apply dressing to back of neck.
Oxygen cannula and tubing	Ears Nose	Apply dressing to external ear. Periodically remove cannula to relieve pressure and inspect for pressure injury (EPUAP/NPIAP/PPPIA, 2019a; Yiğitoğlu & Aydoğan, 2023). Use soft silicone oxygen tubing.
Noninvasive positive-pressure ventilation (NIPPV)/bi-level positive airway pressure (BiPAP)	Forehead Nose/nasal bridge	Pretreat bridge of nose and nasolabial folds with dressing before application of mask. If possible, remove mask for a few minutes.
Drainage tubing	Area immediately next to drainage tube Adjacent area during patient position changes	Apply appropriate dressing around drainage tube. Check tubing placement with each position change. Instruct patient not to lie on the tubing.
Indwelling catheter	Thighs Female: urethra, labia Male: tip of penis	Provide meticulous perineal care. Anchor and secure catheter to reduce pressure.
Orthopedic device	All areas where device comes in contact with patient's skin and tissues	When possible and not contraindicated, inspect under the device.
Neck collar	Neck and occipital region Scalp	Remove hard collars as soon as possible and replace with softer collar (Wang et al., 2020). Inspect scalp daily.
Compression stockings	Calf Behind knee Heel Toes	Verify proper fit. To reduce pressure and risk of injury to skin and underlying tissue, remove stockings twice daily for at least 1 hour (Garcia et al., 2022).
Immobilization device	Wrists Ankles	Apply padding or dressing between patient's skin and immobilizer. Verify space between immobilizer and patient's skin. With assistive personnel present, remove restraints one at a time to inspect skin.

[a]In addition to routine inspection and cleaning of skin under and around medical device.

STEP	RATIONALE
11. Observe patient for preferred positions in bed or chair.	Preferred positions result in weight of body being placed on certain bony prominences. Presence of contractures may result in pressure exerted in unexpected places.
12. Observe ability of patient to initiate and help with position changes.	Potential for friction and shear increases when patient is completely dependent on others for position changes.
13. Assess knowledge and prior experience with pressure injury prevention techniques and feelings about procedure.	Reveals need for patient instruction and/or support.

PLANNING

1. Expected outcomes following completion of procedure: • Risk factors are identified. • Patient experiences no change from baseline skin assessment. • Skin is intact with no evidence of erythema and no signs of breakdown. • Patient and family caregiver learn patient's personal risk factors for pressure injury.	Establishes baseline for future assessment. Prevention guidelines prevent occurrence or worsening of pressure injury. Prevention strategies reduce risk factors. Demonstrates learning.
2. Close room door or pull the curtain around the bed and position the patient so that only the area currently being examined is exposed.	Provides privacy and exposed area for assessment.
3. Prepare and organize equipment. Be sure you have correct risk assessment tool at bedside.	Preparing equipment before the procedure helps to ensure a clean and distraction-free area for organizing procedure-related equipment.
4. Explain procedure(s) and purpose to patient and family caregiver.	Reveals need for patient instruction and/or support.
5. Arrange for extra personnel to help as necessary. Organize supplies at bedside.	Some patients are unable to assume positioning independently for procedure.

IMPLEMENTATION

1. Implement Pressure Injury Prevention guidelines according to agency policy.	Reduces patient's risk for developing pressure injury (Nix & Bryant, 2024).
2. Perform hand hygiene and apply clean gloves.	Reduces transmission of microorganisms.
3. Raise bed to appropriate working height. Raise side rail on opposite side of bed and lower side rail on working side.	Promotes good body mechanics. Use of side rails in this manner promotes patient safety.
4. Following initial assessment, continue to inspect skin at least once a day. a. Observe patient's skin; pay particular attention to bony prominences and areas around and under medical devices and tubes. If you find reddened area, gently press area with gloved finger to check for blanching. If area does not blanch, suspect tissue injury and recheck in 30 minutes to 1 hour. Any discoloration may vary from pink to deep red.	Routine skin inspection is fundamental to risk assessment and in selecting interventions to reduce risk (Nix & Bryant, 2024; TJC, 2022). Persistent redness when lightly pigmented skin is pressed can indicate tissue injury.

Clinical Judgment *Do not massage reddened areas because doing so may cause additional tissue trauma. Reddened areas indicate blood vessel damage, and massaging has the potential to damage underlying tissues (Nix & Bryant, 2024; EPUAP/NPIAP/PPPIA, 2019a).*

b. If patient has darkly pigmented skin, look for color changes that differ from the patient's normal skin color.	Darkly pigmented skin may not blanch. A change in color may occur at the site of pressure; this change in color differs from patient's usual skin color (EPUAP/NPIAP/PPPIA, 2019a; EPUAP/NPIAP/PPPIA, 2019b) (see Box 39.2).
5. Each shift, check all treatment and assistive devices (catheters, feeding tubes, casts, braces) for potential pressure points (see Table 39.2).	Pressure from these devices increases risk for injury on bony prominences and other areas.
a. Verify that device is correctly sized, positioned, and secured.	Incorrect size, placement, and securing of medical device can cause excessive pressure and rubbing by device on underlying skin (Nix & Bryant, 2024; EPUAP/NPIAP/PPPIA, 2019a).
b. Consider shielding underlying at-risk skin with protective dressing (silicone, hydrocolloid).	These dressings absorb moisture from body and reduce pressure to underlying skin (EPUAP/NPIAP/PPPIA, 2019a; WOCN, 2016).

Clinical Judgment *Inspect skin around and beneath orthopedic devices (e.g., cervical collar, braces, or cast). Note any abrasions or warmth in areas where devices can rub against the skin. In addition, a medical device can result in an altered microclimate at the skin-device interface, thus increasing the risks for injury (Nix & Bryant, 2024; EPUAP/NPIAP/PPPIA, 2019a).*

STEP	RATIONALE

6. Remove and dispose of gloves; perform hand hygiene.

Reduces transmission of microorganisms.

7. Review patient's pressure injury risk assessment score.

Risk scores aid in identifying interventions to lessen or eliminate present risk factors.

8. If immobility, inactivity, or poor sensory perception is a risk factor for patient, consider one of the following interventions (WOCN, 2016):

Immobility and inactivity reduce patient's ability or desire to independently change position. Poor sensory perception decreases patient's ability to feel sensation of pressure or discomfort.

   a. Reposition patient based on frequent assessment findings of individual's skin condition and risk factors to identify early signs of pressure damage. If skin changes occur, reevaluate the positioning plan (Nix & Bryant, 2024).

Reduces duration and intensity of pressure. Some patients may require more frequent repositioning (Nix & Bryant, 2024; EPUAP/NPIAP/PPPIA, 2019a; WOCN, 2016).

   b. When patient is in side-lying position in bed, use 30-degree lateral position (see illustration). Avoid 90-degree lateral position.

Reduces direct contact of trochanter with support surface.

   c. Place patient (when lying in bed) on pressure-redistribution surface.

Reduces amount of pressure exerted on tissues.

   d. Place patient (when in chair) on pressure-redistribution device and shift points under pressure at least every hour (Nix & Milne, 2024; WOCN, 2016).

Reduces amount of pressure on sacral and ischial areas.

9. If friction and shear are identified as risk factors, consider the following interventions:

Friction and shear damage underlying skin.

   a. Use safe patient-handling guidelines to reposition patient (see Chapter 11). For example, use slide board to transfer patient from bed to stretcher.

Proper repositioning of patient prevents creating shear from dragging patient along sheets. Slide board provides slippery surface to reduce friction. Use of lift team when appropriate raises patient's skin off sheets.

   b. Ensure that heels are free from bed surface by using a pillow under calves to elevate heels or use a heel-suspension device; knees should be in 5- to 10-degree flexion (EPUAP/NPIAP/PPPIA, 2019a; WOCN, 2016).

"Floating" heels from bed surface offloads the heel completely and redistributes the weight of the leg along the calf without applying pressure on the Achilles tendon (EPUAP/NPIAP/PPPIA, 2019a).

   c. Maintain head of the bed at 30 degrees or lower or at the lowest degree of elevation consistent with patient's condition (do not lower head of bed if patient is at risk for aspiration) (WOCN, 2016).

Decreases potential for patient to slide toward foot of bed and incur shear injury.

10. If patient receives low score on moisture subscale, consider one of the following interventions:

Continual exposure of body fluids on patient's skin increases risk for skin breakdown and pressure injury development.

   a. Apply clean gloves. Clean and dry the skin as soon as possible after each incontinence episode (WOCN, 2016). Apply moisture barrier ointment to perineum and surrounding skin after each incontinence episode.

Friction and shear are enhanced in the presence of moisture. Protects skin from fecal or urinary incontinence.

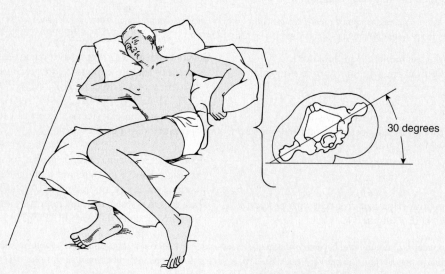

STEP 8b Thirty-degree lateral position with pillow placement.

STEP	RATIONALE
b. If skin is denuded, use protective barrier after each incontinence episode.	Provides barrier between skin and stool/urine, allowing for healing.
c. If moisture source is from wound drainage, consider frequent dressing changes, skin protection with protective barriers, or collection devices.	Removes frequent exposure of wound drainage from skin.
11. If friction and shear are risk factors and patient is chair bound:	Relief of pressure by changing from lying to sitting position is insufficient if sitting lasts a prolonged time. The maximum amount of time a patient can sit before there is a need to reposition is unknown (Nix & Bryant, 2024; WOCN, 2016).
a. Tilt patient's chair seat to prevent sliding forward, and support arms, legs, and feet to maintain proper posture (EPUAP/NPIAP/PPPIA, 2019a).	
b. Limit amount of time patient spends in a chair without pressure relief (EPUAP/NPIAP/PPPIA, 2019a).	
c. For patients who can reposition themselves while sitting, encourage pressure relief every 15 minutes using chair push-ups, forward lean, or side to side (WOCN, 2016).	
12. Educate patient and family caregiver regarding specific pressure injury risk factors and prevention.	Helps patients and family caregiver understand and adhere to interventions designed to reduce pressure injury risk (Nix & Bryant, 2024; Berlowitz et al., 2022).
13. Remove and dispose of gloves; perform hand hygiene.	Reduces transmission of microorganisms.
14. Help patient to a comfortable position.	Restores comfort and sense of well-being.
15. Raise side rails (as appropriate) and lower bed to lowest position, locking into position.	Ensures patient safety and prevents falls.
16. Place nurse call system in an accessible location within patient's reach.	Ensures patient can call for assistance if needed.
17. Perform hand hygiene.	Reduces transmission of microorganisms.

EVALUATION

1. Observe patient's skin for areas at risk for tissue damage, noting change in color, appearance, or texture.	Enables you to evaluate success of prevention techniques.
2. Observe tolerance of patient for position change by measuring level of comfort on pain scale.	Position changes sometimes interfere with patient's sleep and rest pattern.
3. Compare subsequent risk assessment scores and skin assessments.	Provides ongoing comparison of patient's risk level to facilitate appropriateness of plan of care.
4. Use Teach-Back: "I want you to understand why we need to assess your skin on an ongoing basis. Tell me in your own words why we will be checking your skin on a regular basis." Revise your instruction now or develop a plan for revised patient/family caregiver teaching if patient/family caregiver is not able to teach back correctly.	Teach-back is a technique for health care providers to ensure that they have explained medical information clearly so that patients and their families understand what is communicated to them (AHRQ, 2023).

Unexpected Outcomes

1. Skin becomes mottled, reddened, purplish, or bluish.

2. Areas under pressure develop persistent discoloration, induration, or temperature changes.

Related Interventions

- Refer patient to wound, ostomy, continence nurse; dietitian; clinical nurse specialist (CNS); nurse practitioner (NP); and/or physical therapist as needed. Reevaluate position changes and bed surface.

- Refer patient to wound, ostomy, continence nurse; dietitian; CNS; NP; and/or physical therapist as needed.
- Modify patient's positioning and turning schedule.

Documentation

- Document any skin changes, patient's risk score, and skin assessment. Describe positions, turning intervals, pressure-redistribution devices, and other prevention measures. Note patient's response to the interventions.
- Document your evaluation of patient's and family caregiver's understanding of the need for frequent skin and pressure injury assessment education.

Hand-Off Reporting

- Report need for additional consultations for the high-risk patient to health care provider.

Special Considerations
Patient Education

- Help patient and family caregiver understand multiple factors involved in preventing and treating pressure injuries.

- Explain and demonstrate positioning options to achieve pressure redistribution.
- Explain the purpose and maintenance of pressure-redistribution devices (see Chapter 13).
- When teaching patients to change position for pressure redistribution, suggest using television programming and commercial intervals or a watch with an alarm as reminders.

Pediatrics

- Infants and young children in diapers are at risk for skin breakdown.
- Neonatal and pediatric populations have immature skin that is less resistant to pressure and are at risk for pressure injury and MDRPI because medical equipment may not fit properly (Nix & Bryant, 2024).
- Use an agency-approved scale to assess risk and prevention of hospital-acquired pressure injuries in infants and young children (Liao et al., 2018).

Older Adults

- Reevaluate sitting posture and position because body weight and muscle tone change with age.
- In older adults the dermis is not thick. Skin over the legs and forearms is especially thin. There is less subcutaneous tissue,

leading to less padding protection over bony prominences, and the time for epidermal regeneration is diminished, leading to slower healing (Rogers, 2023).

Populations With Disabilities

- Some disabled patients may not have sensation that warns them of impending skin injury due to neurological injuries (e.g., spinal cord injury, after cerebrovascular accident). This population is at great risk for skin injury.

Home Care

- Identify community resources such as neighbors and relatives to provide help if patient needs help with position changes.
- Closely monitor home care patients for pressure injury development if they have any of the following risk factors: wheelchair or bed dependence, incontinence, anemia, fracture, and/or skin drainage.
- Remind patient and family caregiver that position changes need to occur while a patient is sitting in a chair. Consider shifts in position every 15 minutes. Small shifts such as moving or repositioning the legs redistribute pressure over bony prominences (WOCN, 2016).

◆ SKILL 39.2   **Treatment of Pressure Injuries**

 Video Clip

The principles of managing patients with pressure injuries include systematic support of patients, reduction or elimination of the cause of skin breakdown, and management that provides an environment conducive to healing. Once you find the cause of the pressure injury, use clinical judgment to take steps to control or eliminate it. For example, if the injury is related to unrelieved pressure, choose the appropriate pressure-redistribution surface, develop a turning schedule, reposition tubing from medical equipment, or choose the appropriate chair pad. Next, assess the patient's wound-healing abilities: cardiovascular and pulmonary function, nutritional status, and conditions that interfere with wound healing such as diabetes mellitus, steroid administration, and immunosuppression (Al Aboud & Manna, 2023). Wound assessment tools such as the Bates-Jensen Wound Assessment Tool (BWAT) (Gupta et al., 2023) and the Pressure Ulcer Scale for Healing (PUSH) tool can help to determine the individual treatment goals for different pressure injuries.

The best environment for wound healing is moist and free of necrotic tissue and infection. Perform a thorough assessment of the wound and the periwound skin before initiating wound therapy. No specific studies demonstrate the benefit of using one cleanser over another for pressure injuries. In most cases water or saline is sufficient for cleansing a clean wound (WOCN, 2016). Hydrogen peroxide was once widely used but is now known to cause tissue damage. When a wound is contaminated with debris, necrotic tissue, or heavy drainage, use a cleaner that is noncytotoxic to healthy tissue. If the tissue in the wound is devitalized, consult with a patient's health care provider to consider debridement, which is the removal of devitalized tissue. Debridement is accomplished by the choice of dressing and the use of enzyme preparations or surgical techniques. The choice of the type of debridement depends on a patient's overall condition, the condition of the wound, and the type of devitalized tissue (WOCN, 2016).

Choose wound dressings to meet the characteristics of the wound bed (Borchert, 2022; Britto et al., 2023). The type of dressings to use will change as the pressure injury characteristics change; frequent wound assessment is key. The choice of a wound dressing depends on the type of wound tissue in the base of the wound, the amount of wound drainage, the presence or absence of infection, the location of the wound, the size of the wound, the ease of use, cost-effectiveness, and patient comfort. Categories of wound dressings include transparent films, hydrocolloids, hydrogels, foams, calcium alginates, gauze, and antimicrobial dressings (see Chapter 40).

Advanced wound care therapies used in select cases include growth factors, electrical stimulation, and negative-pressure wound therapy (NPWT). Growth factors occur naturally in wound fluid; they regulate cell proliferation and differentiation and are considered in the treatment of stage 3 and 4 pressure injuries that have delayed healing (EPUAP/NPIAP/PPPIA, 2019a). Electrical stimulation induces intermittent muscle contractions and reduces the risk of pressure injury development in individuals with spinal cord injury by increasing muscle mass and improving blood flow and oxygenation (EPUAP/NPIAP/PPPIA, 2019a). In NPWT, subatmospheric (negative) pressure is applied to the wound bed through suction to facilitate healing and collect wound fluid (Nix & Bryant 2022; Netsch, 2022) (see Chapter 39).

Delegation

The skill of treating pressure injuries and dressing changes cannot be delegated to assistive personnel (AP). Instruct the AP to:

- Report immediately to the nurse pain, fever, or any wound drainage
- Report immediately to the nurse any change in skin integrity
- Report any potential contamination to existing dressing, such as patient incontinence or dislodgement of the dressing

Interprofessional Collaboration

- Plan a dressing change with the wound care team to assess the status of the wound together to determine effectiveness of the treatment plan and if the wound is showing progress toward healing.

Equipment

- Protective equipment: clean gloves, goggles, cover gown (if splash is a risk)
- Sterile gloves (optional)
- Plastic bag for dressing disposal
- Wound-measuring device
- Sterile cotton-tipped applicators (check agency policy for use of sterile applicators)
- Normal saline or cleansing agent (as ordered)
- Topical agent or solution (as ordered)
- Dressing of choice based on patient wound characteristics (see Chapter 40, Table 40.1)
- Hypoallergenic tape (if needed)
- Irrigation syringe (optional)
- Scale for assessing wound healing

STEP	RATIONALE

ASSESSMENT

STEP	RATIONALE
1. Identify patient using at least two identifiers (e.g., name and birthday or name and medical record number), according to agency policy.	Ensures correct patient. Complies with The Joint Commission standards and improves patient safety (TJC, 2023).
2. Review patient's electronic health record (EHR), including health care provider's order and nurses' notes. Note previous dressing change for wound assessment, types of topical medications, types of analgesia if needed, and wound care supplies.	Identifies purpose of treatment of pressure injury. Ensures administration of proper medications and treatments for specific wound care needs.

Clinical Judgment *Determine if the order is consistent with established wound care guidelines and outcomes for a patient. If the order is not consistent with guidelines or varies from the identified outcome for a patient, review with the health care team.*

STEP	RATIONALE
3. Review EHR to determine patient's age and history of dehydration, malnutrition, exposure to radiation therapy, underlying chronic conditions (e.g., diabetes mellitus, immunosuppression), and edema of the skin.	Common risk factors for medical adhesive–related skin injury (MARSI) (Fumarola et al., 2020).
4. Assess patient/family caregiver's health literacy.	Determines degree to which individuals have the ability to find, understand, and use information and services to make informed health-related decisions and actions for themselves and others (CDC, 2023).
5. Assess patient's knowledge, prior experience with treatment of pressure injuries, and feelings about procedure.	Reveals need for patient instruction and/or support.
6. Assess character of patient's pain and rate acuity on a pain scale of 0 to 10. If patient is in pain, determine if prn pain medication has been ordered and administer.	Dressing change should not be traumatic for patient; evaluate wound pain before, during, and after wound care management (Britto et al., 2023).
7. Ask patient and check EHR for history of allergies. Check allergy bracelet. Determine if patient has allergies to topical agents.	Topical agents and dressings could contain elements that cause localized skin reactions.
8. Provide privacy and explain procedure.	Protects patient's privacy; reduces anxiety. Promotes cooperation.
9. Position patient to allow dressing removal and position plastic bag for dressing disposal.	Provides an accessible area for dressing change. Proper disposal of old dressing promotes proper handling of contaminated waste.
10. Perform hand hygiene and apply clean gloves. Remove and discard old dressing.	Reduces transmission of microorganisms and prevents accidental exposure to body fluids.
11. Assess patient's wounds using wound parameters and continue ongoing wound assessment per agency policy. **NOTE:** This may be done during wound care procedure.	Determines effectiveness of wound care and guides treatment plan of care (WOCN, 2016).
a. *Wound location:* Describe body site where wound is located.	
b. *Stage of wound:* Describe extent of tissue destruction (see Box 39.1).	Staging is a way of assessing a pressure injury based on depth of tissue destruction.
c. *Wound size:* Length, width, and depth of wound are measured per agency protocol. Use disposable measuring guide for length and width. Use cotton-tipped applicator to assess depth (see illustration).	Injury size changes as healing progresses; therefore longest and widest areas of wound change over time. Measuring width and length by measuring consistent areas provides consistent measurement. Wound size influences therapies needed (Foltynski et al., 2021).
d. *Presence of undermining, sinus tracts, or tunnels:* Use sterile cotton-tipped applicator to measure depth, undermining, or sinus tracts.	Wound depth determines amount of tissue loss.

STEP	RATIONALE

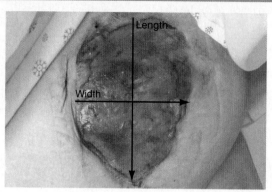

STEP 11c Measuring wound width, length, and undermining of skin. (*From Bryant RA, Nix DP: Acute and chronic wounds: intraprofessionals from novice to expert, ed 6, St. Louis, 2024, Elsevier.*)

e. *Condition of wound bed:* Describe type and percentage of tissue in wound bed.	Approximate percentage of each type of tissue in wound provides critical information on progress of wound healing and choice of dressing. Wound with high percentage of black tissue may require debridement; yellow tissue or slough tissue may indicate presence of infection or colonization; and granulation tissue indicates that wound is moving toward healing (EPUAP/NPIAP/PPPIA, 2019a).
f. *Volume of exudate:* Describe amount, characteristics, odor, and color.	Amount and type of exudate may indicate type and frequency of dressing changes (Bates-Jensen, 2022).
g. *Condition of periwound skin:* Examine skin for breaks, dryness, and presence of rash, swelling, redness, or warmth. Modify assessment based on patient's skin color (see Box 39.2).	Impaired periwound skin indicates progressive tissue damage (EPUAP/NPIAP/PPPIA, 2019a). Maceration on periwound skin shows need to alter choice of wound dressing.
h. *Wound edges:* With a gloved finger, examine wound edges for condition of tissue.	Gives information regarding epithelialization, chronicity, and etiology.
12. Assess periwound skin; check for maceration, redness, or denuded tissue.	Periwound skin is fragile and must be protected from further injury. Skin condition determines if skin barrier is needed (EPUAP/NPIAP/PPPIA, 2019a).
13. Remove gloves and discard in appropriate receptacle. Perform hand hygiene.	Reduces transmission of microorganisms. Repeated hand hygiene is needed as you assess other pressure areas. Different organisms contaminate different wounds.
14. Assess for factors affecting wound healing: poor perfusion, immunosuppression, or preexisting infection.	Factors affect treatment and wound healing.
15. Assess patient's nutritional status (see Chapter 30). Clinically significant malnutrition is present if (1) anemia or (2) decreased serum albumin level occurs; or if (3) body weight decreases by 5% of body weight in 30 days (10% in 180 days), or body mass index (BMI) is less than 22 (Friedrich et al., 2022).	Delayed wound healing occurs in poorly nourished patients (EPUAP/NPIAP/PPPIA, 2019a; Friedrich et al., 2022).

Clinical Judgment *When you suspect malnutrition, consider a nutritional consultation to modify patient's diet to promote wound healing. Decreasing albumin levels occur in inflammatory conditions, liver dysfunction, and so on. A specific albumin level is not an indicator of impaired nutrition (Friedrich et al., 2022).*

16. Assess patient's knowledge, prior experience with prevention, treatment, and feelings about procedure.	Reveals need for patient instruction and/or support.

PLANNING

1. Expected outcomes following completion of procedure: • Wound drainage decreases.	Reflects decrease in inflammatory process and progress toward healing.
• Granulation tissue is present in wound base.	Evidence that wound is moving toward healing.
• Skin surrounding injury remains healthy and intact.	No additional damage is evident; dressing is appropriate to contain wound drainage.
• Nutritional intake meets caloric and nutrient targets.	Nutritional therapy provides adequate protein to support wound healing.

STEP	RATIONALE
• Patient's overall skin remains intact and without further breakdown.	Patient remains at risk for further breakdown while existing injury heals.
• Patient or family caregiver is able to describe signs of wound healing and wound deterioration.	Demonstrates learning.
2. Explain procedure to patient and family caregiver.	Preparatory explanations relieve anxiety, correct any misconceptions about injury and its treatment, and offer an opportunity for patient and family caregiver education.
3. Provide privacy.	Protects patient's privacy.
4. Organize and set up the following equipment and supplies:	Ensures more efficiency when completing an assessment.
a. Wash basin, warm water, equipment, and supplies	
b. Normal saline or other wound-cleaning agent	Clean wound surface before applying topical agents and new dressing.
c. Prescribed topical agent:	
(1) Enzyme debriding agents (Follow specific manufacturer's directions for frequency of application.)	Enzymes debride dead tissue to clean injury surface and do not injure healthy tissue.
Or	
(2) Topical antibiotics	Topical antibiotics decrease bioburden of wound and should be considered for use if no healing is noted after 2 to 4 weeks of optimal care (WOCN, 2016).
d. Select appropriate dressing based on pressure injury characteristics, principles of wound management, and patient care setting. Dressing options include (see Chapter 40):	Dressing should maintain moist environment for wound while keeping surrounding skin dry (Jaszarowsski & Murphee, 2022).
(1) Gauze—Apply as moist dressing, a dry cover dressing when using enzymes or topical antibiotics, or a means to deliver solution to wound (see Chapter 40)	Gauze delivers moisture to wound and is absorptive.
(2) Transparent film dressing—Apply over superficial injuries with minimal or no exudate and skin subjected to friction	Maintains moist environment and offers intact skin protection.
(3) Hydrocolloid dressing	Maintains moist environment to facilitate wound healing while protecting wound base.

Clinical Judgment *Research shows that routine use of a hydrocolloid dressing may not be effective to promote healing of a pressure injury. Use clinical judgment to analyze wound symptoms, clinical experience, patient preference, and the cost of intervention prior to selecting a hydrocolloid product (Kaminska et al., 2020).*

STEP	RATIONALE
(4) Hydrogel—available in sheet or in tube	Maintains moist environment to facilitate wound healing.
(5) Calcium alginate	Highly absorbent of wound exudate in heavily draining wounds.
(6) Foam dressing	Protective and prevents wound dehydration; also absorbs moderate to large amounts of drainage.
(7) Silver-impregnated dressing or gel	Controls bacterial burden in wound.
(8) Wound fillers	Fills shallow wounds, hydrates, and absorbs.
e. Obtain hypoallergenic tape or adhesive dressing sheet	Used to secure nonadherent dressing. Prevents skin irritation and tearing.

IMPLEMENTATION

STEP	RATIONALE
1. Perform hand hygiene.	Reduces transmission of microorganisms.
2. Open sterile packages and topical solution containers (see Chapter 10). Keep dressings sterile. Wear goggles, mask, and moisture-proof cover gown if potential for contamination from spray exists when cleaning wound.	Reduces transmission of microorganisms.
3. Raise bed to appropriate working height. If side rails in use, raise side rail on opposite side of bed and lower side rail on working side.	Promotes good body mechanics. Use of side rails in this manner promotes patient safety.
4. Place waterproof pad under patient.	Prevents soiling bed linen.
5. Arrange patient's gown to expose injury and surrounding skin. Keep remaining body parts draped.	Prevents unnecessary exposure of body parts.
6. Clean wound thoroughly with normal saline or prescribed wound-cleaning agent (see Chapter 40) from least contaminated to most contaminated area. For deep injuries, clean with saline delivered with irrigating syringe as ordered. Remove gloves and discard.	Cleaning wound removes wound exudate, unwanted substances from the skin's surface, and/or dressing residue and reduces surface bacteria (EPUAP/NPIAP/PPPIA, 2019a).
7. Perform hand hygiene and apply clean or sterile gloves. (Refer to agency policy.)	Maintains aseptic technique during cleaning, measuring, and applying dressings.

STEP	RATIONALE
8. Apply topical agents to wound using cotton-tipped applicators or gauze as ordered:	
a. Enzymes	Follow manufacturer's directions for method and frequency of application. Enzymatic debridement is the topical application of enzymes such as collagenase over the necrotic tissue (Bryant & Nix, 2024). Be aware of which solutions inactivate enzymes, such as iodine and silver-based products, and avoid their use in wound cleaning (Ramundo, 2022).
(1) Apply small amount of enzyme debridement ointment directly to necrotic areas in pressure injury. *Do not apply enzyme to surrounding skin, as it may macerate the surrounding skin.*	Thin layer absorbs and acts more effectively than thick layer. Excess medication irritates surrounding skin (Bryant & Nix, 2024). Proper distribution of ointment ensures effective action.

Clinical Judgment *If using an enzymatic debriding agent, do not use iodine, silver-based products, or Dakin solution as wound-cleaning agents. Collagenase and other enzymatic agents are not compatible with these cleansing agents and are rendered ineffective (Ramundo, 2022).*

STEP	RATIONALE
(2) Place moist gauze dressing directly over injury and tape in place. Follow specific manufacturer recommendation for type of dressing material to use to cover a pressure injury when using enzymes. Tape dressing in place.	Protects wound and prevents removal of ointment during turning or repositioning.
b. **Antibacterial** (e.g., bacitracin, metronidazole, and silver sulfadiazine)	Reduces bacterial growth.
9. Apply prescribed wound dressing:	
a. Hydrogel:	Hydrogel dressings are designed to hydrate and donate moisture to wound (Brumberg et al., 2021).
(1) Cover surface of injury with thick layer of amorphous hydrogel or cut sheet to fit wound base.	Provides moist environment to facilitate wound healing.
(2) Apply secondary dressing such as dry gauze; tape in place.	Holds hydrogel against wound surface because amorphous hydrogel (in tube) or sheet form does not adhere to wound and requires secondary dressing to hold it in place.
(3) If using impregnated gauze, pack loosely into wound; cover with secondary gauze dressing and tape.	A loosely packed dressing delivers gel to wound base and allows any wound debris to be trapped in gauze.
b. Alginate, such as **calcium alginate:**	Alginate dressings absorb serous fluid or exudate, forming a nonadhesive hydrophilic gel, which conforms to shape of wound (Han, 2023; Jaszarowsski & Murphee, 2022). Use in heavily draining wounds.
(1) Lightly pack wound with alginate using sterile cotton-tipped applicator or gloved finger.	The dressing swells and increases in size; tight packing can compromise blood flow to the tissues.
(2) Apply secondary dressing and tape in place.	
c. Transparent film dressing, hydrocolloid, and foam dressings (see Chapter 40)	

Clinical Judgment *Use transparent dressings for autolytic debridement of noninfected superficial pressure injuries. Use a hydrocolloid dressing to protect skin from friction. Some brands have custom shapes available for specific anatomical parts such as the heel, elbow, and sacrum.*

STEP	RATIONALE
10. Reposition patient comfortably off pressure injury.	Prevents pressure to injury.
11. Remove and dispose of gloves. Dispose of soiled supplies in appropriate receptacle. Perform hand hygiene.	Reduces transmission of microorganisms.
12. Raise side rails (as appropriate) and lower bed to lowest position, locking into position.	Ensures patient safety and prevents falls.
13. Place nurse call system in an accessible location within patient's reach.	Ensures patient can call for assistance if needed.
14. Perform hand hygiene.	Reduces transmission of microorganisms.

STEP	RATIONALE

EVALUATION

1. Observe skin surrounding injury for inflammation, edema, and tenderness.

2. Inspect dressings and exposed injuries, observing for drainage, foul odor, and tissue necrosis. Monitor patient for signs and symptoms of infection: fever and elevated white blood cell (WBC) count.

3. Compare subsequent injury measurements using one of the scales designed to measure wound healing such as PUSH tool or BWAT.

4. **Use Teach-Back:** "I want to be sure that you understand why we will examine your pressure injury on an ongoing basis. Why will we measure your wound and look at the tissue type and surrounding skin each time we change your dressing?" Revise your instruction now or develop a plan for revised patient/family caregiver teaching if patient/family caregiver is not able to teach back correctly.

Determines progress of wound healing.

Injuries can become infected.

Allows comparison of serial measurements to evaluate wound healing. Provides standard method of data collection that demonstrates wound progress or lack thereof.

Teach-back is a technique for health care providers to ensure that they have explained medical information clearly so that patients and their families understand what is communicated to them (AHRQ, 2023).

Unexpected Outcomes

1. Skin surrounding injury becomes macerated.

2. Injury becomes deeper with increased drainage and/or development of necrotic tissue.

3. Pressure injury extends beyond original margins.

Related Interventions

- Reduce exposure of surrounding skin to topical agents and moisture.
- Select dressing that has increased moisture-absorbing capacity.
- Review current wound care management.
- Consult with interprofessional team regarding changes in wound care regimen.
- Obtain wound cultures (see Chapter 7).
- Monitor for systemic signs and symptoms of poor wound healing such as abnormal laboratory results (WBC count, levels of hemoglobin/hematocrit, serum albumin, serum prealbumin, total proteins), weight loss, and fluid imbalances.
- Assess and revise current turning schedule.
- Consider further pressure-redistribution devices.

Documentation

- Document type of wound tissue present in injury, injury measurements, periwound skin condition, character of drainage or exudate, type of topical agent used, dressing applied, and patient's response.
- Document your evaluation of patient's and family caregiver's understanding of frequent observation and measuring of wound.

Hand-Off Reporting

- Report any deterioration in injury appearance to nurse in charge or health care provider.

Special Considerations

Patient Education

- Discuss treatment and identify individual(s) who will help with care at home.
- Discuss process of wound healing and expected wound appearance. For example, discuss patient's perception about appearance of the pressure injury. Sometimes eschar looks like a scab to a patient, and the patient needs to understand the difference. A scab is caused by exudate, and an eschar is dead tissue that the patient should not remove.
- Discuss with patient and family caregivers perceptions about size of pressure injury. Some wounds, especially after

debridement, may appear larger and are troublesome to patients and support people.
- Discuss with patient and family caregivers perceptions about treatment. Some patients and family caregivers believe that it is cruel for staff to keep turning and positioning a patient on a frequent basis.
- Review prevention guidelines to prevent further breakdown.
- Discuss options for maintaining good nutrition.

Pediatrics

- Immature skin is less resistant to pressure, especially from medical devices.
- It is imperative to consider patient's size and weight before applying a medical device and to ensure that such devices are safe to use in chairs, beds, cribs, and under head, elbows, and heels in pediatric patients (Nix, 2024).

Older Adults

- Wound healing is often slower in older adults (Rogers, 2023).
- The normal reduction in the Langerhans cells in the older adult's epidermis causes a decrease in T-cell function and immunity.
- Because older skin has a slower and less intense inflammatory reaction, monitor older patients more closely for altered responses to skin irritants.

Home Care

- **NOTE:** Before discharge to home, some patients may be discharged to long-term care facilities that specialize in pressure injury and wound care.
- Consider family caregiver time when selecting a dressing. In the home care setting, caregivers may sometimes choose more expensive dressing materials to reduce the frequency of dressing changes.

- Identify clean storage area for dressing supplies. Determine availability of required supplies. Discuss need for home care nurse.
- Discuss need for home pressure-redistribution surface or bed. Identify adaptive equipment needed to care for patient at home.
- Medicare regulations limit reimbursement for some types of support surfaces in the treatment of pressure injuries.

◆ CLINICAL JUDGMENT AND NEXT-GENERATION NCLEX® EXAMINATION–STYLE QUESTIONS

A 72-year-old patient in intensive care has an endotracheal tube (ET) inserted through the mouth for ventilation, a nasoenteral feeding tube, an intravenous (IV) line in place on the back of the hand, and an abdominal incision that is dry and intact. The patient weighs 90.9 kg (200 lb) and is approximately 167.6 cm (5 feet 6 inches) tall. A red, intact, warm area that does not blanch is noted over the sacrum. A skin risk assessment using the Braden Scale was completed with these results: Sensory Perception (4); Moisture (2); Activity (2); Mobility (2); Nutrition (3); and Friction and Shear (1).

1. Which of the following areas does the nurse identify as being at risk for a pressure injury? **Select all that apply.**
   1. Abdomen
   2. Sacrum
   3. Nose
   4. Mouth
   5. Back of the hand

2. The nurse is planning care for the patient based on the Braden Scale results. Select whether the interventions are indicated or not indicated.

Interventions	Indicated	Not Indicated
Develop and implement a turning schedule.		
Massage reddened areas at each position change.		
Place a protective dressing over the sacrum.		
Use iodine following enzymatic debriding.		
Implement safe patient handling to help reposition frequently.		
Consult with the wound clinical nurse specialist (CNS) about the most appropriate bed surface to redistribute pressure.		

3. On further inspection, the patient is found to have a partial-thickness injury tissue on the right heel. How will the nurse document this finding?
   1. Stage 1 pressure injury
   2. Stage 2 pressure injury
   3. Stage 3 pressure injury
   4. Stage 4 pressure injury

4. The nurse reviews the patient's laboratory report and notices an albumin level of 2.9 g/dL (normal range, 3.5–5.4 g/dL). Which order will the nurse request when collaborating with the health care provider?
   1. Decrease in nasoenteral feeding
   2. Antibiotics to treat potential wound infections
   3. Consultation with registered dietitian nutritionist (RDN)
   4. Physical therapy to ambulate the patient daily

5. Several weeks later, the patient is to be discharged to home. The spouse asks what can be done at home to prevent any skin breakdown. Which of the following recommendations will the nurse make? **Select all that apply.**
   1. Encourage intake of protein.
   2. Ambulate several times daily as able.
   3. Report skin changes to the health care provider.
   4. Perform daily skin checks on areas that are prone to pressure.
   5. Immediately place a dressing on any area that appears reddened.

Visit the Evolve site for Answers to Clinical Judgment and Next-Generation NCLEX® Examination–Style Questions.

REFERENCES

Agency for Healthcare Research and Quality (AHRQ): *Teach-back: intervention*, 2023. https://www.ahrq.gov/patient-safety/reports/engage/interventions/teach-back.html.

Al Aboud AM, Manna B: Wound Pressure Injury Management. [Updated 2023 Apr 19]. In: StatPearls [Internet]. Treasure Island (FL), 2023, StatPearls.

Alderden J, et al: Midrange Braden subscale scores are associated with increased risk for pressure injury development among critical care patients, *J Wound Ostomy Continence Nurs* 44(5):420, 2017.

Bates-Jensen, BM: Assessment of the patient with a wound. In *Core curriculum: wound management*, ed 2, Philadelphia, PA, 2022, Wolters Kluwer.

Berlowitz D, et al: *Epidemiology, pathogenesis, and risk assessment of pressure-induced skin and soft tissue injury*, 2022, UpToDate. https://uptodate.com/contents/epidemiology-pathogenesis-and-risk-assessment-of-pressure-induced-skin-and-soft-tissue-injury.

Bohn G, Bryant RA: Wound-healing physiology and factors that affect the repair process. In Bryant RA, Nix DP, editors: *Acute and chronic wounds: current management concepts*, ed 6, St. Louis, 2024, Elsevier.

Borchert K: Pressure injury prevention and maintaining a successful plan and program. In McNichol L, Ostomy, and Continence Nurses Society, et al., editors: *Wound, Ostomy, and Continence Nurses Society (WOCN) core curriculum*, ed 2, Philadelphia, 2022, Wolters Kluwer.

Britto EJ, et al: Wound dressings. [Updated 2023 May 18]. In: *StatPearls* [Internet]. Treasure Island (FL), 2023, StatPearls Publishing.

Brophy S, et al: What is the incidence of medical device-related pressure injuries in adults within the acute hospital setting? A systematic review, *J Tissue Viability* 30(4):489–498, 2021.

Brumberg V, et al: Modern wound dressings: hydrogel dressings, *Biomedicines* 9(9):1235, 2021.

Bryant RA: Skin damage: types and treatment. In Bryant RA, Nix DP, editors: *Acute and chronic wounds: intraprofessionals from novice to expert*, ed 6, St. Louis, 2024, Elsevier.

Bryant RA, Nix DP: Principles of wound healing and topical management In Bryant RA, Nix DP, editors: *Acute and chronic wounds: intraprofessionals from novice to expert*, ed 6, St. Louis, 2024, Mosby.

Centers for Medicare and Medicaid Services: *Hospital-acquired conditions*, 2022. https://www.cms.gov/Medicare/Medicare-Fee-for-Service-Payment/Hospital-AcqCond/Hospital-Acquired_Conditions. Accessed August 30, 2023.

Centers for Disease Control and Prevention (CDC): *What is health literacy?* 2023. https://www.cdc.gov/healthliteracy/learn/index.html. Accessed August 30, 2023.

Chaboyer W, et al: Adherence to evidence-based pressure injury prevention guidelines in routine clinical practice: a longitudinal study, *Int Wound J* 14(6):1290, 2017.

Cox J, et al: Pressure injuries in critical care patients in US hospitals: results of the International Pressure Ulcer Prevalence Survey, *J Wound Ostomy Continence Nurs* 49(1):21–28, 2022.

Doughty DB, McNichol LL: General concepts related to skin and soft tissue injury caused by mechanical factors. In McNichol LL, et al., editors: *Core curriculum: wound management*, ed 2, Philadelphia, PA, 2022, Wolters Kluwer.

Doughty DB, McNichol LL: General concepts related to skin and soft tissue injury caused by mechanical factors. In McNichol LL, et al., editors: *Core curriculum: wound management*, ed 2, Philadelphia, PA, 2022, Wolters Kluwer.

Duerst KJ, et al: Preventing medical device–related pressure injuries due to non-invasive ventilation masks and nasal cannulas. *Crit Care Nurse* 42(5):14–21, 2022. https://doi.org/10.4037/ccn2022783.

European Pressure Ulcer Advisory Panel (EPUAP), National Pressure Injury Advisory Panel (NPIAP), Pan Pacific Pressure Injury Alliance: *Treatment of pressure ulcers/injuries: Clinical Practice Guideline. The International Guideline*, Emily Haesler (editor). 2019a, EPUAP/NPIAP/PPPIA.

European Pressure Ulcer Advisory Panel (EPUAP), National Pressure Injury Advisory Panel (NPIAP), Pan Pacific Pressure Injury Alliance: *Treatment of pressure ulcers/injuries: Quick reference guide*. Emily Haesler (editor). 2019b, EPUAP/NPIAP/PPPIA.

Foltynski P, et al: Wound surface area measurement methods, *Biocybern Biomed Eng* 41(4):1454–1465, 2021.

Friedrich E: Nutritional strategies for wound management. In McNichol LL, et al., editors: *Core curriculum: wound management*, ed 2, Philadelphia, PA, 2022, Wolters Kluwer.

Fumarola S, Allaway R, Callaghan R, et al: Overlooked and underestimated: medical adhesive-related skin injuries. Best practice consensus document on prevention, *J Wound Care* 29(Suppl 3c):S1–S24, 2020.

Garcia M, et al: Pressure injuries related to the use of compression stockings in pediatric surgical patients, *J Pediatr Surg Nurs* 11(2):71–74, 2022.

Gupta S, et al: Wound assessment using Bates Jensen wound assessment tool in acute musculoskeletal injury following low-cost wall-mounted negative-pressure wound therapy application, *Indian J Orthop* 57:948–956, 2023.

Han SK. Interactive Wound Dressings. In: Han S, editor: *Innovations and advances in wound healing*, ed 3, Springer, 2023, Singapore.

Hockenberry MJ, et al: *Wong's nursing care of infants and children*, ed 12, St. Louis, 2024, Elsevier.

Hotaling P, Black J: Ten top tips: honing your pressure injury risk assessment, *Wounds Int* 12(1):8, 2021.

Huang C, Ma Y, Wang C, et al: Predictive validity of the Braden Scale for pressure injury risk assessment in adults: a systematic review and meta-analysis, *Nurs Open* 8:2194–2207, 2021. https://doi.org/10.1002/nop2.972.

Jaszarowski K, Murphee RW: Wound cleaning and dressing selection. In McNichol LL, et al., editors: *Core curriculum: wound management*, ed 2, Philadelphia, PA, 2022, Wolters Kluwer.

Johansen E, et al: ABCD before Everything else—Intensive care nurses' knowledge and experience of pressure injury and moisture-associated skin damage, *Int Wound J* 20:285–295, 2023.

Kaminska MS, et al: Effectiveness of hydrocolloid dressings for treating pressure ulcers in adult patients: a systematic review and meta-analysis, *Int J Environ Res Public Health* 17(21):7881, 2020.

Liao Y, et al: Predictive accuracy of the Braden Q Scale in risk assessment for paediatric pressure ulcer: a meta-analysis, *Int J Nurs Sci* 10:419, 2018.

McNichol L, et al. *Ostomy, and Continence Nurses Society*, ed 2, Philadelphia, PA, 2022, Wolters Kluwer.

Mondragon N, Zito PM: Pressure injury. [Updated 2022 Aug 25]. In: *StatPearls* [Internet]. Treasure Island (FL), 2022, StatPearls.

Netsch D: Refractory wounds. In McNichol LL, et al., editors: *Core curriculum: wound management*, ed 2, Philadelphia, PA, 2022, Wolters Kluwer.

Nix DP: Skin and wound inspection and assessment. In Bryant RA, Nix DP, editors: *Acute and chronic wounds: intraprofessionals from novice to expert*, ed 6, St. Louis, 2024, Elsevier.

Nix, DP; Bryant RA: Fistula Management. In McNichol LL, et al., editors: *Core curriculum: wound management*, ed 2, Philadelphia, PA, 2022, Wolters Kluwer.

Nix DP, Bryant R: Pressure injuries. In Bryant RA, Nix DP, editors: *Acute and chronic wounds: intraprofessionals from novice to expert*, ed 6, St. Louis, 2024, Elsevier.

Nix DP, Milne CT: Pressure redistribution support surfaces. In Bryant RA, Nix DP, editors: *Acute and chronic wounds: intraprofessionals from novice to expert*, ed 6, St. Louis, 2024, Elsevier.

Padula CA, et al: Prevention of medical device-related pressure injuries associated with respiratory equipment use in a critical care unit, *J Wound Ostomy Continence Nurs* 44(2):138, 2017.

Pusey-Reid E, et al: Skin assessment in patients with dark skin tone, *Am J Nurs* 123(3):36–43, 2023.

Ramundo J: Principles and guidelines for wound debridement, In McNichol LL, et al., editors: *Core curriculum: wound management*, ed 2, Philadelphia, PA, 2022, Wolters Kluwer.

Rogers J: *McCance & Huether's pathophysiology*, ed 9, St. Louis, 2023, Elsevier.

Saleh MYN, Ibrahim, EIM: Prevalence, severity, and characteristics of medical device related pressure injuries in adult intensive care patients: a prospective observational study, *Int Wound J* 20(1):109–119, 2023.

Sullivan R, et al: Evaluation of a modified version of the Norton Scale for use as a pressure injury risk assessment instrument in critical care, *WOCN* 47(3):224, 2020.

Thayer DM, et al: Top down injuries: prevention and management of moisture-associated skin damage, medical adhesive–related skin injury and skin tears. In McNichol LL, et al., editors: *Core curriculum: wound management*, ed 2, Philadelphia, PA, 2022, Wolters Kluwer.

The Joint Commission (TJC): *2023 National patient safety goals*, Oakbrook Terrace, IL, 2023, The Joint Commission. https://www.jointcommission.org/standards/national-patient-safety-goals/. Accessed August 30, 2023.

The Joint Commission (TJC): *Preventing pressure injuries*, 2022. https://www.jointcommission.org/resources/news-and-multimedia/newsletters/newsletters/quick-safety/quick-safety-issue-25-preventing-pressure-injuries/preventing-pressure-injuries/. Accessed August 30, 2023.

Wang HN, et al: Pressure injury development in critically ill patients with a cervical collar in situ: a retrospective longitudinal study, *Int Wound J* 17(4):944–956, 2020.

Wound, Ostomy, and Continence Nurses Society (WOCN): *Guideline for prevention and management of pressure ulcers*, WOCN clinical practice guidelines series, Mount Laurel, NJ, 2016, The Society.

Yiğitoğlu E, Aydoğan S: Determination of medical device-related pressure injury in COVID-19 patients: a prospective descriptive study, *J Tissue Viability* 32(1):74–78, 2023.

40 | Dressings, Bandages, and Binders

Skill 40.1 **Applying a Dressing (Dry and Moist Dressings), p. 1166**

Skill 40.2 **Applying a Pressure Bandage, p. 1175**

Skill 40.3 **Applying a Transparent Dressing, p. 1178**

Skill 40.4 **Applying a Hydrocolloid, Hydrogel, Foam, or Alginate Dressing, p. 1181**

Procedural Guideline 40.1 **Applying Rolled Gauze and Elastic Bandages, p. 1187**

Procedural Guideline 40.2 **Applying an Abdominal Binder, p. 1191**

OBJECTIVES

Mastery of content in this chapter will enable you to:
- Apply clinical judgment and assess a wound correctly.
- Explain the purposes and application techniques of dressings, bandages, and abdominal binders.
- Discuss approaches used to reduce risk of infection during dressing and bandage changes.
- Compare and contrast different types of wound dressings selected on the basis of wound characteristics.
- Demonstrate how to apply dry, damp-to-dry, pressure, transparent, and synthetic dressings correctly.
- Demonstrate how to apply an abdominal binder correctly.

MEDIA RESOURCES

- http://evolve.elsevier.com/Perry/skills
- Review Questions
- **NSO** Nursing Skills Online
- Answers to Clinical Judgment and Next-Generation NCLEX® Examination–Style Questions
- Skills Performance Checklists
- Printable Key Points

PURPOSE

Wound healing is an integrated physiological process. The tissue layers involved and their capacity for regeneration determine the mechanism for repair of any wound (Bohn & Bryant, 2024). Duration of treatment and management of wound complications, such as infection; increased impairment in skin integrity; a decline in a patient's immune function; or a decline in a patient's functional status all add to the cost of care (Beitz, 2022).

Effective wound management must (1) control or eliminate causative factors, (2) reduce existing and potential cofactors, and (3) create and maintain a physiologic local wound environment (Bryant & Nix, 2024). To manage a patient's existing wound, use clinical judgment and scientific knowledge to determine the appropriate moisture in the wound bed and proper wound dressing techniques to promote wound healing (Tan et al., 2021).

Dressings, bandages, and binders support underlying tissues and promote wound healing. Selection of the appropriate type of dressing is based on specific characteristics of the wound; the expected outcomes desired; and, for chronic wounds, the practicality and feasibility of performing the dressing changes by family caregivers in the home setting (Box 40.1). Numerous dressings and wound care products are available for managing acute and chronic wounds (Table 40.1). The type and condition of the wound bed, surrounding periwound, and type and amount of drainage determine the type of dressing to use.

PRACTICE STANDARDS

- Berrios-Torres SI, et al., 2017: Centers for Disease Control and Prevention Guideline for Prevention of Surgical Site Infection
- Wound, Ostomy and Continence Nurses Society (WOCN), 2017: Guideline for Prevention and Management of Pressure Ulcers (Injuries), WOCN Clinical Practice Guideline Series
- The Joint Commission (TJC), 2023: National Patient Safety Goals–Patient Identification

SUPPLEMENTAL STANDARDS

- European Pressure Ulcer Advisory Panel (EPUAP), National Pressure Injury Advisory Panel (NPIAP), and Pan Pacific Pressure Injury Alliance (PPPIA), Haesler E, editor, 2019a: *Treatment of Pressure Ulcers/Injuries: Clinical Practice Guideline. The International Guideline.*
- Fumarola S, et al., 2020: Overlooked and Underestimated: Medical Adhesive–Related Skin Injuries. Best Practice Consensus Document on Prevention

PRINCIPLES FOR PRACTICE

- Acute wounds go through a predictive wound-healing process moving through the following stages: hemostasis, inflammation, proliferation (repair), and maturation (remodeling) (Beitz, 2022). Chronic wounds do not heal progressively, often remaining or "stalling" in the repair process (Beitz, 2022; Ermer-Seltun & Rolstad, 2022).

- The Tissue, Infection/inflammation, Moisture imbalance, and Edge of wound (TIME) clinical decision support tool is valuable in selecting wound treatments. The tool identifies barriers, key

clinical assessments, and treatment options for chronic wounds (Blackburn et al., 2022; Munro, 2021, 2017; Ousey et al., 2018):

- **Tissue management:** Removes nonviable, nonhealthy tissue from the wound bed. In addition, tissue management also reduces bioburden of the wound, which impedes wound healing. Wound debridement reduces bioburden and in turn reduces risk for wound infection (Assadian et al., 2018; Stiehl, 2021).
- **Inflammation/infection:** Influenced by the presence of nonviable tissue, high bacterial loads, and impaired leukocytes. The goal is to identify and treat wound infection and inflammation promptly.
- **Moisture:** When a wound surface is too wet or too dry, the repair process is delayed. The goal is to keep a wound surface moist, not wet. Prolonged moisture to the skin causes moisture-associated skin damage (MASD). When caring for patients with acute or chronic wounds, this moisture can be from wound exudate or excessively moist dressings (Earlam & Woods, 2022).
- **Edge:** Affects the integrity of the perimeter of the wound. A closed or compromised wound edge prevents resurfacing and wound repair. The goal is to have a proliferative wound edge.
- Many wounds are colonized or contaminated with low levels of bacteria. Know the cause and type of wound to ensure the proper treatment plan is in place and healing outcomes are achieved. Select dressing material that has characteristics to promote wound healing (Box 40.1).

BOX 40.1

Dressing Characteristics and Outcomes

Characteristics

- Nontraumatic and able to absorb exudate; keeps wound bed moist and surrounding periwound tissues dry and intact
- Appropriate for infected wounds
- Can be removed without trauma, pain, or leaving dressing fragments in the wound
- Conforms to the body part for ease of movement
- Maintains stable physiological wound environment
- Easy to apply and remove with easy-to-follow patient/family caregiver instructions
- Cost-effective

Outcomes

- Reduces volume of exudate and amount of necrotic tissue
- Resolves or prevents periwound erythema
- Reduces wound dimensions or depth of sinus tract
- Reduces pain intensity during dressing changes

Data from McNichol LL, et al., editors: *Wound Ostomy and Continence Nurses Society Core Curriculum: wound management*, ed 2, Philadelphia, 2022, Wolters Kluwer.

TABLE 40.1

Comparison of Wound Care Products

Product Category	Indications for Use	Contraindications	Advantages	Disadvantages	Frequency of Change (per Manufacturer Recommendations)
Gauze Dressings					
Cotton or synthetic material; woven or nonwoven construction; nonwoven gauze is preferred when used as a primary dressing	Protection of surgical incision Maintain a moist wound base (wet-to-moist) Secondary dressing for other wound products Packing wounds	Granulating wounds as primary treatment	Available in many sizes and forms: Sterile and nonsterile Impregnated products—iodinated agents, chlorhexidine gluconate, petroleum, etc	May adhere to healthy tissue and cause injury on removal Loose fibers can become embedded in the wound bed and act as a foreign body, increasing the risk of infection Wet-to-moist dressing requires frequent dressing changes	Usually change 2 or 3 times per day as needed.
Transparent Films					
Hypoallergenic adhesive membrane dressings; waterproof, impermeable to fluids and bacteria; allow oxygen and moisture vapor exchange	Dry to minimally exudative wound Promote autolytic debridement As a secondary dressing to other products such as alginates and foam Selected to allow a 2.5 cm (1 inch) perimeter of intact surrounding skin	Not recommended for acutely infected wounds Third-degree burns	Easy to apply and remove without damage to underlying tissue Permit viewing of wound Create second skin; protect from friction Waterproof Create moist wound that softens thin slough and eschar Protective shield to external fluids and bacteria	May cause moisture-associated skin maceration (MASD) and MARSI; use a liquid skin protectant before application May need to use an adhesive-release product to prevent skin tears and stripping	When used as a primary dressing for a minimally exudative wound, wear time is 3–7 days. If using to facilitate autolytic debridement, change when exudate extends beyond the edges of the wound onto periwound skin.

Continued

TABLE 40.1

Comparison of Wound Care Products—cont'd

Product Category	Indications for Use	Contraindications	Advantages	Disadvantages	Frequency of Change (per Manufacturer Recommendations)
Hydrocolloids					
Adhesive dressings that promote a moist wound environment; they contain gel-forming agents; mold to body contours; considered semiocclusive dressings	Partial- or full-thickness wound; shallow Minimal-to-moderate exudating wounds Clean and noninfected shallow wounds Can be used in combination with absorbent powder or alginate	Infected wounds; wounds with heavy exudate, sinus tracts, or exposed tendons and bones Use with caution in people with diabetes mellitus or arterial disease	Available in many sizes, conforms to body contours Promote autolytic debridement of necrotic tissue Reduce pain Impermeable to fluids/bacteria Thermal insulator Easy to apply and remove	Potential for periwound MASD if dressing left in place too long; correct dressing size should allow for 2.5 cm (1 inch) of intact periwound skin Drainage (gelatinous mass) under dressing often mistaken for pus/infection Adhesive possibly too aggressive for fragile skin	Change every 3–7 days, depending on volume of exudate. If dressing change is required every 3 days or less, an alternative dressing should be considered.
Hydrogel					
Solid sheets that are glycerin- or water-based dressings designed to absorb wound drainage and maintain clean, moist wound	Wounds with minimal or no exudate, minor burns, and some dermatitis; they have a cooling effect, which may provide some pain management	Third-degree burns Wounds with heavy exudate	Nonadherent Cool and soothing Decrease pain Facilitates autolysis Conform to wound	Potential for periwound maceration (MASD) or candidiasis of periwound area	Frequency of dressing change is 1–3 days and is dependent on type of hydrogel preparation, volume of exudate, and characteristics of secondary dressing.
Alginates					
Highly absorbent, non-woven material that forms gel when exposed to wound drainage	Moderate-to-heavily exudating wounds; shallow or deep Full-thickness wounds without depth Leg ulcers, donor sites, traumatic wounds	Dry necrotic wounds Wounds covered with eschar In combination with hydrogels	Nonadhering, nonocclusive Hemostatic properties May be packed into tunneled areas Promote autolytic debridement in exudating wounds	More expensive than gauze or gauze packing strips Not practical for large wounds Gelled material may be mistaken for purulence	Change every 1–3 days depending on the amount of exudate and type of secondary dressing.
Foam Dressings					
Absorbent, nonadherent polyurethane or film-coated layer used to protect wounds and maintain moist healing environment	May be used as preventative dressing for patient with fragile skin to reduce the risk of friction injury Moderate-to-heavily exudating wounds Partial- and full-thickness wounds; shallow and deep Stage 2–4 pressure injuries	Wounds with eschar or dry wounds; third-degree burns	Highly absorbent while maintaining moist wound environment Often used as secondary dressing along with films and absorbers Many nonadherent to wound bed	Nonadhesive foams require secondary dressing Maceration of periwound may occur if dressing left on too long	Change every 24 hours or as needed, which is dependent on the amount of wound exudate and absorptive capacity of the foam dressing.

Data from Jaszarowski K, Murphree RW: Wound cleansing and dressing selection. In McNichol LL et al: *WOCN Core Curriculum Wound Management*, ed 2, Philadelphia, 2022, Wolters Kluwer.

- The key principles of a healthy physiological wound environment are adequate moisture, temperature control, pH, and control of bacterial burden.
- An effective dressing removes excess wound exudate, debrides dead tissue, controls wound moisture, protects the underlying wound, and reduces the spread of infection (Hasatsri et al., 2018; Jaszarowski & Murphree, 2022).
- Primary wound healing occurs when tissue is cut cleanly and margins are reapproximated (i.e., surgical incisions).
- Secondary wound healing occurs when skin is left open, healing from granulation tissue at the base of the wound combined with epithelialization from the sides.
- Know the expected amount and type of wound exudate or drainage (Box 40.2).

Types of Wound Drainage

Serous, which is a clear, watery plasma

Sanguineous, which indicates fresh bleeding; bright red

Serosanguineous, which is a pale, red, more watery drainage than sanguineous drainage

Purulent, which is a thick, yellow, green, tan, or brown drainage

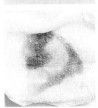

PERSON-CENTERED CARE

- Identify and respect patients' specific cultural or spiritual practices as they relate to the management of wounds (Waters, 2017). Ask patient or family caregiver if there are any special considerations or practices to be aware of before proceeding with wound care.
- Respect and maintain a patient's privacy during dressing changes. Recognize a patient's culturally specific needs, such as the need for gender-congruent caregivers.
- Identify individual measures to minimize a patient's discomfort during a dressing change by understanding a patient's values and beliefs about pain management.
- Patients may attribute different meanings to wounds and trauma, blood loss, and disposal of soiled dressings and linens. To provide patient-centered care, it is important to assess and try to understand the different meanings of blood and wounds and how they affect patients and their families.
- Provide an opportunity for family caregivers to be present during dressing changes (if patient approves). This allows them to see the actual dressing change, and it provides the patient comfort and emotional support (WOCN, 2017).
- A priority in wound care management is patient comfort (Bonham, 2022):
  - Provide patients appropriate analgesic doses 30 minutes before a dressing change to maximize comfort when the dressing and tissues will be manipulated. Recommend pharmacological and nonpharmacological pain-relief measures before dressing changes, even when patients do not request them. These measures include but are not limited to reducing sensory stimulus during dressing change, allowing the patient to perform dressing change, and allowing for "time-outs" during painful dressing changes (Bonham, 2022; Oropallo & Quraishi, 2024).
  - Select dressings that help to reduce pain. For example, moisture-retentive dressings have some ability to reduce wound-related pain and also reduce the number of dressing changes needed (Ermer-Seltun & Rolstad, 2022).
  - Protection of the periwound skin should be routine in care of wounds. The use of liquid skin protectants and moisture barriers are effective in reducing moisture-associated skin damage (MASD) and medical adhesive–related skin injury (MARSI). Periwound MASD occurs when wound exudate, containing proteolytic enzymes, are in prolonged contact

with the patient's skin (Earlam & Woods, 2022). Select dressings that manage exudate and do not allow exudate to pool on the patient's skin (Earlam & Woods, 2022; Ermer-Seltun & Rolstad, 2022).
- Involve family caregiver early in the dressing change education. It is likely that the patient will continue to have the same type of dressing while at home, and the patient and family caregiver need to know proper techniques for changing it and disposing of medical waste (Jaszarowski & Murphree, 2022).

EVIDENCE-BASED PRACTICE

Management of Chronic Wounds

Wound healing is a complicated process and depends on the type of wound. For example, acute wounds occur from unexpected accidents or surgical incisions and have a predictable healing time frame. Chronic wounds commonly result from burns, pressure injury, or leg ulcers and do not follow a predictable healing time frame (Ghomi et al., 2019). Chronic wounds fail to move past the inflammatory phase of wound healing (Ghomi et al., 2019; Munro, 2017, 2021). These wounds often have bacterial bioburden and slough. Infection is the most frequent complication in nonhealing wounds; this factor alone increases health care cost, extends length of stay in health care agencies, and impacts a patient's independence and quality of life (Barrett, 2017). Recent advances in wound care have created several new debriding products used for managing chronic, necrotic wounds (Ghomi et al., 2019). Autolytic debriding products, such as hydrocolloids, transparent films, and hydrogels, are applied directly to the wound bed. These products rehydrate dry devitalized tissue and regulate the wound environment so the body's own proteolytic enzymes and phagocytic cells can debride the necrotic tissues (EPUAP/NPIAP/PPPIA, 2019a).
- Comprehensive wound and periwound assessment aids in the progress of wound healing and promotes early identification of wound infections (EPUAP/NPIAP/PPPIA, 2019b).
- Use the evidence-based practice TIME framework to regularly assess chronic wounds (see principles of practice) (Munro, 2017, 2021; Ousey et al., 2018).
- Ongoing assessment and management of chronic wounds and the periwound area identifies risk factors for and early signs of medical adhesive–related skin injury (MARSI), periwound MASD, and medical device–related pressure injury (MDRPI) (Earlam & Woods, 2022; Oznur et al., 2022)

- Wound and periwound cleansing with topical agents, such as a combination of hypochlorite/hypochlorous agents and antiseptics, reduces the bioburden in chronic wounds (Assadian et al., 2018; EPUAP/NPIAP/PPPIA, 2019a).
- Polyurethane film dressings are effective in promoting a moist wound environment and reducing infection in chronic wounds (Ghomi et al., 2019).
- Silicone or foam dressings on skin around drainage tubes, wound irrigation systems, nasoenteral tubes, etc. reduce the risk for MDRPI and resultant chronic wounds (EPUAP/NPIAP/PPPIA, 2019a; Oznur et al., 2022).

SAFETY GUIDELINES

- A wound is a break in skin integrity that increases a patient's risk for infection. Perform hand hygiene before and after a dressing change. Use appropriate gloves when changing a dressing. Verify wound closure techniques (e.g., sutures, staples, surgical glue), as each of these require specific wound care guidelines. These wound care actions reduce the risk for surgical site infections (Berrios-Torres et al., 2017).
- Surgical glue (cyanoacrylate glue) has several advantages: It provides a waterproof barrier, it is transparent and the wound is easier to inspect, and it reduces time associated with dressing changes. There is some clinical evidence that surgical glue has antimicrobial properties against gram-positive bacteria, which are common surgical site infection (SSI) pathogens (Machin et al., 2019).

- Wounds related to vascular insufficiency, diabetes mellitus, pressure, trauma, and surgery are all very different and must have an individualized treatment plan. Not knowing the cause of a wound can have serious negative effects if you use treatments that are contraindicated for certain types of wounds (Bryant & Nix, 2024).
- Inspect wound and periwound skin at least daily or according to agency policy. Identify and document areas of erythema, blistering, skin tears, etc., which are signs of medical adhesive–related skin injury (MARSI). Identify areas of inflamed skin with irregular borders, rash, or change in skin color, which are signs of moisture-associated skin damage (MASD). Modify frequency of assessment and dressing changes on the basis of the patient's risk factors and/or wound condition.
- Identify appropriate wound-cleaning agents. No agent is ideal for every situation; therefore verify the type and frequency of wound-cleaning agents.
- Determine if wound-drainage devices are present in the wound to prevent their accidental dislocation when you remove the old dressing (see Chapter 38).
- Verify that any wound-drainage devices do not cause pressure on adjacent skin, which can result in medical device pressure–related injury (MDRPI) (EPUAP/NPIAP/PPPIA, 2019b; Parvizi et al., 2023).
- In the home setting, assess the patient's and family caregiver's knowledge of infection control practices and provide patient education as needed.

◆ SKILL 40.1   Applying a Dressing (Dry and Moist Dressings)

Gauze is used for wound cleansing and as a wick, filter, and dressing. It can be moistened with various solutions for wound healing. Gauze dressings are used for wound healing by primary intention with little drainage (Jaszarowski & Murphree, 2022). Dry dressings protect the wound from injury, reduce discomfort, and speed healing. Dry gauze dressings do not interact with wound tissues and cause little wound irritation. These dressings are commonly used for abrasions and nondraining postoperative incisions (see Table 40.1). Telfa gauze dressings contain a shiny, nonadherent surface on one side that does not stick to a wound. Drainage passes through the nonadherent surface to the outer gauze dressing.

Dry dressings are not appropriate for debriding wounds. When gauze adheres to drainage on a wound surface, removal is painful, and the seal can pull off healthy tissue when the gauze is removed (Bryant & Nix, 2024). If the old gauze dressing does adhere to a wound, moisten the dressing with sterile normal saline or sterile water before removing it to minimize wound trauma and pain.

Moist dressings (formerly called *wet-to-dry* or *moist-to-dry*) are gauze moistened with an appropriate solution, most commonly normal saline. A moist dressing has a moist contact dressing layer, which is in contact with the wound bed. The moistened gauze increases the absorptive ability of the dressing to collect exudate and wound debris. When other forms of moisture-retentive dressings are not available, moist gauze is effective to mechanically debride the wound and promote wound healing. It is important to avoid excessively wet dressings on the wound surface, which causes MASD, resulting in maceration of the underlying tissue, periwound skin damages, and further skin injury (EPUAP/NPIAP/PPPIA 2019a; Jaszarowski & Murphree, 2022).

Recent advances in wound care have created several new debriding products used for debriding necrotic wounds. Autolytic debriding products are applied to wounds to allow enzymes to self-digest

dead tissue. Enzymatic debriding agents applied directly to a wound bed act by digesting collagen in necrotic tissue (Assadian et al., 2018; EPUAP/NPIAP/PPPIA, 2019a, 2019b; Ramundo, 2022). Both autolytic and enzymatic products are often used in combination with moist gauze but may also come as prepackaged dressings that do not require any additional gauze (see Table 40.1).

Delegation

The skill of applying dry and moist dressings can be delegated to assistive personnel (AP) if the wound is chronic (see agency policy). The nurse is responsible for wound assessments, care of acute new wounds, wound care requiring sterile technique, and evaluation of wound healing. Instruct the AP about:

- Any unique modifications of the dressing change, such as the need for use of special tape or taping techniques to secure the dressing.
- Reporting any change in the patient's skin near the wound, such as rash, redness, etc.
- Reporting pain, fever, bleeding, or wound drainage to the nurse immediately.
- Reporting any potential contamination to existing dressing (e.g., patient incontinence or other body fluids, a dressing that becomes dislodged).

Interprofessional Collaboration

- Involve a wound, ostomy, and continence nurse (WOCN) or wound care specialist with nonhealing wounds, a medical device–related pressure injury (MDRPI), moisture-associated skin damage (MASD), or other pressure injuries.
- Infection control team is involved with newly infected wounds to determine what, if any, additional infection control measures (e.g., wound cultures, wound vac therapy, isolation) are needed.

Equipment

- Personal protective equipment (PPE) (i.e., gown, goggles, mask) if needed
- Clean and sterile gloves
- Sterile dressing set including sterile scissors and forceps (check agency policy) (Fig. 40.1)
- Sterile drape (optional)
- Necessary dressings as ordered: fine-mesh gauze, 4 × 4–inch gauze, abdominal pads (ABDs); an appropriate cover dressing material that retains moisture
- Sterile basin (optional)
- Antiseptic ointment (as prescribed)
- Wound cleanser (as prescribed)
- Sterile normal saline (or prescribed solution)
- Debriding gel as ordered
- Tape (include nonallergenic tape as needed), Montgomery ties, or bandages as needed
- Skin barrier (optional if using Montgomery ties)
- Adhesive remover, scissors, or hair clipper (optional)
- Protective waterproof underpad

- Biohazard bag
- Additional lighting if needed (e.g., flashlight, treatment light)

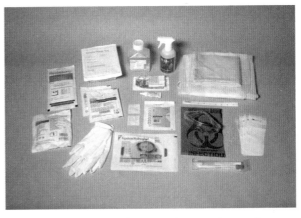

FIG. 40.1 Dressing set with personal protective equipment and wound cleaners.

STEP	RATIONALE

ASSESSMENT

STEP	RATIONALE
1. Identify patient using at least two identifiers (e.g., name and birthday or name and medical record number) according to agency policy.	Ensures correct patient. Complies with The Joint Commission standards and improves patient safety (TJC, 2023).
2. Review patient's electronic health record (EHR), including health care provider's order and nurses' notes. Note previous dressing change, including equipment used and patient response.	Verifies dressing orders and any prior dressing change issues.
3. Review EHR to determine patient's age and history of dehydration, malnutrition, exposure to radiation therapy, underlying chronic conditions (e.g., diabetes mellitus, immunosuppression), edema of the skin, and the presence of erythema, blistering, excoriation, or erosion of skin or a rash under or adjacent to adhesive's securing dressing.	Common risk factors for medical adhesive–related skin injury (MARSI) (Fumarola et al., 2020). Erythema, blistering, and excoriation are signs of MARSI and are related to the skin's reaction to an adhesive (Hitchcock et al., 2021; Thayer et al., 2022). Erosion of underlying or superficial periwound skin or periwound area or rash is an indication of MASD (Earlam & Woods, 2022).
4. Assess patient's/family caregiver's health literacy.	Determines degree to which individuals have the ability to find, understand, and use information and services to make informed health-related decisions and actions for themselves and others (CDC, 2023).
5. Assess patient for allergies, especially antiseptics, tape, or latex. Have patient describe allergic response and acquire specific orders for dressing change.	Reduces risk for localized or systemic allergic reactions to these supplies.
6. Ask patient to describe character of any wound pain and to rate level of wound pain acuity on a pain scale of 0 to 10. Administer prescribed analgesic as needed 30 minutes before dressing change.	Serves as baseline to measure response to dressing therapy. Superficial and chronic wounds with multiple exposed nerves may be intensely painful, whereas deeper wounds with destruction of dermis should be less painful (Bonham, 2022). A comfortable patient is less likely to move suddenly, causing wound or supply contamination.
7. Review EHR to identify patients at risk for poor wound healing, including aging, premature infant, obesity, diabetes mellitus, circulation disorders, nutritional deficit, immunosuppression, radiation therapy, high levels of stress, and use of steroids.	Physiological changes resulting from aging, chronic illness, poor nutrition, medications, and cancer treatments (radiation and chemotherapy) have the potential to affect wound healing (Beitz, 2022).
8. Perform hand hygiene and apply clean gloves. Assess condition of skin around wound and existing dressing and presence of drainage on outer gauze. Remove and dispose of gloves and perform hand hygiene.	Reduces transmission of microorganisms. Provides baseline for comparison with previous dressing changes for condition of skin around wound. Helps to plan for proper dressing type and securement of supplies needed and for whether help is needed during dressing procedure.
9. Assess patient's/family caregiver's knowledge, prior experience with dressing change, and feelings about procedure.	Reveals need for patient instruction and/or support.

STEP	RATIONALE

PLANNING

1. Expected outcomes following completion of procedure:
   - Patient's wound shows evidence of healing by decrease in size and reduced drainage, redness, or swelling.
   - Patient reports decrease in pain after dressing change as compared with pain level noted during assessment.
   - Dressing remains clean, dry, and intact.

   - Patient or family caregiver explains purpose of dressing and method of dressing application.
2. Provide privacy and explain procedure. Explain to patient any sensations (e.g., removal of adhesive and old dressing, cleansing solution in and around the wound) that might be felt during the dressing change.
3. Perform hand hygiene. Organize and set up any equipment needed to perform procedure at bedside.
4. Place biohazard bag within reach of work area. Fold top of bag to make a cuff (see illustration).

Indicates that wound is healing appropriately.

Indicates that patient has appropriate analgesia.

Indicates that proper application and securement are used for dressing.
Indicates understanding and that learning has occurred.

Protects patient's privacy; reduces anxiety. Promotes cooperation.

Ensures more efficiency when completing the procedure.

Ensures easy disposal of soiled dressings. Do not reach across sterile field.

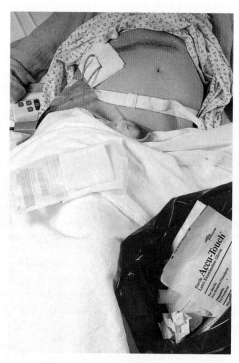

STEP 4 Disposable waterproof bag placed near dressing.

5. Position patient comfortably and drape to expose only wound site. Instruct patient not to touch wound or sterile supplies.

Draping provides access to wound while minimizing exposure. Dressing supplies become contaminated when touched by patient's hand.

IMPLEMENTATION

1. Perform hand hygiene and apply clean gloves. Apply gown, goggles, and mask if risk for splashing exists.
2. Gently remove tape, bandages, or ties. Using two hands, slowly remove adhesive at a low angle, parallel to the patient's skin, while supporting the skin at the skin-tape interface (Thayer et al., 2022). If dressing is over hairy area, remove in direction of hair growth (Hitchcock et al., 2021). Get patient permission to clip or shave area (check agency policy). Remove any adhesive from skin.

Use of PPE reduces transmission of microorganisms.

Pulling tape parallel to the patient's skin and providing support at the skin-tape interface reduces skin tears (Thayer et al., 2022).

STEP	RATIONALE

Clinical Judgment *If a transparent dressing is present, gently pull the edge of the film and allow the film to release and lift from the patient's skin (Thayer et al., 2022).*

Clinical Judgment *If surgical glue was used to close the wound, assess that the glue is intact. Do not remove the glue. Only replace the top dressing as needed.*

3. With gloved hand or forceps, remove dressing one layer at a time, observing appearance of drainage on dressing. Carefully remove outer secondary dressing first, and then remove inner primary dressing in contact with wound bed. If drains are present, slowly and carefully remove dressings (see illustration) and avoid tension on any drainage devices. Keep soiled dressing from patient's sight.

Purpose of primary dressing is to remove necrotic tissue and exudate. Appearance of drainage may be upsetting to patient. Avoids accidental removal of drain.

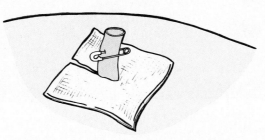

STEP 3 Penrose drain with split gauze.

a. If bottom layer of a moist dressing adheres to wound, gently free dressing while alerting patient of discomfort.

A moist dressing debrides the wound, gently freeing any adhered dressing material prevents trauma to a healing wound surface (Bryant & Nix, 2024).

b. If dry dressing adheres to wound that is not to be debrided, moisten with normal saline first, wait 1 to 2 minutes, and then remove.

Provides easier, nontraumatic dressing removal and prevents injury to wound surface and periwound areas (Ramundo, 2022).

4. Inspect wound and periwound for appearance, color, size (length, width, and depth), drainage, edema, presence and condition of drains, approximation (wound edges are together), granulation tissue, or odor. Use measuring guide or ruler to measure size of wound (see Chapter 38). Inspect periwound area for signs of MARSI and MASD and gently palpate wound edges for bogginess or patient report of increased pain.

Assesses condition of wound and periwound condition. Indicates status of healing. Adhesives used to secure some dressings increase the patient's risk for MARSI (Thayer et al., 2022). The use of moist dressings increases the patient's risk for MASD (Earlam & Woods, 2022).

Clinical Judgment *If signs of MARSI or MASD are present, investigate new adhesive material or other methods to secure dressing and determine whether additional moisture-absorbent dressing materials are needed. A WOCN or wound care specialist can guide wound care revisions.*

Clinical Judgment *If drainage is observed or there is an odor from the wound, verify with health care provider about obtaining a wound culture.*

5. Fold dressings with drainage contained inside and remove gloves inside out. With small dressings, remove gloves inside out over dressing (see illustrations). Dispose of gloves and soiled dressing according to agency policy. Cover wound lightly with sterile gauze pad and perform hand hygiene.

Contains soiled dressings, prevents contact of your hands with drainage, and reduces cross-contamination.

6. Describe appearance of wound and any indicators of wound healing to patient.

Wounds may be unsettling and frightening to patients. It helps a patient to know that wound appearance is as expected and whether healing is taking place.

7. Create sterile field with sterile dressing tray or individually wrapped sterile supplies on over-bed table (see Chapter 10). Pour any prescribed solution into sterile basin.

Sterile dressings remain sterile while on or within sterile surface. Preparation of all supplies before dressing change prevents break in technique during dressing change.

8. Clean wound (see Chapter 38):
   a. Perform hand hygiene and apply clean gloves. Use gauze or cotton ball moistened in saline or antiseptic swab (per health care provider order) for each cleaning stroke or spray wound surface with wound cleaner.

Prevents transfer of organisms from previously cleaned area.

   b. Clean from least to most contaminated area (see Chapter 38) (see illustration).

Cleaning in this direction prevents introduction of organisms into wound.

STEP	RATIONALE

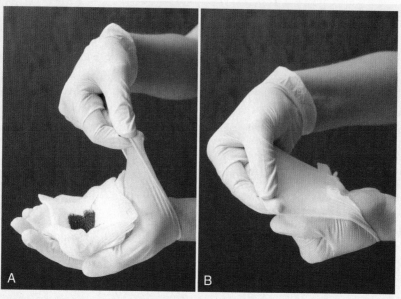

STEP 5 (A) and (B) Dispose of soiled dressings by placing in gloved hand and pulling glove off over dressing and then off hand.

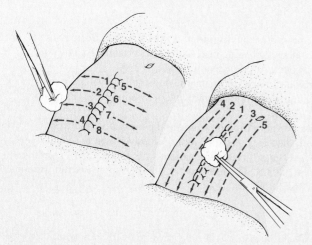

STEP 8b Methods for cleaning a wound, cleaning from least to most contaminated.

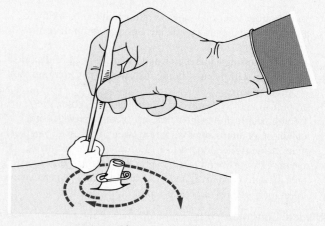

STEP 8c Cleaning around a drain site.

c. Clean around any drain (if present), using circular strokes starting near drain and moving outward and away from insertion site (see illustration) (see Chapter 38).	Correct aseptic technique in cleaning prevents contamination.
d. Use sterile dry gauze to blot wound bed in same manner.	Drying reduces excess moisture, which could eventually harbor microorganisms.
9. Apply antiseptic ointment (if ordered) with sterile cotton-tipped applicator or gauze along wound edges. Dispose of gloves. Perform hand hygiene.	Helps reduce growth of microorganisms.
10. Apply dressing (see agency policy):	
a. Dry sterile dressing	

Clinical Judgment *Dry dressings are not appropriate for debriding wounds. In the presence of drainage, a dry dressing may adhere to the wound bed and surrounding tissue, causing pain and trauma on removal. Dry dressings have the disadvantage of moisture evaporating quickly, which can cause a dressing to dry out. As a result, frequent dressing changes are usually needed and there are increased infection rates when compared with semiocclusive dressings (Thayer et al., 2022).*

(1) Apply clean gloves (see agency policy).	Some health care agencies or the condition of a wound may require sterile gloves.

STEP	RATIONALE

(2) Apply loose woven gauze as contact layer (see illustration).

(3) If drain is present, apply precut, split 4 × 4–inch gauze around drain. — Secures drain and promotes drainage absorption at site.

(4) Apply additional layers of gauze as needed. — Ensures proper coverage and optimal absorption.

(5) Apply thicker woven pad (e.g., Surgipad, abdominal [ABD] pad) for the outermost dressing if needed (see illustration). — This dressing is used on postoperative wounds when there is excessive drainage.

b. Moist dressing: — The moistened gauze increases the absorptive ability of the dressing to collect exudate and wound debris.

Clinical Judgment *For patients at risk for MASD, use a moisture barrier, such as skin sealants, skin barrier ointments or paste, and solid-wafer skin barriers to protect periwound skin (Earlam & Woods, 2022).*

(1) Apply sterile gloves (see agency policy). — Reduces transmission of infection.

(2) Place fine-mesh or loose 4 × 4–inch gauze in container of prescribed sterile solution. Wring out excess solution thoroughly. — Damp gauze absorbs drainage and, when allowed to dry, traps debris.

Clinical Judgment *When using "packing strips," use sterile scissors to cut the amount of dressing that you will use to pack the wound. Do not let the packing strip touch the outside of the bottle. Place packing strip in container of prescribed sterile solution. Wring out excess solution.*

(3) Fluff the damp fine-mesh or open-weave gauze and apply as single layer directly onto wound surface. If wound is deep, gently pack gauze into wound with sterile gloved hand or forceps until all wound surfaces are in contact with damp gauze, including dead spaces from sinus tracts, tunnels, and undermining (see illustration A). Be sure that gauze does not touch periwound skin (see illustration B). — Inner gauze should be moist, not wet, to absorb drainage and adhere to debris. When packing a wound, gauze should conform to base and side of wound (Brace, 2024; Bryant & Nix, 2024). Wound is loosely packed to facilitate wicking of drainage into absorbent outer layer of dressing (Box 40.3). Moisture that escapes dressing often macerates the periwound area (Earlam & Woods, 2022).

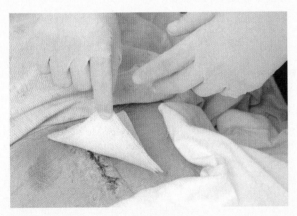

STEP 10a(2) Placing dry gauze dressing over simple wound.

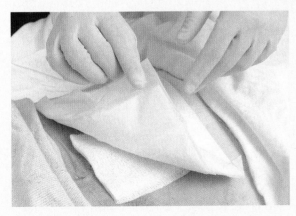

STEP 10a(5) Placing abdominal pad over gauze dressing.

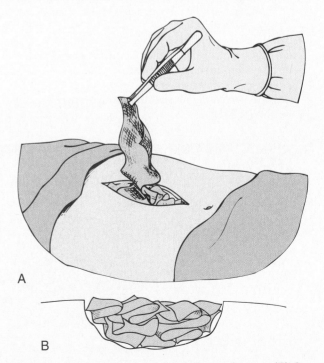

STEP 10b(3) (A) Packing wound with fine-mesh gauze. (B) Cross-section of deep wound packed loosely with gauze roll.

STEP	RATIONALE

BOX 40.3

Principles for Packing a Wound

- Use the wound characteristics to decide which type of packing is appropriate.
- Make sure that the packing material can be safely used to pack a wound.
- Moisten the packing material with a noncytotoxic solution such as normal saline. Never use cytotoxic solutions (e.g., povidone-iodine) to pack a wound.

- If using woven gauze, fluff it before packing it into the wound.
- Loosely pack the wound.
- Do not let the packing material drag or touch the surrounding wound tissue before you put it into the wound.
- Fill all the wound dead space with the packing material.
- Pack the wound until you reach the wound surface; never pack the wound higher than the wound surface.

Clinical Judgment *Count and document the number of pieces of gauze that are packed in the wound, especially deep wounds. This ensures that all gauze is removed from the wound with each dressing change.*

Clinical Judgment *When packing the wound, use loosely woven gauze and do not overpack or underpack (Bryant & Nix, 2024). Packing should fill the wound but should not be above the level of the skin.*

STEP	RATIONALE
(4) Apply dry moisture retentive sterile dressing material over moist gauze.	Dry moisture retentive layer helps to maintain a moist, not wet, inner dressing and helps to reduce MASD (Earlam & Woods, 2022).
(5) Cover with ABD pad, Surgipad, or gauze.	Protects wound from entrance of microorganisms and maintains a dry surface dressing.

Clinical Judgment *The dry surface dressing helps to maintain dry bed linens and reduce exposure of the patient's skin to moisture.*

STEP	RATIONALE
11. Secure dressing:	
a. *Tape:* Apply nonallergenic tape over gauze and 2.5 to 5 cm (1 to 2 inches) beyond dressing.	Supports wound and ensures placement and stability of dressing. Nonallergenic tape reduces the risk for MARSI (Thayer et al., 2022).
b. Montgomery ties (see illustrations):	Prevents skin irritation. Ties allow for repeated dressing changes without removal of tape.
(1) Be sure that skin is clean. Application of skin barrier is recommended (see Chapter 38).	
(2) Expose adhesive surface of tape ends.	
(3) Place ties on opposite sides of dressing over skin barrier.	
(4) Secure dressing by lacing ties across dressing snugly enough to hold it secure but without placing pressure on skin.	Skin barrier (stomahesive) protects intact skin from stretch and tension of adhesive tape, reducing risk of MARSI.
c. For protective window:	
(1) Cut hydrocolloid pad into four strips used to form a "window" around the wound.	A protective window is an alternative to Montgomery ties for smaller wounds. There is less skin irritation by placing tape on window strips.
(2) Use skin barrier to wipe areas of skin where strips will be applied.	

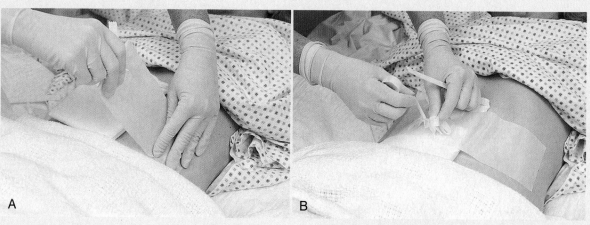

A   B

STEP 11b Montgomery ties. (A) Each tie is placed at side of gauze dressing. (B) Securing ties encloses dressing.

STEP	RATIONALE

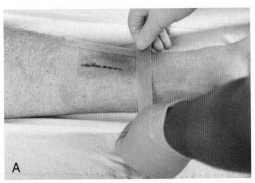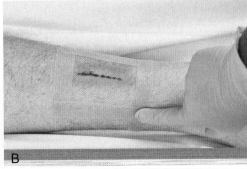

STEP 11c(3) Apply adhesive strips to frame a "window" around wound using four strips.

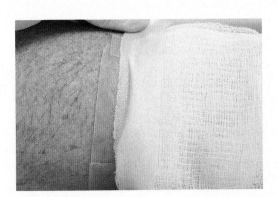

STEP 11c(4) Apply dressing; secure tape ends to adhesive strips.

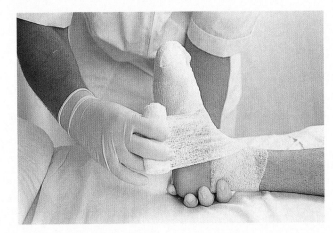

STEP 11d Wrap rolled gauze around extremity to secure dressing.

(3) Apply hydrocolloid dressing strips to frame a "window" around the wound using four strips, one on each side, one on the top, and one on the bottom of the dressing material (see illustrations).

(4) Apply dressing; secure tape ends to stomahesive or hydrocolloid strips (see illustration).

d. For dressing on an extremity, secure with rolled gauze (see illustration) or elastic net. | Rolled gauze conforms to contour of foot or hand.

12. Dispose of all dressing supplies. Remove cover gown and goggles; remove gloves inside out; dispose of all items according to agency policy. Perform hand hygiene. | Reduces transmission of microorganisms. Clean environment enhances patient comfort.

13. Label tape over dressing with your initials and date dressing is changed. | Provides timeline for when next dressing change is to be scheduled.

14. Help patient to a comfortable position. | Restores comfort and sense of well-being.

15. Raise side rails (as appropriate) and lower bed to lowest position, locking into position. | Ensures patient safety and prevents falls.

16. Place nurse call system in an accessible location within patient's reach. | Ensures patient can call for assistance if needed.

EVALUATION

1. Compare observations of the wound and periwound area with previous assessment and observe appearance of wound for healing: measure size of wound; observe amount, color, and type of drainage and periwound erythema, rash, excoriation, or swelling; and observe for signs associated with MARSI and MASD. | Determines rate of healing and any presence of MARSI and MASD.

2. Ask patient to describe character of wound pain and rate acuity on a pain scale of 0 to 10. | Increased pain is often an indication of wound complications such as infection or a result of dressing pulling tissue.

STEP	RATIONALE
3. Inspect condition of dressing at least every shift.	Determines status of wound drainage.
4. **Use Teach-Back:** "I want to be sure I explained why and how often you need to continue these dressing changes when you go home. Tell me why it is important to change your dressing and how often you will do this." Revise your instruction now or develop a plan for revised patient/family caregiver teaching if patient/family caregiver is not able to teach back correctly.	Teach-back is a technique for health care providers to ensure that they have explained medical information clearly so that patients and their families understand what is communicated to them (AHRQ, 2023).

Unexpected Outcomes	Related Interventions
1. Wound appears inflamed and tender, drainage is evident, and/or odor is present.	• Monitor patient for signs of infection (e.g., fever, increased white blood cell count). • Notify health care provider. • Obtain wound cultures as ordered. • If there is yellow, tan, or brown necrotic tissue, notify health care provider to determine need for debridement (Table 40.2).
2. Wound bleeds during dressing change.	• Observe color and amount of bloody drainage. If excessive, may need to apply direct dressing. • Inspect area along dressing and directly underneath patient to determine amount of bleeding. • Obtain vital signs as needed. • Notify health care provider.
3. Periwound area has an erythema rash and is blistered, and excoriation and skin tears are present, all signs of MARSI or MASD.	• Consult a wound care specialist to determine changes in dressing care and adhesives. • Provide topical agents and skin barrier as prescribed.
4. Patient reports sensation that "something has given way under the dressing."	• Observe wound for increased drainage or dehiscence (partial or total separation of wound layers) or evisceration (total separation of wound layers and protrusion of viscera through wound opening). • If dehiscence or evisceration occurs, protect wound. Cover with sterile moist saline dressing. • Instruct patient to lie still. • Stay with patient to monitor vital signs. • Notify health care provider.

TABLE 40.2

Problems Associated With Wounds Requiring Debridement

Problem	Nursing Activities
Solutions used may be irritating to healthy skin around wound.	Protect healthy skin with protective barrier such as stomahesive, or apply topical ointments such as zinc oxide. If zinc oxide is used, it should be removed with mineral oil. Avoid scrubbing the skin because scrubbing can cause harm to the epithelial layer.
Wound becomes excessively dry.	A continually moist dressing (with a health care provider's order) might be tried. Eliminate fine-mesh gauze and lightly pack wound with fluffy gauze dampened with prescribed solution.
Wound is deep, and retention of dressing in cavity is suspected.	Irrigate wound copiously with prescribed solution to loosen dressing for removal. Use continuous "ribbon" or strip of gauze to dress deep wounds.
Wound drainage is damaging healthy tissue.	Protect healthy tissue with skin barrier such as a hydrocolloid. Wounds with large amounts of drainage may benefit from occlusive drainage collection device.
Patient's skin is irritated by tape.	Use hydrocolloid under tape, Montgomery ties as needed, and fabric tape that has multidirectional stretch; secure dressing with binder or wrap with rolled gauze if on extremity.

Documentation

• Document appearance and size of wound, characteristics of drainage, presence of necrotic tissue, type of dressing applied, periwound skin integrity, patient's response to dressing change, and level of comfort.
• Document patient's and family caregiver's understanding through teach-back.

Hand-Off Reporting

• Report any unexpected appearance of wound drainage, accidental removal of drain, or bright red bleeding.
• Report any changes in periwound skin or signs of MARSI or MASD.
• Report any change in wound integrity (e.g., evidence of wound dehiscence or evisceration).

Special Considerations

Patient Education

- Explain expected wound appearance and risks of improper wound care. Provide patient and family caregiver with a written list of signs to report to the health care provider.
- After demonstrating wound care, have patient or family caregiver perform dressing change with and without supervision.

Pediatrics

- Some pediatric patients are fearful of dressing changes. Obtain patient's cooperation and/or have another person available to keep child from moving during dressing change procedure (Hockenberry et al., 2024).
- Older children may need something to do during dressing changes. Listening to music or watching a video helps to relieve some of the boredom or stress during the procedure (Hockenberry et al., 2024).

Older Adults

- Normal aging changes of skin and tissue and the inflammatory response may delay wound healing (Richbourg, 2022).
- Consider risk factors in older-adult patients for impaired skin integrity, such as sensory impairment, dry and dehydrated skin, or impaired nutritional status, that will affect wound healing (Touhy & Jett, 2022).

- Avoid early and frequent removal of hydrocolloid dressing strips to prevent MARSI to surrounding intact skin.
- Adhesive tape may be too irritating to older adults' skin and cause skin tears. Use paper tape, nonallergenic tape, or wraps or mesh to avoid tape contacting a patient's skin (Thayer et al., 2022; Touhy & Jett, 2022).

Populations With Disabilities

- Patients with cognitive disabilities are vulnerable to increased agitation and fear during dressing changes, and a family member or caregiver present during dressing change often helps to reduce agitation and anxiety (Mendes, 2018; Waters, 2017).

Home Care

- When the patient needs dressing changes at home, be sure to educate patient and family caregiver on the proper techniques for using dressing materials and for disposing of medical waste.
- Consider resources within the home, ability of a family caregiver, and the amount of time needed to change a particular dressing when selecting a dressing procedure in the home setting. More expensive dressings may be used to decrease frequency of dressing changes.
- Reimbursement for wound care requires a signed health care provider's order, treatment plan, and documentation of the actual care provided.

✦ SKILL 40.2 Applying a Pressure Bandage

The first step in treating a hemorrhage is to control the bleeding. One method is the application of direct pressure. A pressure bandage is a temporary treatment to control excessive, sudden, unanticipated bleeding (Charlton et al., 2021). Applied with elastic bandages, a pressure dressing exerts localized downward pressure over an actual or potential bleeding site. Hemorrhage may occur during or after diagnostic interventions (e.g., cardiac catheterization, arterial puncture, organ biopsy), surgery, or a life-threatening occurrence related to trauma (stabbing, gunshot). Early application of a tourniquet or pressure dressing can slow the flow of blood and promote clotting at the site (hemostasis) until definitive action can be taken (Bendri et al., 2022). Given the emergent nature of an acute bleeding episode, the aseptic techniques considered essential in most dressing applications are secondary to the goal of halting the bleeding.

Delegation

The skill of applying a pressure dressing in an emergency situation cannot be delegated to assistive personnel (AP). If application requires more than one person, the AP can assist. Instruct the AP to:
- Assist the nurse as directed.

- Observe the pressure dressing during care activities to make sure that it remains in place and that there is no visible bleeding from the site.
- Observe underneath patient for bleeding after dressing has been applied.

Interprofessional Collaboration

- When excessive bleeding occurs. another health care provider, such as a surgeon, is needed to intervene and stop the bleeding. Intervention often requires surgery or invasive procedures.

Equipment

- Clean gloves
- Necessary dressings/equipment: fine-mesh gauze, abdominal (ABD) pads, hemostatic dressings, elastic rolled gauze, chest tube tray
- Adhesive tape; hypoallergenic
- Adhesive remover (optional)
- Personal protective equipment (PPE) (e.g., gown, goggles, mask) as needed
- Equipment for vital signs

STEP	RATIONALE

ASSESSMENT

1. If situation permits, identify patient using at least two identifiers (e.g., name and birthday or name and medical record number) according to agency policy.	Ensures correct patient. Complies with The Joint Commission standards and improves patient safety (TJC, 2023).
2. Perform hand hygiene and apply clean gloves. Anticipate patients at risk for unexpected bleeding, including traumatic injury, arterial puncture, donor graft site, postoperative incision, wounds after surgical debridement, and surgical patient with history of bleeding disorder.	Familiarity with conditions associated with unexpected bleeding allows you to rapidly respond to bleeding.

STEP	RATIONALE
3. Look for visible presence of blood or blood pulsating from arterial site.	These are signs of hemorrhage.

Clinical Judgment *To fully assess the amount of blood loss from a patient who is bleeding from a thoracic or abdominal surgical or traumatic wound, turn patient over and inspect for any blood pooling under the patient.*

4. If situation permits, assess patient for allergies to antiseptics, tape, or latex. If patient is nonresponsive and no history is available, use nonlatex or nonallergenic supplies.	Prevents localized or systemic allergic reaction.
5. Quickly assess patient's anxiety level.	Determines need for education and positive reinforcement during procedure.
6. If possible, review electronic health record (EHR) for patient's baseline vital signs before onset of hemorrhage.	If data are available, baseline vital signs indicate status of circulatory function.
7. After the initial crisis and if the situation permits, assess patient's/family caregiver's health literacy.	Ensures patient and family caregiver have the capacity to obtain, communicate, process, and understand basic health information (CDC, 2023).

PLANNING

1. Expected outcomes following completion of procedure:	
• Patient shows cessation of bleeding and no evidence of hematoma formation.	Hemostasis is achieved.
• Patient maintains stable blood pressure and heart rate.	Hemodynamic stability is achieved with minimal blood loss.
• Distal circulation is maintained with intact pulses (distal to site of injury).	Bandage applied without excessive pressure.
2. Provide privacy and, if possible, explain procedure and what is occurring to the patient.	Protects patient's privacy; reduces anxiety. Promotes cooperation.
3. Perform hand hygiene. Obtain specialized equipment, such as chest tube tray and hemocclusive dressing material.	Reduces transmission of microorganisms. Ensures efficiency during the procedure.
4. If not already present, arrange for extra personnel to help as needed.	Extra personnel assist in positioning the patient, obtaining additional equipment, and escorting family caregivers from the treatment area.

IMPLEMENTATION

Phase I: Immediate Action—First Nurse

1. Perform hand hygiene and apply clean gloves. Identify external bleeding site. You will need to turn patients to observe underneath those who have large abdomens.	Quick identification increases response time to stop bleeding. Maintaining asepsis and privacy are considered only if time and severity of blood loss permit.

Clinical Judgment *Wounds to groin area also can result in large amounts of blood loss, which is not always visible.*

2. Use both hands and press as hard as you can to apply immediate manual pressure to bleeding site.	External pressure over the wound helps control bleeding.
3. Remain with the patient and seek help. Have another person notify patient's health care provider as appropriate.	Situation could be life threatening. Patient should not be left alone.

Clinical Judgment *Find another member of the health care team to insert intravenous catheters, prepare dressings, and prepare for emergency transport to the operating room.*

Phase II: Applying Pressure Bandage—Second Nurse

4. If the situation permits, perform hand hygiene and apply clean gloves. Quickly identify source of bleeding.	Determines method of application and supplies to use.
• *Arterial bleeding* is bright red and gushes forth in waves related to patient's heart rate; if vessel is very deep, flow is steady.	
• *Venous bleeding* is dark red and flows smoothly.	
• *Capillary bleeding* is oozing of dark red blood; self-sealing controls this bleeding.	
5. Elevate affected body part (e.g., extremity) if possible.	Helps slow rate of bleeding.
6. First nurse continues to apply direct pressure as second nurse unwraps elastic rolled bandage and places within easy reach. Second nurse quickly cuts three to five lengths of adhesive tape and places them within reach; *do not clean wound*.	Pressure dressing controls bleeding temporarily. Preparation allows for securing pressure bandage quickly.
7. In simultaneous coordinated actions:	
a. Rapidly cover bleeding area with multiple thicknesses of gauze compresses. The first nurse slips fingers out as other nurse exerts adequate pressure to continue controlling bleeding (see illustration).	Gauze is absorbent. Layers provide bulk against which local pressure can be applied to bleeding site.

STEP	RATIONALE

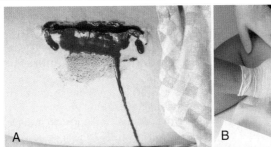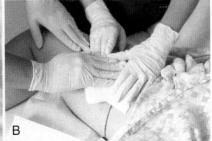

STEP 7a (A) Bleeding wound. (B) Nurses apply pressure dressing.

b. Place adhesive strips 7 to 10 cm (3 to 4 inches) beyond width of gauze dressing with even pressure on both sides of fingers as close as possible to central bleeding source. Secure tape on distal end, pull tape across dressing, and keep firm pressure as proximate end of tape is secured.	Tape exerts downward pressure, promoting hemostasis. To ensure blood flow to distal tissues and prevent tourniquet effect, adhesive tape must not be continued around entire extremity.
c. Remove fingers temporarily and quickly cover center of area with third strip of tape.	Provides pressure to source of bleeding.
d. Continue reinforcing area with tape as each successive strip is overlapped on alternating sides of center strip. **Keep applying pressure**.	Prevents tape from loosening.
e. When pressure bandage is on extremity, apply gauze directly over bleeding site. Then apply elastic rolled bandage over gauze: Apply two circular turns tautly on both sides of fingers that are pressing gauze. Compress over bleeding site. Simultaneously remove finger pressure and apply rolled bandage over center. Continue with figure-eight turns, moving from distal to proximal moving toward the patient's heart. Secure end with two circular turns and strip of adhesive (see Procedural Guideline 40.1).	Elastic rolled bandage acts as pressure bandage, exerting more even pressure over extremity. (**NOTE**: Gauze rolled bandage can be used if elastic is not available.)
8. Once bandage is applied, dispose of any contaminated supplies; remove and dispose of gloves. Perform hand hygiene.	Reduces transmission of microorganisms.
9. If the situation permits, help patient to a comfortable position.	Restores comfort and sense of well-being.
10. Raise side rails (as appropriate) and lower bed to lowest position, locking into position.	Ensures patient safety and prevents falls.
11. Place nurse call system in an accessible location within patient's reach.	Ensures patient can call for assistance if needed.

EVALUATION

1. Observe dressing for control of bleeding.	Effective pressure bandage controls bleeding without blocking distal circulation.
2. Evaluate adequacy of circulation (distal pulse, skin temperature, and color).	Determines level of perfusion to distal body parts.
3. Estimate volume of blood loss (e.g., count number of dressings used, weigh saturated dressing).	Helps to determine blood and fluid replacement needs.
4. Monitor vital signs.	Identifies patient's response to blood loss and early stages of hypovolemic shock.

Unexpected Outcomes

1. There is continued bleeding. Fluid and electrolyte imbalance, tissue hypoxia, confusion, hypovolemic shock, and cardiac arrest develop.

2. Pressure dressing is too tight and occludes circulation.

Related Interventions

- Notify health care provider immediately.
- Reinforce or adjust pressure dressing.
- If bleeding from extremity, elevate affected body part.
- Initiate intravenous (IV) therapy per order.
- Monitor vital signs every 5 to 15 minutes (apical pulse, distal pulses, and blood pressure).
- Inspect areas distal to pressure dressing to ensure that circulation has not been occluded.
- Adjust dressing as needed.

Documentation

- Document location of bleeding, assessment findings, application and type of pressure dressing, and patient response.

Hand-Off Reporting

- Report immediately to health care provider present status of patient's bleeding control, time bleeding was discovered, estimated blood loss, nursing interventions (including effectiveness of applied pressure bandage), apical and distal pulses, blood pressure, mental status, signs of restlessness, and need for health care provider to administer to patient without delay.

Special Considerations

Patient Education

- Explain to patient and family caregiver (if present) need to monitor vital signs.
- Explain need for patient to remain quiet and stay in position to reduce bleeding.

Pediatrics

- If family and health care providers can remain calm, a child may calm down and be more cooperative (Hockenberry et al., 2024).

Older Adults

- Because of the normal changes of aging, the older adult has an increased risk for vascular and tissue changes distal to the pressure dressing. Evaluate skin and pulse distal to the pressure bandage frequently (Touhy & Jett, 2022).

Populations With Disabilities

- This is an emergent situation and requires fast action from several health care professionals. The number of professionals and the noise during this emergent situation can cause a patient with cognitive disabilities to become more agitated and uncooperative. Continue to use a calm voice and explain to the patient what the doctors and nurses are doing to help (Mendes, 2018).

Home Care

- If patient is at risk for hemorrhage, instruct on the following:
  - How family caregiver or patient should apply pressure with clean towels or linen
  - Immediate activation of emergency system (9-1-1)
  - How to position patient by elevating affected body part (if extremity)

Caution: If a puncture wound occurs from a penetrating object (e.g., knife, toy, building materials), instruct family caregivers not to remove the object. Removal will cause more rapid blood loss and may damage underlying structures.

✦ SKILL 40.3   Applying a Transparent Dressing

Transparent film dressing is a thin sheet of polyurethane with a layer of acrylic hypoallergenic adhesive on one side. A transparent dressing is often the dressing of choice over an intravenous (IV) catheter insertion site (see Chapter 28). The adhesive is inactivated by moisture and will not adhere to a moist surface (Jaszarowski & Murphree, 2022). It is a semiocclusive dressing, which will keep the wound moist by retaining moisture lost by the wound.

Once it is applied, a moist exudate forms over the wound surface, which prevents tissue dehydration and allows for rapid, effective healing by speeding epithelial cell growth. The dressings are appropriate for prophylaxis on high-risk intact skin (e.g., high-friction areas) or patient's heels (Jaszarowski & Murphree, 2022).

Transparent film dressings can promote autolytic debridement of eschar if needed. They are available in a variety of sizes and shapes that conform to the body and are more cost efficient than a hydrocolloid dressing in preventing pressure injuries (PIs). The synthetic permeable membrane acts as a temporary second skin, adheres to undamaged skin to contain exudate, minimizes wound contamination, and allows a wound to "breathe" (Armstrong et al., 2023; EPUAP/NPIAP/PPPIA, 2019a).

Delegation

The skill of applying a transparent dressing for select wounds can be delegated to assistive personnel (AP) (refer to agency policy).

The assessment of the wound and care of sterile or new acute wounds cannot be delegated to AP. Instruct the AP by:
- Explaining how to adapt the skill for a specific patient.
- Reporting any signs of bleeding, drainage, infection, or poor wound healing immediately to the nurse.
- Reporting loosening of a dressing.

Interprofessional Collaboration

- When a patient's skin shows signs of poor wound healing or early signs of pressure injury development, a wound care specialist can assist in individualizing dressing care.

Equipment

- Sterile gloves (optional)
- Clean gloves
- Dressing set (optional)
- Sterile saline or other cleansing agent (as ordered)
- Cotton swabs
- Biohazard bag for disposal
- Transparent dressing (size as needed)
- Sterile 4 × 4–inch gauze pads
- Skin-preparation materials (optional)
- Personal protective equipment (PPE) (e.g., gown, goggles, mask) as needed

---

STEP	RATIONALE

ASSESSMENT

1. Identify patient using at least two identifiers (e.g., name and birthday or name and medical record number) according to agency policy.

Ensures correct patient. Complies with The Joint Commission standards and improves patient safety (TJC, 2023).

2. Review patient's electronic health record (EHR), including health care provider's order for frequency and type of dressing change.

Health care provider orders frequency of dressing changes and special instructions.

STEP	RATIONALE
3. Review previous nurses' notes in EHR or chart, noting location, wound assessment, size of wound, and patient response to dressing changes.	Determines type of materials and size of transparent dressing needed for dressing change.
4. Review EHR to determine patient's age and history of dehydration, malnutrition, exposure to radiation therapy, underlying chronic conditions (e.g., diabetes mellitus, immunosuppression), edema of the skin, and the presence of erythema, blistering, excoriation, or erosion of skin or a rash under or adjacent to adhesive's securing dressing.	Common risk factors for medical adhesive–related skin injury (MARSI) (Fumarola et al., 2020). Erythema, blistering, and excoriation are signs of MARSI and are related to the skin's reaction to an adhesive (Thayer et al., 2022). Erosion of underlying or superficial periwound skin or periwound area or rash are indications of moisture-associated skin damage (Earlam & Woods, 2022).

Clinical Judgment *Transparent dressings are applied over clean, debrided wounds that are not actively bleeding.*

STEP	RATIONALE
5. Review EHR for patient's medical history indicating risks for impaired wound healing (e.g., aging, poor nutrition, steroid use).	Physiological changes caused by aging, chronic illness, poor nutrition, medications, and cancer treatments have potential to affect wound healing (Beitz, 2022).
6. Assess patient's/family caregiver's health literacy.	Determines degree to which individuals have the ability to find, understand, and use information and services to make informed health-related decisions and actions for themselves and others (CDC, 2023).
7. Assess patient for allergies, especially antiseptics, tape, or latex. Have patient describe allergic response.	Prevents local or systemic allergic reaction. If information is not available, use nonlatex products and hypoallergenic tape.
8. Ask patient to describe character of any wound pain and to rate severity using pain scale of 0 to 10. Administer prescribed analgesic as needed 30 minutes before dressing change.	Comfortable patient will be less likely to move suddenly, causing wound or supply contamination. Serves as baseline to measure response to dressing therapy.
9. Assess patient's knowledge, prior experience with transparent dressing, and feelings about procedure.	Reveals need for patient instruction and/or support.

PLANNING

STEP	RATIONALE
1. Expected outcomes following completion of procedure:	
• Patient's wound shows evidence of healing by decrease in size and reduced drainage, redness, or swelling.	Indicates that wound is healing appropriately.
• Patient reports decrease in pain after dressing change as compared with pain level noted during assessment.	Indicates that patient has appropriate analgesia.
• Dressing remains clean and intact.	Indicates that proper application and securement are used for dressing.
• Patient or family caregiver explains purpose of dressing and method of dressing application.	Indicates understanding and that learning has occurred.
2. Provide privacy and explain procedure.	Protects patient's privacy; reduces anxiety. Promotes cooperation.
3. Perform hand hygiene. Organize and set up any equipment needed to perform procedure at bedside.	Reduces transmission of microorganisms. Ensures more efficiency when completing an assessment.
4. Place biohazard bag within reach of work area.	Ensures easy disposal of soiled dressing.
5. Position patient comfortably and drape to expose only wound site. Instruct patient not to touch wound or sterile supplies.	Draping provides access to wound while minimizing exposure. Dressing supplies become contaminated when touched by patient's hand.

IMPLEMENTATION

STEP	RATIONALE
1. Perform hand hygiene and apply clean gloves. Apply PPE as needed if there is a risk for splashing.	Reduces transmission of infectious organisms from soiled dressings to your hands.
2. Remove old dressing by stretching film in direction parallel to wound rather than pulling.	Stretching action gently breaks dressing seal and dressing lifts off skin, reducing excoriation, tearing, or irritation of skin. Thus, reduces risk for MARSI (Thayer et al., 2022).
3. Dispose of soiled dressing in waterproof bag, remove gloves by pulling them inside out, dispose of them in waterproof bag, and perform hand hygiene.	Reduces transmission of microorganisms.
4. Prepare dressing supplies. Use sterile supplies for new wounds (check agency policy).	Reduces risk for break in sterile technique.
5. Pour saline or prescribed solution over 4 × 4–inch sterile gauze pads.	Maintains sterility of dressing.
6. Apply clean or sterile gloves (check agency policy).	Allows you to handle dressings.
7. Clean wound and periwound area gently with 4 × 4–inch sterile gauze pads moistened in sterile saline or spray with wound cleaner. Clean in direction from least to most contaminated area (see Skill 40.1).	Reduces introduction of organisms into wound.

STEP	RATIONALE
8. Pat skin around wound in same direction as Step 7; dry thoroughly with dry 4 × 4–inch sterile gauze pads.	Transparent dressing with adhesive backing does not adhere to damp surface (Jaszarowski & Murphree, 2022).
9. Inspect wound for tissue type, color, odor, and drainage; measure size if indicated (see Chapter 38).	Provides baseline for monitoring wound healing.
10. Remove and dispose of gloves and perform hand hygiene.	Reduces transmission of microorganisms.

Clinical Judgment *If wound has a large amount of drainage, do not use a transparent dressing. Instead, choose another dressing that can absorb drainage. You may need to consult with wound care specialist.*

Clinical Judgment *If patient has thin or fragile skin, use a skin barrier on the skin around a wound before dressing application to protect patient's skin from further injury (Ermer-Seltun & Rolstad, 2022).*

STEP	RATIONALE
11. Apply clean gloves and apply transparent dressing according to manufacturer directions. *Do not stretch film during application and avoid wrinkles.*	Wrinkles provide tunnel for exudate drainage.
a. Remove paper backing, taking care not to allow adhesive areas to touch one another.	
b. Place film smoothly over wound without stretching (see illustrations).	Ensures coverage of wound. Prevents shearing of skin from dressing that is too tight. Stretching can also break wound seal.
c. Use your fingers to smooth and adhere dressing.	
12. Discard soiled dressing materials properly. Remove gloves by pulling them inside out and discard in prepared bag. Perform hand hygiene.	Prevents transmission of microorganisms.
13. Label dressing with date, your initials, and time of dressing change on outer label of dressing (see illustration).	Provides record for determining when to next change dressing.
14. Help patient to a comfortable position.	Restores comfort and sense of well-being.
15. Raise side rails (as appropriate) and lower bed to lowest position, locking into position.	Ensures patient safety and prevents falls.
16. Place nurse call system in an accessible location within patient's reach.	Ensures patient can call for assistance if needed.

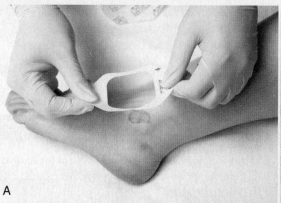 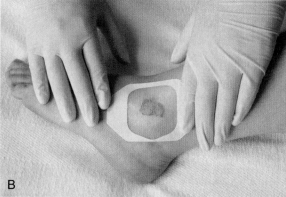

STEP 11b (A) Transparent dressing placed over small wound on ankle. (B) Place film smoothly without stretching.

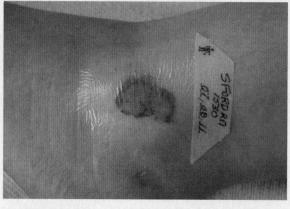

STEP 13 Transparent dressing correctly labeled.

STEP	RATIONALE

EVALUATION

1. Inspect appearance of wound and characteristics and amount of drainage. Measure wound size (see Chapter 38).
2. Inspect condition of periwound areas.
3. Ask patient to describe character of pain and rate severity of wound pain using scale of 0 to 10.
4. **Use Teach-Back:** "I want to be sure you understand how to apply this transparent dressing since you will be using it at home. Show me how you will apply this dressing." Revise your instruction now or develop a plan for revised patient/family caregiver teaching if patient/family caregiver is not able to teach back correctly.

Clear dressing allows you to observe wound and status of wound healing.
Identifies any injury to surrounding skin.
Determines any change in pain during procedure.

Teach-back is a technique for health care providers to ensure that they have explained medical information clearly so that patients and their families understand what is communicated to them (AHRQ, 2023).

Unexpected Outcomes

1. Wound is inflamed, tender. Accumulation of fluid with white, opaque appearance and erythema of surrounding tissue; increased drainage or change in the color of drainage; necrosis; and/or odor is present.

2. Dressing does not stay in place.

Related Interventions

- Remove dressing and obtain wound culture according to agency policy.
- Different type of dressing may be required.
- Notify health care provider.

- Evaluate size of dressing used to be sure it extends over wound margin (2.5 to 3.75 cm [1 to 1.5 inches]).
- Assess for increased drainage from wound.
- Dry patient's skin thoroughly before reapplication
- Try a skin barrier around wound edges.

Documentation

- Document appearance of wound, presence and characteristics of drainage, type of dressing applied, patient's response to dressing change, and level of comfort.
- Document patient's and family caregiver's understanding through teach-back for effective application of dressing.

Hand-Off Reporting

- Report any signs of infection, changes in skin integrity, or signs of pressure injury to the health care provider.

Special Considerations

Patient Education

- Explain need to change dressing should edges loosen.
- Explain to patient and family caregiver that collection of wound fluid under dressing is not "pus" but normal interaction of body fluids with dressing. Caution them to not try to remove fluid (e.g., puncture dressing with a needle).

Pediatrics

- Adhesive backing may cause skin tears on premature infants' immature skin (Hockenberry et al., 2024).
- Children may find this procedure more tolerable if they know that the longer the dressing is left on, the easier it is to remove (Hockenberry et al., 2024).

Older Adults

- Adhesive backing may be too strong for the skin of older adults. Do not use a film dressing that has an adhesive backing with a stronger bond to the epidermis than the epidermis has to the dermis (Thayer et al., 2022).

Home Care

- Wound may be cleaned in shower if approved by health care provider.
- Many types of transparent dressings exist. Explore types with patient and recommend type to which patient has easy access and finds easy to apply.

✦ SKILL 40.4 **Applying a Hydrocolloid, Hydrogel, Foam, or Alginate Dressing**

Achieving the optimal moisture and exudate balance are essential for wound healing (Fletcher & Probst, 2020). The dressings in this section aid in maintaining that delicate moisture balance in healing wounds.

A hydrocolloid dressing is designed to maintain moisture inside a wound without allowing the accumulation of exudate (Valderrama et al., 2021). Because these dressings maintain a moist wound environment, they promote significantly better, cost-efficient wound healing outcomes compared with conventional gauze (Armstrong et al., 2023; Valderrama et al., 2021). These dressings absorb drainage and hydrate and debride wounds. When in contact with wound drainage, the hydrocolloid forms a gel that promotes a moist environment and facilitates autolytic and enzymatic debridement (Bryant & Nix, 2024). The absorption of moisture into a hydrocolloid dressing creates a moisture barrier and reduces the risk for MARSI (Hitchcock et al., 2021). These dressings cushion a wound surface to reduce pain and protect the wound and periwound skin.

Hydrogel dressings are glycerin- or water-based dressings, are moisture retentive, and are designed to hydrate a wound, thus promoting moist wound healing and autolysis (Bryant & Nix, 2024). They have some absorptive properties. These dressings are similar to hydrocolloids and come in the form of sheets, amorphous gels, and impregnated gauze. The gels are nonadherent and less painful to remove.

Foam dressings absorb exudate in superficial or deep wounds, protect friable periwound skin, provide autolytic debridement, and pad high-trauma areas. Foam dressings manage chronic and infected wounds. In addition, multilayered foam dressings aid in preventing heel and sacral pressure injuries (Bryant & Nix, 2024; Haesler, 2017).

Alginate dressings are manufactured from natural substances (seaweed) and are known for their absorptive properties, forming a gel over the wound surface to contain exudate. This dressing may come as a sheet or rope. An alginate dressing protects the wound, creates a moist environment, and promotes autolysis, granulation, and epithelialization of the wound bed (Fletcher & Probst, 2020). You can safely pack deep tracking wounds with calcium-sodium alginate preparation, which allows easy removal with little risk for retained dressing deep in a wound cavity (Bryant & Nix, 2024).

Delegation

The skill of applying a hydrocolloid, hydrogel, foam, or alginate dressing cannot be delegated to assistive personnel (AP). Instruct the AP to:

- Help position patient during dressing application.
- Immediately report to the nurse any pain, fever, bleeding, wound drainage, or slippage of dressing.

Interprofessional Collaboration

- Complicated wounds, such as chronic, infected, or draining wounds require individualized and specialized dressing materials. A WOCN or wound specialist can determine the most effective and efficient dressing protocol to promote wound healing.

Equipment

- Clean gloves
- Sterile gloves (optional)
- Dressing set (optional: items will vary):
  - Sterile scissors
  - Sterile drape
  - Face mask
  - Sterile gloves
  - Tape measure or other measuring guide
  - Tape (nonallergenic paper or adhesive)
  - 4 × 4 gauze squares
  - Dressing change label
  - Antiseptic swabs
- Necessary primary dressings: gauze, hydrocolloid, hydrogel, foam, or alginate
- Secondary dressing of choice
- Montgomery ties
- Sterile saline or other cleaning solution (as ordered)
- Skin barrier wipe
- Biohazard bag
- Adhesive remover
- Debriding gel (as ordered)
- Irrigating solution if ordered (see Skill 40.1)
- Additional personal protective equipment (PPE) (e.g., gown, goggles, mask) as needed

STEP	RATIONALE

ASSESSMENT

1. Identify patient using at least two identifiers (e.g., name and birthday or name and medical record number) according to agency policy.	Ensures correct patient. Complies with The Joint Commission standards and improves patient safety (TJC, 2023).
2. Review patient's electronic health record (EHR), including health care provider's order for frequency and type of dressing change.	Health care provider orders frequency of dressing changes and special instructions.
3. Review EHR to determine patient's age and history of dehydration, malnutrition, exposure to radiation therapy, underlying chronic conditions (e.g., diabetes mellitus, immunosuppression), edema of the skin, and the presence of erythema, blistering, excoriation, or erosion of skin or a rash under or adjacent to adhesive's securing dressing.	Common risk factors for medical adhesive–related skin injury (MARSI) (Fumarola et al., 2020). Erythema, blistering, and excoriation are signs of MARSI and are related to the skin's reaction to an adhesive (Thayer et al., 2022). Erosion of underlying or superficial periwound skin or periwound area or rash are indication of moisture-associated skin damage (Earlam & Woods, 2022).
4. Review patient's EHR, including health care provider's order and nurses' notes, for frequency and type of dressing change. Note possible need to use customized shape or size of dressing to fit difficult body parts (e.g., sacrum, heels, elbows).	Indicates type of dressing or application to use. Customized shapes aid in patient-centered dressing selection and better dressing adherence.

Clinical Judgment *Do not use highly absorptive dressings such as alginate or foam on nonexudative wounds.*

5. Assess patient's/family caregiver's health literacy.	Determines degree to which individuals have the ability to find, understand, and use information and services to make informed health-related decisions and actions for themselves and others (CDC, 2023).
6. Assess for presence of allergies, especially antiseptics, tape, or latex. Have patient describe allergic response.	Prevents localized or systemic reaction to supplies.
7. Ask patient to describe character of wound pain and to then rate severity of pain using scale of 0 to 10. Administer prescribed analgesic as needed 30 minutes before dressing change.	Patient may require pain medication before dressing change. Allows for peak effect of drug during procedure.

STEP	RATIONALE
8. Perform hand hygiene and apply clean gloves. Inspect location, size, and condition of wound. Remove and dispose of gloves and perform hand hygiene.	Determines supplies and level of assistance needed. Reduces transmission of microorganisms.
9. Assess patient's knowledge and prior experience with dressings, and feelings about procedure.	Reveals need for patient instruction and/or support.

PLANNING

STEP	RATIONALE
1. Expected outcomes following completion of procedure:	
• Patient's wound shows evidence of healing as it becomes smaller in size/depth with less drainage, redness, or swelling.	Dressing effective in promoting healing.
• Patient reports relief or reduction of wound pain during and after dressing change.	Pain control achieved during dressing removal and reapplication.
• Dressing remains clean, dry, and intact.	Dressing applied correctly.
• Patient or family caregiver explains procedure correctly.	Indicates that learning has occurred.
2. Provide privacy and explain procedure.	Protects patient's privacy; reduces anxiety. Promotes cooperation.
3. Perform hand hygiene. Organize and set up any equipment needed to perform procedure at bedside.	Reduces transmission of microorganisms. Ensures more efficiency when completing the procedure.
4. Place biohazard bag within reach of work area. Fold top of bag to make a cuff.	Ensures easy disposal of soiled dressings. Nurse should not reach across sterile field.
5. Position patient comfortably and drape to expose only wound site. Instruct patient not to touch wound or sterile supplies.	Draping provides access to wound while minimizing exposure. Dressing supplies become contaminated when touched by patient's hand.

IMPLEMENTATION

STEP	RATIONALE
1. Perform hand hygiene and apply clean gloves. Apply appropriate PPE as needed if there is a risk for splashing.	Reduces transmission of infectious organisms.
2. Drape patient and expose wound site. Instruct patient not to touch wound or sterile supplies.	Draping provides access to wound while minimizing exposure. Dressing supplies become contaminated when touched by patient's hand.
3. Using nondominant hand, gently remove tape, bandages, or ties of existing dressing. Pull tape parallel to skin and toward dressing. If dressing is over hairy areas, remove tape in direction of hair growth (Hitchcock, 2021) and get patient's permission to clip or shave area before applying new dressing (check agency policy). Remove any adhesive from skin.	Pulling tape toward dressing reduces stress on wound edges, irritation, and discomfort.
4. With gloved hand or forceps, remove old dressing one layer at a time. Note amount and character of drainage (see illustration). Use caution to avoid tension on any drains.	Reduces irritation and possible injury to skin. Prevents accidental removal of drain.

Clinical Judgment *Check removal directions for specific brand of dressing used. Some brands need to have old dressing soaked, irrigated, or moistened for removal. If necessary, use adhesive remover to ease off dressing but avoid contact of adhesive remover with the wound.*

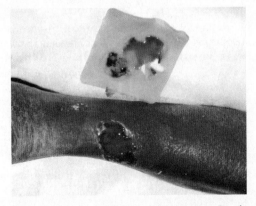

STEP 4 Hydrocolloid dressing after removal from venous injury. Purulent-appearing exudate is present on dressing and wound. This is expected with autolysis under the dressing and is not evidence of infection. (*From Bryant R, Nix D: Acute and chronic wounds: intraprofessionals from novice to expert, ed 6, St Louis, 2024. Elsevier.*)

STEP	RATIONALE
5. Fold dressings with drainage contained inside and remove gloves inside out. With small dressings, remove gloves inside out to enclose dressing (see Skill 40.1). Dispose of gloves and soiled dressing according to agency policy. Cover wound lightly with a sterile 4 × 4–inch gauze pad. Perform hand hygiene.	Contains soiled dressings; prevents contact of your hands with drainage; reduces cross-contamination.

Clinical Judgment *Hydrocolloid dressings interact with wound fluids and form a soft whitish-yellowish gel, which is sometimes hard to remove and may have a faint odor. A residual gel substance occurs in wound beds with some absorption dressings. This is a normal occurrence; do not confuse these findings with pus or purulent exudate, wound infection, or wound deterioration (Bryant & Nix, 2024).*

STEP	RATIONALE
6. Prepare sterile field with sterile dressing kit or individually wrapped sterile supplies on over-bed table (see Chapter 10). Pour prescribed solution into sterile bowl.	Creates sterile work area.
7. Remove gauze cover over wound.	
8. Clean wound:	
a. Apply clean gloves. Sterile gloves are optional (see agency policy). Use 4 × 4–inch gauze cotton ball moistened in saline or an antiseptic swab (per health care provider order) for each cleaning stroke. *Option:* Spray wound surface with wound cleaner (see Chapter 39).	Reduces introduction of organisms into wound. Cleaning and irrigating effectively remove residual dressing gel without injuring newly formed delicate granulation tissue in healing wound bed.
b. Clean in direction from least contaminated to most contaminated (see Skill 40.1).	Cleaning in this direction prevents introduction of organisms into noncontaminated areas.
c. Clean around any drain using circular stroke starting near drain and moving outward away from insertion site (see Skill 40.1).	
9. Use sterile dry gauze to blot dry wound bed and on skin around wound using same direction as Steps 8b and c.	Dressing will not adhere to damp surface. Periwound maceration can enlarge wound and impede healing.
10. Inspect appearance and condition of wound (see Skill 40.1). Measure wound size and depth (see Chapter 38).	Appearance and measurement indicate state of wound healing.

Clinical Judgment *Thoroughly inspect the wound and periwound area and under adhesive material for signs of MARSI or MASD, which include contact dermatitis, maceration, blisters, excoriation, or skin tears (Hitchcock et al., 2021). Observe for subtle signs of infections: increased or altered exudate; friable, bright red granulation tissue; increased odor; increased pain; or localized edema. Any combination of two or more is indicative of a local wound infection, which can be managed with local measures, such as topical antimicrobials or antimicrobial dressings in addition to effective debridement (Ramundo, 2022).*

Clinical Judgment *If signs of MARSI or MASD are present, investigate new adhesive material or other methods to secure dressing, or choose another moisture retentive/absorptive dressing material. A WOCN or wound care specialist can guide wound care revisions.*

STEP	RATIONALE
11. Remove and dispose of gloves and perform hand hygiene. Apply clean gloves. Sterile gloves are optional (see agency policy).	Reduces transmission of microorganisms.
12. Apply dressing (see manufacturer directions).	Ensures proper application of dressing.
	Different brands of dressings require different application techniques.
a. **Hydrocolloid dressings:**	
(1) Select proper size wafer, allowing dressing to extend onto intact periwound skin at least 2.5 cm (1 inch) (Jaszarowski & Murphree, 2022) (see illustration).	These occlusive hydrocolloid sheets maintain a moist wound environment, prevent shear and friction from loosening edges, and circumvent the need for tape along dressing borders (Jaszarowski & Murphree, 2022; Bryant & Nix, 2024).
(2) Apply skin barrier wipe to surrounding skin that will come in contact with any adhesive or gel.	Protects periwound skin. Because of high water content of gels, care must be taken to protect periwound skin from MASD through use of skin barrier (Earlam & Woods, 2022; Jaszarowski & Murphree, 2022).
(3) For deep wound, apply hydrocolloid granules, impregnated gauze, or paste before the wafer.	Functions as filler material to ensure contact with all wound surfaces.
(4) Remove paper backing from adhesive side and place over wound. **Do not stretch and avoid wrinkles or tenting.** Hold dressing in place for 30 to 60 seconds after application.	Dressing molds to wound shape at body temperature (Bryant & Nix, 2024).
(5) If cut from larger piece, tape edges with nonallergenic tape to avoid rolling or adherence to clothing.	

STEP	RATIONALE

Clinical Judgment *Edges may be notched to help mold around wound. Consider using custom shapes to better conform to certain parts of the body, such as heels, elbows, and sacrum.*

b. Hydrogel dressings:

(1) Apply skin barrier wipe to surrounding skin that will come in contact with any adhesive or gel.

Protects periwound skin. Because of high water content of gels, care must be taken to protect periwound skin through use of skin barrier (Jaszarowski & Murphree, 2022; Earlam & Woods, 2022).

(2) Apply gel or gel-impregnated gauze directly into wound, spreading evenly over wound bed (see illustration). Fill wound cavity with gel about one-third to one-half full or pack gauze loosely, including any undermined or tunneled areas. Cover with moisture-retentive dressing or hydrocolloid wafer.

Hydrogels hydrate and facilitate autolytic debridement of wounds. Use caution to avoid overfilling of the wound bed. Partially filling of the wound bed allows for expansion of the hydrogel with absorption of exudate (Jaszarowski & Murphree, 2022).

Clinical Judgment *Hydrogel sheets* **composed of water** *should be cut to size of wound only.*

(3) Cut hydrogel sheet containing glycerin so that it extends 2.5 cm (1 inch) out onto intact periwound skin. Cover with secondary moisture-retentive dressing if needed.

Protects skin around wound from maceration.

(4) Secure dressing with nonallergenic tape if secondary dressing is not self-adhering.

The gel dressings are nonadherent and must be covered with a secondary dressing to hold them in place.

c. Foam dressings:

(1) Know removal and application characteristics of specific brand of foam dressing. This dressing material is not for dry wounds or wounds with eschar (Jaszarowski & Murphree, 2022) (see manufacturer's directions).

Foam dressings collect moderate-to-heavy wound exudate and promote autolytic debridement. Some foam dressings contain an antimicrobial substance to reduce risk for bacterial colonization in wounds (Jaszarowski & Murphree, 2022).

(2) Apply skin barrier wipe to surrounding skin that will come in contact with thin foam dressing adhesive.

Protects periwound skin from maceration or irritation from adhesive.

(3) Cut foam sheet to extend 2.5 cm (1 inch) out onto intact periwound skin. (Verify which side of foam dressing should be placed toward wound bed and which side should be facing away from it; check product instructions.)

Ensures proper absorption and keeps wound exudate away from wound bed (Bryant & Nix, 2024; Jaszarowski & Murphree, 2022).

(4) Cut foam to fit around drain or tube.

(5) Cover with secondary dressing, such as loose gauze, as needed.

Some foam must be covered with secondary dressing (Jaszarowski & Murphree, 2022).

Clinical Judgment *Foam dressings may macerate periwound skin and should be changed before they become overly saturated with exudate (Jaszarowski & Murphree, 2022).*

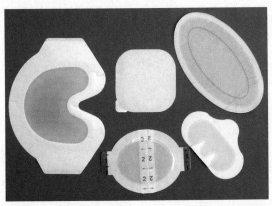

STEP 12a(1) Variety of sizes and shapes of hydrocolloid dressings. (*Courtesy Bonnie Sue Rolstad.*)

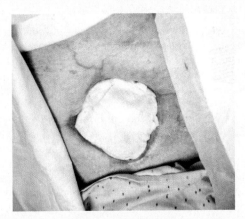

STEP 12b(2) Hydrogel-impregnated gauze used to maintain moist wound bed and fill dead space in this deep abdominal wound with undermining. (*From Bryant R, Nix D: Acute and chronic wounds: intraprofessionals from novice to expert, ed 6, St Louis, 2024, Elsevier.*)

STEP	RATIONALE

d. Alginate dressings:

Clinical Judgment *Before applying new dressing material, fully irrigate the wound to remove all prior dressing residue (Jaszarowski & Murphree, 2022).*

(1) Cut sheet or rope to fit size of wound or loosely pack into wound space (see illustration), filling one-half to two-thirds full.	Alginate dressings expand with absorption of serous fluid or exudate and promote debridement (Bryant & Nix, 2024; Jaszarowski & Murphree, 2022).
(2) Apply secondary dressing, such as transparent film (see illustration) (see Skill 40.3), foam, or hydrocolloid.	Secondary dressing reduces the risk of wound drainage on bed linens and clothing.
13. Label dressing with your initials and date dressing changed.	Provides timeline for next dressing change.
14. Discard soiled dressing materials properly. Remove gloves by pulling them inside out and discard in prepared bag. Perform hand hygiene.	Prevents transmission of microorganisms.
15. Help patient return to a comfortable position.	Restores comfort and sense of well-being.
16. Raise side rails (as appropriate) and lower bed to lowest position, locking into position.	Ensures patient safety and prevents falls.
17. Place nurse call system in an accessible location within patient's reach.	Ensures patient can call for assistance if needed.

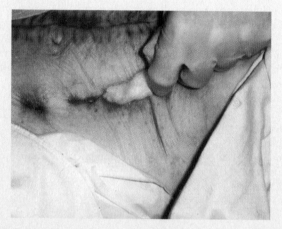

STEP 12d(1) Alginate dressing applied to fill dead space and absorb exudate in full-thickness abdominal wound. (*From Bryant R, Nix D: Acute and chronic wounds: intraprofessionals from novice to expert, ed 6, St Louis, 2024 Elsevier.*)

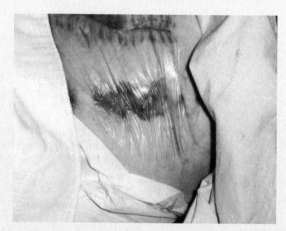

STEP 12d(2) Alginate dressing secured with secondary transparent dressing. (*From Bryant R, Nix D: Acute and chronic wounds: intraprofessionals from novice to expert, ed 6, St Louis, 2024 Elsevier.*)

EVALUATION

1. Compare observations of the wound and periwound area with previous assessment and observe appearance of wound for healing: measure size of wound; observe amount, color, and type of drainage and periwound erythema or swelling; and observe for signs associated with MARSI or MASD. Palpate around wound for tenderness.	Determines rate of healing and any presence of MARSI or MASD.
2. Evaluate patient's level of comfort by having patient describe character of pain and rate severity on scale of 0 to 10.	Documents patient's level of comfort after procedure.
3. Inspect condition of dressing at least every shift or as ordered.	Determines integrity of wound dressing.
4. Use Teach-Back: "I want to be sure I explained why I need to use a foam dressing for your wound. Tell me why this foam dressing material is the best option for your wound." Revise your instruction now or develop a plan for revised patient/family caregiver teaching if patient/family caregiver is not able to teach back correctly.	Teach-back is a technique for health care providers to ensure that they have explained medical information clearly so that patients and their families understand what is communicated to them (AHRQ, 2023).

STEP	RATIONALE

Unexpected Outcomes

1. Wound develops more necrotic tissue and increases in size.

Related Interventions

- In rare instances, some wounds do not tolerate hypoxia induced by hydrocolloid dressings. In these patients, discontinue use. Notify health care provider.
- Evaluate appropriateness of wound care protocol.
- Evaluate for other factors impairing wound healing.
- Consult with wound care specialist.

2. Dressing does not stay in place.

- Evaluate size of dressing used to be sure it extends over wound for adequate margin (2.5 cm [1 inch]), or dry skin more thoroughly before reapplication.
- Consider custom shapes for difficult body parts. "Picture frame" edges of hydrocolloid dressing using tape.
- Dressing may be secured with rolled gauze, tape, transparent dressing, or dressing sheet.

3. Periwound skin show signs of MARSI dermatitis, blistering, maceration, or skin tears.

- Assess moisture control property of dressing.
- Consistently use adhesive remover product when removing old dressing
- Consistent use of skin barrier may reduce irritation.
- Choose a new dressing type with minimal amount of adhesive on patient's skin.
- Gently remove the medical adhesive, keeping it close to the skin and in the direction of hair growth (Hitchcock et al., 2021).

Documentation

- Document size and appearance of wound, characteristics of drainage, presence of necrotic tissue, type of dressings applied, patient's response to dressing change, and level of comfort.
- Document your evaluation of patient learning.

Hand-Off Reporting

- Report location and condition of wound, type of dressings used, and any change in wound management.
- Report signs of infection, necrosis, or deteriorating wound status to health care provider immediately.
- Report any unexpected appearance of wound drainage, bright red bleeding, evidence of wound dehiscence or evisceration, any change in exudate, odor, pain, or localized edema to health care provider.

Special Considerations

Patient Education

- Explain expected wound appearance, fluid or gel accumulation in wound bed, and possible odor with use of specific dressing.

- Because application techniques can vary with different brands, tell patient and family caregiver not to purchase a brand different from the one for which you gave instructions. If a different brand must be used, instruct patient and caregiver to check with you for any additional instructions or modifications in application and removal techniques.

Pediatrics

- See Pediatric Considerations for Skills 40.1, 40.2, and 40.3.

Older Adults

- See Gerontological Considerations for Skills 40.1, 40.2, and 40.3.
- Avoid early and frequent removal of a hydrocolloid dressing to reduce injury to surrounding intact skin.

PROCEDURAL GUIDELINE 40.1 *Applying Rolled Gauze and Elastic Bandages*

Use rolled gauze and elastic bandages to secure or wrap hard-to-cover areas of the body, such as dressings on extremities and amputation stumps. Gauze bandages are lightweight and inexpensive, mold easily around body contours, and permit air circulation to prevent skin maceration.

Elastic bandages apply compression to a body part. Elastic bandages are a secondary dressing, providing protection, pressure, immobilization, and anchoring of underlying dressings or splints. They conform well to body parts and are available in rolls of various widths and materials, including elastic, webbing, elasticized knit, and muslin. Elastic compression to a lower extremity prevents edema by promoting the return of blood from the peripheral to the central circulation. Select a bandage on the basis of the size and shape of the part (e.g., a rolled gauze or elastic bandage on a wrist or ankle would be smaller than a bandage for the upper leg or thigh).

When applying a bandage, select a type of bandage turn (Table 40.3) and width depending on the size and shape of the body part to be bandaged. For example, 7.5-cm (3-inch)–wide bandages are commonly used for the adult leg.

Continued

PROCEDURAL GUIDELINE 40.1 *Applying Rolled Gauze and Elastic Bandages—cont'd*

TABLE 40.3

Types of Bandage Turns

Type	Description	Purpose or Use
Circular turn	Bandage turn overlapping previous turn completely	Anchors bandage at first and final turn; covers small part (finger, toe)
Spiral turn	Bandage ascending body part with each turn overlapping previous one by one-half or two-thirds the width of bandage	Covers cylindrical body parts such as wrist or upper arm
Spiral-reverse turn	Turn requiring twist (reversal) of bandage halfway through each turn	Covers cone-shaped body parts such as forearm, thigh, or calf; useful with non-stretching bandages such as gauze or flannel
Recurrent turn	Bandage first secured with two circular turns around proximal end of body part; half-turn made perpendicular up from bandage edge; body of bandage brought over distal end of body part to be covered, with each turn folded back over on itself	Covers uneven body parts such as head or stump

Delegation

The skill of applying an elastic or rolled gauze bandage cannot be delegated to assistive personnel (AP). A nurse assesses the condition of any wound or dressing before applying a bandage. The skill of applying bandages to secure nonsterile dressings can be delegated to AP (refer to agency policy). Instruct the AP about:
- Modifying the bandage application, such as with special taping.
- Reviewing what to observe and report back to the nurse (e.g., patient's complaint of pain, numbness, or tingling after application or changes in patient's skin color or temperature).

Interprofessional Collaboration

- Physical therapist can verify that a patient's extremity has sufficient support and that the elastic bandage is applied appropriately. This is especially important when an elastic bandage is ordered for an amputated limb (Matthews et al., 2019).

Equipment

Correct width and number of gauze or elastic bandages; clips or adhesive tape; clean gloves if wound drainage is present; *option:* pillow

Steps

1. Identify patient using at least two identifiers (e.g., name and birthday or name and medical record number) according to agency policy (TJC, 2023).
2. Review patient's electronic health record (EHR) for specific orders related to application of rolled gauze or elastic bandage. Note area to be covered, type of bandage required, frequency of change, and previous response to treatment.

Clinical Judgment *If the patient has an underlying dressing, which is secured with adhesive, the patient has a risk for MARSI. Review patient's EHR to determine patient's age and history of dehydration, malnutrition, exposure to radiation therapy, underlying chronic conditions (e.g., diabetes mellitus, immunosuppression), and edema of the skin (Fumarola et al., 2020).*

3. Assess patient's/family caregiver's health literacy.
4. Assess patient's level of comfort by asking patient to describe character of pain and rating severity on a pain scale of 0 to 10. Administer prescribed analgesic 30 minutes before dressing change as needed.
5. Perform hand hygiene. Assess adequacy of circulation by palpating temperature of skin and pulses, presence of edema, and sensation (distal to area to be bandaged). Observe skin color and movement of body part to be wrapped.

Clinical Judgment *Impaired circulation may result in pain, coolness to touch when compared with the opposite side of the body, cyanosis or pallor of skin, diminished or absent pulses, edema or localized pooling, and numbness and/or tingling of body part.*

6. Apply clean gloves. Inspect skin of area to be bandaged. Note alterations in integrity such as presence of abrasion, blistering, discoloration, or chafing. Pay close attention to areas under medical adhesive or over bony prominences.
7. Inspect the condition of any wound for appearance, size, and presence and character of drainage, and be sure that it is covered with a proper dressing. If not, reapply dressing (check agency policy for type of gloves to use). Remove and dispose of gloves and perform hand hygiene.

PROCEDURAL GUIDELINE 40.1 *Applying Rolled Gauze and Elastic Bandages—cont'd*

8. Assess for size of bandage:
   a. *Rolled gauze or basic elastic bandage to secure a dressing:* Assess size of area to be covered. Each successive rolled gauze/elastic should overlap previous layer. Use smaller widths for upper extremities and larger widths for lower extremities.
   b. *Elastic bandage to provide simple compression:* Assess circumference of lower extremity before or shortly after patient gets out of bed in the morning or after patient has been in bed for at least 15 minutes. Select width that will cover and overlap without bulkiness.
9. Assess patient's/family caregiver's knowledge, prior experience with bandaging, and feelings about procedure.

Clinical Judgment *If needed, administer prescribed analgesic 30 minutes before changing or applying bandage.*

10. Perform hand hygiene. Gather and organize supplies at bedside.
11. Provide privacy and explain procedure. Position patient comfortably in an anatomically correct supine position in bed.
12. Perform hand hygiene and apply clean gloves.
13. Apply gauze or elastic bandage to secure dressings:
    a. Elevate dependent extremity for 15 minutes before applying elastic bandage to promote venous return.
    b. Verify that primary dressing over wound is securely in place.
    c. Begin elastic bandage application at the distal body part. Hold elastic bandage in your dominant hand and use other hand to lightly hold beginning layer.
    d. Apply even tension during application and begin with two circular turns to anchor bandage. Continue to maintain even tension and transfer roll to dominant hand as you wrap bandage (see illustration).
    e. Apply bandage from distal point toward proximal boundary (see illustration), using appropriate turns to cover various body parts (see Table 41.3).
       (1) Spiral dressing is often used to cover cylindrical body parts, such as a wrist. Roll gauze, overlapping each layer by one-half to two-thirds the width of the bandage.

   (2) Use figure-eight dressing to cover joint because a snug fit provides support and immobilization to an injured joint. To apply overlap turns, alternate ascending and descending over bandaged part, each turn crossing the previous one to form a figure-eight pattern.

Clinical Judgment *Double-check your tension and ensure that bandage is snug but not tight and that primary dressing or splint is positioned correctly. A tight bandage may cause numbness and tingling from impaired circulation and/or pressure on peripheral nerves.*

   (3) Unroll and slightly stretch bandage.
   (4) Overlap turns by one-half to two-thirds the width of bandage roll.
   (5) Secure bandage with clip before applying additional rolls.
   (6) End bandage with two circular turns; secure end of gauze or elastic bandage to outside layer of bandage, not skin, with tape or clips (see illustration).

Clinical Judgment *Keep toes or fingertips uncovered and visible for follow-up circulatory assessment, except in cases in which toes or fingers are treated because of wounds.*

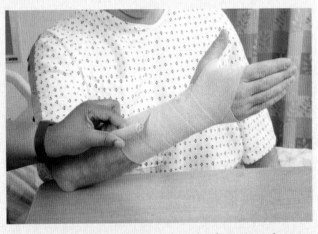

STEP 13e Apply bandage from distal to proximal.

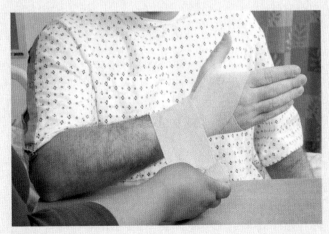

STEP 13d Hold elastic bandage in dominant hand and apply with circular turns.

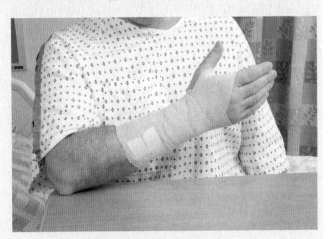

STEP 13e(6) Secure with tape or closure device.

Continued

PROCEDURAL GUIDELINE 40.1 *Applying Rolled Gauze and Elastic Bandages—cont'd*

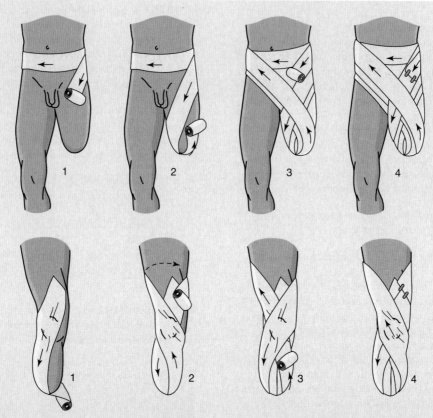

STEP 14 *Top*, Correct method for bandaging midthigh amputation stump. Note that bandage must be anchored around patient's waist. *Bottom*, Correct method for bandaging midcalf amputation stump. Note that bandage need not be anchored around waist. (*From Monahan F, et al: Phipps' medical-surgical nursing: health and illness perspectives, ed 8, St Louis, 2006, Mosby.*)

14. Apply elastic bandage over stump (see illustrations):
    a. Elevate stump with pillow or support it with the help of another person.
    b. Secure bandage by wrapping it twice around proximal end of stump or person's waist (depending on size of stump).
    c. Make half-turn with bandage perpendicular to its edge.
    d. Bring body of bandage over distal end of stump.
    e. Continue to fold bandage over stump, wrapping from distal to proximal points.
    f. Secure with metal clips, self-gripping fastener if provided, or tape.
15. Remove and dispose of gloves if worn and perform hand hygiene.
16. Help patient to a comfortable position.
17. Raise side rails (as appropriate) and lower bed to lowest position, locking into position.
18. Place nurse call system in an accessible location within patient's reach.
19. Assess degree of tightness of bandage, wrinkles, looseness, and presence of drainage.
20. Assess distal extremity circulation when bandage application is complete, at least twice during next 8 hours, and then at least every shift.
    a. Observe skin color for pallor or cyanosis.
    b. Palpate skin for warmth.

    c. Palpate distal pulses and compare bilaterally.
    d. Ask patient to describe character of any pain and to rate severity on a pain scale of 0 to 10. Ask patient to note if any numbness, tingling, or other discomfort is present to evaluate for neurological and vascular changes.
21. Observe mobility of extremity as patient turns or repositions.
22. **Use Teach-Back:** "I want to be sure I explained how to apply the elastic roll to your sprained ankle. Show me how you would apply this elastic roll to your ankle." Revise your instruction now or develop a plan for revised patient/family caregiver teaching if patient/family caregiver is not able to teach back correctly.
23. Document patient's level of comfort, circulation status, type of bandage applied, presence of swelling, and range of motion at baseline and after bandage application on flow sheet in EHR.
24. Report any changes in neurological or circulatory status to health care provider.
25. Hand-off reporting:
    • Immediately report any changes in circulatory status to health care provider and to nurse in charge.
    • Report any changes in wound or skin integrity (e.g., pain, skin irritation, blistering) to nurse in charge.

PROCEDURAL GUIDELINE 40.2 *Applying an Abdominal Binder*

An abdominal binder supports large abdominal incisions that are vulnerable to tension or stress as a patient moves or coughs (Fig. 40.2). Binders support underlying muscles and large incisions, lessening muscle stress, which helps a patient move more freely and provides a noninvasive intervention for enhancing recovery of walk performance, controlling pain, and improving a patient's experience following major abdominal surgery (Gallagher, 2022).

Recent research demonstrates benefits of abdominal binders following major abdominal surgery with midline incisions such as improved postoperative mobility and pain control (Arici et al., 2016; Mizell et al., 2023). Because abdominal binders facilitate early ambulation, patients have fewer postoperative complications related to lack of exercise (e.g., postoperative pneumonia, deep vein thrombosis [DVT]) (Mizell et al., 2023). For some patients, abdominal binders support underlying muscles and large incisions, thus lessening muscle stress, which helps a patient move more freely without additional discomfort (Gallagher, 2022; Gillier et al., 2016). Correctly applied bandages and binders do not cause injury to underlying and nearby body parts or create discomfort for a patient. For example, a chest binder should not be so tight as to restrict chest wall expansion.

Delegation

The skill of applying a binder can be delegated to assistive personnel (AP). However, the nurse must first assess the condition of any incision, the skin, and the patient's ability to breathe before binder application. Instruct the AP about:

- How to modify the skill, such as special wrapping or manner of securing the binder.
- Reporting patient's complaint of pain, numbness, tingling, or difficulty breathing after applying abdominal binder or any changes in patient's skin color or temperature.

Interprofessional Collaboration

- If the patient has an open abdominal wound, a WOCN or wound care specialist can assist in determining how to safely

apply the binder to protect the wound as special dressings may be required.

Equipment

Clean gloves if wound drainage present; gauze bandage as needed; correct type and size of binder; closures for cloth binder

Steps

1. Identify patient using at least two identifiers (e.g., name and birthday or name and medical record number) according to agency policy (TJC, 2023).
2. Review electronic health record (EHR) for order for binder (check agency policy).
3. Review EHR and nurses' notes to identify data regarding size of patient, and select appropriate binder to ensure proper fit (see manufacturer's guidelines).
4. Assess patient's/family caregiver's health literacy.
5. Observe patient who needs support of thorax or abdomen; observe ability to breathe deeply, cough effectively, and turn or move independently.
6. Perform hand hygiene and apply clean gloves. Inspect skin for actual or potential alterations in integrity. Observe for irritation, abrasion, and skin surfaces that come in contact with the binder.

Clinical Judgment *If the patient has an underlying dressing, which is secured with adhesive, the patient has a risk for MARSI. Review patient's EHR to determine patient's age and history of dehydration, malnutrition, exposure to radiation therapy, underlying chronic conditions (e.g., diabetes mellitus, immunosuppression), and edema of the skin (Fumarola et al., 2020).*

7. Inspect any surgical dressing for intactness, presence of drainage, and coverage of incision. Change any soiled dressing before applying binder (using clean gloves). Dispose of soiled dressings in appropriate container, remove and dispose of gloves, and perform hand hygiene.
8. Determine patient's level of comfort by assessing character of pain and measuring acuity on a pain scale of 0 to 10.

Clinical Judgment *If patient reports increased pain, administer prescribed analgesic 30 minutes before binder application.*

9. Assess patient's knowledge of purpose of binder, previous experience, and feelings about procedure.
10. Provide privacy and explain procedure to patient. Prepare supplies at bedside.
11. Perform hand hygiene and apply clean gloves
12. Apply abdominal binder:
    a. Position patient in supine position with head slightly elevated and knees slightly flexed.
    b. Help patient roll on side away from you toward raised side rail while firmly supporting abdominal incision and dressing with hands. Fanfold far side of binder toward midline of binder.
    c. Place binder flat on bed, right side up. Fanfold far side of binder toward midline of binder so that patient can roll over with minimal effort.
    d. Place fanfolded ends of binder under patient.

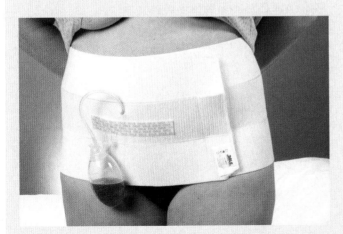

FIG. 40.2. Abdominal binder with Velcro closures. (*Courtesy Dale Medical Products, Plainsville, MA.*)

Continued

PROCEDURAL GUIDELINE 40.2 *Applying an Abdominal Binder—cont'd*

   e. Instruct or assist patient to roll over the folded binder. For overweight patients, have a second nurse or AP assist.

   f. Unfold and stretch ends out smoothly on far side of bed. Then stretch out ends on near side of bed.

   g. Instruct patient to roll back into supine position.

   h. Adjust binder so that supine patient is centered over binder, using symphysis pubis and costal margins as lower and upper landmarks.

   i. If patient is very thin, pad iliac prominences with gauze bandage.

   j. Close binder. Pull one end of binder over center of patient's abdomen. While maintaining tension on that end of binder, pull opposite end of binder over center and secure with Velcro closure tabs or metal fasteners. This provides continuous wound support and comfort.

Clinical Judgment *After binder is in place, assess patient's ability to breathe deeply and cough effectively. When applied correctly, an abdominal binder over midline abdominal incisions should not have any effect on the patient's pulmonary function.*

13. Assess patient's comfort level and adjust binder as needed. Ask patient to describe character of pain and rate severity on a pain scale of 0 to 10.

14. Remove and dispose of gloves and perform hand hygiene.

15. Help patient to a comfortable position. Raise side rails (as appropriate) and lower bed to lowest position, locking into position.

16. Place nurse call system in an accessible location within patient's reach.

17. Remove binder and surgical dressing to assess skin and wound characteristics at least every 8 hours.

18. Evaluate patient's ability to ventilate properly, including deep breathing and coughing, every 4 hours to determine presence of impaired ventilation and potential pulmonary complications.

19. **Use Teach-Back:** "I want to be sure I explained clearly why this binder supports your abdomen, helps control discomfort, and makes it more comfortable to walk, sit in a chair, and deep breathe and cough." Revise your instruction now or develop a plan for revised patient/family caregiver teaching if patient/family caregiver is not able to teach back correctly.

20. Document baseline and post binder condition of skin and wound, integrity of underlying dressing, and patient's comfort level in the EHR.

21. Hand-off reporting: Report any complications (e.g., pain, skin irritation, changes to wound, impaired ventilation) to nurse in charge.

22. Report reduced ventilation (e.g., pulse oximetry) to health care provider immediately.

✦ CLINICAL JUDGMENT AND NEXT GENERATION NCLEX® EXAMINATION–STYLE QUESTIONS

A 75-year-old patient underwent an exploratory laparotomy with a total gastrectomy. On postoperative day 2, the patient develops a fever of 38.5°C (101.3°F) and extreme fatigue. There is purulent, yellow drainage coming from the midline incision and surrounding erythema. Approximately 5 cm (2 inches) of the incision was opened at bedside by staple removal.

1. Which type of supply does the nurse gather to put on the patient's wound?
   1. Wet-to-moist dressing
   2. Pressure bandage
   3. Abdominal binder
   4. Hydrocolloid dressing

2. When performing a wet-to-moist dressing change for the patient, which action will the nurse take **next** after removing the former dressing?
   1. Blot the wound dry.
   2. Clean the wound with saline-moistened gauze.
   3. Inspect the appearance and condition of the wound.
   4. Loosely pack the wound with moistened gauze.

3. Choose the **most likely** options for the information missing from the statement below by selecting from the list of word choices provided.

   After dressing the wound, the nurse will **[Word Choice]** and **[Word Choice]**.

Word Choices
Ensure that the next meal tray will be delivered on time
Apply a transparent dressing over the wet-to-moist dressing
Assess the patient's pain level
Review the patient's laboratory findings
Teach the patient how to care for the wound at home
Request an order for an abdominal x-ray

4. On postoperative day 3, the nurse notices a large amount of bright red blood coming from the base of the open wound. Which supply will the nurse use at this time?
   1. Wet-to-moist dressing
   2. Pressure bandage
   3. Abdominal binder
   4. Hydrocolloid dressing

5. The patient is noted to have a shallow wound with minimal exudate. Which dressing type would the nurse select? **Select all that apply.**
   1. Dry gauze dressing
   2. Calcium alginate dressing
   3. Hydrogel dressing
   4. Transparent film dressing
   5. Hydrocolloid dressing

Visit the Evolve site for Answers to Clinical Judgment and Next Generation NCLEX® Examination—Style Questions.

REFERENCES

Agency for Healthcare Research and Quality (AHRQ): *Teach-back: intervention*, 2023. https://www.ahrq.gov/patient-safety/reports/engage/interventions/teachback.html. Accessed September 1, 2023.

Arici A, et al: The effect of using an abdominal binder on postoperative gastrointestinal function, mobilization, pulmonary function, and pain in patients undergoing major abdominal surgery: a randomized controlled trial, *Int J Nurs Stud* 62:108, 2016.

Armstrong D, et al: *Basic principles of wound management*, 2023, UpToDate. https://www.uptodate.com/contents/basic-principles-of-wound-management, Accessed September 1, 2023.

Assadian O, et al: Use of wet-to-moist cleansing with different irrigation solutions to reduce bacterial bioburden in chronic wounds, *J Wound Care* 27(Suppl 10):S10, 2018.

Barrett S: Wound-bed preparation: a vital step in the healing process, *Br J Nurs* 26(12):S24, 2017.

Bendri H, et al: Tourniquet application for bleeding control in a rural trauma system: outcomes and implications for prehospital providers, *Prehosp Emerg Care* 26(2):246, 2022.

Berrios-Torres SI, et al: Centers for Disease Control and Prevention guideline for the prevention of surgical site infection, *JAMA Surg* 152(8):784, 2017.

Beitz J: Wound healing. In McNichol LL, et al., editors: *Wound, Ostomy, and Continence Nurses Society core curriculum: wound management*, ed 2, Philadelphia, 2022, Wolters Kluwer.

Blackburn J, et al: Reviewing the use of the aetiology-specific T.I.M.E. clinical decision support tools to promote consistent holistic wound management and eliminate variation in practice, *Wounds Int* 13(1):48, 2022.

Bohn G, Bryant RA: Wound-healing physiology and factors that affect the repair process. In Bryant RA, Nix DP, editors: *Acute and chronic wounds: intraprofessionals from novice to expert*, ed 6, St. Louis, 2024, Elsevier.

Bonham P: Assessment and management of patients with wounds due to lower extremity arterial disease (LEAD). In McNichol LL, et al., editors: *WOCN core curriculum wound management*, ed 2, Philadelphia, 2022, Wolters Kluwer.

Brace JA: Wound debridement. In Bryant RA, Nix DP, editors: *Acute and chronic wounds: intraprofessionals from novice to expert*, ed 6, St. Louis, 2024, Elsevier.

Bryant RA, Nix DP: Principles of wound healing and topical management. In Bryant RA, Nix DP, editors: *Acute and chronic wounds: intraprofessionals from novice to expert*, ed 6, St. Louis, 2024, Mosby.

Centers for Disease Control and Prevention (CDC): *What is health literacy?* 2023. https://www.cdc.gov/healthliteracy/learn/index.html. Accessed September 1, 2023.

Charlton NP, et al: Control of severe, life-threatening external bleeding in the out-of-hospital setting: a systematic review, *Prehosp Emerg Care* 25(2):235, 2021.

Earlam AS, Woods L: Moisture-associated skin damage: the basics, *Am Nurse J* 17(10):6, 2022.

Ermer-Seltun J, Rolstad BS: General principles of topical therapy. In McNichol LL, et al., editors: *Wound, Ostomy, and Continence Nurses Society core curriculum: wound management*, ed 2, Philadelphia, 2022, Wolters Kluwer.

European Pressure Ulcer Advisory Panel (EPUAP) and National Pressure Injury Advisory Panel (NPIAP), and Pan Pacific Pressure Injury Alliance: *Treatment of pressure ulcers/injuries: Clinical Practice Guideline. The International Guideline*, Emily Haesler (ED), EPUAP/NPIAP/PPPIA, 2019a.

European Pressure Ulcer Advisory Panel (EPUAP) and National Pressure Injury Advisory Panel (NPIAP), and Pan Pacific Pressure Injury Alliance: *Treatment of pressure ulcers/injuries: Quick Reference Guide*, Emily Haesler (ED), EPUAP/NPIAP/PPPIA, 2019b.

Fletcher F, Probst A: Managing dry wounds in a clinical practice: challenges and solutions, *Wounds Int* 11(2):47, 2020.

Fumarola S, et al: Overlooked and underestimated: medical adhesive-related skin injuries. Best practice consensus document on prevention, *J Wound Care* 29(Suppl 3c):S1–S24, 2020.

Gallagher S: Skin and wound care for the bariatric population. In McNichol LL, et al., editors: *WOCN Core curriculum wound management*, ed 2, Philadelphia, 2022, Wolters Kluwer.

Ghomi ER, et al: Wound dressings: current advances and future directions, *J Appl Polym Sci* 136(27):47738, 2019.

Gillier CM, et al: A randomized controlled trial of abdominal binders for the management of postoperative pain and distress after cesarean delivery, *Int J Gynaecol Obstet* 133:188, 2016.

Haesler E: Evidence summary: pressure injuries: preventing heel pressure injuries with prophylactic dressings, *Wound Pract Res* 25(94):210, 2017.

Hasatsri S, et al: Comparison of the morphological and physical properties of different absorbent wound dressings, *Dermatol Res Pract* 2018:9367034, 2018.

Hitchcock J, et al: Preventing medical adhesive-related skin injury (MARSI), *Br J Nurs* 30(15):S48, 2021.

Hockenberry MJ, et al: *Wong's nursing care of infants and children*, ed 12, St. Louis, 2024, Mosby.

Jaszarowski K, Murphree RW: Wound cleansing and dressing selection. In McNichol LL, et al., editors: *WOCN Core curriculum wound management*, ed 2, Philadelphia, 2022, Wolters Kluwer.

Machin M, et al: Systematic review of the use of cyanoacrylate glue in addition to standard wound closure in the prevention of surgical site infection, *Int Wound J* 16:387, 2019.

Matthews CN, et al: Does an elastic compression bandage provide any benefit after primary TKA? *Clin Orthop Relat Res* 477(1):134, 2019.

Mendes A: Meeting the care needs of a person with dementia who is distressed, *Br J Nurs* 27(4):219, 2018.

Mizell J, et al: *Complications of abdominal surgical incisions*, 2023, UpToDate. https://www.uptodate.com/contents/complications-of-abdominal-surgical-incisions#!. Accessed September 1, 2023.

Munro G: Barriers and enablers for effective implementation of the TIME framework for chronic wounds in a district nursing service, *Wounds Int* 12(1):26, 2021.

Munro G: Causes and consideration with chronic wounds: a narrative review of the evidence, *Wound Pract Res* 25(2):88, 2017.

Oropallo A, Quraishi W: Wound pain. In Bryant RA, Nix DP, editors: *Acute and chronic wounds: intraprofessionals from novice to expert*, ed 6, St. Louis, 2024, Mosby.

Ousey K, et al: Understanding clinical practice challenges: a survey performed with wound care clinicians to explore wound assessment frameworks, *Wounds Int* 9(4):58, 2018.

Oznur ED, et al: Incidence, characteristics, and risk factors of medical device-related pressure injuries: an observational study, *Intensive Crit Care Nurs* 69:103180, 2022. https://doi.org/10.1016/j.iccn.2021.103180.

Parvizi A, et al: A systematic review of nurses' knowledge and related factors towards the prevention of medical device-related pressure ulcers, *Int Wound J* 20(7):2843-2854, 2023.

Ramundo JM: Principles and guidelines for wound debridement. Wound debridement. In McNichol LL, et al., editors: *WOCN Core curriculum wound management*, ed 2, Philadelphia, 2022, Wolters Kluwer.

Richbourg L: Skin and wound care for the geriatric population. In McNichol LL, et al., editors: *WOCN Core curriculum wound management*, ed 2, Philadelphia, 2022, Wolters Kluwer.

Stiehl JB: Early wound bed preparation: irrigation and debridement, *J Wound Care* 30(9):S8–S16, 2021.

Tan NM, et al: Use of hydrocolloid protective sheets to protect skin against direct contact from body secretions, *WCET J* 2021;41(4):18–21.

The Joint Commission (TJC): *2021 National patient safety goals*, Oakbrook Terrace, IL, 2022, The Joint Commission. https://www.jointcommission.org/standards/national-patient-safety-goals/. Accessed September 1, 2023.

Thayer D, et al: Prevention and management of moisture-associated skin damage (MASD), medical adhesive-related skin injury (MARSI), and skin tears. In McNichol LL, et al., editors: *WOCN Core curriculum wound management*, ed 2, Philadelphia, 2022, Wolters Kluwer.

Touhy TA, Jett K: *Ebersole and Hess' gerontological nursing & healthy aging*, ed 6, St. Louis, 2022, Elsevier.

Valderrama OM, et al: Successful management of the open abdomen with hydrocolloid dressing in a resource-constrained setting, *Hernia* 25:1519, 2021.

Waters N: From ancient wisdom to modern science: retracing knowledge of mind-body connections in wound healing, *Wounds Int* 8(1):16, 2017.

Wound, Ostomy, and Continence Nurses Society (WOCN): *Guideline for prevention and management of pressure ulcers (injuries)*, WOCN Clinical Practice Guideline Series, Mount Laurel, NJ, 2017, The Society.

PHASE 1

QUESTION 1.
The nurse is performing an assessment of a client admitted to a long-term care agency following hospitalization.

Highlight the findings that require further assessment by the nurse.

History and Physical	Nurses' Notes	Vital Signs	Laboratory Results
1400: 80-year-old client admitted today from the hospital after being on a ventilator with COVID-19 for a prolonged time. Here for rehabilitation before returning to assisted living, where she normally resides with her 82-year-old spouse. Medical history of depression and anxiety well-controlled with medication. Patient is 167.7 cm (5 ft 6 in), weighs 46.2 kg (102 lb). Alert and oriented × 4. Admits to being very tired after the hospitalization. Denies pain. Vital signs: T 36.8°C (98.2°F); HR 78 beats/min; RR 14 breaths/min; BP 128/74 mm Hg; SpO₂ 99% on RA. PERRLA, cranial nerves intact. Lungs clear to auscultation, heart regular rate and rhythm with no murmurs, and a soft, nontender abdomen. In bed, has difficulty turning onto side by self. Muscle strength arms 2-3 on scale of 5. ROM normal in upper and lower extremities. Full skin assessment reveals reddened areas on the sacrum and heels.			

QUESTION 2.
The nurse reviews documentation for this client.

Complete the following sentence by selecting from the list of word choices below.

Based on the history, the nurse notes that the client is at high risk for developing [Word Choice].

Word Choices
Sepsis
Urticaria
Pruritus
Pressure injuries

PHASE 2

QUESTION 3.
Upon further assessment, the nurse notes that the injury to the sacrum is very shallow and measures 2 cm × 3 cm in circumference. The area is nonblanchable. There are small blisters present. No oozing or drainage is noted.

Complete the following sentence by selecting from the list of word choices below.

The nurse will provide *prioritized* teaching and intervention to address a [Word Choice] pressure injury.

Word Choices
Stage 1
Stage 2
Stage 3
Stage 4

QUESTION 4.
The nurse begins to plan care.

With which member of the interprofessional health care team will the nurse plan to collaborate to care for the client? **Select all that apply.**

- SANE nurse
- Wound care nurse
- Speech therapist
- Physical therapist
- Health care provider
- Registered dietitian nutritionist

PHASE 3

QUESTION 5.

The nurse is implementing interventions to address the wounds on the sacrum and heels.

Which **3** actions will the nurse take at this time?

○ Massage the affected areas.
○ Rub lotion into the heels and sacrum.
○ Place a friction-reducing sheet underneath the client.
○ Encourage intake of a diet high in protein.
○ Remind and assist the client to turn or move every 3 hours.
○ Apply ointment and an occlusive dressing to reddened areas.
○ Obtain a specialized air mattress for the client's bed.

QUESTION 6.

A week later, the nurse is assessing the client's skin.

Highlight the assessment findings that indicate that the client's condition is declining.

History and Physical	Nurses' Notes	Vital Signs	Laboratory Results

1524: Complete skin assessment performed. Area on sacrum measures 3 cm × 4 cm. Very small open area noted with yellowish drainage. Heels have no redness nor breakdown bilaterally. Tender, reddened area noted on the back of the skull; measures 1 cm × 1 cm. Vital signs: T 38.5°C (101.3°F); HR 76 beats/min; RR 16 breaths/min; BP 126/78 mm Hg; SpO₂ 97% on RA.

UNIT 15
Home Care

Clients who require home care depend on nurses to critically assess and identify all the factors within the home that could affect their safety and health outcomes. Use a client-centered, systematic, ongoing process to assess a client's health status and needs. Home health nurses manage clients' problems, often over several weeks. Establishing an initial database of a client's health status and home environment is essential in order to monitor for change. Once problems and needs have been identified, a home health nurse discusses them with the client, family, and other caregivers. Together, they determine outcomes that reflect the client's desires, priorities, cultural values, and preferences. The two greatest priorities in home health care are client safety and education to enable clients to perform self-care or assist the family caregivers who provide care.

Client safety in the home begins with a home environment assessment so that you can make adaptations to the home to minimize the effects of a client's limitations or deficiencies. It also allows for maximizing any client strengths. If a client returns home with an unsteady gait or poor balance, an assessment of the condition of stairs and common walkways leads you to recommend alterations such as installing railings along stairs, removing objects or rugs that can cause tripping, and repairing uneven walking surfaces. The same client will require clinical judgment regarding which strategies are appropriate for fire safety. A recurring principle is to be sure your recommendations are accepted by clients and family members and that resources (e.g., economic, people, time) are available so that they can make the changes in the home that are necessary.

Clients who have cognitive deficits pose special challenges to keep them safe in the home. Your assessment focuses on the level of deficit a client is experiencing, the level of family caregiver support available, and any hazards existing in the home. You will critically apply your assessment findings to provide interventions that maximize a client's abilities by simplifying tasks and providing consistency in daily activities. Often a family caregiver has found ways to manage a client with cognitive deficits by minimizing anxiety, reducing wandering, and keeping the client engaged. When successful interventions exist, use them in your plan of care. Your knowledge of cognitive deficits offers guidance in helping family caregivers anticipate the progression of the disease.

The list of nursing skills that a client and/or family caregiver may need to perform in the home has become lengthy as more emphasis has been placed on the early discharge of clients from health care agencies. In all cases, client safety and education are necessary so that clients know not only how to perform skills correctly but also what problems or complications to anticipate and when to contact a health care provider. When you instruct a client or family caregiver on performing a skill, follow the same basic steps that you would use. However, adapt the steps of a skill so that the client can follow infection control and safety principles and use equipment that can be obtained for the home. Also plan skills at times convenient for clients (when possible). Do not use shortcuts but make evidence-based adaptations. The use of therapeutic communication and education principles promotes trusting relationships with a client and family caregiver. When you gain that trust, a client acquires confidence in you and the ability to perform self-care. A client needs to be competent in performing a skill and know when to seek help from a health care provider.

Home Care Safety

SKILLS AND PROCEDURES

Skill 41.1 **Home Environment Assessment and Safety, p. 1200**

Skill 41.2 **Adapting the Home Setting for Clients With Cognitive Deficits, p. 1209**

Skill 41.3 **Medication and Medical Device Safety, p. 1216**

OBJECTIVES

Mastery of content in this chapter will enable you to:

- Identify clients at risk for safety problems and possible accidents in the home.
- Support the self-care of clients in the home.
- Explain the factors within a home environment that create risks for client injury.
- Demonstrate how to perform a home safety risk assessment.

- Identify interventions that modify the home environment for physical safety.
- Identify interventions to reduce safety risks for clients with sensory, cognitive, and mental status alterations.
- Recommend strategies to ensure safe medication administration within the home.
- Demonstrate how to perform a geriatric fall risk assessment.

MEDIA RESOURCES

- http://evolve.elsevier.com/Perry/skills
- Review Questions
- Answers to Clinical Judgment and Next-Generation NCLEX® Examination–Style Questions

- Skills Performance Checklists
- Printable Key Points

PURPOSE

A safe and healthy home is a cornerstone to independent living. The National Center for Healthy Housing (NCHH, 2022) describes a healthy home as one that can and should support good health. However, 40% of homes in the United States have at least one health or safety hazard, such as exposure to mold or toxic chemicals, entry steps without handrails, and missing smoke detectors (NCHH, 2021). Mobility is an essential part of remaining independent and provides many health benefits, but immobility increases clients' risk for isolation and physical risks such as falls. Anticipating and preventing injuries in the home is essential to clients' welfare. Injuries and violence have an impact on one's sense of security and can affect an individual, the family, and the community. *Healthy People 2030* identifies injury prevention as a health behavior, with objectives geared toward preventing unintentional injuries (Office of Disease Prevention and Health Promotion [ODPHP], n.d.). Home care safety begins before a client is discharged from a health care agency. A home care nurse and interprofessional team collaborate with the client and family caregiver to assess the home environment for risks, with a goal to select appropriate interventions for preventing unintentional injuries.

PRACTICE STANDARDS

- National Institute on Aging (NIA), 2022: Taking Medications Safely As You Age—Medication safety program for older adults

- The Joint Commission (TJC), 2023: Home Care National Patient Safety Goals—Home care, client identification

PRINCIPLES FOR PRACTICE

- The term "client" is used in home care settings due to the collaborative relationship with the interprofessional team.
- Home care safety involves communication and collaboration among a client, family caregivers, and interprofessional home care providers.
- The ultimate goal of home care safety is to create an environment in which a client and family caregiver can provide self-care safely and effectively.
- Insurance coverage, including Medicare, can be limited for home care. Therefore the time spent in the home with the client must be well planned and used to the fullest.
- Clients living in socioeconomically disadvantaged areas may be at increased risk for injury as a result of environmental hazards, violence, or poor living conditions.
- Fall prevention is a critical aspect of care for older adults, especially in the community. Even without injury, falls cause a loss of confidence that results in reduced physical activity, increased dependency, and social withdrawal (Touhy & Jett, 2022).
- More than one-third of community-living adults over age 65 fall at least once a year; half of them experience multiple falls. Approximately 10% of falls result in a major injury such as a fracture, and falls are one of the principal causes of death and disability in older persons (Piau et al., 2020).

PERSON-CENTERED CARE

- Respect a client's home. When providing home care nursing, you are a guest. Take time to listen to a client's health concerns and apply clinical judgment to understand which interventions within the home are likely to be consistent with the client's and the family caregiver's values and preferences.
- Communication is essential in home care and is a continuous process between you and a client. At the first meeting, introduce yourself, explain how you would like the client to address you, and ask the client and family caregiver how you should address them. If a language barrier exists, have a professional interpreter assist you.
- Collaborate with clients in assessing their home environments. Ask them if they are willing to give you a tour of their home, and explain how a home assessment can reduce the risk for falls or injuries. Do not focus on what is wrong (e.g., barriers or features in disrepair); point out why safety is an issue for the client (based on health condition) and explain why a change in a feature of the home will make the client safer and promote independent living.
- Assess for culture-specific health-related beliefs that may affect a client's willingness to use home care services.
- When assessing the availability of family caregivers in the home, recognize that clients can value the role of caregivers in different ways. With the client's permission, include these family caregivers when performing the home safety assessment and making home adaptations.
- Assess and provide support for informal and family caregivers; the presence or absence of these could be the difference between a client remaining in the home or being readmitted to an acute care facility (Touhy & Jett, 2022).

EVIDENCE-BASED PRACTICE

Using Telehealth to Support Clients and Family Caregivers

Older adults with dementia living in the community often require support services to help them maintain their independence and functioning, as well as assistance from family caregivers (Alzheimer's Association, 2022a). In the past several years the use of telehealth has gained popularity as a means to provide services and also support family caregivers. Virtual care, or telehealth, has been defined as any interaction between clients and/or family caregivers occurring remotely using any forms of communication or information technologies, with the aim of facilitating or maximizing the quality and effectiveness of client care (Gosse et al., 2021). Nurses can assist clients and family caregivers in using telehealth to help provide care and as a means of support to lessen stress and feelings of isolation.

- Video teleconferencing has successfully been used to remotely assess, diagnose, and manage clients with dementia (Gosse et al., 2021).
- Telemedicine programs often have access to supplemental clinical information to aid in diagnosis and involve interprofessional teams to manage client complexity (Gosse et al., 2021).
- The Telephone Interview for Cognitive Status (TICS) was modeled after the Mini-Mental State Examination (MMSE) and can be used for dementia screening. Other validated instruments for cognitive screening include telephone-based MMSE

instruments and the telephone Montreal Cognitive Assessment (T-MoCA) (Gosse et al., 2021).
- Obstacles to accessing in-person care arise with dementia progression (declining mobility, increasing disorientation with schedule changes, worsening neuropsychiatric symptoms, and an increasing reliance on caregivers); virtual care may minimize the disruptions that in-person visits pose (Gosse et al., 2021).
- A recent study examined caregivers' perceptions of using telehealth to help care for a person with dementia. Barriers included concerns that technology gets hacked, difficulty using technology, difficulty for the person with dementia in being engaged in the virtual conversation, and need for examination to be conducted in person, especially on "bad days" (Gately et al., 2022).
- Findings to support the use of telehealth by caregivers included not having to take the older adult outside the home for a follow-up visit; potential to reduce the need for travel, in terms of both distance and traffic; increased access; and decreased stress for both the caregiver and the person with AD (Gately et al., 2022).
- A study that examined benefits of caregivers of clients with dementia who used video support versus telephone support found that caregivers had improved confidence and reduced frequency and severity of all types of priority care challenges. Priority care challenges included managing behavioral and psychological symptoms of dementia, understanding disease expectations, and performing activities of daily living care (Shaw et al., 2020).

SAFETY GUIDELINES

- Have a client's vision and condition of feet checked annually by a qualified health care provider (Touhy & Jett, 2022).
- TJC safety goals for the home include a focus on fall prevention, identification of risks for clients who use oxygen, handcleaning guidelines to prevent infection, and safe use of medications (TJC, 2023).
- Accident prevention begins with making timely and adequate home repairs (e.g., replacing loose floor tiles and torn rugs, securing railings on stairwells). When clients do not have the resources for maintaining a safe home environment, a nurse's role is to help identify appropriate resources or services in the community.
- When helping clients change the home environment, retain as much of their independence and ability to provide self-care as possible.
- Make modifications to the home environment only after considering a client's physical strengths, remaining functional abilities, and resources for making a change.
- Collaborate with clients, family caregivers, and health care providers in the community in finding the best approaches for meeting a client's safety needs.
- Have family caregivers encourage clients to keep moving. Activities that improve balance and strengthen legs (e.g., tai chi, Pilates) can prevent falls (Touhy & Jett, 2022).
- Ask clients if they worry about falling or feel unsteady when standing or walking (Touhy & Jett, 2022).
- Frequently ask if client and family caregiver have concerns or questions about safety and if they have any suggestions to improve safety (Hoffman et al., 2019).

✦ SKILL 41.1   Home Environment Assessment and Safety

The home environment should be a place where individuals feel healthy, comfortable, and safe. People want to be able to move about freely within their homes, regardless of the size of the home, and to have a sense of control over daily living routines. This requires maintaining personal space and a sense of privacy. As the home care nurse, you can help a client maintain independence and reduce risk in the home environment by conducting a safety assessment.

Clients requiring home care often experience physical alterations (e.g., progressive physical changes of aging) that require changes in their home environment. For example, if a client has poor balance but good upper-arm strength, you may need to make modifications (e.g., install handrails on both sides of a staircase and in bathroom areas) so that the client can safely walk or move throughout the house, ascend and descend stairs, and enter and exit a bathtub or shower. Teaching a client to safely use assistive devices (e.g., walker or cane) (see Chapter 12) helps increase mobility and maintain independence (Fig. 41.1).

Respect the concept of personal space. Making changes too rapidly without a client's consent causes more problems than benefits. Appreciate the arrangement of a client's space within the home and do not move things or suggest modifications without permission. Provide a rationale to the client as to why the changes are beneficial and/or needed; explain in relationship to the client's specific fall risk. Knowing the rooms that a client uses most frequently helps in making the right adjustments to create a safe environment.

Delegation

The skill of conducting an initial home safety assessment cannot be delegated to assistive personnel (AP). Instruct the AP to:
• Suggest ways to make the home safer

Interprofessional Collaboration

• Work with the family caregiver and client to complete the initial home safety assessment. A physical therapist (PT) or occupational therapist (OT) can assist in identifying risks to mobility and self-care maintenance.

Equipment

• Home safety checklist

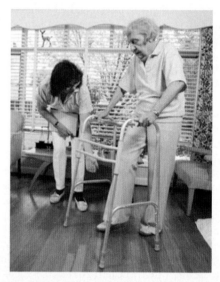

Fig. 41.1   Use of walker may help client remain mobile.

STEP	RATIONALE

ASSESSMENT

1. Identify client using at least two identifiers (e.g., name and birthday or name and medical record number) according to agency policy.

2. Assess client's and family caregiver's health literacy level and knowledge of safety risks.

3. Review risk factors that predispose clients to accidents within the home (share these with client and family caregiver during assessment):
   a. Reduced visual acuity (see Chapter 6)

   b. Hearing impairment (see Chapter 6)

   c. Neuromuscular alterations (e.g., lower extremity weakness, unsteady gait, impaired balance, poor ankle dorsiflexion). If client has lower extremity weakness or unsteady gait, administer the Banner Mobility Assessment Tool (BMAT 2.0) (Boynton et al., 2020; Matz, 2019) (see Chapter 12).

Ensures client safety. Complies with The Joint Commission standards and improves client safety (TJC, 2023).

Determines degree to which individuals have the ability to find, understand, and use information and services to make informed health-related decisions and actions for themselves and others (Centers for Disease Control and Prevention [CDC], 2023).
Elimination of risk factors will be focus of interventions (Touhy & Jett, 2022).

Reduced visual function such as reduced acuity, depth perception, adaptation to dark or glaring light, and visual motion perception places client at risk for falling (Touhy & Jett, 2022).
Prevents client from hearing normal environmental sounds (e.g., call out by family member) clearly as source of orientation. Prevents clear perception of home-installed alarms (e.g., smoke alarm).
Interferes with communication for clients to hear and interpret what you are saying (Touhy & Jett, 2022).
Factors predispose clients to falls. Recurrent falls are associated with difficulty in standing up from chair.

STEP	RATIONALE
d. Reduced energy or fatigue	Predisposes clients to falls.
e. Incontinence or nocturia	Frequent trips to bathroom often cause client with other deficits to accidentally trip or fall over barriers. Dementia does not cause incontinence, but it affects a client's ability to find bathroom and recognize need to void (Touhy & Jett, 2022).
f. History of stroke, parkinsonism, delirium, seizures, dementia, or syncope	These conditions present multiple risks for falls, including impaired gait and coordination, visual changes, diminished cognition, pain, muscle weakness, and polypharmacy (Frith et al., 2019). Age-related changes of neurological system include slowing of reaction time (Meiner, 2019).
g. Cardiopulmonary conditions: postural hypotension, arrhythmias, palpitations, difficulty breathing, or shortness of breath	Dizziness, fatigue, and light-headedness predispose to falls and cause client to be unsteady and compensate for difficulties.
h. Medication usage and history, including polypharmacy and use of sedatives, antihypertensives, antidepressants, and diuretics	Use of multiple medications has been associated with falls (Zaninotto et al., 2020). Medications that alter sensorium affect balance and judgment (Frith et al., 2019).
i. History of previous fall—obtain detailed description of previous fall: determine nature of the fall and if client had other injuries within home. Be specific in your assessment. Use mnemonic SPLATT (Ritchey et al., 2022): • Symptoms at time of fall • Previous fall • Location of fall • Activity at time of fall • Time of fall • Trauma after fall	Increases risk for future fall (Piau et al., 2020). Key symptoms are helpful in identifying cause of fall. Onset, location, and activity associated with fall provide further details on causative factors and how to prevent future falls. SPLATT test allows client to explain symptoms in own words; it is important to understand circumstances around fall (Ritchey et al., 2022).
4. Instruct client who has had a near fall or actual fall to maintain a fall diary (Box 41.1).	Information in fall diary is helpful in determining factors before fall and consequences of falling (Meiner, 2019).
5. Determine if client is afraid of falling using the Falls Efficacy Scale (FES-1) or the Activities-specific Balance Confidence (ABC) scale, which measures a client's confidence with doing specific activities of daily living without falling or losing their balance (Soh, 2021).	Fear of falling is significantly associated with falls in community dwelling older adults, especially in individuals with more than one fall in the past year (Asai et al., 2022; Appeadu & Bordini, 2023).

Clinical Judgment *In addition to client, include family caregivers as a resource in assessments because they may witness accident trends or patterns.*

STEP	RATIONALE
6. Share with client and family caregiver any risk factors identified in initial assessment and how these affect mobility in the home. For example: **a.** Gait alteration will require even floor surfaces for walking. **b.** Visual alteration will require marked steps and less glare.	Increases client understanding of need to assess home safety and how risks directly affect safety (Hoffman et al., 2019).
7. Partner with client and family caregivers to conduct **home safety assessment**:	Provides comprehensive review of all areas within home that pose hazardous situations (Hoffman et al., 2019). Home risk assessment and modification are effective for reducing the number of falls and fallers in community-dwelling older adults, mostly among those who are classified as having a high risk of falling (Campani et al., 2021).
a. Front and back entrances: **(1)** Are walkways to front/back door even and free from holes or cracks?	Entrances pose barriers in surfaces over which client must walk. Uneven pavement and holes may not be seen by client, causing tripping and falls. Creates risk for client with stumbling gait.
(2) Are home entrances, including walkways, well lit?	Poorly lit areas prevent individuals from seeing variations in walking surface.

BOX 41.1

Fall/Near-Fall Diary

- Keep a notebook and create across the longest edge of the paper these headings: "Date," "Time of Fall," "Activity at Time of Fall," "Symptoms," and "Injury."
- As soon as possible after a fall, have client or family caregiver complete information under each heading.
- List emergency contact numbers at the bottom of the fall diary for client to call in case a fall results in serious injury.
- Instruct client to bring the diary to the health care provider's office at the next scheduled visit or share information with home care nurse on next home visit.

Adapted from Meiner SE: *Gerontologic nursing,* ed 6, St. Louis, 2019, Mosby.

STEP	RATIONALE
(3) Does client have nonskid strips/safety treads or bright-colored paint on outdoor steps? Which colors are most easily seen by client? Are these colors used?	Nonskid surfaces cause fewer slips on stairs. Color on steps permits individual to see edges, accommodating for any reduced depth perception.
(4) Are doormats in good repair with nonskid backing and tapered edge?	Raised edges pose risk for tripping. Doormats without nonskid backing slide when stepped on, causing client to lose balance.
(5) Are doors in good repair, and do they open and close easily? Can client open and close all doors easily? Are the doors and window locks in good condition? Are there deadbolt locks?	Act of opening and closing door is difficult if grasp is weak. Tripping may occur during opening and cause a fall. Opening and closing doors and windows are essential for safety in the event of fire. Deadbolts provide additional safety but must be easy for the client to use.
(6) Is there a sturdy handrail on both sides of stairs leading to entrance?	Handrails provide greater support while ascending and descending stairs.
(7) Are steps in good condition with even, flat surfaces?	Uneven surfaces predispose to tripping.
(8) Are doorways and stairs free of clutter?	Reduces risk for tripping and/or falling.
b. Kitchen:	Kitchen is one of most hazard-oriented rooms in home. Poses serious hazards for fire.
(1) Does client wear clothing with short or close-fitting sleeves when cooking?	Short or close-fitting sleeves are less likely to accidentally catch fire when person works at stove.
(2) Does client always stay in kitchen when cooking?	Lack of attention when using fire is risk.
(3) Does client have loud timer to signal when food is cooked?	Prevents burning food and risk for fire.
(4) Does client keep stovetop and oven clean and grease free?	Grease is highly flammable.
(5) Are stove control dials easy to see and use?	Client may accidentally use higher flame than is necessary for cooking safely.
(6) Is charged, easy-to-use fire extinguisher close at hand?	Extinguisher should be in working order and ready for use at all times.

Clinical Judgment *Have client demonstrate steps of how to use fire extinguisher (see Chapter 14).*

STEP	RATIONALE
(7) Are emergency numbers for police, fire, and poison control posted on or near telephone? Is a copy of living will stored in accessible location?	Emergency phone numbers and extinguisher ensure quick response if fire occurs. Emergency medical technicians (EMTs) who respond to emergency look for advance directives.
(8) Can items in kitchen cabinets and shelves be reached without climbing on stool or chair?	Climbing on step stools or chairs creates risks for falls.
(9) Is there adequate lighting over sink, stove, and work areas?	Poor lighting makes it difficult to see control knobs or dials and provides inadequate illumination when using sharp knives or utensils (Touhy & Jett, 2022).
(10) Are kitchen throw rugs and mats slip resistant?	Rugs or mats that are not slip resistant can easily slide on tile or wood floors.
(11) Assess food safety: Are perishable foods in refrigerator and nonperishable foods safe to eat? Does client wash hands properly before food preparation? Is food stored appropriately, kept separate, and at right temperature? Have expiration dates passed? Is there evidence that food has spoiled? Does client know how to prepare and store food safely?	Proper food storage and preparation can prevent foodborne illnesses. One basic of food safety is cooking food to its proper temperature. Foods are properly cooked when they are heated for long enough time and at high enough temperature to kill harmful bacteria that cause foodborne illness (CDC, 2022). Eating foods that have spoiled or with expiration dates that have passed puts client at risk for foodborne illness (e.g., food poisoning).
c. Bathroom:	
(1) Can client unlock bathroom door from both sides of door?	Functional locks prevent person from being trapped in bathroom.
(2) Is tub or shower equipped with nonskid mats, abrasive strips, or surfaces that are not slippery?	Bathrooms are hazardous. Wet floors and tub or shower bottoms can be slippery, creating risk for falls.
(3) Does bathroom floor have nonslip surface or rug with nonskid backing?	Slippery tile predisposes to falls (Touhy & Jett, 2022).
(4) Does client use bath oils when bathing?	Use of bath oils makes tub surface slippery and increases risk for falls.
(5) Do bathtub and shower have at least one grab bar or handrail placed where client can reach it?	Grab bars provide extra support while maneuvering into and out of tubs or showers. Grab bars placed correctly where client can safely reach them help to steady balance and gait and lessen chance of falls (Meiner, 2019).
(6) Is client careful not to place towels on grab bars?	Some clients accidentally grab towel instead of bar when needing support. Towel can slip off bar.

STEP	RATIONALE
(7) Does shower have stable stool or chair and handheld sprayer? Is shower easy to access (walk-in versus step-in tub area)?	Shower stool allows client to sit while showering.
(8) Are cold and hot water faucets clearly marked, and is temperature on water heater 48.8°C (120°F) or lower?	Accidental burns can occur from exposure to hot water (Touhy & Jett, 2022).
d. Bedroom:	
(1) Is night-light placed in bedroom and/or bath?	Older adults have altered night vision.
(2) Is working smoke detector just outside bedroom door?	Alarm situated just outside bedroom can awaken person early enough to escape fire.
(3) Can client turn on light without having to get out of bed in dark? Is flashlight available at bedside? Flashlight can be attached to walker or cane (Touhy & Jett, 2022).	Getting out of bed without proper lighting or ability to adjust to light changes and reaching for necessary objects puts client at risk for falls.
(4) Is furniture arranged to provide clear path from bed to bathroom?	Obstructed path creates barrier that causes tripping and falls.
(5) Is phone with emergency numbers within easy reach of bed?	If clients develop physical symptoms while in bed, they need to be able to reach phone without having to get out of bed.
(6) Are other alarm systems available? Push buttons that call for help? Nursery listening devices for cognitively impaired or nonambulatory clients?	Alarm systems placed in readily accessible location can alert family caregivers when person requires immediate help. Bedside phone, cordless phone, intercom buzzer, or lifeline can be placed in readily accessible location. Medical alert systems provide wearable devices to notify Emergency Medical Services (EMS) system of falls (Touhy & Jett, 2022).
e. Living room/family room:	
(1) Are electrical or extension cords removed from under furniture and carpeting? Kept out of way of traffic?	Clients can easily trip or fall over electrical cords. Hidden cords are trip and fire hazards.
(2) Can client turn on light without having to walk into dark room?	Darkened room can disorient and prevent client from seeing uneven surfaces.
(3) Are hallways and walkways free from objects and clutter?	Objects and clutter in common walkway can cause client to trip, resulting in falls.
(4) Are loose area rugs securely attached to floor and not placed over carpeting? (For best safety, consider removing throw rugs.)	Loose edges of rugs are easy for persons to trip over (Touhy & Jett, 2022).
(5) Is furniture arranged in each room so that client can walk around easily?	Furniture creates obstacles to walking in room.
(6) Is all furniture steady and without sharp edges?	Clients often use edge of furniture for support when standing.
f. Around the house:	
(1) Are all living areas and stairways well lit?	Adequate lighting helps people see any barriers or uneven walking surfaces.
(2) Is flooring or carpeting throughout house in good repair?	Frayed carpet or irregular surfaces can cause tripping and result in fall.
(3) Are all thresholds between rooms level with floor or beveled and no more than 1.27 cm (½ inch) in height (American Occupational Therapy Association [AOTA], n.d.)?	Uneven thresholds can cause tripping.
(4) Is light switch at both top and bottom of stairs?	Prevents individual from having to walk part of stairs in dark.
(5) Does lighting produce glare or shadows on stairs or floor surfaces?	Older adults are sensitive to glare because their visual pathway becomes distorted.
(6) Do handrails run continuously from top to bottom of flights of stairs?	Handrails provide source of physical support when ascending and descending stairs.
(7) Are handrails securely attached to wall along stairs?	Handrails should be installed at least on one side of stairwell, but preferably both (Touhy & Jett, 2022; AOTA, n.d.).
(8) Are step coverings in good condition?	Loosened covering can cause tripping.
(9) Are guns kept in house? Are trigger locks installed on all guns? Are guns stored unloaded? Is ammunition in secure location?	Following gun safety standards decreases risk for injury and death related to gun use (National Rifle Association [NRA], 2023).
g. General fire safety:	
(1) Does client have properly working smoke detectors with fresh batteries?	In 2014 through 2018, almost three of every five home fire deaths resulted from fires in homes with no smoke alarms (41%) or no working smoke alarms (16%) (National Fire Protection Association [NFPA], 2022a).

Clinical Judgment *Check to see when smoke alarm battery was last changed; battery should be changed every 6 months. For those who live in daylight saving time zones, change with each time change (NFPA, 2022a).*

STEP	RATIONALE
(2) Does client have several emergency exit plans in case of fire?	Exit plan helps people anticipate route of escape when fire does occur. Exit should not have locks that are difficult to open or any physical barriers.
(3) Has family determined meeting place in event of emergency, such as at mailbox in front of home?	Use of common emergency meeting location is efficient method for determining that all family members are safely out of house.
(4) Does client use portable space heaters? Are they kept at least 1 m (3 feet) away from flammable items?	Heaters, furnaces, and chimneys pose risks for fire. Fires in which the heat source was too close to combustibles were associated with the largest shares of civilian deaths, civilian injuries, and direct property damage (NFPA, 2022b).
(5) Is furnace area free of things that can catch fire?	Keeping area clear of flammable materials can lower risk of fire.
(6) Does qualified professional check furnace and chimney annually?	Buildup of creosote within chimney can catch fire. Overheated motor in furnace can burn out and possibly cause fire. Heating is the second leading cause of home fires and home fire injuries and the third leading cause of home fire deaths (NFPA, 2022b).
(7) Does client who smokes report smoking in bed?	Smoking materials, including cigarettes, pipes, and cigars, started an estimated 17,200 home structure fires reported to U.S. fire departments in 2014 (NFPA, 2022b). Smoking in bed has added risk of client falling asleep while cigarette is lit.
h. General electrical safety:	
(1) Are electrical cords in good condition (i.e., not frayed, spliced, or cracked)?	Damaged cords can short circuit and lead to fire.
(2) Are electrical cords kept away from water?	Use of any appliance or device that is exposed to water creates risk for electrical shock.
(3) Does client use extension cord/outlet extenders with built-in circuit breaker or fuse?	Prevents overloading of circuit that can lead to fire.
(4) Do all wall outlets and switches have cover plates?	Prevents physical contact with wiring.
(5) Does client use light bulbs of correct wattage for each fixture?	Use of excessive wattage can lead to fire.
(6) Is main electrical fuse box for home easily accessible and clearly labeled?	In event of emergency, fuse box should be easy to access so that proper circuit can be cut off.
i. Carbon monoxide prevention:	
(1) Are furnace flues checked regularly for patency?	Obstructed flues are common cause of carbon monoxide toxicity.
(2) Is there working carbon monoxide (CO) detector in home?	CO alarms should be installed in a central location outside each sleeping area and on every level of the home and in other locations where required by applicable laws, codes, or standards (NFPA, 2022c).
8. Assess client's financial resources; determine monthly income used for ongoing expenses.	Determines potential for making repairs to home. Reveals need for low-cost community service support.
9. Assess client's and family caregiver's willingness to make changes. Has client accepted limitations that pose risk for injury? Determine how important functional independence is for client.	Some clients perceive attempts to improve safety within home as intrusive. If you show that necessary revisions to home environment will preserve independence, client will participate more willingly.
10. Assess the client's goals or preferences for how suggested home modifications will be implemented. Assess family caregiver's perceptions as well.	Ensures that client is an active part of decision making.

PLANNING

1. Expected outcomes following completion of procedure:	
• Client and/or family/caregiver describe client's fall risks and associated environmental risks within home that predispose to accidents.	Demonstrates client's and family caregiver's recognition of safety risks that are of greatest concern.
• Client and/or family caregiver initiate actions to correct environmental risks, making home safer.	Client sees value in altering living environment.
• Client remains free of injury.	Environmental barriers are reduced or removed to minimize injuries.
2. Prioritize with client and family caregiver environmental barriers that pose greatest risk.	Client's own physical and/or cognitive deficits make certain environmental risks more hazardous. Prioritization helps client make best choices.
3. Recommend calling in reliable contractor if major home repairs are necessary and acceptable to client and family.	Ensures that repairs are made safely and correctly.

STEP	RATIONALE

IMPLEMENTATION

1. General home safety:
   a. Provide direct light source in areas where client reads, cooks, uses tools, or conducts hobby work. High-intensity light on object or surface that is involved works best. | Visual impairment in older adults is usually the result of cataracts, macular degeneration, glaucoma, or diabetic retinopathy (Touhy & Jett, 2022).

Clinical Judgment *Avoid fluorescent lighting because it creates excessive glare.*

   b. Consider satin and nonglossy finishes for walls, cabinets, and countertops in kitchen. Have sheer curtains or adjustable shades in other living areas. | Reduces glare for older adults.

   c. Apply colored tape or paint to color-code controls of stove, oven, dryer, toaster, and other appliances. | Clients with reduced visual acuity may adjust appliance to wrong setting, creating potential risk for fire or burning (Touhy & Jett, 2022).

   d. Consider installing rotating tray or pull-out drawers with glide mechanisms in kitchen cabinets. Install C-ring handles in lower cabinets. | Makes access to food and kitchen supplies easier.

   e. Install automatic door openers, level doorknob handles, and hook-and-chain locks. | Devices may be easier to grasp and use. Remote-controlled door locks can also provide additional security (Touhy & Jett, 2022).

2. Fall prevention steps:
   a. Paint edges of concrete stairs bright yellow, orange, or white. | Client can see edge of stairs more clearly.

   b. Install treads with uniform depth of 22.5 cm (9 inches) and 22.5-cm (9-inch) risers (vertical face of steps). | If stairs are of uniform size, client does not have to continually adjust vision or stride.

   c. Rearrange furniture to open up space through hallways and major rooms. | Creates unobstructed pathway for ambulation.

   d. Reduce clutter within living areas (e.g., footstools, flower pots, extension cords, children's toys, stacked newspapers or magazines). | Mobility hazards resulting from clutter are especially risky at night.

   e. Secure all carpeting, mats, and tile; place nonskid backing under small rugs and doormats. Remove throw rugs/mats in nonessential (dry) areas. | Reduces chance of client slipping when stepping on rug surface (Touhy & Jett, 2022).

   f. Pad floor and use specialized tile that absorbs impact of falls. | Cushions person's fall.

   g. Use low-rise beds, futon beds, or mattress on floor if not contraindicated. | Lowers distance to floor surface.

Clinical Judgment *Clients with arthritis of the knees or hips can have difficulty rising from a bed or toilet that is too low. Assess bed height for client's comfort and safety. Use of a toilet seat riser has been found to reduce falls (Donohue et al., 2021).*

   h. Have enough electrical outlets installed to be able to plug light or electronic device (e.g., television, video) into nearby outlet. Secure electrical cords against baseboards. | Prevents need to run extension cords across walkways.

   i. Install nonskid strips on surface of bathtub and/or shower stall. Be sure that floor is clean and dry. | Reduces chances of slipping on tub/shower stall surface.

   j. Have grab bar installed in studs at tub, toilet, and/or shower (see illustration). Have client select vertical or horizontal placement if choice available. Be sure that bar is different color than wall and easy to see. | Bar provides stability for maneuvering in bathroom (Touhy & Jett, 2022). Grab bars placed in correct place where client can safely reach them help to steady stance and gait and lessen chance of falls (King, 2019; Meiner, 2019).

   k. Have handrails installed along side of any stairway (see illustration). Be sure that stairways are well lit, with switches at top and bottom of steps. | Ideally, handrails on both sides of stairwell provide greatest stability for client. If entrance space does not allow this, install at least on one side to prevent fall from imbalance (Touhy & Jett, 2022). Older adults have difficulty seeing edges of stairs.

   l. Install appropriate broad-beam lighting for outside walkways. | Provides full illumination.

   m. Keep lighted phone easily accessible next to client's bed. | Prevents client from having to get up out of bed, often in dark.

   n. Install motion-sensor exterior lighting for walkways/driveway. | Reduces risk for client falls caused by dark surroundings.

   o. Offer option for client to use padding or types of clothing that will cushion bony prominences, especially high-risk bony prominences (e.g., hips). Specially designed hip protectors are available (see illustration). | When worn correctly, hip protectors have been found to be effective in reducing the risk of hip fractures in a high-risk population (Nolan et al., 2022).

STEP	RATIONALE

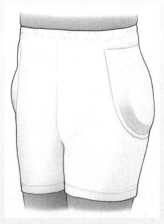

STEP 2j Grab bars and safety seat installed in shower. (*From iStock.com/nazdravie.*)

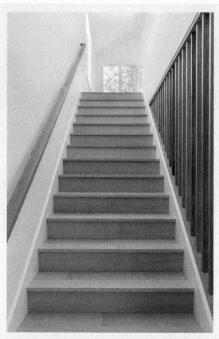

STEP 2k Handrails installed along stairways provide security for clients with visual, balance, and coordination problems. (*From iStock.com/dpproductions.*)

STEP 2o Padded clothing may reduce risk for pressure injuries. (*From Sorrentino SA, Remmert LN: Mosby's textbook for nursing assistants, ed 10, St. Louis, 2021, Elsevier.*)

3. Prevent foodborne illness:
   a. Teach client and family caregiver cleaning practices to prevent spread of infection.
   b. Instruct client not to share eating and drinking utensils.
   c. Instruct client to clean appliances and surfaces daily.

   d. Instruct client in safe food preparation and storage. Refer to guidelines at https://www.cdc.gov/foodsafety/. For example:
   • 4–12 lb turkey can be thawed safely in refrigerator for 1–3 days or in cold water for 6–12 hours; cook poultry to 165°F.
   • Bacon can be stored in refrigerator for 7 days and freezer for 1 month; hamburger and other ground meats can be stored in refrigerator for 1–2 days and in freezer for 3–4 months.

4. Fire safety:
   a. Have smoke detectors installed near each bedroom, in kitchen, and in home basement. Be sure that detector is on each floor of home. Alarm should be close in order to alert client and family when sleeping.
   b. Have client select fire extinguisher that is easy to handle and manipulate (see illustration). Ask client to read instructions and demonstrate its proper use.

Ensures more consistent infection control practices in the home.
Some infections are spread by saliva.
Regular cleaning prevents risk for contamination from food and spread of infection.

Ensures safe thawing and cooking of foods (CDC, 2022).

Safe storage times for food in refrigerator and freezer help prevent foodborne illnesses (CDC, 2022).

Fires most frequently start in basement near furnace, dryer, or electrical wiring; kitchen; or living areas where there is extensive wiring.

Some older adults or clients with disabilities have difficulty gripping mechanisms on certain extinguishers.

STEP	RATIONALE

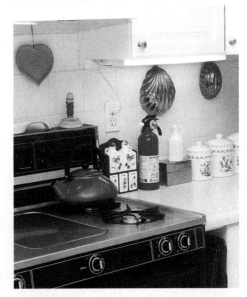

STEP 4b Fire extinguisher accessible in kitchen.

c. Have area around furnace cleared of any flammable items.

Reduces risk for fire.

d. Instruct client to be sure that portable space heater has a thermostat, overheat protection, and auto shutoff in case the heater tips over and that equipment housing and electrical cords are intact (Meiner, 2019).

Space heaters can be overturned by accident, which can cause fire; safety mechanism on newer models will turn unit off immediately (Meiner, 2019). Space heaters are a fire risk (U.S. Consumer Product Safety Commission [CPSC], 2023).

e. Have client make appointments for maintenance of furnace and chimney cleaning in appropriate season.

Furnace maintenance prevents short circuits and fires. Accumulation of creosote on chimney walls can lead to fire.

f. Have client check light bulb wattage in all fixtures.

Ensures proper wattage being used; wattage that exceeds recommendation can cause fire.

g. Have client establish routine during cooking that keeps client in kitchen. Be sure that cooking range is clean and items such as potholders and towels are away from burners.

Food cooking on stove can easily boil over or begin to burn when unattended.

h. If client is a smoker, review need to keep ashtrays clean and emptied. Placing small amount of water or sand in bottom of ashtray is useful if client is visually impaired.

Clients with reduced vision may be unable to tell if cigarette, cigar, or match has extinguished (Touhy & Jett, 2022).

i. Strongly discourage smoking in bed, smoking in chair when there is possibility of falling asleep, smoking near oxygen source, and smoking after taking medication that diminishes alertness. Instruct client/family caregiver to put cigarette or cigar out all the way at first sign of feeling drowsy (Meiner, 2019; U.S. Fire Administration, 2023).

Risks factors for burns and fire. Client's reaction time may be slower when tired.

j. Warn clients to not charge e-cigarettes with phone or tablet charger; don't charge an e-cigarette overnight; store loose batteries in a case (U.S. Fire Administration 2023).

Risk factors for fire from e-cigarettes.

k. Recommend that client install power strips or surge protectors for plugging in multiple appliances/devices.

Prevents risk for electrical short, which can cause fire.

5. Burn safety:

a. Ideal temperature for a hot water heater setting depends on several factors. If children or elderly live in the home, set the thermostat at 48.8° C (120°F). The ideal temperature for domestic hot water in households with immunocompromised persons is 60° C (140°F) (USA Water Quality, 2023).

Lower temperature setting prevents scalding burns (Meiner, 2019).

b. Instruct client to always turn cold water on first.

Prevents direct exposure to hot water.

c. Install touch pads on lamps.

Light is easy to turn on without risk of touching hot light bulb.

d. Use color codes of red for hot and blue for cold on water faucets. (If client has difficulty distinguishing these colors, choose two that are easily distinguished.)

Prevents accidental burning from turning on wrong faucet.

STEP	RATIONALE

6. Carbon monoxide safety:

    a. Have condition of furnace venting checked annually just before turning on furnace.

    Improper venting prevents escape of carbon monoxide, a poisonous gas that alters hemoglobin to prevent formation of oxyhemoglobin and reduces oxygen supply to tissues.

    b. Caution clients against using gas stove or barbecue grill for heating inside home.

    Both are sources of carbon monoxide (Meiner, 2019).

    c. Have battery-operated carbon monoxide detector installed in home; check or replace battery when you change your clocks in fall and spring (see illustration).

    Detector alarms when carbon monoxide reaches unsafe levels. Battery operation is not affected by power outages (Meiner, 2019).

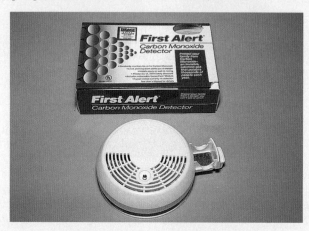

STEP 6c Carbon monoxide detector.

7. Firearm safety:

    a. Teach client about dangers associated with keeping guns in home.

    Risk of suicide increases in homes with firearms (Miller, 2019).

    b. If guns are in home, teach client how to safely store a firearm (e.g., cable or trigger lock, gun case, lock box), to install trigger locks, and to store guns unloaded in locked cabinet (CDC, 2022). Teach client to store ammunition in secured area separate from guns. Store keys in place inaccessible to children.

    The CDC (2022) recommends the publication *Suicide Prevention is Everyone's Business: A Toolkit for Safe Firearm Storage in Your Community*. Following gun safety standards decreases risk of injury and death related to gun use (Miller, 2019).

EVALUATION

1. Have client and family caregiver(s) identify safety risks revealed in home safety assessment.

Demonstrates what client recognizes as an injury risk and its relative importance for changing home environment.

2. During follow-up visit or call to home, ask client to discuss plans for making any modifications and observe changes client has implemented.

Evaluates extent to which client sees risks as potentially harmful and adheres to suggested changes.

3. During follow-up visits or calls, ask if client has experienced any falls or other injuries within home.

Reveals if risks have been eliminated, depending on client's previous history of injury.

4. During subsequent home visits, reassess for progression of dementia if applicable.

Evaluates for potential new risks to client and family caregiver.

5. **Use Teach-Back:** "I want to be sure I explained why you need to make modifications in your home. Tell me why this is important." Revise your instruction now or develop a plan for revised client/family caregiver teaching if client/family caregiver is not able to teach back correctly.

Teach-back is a technique for health care providers to ensure that they have explained medical information clearly so clients and their families understand what is communicated to them (Agency for Healthcare Research and Quality [AHRQ], 2023).

Unexpected Outcomes	Related Interventions
1. Client and family caregiver do not acknowledge risks identified from home safety assessment.	• Determine reason client is reluctant to make changes. Consider limited resources, disbelief concerning need to make changes, fear of loss of autonomy, or other reasons. • Review implications of risks to client's safety and welfare.

STEP	RATIONALE
2. Client fails to make changes agreed on in previous plan.	• Determine reason for failure to make changes. • Help prioritize greatest risks. • Suggest making a single change and gauge client's response.
3. Client falls or sustains burn within home.	• Conduct assessment of contributing factors and conditions in environment at time of injury. • Make revisions based on assessment findings.

Documentation

- Retain copy of home safety assessment in client's home care record.
- Document any instruction provided, client's and family caregiver's response, and changes made within environment.

Special Considerations

Client Education

- Family caregivers will benefit from learning how to safely help client ambulate or transfer from bed to chair or wheelchair to chair, depending on client's mobility limitations (see Chapter 11).
- Instruct client and family caregiver about what to do in case client falls, including access to emergency help and how to prevent further injury.
- When appropriate, teach family caregiver and client how to use any emergency assistive devices (e.g., devices that are worn around client's neck and a special monitor connected to client's telephone). Clients summon help by pressing button on device if phone is inaccessible. Refer the family caregiver to local health care agencies and Department of Aging for options.
- Reinforce the importance of preserving client autonomy as much as possible with family caregivers.

Pediatrics

- Caution parents when working in the kitchen to never pour hot liquids when an infant or young child is nearby.
- Remove all crib toys that are strung across crib or playpen when child begins to push up on hands or knees (4–7 months) (Hockenberry et al., 2022).

- Install safety measures appropriate to developmental level (e.g., cabinet locks and gates).
- Do not let young children use the sink or tub without adult help; when child is in tub, stay with child.

Older Adults

- Use "aging in place" resources and designs to accommodate the needs of seniors or disabled individuals without having to completely redesign the home. Resources include community and government agencies and initiatives such as local councils on aging and AARP. Resources also focus on helping older adults to continue to live in the home of their choice, with a focus on quality of life. For example, install grab bars in bathrooms, movable cabinets under the sink so that someone in a wheelchair can use the space, and light switches and electrical outlets at heights that can be reached easily.
- Place a bedside commode (with bedpan removed) over a conventional toilet seat. Commode level is usually higher than toilet level and can also be moved near the bed for nighttime use.

Populations With Disabilities

- People with disabilities need to adapt their homes so that occupants can reside safely, perform tasks more easily, and live independently despite their physical limitations. Home access modifications can be as simple as adding grab bars or may entail extensive structural alterations including replacing a stairway, adding stair lifts, having a wheelchair ramp, or removing a bathtub and replacing it with a walk-in shower.
- Some home improvements for disabilities may require adherence to standards such as those specified in the Americans With Disabilities Act.

♦ **SKILL 41.2** **Adapting the Home Setting for Clients With Cognitive Deficits**

Clients with cognitive impairments and their family caregivers need special assistance in making adaptations to preserve the clients' abilities to function safely within their homes. An important aspect of safety is a person's ability to perform routine activities of daily living (ADLs) and instrumental activities of daily living (IADLs). This requires a client to make correct decisions about home-management activities. ADLs include a client's ability to bathe, dress, go to the toilet, transfer, and feed oneself. IADLs include the ability to use a telephone, prepare meals, travel, do housework, take medication, and shop. When there are cognitive limitations, a person's independence is threatened. Family caregivers often do not understand changes in a client's cognition or how it might progress and thus require help to determine whether a client is competent to stay at home safely.

Two common cognitive conditions affecting clients in the home are dementia and depression. Depression often results from

social isolation (e.g., an older adult becomes homebound and has few relatives who can offer assistance, or lives alone with few visitors). Major depression is common among elderly adults receiving home health care and is characterized by greater medical illness, functional impairment, and pain (Steele, 2023). Clients with depression are less likely to adhere to medical regimens and do not properly care for themselves (e.g., poor diet, limited activity or exercise). Compared with other home health care clients, depressed clients have been shown to have higher risk of hospitalization, more injury-producing falls, and higher health care costs (Touhy & Jett, 2022).

Dementia is a chronic generalized impairment of intellectual functioning that leads to a decline in the ability to perform basic ADLs and IADLs. It is characterized by a gradual, progressive, irreversible cerebral dysfunction. Alzheimer disease (AD) is the most common form of dementia; worldwide there are 55 million people living with AD and other dementias (Alzheimer's Association, 2022a). As it progresses, older adults become more dependent on family caregivers for help.

AD causes problems with memory, thinking, and behavior. Some individuals with AD are at risk for wandering (Alzheimer's Association, 2022a). Wandering refers to moving about without having a definite place to go or a purpose. A wandering client may walk around the house trying repeatedly to carry out a task independently or try to leave the place of residence, necessitating family caregiver intervention to stop them. Family caregivers need to learn how to make the home safe to discourage wandering and prevent clients from leaving their homes unattended.

Delegation

The skill of making adjustments to the home environment for clients with cognitive deficits can be delegated to assistive personnel (AP). However, the nurse is responsible for the assessment of cognitive function and determination of appropriate modifications. Direct the AP to:

- Inform the nurse when there is a change in client's mood, memory, and ability to maintain the home or perform self-care.

Interprofessional Collaboration

- Collaborate with the health care provider in sharing findings when changes in a client's mental status have been assessed.
- Consider consultation with occupational therapists (OTs), homemaker services, or respite care providers for client and support of family caregiver.

Equipment

- Mini-Mental State Examination (MMSE)
- Geriatric Depression Scale Short Form (GDS-SF)
- Beck Depression Inventory (BDI)
- Calendar
- Paper for making lists
- Medication organizer (optional)
- Bulletin board or posterboard (optional)
- Motion detector (optional)

STEP	RATIONALE

ASSESSMENT

1. Identify client using at least two identifiers (e.g., name and birthday or name and medical record number) according to agency policy.

Ensures client safety. Complies with The Joint Commission standards and improves client safety (TJC, 2023).

2. Assess client over several short periods of time and be ready to adapt assessment if client has sensory disabilities. If client does not speak English, have a professional interpreter assist.

Respects human dignity of client. Improves likelihood of gathering relevant data.

3. Assess client's/family caregiver's health literacy and knowledge of adapting the home environment. It may be necessary to assess only family caregiver.

Determines degree to which individuals have the ability to find, understand, and use information and services to make informed health-related decisions and actions for themselves and others (CDC, 2023).

4. Determine if client has family caregiver who helps with self-care or home-management responsibilities. Consider the following questions:
   - What level of support does the family caregiver provide? Sporadic assistance, household tasks, self-care tasks, monitoring, end-of-life care?
   - How frequently is the family caregiver available?
   - Does the client perceive satisfaction in the family caregiver's support?
   - What level of satisfaction does the family caregiver perceive?
   - Does the family caregiver have access to and/or take advantage of respite care?

Relationship between family caregiver and client helps define how difficult it is to provide caregiving support. Role of family caregiver is often stressful, particularly if individual has other responsibilities such as parenting, work, or school. Determines availability of resource to client and quality of that support. With increasing care recipient disability and need for care, the caregiver's role becomes more labor and time intensive, more complex, and increasingly stressful (Schulz et al., 2020).

5. Be sure that the room in which you meet with the client and family caregiver is well lit with minimal outside noises or interruptions. Listen carefully and speak clearly and in normal tone of voice.

Optimal environment for assessment of client's cognitive and mental status provides more valid assessment.

6. Ask the client to describe own level of health and describe how it affects ability to perform ADLs and IADLs. Ask family caregiver (if available) to confirm description. Screen for risky behaviors (e.g., medication nonadherence, unsupervised use of stove).

Question requires client to focus on one topic. Allows you to assess attention and concentration. Also determines if client is fully perceptive of physical and cognitive capabilities.

Clinical Judgment *Be aware of your communication with the client and family caregivers. Do not make the client think that you are not listening to the client's views. The additional person supplements answers with client's consent, but the client remains the focus of the interview.*

STEP	RATIONALE
7. Ask how the client is handling home-management responsibilities: "Tell me which bills you pay each month. Can you tell me what each one is for?" *Ability to perform ADLs:* "Can you tell me about your normal day? When do you get up, eat meals, dress? Tell me what you do to dress or bathe each morning."	Provides good comparison of client and family caregiver's perceptions. Interaction helps to measure short-term memory, judgment, and problem solving (Frith et al., 2019).
8. Assess client's medication history and adherence to taking medications. Review number and type of medications prescribed compared with those being taken, client's understanding of purpose as prescribed (or as chosen for over-the-counter [OTC] medications), time of day taken, and dosages. Conduct pill count over course of a week (family caregiver may need to help). Also assess where client stores medications. Give special attention to pain medications, anticonvulsants, antihypertensives (especially beta-adrenergic blockers), diuretics, digoxin, aspirin, and anticoagulants.	Depression and dementia can lead to poor medication adherence. Older adults frequently experience medication interactions from polypharmacy (i.e., concurrent prescriptions for multiple medications). Some medications and/or combinations of medications place client at risk for side effects that increase chances of injury as result of physical or cognitive changes. Client-related factors such as disease-related knowledge, health literacy, and cognitive function; medication-related factors such as adverse effects and polypharmacy; and other factors, including client-provider relationship, are barriers to medication adherence.
9. During discussion, observe client's dress, nonverbal expressions, appearance, and cleanliness.	Conditions such as depression and dementia can result in client's inability to attend to personal appearance (Steele, 2023).

Clinical Judgment *Do not confuse behavioral changes with lack of available resources to maintain hygiene. Also be aware of signs and symptoms of abuse or neglect (see Chapter 6). Report suspected abuse to appropriate social service agency.*

STEP	RATIONALE
10. Observe immediate home environment.	Behavioral changes associated with cognitive dysfunction are evident by the appearance of a disorderly home and inappropriate placement of objects (e.g., piles of bills or unwashed clothes, carton of orange juice placed inside kitchen cabinet instead of in refrigerator).

11. If you suspect a cognitive or mental status change:
 	
a. Complete Mini-Mental State Examination (MMSE) or the Mini-Cog for dementia. For the MMSE, you ask a client a series of questions designed to test a range of everyday mental skills. The maximum MMSE score is 30 points. A score of 20 to 24 suggests mild dementia, 13 to 20 suggests moderate dementia, and less than 12 indicates severe dementia (Alzheimer's Association, 2022b).
Using the Mini Cog, ask client to complete two tasks:
  1. Ask to remember names of three common objects, then a few minutes later have client repeat the names.
  2. Draw a face of a clock showing all 12 numbers in the right places and a time specified by the examiner (Alzheimer's Association, 2022b).
	Tests give an overall sense of whether a person is aware of symptoms; knows the date, time, and where they are; can remember a short list of words; can follow instructions; and can do simple calculations (Alzheimer's Association, 2022b). On average, the MMSE score of a person with Alzheimer declines about 2 to 4 points each year (Alzheimer's Association, 2022b).
	
	Mini-Cog is a quick screen for determining if further assessment is needed.

b. Complete Geriatric Depression Scale Short Form (GDS-SF) for depression. (**NOTE:** Other depression scales such as the Beck Depression Inventory [BDI] are available.)	GDS-SF scores greater than 5 indicate a need for further evaluation. The GDS was developed specifically to screen older adults; the Cornell Scale for Depression in Dementia (CSDD) is the recommended assessment for older adults with dementia (Touhy & Jett, 2022).
c. When client demonstrates signs of dementia, conduct a Home Safety Inventory (HSI).	The HSI is a clinical assessment tool to evaluate potential safety issues with individuals and family caregivers of people with dementia (Lach, 2019).
12. If you suspect that client is at risk for wandering or is wandering, observe for the following behaviors (family caregivers might provide information as well) (Alzheimer's Association, 2022c): • Repeated shadowing or seeking whereabouts of family caregiver • Wanting "to go home" even when at home • Inability to locate familiar places (bathroom, kitchen) or getting lost in familiar setting • Going into unauthorized or private places • Searching for "missing" people or places • Walking with no apparent destination or purpose • Haphazard or continuous moving, restless walking, or pacing • Walking that cannot easily be redirected	Alerts family and caregivers to potential safety risks. When wandering extends outside safe environment, client is at increased risk for injury or death.

STEP	RATIONALE
13. Assess whether the client is right- or left-handed.	Wandering generally follows the direction of the dominant hand (Alzheimer's Association, 2022c).
14. Assess which current environmental strategies family caregivers are using to deal with wandering (e.g., latches and alarms on doors, visual cues such as STOP signs, constant supervision, and identification band worn by client). How effective have they been?	Helps to determine level of intervention necessary. Allows for assessment of how family is dealing with issues of wandering and need for additional outside support.
15. Assess family caregiver for signs and symptoms of stress: • Withdrawal from friends and family • Loss of interest in activities previously enjoyed • Feeling irritable, hopeless, and helpless • Changes in appetite, weight, or both • Changes in sleep patterns • Getting sick more often • Feelings of wanting to hurt self or the person for whom the individual is caring • Emotional and physical exhaustion • Irritability	Family caregiver burden is a state of physical, emotional, and mental exhaustion, which may be accompanied by a change in attitude, from positive and caring to negative and unconcerned (Cleveland Clinic, 2023). Addressing the needs of family caregivers of those with dementia improves quality of care for clients with dementia, while reducing health care costs (Touhy & Jett, 2022).

PLANNING

1. Expected outcomes following completion of procedure: • Client is able to complete home management responsibilities within existing limitations. • Client receives appropriate combination of medications for diagnosed conditions. • Client is able to perform self-care activities or receives appropriate help. • Family caregivers implement steps to take to minimize wandering. • Client experiences fewer episodes of wandering. • Family caregiver identifies community resources for support: respite care, adult day care programs, and support groups.	Modifications that help client apply remaining cognitive functions are made. Assistive devices enable client to adhere to prescribed medication regimen. Interventions preserve client's autonomy and maximize functionality. Instruction prepares family caregivers with wandering-management strategies. Wandering-management strategies are effective. Services available for support required by client.
2. If client has difficulty with self-care or fine-motor skills, refer family caregiver to OT, homemaker services, or respite care provider as appropriate.	Occupational therapists provide assistive devices and recommend self-care adaptations. Homemaker services provide added resource for meal preparation and home cleaning. Respite care provides family caregiver temporary rest away from continuous responsibilities.
3. Consider client's level of cognitive impairment when making changes in the living environment. Some clients may require only minor adaptations, and others will depend more on help of family caregivers.	Retention of client's independence and autonomy is ultimate outcome.
4. Determine best time of day for approaches that result in desired response.	Some clients are more alert and responsive in morning versus afternoon or vice versa.

IMPLEMENTATION

1. If client has difficulty remembering when to perform tasks (e.g., paying bills, making appointments), help to create lists or post reminder notes in conspicuous location (e.g., bulletin board, front of refrigerator).	Lists and organizers help client cope with memory loss and still safely perform activities.
2. If client has difficulty remembering when to take medicines, involve family caregiver in finding best solutions: reinforcement with a reminder list or note, provide medication container organized by days of week, or recommend wristwatch with alarm or schedule of text messages to signal medication administration times.	Poor cognitive function is a risk factor of medication nonadherence. Family caregivers are important in assisting with medication adherence (Touhy & Jett, 2022). Reminder systems are beneficial if client or family caregiver is motivated and/or has desire to adhere to them. New text messaging systems can alert clients to take their medications (NIA, 2022).
3. When client has difficulty completing tasks such as writing checks for bills or bringing groceries into home from store, reduce steps it takes to complete task. Consolidate steps or simplify task.	Prevents frustration in completing task and/or forgetting step that leads to task being unfinished.

STEP	RATIONALE

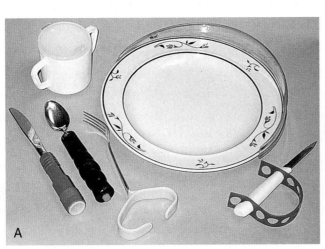 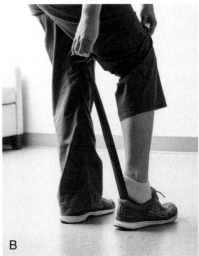

STEP 4 (A) Assistive devices for self-feeding. (B) Assistive device to help put on shoes. (*A from Sharma SK, Stockert PA, Perry AG, et al: Potter and Perry's essentials of nursing foundation, South Asia Edition, St. Louis, 2021, Elsevier. B courtesy ArcMate Manufacturing Corporation. All rights reserved.*)

4. If client has difficulty bathing, dressing, writing, and feeding, offer assistive devices (see Chapter 30) (see illustration).

Assistive eating devices have larger handles, cup handles, or plate edges to help with meals. Assistive dressing devices use Velcro, large zippers, and elastic to facilitate independence when dressing.

5. Help client and family caregiver determine routine schedule for ADLs such as eating, bathing, daily exercise, home cleaning, and napping. Have large calendar posted in conspicuous area to write in appointments or special planned events.

Consistency creates sense of security and keeps client oriented to daily activities. Routines are important in providing security, but client also needs to have option of making changes as needed (Touhy & Jett, 2022).

6. Instruct family caregiver to focus on client's abilities rather than disabilities. Use abilities in modifying approaches to perform daily activities (e.g., if client has limited use of right hand, try approaches that maximize use of left hand).

Retains client's autonomy and sense of self-worth.

7. Consider different activities the person can do to stay active, such as household chores, cooking and baking, exercise, and gardening. Match the activity to what the person can do.

Promotes active lifestyle for person with dementia (Alzheimers.gov, n.d.).

8. Have family caregiver help set up activities so that client can complete tasks (e.g., chopping vegetables before cooking, placing wash basin on table in bedroom for sponge bath, placing clothes to wear for day on bed, unpacking groceries on countertop for eventual storage, arranging food on plate with items in clockwise orientation [e.g., vegetables at 9, salad at 3, meat at 6]).

Helps client master task even though unable either physically or cognitively to perform all steps.

9. Discuss with client, family caregiver, pharmacist, and health care provider options for making medication self-administration safer, including scheduling multiple medications:

Medications sometimes cause physiological changes that create risk for injury.

a. Make sure client can read and understand the name of the medicine, as well as the directions on the container and on the color-coded warning stickers on the bottle. If a label is hard to read, ask pharmacist to use larger type (NIA, 2022).

Unclear or confusing medication labels can create risk for administration errors.

b. Have medications that are likely to cause confusion prescribed to be given at bedtime.

Reduces risk for confusion during waking hours that contributes to disorientation and risk for falling.

Clinical Judgment *Do not recommend bedtime medication administration if client has nocturia because client will be at greater risk for falling.*

c. Space antihypertensives and antiarrhythmics at different times to minimize side effects.

These medications cause blood pressure changes and dizziness, thus increasing risk for falls.

d. When possible, reduce number of pain medications used.

Medications create sedative effects, increasing risk for falls.

e. Have diuretics taken early in day and not at night.

Diuretic effect occurs during day while client is awake.

f. Discuss with health care provider possibility of taking medications at same time.

If safe and appropriate, taking medications at same time will alleviate problem of client remembering multiple administration times (Frith et al., 2019).

STEP	RATIONALE
g. Discuss use of medication organizer and dispenser (see illustrations).	Organizing medication in daily dispenser may help client and family caregiver avoid medication errors of duplicating or missing medications.

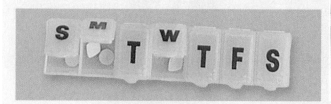

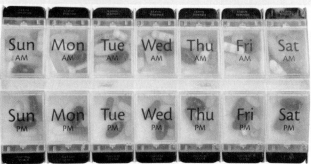

STEP 9g Weekly medication organizers. (A) Single week. (B) Multiple weeks. (*B copyright © Thinkstock.com.*)

STEP	RATIONALE
10. Teach family caregiver how to use simple and direct communication:	Relays care and support through therapeutic communication techniques.
a. Sit or stand in front of client in full view.	Promotes reception of verbal and nonverbal messages.
b. Face client with hearing impairment while speaking; do not cover mouth and do not speak in a loud tone.	Client can see speaker's lips. Prevents voice distortion.
c. Use calm and relaxed approach. Respect personal space.	
d. Use eye contact and touch.	Helps to reinforce messages.
e. Speak slowly, in simple words and short sentences.	Enhances understanding of messages.
f. Remind the person who you are if client doesn't remember, but try not to say, "Don't you remember?" Encourage a two-way conversation for as long as possible.	Avoids potentially causing client to become angry (Alzheimers.gov, n.d.). Helps client feel in control.
g. Use nonverbal gestures that complement verbal messages.	Provides clear messages.
11. Place clocks, calendars, and personal mementos (e.g., pictures, scrapbooks) throughout rooms within home. Enhance environment with addition of tactile boards or three-dimensional art.	Maintaining familiar surroundings maximizes cognitive function.
12. Have family caregiver routinely orient client to who family caregiver is and which activities are going to be completed.	This strategy is useful in clients with progressive dementia. Behavioral symptoms in later stages include delusions, agitation, and hallucinations (Alzheimer's Association, 2022a).
13. Be sure that client has regular naps or rest periods during day.	Fatigue adds to any mental status changes. Provides client energy to perform planned activities.
14. Have family caregiver encourage and support frequent visits by family and friends. Teach family caregiver how to use humor and reminiscing about favorite stories to promote social interaction.	Participation in social activities prevents boredom and restlessness.
15. Provide safe place for person to wander (e.g., large family room or fenced yard).	Reduces risk for injury and leaving residence (Touhy & Jett, 2022).
16. Recommend that family of wandering client install door locks or electronic guards.	Reduces chance of client exiting home unsupervised.
17. Create calm, safe setting that is appropriate for client's abilities (Alzheimer's Association, 2022a).	Prevents falls and minimizes behavioral symptoms.
18. Regularly monitor client for personal comfort (e.g., hunger, thirst, constipation, full bladder, and comfortable temperature) (Alzheimer's Association, 2022a).	Reduces stimuli that prompt wandering.
19. Consider having client wear Global Positioning System (GPS) device to help manage location. Install motion detector near exit site, with portable alarm that can accompany family caregiver.	Alerts family caregiver to client's attempt to exit residence (Alzheimer's Association, 2022a).
20. Collaborate with family caregiver to consider need for full-time care.	Caregiver burden can lead to detrimental outcomes for a client. Consideration of long-term care can be more beneficial for client's safety and well-being and family caregiver's health.

STEP	RATIONALE

EVALUATION

1. During follow-up visits, ask client to review home-management activities completed the morning of that day and previous day.

Determines client's ability to recall events and evaluates if client completed planned activities.

2. Review with client and family caregiver revised schedule for medication administration.

Evaluates understanding of regimen.

3. Check pill count you asked client/family caregiver to maintain for a week.

Tracking doses confirms if client is adherent to regimen.

4. Ask family caregiver to describe ways that will increase client's success in completing home-management and self-care activities.

Measures learning.

5. Have family caregiver show schedules of daily routines and review specific approaches used. Observe environment for presence of reality orientation cues.

Determines family caregiver's success in applying information and making environmental changes.

6. Have family caregivers describe options for minimizing wandering.

Measures learning.

7. Have family caregivers report number of occurrences of wandering.

Determines if reduction in wandering has occurred.

8. **Use Teach-Back:** "I want to be sure I explained how you can help reduce the number of times your husband wanders. Tell me some ways you can do this." Revise your instruction now or develop a plan for revised family caregiver teaching if family caregiver is not able to teach back correctly.

Teach-back is a technique for health care providers to ensure that they have explained medical information clearly so clients and their families understand what is communicated to them (AHRQ, 2023).

Unexpected Outcomes

1. Client is unable to complete ADLs and IADLs as planned.

2. Family caregiver is unable to describe or implement techniques that will improve client's orientation and ability to complete activities.

3. Client's wandering increases.

4. Client misses medication doses or takes wrong dosage.

Related Interventions

- Further modifications are sometimes necessary.
- Reassess what occurred when task was not completed.
- Have family caregiver offer suggestions.
- Reinstruction and discussion are necessary.
- Support for family caregiver is sometimes necessary before caregiver can learn how to support someone else.
- Consider that family caregiver is not able to provide necessary support; need to analyze other options.
- Reinstruction and discussion are necessary.
- Family caregiver may not have resources available to adapt environment.
- Review list of medications and method for administering (e.g., medication dispenser).
- Reconsider strategies to organize and schedule medications.
- Assess client for adverse effects (NIA, 2022).

Documentation

- Document all assessment findings, including client's functional, cognitive, and mental status; availability of family caregiver; recommended interventions; and client's and family caregiver's response.

Reporting

- Report to health care provider any change in client's behavior that reflects a decline in cognitive or mental status.

Special Considerations

Client Education

- Instruct family caregiver in signs and symptoms of dementia and depression. If client's functionality continues to decline, family caregiver may choose to learn more ADL support skills (e.g., how to help with hygiene, dressing, transfer and turning, toileting).
- Have client or family caregiver keep updated list of medications that can be brought to emergency department if needed.

- For clients with dementia, teach family caregivers about developing an emergency plan (Alzheimer's Association, 2022c):
  - Have a plan in place before a client wanders so that all family members know what to do in case of an emergency.
  - Keep a list of people to call on for help. Have telephone numbers easily accessible.
  - Ask neighbors, friends, and family to call if they see the client alone.
  - Keep a recent, close-up photo and updated medical information on hand to give to police.
  - Know your neighborhood. Pinpoint dangerous areas near the home, such as bodies of water, open stairwells, dense foliage, tunnels, bus stops, and roads with heavy traffic.
  - Keep a list of places where the person may wander or has wandered previously. This could include past jobs, former homes, places of worship, or a restaurant.

Pediatrics

- Often, children with cognitive impairment are not aware of inherent dangers during play and other activities. Parental supervision is critical.

Older Adults

- Early diagnosis of the cause of dementia is best for the client and family caregiver so that prompt treatment can begin, the client can be included in treatment decisions as much as possible, and the family caregiver has an understanding of the behavior (Alzheimer's Association, 2022a).
- Family caregivers will need access to respite programs, which will allow them planned time away from their caregiving role.
- Consider that clients may not have family caregivers who are able or willing to care for them. Additional help of a contracted caregiver may be required if available; this may also affect client's ability to stay in the home and not be placed in assisted or skilled care.
- If wandering is an ongoing problem, recommend enrolling client in the national MedicAlert + Alzheimer's Association Safe Return program, which provides 24-hour emergency and wandering response services and support services for family and caregivers (Alzheimer's Association, 2022a). Local resources of informal caregivers (e.g., neighbors and members of the spiritual community) can also be explored to ensure safety for the client inside and outside of the home.
- Additional caregiver support resources: AARP (aarp.org, 877-333-5885); Family Caregiver Alliance (caregiver.org, 800-445-8106); National Alliance for Caregiving (caregiving.org, 202-918-1013); Well Spouse Association (wellspouse.org, 732-577-8899).

♦ SKILL 41.3   Medication and Medical Device Safety

The older people become, the more prescription medications they are likely to take. It becomes your responsibility in the care of any client taking prescription medications to assist the client in following the ordered medication regimen correctly. The first time you visit a client's home, you will review and list all of a client's medications and inspect medication bottles. It is important to note medication name, dosage, frequency, and route and to compare your list with any previous lists (e.g., known medications ordered by primary health care provider or other physicians and hospital discharge instructions). This process is known as *medication reconciliation*; the goal is to ensure that there are no errors or omissions in a client's medication regimen while also assessing if there is any need for change in medications (NIA, 2022).

Clients in the home frequently manage the administration of medications and the use of medical devices such as syringes, blood glucose monitoring equipment, dressing supplies, and even intravenous (IV) devices. This includes administration, storage, and disposal of medications and medical devices. It is critical that a client administers medications correctly, uses devices properly, cleans equipment, and removes waste properly. Infection control is just one safety principle that a client and/or family caregiver must learn for the home setting. Make sure that clients know regulations regarding waste disposal and follow the procedures consistent with local and federal laws (e.g., place soiled dressings in securely fastened plastic bags before adding to regular trash and use trash containers with tight lids to avoid attracting animals).

Be prepared to care for a client with sensory, mobility, or cognitive deficits. Clients who require special consideration include those with acute sensory or neurological impairment; those with chronic illness such as diabetes mellitus or arthritis; and older adults, who frequently have physical limitations that make manipulating medical devices and dispensing medications difficult. For example, clients with arthritic hands are often unable to open medication containers because of weakness in the hands and the pain created by pressure on the joints.

Delegation

The skill of assessing for and monitoring medication and medical device safety cannot be delegated to assistive personnel (AP). Direct the AP to:
- Make suggestions that further ensure client safety regarding the use of basic infection control practices.
- Make suggestions as to how to properly dispose of sharps, needles, and contaminated supplies in the home.

Equipment

- Colored marking pens
- Labels
- Puncture-resistant sharps container or 2-L hard plastic bottle with cap
- Duct, masking, or adhesive tape
- Assistive devices (e.g., syringe magnifier)
- Medication organizers

STEP	RATIONALE

ASSESSMENT

1. Identify client using at least two identifiers (e.g., name and birthday or name and medical record number) according to agency policy.

2. Assess client's and family caregiver's health literacy level and knowledge of medication and medication devices (e.g., ask them to read a medication label out loud to you, read instructions on use of glucose meter).

3. Assess client's sensory, musculoskeletal, and neurological function (see Chapter 6), specifically hand strength, ability to read doses on syringe, ability to prepare medicine in a syringe, and ability to open medication container. If cognitive deficit exists, see Skill 41.2.

Ensures client safety. Complies with The Joint Commission standards and improves client safety (TJC, 2023).

Determines degree to which individuals have the ability to find, understand, and use information and services to make informed health-related decisions and actions for themselves and others (CDC, 2023).

Reveals any deficits that will affect preparation and use of medications or medical devices.

STEP	RATIONALE
4. Determine if client has family caregiver who helps with self-care or home-management responsibilities (see Skill 41.2). Does family caregiver have any functional limitations affecting their ability to assist client? If family caregiver provides routine help, ask family caregiver if there are any concerns about being able to care for client.	Determines if client has resource in form of family caregiver. Assesses family caregivers' health and ability to assist. Can help educate family caregivers as to need for assistance and provide information to avoid injury.
5. Assess client's medication regimen and length of time that client has been receiving each medication. Ask client to describe doses taken daily for each medication. Query family caregiver if necessary.	Determines complexity of medication regimen and how familiar client or family caregiver is with regimen.

Clinical Judgment *Be sure that medication labels are not confusing for a client. For example, the Spanish word for "eleven" is written as "once." A Spanish-speaking client could confuse a medication direction that requires them to take a medication 1 time a day as 11 times a day.*

STEP	RATIONALE
6. Ask client to show you where medications are stored in home. Look at each container.	Determines condition and labeling of containers.
7. Assess temperature of storage area.	Medication should not be stored in extreme heat. Insulin should not be stored near extreme heat or cold (American Diabetes Association [ADA], 2023).
8. Assess client's daily schedule for medication administration. Ask client to describe schedule and whether there are any problems in following that schedule. Use family caregiver as resource, if appropriate.	Helps to reveal client's adherence to or misunderstanding of instructions.
9. If client self-administers injections, ask to see where client stores supplies and what is used to dispose of used syringes and needles.	Determines sterility of stored equipment and whether method of disposal creates risk to client or family for needlestick injuries.
10. If client uses glucose-monitoring device, ask to see where monitor, lancets, and glucose strips are stored. Also ask about how client disposes of lancets.	Allows you to examine cleanliness of equipment, sterility of lancets, and condition of glucose strips. Sharps should be disposed of in puncture-proof container.

PLANNING

1. Expected outcomes following completion of procedure:	
• Client and family caregiver discuss principles of medication safety.	Client education includes information and techniques for safe medication administration.
• Client and family caregiver prepare and administer medications independently.	Adaptations successfully accommodate client's and/or family caregiver's deficits in handling and manipulating equipment.
• Client and family caregiver identify correct conditions for storing medications, medical devices, and supplies.	Instruction focuses on ensuring infection control measures (Medline Plus, 2022).
• Client and family caregiver dispose of used medical equipment and supplies correctly.	Appropriate receptacles and methods for disposal are made available and used.

IMPLEMENTATION

STEP	RATIONALE
1. Teach client and family caregiver the following principles of safe medication use:	
a. Never take medicine prescribed for another person (NIA, 2022).	Medications must be of full strength and used for appropriate pharmacological reason to have therapeutic benefit.
b. Do not take any medicine more than 1 year old or after expiration date on container (NIA, 2022).	Expired medication is sometimes toxic or no longer effective.
c. Always keep medicines in original container (Medline Plus, 2022).	Prevents accidental "mix-up" of medications and medication errors.
d. Always finish prescribed medication (NIA, 2022); do not save for future illness.	Prevents underdosing or inappropriate dosing.
e. Do not take medicine that has changed color, texture, or smell, even if it has not expired.	Medication will be inactive.
f. Wash hands before and after administering/taking medication.	Contaminated hands are source of infection transmission.
2. Recommend approaches for safe preparation of medications:	
a. For clients with weakened grasp or pain in hands and fingers, have local pharmacist place medications in screw-top container.	Tops of childproof containers are difficult to remove, especially if hand and finger grasp is weakened.

Clinical Judgment *If client has children or grandchildren who have easy access to medication storage area or client's purse, be sure that medications are stored in secure place (Medline Plus, 2022).*

STEP	RATIONALE
b. For clients with visual alterations, have pharmacy type larger labels on all medication containers.	Ensures that client is able to read drug name and dosage schedule clearly.
c. For clients who are legally blind, have Braille labels placed on medication containers.	Labels embossed with medication name, strength, and prescription numbers are easy to read for client trained in use of Braille (Shetty et al., 2021).
d. For clients taking multiple medications, ask if they wish to try to introduce a color-coding system. Use same color for medications that client needs to take at same time. Mark tops of bottle caps with colored marking pen.	Technique helps client take correct medications and doses at correct times of day. Best used when client is reliable in self-administration.
e. Provide specially designed syringes with large numerals or syringe magnifier for clients with visual alterations (see illustration).	Ensures that accurate dose of medication is prepared in syringe.

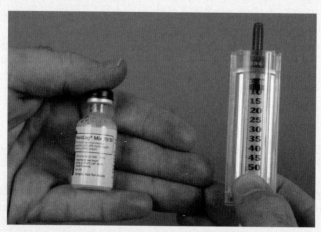

STEP 2e Syringe with magnifier.

f. For clients who have difficulty manipulating syringes, offer spring-loaded needle insertion aid.	Delivers injection safely without manipulation of plunger.

Clinical Judgment *Teach family caregivers what to do following a needlestick injury. Wash the affected area thoroughly with soap and water and dry. If client has acquired immunodeficiency syndrome (AIDS), hepatitis, or other communicable disease, family caregivers should pursue appropriate laboratory testing.*

g. Teach family caregivers how to properly draw up prescribed volume of medication into syringe. When necessary, have family caregiver prepare extra prefilled syringes for client's use when family caregiver is absent.	Ensures that family caregiver knows proper preparation techniques and that client has access to injections. Watch client and/or family caregiver draw up and dispense medications to determine if more teaching is needed.
3. Recommend approaches for safe medication and supply storage:	
a. Store medications in safe, dry place, preferably in dresser drawer or a kitchen cabinet away from the stove, sink, and any hot appliances. *Option:* Store medicine in a storage box, on a shelf, or in a closet.	Moisture in bathroom may cause medications to decompose.
b. Keep liquid medications and parenteral medications, especially insulin, in cool place.	Prevents decomposition of medication.

Clinical Judgment *Although manufacturers recommend storing insulin in the refrigerator, injecting cold insulin can sometimes make the injection more painful. To avoid this, store the bottle of insulin being used at room temperature. Insulin kept at room temperature will last approximately 1 month. However, remember to store extra bottles in the refrigerator if a client buys more than one bottle at a time to save money (ADA, 2023). If insulin is stored in refrigerator, be sure that medication is in a bin or container, away from food.*

c. Keep medical supplies such as syringes, dressing supplies, and glucose meter in airtight container (e.g., plastic storage bin) and store in cool place such as bedroom closet.	Ensures that supplies are not exposed to moisture or other contaminants.
d. Instruct client and family caregiver to use new needle with each medication administration.	Multiple use of same needle puts client at risk for infection.

STEP	RATIONALE
4. Review with client and family caregiver proper techniques for disposal of unused parts of medications or outdated medications properly using these guidelines:	Proper practices necessary to prevent client injury.
a. The best way to dispose of most types of old, unused, unwanted, or expired medicines (both prescription and over the counter) is to drop off the medicine at a medication take-back site, location, or program immediately (U.S. Food and Drug Administration [FDA], 2020).	Professionals will dispose of medications without risk of access to others.
b. DO NOT FLUSH unused medications. However, the FDA (2020) has determined that certain medications should be flushed **if a medication take-back site is not available** because of their abuse potential. Read the instructions on the medication and talk to a pharmacist or go to the FDA (2020) website for a list of medications that can be flushed.	FDA recognizes that the recommendation to flush certain potentially dangerous medicines **only when a take-back option is not readily available** raises questions about the impact of the medications on the environment and the contamination of surface and drinking water supplies (FDA, 2020).
c. Many medicines, except those on the FDA flush list (see above), can be thrown into household trash. Follow these steps:	
(1) Remove the medications from their original containers and mix them with something undesirable, such as used coffee grounds, dirt, or cat litter.	This makes the medicine less appealing to children and pets and unrecognizable to someone who might intentionally go through the trash looking for medications.
(2) Put the mixture in something you can close (a resealable zipper storage bag, empty can, or other container).	Prevents medication from leaking or spilling out.
(3) Throw the container in the garbage.	
(4) Scratch out or remove the label containing all personal information on the empty medicine packaging. Throw the packaging away.	Protects client's identity and privacy.
d. Check for approved state and local collection programs or with area hazardous waste facilities.	In certain states you may be able to take your unused medications to your community pharmacy (FDA, 2020).
5. Review with client and family caregiver proper techniques for disposal of sharps and disposable medical supplies:	
a. Obtain sharps container from medical supply store or IV equipment supplier. (If finances are limited, have client use small-neck plastic bottle such as soda bottle.) Dispose of all needles and lancets in container.	Puncture-proof container prevents exposure to contaminated needlestick. Small-neck container makes it difficult for anyone to easily retrieve used needle or sharp.
b. Caution against filling sharps container to point where needles protrude out of opening. Discard when three-fourths full, securing top with duct tape or adhesive tape.	Prevents needlesticks.
c. Store sharps container in area inaccessible to children.	Prevents injury to child.
d. Dispose of soiled dressings, used glucose testing reagent strips, and IV tubing in separate, sealed, plastic garbage bag. Place in second plastic bag (double bagged) and discard appropriately as trash.	Prevents contamination with other items in home. Minimizes chances of family caregiver being exposed to infectious waste.
e. Consult local public health department or community authorities regarding proper way to dispose of waste.	Most communities have strict guidelines for waste disposal.

EVALUATION

1. Have client and/or family caregiver describe steps to take to ensure that medications are safe to use.	Demonstrates learning.
2. Observe client and/or family caregiver prepare and administer medication dose.	Evaluates ability to physically manipulate medications and necessary equipment.
3. Observe home setting for location of medications and supplies.	Evaluates client's and/or family caregiver's adherence to recommendations.
4. Have client describe how sharps or medical equipment is discarded.	Demonstrates learning.
5. Perform pill counts (pills remaining in containers) at successive intervals such as twice a week for 2 weeks.	Helps to verify that client takes correct number of medications over period of time.

STEP	RATIONALE
6. **Use Teach-Back:** "I want to be sure I explained the importance of throwing away your lancets and needles the right way. Tell me how to dispose of your lancets correctly and why this is important." Revise your instruction now or develop a plan or revised client/family caregiver teaching if client/family caregiver is not able to teach back correctly.	Teach-back is a technique for health care providers to ensure that they have explained medical information clearly so that clients and their families understand what is communicated to them (AHRQ, 2023).

Unexpected Outcomes	Related Interventions
1. Client and/or family caregiver is unable to recall principles for safe use of medications.	• Reinstruction necessary, or client and family caregiver need chance to ask more questions regarding benefit of precautions. • Offer simple, plain language and/or written instructions.
2. Client and/or family caregiver has difficulty or is unable to prepare and self-administer medication.	• Offer further help to set up equipment. • Offer assistive aids. • Reinstruct in steps used to prepare medication.
3. Medications, sharps, and/or medical devices are not disposed of or stored properly.	• Assess whether client chooses to store items conveniently rather than safely or has limited resources. • Reinstruction and discussion are necessary.
4. Excess or insufficient number of pills found during pill count.	• Review with client and family caregiver daily medication prescribed. • Reevaluate use of dosage reminders. • Notify health care provider.

Documentation

• Document assessment findings, instructions, and recommendations to client and family caregiver and results of return demonstrations.

Reporting

• Report to health care provider any unsafe situation found within the home.

Special Considerations

Teaching

• Instruct clients in care of linens. Instruct the client or family caregiver to avoid agitating the soiled linens and to handle them as little as possible (CDC, 2019).

• If linens are contaminated with microorganisms, they should be decontaminated by washing with soap/detergent and hot water. Commercial washers may reach a temperature of 160°F; normal washing cycles using laundry chemicals suitable for lower temperatures in the home are usually adequate to clean linens (CDC, 2019).

Pediatrics

• It is vital to keep medications and other equipment such as cleaning products out of the reach of children (Hockenberry et al., 2022).
• All medicines and cleaning products should have child safety caps (Hockenberry et al., 2022).
• If teaching self-management skills, include adult supervision and input. Never refer to medications as "candy."

✦ CLINICAL JUDGMENT AND NEXT-GENERATION NCLEX® EXAMINATION–STYLE QUESTIONS

The home health care nurse receives a referral for a 79-year-old client recently hospitalized for 1 night after a fall at home. Diagnostic tests revealed no acute injuries. Medical history includes rheumatoid arthritis and mild dementia. The client takes donepezil at night to slow the process of dementia and an NSAID as needed for joint pain. He lives in a split-level four-bedroom home with his 70-year-old sibling who provides assistance with ADLs as needed. The referral is meant to assess the client's home situation and identify any health needs.

1. After reviewing the referral history, which of the following factors should the nurse assess to determine the client's fall risk? **Select all that apply**.
   1. Degree of agitation
   2. Implications of joint pain
   3. Cognitive changes that have taken place
   4. Amount of depth perception
   5. Steadiness of gait

2. The nurse observes how the client and caregiver organize the client's medications. Which assessment finding requires the nurse to intervene?
   1. Pill organizer has medications inserted based on the time of day to be taken.
   2. Medication bottles are labeled with pharmacy warning stickers.
   3. Client demonstrates the ability to open medication bottles without difficulty.
   4. Medications are stored in the kitchen and in the client's bathroom.

3. The nurse conducts a home assessment. Which finding will the nurse discuss with the client and caregiver?
   1. Handrails are located on the staircase to upper level of home.
   2. Lights are present over the sink, stove, and kitchen table.
   3. Decorative throw rugs are placed throughout the home.
   4. Phone with emergency numbers is within reach on a nightstand.

4. When the nurse visits the client again 2 weeks later, it is reported that several doses of medication have been missed recently. Which caregiver characteristic is **most** important for the nurse to assess to determine the caregiver's ability to assist the client with taking medication?
   1. Health literacy level
   2. Functional ability
   3. Transportation accessibility
   4. Financial means to pay for medication

5. At a subsequent visit, the caregiver reports that it is becoming more difficult to communicate well with the client when it is time to take medication.

Complete the following sentence by selecting from the list of options below.

The nurse will teach the caregiver to **1 [Select]** and **2 [Select]** to enhance communication.

Options for 1	Options for 2
Avoid nonverbal gestures	Speak quickly
Talk very loudly	Repeat phrases if necessary
Stand or sit in front of the client	Place the client in a nursing home
Give medications without talking	Only smile infrequently

Visit the Evolve site for Answers to Clinical Judgment and Next-Generation NCLEX® Examination–Style Questions.

REFERENCES

Agency for Healthcare Research and Quality (AHRQ): *Teach-back: intervention,* 2023. https://www.ahrq.gov/patient-safety/reports/engage/interventions/teach-back.html.

Alzheimer's Association: *Alzheimer's and dementia safety and injury prevention,* 2022a. https://www.alz.org/professionals/public-health/core-areas/safety-and-injury-prevention. Accessed November 6, 2023.

Alzheimer's Association: *Medical tests,* 2022b. https://www.alz.org/alzheimers-dementia/diagnosis/medical_tests. Accessed November 6, 2023.

Alzheimer's Association: *Wandering,* 2022c. https://alz.org/help-support/caregiving/stages-behaviors/wandering. Accessed November 6, 2023.

Alzheimers.gov: *Tips for caregivers and families of people with dementia,* n.d. https://www.alzheimers.gov/life-with-dementia/tips-caregivers. Accessed August 5, 2023.

American Diabetes Association (ADA): *Insulin storage and syringe safety,* 2023. https://www.diabetes.org/healthy-living/medication-treatments/insulin-other-injectables/insulin-storage-and-syringe-safety. Accessed August 5, 2023.

American Occupational Therapy Association (AOTA): *Rebuilding together: safe at home checklist,* n.d. https://www.aota.org/-/media/corporate/files/practice/aging/rebuilding-together/rt-aging-in-place-safe-at-home-checklist.pdf. Accessed November 6, 2023.

Appeadu MK, Bordini B: *Falls and fall prevention in the elderly,* StatPearls, updated February 20, 2023. https://www.ncbi.nlm.nih.gov/books/NBK560761/.

Asai T, et al: The association between fear of falling and occurrence of falls: a one-year cohort study, *BMC Geriatrics* 22:393, 2022.

Boynton T, et al: *The bedside mobility assessment tool 2.0,* The American Nurse, 2020 https://www.americannurse.com/the-bedside-mobility-assessment-tool-2-0/. Accessed July 12, 2023.

Campani D, et al: Home and environmental hazards modification for fall prevention among the elderly, *Public Health Nurs* 38(3):493–501, 2021.

Centers for Disease Control and Prevention (CDC): *Laundry: washing infected material,* 2019, https://www.cdc.gov/mrsa/community/environment/laundry.html. Accessed November 6, 2023.

Centers for Disease Control and Prevention (CDC): *Four steps to food safety,* 2022. https://www.cdc.gov/foodsafety/. Accessed November 24, 2023.

Centers for Disease Control and Prevention (CDC): *Fast facts: firearm violence protection,* 2022. https://www.cdc.gov/violenceprevention/firearms/fastfact.html. Accessed August 3, 2023.

Centers for Disease Control and Prevention (CDC): *What is health literacy?* 2023. https://www.cdc.gov/healthliteracy/learn/index.html.

Cleveland Clinic: *Caregiver burnout,* 2023. https://my.clevelandclinic.org/health/diseases/9225-caregiver-burnout. Accessed November 6, 2023.

Donohue K, et al: Fall prevention among veterans in a skilled nursing facility, *J Am Geriatr Soc* 69(Suppl 1):S11, 2021.

Frith KH, et al: A longitudinal fall prevention study for older adults, *J Nurse Pract* 15:295–300, 2019.

Gately ME, et al: Factors influencing barriers and facilitators to in-home video telehealth for dementia management, *Clin Gerontol* 45(4):1020–1033, 2022.

Gosse PJ, et al: Virtual care for patients with Alzheimer disease and related dementias during the COVID-19 era and beyond, *CMAJ* 193:E371–E377, 2021.

Hockenberry MJ, et al: *Wong's essentials of pediatric nursing,* ed 11, St. Louis, 2022, Elsevier.

Hoffman G, et al: Caregivers' view of older adult fall risk and prevention during hospital to home transitions, *Appl Nurs Res* 47:10–15, 2019.

King EC, et al: Assisting frail seniors with toileting in a home bathroom: approaches used by home care providers, *J Appl Gerontol* 38(5):717–749, 2019.

Lach H: Try This: *Best practices in nursing care to older adults with dementia: home safety inventory for older adults with dementia, D12,* Revised 2019. https://hign.org/consultgeri/try-this-series/home-safety-inventory-older-adults-dementia. Accessed November 6, 2023.

Matz M: *Patient handling and mobility assessments,* ed 2, 2019, The Facility Guidelines Institute. https://www.fgiguidelines.org/wp-content/uploads/2019/10/FGI-Patient-Handling-and-Mobility-Assessments_191008.pdf. November 6, 2023.

Medline Plus: *Storing your medicines,* 2022, U.S. National Library of Medicine. https://medlineplus.gov/ency/patientinstructions/000534.htm. Accessed August 3, 2023.

Meiner SE: Safety. In Meiner SE, editor: *Gerontologic nursing,* ed 6, St. Louis, 2019, Mosby.

Miller K: Gun ownership and older adults—when is it time to take action? *Todays Geriatr Med* 12(3):10–13, 2019.

National Center for Healthy Housing (NCHH): *United States 2020 healthy housing fact sheet,* 2021. https://nchh.org/resource-library/fact-sheet_state-healthy-housing_usa.pdf. Accessed November 6, 2023.

National Center for Healthy Housing (NCHH): *State of healthy housing,* 2022. https://nchh.org/. Accessed November 6, 2023.

National Fire Protection Association (NFPA): *Smoke alarms,* 2022a. https://www.nfpa.org/Public-Education/Staying-safe/Safety-equipment/Smoke-alarms. Accessed November 6, 2023.

National Fire Protection Association (NFPA): *Top fire causes,* 2022b. https://www.nfpa.org/Public-Education/Fire-causes-and-risks/Top-fire-causes. Accessed November 6, 2023.

National Fire Protection Association (NFPA): *Public education: carbon monoxide alarms,* 2022c. https://www.nfpa.org/Public-Education/Staying-safe/Safety-equipment/Carbon-monoxide. Accessed November 6, 2023.

National Institute on Aging (NIA): *Taking medications safely as you age,* 2022. https://www.nia.nih.gov/health/taking-medicines-safely-you-age. Accessed August 3, 2023.

National Rifle Association (NRA): *NRA gun safety rules,* 2023. https://gunsafetyrules.nra.org/. Accessed November 6, 2023

Nolan P, et al: A description of novel uses of hip protectors in an elderly hip fracture population: a technical report, *Cureus* 14(1):e21028, 2022.

Office of Disease Prevention and Health Promotion: *Injury prevention. Healthy People 2030,* n.d., U.S. Department of Health and Human Services. https://health.gov/healthypeople/objectives-and-data/browse-objectives/injury-prevention. Accessed November 6, 2023.

Piau A, et al: When will my patient fall? Sensor-based in-home walking speed identifies future falls in older adults, *J Gerontol* 75(5)968–973, 2020.

Ritchey KC, et al: "Falls". In Gonzales-Fernandez M, Schaaf S, editors: *Handbook of physical medicine and rehabilitation,* New York, 2022, Springer Publishing Co., p 399.

Schulz R, et al: Family caregiving for older adults, *Annu Rev Psychol* 71:635–659, 2020.

Shaw CA, et al: Effects of a video-based intervention on caregiver confidence for managing dementia care challenges: findings from the FamTechCare clinical trial, *Clin Gerontol* 43(5):508–517, 2020.

Shetty S, et al: Empowering the visually impaired by customized Braille prescription and thus reducing medication errors, *Indian J Ophthalmol* 69:1388–1390, 2021.

Soh SL, et al: Falls efficacy: extending the understanding of self-efficacy in older adults towards managing falls. *J Fragil Sarcop Falls* 6(3):131, 2021.

Steele D: *Keltner's psychiatric nursing,* ed 9, St. Louis, 2023, Elsevier.

The Joint Commission (TJC): *Home care national patient safety goals,* 2023. https://www.jointcommission.org/standards/national-patient-safety-goals/home-care-national-patient-safety-goals/.

Touhy TA, Jett KF: *Ebersole and Hess' gerontological nursing & health aging,* ed 6, St. Louis, 2022, Elsevier.

USA Water Quality: *What temperature should a hot water heater be set at?* 2023. https://www.usawaterquality.org/temperature-should-hot-water-heater-be-set/. Accessed August 3, 2023.

U.S. Consumer Product Safety Commission (CPSC): *CPCS warns consumers to be cautions when using space heaters, furnaces, and fireplaces this winter,* 2023. https://www.cpsc.gov/Newsroom/News-Releases/2023/CPSC-Warns-Consumers-to-be-Cautious-When-Using-Space-Heaters-Furnaces-and-Fireplaces-This-Winter. Accessed August 3, 2023.

U.S. Fire Administration: *Smoking fire safety,* 2023. https://www.usawaterquality.org/temperature-should-hot-water-heater-be-set/https://www.usfa.fema.gov/prevention/home-fires/at-risk-audiences/smoking/. Accessed August 3, 2023.

U.S. Food and Drug Administration (FDA): *Drug disposal: FDAs flush list for certain medicines,* 2020. https://www.fda.gov/drugs/disposal-unused-medicines-what-you-should-know/drug-disposal-flush-potentially-dangerous-medicine#FlushList. Accessed August 3, 2023.

Zaninotto P, et al. Polypharmacy is a risk factor for hospital admission due to a fall: evidence from the English Longitudinal Study of Ageing, *BMC Public Health* 20:1804, 2020. https://doi.org/10.1186/s12889-020-09920-x.

SKILLS AND PROCEDURES

Skill 42.1 **Teaching Clients to Measure Body Temperature, p. 1224**

Skill 42.2 **Teaching Blood Pressure and Pulse Measurement, p. 1227**

Skill 42.3 **Teaching Intermittent Self-Catheterization, p. 1232**

Skill 42.4 **Using Home Oxygen Equipment, p. 1236**

Skill 42.5 **Teaching Home Tracheostomy Care and Suctioning, p. 1243**

Skill 42.6 **Teaching Medication Self-Administration, p. 1248**

Skill 42.7 **Managing Feeding Tubes in the Home, p. 1253**

Skill 42.8 **Managing Parenteral Nutrition in the Home, p. 1257**

OBJECTIVES

Mastery of content in this chapter will enable you to:
- Identify factors that influence clients' and family caregivers' abilities to learn and care for clients at home.
- Discuss the collaborative nature of home care teaching with the client and/or family caregiver.
- Assess for safety factors that may impair or prohibit a client's ability to perform skills in the home setting.
- Discuss situations that require a client and/or family caregiver to learn skills that support health maintenance.
- Choose evidence-based teaching strategies to use in the home setting.
- Evaluate evidence-based learning strategies that support clients' ability to care for themselves in the home.
- Discuss how to evaluate clients' and family caregivers' ability to perform self-care skills in the home.

MEDIA RESOURCES

- http://evolve.elsevier.com/Perry/skills
- Review Questions
- Audio Glossary
- Answers to Clinical Judgment and Next-Generation NCLEX® Examination–Style Questions
- Skills Performance Checklists
- Printable Key Points

PURPOSE

Many clients recover from or are treated for illnesses in their homes. In these situations, clients assume greater responsibility for managing their own care and are supported by home care nurses and family caregivers. Home care nurses provide health education and resources by collaborating with a client or family caregiver to address the client's health needs, preferences, and values and incorporating their strengths, skills, and capacity (Nies & McEwen, 2019).

PRACTICE STANDARDS

- American Nurses Association (ANA), 2020: Nursing: Scope and Standards of Practice—Teaching home care
- The Joint Commission (TJC), 2023: National Patient Safety Goals—Home Care

SUPPLEMENTAL STANDARDS

- Centers for Disease Control and Prevention (CDC), 2020: Medication Safety Program
- Healthcare Infection Control Practices Advisory Committee (HICPAC), 2019: Guidelines for Prevention of Catheter-Associated Urinary Tract Infections

PRINCIPLES FOR PRACTICE

- Home care nurses thoroughly assess factors that affect a client's and family caregiver's abilities and willingness to manage self-care. Determine what the client and family caregiver want to know, how they learn, and what motivates them to learn new information (ANA, 2020).
- Client teaching is an essential part of nursing practice. Information needs to be relevant, current, and clearly presented for the client and family caregivers to learn skills in the home (Nies & McEwen, 2019).
- Home care nurses creatively adapt teaching strategies to meet each client's unique physical, psychosocial, and cultural needs (Lay et al., 2019; Okwose et al., 2020).
- For collaboration to be successful, home care nurses identify who is involved in the client's care and establish mutual trust and respect through open and honest communication

(Nies & McEwen, 2019). Collaboration should begin prior to the client leaving the health care agency.

- Consider principles of diversity when caring for clients in their homes. Respect each individual's religious and cultural background and beliefs.
- Health education resources for clients and research initiatives for health care providers are available as part of the Research Institute for Home Care (2023) website. Best-practice intervention packages use a variety of media sources such as webinars, podcasts, and blogs to improve care delivery and outcomes to meet different clients' and family caregivers' learning needs (Research Institute for Home Care, 2023).

PERSON-CENTERED CARE

- Engage the client and/or family caregiver(s) as participants in care (Lay et al., 2019).
- Clients must understand how to manage their health and illnesses, take discharge medications correctly and safely, and perform related care at home. In home care, nurses help clients and family caregivers make well-informed decisions about their health practices (Ruel, 2021).
- Respectful communication includes addressing a client in an appropriate manner and using acceptable body language (Touhy & Jett, 2022).
- Determine the client's or family caregiver's preferred method of learning, such as written, verbal, or demonstration. Consider the latest technologies such as smartphones for text messaging, mHealth applications, and web-based on-demand education with other options such as video conferencing or face-to-face sessions (Doorenbos et al., 2020).
- Reinforce verbal instructions with printed, client education information in preferred reading level language, and use other alternative materials such as pictures or illustrations when possible. Evaluate the effectiveness of teaching by using varied methods such as asking questions about the content or return demonstration using technology such as smartphone applications (Doorenbos et al., 2020).

EVIDENCE-BASED PRACTICE

Health Education

The nurse's role in client health education includes errorless teaching and learning (ETL). ETL refers to evidence-based teaching strategies such as content chunking, verbal and written cues, images, and repetition of content that can prevent clients from making errors in their care (Patiag et al., 2020). As the client transitions to home care, the home care nurse collaborates with the interprofessional team, client, and family caregivers to promote effective education for self-management of the client's disease(s).

- A trusting relationship between the nurse and client and family caregiver is essential because the nurse may be the only health care provider in the home (ANA, 2020). The nurse focuses on trust and inclusion as an essential first step in building a client-nurse relationship (Nies & McEwen, 2019).
- Self-management empowers a client or family caregiver to manage their disease to sustain the highest quality of life (Hermanns et al., 2020).
- Health literacy and eHealth are important principles of evidence-based teaching. Clients are empowered to self-manage their disease(s) when using smart device applications for aspects of their care such as medication adherence (Mikulski et al., 2022; Tabi et al., 2019).

- The home care nurse identifies factors in the home that can affect the client's and family caregiver's learning. Environmental factors such as Internet access, lighting, heating, and noise may affect the ability of the nurse to teach and the client and family caregiver to learn (Bastable & Gonzalez, 2019). Other readiness factors can include the client's and family caregiver's physical readiness, such as the client's health status, complexity of the skills, and emotional readiness (Kitchie, 2019; Qiao et al., 2020).
- Recognizing the multiple roles clients and family caregivers may have in their home setting is part of the home care nurse's role. Assess for alterations in family coping that may impact the effectiveness of teaching (Imperial-Perez & Heilemann, 2019).
- eHealth refers to electronic and digital processes used to improve health such as texting health reminders and using health applications with smart devices (Doorenbos et al., 2020).
- Clients and family caregivers have different learning styles. Incorporate varied teaching methods including eHealth processes (Doorenbos et al., 2020).
- Use of pictorial medication cards with plain language improves clients' and family caregiver's understanding of medications. Pictures of medications may reduce the chance of the client mistakenly taking the wrong medication (Patiag et al., 2020).
- Smart phone applications for client education support the teaching strategies of chunking, repetition, and cues for self-management of medications (Mikulski et al., 2022) and self-management of chronic diseases (Hermanns et al., 2020).
- Use Teach-Back and ask clients and family caregivers to explain, in their own words, what has been learned. When the client or family caregiver cannot recall or misunderstands, the nurse can reexplain or demonstrate the content (Agency for Healthcare Research and Quality [AHRQ], 2023).
- During Teach-Back, ask nonthreatening questions such as, "I want to be sure you know how to dispose of your needles and medical waste correctly in your home. Can you tell me what container you will use to throw out your needles? Which of your medical products and waste need to go in special medical waste containers in your home?" (Prochnow et al., 2019).

SAFETY GUIDELINES

- Assess if a client in the home setting is able to safely perform a skill. If the client cannot execute a skill independently, identify a family caregiver who will provide it safely in the home setting.
- Assess and determine if the client has home medical equipment and knows how to use it properly for safe and successful self-care management.
- Include teaching interventions for other people in the household who positively or negatively influence the client's self-care.
- Explain to the client and family caregiver(s) that individuals who are ill can struggle with understanding, remembering, and using health education information regardless of their previous health literacy level (Network of the National Library of Medicine [NNLM], n.d.).
- Informal cues of potentially low literacy in clients and/or family caregivers include misreading prescription labels and not following a health care provider's directions (Office of Disease Prevention and Health Promotion [ODPHP], 2020).
- Provide an opportunity for client and/or family caregiver to demonstrate skill.
- Assess the environment and teach appropriate disposal of client care medical products. For example, after clients use needles and other sharps, place the items in sharps disposal containers. Containers are to be placed at a height that is not accessible to children and pets.

✦ SKILL 42.1   Teaching Clients to Measure Body Temperature

An elevation in body temperature may be an early warning sign of serious health problems. Clients susceptible to temperature alterations (e.g., immunosuppressed clients) or their family caregivers need to know how to measure temperature correctly so that clients can seek medical attention earlier. Parents need to know how to measure their children's temperature because children can develop high fevers quickly; older adults or their family caregivers need to know the techniques for temperature measurement because older adults have impaired temperature-control mechanisms. Teach clients and family caregivers the skills of measuring body temperature and techniques to lower temperature when a fever occurs at home.

A variety of body temperature thermometers are currently available, including disposable single-use, electronic digital, temporal artery, and tympanic thermometers. The Environmental Protection Agency (EPA, 2023) recommends the use of nonmercury thermometers, and most states have banned the sale of mercury fever thermometers. If a mercury thermometer breaks or is not disposed of properly, the mercury vapor gets into the air, posing a major health risk in the home and community (see Box 42.1) (EPA, 2023). Educate clients about the environmental hazards associated with mercury in the home and encourage them to purchase mercury-free thermometers.

Help a client choose the most appropriate thermometer to use in the home on the basis of their normal dexterity, vision, and financial resources. For example, a client with visual impairment from glaucoma or retinopathy is able to read a thermometer with a large digital display more easily. The need for an oral, rectal, or axillary temperature depends on the client's age and health status (see Chapter 5).

Delegation

The skill of teaching clients to measure body temperature cannot be delegated to assistive personnel (AP). Instruct the AP to:

- Inform the nurse of client or family caregiver concerns about measuring body temperature

Interprofessional Collaboration

- Parameters to report abnormal body temperature are decided upon by the health care provider and nurse.

Equipment

- Thermometer
- Disposable probe cover (if needed)
- Water-soluble lubricant (for rectal measurements)
- Paper and pencil or pen or computer if frequent measurements are to be taken
- Disposable clean gloves (for rectal temperature taken by a family caregiver)

BOX 42.1

Steps to Take in the Event of a Thermometer Mercury Spill

- If possible, close the room off from the rest of the house and increase ventilation in the affected room by opening windows or turning on a fan.
- Put on rubber, nitrile, or latex gloves. Do not touch mercury. Do not allow children to help clean up the spill. Remove all pets from the area.
- Pick up glass pieces, place them in a folded paper towel, and place glass and towel into plastic zipper bag.
- Use a squeegee or cardboard to gather mercury beads. Use an eyedropper to collect or draw up visible mercury beads. Slowly and carefully squeeze mercury onto a damp paper towel. Place the paper towel in a plastic zipper bag and secure. Then put shaving cream on a small brush and "dot" the area or press duct tape in area to pick up smaller beads.
- Place mercury, material used to pick up mercury, and broken glass in a plastic zipper bag. Triple bag the contaminated objects (place in a total of three sealed bags).
- Place gloves, mercury, and all other waste into a trash bag. Secure and label the bag.
- Call local health department to determine where to dispose of mercury safely.
- If possible, keep windows open and room well ventilated for at least 24 hours after cleanup.
- Instruct client not to use a vacuum cleaner, a broom, or household cleaners when cleaning up mercury spill. Also instruct client not to put mercury down the drain or place contaminated clothing into the washing machine.

Data from Environmental Protection Agency: What to do if a mercury thermometer breaks, 2023. https://www.epa.gov/mercury/what-do-if-mercury-thermometer-breaks. Accessed October 26, 2023.

STEP	RATIONALE

ASSESSMENT

1. Identify client using at least two identifiers during first visit according to agency policy. Confirmation of the address also occurs in the home setting and can be used as one of the two identifiers. Facial recognition can be used as one of the two identifiers for ongoing visits (TJC, 2023).

Ensures client safety. Complies with The Joint Commission standards and improves client safety (TJC, 2023).

2. Assess client's electronic health record (EHR) including health care provider's orders and nurses' notes. Note previous teaching sessions (if any) about body temperature measurement and client's/family caregiver's response to teaching.

Identifies focus for instruction and potential difficulty with teaching how to measure body temperature.

3. Assess client's/family caregiver's health literacy.

Determines degree to which individuals have the ability to find, understand, and use information and services to make informed health-related decisions and actions for themselves and others (CDC, 2023).

STEP	RATIONALE
4. Assess client's/family caregiver's ability to manipulate and read thermometer. Have client put on eyeglasses if necessary.	Physical restrictions in handling or reading thermometer prevent client from being able to read thermometer and often require teaching the family caregiver instead of the client.
5. Assess client's/family caregiver's knowledge of normal temperature range for client, symptoms of fever and hypothermia, and client's risk for body temperature alterations.	Identifies client's/family caregiver's ability to recognize alterations in body temperature and to initiate preventive health measures.
6. Assess client's/family caregiver's ability to determine appropriate type of thermometer to be used in varying situations (see Chapter 5).	Determines knowledge of age-related or medical conditions that determine selection of thermometer.
7. Assess client's/family caregiver's learning readiness and ability to concentrate; consider presence of pain, nausea, or fatigue and client's interest in instruction.	Presence of significant illness, frailty, or confusion affects client's ability to attend to teaching plan. Indicates need to rely on family caregiver for learning and implementation (if available) on short- or long-term basis.
8. Assess client's/family caregiver's goals or preferences for how skill is to be performed or what is expected.	Allows care to be individualized for client.
9. Assess knowledge and experience of client's/family caregiver's skill to be performed and feelings about procedure.	Reveals need for client/family caregiver instruction or support.

PLANNING

1. Expected outcomes following completion of procedure: • Client/family caregiver is able to correctly measure body temperature.	Indicates that skills have been learned.
2. Select setting in home where client is most likely to measure temperature and is a good location for teaching session: a. Select room that is well lit with comfortable seating.	Allows care to be individualized to client. Improves likelihood of client and family caregiver being attentive to instruction. Lighting of room improves visualization of skill. Teaching is more effective when the environment is conducive to learning.
b. Provide privacy and prepare and organize equipment.	Ensures an organized procedure for teaching body temperature measurement. Minimizes embarrassment. Helps client relax.
c. Be sure that client is close and can see nurse clearly.	Visualization of the nurse's techniques and the actual thermometer reading requires proximity to the nurse.
d. Control sources of noise and distractions (ask if children can be taken to another room; pets taken outside; audio noises turned off).	Room environment needs to minimize existing sensory alterations. Comfortable environment free of distractions promotes client's attention.
3. Discuss with client/family caregiver normal temperature ranges for client and demonstrate how to measure body temperature.	Promotes client cooperation. Clients are often curious about their temperatures and should be cautioned against prematurely removing thermometer to read.

IMPLEMENTATION

1. Demonstrate steps of thermometer preparation, insertion, and reading. Provide rationale for steps to client/family caregiver.	Providing demonstration to clients first is part of teach-back (Cutilli, 2020).
a. Instruct client to take oral temperature 20 to 30 minutes after smoking or ingesting hot or cold liquids or foods and to wait at least an hour after hot bath or vigorous exercise. Explain indications for selecting temperature site other than oral.	Waiting at least 20 minutes after drinking hot or cold liquids or foods improves accuracy of temperature reading (United States National Library of Medicine [USNLM], 2023b).
b. Perform hand hygiene (apply gloves if needed). Instruct family caregiver to wear clean, disposable gloves if in contact with body fluids.	Reduces transmission of microorganisms. Client and family caregiver must be knowledgeable about infection-prevention techniques.
c. Teach client/family caregiver proper way to position client for temperature measurement (see Chapter 5).	Improves accuracy of readings.
d. Demonstrate temperature measurement technique and have client/family caregiver perform each step with guidance. Do not rush the client.	Allows for correction of errors in technique as they occur and for discussion of potential consequences of errors.
e. Explain any special precautions in using thermometers: oral thermometer must be placed in sublingual pocket; rectal thermometers must be lubricated with water-soluble lubricant; use rectal thermometer only for measuring rectal temperatures; never force rectal thermometer into rectum.	Ensures accurate reading and avoidance of injury to client.

STEP	RATIONALE
f. Discuss typical time frame needed for each type of temperature to register (based on thermometer type) and how to take reading.	Ensures accurate reading.
g. Teach proper method for removing, cleaning, and storing thermometer (when applicable) and select suitable storage location.	Prevents transmission of infection. Thermometer is stored properly so that it does not break or become inaccurate when not in use.
h. Remove and dispose of gloves in appropriate receptacle and perform hand hygiene.	Reduces transmission of microorganisms.
2. Discuss common symptoms of fever: warm, dry, flushed skin; feeling warm; chills; piloerection; malaise; and restlessness.	Client/family caregiver needs to recognize onset of fever in self or family member for early detection and intervention.
3. Discuss common signs and symptoms of hypothermia: cool skin, uncontrolled shivering, loss of memory, and signs of poor judgment. Explain that people with inadequate home heating, older adults, or those unaware of potential dangers of cold conditions are at risk.	Client/family caregiver needs to recognize onset of hypothermia in self or family member for early detection and intervention (Touhy & Jett, 2022).

Clinical Judgment *Teach client to take temperature after chills/shivering subsides to obtain an accurate temperature. However, an axillary temperature can give needed information regarding temperature even when chills or shivering is present.*

STEP	RATIONALE
4. Discuss importance of notifying health care provider when temperature elevations occur. Collaborate with health care provider on the range of acceptable temperature readings for the specific client and when notification should be done. Review common therapies for temperature reduction that are safe to perform at home, including using antipyretics; exposing skin to air; reducing room temperature; increasing air circulation; applying cool, moist compresses to skin (e.g., forehead); and drinking fluids (Touhy & Jett, 2022).	Treating fever enhances client comfort (Hockenberry et al., 2024).
5. Provide set of written guidelines for client and family caregiver's reference at appropriate level of health literacy.	Recognizes degree to which individuals have the ability to find, understand, and use information and services to make informed health-related decisions and actions for themselves and others (CDC, 2023).
6. Give client/family caregiver paper or digital logbook to time and record temperature if frequent monitoring is required. Instruct client to use written record to report temperatures to health care provider.	Keeping organized record of temperatures helps client validate and report temperature fluctuations to health care provider.
7. Help client assume comfortable, safe position.	Restores comfort and sense of well-being.
8. Remove gloves if worn and dispose in appropriate receptacle. Perform hand hygiene.	Reduces transmission of microorganisms.

EVALUATION

1. Have client/family caregiver independently demonstrate technique for temperature measurement, including body placement and ability to read thermometer three separate times.	When psychomotor skill is performed with confidence and correctly, it demonstrates mastery of skill.
2. Ask client/family caregiver to identify normal temperature range and influence of smoking and hot and cold liquids or foods on oral readings; discuss safety implications for temperature measurement.	Measures cognitive learning and confirms understanding of information.
3. Have client/family caregiver describe common signs and symptoms of fever and hypothermia and methods for control.	Measures cognitive learning.
4. Watch client/family caregiver clean and store equipment.	Proper cleaning prevents bacterial growth, and proper storage preserves accuracy of thermometer.
5. Watch client record temperature values and times in log. Review client's log periodically to ensure that temperatures are being recorded correctly.	Health care providers make changes in client care based on information provided by client. To ensure that changes are made appropriately, client needs to record accurate information.
6. Use Teach-Back: "I want to be sure I explained the importance of measuring your temperature. Explain in your own words why it is important to know how to take your own temperature." Revise your instruction now or develop a plan for revised client/family caregiver teaching if client/family caregiver is not able to teach back correctly.	Teach-back is a technique for health care providers to ensure that they have explained medical information clearly so that clients and their families understand what is communicated to them (Agency for Healthcare Research and Quality [AHRQ], 2023).

STEP	RATIONALE

Unexpected Outcomes

1. Client/family caregiver is unable to measure temperature, clean and store thermometer correctly, or verbalize knowledge about fever and temperature measurement.

2. Client reports breaking mercury glass thermometer.

Related Interventions

- Ask client/family caregiver to describe difficulties experienced while performing temperature measurement.
- Use a different teaching strategy.
- Plan for client to perform another return demonstration during next scheduled home care visit or plan to teach family caregiver.
- Teach client steps to dispose of thermometer safely (Box 42.1).

Documentation

- Document client's temperature and information taught and client's and family caregiver's return demonstration.

Hand-Off Reporting

- Report location of session, who participated, type of thermometer used, content discussed, client's and/or family caregiver's response to procedures, and evaluation of client learning.
- Report to health care provider any high and low temperatures.

Special Considerations

Client Education

- Teach client or family caregiver to never force thermometer into rectum or use rectal thermometer after rectal surgery, when the client has a rectal disorder such as a tumor or severe hemorrhoids, when the client has a low platelet count, or when it is difficult to position client for proper thermometer placement.
- Use caution in recommending aspirin or any other over-the-counter (OTC) drug or antipyretic medicine in clients whose conditions contraindicate their use (e.g., gastric ulcer, bleeding tendencies, allergic reactions, medication interactions, liver or kidney dysfunction). Encourage client to contact health care provider before using OTC antipyretics.
- Always leave a phone number and instructions about how to reach home care nurse if needed.

Pediatrics

- Stage of growth and development of child will determine site of measurement and type of equipment used (see Chapter 5).
- Different types of thermometers are available for use with children (e.g., temporal artery, tympanic). Reliability of these different thermometers varies; ensure that parents know how to use the equipment correctly and detect the signs and symptoms of a fever (Hockenberry et al., 2024).
- Teach parents that sponging is recommended for elevated hyperthermia. Ice water and alcohol are not to be used and are potentially dangerous (Hockenberry et al., 2024). Ice water or alcohol can cause shivering when placed on the skin. Shivering increases body temperature.
- Avoid aspirin in people younger than the age of 19 to prevent Reye syndrome.
- Instruct client that environmental measures can be used as a supplement to reduce fever if the child tolerates them and if they do not induce shivering. Examples of such measures include reducing room temperature and increasing room circulation (Hockenberry et al., 2024).

Older Adults

- Normal temperatures in older adults often range below 36.1°C (97°F); therefore a normal temperature range for adults sometimes reflects a fever in the older adult (Touhy & Jett, 2022).
- Altered internal temperature regulation or dehydration occurs frequently in frail, debilitated clients. Temperature measurement becomes important to prevent severe states of hypothermia or hyperthermia.
- Consider common age-related sensory changes in the older adult and direct teaching strategies to compensate for any alterations (e.g., a magnifying glass to read thermometer).

Populations With Disabilities

- Consider a multisession education model when working with clients with an intellectual disability (Taylor, 2021).

◆ SKILL 42.2 Teaching Blood Pressure and Pulse Measurement

Clients with a variety of illnesses such as cardiac, kidney, or vascular diseases are susceptible to wide variations in their blood pressure (BP) and pulse. They benefit from knowing how to assess their own BP and pulse because they are able to seek medical attention early when readings vary from their acceptable ranges. In addition, healthy people who exercise learn how their body responds to exercise and are able to determine appropriate exercise plans based on knowing what their BP and pulse are before, during, and after exercise.

Research related to home monitoring of BP has illustrated the importance of regular monitoring outside of acute care settings and health care offices so that the health care provider can treat clients with hypertension appropriately (Aungsuroch et al., 2022). If treatment is based on single readings during an office visit, health care providers do not see an accurate picture of a client's health. To gather this essential information about clients living at home, you will teach them to measure their BP and pulse regularly and report readings that are outside of their individualized normal values. For example, teach clients about factors that affect the accuracy of BP readings such as cuff placement, movement of the tubing, speaking during measurement, and position and movement of the extremity or body.

Aneroid sphygmomanometers are available to measure BP in the home (see Chapter 5). Aneroid manometers are safe, lightweight, compact, and portable. In the home, many clients choose to use commercial automatic electronic BP devices. These devices may measure pulse rate and produce a BP measurement without the need to use a stethoscope. The devices involve placing a cuff around the arm, the wrist, or a fingertip (Fig 42.1). A reading is displayed electronically for the client. Electronic BP monitors are often easier to use, but their accuracy compared with manual BP monitoring is still a focus of debate. However, home monitoring of BP is still recommended because of the increased number of BP readings that can be obtained (Lindros et al., 2019). It is essential for clients to keep a record of all of their BP readings and compare those obtained by a health care provider with those obtained with their electronic monitor to assess the accuracy of readings.

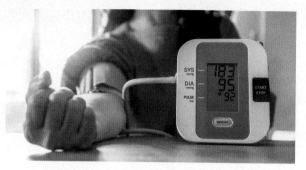

FIG. 42.1 Home blood pressure electronic monitoring device. (*From iStock.com/Chinnapong.*)

Additional factors that affect the accuracy of BP monitoring are cuff size and placement (Park et al., 2022). Have clients learn to place a cuff directly on their skin. BP cuffs that are too small tend to overestimate BP, whereas cuffs that are too large tend to underestimate it (Park et al., 2022). Not all electronic home BP monitors come with interchangeable cuff sizes, which can complicate BP monitoring at home. Help clients and family caregivers determine cuff size, calibration, and accuracy of electronic equipment before they determine which type of BP monitor to purchase.

Delegation

The skill of teaching clients to measure BP and pulse cannot be delegated to assistive personnel (AP). Instruct the AP to:
- Report concerns related to BP (e.g., episodes of suspected orthostatic hypotension) and measurements to the nurse

Interprofessional Collaboration

- Parameters to report abnormal BP results are discussed with the health care provider.

BOX 42.2

Guidelines for Blood Pressure Cuff Size

Adult Sizes
- For "small adult" size: 10 × 24 cm (4 × 9.5 inches)
- For "adult" size: 13 × 30 cm (5 × 11.8 inches)
- For "large adult" size: 16 × 38 cm (6.3 × 15 inches)
- For "adult thigh" size: 20 × 42 cm (7.8 × 16.5 inches)

Pediatric Sizes
- For newborn or premature infants, use "newborn" size: 4 × 8 cm (1.5 × 3 inches)
- For infants, use "infant" size: 6 × 12 cm (2.3 × 4.7 inches)
- For older children, use "child" size: 9 × 18 cm (3.5 × 7 inches)
- A standard adult cuff, a large adult cuff, and a thigh cuff for use in children with large arms may be needed.

Pediatric sizes data from Hockenberry MJ, et al: *Wong's nursing care of infants and children* ed 12 , St. Louis, 2024, Elsevier.

Equipment

For Blood Pressure
- Sphygmomanometer or electronic BP reading device (Fig. 42.1) with bladder and cuff: Bladder should completely encircle arm without overlapping; cuff should be secure and fit snugly (Box 42.2).
- Stethoscope (two-headed teaching stethoscope is ideal) if using sphygmomanometer. This enables the nurse teaching the skill to know if the person learning how to take a BP obtains a correct BP reading.

For Pulse
- Wristwatch or clock with a second hand

For Both Blood Pressure and Pulse
- Log

STEP	RATIONALE

ASSESSMENT

1. Identify client using at least two identifiers during first visit according to agency policy. Confirmation of the address also occurs in the home setting and can be used as one of the two identifiers. Facial recognition can be used as one of the two identifiers for ongoing visits (TJC, 2023).

Ensures client safety. Complies with The Joint Commission standards and improves client safety (TJC, 2023).

2. Assess client's electronic health record (EHR) including health care provider's orders and nurses' notes. Note previous teaching sessions (if any) about BP and pulse measurement and client's/family caregiver's response to teaching.

Identifies focus for instruction and potential difficulty with teaching how to measure BP and pulse.

3. Assess client's/family caregiver's health literacy.

Determines degree to which individuals have the ability to find, understand, and use information and services to make informed health-related decisions and actions for themselves and others (CDC, 2023).

4. Assess client's/family caregiver's psychomotor function: visual (see dial and clock) and auditory (hear Korotkoff sounds) acuity, ability to manipulate BP monitoring equipment, and ability to feel pulse.

Vision or hearing problems necessitate use of equipment that has been adapted for these conditions (e.g., larger print) (Touhy & Jett, 2022). Other deficits may require family caregiver to perform skills.

5. Assess client's/family caregiver's knowledge of normal BP and pulse range for client and the symptoms of high or low readings. (Consult with health care provider regarding normal range desired.)

Identifies client's/family caregiver's ability to know when to initiate preventive health measures and recognize alterations in BP and pulse.

6. Assess client's/family caregiver's knowledge of what BP and pulse measure, specific medical issues that affect them, and why awareness of variations is important to client's health.

Identifies client's/family caregiver's understanding of potential cause-and-effect relationships between variations in BP and pulse and health status.

STEP	RATIONALE
7. Assess client's/family caregiver's learning readiness and ability to concentrate; consider presence of pain, nausea, or fatigue and client's interest in instruction.	Presence of significant illness, frailty, or confusion affects client's ability to attend to teaching plan. Indicates need to rely on family caregiver for learning and implementation (if available) on short- or long-term basis.
8. Assess home environment for favorable place to measure BP and pulse (e.g., quiet room with comfortable place to sit). Assess the quality of home BP equipment (Balanis & Sanner, 2021).	Ensures more accurate measurement (Balanis & Sanner, 2021).
9. Assess client's/family caregiver's knowledge and experience in measuring BP and pulse.	Reveals need for client/family caregiver instruction or support.
10. Assess client's/family caregiver's goals or preferences for how skill is to be performed or what is expected.	Allows care to be individualized for client.

PLANNING

1. Expected outcomes following completion of procedure:	
• Client/family caregiver accurately measures BP and pulse.	Learning has occurred.
• Client/family caregiver explains importance of measuring BP and pulse, common causes for changes, best time for measurement, and when to communicate with health care provider to evaluate changes in treatment regimen.	Measures cognitive learning.
• Client/family caregiver demonstrate proper care of equipment.	Measures psychomotor learning.
2. Select setting in home where client is most likely to measure temperature and is a good location for teaching session:	Allows care to be individualized to client. Improves likelihood of client and family caregiver being attentive to instruction.
a. Select room that is well lit with comfortable seating.	Lighting of room improves visualization of skill. Teaching is more effective when the environment is conducive to learning.
b. Provide privacy and prepare and organize equipment.	Ensures an organized procedure for teaching body temperature measurement. Minimizes embarrassment.
c. Be sure that client is close and can see nurse clearly.	Visualization of the nurse's techniques and the actual thermometer reading requires proximity to the nurse.
d. Control sources of noise and distractions (ask if children can be taken to another room; pets taken outside; audio noises turned off).	Room environment needs to minimize existing sensory alterations. Comfortable environment free of distractions promotes client's attention.
3. Encourage client/family caregiver to perform measurements on routine schedule for long-term monitoring plan.	Daily activities and many extrinsic and intrinsic factors affect measurement fluctuations. Routine schedule allows for daily comparisons.
4. Encourage client to avoid exercise, caffeine, and smoking for 30 minutes before assessment to avoid inaccuracy. Recommend the client sit quietly without any distractions such as reading for 5 minutes before taking the measurement.	These factors cause elevations in BP and pulse (American Heart Association [AHA], 2022).
5. Prepare for client/family caregiver perform measurement in comfortable position, with arm supported at heart level and feet flat on floor and in warm and quiet environment.	Maintains client's comfort during measurement. Systolic and diastolic BP increase with crossed-leg position (AHA, 2022).

IMPLEMENTATION

1. **BP measurement:**	
a. Perform hand hygiene.	Reduces transmission of microorganisms. Client and family caregiver must be knowledgeable about infection-prevention techniques.
b. Explain importance of having client sit quietly for 5 minutes with back supported and feet on floor before measurement. If client cannot sit in this position, select position that client can maintain. Separate repeat blood pressure readings by at least 1 minute.	Reduces anxiety that can falsely elevate BP readings. It is important for client to maintain same position for each reading and separate repeat blood pressure readings by at least 1 minute to avoid false readings (AHA, 2022).
c. Discuss with client/family caregiver best sites for assessing BP. For self-measurement, brachial artery is almost always used. If client cannot sit in this position, select position that client can maintain. Explain to avoid applying cuff to arm with: • Intravenous (IV) catheter with or without fluids infusing • Arteriovenous shunt • Breast or axillary surgery • Trauma, inflammation, or disease	Most accessible sites are easiest to measure for accuracy of assessment. Appropriate site selection promotes accuracy in reading and minimizes potential for trauma. It is important for client to maintain same position for each reading. Application of pressure from inflated bladder temporarily impairs blood flow and compromises circulation in extremity that already has impaired circulation.

STEP	RATIONALE
d. Demonstrate steps for measuring BP (see Chapter 5):	Allows for correction of errors in technique as they occur and for discussion of potential consequences of errors.
(1) Use of sphygmomanometer and stethoscope:	
(a) Teach palpating artery, positioning cuff, wrapping cuff, placing stethoscope, inflating and releasing cuff, and listening for Korotkoff sounds.	Prepares client/family caregiver for measuring BP.
(b) Describe sounds of measurement and relationship to observation of gauge during BP reading. Caution client/family caregiver about level and length of time appropriate for cuff inflation.	Ensures accurate reading. Prolonged inflation of cuff impairs circulation to extremity.
(c) Teach client/family caregiver to routinely clean diaphragm and earpieces of stethoscope with rubbing alcohol or damp cloth between uses.	Stethoscopes are frequently contaminated with microorganisms. Cleaning stethoscope routinely prevents transmission of microorganisms.

Clinical Judgment *Upper arm self-measure BP monitoring devices are preferred over wrist devices (Shimbo et al., 2020). If client/family caregiver needs to use stethoscope to take BP, use double-headed teaching stethoscope to verify accuracy of reading or read BP at least 1 minute after client's attempt to verify accuracy. If client is having difficulty hearing Korotkoff sounds, ensure that the cuff has been applied appropriately and the correct size cuff is used. Also determine correct use of equipment (e.g., cuff may have been deflated too quickly or too slowly; cuff may not have been pumped high enough for systolic readings).*

STEP	RATIONALE
(2) Use of electronic BP monitor:	
(a) Teach correct placement of cuff and use of electronic equipment for proper cuff inflation (follow manufacturer's directions).	Using electronic equipment correctly helps ensure accurate BP readings. Wrist devices can increase risk of inaccurate BP readings because of client positioning (Shimbo et al., 2020).
2. Pulse measurement:	
a. Discuss with client/family caregiver best sites for assessing pulse: radial and carotid.	Radial and carotid sites are accessible and usually easiest to palpate. Constricted vessels in the family caregiver's fingers can cause a decrease in sensation, making it more difficult to feel the pulse sensation.
b. Reinforce need for the family caregiver's fingers to be warm enough to accurately assess the pulse.	

Clinical Judgment *The carotid pulse is not a preferred site to count the pulse. The carotid pulse is used only to determine if a pulse is present because of the risk of stimulating the carotid sinus.*

STEP	RATIONALE
c. Demonstrate steps for palpating pulse (see Chapter 5): position of artery on wrist or neck, how to locate artery, using fingertips for palpation, compressing artery, palpating pulse before counting, counting pulse, and calculating pulse rate (see illustration).	Allows for correction of errors in technique as they occur and for discussion of potential consequences of errors.
(1) Instruct in use of gentle pressure; reinforce not to press hard over pulse site.	Pressing too hard occludes artery.
(2) Instruct in use of watch or clock with second hand to count pulse.	Ensures correct timing of pulse.

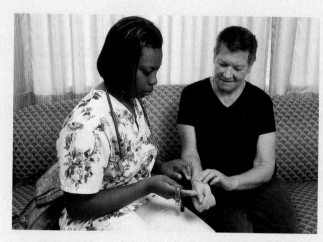

STEP 2c Nurse observing client checking radial pulse.

STEP	RATIONALE
(3) Instruct to count for full 60 seconds, starting with second hand at 12-o'clock position.	Consistent timing of procedure reduces confusion or forgetfulness about time period or starting point used for pulse measurement. Full 60-second count increases accuracy of measure.
3. Educate client/family caregiver about normal desired BP and pulse ranges, purposes for monitoring, and when to take measurements (e.g., before and after taking cardiac or antihypertensive medications; before, during, and after exercise; during any episode of chest pain).	Client/family caregiver needs to be able to determine when values are not in desired ranges and when measurements need to be taken.
4. Describe symptoms that indicate need to perform BP and/or pulse measurement.	Promotes understanding of health status alterations that need medical intervention.

Clinical Judgment *Discuss importance of notifying health care provider and withholding medications when abnormal values in BP or pulse occur (e.g., hypotension or bradycardia). Client needs to understand preventive measures to take and follow health care provider's directions if alterations develop.*

STEP	RATIONALE
5. Have client/family caregiver attempt each step of skill on you or family member.	Chunking content into smaller parts is effective for learning (Kapadia et al., 2020). You can correct any errors in technique as they occur.
6. Observe client/family caregiver demonstrate techniques to measure BP and pulse. When measuring BP, do not allow multiple repetitive BP attempts on any one limb.	After developing confidence in measuring values in others, client is ready to measure own values. Making multiple repetitive BP attempts restricts circulation and results in inaccurate measurement.
7. Teach client/family caregiver to monitor BP and pulse even if they remain within normal range.	Continuous monitoring provides important information that evaluates effectiveness of medications or other treatments.
8. Provide client/family caregiver with printed instructions with written or pictorial guide or an electronic format for demonstration of procedure if possible.	Clients and family caregivers can have different learning styles. Incorporate varied teaching methods such as digital media and images with words to improve understanding and skill (Chandar et al., 2019; Goessl et al., 2019).
9. Give client/family caregiver log to record BP and pulse and time they were taken. In addition, client documents whether or not medications that affect BP or pulse were taken. Instruct client to bring written record to follow-up appointments to report readings to health care provider.	Keeping organized record of BP and pulse readings and medications empowers client and provides accurate information to health care providers.
10. Instruct client/family caregiver in proper care of equipment (e.g., storage, cleaning, and battery care).	Improper care and storage of equipment affects accuracy of measurement.
11. Help client assume comfortable and safe position.	Restores comfort and sense of well-being.
12. Perform hand hygiene.	Reduces transmission of microorganisms.

Clinical Judgment *If in the home setting the client has blood pressure fluctuations with positional changes, instruct family caregiver to remain with client and observe client for light-headedness or dizziness when assisting client to comfortable position.*

EVALUATION

1. Observe client/family caregiver demonstrate technique for BP and/or pulse measurement on at least three different occasions and verify that client adds information to logbook correctly.	When psychomotor skill is performed with confidence and correctly, it demonstrates mastery of skill.
2. Ask client/family caregiver if readings are within desired range and when to report abnormal readings to health care provider.	Determines client's/family caregiver's ability to know when readings are within proper range and what to do when abnormal readings are obtained.
3. Ask client/family caregiver to describe reason for BP and pulse monitoring and any related medications (e.g., antihypertensives, antidysrhythmics) or treatment (e.g., diet and exercise).	Determines if client/family caregiver understands monitoring and related therapies.
4. Have client/family caregiver demonstrate proper care of equipment.	Demonstrates learning.
5. **Use Teach-Back:** "I want to be sure I explained the importance of measuring your BP. Explain to me how your medications can affect your BP readings." Revise your instruction now or develop a plan for revised client/family caregiver teaching if client/family caregiver is not able to teach back correctly.	Teach-back is a technique for health care providers to ensure that they have explained medical information clearly so that clients and their families understand what is communicated to them (AHRQ, 2023).

STEP	RATIONALE

Unexpected Outcomes

1. Client/family caregiver is unable to measure BP or pulse (e.g., inability to manipulate equipment, see numbers on equipment or clock, or hear BP sounds).

Related Interventions

- Alter teaching plan to accommodate client's problems (e.g., use other types of equipment that are easier to manipulate, see, or hear).
- Reinforce information taught and continue return demonstrations until client is able to perform skill.
- Teach skill to different family caregiver.

2. Client/family caregiver has difficulty explaining purposes of measurement or implications of therapy.

- Review and reinforce information that client/family caregiver does not understand. Repeat teach-back for content.

Documentation

- Document BP and pulse and teaching, client and family caregiver responses, and demonstration.

Hand-Off Reporting

- Report location of teaching session for BP and pulse, who participated, equipment used, content discussed, and client's and/or family caregiver's response to procedure and evaluation of client learning.
- Report abnormal readings of BP and/or pulse to health care provider.

Special Considerations

Client Education

- Educate client about risks for hypertension, hypotension, or change in pulse rate (see Chapter 5).
- Ensure that client understands health care provider's recommendations for treatment regimen, including potential side effects and interactions of any medication therapies (e.g., clients taking thyroid medications might need to withhold them when BP is above normal range or pulse is above 100 beats/min). Confirm specific guidelines for BP and pulse with health care provider; document information in home care record; and provide clear, written instructions for the client.
- Always leave a phone number and instructions about how to reach home care nurse if needed.

Pediatrics

- Readings (BP or pulse) are often inaccurate if an infant or child is anxious and uncooperative. BP is also inaccurate when the

cuff size is inappropriate. Having others divert the child's attention or taking a BP or pulse while the child is seated on the parent's lap usually helps calm the child (Hockenberry et al., 2024).
- Young children will be more likely to cooperate if allowed to touch and/or play with equipment before procedure. Consider performing the procedure first on the parent or another person significant to child. This allows the child to observe that the procedure is safe.
- Use the radial pulse in children older than 2 years. The apical pulse is more reliable for infants and young children. Use a stethoscope to obtain the apical heart rate (Hockenberry et al., 2024).

Older Adults

- Musculoskeletal changes such as arthritis or other joint conditions may impair a client's ability to position limb comfortably and/or perform fine-motor skills required to measure BP and pulse (Touhy & Jett, 2022).
- Older adults, especially those who are frail or who have lost upper-arm mass, require a smaller BP cuff.
- Home BP monitoring is not a replacement for BP monitoring by health care providers in older adults, but it can serve to provide more information to ensure the best treatment.

Populations With Disabilities

- Consider a multisession education model when working with clients with an intellectual disability (Latteck & Bruland, 2020).

♦ SKILL 42.3 **Teaching Intermittent Self-Catheterization**

Clients who cannot empty bladders may be taught intermittent self-catheterization. Self-catheterization is performed to empty the bladder at periodic intervals throughout a 24-hour day (Balhi & Arfaoui, 2021). Infections in the bladder or kidneys and damage to the kidneys sometimes result from incomplete emptying of the bladder. Clean intermittent self-catheterization (CISC) is a safe and effective way to empty the bladder. The client performs self-catheterization with clean technique, eliminating the need to wear gloves. Clients who use CISC have a variety of health problems that affect the neuromuscular control of the bladder (Balhi & Arfaoui, 2021; Sassani et al., 2019). Current practice supports CISC for use in the home to provide a means to completely empty the bladder, prevent urinary tract infections (UTIs), and, when feasible, return more quickly to normal voiding (Sassani et al., 2019). Inadequate or excessive fluid intake, poor catheterization technique

and catheter care, and traumatic catheterization can cause UTIs. Teaching proper self-catheterization technique is crucial in preventing infections (Balhi & Arfaoui, 2021).

Using CISC helps clients believe that there is more control of daily needs, which enhances quality of life. It helps some clients become continent, maintain a positive body image, and experience less anxiety and embarrassment. In addition, CISC allows clients to express sexuality and sustain satisfying relationships. However, the skill requires physical and manual dexterity, and clients must adhere to a regular schedule for it to be successful (Balhi & Arfaoui, 2021). When the client is unable to perform CISC independently, teach the family caregiver how to perform the skill. For clients with certain medical conditions (e.g., cognitive disorders), teaching the client's caregiver how to perform intermittent catheterization is recommended (Balhi & Arfaoui, 2021).

Delegation

The skill of teaching intermittent self-catheterization cannot be delegated to assistive personnel (AP). Instruct the AP to:
- Document the amount of urine on the paper or digital logbook if the client is unable
- Report to the nurse cloudy urine or changes in the color, odor, and/or amount of urine

Interprofessional Collaboration

Urology services and an advanced practice nurse can provide clinical expertise with intermittent self-catheterization.

Equipment

- Soap, water, and clean washcloth
- Mirror (optional)
- Urethral catheter (smallest size that is able to pass easily into the bladder and completely drain client's urine)
- Lubricant (e.g., water-soluble jelly) if catheter is uncoated
- Container for collection of urine (e.g., urinal)—not needed for clients emptying urine directly into toilet
- Mild soap (e.g., Ivory)
- Disposable item or container (e.g., brown paper bag, clean towel)
- Disposable clean gloves (for family caregiver)
- Logbook (optional)

STEP	RATIONALE

ASSESSMENT

1. Identify client using at least two identifiers during first visit according to agency policy. Confirmation of the address also occurs in the home setting and can be used as one of the two identifiers. Facial recognition can be used as one of the two identifiers for ongoing visits (TJC, 2023).

Ensures client safety. Complies with The Joint Commission standards and improves client safety (TJC, 2023).

2. Assess client's electronic health record (EHR) including health care provider's orders and nurses' notes. Note if any previous teaching session on CISC was performed and client's/family caregiver's response to teaching.

Identifies focus for instruction and potential difficulty with teaching how to perform CISC.

3. Assess client's/family caregiver's health literacy.

Determines degree to which individuals have the ability to find, understand, and use information and services to make informed health-related decisions and actions for themselves and others (CDC, 2023).

4. Ask client and check EHR for history of allergies.

Catheter of different material is needed if client has latex allergy.

5. Perform hand hygiene. Assess client's/family caregiver's knowledge about CISC and observe performance of CISC if client has performed previously. If family caregiver will perform CISC, have individual also perform hand hygiene and then put on clean gloves.

Reduces transmission of microorganisms. Client and family caregiver must be knowledgeable about infection-prevention techniques. Reveals need for client/family caregiver instruction and/or support.

6. Assess client's/family caregiver's ability to manipulate and handle the catheter and reach the perineum.

Physical restrictions in handling or manipulating the catheter and reaching the perineum may prevent client from being able to perform CISC and often necessitate teaching family caregiver instead of client (Balhi & Arfaoui, 2021).

7. Assess client's/family caregiver's goals or preferences for how skill is to be performed or what is expected.

Allows care to be individualized for client.

PLANNING

1. Expected outcomes following completion of procedure:
   - Client/family caregiver states signs and symptoms that indicate need for CISC.

Indicates ability to identify appropriate times to use CISC.

   - Client/family caregiver correctly demonstrates how to perform CISC and clean and store equipment.

Demonstration of skills with return demonstration is an effective method for client/family caregiver to learn (Logan, 2020).

   - Client/family caregiver verbalizes signs and symptoms of complications of CISC such as UTI, strictures, and urethral bleeding (Saadat et al., 2019).

Urinary complications such as UTI can result in clients who use CISC (Gray et al., 2019). Verbalization of signs and symptoms of complications helps clients or family caregivers identify potential problems early and seek appropriate care.

2. Help client/family caregiver select catheter that is easiest to use, causes least amount of trauma, and is most comfortable.

Different types of catheters are currently available (Balhi & Arfaoui, 2021).

3. Select setting in home that client/family caregiver will most likely use when performing CISC and is a good place for teaching session.

Allows care to be individualized to client. Improves likelihood of client being attentive to instruction.

4. Explain procedure to client/family caregiver.

Promotes cooperation.

5. Provide privacy. Organize and set up equipment needed to perform procedure.

Protects client's privacy; reduces anxiety. Ensures more efficiency when completing an assessment.

STEP	RATIONALE

IMPLEMENTATION

1. Have client/family caregiver perform appropriate hand hygiene using soap and water. If family caregiver is performing skill, instruct how to apply pair of disposable clean gloves.

2. Perform hand hygiene. Help client get into comfortable position. Some men prefer to stand, whereas others prefer to sit. Female clients often need to try different positions to decide which position is most effective and comfortable. Position client in place that has adequate lighting.

3. Teach client/family caregiver how to clean urethral meatus:

   a. *For women:* Have client spread labia with one hand. Use other hand to clean urethral opening with a washcloth containing warm soapy water, and then use a clean, moist washcloth to rinse. Have female clean in direction from urethral meatus toward rectum. If menses are present, have client/family caregiver cleanse the perineum using a different washcloth. Clean and dry before beginning inserting catheter.

   b. *For men:* If client has not been circumcised, teach him to retract foreskin to expose urethral meatus. Teach client to hold penis perpendicular to body with one hand, use other hand to clean urethral opening with a washcloth containing warm soapy water, and then use a clean moist washcloth to rinse. Have male clean in circular motion from meatus outward.

4. Teach female client/family caregiver how to insert catheter:

   a. Catheter selection often depends on client preference.

   b. Using mirror, help client locate meatus. Explain that it is just below clitoris and just above vaginal opening.

Clinical Judgment *The woman's position impacts the success of CISC. Many women find standing with one foot on the toilet the easiest position to use. Confirm the client can balance safely in this position before proceeding. Hand hygiene is performed before positioning for the self-catheterization. After cleaning the vulva area, the client takes their nondominant hand to expand the labia using the second and fourth fingers. The client's middle finger locates the urethral opening after confirming the landmarks of the clitoris and vagina. The catheter is inserted toward the umbilicus (Shaeffer, 2023).*

   c. If an uncoated catheter is selected, have client lubricate tip of catheter with water-soluble jelly by rotating tip to spread lubricant around bottom 2.5 to 5 cm (1–2 inches) of catheter. Coated catheters do not require use of separate lubrication.

   d. Place outflow end of catheter into urine collection container or let hang over toilet bowl. Slowly and gently insert tip of catheter 5 to 10 cm (2–4 inches) into meatus until urine begins to flow.

Clinical Judgment *If client feels resistance at the internal sphincter, teach her to bear down gently and slowly insert catheter (Reber, 2020).*

5. Teach male client/family caregiver how to insert catheter:

   a. Catheter selection depends on client preference and other factors such as ability to learn the skill.

   b. Lubricate tip of uncoated catheter with water-soluble jelly by rotating tip to spread lubricant around bottom 13 to 18 cm (5–7 inches) of catheter. Coated catheters do not require separate lubricant (Orlandin et al., 2020).

   c. Place outflow end of catheter into urine collection container or let hang over toilet bowl. Slowly and gently insert tip of catheter 15 to 20 cm (6–8 inches) into meatus until urine begins to flow. For uncircumcised male, retract foreskin before inserting catheter. Tell client that catheter often needs to be inserted all the way for urine to begin to flow. Pull foreskin back to normal position when catheterization is complete.

Rationale column

Reduces transmissions of microorganisms.

Reduces transmission of infection. Adequate lighting improves visualization of meatus and equipment and accuracy of insertion.

Clients using clean technique do not need to wear gloves. Family caregivers performing the procedure should wear clean gloves (Gray et al., 2019).

Retraction of labia allows for female urethral meatus to be cleaned, reducing risk for infection (Reber, 2020). Reduces transmission of infection from rectal area to meatus. An additional washcloth for menses provides mechanism to remove menstrual blood.

Ensures cleaning of meatus and reduces risk for infection (Reber, 2020).

Client preference is dependent on many factors such as expertise of nurse teaching and client comfort and handling of the catheter (Hentzen et al., 2020).

Mirror helps visualize anatomy for the client (Balhi & Arfaoui, 2021).

Lubrication reduces urethral trauma (Orlandin et al., 2020).

Appearance of urine indicates that catheter tip is in bladder.

A variety of catheters are currently available. Single-use catheters are recommended for clients at home (Saadat et al., 2019).

Lubrication reduces urethral trauma (Orlandin et al., 2020).

Male urethra is longer than female urethra. Flow of urine indicates that catheter tip is in bladder.

STEP	RATIONALE

Clinical Judgment *Men may experience some resistance when the catheter reaches the prostatic urethra or the neck of the bladder. If client feels resistance, do not pull the catheter in and out. Teach to bear down as if to void (Reber, 2020).*

6. Instruct client/family caregiver to hold catheter in place while urine flows into container or toilet.	Release of catheter during procedure often causes catheter to accidentally come out before bladder is completely emptied.
7. When urine stops, slowly remove the catheter. Pinch the catheter end closed.	Slow removal of catheter allows urine to drain. Pinch the end closed to avoid getting wet (U.S. National Library of Medicine [USNLM], 2023a).
8. Single-use catheters are discarded after self-catheterization is complete (Balhi & Mrabet, 2020).	Minimizes risk of UTIs.
9. Help client to assume comfortable position.	Restores comfort and sense of well-being.
10. Remove and dispose of gloves. Perform hand hygiene.	Reduces transmission of microorganisms. Client and family caregiver must be knowledgeable about infection-prevention techniques.
11. Give client log to record amount of urine if needed.	Some clients need to keep track of urinary output.

EVALUATION

1. Observe while client/family caregiver independently demonstrates technique for CISC.	Feedback through return demonstration of psychomotor skill is best means of evaluating learning of skill.
2. Ask client to identify plan for timing of CISC and steps to take when problems arise.	Measures client's cognitive learning and ability to problem solve.
3. Review client's logbook and watch client enter information about urine output if indicated.	Confirms that client understands record keeping and importance of tracking urine output.
4. **Use Teach-Back:** "I want to be sure I explained the steps clearly for how to open the catheter's package. Explain to me how you will open the package." Revise your instruction now or develop a plan for revised client/family caregiver teaching if client/family caregiver is not able to teach back correctly.	Teach-back is a technique for health care providers to ensure that they have explained medical information clearly so that clients and their families understand what is communicated to them (AHRQ, 2023).

Unexpected Outcomes

1. Client is unable to easily pass catheter into bladder.

2. Client reports having symptoms of UTI (e.g., intense urge to urinate, flank or abdominal pain, malaise, fever, chills).

Related Interventions

- Teach client not to force catheter into bladder.
- Tell client to go to nearest urgent care center or emergency department if bladder is full and client is unable to insert catheter.
- Consider initiating consultation with urologist.

- Inform client's health care provider of symptoms and anticipate treatment with antibiotic.

Documentation

- Document teaching, client and family caregiver responses, and demonstration.
- Document urine output in home care record and home documentation system (e.g., logbook).

Hand-Off Reporting

- Report signs and symptoms of UTIs and difficulty performing CISC to health care provider.

Special Considerations

Client Education

- Discuss with client realistic expectations to become independent with CISC. Clients may perceive that the procedure will be easy to learn and painless. Lack of client motivation is the most common reason for failure with CISC (Balhi & Mrabet, 2020).

- Always leave a phone number and instructions about how to reach home care nurse if needed.

Pediatrics

- Assessment of a child's motivation and physiological and developmental readiness is important to the success of CISC (Bradley, 2020).
- When teaching children to perform CISC, use developmentally appropriate teaching strategies. Urinary diversion requires special care (see Chapter 33).
- Concerns of children and adolescents who use CISC include leakage and being wet. They are also often concerned about what peers know. Allow children to voice concerns and help them problem solve what to do in a variety of situations.

Older Adults

- CISC is effective in older adults because it helps restore continence, decreases urinary urge and nocturia, and improves quality of life.

- Older adults may have difficulty performing CISC because of limited manual dexterity, musculoskeletal issues, and neurological issues. Individualize care for a client's needs and functional abilities (Touhy & Jett, 2022).

Populations With Disabilities

- Consider a multisession education model when working with clients with an intellectual disability (Latteck & Bruland, 2020).

◆ SKILL 42.4   Using Home Oxygen Equipment

Medical oxygen is classified by the Food and Drug Administration (FDA) as a drug; therefore a prescription from a health care provider is required for home use (Centers for Medicare and Medicaid Services, n.d.). The prescription includes the following components: drug/apparatus, dose, route of administration, and duration. The route of administration of oxygen in the home may include nasal cannula, face mask, tracheal mask, or tracheal catheter. Equipment selection needs to support as much client independence as feasible (Branson et al., 2019).

Oxygen-conserving devices (OCDs) were introduced to reduce the weight of portable oxygen systems and extend operating time by not wasting oxygen through continuous flow. There are three types of OCDs:

- *Reservoir nasal cannula:* Stores oxygen in a small chamber during exhalation for subsequent delivery during early-phase inhalation.

- *Demand pulsing oxygen-delivery systems:* Deliver a burst of oxygen at the onset of inspiration; small oxygen pulses are effective in oxygenating a client.
- *Transtracheal oxygen catheter:* Delivers oxygen directly to the trachea through a catheter placed through the anterior neck, bypassing the upper airway (Weekley & Bland, 2023). (Table 42.1).

Oxygen sources in the home include liquid oxygen systems, compressed oxygen in tanks, or oxygen concentrators (Fig. 42.2A) (Harding et al., 2020). Some oxygen tanks (e.g., compressed) are large and stationary. Portable tanks weighing more than 10 lb are not designed to be carried and deliver oxygen for about 5 hours at 2 L/min. Ambulatory tanks weigh less than 10 lb, are designed to be carried (Fig. 42.2B), and deliver oxygen for at least 4 hours at 2 L/min. Table 42.2 describes types of home oxygen therapy for adults with chronic lung disease.

TABLE 42.1

Oxygen Flow and Appropriate Uses for Oxygen-Delivery Devices

Device	Flow (L/min)	FiO$_2$ Range (%)	Uses
Nasal cannula	1–6	24–44	Clients who require low concentrations of oxygen therapy
Simple face mask	6–12	35–50	Clients who require short-term oxygen therapy with moderate FiO2 needs
Oxygen-conserving cannula	8	Up to 30–50	Clients in need of long-term home therapy
Partial and nonrebreather mask	10–15	60–90	Clients in acute respiratory failure or in emergency situations

Data from Harding M, et al: *Lewis's medical-surgical nursing: assessment and management of clinical problems*, ed 11, St Louis, 2020, Elsevier.

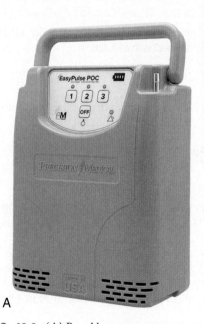
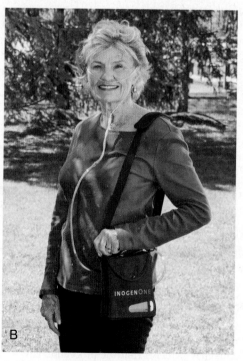

FIG. 42.2 (A) Portable oxygen concentrator for home use. (B) Ambulatory tank is small enough to be carried easily. (A, *Image courtesy Precision Medical, Inc.* B, *From Ignatavicius D, et al: Medical-surgical nursing: concepts for interprofessional collaborative care, ed 10, St Louis, 2021, Elsevier.*)

TABLE 42.2

Description of Home Oxygen Therapy for Adults With Chronic Lung Disease

Home Oxygen Therapy	Description of Oxygen Therapy
Ambulatory oxygen	Oxygen therapy during a client's exercise or activities of daily living.
Continuous oxygen	Oxygen therapy ordered for 24 h/day.
Home oxygen	Oxygen therapy occurring at the client's place of residence (e.g., home environment). Home oxygen can be additionally categorized such as ambulatory, continuous, or long-term oxygen.
Long-term oxygen	Oxygen ordered for clients diagnosed with chronic hypoxemia. Health care provider prescription for oxygen is usually for at least 15 to 18 h/day and for a long duration of time.
Nocturnal oxygen	Oxygen therapy for sleep only.
Palliative oxygen	Oxygen provided to alleviate a client's dyspnea. Frequency of the health care provider's order for oxygen may include continuous, ambulation, or nocturnal.
Short-burst oxygen	As-needed delivery of oxygen for activities such as before or after exercise. Client does not have a diagnosis of hypoxemia.

Adapted from Jacobs SS, et al: Home oxygen therapy for adults with chronic lung diseases: an official American Thoracic Society clinical practice guidelines, *Am J Respir Crit Care* 202(10):e125, 2020; Lacasse Y, et al: Home oxygen in chronic obstructive pulmonary disease, *Am J Respir Crit Care Med* 197(10):1255, 2018.

Compressed oxygen requires a regulator and flowmeter. The client receives delivery of several large oxygen tanks to the home. The size of the tank and flow rate determine how long compressed oxygen tanks will last. Liquid systems take up less space because oxygen is stored in a liquid state. Liquid oxygen is stored at or below −183°C (−297°F) and requires the use of a small ambulatory tank that is filled from a reservoir in the home (Fig. 42.3). The oxygen concentrator method extracts oxygen from room air and supplies oxygen to the client at prescribed flow rates. Oxygen concentrators deliver a lower percentage of oxygen to the flowmeter. Therefore if a client is switched to a concentrator, the flow rate usually needs to be adjusted. The client who uses a concentrator needs to have a backup system such as a portable oxygen tank in case of power failure. The oxygen provider who provides the therapy equipment will also instruct the client and family caregiver on equipment care. Regardless of the equipment used, clients are taught concepts to reduce the risk of infection from oxygen therapy. Box 42.3 presents a client and family caregiver teaching guide to reduce risk of infection.

Home oxygen equipment and supplies are designated as durable medical equipment (DME) by Medicare; a certificate of medical necessity (CMN) is required for clients who receive services from Medicare and Medicaid (CMS, n.d.). Governmental or private insurance often pays for home oxygen therapy if there is a written order from the health care provider.

Clients and their family caregivers need extensive teaching to use oxygen therapy correctly and safely. Instruct a client to have an all-purpose fire extinguisher nearby and learn how to use it and to keep the oxygen supplier's number handy. In addition, provide client education about the safe use of oxygen in the home (Box 42.4). When initiating and managing ongoing oxygen therapy, collaborate with the client, health care provider, family caregivers, DME provider, and payer.

Delegation

- The skill of teaching clients how to use home oxygen equipment cannot be delegated to assistive personnel (AP). Instruct the AP to:
- Inform the nurse of concerns regarding use or storage of oxygen therapy.

Interprofessional Collaboration

- DME home oxygen vendors provide oxygen equipment in the home.

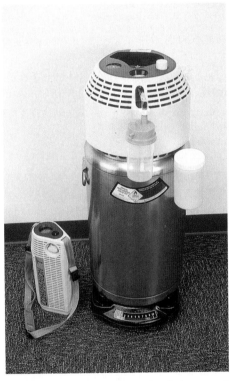

FIG. 42.3 Oxygen reservoir and ambulatory tank.

BOX 42.3

Client and Family Caregiver Teaching: Decreasing Risk for Infection

- Brush teeth or use mouthwash several times a day.
- Wash nasal cannula (prongs) with a liquid soap and thoroughly rinse once or twice a week.
- Replace nasal cannula every 2–4 weeks.
- If you have a cold, replace the cannula after your cold symptoms have passed.
- Always remove secretions that are coughed out.
- If you use an oxygen concentrator, unplug the unit, wipe down the cabinet with a damp cloth, and dry it on a daily basis.
- Change the filter per the vendor's directions.

From Harding M et al: *Lewis's medical-surgical nursing: assessment and management of clinical problems*, ed 11, St Louis, 2020, Elsevier.

Safe Home Oxygen Therapy

Fire Safety

Although oxygen is not flammable, it will burn if it comes in contact with fire; therefore:

- Use and store oxygen in a well-ventilated area.
- Do not use flammable liquids such as paint thinners, gasoline, or aerosol sprays while using oxygen.
- Do not use open flames (e.g., matches, fireplaces, stoves, space heaters, candles) when oxygen is in use.
- Do not allow smoking in the house. Post "No Smoking" signs inside and outside the house (Patient Safety Network, 2019).
- Install smoke detectors and have a fire extinguisher available in the home. Test smoke detectors twice a month.
- Help client/family caregiver plan a fire evacuation route. Have two routes out of every room and an outside meeting place.

Oxygen Storage and Handling

- Store oxygen tanks upright in carts or stands to prevent tipping or falling or place tanks flat on the floor when not in use.

- Do not store oxygen tanks in the trunk of a car.
- When transporting oxygen in a vehicle, ensure that tanks are secured properly in the passenger area with the windows opened 5 to 7.5 cm (2–3 inches) to allow adequate ventilation.

Concentrator Safety

- Plug concentrators into properly grounded outlets.
- Do not use extension cords, power strips, or multioutlet adapters with concentrators.
- Ensure that power supply or circuit meets or exceeds the amperage requirements of the concentrator.

Liquid Oxygen Safety

- Avoid direct contact with liquid oxygen because it can cause frostbite. The vapors are also extremely cold and can damage delicate tissues such as eyes.
- Do not touch connectors that are frosted or icy.
- Keep ambulatory tanks upright; do not lay them down or place on their side.

Adapted from Harding M, et al: *Lewis's medical-surgical nursing: assessment and management of clinical problems,* ed 11, St Louis, 2020, Elsevier; American Lung Association: *Oxygen therapy,* 2023. https://www.lung.org/lung-health-diseases/lung-procedures-and-tests/oxygen-therapy; and United States National Library of Medicine (USNLM): *Oxygen safety,* 2022b. https://medlineplus.gov/ency/patientinstructions/000049.htm.

Equipment

- Nasal cannula, oxygen mask (see Chapter 23), OCD or other prescribed delivery device
- Oxygen tubing

- Home oxygen-delivery system (compressed oxygen, oxygen concentrator, or liquid oxygen) with all required equipment (varies with supplier and system used)
- "No Smoking/Oxygen in Use" sign for each entrance to the home

STEP	RATIONALE
ASSESSMENT	
1. Identify client using at least two identifiers during first visit according to agency policy. Confirmation of the address also occurs in the home setting and can be used as one of the two identifiers. Facial recognition can be used as one of the two identifiers for ongoing visits (TJC, 2023).	Ensures client safety. Complies with The Joint Commission standards and improves client safety (TJC, 2023).
2. Assess client's electronic health record (EHR) including health care provider's orders and nurses' notes. Note previous teaching sessions about home oxygen therapy and client's/family caregiver's response to teaching.	Identifies focus for instruction and potential difficulty with teaching how to manage oxygen equipment in the home.
3. Determine appropriate backup systems for compressor in event of power failure (e.g., notify local emergency medical services [EMS]). Have spare oxygen tank available for emergency use.	Many municipalities require that clients who have home oxygen equipment notify EMS before putting equipment in home. In case of power outage, EMS will call home and, in some cases, home is on priority list for having power restored.
4. Assess client's/family caregiver's health literacy.	Determines degree to which individuals have the ability to find, understand, and use information and services to make informed health-related decisions and actions for themselves and others (CDC, 2023).
5. Complete a risk assessment that includes assessment of client and household member(s) smoking status and other household risks of fire, trips, and falls (Jacobs et al., 2020).	Ensures safe, continuous delivery of home oxygen.
6. Assess client's/family caregiver's knowledge and experience with home oxygen.	Reveals need for client/family caregiver instruction and/or support.
7. Assess client's/family caregiver's learning readiness and ability to concentrate; consider presence of pain, nausea, or fatigue and client's interest in instruction.	Presence of significant illness, frailty, or confusion affects client's ability to attend to teaching plan. Indicates need to rely on family caregiver for learning and implementation (if available) on short- or long-term basis.
8. Assess client's/family caregiver's goals or preferences for how skill is to be performed or what is expected.	Allows care to be individualized for client.

STEP	RATIONALE

PLANNING

1. Expected outcomes following completion of procedure:
- Client receives oxygen at prescribed rate.
- Client/family caregiver verbalizes purpose and correct use of home oxygen.
- Client/family caregiver demonstrates how to apply, regulate, and maintain oxygen system.
- Client/family caregiver states indications for calling DME supplier to replenish oxygen supply and reorder oxygen-delivery supplies.
- Client/family caregiver verbalizes safety guidelines for oxygen use.
- Client/family caregiver verbalizes emergency plan of care (Commonwealth of Massachusetts, 2023).

Oxygen system set up correctly.
Provides measurable criteria to determine level of understanding.

Indicates learning has occurred.

Client needs constant supply of oxygen at home.

Provides measure of understanding of oxygen use.

Ensures safe, continuous delivery of home oxygen.

2. Select setting in home where client is most likely to use oxygen equipment and that is conducive to a teaching session:
- **a.** Select a room that is well lit with comfortable seating.

- **b.** Be sure that client is close and can see nurse clearly.

- **c.** Control sources of noise and distractions.

- **d.** Provide privacy and prepare and organize equipment.

Practicing in same environment where skill is routinely performed facilitates comprehension and learning.
Lighting of room improves visualization of skill. Teaching is more effective when the environment is conducive to learning.
Visualization of the nurse's techniques requires proximity to the nurse.
Room environment needs to minimize existing sensory alterations. Comfortable environment free of distractions promotes client's attention.
Minimizes embarrassment.

IMPLEMENTATION

1. Teach client/family caregiver how to perform hand hygiene before handling oxygen equipment.

2. Place oxygen-delivery system in clutter-free environment that is well ventilated; away from walls, drapes, curtains, bedding, and combustible materials; and at least 2.4 m (8 feet) from heat sources.

Reduces transmission of microorganisms.

Keeps system balanced and prevents injury.

Clinical Judgment *Do not place oxygen delivery system in a closet. Keep grease, oil, and petroleum away from equipment. Turn off the equipment when not in use (American Lung Association, 2023).*

3. Demonstrate steps for preparation and maintenance of oxygen therapy:
- **a.** Compressed oxygen system:
  - **(1)** Turn cylinder valve counterclockwise two to three turns with wrench.
  - **(2)** Check cylinders by reading amount on pressure gauge.
  - **(3)** Store wrench with oxygen tank or in other safe place near the tank.
- **b.** Oxygen concentrator system:
  - **(1)** Plug concentrator into appropriate outlet.
  - **(2)** Turn on power switch. Alarm will sound for a few seconds.

- **c.** Liquid oxygen system:
  - **(1)** Check liquid system by depressing button at lower right corner and reading dial on stationary oxygen reservoir or ambulatory tank.
  - **(2)** Collaborate with DME provider to provide instruction in refilling ambulatory tank when it becomes empty.

Demonstration is reliable technique for teaching psychomotor skill and enables client to ask questions.

Turns on oxygen.

Verifies adequate oxygen supply for client use.
Storing wrench in safe place ensures that it is available whenever needed.

Provides power safely to concentrator.
Starts concentrator motor.
Alarm turns off when desired pressure inside concentrator is reached.

Verifies adequate oxygen supply for client use.

Ensures that continuous oxygen therapy is not interrupted.

Clinical Judgment *There are numerous options for home oxygen equipment available to clients. Education about the oxygen equipment and oxygen safety, including smoking cessation, fire prevention, and fall hazards, are best practice for home oxygen therapy (Jacobs et al., 2020). Discuss with client the need for backup emergency power in the event of power loss (Jacobs et al., 2020).*

STEP	RATIONALE

(3) To refill liquid oxygen tank:

(a) Wipe both filling connectors with clean, dry, lint-free cloth.

Removes dust and moisture from system.

(b) Turn off flow selector of ambulatory unit.

(c) Attach ambulatory unit to stationary reservoir by inserting female adapter from ambulatory tank into male adapter of stationary reservoir (see illustration).

Secures connection between oxygen reservoir and ambulatory tank.

(d) Open fill valve on ambulatory tank (e.g., lever, button, key) and apply firm pressure to top of stationary reservoir (see illustration). Stay with unit while it is filling. You will hear a loud hissing noise. Tank should be filled in about 2 minutes.

Prevents leakage of oxygen during filling process. If oxygen leaks during filling process, connection between ambulatory tank and reservoir potentially ices up, and ambulatory and reservoir tanks stick together.

(e) Disconnect ambulatory unit from stationary reservoir when hissing noise changes and vapor cloud begins to form from stationary unit.

Overfilling causes ambulatory unit to malfunction as a result of high pressure in tank.

Clinical Judgment *If ambulatory unit does not separate easily, valves from reservoir and ambulatory unit are frozen together. Wait until valves warm to disengage (about 5–10 minutes). Do not touch any frosted areas because contact with skin causes skin damage from frostbite.*

(f) Wipe both filling connectors with clean, dry, lint-free cloth.

Ice often forms during filling process. Removes moisture from oxygen system.

4. Connect oxygen-delivery device (e.g., nasal cannula) to oxygen-delivery system (see Chapter 23) (see illustration).

Connects oxygen source to delivery method.

5. Adjust oxygen flow rate (L/min) to ordered rate.

Ensures that ordered oxygen dose is delivered.

6. Have client/family caregiver apply oxygen-delivery device (e.g., nasal cannula) correctly (see Chapter 23). Ensure that client has two sets of oxygen-delivery devices and tubing.

Delivers oxygen to client. Extra set of equipment is used when equipment is cleaned or in case of equipment malfunction.

7. Instruct client and family caregiver not to change oxygen flow rate.

Exceeding prescribed amount of oxygen is sometimes harmful (e.g., in client with chronic obstructive pulmonary disease [COPD]).

8. Have client/family caregiver perform each step with guidance. Provide written material at appropriate health literacy level for reinforcement and review.

Allows for correction of any errors in technique and discussion of their implications.

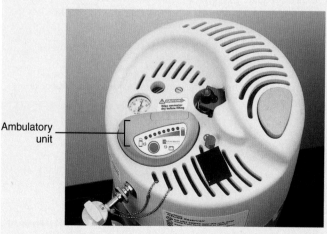

STEP 3c(3)(c) Top view of stationary reservoir.

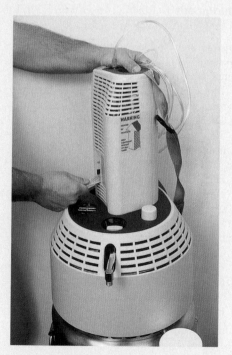

STEP 3d(3)(d) Fill valve on ambulatory tank is opened while applying firm pressure to top of ambulatory tank.

Ambulatory unit

STEP	RATIONALE

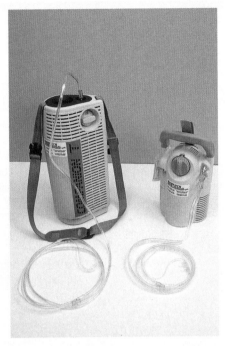

STEP 4 Oxygen-delivery device (nasal cannulas) and tubing attached to ambulatory oxygen tanks.

9. Instruct client/family caregiver to notify health care provider if signs or symptoms of hypoxia occur, including apprehension, anxiety, decreased ability to concentrate, decreased levels of consciousness, increased fatigue, dizziness, behavioral changes, increased pulse, increased respiratory rate, pallor, and cyanosis or respiratory tract infection (e.g., fever, increased sputum, change in color of sputum, foul sputum odor).

Hypoxia sometimes occurs at home when client uses oxygen. Possible causes of hypoxia include poor tubing connections; use of long oxygen tubing; or worsening of client's physical problem, with change in respiratory status.

Respiratory tract infections increase oxygen demand and often affect oxygen diffusion from pulmonary capillaries to alveoli, creating exacerbation of client's pulmonary disease.

10. Discuss emergency plans for power loss, natural disaster, and acute respiratory distress. Have client/family caregiver call 9-1-1 and notify health care provider and home care agency.

Ensures appropriate response and can prevent worsening of client's condition.

11. Instruct client and family caregiver in safe home oxygen practices, including placing "No Smoking/Oxygen in Use" signs at each entrance to home, not allowing smoking in house, keeping oxygen tanks 2.4 m (8 feet) away from open flames, potential trip hazards of tubing and cylinders, and storing oxygen tanks upright.

Ensures safe use of oxygen in home and prevents injury to client and family (Suntharalingam et al., 2018).

12. Help client assume safe and comfortable position.

Restores comfort and sense of well-being.

13. Place a bell or other type of sound-making device in a location within client's reach.

Ensures client can call for assistance if needed and promotes safety.

14. Remove and dispose of any extraneous supplies. Perform hand hygiene.

Reduces transmission of microorganisms. Client and family caregiver must be knowledgeable about infection-prevention techniques.

EVALUATION

1. Monitor rate at which oxygen is being delivered during each home visit.

Determines if client/family caregiver is regulating oxygen at prescribed rate.

2. Ask client/family caregiver about ease of use or problems associated with home oxygen.

Determines ability of client/family caregiver to deal with stressors associated with home oxygen use. Also indicates client's risk for inappropriate oxygen use.

3. Ask client/family caregiver to state safety guidelines, emergency precautions, and emergency plan.

Determines client's/family caregiver's knowledge of what to do if power fails, there is a failure in equipment, or client's status worsens.

STEP	RATIONALE
4. Use Teach-Back: "I want to be sure I explained the importance of oxygen. Tell me in your own words why you need oxygen and the signs and symptoms of decreased oxygen levels." Revise your instruction now or develop a plan for revised client/family caregiver teaching if client/family caregiver is not able to teach back correctly.	Teach-back is a technique for health care providers to ensure that they have explained medical information clearly so that clients and their families understand what is communicated to them (AHRQ, 2023).

Unexpected Outcomes	Related Interventions
1. Client has signs and symptoms associated with hypoxia.	• Determine if oxygen-delivery device and oxygen source are delivering oxygen properly. • Determine if prescribed oxygen flow rate is set properly. • Assess client for change in respiratory status such as airway plugging, respiratory tract infection, or bronchospasm. • Teach client/family caregiver when to notify health care provider or activate EMS because of signs of hypoxia.
2. Client uses unsafe practices with oxygen therapy, uses oxygen around fire or cigarette smoking, or sets incorrect flow rate.	• Reinforce client education and perform follow-up reassessment (see Box 42.4). • Include family caregiver in instruction and set up problem-solving exercises with client.
3. Client is unable to fill ambulatory system.	• Identify and instruct family caregiver who can help client fill tank.

Documentation

- Document teaching plan, information provided to client, and client's and family caregiver's ability to discuss information.
- Document oxygen-delivery system, related supplies, and prescribed oxygen flow rate.

Hand-Off Reporting

- Report reason for oxygen, type of equipment, contact information for supplier, safety measures in the home, client's or family caregiver's response to teaching, and evaluation of client or family caregiver learning.
- Report respiratory complications/concerns to health care providers involved in client's care.

Special Considerations

Client Education

- Potential for oxygen desaturation and decreased oxygen delivery to brain impairs client's ability to remember previous learning. Provide frequent teaching sessions and written or pictorial instructions to reinforce previous learning of teaching plan.
- Teach client or family caregiver that there is considerable risk of fire or injury if anyone smokes around oxygen. This risk includes e-cigarettes, commonly called vaping (Jacobs et al., 2020). Explain to client and family caregiver signs of hypoxia. Hypoxia sometimes occurs at home when client uses oxygen. Possible causes of hypoxia include poor tubing connections, use of long oxygen tubing, or worsening of client's physical problem with change in respiratory status.
- Teach the client or family caregiver not to smoke within the home for the safety of all occupants. Post "Oxygen in Use" signs on all exterior doors and on bedroom door.
- Instruct client or family caregiver in appropriate cleaning, disinfecting, and maintenance of all oxygen-delivery systems and supplies. Verify instructions with manufacturer guidelines and DME supplier's instructions.
- Instruct client or family caregiver to check mask and tubing by placing hands or face over mask or cannula to feel airflow and check that mask is not too tight; tight masks often leave marks on skin and cause pressure injuries.
- Always leave a phone number and instructions about how to reach home care nurse if needed.

Pediatrics

- Keep equipment out of reach of any children in home. Do not allow children to handle or operate home oxygen equipment.
- The developmental stage of the client along with the equipment size and flow rate should be considered for this population (Hayes et al., 2019).
- Keep children away from fire and flames at all times; as appropriate, educate about dangers of oxygen coming into contact with fire (Kaviany & Collaco, 2019).

Older Adults

- Older adults have less efficient respiratory systems and less surface area for gas exchange; thus they are at greater risk for cerebral anoxia and confusion when experiencing decreased oxygen levels. They may be unable to recognize respiratory problems or problems with their oxygen-delivery system; therefore older adults need frequent contact with a designated family caregiver.
- Check on the position of the oxygen delivery device because it can become dislodged or placed on top of the head or on the floor without the client's awareness.

Populations With Disabilities

- It is important to consider previous life experiences that may influence the readiness to learn and knowledge acquisition of people with intellectual disabilities (Geukes et al., 2019).

✦ SKILL 42.5   Teaching Home Tracheostomy Care and Suctioning

Performing tracheostomy care and suctioning in the home is similar to performing them in the hospital except for one key variable: the use of *medical asepsis* or *clean technique*. The home environment has fewer germs than hospitals; therefore clean technique can be used. Aseptic technique is used in the hospital because the client is more susceptible to infection and more virulent or pathogenic microorganisms are usually present. In the home setting, the majority of clients use clean technique. Use clinical judgment in choosing the correct technique for each client (e.g., use aseptic technique with clients who are immunocompromised; are infected [not colonized]; or have family caregivers infected with viral, bacterial, or fungal microorganisms). Clients living in unclean conditions also need to be suctioned with aseptic technique whenever possible to try to prevent infection. All family caregivers need to use Standard Precautions when suctioning with either clean or aseptic technique.

Caring for a tracheostomy at home begins in the hospital (see Chapter 24) with teaching and return demonstration. The client/family caregiver usually learn better when instructed in less invasive techniques. For example, tracheal stoma care precedes more invasive techniques such as inner cannula care and suctioning. Continually develop, implement, and evaluate the teaching plan based on client/family caregiver performance. It is imperative that clients and family caregivers have the ability to practice suctioning frequently before discharge to develop confidence with skill performance; otherwise, arrangements to provide 24-hour care are necessary before discharge.

Delegation

The skill of teaching home tracheostomy care and suctioning cannot be delegated to assistive personnel (AP). Instruct the AP to:
- Report changes in client's level of consciousness, irritability, vital signs, or decreased pulse oximetry
- Report increased airway secretions

Interprofessional Collaboration
- Respiratory services, health care provider, and DME are frequently used in the management of home tracheostomy and suctioning.

Equipment
- Suction machine with connecting tube
- Clean or sterile gloves
- Three small basins
- Hydrogen peroxide
- Normal saline
- Appropriate-size sterile or clean and disinfected suction catheter (diameter no greater than half the diameter of the tracheostomy tube [e.g., if tracheostomy tube is 8 mm (0.3 inches), use 16-Fr or smaller suction catheter])
- Tracheostomy care kit or clean 4 × 4–inch gauze pads (non-shredding)
- Small nylon bottle brush or pipe cleaners or disposable inner cannula
- Cotton-tipped applicators
- Tracheostomy ties (twill tape [⅛-inch preferably] or hook-and-loop–type tie holders)
- Mirror
- Wet washcloth or paper towel (optional)
- Dry cloth, towel, or paper towel (optional)
- Protective eyewear (optional)
- Trash bag (plastic, leak-proof preferred)
- Disposable apron (optional)
- Bag-valve-mask (BVM) with oxygen supply (optional)

STEP	RATIONALE

ASSESSMENT

1. Identify client using at least two identifiers during first visit according to agency policy. Confirmation of the address also occurs in the home setting and can be used as one of the two identifiers. Facial recognition can be used as one of the two identifiers for ongoing visits (TJC, 2023). | Ensures client safety. Complies with The Joint Commission standards and improves client safety (TJC, 2023). |

2. Assess client's electronic health record (EHR) including health care provider's orders and nurses' notes. Note previous teaching sessions about tracheostomy care and suctioning and client's/family caregiver's response to teaching. | Identifies focus for instruction and potential difficulty with teaching how to care for and suction a tracheostomy. |

3. Assess client's/family caregiver's health literacy. | Determines degree to which individuals have the ability to find, understand, and use information and services to make informed health-related decisions and actions for themselves and others (CDC, 2023). |

4. Assess client's/family caregiver's vision and fine motor function for ability to perform tracheostomy care and suctioning properly. Also assess client's level of consciousness and ability to problem solve. Ask client/family caregiver to explain what to do for the following: | Instructing family caregiver is essential if client's physical and cognitive impairment prevents ability to perform tracheostomy care and suctioning. Emergency situations usually require family caregiver to suction. |

   a. Tracheostomy care: observing excess peristomal secretions, excess intratracheal secretions, and soiled or damp tracheostomy dressing/ties | Knowledge needed for client/family caregiver to accurately assess need to provide tracheostomy care. Signs and symptoms are related to presence of secretions at stoma site or within tracheostomy tube. |

STEP	RATIONALE
b. Suctioning: assessment of client's perceived need for suctioning, presence of gurgling, wheezes on inspiration or expiration, restlessness, ineffective coughing, tachypnea, cyanosis, acutely decreased level of consciousness, tachycardia or bradycardia, acutely shallow respirations, or acute dyspnea	Knowledge allows client/family caregiver to accurately determine need to perform tracheostomy tube suctioning. Physical signs and symptoms result from lower-airway obstruction and tissue hypoxia.
5. Assess client's/family caregiver's ability to assess pulse rate and respirations.	Skill needed for client/family caregiver to monitor physiological change during tracheostomy care.
6. Assess client's learning readiness and ability to concentrate; consider presence of pain, nausea, or fatigue and client's interest in instruction.	Presence of significant illness, frailty, or confusion affects client's ability to attend to teaching plan. Indicates need to rely on family caregiver for learning and implementation (if available) on short- or long-term basis.
7. Perform hand hygiene.	Reduces transmission of microorganisms. Client and family caregiver must be knowledgeable about infection-prevention techniques.
8. Assess client's/family caregiver's goals or preferences for how skill is to be performed or what client expects.	Allows care to be individualized to client.

PLANNING

1. Expected outcomes following completion of procedure:	
• Client/family caregiver identifies signs and symptoms indicating need for tracheostomy care and suctioning.	Client/family caregiver is able to institute preventive means to maintain airway.
• Client/family caregiver states factors that influence tracheostomy airway functioning.	Tracheostomy often impairs normal airway clearance, humidification, and gas exchange.
• Client/family caregiver correctly demonstrates complete tracheostomy tube care and suctioning in controlled setting.	Provides validation of ability to perform procedure.
• Client/family caregiver identifies signs of stoma inflammation or respiratory tract infection and when to notify health care provider.	Measures cognitive learning.
• Lower and upper airways are cleared of secretions, as evidenced by absent or diminished wheezes and gurgles in large airways, normalization of pulse and respiratory rate, increased depth of respirations, absence of cyanosis, improved color, and decreased dyspnea.	Suctioning by client/family caregiver is successful.
• Stoma site is clean and free of an infection and transesophageal fistula. Signs of transesophageal fistula include frequent coughing when eating, aspiration, and/or fever.	Tracheostomy care is successful.
• Inner cannula is free of secretions.	
2. Select setting in home in which client/family caregiver is most likely to perform tracheostomy tube care and that is conducive to teaching.	Practicing skill in same setting where skill will be routinely performed facilitates comprehension and learning.
a. Select room that is well lit with comfortable seating.	Lighting of room improves visualization of skill. Teaching is more effective when the environment is conducive to learning.
b. Be sure that client is close and can see nurse clearly.	Visualization of the nurse's techniques requires proximity to the nurse.
c. Control sources of noise and distractions.	Comfortable environment free of distractions promotes client's attention.
d. Provide privacy and prepare and organize supplies.	Minimizes embarrassment.
3. Perform hand hygiene and apply clean gloves.	Reduces transmission of microorganisms.
4. Demonstrate to client and family caregiver how to organize and set up any equipment needed to perform procedure.	Promotes cooperation.
5. Discuss and demonstrate with client/family caregiver proper position for procedure (high Fowler position in front of mirror).	Promotes understanding of comfort and safety principles and facilitates visibility.

STEP	RATIONALE

IMPLEMENTATION

1. Suctioning:

a. Verify health care provider's orders for suctioning. Ensure that client and family caregiver understand suctioning order.

Invasive procedure requires order.

Order may be written for as-needed suctioning; ensures that client and family caregiver understand what this means.

b. Teach client/family caregiver techniques for hand hygiene and application of clean gloves.

Reduces transmission of microorganisms. Client and family caregiver must be knowledgeable about infection-prevention techniques.

c. Explain and demonstrate step-by-step preparation and completion of tracheostomy tube suctioning using either open or closed suctioning (see Chapter 24) (see illustration).

Demonstration is reliable technique for teaching psychomotor skill and enables client/family caregiver to ask questions throughout procedure. Steps used to suction clients in hospital are also used in home.

Clinical Judgment *Instillation of normal saline before suctioning, once a common practice, is no longer recommended. Use of normal saline adversely affects arterial and tissue oxygenation (Meister et al., 2021).*

d. After client/family caregiver suctions tracheostomy, teach how to suction nasal and oral pharynx and perform mouth care. Encourage client/family caregiver to brush teeth with small soft toothbrush 2 times a day and use mouth moisturizer to moisturize lips every 2 to 4 hours.

Suctioning removes secretions from trachea and lower airway that clients are not able to clear by coughing (Meister et al., 2021). Dental plaque harbors microorganisms.

e. At conclusion of procedure, have client take two or three deep breaths; reassess status of breathing.

Deep breathing reduces oxygen loss and prevents hypoxia. Expect client's respiratory status to improve following suctioning.

f. Demonstrate how to disconnect suction catheter and coil and discard catheter in appropriate receptacle. If catheter is to be cleaned and disinfected, set aside. Have client/family caregiver remove soiled gloves and dispose of in appropriate container; perform hand hygiene.

Reduces transmission of microorganisms. Client and family caregiver must be knowledgeable about infection-prevention techniques.

2. Tracheostomy care:

a. Have client sit at table with mirror. Instruct client/family caregiver how to perform hand hygiene and apply clean gloves with you. Teach techniques for cleaning stoma and tracheostomy tube and changing tracheostomy ties and dressing (see illustrations and Chapter 24). *Exception:* Clean inner cannula with approved cleaning solution such as hydrogen peroxide and small brush (CDC, 2019).

Prevents transmission of microorganisms. Steps used to provide tracheostomy care in hospital are also used in home.

Reusable equipment may be disinfected by immersion in 3% hydrogen peroxide for 30 minutes (CDC, 2019) and then rinsed with water. **Hydrogen peroxide should not be used on client's tissues.**

Clinical Judgment *During tracheostomy care, a client is at risk for the tracheostomy tube coming out. Instruct client/family caregiver to never remove the old tracheostomy tube ties until the new ties are secured properly. The obturator of the tube set currently inserted should be readily available in the event the tracheostomy tube slips out. Keep two tracheostomy tubes, one the same size as the client's and one a size smaller, accessible to the client so that the client or family caregiver can insert a new tube if the tube comes out. Provide a checklist of required supplies to safely care for a tracheostomy. Instruct the client/family caregiver to check daily for the supplies (National Tracheostomy Safe Project [NTSP], 2023).*

b. Have client/family caregiver remove and dispose of gloves. Perform hand hygiene.

Reduces transmission of microorganisms.

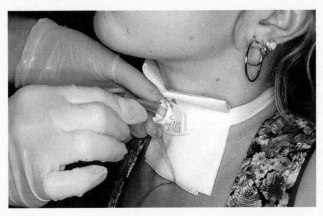

STEP 1c Insertion of suction catheter into tracheostomy tube.

STEP	RATIONALE

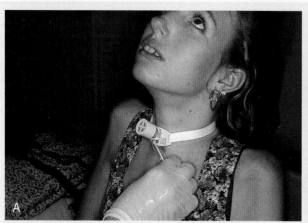 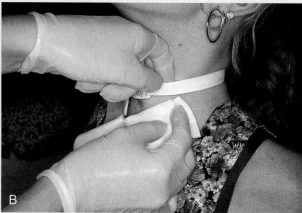

STEP 2a (A) Cleaning area around tracheal stoma. (B) Applying clean tracheostomy dressing.

c. Instruct client/family caregiver to apply clean gloves. Demonstrate technique for cleaning reusable supplies in warm soapy water. Rinse thoroughly and dry between two layers of clean paper towels. Store supplies in loosely closed clear plastic bag; label bag.	Prevents transmission of microorganisms. Air must circulate, or humidity in bag can promote microorganism growth.
d. Have client/family caregiver remove and dispose of gloves. Perform hand hygiene.	Reduces transmission of microorganisms.
3. Disinfecting supplies:	
a. Explain procedure for disinfecting reusable supplies. To disinfect supplies, use one of following methods after performing hand hygiene and donning gloves:	Removes organisms and reduces risk for infection.
(1) *Method 1:* Soak reusable supplies that touch membranes in prepared solution of 3% hydrogen peroxide for 30 minutes (CDC, 2019).	
(2) *Method 2:* Soak reusable supplies that touch membranes in prepared solution of 70% isopropyl for 5 minutes (CDC, 2019). Rinse usable supplies in saline or sterile saltwater (Johns Hopkins Medicine, n.d.).	
(3) *Method 3:* Soak reusable supplies that touch membranes in 1:50 prepared dilution of 5.25% to 6.15% sodium hypochlorite (household bleach) for 5 minutes (CDC, 2019). Rinse reusable supplies in saline or sterile saltwater (Johns Hopkins Medicine, n.d.).	
4. Have client/family caregiver perform each step with guidance from you.	Adults learn psychomotor skills best by active participation; you can correct any errors in technique as they occur and discuss their implications.
5. Help client assume comfortable position.	Restores comfort and sense of well-being.
6. Teach client/family caregiver signs and symptoms of the following:	Client/family caregiver must be able to recognize onset of complications associated with long-term tracheostomy use early so that medical treatment can begin, reducing risk for more serious negative outcomes (Karaca et al., 2019). Emphasize importance of notifying health care provider when signs and symptoms of complications occur.
a. Stoma infection (redness, tenderness, drainage)	
b. Respiratory tract infection (fever, increased sputum, change in color of sputum, foul sputum odor, increased cough, chills, night sweats)	
c. Transesophageal fistula (air leaking through stoma, nose, or mouth with cuff properly inflated; more air needed to inflate cuff; aspiration of food or liquid during suctioning; excessive belching; coughing when swallowing)	
7. Place a bell or other type of sound-making device in an accessible location within client's reach.	Ensures client can call for assistance to promote safety.
8. Remove and dispose of gloves. Perform hand hygiene.	Reduces transmission of microorganisms. Client and family caregiver must be knowledgeable about infection-prevention techniques.

STEP	RATIONALE

EVALUATION

1. Observe as client/family caregiver demonstrates technique for tracheostomy tube care and suctioning.
2. Ask client/family caregiver to describe signs and symptoms indicating need for tracheostomy care and suctioning and the factors that influence tracheostomy airway functioning.
3. Have client and family caregiver explain the problems that need to be reported to their health care provider.
4. Ask client/family caregiver to describe how to clean and disinfect reusable supplies.
5. **Use Teach-Back:** "I want to be sure I explained how you will feel and what you may see if you develop problems or complications with your tracheostomy. Tell me the signs and symptoms for needing to suction your tracheostomy." Revise your instruction now or develop a plan for revised client/family caregiver teaching if client/family caregiver is not able to teach back correctly.

Feedback through independent demonstration of psychomotor skill is reliable method to evaluate learning.

Demonstrates learning and client's and family caregiver's ability to respond when airway problems develop.

Demonstrates client's ability to take steps for emergent care.

Correct techniques will reduce risk for infection.

Teach-back is a technique for health care providers to ensure that they have explained medical information clearly so that clients and their families understand what is communicated to them (AHRQ, 2023).

Unexpected Outcomes

1. Stoma site is reddened or hard, with or without foul drainage.

2. Copious colored secretions are present around stoma or when client/family caregiver suctions tracheostomy.

3. Bloody secretions or change in color from clear or light yellow to green when client suctioned.

4. No secretions are suctioned.

5. Skin breakdown is present at stoma site.

Related Interventions

- Evaluate client's/family caregiver's technique.
- Increase frequency of tracheostomy care.

- Have client use sterile technique for suctioning and tracheostomy care.
- Secretions may be pink, rust colored, or blood tinged, depending on problem; documenting color helps health care provider diagnose problem.
- Evaluate for adequate humidity (use room humidifier or tracheostomy collar humidity, if needed) (see Chapter 24).
- Notify health care provider.

- Evaluate suctioning technique, suctioning frequency, and size of catheter used. Usual length to insert catheter is length of tracheostomy tube plus ¼ inch.
- Assess for signs of infection.
- Assess client for use of anticoagulant medications.

- Evaluate client's fluid status and need for increased humidity.
- Determine if appropriate-size suction catheter is used.
- Reassess need to suction.

- Assess site for pressure areas or site infection.
- Remove pressure source.

Documentation

- Document client instruction and client's and family caregiver's ability to demonstrate tracheostomy care, suctioning skills, and disinfecting skills.
- Develop a system of documenting for client or family caregiver to describe appearance of trach and secretions, client tolerance, and tracheostomy care provided.

Hand-Off Reporting

- Report location of tracheostomy teaching session, who participated, content discussed, client's and/or family caregiver's response to procedure, and evaluation of client learning.
- Report any unexpected outcomes or concerns, such as a hardened or reddened stoma, to health care providers involved in client's care.

Special Considerations

Client Education

- The nose and mouth normally provide warmth, filtering, and moisture for the air we breathe. A tracheostomy tube bypasses

these mechanisms. Humidification must be provided to keep secretions thin and to avoid mucus plugs.
- Always leave a phone number and instructions about how to reach home care nurse if needed.

Pediatrics

- Encourage parents to give tracheostomy care as soon as child is stable in the hospital. The more time there is to practice these skills, the more comfortable parents become in caring for the child at home.
- Use simulation to teach best practices for tracheostomy care in children (McCoy et al., 2021).
- Children with tracheostomies need to socialize and play with other children who are close to their own age (Hockenberry et al., 2024).
- To prevent hypoxia, teach family caregivers that suctioning needs to last no more than 5 seconds in infants and 10 seconds in children.
- Teach family caregivers pediatric cardiopulmonary resuscitation and situational awareness for circumstances such as a dropped cannula when its replacement is not within immediate reach (Prickett et al., 2019).

Older Adults
- Older adults lose some properties of elastic recoil and often have greater difficulty clearing airway secretions through cough. As a result, they require more suctioning and airway care and have increased risk for infection (Touhy & Jett, 2022).
- Assess for cognitive, mobility, or sensory impairments that impair ability to manage artificial airway at home, and teach family caregiver if client is unable to manage airway independently.

- Anxiety accompanies decreased ability to breathe and may cause the older adult to become too nervous to perform suctioning independently.

Populations With Disabilities
- Consider a multisession education model when working with clients with an intellectual disability (Latteck & Bruland, 2020).

✦ SKILL 42.6   Teaching Medication Self-Administration

Nurses teach clients and family caregivers how to safely administer medications in the home. The term *compliance* was used in the past to describe if clients' behaviors matched health care providers' recommendations when it came to taking prescribed medications or adhering to prescribed treatments (Jeminiwa et al., 2019). Recent literature supports the term *adherence*, which emphasizes a client's role in decision making, taking into account freedom of choice (Jeminiwa et al., 2019). Medication adherence for a client includes distinct phases of 1) taking the first dose as prescribed and then 2) continuing to take medications as prescribed (Pino et al., 2021). When a client chooses to stop taking a prescribed medication, the phase is referred to as discontinuation (Pino et al., 2021). One method that has been identified to increase adherence is to understand and then support clients' decisions regarding how to take their medications. Use teaching methods that incorporate active listening so that you can adapt clients' needs and concerns into their medication regimen.

Some barriers to medication adherence include fear of adverse reactions from medications, belief that a medication does not help, inconvenience of taking medication, cost of medication, inadequate knowledge, forgetfulness, and relationship with health care provider (Lee et al., 2019). Considering these potential barriers, you can provide information and support to ensure that a client or family caregiver is making a well-informed decision when it comes to whether or not to take a medication. Once a client has mastered the skill of administering medications, you must continue to validate that the skill is being performed correctly and assess for new issues and concerns.

Delegation
The skill of teaching clients medication self-administration cannot be delegated to assistive personnel (AP). Instruct the AP to:
- Communicate to the nurse problems that the client or family caregiver reports having with medication administration.

Interprofessional Collaboration
- Pharmacists and health care provider are frequently contacted when client or family caregiver report difficulty with medication self-administration, such as pill size, availability of medication, or side effects.

Equipment
- Medication
- Liquid to take with medication
- Medication administration record or other up-to-date list of current medications from health care provider
- Medication log
- Container for daily or weekly preparation
- Measuring devices as needed (e.g., medicine cup, teaspoon)
- Teaching tools (e.g., charts, written instructions, color codes for medicine containers)

STEP	RATIONALE

ASSESSMENT

1. Identify client using at least two identifiers during first visit according to agency policy. Confirmation of the address also occurs in the home setting and can be used as one of the two identifiers. Facial recognition can be used as one of the two identifiers for ongoing visits (TJC, 2023).

Ensures client safety. Complies with The Joint Commission standards and improves client safety (TJC, 2023).

2. Assess client's electronic health record (EHR) including health care provider's orders and nurses' notes. Note previous teaching sessions about medication self-administration and client's/family caregiver's response to teaching.

Identifies focus of instruction and potential difficulty with learning medication self-administration.

3. Assess client's/family caregiver's health literacy.

Determines degree to which individuals have the ability to find, understand, and use information and services to make informed health-related decisions and actions for themselves and others (CDC, 2023).

4. Ask client and check EHR for history of allergies. If client has allergies, check with pharmacist if any of the prescribed medications could cause an allergic reaction.

Verification of allergies is a critical step in client safety and must be performed before any medications are administered.

5. Assess client's/family caregiver's learning readiness and ability to concentrate (consider presence of pain, nausea, or fatigue and client interest in instruction) and learning style preference.

Presence of significant illness, frailty, or confusion affects person's ability to attend to teaching plan. Indicates need to rely on family caregiver for learning and implementation (if available) on short- or long-term basis. Learning style affects choice of teaching resources.

STEP	RATIONALE
6. Assess client's/family caregiver's belief in need for medication therapy. Consider prior experiences, ethnic values, religious beliefs, personal experiences with medications, and family caregivers' values about medications.	Many factors influence client's willingness to follow drug regimen.
7. Assess client's prescribed and over-the-counter (OTC) medications, including use of herbal supplements: Has more than one health care provider prescribed medications? Are labels clearly marked? Are time schedules confusing? Do different drugs look alike? Does client store medications together or out of original containers? Are expiration dates on bottles still current?	Determines sources of confusion affecting client's adherence. Adherence with medication therapy (especially in older adults) is often complicated by polypharmacy (multiple chronic conditions are often treated with multiple medications, sometimes prescribed by more than one health care provider). Adherence is more complicated when medication regimens are complex.
8. Be sure that family caregiver knows client's drug allergies and type of allergic response.	As new drugs are prescribed, the family caregiver often becomes the one to monitor for inappropriate drug prescription.
9. Consult with health care provider to review medications that client is receiving and simplify regimen if possible.	Review of medications helps minimize risk for drug interactions from multiple medications and ensures accuracy of medication regimen. Simplification of regimen improves adherence, particularly related to daily frequency of prescribed doses.
10. Assess client's/family caregiver's goals or preferences for how skill is to be performed or what client expects.	Allows care to be individualized to client.

PLANNING

1. Expected outcomes following completion of procedure:	
• Client/family caregiver is able to state purpose of each medication and why it is beneficial. If medication has been discontinued, client/family caregiver correctly explains why this was done.	Demonstrates cognitive learning.
• Client/family caregiver identifies common adverse effects and relief measures.	Encourages adherence to medication therapy.
• Client/family caregiver is able to state when to notify health care provider about medication problems.	Empowers client/family caregiver to participate in care.
• Client/family caregiver reads each label and explains when each medication should be taken.	Prevents medication administration errors.
• Client/family caregiver demonstrates self-administration of medication by prescribed route.	Demonstrates skill achieved.
2. Select setting in home in which client/family caregiver is likely to prepare and administer medications:	Practicing skill in same setting in which skill is to be performed facilitates comprehension and learning.
a. Select room that is well lit and offers comfortable seating.	Lighting of room improves visualization of skill. Teaching is more effective when the environment is conducive to learning.
b. Be sure that client is close and can see nurse clearly.	Visualization of the nurse's techniques requires proximity to the nurse.
c. Control sources of noise and distractions.	Room environment needs to minimize existing sensory alterations. Comfortable environment free of distractions promotes client's attention.
3. Prepare teaching materials:	Teaching materials can support client and family caregiver engagement and family-centered, high-quality care (Rojas-Ocana et al., 2021).
a. Plan approach that matches client's/family caregiver's learning preference (visual, auditory, reading/writing, kinesthetic):	Using an instructional approach that matches client's/family caregiver's learning style in the context in which learning occurs allows for an individualized approach that incorporates teaching modalities to maximize client learning (Wood et al., 2019).
(1) Written materials printed in large bold letters (set in 14-point or larger type)	Assists clients with visual limitations.
(2) DVD or Internet instructional programs	
(3) Illustrations of medication safety guidelines	
(4) Handling equipment and supplies	
4. Consider mobile health (mHealth) applications delivered through smart phones or tablet devices.	Health applications provide alternatives to formats such as print copies or DVD (Doorenbos et al., 2020).
5. Ensure that client is wearing glasses or hearing aids if needed during teaching session.	Use of glasses or hearing aids increases client's sensory perception and likelihood of attending to teaching session and understanding content.
6. Arrange teaching time to allow participation of client with family caregivers (see illustration).	Family caregiver can serve as positive resource to client and often reinforces information provided (Doorenbos al., 2020).

STEP	RATIONALE

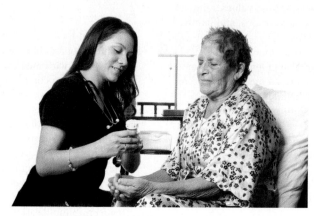

STEP 6 Client participates in medication self-administration teaching program. (*From iStock.com/ phakimata.*)

IMPLEMENTATION

1. Instruct client/family caregiver about importance of performing hand hygiene before medication self-administration.

Reduces transmission of microorganisms.

2. Present information clearly and concisely:
  a. Face learner in well-lit room.

Allows visualization of client's nonverbal responses to education. Client with hearing loss or visual problem is able to see your expressions, read written information, and hear your voice more clearly.

  b. Use short sentences and speak in slow, low-pitched voice.

Enhances understanding of information.

  c. Provide descriptions in understandable terms.

Use plain language when teaching clients and family caregivers. Medication content written in plain language can reduce confusion and improve comprehension about medications (Tyson et al., 2021).

  d. *Option:* Provide tables for explaining actions, side effects, or schedules; offer bar charts to show when medications reach peak effects.

Data show that clients prefer charts to present clinical data, while tables improve clients' understanding (CDC, 2022).

3. Frequently pause during instruction so that client/family caregiver can ask questions and express understanding of content.

Increases learner participation. Ongoing feedback ensures that client is acquiring information.

4. Instruct client/family caregiver on following content: purpose of regularly scheduled and prn (as needed) medications and their desired effects, how medication works and why it helps, dosage schedules and rationale, common side effects, what to do to relieve side effects, what to do if dose is missed, when to call health care provider with problems, whom to call with problems, medication safety guidelines, and implications when medications are not taken.

Provides client/family caregiver with sufficient information to understand and take medications safely at home.

5. Instruct client/family caregiver in appropriate route of medication delivery.

Client needs to be proficient in all routes of medication administration. Adverse effects often occur if medications are administered incorrectly.

6. Provide frequent, short teaching sessions. Plan to have several teaching sessions, especially if client needs to take multiple medications.

Frequent sessions improve client's attention and retention of information discussed.

7. Provide teaching about OTC medications and herbal supplements.

Clients may not understand effects of OTC and herbal supplements (Kim et al., 2022).

8. Provide client with written schedules or individualized instruction sheets for review. Offer special charts, diagrams, learning aids, written information, weekly pill organizers, and Internet/Intranet resources (see illustration).

Clear written information, charts, and other resources such as media sources enhance client learning (Research Institute for Home Care, 2023).

9. Offer help as client practices preparing medication (e.g., "Let's prepare the medications you will take with your meals or the medicines you take first in the morning").

Allows for observation of client's ability to read labels correctly and prepare all medications for prescribed times.

STEP	RATIONALE

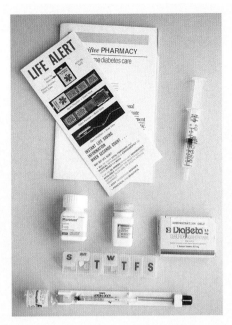

STEP 8 Examples of aids for client self-administration of medication.

10. Have pharmacy provide clear, large-print labels for medication bottles and medication teaching handouts if appropriate.	Improves client's ability to read and follow directions.
11. Have pharmacy provide containers that client can open independently if manual dexterity is limited.	Most pharmacies dispense pills in "childproof" containers, which clients with limited mobility of fingers or hands often find difficult to manipulate or open.

Clinical Judgment *If there are pets or small children in the home or children who frequently visit the home, help client establish a "safe place" for medication storage to reduce risk for accidental ingestion by pets or children.*

12. Facilitate arrangements for pharmacy to receive written prescriptions in timely fashion if required for dispensing. Arrange for pharmacy to deliver medications to home if client is unable to arrange for transportation to pharmacy.	Availability of drugs influences adherence.
13. Discuss with client/family caregiver how to dispose of discontinued or expired medications.	Ensures safe disposal.
14. Help client assume comfortable position.	Restores comfort and sense of well-being.

EVALUATION

1. Ask client/family caregiver to explain information about each drug: purpose; actions; routes; timing of medications and maximum frequency of use of either prescribed or OTC medications; side effects and interactions; and foods, herbals, or OTC medications to avoid.	Clients and family caregivers need to be able to understand information received, remember it, and apply it (Prochnow et al., 2019; Wood et al., 2019).
2. Ask client/family caregiver to describe when to call health care provider or refer to printed information for resources.	Developing techniques to gain information and support self-efficacy helps client adherence to medications (Taba et al., 2022).
3. Have client/family caregiver prepare and administer doses for all prescribed medications.	Indicates understanding of medication dosages and schedules.
4. **Use Teach-Back:** "I want to be sure I explained how to safely dispose of medicines you are no longer taking. Tell me in your own words the correct way to dispose of your tablets here in the home." Revise your instruction now or develop a plan for revised client/family caregiver teaching if client/family caregiver is not able to teach back correctly.	Teach-back is a technique for health care providers to ensure that they have explained medical information clearly so that clients and their families understand what is communicated to them (AHRQ, 2023).

STEP	RATIONALE
Unexpected Outcomes	**Related Interventions**
1. Client/family caregiver makes errors in preparing medications or is unable to recall and/or explain information discussed in teaching sessions.	• Provide additional instruction and/or teaching materials for consultation when information is forgotten or unclear.
	• Ensure that written instructions are at client's level of understanding. Some commercially prepared booklets contain instructions that are too complex or contain medical jargon that is difficult to understand.
	• Consider use of different pictures, color coding, diagrams, and tape-recorded instructions for clients with a visual impairment or a reading disability.
	• Consider use of weekly pill organizers.
	• Periodically observe client/family caregiver preparing and administering medications.
2. Medication self-administration plan is not possible because of client's self-care deficits. This is common when client develops cognitive changes.	• Develop alternative plan, which often relies on family caregivers to safely administer home medication regimen.
3. Client refuses to take medications as prescribed.	• Explore and identify reasons for nonadherence, which often include the following: cost, side effects, complexity of regimen, problems with swallowing or other side effects, and cultural preferences.
	• See Box 42.5.

BOX 42.5

Evidence-Based Nursing Interventions to Enhance Adherence to Medication Therapy

• Involve clients as partners in collaboration. Encourage them to express their views and share in the decision making with you.
• Use of interactive software on electronic portable devices to promote learning and improve client confidence can be effective across generations.
• Encourage clients to take medications by explaining benefits.
• Use electronic medication reminders such as medication adherence apps.
• Use pill organizers such as pill boxes, patches, or fobs.
• Be empathetic regarding clients' feelings.
• Encourage a sense of control for the client by providing information about diagnosis and treatment.
• Recognize family caregiver needs and provide information and support. Understand that family caregiver may have competing responsibilities (e.g., employment, other dependents).

Adapted from Ali EE, et al: User acceptance of an app-based adherence intervention: perspectives from patients taking oral anticancer medications, *J Oncol Pharm Pract* 25(2):394–395, 2019; Centers for Disease Control and Prevention (CDC): *Health literacy medications,* 2022.

Documentation

• Document instruction provided and learning outcomes achieved by client and family caregiver.
• Develop a system of recording (client diary) for client or family caregiver to use to document adherence to dosage schedules and self-monitoring of any problems.
• Always leave a phone number and instructions about how to reach home care nurse if needed.

Hand-Off Reporting

• Report location of session, who participated, content discussed, client's and/or family caregiver's response to procedure, and evaluation of client learning.

Special Considerations

Client Education

• See Chapter 41 for guidelines for medication safety.
• If it is difficult to plan a separate teaching session, teach client while administering medications.
• Examples of learning aids include homemade calendars for each week that contain plastic bags containing medications to take at specific times, egg cartons divided into color-coded sections with medications for the day, clock faces for clients who cannot read or see clearly, color-coding for drug types (e.g., blue for sedative, red for pain pill), and pillboxes that identify days of the week and times of day.

Pediatrics

• Children with chronic illness are at higher risk for medication errors, especially with liquid medications and complex medication schedules (Yin et al., 2021). Instruct adults to keep all medications locked and securely out of reach of children.
• Encourage family caregivers not to tell children that medications are treats because this increases the risk for child overdosing by mistaking medicine for candy.
• Successful medication teaching involves the child's parents or other family caregivers and the child and siblings whenever possible. To provide effective medication teaching to children, take the child's developmental and cognitive abilities into consideration when planning teaching sessions (Hockenberry et al., 2024).
• Offer alternative teaching strategies such as Internet-based learning modules to family caregivers and children (Fenske, 2019).
• Family caregivers need to supervise older children as they begin taking responsibility for their own treatment.

Older Adults

• Capacity for learning new information remains as people age (in the absence of dementia); however, older clients often need additional time to accomplish learning. Allow adequate time and number of teaching sessions to support successful learning (Touhy & Jett, 2022).

- Engage clients to ask questions about their ambivalence toward taking medications. Use open-ended questions to explore potential medication belief discrepancies, and stress the benefits of medications (Qiao et al., 2020).
- Effective teaching strategies for older adults include memory aids, information written in large letters, involvement of family caregiver, follow-up teaching sessions either over the telephone or in person, and computer-assisted teaching guides.
- Cognition problems coupled with complexity of medication regimens have a negative effect on older adults' ability to self-administer medication safely. Try to decrease the complexity of medication regimens in clients with cognitive deficits whenever possible to promote safe medication self-administration practices.
- If client or family caregiver does not have English as the primary language, evaluate the need for translation by an appropriate medical translator.

- Older adults often have to take medications in multiple routes (e.g., oral, inhaled, injections). Problems with physical dexterity, eyesight, cognitive skills, and memory negatively often affect adherence to medication schedules. Establish a therapeutic nurse-client relationship to help clients overcome these barriers to adherence.

Populations With Disabilities

- Consider a multisession education model when working with clients with an intellectual disability (Latteck & Bruland, 2020).
- It is important to consider that previous life experiences may influence the readiness to learn and knowledge acquisition of people with intellectual disabilities (Geukes et al., 2019).

◆ SKILL 42.7 Managing Feeding Tubes in the Home

The number of clients receiving enteral feedings at home in the United Kingdom and the world is dramatically increasing (Ojo et al., 2019). Clients benefit when they are able to see tube-feeding equipment and devices when learning how to administer home enteral nutrition. Provide hands-on experience and client involvement with decision making about home enteral nutrition whenever possible. Enteral nutrition therapy in the home setting is usually offered when a client is unable to meet their nutrition requirements through eating but has a functioning gastrointestinal tract and is medically stable (Bischoff et al., 2020). The client or family caregiver is able to administer feedings, and there is sufficient time in a controlled environment to learn the skill.

This procedure in the home setting follows the guidelines and skills described in Chapter 31. Most clients who receive enteral nutrition in the home have either gastrostomy or jejunostomy tubes. This skill focuses on teaching the client or family caregiver how to administer such feedings in the home. Frequently in the home setting, the nurse is responsible for reinsertion of gastrostomy feeding tubes, and the health care provider is responsible for reinsertion of jejunostomy tubes.

Delegation

The skill of teaching clients and family caregivers how to manage feeding tubes in the home cannot be delegated to assistive personnel (AP). Instruct the AP to:
- Report when client has difficulty with feeding, coughing, gagging, respiratory distress, discomfort, or vomiting

Interprofessional Collaboration

- The health care provider, registered dietitian, and speech and occupational therapists are frequently part of the management of enteral feedings (American Society for Parenteral and Enteral Nutrition [ASPEN], 2023).

Equipment

See Skills 31.1 through 31.4 and Procedural Guideline 31.1 for lists of equipment.
- Log to record daily weights, intake and output (I&O), temperature, and feeding residuals

---

STEP	RATIONALE

ASSESSMENT

1. Identify client using at least two identifiers during first visit according to agency policy. Confirmation of the address also occurs in the home setting and can be used as one of the two identifiers. Facial recognition can be used as one of the two identifiers for ongoing visits (TJC, 2023).	Ensures client safety. Complies with The Joint Commission standards and improves client safety (TJC, 2023).
2. Assess client's electronic health record (EHR) including health care provider's orders and nurses' notes. Note previous teaching sessions about enteral feedings and client's/family caregiver's response to teaching.	Identifies focus of instruction and potential difficulty with managing feeding tubes.
3. Assess client's/family caregiver's health literacy.	Determines degree to which individuals have the ability to find, understand, and use information and services to make informed health-related decisions and actions for themselves and others (CDC, 2023).
4. Assess client's and family caregiver's physical (visual, fine motor) function. Also assess emotional, financial, and community resources.	Determines client's and family caregiver's ability to manipulate equipment. Availability of resources increases ability for self-care home management.

STEP	RATIONALE
5. Assess environmental conditions of home (sanitation, storage of equipment, work area, supplies, and power source).	Determines if home environment is safe for enteral feeding, with minimal risks for infection and complications.
6. Assess client's/family caregiver's understanding of purpose of enteral feedings and positive expected outcomes.	Understanding rationale of treatment is critical to enhancing participation and cooperation in care.
7. Assess client's/family caregiver's understanding of storage and management of equipment and supplies as well as where and how to obtain supplies.	Ensures safe home management and decreases risk for complications. Home care delivery companies usually deliver a month's supply at a time. Garage is not a good storage place during hot weather; use space where the supplies will be kept at temperature recommended by the manufacturer.
8. Assess client's learning readiness and ability to concentrate (consider presence of pain, nausea, or fatigue and client interest in instruction) and learning style preference.	Presence of significant illness, frailty, or confusion affects client's ability to attend to teaching plan. Indicates need to rely on family caregiver for learning and implementation (if available) on short- or long-term basis. Learning style affects choice of teaching resources.
9. Perform hand hygiene.	Reduces transmission of microorganisms. Client and family caregiver must be knowledgeable about infection-prevention techniques.
10. Observe client/family caregiver administer an enteral feeding (when previously ordered).	Determines which specific components of skill client/family caregiver can complete easily and which are more difficult and require reinforcement.
11. Assess client's/family caregiver's knowledge and experience in managing a feeding tube.	Reveals need for client/family caregiver instruction or support.
12. Assess client's/family caregiver's goals or preferences for how skill is to be performed or what is expected.	Allows care to be individualized for client.

PLANNING

1. Expected outcomes following completion of procedure: • Client/family caregiver verbalizes purpose of enteral feedings and enhanced nutritional health. • Client/family caregiver demonstrates proper use of equipment and handling of formulas. • Client/family caregiver demonstrates accurate administration of enteral feedings and medications. • Client/family caregiver verbalizes understanding of signs, symptoms, and management of complications of feeding such as nausea, vomiting, and tube obstruction or dislodgment.	Provides measurable criteria to determine level of cognitive understanding. Provides demonstration of skills needed to manage home enteral nutrition. Provides demonstration of skills needed to administer home enteral nutrition and medications. Confirms that client/family caregiver has knowledge needed to respond when problems with feedings develop.
2. Select setting in home in which client/family caregiver is likely to prepare and administer enteral feedings: a. Select room that is well lit with comfortable seating. b. Be sure that client is close and can see nurse clearly. c. Control sources of noise and distractions.	Improves likelihood of client and family caregiver being attentive to instruction. Lighting of room improves visualization of skill. Teaching is more effective when the environment is conducive to learning. Room environment needs to minimize existing sensory alterations. Comfortable environment free of distractions promotes client's attention.
3. Provide privacy and prepare and organize equipment and supplies.	Ensures an organized procedure. Protects client's privacy; reduces anxiety. Ensures more efficiency when completing an assessment.

IMPLEMENTATION

1. Perform hand hygiene. Instruct family caregiver to wear clean, disposable gloves.	Reduces transmission of microorganisms. Client and family caregiver must be knowledgeable about infection-prevention techniques.
2. Help client/family caregiver determine feeding schedule that will maintain nutritional requirements, fit within client's or family's schedule, and fit health care provider's order.	Promotes adherence to enteral nutrition therapy. Initiate education with the client/family caregiver early to identify potential issues (Pars & Soyers, 2020).

Clinical Judgment *Explain that family caregiver needs to communicate to the nurse or health care provider any changes in feeding schedules made to fit daily routine.*

STEP	RATIONALE
3. Have client/family caregiver apply clean gloves with you. If a client has a nasoenteral tube, demonstrate how to identify placement of feeding tube: aspirating gastric fluid, checking pH of gastric fluid, and acceptable pH range (see Skill 31.2).	Reduces transmission of microorganisms. Complete pH testing periodically (Chauhan et al., 2021). Studies support the sensitivity and specificity of pH testing for tube placement as a first-line measure to confirm tube placement. Testing of pH is more reliable when tube feeding can be stopped 1 hour before testing (Judd, 2020). Acceptable value range is a pH of 5.0 or less (Judd, 2020).

Clinical Judgment *Instruct client/family caregiver to avoid administration of all feedings, flushes, or medications if there is any doubt as to placement of enteral feeding tube (Anderson, 2019; Judd, 2020).*

STEP	RATIONALE
4. Observe as client/family caregiver demonstrates how to check correct placement of nasally placed tube.	Return demonstration identifies if there are areas for further teaching.
5. When client has a gastrostomy tube, watch client/family caregiver check for gastric residual volume by aspirating gastric contents.	Automatic cessation of feeding should not occur for gastric residual volume less than 500 mL in the absence of other signs of intolerance such as nausea or abdominal distention (Yasuda et al., 2021).
6. Discuss use of medical asepsis in setting up and changing administration sets, mixing formulas (do not add formula to hanging bag), refrigerating unused formula, limiting amount of formula "hung" at one time to amount that can be infused in 4- to 6-hour period (less time in warmer weather), and maintaining and caring for bag.	Medical aseptic technique minimizes risk for microorganism contamination. Refrigeration and limiting "hang" time reduce microorganisms. Changing administration sets every 24 hours reduces microorganism growth (USNLM, 2022a).
7. Instruct client/family caregiver that client needs to sit up in chair or have head of bed elevated at least 30 degrees, preferably 45 degrees, while receiving feedings or medications or when tube is flushed.	Decreases risk for aspiration. Aspiration is indicated by increased coughing, difficulty in breathing, or increased sputum (Bischoff et al., 2020).
8. Observe client/family caregiver mixing, administering, and storing formulas. Discuss flushing of tube after administration of feedings or medications.	Identifies competence and if there is a need for further teaching. Regular flushing of tube prevents clogging.
9. Watch client/family caregiver change administration sets and clean bags. Have them dispose of supplies, remove and dispose of gloves, and perform hand hygiene.	Demonstrates proper techniques for reducing transmission of microorganisms. Client/family caregiver must know proper infection prevention techniques.
10. Observe client/family caregiver administering medications and flushing tube (see Skill 21.2).	Ensures that medications are given correctly (Anderson, 2019).

Clinical Judgment *Verify the written health care provider orders to administer specific medications via enteral tubes. Check with the health care provider if the client can take the medications orally even with a feeding tube. Speak with the pharmacist about which medications can be safely crushed or dissolved and if sterile water is preferred solution (Institute for Safe Medication Practices [ISMP], 2022).*

STEP	RATIONALE
11. Discuss and observe use of infusion pump if client is receiving continuous feeding (see Chapter 31).	Use of tube-feeding infusion pumps is complex and requires reinforcement.
12. Discuss measures to stabilize feeding tube in clients with abdominal tubes and to clean and protect skin insertion site (see Chapter 31).	Prevents tube from dislodging and skin breakdown.
13. Provide contact information for ordering equipment and supplies or whom to call in case of equipment failure.	Ensures that family caregiver is able to respond in an emergency.
14. Place a bell or other type of sound-making device in an accessible location within client's reach.	Ensures client can call for assistance if needed and promotes safety.
15. Discuss emergency plan and actions to take for signs and symptoms of aspiration such as elevating head of bed, oral suctioning, and calling health care provider.	Ensures understanding of management of equipment, supplies, emergency plan, and collaboration.
16. Discuss whom to contact and when for signs of diarrhea, constipation, or weight loss.	Provides support to client/family caregiver.
17. Remove and dispose of gloves. Perform hand hygiene.	Reduces transmission of microorganisms.

STEP	RATIONALE

EVALUATION

1. Ask client/family caregiver to state purpose of home enteral nutrition therapy, feeding schedule, and signs and symptoms of complications.

Demonstrates cognitive learning.

2. Observe client/family caregiver performing medical asepsis techniques, checking tube placement, aspirating residuals, administering medications and feedings, and using and cleaning equipment.

Demonstrates psychomotor learning.

3. Ask client/family caregiver to state measures used to prevent complications (e.g., verification of tube position before each feeding, elevation of client's head during feeding, stabilization and flushing of tubing).

Ensures safe home management and identification of areas for teaching.

4. Ask client/family caregiver how to care for open formula cans.

5. **Use Teach-Back:** "I want to be sure I explained how to manage complications that can occur with your tube feedings. Tell me how to manage nausea, stomach fullness or distention, and diarrhea." Revise your instruction now or develop a plan for revised client/family caregiver teaching if client/family caregiver is not able to teach back correctly.

Ensures safe home management for preventing foodborne illness. Teach-back is a technique for health care providers to ensure that they have explained medical information clearly so that clients and their families understand what is communicated to them (AHRQ, 2023).

Unexpected Outcomes	Related Interventions
1. Feeding tube becomes displaced.	• Instruct client/family caregiver to stop feeding and notify home care nurse. • Nurse or health care provider will reposition feeding tube and verify placement before initiating any enteral feeding.
2. Signs and symptoms of aspiration are present.	• Stop feeding. Raise head of bed. • Verify tube position. • Notify health care provider.
3. Client develops diarrhea.	• Notify health care provider. • Collaborate with registered dietitian and health care provider to consider change in strength, type, or rate of enteral feeding, or temperature of feeding (Johnson et al., 2019).
4. Skin surrounding stoma breaks down, or drainage around insertion site develops.	• Clean stoma area more frequently. • Apply antibiotic ointment around stoma as ordered. • Contact health care provider.

Documentation

• Document instructions given to client and family caregiver and their response.
• Document specifics of enteral feeding plan, including type and size of tube in home, formula, and amounts to be administered in specific time frames.
• Clients or family caregivers need to record I&O, daily weights, amount of gastric fluid aspirated before each feeding (or every 4 hours if receiving continuous feeding), date and time of feedings, amount and type of formula, any additives, and date and time that administration sets are changed.

Hand-Off Reporting

• Report reason for enteral feeding, type of tube and equipment, contact information for supplier, client's or family caregiver's response to teaching, and evaluation of client or family caregiver learning.
• Report complications and concerns to health care providers involved in client's care.

Special Considerations

Client Education

• Performing skill without nurse in attendance may provoke anxiety. Always leave a phone number and instructions about how to reach home care nurse if needed.

• Teach client and family caregiver the maximum hang time for any enteral feeding. After a can of formula has been opened, it should remain at room temperature for no longer than 8 to 12 hours.
• Educate client and family caregiver that routine water flushing before and after feeding is usually recommended to prevent tube obstruction (Bischoff et al., 2020).

Pediatrics

• Medications should not be mixed with enteral formula. Pharmacists should be consulted prior to administering medications through a feeding tube to confirm the therapeutic effectiveness (Cober & Gura, 2019).
• Children who receive long-term home enteral feedings often experience developmental and growth delays. Other common problems include sleep disturbance, tube blockages, problems with delivery of equipment, and equipment malfunction. Therefore these children require close follow-up and frequent nutritional monitoring.
• Teach family caregiver to position children who cannot sit up during or after a tube feeding on their right side during the tube feeding and for approximately 1 hour after it (Hockenberry et al., 2024).

Older Adults
- Assess for changes and limitations in sensory function, mobility, or dexterity that indicate a need to teach a family caregiver how to administer feedings.
- Clients with dementia who are receiving enteral tube feeding are at higher risk for incidence of removal of the tube (Bischoff et al., 2020).

Populations With Disabilities
- Using enteral tubes to administer medications to clients at residential facilities increases the risk of multiple medications being administered at one time, increasing risk of drug interactions (Bishcoff et al., 2020).

◆ SKILL 42.8   Managing Parenteral Nutrition in the Home

Parenteral nutrition (PN) in the home is indicated for clients who cannot take adequate nutrition by mouth and when enteral feedings are contraindicated (e.g., cancer, renal failure, motor neuron disorders, cardiac disease, chronic respiratory or gastrointestinal disorders) (Bischoff et al., 2020). Nurses who manage PN in the home collaborate frequently with registered dietitians and other health care providers to ensure that clients receive sufficient calories, protein, and fluid. PN is administered through a long-term central venous catheter (CVC) such as a tunneled CVC (e.g., Groshong or Hickman catheter), an implantable port, or a peripherally inserted central catheter (PICC) (see Chapter 28). Potential complications are associated with PN infusion, including intravenous (IV)-related blood clots and bloodstream infection.

PN is individually formulated and includes a mixture of amino acids, dextrose, fat emulsions, vitamins, electrolytes, minerals, and trace elements (Iacone et al., 2020). Administering PN in the home requires an interprofessional approach and a client and/or family caregiver who demonstrates competency in its preparation and administration (Pironi et al., 2020).

Usually, administration of PN in the home takes about 12 hours; thus many clients choose to receive their PN during the night. Because of the risks involved with PN and because management in the home is complex, clients receive their first infusion in an acute care setting. After discharge, a home care nurse visits frequently. The home care nurse will need to carefully assess the reaction of the client or family caregiver to the use of the technology needed to administer PN at home and provide emotional support. Although administering PN in the home increases clients'

autonomy, it often interferes with their ability to maintain their normal routines. Work with the client or family caregiver to stress the benefits and offer support in dealing with related issues.

Delegation
The skill of managing PN in the home cannot be delegated to assistive personnel (AP). Instruct the AP to:
- Report findings of fingerstick blood glucose monitoring
- Report vital signs outside of normal range to nurse
- Report client complaints of shortness of breath, headache, weakness, or discomfort
- Report if the catheter dressings are wet or if there is bleeding at the site

Interprofessional Collaboration
- The health care provider, nutritional specialist, and/or nutrition service are frequently involved in the management of PN in the home.

Equipment
- IV solution of PN
- IV tubing with optional filter
- Electronic IV infusion pump with alarms and protection from free flow
- Home blood glucose monitoring equipment
- Antiseptic swabs
- Clean gloves
- Log

STEP	RATIONALE
ASSESSMENT	
1. Identify client using at least two identifiers during first visit according to agency policy. Confirmation of the address also occurs in the home setting and can be used as one of the two identifiers. Facial recognition can be used as one of the two identifiers for ongoing visits (TJC, 2023).	Ensures client safety. Complies with The Joint Commission standards and improves client safety (TJC, 2023).
2. Assess client's electronic health record (EHR) including health care provider's orders and nurses' notes. Note any previous teaching sessions for parental nutrition and client's/family caregiver's response to teaching.	Identifies focus of instruction and potential difficulty with teaching how to perform parental nutrition in the home.
3. Assess client's/family caregiver's health literacy.	Determines degree to which individuals have the ability to find, understand, and use information and services to make informed health-related decisions and actions for themselves and others (CDC, 2023).
4. Assess client's fluid and electrolyte levels, serum albumin, total protein, transferrin, prealbumin, triglycerides, and glucose levels. Assess body composition and consult with registered dietitian nutritionist.	Provides additional baseline assessment data (Pironi et al., 2020). Body composition assessment is evaluated with varied tests such as ultrasonography and computed tomography (Sheean et al., 2019). The PN mixture will vary depending on client factors such as nutritional status, organ functioning, and underlying disease (Iacone et al., 2020).

STEP	RATIONALE
5. Perform hand hygiene. Instruct family caregiver to apply clean gloves.	Reduces transmission of microorganisms. Client and family caregiver must be knowledgeable about infection-prevention techniques.
6. Have family caregiver observe while you assess client's venous access device for edema, drainage, tenderness, and signs of inflammation (see Chapter 28). Measure circumference of upper arm if client has peripherally inserted central catheter (PICC); mark place on arm where measurement was taken.	Infection is common complication when client has venous access device. Measurement of arm helps detect infiltration of PICC. Mark on arm ensures consistent measurements over time.
7. Remove and dispose of gloves and perform hand hygiene.	Reduces transmission of microorganisms. Client and family caregiver must be knowledgeable about infection-prevention techniques.
8. Verify health care provider's order for PN, including amino acids, dextrose, fat emulsions, vitamins, minerals, trace elements, electrolytes, and flow rate.	Ensures safe and accurate PN administration.
9. Assess client's learning readiness, anxiety and ability to concentrate (consider presence of pain, nausea, or fatigue and client interest in instruction), and learning style preference.	Presence of significant illness, frailty, or confusion affects client's ability to attend to teaching plan. Indicates need to rely on family caregiver for learning and implementation (if available) on short- or long-term basis. Learning style affects choice of teaching resources.
10. Assess client's/family caregiver's previous knowledge and experience in managing PN in home. Have client/family caregiver perform return demonstration if able to perform skill.	Determines level of understanding before beginning teaching session.
11. Assess client's/family caregiver's goals or preferences for how skill is to be performed or what is expected.	Allows care to be individualized to client.

PLANNING

1. Expected outcomes following completion of procedure: • Client/family caregiver is able to administer PN correctly. • Client/family caregiver demonstrates proper care of central venous catheter (CVC). • Client/family caregiver explains how to properly store and maintain formulas for feeding. • Client/family caregiver states signs and symptoms of alterations that need to be reported to health care provider. • Client/family caregiver demonstrates correct measurement of blood glucose.	Indicates that skills have been effectively learned. Prevents infection and ensures patency of venous access device. Knowledge of infection control principles prevents foodborne illness. Ensures safe administration of PN in home. Necessary for safe monitoring of client's response to PN therapy.
2. Select setting in home where client is most likely to administer PN and that is conducive to a teaching session.	Practicing in same environment where skill is routinely performed facilitates comprehension and learning. Teaching is more effective when the environment is conducive to learning.
a. Select room that is well lit with comfortable seating.	Lighting of room improves visualization of skill.
b. Organize supplies.	Ensures more efficiency during teaching session.
c. Be sure that client is close and can see nurse clearly.	Visualization of the nurse's techniques requires proximity to the nurse.
d. Control sources of noise and distractions.	Room environment needs to minimize existing sensory alterations. Comfortable environment free of distractions promotes client's attention.
e. Explain procedure to client.	Promotes cooperation.

IMPLEMENTATION

1. Provide name and phone number of people or resources available 24 hours a day, 7 days a week in case problems arise.	Provides reassurance and allows client/family caregiver to troubleshoot problems and answer questions.
2. Explain type/name of infusion, volume and infusion rate, expected outcomes, and components of PN. Explain that PN needs to be stored in refrigerator.	Allows client/family caregiver to verify that correct PN is infused and that client/family caregiver understands expected outcomes of care. Refrigeration maintains integrity of PN.
3. Have client/family caregiver perform each of the following steps with guidance from nurse. Do not rush client.	Allows you to correct errors in technique as they occur and discuss implications.

STEP	RATIONALE
4. Instruct client/family caregiver to inspect the IV solution bag label, ensure that client's name is on label, ensure that solution has not expired, and check bag for leaks.	Ensures that client/family caregiver knows how to check pharmacy-prepared solution to ensure right client receives right PN. Bag needs to be intact to maintain closed system and ensure that client receives all prescribed nutrients.
5. Suggest taking PN solution out of refrigerator for 30 to 60 minutes before scheduled infusion time.	Chilled solution often causes discomfort; allowing solution to warm enhances comfort during infusion.
6. Explain need to inspect fluid in bag for color and precipitates.	Changes in color or precipitates in bag indicate disruption in PN.

Clinical Judgment *If precipitate appears, components of mixture are separated, or color changes, explain that solution needs to be discarded. To decrease chance of waste, calculate the amount of PN needed for a specified period of time so there is enough but not too much.*

STEP	RATIONALE
7. Have client/family caregiver perform hand hygiene and apply clean gloves with you. Demonstrate how to attach IV tubing to bag, how to attach filter to IV tubing (optional), how to prime IV tubing, and how to load IV tubing into electronic infusion pump (see Chapter 28).	Reduces spread of microorganisms. Prepares PN solution for IV administration.
8. Wipe CVC port with alcohol and show how to flush CVC and connect IV tubing to port (see Chapter 28). Use needleless system whenever possible.	CVC needs to be patent, and IV tubing needs to connect to CVC to allow PN to be administered. Needleless systems prevent needlestick injuries.
9. Explain how to determine appropriate rate of infusion and program infusion pump (see Skill 28.2). Caution client and family caregiver against changing rate to "catch up."	Ensures that PN is administered at appropriate rate.
10. Have client and family caregiver remove and dispose of gloves; perform hand hygiene.	Reduces spread of microorganisms.
11. When infusion is completed, explain and demonstrate how to disconnect IV tubing and flush CVC (see Chapter 28). Ensure that client/family caregiver performs hand hygiene before and after disconnecting line.	Flushing CVC following infusion maintains patency of vascular access device. Meticulous hand hygiene prevents infection.
12. Describe appropriate use and storage of infusion pump and supplies. Explain appropriate tubing replacement schedules.	Maintains integrity of equipment; appropriate timing of tubing changes reduces risk of infection.
13. Help to develop plan for appropriate disposal of supplies, including needles, syringes, and unused medications or solutions, using principles of Standard Precautions.	Implementation of Standard Precautions is necessary to prevent transmission of communicable diseases and needlestick injuries. Check government recommendations by location for proper disposal of needles in a home setting. Recommendations may include medically approved sharps container or a strong plastic container with lid (SafeNeedleDisposal.org, 2023).
14. Demonstrate appropriate care of CVC site; discuss how to change dressings, frequency of dressing changes, and signs of infection (see Skill 28.6).	Reduces risk of infection at CVC insertion site.
15. Teach client and/or family caregiver about signs and symptoms that indicate potential complications from PN therapy (e.g., infection and phlebitis at CVC site, refeeding syndrome, hyperglycemia, hypernatremia, hypophosphatemia, hypokalemia, hypomagnesemia) and when to call for help.	Knowledge of complications of PN therapy allows for early detection and appropriate action.
16. Demonstrate how to use a glucose monitor for testing and monitoring blood glucose. Explain frequency of testing, normal glucose values, and what to do if values fall outside of expected range (see Chapter 7).	PN increases blood glucose levels, which negatively affects client outcomes. Frequent monitoring of glucose level helps detect problems early. Expect testing frequency to decrease as client's condition and response to PN stabilize.
17. Help client to a comfortable position.	Restores comfort and sense of well-being.
18. Place a bell or other type of sound-making device in an accessible location within client's reach.	Ensures client can call for assistance if needed and promotes safety.
19. Remove and dispose of gloves. Perform hand hygiene.	Reduces transmission of microorganisms. Client and family caregiver must be knowledgeable about infection-prevention techniques.
20. Provide client with logbook to document administration of PN, weights, intake and output (I&O), and blood glucose levels.	Allows health care providers and clients to evaluate outcomes and detect adverse effects of nutritional therapy.
21. Help client develop plan to reorder supplies, PN fluid, and prescribed additives; for emergencies (e.g., what to do if electricity goes out); and for home safety (e.g., how to get to bathroom without tripping over IV tubing).	Plans allow for continuous, safe, and effective administration of PN.

STEP	RATIONALE

EVALUATION

1. Have client/family caregiver independently demonstrate initiation, infusion, and discontinuation of PN infusion and CVC site care.
2. Watch client/family caregiver clean and store PN, equipment, and supplies.
3. Ask client/family caregiver to identify expected outcomes of nutritional therapy.
4. Have client/family caregiver independently demonstrate blood glucose monitoring and documentation.
5. Watch client/family caregiver document information in log. Review client's/family caregiver's log periodically to ensure that information is being documented correctly.

6. *Use Teach-Back:* "I want to be sure I explained the common signs and symptoms of infection and other potential complications of PN. Tell me the signs and symptoms of infection." Revise your instruction now or develop a plan for revised client/family caregiver teaching if client/family caregiver is not able to teach back correctly.

Feedback through return demonstration of psychomotor skill is best means of evaluating mastery of skill.

Proper cleaning and storage reduce risk of bacterial growth.

Measures client cognitive learning and confirms understanding of information.
Ensures mastering of skill needed for effective evaluation of client status.
Health care providers make changes in client care based on information provided by client. To ensure that changes are made appropriately, client needs to document accurate information.
Teach-back is a technique for health care providers to ensure that they have explained medical information clearly so that clients and their families understand what is communicated to them (AHRQ, 2023).

Unexpected Outcomes

1. Client/family caregiver is unable to manage home PN therapy or verbalize information that was taught.

2. Client/family caregiver reports signs and symptoms of complications from PN or CVC.

Related Interventions

- Ask client/family caregiver to describe difficulties experienced while performing skill.
- Use different teaching strategy.
- Teach family caregiver further and evaluate need to increase frequency of home visits to ensure safe administration of PN at home.
- Inform health care provider.
- Tell client/family caregiver to call emergency medical services (EMS) if signs and symptoms are severe.

Documentation

- Document information taught, client's and family caregiver's response, and outcomes of PN therapy (e.g., weight, electrolyte and glucose levels, physical assessment findings) in home care log.
- Document appearance of CVC site, infusions, glucose monitoring results, and client's weight in home care log.

Hand-Off Reporting

- Report location of PN teaching session, who participated, content discussed, client's and/or family caregiver's response to PN procedure, and evaluation of client learning.
- Report any signs and symptoms of complications from PN or CVC to health care providers involved in client's care.

Special Considerations
Client Education

- Assess client's psychosocial status while providing information. Many clients experience a decrease in the quality of life when PN feedings are started in the home, which often increases anxiety and decreases comprehension of information.
- Eating is often a social event. When clients do not eat, they tend to feel socially isolated. Teach clients and family caregivers the importance of maintaining social relationships and enhancing social support during PN therapy. Refer client to support groups and other resources such as the Oley Foundation (https://oley.org/page/SupportGroups).

- Telemedicine is available for home PN clients (Folwarski et al., 2021).
- Always leave a phone number and instructions about how to reach home care nurse if needed.

Pediatrics

- The risk for displacement of the CVC increases as the child grows. Ensure that the placement of the venous access device is confirmed with x-ray film examination as the child grows.
- Teach the family caregiver to socialize child with other children to enhance development (Hockenberry et al., 2024).
- Composition and volume of PN solution are based on the child's nutritional requirements and growth (Goulet et al., 2021).

Older Adults

- Frail older adults are at high risk for electrolyte disturbances. Frequently assess and monitor their response to PN and their laboratory values.
- Carefully assess client's ability to perform skill. Management of PN at home is complex and requires manual dexterity, visual acuity, and high-level critical thinking and decision-making skills. Include family caregiver in teaching plan to help with management of home PN.

Populations With Disabilities

- It is important to consider that previous life experiences may influence the readiness to learn and knowledge acquisition of people with intellectual disabilities (Geukes et al., 2019).

✦ CLINICAL JUDGMENT AND NEXT-GENERATION NCLEX® EXAMINATION–STYLE QUESTIONS

The home health care nurse is scheduled for an initial visit with a 77-year-old client who lives in a private home with a 71-year-old spouse. The client has cognitive decline due to dementia and is currently hospitalized with a new diagnosis of COPD. He is to be discharged in 24 hours. Enteral tube feedings that were initiated in the hospital are to continue at home. The client is also to receive home oxygen therapy.

1. Which home assessments will the nurse perform in advance of home oxygen being delivered for the client? **Select all that apply.**
   1. Presence of smoke detectors
   2. Access to fire extinguishers
   3. Sources of heating
   4. Smoking status of people in the home
   5. Available electric outlets

2. The nurse is preparing for an initial teaching session with the caregiver about management of the client's enteral tube feedings. Which steps need to be completed before the nurse begins teaching? **Select all that apply.**
   1. Review health care provider's orders and nurses' notes.
   2. Determine health literacy level of the caregiver.
   3. Assess caregiver's understanding of the enteral feeding process.
   4. Evaluate availability of space in home to prepare feedings and store supplies.
   5. Gather information about sterile technique that is needed for feedings.

3. After teaching, the caregiver says, "I will crush up all the medications and give them in the tube feeding." Which nursing response is appropriate?
   1. "That is a very efficient way to administer medication."
   2. "Do you have a pill crusher that is available?"
   3. "It is better to dissolve medications instead of crush them."
   4. "There are medications that cannot be crushed."

4. The client will also have a home health care aide (assistive personnel) who visits the home. Which care will the nurse delegate to AP?
   1. Teaching the caregiver about the feeding tube
   2. Assessing the client's nutrition status
   3. Evaluating the need for more home care equipment
   4. Providing ongoing hygiene and oral care

5. At a subsequent visit, the caregiver reports that the client's nephew visits often and vapes inside the home.

   Determine whether each nursing health teaching statement below is indicated or not indicated.

Nursing Health Teaching	Indicated	Not Indicated
"Vaping devices are combustible around oxygen. Persons can be seriously injured when vaping devices are used in homes with oxygen therapy."		
"After turning off the oxygen for 2-3 minutes, it is safe to use the vaping device in the home."		
"I would notify the fire company that someone is vaping in the home so that they can tell you if it is safe or not."		
"If anyone vapes in the home, you and your spouse are at serious risk of experiencing a home explosion and fire."		
"As long as you are vaping in a room away from the oxygen, there is no need to be concerned."		
"Which type and brand of vaping device are you using?"		

Visit the Evolve site for Answers to Clinical Judgment and Next-Generation NCLEX® Examination–Style Questions.

REFERENCES

Agency for Healthcare Research and Quality (AHRQ): *Teach-back: intervention,* 2023. https://www.ahrq.gov/patient-safety/reports/engage/interventions/teachback.html.

American Heart Association (AHA): *Monitoring blood pressure at home can be tricky. Here's how to do it right,* 2022. https://www.heart.org/en/news/2022/05/23/monitoring-blood-pressure-at-home-can-be-tricky-heres-how-to-do-it-right. Accessed August 24, 2023.

American Lung Association: *Oxygen therapy,* 2023. https://www.lung.org/lung-health-diseases/lung-procedures-and-tests/oxygen-therapy. Accessed August 24, 2023.

American Nurses Association (ANA): *Nursing: scope and standards of practice,* ed 4, Silver Spring, MD, 2020, The Association.

American Society for Parenteral and Enteral Nutrition (ASPEN): *Resources for patient populations or healthcare management,* 2023. https://www.nutritioncare.org/Guidelines_and_Clinical_Resources/Resources_for_Patient_Populations_or_Healthcare_Management/. Accessed August 29, 2023.

Anderson L: Enteral feeding tubes: an overview of nursing care, *Br J Nurs* 28(12):753, 2019.

Aungsuroch Y, et al: Management program affects blood pressure among Indonesians with hypertension: a quasi-experimental study, *Iran J Nurs Midwifery Res* 27(3):234, 2022.

Balanis T, Sanner B: Detection of atrial fibrillation using a home blood pressure monitor, *Vasc Health Risk Manag* 17:408, 2021.

Balhi S, Arfaoui R: Barriers affecting patient adherence to intermittent self-catheterisation, *Br J Community Nurs* 26(9):444–448, 2021.

Balhi S, Mrabet MK: Teaching patients clean intermittent self-catheterisation: key points, *Brit J Community Nurs* 25(12):590, 2020.

Bastable S, Gonzalez KM: Overview of education in healthcare. In Bastable S, editor: *Nurse as educator principles of teaching and learning for nursing practice,* ed 5, Burlington, MA, 2019, Jones & Bartlett.

Bischoff SC, et al: ESPEN guideline on home enteral nutrition, *Clin Nutr* 39(1): 5–22, 2020.

Bradley E: Achieving independence in toileting: self-catheterization efficacy and the role of the school nurse, *NASN Sch Nurse* 35(6):314, 2020.

Branson RD, et al: Home oxygen therapy devices: providing the prescription, *Respir Care* 64(2):230–232, 2019.

Centers for Disease Control and Prevention (CDC): *Disinfection in ambulatory care*, 2019. https://www.cdc.gov/infectioncontrol/guidelines/disinfection/healthcare-equipment.html#DisinfectionAmbulatory. Accessed August 22, 2023.

Centers for Disease Control and Prevention (CDC): *Medication safety program*, 2020. https://www.cdc.gov/medicationsafety/campaign_initiatives.html. August 22, 2023.

Centers for Disease Control and Prevention (CDC): *Health literacy numeracy*, 2022. https://www.cdc.gov/healthliteracy/researchevaluate/numeracy.html. August 22, 2023.

Centers for Disease Control and Prevention (CDC): *What is Health Literacy?* 2023. https://www.cdc.gov/healthliteracy/learn/index.html. August 22, 2023.

Centers for Medicare and Medicaid Services: n.d. Home page: www.cms.gov.

Chandar JJ, et al: Assessing the link between modified 'teach back' method and improvement in knowledge of the medical regimen among youth with kidney transplants: the application of digital media, *Patient Educ Couns* 102:1035, 2019.

Chauhan D, et al: Nasogastric tube feeding in older patients: a review of current practice and challenges faced, *Curr Gerontol Geriatr Res* 2021:6650675, 2021.

Cober MP, Gura KM: Enteral and parenteral nutrition considerations in pediatric patients, *Am J Health Syst Pharm* 76(19):1506, 2019.

Commonwealth of Massachusetts: *Home oxygen safety*, 2023. https://www.mass.gov/service-details/home-oxygen-safety. Accessed August 24, 2023.

Cutilli CC: Excellence in patient education: evidence-based education that "sticks" and improves patient outcomes, *Nurs Clin North Am* 55(2):279–280, 2020.

Doorenbos A, et al: eHealth education: Methods to enhance oncology nurse, patient, and caregiver teaching, *Clin J Onc Nurs* 24(3):43–45, 2020.

Environmental Protection Agency (EPA): *Mercury thermometers*, 2023. https://www.epa.gov/mercury/mercury-thermometers. August 22, 2023.

Fenske RF: Tablet computer use at the bedside in a new patient/family education program, *J Hosp Librariansh* 19(2):110–128, 2019.

Folwarski M, et al: Organizational issues of home parenteral nutrition during COVID-19 pandemic: results from multicenter, nationwide study, *Nutri* 86:2, 2021.

Geukes C, et al: Health literacy and people with intellectual disabilities: What we know, what we do not know, and what we need: a theoretical discourse, *Int J Environ Res Public Health* 16(3):E463, 2019.

Goessl C, et al: Effectiveness of DVD vs. group-initiated diabetes prevention on information uptake for high & low literacy participants, *Patient Educ Couns* 102(5):968–969, 2019.

Goulet O, et al: Pediatric home parental nutrition in France: a six years national survey, *Clin Nutr* 40(10):5280, 2021.

Gray M, et al: Nursing practice related to intermittent catheterization, *J Wound Ostomy Continence Nurs* 46(5):418, 2019.

Harding MM, et al: *Lewis's medical-surgical nursing: assessment and management of clinical problems*, ed 11, St. Louis, 2020, Elsevier.

Hayes D, et al: Home oxygen therapy for children, *Am J Respir Crit Care Med* 199:1:e5–e6, 2019.

Healthcare Infection Control Practices Advisory Committee (HICPAC): *2019 Guidelines for prevention of catheter-associated urinary tract infections.* https://www.cdc.gov/infectioncontrol/pdf/guidelines/cauti-guidelines-H.pdf. Accessed August 25, 2023.

Hentzen C, et al: What criteria affect a patient's choice of catheter for self-catheterization? *Neurol Urodyan* 39(1):412, 2020.

Hermanns N, et al: Trends in diabetes self-management education: Where are we coming from and where are we going? A narrative review, *Diabet Med* 37(3):436, 2020.

Hockenberry MJ, et al: *Wong's nursing care of infants and children*, ed 12, St. Louis, 2024, Elsevier.

Iacone R, et al: Macronutrients in parenteral nutrition: amino acids, *Nutrients* 12(3):772–773, 2020.

Imperial-Perez F, Heilemann MV: Having to be the one: mothers providing home care to infants with complex cardiac needs, *Am J Crit Care* 28(5):354, 2019.

Institute for Safe Medication Practices (ISMP): Preventing errors when preparing and administering medications via enteral feeding tubes, *Acute care ISMP medication safety alert!* 27(23):1–5, 2022. https://www.nutritioncare.org/uploadedFiles/Documents/Guidelines_and_Clinical_Resources/ISMP%20Safety%20Alert_Medications%20and%20Enteral%20Feeding%20Tubes.pdf Accessed August 29, 2023.

Jacobs SS, et al: Home oxygen for adults with chronic lung disease: an official American Thoracic Society clinical practice guide, *Am J Respir Crit Care* 202(10):e122–e137, 2020.

Johns Hopkins Medicine: *Cleaning and caring for tracheostomy equipment*, n.d. https://www.hopkinsmedicine.org/tracheostomy/living/equipment_cleaning.html#trach. Accessed August 24, 2023.

Johnson TW, et al: Addressing frequent issues of home enteral nutrition patients, *Nutr Clin Pract* 34(2):189–190, 2019.

Judd M: Confirming nasogastric tube placement in adults, *Nurs 2020* 50(4):46, 2020.

Kapadia MR, et al: Teaching patient-related communication to surgical residents in brief training sessions, *J Surg Educ* 77(6):1496, 2020.

Karaca T, et al: Caring for patients with a tracheostomy at home: a descriptive, cross-sectional study to evaluate health care practices and caregiver burden, *Ostomy Wound Manage* 65(3):22, 2019.

Kaviany P, Collaco JM: Oxygen delivery in the home setting: Supplemental oxygen can be delivered safely to patients in their home, *Contemp Pediatr* 36(9):14, 2019.

Kim M, et al: Health literacy level and comprehension of prescription and nonprescription drug information, *Int J Environ Res Public Health* 19(11):6665, 2022.

Kitchie S: Readiness to learn. In Bastable S, editor: *Nurse as educator principles of teaching and learning for nursing practice*, ed 5, Burlington, MA, 2019, Jones & Bartlett, pp 131–139.

Jeminiwa R, et al: Impact of eHealth on medication adherence among patients with asthma: a systematic review and meta-analysis, *Respir Med* 149:61, 2019.

Lacasse Y, et al: Home oxygen in chronic obstructive pulmonary disease, *Am J Respir Crit Care Med* 197(10):1255, 2018.

Latteck ÄD, Bruland D: Inclusion of people with intellectual disabilities in health literacy: Lessons learned from three participative projects for future initiatives, *Int J Environ Res Public Health* 17(7):8, 2020.

Lay S, et al: Home care program increases the engagement in patients with heart failure, *Home Health Care Manag Pract* 31(2):99, 103, 2019.

Lee S, et al: Effects of the chronic disease self-management program on medication adherence among older adults, *Transl Behav Med* 9(2):380–382, 2019.

Lindroos AS, et al: Agreement between ambulatory and home blood pressure monitoring in detecting nighttime hypertension and nondipping patterns in the general population, *Am J Hypertens* 32(8):734, 2019.

Logan K: An exploration of men's experiences of learning intermittent self-catheterisation with a silicone catheter, *Brit J Nurs* 29(2):84, 2020.

McCoy JL, et al: Pediatric tracheostomy care simulation: real-life scenarios in a safe learning environment, *Respir Care* 67(1):42–43, 2021.

Meister KD, et al: Multidisciplinary safety recommendations after tracheostomy during COVID-19 pandemic: state of the art review, *Otolaryngol Head Neck Surg* 164(5):8, 2021.

Mikulski BS, et al: Mobile health applications and medication adherence of patients with hypertension: a systematic review and meta-analysis, *Am J Prev Med* 62(4):626, 2022.

National Tracheostomy Safe Project (NTSP): *Cleaning or changing the inner cannula*, 2023. http://www.tracheostomy.org.uk/healthcare-staff/basic-care/inner-cannula-care. Accessed August 24, 2023.

Network of the National Library of Medicine (NNLM): *An introduction to health literacy*, n.d. https://nnlm.gov/guides/intro-health-literacy. Accessed August 24, 2023.

Nies MA, McEwen M: *Community public health nursing*, ed 7, St. Louis, 2019, Elsevier.

Office of Disease Prevention and Health Promotion (ODPHP): *Healthy People 2020*, 2020. https://www.healthypeople.gov/2020/topics-objectives/topic/social-determinants-health/interventions-resources/health-literacy. Accessed August 22, 2023.

Ojo O, et al: The effect of enteral tube feeding on patients' health-related quality of life: a systematic review, *Nutr* 11(5):1, 2019.

Okwose NC, et al: Overcoming barriers to engagement and adherence to a home-based physical activity intervention for patients with heart failure: a qualitative focus group study, *BMJ Open* 10(9):e036382, 2020.

Orlandin L, et al: Difficulties of patients and caregivers in performing clean intermittent catheterization, *J Enterostomal Ther* 18 (e1520):2, 2020.

Park L, et al: A guide to undertaking and understanding blood pressure measurement, *Brit J Nurs* 31(7):360–361, 2022.

Pars H, Soyer T: Home gastrostomy feeding education program: Effects on the caregiving burden, knowledge, and anxiety level of mothers, *JPEN J Parenter Enteral Nutr* 44(6):1029, 2020.

Patiag MC, et al: Do errorless methods improve discharge medication instruction and adherence? *Rehabil Nurs* 45(6):358–359, 2020.

Patient Safety Network: *E-cigarette explosion in a patient room*, 2019. https://psnet.ahrq.gov/webmm/case/474/E-cigarette-Explosion-in-a-Patient-Room. Accessed August 25, 2023.

Pino S, et al: Improving medication adherence in hypertensive patients: a scoping review, *Prev Med* 146(2021):1, 2021.

Pironi L, et al: ESPEN guideline on home parenteral nutrition, *Clin Nutr* 39(6):1645–1666, 2020.

Prickett K, et al: Simulation-based education to improve emergency management skills in caregivers of tracheostomy patients, *Int J Pediatr Otorhinolaryngol* 120:159, 2019.

Prochnow JA, et al: Improving patient and caregiver new medication education using an innovative teach-back toolkit, *J Nurs Care Qual* 34(2):101–102, 2019.

Qiao X, et al: The association between frailty and medication adherence among community-dwelling older adults with chronic diseases: medication beliefs acting as mediators, *Patient Educ Couns* 103(12):2554, 2020.

Reber CR: Urinary elimination. In Perry AG, et al., editors: *Nursing interventions & clinical skills*, ed 7, St. Louis, 2020, Elsevier, pp 499–506.

Rojas-Ocana MJ, et al: Educational interventions by nurses in caregivers with their elderly patients at home, *Prim Health Care Res Dev* 22(e26):7, 2021.

Ruel J: Home health care nursing impacts on emergency department utilization, *Adv Emer Nurs J* 43(4):325, 2021.

Research Institute for Home Care: *About*, 2023. https://researchinstituteforhomecare.org/about/. Accessed August 22, 2023.

Saadat SH, et al: Clean intermittent catheterization: Single use vs. reuse, *Can Urol Assoc J* 13(2):64–65, 2019.

SafeNeedleDisposal.org: *Sharps management*, 2023. https://safeneedledisposal.org/. Accessed August 25, 2023.

Sassani JC, et al: Variables associated with an inability to learn clean intermittent self-catheterization after urogynecologic surgery, *Int Urogynecol J* 5:1, 2019.

Shaeffer AJ: *Placement and management of urinary bladder catheters in adults*, 2023, UpToDate. https://www.uptodate.com/contents/placement-and-management-of-urinary-bladder-catheters-in-adults. Accessed August 25, 2023.

Sheean P, et al: American Society for Parenteral and Enteral Nutrition clinical guidelines: the validity of body composition assessment in clinical populations, *JPEN J Parenter Enteral Nutr* 6:1, 2019.

Shimbo D, et al: Self-measured blood pressure monitoring at home: a joint policy statement from the American Heart Association and American Medical Association, *Circulation* 142(4):e46–e47, 2020.

Suntharalingam J, et al: British Thoracic Society quality standards for home oxygen use in adults, *BMJ Open Respir Res* 18:4(1):e000223, 2018.

Taba M, et al: Adolescents' self-efficacy and digital health literacy: a cross-sectional mixed methods study, *BMC Public Health* 22(1):10–11, 2022.

Tabi K, et al: Mobile apps for medication management: review and analysis, *JMIR Mhealth Uhealth* 7(9):e2, 2019.

Taylor K: Enabling patients with learning disabilities to self-manage lower limb lymphoedema, *Brit J Nurs* 30(13):825, 2021.

The Joint Commission (TJC): *2022 National patient safety goals for the home care program*, Oakbrook Terrace, IL, 2021, The Joint Commission. https://www.jointcommission.org/-/media/tjc/documents/standards/national-patient-safety-goals/2022/npsg_chapter_ome_jan2022.pdf. Accessed August 24, 2023.

Touhy TT, Jett KF: *Ebersole and Hess' toward healthy aging: human needs and nursing response*, ed 6, St. Louis, 2022, Elsevier.

Tyson DM, et al: Understanding cancer survivors' educational needs about prescription opioid medications: Implications for cancer education and health literacy, *J Cancer Educ* 36(2):215, 2021.

United States National Library of Medicine (USNLM): *Gastrostomy feeding tube – pump – child*, 2022a. https://medlineplus.gov/ency/patientinstructions/000333.htm. Accessed August 24, 2023.

United States National Library of Medicine (USNLM): *Oxygen safety*, 2022b. https://medlineplus.gov/ency/patientinstructions/000049.htm. Accessed August 24, 2023.

United States National Library of Medicine (USNLM): *Self catheterization – male*, 2023a. https://medlineplus.gov/ency/patientinstructions/000143.htm. Accessed August 24, 2023.

United States National Library of Medicine (USNLM): *Temperature measurement*, 2023b. https://medlineplus.gov/ency/article/003400.htm. Accessed August 24, 2023.

Weekley MS, Bland LE: *Oxygen administration*, 2023, Stat Pearls (Internet). https://www.ncbi.nlm.nih.gov/books/NBK551617/. Accessed August 29, 2023.

Wood LS, et al: Immune checkpoint inhibitor therapy: key principles when educating patients, *Clin J Oncol Nurs* 23(3):272–274, 277–278, 2019.

Yasuda H, et al: Monitoring of gastric residual volume during enteral nutrition, *Cochrane Database Syst Rev* 9(9):CD013335, 2021.

Yin HS, et al: Preventing home medication administration errors, *Pediatr* 148(6):1, 2021.

UNIT 15
Home Care:
Next-Generation NCLEX® (NGN)–Style Unfolding Case Study

PHASE 1

QUESTION 1.

The home health nurse is visiting a client who has been recently discharged back to home after a prolonged hospitalization.

Highlight the findings that would concern the nurse.

History and Physical	Nurses' Notes	Vital Signs	Laboratory Results

1400: 77-year-old client seen in the home today following discharge yesterday after a 3-week hospitalization for pneumonia. Medical history of osteoporosis and two hip fractures over the past 3 years. Has lived in this house for 30+ years. Spouse died last year; no one else resides here. Three cats are noted going inside and outside via small pet door. The client is alert and oriented × 4 and expresses happiness at being home. Reports "I may be tired, but I am glad to be home." Denies pain. Vital signs: T 37.2°C (98.9°F); HR 68 beats/min; RR 14 breaths/min; BP 110/68 mm Hg; Spo₂ 98% on RA. Assessment reveals a frail client. PERRLA, cranial nerves intact. Lungs clear to auscultation, heart regular rate and rhythm with no murmurs, and a soft, nontender abdomen. Full range of motion in upper and lower extremities. No skin abnormalities noted. Gait somewhat shuffled.

QUESTION 2.

The nurse further assesses the client's house.

Complete the following sentence by selecting from the list of word choices below.

The nurse notes that the client is at high risk for falls as evidenced by the findings of **[Word Choice]**, **[Word Choice]**, and **[Word Choice]**.

Word Choices
Rugs on floors
Cordless phone on nightstand by bed
Glasses and plates on top shelves of cabinets
Stairs going to the second floor
Walk-in shower with hand bars
Elevated toilet seat
Walker

PHASE 2

QUESTION 3.

The nurse must prioritize fall risks for this client.

Complete the following sentence by selecting from the list of word choices below.

The nurse *prioritizes* addressing **[Word Choice]** to improve the client's safety by minimizing the risk for falls.

Word Choices
Rugs on the floor
Glasses and plates on top shelves of cabinets
Stairs going to the second floor

QUESTION 4.

The nurse plans to perform a further assessment of the home and the client's living arrangements the next day.

Which assessments will the nurse plan to perform at that time? **Select all that apply.**

- Type of stove
- Safe use of walker
- Presence of smoke detectors
- Amount and kind of food in refrigerator
- Ability to self-bathe and get dressed
- Medication administration practices

PHASE 3

QUESTION 5.

The next week, the nurse arrives to evaluate the client. During the past week, the client developed shortness of breath and was placed on home oxygen therapy. Also, the client's daughter arrived from out of town and reports that she will be staying with the client for the next few weeks. The nurse teaches the daughter and client about oxygen therapy.

Which **2** statements by the client's daughter indicate that teaching was effective?

○ "Extra oxygen tanks can be stored in the kitchen."
○ "Oxygen tanks must be kept at least 4 feet from open flames."
○ "I bought No Smoking/Oxygen in Use signs for each doorway."
○ "We should report any signs of dizziness to the health care provider."
○ "If my mother gets shorter of breath, I will increase the oxygen flow rate."
○ "My husband may visit while I am here with my mother, but he will smoke in another room."

QUESTION 6.

Several days later, the nurse checks on the client.

Highlight the assessment findings that indicate that the client is safe at home.

History and Physical	Nurses' Notes	Vital Signs	Laboratory Results

1400: Home assessment performed. Client is eating a meal of fish and potatoes with daughter. Client's son-in-law is visiting; daughter states he has gone for a drive so that he can smoke. Stove is off and not in use. Refrigerator is full of fresh produce. Client's daughter purchased an extra-long tube for oxygen so that the client can walk around her home easily. No Smoking/Oxygen in Use signs are placed at each doorway.

Appendix A

TERMINOLOGY/COMBINING FORMS: PREFIXES AND SUFFIXES

Medical terminology is similar to a foreign language. Many medical terms are derived from Latin and Greek sources. They often consist of two or more simple words or word elements. A word root or *combining form* may be put together with a *prefix* and a *suffix*.

Root—the basis of a word
Example: *nephr*/o/tic (degenerative changes in the kidney)
Root: nephr- (kidney)

Linking vowel—a vowel that joins the combining form to the suffix or another combining form
Example: nephr/*o*/sis (disease of the kidneys)
Linking vowel: o

Prefix—the beginning of a word
Example: *hyper*/active (excessively active)
Prefix: hyper- (excessive)

Suffix—the ending of a word
Example: nephr/*itis* (inflammation of the kidney)
Suffix: -itis (inflammation)

Combining form—the union of a word root with a linking vowel
Example: *hepato*/megaly (enlargement of the liver)
Combining form: hepato- (liver)

The following table provides some of the most commonly used terminology for your reference.

COMMON PREFIXES

Prefix	Definition
a-	without
ab-	away from
abd-	abdominal
acu-	sharp
ad-	toward
adip-	fat
ad lib-	freely, as wanted
aero-	air, gas
al-	toward
ambi-	both
an-	not
ana-	up
ante-	before, in front of
anti-	against
arteri-	artery
arthro-	joint
auto-	self
bi-	two
brady-	slow
cata-	down
chole-	bile
cili-	eyelid
circum-	around
co-	with, together
cogni-	know
colo-	colon
con-	with, together

Prefix	Definition
contra-	against
crani-	skull
cut-	skin
cyt-	cell
de-	from, lack of
demi-	half
dent-	tooth
derm-	skin
dia-	through, across
diplo-	double, twofold
dis-	to free or undo
dors-	back
dur-	hard
dy-	two
dys-	bad, painful, difficult, abnormal
ec-	out, out from
ecto-	outside
em-	in
embol-	to insert
encephalo-	brain
endo-	in, within
entero-	intestine
epi-	above, on
erythro-	red
eso-	within, inward
et-	and
eu-	good, normal
ex-	out, away from
exo-	outside
extra-	outside
faci-	face
fiss-	split, cleft
fore-	before, in front of
gastro-	stomach
glosso-	relating to the tongue
glyco-	sugar
haplo-	simple, single
heme-	iron-based
hemi-	one half
hepat-	liver
hetero-	different
histo-	tissue
homo-	same
hydro-	wet, water
hyper-	excessive, above normal
hypo-	under, below
im-	not
in-	in, not
infra-	under, below
inter-	between
intra-	in, within
isch-	deficiency
iso-	equal, alike
lapis-	stone
lapra-	loin or flank, sometimes abdomen
latero-	side
macro-	large

Prefix	Definition
mal-	bad
meato-	opening
medi-	middle
melano-	black
mesa-	middle
meso-	middle
meta-	beyond, change
micro-	small
mono-	one
morpho-	form, structure
multi-	many, much
neo-	new
nephro-	kidney
oculo-	eye
onco-	tumor
oro-	mouth
osteo-	bone
pan-	all
para-	beside, beyond
per-	through, by
peri-	around
phago-	eating
poly-	many, much
post-	after, behind
pre-	before, in front of
primi-	first
pro-	before, in front of
pseudo-	false
quadri-	four
re-	again, backward
retro-	backward, behind
rhabdo-	rod-shaped, striated
rhodo-	red
scler-	hardening
semi-	one half
stetho-	chest
sub-	under, below
super-	above, excessive
supra-	above, excessive
sym-	together
syn-	union, together, joined
tachy-	rapid
tetra-	four
therm-	heat
trans-	through, across
tri-	three
ultra-	beyond, excess
uni-	one
vas-	vessel or duct
xantho-	yellow
xero-	dry

COMMON SUFFIXES

Suffix	Definition
-ac	pertaining to
-agra	excessive pain
-al	pertaining to
-algia	painful condition, pain
-apheresis	removal
-ar	pertaining to
-ary	pertaining to
-ase	enzyme
-bi	two, double
-blast	developing cell
-cele	hernia, swelling, sac
-centesis	puncture of a cavity
-clasis	break, fracture

Suffix	Definition
-clysis	irrigation, washing
-coccus	berry shaped
-crit	to separate
-cyte	cell
-desis	fusion, binding, fixation
-drome	to run
-dynia	pain
-ectasis	expansion, dilation
-ectomy	excision, removal of a body part
-emesis	vomiting
-emia	blood
-er	one who
-gen	forming, producing, origin
-genesis	forming, producing, origin
-genic	origin, formation
-grade	to go
-gram	the record made, mark
-graph	instrument for recording, machine
-graphy	the process, process of recording
-ia	condition
-iasis	morbid condition
-iatry	treatment, medicine
-ic/-ical	pertaining to
-icle	small, minute
-ism	condition
-ist	one who specializes in, specialist
-itis	inflammation
-lith	stone, calculus
-logist	specialist in the study of
-logy	process of study
-lysis	dissolution, setting free
-malacia	softening, soft
-megaly	enlargement
-meter	instrument for measuring
-metry	act of measuring
-odynia	pain
-oid	form, shape
-ole	small, minute
-ology	study or science of
-oma	tumor
-opsy	to view
-or	one who
-orrhea	flow, discharge
-osis	condition or state
-ous	pertaining to
-para	to bear (offspring)
-paresis	partial paralysis
-pathy	disease, suffering
-penia	deficiency, lack of, decrease
-pexy	fixation
-phagia	eating, swallowing
-phasia	speech
-philia	attraction for
-phobia	fear
-physis	to grow
-plasia	formation, growth
-plasm	growth, formation
-plasty	mold, shape, repair
-plegia	paralysis
-poiesis	formation, production
-ptosis	downward displacement, falling
-ptysis	spitting
-rrhage	bursting forth, rupture
-rrhaphy	suturing in place
-rrhea	flow, discharge
-rrhexis	rupture
-scope	instrument to visually examine
-scopy	process of examining, visual examination

Suffix	Definition
-sepsis	infection
-sis	state of, condition
-spasm	involuntary spasm
-stalsis	constriction
-stasis	control, constant level, stop
-stenosis	narrowing, stricture
-stomy	creation of an opening
-therapy	treatment
-tic	pertaining to

Suffix	Definition
-tome	instrument for cutting
-tomy	process of cutting, incision
-toxic	poison
-tresia	opening
-tripsy	surgical crushing
-trophy	nourishment
-ula	small, minute
-ule	small, minute
-y	process

Answers to Clinical Judgment and Next-Generation NCLEX® Examination–Style Questions

CHAPTER 1

1. Answer:

Health History	Nurses' Notes	Vital Signs	Laboratory Results

1634: Patient in bed, reporting pain of 5 on a 0-to-10 scale, which she says is "about what it always is." Height: 163 cm (64 inches); weight: 45.8 kg (101 lb). VS: T 37.2°C (99.0°F); HR 62 beats/min; RR 14 breaths/min; BP 102/68 mm Hg. Spo₂ 98% on RA. Spouse reports patient did not eat anything for breakfast or lunch today, stating, "I'm just not hungry."

The patient with cancer may have a baseline level of pain; however, the nurse will always further assess to explore other contributing or causative factors. The nurse will also further assess the patient's nutrition status because the patient has not eaten today. This may be an isolated event, or it may be an ongoing concern that further compromises the patient. Other findings are within expected parameters and do not require immediate further assessment.

2. Answer: The patient is at high risk for **dehydration** as evidenced <u>by decreased fluid intake</u>.
The patient's risk for dehydration is high, given that she has not had intake aside from 4 ounces of water earlier in the day. At this time, there are no indications of risk for lymphedema, sepsis, or skin dryness. Other options do not provide a rationale for dehydration.

3. Answer: The priority for the patient at this time is to **manage pain** and **facilitate fluid intake**.
The patient's pain of 6 on a 0-to-10 scale merits prioritization, as does the fact that she has not consumed enough fluids. Although moisturizing skin is a favorable action, this is not a priority. Helping the patient to walk is only necessary if that is the patient's desire. Because she is on hospice, this is unlikely to be a priority need. Although prevention of further metastasis is a goal of cancer treatment, it is not a goal of hospice care. The goal of hospice care is to provide a peaceful, comfortable death with dignity.

4. Answer:

X Continue to administer oxycodone as prescribed.
○ Require the patient to perform hygiene care for exercise.
X Ask patient to identify favorite nonalcoholic beverages.
○ Encourage regular ambulation several times daily.
X Monitor vital signs at every nursing visit.
○ Contact the health care provider to admit patient to hospital.
○ Teach spouse about the pathophysiology of ovarian cancer.

To meet the patient's priority needs of pain management and fluid intake, the nurse will continue to administer oxycodone, which should decrease pain. The nurse will also ask about favorite nonalcoholic beverages, which can encourage fluid intake if the patient likes the taste of something specific. It is important to continue monitoring vital signs at every visit to further assess for indications of an increase in pain or dehydration.

The nurse does not need to make the patient perform hygiene care for exercise or ambulate several times daily; she is on hospice care, so the care provided is strategized to provide comfort (not exhaustion). There is no need to call the health care provider to admit the patient to the hospital, as she has DNR orders in place; the goal of hospice care is palliative, not curative. At this time, it is unnecessary to provide pathophysiological teaching about ovarian cancer to the spouse. Focus is placed at this time on comfort and death with dignity rather than on education about a condition that the patient has had for more than a year.

5. Answer:
○ "Why do you think your spouse has depression?"
X "It sounds like you care about your spouse very much."
○ "If I were you, I would tell him to get a job to get out of the house."
X "I can understand why you are concerned about your spouse."
○ "Can you explain how you have made peace with dying?"
○ "I am sure he will grieve, but eventually he will be okay."
○ "We can talk about this after we finish your hygiene care."
○ "I think you should tell your spouse how concerned you are."

The nurse will respond to the patient's statements by verbalizing what is implied: that the patient cares deeply about her spouse. The nurse can also acknowledge the patient's concerns by stating an understanding of those concerns. It is not appropriate for the nurse to attempt to solve the patient's problems; it is, however, appropriate for the nurse to be present in the moment and allow the patient to express her feelings.

The nurse will refrain from asking "why"; this is nontherapeutic. It is also highly likely that the patient's husband is sad about his wife dying, so further investigation (unless the spouse appears to be at risk for harming self or others) is unnecessary. It is inappropriate for the nurse to give advice by telling the patient what the nurse would do in the same situation or telling the patient what the nurse thinks should be done. Asking if the patient can explain how she made peace with death takes the focus off of her concern, which is her spouse. It is nontherapeutic to state that the spouse will eventually be okay; this minimizes the patient's concern. Telling the patient that she and the nurse can talk after hygiene care also minimizes the patient's concern and closes the avenue for communication.

6. Answer:

Previous Patient Finding	Current Patient Finding	Effective	Not Effective
Pain rated at 5 on 0-to-10 scale	Pain rated at 5 on 0-to-10 scale		X
Had consumed very few oral fluids	Spouse confirms patient is drinking several glasses of water daily	X	
Expressed concern about spouse	States, "I talked with my spouse about how I feel."	X	
Ate half of scrambled egg before becoming nauseated	Reports eating one scrambled egg daily	X	
Skin thin and transparent	Skin dry		X

Assessment findings that have improved since the last visit demonstrate that treatment was effective. These include an increase in food and fluid intake and the patient's verbalization of talking to her spouse about how she feels. Assessment findings that are the same or unimproved demonstrate that treatment was not effective. These include having the same degree of pain and ongoing skin concerns such as dryness.

CHAPTER 2

1. **Answer: 2, 4, 6, 7.** The nurse will immediately communicate the heightened confusion, mood changes, holding of left arm, and new behavior to the health care provider. These are the findings that provide context to the patient's mental status at the moment. There has been a progressive mood shift, which culminated in even more confusion today and a physical altercation. In addition, there could be a significant injury to the arm, such as a fracture, that would require immediate attention. This information helps the health care provider to formulate a working diagnosis and order treatment. The nurse will communicate that the patient has a bruised right eye and a superficial laceration of the head secondarily to the provider. These are not life-threatening injuries, so they can be addressed after the nurse has provided the priority information. Last, the nurse can explain that the daughter is involved in the patient's care and that she is understandably distraught about the situation. This is the least important information to provide at this time, as it does not affect the immediate management of the patient's condition.

2. **Answer: 1, 2, 3, 5.** It is appropriate for the nurse to engage in active listening; this demonstrates respect and interest in the patient's condition. The nurse can gather important information that will affect the plan of care while engaging in active listening. The nurse will also repeat sentences calmly as needed and allow the patient time to respond. These actions also demonstrate respect and interest, and provide the patient with time to process the information and formulate a response if able. Patients with dementia often need a longer period of time to interact, so the nurse will provide an open and caring environment to facilitate communication. The nurse will stand in front of the patient instead of at the side; the patient cannot see the nurse well at the side, and it may also be startling to him if he has not seen the nurse with his peripheral vision. This can provoke an unwanted reaction if the patient becomes combative due to fear. The nurse will not give the patient an electronic device to use when talking. This can be very difficult for patients with dementia. The best information the nurse will collect will be from the patient himself and the patient's daughter.

3. **Answer: 4, 5.** The nurse provides therapeutic communication when stating, "I can empathize with how you're feeling." This demonstrates

that the nurse has compassion for the patient's daughter. It is also therapeutic for the nurse to say, "Let's sit together so I can answer your questions." This provides the patient's daughter with time to ask questions and receive responses. By the nurse offering to sit together, a therapeutic and welcoming environment has been created where the conversation will not be rushed.

4. **Answer: 1, 5.** The nurse will respect the patient's personal space, as this promotes dignity and respect for the patient. The nurse will speak kindly, even if the patient is verbally unkind, and refrain from overreacting to the patient's behavior. People with dementia may be unaware of their actions, and the nurse recognizes this and does not respond inappropriately. Scolding is very inappropriate and could escalate the patient's behavior. When the patient is in this acute phase, it would not be safe for the family caregiver to intervene; the health care team needs to take control of this situation and attempt to de-escalate the situation. Respecting the patient's personal space, ignoring challenges, and avoiding overreacting all assist in de-escalation.

5. **Answer: 4.** The nurse will respond therapeutically by recognizing the daughter's feeling. Acknowledging that this must be a difficult situation for her shows respect and empathy. It is inappropriate to state that the patient would talk more if the daughter talked to him; patients with Alzheimer's disease often lose communication skills progressively regardless of the interaction between them and others. Although that is an expected progression, it is nontherapeutic to respond immediately by reminding the daughter that reduced communication was expected. Asking the daughter if she did something to make the patient talk less is inappropriate; this is confrontational and sounds like the nurse may be accusing the daughter of wrongdoing.

CHAPTER 3

1. **Answer:** The nurse will first address the patient's confusion. It is important to determine whether confusion is related to a head injury, memory deficit, anxiety, or other condition. Then the nurse will address the patient's shoulder pain. Pain can contribute to cognitive processing if the pain is unbearable. The stage 1 pressure injury can be addressed after the patient is stabilized. It is not unusual for a patient with uncontrolled type 2 diabetes mellitus to have a blood sugar of 122; this can actually be a more favorable value for patients who have uncontrolled diabetes and are attempting to reestablish control. Mobility has been established at baseline and can be further evaluated later. The nurse will not want to ambulate a confused patient. Nutrition status can be evaluated later, as can the blood pressure and hand tremors. The blood pressure value is not unusual for a patient with hypertension, and hand tremors are associated with Parkinson disease.

2. **Answer: 2, 4.** Medication reconciliation is done on admission and must be complete if a patient is transferred to another unit in the agency or to a different agency. It is also part of the discharge process to ensure the patient's list of medications is correct. This process is not performed each time a medication is given, at the change of every shift, or once every 24 hours.

3. **Answer: 2.** The nurse will report that the patient ate cookies the spouse brought. Patients are to be "NPO" (taking nothing by mouth) for a prescribed amount of time before surgery. Eating or drinking certain things can be cause to delay the surgery so that the stomach is empty. Blood pressure of 140/90 is not dangerously elevated; the shoulder pain and limited range of motion in the affected arm are expected due to the shoulder injury. These can be communicated to the surgeon after discussing the cookies.

4. **Answer: 3, 4.** The nurse will delegate oral and denture hygiene and documentation of intake and output to assistive personnel (AP). These tasks are within the skill set of AP. Assessment (such as of neurological status), administration of opioid medication, and treatments such as dressing changes (which require nursing assessment of a condition) are within the scope of nursing practice and are the responsibility of a registered nurse. Skills of assessment and dressing change cannot be delegated to AP.

5. **Answer: 1.** The nurse needs to intervene when the patient states that extra pain medication will be taken if the discomfort increases. Medication should be taken only as prescribed. If opioid medication

is given, risks for side effects like extreme constipation and respiratory depression increase if more than the prescribed dose is taken. The nurse will redirect the patient to contact the surgeon if the pain is not adequately controlled. All other patient statements are appropriate at the time of discharge and do not require nursing intervention.

CHAPTER 4

1. **Answer: 1.** The nurse will document the patient's response objectively by citing only the facts, which include that the patient refused acetaminophen, the provider was notified, and ondansetron was given. It is inappropriate to subjectively document the patient's refusal. Patients who request a stronger medication are not always seeking drugs. Documenting only the ondansetron administration leaves out a key part of the situation. Documenting that the patient is uncooperative is subjective and unprofessional.

2. **Answer: 1, 2, 3, 4, 7.** It is important for the nurse to provide immediate care and to follow policy and procedure for how falls are handled. First, the nurse will determine if there are other injuries aside from the wrist. Once that assessment is complete, the nurse will ensure the patient is safe and then begin contacting individuals who need to be involved in ongoing care. The nurse will report the fall to the nurse manager of the unit; contact the provider with notification of the situation and to request a wrist x-ray order; complete an incident report (however, an incident report is *not* documented or filed in the patient's electronic health record); and document the sequence of events that took place before and after the fall. The nurse will not scold the patient for getting up without using the nurse call system; rather, the nurse will reteach the importance of using the nurse call system before attempting to get out of bed.

3. **Answer: 4.** Nurses are legally obligated to keep information about patients confidential. The patient must give consent before any health records are shared with others. It is inaccurate and inappropriate to state that the family caregiver can see the records because they are the nearest living relative or that the health record will be available after the patient's discharge. Although the nurse can ask the family caregiver to discuss concerns, it is not appropriate to introduce this phrase until it has been made clear that the health record cannot be shared without the patient's consent. It is also nontherapeutic to ask "why" questions; this places the patient and family caregiver in a defensive position.

4. **Answer: 2.** The nurse will document objective facts, such as the patient's level of activity and any care provided during the last observation. It is inappropriate to document subjective or critical comments about a patient, the family caregiver, care by other health care professionals, or actions by support staff. Although an incident report is an appropriate document to complete, it is not filed with the patient's health record, nor does the nurse document that this form was filled out.

5. **Answer: 2, 3, 5.** Indications that nursing actions from the prior evening and night were effective include verbalization of the understanding to use the nurse call system before getting out of bed, decreased swelling in the affected wrist and hand, and acknowledgement that wearing a soft brace will provide stabilization for comfort over the coming days. Wrist pain of 7 on a 0-to-10 scale and asking if it is time for the next dose of pain medication (which implies that pain is still being experienced) indicate that nursing actions were not effective.

CHAPTER 5

1. **Answer: 2.** Opioid medications can cause respiratory depression. The nurse will report respirations that are 8 breaths/min, as this is lower than the normal 12 to 20 breaths/min. All other findings are within normal limits and do not need to be reported.

2. **Answer: 4.** A decrease in blood pressure and widening of pulse pressure indicate inadequate cardiac output. The changes in oxygenation, respiratory rate, and heart rate are all still within normal limits.

3. **Answer: 1, 3, 4, 5.** See Box 5.6.

4. **Answer: 1.** Fevers cause an increase in oxygen demand, which is reflected by a higher respiratory rate. Fevers should not cause oxygenation to drop that low without other symptoms present. The increased oxygen demand causes the heart rate and blood pressure to rise, not fall.

5. **Answer: See table.** The report of pain as 6 on a scale of 0-to-10 indi-

cates ineffective pain management. Verbalizing how to prepare nutritionally balanced liquids (because the patient's jaw is wired shut), acknowledging the need to increase ambulation, and verbalizing how to maintain oral hygiene measures are all indicators of effective nursing and collaborative interventions.

Assessment Finding	Effective	Not Effective
Patient and family caregiver verbalize how to prepare nutritionally balanced liquids.	X	
The patient reports pain in jaw at 6 on a scale of 0 to 10.		X
Patient and family caregiver state they will increase ambulation as per home physical therapy recommendations.	X	
Family caregiver verbalizes how to maintain oral hygiene measures.	X	

CHAPTER 6

1. **Answer: 1, 4, 5, 7, 8.** The patient with heart failure is experiencing fluid overload. Signs and symptoms include increased respirations, crackles in the lungs, pitting edema in extremities, sudden weight gain (such as 0.8 kg [2 pounds] overnight), and decreased perfusion (slow capillary refill). These symptoms must be reported to the health care provider. The nurse can use therapeutic communication to interact with the patient who expresses sadness over losing a spouse; also, eating a diet high in fiber and drinking water instead of juice are healthy choices. These findings do not need to be reported to the health care provider.

2. **Answer: 4.** The most objective measure of fluid accumulation related to heart failure is the finding of rapid increase of weight overnight. A rapid weight increase indicates the objective presence of fluid accumulation. Further assessment of the amount of water the patient drinks instead of juice can help to explain fluid accumulation but, by itself, is not the best type of assessment to indicate that the patient is experiencing heart failure. Self-reported shortness of breath can be related to many conditions, not just heart failure, so this is not the best type of assessment for the nurse to use to anticipate that the patient is experiencing heart failure. Having a history of renal failure can indicate that the patient has problems with elimination and perfusion, yet this is not the best type of assessment to use to anticipate that the patient is experiencing heart failure.

3. **Answer: 1.** It is within the scope of assistive personnel (AP) to measure intake and output. The nurse will delegate this task, provide education to the AP about what needs to be done, and remain responsible for supervision. Teaching, evaluating, and assessing are nursing roles; these cannot be done by an AP.

4. **Answer: 2, 3, 4.** Walkers are used to promote safety for a patient who has gait difficulty—like a shuffling gait—or other symptoms that may impair mobility such as cognitive changes or peripheral neuropathy. The patient with cognitive changes may not be able to react quickly when walking, so the walker provides stability. The patient with peripheral neuropathy may not have full sensation in the extremities, which can affect gait if the patient does not adequately feel the ground underneath. Again, the walker provides stability in this case. Pedal edema, in isolation, is not a reason to use a walker. An oxygen saturation of 96% on room air is normal and does not imply that a walker is needed.

5. **Answer: 2.** A reduction in crackles in the lungs demonstrates that furosemide treatment is effective. Furosemide works to move fluid; if fluid is reduced, the lungs will sound clearer. The oxygen saturation, temperature, and pulse rate were normal in the nurse's initial assessment and are normal now; therefore these do not indicate that treatment was effective.

CHAPTER 7

1. **Answer: 1, 3, 4, 5.** The nurse anticipates the health care provider will first order a urine culture and sensitivity (because the urine is dark, cloudy, and foul smelling, which are signs of infection); blood cultures due to the elevated temperature, low blood pressure, and elevated pulse rate (which are signs of sepsis); a white blood cell count (to assess for the presence and degree of infection); and electrolytes (to evaluate fluid and electrolyte status due to the cognitive change, low blood pressure, and increased heart rate). There are no data in the case to anticipate that a stool specimen will be ordered. Urethral and throat cultures may be considered later but are not indicated initially at this time.

2. **Answer: 1.** This procedure must be done with sterile technique, so the experienced nurse will intervene if the new nurse dons clean gloves. All other actions are appropriate and do not require the experienced nurse to intervene.

3. **Answer: 4.** A throat culture must be collected from the tonsils after the swab has been inserted without touching the lips, teeth, tongue, or cheeks. This technique prevents contamination with organisms of the oral cavity. The tonsils are swabbed, not the uvula. The head of the bed must be elevated to at least 45 degrees, not 30 degrees. The swab should not touch the tongue en route to the tonsils.

4. **Answer: 4.** The nurse will notify the health care provider of a potential source of infection—fingertips that are red and painful, especially those that are draining pus. It would be extremely painful to soak the fingertips in alcohol. Placing bandages over the fingertips could seal in infection. There is no need to culture each fingertip separately.

5. **Answer: 3.** To function accurately and properly, the code for the test strips used for blood glucose samples must match the code on the glucometer. The nurse will always compare these codes prior to obtaining a blood sample. Glucometers often are charged by being connected to a power supply, but they do not need to be connected to that supply to function. Finger lancets made by any manufacturer for the purpose of blood glucose collection can be used; they do not need to be from the same manufacturer as the glucometer. Glucometers are cleaned, not autoclaved.

CHAPTER 8

1. **Answer: 3, 4.** Possible herniation compresses the brainstem, which contains the vital cardiac, respiratory, and vasomotor centers; sudden death can occur.

2. **Answer: 2.** A manometer is used to measure spinal pressure, so the nurse will gather this before the lumbar puncture. An otoscope is used to examine the ears. A tuning fork is used to assess hearing. An ophthalmoscope is used to examine the eyes.

3. **Answer: 2.** The nurse will place the patient into lateral recumbent position for the lumbar puncture. This provides easy access to the spine. Semi-Fowler, lithotomy, and supine positions are incorrect because they do not allow access to the spine.

4. **Answer: 1, 5.** The nurse will monitor the patient for fluid loss, especially for any leaking cerebrospinal fluid that may have occurred as a result of the procedure. The nurse will administer pain medication rather than withhold it. A chest x-ray is not indicated, given the patient's current symptoms. The patient needs to rest after a lumbar puncture because increased intracranial pressure can develop; therefore the nurse will not ambulate the patient as soon as the procedure ends.

5. **Answer: 3.** The nurse will report that the patient has a headache of 8 on a 0-to-10 scale to the health care provider. This is called a "postprocedure headache" and is not uncommon after a lumbar puncture. It occurs due to leakage of fluid out of the hole created by the fine needle that was used to perform the lumbar puncture. The hole usually closes on its own postprocedure; however, if it does not, the health care provider can place an epidural blood patch to seal it. A pulse rate of 90 beats/min is normal. Tenderness at the puncture site is not uncommon and does not need to be reported. A continued temperature is expected because the patient had this symptom when care was sought.

CHAPTER 9

1. **Answer: dizziness, pulse 58 beats/min, open wound to coccyx.** The pulse rate of 54 beats/min is of concern because it is low, which can contribute to the patient's dizziness. The low pulse rate and dizziness can explain one reason for the patient's fall earlier in the day. The dosage of metoprolol and digoxin may need to be adjusted because of the low pulse rate. The open wound on the coccyx needs to be cleaned and dressed to decrease the risk of infection. Skin barrier and skin protection measures need to be implemented to prevent the wound from increasing in size. The patient's blood pressure and oxygen saturation are within normal limits and do not need to be addressed. The small open wound on the elbow can be addressed at a later point. The urinary incontinence is an ongoing problem and can be addressed after addressing the priority concerns. The temperature is not elevated enough to be a priority at this time.

2. **Answer: 3.** Wash hands with soap and water before performing wound care. Washing hands for at least 20 seconds provides enough time for microorganisms to be removed. Hot water should not be used for handwashing as it causes excessive dryness and possible cracking of the skin. Do not clean hands with betadine, rub alcohol wipes over the hands, or perform a surgical scrub. Betadine and alcohol are not recommended as ways of washing hands. Performing a surgical scrub is done before a surgical procedure.

3. **Answer: 1.** Enact Contact Precautions. This is done to prevent direct contact between the source of infection and you, other members of the interprofessional team, or visitors. Droplet Precautions are instituted when an infection spread by oral secretions larger than 5 microns is diagnosed or suspected (e.g., rubella, streptococcal pharyngitis, pneumonia). Airborne Precautions are instituted when an infection that is spread by oral secretions smaller than 5 microns is diagnosed or suspected (e.g., measles, varicella, tuberculosis). Standard Precautions is followed for all patients.

4. **Answer: 1.** The first thing you will do is remove gloves, one at a time, while not touching the outside of a glove with your bare hand and discard. This is followed by removing eyewear, face shield, or goggles; untying the neck string and then untying the back strings of the gown; allowing the gown to fall off the shoulders; removing the hands from the gown sleeves without touching the outside of the gown; holding the gown inside at the seams and folding it inside out into a bundle before discarding it; removing the mask; and performing hand hygiene.

5. **Answer: 3.** Airborne Precautions because tuberculosis is an infection that is spread by oral secretions smaller than 5 microns. Contact Precautions were already instituted when the patient was diagnosed with MRSA. Droplet Precautions are instituted when an infection that is spread by oral secretions larger than 5 microns is diagnosed or suspected (e.g., rubella, streptococcal pharyngitis, pneumonia). Standard Precautions will not protect you or others from potential infection due to direct contact.

CHAPTER 10

1. **Answer:** A 68-year-old patient is admitted to the hospital for lung surgery related to a tumor in the lower lobe of the left lung. The patient has a 40 pack-year history of smoking and a history of hypertension, history of angina, and myocardial infarction. The patient has an indwelling Foley catheter with dark, foul-smelling urine. The patient confides in the nurse about anxiety over the upcoming surgery and possible diagnosis of cancer. VS include BP 106/74 mm Hg, HR 110 beats/min, RR 22 breaths/min, T 38.2°C (100.8°F), and SPO₂ 98% on room air. The nurse notices that the patient seems restless during the assessment, which reveals crackles in the lungs bilaterally. A chest x-ray shows bilateral infiltrates in the bases of both lungs.

   The nurse will focus on addressing signs of infection, which include foul-smelling urine; an elevation in the pulse, respirations, and temperature; crackles in the lungs; and noted infiltrates. The surgeon may choose to delay surgery if the patient is diagnosed with an infection. Other findings, such as the patient's restlessness, can be addressed after determining the cause for the symptoms associated with infection.

2. **Answer: 1, 3, 4.** The patient has reported a finding that may be associated with a latex allergy. Exploring existing or potential allergies is critical to maintain patient safety. The nurse will report this finding to the surgeon; surgery may be delayed if a latex-free environment is not available. The nurse will also ask if other symptoms occur when the patient is exposed to rubber (latex) to determine whether the allergy affects the respiratory system. The nurse will also document the information in the electronic health record so that other members of the interprofessional team will know about the patient's allergy. This is not a normal reaction, so the nurse will refrain from saying this. It is also unnecessary to state that the patient will not be washing dishes during hospitalization. Although this is true, the response is nontherapeutic.

3. **Answer: 1, 2, 4.** The nurse will take action to protect the safety of the patient. This involves performing hand hygiene to decrease the risk for infection transmission, confirming the patient's known allergy so that all latex can be avoided, and assuring that all equipment needed is present so that the nurse does not have to step away from the sterile field once surgery begins. The nurse will not confirm the patient's identity with one identifier. Two identifiers must be used. The nurse will place the sterile kit at a level just above the waist—not the hip.

4. **Answer: 1.** The nurse must recognize that because the instrument touched the edge of the drape, it is now considered contaminated. Because the instrument is contaminated, a new sterile instrument must be obtained. Wiping the instrument with alcohol does not restore sterility. The instrument cannot be used because it is now contaminated. The nurse can take independent action to obtain a new sterile instrument; the surgeon does not need to be asked what to do.

5. **Answer: 4.** It is critical to maintain surgical asepsis to protect the patient during surgery. The nurse will remove the current gloves, perform hand hygiene, and don new sterile gloves. It is inappropriate to apply a new sterile glove over the one with a hole, to continue the procedure, or to only use the hand with the glove that does not have a hole. These actions increase the risk for infection to the patient.

CHAPTER 11

1. **Answer: 2, 3, 4, 5.** Prior to transfer, the nurse will assess the patient's balance and ability to sit up (BMAT score), orientation to determine if the patient is able to be transferred safely, current blood pressure so that another measurement can be obtained when sitting (to screen for postural hypotension), and weight (which determines the best and safest method for a transfer). It is not necessary to obtain a dietary history, as this will not affect the transfer. It is also not necessary to assess the patient's activity tolerance prior to the CVA, as only a transfer is being planned—not a full activity.

2. **Answer: 1, 3, 5.** The patient is experiencing a reduced nutritional intake. This can contribute to injury during transfer if the patient is weak from lack of nutrition. A cerebrovascular accident will cause reduced sensation as well as reduced mobility in affected extremities. The impairment of function in the left leg and arm are conducive to contractures and pressure injury (as a result of reduced overall mobility). There is no indication that the patient has a condition causing reduced circulation. The blood pressure is not significantly elevated; this should not cause a problem during transfer.

3. **Answer: 3.** Before transferring the patient, the nurse will make sure the gait belt fits appropriately. This will be used for stabilization during the transfer. A gait belt that does not fit can increase the risk for falls, as the device cannot be used as intended if it is the wrong size. The patient should be wearing nonskid socks or shoes—not slippers. The wheelchair must be placed at a 45- to 60-degree angle to the bed (not a 90-degree angle). Family members should not perform transfers in the inpatient setting. This task should be accomplished by trained staff to reduce the risk for falls.

4. **Answer: 1.** The nurse can delegate the task of transferring the patient to a wheelchair for discharge. It is within the scope of assistive personnel (AP) to perform the transfer. The nurse will delegate this task, provide education to the AP about what needs to be done, and remain responsible for supervision. Assessing, teaching, and evaluating are nursing roles; these cannot be done by AP.

5. **Answer: 2.** Although the current nurse will report all of these findings to the oncoming nurse, the priority is to communicate that the patient experienced orthostatic hypotension during the transfer process. This alerts the oncoming nurse so that careful attention to safety during transfers can be reinforced. Noting that the patient sat in a chair for 30 minutes, that the physical therapist came, and that a walker was replaced can all be communicated after the priority information has been shared; these factors demonstrate resolution of an event, whereas the priority information pertains directly to safety during upcoming transfers.

CHAPTER 12

1. **Answer: 1, 3.** Dyspnea and dizziness are signs that indicate that the patient should not be ambulated at this time. If the patient is short of breath or dizzy, the risk for falls increases. Even if the patient is not short of breath or dizzy when ambulation starts, stop ambulation if dizziness lasts 60 seconds or fainting or diaphoresis occurs or if change in breathing patterns or dyspnea with a respiratory rate greater than baseline by more than 20 breaths/min develops. The patient is expected to have pain, a reduced range of motion in the left knee, and concern about an increase in pain; these are not reasons to delay ambulation.

2. **Answer: 4.** First calculate the patient's maximum heart rate by subtracting the patient's age from 220 (220 − 70 = 150). Seventy-five percent of the maximum rate is 112 beats/in—the target rate during exercise.

3. **Answer: 3.** To begin to use a walker safely, the nurse will instruct the patient to balance in the center of the walker first. The nurse will teach the patient to move the walker forward about 6 to 8 inches and then take a step forward with the weaker leg by moving the center of gravity toward the walker.

4. **Answer: 4.** The family member who states that walkers can be used inside and outside the home, as well as on inclines, has demonstrated that teaching by the nurse was effective. Further teaching is needed if the family member says golf balls can be used on the walker's rubber tips (tennis balls should be used), that it is important to take the walker into a shower (the walker should never be taken into a shower), or that the walker can be used for balance when getting up from a chair (it should not be used this way because it is not stable enough).

5. **Answer:**

Patient Statement	Demonstrates Understanding	Requires Nursing Intervention
"I will use my walker only if I feel weak."		X
"All four feet of the walker need to stay on the floor."	X	
"I can use my walker when I need to go upstairs."		X
"The first step I take needs to be with my affected leg."	X	
"I should never lean over my walker."	X	

    The patient has demonstrated an understanding of nursing teaching when confirming that all four feet of the walker need to stay on the floor, the first step is taken with the affected leg, and leaning over the walker should never be done. Keeping the feet of the walker on the floor, leading with the affected leg, and no leaning over the walker are actions that promote safe use of this type of device. The patient needs further teaching via nursing intervention if stating that the walker will be used only while feeling weak; this is inaccurate, as the patient should be using the walker consistently until the health care provider indicates differently. The patient also needs further teaching if stating that the walker can be used to go upstairs. Using the walker in this manner increases the risk for falls.

CHAPTER 13

1. **Answer:**

Nursing Action	Indicated	Not Indicated
Perform a full skin assessment	X	
Modify existing repositioning schedule	X	
Verify that the bed is working properly	X	
Request a consultation with a wound care specialist nurse	X	
Avoid cleansing the skin around the injury to minimize tissue trauma		X

See Skill 13.2. A complete skin assessment (including assessment of the areas reported by the AP) is essential when patients are at risk for or have developed pressure injuries (PIs). This is important for all patients and not only those using support mattresses. An air-suspension lateral rotation bed or any support surface mattress does not take the place of repositioning, so the nurse will modify the existing repositioning schedule to relieve pressure on the areas that are developing PIs. It is always appropriate to verify that equipment is working properly. A wound care specialist can help design a skin-care plan to treat existing wounds and prevent further injuries. The nurse will not avoid cleaning the skin around the injury. This area needs frequent cleaning to avoid infection and worsening of the existing wound.

2. **Answer: 1, 2, 4, 5.** A Braden score of 12 indicates that the patient is at risk for PI development; a score of less than or equal to 16 is a risk for pressure injury. Hypotension decreases the delivery of oxygen and nutrients to the tissues, thus increasing the risk for injury. When anemia is present, there is a decrease in the blood's oxygen-carrying capacity. This further decreases the delivery of oxygen to the tissues, increasing the risk for injury. Urine and feces contain enzymes that are caustic to a patient's skin and increase the risk for injury. A healed PI from more than 12 months ago is not considered a PI risk.

3. **Answer: 2, 5.** The nurse can delegate regular turning and repositioning to the AP. A support surface does not negate the need for regular turning and positioning, and performing these tasks is within the scope of what an AP can do. Patients on certain support surfaces may demonstrate disorientation and behavior changes; the AP can *report* these changes to the nurse, but the nurse must assess the changes and compare with baseline patient assessment. Assessment of an area of redness and determination of the support surface's function are nursing responsibilities that cannot be delegated. It is the nurse's responsibility to collaborate with the interprofessional team to select the appropriate support surface.

4. **Answer: 2, 3, 4, 5.** Dehydration can become a problem because the air circulating around the patient is warm. Moving a patient out of an air-fluidized bed can be difficult because of the high edges and the fact that the patient is submerged in the bed. Use of this device should facilitate management of ongoing episodes of incontinence. The air-fluidized bed is large and heavy, making it difficult to transport. The nurse will not need to assess for back pain; this type of device envelops the patient while reducing pressure.

5. **Answer: 3.** The patient has demonstrated an improvement in blood pressure. Hypotension decreases the delivery of oxygen and nutrients to the tissues, thus increasing the risk for injury. When the blood pressure normalizes, it is an indication that nurse care was effective. Continuing redness on the buttocks and left hip and a reduction in the Braden Scale calculation do not indicate that nursing care has been effective. If the redness is still present and the Braden Scale calculation has decreased since admission, nursing care may not have been instituted properly. Although a respiratory rate of 18 breaths/min is normal, this does not represent a change that indicates that nursing care has been effective in reducing skin injury.

CHAPTER 14

1. **Answer: Cognitive status, hip.** The nurse will first address the patient's cognitive status to determine if there could possibly be changes in level of consciousness or any other indication that there may be a head injury sustained during the fall. This assessment can also provide information about whether there may have been a medical reason for the fall (e.g., syncope, stroke). The nurse will then assess the patient's hip. Although the patient does not indicate that she is in pain, there could still be a musculoskeletal injury sustained during the fall. The nurse can perform any other assessments, such as blood pressure, oxygen saturation, evaluation of urinary status, and blood glucose level, after the primary assessments are done.

2. **Answer: 4.** It is reasonable to request that the diuretic drug be given in the morning so that the patient can urinate more frequently during the day rather than getting up at night. The nurse can put additional reasonable fall precautions in place without requiring a sitter for the patient. Placing the patient in a geri chair is a type of restraint that does not need to occur at this time. Although a hip protector can provide some padding in case of a fall, the better approach is to prevent the fall.

3. **Answer: 2, 3, 5.** Placing a pad alarm on the chair and using a method of diversion (such as music) are actions that can be delegated to AP. Reporting patient behaviors, such as wandering or attempting to get out of bed without assistance, is appropriate to delegate. As with any task that is delegated, the nurse will provide education to the AP about what needs to be done and remain responsible for supervision. Determining the patient's orientation is a form of assessment, which is the nurse's role and cannot be delegated to AP. The AP also cannot select the type of restraint-free intervention. This is the nurse's role, as it is a part of formulating a plan of care.

4. **Answer: 2.** Because the patient fell at night after getting out of bed unsupervised, the nurse will prioritize asking if the patient has a specific bedtime routine. Familiar routines can help people fall asleep faster and stay asleep. This can reduce the risk for falls if the patient is not trying to get up at night. Asking about the patient's communication style, cues that indicate hunger, and activities the patient did at home are all valid questions to design a comprehensive plan of care. These can be asked after the initial question is asked to promote the patient's safety.

5. **Answer: 1.** The first step to take when a chemotherapy spill occurs is to obtain a spill kit. If the nurse suspects direct exposure to the liquid, the other steps should be taken.

CHAPTER 15

1. **Answer:**

Body System	Findings
Neurological	PERRLA; reports feeling dizzy and says, "I'm sure it's because I'm upset about losing our home."
Pulmonary	Lungs clear to auscultation bilaterally
Cardiovascular	Pulses 2+ in all extremities; capillary refill 2 seconds; reports left-sided chest pain that is "sharp"
Gastrointestinal	Bowel sounds present × 4 quadrants; abdomen soft and round, nontender to touch; reports mild nausea

The nurse will follow up on symptoms of feeling dizzy, left-sided chest pain, and mild nausea. Together, these symptoms can be indicative of a myocardial infarction. Other findings are within expected limits and do not require immediate follow-up.

2. **Answer: 3.** The grandparent requires a red tag because of the need for immediate intervention related to chest pain. The mother would require a green tag because she appears uninjured. The father and child require yellow tags because they have injuries that are not life

threatening. Someone who died or was expected to die would receive a black tag.

3. **Answer: 2, 4.** A child who has experienced a disaster needs to stay with family member(s) as long as there are no indications that harm could come to the child due to family actions. A complete head-to-toe assessment is always needed after a disaster to ensure that there are no other physical problems. The nurse will not take the child to be examined alone; this could cause fear or trauma in the child. The nurse will not speak only to the parents; an 8-year-old child is capable of interacting with health care providers. There is no evidence that social services needs to be present during the assessment.

4. **Answer: 4.** The patient who states, "I will take all of the antibiotics the provider gave me even if my leg looks better" has demonstrated that teaching from the nurse was effective. The bandage should not be left on for a week because this could increase the risk for infection. Clean technique, not sterile technique, is needed when a patient cares for this type of wound at home. The laceration should not be cleaned with alcohol or it will damage tissue integrity. Saline or mild soap is recommended for cleansing purposes.

5. **Answer: 1, 4, 5.** The nurse will refer the family to Ready.gov, the nearest community health center, and the Centers for Disease Control and Prevention website. All of these entities have information about prevention and mitigation of disasters. The American Nurses Association and the American Medical Association are professional organizations. They provide guidance for health care providers who respond to disasters but are not preferred resources for the family.

CHAPTER 16

1. **Answer:** The patient most likely has a **broken hip** as evidenced by **excruciating pain**.

    The patient's report of pain began after falling. It was rated at a 9 on a 0-to-10 scale at the time the patient was moved to the stretcher. Given that the patient fell, it is most likely that the patient has a hip fracture as evidenced by the excruciating pain. There is no evidence of having a panic attack, elevated blood glucose, or infection related to any other option.

2. **Answer:**

System	Potential Nursing Intervention
Constitutional (pain)	○ Massage the affected hip **X** Administer IV morphine as prescribed ○ Remind patient that pain will pass and is not serious
Integumentary	**X** Gently cleanse abrasion and laceration with saline ○ Place an occlusive dressing over the abrasion and laceration ○ Prioritize care for abrasion and laceration over other patient needs
Psychosocial	○ Tell the patient that their spouse is likely fine **X** Offer to call the patient's spouse and check in ○ Tell the patient that the focus should be on their own health problems currently

The nurse will administer IV morphine as needed to alleviate the excruciating pain. It is inappropriate to massage the affected hip, as this will increase pain. It is nontherapeutic to state that the pain will go away. First, it likely will not be relieved until pain medication is given. Second, this type of response negates the patient's report of severe pain.

The nurse will gently clean the abrasion and laceration with saline. This solution is gentle and will not increase pain in those areas. An occlusive dressing will keep air from reaching the abrasion and laceration, which can increase the risk for infection if bacteria are present. Care for the abrasion and laceration can be completed after addressing the patient's pain, which is the priority.

The nurse will offer to call the patient's spouse and check in. This is a patient-centered intervention because the client is worried about their spouse. It is nontherapeutic to tell the patient that their spouse is likely fine, as this minimizes concern. It is inappropriate to tell the patient to focus on their own health problems, as this statement also negates concern.

3. **Answer: 1, 3, 4, 5.** The nurse will gather assessment data on the patient's cognition, pain rating, IV catheter patency, and any history of obstructive sleep apnea. The patient must have orientation and cognition to press the button on the PCA device correctly. The patient's pain score in recovery is important, as it allows the nurse to compare ongoing perception of pain while the patient is on PCA. The IV catheter must be patent for the PCA medication to infuse freely. Assessment for a history of obstructive sleep apnea is important, as it is a risk factor for oversedation and respiratory depression. No one other than the patient is to initiate a PCA dose; the nurse will teach any visitors that they are not to touch the PCA device or button.

4. **Answer: 1.** According to the American Society for Pain Management, patients have the right to be treated with dignity, respect, and high-quality pain assessment and management. The nurse will explain that addiction is unlikely, as morphine has been safely prescribed postoperatively when dosed correctly and monitored appropriately. The nurse will further state that soon the patient will be changed to a nonopioid drug for pain management. This information directly addresses the patient's concern. Stating that the patient will not become addicted because the patient does not have a history of drug addiction is nontherapeutic, as this dismisses the patient's concern. The patient should not be discouraged from using the PCA device, as it is carefully dosed and monitored in the early postoperative phase. Asking the patient "Why" is demanding and nontherapeutic; the nurse's role is to address the concern the patient has voiced rather than ask for an explanation for the concern.

5. **Answer: 2.** The nurse will confirm that the patient should take medication about 30 minutes before walking. This gives the medication time to become effective so that pain during walking is minimized. It is inappropriate to tell the patient to take medication only if the pain is unbearable; the pain needs to be progressively managed during recovery. It is also inappropriate to tell the patient to double the medication prescribed; the patient should take only the prescribed amount. It is untrue that there are very few side effects associated with pain medication.

CHAPTER 17

1. **Answer:**

Health History	Nurses' Notes	Vital Signs	Laboratory Results

1634: Patient in bed, reporting pain of 7 on a 0–10 scale, which she says is "about what it always is." Height: 64 in (163 cm); weight: 101 lb (45.8 kg). VS: T = 99.2°F (37.3°C); HR = 86 beats/min; RR = 22 beats/min; BP = 110/66 mm Hg; SpO₂ 96% on RA. No advance directives on file. Patient expresses desire to forego any aggressive therapy; states, "Just make me comfortable." Family in the room expressing various viewpoints on which kind of care should be given if the patient declines.

The nurse will be concerned about the patient's pain. Although metastatic bone cancer is tremendously painful, the nurse will still attempt to address this discomfort to make the patient more comfortable. The nurse will also be concerned that there are no advance directives on file and that the family wants something different than what the patient has expressed. The nurse's responsibility is to the patient; however, it is preferable that an advance directive be in place so that there is legal documentation of the patient's wishes.

2. **Answers: 1, 2, 4, 5.** The nurse will explain that palliative care is a family-centered approach meant to improve the quality of life for patients and families who are facing problems associated with a life-threatening condition. Actions include addressing the patient's pain and other symptoms, creating and maintaining a therapeutic environment, helping

family cope with the current situation, and enhancing the patient's quality of life at the current time. This approach to care does not hasten or postpone death or dying.

3. **Answers: 1, 5.** The nurse will expect the patient to have increased respirations as she attempts to draw in air and restlessness due to lack of oxygenation. The nurse will anticipate cool skin (not warm), an increase in blood pressure (not a decrease) as the body works to facilitate gas exchange, and audible (quiet) inhalation and exhalation.

4. **Answers: 2, 4.** The purpose of an advance directive is to allow the patient who is oriented to make decisions about what kind of care is and isn't desired in case of inability to speak. It is a legally binding document; however, the patient who is oriented can make changes to the advance directive at any time. The health care provider does not decide which interventions are necessary; the patient declares in an advance directive which interventions are and aren't wanted. A DNR order means that cardiopulmonary resuscitation (CPR) will not be administered in cases of cardiac and/or pulmonary arrest; it does not mean that pain medication and all other treatment will be withheld. The advance directive exists to allow the patient to communicate while able; the family cannot change this directive if the patient becomes unconscious.

5. **Answer: 3.** The nurse will thank the granddaughter for the privilege of caring for the grandmother. At this time, it is therapeutic to allow the family to be with the body and share emotions that follow the death of a loved one. Saying it is wrong to be "joyful" when someone dies is nontherapeutic and judgmental. Therapeutic communication keeps the focus on the patient and caregivers; the nurse should not bring personal experience into the conversation. It is nontherapeutic and abrupt to ask the granddaughter to leave the room so that the body can be prepared. The nurse can prepare the body after the family has spent the desired time in the room following the death.

CHAPTER 18

1. **Answers: 1, 3, 4, 5.** All actions are correct when the nurse is making an unoccupied bed, with the exception of placing used, soiled linens on the floor. They should be placed in a linen bag to minimize the spread of any infectious agents.

2. **Answers: 2, 4, 5.** Clean the urethral meatus first in a circular motion to avoid cross-contamination of microorganisms from other areas of the perineum. Tension from an indwelling catheter can cause damage to the urethral sphincter; therefore, avoid placing tension on it. The scrotum has multiple skinfolds, and it is important to remove any body fluids or microorganisms from the area. The foreskin should be replaced rather than left retracted after cleansing. Leaving the foreskin retracted impedes blood supply to the penis and over time causes ischemia. The shaft and scrotum can be cleansed after the urethral meatus.

3. **Answer: 2.** The first action the nurse will take to assist with oral care is to perform hand hygiene and apply clean gloves. This helps to minimize the chance for transferring infectious agents. Other steps can be completed after handwashing and application of clean gloves.

4. **Answer:** See Skill 18.4 Patient Education section. It is important for patients with diabetes mellitus to check bare feet daily to identify any problems that may indicate the beginning or presence of infection. Patients should not walk barefoot, as peripheral neuropathy could prevent feeling sensations when stepping on something that could precipitate an infection. Patients should wear well-fitting shoes and move their feet daily to encourage perfusion. Application of heat (e.g., heating pads) is contraindicated in people with diabetes mellitus because when peripheral neuropathy is present, patients cannot always perceive excessive heat and move their feet away from the source. As a result, tissue damage to the feet and toes can occur. The use of alcohol causes drying of the skin, increasing a person's risk for skin injury, so cleansing should only be done with mild soap and water. Toenails are trimmed as needed on the basis of nail growth. Too-frequent nail trimming increases the risk of injuring the skin surrounding the nail. Nail polish on toes is permitted and does not harm the nail.

Health Teaching	Indicated	Not Indicated	Non-Essential
Observe bare feet daily for red spots, cuts, swelling, and blisters.	X		
Never walk barefoot.	X		
Use a heating pad to relax aching feet.		X	
Get measured for well-fitting shoes, especially exercise shoes.	X		
Move your toes and ankles up and down several times a day.	X		
Avoid nail polish on toes.			X
Use alcohol wipes or cotton balls saturated with alcohol on feet before foot care.		X	
Trim toenails weekly.		X	

5. **Answers: 1, 2, 3, 4, 5.** Factors that place a patient at risk for incontinence-associated dermatitis (IAD) include incontinence of urine and/or stool, impaired mobility, prolonged fever, impaired tissue integrity, and reduced nutrition intake.

CHAPTER 19

1. **Answers: 2, 3.** Several communication strategies can be used when interacting with older adults with a hearing impairment. Ask the patient to identify communication techniques that work best for them. Additionally, the nurse will talk slowly in a normal tone and stand so that the patient can see the nurse's face (as many patients benefit from watching lips move). There is no need to speak much more loudly than usual. This can make it more difficult for the patient to understand. Obtaining the use of an interpreter (as long as the patient fluently speaks the same language as the nurse) and speaking only to the spouse are inappropriate.

2. **Answer: 3.** After performing hand hygiene and donning clean gloves, the nurse will obtain the hearing aid from the patient and make sure it is turned off. Next, the holes in the device can be cleaned. All other actions can be taken subsequently.

3. **Answers: 2, 3, 4, 5.** It is appropriate for the nurse to ask questions about the patient's sight to help to identify reasons the patient may not have seen the stop sign and car ahead of her. These questions include asking whether the patient has had recent new vision changes, if the patient wears corrective lenses normally, whether the patient's eyes have been dryer than normal recently, and whether the patient has had any eye injuries. It is inappropriate to ask "why" questions; this places the patient in a defensive position. At this moment, it is important to determine if there is a visual problem rather than identify the patient's reason for driving.

4. **Answer: 4.** The nurse will intervene to ask more questions when the patient states that her left eye is starting to get blurry like her right eye. This could be a developing infection, another cataract, or signs of another health condition. The other statements do not require further intervention. Cleaning from the inner to outside portion of the eye is appropriate. Using eye drops as directed by the optometrist is appropriate. Seeing the doctor for the upcoming cataract surgery is appropriate.

5. **Answers: 1, 3, 5, 6.** This nurse will provide information about hearing aids and hearing by communicating that it is helpful to tell family members the ways in which the patient can best hear; to protect the hearing aids by storing them away from children and pets; to avoid using a hair dryer near the hearing aids as the heat can cause damage to

the devices; and to reduce background noise or move to a quiet area to hear best when talking with others. The nurse will encourage the patient to stay closer to someone—not at least 5 feet away—when listening to them. The nurse will clarify that hearing aids should not cause discomfort. The nurse will state that batteries will need to be changed periodically, but not every week, and that hearing aids should be removed for cleaning and inspection.

CHAPTER 20

1. **Answer: 4.** Many medications have the potential to cause dizziness and weakness. Considering that metoprolol is a beta blocker that has these side effects and that it is the newest medication the patient has been given, it is most likely that this has caused dizziness and weakness. The nurse will contact the health care provider to discuss this finding, as metoprolol has likely caused the patient's blood pressure to drop, resulting in these symptoms. The patient has been regularly taking sertraline, levothyroxine, and docusate; these are much less likely to induce the new symptoms of dizziness and weakness.

2. **Answer: 1, 2, 3, 4, 5.** The nurse will ask all of these questions, as they can provide meaningful information about why the patient is experiencing weakness and dizziness. It is important to confirm how much medication the patient is taking, especially because the pharmacy filled the metoprolol prescription with 150 mg tablets. It is important to quantify how often the dizziness and weakness are occurring and how long episodes typically last. To determine if the dizziness and weakness are related to metoprolol, the nurse will ask if there is a connection between the length of time after taking this drug and the onset of symptoms. It is also possible that the herbal preparation is responsible for, or contributing to, these symptoms; the nurse will ask for more information about what is in the herbal preparation.

3. **Answer: 1, 2, 3, 4.** "Timoptic .25% solution 1 drop OD BID" has a "naked" decimal point, and it is unclear whether OD means right eye or right ear. "Metoprolol 12.50 mg QD" has a trailing zero, and it is unclear whether the dosage is to be 12.5 mg or 1250 mg; the route of administration is also missing, and the order should indicate PO. "Insulin glargine 6 u SC twice a day" includes the letter *u*, which makes it unclear whether this means unit or if it is a 0 or a 4, and SC could be mistaken as SL or 65 every day. "Enalapril 2.5 mg. PO 3 times a day, hold for systolic blood pressure <100" has a period after mg, which could be mistaken as the number 1, and the < sign could be mistaken as "greater than." The order that states "Baby aspirin, 81 mg, one chewable tablet by mouth one time daily in the morning" is clear; it provides all of the information needed so the patient can safely take this medication.

4. **Answer: 1, 2, 5.** Setting up a pill-dispensing system can ensure safe medication administration in the older adult. Larger-print medication labels and/or pamphlets can be facilitated through the pharmacy. The use of teach-back ensures that the patient understands the medications and increases safety. Use of a magnifying glass is appropriate; however, this is not the only thing that can be done to help the patient visualize labels. There are actions that can be taken rather than having a home health care nurse come to dispense daily medication.

5. **Answer: 1, 3.** The nurse will teach the patient that setting a smartphone alarm for taking each dose of medication can be helpful, as this can prevent missed doses. The nurse will also discuss color-coding medication bottles so that they are easily identifiable and do not get easily mixed up. The nurse will not teach that the patient should double a missed dose of medication; this can cause undesirable side effects. Rather, the nurse should explain what to do for each medication if a dose is missed. It is not practical for this patient to rely on caregivers to give all of the medication; there is nothing that indicates that the patient is incapable of administering the patient's own doses. Although the pharmacy is a good resource, this is not the only way the patient can get information about medication. The nurse will advise the patient to contact the health care provider, the nurse, or the pharmacy about medication rather than searching for information online. Many online pieces of information are not credible and may provide wrong information. The nurse will discuss when each medication must be taken; not all medications are to be given at night.

CHAPTER 21

1. **Answer:**
   The patient reports feeling dizzy, having a cough, and chest soreness upon inspiration. The patient also states, "I'm not really hungry, and I don't feel much like eating." While listening to breath sounds, which include rhonchi, the nurse notes that there are three nitroglycerin transdermal patches on the patient's chest. VS: T 38.6°C (101.4°F); HR 90 beats/min; RR 20 breaths/min; BP 170/98 mm Hg; SpO$_2$ 92% on RA.

   The nurse notes these assessment findings that require follow-up:
   - Dizziness
   - Cough
   - Chest soreness upon inspiration
   - Anorexia and no desire to eat
   - Three nitroglycerin transdermal patches on the chest
   - Fever
   - Increased blood pressure
   - Reduced oxygen saturation

   All of these findings are abnormal and require further nursing assessment and intervention.

2. **Answer: 1.** The nurse will communicate that layering medication increases the risk for infection. By not cleansing the wound and applying fresh medication, the wound may retain bacteria that is in or around it. The nurse will explain the reason for gently cleaning the wound with warm soap and water and reapplying new medication as often as ordered by the health care provider. The nurse will not acknowledge that this is a good way to save money on medication because it could increase health care costs if the wound is further infected. The nurse will not state that the wound needs to be cleaned with alcohol and hot water because this could further damage tissue integrity. The normal healing process does not include buildup of crusts.

3. **Answers: 1, 2, 5.** The nurse will teach the patient that cleaning the application site removes any residual medication from the previous dose. The nurse will confirm that gloves must be worn to apply the ointment and to discard used ointment wrappers to reduce the risk of accidental exposure to medication and systemic reaction to the nitroglycerin (e.g., vasodilation, hypotension). The nurse will not recommend allowing a caregiver to apply the medication without gloves; this increases the risk to the caregiver for developing a systematic reaction. The nurse will also not state that laboratory appointments need to be kept; this type of medication does not require laboratory testing for therapeutic drug values.

4. **Answers: 3, 4, 5.** An enteral tube syringe is necessary to avoid dangerous misconnections and accidently administering the medications through another tube. Flushing the tubing after medication administration clears it of any residual medication and ensures that the tube remains patent. If gastric residuals are high, the absorption of the enteral tube medication is reduced. Verification of tube placement is essential before—not after—administering anything via a nasogastric tube. This must be done via radiograph. Medications are given separately to avoid any drug-to-drug interactions that could clog the feeding tube.

5. **Answer: 1.** See Skill 21.7. It is critical to perform a respiratory assessment before inhaler use. This provides baseline information about the patient's breath sounds and lung expansion. Following the assessment, other steps can be taken to administer the medication.

CHAPTER 22

1. **Answer: 1.** The nurse can direct the AP to notify the nurse of any signs of bleeding such as blood in the urine or stool or any noted blood oozing from a puncture or IV site. The nurse cannot delegate assessment of response to heparin, comparison of medication orders with the dispensed heparin, or drawing up medication; these are all functions within the role of the nurse.

2. **Answer: 3.** After cleaning the site, the nurse will use the nondominant hand and stretch the skin over the site with a forefinger. The needle is then inserted at a 5- to 15-degree angle into the skin until resistance is

felt. The needle is advanced through the epidermis to 3 mm, and the injection commences until a bleb is noted.

3. **Answer: 1, 7.** The experienced nurse will intervene if the new nurse prepares to use the filter needle for administration. This needle is used to aspirate medication and to prevent glass particles from being drawn into the syringe. It must be discarded and a new needle attached before administration. The experienced nurse will also intervene if the new nurse returns the ampule to the medication bin after drawing up a dose. Ampules contain single doses of medication and should not be reused. All other actions are appropriate and do not require intervention by the experienced nurse.

4. **Answer: 3.** The nurse will select the injection port of IV tubing closest to the patient. Then the injection port will be cleaned with an antiseptic swab. The syringe is then connected to the port of the IV line. The IV line is then occluded by pinching tubing just above the injection port. The nurse will then pull back gently on the syringe plunger to aspirate blood return. The tubing is then released, and the medication is injected as per a medication reference manual. Finally, the syringe is withdrawn from the port of the IV line.

5. **Answer: 2.** The nurse will teach the patient that periodic laboratory work will be required while using heparin. Coagulation blood tests are performed periodically so that the health care provider can monitor the patient for the desired therapeutic range for heparin. Minimal bruising is expected with heparin. A soft toothbrush—not a hard one—should be used to gently clean the teeth while on heparin therapy. Numerous supplements interact with heparin and can lead to bleeding or hemorrhage. The patient should talk with a health care provider before taking any over-the-counter supplements.

CHAPTER 23

1. **Answers: 1, 2, 4, 6, 9.** The nurse can delegate activities that are within the skill set of assistive personnel (AP). These activities include obtaining vital signs, assisting with transfers, changing the patient's position when in bed, reporting changes in pulse oximetry when ambulating, and assisting with hygiene. The nurse will delegate these tasks, provide education to the AP about what needs to be done, and remain responsible for supervision. Assessing (lung sounds), teaching (cough and deep breathing exercises), evaluating (skin for pressure), and treatments (such as nasotracheal suctioning) are nursing roles; these cannot be done by an AP.

2. **Answer: 3.** An oxygen saturation of 88% on 2 L of oxygen demonstrates that the plan of care is ineffective at this time. Ideally, this finding should be 95% or above. All other findings are within expected parameters and demonstrate efficacy of the plan of care.

3. **Answer: 3.** Any change in the level of consciousness (LOC) requires the nurse to intervene. LOC changes can indicate hypoxia. A decrease in the work of breathing, improved lung expansion, and an SpO_2 of 94% are favorable findings that do not require the nurse to intervene.

4. **Answers: 1, 2, 4, 5.** The patient who knows that candles cannot be used around oxygen (due to the fire hazard), that signs are required to notify people of where oxygen is used in a home, that no one can smoke around oxygen, and that gas stoves should be avoided near oxygen (again, due to environmental hazards) has demonstrated that teaching has been effective. If a patient believes that incense can be burned instead of using candles, more education is needed; anything that burns can be a fire or combustive hazard if used near oxygen.

5. **Answer: 1.** For adults with COVID-19 and acute hypoxemic respiratory failure despite conventional oxygen therapy, high-flow nasal cannula (HFNC) oxygen is recommended. The other methods of delivery will not be anticipated at this time.

CHAPTER 24

1. **Answer: 2.** The nurse needs to clear the airway by oropharyngeal suctioning because that is the primary problem affecting the patient's ability to oxygenate. The patient may require oxygen, but the airway needs to be cleared first so that oxygen can move. If continuing intervention is needed, the nurse can contact respiratory therapy and prepare for insertion of an endotracheal tube.

2. **Answers: 1, 2, 3, 4, 5.** It is appropriate for the nurse to perform all of these further assessments to determine the patient's ongoing status. Gurgling on inspiration or expiration and drooling may indicate the need to continue suctioning. Restlessness may indicate hypoxia. Chest wall motion can indicate respiratory effort. Lung auscultation demonstrates whether lungs are clear or with adventitious lung sounds that may indicate further respiratory concern.

3. **Answer:**

Body System	Findings
Neurological	PERRLA. Moves extremities equally yet weakly.
Pulmonary	Lungs clear to auscultation. Remains tachypneic.
Cardiovascular	Heart sounds regular without murmur. Capillary refill 4 seconds. All extremities cool to the touch. Pulses +1 in lower extremities.
Gastrointestinal	Abdomen round and soft to gentle touch. Bowel sounds present in all 4 quadrants.

Abnormal findings that require further nursing follow-up include weak extremity movement, ongoing tachypnea, capillary refill of 4 seconds, cool extremities, and +1 pulses in the lower extremities. These findings indicate potential ongoing hypoxia and reduced perfusion. Other findings are within expected parameters and do not require further nursing follow-up.

4. **Answer: 1.** At this time, the nurse will contact the health care provider because nursing interventions have not facilitated easier breathing. There is no indication that a sputum culture is needed because no signs of infection are present. The head of the bed should be raised to facilitate breathing, not lowered. Discontinuation of suctioning is inappropriate because that will increase difficulty breathing as secretions increase.

5. **Answer: 4.** Teeth of patients with endotracheal tubes (ETTs) in place should be brushed at least twice a day; oral care should be performed every 2 to 4 hours to decrease the risk for ventilator-associated pneumonia. Saline should not be instilled in the ETT when suctioning is performed—that is no longer a recommended practice. Adhesive tape remover should not be used when cleaning the endotracheal tube (ETT) because the commercial tube holder will not stick to the ETT, which then increases risk of tube dislodgment. The ETT cuff pressure should be between 2 and 25 mm Hg.

CHAPTER 25

1. **Answer: 2.** Although all of these tests may be eventually ordered, the nurse anticipates that the electrocardiogram will be ordered initially. The patient has a history of myocardial infarction and has an elevated pulse and respiratory rate coupled with a decrease in blood pressure. These findings allude to a cardiovascular concern.

2. **Answer: 1, 2, 3, 4, 5.** An electrocardiogram can be used to evaluate for suspected acute coronary syndromes, implanted defibrillators and pacemakers, syncope, metabolic disorders, and effects and side effects of pharmacotherapeutics.

3. **Answer: 4.** V_1 is placed at the fourth intercostal space (ICS) at the right sternal border. V_3 is placed midway between V_2 and V_4. V_4 is placed at the fifth ICS at the midclavicular line. V_5 is placed at the left anterior axillary line at the level of V_4 horizontally.

4. **Answer:** The *priorities* of care for the patient at this time are to **determine origin of nausea and vomiting** and **manage perfusion**. The patient has a history of myocardial infarction and has an elevated pulse and respiratory rate coupled with a decrease in blood pressure. These findings allude to a cardiovascular concern. Therefore the origin of the nausea and vomiting (which may be related to a cardiac concern) and management of perfusion are the priorities of care. A pain rating of 4 on a 0-to-10 scale following surgery is expected; this can be addressed after the care priorities. Assessment of the surgical incision and contacting family members can be done after addressing the cardiac concerns.

5. **Answer: 3, 5.** The nurse will troubleshoot this finding by cleansing the skin with soap and water (not alcohol) and wiping it dry with a washcloth. Rubbing the skin with a washcloth before electrode placement helps to enhance electrical transfer to signals. The nurse will also inspect the electrodes to make sure they are securely placed. The nurse will refrain from moving electrodes to different locations, as correct placement is required for accuracy of readings. The nurse will not use alcohol on the electrodes, as this is not recommended for good electrical conduction. Electrodes should be changed at least daily and as needed if soiled or dysfunctional.

CHAPTER 26

1. **Answer: 2.** The sudden drainage is most likely related to the position change from moving from the bed to a chair, which allowed a pocket of fluid to drain. The fluid is dark red because it is likely old blood from a pocket in the chest cavity that was not close to an eyelet on the chest tube. In most cases this is a normal finding. The nurse will take vital signs, assess cardiopulmonary status, and monitor the chest tube drainage to be sure that the volume does not increase to over 50 to 150 mL/h. There is no need to contact the Rapid Response Team or to notify the surgeon (as this finding does not indicate hemorrhage). The nurse should not disrupt the chest tubes.

2. **Answer: 3.** The nurse will first disconnect the tubing from the drainage system and then insert the tubing below the surface of a bottle of sterile water or sterile saline to regain a water seal. A new system needs to be obtained. Finally, the nurse can notify the health care provider of the event.

3. **Answer: 4.** Sudden cessation of bleeding may suggest chest tube occlusion, which increases the risk of accumulating a hemothorax; this finding requires nursing intervention. All other findings are expected and do not require nursing intervention.

4. **Answer: 1, 2, 3, 4, 5, 6.** The nurse will perform all actions when assisting with chest tube removal. This includes gathering supplies prior to removal, premedicating the patient with pain medication (as removal can be painful), and placing the patient in semi-Fowler position to facilitate comfort and lung expansion. Respiratory mechanics of deep breathing, exhaling, and bearing down will help to facilitate lung expansion. Once the removal process begins, the nurse will apply a petroleum gauze over the site where the tube was removed, stay with the patient, and provide emotional support. Alcohol should not be used to clean the site where the drain was located; this can damage tissue integrity and be quite painful.

5. **Answer: 1.** Clear breath sounds on auscultation indicate that hospital nursing and collaborative interventions were effective. Findings of an SpO₂ of 91%, pus at the chest tube insertion site, and respiratory rate of 24 breaths/min are abnormal and demonstrate that interventions were ineffective.

CHAPTER 27

1. **Answer: 2.** The nurse will stay with the patient and call for help first. It is critical to remain with the patient once unresponsiveness is established. After calling for help, the nurse can complete the other actions.

2. **Answers: 1, 4.** Minimizing interruptions and providing adequate depth and rate of compressions are the two strategies that the nurse will use to ensure high-quality CPR. Avoiding full chest recoil would hinder the quality by not allowing the full release to provide optimal filling of the heart. Giving more ventilations than recommended would increase the intrathoracic pressure, which would also cause suboptimal filling of the heart. Pausing chest compression before defibrillation (while the defibrillator is being prepared) adds interruption of CPR of more than 10 seconds, which decreases cerebral and coronary perfusion during this time frame.

3. **Answer: 3.** The nurse will instruct the other nurse to apply the automated external defibrillator (AED). Then, the area will be cleared for the AED to be initiated. After the AED delivers a shock, the nurse will check for a pulse and then resume providing chest compressions.

4. **Answers: 1, 2, 3, 4, 5.** Using the SBAR method of communication, the nurse will report the situation (found patient on the floor), background (hospitalized for acute kidney injury), assessment (no pulse when found

on the floor), and response (how long CPR has been administered and how many shocks have been delivered by the AED).

5. **Answer:**

System	Possible interventions
Cardiovascular	**X** Document blood pressure **X** Apply cardiac monitor ○ Discuss cardiac rehabilitation with the patient
Respiratory	○ Explain the cause of infection **X** Assess lung sounds every 2 hours **X** Monitor continuous pulse oximetry
Neurological	**X** Assess for changes in cognition ○ Ask to count backwards from 100 by 7s ○ Tell three words to the patient; ask patient to repeat the words 5 minutes later

The nurse will document the patient's blood pressure and apply a cardiac monitor so that perfusion and the heart's rhythm can be monitored. The nurse will assess lung sounds every 2 hours (or more as needed) and monitor continuous pulse oximetry to ensure that the patient is properly exchanging gas. The nurse will also assess for any changes in cognition, which can accompany hypoxia. There is no need to discuss cardiac rehabilitation; this is a program for patients who have had a myocardial infarction, heart failure, angioplasty, or heart surgery. There is no need to explain a cause of infection because there is nothing that indicates infection is present. There is no need to ask the patient to count backwards or to remember three words. These are tasks associated with a mental status examination to determine if the patient has organic and progressive cognitive impairment.

CHAPTER 28

1. **Answer: 1, 2, 3, 4, 5.** The nurse will assess for clinical markers of vascular and interstitial volume for FVE. There may be an increase in weight, an increase in urine volume, distended neck veins, adventitious lung sounds on auscultation, and dependent edema from increased fluid volume. Although FVE could be a likely cause of difficulty breathing, other conditions could also be the causative agent.

2. **Answer: 3.** The nurse will anticipate a change to an isotonic fluid such as 0.9% saline. Isotonic fluids are given to maintain or increase the extracellular fluid volume as in cases of dehydration. Hypotonic solutions such as 0.45% saline are given when cells are dehydrated and fluids need to be reestablished intracellularly. Hypertonic fluids such as D10W and 5% dextrose in lactated Ringer's are given to increase intravascular fluid volume.

3. **Answer: 4.** After performing hand hygiene, donning gloves and mask, removing the old dressing, and cleaning the catheter site, the nurse will apply a labeled integrated securement device or transparent semipermeable membrane (TSM) dressing.

4. **Answer: 1, 2, 4, 5.** All actions are appropriate except for placing the thumb proximal to the insertion point. This action would not allow for adequate stabilization of the vein and could increase the risk for the nurse to be stuck by the needle. The vein should be stabilized by placing the thumb distal to the insertion site and stretching the skin against the direction of insertion.

5. **Answer: 2, 5.** These findings indicate possible phlebitis and require nursing intervention, as they are unexpected developments following the insertion of a peripheral IV line. All other findings are normal and do not require the nurse to intervene.

CHAPTER 29

1. **Answer: Blood in stool, hematocrit.** These findings indicate blood loss and must be addressed as priorities of care. The patient's heart rate, blood pressure, respiratory rate, and blood glucose are within normal limits; therefore the nurse will continue to monitor these parameters, but they are not concerning at this moment. The nurse can address the patient's question about autologous blood donation after responding to

the priorities of care. Fatigue should resolve after treatment for the priorities of care that indicate blood loss.

2. **Answer: 2.** The PRBCs should be returned to the blood bank because blood transfusions must be initiated within 30 minutes after release from laboratory or blood bank. All other actions are inappropriate.

3. **Answer: 1, 2, 3, 4, 5.** All of these steps are appropriate actions to take to verify at the patient's bedside that the correct blood component is to be transfused to the correct patient.

4. **Answer: 1, 2, 3, 5.** Choices 1, 2, 3, and 5 include the information required to verify and actions to take to ensure that the right blood product is safely given to the right patient. Although vital signs should be taken before transfusion, 15 minutes after beginning the transfusion, and at the completion of the transfusion, PRBCs should be administered over 4 hours, not 2 hours.

5. **Answer: 2.** If a patient exhibits symptoms of an acute hemolytic transfusion reaction, the nurse will stop the infusion of blood, as this is what has caused the problem. Allowing more blood to infuse can exacerbate the symptoms, which in some cases may be fatal. After the transfusion is stopped, the nurse can obtain vital signs, contact the blood bank, and notify the health care provider.

CHAPTER 30

1. **Answer: Aspiration, diminished gag reflex.** The highest risk for the patient at this time is aspiration, as evidenced by a diminished gag reflex, slow swallowing, frequent coughing when swallowing, and inability to swallow all food and liquids, which leak from the corners of the mouth. Although the patient may have some risk for dehydration, malnutrition, or sepsis, these are not the highest risk factors present. The patient is able to consume intake, so dehydration and malnutrition are less likely. The patient is also being treated with antibiotic therapy for pneumonia, so sepsis is less likely. Reduced strength in the hands is not a risk factor for aspiration. Decreased lung sounds and the pulse oximetry of 92% are likely related to pneumonia.

2. **Answer: 2, 4, 5.** The nurse can delegate weight and height measurement to the AP. Assisting a patient to the bathroom and ordering meals are within the skill set of the AP. The nurse will delegate these tasks, provide education to the AP about what needs to be done, and remain responsible for supervision. The remaining elements of collecting a medication history and completing a nutrition screening are nursing roles associated with assessment; these cannot be done by an AP.

3. **Answer: 3, 5.** To improve the patient's intake, the nurse can assess whether the patient is in pain. Experiencing pain can reduce the patient's desire or functional ability to eat. The nurse will also provide between-meal snacks, as this can increase the ability of the patient to eat throughout the day instead of only at mealtime. The patient might require food served at times closer to the normal mealtime rather than on the hospital's schedule. Reminding the patient of the need to eat to heal is nontherapeutic; this action does not address the reasons that the patient may have difficulty eating. Small, frequent servings are usually more tolerable than larger servings for patients who have difficulty eating.

4. **Answer: 1, 2, 3.** Risk factors for malnutrition include difficulty feeding self, poor appetite, and institutionalized living. A BMI of 21 is normal. Family members who take the patient out to eat do not increase the risk for malnutrition, as they can go where the patient enjoys eating and can provide socialization.

5. **Answer: 2, 4.** A minced and moist diet includes finely minced or ground tender meats served in extremely thick, smooth, nonpouring sauce or gravy; mashed potatoes; mashed fruits; and thick cereals. A liquid, moderately thick diet includes runny rice cereal, runny pureed fruit, sauces and gravies, and honey-thickened beverages. A soft and bite-sized diet includes soft, cooked meat cut in small pieces; flakey fish; casseroles; stews; soft, cooked vegetables in bite-sized pieces; and mashed fruits.

CHAPTER 31

1. **Answer: 4.** According to the American Society for Parenteral and Enteral Nutrition (ASPEN), the gold standard for verifying the placement of a blindly inserted feeding tube is to obtain a radiographic film of the abdomen. This helps to ensure that the tip of the tube is resting in the stomach or the intestinal tract. Auscultation of insufflated air is not a reliable indicator of tube placement. Inspecting the character of gastric fluid and checking pH are helpful ongoing measures for confirming tube placement.

2. **Answer: 3, 4, 5.** The feeding has been running at 55 mL/h for 4 hours. This is below the 220 mL that has infused, and patient does not demonstrate any other symptoms of feeding intolerance. The nurse will continue the tube feeding as ordered, refeed the aspirate back to the patient so no caloric intake is lost, and continue to assess for feeding tolerance. There is no need to contact the RDN or to stop the feeding.

3. **Answer: 4.** To prevent the enteral feeding tube from becoming clogged or obstructed and the patient from becoming dehydrated, the nurse should flush the enteral feeding tube every 4 hours during a continuous feeding. Enteral feeding formula should be kept at room temperature to prevent gastric cramping and discomfort. To prevent aspiration of the feeding, the patient should have the head of the bed elevated to at least 30 degrees; 20 degrees is too low. Capillary blood glucose testing is typically done with parenteral feedings, not enteral feedings.

4. **Answer:** The assessment findings the nurse needs to follow up on immediately include the pulse oximetry of 91%; the hard, distended abdomen; and bilateral crackles throughout the lung fields. Pulse oximetry below 93% indicates possible hypoxia. The hard, distended abdomen is indicative of a potential problem with peristalsis and bowel activity. The abdomen should be soft and nondistended, with bowel sounds. The crackles throughout the lung fields need follow-up to ensure that the patient is not developing atelectasis or pneumonia. Left-sided paralysis is already known due to the stroke. The blood pressure, GRV, and respirations are within normal and expected parameters.

5. **Answer: 3.** Following the insertion of a feeding tube, the nurse will document the size and type of the tube, the status of the naris that tube was inserted into, the patient's tolerance of the procedure, and x-ray confirmation of the placement of the tip of the tube. Each of the other documentation examples are missing elements that are important.

CHAPTER 32

1. **Answer: 1, 3, 4, 5.** Assessment of vital signs, weight, lung sounds, and blood glucose are essential to provide a baseline for monitoring a patient's response to fluid infusion. Vital signs will reveal early cardiovascular response. Crackles in the lungs are an early indication of fluid volume excess. Weight gain can occur if fluids are retained. Infusion of fluids too rapidly can cause glucose changes. Level of consciousness is not an anticipated change when CPN is first initiated. Due to the calorie additives (e.g., carbohydrates, fats), the patient's blood glucose can change quickly

2. **Answer: 3.** After applying clean gloves, the nurse will attach the appropriate filter to IV tubing and prime the tubing with the CPN solution, making sure no air bubbles remain. Other actions are taken subsequently: The end of the CVAD is scrubbed with an alcohol swab. The syringe of 0.9% NS solution is attached to the needleless port and flushed with saline. The Luer-Lok end of the CPN IV tubing is connected to the end port of the CVAD, and the IV tubing is placed in the EID. Finally, the flow rate is set and regulated as ordered.

3. **Answer: Central line–associated bloodstream infection (CLABSI), newly inserted central line.** The patient is at risk for CLABSI due to the presence of the newly inserted central line. Fever and malaise are signs of infection. There is no indication that the patient is at high risk for dehydration, chronic fatigue syndrome, kidney failure, or ileus. There is no evidence that the patient has a dietary deficiency. An exacerbation of Crohn disease does not increase the patient's risk for CLABSI, nor does a history of asthma or weight loss.

4. **Answer: 1, 3, 4, 5.** The nurse will monitor closely for signs of evolving infection, which include change in temperature (fever is an indication of infection), change in appearance of the catheter insertion site (redness and/or drainage of pus can indicate infection), change in pulse rate (pulse rate is often elevated in the presence of infection), and signs of chills (which often occur when a patient has an infection). Weight loss can occur in the presence of infection but not during the early phase of an infection. Lung sounds are not indicative of CLABSI.

5. **Answer: 2, 4, 5.** Weight gain in excess of 0.5 kg (1.1 lb) per day can be indicative of fluid retention. The nurse will palpate the lower extremities for edema (which can accumulate if there is fluid retention), auscultate lungs for any adventitious sounds (which may occur if there is fluid retention), and check intake and output (which can also help to substantiate whether the patient has fluid retention). Intake greater than output per each 24-hour period indicates fluid retention from poorly regulated CPN infusion. Reflex responses and serum protein levels will not give important information about the possibility of fluid retention.

CHAPTER 33

1. **Answer: 4.** The nurse will drape the patient, prepare the sterile field, lubricate the catheter, clean the urethral meatus, insert and advance the catheter, advance further when urine appears, inflate the catheter balloon, gently pull until resistance is felt, and attach the drainage tube. See Skill 33.1.

2. **Answer:**

Nursing Action	Indicated	Not Indicated
Cleanse the urinary meatus with alcohol daily.		X
Hang the urinary drainage bag below the level of the bladder.	X	
Change the urinary drainage bag daily.		X
Irrigate the catheter daily with normal saline.		X
Eliminate any kinking in urinary drainage tubing.	X	
Use sterile technique each time emptying the drainage bag.		X

Evidence shows that maintaining flow of urine (e.g., eliminating kinks in tubing) and hanging the urinary drainage bag below the level of the bladder are helpful in prevention of CAUTI. These actions prevent the urine from backflowing. The nurse will not cleanse the urinary meatus with alcohol; this is drying and abrasive and can compromise skin integrity, which can lead to infection. The urinary drainage bag does not need to be changed daily. Irrigation is inappropriate. Clean technique—not sterile—is to be used when emptying the drainage bag.

3. **Answers: 1, 2, 3, 4, 5.** The nurse will report all of these findings to the health care provider, as they can be indicators of a catheter-associated urinary tract infection (CAUTI). It is especially important to remember that older adults may exhibit atypical signs and symptoms of CAUTI, such as a change in mental status, which is wrongly attributed to delirium. A change in mental status may include confusion, agitation, or lethargy. Other symptoms may include cloudy and/or foul-smelling urine and new onset of lethargy.

4. **Answer: 3.** The nurse will intervene if the AP is applying petroleum jelly to the catheter tubing for comfort. Lubrication upon insertion of the catheter should only be done with a water-based lubricant, and any discomfort afterwards should be brought to the attention of the nurse rather than addressed by the AP. Petroleum jelly can prevent air from circulating and creates an environment where bacteria can congregate and contribute to infection. Other actions are appropriate and do not require intervention by the nurse.

5. **Answer: 2.** The nurse needs to provide further teaching when the patient states that bladder spasms are to be expected while the indwelling catheter is present. While spasms may occur, they need to be reported to the health care provider right away. Other patient statements are appropriate and demonstrate that nursing teaching was effective.

CHAPTER 34

1. **Answer:**

Nursing Action	Indicated	Not Indicated
Uses castile soap to prepare the SSE.	X	
Uses cold water to mix with soap to prepare the SSE.		X
Assists patient to a side-lying position.	X	
Primes tubing so it is filled with solution before administering SSE.	X	
Inserts tip of rectal tube 4–5 inches into rectum.		X
Raises enema container to approximately 12 inches above the anus to be instilled.	X	

Castile soap and warm—not cold—water are used to prepare the SSE. The patient is placed into a side-lying position. Tubing is primed so that it is filled with solution before administration. The rectal tube is inserted 6 to 8 cm (2½ to 3 inches; not 4 to 5 inches, which could be painful and disrupt the rectal mucosa), the clamp is opened, and the enema container is raised 30 cm (12 inches) above the anus for a regular enema.

2. **Answer: 3.** As the patient reported constipation before surgery and has been taking opioid medication afterward (which causes constipation), the nurse will anticipate that a fecal impaction is most likely the cause of the failed administration. After attempting the procedure 3 times, the nurse will have assessed and ruled out a variety of potential problems. At this time, it is less likely that the problem is faulty tubing, a broken clamp, or clenching of the patient.

3. **Answer: 2.** The first thing that must be done, with the health care provider's order, is to remove the fecal impaction. Other measures may be needed after the removal to prevent a future fecal impaction.

4. **Answer: 4.** After verifying the order, performing hand hygiene and donning gloves, and confirming the patient's identity, the nurse will measure and mark the tube to determine the correct tubing length. Then the nurse will instruct the patient to flex head forward and swallow while the tube is advanced. The nurse will pass the tube along the floor of nasal passage, then just past the nasopharynx. Once in place, the tube will be taped to the nose for stability.

5. **Answers: 1, 5.** Increasing intake of fiber and fluids can decrease constipation, as can incorporating movement (exercise) into the daily routine. The nurse will not teach the patient to use an enema daily, nor to take laxatives daily. Doing so can make the patient reliant on one or both means to have a bowel movement. Avoidance of gluten is not associated with managing chronic constipation.

CHAPTER 35

1. **Answer: 2.** Although the nurse can collaborate with many members of the interprofessional team, the wound, ostomy, continence nurse will have the most experience and information to provide to address the patient's fear. The surgeon and primary care provider are more likely to provide support by discussing the physiological aspects of the ostomy. The registered dietitian nutritionist is more likely to provide support by discussing foods that create less output and gas.

2. **Answer: 1, 3, 4.** The nurse will assess the urine appearance, temperature, and patient's report of discomfort. Cloudy or dark urine can be indicative of a potential urinary tract infection, as can an elevated temperature or the patient's degree of lower abdominal pain. Intake of solid food will provide information about nutrition status and bowel habits. The peristomal skin condition will provide information about whether the stoma is healthy, functional, or compromised.

3. **Answer:**

Health Teaching	Indicated	Not Indicated
"Empty ostomy pouches when they are one-third to one-half full to avoid leakage."	X	
"Only change the pouch if you notice leakage from under the wafer."		X
"The stoma will normally be red and moist."	X	
"The skin around the stoma is normally intact with some reddening after the adhesive wafer is removed."	X	
"If you notice blisters on the skin around your stoma, scrub them well to make sure the skin is clean."		X
"Pouches should be changed every 3 to 7 days."	X	
"Use alcohol- or acetone-based products to clean stoma thoroughly."		X

It is appropriate for the nurse to provide evidence-based information about stoma, skin, and pouch care following the creation of an ileostomy. Appropriate information includes instructing to empty the pouch when it is one-third to one-half full to avoid leakage, noting that the stoma will be red and moist, stating that the skin surrounding the stoma may have some reddening after the adhesive wafer is removed, and stating the need to change the pouch every 3 to 7 days as needed. It is incorrect and contraindicated for the nurse to tell the patient to only change the pouch if it leaks. To maintain hygiene, this should be done every 3 to 7 days as needed. It is contraindicated to recommend scrubbing blisters and using alcohol- or acetone-based products. Tissue integrity can be compromised, which raises the risk for infection.

4. **Answer: 3.** Once the pouch has been removed, the nurse will teach the patient to observe the stoma and surrounding skin. Any signs of infection or other abnormalities should be noted at this time. Other actions can take place once the patient has performed this assessment.

5. **Answer: 2, 3, 5.** These are appropriate actions to take to prevent recurrence of leakage and protect the peristomal skin. Consulting a wound, ostomy, continence nurse can be helpful, as this expert can help the patient become more proficient in self-care. Reviewing the importance of emptying the pouch before it is half full is appropriate; this will prevent overfilling. Measuring the stoma again is important, as it can change size as it heals following surgery. The nurse will not use alcohol to help dry the skin; this would further damage tissue integrity. The opening in the skin barrier may need to be cut smaller, not larger, than the last one if the stoma size has changed. This also increases vulnerability to further exposure and continued skin breakdown.

CHAPTER 36

1. **Answer:**

Body System	Possible Tasks to Delegate to Assistive Personnel (AP)
General	○ Evaluate for postoperative pain ○ Perform initial assessment upon arrival to unit X Provide repositioning every 2 hours

Body System	Possible Tasks to Delegate to Assistive Personnel (AP)
Integumentary	○ Monitor IV site for infiltration or signs of infection X Provide general hygiene and oral care AS and PM ○ Assess incision site twice per shift
Respiratory	X Document pulse oximetry reading every 4 hours ○ Assess lung sounds every 2 hours ○ Teach how to cough and deep breathe
Renal	X Empty Foley catheter bag X Provide perineal care twice daily ○ Assess kidney function for signs of infection

It is within the scope of assistive personnel (AP) to provide repositioning, to provide general hygiene and oral care, to document pulse oximetry readings, to empty a Foley catheter bag, and to provide perineal care. The nurse will delegate these tasks, provide education to the AP about what needs to be done, and remain responsible for supervision. Assessing, evaluating, monitoring, and teaching are nursing roles; these cannot be done by an AP.

2. **Answer: 3.** After major surgery, patients are often given patient-controlled analgesia (PCA), an opioid medication that can be delivered at the patient's indication. Although PCAs are set to have a lock-out so that the patient does not become overmedicated, it is most likely that the opioid medication is preventing the patient from staying awake. The patient's temperature is slightly elevated but not enough to induce sleepiness. The patient's blood pressure is low but not dangerously low to induce sleepiness. Fatigue after surgery is expected, but this is not usually what causes a patient to have difficulty staying awake when they are being prescribed opioid medication.

3. **Answer: 3.** Auscultation of normal bowel sounds after surgery is the earliest indicator that gastrointestinal function has returned. Other findings come later.

4. **Answers: 1, 2, 3.** Coughing and deep breathing, moving regularly, and using an incentive spirometer will enhance the postsurgical patient's pulmonary status. The patient should not take an antihistamine if breathing is difficult; emergency care should be sought. Splinting the abdomen when rising from bed will minimize pain but not enhance pulmonary status.

5. **Answer: 4.** The nurse will report the patient's temperature of 100.0°F (37.8°C) to the health care provider. Although this may not be an exclusion for discharge, the health care provider needs to determine if further intervention is needed before releasing the patient. All other findings are expected and do not need to be reported.

CHAPTER 37

1. **Answers: 1, 2, 3, 5.** All of these pieces of information need to be confirmed with the patient during the preprocedure time. The nurse will also verify consent in the electronic health record (EHR), ensure that the site has been marked with the surgeon, perform a brief history and physical, review diagnostic and radiologic test results, determine if blood products are acceptable to the patient or if these products are declined, and ask the patient about any special equipment/devices/implants. The name of the person driving the patient home in 48 hours is not necessary; this will be confirmed by the medical surgical nurse before discharge.

2. **Answer: 1.** In the early steps of surgical hand asepsis, the nurse will inspect fingernails and cuticles for any cuts or abrasions that could be a source of infection. Other actions take place following that inspection.

3. **Answers: 1, 2, 3, 4, 5 (all of the above).** TJC (2023) recommends to clean hands before touching a patient, before clean/aseptic procedures, after body fluid exposure/risk, after touching a patient, and after touching patient surroundings.

4. **Answer: Patient identity, correct location of surgery.** The purpose of a time-out is to confirm that the surgery involves the correct patient, correct procedure, correct site, and correct side. Other factors, such as confirming the presence of advance directives, identifying the unit the patient will be transferred to after PACU, identifying the patient's next of kin, and reviewing insurance coverage for surgery are performed outside of the operating suite by other individuals.

5. **Answer: 3.** A principle of sterile technique is that surgical gowns should be an adequate size to wrap around and completely cover the scrubbed team member's body. The back of the gown is not sterile. Unscrubbed team members must stay at least 30.5 cm (12 inches) away from the sterile field while keeping it in constant view. Table drapes are sterile only at table level—not to the floor.

CHAPTER 38

1. **Answers: 1, 2, 3, 4, 5, 6, 7.** All of these assessments must be performed by the nurse when the patient is returned to the medical surgical unit following PACU. This provides a baseline assessment for many factors, which will be used for comparison throughout the patient's stay at the hospital.

2. **Answers: 1, 3, 4, 5.** These are signs of a possible wound infection, which will delay wound healing. Because of the excessive amount of wound drainage, the patient's wound might be infected, causing an elevated temperature and pulse rate. A strong odor, yellow or unusual color of drainage, and warmth and redness of the periwound skin are common indicators of a wound infection. The baseline blood pressure is not indicative of a wound infection.

3. **Answer: 4.** The drain should be emptied, as it is nearly full. The bulb should not be shaken. There is no need to contact the surgeon. The drain should be secured below the level of the wound.

4. **Answer: 1.** Now that the slough (necrotic tissue) has been removed from the wound bed, the nurse anticipates the health care provider will order NPWT. It is unlikely that the wound will be left open to air at this time. There is no need for further wound suturing. Antifungal medication therapy is not anticipated.

5. **Answer: 2.** Typically NPWT is ordered at a pressure of −75 to −125 mm Hg. The nurse will contact the health care provider to clarify the order. Application at a pressure of 200 mm Hg is contraindicated; this is a high pressure and may cause the patient a large amount of pain. The nurse should not fill the wound bed and proceed nor should the nurse contact the manufacturer; the health care provider needs to be contacted to get the order clarified.

CHAPTER 39

1. **Answers: 2, 3, 4.** Because the patient is intubated and on a ventilator, the head of the bed needs to be at a 30-degree angle, making the patient's sacrum at risk for skin breakdown. The nasoenteral feeding tube has the potential to cause a medical device–related pressure injury (MDRPI) on the nares. To reduce this risk, use measures to move pressure away from the tip of the nose. Because the ET tube is secured in place, pressure could be placed on the skin, causing a MDRPI. To reduce this risk, the ET tube should be moved to the other side of the mouth daily. It is unlikely that the abdomen or back of the hand will develop a pressure injury, as they are not experiencing friction, pressure, or shear.

2. **Answer:**

Interventions	Indicated	Not Indicated
Develop and implement a turning schedule.	X	
Massage reddened areas at each position change.		X
Place a protective dressing over the sacrum.	X	
Use iodine following enzymatic debriding.		X
Implement safe patient handling to help reposition frequently.	X	
Consult with the wound clinical nurse specialist (CNS) about the most appropriate bed surface to redistribute pressure.	X	

A person-centered turning schedule helps to reduce pressure on sensitive areas and reduces the risk for pressure injuries or progression of an existing injury. A dressing will aid in protecting early-stage pressure injuries. The use of safe patient-handling principles protects the patient and the nurse from injury. Because the patient has several risk factors and has developed a stage 1 pressure injury, a consultation with the wound CNS would be appropriate to obtain and use the best redistribution surface. Massaging of reddened areas increases the risk for injury and superficial vessel damage to the underlying tissue. Iodine is contraindicated with enzymatic debridement, as this can render the debriding agent ineffective.

3. **Answer: 1.** A stage 1 pressure injury involves nonblanchable erythema of intact skin. All other stages of pressure injuries have further involvement.

4. **Answer: 3.** If malnutrition is suspected, a consultation with the registered dietitian nutritionist (RDN) can be helpful to discuss modification to the patient's diet that could promote wound healing. The nurse will not request a decrease in feeding; nutrition is needed for wound healing. Antibiotics are not needed. The patient cannot be ambulated while on a ventilator.

5. **Answer: 1, 2, 3, 4.** The nurse will recommend that the patient consume protein to facilitate wound healing, ambulate several times daily to reduce ongoing pressure on any body sites, report any skin changes to the health care provider so deterioration does not progress, and perform daily skin checks on areas prone to pressure to observe for changes. There is no need to immediately place a dressing on a reddened area; the change in appearance should be reported to the health care provider, who can recommend whether any treatment is necessary.

CHAPTER 40

1. **Answer: 1.** A wet-to-moist dressing is appropriate for this patient. Wet-to-moist dressings are gauze moistened with an appropriate solution. The primary purpose is to mechanically debride wounds, specifically full-thickness wounds healing by secondary intention and wounds with necrotic tissue. A wet-to-moist dressing has a moist contact dressing layer that touches the wound surface. The dampened gauze increases the absorptive ability of the dressing to collect exudate and wound debris. This layer dries and adheres to dead cells, thus debriding the wound when removed. Other dressing types are not appropriate for this type of wound.

2. **Answer: 2.** The nurse will clean the wound with saline-moistened gauze so that it can be appropriately visualized after being blotted dry. After these steps, application of a new dressing begins.

3. **Answer:** After dressing the wound, the nurse will **assess the patient's pain level** and **review the patient's laboratory findings.**

Ongoing assessment of the patient's pain level provides information regarding the need for analgesia before dressing changes or ambulatory activities. Reviewing the patient's laboratory findings is important to assess for blood culture results and the white blood cell count. Ensuring the next meal tray will be delivered on time will not provide meaningful intervention to the patient's healing process at the moment. Applying a transparent dressing over the wet-to-dry dressing is inappropriate. These are two different kinds of treatments, each having its own purpose. The patient is extremely fatigued and has a fever; this is not the time to provide patient teaching. An abdominal x-ray is unnecessary.

4. **Answer: 2.** A pressure bandage is needed to treat this wound. This is a type of temporary treatment used to control excessive, sudden, unanticipated bleeding. Hemorrhage may occur during surgical intervention (e.g., cardiac catheterization, arterial puncture, organ biopsy) or after surgery, or it may be a life-threatening occurrence related to accidental trauma (e.g., stabbing, suicide attempt). Pressure dressings are essential to stopping the flow of blood and promoting clotting at the site until definitive action can be taken to stop the source. Once the dressing has been applied, the nurse will notify the surgical team immediately of these findings and intervention. Other dressing types are not appropriate for this type of wound.

5. **Answers: 4, 5.** Transparent film dressings have absorbent capacity and are indicated as a primary dressing for superficial wounds with minimal or no exudate. Hydrocolloid dressings contain gel-forming agents and are indicated as a primary wound dressing with minimal to moderate exudate and without depth. A dry dressing is not appropriate for an exudative wound as it may cause traumatic debridement, thus impeding wound healing. Calcium alginate and hydrogel dressings are used for wounds with large amounts of exudate. They are expensive and not the first choice for a shallow wound with minimal exudate.

CHAPTER 41

1. **Answer: 1, 2, 3, 4, 5.** Agitation can be a risk factor for falls if the client is not cooperating with the caregiver or is not following health instructions. The degree of joint pain is important to know, as this can influence whether the client is safe when ambulating and performing ADLs; it is not unusual for people to deviate from safe practices if those practices cause pain. Cognitive changes can influence the risk for falls; the more confused the client becomes, the higher the fall risk. Depth perception is important to know; if the client's depth perception is impaired, the client may miss important safety cues when stepping (e.g., around furniture, on stairs). Steadiness of gait is important to assess; an unsteady gait increases the risk for falls.

2. **Answer: 4.** Medications should not be stored in various locations; they should be kept together. They also should not be kept in humid environments such as bathrooms, so the nurse will intervene to provide teaching about how to store medications properly. All other actions are appropriate and do not require the nurse to intervene.

3. **Answer: 3.** The nurse will discuss the presence of decorative throw rugs throughout the house. These can increase the risk for falls, as they are easy to trip over. All other findings enhance home safety and do not require discussion.

4. **Answer: 2.** The caregiver must first have the functional ability—the physical and mental capacity—to assist the client. If this is present, the nurse can tailor teaching and referrals to the caregiver's needs based on health literacy level, transportation accessibility, and financial needs.

5. **Answer: Stand or sit in front of the client, repeat phrases if necessary.** To engage in safe medication practices, the caregiver needs to communicate as well as possible with the client. Especially when working with clients with dementia, it is important to stand or sit in front of them when talking so that they can see they are being addressed. It is also important to repeat phrases if necessary, as these clients may often forget what they have been told. Other actions listed are nontherapeutic or ineffective and do not facilitate communication.

CHAPTER 42

1. **Answers: 1, 2, 3, 4, 5.** Assessments of all of these factors should take place before delivery of home oxygen. Smoke detectors and fire extinguishers should be present and accessible in the home. Sources of heat must be evaluated, as devices like space heaters should not be used around oxygen due to the potential for combustion. The nurse will need to know the smoking status of anyone in the home; oxygen cannot be used around smoke, fire, or flame. The number and availability of electric outlets is important so that there is assurance the patient can always plug in the home oxygen when moving from room to room.

2. **Answers: 1, 2, 3, 4.** Before teaching, the nurse needs to review the health care provider's orders and nurses' notes. This provides a baseline for what teaching will be required. The health literacy level of the caregiver informs the nurse about which resources and teaching methods to use. Knowing the caregiver's current understanding of the enteral feeding process helps the nurse to determine where to begin teaching and informs the nurse if misconceptions need to be corrected before other teaching takes place. Evaluating the home environment is helpful so that the nurse can discuss exact locations for processes involved in enteral feeding when working with the caregiver. Gathering information about sterile technique is not necessary because medical aseptic technique is used for feedings.

3. **Answer: 4.** The nurse will respond by clarifying that there are some medications that cannot be crushed or given together. The nurse will then review all of the current medications ordered and confirm which medications can and cannot be crushed, as well as which ones must be given at which times. Further teaching will include the caregiver verifying how to administer any new medication with the nurse or pharmacist. Other responses are inappropriate, as they do not provide important information about the fact that some medications cannot be crushed or given together.

4. **Answer: 4.** It is within the scope of assistive personnel (AP) to provide ongoing hygiene and oral care. The nurse will delegate this task, provide education to the AP about what needs to be done, and remain responsible for supervision. Teaching, assessing, and evaluating are nursing roles; these cannot be done by an AP.

5. **Answer:**

Nursing Health Teaching	Indicated	Not Indicated
"Vaping devices are combustible around oxygen. Persons can be seriously injured when vaping devices are used in homes with oxygen therapy."	X	
"After turning off the oxygen for 2–3 minutes, it is safe to use the vaping device in the home."		X
"I would notify the fire company that someone is vaping in the home so that they can tell you if it is safe or not."		X
"If anyone vapes in the home, you and your spouse are at serious risk of experiencing a home explosion and fire."	X	
"As long as you are vaping in a room away from the oxygen, there is no need to be concerned."		X
"Only the flavored types of vaping supplies are problematic."		X

Vaping is a form of smoking that has risk factors associated with home oxygen therapy comparable to smoking cigarettes or cigars. The nurse will clarify that vaping is combustible around oxygen, which can cause serious injury (or death). It is inaccurate to state that turning off the oxygen for 2 to 3 minutes before vaping ensures safety. This is not true. This action would also compromise the oxygen supply to the patient. Referring the spouse to the fire company minimizes and delays intervening to prevent an explosion and/or fire in the home with oxygen; the nurse has the knowledge and resources to provide the needed education. Vaping should not be done anywhere in the home, so it is inaccurate to state that it is safe if done in a room away from oxygen. All types of vaping supplies are combustible, not just flavored ones.

Answers to Next-Generation NCLEX® (NGN)–Style Unfolding Case Studies

UNIT 1: SUPPORTING THE PATIENT THROUGH THE HEALTH CARE SYSTEM

QUESTION 1.

Answer:

History and Physical	Nurses' Notes	Vital Signs	Laboratory Results
1008: Client is here for an annual examination. States they are concerned about having some type of disorder and are afraid of what today's examination might reveal. About 8 months ago, client reports finding blood in their stool and occasional drops of blood in the toilet. No change in diet. Denies abdominal pain or tenderness but states, "Sometimes it burns when I urinate." States that passing stool is difficult at least 2 to 3 times weekly. Has been taking an opioid pain reliever for several weeks following a knee replacement. Has a family history of colon cancer. Alert and oriented × 4; lung sounds clear to auscultation; S_1S_2 present with no murmur heard; bowel sounds present × 4 quadrants; strength in all extremities equal. Vital signs: T 36.8°C (98.2°F); HR 102 beats/min; RR 22 breaths/min; BP 148/86 mm Hg; SpO_2 99% on RA.			

Rationale: Findings that require immediate follow-up by the nurse include blood in the stool and toilet, difficulty passing stool, taking an opioid drug, and having a family history of colon cancer. As the client is having bowel symptoms, all of these findings could be relevant and require further assessment to gather a full understanding of the client's history and concern. Other findings at this time, which include the client's concern about a potential diagnosis, occasional urinary burning, and a mildly elevated heart rate and blood pressure, can be followed up later. Further findings are within expected parameters and do not require follow-up.

QUESTION 2.

Answer:

Client Assessment Finding	Colon Cancer	Constipation	Hemorrhoids
Blood in stool	X	X	X
Drops of blood in toilet	X	X	X
Hard to pass stool		X	X
Taking an opioid drug		X	

Rationale: Blood in stool and drops of blood in the toilet can be associated with colon cancer, constipation, or hemorrhoids. Diagnostic testing and a physical examination by the health care provider will reveal more information about which of these conditions it most likely represents. Difficulty passing stool is characteristic of constipation as well as hemorrhoids. Depending on the size and location of the hemorrhoid(s), it can make passing stool

challenging. Taking an opioid drug is also associated with contributing to constipation.

QUESTION 3.

Answer:
The *priority* at this time is to address the **blood in stool** and the **drops of blood in toilet**.

   Rationale: Due to the potential association with colon cancer, the priority at this time is to address the client's reported blood in stool and drops of blood in the toilet.

QUESTION 4.

Answer:

Client Concern	Indicated	Not Indicated
Blood pressure 148/86 mm Hg		X
Report of blood in stool	X	
Taking an opioid drug	X	
History of knee replacement		X
Respiratory rate 22 breaths/min		X
Difficulty passing stool	X	

   Rationale: It is indicated for the nurse to report right away to the health care provider the patient's report of blood in stool, the patient's use of an opioid drug, and the difficulty in passing stool. Blood in the stool can be associated with colon cancer, so this is a priority. Taking an opioid drug is relevant, as this may be a causative agent. Having difficulty passing stool is important, as this could be related to taking the opioid medication, which causes constipation, or the presence of a rectal tumor. The blood pressure is not significantly elevated, so reporting this can wait. The history of a knee replacement is not relevant to the immediate concern (although taking the opioid drug is relevant). The respiratory rate is only mildly elevated above normal parameters and does not need to be reported at this time.

QUESTION 5.

Answer:
- o   Confirm that blood in stool is a common finding.
- o   Discourage the addition of whole grains to the diet.
- X   Provide information about preparation for colonoscopy.
- X   Increase intake of water to at least eight (8-ounce) glasses daily.
- o   Explain that an antiinflammatory drug will be given for urinary burning.
- X   Report an increase in blood in the stool or toilet to the health care provider immediately.
- o   Be certain to take temperature at lseast twice daily to monitor for infection.
- o   Reassure that there is no reason to be concerned about an unfavorable diagnosis.

   Rationale: Because the client has blood in the stool, it is highly likely that the health care provider will order a colonoscopy. The nurse will provide teaching about the preparation for this diagnostic test. To facilitate easier bowel movements, the nurse will teach the client to consume at least eight 8-ounce glasses of water daily. The nurse will also teach the client to report an increase in blood in the stool or toilet to the provider immediately, as this could indicate a declining condition. The nurse will not confirm that blood in stool is a common finding, as that is untrue. The nurse will not discourage the addition of whole grains to the diet; in fact, whole grains will be encouraged as they can facilitate better elimination. An antiinflammatory drug will not be given for urinary burning; if an infection is suspected, an antibiotic will be given. It is not necessary to obtain temperature readings twice daily. It is inappropriate and nontherapeutic to give the client false hope by reassuring them that there is no need to be concerned about an unfavorable diagnosis.

QUESTION 6.
Answer:

Current Client Findings	Document as Improvement	Document as Unchanged
Blood pressure 118/70 mm Hg	X	
Temperature 36.8°C (98.2°F)		X
Notes drops of blood in toilet		X
Reports relief from fear of an unfavorable diagnosis	X	
Easy stool passage most days of the week	X	

Rationale: Findings that indicate improvement in the client's condition include a lower blood pressure than in the initial encounter, relief of fear, and easy stool passage for most of the week. The client's temperature is unchanged, as is the client's report that there are drops of blood in the toilet. These were initial findings in the original assessment that are unchanged at this time.

UNIT 2: VITAL SIGNS AND PHYSICAL ASSESSMENT

QUESTION 1.
Answer:

History and Physical	Nurses' Notes	Vital Signs	Laboratory Results

1204: Client is here to report "heartburn" that is increasing in frequency. Client states, "The older I get, the more I have this burning in my chest after I eat." Reports no recent changes in diet and no traveling in or out of the country. Works as a long distance truck driver, smokes 2 packs of cigarettes a days, and often eats at fast-food restaurants. The client is 52 years old and weighs 200 pounds (90.7 kg). Denies other symptoms, including abdominal discomfort or bloating, changes in bowel or bladder habits, chest pain, and respiratory difficulty or shortness of breath. Alert and oriented × 4; lung sounds clear to auscultation; S_1S_2 present without murmur; bowel sounds present × 4 quadrants; strength in all extremities equal. Vital signs: T 36.9°C (98.4°F); HR 72 beats/min; RR 14 breaths/min; BP 190/90 mm Hg; Spo₂ 98% on RA.

Rationale: Findings that require immediate follow-up by the nurse include the report of "heartburn" increasing in frequency after eating, eating in fast-food restaurants often, and the elevated blood pressure of 190/90 mm Hg. These signs and symptoms are all abnormal and require further assessment. Other findings are within expected parameters or do not require immediate follow-up.

QUESTION 2.
Answer:
The client is at highest risk for health complications based on the findings of **BP 190/90 mm Hg** and **burning in chest after eating**.

Rationale: Findings that are abnormal that concern the nurse include an elevation in blood pressure and a burning sensation in the chest after eating. These findings could indicate health complications such as hypertension (based on the elevated blood pressure) and gastrointestinal or cardiac concerns based on the burning chest sensation. All other findings listed are expected and do not place the client at the highest of risks for health complications.

QUESTION 3.
Answer:
The nurse is concerned about the client's **temperature** and **blood pressure**.

Rationale: The client's temperature is above normal for this client, and the client's blood pressure is very high; therefore, these findings concern the nurse. The client's heart rate, respiratory rate, and oxygen saturation are within expected parameters and do not concern the nurse at this time.

QUESTION 4.
Answer:
- ○ Abnormal heart rate
- X Overweight
- ○ Burning sensation in chest
- X Smokes cigarettes
- X Limited opportunity to exercise
- ○ Eats a low-fat diet

Rationale: The nurse will teach the client about his risk factors for hypertension, including being overweight, smoking cigarettes, and having limited opportunity to exercise because of his occupation. Currently his heart rate is normal, and he does not have a history of eating low fat foods since he relies on eating at fast food restaurants.

QUESTION 5.
Answer:

System	Potential Interventions
Cardiovascular	X Document blood pressure. X Apply cardiac monitor. ○ Discuss cardiac rehabilitation with the client.
Respiratory	X Auscultate lungs. X Monitor oxygen saturation. ○ Teach cough and deep breathing exercises.
General	○ Prepare to administer antibiotic for fever. X Stay with the client. X Document temperature.

Rationale: The client is experiencing anaphylaxis, a type of allergic reaction that can occur when exposed to allergens. The nurse will document the blood pressure and apply a cardiac monitor to monitor the heart rhythm. The nurse will auscultate the lungs to assess for wheezes and will monitor the client's oxygen saturation with the anticipation that it should increase after treatment. The nurse will stay with the client and document the temperature. There is no need to discuss cardiac rehabilitation or teach cough and deep breathing exercises; the priority is to facilitate breathing. There is no need to give an antibiotic. The slight elevation in temperature is likely due to the client's fight-or-flight response rather than an infection.

QUESTION 6.

Answer:

Current Client Findings	Document as Improvement	Document as Unchanged
Temperature 99.2°F (37.3°C)		X
Blood pressure 118/70 mm Hg	X	
Spo₂ 99%	X	
Lungs clear to auscultation	X	
RR 18 breaths/min		X

Rationale: Findings that indicate improvement in the client's condition include a lower blood pressure, a much higher oxygen saturation, and clear lungs. The client's temperature and respiratory rate are unchanged. These were initial findings when the client reported to the emergency department, and they are the same at this time.

UNIT 3: SPECIAL PROCEDURES

QUESTION 1.

Answer:

History and Physical	Nurses' Notes	Vital Signs	Laboratory Results

1228: Client reports to urgent care reporting 3 days of worsening pain upon urination, abdominal discomfort, and fatigue. The urinary pain is described as "burning" in nature and occurring with each urination. The patient states, "I constantly feel as if I have to urinate, but when I go to the bathroom, very little urine will come out." The patient also states she has experienced a thick vaginal discharge for the past 2 days that "smells awful" and is yellowish-green in color. Sexual history reveals unprotected intercourse with partner and one other individual recently. Alert and oriented × 4; lung sounds clear to auscultation; S₁S₂ present without murmur; bowel sounds present × 4 quadrants; strength in all extremities equal. Lower abdominal tenderness in the LLQ and RLQ upon gentle palpation. Vital signs: T 38.4°C (101.2°F); HR 78 beats/min; RR 20 breaths/min; BP 124/78 mm Hg; SpO₂ 98% on RA.

Rationale: Findings that require immediate follow-up by the nurse include 3 days of pain upon urination, abdominal discomfort, fatigue, feelings of having to urinate, little urine being produced, thick and foul-smelling vaginal discharge, lower abdominal tenderness, and fever. These signs and symptoms are all abnormal and require further assessment. These symptoms could be related to numerous conditions; however, it may be significant that the client has recently had unprotected intercourse with someone new; this must also be followed up on immediately by the nurse. Other findings are within expected parameters and do not require immediate follow-up.

QUESTION 2.

Answer:
The nurse determines the patient's priorities and prepares to perform the following: **clean voided urine sample** and **vaginal discharge specimen**.

Rationale: The nurse will prepare for the collection of a clean voided urine sample and a vaginal discharge swab. Both need to be collected to test for possible microorganisms because of the patient likely having pelvic

inflammatory disease. Assessment of fatigue is not an immediate priority. A neurologic and breast exam are not necessary based on patient's presenting findings.

QUESTION 3.

Answer:
The client needs that the nurse will *prioritize* communicating to the health care provider include **qualities of vaginal discharge** and **temperature.**

Rationale: The two findings with the highest combined risk for poor outcomes include the combination of foul-smelling vaginal discharge and fever, which are indicative of a likely infection. Infections can lead to multiple poor outcomes, so the nurse will prioritize communication of these findings. The other findings can be reported to the health care provider secondarily.

QUESTION 4.

Answer:
The nurse anticipates that the health care provider will order diagnostic testing of **urinalysis** and **vaginal discharge culture.**

Rationale: A urinalysis and vaginal discharge culture are anticipated; the client's current signs and symptoms most closely align with prioritization of evaluating the renal and reproductive systems for infection. Other tests are not anticipated, as they do not align with the client's current signs and symptoms.

QUESTION 5.

Answer:
- ○ Mpox
- ○ Syphilis
- ○ Hepatitis
- X Gonorrhea
- X Chlamydia
- ○ Genital herpes
- ○ Human immunodeficiency virus

Rationale: Vaginal discharge cultures obtained during a pelvic examination are tested for gonorrhea and chlamydia. Evaluation for mpox is done after collecting a tissue sample from an open lesion. Evaluation for syphilis and human immunodeficiency virus is done via a blood sample. Evaluation for genital herpes is done via a culture of fluid gathered from a herpes lesion.

QUESTION 6.

Answer:
- X "Prior to the test, you will check my neurologic status."
- X "I will lie on my side during the test."
- X "My lower leg strength will be evaluated before the test."
- X "Before the test, I must go to the bathroom to empty my bladder."
- ○ "It is important that you help me sit up and get in a chair after the puncture is done."
- X "I can expect that my headache may get worse after this lumbar puncture is done."
- X "A needle is going to be placed in an area around the spinal cord during the lumbar puncture."

Rationale: All of these statements, other than stating that there is a need to get up in a chair after the procedure, are evaluated by the nurse as showing that the client has understood the teaching. The client will be instructed to remain flat after the test, not to be transferred upright and to a chair.

UNIT 4: INFECTION CONTROL

QUESTION 1.
Answer:

History and Physical	Nurses' Notes	Vital Signs	Laboratory Results

0248: Client in the emergency department after returning from a vacation. States, "I started to feel unwell while flying home yesterday." This morning, the client awoke with a productive cough, chills, fever, diarrhea, weakness, and vomiting. Alert and oriented × 4; lung sounds with rhonchi; S_1S_2 present without murmur; bowel sounds present × 4 quadrants; tenderness noted near the umbilicus; strength diminished yet equal in all extremities. Vital signs: T 39.6°C (103.2°F); HR 86 beats/min; RR 18 breaths/min; BP 134/98 mm Hg; SpO$_2$ 93% on RA.

Rationale: Findings that may indicate a respiratory infectious process include productive cough, chills, fever, rhonchi, weakness, and diminished oxygen saturation. Findings that may indicate a gastrointestinal infectious process include chills, fever, diarrhea, weakness, vomiting, and umbilical tenderness. Other findings are within normal parameters.

QUESTION 2.
Answer:
Before entering the client's room, the triage nurse dons **clean gloves** and **a mask.**

Rationale: Standard Precautions when there is a risk of coming in contact with any secretions (e.g., mucus) requires clean gloves. If the patient is coughing, the risk of contacting aerosolized microorganisms is decreased by wearing a mask. These help the nurse to avoid contact with potential secretions or respiratory inhalants. A gown, a cap, and a pair of goggles would be donned if the nurse anticipated assisting with a procedure in which they may encounter splatter or soiling. Sterile gloves are not needed for a basic evaluation.

QUESTION 3.
Answer:
The client needs that the nurse will address include following **Contact Precautions** and **washing hands regularly.**

Rationale: The diagnosis of *C. difficile* requires the nurse to initiate Contact Precautions and to wash hands regularly. These are two evidence-based ways of preventing transmission of an organism by contact. Standard Precautions should have been initiated when the client first presented to the emergency department. Airborne Precautions and Droplet Precautions are unnecessary, given that the client is negative for COVID-19 and influenza. Explaining how to avoid *C. difficile*, encouraging fluids, and collecting repeat vital signs are not client needs at this moment; they can be accomplished later after infection control actions have been instituted.

QUESTION 4.
Answer:

Client Concern	Indicated	Not Indicated
Blood pressure 90/60 mm Hg	X	
Urinary output <30 mL/hr	X	
Family at the bedside		X
Several episodes of watery diarrhea		X
Respiratory rate 12 breaths/min		X

Rationale: The nurse will plan to report the low blood pressure and reduced urinary output to the health care provider; these are concerning signs that could indicate deterioration in the client's condition. It is not indicated for the nurse to plan to report to the provider that the family is at the bedside; this does not give context to the client's condition. It is also not indicated to report several episodes of watery diarrhea, as this is an expected finding associated with *C. difficile* infection and part of the patient's history, nor to report the respiratory rate, which is within normal parameters.

QUESTION 5.
Answer:
X Perform hand hygiene.
X Apply glove to dominant hand first.
○ Roll cuff of applied glove over the wrist.
○ Hold gloved hands close to body after application.
X Slip hand underneath cuff of second glove after first glove is applied.
○ Lay unopened package of sterile gloves on chest-high flat surface.
X Grab glove for dominant hand by touching the glove's inside surface or cuff.

Rationale: Correct actions the nurse will take when donning sterile gloves include performing hand hygiene, grabbing the glove for the dominant hand by touching the glove's inside surface or cuff, applying a glove to the dominant hand first, slipping the dominant hand underneath the cuff of the second glove, and then applying the second glove. The nurse will not roll the cuff of the applied glove over the wrist; the glove should remain smooth. The nurse will hold gloved hands away from the body after application to reduce the risk for contamination. The nurse will initially lay the unopened package of sterile gloves on a waist-high flat surface.

QUESTION 6.
Answer:

Current Client Findings	Improved	Declined
Blood pressure 120/82 mm Hg	X	
Temperature 37.7°C (99.9°F)	X	
No watery diarrhea in 24 hours	X	
No abdominal tenderness	X	
Mucus with tinges of blood		X

Rationale: Findings that indicate an improvement in the client's condition include today's blood pressure and temperature, which are reduced from admission; the lack of watery diarrhea for 24 hours; and no abdominal tenderness. The new finding of mucus with tinges of blood shows a decline in condition, as this is a new and abnormal symptom.

UNIT 5: ACTIVITY AND MOBILITY

QUESTION 1.
Answer:

History and Physical	Nurses' Notes	Vital Signs	Laboratory Results

1341: 50-year-old client brought to the emergency department by spouse, who reports client has experienced progressive weakness over the past few days. History positive for multiple sclerosis. Over the past few months, client has experienced an increase in peripheral neuropathy and has been sitting in a wheelchair more often. Client appears sleepy yet is able to be awakened upon command; lung sounds clear; S_1S_2 present without murmur; bowel sounds present × 4 quadrants; strength weak yet equal in all extremities. 5-cm (2-inch) reddened and nonblanchable area on sacrum; no breakdown noted. Vital signs: T 39.0°C (102.2°F); HR 62 beats/min; RR 12 breaths/min; BP 110/70 mm Hg; SpO$_2$ 98% on RA.

Rationale: The nurse will follow up on findings that could contribute to a decline in the client's health, including progressive weakness (as evidenced by the sleepiness yet ability to be awakened, weak extremities, and the need to sit in a wheelchair more often), increase in peripheral neuropathy, a nonblanchable area on the sacrum, and fever. Other findings do not require follow-up at this time. It is also important that the nurse follow up on the client's history of multiple sclerosis. A baseline will be important as the nurse compares those findings to today's findings.

QUESTION 2.
Answer:
The nurse anticipates that the client is at high risk for **falls** due to **peripheral neuropathy.**

Rationale: Multiple sclerosis can be accompanied by peripheral neuropathy; the client may have numbness in the extremities. If clients cannot feel their feet, this places them at a high risk for falls. The client is not at risk for appendicitis; the bowel sounds are within expected parameters. The client is not at risk for hypertensive crisis; the blood pressure is within expected parameters. The client is not at risk for respiratory distress; the respiratory rate is within expected parameters.

QUESTION 3.
Answer:
The nurse will obtain a **fall risk arm band** and **gait belt** to increase client safety.

Rationale: The client is at a high risk for falls. Therefore, the nurse will gather a fall risk arm band and a gait belt, which will be used for transferring. There is no need for a cervical collar or lumbar brace at this time, and there is no indication a drug allergy arm band is needed. Splints for the feet would not serve any purpose.

QUESTION 4.
Answer:

Potential Nursing Action	Indicated	Not Indicated
Delegate teaching of range-of-motion (ROM) exercises to assistive personnel (AP).		X
Monitor oxygen saturation during any activity.	X	
Perform an assessment using the Braden Scale.	X	
Obtain foam overlay for bed.	X	
Massage nonblanchable area on sacrum.		X

Rationale: The nurse will monitor oxygen saturation with any activity to determine whether the client is oxygenating appropriately. The nurse will also perform a skin assessment using the Braden Scale to determine the client's risk for pressure injury. Because the client has a 5-cm (2-inch) nonblanchable area of skin on the sacrum, the nurse will obtain a foam overlay to relieve pressure. The nurse will not delegate teaching about ROM exercises; teaching requires the scope of practice of a nurse instead of AP. The nurse will refrain from massaging the nonblanchable area on the sacrum, as this could impair tissue integrity and predispose the area to breakdown.

QUESTION 5.
Answer:
X   Perform hand hygiene.
X   Use a gait belt during the transfer process.
X   Assess range of motion before transferring.
X   Determine client's level of consciousness before moving.
○   Instruct client to avoid using wheelchair armrests to rise.
○   Move client as quickly as possible to bed after standing from chair.
○   Adjust bed height 5 cm (2 inches) below the wheelchair seat height prior to transfer.

Rationale: Correct actions the nurse will take when transferring the client from the wheelchair to the bed include performing hand hygiene, using a gait belt, and assessing the client's range of motion (ROM) and level of consciousness before moving them. All of these actions assist the nurse in performing a safe transfer. The nurse will not discourage the client from using the armrests to rise; rather, the nurse will tell the client to place their hands on the armrests and use those to push off when attempting to stand. The nurse will allow the client to sit on the edge of the bed for a moment after transfer rather than moving as quickly as possible when transferring. This helps the client to maintain orientation. The bed height will be positioned at the level of the wheelchair seat, not 5 cm (2 inches) below it.

QUESTION 6.
Answer:

System	Client Assessment Findings
Cardiovascular	○ Blood pressure 80/50 mm Hg X Pulse 74 beats/min X Heart regular rate and rhythm
Respiratory	X Oxygen saturation 96% on RA X Respiratory rate 12 breaths/min X Lungs clear bilaterally
General	○ Reports feeling weak ○ States, "I am dizzy" X Temperature 37.1°C (98.8°F)

Rationale: Findings that indicate a successful transfer include pulse 74 beats/min, heart regular rate and rhythm, oxygen saturation 96% on RA, respiratory rate of 12 breaths/min, clear lungs, and temperature 37.1°C (98.8°F). These are findings within expected parameters. A very low blood pressure, weakness, or dizziness may mean that the client became hypotensive during transfer.

UNIT 6: SAFETY AND COMFORT

QUESTION 1.
Answer:
○   19-year-old who is walking around and hysterically looking for their sister
○   24-year-old with a displaced fracture of the femur
○   36-year-old with first-degree injuries to 50% of the body
X   40-year-old with a tourniquet around a traumatic leg amputation
○   58-year-old who is sitting upright and appears confused

Rationale: Triage is the process of sorting individuals by the seriousness of their condition and their likelihood of survival. Victims are issued a colored tag by the triage nurse upon initial assessment. People issued a green tag have no injuries or minor injuries; they are able to walk and are unlikely to deteriorate in physical condition over the coming days. People given a yellow tag can be delayed for treatment. They will need to be seen by a health care provider for treatment, but they can wait for 2 to 3 hours before assessment. People given a red tag need immediate care; they usually have an airway or circulatory injury but can probably be saved with immediate intervention and transport. Medical attention is needed within minutes up to 1 hour. People issued a black or gray tag have died or are expected to die. They are unlikely to survive given the severity of their injuries. When possible, palliative care should be implemented.

QUESTION 2.
Answer:
The emergency nurse anticipates that the client is at high risk for **hemorrhage** due to **presence of a tourniquet.**

Rationale: A client who has had a tourniquet applied most likely has a risk for hemorrhage. Tourniquets are applied to control bleeding. The remaining conditions are unlikely, given the client's presentation. The client is more likely to experience hyperventilation than hypoventilation, as evidenced by screaming. The client is more likely to experience hypotension due to hemorrhage than to be at risk for hypertension. Fluid deficit—not fluid overload—is likely if a client hemorrhages. Oxygen saturation of 95% is within an expected parameter. Multiple lacerations do not place the client at a high risk for anything at this time.

QUESTION 3.
Answer:
The nurse will **page the trauma surgery team** and **stay with the client** to increase client safety at this time.

   Rationale: The client has a traumatic injury that requires immediate evaluation by the trauma surgery team. The nurse will not administer hypotonic IV fluids; this could exacerbate the hypovolemia and the hypotension related to the traumatic injury and induce cardiovascular collapse. The nurse will not remove the tourniquet, as hemorrhage could occur. The nurse will stay with the client to provide monitoring and support while waiting for the trauma surgery team to arrive. Assessment and monitoring are never to be delegated to AP. Locating a family member is not a priority of care at this time.

QUESTION 4.
Answer:

Potential Nursing Action	Indicated	Not Indicated
Delegate fall risk assessment to assistive personnel (AP).		X
Apply restraints prophylactically.		X
Arrange for a sitter to be present in the room.		X
Administer morphine per health care provider's "prn-as needed" order every 2-4 hours		X
Monitor vital signs every 15 minutes for the first hour.	X	

   Rationale: At this time, the only action from this list that is indicated is to monitor the client's vital signs every 15 minutes for the first hour. This provides the nurse with important assessment data in the client's early period of recovery. The nurse will provide this monitoring as well as assessing the incision regularly. Assessment of fall risk is to be performed by the nurse, who has the education and experience to perform this task and to implement interventions if something abnormal or unexpected occurs; it is not a task that can be delegated to AP. The client is sleepy and lethargic following surgery, which is probably related to anesthesia. There is no need to apply restraints prophylactically (which would be illegal) or to have a sitter present. There is also no need at this time to administer morphine, as the client is not exhibiting signs or behaviors of pain and is still lethargic.

QUESTION 5.
Answer:
○ Remove surgical dressings to facilitate comfort.
○ Reassure the client that postsurgical pain of this intensity is normal.
X Assess character of pain and ask client to rate severity on a scale of 0 to 10.
X Prepare to administer pain medication as ordered and on time.
X Evaluate the medication record for regular and PRN pain medication.
○ Tell the client to try to relax to regain control, as crying will exacerbate the pain level.
○ Ask family members whether the client would like to have a chaplain come to the room.
   Rationale: The nurse will ask the client to describe the pain and quantify the pain severity; this helps the nurse to understand how the client perceives the pain in terms of severity. The nurse will administer pain medications regularly and on time; this facilitates pain control around the

clock. The nurse will also evaluate the medication record to be certain that regular and PRN (as needed) pain medications are ordered; this increases the timeliness of pain management. It is inappropriate to remove the surgical dressings; this could introduce infection into the wound or disrupt the surgical repair. The nurse will not state that this type of pain intensity is normal; the nurse is to listen to the client's perception of pain without minimizing their experience. Telling the client to regain control is inappropriate and nontherapeutic. The nurse should not ask family members whether the client wants to have a chaplain visit; if asked, this question should be addressed to the client.

QUESTION 6.
Answer:
X "I have lived a wonderful life."
○ "My pain level is an 8 on a 0-to-10 scale."
○ "I am sure that if I have enough faith, I will be cured."
X "The family and I have spent a lot of time together lately."
X "My spouse and I made funeral arrangements earlier this week."
X "I have been using aromatherapy to decrease my pain levels."
X "My priest stops by several times a week to see how I am doing."
   Rationale: Client statements that indicate that nursing interventions undertaken by the hospice nurse have provided comfort at the end of life include: genuine and positive reflection on the life that has been lived, spending time with family, acknowledging that death is imminent (e.g., making their own funeral arrangements), seeking self-care actions that provide comfort (e.g., using aromatherapy), and engaging with family, spiritual leaders, and friends as desired. A high pain level and lack of recognition of the finality of a terminal diagnosis do not indicate that nursing interventions were effective in providing comfort at the end of life.

UNIT 7: HYGIENE

QUESTION 1.
Answer:

History and Physical	Nurses' Notes	Vital Signs	Laboratory Results

1544: Client admitted after a 3-day stay on the intensive care unit (ICU) for diabetic ketoacidosis. History of type 1 diabetes mellitus and glaucoma. Client is very weak; awakes when hearing name and then falls back asleep quickly. Lung sounds clear. S_1S_2 present without murmur. Bowel sounds present × 4 quadrants. Strength diminished and weak, yet equal in all extremities. No skin breakdown noted. Upon assessment, the client has been incontinent of urine. Blood glucose 1 hour after last meal is 140 mg/dL. Vital signs: T 37.6°C (99.6°F); HR 68 beats/min; RR 12 breaths/min; BP 108/72 mm Hg; SpO₂ 99% on RA.

   Rationale: A client who has been in intensive care for 3 days is likely to be very weak upon presentation. Diabetic ketoacidosis is a serious and potentially life-threatening condition, so this history helps to establish why the client is so weak. It is also significant that the client has glaucoma, which could indicate a visual deficit. It would not be safe to get this client up to the shower. Also, a client who falls back to sleep quickly while in bed would be unlikely to be able to finish their own bath. Any time a client is incontinent of urine or stool, they should be cleaned, and the bed should be changed.

QUESTION 2.
Answer:
The nurse identifies that the client is at high risk for **skin breakdown** due to **incontinence**.
   Rationale: At this time, the client's health record indicates that there is a risk for skin breakdown due to incontinence of urine. There is no evidence that the client is at high risk for urinary tract infection or sepsis, as their temperature is elevated only slightly. There is no evidence of risk for ongoing diabetic ketoacidosis related to type 1 diabetes mellitus, as the client was already discharged from ICU and has a blood glucose level of

140 mg/dL. The blood glucose would need to be much higher to be a cause for immediate concern.

QUESTION 3.
Answer:
The nurse will <u>change the bed</u> and <u>provide the client with a bath</u> as the priorities of care at this time.

Rationale: The client needs to be cleaned and the bed changed as priorities of care to decrease the risk for skin breakdown. Afterward, the nurse can provide further assessment by obtaining the temperature, performing a subsequent blood glucose test, and auscultating the lungs. An absorbent pad should be placed beneath the client after a bath and bed change.

QUESTION 4.
Answer:

Potential Nursing Action	Indicated	Not Indicated
Perform a full skin assessment during the bed bath.	X	
Delegate a full bed bath and linen change to assistive personnel (AP).	X	
Have the client sit in a chair while the linens are changed.		X
Contact the health care provider.		X
Determine whether the client uses eyedrops for glaucoma.	X	

Rationale: Within the plan of care, it is appropriate for the nurse to delegate a full bed bath and linen change to assistive personel (AP). These tasks are within the skill set of an AP. While the AP is providing a bath, the nurse can perform a full assessment of the skin. The nurse will also check the medication record to determine whether the client uses eyedrops for glaucoma. These types of eyedrops are available only by prescription and must be used regularly to be effective. It is not indicated for the nurse to have the client sit in a chair while linens are changed; the client is too weak for this. It is also not indicated to contact the health care provider; the client's current needs can be addressed by the nurse.

QUESTION 5.
Answer:
○ Don sterile gloves prior to administration.
○ Identify the client with one form of identification.
○ Wipe each eye from the outer to the inner canthus.
X Assess the eyes for redness, drainage, irritation, and lesions.
○ Stabilize the eyedropper against the inner canthus of each eye.
X Explain the procedure to the client before administering eyedrops.
X Observe the pupils for equality in reaction to light and accommodation.

Rationale: The nurse will assess the eyes, observe the pupils, and explain the procedure of administering eyedrops for glaucoma to the client. These are actions that are required for safe medication administration. The nurse will don clean—not sterile—gloves. The client must be identified with two forms of identification, not one. Eyes are wiped from the inner to the outer canthus. The eyedropper is positioned over the eye, not stabilized against the inner canthus. Doing so could introduce microorganisms to the eyedropper.

QUESTION 6.
Answer:
○ "My skin feels rough and dry."
X "I feel like sitting up in bed at this time."
X "I haven't experienced skin breakdown since I was hospitalized."
○ "All of the movement I had to do during my bath made me nauseated."
○ "I noticed that I have some little blisters on the backs of both of my heels."
X "My spouse and I are planning to make a healthy menu plan when I am discharged."

Rationale: Favorable findings that indicate that nursing interventions were effective include an increase in energy (e.g., feeling like sitting up in the bed), experiencing no skin breakdown while hospitalized, and having a desire to make a healthy eating plan after hospitalization for diabetic ketoacidosis. Having rough and dry skin, feeling nauseated after movement from a bath, and finding blisters on the heels are findings that indicate that nursing interventions were not effective.

UNIT 8: MEDICATION ADMINISTRATION

QUESTION 1.
Answer:
○ Has no history of chronic health problems except diabetes mellitus
○ Small amount of serosanguineous drainage present on surgical dressing
X Reports left hip pain of 8 on a 0-to-10 pain intensity scale
○ Easily arousable
○ Heart rate = 88 beats/min
X Blood pressure = 152/90 mm Hg
X Current blood sugar is 140 mg/dL

QUESTION 2.
Answer:
Based on the client's assessment data, the nurse determines that the client's vital sign findings are due to <u>incisional infection</u> and <u>recent movement in bed</u>. The client's blood sugar reading is caused by <u>IV D5 ½NS</u> and the blood pressure reading is due to <u>postoperative pain</u>.

QUESTION 3.
Answer:
X Deep vein thrombosis
X Incisional infection
X Hypoglycemia
X Bleeding
○ Hypotension
X Constipation
○ Urinary tract infection
○ Anxiety
X Hyperglycemia

QUESTION 4.
Answer:

Client Questions	Appropriate Nurse's Response for Each Client Question
"How long am I going to need this injection in my stomach?"	"Since you are not yet up and walking, you need to keep your blood moving in your body."
"Will I need to have these injections at home?"	"You will not need any medications to prevent clots at home as long as you are able to move and walk and remain mobile."
"My neighbor had a broken leg and stayed in bed to prevent clots from moving from her legs. So why do I need to move?"	"You need to move and exercise your hip to help prevent clots."
"Can I take a bath when I get home?"	"You may bathe or shower when you are up to it as long as you cover your incision to prevent moisture."
"When will I be able to bear weight on this hip?"	"You will be able to move and walk with a walker for a while until the physical therapist tells you not to use it any longer."

QUESTION 5.
Answer:

Health Teaching	Indicated	Not Indicated	Non-Essential
"Do not mix the glargine and regular insulin in the same syringe."	X		
"You may store the insulin in the refrigerator if not in use."	X		
"Inject the insulin when it is cold from the refrigerator."		X	
"Rotate the insulin injection sites between the abdomen and outer thigh."		X	
"There is no need to check your urine or stool for blood."		X	
"Be careful with OTC medications such as aspirin and herbal additions such as garlic and ginger."	X		
"Inspect your injection sites every day for increased redness, heat, or drainage; if any of these are present, call your surgeon immediately."	X		

QUESTION 6.
Answer:

Evaluation Finding	Effective	Not Effective	Unrelated
Injection sites show no sign of infection	X		
Reports increased pain in her left hip		X	
Draws up both insulin glargine and regular in same syringe		X	
Uses different sites for insulin injections	X		
Reports having periods of anxiety			X
States that cannot see the markings on the insulin syringe		X	

UNIT 9: OXYGENATION

QUESTION 1.
Answer:

History and Physical	Nurses' Notes	Vital Signs	Laboratory Results

2234: Client brought to the emergency department by roommate. The roommate states, "We live across the street from the hospital, and I made her come here. We were at a party and ate some cookies, and then she broke out in this weird rash." Medical history in the electronic health record (EHR) reveals a history of depression, which is controlled with sertraline by mouth daily, and anxiety, which is treated as needed with hydroxyzine by mouth PRN. Assessment reveals lung sounds with mild stridor and mildly decreased breath sounds, facial swelling, and urticaria on the neck and chest. Client reports, "I feel as if I am swallowing over something, but nothing is in my throat, and my heart feels as if it is going to beat out of my chest. I'm really scared!" S_1S_2 present without murmur. Bowel sounds present × 4 quadrants; strength equal in all extremities. Vital signs: T 37.6°C (99.6°F); HR 120 beats/min; RR 26 breaths/min; BP 168/100 mm Hg; SpO2 89% on RA.

Rationale: The nurse will follow up on findings that are consistent with an allergic reaction to food—impaired lung sounds; facial swelling; urticaria; the sensation of swallowing over something (which can indicate that the throat is closing); palpitations; elevations in the heart rate, blood pressure, and respiratory rate; and a decreased oxygen saturation. It is often also accompanied by a foreboding sense of doom.

QUESTION 2.
Answer:
The nurse anticipates that the client is most likely experiencing **anaphylaxis** due to **food allergy.**

Rationale: The nurse anticipates that the client is most likely experiencing anaphylaxis due to a food allergy. The client ate cookies at a party, which could have included ingredients to which the client had an allergy. Allergic reactions to food often include the development of urticaria and facial or lip swelling. Anaphylaxis is characterized by laryngeal edema, decreased oxygen saturation, and often a foreboding feeling of doom.

QUESTION 3.
Answer:
The nurse will *first* address the client's **oxygen saturation**.

Rationale: The client's airway is compromised, so the priority is to address oxygen saturation. All other factors, including what may have been in the cookie that the client consumed, can be addressed subsequently.

QUESTION 4.
Answer:
The nurse will prepare for the following interventions: **avoid airway collapse** and **prevent respiratory arrest**.

Rationale: To minimize the client's risks, the nurse will prepare for interventions that are meant to avoid airway collapse and prevent respiratory arrest. The client's presenting signs and symptoms were escalating, from an initial rash to the development of difficulty in swallowing; these factors often precede loss of the airway. There is no indication of risk for venous thromboembolism at this moment. Diphenhydramine is not indicated as first-line therapy for anaphylaxis. There is no indication that the client's reaction is to sertraline, a drug that is taken daily per the medical history. Further increasing the heart rate is contraindicated, as it is already elevated.

QUESTION 5.

Answer:

- ○ Apply wrist restraints.
- **X** Prepare for intubation.
- **X** Administer epinephrine.
- ○ Contact the client's family.
- ○ Place in Trendelenburg position.
- ○ Inform the roommate of what is happening.
- **X** Initiate rapid bolus infusion of 1000 mL normal saline.

Rationale: The nurse will simultaneously prepare for intubation, as the client may be losing their airway; administer epinephrine, which is first-line therapy for anaphylaxis; and initiate a rapid bolus infusion of 1000 mL normal saline to compensate for fluid shifts associated with severe loss of intravascular volume. Wrist restraints are not indicated unless the client poses a danger to self or others. Contacting the client's family can wait. The client should be placed in recumbent position, not Trendelenburg position. Informing the roommate of what is happening could violate HIPAA unless the roommate is the client's next of kin or power of attorney. That relationship can be investigated later.

QUESTION 6.

Answer:

History and Physical	Nurses' Notes	Vital Signs	Laboratory Results

0422: Client in ICU following stabilization after anaphylaxis in the emergency department. Resting comfortably. Cardiac monitor shows sinus rhythm at 72 beats/min. Other vital signs: T 37.2°C (99.0°F); RR 18 breaths/min; BP 128/88 mm Hg; SpO$_2$ 97%. Opens eyes to stimuli; PERRLA. Lung sounds clear bilaterally. S$_1$S$_2$ present without murmur.

Rationale: Findings that indicate that the client is progressing favorably include the following: resting comfortably; heart rate in sinus rhythm at 72 beats/min and no murmur noted; temperature, respiratory rate, and blood pressure lower than initial presentation; normal oxygenation; and clear lung sounds. The client is neurologically intact, as she opens eyes to stimuli, and eyes are PERRLA.

UNIT 10: FLUID BALANCE

QUESTION 1.

Answer:

History and Physical	Nurses' Notes	Vital Signs	Laboratory Results

0902 52-year-old client here for transfusion today. History of seasonal allergies to pollens. Was recently seen at urgent care after twisting their ankle while walking. Client is scheduled in several weeks for elective rhinoplasty surgery to reduce the size of their nose. Has a history of hemophilia. Preoperative hemoglobin is 7 g/dL and hematocrit is 32%. Vital signs: T 37.2°C (99°F); HR 72 beats/min at rest; RR 18 breaths/min; BP 132/78 mm Hg.

Rationale: Transfusion therapy can be indicated for clients who have low hemoglobin and hematocrit. It is important for a client to be as healthy as possible prior to surgery, even if it is elective. This is especially important in patient with a history of hemophilia.

QUESTION 2.

Answer:

The nurse anticipates that the client is most likely to be prescribed an infusion of <u>red blood cells</u> and <u>clotting factor concentrates.</u>

Rationale: The nurse anticipates that the client is most likely to be prescribed an infusion of red blood cells (RBCs) to raise the hemoglobin and hematocrit level, especially prior to elective surgery. Because the patient has hemophilia, the transfusion of clotting factors is likely needed. Colloid components–albumin 5% pooled are used to treat hypoproteinemia in burns and hypoalbuminemia in shock and ARDs and/or to support blood pressure in dialysis and acute liver failure. Whole blood contains RBCs, but this patient does not require the increased volume of plasma. Cryoprecipitate is given often in the presence of massive blood loss.

QUESTION 3.

Answer:

Prior to administering RBCs, the nurse will *first* <u>verify the health care provider's order for transfusion</u>.

Rationale: The nurse will verify the health care provider's order first. If there is any question about this order, the other steps are irrelevant. The nurse will assure that the order is present with a date, time to begin transfusion, any special instructions noted, duration of infusion, and inclusion of any pretransfusion or posttransfusion medications that must be administered.

QUESTION 4.

Answer:

Once the blood arrives, the nurse plans to initially <u>inspect the bag for any signs of contamination</u> and <u>compare the blood product with the client's identifiers with another nurse.</u>

Rationale: To minimize infusion risks, the nurse will first perform safety checks. These include inspecting the bag for any signs of contamination or compromise and verifying the client's identity and the prescribed blood product with another nurse. If there are any discrepancies or concerns with these two actions, subsequent actions cannot take place. If these two actions demonstrate no problem with the bag of blood or with the confirmation of the blood product with the client's identifiers, then further actions to administer the blood can be taken.

QUESTION 5.

Answer:

- **X** Stop the infusion.
- ○ Offer sips of water.
- ○ Restart the infusion at a faster rate.
- ○ Set the infusion to deliver more slowly.
- ○ Provide reassurance that this is a normal feeling.
- ○ Delegate monitoring of vital signs to assistive personnel.
- ○ Give the client a magazine to read to provide distraction.

Rationale: The critical action the nurse must take at the first sign of a reaction is to stop the infusion. The symptoms the client is experiencing are consistent with a mild to moderate allergic reaction. After stopping the transfusion, the nurse will change the administration set and administer 0.9% sodium chloride at a rate to maintain patent IV access. The nurse will then notify the health care provider and blood bank, administer antihistamines as ordered, and monitor and document vital signs every 15 minutes. The transfusion may be restarted if fever, dyspnea, and wheezing are not present. The nurse will not offer sips of water, restart the infusion faster (before going through the actions just noted), simply slow the infusion, provide reassurance that this feeling is normal, delegate monitoring to assistive personnel, or distract the client with a magazine. The client's symptoms could rapidly progress, so it is critical to stop the infusion.

QUESTION 6.
Answer:

History and Physical	Nurses' Notes	Vital Signs	Laboratory Results
1355: Client resting comfortably in chair as RBCs infuse. Vital signs include T 37.0°C (98.6°F); RR 16 breaths/min; HR 76 beats/min; BP 118/72 mm Hg; SpO₂ 99%. Alert and oriented × 4. Lung sounds clear bilaterally. S₁S₂ present without murmur.			

Rationale: Findings that indicate that the client is progressing favorably include the following: resting comfortably without restlessness, normal vital signs, alertness with full orientation, clear lung sounds, and regular heart sounds.

UNIT 11: NUTRITION

QUESTION 1.
Answer:

History and Physical	Nurses' Notes	Vital Signs	Laboratory Results
1442: 91-year-old client admitted from long-term care agency with weakness and failure to thrive. Client has reportedly lost 5 kg (11 lb) in the past 3 months. Assessment reveals a cachectic individual with brittle hair, dry skin, red mucous membranes, lungs clear to auscultation, heart rate regular at 64 beats/min, and lower extremities with poor tone. Height 177.8 cm (70 inches), weight 56.2 kg (124 lb). BMI 17.8.			

Rationale: Signs and symptoms associated with malnourishment include weakness, failure to thrive, losing more than 4.5 kg (10 lb) in 3 months, brittle hair, dry skin, red (instead of pink) mucous membranes, extremities with poor tone, and a BMI under 18.5.

QUESTION 2.
Answer:
The nurse anticipates that the client is at highest risk for **dehydration.**
Rationale: Clients with malnourishment are at high risk for dehydration, especially if they are not consuming or receiving fluid hydration. There is no imminent risk for fluid retention, especially since the client is not drinking much. At this time, based on the client's symptoms, there is no indication that the client is at high risk for dysphagia or reflux.

QUESTION 3.
Answer:
The nurse *prioritizes* facilitating the client's intake of **fluids**.
Rationale: Oral intake is always preferred over enteral and parenteral nutrition. The nurse will prioritize intake of fluids to prevent dehydration. If the client can consume fluids by mouth, the registered dietitian nutritionist (RDN) can suggest nutritional options that optimally deliver calories and nutrients. Fats, proteins, and carbohydrates are usually included in drinkable nutritional supplements.

QUESTION 4.
Answer:
X 60-mL ENFit syringe
X Skin barrier protectant
X Water-soluble lubricant
X Emesis basin
X Tongue blade
O Sterile gloves
X Hypoallergenic tape

Rationale: Before the insertion of a small-bore feeding tube, the nurse will plan to gather all of the supplies listed except for sterile gloves. The nurse will plan to gather clean gloves rather than sterile ones.

QUESTION 5.
Answer:
O Maintain head-of-bed elevation at 20 degrees.
X Document how the client tolerated the procedure.
X Print the date and time on the nasal portion of the tape.
O Immediately begin feeding through the newly placed tube.
X Fasten the end of the tube to the client's gown using a clip or tape.
O Clean tubing at the nostril with a cotton pad dipped in alcohol.
X Ensure that an order for an x-ray of the chest/abdomen has been placed.
Rationale: Once the small-bore feeding tube has been inserted, the nurse will perform all actions with the exception of maintaining the head of bed elevation at 20 degrees, immediately beginning the feeding, and cleaning the tubing at the nostril with a cotton pad dipped in alcohol. Instead, the nurse will maintain the head of bed elevation at 30 degrees (preferably 45 degrees) unless contraindicated. Feeding is contraindicated until the chest/abdomen x-ray has been confirmed tube placement. The nurse will clean the tubing at the nostril with a soft washcloth dampened in mild soap and water so that alcohol does not dry the skin.

QUESTION 6.
Answer:

History and Physical	Nurses' Notes	Vital Signs	Laboratory Results
0808: Client sitting up in bed taking sips of water. Client reports being tired but "feeling better." Mucous membranes pink and moist. Lung sounds clear; S₁S₂ present without murmur; bowel sounds present × 4 quadrants. No skin breakdown noted. Vital signs: T 36.9°C (98.4°F); HR 70 beats/min; RR 14 breaths/min; BP 108/68 mm Hg; SpO₂ 99% on RA. Height 177.8 cm (70 inches), weight 59.0 kg (130 lb). BMI 18.7.			

Rationale: Findings that indicate that the client's nutritional status has improved include sitting up, taking sips of water, feeling better, pink mucous membranes (instead of red), and an increase in weight and BMI.

UNIT 12: ELIMINATION

QUESTION 1.
Answer:

History and Physical	Nurses' Notes	Vital Signs	Laboratory Results
1300: 88-year-old client of female gender identity with history of dementia admitted from long-term care agency. Long-term care agency nurse states that the client began to decline this morning and has experienced intermittent hallucinations after developing a fever of 40°C (104.0°F). Other vital signs include HR 90 beats/min; RR 20 breaths/min; BP 150/92 mm Hg; SpO₂ 98% on RA. Assessment reveals a well-nourished individual with PERRLA, lungs clear to auscultation, regular heart rate with no murmurs, and a soft, nontender abdomen. Not oriented to person, time, location, or situation, which the agency nurse states is the client's baseline. The client has an indwelling urinary catheter present. Urine is cloudy and dark colored. The long-term care nurse reports the catheter has been in place for 10 days.			

Rationale: The nurse will immediately follow up on signs and symptoms that may indicate infection, which include intermittent hallucinations and high fever. These are common findings in older adults who have a urinary tract infection. The nurse will also immediately assess the condition of the indwelling catheter, as it is a possible source of infection, particularly since it has been in place for 10 days. Cloudy, dark-colored urine is an indication of infection. Disorientation does not require immediate follow-up, as the client has a history of dementia. Other findings are within expected parameters and do not require further assessment at this time.

QUESTION 2.
Answer:
The nurse will contact the long-term care agency nurse to inquire about the client's <u>amount and type of usual fluid intake</u> and <u>client's ability to feed self.</u>

    Rationale: The nurse will need to know about the client's usual fluid intake; changes in fluid intake can affect fluid balance, which can affect urinary elimination. Also, if the patient is unable to feed self without assistance, this must be a consideration in any effort to increase oral fluids. It will be helpful for the nurse to know if the client's usual patterns of fluid intake have changed recently or have remained the same. The client's current weight is not necessary, as the assessment demonstrates that the client is well-nourished. Also, weight can be collected at the hospital and is not a factor regarding the patient's possible infection. A psychiatric history is not needed currently. The intermittent hallucinations the client is experiencing, when coupled with a high fever, are more indicative of a possible infection in an older adult than a psychiatric concern. Food preferences are not necessary at this time; the client is well-nourished so food intake is not a primary concern.

QUESTION 3.
Answer:
The nurse will prioritize communicating to the health care provider about the client's temperature of <u>40°C (104.0°F)</u> and <u>indwelling urinary catheter with dark cloudy urine.</u>

    Rationale: Due to the likelihood that the client is experiencing CAUTI, the nurse will prioritize communicating to the health care provider the client's temperature and presence of an indwelling urinary catheter draining dark, cloudy urine. These are two important factors in understanding the client's condition, which the health care provider will need to know about initially. The nurse can communicate the client's disorientation later, as this is likely related to their history of dementia, and the slightly elevated blood pressure value, which is not of priority concern.

QUESTION 4.
Answer:
X Soap
X Washcloth
X Clean gloves
X Sterile gloves
X Drainage bag
X Waterproof absorbent pad
X Syringe prefilled with sterile water
    Rationale: The nurse will plan to gather all of these supplies. They will all be used in the insertion of an indwelling urinary catheter.

QUESTION 5.
Answer:
X Separate labia with nondominant hand.
o Don sterile gloves and cleanse perineum.
o Place sterile drape under client with shiny side up.
o Lubricate catheter tip before insertion with petroleum jelly.
o Cleanse labia and urinary meatus from anus toward clitoris.
X Inflate catheter balloon by using syringe prefilled with sterile water.
    Rationale: The nurse prepares to cleanse the perineum of a female patient by separating the labia with the nondominant hand. The hand stays in that position throughout catheterization. The nurse will inflate the catheter balloon by using the syringe prefilled with sterile water. All other actions require modification to maintain safe, sterile technique. The perineum should be cleaned by using clean gloves before the sterile technique begins. The sterile drape should be placed with the shiny side

down under the client. The catheter tip should be lubricated with a water-based type of lubricant instead of petroleum jelly. The labia and urinary meatus should be cleansed from the clitoris toward the anus to minimize the chance of introducing infection into the vagina and urethra.

QUESTION 6.
Answer:
o The meatus is chafed.
o The client is restless.
X A bladder scan reveals no urine in the bladder.
o Bladder palpation reveals distention.
o Urine leaks around the tubing connection.
X The bag is noted to have 80 mL of urine collected.
    Rationale: Findings that indicate that the procedure was completed accurately include the bladder scan showing no urine in the bladder and the presence of urine in the collection bag. The meatus should not be chafed during insertion of an indwelling urinary catheter. Bladder palpation should not reveal distention; distention should be relieved when the urine drains into the collection bag. Urine should not leak around the tubing connection. A restless patient could indicate fullness of the bladder but would be difficult to assess in a disoriented patient.

UNIT 13: CARE OF THE SURGICAL PATIENT

QUESTION 1.
Answer:

History and Physical	Nurses' Notes	Vital Signs	Laboratory Results
1030: 76-year-old client scheduled for knee replacement surgery in 2 weeks. Medical history includes type 2 diabetes mellitus, hypercholesterolemia, and hypertension. Medication history includes metformin 500 mg by mouth twice daily, lovastatin 20 mg by mouth every night, and amlodipine 5 mg by mouth at night. Has recently been on a prednisone oral dose pack when the client's jaw became very inflamed following a dental procedure. Family history positive for malignant hyperthermia. Vital signs: T 36.8°C (98.2°F); HR 74 beats/min; RR 16 breaths/min; BP 160/98 mm Hg; SpO$_2$ 98% on RA. Assessment reveals a well-nourished client. PERRLA, cranial nerves intact. Skin without lesions. Lungs clear to auscultation, heart regular rate and rhythm with no murmurs, and a soft, nontender abdomen. Alert and oriented × 4.			

    Rationale: The nurse will follow up on findings that may place the client at risk for complications related to surgery. These include a history of type 2 diabetes mellitus (which can be associated with impaired healing), hypercholesterolemia and hypertension (which can increase cardiovascular risk during and after surgery), the recent use of a prednisone dose pack (which can depress the immune system), and the family history of malignant hyperthermia, which is an inherited condition.

QUESTION 2.
Answer:
Based on the history, the nurse notes that the client is at high risk for developing **malignant hyperthermia.**
    Rationale: The client's history is positive for a family history of malignant hyperthermia. This is an inherited tendency in which an individual has a reaction to certain drugs that are used in anesthesia during surgery. The client develops a high body temperature, rigid muscles or spasms, and a rapid heart rate; without treatment, this condition can be fatal.

QUESTION 3.

Answer:

The nurse will provide *prioritized* teaching to the client about <u>malignant hyperthermia</u>.

    Rationale: Because malignant hyperthermia can be fatal, the nurse will prioritize this teaching. All other teaching can be completed afterward.

QUESTION 4.

Answer:

○ Percuss liver.
X Auscultate lungs.
X Evaluate mental status.
○ Palpate surgical knee.
X Observe cardiac monitor.
X Record output in urinary catheter bag.

    Rationale: The nurse will plan to perform assessments that provide information about the client's postsurgical status, including auscultation of lungs, evaluation of mental status, observation of the cardiac monitor, and documentation of the amount of output in the urinary catheter bag. The nurse will not percuss the liver or any other organs; percussion is done by the health care provider. The nurse will not palpate the surgical knee, as this is likely to induce pain and could disrupt the wound.

QUESTION 5.

Answer:

X Ask the client to quantify the pain on a 0-to-10 scale.
○ Explain that pain medication must be reserved for severe pain.
○ Tell the spouse to push the patient-controlled anesthesia (PCA) button if the client is too tired to do so.
X Prepare to administer the next dose of pain medication as ordered.
X Provide teaching on how to use the PCA pump.
○ Teach that nonpharmacologic methods of pain control are preferable to opioids.

    Rationale: The client who has just returned from surgery will require pain management. Opioid medication is usually administered via a PCA pump. The client may also be prescribed other pain medication that the nurse administers. The nurse will first ask the client to rate the pain on a 0-to-10 scale. This provides a way for the nurse to evaluate later, after pain medication has been given, whether pain management methods were effective. The nurse will also prepare to administer the next dose of pain medication and will teach the client how to use the PCA so that they can provide their own pain relief (on a timed and locked-dose basis). The nurse will not state that pain medication is reserved only for severe pain. Pain should be controlled so that it does not escalate in severity. The nurse will not teach the spouse to push the PCA button; only the client is permitted to do this. The nurse will not teach that nonpharmacologic methods of pain control are preferred to opioids. In the immediate postsurgical phase, opioid medication is an important method of pain relief.

QUESTION 6.

Answer:

History and Physical	Nurses' Notes	Vital Signs	Laboratory Results
1313: 76-year-old client returned 4 hours ago from right knee replacement surgery. Family at bedside. Vital signs: T 37.1°C (98.8°F); HR 72 beats/min; RR 18 breaths/min; BP 122/78 mm Hg. Client initially rated pain at 7 on 0-to-10 scale; now rates pain at 3. Skin flushed and red. Appears to be drifting off to sleep.			

    Rationale: Findings that indicate that pain was effectively managed include all vital signs within expected parameters, a decrease in the subjective rating of pain on a 0-to-10 scale, and being comfortable enough to appear to drift off to sleep.

UNIT 14: DRESSINGS AND WOUND CARE

QUESTION 1.

Answer:

History and Physical	Nurses' Notes	Vital Signs	Laboratory Results
1400: 80-year-old client admitted today from the hospital after being on a ventilator with COVID-19 for a prolonged time. Here for rehabilitation before returning to assisted living, where she normally resides with her 82-year-old spouse. Medical history of depression and anxiety well-controlled with medication. Patient is 167.7 cm (5 ft 6 in), weighs 46.2 kg (102 lb). Alert and oriented × 4. Admits to being very tired after the hospitalization. Denies pain. Vital signs: T 36.8°C (98.2°F); HR 78 beats/min; RR 14 breaths/min; BP 128/74 mm Hg; SpO₂ 99% on RA. PERRLA, cranial nerves intact. Lungs clear to auscultation, heart regular rate and rhythm with no murmurs, and a soft, nontender abdomen. In bed, has difficulty turning onto side by self. Muscle strength in arms 2-3 on scale of 5. ROM normal in upper and lower extremities. Full skin assessment reveals reddened areas on the sacrum and heels.			

    Rationale: The nurse will follow up on findings that focus on the patient's mobility and skin condition. These findings include a recent history of being on a ventilator for COVID-19 (requiring bed rest), patient being underweight for height, reduced ability to turn self, and reddened areas on the sacrum and heels. The nurse will need to gather further information on how debilitated the client was while suffering from COVID-19 and the length of the hospital stay and time on a ventilator. Was the patient on a mobility protocol while in the hospital? This information can give context to the reddened areas on the sacrum and heels. These skin findings need further assessment to determine how compromised these areas are.

QUESTION 2.

Answer:

Based on the history, the nurse notes that the client is at high risk for developing <u>pressure injuries</u>.

    Rationale: The client's history of prolonged use of a ventilator, nutritional status, mobility limitations, and the reddened areas on the sacrum and heels place the client at high risk for developing pressure injuries. There is no evidence that the client is at high risk for sepsis; vital signs, including temperature, are normal, and there are no other immediate signs of infection. Urticaria often results from exposure to an allergen; there is no evidence that wheals are present on the skin. Pruritus is itching, and there is no evidence that the client has been exposed to anything that would result in itching.

QUESTION 3.

Answer:

The nurse will provide *prioritized* teaching and intervention to address a <u>Stage 2</u> pressure injury.

    Rationale: The assessment findings of an injury that is shallow, nonblanchable, and with blisters are consistent with a stage 2 pressure injury. Stage 1 injuries are red or pink in clients with light skin or modified in color from surrounding skin for clients with dark skin. There may be temperature differences noted in that area from the surrounding skin; however, there is no open wound. A stage 3 pressure injury extends into the fat layer of the skin. A stage 4 pressure injury extends through all layers of skin and can include exposed bone, tendons, or muscle.

QUESTION 4.

Answer:

○ SANE nurse
X Wound care nurse
○ Speech therapist
X Physical therapist
X Health care provider
X Registered dietitian nutritionist

Rationale: The nurse will plan to collaborate with the wound care nurse, physical therapist, health care provider, and registered dietitian nutritionist. The wound care nurse can provide information on specialized care for this type of wound. The physical therapist can help with improving mobility, which takes pressure off the sacrum. The health care provider will oversee the overall plan of care and will place prescription and consult orders. The registered dietitian nutritionist can evaluate the client's diet and make recommendations for nutrition intake that facilitates wound healing. A SANE nurse is a forensic nurse examiner. There is no need for those services or the services of a speech therapist at this time.

QUESTION 5.

Answer:

○ Massage the affected areas.
○ Rub lotion into the heels and sacrum.
X Place a friction-reducing sheet underneath the client.
X Encourage intake of a diet high in protein.
○ Remind and assist the client to turn or move every 3 hours.
○ Apply ointment and an occlusive dressing to reddened areas.
X Obtain a specialized air mattress for the client's bed.

Rationale: The nurse will implement interventions that are targeted to relieve pressure and encourage wound healing. Placing a friction-reducing sheet under the client makes it easier for two people to move the client up in bed as needed. This reduces shear and friction on the skin. Encouraging a diet high in protein is helpful, as protein can facilitate quicker wound healing. Obtaining a specialized air mattress for the client's bed is helpful, as this can minimize pressure on the affected areas. The wound areas should not be massaged, as this can facilitate skin breakdown. A client with a pressure injury should not have lotion rubbed in, nor should an ointment and occlusive dressing be used; rather, the skin should be kept very clean and dry. Moisture can increase the risk for bacterial invasion. The client should not be turning or moving every 3 hours; this should occur every 1 to 2 hours at the minimum.

QUESTION 6.

Answer:

History and Physical	Nurses' Notes	Vital Signs	Laboratory Results

1524: Complete skin assessment performed. Area on sacrum measures 3 cm × 4 cm. Very small open area noted with yellowish drainage. Heels have no redness or breakdown bilaterally. Tender, reddened area noted on the back of the skull; measures 1 cm × 1 cm. Vital signs: T 38.5°C (101.3°F); HR 76 beats/min; RR 16 breaths/min; BP 126/78 mm Hg; SpO₂ 97% on RA.

Rationale: Findings that indicate that the client's condition has deteriorated include enlargement of the initial sacral wound, an opening on the wound, and yellowish drainage present. The fever indicates that infection may be present. The presence of a new tender, reddened area on the back of the skull measuring 1 cm × 1 cm suggests that the client may not have been turned or moved regularly. All other findings are within expected parameters.

UNIT 15: HOME CARE

QUESTION 1.

Answer:

History and Physical	Nurses' Notes	Vital Signs	Laboratory Results

1400: 77-year-old client seen in the home today following discharge yesterday after a 3-week hospitalization for pneumonia. Medical history of osteoporosis and two hip fractures over the past 3 years. Has lived in this house for 30+ years. Spouse died last year; no one else resides here. Three cats are noted going inside and outside via small pet door. The client is alert and oriented × 4 and expresses happiness at being home. Reports "I may be tired, but I am glad to be home." Denies pain. Vital signs: T 37.2°C (98.9°F); HR 68 beats/min; RR 14 breaths/min; BP 110/68 mm Hg; Spo₂ 98% on RA. Assessment reveals a frail client. PER-RLA, cranial nerves intact. Lungs clear to auscultation, heart regular rate and rhythm with no murmurs, and a soft, nontender abdomen. Full range of motion in upper and lower extremities. No skin abnormalities noted. Gait somewhat shuffled.

Rationale: The home health care nurse assesses clients for safety and adherence to treatment. Part of the assessment includes observation of the home environment. The nurse is concerned that the client has just been discharged after a 3-week hospitalization for pneumonia, which has left the client tired. The history of frailty, osteoporosis, and hip fractures and the client's shuffled gait alert the nurse to a concern for falls. The nurse is also concerned that the client lives alone; if something is needed immediately, it may be challenging for the client's needs to be met. The presence of pets can often be therapeutic; however, having three cats that are constantly moving can increase the risk for falls. Also, since the cats go outside the home, they can introduce sources of infection into the house.

QUESTION 2.

Answer:

The nurse notes that the client is at high risk for falls as evidenced by the findings of <u>rugs on floors</u>, <u>glasses and plates on top shelves of cabinets,</u> and <u>stairs going to the second floor.</u>

Rationale: The client's risk for falls is evident in several risk factors. Rugs on the floor are easy to trip over. Keeping frequently used items on high shelves may require the client to reach and lose their balance or to use a step stool or ladder, which can lead to falls. The use of stairs increases the fall risk, as clients may have visual or perceptual deficits as they age, especially after a long hospitalization when they are not fully recovered. The remaining choices do not present a high risk for falls.

QUESTION 3.

Answer:

The nurse *prioritizes* addressing <u>rugs on the floor</u> to improve the client's safety by minimizing the risk for falls.

Rationale: The nurse will prioritize addressing the rugs on the floor. First, rugs are one of the most common causes of falls in the home. Second, this problem is easy to address because the rugs can simply be removed. Rearranging glasses and plates takes longer and can be a secondary priority. Determining how to navigate stairs, or whether going up the stairs is even necessary, can be addressed secondarily also.

QUESTION 4.

Answer:

X Type of stove
X Safe use of walker
X Presence of smoke detectors
X Amount and kind of food in refrigerator
X Ability to self-bathe and get dressed
X Medication administration practices

Rationale: The nurse will plan to evaluate all of these factors. The client's safety is evaluated in the way the home is laid out, in the safety mechanisms (such as smoke detectors and carbon monoxide detectors) placed (or missing) in the home, and in the ways the client performs self-care in the home environment. All of these factors are important in the full evaluation of client safety.

QUESTION 5.
Answer:
- ○ "Extra oxygen tanks can be stored in the kitchen."
- ○ "Oxygen tanks must be kept at least 4 feet from open flames."
- X "I bought No Smoking/Oxygen in Use signs for each doorway."
- X "We should report any signs of dizziness to the health care provider."
- ○ "If my mother gets shorter of breath, I will increase the oxygen flow rate."
- ○ "My husband may visit while I am here with my mother, but he will smoke in another room."

Rationale: Teaching has been effective when the client's daughter states that she has purchased signs that read No Smoking/Oxygen in Use for each doorway, as these must be displayed. Teaching has also been effective when she states that any dizziness should be reported to the health care provider, as this could be a sign of hypoxia. Oxygen tanks should be stored in areas where there is a minimal risk for fire; the kitchen is not a safe place to store them. Oxygen tanks must be kept at least 8 feet—not 4 feet—away from open flames. The client and family should never increase the oxygen rate without the direction of a health care provider. Anyone who is in the house should refrain from smoking at all times; it is unsafe to smoke even in the next room when oxygen is in use.

QUESTION 6.
Answer:

History and Physical	Nurses' Notes	Vital Signs	Laboratory Results

1400: Home assessment performed. Client is eating a meal of fish and potatoes with daughter. Client's son-in-law is visiting; daughter states he has gone for a drive so that he can smoke. Stove is off and not in use. Refrigerator is full of fresh produce. Client's daughter purchased an extra-long tube for oxygen so that the client can walk around her home easily. No Smoking/Oxygen in Use signs are placed at each doorway.

Rationale: Findings that indicate that the client is safe at home include the observation of the client having a nutritious meal, with fresh produce in the refrigerator; the daughter's husband being away from the house to smoke rather than doing so in a nearby room; and the presence of No Smoking/Oxygen in Use signs at each doorway. The use of an extra-long tube for oxygen is discouraged, as this can increase the risk for falls; the presence of this device does not demonstrate client safety at home.

Index

A

Abbreviations
  "do not use" list of, 597
  in documentation, 52
Abdomen
  concave, 154
  flat, 154
  landmarks in, 154
  quadrants of, 155f
  round, 154
Abdominal assessment, 151–157
  anatomy, 152f
  delegation in, 152
  in disabled patient, 157
  documentation in, 157
  equipment for, 152–153
  evaluation in, 156
  hand-off reporting in, 157
  implementation in, 154
  interprofessional collaboration in, 152
  in older adults, 157
  patient education in, 157
  in pediatric patient, 157
  planning in, 153
Abdominal binder, 1191b, 1191f
Abdominal distention, 154
Abdominal girth, 154, 155f
Abdominal pain, 151, 151–152t
Abdominal paracentesis, 240–246
Abducens nerve, 168
Abduction pillow, 355, 356t
ABO system, 896–897, 897t
Abrasion, 522–523t, 523f
Absorption, medication, 587, 589t
Abuse, assessment of, 111
Accountability, 11, 11t
Acid mantle, 1110
Acne, 522–523t, 522f
Acoustic stethoscope, 86f
Active listening, 20b
Active motion, 166
Activities of daily living (ADLs)
  in home setting, for cognitive deficits, 1209
  range-of-motion exercises incorporated
    into, 332t
Actual body weight (ABW), 921
Acuity records, 59–60
Acute hemolytic transfusion reaction (AHTR),
  898–899t, 908
Acute pain, definition of, 444
Administration sets
  for blood transfusions, 905f
  for intravenous therapy, 857f, 871t
Admission, 40–51
  admitting process, 42–45
  assessment, 44–45
  evidence-based practice of, 41
  nurse role in, 43–44
  person-centered care of, 41
  practice standards, 40
  principles for practice, 40–41

Admission (Continued)
  purpose of, 40
  safety guidelines of, 41
  special considerations for, 45
  supplemental standards, 40
Admission personnel, role of, 42–43
Adolescents. see also Pediatric patients
  physical assessment of, 116–117
Advance care planning (ACP), 43
Advance directives, 43b, 823
Adventitious sounds, 133, 133–134t
Adverse drug reactions (ARD), medication
  action, 589–590
Adverse event reporting, 63–64, 64b
Adverse transfusion reactions, monitoring for,
  908–911
  assessment in, 908
  in children, 911
  delegation in, 908
  documentation in, 911
  equipment for, 908–911
  evaluation in, 911
  in home care, 911
  implementation in, 910
  interprofessional collaboration in, 908
  in older adults, 911
  patient education in, 911
  planning in, 909
AED. see Automated external defibrillator
Aerobic culture, 205
Aerosol sprays, 588t, 627
Aging. see Older adults
AHTR. see Acute hemolytic transfusion reaction
Air embolism, 891–892t, 969–970t
Air mattress, 369, 369f
Airborne precautions, 268t
Air-filled cushion, for wheelchair, 368f
Air-fluidized beds, 363–364t, 373
Air-suspension beds, 373
Airway management, 753–788
  artificial airway, 759–770, 763f, 764f, 766f
    assessment, 761
    in children, 768
    delegation in, 760
    documentation in, 768
    endotracheal tubes, 760, 760f
    equipment for, 760–768
    evaluation, 767
    hand-off reporting in, 768
    home care in, 768–770
    implementation, 763
    interprofessional collaboration for, 760
    in older adults, 768
    patient education in, 768
    planning, 762
    in populations with disabilities, 768
    tracheostomy tubes, 760
  closed (in-line) suction, 769–770b, 769f
  endotracheal tube care, 770–777, 771f, 775b, 776f
    assessment, 772
    in children, 777
    delegation in, 771
    documentation in, 777
    equipment for, 771–777
    evaluation, 776

Airway management (Continued)
    hand-off reporting in, 777
    implementation, 773
    interprofessional collaboration for, 771
    in older adults, 777
    patient education in, 777
    planning, 773
  evidence-based practice for, 754
  nasotracheal/pharyngeal suctioning, 759–770,
    763f, 764f, 766f
    assessment, 761
    in children, 768
    delegation in, 760
    documentation in, 768
    equipment for, 760–768
    evaluation, 767
    hand-off reporting in, 768
    home care in, 768–770
    implementation, 763
    interprofessional collaboration for, 760
    in older adults, 768
    patient education in, 768
    planning, 762
    in populations with disabilities, 768
  oropharyngeal suctioning, 755–759, 755f
    assessment, 756
    delegation in, 755
    documentation in, 759
    equipment for, 755–758
    evaluation, 758
    hand-off reporting in, 759
    home care in, 759
    implementation, 757
    interprofessional collaboration for, 755
    in older adults, 759
    patient education in, 759
    planning, 756
    in populations with disabilities, 759
  person-centered care for, 754
  practice standards for, 753
  principles for practice in, 753
  purpose of, 753
  safety guidelines for, 754–755
  supplemental standards for, 753
  tracheostomy care, 778–787, 778f, 779b, 779t,
    782f, 783f, 784f, 785f
    assessment, 780
    in children, 787
    delegation in, 779
    documentation in, 786
    equipment for, 779–786
    evaluation, 786
    hand-off reporting in, 786
    home care in, 787
    implementation, 781
    interprofessional collaboration
      for, 779
    in older adults, 787
    patient education in, 786
    planning, 780
    in populations with disabilities, 787
Alarm fatigue, 789–790
  reduction of, 794b
Albumin, 900t
Alcohol-based hand sanitizers, 262

Page numbers followed by *b* indicates boxes,
f indicates illustrations, and *t* indicates tables.

Alginate dressing, 1118t, 1163–1164t
  application of, 1181–1192, 1186f
    assessment, 1182
    in children, 1187
    delegation in, 1182
    documentation in, 1187
    equipment for, 1182–1187
    evaluation, 1186
    hand-off reporting in, 1187
    implementation, 1183
    interprofessional collaboration in, 1182
    in older adults, 1187–1192
    patient education in, 1187
    in pediatrics, 1187
    planning, 1183
Allergic reactions
  medication action, 590, 590f, 590t
  to transfusions, 898–899t
  type IV, 288b
All-hazards event, 418b
All-hazards preparedness, 418b
Alopecia, 547–548t
Alzheimer's disease, 1209–1210
Ambulation, assisting with, 342–345b
  delegation in, 342
  equipment for, 342
  step of, 342–345, 343f, 344f, 345f
Ambulatory oxygen, 1237t
Ambulatory Surgery Discharge Criteria, 1085b
Ambulatory tank, 1240f
American Nurses Association (ANA), 53
Amplifier, in hearing aids, 577
Ampules, 664–673, 665f, 667f, 668f, 669f
  assessment, 666
  delegation in, 665
  equipment for, 665–673
  evaluation, 670
  interprofessional collaboration, 665
  planning, 666
Anaerobic culture, 205
Analgesia
  epidural, 445–446, 472–479, 472f, 473f
    assessment, 474
    delegation in, 473
    documentation in, 478
    equipment for, 473–478
    evaluation, 477
    hand-off reporting in, 478
    home care and, 478–479
    implementation, 475
    interprofessional collaboration of, 473
    in older adults, 478
    patient education in, 478
    in pediatrics, 478
    planning, 475
  local anesthetic infusion pump for, 479–482, 479f
    assessment, 479
    delegation in, 479
    documentation in, 482
    equipment for, 479–482
    evaluation, 481
    hand-off reporting in, 482
    home care and, 482
    implementation, 480
    interprofessional collaboration of, 479
    in older adults, 482
    patient education in, 482
    in pediatrics, 482
    planning, 480
  patient-controlled, 466–472, 466b
    assessment, 467
    delegation in, 467
    discontinue, 470
    documentation in, 471
    epidural, 473
    equipment for, 467–471
    evaluation, 471
    hand-off reporting in, 471–472
    home care and, 472

Analgesia (Continued)
    implementation, 468, 469f
    interprofessional collaboration of, 467
    in older adults, 472
    patient education in, 472
    in pediatrics, 472
    planning, 468
Analog hearing aid, 578
Aneroid manometers, 1227
Aneroid sphygmomanometers, 1227
Anesthesia, 1080t
Anger
  definition of, 26
  violence associated with, 26
Angioedema, 590t
Angle of Louis, 132–133, 142
Ankles, range-of-motion in
  assessment of, 167t
  exercise for, 332t, 333–336t
Antecubital veins, location of, 209f
Anterior thorax, 138, 138f
Anthrax, 425–426t
Anticipatory grief, 500–501
Antimicrobial soap, for handwashing, 264
Antisepsis, surgical hand, 1098–1101, 1099f, 1100f
Antiseptic hand rub, 263, 264, 264f
Anxiety
  behavioral manifestations of, 26b
  separation, 45
Apical impulse, 88, 88f, 143
Apical pulse, 82t, 86–90, 144
  assessment of, 87
  delegation in, 87
  documentation in, 90
  equipment, 87–90
  evaluation of, 90
  hand-off reporting in, 90
  home care in, 90
  implementation, 88
  interprofessional collaboration, 87
  in older adults, 90
  patient education in, 90
  in pediatric patient, 90
  planning of, 88
Apnea, obstructive sleep, 734, 744t, 1061
Apocrine glands, 522
Appendicitis, 151–152t
Aquathermia heating pad, 487, 487f
Aqueous solution, 588t
Aqueous suspension, 588t
Arterial blood gas measurements
  arterial specimen for, 220–225, 221f, 223f, 224f
  in children, 225
  description of, 220
  in disabled patient, 225
  equipment for, 220–224
  in older adults, 225
  patient education on, 225
Arterial insufficiency, 146t
Arterial specimen, for blood gas measurement,
    220–225, 221f, 223f, 224f
Arteriogram, 234–240, 234f
Artificial airway, 759–770, 763f, 764f, 766f
  assessment, 761
  in children, 768
  delegation in, 760
  documentation in, 768
  endotracheal tubes, 760, 760f
  equipment for, 760–768
  evaluation, 767
  hand-off reporting in, 768
  home care in, 768–770
  implementation, 763
  interprofessional collaboration for, 760
  in older adults, 768
  oxygen therapy in, 727–730, 727f
    assessment, 728
    delegation in, 727
    documentation in, 730

Artificial airway (Continued)
    equipment, 727–730
    evaluation, 730
    hand-off reporting in, 730
    home care in, 730
    implementation, 729
    interprofessional collaboration, 727
    patient education in, 730
    planning, 728
  patient education in, 768
  planning, 762
  in populations with disabilities, 768
  tracheostomy tubes, 760
Ascending stairs, with crutches, 352, 352f
Aspiration
  protecting patient from, 612b
  skill procedures for, 240–243
    assessment of, 243
    in children, 246
    delegation in, 240
    in disabled patient, 246
    documentation in, 246
    equipment for, 242
    evaluation of, 245
    hand-off reporting in, 246
    home care in, 246
    implementation of, 244
    in older adults, 246
    patient education in, 246
    planning of, 243
Aspiration pneumonia, 932
Aspiration precautions, 931–937, 932b
  assessment in, 934
  in children, 937
  delegation in, 932–933
  documentation in, 936
  dysphagia management, 932
  equipment for, 933–936
  evaluation in, 936
  hand-off reporting in, 936
  in home care, 937
  implementation in, 934
  interprofessional collaboration in, 933
  in older adults, 937
  patient education in, 937
  planning in, 934
  in populations with disabilities, 937
Assessment
  abdominal, 151–157
    anatomy, 152f
    delegation in, 152
    in disabled patient, 157
    documentation in, 157
    equipment for, 152–153
    evaluation in, 156
    hand-off reporting in, 157
    implementation in, 154
    interprofessional collaboration in, 152
    in older adults, 157
    patient education in, 157
    in pediatric patient, 157
    planning in, 153
  cardiovascular, 140–151
    delegation in, 140
    documentation in, 150
    equipment for, 140
    hand-off reporting in, 150
    home care, 151
    implementation in, 142
    in older adults, 151
    patient education in, 150–151
    in pediatric patient, 151
    planning in, 141
  genitalia, 157–162
    in children, 162
    delegation in, 157
    documentation in, 162
    equipment for, 158–162
    evaluation in in, 161

Assessment (*Continued*)
  female, 158, 160
    hand-off reporting in, 162
    implementation in, 160
    interprofessional collaboration in, 158
    male, 159, 161
    in older adults, 162
    patient education in, 162
    planning in, 160
  head and neck, 126–132
    delegation in, 126
    in disabled patient, 132
    documentation in, 131
    equipment for, 126
    evaluation in, 131
    hand-off reporting in, 131
    home care in, 132
    implementation in, 127, 128f
    interprofessional collaboration in, 126
    in older adults, 132
    patient education in, 131–132
    in pediatric patient, 131–132
    planning in, 127
  musculoskeletal and neurological,
      162–172
    delegation in, 163
    in disabled patient, 170–172
    documentation in, 170
    equipment for, 163–169
    evaluation in, 169
    hand-off reporting in, 170
    implementation in, 164
    interprofessional collaboration in, 163
    in older adults, 170
    patient education in, 170–172
    in pediatric patient, 170
    planning in, 164
  pain, 443–497, 452t
    assessment, 446, 449f
    basic comfort measures and, 446–453
    delegation in, 446
    documentation in, 451
    equipment for, 446–451
    evaluation, 451
    evidence-based practice of, 445
    hand-off reporting in, 451
    home care and, 453
    implementation, 450, 450f
    interprofessional collaboration of, 446
    in nonverbal patients, 447b
    in older adults, 452–453
    patient education in, 451–452
    in pediatrics, 452
    person-centered care of, 444–445
    planning, 449
    in populations with disabilities, 453
    practice standards of, 444
    principles for practice, 444
    purpose of, 443–444
    safety guidelines for, 445–446
    supplemental standards of, 444
  thorax and lung, 132–140, 132f
    in children, 139–140
    delegation in, 134
    documentation in, 139
    equipment for, 134
    evaluation in, 139
    hand-off reporting in, 139
    implementation in, 135
    interprofessional collaboration
        in, 134
    in older adults, 140
    patient education in, 139–140
    in pediatric patient, 139–140
    planning in, 135
  wound, 1114–1116b, 1116f
Assist control (AC) ventilation, 742t
Assist devices, types of, 346t
Assistive devices, for self-feeding, 1213f

Assistive personnel (AP)
  in communication, 26
  moving and positioning patients in bed by, 313
  transferring patients by, 298–299
Association of Perioperative Registered Nurses
    (AORN), 1098
Asthma action plan, 741f
Athlete's foot, 551–552t, 551f
Atrial fibrillation, 145t, 822f
Atrophy, 124b
Auscultation, 114–115
  of bowel sounds, 155
  for carotid artery bruit, 146f
  of heart sounds, 143, 144f, 144t
  stethoscope for, 114–115, 114b
Autolytic debridement, 1113–1114
Automated external defibrillator (AED),
    827–830, 827f, 829f
  assessment, 828
  in children, 830
  delegation in, 827
  documentation in, 830
  equipment for, 827–830
  evaluation, 829
  hand-off reporting in, 830
  home care in, 830
  implementation, 828
  interprofessional collaboration of, 827
  patient education in, 830
  planning, 828
Automated medication dispensing system, 593, 593f
Autopsy, of body after death, 510
Autotransfusion, of chest tube drainage, 817–819
  assessment, 817
  documentation in, 819
  evaluation, 819
  hand-off reporting in, 819
  implementation, 818
  in older adults, 819
  patient education in, 819
  planning, 818
Axilla, body temperature measurement, 73b, 78, 78f

B

Bacillus anthracis, 425–426t
Bacteremia, 969–970t
Bacterial phlebitis, 859
Bag-valve mask device, 834f
BAI. *see* Breath-actuated inhaler
Bandage turns, types of, 1188t
Bandages
  elastic
    application of, 1187–1190b, 1189f
    on midthigh amputation stump, 1190f
    secure, 1189f
  gauze, 1163–1164t
    application of, 1187–1190b
    on midthigh amputation stump, 1190f
Banner Mobility Assessment Tool (BMAT), for
    transferring patients, 299
Bar-coding, 594–595
Bariatric bed, 373, 373f
Bariatric lift, for transferring patients, 310f
Basement membrane zone, 1111, 1111f
Basic comfort measures, pain assessment and,
    446–453
Basic disaster supply kit, 430b
Basilic vein, 852f
Bates-Jensen Wound Assessment Tool
    (BWAT), 1154
Bathing cloths, 537–538, 537f
Baths, types of, 525b
Bed
  air-fluidized, 363–364t, 373
  air-suspension, 373
  bariatric, 373, 373f
  Fowler position in, 316
  high-air-loss, 373
  low-air-loss, 363–364t, 373

Bed (*Continued*)
  moving and positioning patients in, 313–321
    assessment in, 313
    in children, 321
    delegation in, 313
    documentation in, 321
    equipment for, 313–321
    hand-off reporting in, 321
    in home care, 321
    interprofessional collaboration of, 313
    in older adults, 321
    patient education in, 321
    planning in, 314
    using friction-reducing device, 315f
  positions of, 557–558t
  semi-Fowler position in, 316, 316f, 317f
  special, 362–380, 363–364t
  supine position in, 317, 317f
  30-degree lateral side-lying position in, 318,
      318f, 319f, 1152f
Bed bath, complete or partial, 524–534, 525b
  assessment, 525
  delegation in, 525
  documentation in, 533
  equipment for, 525–533
  evaluation, 533
  hand-off reporting in, 533
  home care and, 534
  implementation, 527, 528f, 529f, 530f, 531f, 532f
  interprofessional collaboration of, 525
  in older adults, 534
  patient education in, 534
  planning, 527
  in populations with disabilities, 534
Bed making, 519–564
  occupied, 557–558t, 557–562b
    delegation in, 558
    equipment for, 558
    interprofessional collaboration of, 558
    steps in, 559–562, 559f, 560f, 561f
  unoccupied, 561–562b
Bedpan, 1020b, 1020f, 1021f
Behind-the-ear (BTE) hearing aids, 577f, 577t
Belt restraint, self-releasing roll, 401, 402f
Bereavement, 500
Beta-adrenergic blockers, 755
Bilevel positive airway pressure (BiPAP), 734, 734f
Binder, abdominal, 1191b, 1191f
Biohazard bag, for specimen collection, 272f
Biological exposure, patient care after, 424–429,
    424b, 424f, 425–426t
  assessment, 426
  delegation in, 424
  documentation in, 429
  equipment for, 426–428
  evaluation, 428
  hand-off reporting in, 429
  home care and, 429
  implementation, 427
  interprofessional collaboration of, 426
  in older adults, 429
  patient education in, 429
  in pediatrics, 429
  planning, 427
  in populations with disabilities, 429
Biological warfare agents, 425–426t
Bioterrorism agents/diseases, 424b
Biotransformation, 587
Biot's respiration, 94b
Bladder scan, 1003–1004b, 1003f, 1004f
Blanket suture, 1122f, 1126
Blinking reflex, 566–567b
Blood
  occult, measurement
    in gastric secretions (Gastroccult),
        190–192, 191f
    in stool, 187–190, 187f, 189f
  warming of, 901, 901f
  whole, 900t

Blood gas measurements
  arterial specimen for, 220–225, 221f, 223f, 224f
  in children, 225
  description of, 220–225
  equipment for, 220–224
  in older adults, 225
  patient education on, 225
Blood glucose monitoring, 215–219, 215f, 217f, 218f
  assessment, 216
  in children, 219
  delegation in, 215
  description of, 215
  equipment for, 216
  evaluation, 219
  implementation, 216
  interprofessional collaboration in, 215
  monitor, 215f
  in older adults, 219
  patient education on, 219
  planning, 216
  reflectance meters for, 215
Blood pressure
  client teaching on, 1227–1232, 1228f
  cuff size, 1228b
  definition of, 95
  equipment, 96
  measurement of
    advantages and limitations of, 97b
    arterial, 95–107, 95f
    assessment, 97
    by auscultation, 95
    brachial artery, 100f
    cuffs, 96, 96f, 104f, 104t
    delegation in, 97
    direct method of, 96
    documentation in, 103
    Doppler ultrasonic stethoscope for, 102f
    electronic, 104–105b, 104f, 105f
    equipment for, 97–103
    evaluation, 102
    hand-off reporting in, 103
    home care in, 103–107
    implementation, 99, 99f
    interprofessional collaboration, 97
    mistakes in, 97b
    in older adults, 103
    by palpation, 101
    in pediatric patient, 103
    planning, 98
Blood products, 895, 896f, 900t
Blood specimens
  central venous catheter collection of, 212, 212f, 213f
  skin puncture for, 206
  syringe method for, 209, 210f, 211f
  transfer device, 888f
  Vacutainer system for, 210, 211f, 212f
  venipuncture collection of, 206–214, 209f, 210f, 211f, 212f, 213f
Blood therapy, 895–914
Blood transfusion
  ABO system, 896–897, 897t
  administration set for, 905f
  adverse events, 896
  allogeneic, 896
  autologous, 896
  blood products, 895, 896f, 900t
  definition of, 895
  evidence-based practice, 897–898
  human leukocyte antigen system, 897
  indications for, 900–901
  initiation of, 900–908, 901f
    assessment in, 901
    in children, 908
    delegation in, 901
    documentation in, 907
    equipment for, 901–907
    evaluation in, 907
    hand-off reporting in, 907

Blood transfusion (*Continued*)
    in home care, 908
    implementation in, 903
    interprofessional collaboration of, 901
    in older adults, 908
    patient education in, 907–908
    planning in, 903
  labelling of blood, 903f, 904f
  person-centered care, 897
  platelets, 896f, 900t
  reactions
    acute hemolytic, 898–899t
    adverse, 908–911
    allergic, 898–899t
    circulatory overload, 898–899t
    febrile, nonhemolytic, 898–899t
    hemolytic, 898–899t, 908
    monitoring for, 908–911
    prevention of, 897–898
    types of, 898–899t
  Rh system, 897
  safety guidelines, 898–899t, 898–900
  warming of blood, 901f, 905
  whole blood, 900t
Bloodborne pathogens, 845b
BMAT. *see* Banner Mobility Assessment Tool
Body alignment, 313
Body lice, 547–548t
Body mass index (BMI), 118, 921, 922b, 922f
Body mechanics, 297b
Body temperature
  definition of, 72
  evaluation of, 81
  factors affecting, 72
  implementation, 76, 76f, 77f
  measurement of, 72–82
    assessment in, 75
    axillary, 73b, 78, 78f
    client teaching on, 1224–1227
    delegation in, 72–73
    documentation in, 81
    equipment for, 73–81
    evaluation in, 81
    hand-off reporting in, 81
    home care in, 82
    implementation in, 76
    in older adults, 82
    oral, 73b, 76
    patient education in, 81
    in pediatric patients, 81–82
    planning in, 76
    rectal, 73b, 77, 78f
    sites for, 72, 72b, 73b
    skin, 73b
    temporal artery, 73b, 80, 80f
    thermometers for, 72
    tympanic membrane, 73b, 79, 79f
  planning, 76
  range of, 72, 72f
Bone demineralization, 170
Bone marrow aspiration/biopsy, 240–246, 241–242t, 242f
Botulism, 425–426t
Bowel elimination, 1018–1037
  bedpan for, 1020b, 1020f, 1021f
  enema, 1024–1029, 1024t, 1025f, 1027f
  evidence-based practice in, 1019
  fecal impaction
    Bristol Stool Form Scale, 1023f
    remove, digitally, 1022–1024b, 1023b, 1023f
    symptoms of, 1022
  person-centered care for, 1019
  practice standards for, 1018
  principles for practice, 1018–1019
  purpose of, 1018
  safety guidelines for, 1019–1024
Bowel sounds, 155
Braces, 356t

Brachial artery, palpation of, blood pressure measurement using, 100f
Brachial pulse, 82t, 148, 148f
Braden Scale, for pressure injuries, 1147, 1147t
Bradypnea, 94b
Brain death, 510
Brand name, 587
Breath sounds. *see also* Respirations
  adventitious, 133, 133–134t
  auscultation of, 137, 137f
  normal, 138t
Breath-actuated inhaler (BAI), 643f
Breathing
  accessory muscles of, 138
  rate and rhythm of, 136
Briggs adapter, 727
Bristol stool form scale, 1023f
Broad openings, 20b
Bronchoscopy, 246–250, 247f
  assessment of, 247
  in children, 250
  delegation in, 247
  in disabled patients, 250
  documentation in, 250
  equipment for, 247–250
  evaluation of, 249
  hand-off reporting in, 250
  home care in, 250
  implementation of, 248
  interprofessional collaboration of, 247
  in older adults, 250
  patient education in, 250
  planning of, 248
Brushing, of teeth, 538, 540f
Burn safety, in home environment, 1207
Butterfly needle, 846f
Buttocks lift, 1068f

C

Calcium, 170
Callus, 551–552t, 551f
Cancer
  cervical, 159
  colorectal, 160
  endometrial, 159
  lung, 134
  ovarian, 159
  prostate, 159
Canes, use of, 345–355, 346f, 346t
  assessment in, 347
  in children, 355
  delegation in, 347
  documentation in, 355
  equipment for, 347
  evaluation, 354
  hand-off reporting in, 355
  home care and, 355
  implementation, 348, 350f, 351f, 352f, 353f
  interprofessional collaboration of, 347
  in older adults, 355
  patient education in, 355
  planning in, 347
  in populations with disabilities, 355
Cannula
  nasal, for oxygen delivery, 720–722, 721–722t, 721f
  oxygen-conserving, 721–722t, 722
  oxygen-reserving, 721–722t, 722f
  reservoir nasal, 1236
Cap, applying and removing, 279–282, 280f
Capillary refill, 147
Caplet, 588t
Capnography, 771, 941
Capsules, 588t
Carbon dioxide detectors, 941
Carbon monoxide (CO) safety, in home environment, 1204, 1208, 1208f

Cardiac care, 789–798
 cardiac monitor, 794–797, 794b, 796f
 evidence-based practice for, 789–790
 person-centered care for, 789
 practice standards for, 789
 principles for practice in, 789, 790t
 purpose of, 789
 safety guidelines for, 791
 supplemental standards for, 789
 12-lead electrocardiogram, 791–794, 793f
Cardiac catheterization, 234–240, 234f
Cardiac monitor, 794–797, 794b, 796f
 assessment, 795
 in children, 797
 delegation in, 795
 documentation in, 797
 equipment for, 795–797
 evaluation, 796
 hand-off reporting in, 797
 implementation, 795
 indications for, 794b
 interprofessional collaboration of, 795
 in older adults, 797
 patient education in, 797
 planning, 795
 in populations with disabilities, 797
Cardiac rhythms, 789, 790t
Cardiopulmonary arrest, 821
Cardiopulmonary resuscitation (CPR), 823–824,
  830, 833t
 in palliative care, 499
Cardiovascular assessment, 140–151
 delegation in, 140
 documentation in, 150
 equipment for, 140
 hand-off reporting in, 150
 home care, 151
 implementation in, 142
 in older adults, 151
 patient education in, 150–151
 in pediatric patient, 151
 planning in, 141
Care plans, standardized, 60
Caregiver, needs of, 500
Carotid artery
 anatomy of, 145f
 assessment of, 145
 bruit, auscultation for, 146f
 palpation of, 145, 145f
Carotid pulse, 82t
Casualty, 418b
Catheter(s)
 central venous
  blood specimen collection from, 212,
   212f, 213f
  triple-lumen, 212f
 damage, 891–892t
 latex, 1008
 migration, 891–892t
 nontunneled, discontinuation of, 882–892
 over-the-needle, 846, 846f, 846t
 peripheral intravenous, discontinuing, 878, 879f
 peripherally inserted central, 279, 880t, 881f
 single-use straight, 987, 988f
 size of, 987–988, 988f
 straight or indwelling, 987
 transtracheal oxygen, 1236
 urinary, indwelling
  care for, 998–1004
  documentation in, 997
  in females, 991, 991f
  hand-off reporting in, 997
  insertion of, 987–998, 987b, 988f, 989f, 992f,
   993f, 994f, 995f, 996f
  in males, 990, 991f
  in older adults, 997
  patient education, 997, 1008
  in pediatrics, 997
  removal of, 998–1004, 1000f

Catheter(s) (Continued)
 UTI and, 987
 Yankauer suction, 755
Catheterization
 urinary, 987
  drape for, 992f
  equipment for, 988–989, 989f
  of urinary diversion, 1050–1052
Catheter-related bloodstream infection
  (CRBSI), 843
Catheter-related sepsis, 969–970t
CEI. see Continuous epidural infusion
Ceiling lift, for transferring patients, 306f
Celiac disease, 151–152t
Centers for Disease Control and Prevention,
  isolation guidelines, 268t
Centers for Medicare and Medicaid, patients'
  rights provided by, 42–43, 42–43b
Central line-associated bloodstream infections
  (CLABSI), 844
Central parenteral nutrition, 970–975, 970t, 973f
 assessment, 971
 delegation in, 970
 documentation in, 974
 equipment for, 971–974
 evaluation, 974
 hand-off reporting in, 974
 home care in, 975
 implementation, 972
 interprofessional collaboration, 971
 in older adults, 975
 patient education in, 975
 in pediatrics, 975
 planning, 972
Central vascular access devices (CVAD),
  879–893, 880f, 880t, 888f, 891–892t, 973f
 assessment, 882
 blood sampling in, 882
 changing the injection cap in, 882
 in children, 893
 delegation in, 881
 discontinuation of a nontunneled catheter in,
  882–892
 documentation in, 892–893
 equipment for, 881–892
 evaluation, 890
 hand-off reporting in, 893
 home care in, 893
 implementation, 884
 insertion and dressing care, 881–882
 interprofessional collaboration for, 881
 in older adults, 893
 patient education in, 893
 planning, 883
 site care and dressing change, 882, 882f
Central venous catheter
 blood specimen collection from, 212, 212f, 213f
 triple-lumen, 212f
Cephalic vein, 852f
Cerebrospinal fluid (CSF), 240
Cervical cancer, 159
Cervical spine, range-of-motion in, exercise for,
  333–336t
Chain of infection, 261, 261f, 261t
Charting by exception (CBE), 61
Cheilitis, 529
Chemical dot single-use thermometer, 74b, 74f
Chemical exposure, patient care after, 430–434,
  431f, 431t
 assessment, 431
 delegation in, 431
 documentation in, 434
 equipment for, 431–434
 evaluation, 433
 hand-off reporting in, 434
 home care and, 434
 implementation, 432
 interprofessional collaboration of, 431
 in older adults, 434

Chemical exposure, patient care after (Continued)
 patient education in, 434
 in pediatrics, 434
 planning, 432
 in populations with disabilities, 434
Chemical injuries, to eye, 570
Chemical name, 587
Chemical phlebitis, 859
Chemical safety, 405–406b, 406b, 407f
Chemical warfare agents, 431t
Chemotherapy medications, handling, 594, 595f
Chest
 excursion of, 138
 landmarks of, 132–133, 132f
Chest cavity, 799
Chest compressions, 833t
Chest tubes, 800
 drainage. see also Closed chest drainage systems
  autotransfusion of, 817–819
  measurement of, 172f
 insertion of, 804, 805
 mediastinal, 800–801, 801f
 milking of, 802
 placement, 800, 801f
 removal of, 813–816
 solving problems related to, 810t
 stripping of, 802
Cheyne-Stokes respiration, 94b
CHG. see Chlorhexidine gluconate
Children. see Pediatric patients
Chin-down position, 935
Chlorhexidine, 853f
Chlorhexidine gluconate (CHG), bathing, 521,
  525b, 536–538b, 537f
Cholecystitis, 151–152t
Chronic lung disease, home oxygen therapy
  for, 1237t
Chronic obstructive pulmonary disease (COPD),
  oxygen therapy for, 720, 730, 734
Chronic pain, definition of, 444
Circular turn, of bandage, 1188f, 1188t
Circulating nurse, 1095, 1096b
Circulatory overload, 898–899t
Circulatory system, assessment of, 140
CLABSI. see Central line-associated bloodstream
  infections
Clarification, 20b
Clean intermittent self-catheterization
  (CISC), 1232
Clean-voided urine specimen, 180
Clear-liquid diet, 926t
Clinical decision making, 2–3, 4f, 6–7, 7b
Clinical information system (CIS), 53b, 56
Clinical judgment
 defined, 2–3
 evaluation of, 13–14
 in nursing practice, 2–3
Clinical judgment model, 3, 3f
Closed chest drainage systems, 799–820
 autotransfusion of chest tube drainage, 817–819
 disposable systems, 801
 evidence-based practice for, 802
 managing of, 803–812, 807f, 808f, 810t
  assessment, 805
  in children, 812
  documentation in, 812
  dry suction water-seal systems, 803f,
   804–812, 804t
  evaluation, 811
  hand-off reporting in, 812
  home care in, 812
  implementation, 806
  in older adults, 812
  patient education in, 812
  planning, 806
  in populations with disabilities, 812
  wet suction water-seal systems, 803–804, 804t
 person-centered care for, 802
 Pleur-evac, 807f, 810t

Closed chest drainage systems (*Continued*)
  practice standards for, 799
  principles for practice of, 799–802, 800f
  purpose of, 799
  removal of chest tubes, 813–816
  safety guidelines for, 802–803
  supplemental standards for, 799
Closed gloving, 1102–1105, 1103f, 1104f
Closed (in-line) suction, 769–770b, 769f
Closed-system transfer device, 595f
Clostridium botulinum toxin, 425–426t
Clostridium difficile infection, 267
CMV. *see* Continuous mandatory ventilation
Code team, 830
Cognitive deficits
  communication with patients with, 31
  home setting for, 1209–1216, 1213f, 1214f
    assessment for, 1210
    in children, 1216
    client education in, 1215
    delegation in, 1210
    documentation in, 1215
    equipment for, 1210–1215
    evaluation in, 1215
    implementation in, 1212
    interprofessional collaboration in, 1210
    in older adults, 1216
    planning in, 1212
    reporting in, 1215
  older adults with, 30
Cold application, 483t, 489–493
  assessment, 490
  delegation in, 489
  documentation in, 493
  equipment for, 489–492
  evaluation, 492
  hand-off reporting in, 493
  home care and, 493
  implementation, 491
  interprofessional collaboration of, 489
  in older adults, 493
  for pain, 483t, 489
  patient education in, 493
  in pediatrics, 493
  planning, 490
  in populations with disabilities, 493
Collagen, 1111
Colleagues, meeting with, in clinical judgment, 14
Colonoscopy, 250, 251f
Colorectal cancer, 160
Colostomy
  pouching, 1039f, 1040–1050, 1041f, 1044f
  sigmoid, 1039f
Comatose patients, eye care for, 566–567b
Combing, hair, 547–550b, 549f
Communication
  assistive personnel, 21
  barriers to, 19
  with cognitively impaired patients, 31–33
    assessment of, 31
    in children, 33
    delegation in, 31
    in disabled patients, 33
    documentation in, 33
    evaluation, 32
    hand-off reporting in, 33
    home care, 33
    implementation, 32
    interprofessional collaboration, 31–33
    in older adults, 33
    patient education, 33
    planning, 32
  with colleagues, 33–35
    assessment of, 34
    delegation in, 34
    evaluation, 35
    implementation, 34
    interprofessional collaboration, 34–35
    planning, 34

Communication (*Continued*)
  definition of, 17, 18f
  in discharge planning, 48
  empathy in, 21
  evidence-based practice and, 19
  for home care safety, 1199
  nonverbal, 17–18
  nurse-patient relationship in, 20–25
    assessment, 21, 22f
    in children, 25
    delegation in, 21
    in disabled patients, 25
    documentation in, 25
    evaluation, 24
    hand-off reporting in, 25
    in home care, 25
    implementation, 23
    interprofessional collaboration, 21–25
    in older adults, 25
    planning, 23
  with patients who have difficulty coping,
      26–30
    assessment of, 26
    in children, 30
    delegation in, 26
    in disabled patients, 30
    documentation in, 30
    evaluation, 29
    hand-off reporting in, 30
    home care in, 30
    implementation, 28
    interprofessional collaboration, 26–30
    in older adults, 30
    patient education, 30
    planning, 27
  person-centered care, 18–19, 18b, 19f
  planning, 27
  practice standards, 17
  principles for practice, 17–18
  purpose, 17
  safety guidelines for, 19
  supplemental standards, 17
  therapeutic, 17, 18, 20b, 22f
Competencies, in critical thinking, 4–7
Complete blood count (CBC), 92
Complete Geriatric Depression Scale Short Form
      (GDS-SF), 1211
Completely-in-canal (CIC) aids, 577f, 577t
Complex critical thinking, 8
Complicated grief, 500–501
Compressed oxygen system, 1239
Computerized provider order entry (CPOE), 53b,
      63, 593
Concentrator safety, 1238b
Condom-type external catheter, 1008, 1010f
Confidence, 10, 11t
Confidentiality, 55–56
Conscious sedation, 1080t
ConstaVac drainage system, 1128
Constipation, 151–152t
  causes of, 1019b
  functional, 1022
Contact dermatitis, 522–523t, 523f
Contact lenses, care of, 567–569b, 569f
Contact precautions, 268t
Continent urinary diversion, 1039f
Continuous epidural infusion (CEI), 473
Continuous IV infusion, 871
Continuous mandatory ventilation
      (CMV), 742t
Continuous oxygen, 1237t
Continuous positive airway pressure (CPAP), 734,
      734f, 742t
Continuous subcutaneous infusion (CSQI),
      705–711, 705b, 705f, 708f, 710b
  assessment, 706
  in children, 710
  delegation in, 706
  documentation in, 710

Continuous subcutaneous infusion (*Continued*)
  equipment for, 706–710
  evaluation, 709
  hand-off reporting in, 710
  home care in, 711
  implementation, 707
  interprofessional collaboration, 706
  in older adults, 710
  patient education in, 710
  planning, 707
  in populations with disabilities, 710
Continuous suture, 1122f, 1126
Contrast media studies, 234–240
  assessment of, 235
  in children, 239
  delegation in, 234–235
  in disabled patients, 239
  documentation in, 239
  equipment for, 235
  evaluation of, 238
  hand-off reporting in, 239
  home care in, 240
  implementation of, 237
  interprofessional collaboration of, 235
  in older adults, 239
  patient education in, 239
  planning of, 236
Controlled coughing, 1070, 1070f
Controlled release medication, 588t
Controlled substance, 613
Controlled Substances Act, 603
Convalescent phase (Phase III) recovery,
      1087–1093, 1091f
Corns, 551–552t, 551f
Coronavirus disease (COVID-19), 419b, 422
  applying masks during, 279
Costal angle, 138
"Cough hygiene practices," 263
Coughing, controlled, 1070, 1070f
COVID-19. *see* Coronavirus disease
CPR. *see* Cardiopulmonary resuscitation
Crab lice, 547–548t
Crackles, 133, 133–134t
Cranial nerves, assessment of, 162–163
CRBSI. *see* Catheter-related bloodstream
      infection
Creativity, 11t, 12
Critical pathways, 60–61, 60f
Critical thinking, 3–4
  attitudes, 10–12, 11t
    confidence, 10, 11t
    creativity, 11t, 12
    curiosity, 11t, 12
    discipline, 11t, 12
    fairness, 11, 11t
    humility and self-awareness, 11t, 12
    integrity, 11t, 12
    perseverance, 11t, 12
    responsibility and accountability, 11, 11t
    risk taking, 11–12, 11t
    thinking independently, 10–11, 11t
  basic, 7
  clinical decision making, 6–7
  commitment, 8
  competencies, 4–7
  complex, 8
  components of, 8–13
    competence, 8
    environment, 10
    experience, 10
    knowledge base, 8–10
    standards for, 12–13
  diagnostic reasoning, 5–6
  evolving case study, 3–4
  general, 4–5
  levels of, 7–8, 8b
  standards for, 12–13
  synthesis, 14, 14f
Crohn disease, 151–152t

Crutches
  ascending stairs with, 352, 352f
  descending stairs with, 353, 353f
  use of, 345–355, 346t, 347f
    assessment in, 347
    in children, 355
    delegation in, 347
    documentation in, 355
    equipment for, 347
    evaluation, 354
    hand-off reporting in, 355
    home care and, 355
    implementation, 348, 350f, 351f, 352f, 353f
    interprofessional collaboration of, 347
    in older adults, 355
    patient education in, 355
    planning in, 347
    in populations with disabilities, 355
Cryoprecipitate, 900t
Culture
  blood, 212
  nose and throat specimens, 192–196, 194f, 195f
Culture and sensitivity
  of sputum specimens, 199
  of urine, 180
Curiosity, 11t, 12
CVAD. see Central vascular access devices

D
Dandruff, 547–548t
Databases, patient, 61
Death, body after, care of, 510–513
  assessment, 510
  delegation in, 510
  documentation in, 513
  equipment for, 510
  evaluation, 513
  home care and, 513, 514t
  implementation, 511, 513f
  interprofessional collaboration of, 510
  in older adults, 513
  in pediatrics, 513
  planning, 511
Debridement, 1113
Decision making, critical thinking and, 5
Deconditioning, 325
Deep breathing, progressive relaxation with, 457
Deep palpation, 113, 114f
Deep sedation, 229, 232t
Deep tendon reflexes, assessment of, 169
Deep vein thrombosis (DVT), risk factors for, 337b
Deep-breathing exercise, 1068f
De-escalation, of anger, 26
Defibrillation
  automated external defibrillator for, 827, 833t
  pad placement for, 835f
Delayed primary intention, 1112
Deltoid muscle, 687, 688f
Demand pulsing oxygen-delivery systems, 1236
Dementia, 118b, 1209–1210
Dental caries, 529
Dental diet, 926t
Dentin, 524, 524f
Dentures, 129
  care of, 542–543b, 543f
Depression
  communication in patients with, 31
  definition of, 26
  interprofessional collaboration, 26–30
  in pediatric patients, 30
  from social isolation, 1209
  symptoms of, 26b
Dermis, 1111, 1111f
Dermoepidermal junction, 1111, 1111f
Descending stairs, with crutches, 353, 353f
Dextrose
  in saline solutions, 843t
  in water solutions, 843t
Diabetic diet, 926t

Diagnostic procedures, 227–258
  arteriogram, 234–240, 234f
  aspiration, 240–243
  bone marrow aspiration/biopsy, 240–246, 241–242t, 242f
  bronchoscopy, 246–250, 247f
  cardiac catheterization, 234–240, 234f
  contrast media studies, 234–240
  evidence-based practice, 228
  intravenous moderate sedation, 229–233
  intravenous pyelogram, 234–240
  lumbar puncture, 240–246, 241–242t
  paracentesis, 240–246, 241–242t
  person-centered care, 228
  practice standards in, 227
  principles for practice, 227–228, 228b
  purpose of, 227
  safety guidelines, 228–229
  supplemental standards, 227
  thoracentesis, 240–246, 241–242t
  undergoing endoscopy, 250–254
Diagnostic reasoning, 5–6
Diaphoresis, 373
Diastolic pressure, 95
Dietary guidelines, 925
Dietary Guidelines for Americans, 917
Diets, 926t
Digital hearing aid, 578
Dimensional analysis method, 601–602, 601b
Disabilities, populations with
  abdominal assessment in, 157
  administering enema in, 1029
  applying physical restraints in, 405
  arterial blood gas measurements in, 225
  artificial airway in, 768
  aspiration precautions in, 937
  aspiration procedures in, 246
  assist devices and, 355
  assisting adults with oral nutrition in, 931
  blood pressure and pulse measurement in, 1232
  body temperature measurements in, 1227
  bronchoscopy in, 250
  canes in, 355
  cardiac monitor in, 797
  closed chest drainage systems in, 812
  cold application in, 493
  complete or partial bed bath in, 534
  continuous subcutaneous infusion in, 710
  contrast media studies in, 239
  crutches in, 355
  dry dressing in, 1175
  ear medications in, 638
  end-of-life care in, 509
  fall prevention in, 393–394
  feeding tubes in
    administration of, 623
    management of, 1257
  gastrointestinal endoscopy, 254
  general survey for, 126
  head and neck assessment in, 132
  home environment assessment and safety in, 1209
  home oxygen therapy in, 1242
  incontinence device in, 1012
  intermittent self-catheterization in, 1236
  intradermal injections in, 677
  intramuscular injections in, 692
  intravenous moderate sedation, 233
  intravenous push in, 698
  medication self-administration, 1253
  metered-dose inhalers in, 649
  moist and dry heat applications in, 489
  mouth care in, 547
  musculoskeletal assessment in, 170–172
  nail and foot care in, 556
  nasal instillations in, 642
  nasotracheal/pharyngeal suctioning in, 768
  noninvasive positive pressure ventilation, 739
  nonpharmacological pain management in, 460

Disabilities, populations with (*Continued*)
  nose and throat specimens from, 196
  nurse-patient relationship in, 25
  nutrition screening in, 925
  ophthalmic medications in, 634
  oral hygiene in, 542
  oral medications in, 618
  oropharyngeal suctioning in, 759
  oxygen therapy, 727
  pain assessment in, 453
  parenteral nutrition in, 1260
  patient care for
    after biological exposure, 429
    after chemical exposure, 434
    after natural disaster, 441
    after radiation exposure, 438
  peripheral intravenous device, 861
  pharmacological pain management in, 466
  piggyback infusion in, 705
  pouching a urostomy in, 1050
  pressure bandage in, 1178
  promoting early activity and exercise and, 331
  small-bore feeding tube in, 949
  small-volume nebulizers in, 653
  special beds and, 377
  subcutaneous injections in, 685
  support surfaces and, 373
  supporting patients and families in grief, 504
  symptom management at end of life in, 509
  syringe pumps in, 705
  tracheostomy care and suctioning in, 1248
  transferring, 311
  urine specimen collection in, 185
  vaginal or urethral discharge specimens in, 199
  walkers in, 355
  wound irrigation in, 1122
Disaster
  definitions and types of, 418b
  potential hazards at the scene of, 423b
Disaster preparedness, 417–442
  evidence-based practice of, 422
  person-centered care of, 421–422
  practice standards of, 417
  principles for practice, 418–420, 418b, 419b, 419f, 420f
  purpose of, 417
  safety guidelines for, 422–424, 422b, 423b, 423f
  supplemental standards of, 417
  triage categories, 421, 421b
Discharge planning, 40–51
  admitting process, 42–45
  assessment, 44–45
  communication in, 48
  day of discharge, 48–49, 49b
  evidence-based practice of, 41
  goal of, 47
  nurse role, 48
  pediatric patients, 49
  person-centered care of, 41
  practice standards, 40
  principles for practice, 40–41
  purpose of, 40
  safety guidelines of, 41
  special considerations for, 45, 49–50
  supplemental standards, 40
Discharge process, 47–50, 47b
Discharge summaries, 61, 61b
Discipline, 11t, 12
Disinfecting supplies, 1246
Disposable bed bath, 525b
Disposable closed chest drainage systems, 801, 801f, 808f
Disposable injection units, 664, 664f
Disposable washcloths, 536–538b, 537f
Distraction, 453, 458
Disuse syndrome, 324
"Do not resuscitate" (DNR) status, 499

Documentation, 52–68
  abbreviations used in, 52
  in abdominal assessment, 157
  accuracy of, 57
  in administering enema, 1028
  adverse event reporting, 63–64, 64b
  in adverse transfusion reactions, 911
  in arterial blood gas measurements, 224
  in artificial airway, 768
  in aspiration precautions, 936
  in assisting adults with oral nutrition, 930
  in automated external defibrillator, 830
  in autotransfusion of chest tube drainage, 819
  in biological exposure, patient care after, 429
  in blood glucose monitoring, 219
  in blood pressure measurement, 103, 1232
  in blood specimen collection, 214
  in blood transfusion, 907
  in body temperature measurement, 81, 1227
  in bronchoscopy, 250
  in cardiac monitor, 797
  in cardiovascular assessment, 150
  in central parenteral nutrition, 974
  in central vascular access devices (CVAD),
      892–893
  charting by exception, 61
  in chemical exposure, patient care after, 434
  in closed chest drainage systems, 812
  in cold application, 493
  in communication
      with cognitively impaired patients, 33
      with patients who have difficulty coping, 30
  complete, 57, 57t
  computerized, 53f
  concise, 57
  confidentiality, 55–56
  in continuous subcutaneous infusion, 710
  in contrast media studies, 239
  current, 57–58
  in dry dressing application, 1174
  in dysphagia, 936
  in ear irrigation, 576
  in ear medications, 638
  electronic health records for, 45, 52, 53b, 58–61
  in end-of-life care, 509
  in epidural analgesia, 478
  evidence-based practice for, 55, 55b
  in eye irrigation, 573
  factual, 57
  in fall prevention, 393
  in feeding tubes, 953, 1256
  in foam dressing application, 1187
  format, 61–62
  in gastrointestinal endoscopy, 254
  in general survey, 125
  in genitalia assessment, 162
  hand-off reports, 54, 62–63b
  in head and neck assessment, 131
  in hearing aids care, 580
  in heat applications, 488
  high-quality, 57–58
  home care, 64, 65b
  in home environment assessment and
      safety, 1209
  in home oxygen therapy, 1242
  in home setting for cognitive deficits, 1215
  in hydrocolloid dressing application, 1187
  in hydrogel dressing application, 1187
  in immobilization devices, 359
  in incentive spirometry, 734
  in incontinence device, 1012
  in indwelling urinary catheter, 997
  in intermittent self-catheterization, 1235
  in intradermal injections, 677
  in intramuscular injections, 691
  in intravenous flow rates, 866
  in intravenous moderate sedation, 233
  in intravenous push, 698
  in intravenous solutions, 870

Documentation (Continued)
  in isolation precautions, 274
  legal guidelines for, 56–57, 56t
  in local anesthetic infusion pump, 482
  in long-term health care, 65
  in mechanical ventilation, 750
  in medical device safety, 1220
  in medication and medical device safety, 1220
  in medication self-administration, 1252
  in metered-dose inhalers (MDI), 648
  methods of, 58
  in mouth care, 547
  in musculoskeletal assessment, 170
  in nail and foot care, 556
  narrative, 61
  in nasal instillations, 642
  in negative-pressure wound therapy, 1138
  in nonpharmacological pain management, 459
  in nose and throat specimen collection, 196
  in nurse-patient relationship, 25
  in nutrition screening, 924
  occult blood
      in gastric secretions, 192
      in stool specimen, 189
  in ophthalmic medications, 634
  in oral hygiene, 542
  in oral medications, 617
  in oral nutrition, 924
  in pain assessment, 451
  in parenteral nutrition, 974, 1260
  in patient-controlled analgesia, 471
  in peripheral intravenous device, 860
  person-centered care, 54–55, 54f
  in pharmacological pain management, 466
  in physical restraints, 405
  in piggyback infusion, 704
  plan of care, 62
  in positioning patients, 321
  practice standards, 52
  in pressure bandage, 1178
  principles for practice, 53–54, 54b
  problem-oriented medical records, 61–62
  progress notes, 62
  in pulse measurement, 1232
  purpose, 52
  in radiation exposure, patient care after, 437
  in restraint-free environment, 398
  in resuscitation management, 837
  safety guidelines, 55
  SBAR, 62
  in seizure precautions, 413
  in small-volume nebulizers, 653
  in special beds, 377
  in sputum specimens, 203
  in staple removal, 1127
  in sterile field preparation, 287
  in sterile gloving, 291
  in subcutaneous injections, 685
  supplemental standards, 53
  in support surfaces, 372
  in suprapubic catheter care, 1016
  in surgical hand antisepsis, 1101
  in suture removal, 1127
  in syringe pumps, 704
  in thorax and lung assessment, 139
  in topical medications, 628
  in tracheostomy care and suctioning, 1247
  in transferring patients, 311
  in transparent dressing, 1181
  in 12-lead electrocardiogram, 794
  in urine specimen collection, 185
  in vaginal or urethral discharge specimens, 198
  in workplace violence and safety, 38
  in wound drainage, 206, 1132
  in wound irrigation, 1122
Doppler instrument, for pulse palpation, 149, 149f
Doppler ultrasonic stethoscope, 102f
Dorsal metacarpal vein, 852f
Dorsal recumbent position, 116t

Dorsalis pedis pulse, 82t, 148, 148f
Douche, 653, 655
DPI. see Dry powder inhaler
Drainage
  sterile, 989, 989f
  wound, 1128–1132, 1128f
      assessment, 1129–1132
      in children, 1132
      closed-drain system in, 1128
      delegation in, 1128
      documentation in, 1132
      equipment for, 1128
      evaluation, 1132
      hand-off reporting in, 1132
      Hemovac drain, 1130f
      home care in, 1132
      implementation, 1129
      Jackson-Pratt drain in, 1131f
      measurement of, 172f
      in older adults, 1132
      open-drain system in, 1128
      patient education in, 1132
      in pediatrics, 1132
      Penrose drain in, 1128, 1128f, 1169f
      planning, 1129
      types of, 1165b
Drapes, sterile, 282
  in female, 992f
  in male, 992f
  preparation of, 285, 285f
Dressings, 1162–1196
  alginate, 1163–1164t
      application of, 1181–1192, 1186f
  category of, 1163–1164t
  characteristics of, 1163b
  disposal of, 1170f
  dry and moist, 1166–1175, 1167f, 1168f, 1169f,
      1170f
  evidence-based practice, 1165–1166
  foam, 1163–1164t, 1181–1192
  gauze, 1163–1164t, 1187–1190b
  hydrocolloid, 1163–1164t
      application of, 1181–1192, 1183f, 1185f
  hydrogel, 1163–1164t
      application of, 1181–1192, 1185f
  moist, 1166–1175, 1167f, 1168f, 1169f, 1170f,
      1171f, 1172f, 1173f
  outcomes of, 1163b
  person-centered care in, 1165
  practice standards in, 1162
  principles for practice in, 1162–1164
  problems associated with, 1174t
  purpose of, 1162
  safety guidelines for, 1165b, 1166
  secure, 1172f, 1173f
  selection of, 1163
  transparent, 1163–1164t
      application of, 1178–1181, 1180f
Droplet precautions, 268t
Dry dressing, application of, 1166–1175, 1167f,
      1168f, 1169f, 1170f, 1171f, 1172f, 1173f
  assessment, 1167
  in children, 1175
  delegation in, 1166
  documentation in, 1174
  equipment for, 1167–1174
  evaluation, 1173
  hand-off reporting in, 1174
  home care in, 1175
  implementation, 1168
  in older adults, 1175
  patient education in, 1175
  in pediatrics, 1175
  planning, 1168
  in populations with disabilities, 1175
Dry powder inhaler (DPI), 643f
  placement of, 647f
Dry skin, 522–523t, 522f
Dry suction water-seal systems, 803f, 804–812, 804t

Dual sensory impairment (DSI), 566
Duodenal ulcer, 151–152t
Durable medical equipment (DME), 1237
DVT. *see* Deep vein thrombosis
Dysphagia
 causes of, 932b
 in children, 937
 diet for, 932, 933t
 documentation in, 936
 equipment for, 933–936
 in home care, 937
 interprofessional collaboration in, 933
 management of, 932
 in older adults, 937
 referral criteria for, 932b
 symptoms of, 931

E

Ear(s). *see also* Hearing aids
 care of, 565–584
  for comatose patients, 566–567b
  evidence-based practice, 566
  person-centered care, 565–566
  practice standards, 565
  principles for practice, 565
  purpose of, 565
  safety guidelines of, 566–569
 irrigation, 573–576
  assessment in, 574
  in children, 576
  delegation in, 573
  documentation in, 576
  equipment for, 573–576
  evaluation in, 576
  hand-off reporting in, 576
  in home care, 576
  implementation in, 575, 575f
  interprofessional collaboration in, 573
  patient education in, 576
  planning in, 574
 medications, 635–638, 637f
  assessment, 635
  in children, 638
  delegation in, 635
  documentation in, 638
  equipment for, 635
  evaluation, 637
  hand-off reporting in, 638
  implementation, 636
  interprofessional collaboration for,
   635–638
  planning, 636
  in populations with disabilities, 638
Eardrops, 635
Early activity, promotion of, 326–345
Ebola virus disease (EVD), 418b
Eccrine glands, 522
ECG. *see* Electrocardiogram
Eczema, 590t
Effleurage, 455, 455f
Egg-crate foam overlay, 368, 369f
Elastic bandages
 application of, 1187–1190b, 1189f
 on midthigh amputation stump, 1190f
 secure, 1189f
Elastic stockings. *see* Graduated compression
   stockings
Elbow, range-of-motion in
 assessment of, 167t
 exercise for, 332t, 333–336t
Elbow restraint, 401, 401f
Elder abuse, 121
Electrical safety, 405–406b, 406b, 407f, 1204
Electrocardiogram (ECG), 12-lead,
   791–794, 793f
 assessment, 791
 in children, 794
 delegation in, 791
 documentation in, 794

Electrocardiogram (*Continued*)
 equipment for, 791–793
 evaluation, 793
 hand-off reporting in, 794
 home care in, 794
 implementation, 792
 interprofessional collaboration of, 791
 lead placement for, 793f, 796f
 in older adults, 794
 patient education in, 794
 planning, 792
Electronic health records (EHR), 45, 52, 53b,
   58–61
 discharge summaries, 61, 61b
 flow sheets, 58–59
 graphic records, 58–59, 59f
 nursing history, admission, 58
 patient care summary, 59
 patient education record, 59
 standardized care plans, 60
Electronic infusion device (EID), in blood
   transfusion, 905
Electronic thermometer, 74b
Elixir, 588t
Emergency Medical Treatment and Labor Act
   (EMTALA), 46
Emergency resuscitation cart, 831f
Empathy, 21
Enamel, 524, 524f
End-of-life care, 498–518
 evidence-based practice of, 500
 person-centered care of, 499
 practice standards of, 498
 principles for practice, 498–499
 purpose of, 498, 499b, 499f
 safety guidelines for, 500
 symptom management at, 504–509, 504f
  assessment of, 504
  delegation in, 504
  documentation in, 509
  equipment for, 504–509
  evaluation, 508
  hand-off reporting in, 509
  home care and, 509
  implementation, 506
  interprofessional collaboration of, 504
  in older adults, 509
  patient education in, 509
  in pediatrics, 509
  planning, 506
  in populations with disabilities, 509
Endometrial cancer, 159
Endoscopic retrograde cholangiopancreatography
   (ERCP), 250
Endoscopy, gastrointestinal, 250–254
 assessment of, 251
 in children, 254
 delegation in, 250
 in disabled patients, 254
 documentation in, 254
 equipment, 251–254
 evaluation of, 253
 hand-off reporting in, 254
 home care in, 254
 implementation of, 252
 interprofessional collaboration of, 251
 in older adults, 254
 patient education in, 254
 planning of, 252
Endotracheal tube, 770–777, 771f, 775b, 776f
 assessment, 772
 in children, 777
 evaluation, 776
 implementation, 773
 in older adults, 777
 patient education in, 777
 planning, 773
Endotracheal (ET) tube, 720, 727, 742–743
End-tidal CO$_2$ detector, 771, 771f

Enema
 administering, 1024–1029, 1025f, 1027f
  assessment, 1025
  delegation in, 1024
  documentation in, 1028
  equipment for, 1024–1028
  hand-off reporting in, 1028
  implementation, 1026, 1028
  in older adults, 1029
  in pediatrics, 1028
  planning, 1025
  in populations with disabilities, 1029
 medicated, 1024
 oil-retention, 1024
 types of, 1024t
Enema bag, 1025
ENFit connection system, 618f
Enteral connector, 618f
Enteral nutrition, 940–965
 administering, 955–963, 957f, 959f, 960f
 combination tubes for, 962, 962f
 definition of, 940
 evidence-based practice, 941
 feeding tubes, 940
  delegation in, 950
  dislocation of, 949–950
  documentation in, 953
  equipment for, 950–952
  gastric aspirate obtained using, 949f, 952f
  hand-off reporting in, 953
  home care in, 953
  home care teaching, 1253
  interprofessional collaboration in, 950
  irrigating, 953–955
  nasointestinal, 955–963
  in older adults, 953
  patient education, 953
  in pediatrics, 953
  safety guidelines, 941
  verifying placement of, 949–953
 gastrostomy tube for
  care of, 962–963b, 962f
  percutaneous endoscopic, 962, 962f
  technique, 955–963
 home care in, 961–963, 1253
 intermittent feeding, 958f
 jejunostomy tube for
  care of, 962–963b
  endoscopic insertion of, 963f
  technique, 955–963
 in older adults, 961
 patient education, 961
 person-centered care, 941
 technique, 955–963, 957f, 959f, 960f
Enteric-coated medications, 588t
Environment, 41
Environmental factors, in critical thinking, 10
Enzymatic debridement, 1113
Epidermis, 522, 1111, 1111f
Epidural analgesia, 445–446, 472–479, 472f, 473f
 assessment, 474
 delegation in, 473
 documentation in, 478
 equipment for, 473–478
 evaluation, 477
 hand-off reporting in, 478
 home care and, 478–479
 implementation, 475
 interprofessional collaboration of, 473
 in older adults, 478
 patient education in, 478
 in pediatrics, 478
 planning, 475
Epidural anesthesia, 1080t
Epidural space, 472, 472f, 473f
EPUAP. *see* European Pressure Ulcer Advisory
   Panel
Erb's point, 143
Errorless teaching and learning (ETL), 1223

Eschar, 1112t
Esophagogastroduodenoscopy (EGD), 250
European Pressure Ulcer Advisory Panel
　(EPUAP), 524–525
EVD. *see* Ebola virus disease
Evidence-based practice (EBP)
　admitting process, 41
　airway management, 754
　blood transfusion, 897–898
　bowel elimination, 1019
　cardiac care, 789–790
　catheterization, 985
　closed chest drainage systems, 802
　communication and, 19
　in critical thinking, 8–9, 9t
　diagnostic procedures, 228
　disaster preparedness, 422
　discharge planning, 41
　documentation in, 55, 55b
　dressings, 1165–1166
　end-of-life care, 500
　enteral nutrition, 941
　exercise, 325–326
　eye care, 566
　health assessment, 111–112
　home care safety, 1199
　home care teaching, 1223
　intraoperative care, 1097
　life support, 823–824
　medical asepsis, 262
　nonparenteral medications, 609
　oral nutrition, 918–919
　ostomy care, 1040
　pain assessment, 445
　for parenteral medications, 660
　parenteral nutrition, 968
　patient safety, 383–384
　personal hygiene, 521
　postoperative care, 1060
　preoperative care, 1060
　pressure injuries, 1145–1146
　safe medication preparation, 603
　safe patient handling and mobility (SPHM),
　　297–298
　specimen collection, 179
　sterile technique, 278
　support surfaces, 365
　transfer process, 41
　urinary elimination, 985
　vital signs, 71
　wound care and irrigation, 1113–1114
Evisceration, of wound, 1114
Exercise, 324–361
　early, promotion of, 326–345
　　assessment in, 327
　　in children, 331
　　delegation in, 326–327
　　documentation in, 331
　　equipment for, 327
　　evaluation, 330
　　hand-off reporting in, 331
　　home care and, 331–345
　　implementation, 329
　　interprofessional collaboration of, 327
　　in older adults, 331
　　patient education in, 331
　　planning, 328
　　in populations with disabilities, 331
　evidence-based practice of, 325–326
　person-centered care in, 325
　practice standards of, 325
　principles for, 325
　purpose of, 324–325
　range-of-motion
　　activities of daily living incorporation of, 332t
　　delegation in, 332
　　equipment for, 332
　　interprofessional collaboration of, 332
　　performing, 331–337b

Exercise (*Continued*)
　　step of, 332–337, 333–336t
　　support during, 333f
　safety guidelines for, 326
Exhaled minute ventilation (VE), 743t
Expectoration, sputum collection by, 199b
Experience
　in clinical decision making, 6
　in critical thinking, 10
Expiration, 91, 91f
External tunneled catheter, 880t, 881f
Extract, 588t
Extravasation, 891–892t
Extremity (ankle or wrist) restraint, soft, 402, 402f
Eye(s)
　assessment of, 127
　care of, 565–584
　　evidence-based practice, 566
　　person-centered care, 565–566
　　practice standards, 565
　　principles for practice, 565
　　purpose of, 565
　　safety guidelines of, 566–569
　irrigation, 570–573
　　assessment in, 570
　　in children, 573
　　delegation in, 570
　　documentation in, 573
　　equipment for, 570–573
　　evaluation in, 572
　　hand-off reporting in, 573
　　in home care, 573
　　implementation in, 571, 572f, 577f
　　interprofessional collaboration in, 570
　　patient education in, 573
　　planning in, 571
Eyedrops, 631, 634
Eyewear, applying and removing, 279–282, 280f

F

Facial nerve, 168
Fairness, 11, 11t
Fall(s)
　in older adults, 1199
　prevention of, 383–384
　　assessment, 386, 388f
　　delegation in, 386
　　documentation in, 393
　　equipment for, 386–393
　　evaluation, 392
　　hand-off reporting in, 393
　　in health care settings, 384–394, 385t
　　home care and, 394
　　in home environment, 1205, 1206f
　　implementation, 389, 389f, 390f
　　in older adults, 393
　　patient education in, 393
　　in pediatrics, 393
　　planning, 388
　　in populations with disabilities, 393–394
　　wheelchair for, 391, 392f
Fall/near-fall diary, 1201b
Fat-modified diet, 926t
Fecal impaction
　Bristol Stool Form Scale, 1023f
　removal, 1022–1024b, 1023b, 1023f
　symptoms of, 1022
Feeding tubes
　administering medications through, 618–623
　　assessment, 619
　　in children, 623
　　delegation in, 618
　　documentation in, 623
　　equipment for, 618–622
　　evaluation, 622
　　hand-off reporting in, 623
　　implementation, 620
　　interprofessional collaboration for, 618
　　in older adults, 623

Feeding tubes (*Continued*)
　　patient education in, 623
　　planning, 620
　　in populations with disabilities, 623
　blocked, 623b
　definition of, 940
　dislocation of, 949–950
　documentation in, 953
　gastric aspirate obtained using, 949f, 952f
　gastrostomy
　　care of, 962–963b, 962f
　　percutaneous endoscopic, 962, 962f
　　technique, 955–963
　hand-off reporting in, 953
　home care in, 953
　home care teaching, 1253–1257
　irrigating, 953–955
　jejunostomy
　　care of, 962–963b
　　endoscopic insertion of, 963f
　　technique, 955–963
　nasogastric. *see* Nasogastric feeding tubes
　nasointestinal, 955–963
　in older adults, 953
　patient education, 953
　in pediatrics, 953
　safety guidelines, 941
　verifying placement of, 949–953
Female health teaching, 162
Female urinal, 986f
Femoral pulse, 82t, 149, 149f
Fentanyl, 473
Fingers, range-of-motion in, exercise for, 332t,
　333–336t
Fire extinguisher, 1207f, 1237
Fire safety, 405–406b, 406b, 407f, 1203, 1206,
　1207f, 1238b
Firearm safety, in home environment, 1208
Flat position, 557–558t, 558f
Flossing, of teeth, 538
Flotation pad, 368
Flow sheets, 58–59
Flow-oriented incentive spirometer, 730, 731f
Foam dressings, 1118t, 1163–1164t
　application of, 1181–1192
　　assessment, 1182
　　in children, 1187
　　delegation in, 1182
　　documentation in, 1187
　　equipment for, 1182–1187
　　evaluation, 1186
　　hand-off reporting in, 1187
　　implementation, 1183
　　interprofessional collaboration in, 1182
　　in older adults, 1187–1192
　　patient education in, 1187
　　in pediatrics, 1187
　　planning, 1183
Foam mattress, 368
Foam overlay, indications for, 363–364t
Food disaster supply kit, guidelines for, 430b
Food safety, 919b
Food safety tips, 919b
Foot
　care of, 551–562
　　assessment, 552
　　delegation in, 552
　　equipment for, 552–556
　　evaluation, 555
　　hand-off reporting in, 556
　　home care and, 556–562
　　implementation, 554, 555f
　　interprofessional collaboration of, 552
　　in older adults, 556
　　patient education in, 556
　　in pediatrics, 556
　　planning, 554
　　in populations with disabilities, 556
　　range-of-motion in, exercise for, 333–336t

Foot circles, 1072f
Foot odors, 551–552t
Forearm, range-of-motion in, exercise for, 333–336t
Forearm crutch, 346t, 347f
Formula method, 601, 601b
Four-point gait, 349, 350f
Fowler position, 316, 557–558t, 557f, 943
Fraction of inspired oxygen (FiO₂), 743t
Francisella tularensis, 425–426t
FRDs. *see* Friction-reducing devices
Freedom splint, 401, 401f
Fresh frozen plasma, 900t
Friction
    pain from, 456
    in pressure injuries, 1147, 1151, 1152
Friction-reducing devices (FRDs), for transferring
        patients, 298, 308f
Full-liquid diet, 926t
Full-thickness wounds, 1111b, 1113
Functional constipation, 1022

G

Gag reflex, 544
Gait
    assessment of, 165
    four-point, 349, 350f
    inspection of, 165
    swing-through, 350
    swing-to, 351, 351f
    three-point, 349, 351f
    two-point, 350, 351f
Gait belt, 342, 391
    for transferring patients, 303, 304f
Gamma rays, 434
Gastric aspirate, 949f, 952f
Gastric decompression, nasogastric tube for,
        1029–1036, 1031f, 1032f, 1033f, 1034f
    assessment, 1030
    in children, 1036
    documentation in, 1036
    equipment for, 1029–1036, 1029f
    evaluation, 1036
    hand-off reporting in, 1036
    implementation, 1030
    in older adults, 1036
    planning, 1030
    in populations with disabilities, 1036
Gastric distention, 735t
Gastric residual volume (GRV), 621, 941
Gastric secretions, occult blood measurements in,
        190–192, 191f
Gastric ulcer, 151–152t
Gastroccult testing, 190–192, 191f
Gastroenteritis, 151–152t
Gastrostomy tube
    care of, 962–963b, 962f
    percutaneous endoscopic, 962, 962f
    technique, 955–963
Gauze bandages, 1163–1164t
    application of, 1187–1190b
    on midthigh amputation stump, 1190f
Gauze dressing, 1118t
Gel overlay, indications for, 363–364t
General anesthesia, 1080t
General survey, 117–126
    assessment in, 117
    delegation in, 117
    in disabled patients, 126
    documentation in, 125
    equipment for, 117–125
    hand-off reporting in, 125
    home care, 126
    implementation in, 120
    interprofessional collaboration in, 117
    in older adults, 126
    patient education in, 125–126
    in pediatric patient, 126
    planning in, 119
Generic name, 587

Genitalia, assessment, 157–162
    in children, 162
    delegation in, 157
    documentation in, 162
    equipment for, 158–162
    evaluation in in, 161
    female, 158, 160
    hand-off reporting in, 162
    implementation in, 160
    interprofessional collaboration in, 158
    male, 159, 161
    in older adults, 162
    patient education in, 162
    in pediatric patient, 162
    planning in, 160
Gingivae, 524
Gingivitis, 529
Glossopharyngeal nerve, 168
Gloves
    applying and removing, 281, 281f
    clean, 270
    over gown sleeves, 270f
    removal of, 273f
Gloving
    closed, 1102–1105, 1103f, 1104f
    sterile, 287–291, 289f, 290f
Glucose
    blood. *see* Blood glucose monitoring
    urine screening for, 185–186b
Gown, sterile, 1102–1105, 1103f, 1104f
Grab bars, 1206f
Graduated compression (elastic) stockings,
        337–342b, 338f
    delegation in, 338
    equipment for, 338
    step of, 338–342, 339b, 339f, 340f, 341f
Granulation tissue, 1112
Graphic records, 58–59, 59f
Grief, supporting patients and families in,
        500–504
    assessment, 501
    delegation in, 501
    documentation in, 503
    evaluation, 503
    hand-off reporting in, 503
    home care and, 504
    implementation, 502
    interprofessional collaboration of, 501–503
    maternal-child health in, 503
    in older adults, 503–504
    patient education in, 503
    in pediatrics, 503
    planning, 502
    in populations with disabilities, 504
GRV. *see* Gastric residual volume
Guided imagery, of nonpharmacological pain
        management, 458
Gums, 524

H

Hair
    combing, 547–550b, 549f
    loss of, 547–548t
    personal hygiene of, 524
    problems of, 547–548t
    shampooing, 550b, 550f
    shaving, 547–550b, 549f
Hair follicle, 524, 524f
HAIs. *see* Health care-associated infections
Halitosis, 529
Hand(s)
    antisepsis, surgical, 1098–1101, 1099f, 1100f
    grasp strength, 165, 165f
    range of motion in, assessment of, 167t
Hand hygiene, 262, 263–266
    in aspiration precautions, 934
    in assisting adults with oral nutrition, 926
    in blood transfusion, 904
    factors affecting, 263

Hand hygiene *(Continued)*
    guidelines for, 263
    handwashing, 263
    home care in, 266
    in nutrition screening, 921
    in older adults, 266
    in parenteral nutrition, 1258
    patient education in, 266
    for sterile field, 283
Hand scrub, 1098
Hand-off reporting
    in abdominal assessment, 157
    in administering enema, 1028
    in alginate dressing application, 1187
    in apical pulse, 90
    in arterial blood gas measurements, 224
    in artificial airway, 768
    in aspiration precautions, 936
    in automated external defibrillator, 830
    in autotransfusion of chest tube drainage, 819
    in biological exposure, patient care after, 429
    in blood glucose monitoring, 219
    in blood pressure measurement, 103
    in blood specimen collection, 214
    in blood transfusion, 907
    in body temperature measurement, 81
    in bronchoscopy, 250
    in cardiac monitor, 797
    in cardiovascular assessment, 150
    in catheterizing a urinary diversion, 1052
    in central parenteral nutrition, 974
    in central vascular access devices, 893
    in chemical exposure, patient care after, 434
    in closed chest drainage systems, 812
    in cold application, 493
    in communication, 54, 62–63b
        with cognitively impaired patients, 33
        in nurse-patient relationship, 25
        with patients who have difficulty coping, 30
    in continuous subcutaneous infusion, 710
    in contrast media studies, 239
    in dry dressing application, 1174
    in ear irrigation, 576
    in ear medications, 638
    in electrocardiogram, 12-lead, 794
    in end-of-life care, 509
    in endotracheal tube care, 777
    in epidural analgesia, 478
    in eye irrigation, 573
    in fall prevention, 393
    in feeding tubes, 953
    in foam dressing application, 1187
    in gastrointestinal endoscopy, 254
    in general survey, 125
    in genitalia assessment, 162
    in head and neck assessment, 131
    in hearing aids, 580
    in heat applications, 488
    in home oxygen therapy, 1242
    in hydrocolloid dressing application, 1187
    in hydrogel dressing application, 1187
    in immobilization devices, 359
    in incentive spirometry, 734
    in incontinence device, 1012
    in indwelling urinary catheter, 997
    in intradermal injections, 677
    in intramuscular injections, 691
    in intravenous flow rates, 867
    in intravenous moderate sedation, 233
    in intravenous push, 698
    in intravenous solutions, 871
    in isolation precautions, 274
    in local anesthetic infusion pump, 482
    in mechanical ventilation, 750
    in metered-dose inhalers, 649
    in moist dressing, 1174
    in musculoskeletal assessment, 170
    in nail and foot care, 556
    in nasal instillations, 642

Hand-off reporting (*Continued*)
  in nasotracheal/pharyngeal suctioning, 768
  in natural disaster, patient care after, 440
  in negative-pressure wound therapy, 1138
  in noninvasive positive pressure ventilation, 739
  in nonpharmacological pain management, 459
  in nose and throat specimen collection, 196
  in nutrition screening, 924
  occult blood
    in gastric secretions, 192
    in stool specimen, 189
  in ophthalmic medications, 634
  in oral hygiene, 542
  in oral medications, 617
  in oropharyngeal airway, 827
  in oropharyngeal suctioning, 759
  in pain assessment, 451
  in patient-controlled analgesia (PCA), 471–472
  in peripheral intravenous device, 860
  in peripheral intravenous dressing, 878
  in pharmacological pain management, 466
  in physical restraints, 405
  in piggyback infusion, 704
  in positioning patients, 321
  in pouching a colostomy, or ileostomy, 1046
  in pouching a urostomy, 1050
  in pressure bandage application, 1178
  in radiation exposure, patient care after, 437
  in respiration assessment, 94
  in restraint-free environment, 398
  in resuscitation management, 837
  in small-volume nebulizers, 653
  in special beds, 377
  sputum specimens, 203
  in staple removal, 1127
  in sterile gloving, 291
  in subcutaneous injections, 685
  in support surfaces, 372
  in suprapubic catheter care, 1016
  in surgical hand antisepsis, 1101
  in suture removal, 1127
  in syringe pumps, 704
  in topical medications, 628
  in tracheostomy care, 786
  in transferring patients, 311
  in transparent dressing application, 1181
  in urine specimen collection, 185
  in vaginal or urethral discharge specimens, 198
  in workplace violence and safety, 38
  in wound drainage, 206, 1132
  in wound irrigation, 1122
Hand-offs, 41
Handrails, 1206f
Handwashing
  equipment for, 263
  using regular or antimicrobial soap, 264, 264f, 265f
Harris flush enema, 1024t
Head and neck
  assessment, 126–132
    delegation in, 126
    in disabled patient, 132
    documentation in, 131
    equipment for, 126
    evaluation in, 131
    hand-off reporting in, 131
    home care in, 132
    implementation in, 127, 128f
    interprofessional collaboration in, 126
    in older adults, 132
    patient education in, 131–132
    in pediatric patient, 131–132
    planning in, 127
  inspection of, 129
  lymph nodes of, 130, 130f
Head lice, 547–548t
Head tilt-chin lift, 833f
Headaches, in children, 132

Health assessment, 110–176
  of adolescents, 116–117
  assessment techniques, 113–115
  of children, 116–117
  evidence-based practice in, 111–112
  general survey for, 117–126
  of older adults, 117
  patient preparation for, 115–116, 116t
  person-centered care in, 111
  practice standards, 111
  preparation for, 115–116
  principles for practice, 111
  purpose of, 110–111, 111t
  safety guidelines for, 112–113
  supplemental standards, 111
  techniques for, 113–115
    auscultation, 114–115
    inspection, 113
    palpation, 113, 114f
    percussion, 114
  of transgender and gender-diverse patients, 111–112
Health care agency, 63, 63b
Health care-associated infections (HAIs), reduction of, 521
Health information system (HIS), 53b
Health Insurance Portability and Accountability Act (HIPAA)
  confidentiality, 55–56
  description of, 43
  security rule of, 54
Health literacy, 21, 1223
Healthy eating style, 924b
Healthy People 2030, 325
Hearing aids, care of, 577–581
  assessment in, 578
  in children, 581
  delegation in, 578
  documentation in, 580
  equipment for, 578–580
  evaluation in, 580
  hand-off reporting in, 580
  in home care, 581
  implementation in, 579
  interprofessional collaboration in, 578
  in older adults, 581
  patient education in, 581
  planning in, 579
Hearing impairment, 577
Heart
  assessment of, 140, 142f
  murmurs, 141
  rhythms of, 790t
Heart sounds, auscultation of, 143, 144f
Heat applications, moist and dry, 482–489, 483f, 483t
  assessment, 484
  delegation in, 483
  documentation in, 488
  equipment for, 483–488
  evaluation, 488
  hand-off reporting in, 488
  home care and, 489
  implementation, 485, 487f
  interprofessional collaboration of, 483
  in older adults, 489
  patient education in, 488
  in pediatrics, 489
  planning, 485
  in populations with disabilities, 489
Heated high-flow nasal cannula (HHFNC), 719, 721–722t, 721f, 722
Heatstroke, 81
Heimlich chest drain valve, 801f, 810t
Hematocrit, 92
Hematomas, 891–892t
Hemiplegic patient, in supine position, 317
Hemoccult testing, 187, 187f, 189f

Hemothorax, 800
  in vascular access devices, 891–892t
Hemovac drain, 1128
  empty, 1130f
Heparin, subcutaneous injection of, 679b
HFJV. *see* High-frequency jet ventilation
HFNC. *see* High-flow nasal cannula
HFOV. *see* High-frequency oscillatory ventilation
HHFNC. *see* Heated high-flow nasal cannula
High-air-loss beds, 373
High-efficiency particulate masks, 267b
High-fiber diet, 926t
High-flow nasal cannula (HFNC), 719, 721–722t, 721f, 722
High-frequency jet ventilation (HFJV), 742t
High-frequency oscillatory ventilation (HFOV), 742t
Hips
  movements, 1072f
  range-of-motion in
    assessment of, 167t
    exercise for, 332t, 333–336t
Hirsutism, 522–523t, 523f
Hives, 590t
Home care
  adverse transfusion reactions, 911
  after biological exposure, 429
  after chemical exposure, 434
  after natural disaster, 441
  after radiation exposure, 438
  apical pulse measurement in, 90
  applying physical restraints and, 405–408
  artificial airway, 768–770
  aspiration, 246
  aspiration precautions in, 937
  assist devices and, 355
  automated external defibrillator, 830
  blood glucose monitoring, 219
  blood pressure assessment in, 103–107
  blood transfusion in, 908, 911
  body temperature measurement in, 82
  bronchoscopy, 250
  cardiovascular assessment, 151
  care of body after death, 513, 514t
  central parenteral nutrition, 975
  central vascular access devices, 893
  closed chest drainage systems, 812
  cold application, 493
  in communication
    with cognitively impaired patients, 33
    with patients who have difficulty coping, 30
  complete or partial bed bath and, 534
  continuous subcutaneous infusion, 711
  contrast media studies, 240
  documentation in, 64, 65b
  dry dressings, 1175
  dysphagia in, 937
  ear irrigation, 576
  electrocardiogram, 794
  enteral nutrition, 961–963
  eye irrigation, 573
  fall prevention, 394
  feeding tubes, 953
  gastrointestinal endoscopy, 254
  general survey, 126
  hand hygiene, 266
  head and neck assessment, 132
  hearing aids in, 581
  in heat applications, 489
  immobilization devices, 359
  in incontinence device, 1012
  in indwelling urinary catheter irrigation, 1008
  infusion tubing, 874
  intramuscular injections, 692
  intravenous flow rates, 867
  intravenous moderate sedation, 233
  intravenous push, 698
  intravenous pyelogram, 240
  intravenous solutions, 871

Home care (*Continued*)
   isolation precautions, 275
   local anesthetic infusion pump, 482
   mechanical ventilation, 751
   metered-dose inhalers, 649
   moist and dry heat applications, 489
   moist dressing application, 1175
   mouth care, 547–550
   nail and foot care, 556–562
   nasogastric feeding tubes, 949
   nasotracheal/pharyngeal suctioning, 768–770
   negative-pressure wound therapy, 1138
   noninvasive positive pressure ventilation,
      739–740
   nonpharmacological pain management, 460
   nurse-patient relationship in, 25
   nutrition screening in, 925
   occult blood
      in gastric secretions, 192
      in stool specimen, 190
   ophthalmic medications, 634
   oral hygiene, 542–543
   oral medications, 618
   oropharyngeal suctioning, 759
   oxygen therapy, 727, 730
   pain assessment, 453
   patient-controlled analgesia, 472
   peripheral intravenous device, 861
   peripheral intravenous dressing, 878
   pharmacological pain management, 466
   physical restraints, 405–408
   piggyback infusion, 705
   positioning patients, 321
   pouching a urostomy, 1050
   preparing sterile field in, 287
   pressure bandage in, 1178
   for pressure injuries, 1154, 1160
   promoting early activity and exercise, 331–345
   respiratory assessment in, 95
   restraint-free environment, 398
   resuscitation management, 837
   seizure precautions and, 413
   for small-volume nebulizers, 653–657
   special beds, 377
   for subcutaneous injections, 685
   support surfaces and, 373
   supporting patients and families in grief
      and, 504
   symptom management at end of life and, 509
   syringe pumps, 705
   topical medications, 628
   tracheostomy care, 787
   transferring patients in, 311–312
   transparent dressings in, 1181
   urine specimen collection, 185–186
   wound drainage in, 1132
   wound irrigation, 1122
Home care safety, 1197–1221
   evidence-based practice for, 1199
   home environment assessment and, 1200–1209,
      1200f, 1201b, 1206f, 1207f, 1208f
   home setting, for cognitive deficits, 1209–1216,
      1213f, 1214f
   medication and medical device, 1216–1220,
      1218f
   person-centered care for, 1199
   practice standards for, 1198
   principles for practice of, 1198
   purpose of, 1198
   safety guidelines for, 1199
Home care teaching, 1222–1265
   blood pressure and pulse measurement,
      1227–1232, 1228f
      assessment in, 1228
      in children, 1232
      client education in, 1232
      delegation in, 1228
      documentation in, 1232
      equipment for, 1228–1232

Home care teaching (*Continued*)
      evaluation in, 1231
      hand-off reporting in, 1232
      implementation in, 1229, 1230f
      interprofessional collaboration in, 1228
      in older adults, 1232
      planning in, 1229
      in populations with disabilities, 1232
   body temperature measurements, 1224–1227
      assessment in, 1224
      in children, 1227
      client education in, 1227
      delegation in, 1224
      documentation in, 1227
      equipment for, 1224–1227
      evaluation in, 1226
      hand-off reporting in, 1227
      implementation in, 1225
      interprofessional collaboration in, 1224
      in older adults, 1227
      planning in, 1225
      in populations with disabilities, 1227
   evidence-based practice of, 1223
   feeding tubes in, 1253–1257
      in children, 1256
      client education in, 1256
      delegation in, 1253
      documentation in, 1256
      equipment for, 1253–1256
      evaluation in, 1256
      hand-off reporting in, 1256
      implementation for, 1254
      interprofessional collaboration in, 1253
      in older adults, 1257
      planning for, 1254
      in populations with disabilities, 1257
   intermittent self-catheterization, 1232–1236
      assessment in, 1233
      in children, 1235
      client education in, 1235
      delegation in, 1233
      documentation in, 1235
      equipment for, 1233–1235
      evaluation in, 1235
      hand-off reporting in, 1235
      implementation in, 1234
      interprofessional collaboration in, 1233
      in older adults, 1235–1236
      planning in, 1233
      in populations with disabilities, 1236
   medication self-administration, 1248–1253
      assessment in, 1248
      in children, 1252
      client education in, 1252
      documentation in, 1252
      evaluation in, 1251
      hand-off reporting in, 1252
      implementation in, 1250, 1251f
      in older adults, 1252–1253
      planning in, 1249, 1250f
      in populations with disabilities, 1253
   oxygen-delivery devices, 1236t, 1241f
   parenteral nutrition, 1257–1260
      assessment in, 1257
      in children, 1260
      client education in, 1260
      delegation in, 1257
      documentation in, 1260
      equipment for, 1257–1260
      hand-off reporting in, 1260
      implementation in, 1258
      interprofessional collaboration in, 1257
      in older adults, 1260
      planning in, 1258
      in populations with disabilities, 1260
   person-centered care, 1223
   practice standards, 1222
   principles for practice of, 1222–1223
   purpose of, 1222

Home care teaching (*Continued*)
   safety guidelines for, 1223
   tracheostomy care and suctioning, 1243–1248
      assessment in, 1243
      in children, 1247
      client education in, 1247
      delegation in, 1243
      documentation in, 1247
      equipment for, 1243–1247
      evaluation of, 1247
      hand-off reporting in, 1247
      implementation in, 1245, 1245f, 1246f
      interprofessional collaboration in, 1243
      in older adults, 1248
      planning in, 1244
      in populations with disabilities, 1248
Home environment, assessment and safety of,
      1200–1209, 1200f, 1206f, 1207f, 1208f
   bathroom, 1202
   bedroom, 1203
   in children, 1209
   client education in, 1209
   delegation in, 1200
   documentation in, 1209
   equipment for, 1200–1209
   evaluation in, 1208
   fall/near-fall diary in, 1201b
   front and back entrances, 1201
   implementation in, 1205, 1206f, 1207f, 1208f
   interprofessional collaboration in, 1200
   kitchen, 1202
   living room, 1203
   in older adults, 1209
   planning in, 1204
   in populations with disabilities, 1209
Home oxygen therapy
   assessment for, 1238
   in children, 1242
   client education in, 1242
   delegation in, 1237
   delivery systems, 1239
   description of, 1237t
   documentation in, 1242
   equipment for, 1236–1242, 1240f, 1241f
   evaluation of, 1241
   hand-off reporting in, 1242
   implementation in, 1239
   interprofessional collaboration in, 1237
   in older adults, 1242
   planning in, 1239
   in populations with disabilities, 1242
   safety of, 1238b
Home Safety Inventory (HSI), 1211
Hospice care, 498
Hospital Consumer Assessment of Healthcare
      Providers and Systems (HCAHPS) tool, 48
Household measurement, 595, 596t
"Huff" coughing, 1069
Human leukocyte antigen, 897
Human papillomavirus (HPV) vaccine, 159
Humility, 11t, 12
Humor, 20b
Humulin 70/30, 679t
Hydraulic lift, for transferring patients, 306f
Hydrocolloid dressings, 1163–1164t
   application of, 1181–1192, 1183f, 1185f
      assessment, 1182
      in children, 1187
      delegation in, 1182
      documentation in, 1187
      equipment for, 1182–1187
      evaluation, 1186
      hand-off reporting in, 1187
      implementation, 1183
      interprofessional collaboration in, 1182
      in older adults, 1187–1192
      patient education in, 1187
      in pediatrics, 1187
      planning, 1183

Hydrocolloids, 1118t
Hydrogel dressings, 1118t, 1163–1164t
  application of, 1181–1192, 1185f
    assessment, 1182
    in children, 1187
    delegation in, 1182
    documentation in, 1187
    equipment for, 1182–1187
    evaluation, 1186
    hand-off reporting in, 1187
    implementation, 1183
    interprofessional collaboration in, 1182
    in older adults, 1187–1192
    patient education in, 1187
    in pediatrics, 1187
    planning, 1183
Hydromorphone, 473
Hydrothorax, 891–892t
Hygiene. see also Personal hygiene
  hand, 262, 263–266
    factors affecting, 263
    guidelines for, 263
    handwashing, 263
    home care in, 266
    in older adults, 266
    patient education in, 266
  oral, 538–543
    assessment, 538
    delegation in, 538
    documentation in, 542
    equipment for, 538–541
    evaluation, 541
    hand-off reporting in, 542
    home care and, 542–543
    implementation, 540, 540f
    in older adults, 542
    patient education in, 542
    in pediatrics, 542
    planning, 539
    in populations with disabilities, 542
  personal, 519–564
    evidence-based practice of, 521
    of hair, 524
    person-centered care of, 521
    practice standards of, 520–521
    principles for practice, 521
    purpose of, 520
    safety guidelines for, 521–522
    of skin, 522, 522–523t
    supplemental standards of, 521
Hypercapnia, 735t
Hyperglycemia, 969–970t
Hyperpnea, 94b
Hypertension, 95–96, 96t
Hyperthermia, 75
Hypertonic solutions, 844, 1024t
Hyperventilation, 94b
Hypoglycemia, 969–970t
Hypotension, 96
Hypothermia, 81
Hypotonic solutions, 844
Hypoventilation, 94b
Hypoxia, 718, 719b

I
Ideal body weight (IBW), 921
Identification bracelet, 590f
Idiosyncratic reactions, medication action, 591
I:E ratio, 743f
IgE-mediated allergic reaction, 288b
Ileal pouch anal anastomosis, 1039f
Ileostomy, 1039f
  pouching, 1039f, 1040–1050, 1041f, 1044f
Immobilization device-related pressure
    injuries, 1150t
Immobilization devices, 324–361
  patient with, care for, 355–359, 356f, 356t
    assessment in, 357
    in children, 359

Immobilization devices (Continued)
    delegation in, 356
    documentation in, 359
    equipment for, 356–359
    evaluation, 358, 359f
    hand-off reporting in, 359
    home care and, 359
    implementation, 357
    interprofessional collaboration of, 356
    in older adults, 359
    patient education in, 359
    planning, 357
Immobilizers, 355, 356f, 356t
Implanted venous ports, 880, 880t, 881f
Incentive spirometers, 1069f
Incentive spirometry, 730–734, 731f, 732f
    assessment, 731
    in children, 734
    delegation in, 731
    documentation in, 734
    equipment for, 731–733
    evaluation, 733
    hand-off reporting in, 734
    implementation, 732
    interprofessional collaboration for, 731
    in older adults, 734
    patient education in, 734
    planning, 732
Incontinence device, applying, 1008–1012,
    1008f, 1010f
    assessment, 1009
    in children, 1012
    delegation in, 1008–1009
    documentation in, 1012
    equipment, 1009–1012
    evaluation, 1011
    hand-off reporting in, 1012
    home care in, 1012
    implementation, 1009
    interprofessional collaboration, 1009
    in older adults, 1012
    patient education in, 1012
    planning, 1009
    in populations with disabilities, 1012
Incorrect placement, 891–892t
Indwelling urinary catheter
    care of, 998–1004
    closed continuous irrigation of, 1004f,
      1005–1008, 1006f
    closed intermittent irrigation of, 1005
    documentation in, 997
    in females, 991f
    hand-off reporting in, 997
    insertion of, 987–998, 987b, 988f, 989f, 992f,
      993f, 994f, 995f, 996f
    irrigation, 1004–1008, 1004f, 1006f
    in males, 991f
    in older adults, 997
    patient education, 997, 1008
    in pediatrics, 997
    removal of, 998–1004, 1000f
Infection
    chain of, 261, 261f, 261t
    localized, 969–970t
    risk of, in home oxygen equipment, 1237b
    spread of, prevention of, in home
      environment, 1205
    urinary tract, catheter-associated, 987
    in vascular access devices, 891–892t
Infiltration, 891–892t
Informed consent, 228, 1076t
Informing, 20b
Infusion Nurses Society (INS), 845
    standards, 845b
Infusion therapy, 844
Infusion tubing, for intravenous therapy, 871–874,
    871t, 873f
    assessment, 871
    delegation in, 871

Infusion tubing, for intravenous therapy
    (Continued)
    documentation in, 874
    equipment for, 871–874
    evaluation, 874
    hand off-reporting for, 874
    home care in, 874
    implementation, 872
    patient education in, 874
    planning, 872
Ingrown nails, 551–552t, 552f
Inhalers
    breath-actuated, 643f
    dry powder, 643f
      placement of, 647f
    metered-dose, 642–649, 643b, 643f, 645f,
      646f, 647f
    pressurized metered-dose, 642
    types of, 643f
Injection
    intradermal, 673–677, 675f
    intramuscular, 685–692, 686f
    pens, 664
    subcutaneous, 677–685, 678f, 682f, 683f, 684f
INS. see Infusion Nurses Society
Inspection, 113
Inspiration, 91, 91f
Institute for Safe Medication Practices
    (ISMP), 659
Instrumental activities of daily living (IADLs), in
    home setting, for cognitive deficits, 1209
Insulin, subcutaneous injection of, 678–679, 679t
Insulin aspart, 679t
Insulin detemir, 679t
Insulin glargine, 679t
Insulin glulisine, 679t
Insulin lispro, 679t
Insulin syringe, 663, 663f
Intake and output monitoring, 170–172b, 171f,
    171t, 172f
Integrated bed system, 369
Integrated securement device dressings, 874
Integrity, 11t, 12
Intellectual standards, for critical thinking,
    12–13, 12b
Intercostal spaces, 132–133
Intermittent extension set, 871–874
Intermittent self-catheterization, teaching,
    1232–1236
Intermittent suture, 1122f
International Dysphagia Diet, 932, 933t
Interrupted sutures, removal of, 1125f
In-the-ear (ITE) hearing aids, 577f, 577t
Intracranial pressure (ICP), increased, 240
Intradermal (ID) injections, 673–677, 675f
    assessment, 673
    in children, 677
    delegation in, 673
    documentation in, 677
    equipment for, 673–677
    evaluation, 676
    hand-off reporting in, 677
    implementation, 674
    interprofessional collaboration, 673
    in older adults, 677
    patient education in, 677
    planning, 674
    in populations with disabilities, 677
Intramuscular (IM) injections, 685–692, 686f
    all injections, 688–691
    assessment, 688
    in children, 692
    delegation in, 687
    deltoid muscle, 687, 688f
    documentation in, 691
    equipment for, 687–688
    evaluation, 691
    hand-off reporting in, 691
    home care in, 692

Intramuscular (IM) injections (*Continued*)
  implementation, 689
  injection sites, 686
  interprofessional collaboration, 687
  in older adults, 692
  patient education in, 691–692
  planning, 689
  in populations with disabilities, 692
  vastus lateralis muscle, 686–687, 687f
  ventrogluteal site, 686
Intraocular disk, 588t, 629, 633f
Intraoperative care, 1095–1108
  closed gloving in, 1102–1105, 1103f, 1104f
  evidence-based practice in, 1097
  person-centered care in, 1096
  practice standards in, 1095
  principles for practice of, 1095–1096, 1096b
  purpose of, 1095
  safety guidelines in, 1097–1098
  sterile gown in, 1102–1105, 1103f, 1104f
  surgical hand antisepsis in, 1098–1101, 1099f, 1100f
  surgical safety checklist in, 1096, 1097f
Intravenous and vascular access therapy, 841–894
  central vascular access devices, 879–893, 880f, 880t, 888f, 891–892t
  evidence-based practice, 844
  infusion tubing, changing of, 871–874, 871t, 873f
  intravenous flow rates, 861–867, 862f, 864f, 865f
  intravenous solutions, 867–871, 869f
  peripheral intravenous device
    dressing, 874–878, 876f
    insertion of, 846–861, 846f, 846t, 850f, 851f, 852f, 853f, 854f, 857f, 858f, 860t
  person-centered care, 844
  practice standards for, 842
  purpose of, 842
  safety guidelines for, 844–845, 845b
  supplemental standards for, 842–843
Intravenous flow rates, 861–867, 862f, 864f, 865f
  assessment, 862
  in children, 867
  delegation in, 862
  documentation in, 866
  equipment for, 862–866
  evaluation, 866
  hand-off reporting in, 867
  home care in, 867
  implementation, 864
  in older adults, 867
  patient education in, 867
  planning, 863
Intravenous moderate sedation, 229–233
  assessment of, 230
  in children, 233
  delegation in, 229
  in disabled patients, 233
  documentation in, 233
  equipment for, 229–230
  evaluation of, 232
  hand-off reporting in, 233
  home care in, 233
  implementation of, 231
  interprofessional collaboration of, 229
  in older adults, 233
  patient education in, 233
  planning, 231
Intravenous push, 692–698, 692b, 693b, 695f, 696f
  assessment, 693
  in children, 698
  delegation in, 693
  documentation in, 698
  equipment for, 693–698
  evaluation, 697
  hand-off reporting in, 698
  home care in, 698
  implementation, 694

Intravenous push (*Continued*)
  interprofessional collaboration, 693
  in older adults, 698
  patient education in, 698
  planning, 694
  in populations with disabilities, 698
Intravenous pyelogram, 234–240
Intravenous (IV) solutions, 843–844, 843t, 867–871, 869f
  assessment, 867
  delegation in, 867
  documentation in, 870
  equipment for, 867–870
  evaluation, 870
  hand-off reporting in, 871
  home care in, 871
  implementation, 868
  patient education in, 871
  planning, 868
Intubation. *see* Artificial airway
Intuition, defined, 5
Iron overload, 898–899t
Irradiated red blood cells (RBCs), 900t
Irrigation
  ear, 573–576
    assessment in, 574
    in children, 576
    delegation in, 573
    documentation in, 576
    equipment for, 573–576
    evaluation in, 576
    hand-off reporting in, 576
    in home care, 576
    implementation in, 575, 575f
    interprofessional collaboration in, 573
    patient education in, 576
    planning in, 574
  eye, 570–573
    assessment in, 570
    in children, 573
    delegation in, 570
    documentation in, 573
    equipment for, 570–573
    evaluation in, 572
    hand-off reporting in, 573
    in home care, 573
    implementation in, 571, 572f, 577f
    interprofessional collaboration in, 570
    patient education in, 573
    planning in, 571
  feeding tubes, 953–955
    assessment, 953
    delegation in, 953
    documentation in, 955
    equipment for, 953–955
    evaluation, 954
    hand-off reporting in, 955
    implementation, 954
    interprofessional collaboration, 953
    in pediatrics, 955
    planning, 954
  indwelling urinary catheter, 1004–1008, 1004f, 1006f
    assessment for, 1005
    delegation in, 1004
    documentation in, 1008
    equipment for, 1005–1008
    evaluation, 1007
    hand-off reporting in, 1008
    home care in, 1008
    implementation, 1006
    interprofessional collaboration, 1005
    patient education in, 1008
    planning, 1005
  wound, 1117–1122, 1117f, 1117t
    in children, 1122
    delegation in, 1117
    documentation in, 1122
    equipment for, 1117

Irrigation (*Continued*)
    hand-off reporting in, 1122
    home care in, 1122
    patient education in, 1122
    patient position for, 1119f
    in pediatrics, 1122
    in populations with disabilities, 1122
Irritant contact dermatitis, 288b
ISMP. *see* Institute for Safe Medication Practices
Isolation gown, 270f
Isolation guidelines, for tuberculosis, 267b
Isolation precautions, caring for patients under, 266
  assessment for, 269
  delegation in, 269
  documentation in, 274
  equipment for, 269
  hand-off reporting in, 274
  home care in, 275
  interprofessional collaboration in, 269
  in older adults, 275
  patient education for, 274
  pediatric considerations for, 274–275
  personal protective equipment for
    applying, 270, 270f
    removal of, 272, 273f
Isophane insulin suspension (NPH), 679t

J

Jackson-Pratt wound drainage system, 172f, 1091f, 1128f, 1131f
Jaw thrust, 833f
Jejunostomy tube
  care of, 962–963b
  endoscopic insertion of, 963f
  technique, 955–963
Jet injection system, 678, 678f
Joint Commission Universal Protocol, diagnostic procedures, 231b

K

Ketones, urine screening for, 179
Knee
  movements of, 1072f
  range-of-motion in
    assessment of, 167t
    exercise for, 332t, 333–336t
Knee-chest position, 116t
Korotkoff phases, 95f
Kussmaul respiration, 94b
Kyphosis, 166f

L

Lateral recumbent position, 116t
Lateral rotation bed, 374, 374f
Lateral thorax, 137, 138f
Lateral transfer, from bed to stretcher, 307, 308f, 309f, 310f
Latex allergy, 282, 288b
Latex gloves, applying, 288
Leukocyte-poor red blood cells (RBCs), 900t
Level of consciousness, 118
Levin tube, 1029, 1029f
Life support, emergency measures for, 821–840
  automated external defibrillator, 827–830, 827f, 829f
  evidence-based practice for, 823–824
  oropharyngeal airway, inserting of, 824–827, 824f, 824t, 825f
  person-centered care, 821–823
  practice standards for, 821
  principles for practice in, 821, 822–823t
  purpose of, 821
  resuscitation management, 830–837, 831f, 832f, 833f, 833t, 834f, 835f
  safety guidelines for, 824
  supplemental standards for, 821
Light palpation, 113, 114f
Linen-wrapped package, sterile, 284, 285f
Liniment, 588t

Liquid medication, 610, 614f, 617
Liquid oxygen, 1237, 1238b, 1239
Listening, active, 20b
Lithotomy position, 116t
Local anesthesia, 1080t
Local anesthetic infusion pump, 479–482, 479f
    assessment, 479
    delegation in, 479
    documentation in, 482
    equipment for, 479–482
    evaluation, 481
    hand-off reporting in, 482
    home care and, 482
    implementation, 480
    interprofessional collaboration of, 479
    in older adults, 482
    patient education in, 482
    in pediatrics, 482
    planning, 480
Lofstrand crutch, 346t, 347f
Logrolling, positioning patients, 319, 320f
Long-term care
    documentation in, 65
    resident assessment instrument, 47
Long-Term Care Facility Resident Assessment
        Instrument, 65
Long-term oxygen, 1237t
Lordosis, 166f
Lotion, 588t
Low-air-loss beds, 363–364t, 373
Low-air-loss overlay, indications for,
        363–364t
Lower extremities, range of motion in, assessment
        of, 167t
Lower gastrointestinal endoscopy, 254
Low-fiber diet, 926t
Low-pressure seat cushion, 369, 369f
Low-residue diet, 926t
Luer-Lok syringes, 183, 662–663, 663f
Lumbar puncture, 240–246, 241–242t
Lung cancer, 134
Lungs
    anatomy, 799, 800f
    assessment of, 132–140
    lobes of, 132–133, 133f
Lymph nodes, of head and neck, 130, 130f

M
Maceration, 551
Macule, 124b
Male health teaching, 162
Male urinal, 986f
Malignant melanoma, 122b, 122f
Malnutrition, 916
Malnutrition Screening Tool (MST), 919, 920b
Manmade disasters, 418b
Manual intermittent bolus, 473
Mask
    applying and removing, 273f, 279–282,
        280f, 281f
    partial nonrebreather, 721–722t
    for patients under isolation precautions, 263
    simple face, 721–722t, 721f, 722, 1236t
    Venturi, 720f, 721–722t, 722
Mass casualty incident or event (MCI), 418b
Massage, 453, 456, 456f
Maternal-child health, in supporting patients and
        families in grief, 503
Mattress
    air, 369, 369f
    alternating pressure, 365
    foam, 368
MCDs. see Mobile compression devices
MCI. see Mass casualty incident or event
MDI. see Metered-dose inhalers
Measles, outbreaks of, 418b
Mechanical debridement, 1113
Mechanical diet, 926t
Mechanical phlebitis, 859

Mechanical ventilation, 742–751, 742t, 743f
    alarms and settings, 743t, 744t
    assessment, 745
    in children, 750–751
    delegation in, 744–745
    documentation in, 750
    in endotracheal tube care, 770–771
    equipment for, 745–750
    evaluation, 749
    hand-off reporting in, 750
    home care in, 751
    implementation, 747
    interprofessional collaboration for, 745
    in older adults, 751
    patient education in, 750
    planning, 747
    ventilator-associated events,
        744, 745b
Median cubital vein, 852f
Mediastinal chest tubes, 800–801, 801f
Medical asepsis, 259–276
    evidence-based practice of, 262
    person-centered care in, 262
    practice standards for, 260
    principles for practice in, 260–262
    purpose of, 260
    safety guidelines for, 262–263
Medical device safety, 1216–1220, 1218f
    assessment for, 1216
    in children, 1220
    client teaching in, 1220
    delegation in, 1216
    documentation in, 1220
    equipment for, 1216–1220
    evaluation in, 1219
    implementation in, 1217
    planning in, 1217
    reporting in, 1220
Medical device-related pressure injuries, strategies
        to prevent, 1150t
Medical disasters, 418b
Medical oxygen, 1236
Medicated enemas, 1024
Medication(s)
    absorption, 589t
    adherence to, 1252b
    administration of, 596–600, 596b
        in nursing process, 603–605
        right documentation, 599–600
        right dose, 598
        right medication, 597–598
        right patient, 598, 598f, 599f
        right route, 598–599
        right time, 599
        in transmission-based precautions, 271
    organizer, 1214f
    parenteral. see Parenteral medications
    reconciliation, 44–45, 1216
    safety, 1216–1220, 1218f
        assessment for, 1216
        in children, 1220
        client teaching in, 1220
        delegation in, 1216
        documentation in, 1220
        equipment for, 1216–1220
        evaluation in, 1219
        implementation in, 1217
        planning in, 1217
        reporting in, 1220
    sedation uses of, 228
    self-administration of, 1248–1253, 1250f
    topical. see Topical medications
Medication errors, 598
    prevention, 603, 603b
    reporting, 605
Medication interactions, medication
        action, 591
Medication labels, 600, 600f
Medication orders, 597–598, 597b

Medication preparation, 600–602
    dosage calculation, 600–602
    interpreting medication labels, 600
Melanocytes, 1110
Melanoma, ABCDE rule of, 122b, 122f
Menarche, 157
Men's Liberty Acute Male Incontinence Device,
        1010f
Mercury spill, 1224b
Message, 41
Metered-dose inhalers (MDI), 642–649, 643b,
        643f, 645f, 646f, 647f
    assessment, 643
    in children, 649
    delegation in, 643
    documentation in, 648
    equipment for, 643–648, 643f
    evaluation, 648
    hand-off reporting in, 649
    home care in, 649
    implementation, 644
    interprofessional collaboration for, 643
    in older adults, 649
    patient education in, 649
    planning, 644
    in populations with disabilities, 649
Methicillin-resistant *Staphylococcus aureus*
        (MRSA), 267
Metric system, 595
Microphone, in hearing aids, 577
Midstream (clean-voided) urine specimen,
        179–186, 180f, 182f, 183f
Military time clock, 58f
Mini-Cog, 1211
Mini-infusion pump, 699
Minimal sedation (anxiolysis), 232t
Mini-Mental State Examination (MMSE), 1211
Minimum effective concentration (MEC), 588–589
Misconceptions, pain, 452t
Mitten restraint, 401, 401f
Mobile compression devices (MCDs), application
        of, 340–341, 341f
Mobility, 324–361
Moderate sedation, intravenous, 229–233
    assessment of, 230
    in children, 233
    delegation in, 229
    in disabled patients, 233
    documentation in, 233
    equipment for, 229–230
    evaluation of, 232
    hand-off reporting in, 233
    home care in, 233
    implementation of, 231
    interprofessional collaboration of, 229
    in older adults, 233
    patient education in, 233
    planning, 231
Moderate sedation/analgesia (conscious
        sedation), 232t
Modified Ramsay Sedation Scale, 232t
Moist dressing, application of, 1166–1175, 1167f,
        1168f, 1169f, 1170f, 1171f, 1172f, 1173f
    assessment, 1167
    in children, 1175
    delegation in, 1166
    documentation in, 1174
    equipment for, 1167–1174
    hand-off reporting in, 1174
    home care in, 1175
    implementation, 1168, 1173
    interprofessional collaboration in, 1166
    in older adults, 1175
    patient education in, 1175
    planning, 1168
    in populations with disabilities, 1175
Moisture-impervious bags, 272, 272f
Molded splints, 356t
Mouth, assessment of, 129, 129f

Mucositis, 539
Multidrug-resistant organisms (MDROs), caring for patients with, 267
Multimodal analgesia, 444
Multiple electrolyte solutions, 843t
Musculoskeletal assessment, 162–172
  delegation in, 163
  in disabled patient, 170–172
  documentation in, 170
  equipment for, 163–169
  evaluation in, 169
  hand-off reporting in, 170
  implementation in, 164
  interprofessional collaboration in, 163
  in older adults, 170
  patient education in, 170–172
  in pediatric patient, 170
  planning in, 164
Mustache care, equipment for, 548
Mydriatics, 634
MyPlate, 918f, 932

N
Nail(s)
  care of, 551–562
    assessment, 552
    delegation in, 552
    documentation in, 556
    equipment for, 552–556
    evaluation, 555
    hand-off reporting in, 556
    home care and, 556–562
    implementation, 554, 555f
    interprofessional collaboration of, 552
    in older adults, 556
    patient education in, 556
    in pediatrics, 556
    planning, 554
    in populations with disabilities, 556
  personal hygiene of, 524
  problems of, 551–552t
Nail bed, 524
Naloxone, administration of, 461b
Narrative documentation, 61
Narrative note, 62
Nasal cannula, 720–722, 721–722t, 721f, 1236t, 1241f
Nasal instillations, 638–642, 640f, 641f
  assessment, 638
  in children, 642
  delegation in, 638
  documentation in, 642
  equipment for, 638–642
  evaluation, 641
  hand-off reporting in, 642
  implementation, 639
  interprofessional collaboration for, 638
  patient education in, 642
  planning, 639
  in populations with disabilities, 642
Nasal spray, 638, 640, 641f
Nasogastric feeding tubes, 1029
  enteral nutrition using, 940
  gastric aspirate obtained using, 952f
  for gastric decompression, 1029–1036, 1029f, 1031f, 1032f, 1033f, 1034f
  Levin tube, 1029, 1029f
  in older adults, 1036
  Salem sump tube, 1029, 1029f
Nasointestinal feeding tubes, enteral nutrition administered using, 955–963
Nasopharyngeal suctioning, 759–770, 763f, 764f, 766f
  assessment, 761
  in children, 768
  evaluation, 767
  home care in, 768–770
  implementation, 763
  in older adults, 768

Nasopharyngeal suctioning (Continued)
  patient education in, 768
  planning, 762
  in populations with disabilities, 768
Nasotracheal catheter, 764f
Nasotracheal suctioning, 759–770, 763f, 764f, 766f
  assessment, 761
  in children, 768
  evaluation, 767
  home care in, 768–770
  implementation, 763
  in older adults, 768
  patient education in, 768
  planning, 762
  in populations with disabilities, 768
National Pressure Injury Advisory Panel (NPIAP), 524–525
National Terrorism Advisory System, overview of, 419f
Natural disaster, patient care after, 438–441, 438f
  assessment, 438
  delegation in, 438
  documentation in, 440
  equipment for, 438–440
  evaluation in, 440
  hand-off reporting in, 440
  home care and, 441
  implementation, 439
  interprofessional collaboration of, 438
  in older adults, 441
  patient education in, 440
  in pediatrics, 440–441
  planning, 439
  in populations with disabilities, 441
Natural/environmental disasters, 418b
Nebulizers, small-volume, 649–657, 651f
  assessment, 650
  in children, 653
  delegation in, 649
  documentation in, 653
  equipment for, 649–652
  evaluation, 652
  hand-off reporting in, 653
  home care in, 653–657
  implementation, 651
  interprofessional collaboration for, 649
  in older adults, 653
  patient education in, 653–657
  planning, 650
  in populations with disabilities, 653
Neck, range-of-motion in
  assessment of, 167t
  exercise for, 332t, 333–336t
Necrotizing osteochondritis, 219
Needleless systems, 662, 662b, 662f
Needles, 663, 663f
Needlestick prevention, 661–662
Needlestick Safety and Prevention Act, 661–662
Negative-pressure wound therapy (NPWT), 1133–1138, 1133f
  assessment, 1134
  in children, 1138
  delegation in, 1133
  documentation in, 1138
  equipment for, 1133–1138
  evaluation, 1137
  hand-off reporting in, 1138
  home care in, 1138
  implementation, 1134
  in older adults, 1138
  patient education in, 1138
  in pediatrics, 1138
  planning, 1134
  seal with, maintaining, 1137b
Neurological assessment, 162–172
Neuropathic pain, definition of, 444
Nociceptive pain, definition of, 444
Nocturnal oxygen, 1237t

Nodule, 124b
Noninvasive positive pressure ventilation (NIPPV or NPPV), 734–740, 734f, 735t
  assessment, 736
  in children, 739
  delegation in, 735
  documentation in, 739
  equipment for, 735–738
  evaluation, 738
  hand-off reporting in, 739
  home care in, 739–740
  implementation, 737
  interprofessional collaboration for, 735
  patient education in, 739
  in patients with disabilities, 739
  planning, 736
Noninvasive ventilation (NIV). see Noninvasive positive pressure ventilation
Non-Luer-Lok syringes, 662–663, 663f
Nonparenteral medications, 608–658
  ear medications, 635–638, 637f
  evidence-based practice for, 609
  feeding tube, administration through, 618–623, 623b
  metered-dose inhalers, 642–649, 643b, 643f, 645f, 646f, 647f
  nasal instillations, 638–642, 640f, 641f
  ophthalmic medications, 629–634, 631f, 632f, 633f
  oral medications, 609–618, 612b, 613f, 614f, 616f
  person-centered care for, 609
  practice standards for, 608
  principles for practice in, 609, 609b
  purpose of, 608
  rectal suppositories, 655–657b, 656f
  safety guidelines for, 609–610
  small-volume nebulizers, 649–657, 651f
  supplemental standards for, 609
  topical medications, 623–628, 626f
  vaginal medications, 653–655b, 653f, 654f, 655f
Nonpharmacological pain management, 453–460
  assessment, 454
  delegation in, 453
  documentation in, 459
  equipment for, 453–459
  evaluation, 459
  hand-off reporting in, 459
  home care and, 460
  implementation, 455, 455f, 456f
  interprofessional collaboration of, 453
  in older adults, 460
  in pediatrics, 459–460
  planning, 454
  in populations with disabilities, 460
Nonpowdered gloves, 288
Nonpowered air-filled overlay, indications for, 363–364t
Nontunneled percutaneous catheter, 880t
Nonverbal communication, 17–18
Nonviable tissue, in wound, 1113
Normal sinus rhythm, 790t
Norton Scale, 1146
Nose, inspection of, 129, 129f
Nose drops, 640, 640f
Nose specimens, for culture, 192–196, 194f, 195f
Novolin 70/30, 679t
Novolog Mix 70/30, 679t
NPIAP. see National Pressure Injury Advisory Panel
Nurse
  admission personnel by, 42–43b, 43–44
  at risk for incivility and bullying, 19
Nurse-patient relationship, establishing of, 20–25
Nursing history, admission, 58
Nursing information system (NIS), 53b, 58
Nursing Interventions Classification (NIC), 58
Nursing Outcomes Classification (NOC), 58
Nursing practice, clinical judgment in, 2–3

Nutrition
  enteral, 940–965
    administering, 955–963, 957f, 959f, 960f
    combination tubes for, 962, 962f
    definition of, 940
    evidence-based practice, 941
    feeding tubes, 940
    home care in, 961–963, 1253
    intermittent feeding, 958f
    in older adults, 961
    patient education, 961
    person-centered care, 941
    safety guidelines, 941
    technique, 955–963, 957f, 959f, 960f
  parenteral, 966–982
    catheter for, 967f
    central, 970t, 971
    central venous catheter for, 967f
    complications of, 969–970t
    documentation in, 974
    evidence-based practice for, 968
    home care teaching, 1257–1260
    indications for, 967b
    monitoring and laboratory orders for, 968b
    in older adults, 975, 979
    patient education for, 975
    in pediatrics, 979
    peripheral, 970t, 975–979
    peripherally inserted central catheter
      for, 967f
    person-centered care for, 968
    practice standards for, 966
    principles for practice, 966–968
    purpose of, 966
    safety guidelines for, 968–970
    via infusion pump, 973f
  problems, risk factors for, 917, 917b
  screening of, 919–925, 920b
Nutrition Risk Screening (NRS), 919, 920b
Nutrition screening, 919–925
  assessment in, 921
  body mass index, 921, 922b, 922f
  in children, 924
  delegation in, 920
  documentation in, 924
  equipment for, 921
  evaluation in, 923
  hand-off reporting in, 924
  history, 923
  in home care, 925
  implementation in, 923
  interprofessional collaboration of, 921
  in older adults, 924–925
  patient education in, 924, 924b
  physical examination, 920, 920t
  planning, 922
  in populations with disabilities, 925
Nutritional status
  physical signs of, 920t
  weight changes as indicator of, 922t

O
Obstructive sleep apnea (OSA), 734, 744t, 1061
Occlusion
  prevention of, 802
  in vascular access devices, 891–892t
Occlusive dressing, 890
Occult blood
  in gastric secretions (Gastroccult), 190–192, 191f
  in stool, 187–190, 187f, 189f
Occupied bed, making of, 557–558t, 557–562b
  delegation in, 558
  equipment for, 558
  interprofessional collaboration of, 558
  steps in, 559–562, 559f, 560f, 561f
OCDs. see Oxygen-conserving devices
Oculomotor nerve, 168
Oil-retention enema, 1024, 1024t
Ointment, 588t

Older adults
  abdominal assessment in, 157
  abuse of, 121
  alginate dressing in, 1187–1192
  anger in, 30
  applying physical restraints in, 405
  arterial blood gas measurements in, 225
  artificial airway in, 768
  aspiration procedures in, 246
  assist devices and, 355
  assisting adults with oral nutrition in, 931
  autotransfusion of chest tube drainage in, 819
  blood glucose monitoring in, 219
  blood pressure and pulse measurement in, 1232
  blood pressure assessment in, 103
  blood specimen collection in, 214
  blood transfusion in, 908, 911
  body temperature measurement in, 82, 1227
  bronchoscopy in, 250
  cardiac monitor in, 797
  cardiovascular assessment in, 151
  cardiovascular system in, 1074t
  care of body after death in, 513
  central vascular access devices in, 893
  cognitively impaired, communication with, 33
  cold application in, 493
  complete or partial bed bath in, 534
  continuous subcutaneous infusion in, 710
  contrast media studies in, 239
  dry dressings in, 1175
  dysphagia in, 937
  electrocardiogram in, 794
  endotracheal tube care in, 777
  enema in, 1029
  enteral nutrition, 961
  epidural analgesia in, 478
  fall prevention in, 393
  feeding tube administration in, 623
  feeding tubes in, 1257
  foam dressings in, 1187–1192
  gastrointestinal endoscopy in, 254
  general survey for, 126
  hand hygiene in, 266
  head and neck assessment in, 132
  hearing aids in, 581
  home care in, 478–479
  home environment assessment and safety
    in, 1209
  home oxygen equipment for, 1242
  home setting, for cognitive deficits in, 1216
  hydrocolloid dressings in, 1187–1192
  hydrogel dressings in, 1187–1192
  immobilization devices in, 359
  incentive spirometry in, 734
  indwelling urinary catheter insertion in, 997
  integumentary system in, 1074t
  intermittent self-catheterization in, 1235–1236
  intradermal injections in, 677
  intramuscular injections in, 692
  intravenous flow rates in, 867
  intravenous moderate sedation in, 233
  intravenous push in, 698
  isolation precautions for, 275
  local anesthetic infusion pump in, 482
  mechanical ventilation in, 751
  medication self-administration in, 1252–1253
  metabolic system of, 1074t
  metered-dose inhalers in, 649
  moist and dry heat applications in, 489
  mouth care in, 547
  musculoskeletal assessment in, 170
  nail and foot care in, 556
  nasogastric tube in, 1036
  nasotracheal/pharyngeal suctioning in, 768
  negative-pressure wound therapy in, 1138
  neglect of, 121
  neurological system of, 1074t
  nonpharmacological pain management in, 460
  nose and throat specimens from, 196

Older adults (Continued)
  nurse-patient relationship in, 25
  nutrition screening in, 924
  ophthalmic medications in, 634
  oral hygiene in, 542
  oral medications in, 617–618
  oropharyngeal suctioning in, 759
  oxygen therapy in, 727
  pain assessment in, 452–453
  parenteral nutrition in, 975, 979, 1260
  patient care in
    after biological exposure, 429
    after chemical exposure, 434
    after natural disaster, 441
    after radiation exposure, 438
  patient positioning in, 321
  patient preparation for surgery of, 1079
  patient-controlled analgesia in, 472
  peripheral intravenous device in, 861, 861f
  peripheral intravenous dressing in, 878
  pharmacological pain management in, 466
  physical assessment of, 117
  piggyback infusion in, 704–705
  pouching a colostomy, or ileostomy for, 1046
  pouching a urostomy in, 1050
  preoperative assessment for, 1065
  preoperative teaching for, 1073–1075, 1074t
  pressure bandage in, 1178
  pressure injuries in, 1154, 1159
  promoting early activity and exercise and, 331
  pulmonary system in, 1074t
  pulse measurement in, 1232
    apical, 90
    radial, 86
  removing sutures and staples in, 1128
  renal system in, 1074t
  respiratory assessment in, 95
  restraint-free environment in, 398
  resuscitation management in, 837
  seizure precautions in, 413
  small-volume nebulizers in, 653
  special beds and, 377
  subcutaneous injections in, 685
  support surfaces and, 373
  supporting patients and families in grief in,
    503–504
  symptom management at end of life in, 509
  syringe pumps in, 704–705
  thorax and lung assessment in, 140
  topical medications in, 628
  tracheostomy care in, 787, 1248
  transferring in, 311
  transparent dressings in, 1181
  urine specimen collection in, 185
  vaginal or urethral discharge specimens in, 199
  who have difficulty coping, communication
    with, 30
  wound drainage in, 1132
Olfaction, 115, 115t
ONC. see Over-the-needle catheter
OPA. see Oropharyngeal airway
Open-drain system, 1128
Ophthalmic medications, 629–634, 631f, 632f, 633f
  assessment, 629
  in children, 634
  delegation in, 629
  documentation in, 634
  equipment for, 629–634
  evaluation, 634
  hand-off reporting in, 634
  home care in, 634
  implementation, 630
  interprofessional collaboration for, 629
  in older adults, 634
  patient education in, 634
  planning, 630
Opioids, 460–461, 461b
  side effects of, 755
Oral cavity, 523–524

Oral hygiene, 538–543
  assessment, 538
  delegation in, 538
  documentation in, 542
  equipment for, 538–541
  hand-off reporting in, 542
  home care and, 542–543
  implementation, 540, 540f
  in older adults, 542
  patient education in, 542
  in pediatrics, 542
  planning, 539
  in populations with disabilities, 542
Oral measurement, of body temperature, 73b, 76
Oral medications, 609–618, 612b, 613f, 614f, 616f
  assessment, 611
  in children, 617
  delegation in, 610
  documentation in, 617
  equipment for, 611–617
  evaluation, 617
  hand-off reporting in, 617
  home care in, 618
  implementation, 612
  interprofessional collaboration for, 610
  in older adults, 617–618
  patient education in, 617
  planning, 612
  in populations with disabilities, 618
Oral nutrition, 915–939
  aspiration precautions, 931–937, 932b
  assisting adults with, 925–931, 926t
  clock setup, 929f
  documentation in, 924
  evidence-informed practice, 918–919
  Malnutrition Screening Tool, 920b
  mealtime adaptive equipment for, 928f
  MyPlate, 918f, 932
  person-centered care, 917–918, 918f
  physical examination in, 920, 920t
  problems with, risk factors for, 917b
  safety guidelines, 919, 919b
  screening of, 919–925, 920b
Organ donation, 510
Organization, in clinical decision making, 6
Oropharyngeal airway (OPA), insertion, 824–827, 824f, 824t, 825f
  assessment, 825
  in children, 827
  delegation in, 824
  documentation in, 827
  equipment for, 824–827
  evaluation, 826
  hand-off reporting in, 827
  implementation, 826
  interprofessional collaboration of, 824
  planning, 825
Oropharyngeal suctioning, 755–759, 755f
  assessment, 756
  evaluation, 758
  home care in, 759
  implementation, 757
  in older adults, 759
  patient education in, 759
  planning, 756
  in populations with disabilities, 759
Orthostatic hypotension, 96, 342
Orthotic devices, 355
OSA. see Obstructive sleep apnea
Ostomy care, 1038–1056
  evidence-based practice for, 1040
  person-centered care for, 1039–1040
  practice standards for, 1038
  principles for practice of, 1038
  purpose of, 1038
  safety guidelines for, 1040
  stoma
    budded, 1041f
    measurement of, 1044f

Ostomy care (Continued)
    retracted, 1041f
    skin barrier for, 1040
Ovarian cancer, 159
Overexertion injuries, 296, 297f
Overlays, 363–364t
Over-the-needle catheter (ONC), 846, 846f, 846t
Oxygen concentrator system, 1239, 1240f
Oxygen-conserving cannula, 721–722t, 722, 1236t
Oxygen-conserving devices (OCDs), 1236
Oxygen-delivery devices, 720–727, 720f, 721–722t, 721f, 722f
  assessment, 723
  in children, 726
  delegation in, 722
  documentation in, 726
  equipment, 723–726
  evaluation, 726
  hand-off reporting in, 726
  home care in, 727, 1236t, 1241f
  implementation, 724
  interprofessional collaboration, 723
  in older adults, 727
  patient education in, 726
  in patients with disabilities, 727
  planning, 724
Oxygen delivery systems
  demand pulsing, 1236
  devices, 1236t
  flow rates for, 1236t
Oxygen flowmeter, 720, 722f
Oxygen mask, 721f, 722
Oxygen-reserving cannula, 721–722t, 722f
Oxygen reservoir, 1240, 1240f
Oxygen saturation, 105–107b, 107f
Oxygen storage and handling, 1238b
Oxygen therapy, 717–752
  in artificial airway patients, 727–730, 727f
  evidence-based practice, 719
  incentive spirometry, 730–734, 731f, 732f
  mechanical ventilator, 742–751, 742t, 743f
  noninvasive positive pressure ventilation, 734–740, 734f, 735f
  oxygen-delivery devices, 720–727, 720f, 721–722t, 721f, 722f
  peak flowmeter, 739–740b, 740f, 741f
  person-centered care, 719
  practice standards for, 718
  principles for practice, 718–719, 719b
  purpose of, 718
  safety guidelines for, 719–720, 720b
  supplemental standards for, 718

P
Pain
  definition of, 443
  management of, evidence-based, 445
  misconceptions, 452t
  musculoskeletal, 164
  rating scale of, 449f
Pain assessment, 443–497, 452t
  assessment, 446, 449f
  basic comfort measures and, 446–453
  delegation in, 446
  documentation in, 451
  equipment for, 446–451
  evaluation, 451
  evidence-based practice of, 445
  hand-off reporting in, 451
  home care and, 453
  implementation, 450, 450f
  interprofessional collaboration of, 446
  in nonverbal patients, 447b
  in older adults, 452–453
  patient education in, 451–452
  in pediatrics, 452
  person-centered care of, 444–445
  planning, 449
  in populations with disabilities, 453

Pain assessment (Continued)
    practice standards of, 444
    principles for practice, 444
    purpose of, 443–444
    safety guidelines for, 445–446
    supplemental standards of, 444
Pain control, noninvasive approaches to, 228
Pain management
  nonpharmacological, 453–460
    assessment, 454
    delegation in, 453
    documentation in, 459
    equipment for, 453–459
    evaluation, 459
    hand-off reporting in, 459
    home care and, 460
    implementation, 455, 455f, 456f
    interprofessional collaboration of, 453
    in older adults, 460
    in pediatrics, 459–460
    planning, 454
    in populations with disabilities, 460
  pharmacological, 460–466
    assessment, 462, 463b
    delegation in, 461
    documentation in, 466
    equipment for, 461–465
    evaluation, 465
    hand-off reporting in, 466
    home care and, 466
    implementation, 464
    interprofessional collaboration of, 461
    in older adults, 466
    opioids, 460–461, 461b
    patient education in, 466
    in pediatrics, 466
    planning, 463
    in populations with disabilities, 466
Palliative care, 498, 499b, 499f
Palliative oxygen, 1237t
Palpation, 113, 114f
  of abdomen, 153, 156f
  of carotid arteries, 145, 145f
Pan Pacific Pressure Injury Alliance National Pressure Ulcer Advisory Panel, 524–525
Pancreatitis, 151–152t
Pandemic, 418b, 422
Papule, 124b
Paracentesis, 240–246, 241–242t
Paralytic ileus, 151–152t
Parens patriae, 897
Parenteral medications, 659–716
  ampules, 664–673, 665f, 667f, 668f, 669f
  continuous subcutaneous infusion, 705–711, 705b, 705f, 708f
  evidence-based practice for, 660
    subcutaneous injection technique, 660
  intradermal injections, 673–677, 675f
  intramuscular injections, 685–692, 686f
  intravenous push, 692–698, 692b, 693b, 695f, 696f
  mixing of, in one syringe, 671b, 671f, 672f
  person-centered care, 660
  piggyback and syringe pumps, 699–705, 701f, 703f
  practice standards for, 659–660
  principles for practice, 660
  purpose of, 659
  safety guidelines for, 660–664, 661f, 661t
    equipment, 662–664
    needlestick prevention, 661–662, 662b, 662f
  subcutaneous injections, 677–685, 678f, 682f, 683f, 684f
  supplemental standards for, 660
  vials, 664–673, 665f, 667f, 668f, 669f
Parenteral nutrition, 966–982
  catheter for, 967f
  central, 970t, 971
  central venous catheter for, 967f

Parenteral nutrition (*Continued*)
complications of, 969–970t
documentation in, 974
evidence-based practice for, 968
home care teaching, 1257–1260
indications for, 967b
monitoring and laboratory orders for, 968b
in older adults, 975, 979
patient education for, 975
in pediatrics, 975, 979
peripheral, 970t, 975–979
peripherally inserted central catheter for, 967f
person-centered care for, 968
practice standards for, 966
principles for practice, 966–968
purpose of, 966
safety guidelines for, 968–970
via infusion pump, 973f
Parietal pleura, 799
Paronychia, 551–552t, 552f
Partial nonrebreather mask, 1236t
Partial-thickness wounds, 1113
Pasero Opioid Sedation Scale (POSS), 445, 463b
Passive motion, 166
Paste, 588t
Patient, rights of, 42–43, 42–43b
Patient care summary, 59
Patient-centered database, 9–10
Patient-controlled analgesia (PCA), 466–472, 466b
assessment, 467
delegation in, 467
discontinue, 470
documentation in, 471
epidural, 473
equipment for, 467–471
evaluation, 471
hand-off reporting in, 471–472
home care and, 472
implementation, 468, 469f
interprofessional collaboration of, 467
in older adults, 472
patient education in, 472
in pediatrics, 472
planning, 468
Patient-controlled epidural analgesia (PCEA), 473
Patient education
alginate dressing, 1187
arterial blood gas measurements, 225
artificial airway, 768
aspirations, 246
assist devices, 355
assisting adults with oral nutrition, 930–931
automated external defibrillator, 830
blood glucose monitoring, 219
blood pressure and pulse measurement, 1232
blood pressure assessment, 103
blood specimen collection, 214
blood transfusion, 907, 911
body temperature, 81, 1227
bronchoscopy, 250
cardiac monitor in, 797
catheterizing a urinary diversion, 1052
central vascular access devices, 893
closed chest drainage systems, 812, 816, 819
cold application, 493
communication by, 25, 30
complete or partial bed bath, 534
continuous subcutaneous infusion, 710, 710b
contrast media studies, 239
dry dressings, 1175
electrocardiogram, 794
for endotracheal tube care, 777
enteral nutrition, 961
epidural analgesia, 478
eye irrigation, 573
fall prevention, 393
feeding tubes
administration, 623
management, 1256

Patient education (*Continued*)
foam dressings, 1187
gastrointestinal endoscopy in, 254
hand hygiene, 263
hearing aids, care of, 581
home environment assessment and safety, 1209
home oxygen equipment, 1242
home setting, for cognitive deficits, 1215
hydrocolloid dressings, 1187
hydrogel dressings, 1187
immobilization devices, 359
incentive spirometry, 734
indwelling urinary catheter, 997, 1008
infusion tubing, 874
intermittent self-catheterization, 1235
intradermal injections, 677
intramuscular injections, 691–692
intravenous flow rates, 867
intravenous moderate sedation, 233
intravenous push, 698
intravenous solutions, 871
isolation precautions, 274
local anesthetic infusion pump, 482
lumbar puncture, 246
managing wound drainage evacuation, 1132
mechanical ventilation, 750
medication self-administration, 1252
metered-dose inhalers, 649, 649b
moist and dry heat applications, 488
mouth care, 547
nail and foot care, 556
nasal instillations, 642
nasotracheal/pharyngeal suctioning, 768
negative-pressure wound therapy, 1138
noninvasive positive pressure ventilation, 739
nose and throat specimens, 196
nutrition screening, 924, 924b
ophthalmic medications, 634
oral hygiene, 542
oral medications, 617
oropharyngeal suctioning, 759
oxygen therapy, 726–727, 730
pain assessment, 451–452
parenteral nutrition, 1260
patient care
after biological exposure, 429
after chemical exposure, 434
after natural disaster, 440
after radiation exposure, 437
patient-controlled analgesia, 472
peripheral intravenous device, 860
peripheral intravenous dressing, 878
pharmacological pain management, 466
physical restraints, 405
piggyback infusion, 704
positioning patients, 321
pouching a colostomy, or ileostomy, 1046
pouching a urostomy, 1050
pressure bandage, 1178
pressure injuries, 1153–1154
promoting early activity and exercise, 331
pulse measurement, 1227–1232
apical, 90
radial, 86
record, 59
removing sutures and staples, 1127
respiratory assessment in, 94–95
restraint-free environment, 398
resuscitation management, 837
seizure precautions, 413
small-bore feeding tube, 948
small-volume nebulizers, 653
special beds, 377
sputum specimens, 203
sterile gloving, 291
subcutaneous injections, 685
support surfaces, 372
supporting patients and families in grief, 503
suprapubic catheter care, 1016

Patient education (*Continued*)
symptom management at end of life, 509
syringe pumps, 704
topical medications, 628
tracheostomy care, 786, 1247
transferring patients, 311
transparent dressings, 1181
urinary catheterization, 997, 1008
urine specimen collection, 185–186
vaginal or urethral discharge specimens, 199
wound drainage specimens, 206
wound irrigation, 1122
Patient preparation, for surgery, 1075–1079
Patient safety, 382, 384f
evidence-based practice of, 383–384
person-centered care of, 383
practice standards of, 383
principles for practice, 383
purpose of, 382
safety guidelines for, 384
supplemental standards of, 383
Patient status, in clinical decision making, 6–7
Patient transitions, errors in, 41
PCA. *see* Patient-controlled analgesia
PCEA. *see* Patient-controlled epidural analgesia
Peak concentration, 589
Peak expiratory flow rate (PEFR), 739
Peak flowmeter, 739–740b, 740f, 741f
Peak pressure, 95
Pediatric patients
abdominal assessment in, 157
admission of, 49
alginate dressing in, 1187
anxiety in, 30
applying physical restraints in, 405
arterial blood gas measurements in, 225
artificial airway in, 768
aspiration precautions in, 937
aspiration procedures in, 246
assist devices in, 355
assisting adults with oral nutrition in, 931
automated external defibrillator in, 830
blood glucose monitoring in, 219
blood pressure and pulse measurement in, 1232
blood pressure assessment in, 103
blood specimen collection in, 214
blood transfusion in, 908, 911
body temperature measurements in, 81–82, 1227
bronchoscopy in, 250
cardiac monitor in, 797
cardiovascular assessment in, 151
care of body after death in, 513
central vascular access devices in, 893
closed chest drainage systems in, 812, 816
cognitively impaired, communication with, 33
cold application in, 493
complete or partial bed bath in, 534
continuous subcutaneous infusion in, 710
contrast media studies in, 239
depression in, 30
dry dressings in, 1175
ear irrigation in, 576
ear medications in, 638
electrocardiogram in, 794
endotracheal tube care in, 777
enema in, 1028
enteral nutrition in, 953
epidural analgesia in, 478
eye irrigation in, 573
fall prevention in, 393
feeding tubes in
administration of, 623
management of, 953, 1256
foam dressings in, 1187
gastrointestinal endoscopy in, 254
general survey for, 126
head and neck assessment in, 131–132
headaches in, 132
hearing aids, care of, 581

Pediatric patients (*Continued*)
  home environment assessment and safety in, 1209
  home oxygen equipment for, 1242
  home oxygen therapy for, 1242
  home setting, for cognitive deficits in, 1216
  hydrocolloid dressings in, 1187
  hydrogel dressings in, 1187
  immobilization devices in, 359
  incentive spirometry in, 734
  indwelling urinary catheter insertion in, 997
  intermittent self-catheterization in, 1235
  intradermal injections in, 677
  intramuscular injections, 692
  intravenous flow rates in, 867
  intravenous moderate sedation in, 233
  intravenous push in, 698
  isolation precautions for, 274–275
  local anesthetic infusion pump in, 482
  managing wound drainage evacuation in, 1132
  mechanical ventilation in, 750–751
  medication and medical device safety in, 1220
  medication self-administration in, 1252
  metered-dose inhalers in, 649
  moist and dry heat applications in, 489
  mouth care in, 547
  musculoskeletal assessment in, 170
  nail and foot care in, 556
  nasal instillations in, 642
  nasogastric tube for, 1036
  nasotracheal/pharyngeal suctioning in, 768
  negative-pressure wound therapy in, 1138
  noninvasive positive pressure ventilation in, 739
  nonpharmacological pain management in,
    459–460
  nose and throat specimens from, 196
  nurse-patient relationship in, 25
  nutrition screening in, 924
  occult blood
    in gastric secretions, 192
    in stool specimen, 189–190
  ophthalmic medications in, 634
  oral hygiene in, 542
  oral medications in, 617
  oropharyngeal airway in, 827
  oropharyngeal suctioning in, 759
  oxygen therapy in, 726
  pain assessment in, 452
  parenteral nutrition in, 975, 979, 1260
  patient care in
    after biological exposure, 429
    after chemical exposure, 434
    after natural disaster, 440–441
    after radiation exposure, 437
  patient preparation for surgery of, 1079
  patient-controlled analgesia in, 472
  peripheral intravenous device in, 860–861
  peripheral intravenous dressing in, 878
  pharmacological pain management in, 466
  physical assessment of, 116–117
  piggyback infusion in, 704
  positioning, 321
  pouching a colostomy, or ileostomy in, 1046
  pouching a urostomy in, 1050
  preoperative assessment for, 1065
  preoperative teaching for, 1073
  pressure bandage in, 1178
  pressure injuries in, 1154, 1159
  promoting early activity and exercise in, 331
  pulse measurement in
    apical, 90
    radial, 86
  respiratory assessment in, 95
  resuscitation management in, 837
  seizure precautions in, 413
  separation anxiety in, 45
  small-bore feeding tube in, 948
  small-volume nebulizers in, 653
  special beds in, 377
  sputum specimens in, 203

Pediatric patients (*Continued*)
  subcutaneous injections in, 685
  support surfaces in, 372–373
  supporting patients and families in grief in, 503
  suture removal in, 1128
  symptom management at end of life in, 509
  syringe pumps in, 704
  thorax and lung assessment in, 139–140
  tracheostomy care in, 787, 1247
  transferring, 311
  transparent dressings in, 1181
  urine specimen collection in, 185, 185f
  vaginal or urethral discharge specimens in, 199
  who have difficulty coping, communication
    with, 30
  wound drainage specimens in, 206
  wound irrigation in, 1122
Pediculosis capitis, 547–548t
Pediculosis corporis, 547–548t
Pediculosis pubis, 547–548t
PEEP. *see* Positive end-expiratory pressure
PEFR. *see* Peak expiratory flow rate
Penrose drain, 1128, 1128f, 1169f
Peptic ulcers, 151–152t
Perception, sharing, 20b
Percutaneous endoscopic gastrostomy (PEG) tube,
    618, 962–963b, 962f
Perineal care, 534–535b
  clean, before urinary catheterization, 993f
  for female, 535f
  for male, 535f
Periodontal membrane, 524
Periodontitis, 529
Peripheral arteries, palpation of, 147
Peripheral intravenous device, 846–861, 846f,
    846t, 850f, 851f, 852f, 853f, 854f, 857f,
    858f, 860t
  assessment, 847
  in children, 860–861
  delegation in, 846
  discontinuing, 878, 879f
  documentation in, 860
  equipment for, 846–860
  evaluation, 858
  hand-off reporting in, 860
  home care in, 861
  implementation, 848
  in older adults, 861
  patient education in, 860
  in patients with disabilities, 861
  planning, 848
Peripheral intravenous dressing, 874–878, 876f
  assessment, 875
  in children, 878
  delegation in, 875
  documentation in, 878
  equipment for, 875–878
  evaluation, 878
  hand-off reporting in, 878
  home care in, 878
  implementation, 876
  in older adults, 878
  patient education in, 878
  planning, 875
Peripheral parenteral nutrition, 970t
  with lipid (fat) emulsion, 975–979
    assessment in, 976
    documentation in, 979
    evaluation, 978
    hand-off reporting in, 979
    implementation, 977
    in older adults, 979
    patient education for, 979
    in pediatrics, 979
    planning, 976
Peripheral vascular access device, 846t
Peripherally inserted central catheters (PICCs),
    279, 880t, 881f, 967f
Perseverance, 11t, 12

Personal hygiene, 519–564
  evidence-based practice of, 521
  of hair, 524
  of nail, 524
  person-centered care of, 521
  practice standards of, 520–521
  principles for practice, 521
  purpose of, 520
  safety guidelines for, 521–522
  of skin, 522, 522–523t
  supplemental standards of, 521
Personal protective equipment (PPE), 423, 423f
  application of, 270, 270f
  for isolation precautions, 269
  for patients under isolation precautions, 267
  removal of, 272, 273f
  for sterile field, 283
  for transmission-based precautions, 270f
Personal self-disclosure, 21
Person-centered care
  blood transfusion, 897
  in bowel elimination, 1019
  diagnostic procedures, 228
  in dressings, 1165
  enteral nutrition, 941
  for home care safety, 1199
  home care teaching, 1223
  in intraoperative care, 1096
  in medical asepsis, 262
  nutrition screening, 917–918, 918f
  for ostomy care, 1039–1040
  for parenteral nutrition, 968
  for postoperative care, 1060
  specimen collection, 179
  for urinary elimination, 985
Pétrissage, 455, 455f
pH, urine screening for, 179
Pharmacokinetics, 587–588
Pharmacological pain management, 460–466
  assessment, 462, 463b
  delegation in, 461
  documentation in, 466
  equipment for, 461–465
  evaluation, 465
  hand-off reporting in, 466
  home care and, 466
  implementation, 464
  interprofessional collaboration of, 461
  in older adults, 466
  opioids, 460–461, 461b
  patient education in, 466
  in pediatrics, 466
  planning, 463
  in populations with disabilities, 466
Phlebitis, 859
Physical Activity Guidelines for Americans,
    325–326
Physical assessment
  of adolescents, 116–117
  of children, 116–117
  of older adults, 117
Physical dependence, 591
Physical examination, in nutrition screening,
    920, 920t
Physical restraints
  application of, 398–408, 399b
    assessment, 394, 399
    delegation in, 399
    documentation in, 405
    equipment for, 399–404
    evaluation in, 404
    hand-off reporting in, 405
    home care and, 405–408
    implementation, 400, 401f, 402f, 403f
    interprofessional collaboration of, 399
    in older adults, 405
    patient education in, 405
    in pediatrics, 405
    in populations with disabilities, 405

Physical restraints (Continued)
belt restraint, self-releasing roll, 401, 402f
elbow restraint, 401, 401f
mitten restraint, 401, 401f
soft extremity (ankle or wrist) restraint, 402, 402f
Physiological normal saline, 1024t
PICCs. see Peripherally inserted central catheters
PIEB. see Programmed intermittent epidural bolus
Piggyback infusion, 699–705, 701f, 703f
assessment, 699
in children, 704
delegation in, 699
documentation in, 704
equipment for, 699–704
evaluation, 704
hand-off reporting in, 704
home care in, 705
implementation, 700
interprofessional collaboration, 699
in older adults, 704–705
patient education in, 704
planning, 700
in populations with disabilities, 705
Pill-crushing device, 614f
Pillow placement, 1152f
Pinch-off syndrome, 891–892t
Pitting edema, 147, 147f
Plague, 425–426t
Plantar flexion, 1071
Plantar warts, 551–552t, 551f
Plastic face mask with reservoir bag, 721f
Platelets, 896f, 900t
Pleura, 799
Pleural effusion, 799, 800
Pleural friction rub, 133, 133–134t
Pleural space, 799
Pleur-evac drainage system, 807f, 810t
Pneumonia, 720
aspiration, 932
ventilator-associated, 742–743, 744, 745b, 754
Pneumothorax, 799, 800, 969–970t
tension, 800, 810t
traumatic, 800
in vascular access devices, 891–892t
Pocket mask, 834f
Point of maximal impulse (PMI), 88, 88f, 89f, 141, 143f
Polypharmacy, 466
Popliteal pulse, 82t, 148, 149f
Positioning patients
assessment in, 313
in bed, 313–321
body mechanics during, 297b
in children, 321
delegation in, 313
documentation in, 321
equipment for, 313–321
hand-off reporting in, 321
in home care, 321
implementation in, 314
interprofessional collaboration of, 313
logrolling, 319, 320f
in older adults, 321
patient education in, 321
planning in, 314
using friction-reducing device, 315f
for wound irrigation, 1119f
Positive end-expiratory pressure (PEEP), 743t
Positive expiratory pressure (PEP) device, 1070f
Positive pressure ventilation, 742–743, 743f see also Mechanical ventilation
POSS. see Pasero Opioid Sedation Scale
Postanesthesia care unit (PACU)
Aldrete score for, 1081t
immediate anesthesia recovery in, 1079–1087, 1080t, 1082f, 1083f, 1085b
Postanesthetic Discharge Scoring System (PADSS), 231t, 1081t
Posterior thorax, 136, 136f, 137f

Posterior tibial pulse, 82t, 148, 149f
Postoperative care, 1057–1094
convalescent phase (Phase III) recovery, 1087–1093
discharge criteria for, 1085b
early, 1087–1093
evidence-based practice for, 1060
immediate anesthesia recovery in, 1079–1087, 1080t, 1082f, 1083f, 1085b
person-centered care for, 1060
practice standards for, 1059
principles for practice, 1060
purpose of, 1059
safety guidelines, 1060–1061
splinting incisions, 1071f
Postural alignment, 166
Postural hypotension, 342
Posture, assessment of, 121, 121f
Pouching
of colostomy, 1039f, 1040–1050, 1041f, 1044f
of ileostomy, 1039f, 1040–1050, 1041f, 1044f
of urostomy, 1046–1050, 1047f
Powder, 588t, 623
Power source, in hearing aids, 577
PPE. see Personal protective equipment
Premature ventricular contractions (PVCs), 145t, 790t
Preoperative care, 1057–1094
assessment for, 1061–1065, 1063f
evidence-based practice for, 1060
person-centered care for, 1060
practice standards for, 1059
preoperative teaching on, 1065–1075, 1068f, 1069f, 1070f, 1071f, 1072f
principles for practice, 1060
purpose of, 1059
safety guidelines, 1060–1061
Preoperative teaching, 1065–1075, 1068f, 1069f, 1070f, 1071f, 1072f
Prepackaged enema container, 1025f
Pressure bandage, application of, 1175–1178, 1177f
assessment, 1175
in children, 1178
documentation in, 1178
evaluation, 1177
hand-off reporting in, 1178
home care in, 1178
implementation, 1176t
in older adults, 1178
patient education in, 1178
in pediatrics, 1178
planning, 1176
in populations with disabilities, 1178
Pressure injuries, 362
bony prominences in, 1142, 1142f
Braden Scale for, 1147
contributing factors for, 362
definition of, 1141
evidence-based practice for, 1145–1146
friction in, 1147, 1151, 1152
immobilization device-related, strategies to prevent, 1150t
medical device-related, strategies to prevent, 1150t
in older adults, 1154, 1159
in pediatrics, 1154, 1159
person-centered care in, 1145, 1145b
practice standards of, 1141
prevention and care, 365, 1141–1161
prevention strategies for, 1146–1154, 1147t, 1150t, 1152f
principles for practice in, 1141–1145
purpose of, 1141
risk assessment for, 1146–1154, 1147t, 1150t, 1152f
safety guidelines for, 1146
sites for, 1142
skin assessment for, 1146–1154, 1147t, 1150t, 1152f

Pressure injuries (Continued)
staging of, 1143–1144b
treatment of, 1154–1160, 1156f
Pressure redistribution support surface, 365–368b, 367f
Pressure support ventilation (PSV), 742t
Pressure Ulcer Scale for Healing (PUSH) tool, 1154
Pressure-regulated volume-control ventilation (PRCV or PRVC), 742t
Pressurized metered-dose inhalers (pMDIs), 642
Primary wound healing, 1111, 1164
Problem list, 61–62
Problem solving
critical thinking in, 4–5
effective, 5
Problem-oriented medical records, 61–62
Professional standards, for critical thinking, 13
Programmed intermittent epidural bolus (PIEB), 473
Progress notes, 62
Progressive diet, 926t
Progressive relaxation, with deep breathing, 457
Prone position, 116t
Prostate cancer, 159
Protected health information (PHI), 43
Protein screening, in urine specimen, 179
Pruritus, 590t
Psychological dependence, 591
Pulp, of teeth, 524f
Pulse
apical, 144
measurement, 1230
client teaching on, 1227–1232
home care teaching, 1227
radial, 82–86, 82t, 83f, 1230f
sites for, 82t
Pulse deficit, 90
Pulse oximetry, 92, 106b, 107f
Pulsed lavage, 1117
Pupillary reflexes, 128, 128f
Pupils, inspection of, 128
Pureed diet, 926t
Purulent wound drainage, 1165b
Pustule, 124b
PVCs. see Premature ventricular contractions

Q
Quad cane, 346f

R
Radial pulse, 147, 148f, 1230f
assessment, 83
delegation in, 83
in disabled patients, 86
documentation in, 85
equipment, 83–85
evaluation, 85
hand-off reporting in, 86
implementation, 84, 84f
interprofessional collaboration, 83
in older adults, 86
patient education in, 86
in pediatric patients, 86
planning, 84
Radiation exposure, patient care after, 434–438
assessment, 435
delegation in, 435
documentation in, 437
equipment for, 435–437
evaluation, 437
hand-off reporting in, 437
home care and, 438
implementation, 436
interprofessional collaboration of, 435
in older adults, 438
patient education in, 437
in pediatrics, 437
planning, 436
in populations with disabilities, 438

Range-of-motion (ROM)
    assessment of, 166, 167t
    exercises
        activities of daily living incorporation of, 332t
        delegation in, 332
        equipment for, 332
        interprofessional collaboration of, 332
        performing, 331–337b
        step of, 332–337, 333–336t, 337b
        support during, 333f
Rapid Estimate of Adult Literacy in Medicine, 21
Rash, 590t
Ratio-and-proportion method, 601b, 602
Reactive hyperemia, 123
Read-back, 63
Receiver
    in communication process, 41
    in hearing aids, 577
Records
    electronic health, 45, 52, 53b, 58–61
    problem-oriented medical, 61–62
Rectal measurement, of body temperature, 73b, 77, 78f
Rectal suppositories, 655–657b, 656f
Rectum assessment, 157–162
Recurrent turn, of bandage, 1188f, 1188t
Red blood cells (RBCs), 900t
    count, 91
Refeeding syndrome, 970
Reflection, 20b
    in clinical judgment, 13–14, 13b
Refocusing, 20b
Relaxation, 453
Rescue breathing, 833t
Reservoir nasal cannula, 1236
Resident assessment instrument (RAI), 47
RESPECT model, 111, 112f
Respirations, assessment of, 91–95, 91f, 94b
    delegation in, 91
    documentation in, 94
    equipment for, 91–94
    evaluation, 94
    hand-off reporting in, 94
    home care in, 95
    implementation, 93
    interprofessional collaboration, 91
    in older adults, 95
    patient education in, 94–95
    in pediatric patients, 95
    planning, 92
Respirator masks, fit-testing for, 270, 271b
Respiratory depression, 465
Respiratory rate (R or RR), 743t
Responsibility, 11, 11t
Restating, 20b
Restraint-free environment, 394–398, 394b
    assessment, 394
    delegation in, 394
    documentation in, 398
    equipment for, 394–397
    evaluation, 397
    hand-off reporting in, 398
    home care and, 398
    implementation, 396
    interprofessional collaboration of, 394
    in older adults, 398
    patient education in, 398
    planning, 395
Restraints
    patients' rights regarding, 42–43b
    physical
        application of, 398–408, 399b
        belt restraint, self-releasing roll, 401, 402f
        elbow restraint, 401, 401f
        mitten restraint, 401, 401f
        soft extremity (ankle or wrist) restraint, 402, 402f
Restricted fluids diet, 926t

Resuscitation management, 830–837, 831f, 832f, 833f, 833t, 834f, 835f
    assessment, 831
    in children, 837
    delegation in, 830
    documentation in, 837
    equipment for, 831–837, 831f
    evaluation, 836
    hand-off reporting in, 837
    home care in, 837
    implementation, 832
    interprofessional collaboration of, 830–831
    in older adults, 837
    patient education in, 837
    planning, 831
Retainers, 129
Reusable thermometer, 74b
Reverse Trendelenburg position, 557–558t, 558f
Rh system, 897
Rhinitis, 590t
Rhonchi, 133, 133–134t
Rigid gas permeable (RGP) lens, 567–569b
Rinsing, of teeth, 538
Risk taking, 11–12, 11t
ROHO cushion, for wheelchair, 368f
Romberg's test, 169
Rotation therapy, indications for, 363–364t
Routes of administration, for medication, 591, 591t, 592t

S
Safe medication preparation, 585–607
    dosage calculation, 600–602
        conversions within one system, 600
        dimensional analysis method, 601–602, 601b
        formula method, 601, 601b
        in older adults, 602, 602b
        pediatric doses, 602
        ratio-and-proportion method, 601b, 602
    evidence-based practice in, 603
    interpreting medication labels, 600, 600f
    medication action, 589–591
        adverse drug reactions, 589–590
        allergic reactions, 590, 590f, 590t
        idiosyncratic reactions, 591
        medication interactions, 591
        medication misuse, 591
        medication tolerance and dependence, 591
        side effects, 590–591
        therapeutic effects, 589
        toxic effects, 591
    medication administration in, 596–600, 596b
        right documentation, 599–600
        right dose, 598
        right medication, 597–598
        right patient, 598, 598f, 599f
        right route, 598–599
        right time, 599
    medication distribution in, 593–595
        automated medication dispensing system, 593, 593f
        bar-coding, 594–595
        computerized provider order entry, 593
        distribution systems, 593
        handling chemotherapy medications in, 594, 595f
        special handling of controlled substances, 593–594, 594b, 594f
        unit dose, 593
    medication dose responses, 588–589, 589f
    medication errors
        prevention, 603, 603b
        reporting, 605
    medication measurement systems in, 595
        household measurement, 595, 596t
        metric system, 595
        solutions, 595
    nursing process in, 603–605
        assessment, 603–604

Safe medication preparation (Continued)
        evaluation, 604–605
        implementation, 604
        medication administration, 604
        planning, 604
        preadministration activities, 604
    patient and family caregiver teaching in, 605
    person-centered care, 596–602
    pharmacological concepts in
        classification, 587
        medication forms, 587, 588t
        medication names, 587
        pharmacokinetics, 587–588
    practice standards in, 587
    principles for practice, 587–595
    routes of administration, 591, 591t, 592t
Safe patient handling and mobility (SPHM), 295–323
    algorithm for, 301f
    evidence-based practice of, 297–298
    person-centered care in, 297
    practice standards of, 296
    principles for, 296–297
    programs, efficacy of, 297–298
    purpose of, 296, 297b, 297f
    safety guidelines for, 298
    supplemental standards of, 296
Safety guidelines
    for airway management, 754–755
    for blood transfusion, 898–899t, 898–900
    for bowel elimination, 1019–1024
    for cardiac care, 791
    for catheterization, 985–987, 985b
    for closed chest drainage systems, 802–803
    for communication, 19
    for community, 1199
    for diagnostic procedures, 228–229
    for disaster preparedness, 422–424, 422b, 423b, 423f
    for discharge planning, 41
    for documentation, 55
    for dressings, 1165b, 1166
    for end-of-life care, 500
    for enteral nutrition, 941
    for exercise, 326
    for eye care, 566–569
    feeding tubes, 941
    for health assessment, 112–113
    for home care safety, 1199
    for intraoperative care, 1097–1098
    for life support, 824
    for medical asepsis, 262–263
    for nonparenteral medications, 609–610
    for oral nutrition, 919, 919b
    for ostomy care, 1040
    for oxygen therapy, 719–720, 720b
    for pain assessment, 445–446
    for parenteral medications, 660–664, 661f, 661t
    for parenteral nutrition, 968–970
    for patient safety, 384
    for personal hygiene, 521–522
    for postoperative care, 1060–1061
    for preoperative care, 1060–1061
    for pressure injuries, 1146
    for specimen collection, 179
    for sterile technique, 278
    for support surfaces, 365–368
    for transfer process, 41
    for urinary elimination, 985–987
    for vital signs, 71–72
    for wound care and irrigation, 1114–1116, 1114f
Salem sump tube, 1029, 1029f
Saline flush, 696
Saline lock, 693
Saline solutions, 843t
Saliva, 523–524
Sanguineous wound drainage, 1165b
SBAR documentation, 45–46, 62
Scalp, problems of, 547–548t

Scar tissue formation, 891–892t
Scientific method, 4, 5t
Scoliosis, 166f, 170
Scrub nurse, 1096b
Sebum, 522
Seclusion, 42–43b
Secondary wound healing, 1111, 1164
Sedation scales, 445
Seizure, precautions, 408–413, 408b, 409b, 410f
   delegation in, 408
   documentation in, 413
   equipment for, 409
   hand-off reporting in, 413
   home care and, 413
   interprofessional collaboration of, 409
   in older adults, 413
   patient education in, 413
   in pediatrics, 413
Self-administration, of medications, 1248–1253, 1250f
Self-awareness, 11t, 12
Self-catheterization, intermittent, teaching, 1232–1236
Self-disclosure, personal, 21
Semi-Fowler position, 316, 316f, 317f, 557–558t, 557f
Sender, 41
Separation anxiety, 45
Sepsis, 891–892t
   catheter-related, 969–970t
Sequential compression device (SCD), 337–342b, 338f
   delegation in, 338
   equipment for, 338
   step of, 338–342, 339b, 339f, 340f, 341f
Serosanguineous wound drainage, 1165b
Serous wound drainage, 1165b
Sexually transmitted infection (STI), 196
Shampooing, hair, 550b, 550f
Sharp debridement, 1113
Shaving, hair, 547–550b, 549f
Short-burst oxygen, 1237t
Shoulders, range-of-motion in
   assessment of, 167t
   exercise for, 332t, 333–336t
Shower, 525b, 536–538b, 537f
Side effects, 590–591
Sigmoid colostomy, 1039f
Silence, 20b
Silent aspiration, 932
Simple face mask, 1236t
SIMV. see Synchronized intermittent mandatory ventilation
Single (one-time) orders, 597
Single-lumen catheters, 987–998, 988f
Sinus arrhythmia, 145t
Sinus bradycardia, 145t, 790t, 822f
Sinus rhythm, normal, 790t
Sinus tachycardia, 145t, 790t, 822f
Sinuses, inspection of, 129
Sitting position, 116t
Situation awareness, in clinical decision making, 7
Sitz bath, 486, 487f, 525
Skeletal vertebra, 472f
Skin
   barrier, 1040
   color variations, 119t
   erosion, 891–892t
   layers of, 1110, 1111f
   lesions, 124b
   personal hygiene of, 522, 522–523t
   rashes, 522–523t, 523f
   turgor, assessment of, 123, 123f
Skin puncture
   for blood glucose monitoring, 215
   for blood specimen collection, 206
Slide board, for transferring patients, 307, 308f
Slide clamps, for CVAD, 888f

Small-bore feeding tube
   assessment, 942
   delegation in, 942
   dislocation of, 949–950
   documentation in, 948
   equipment for, 942–948
   evaluation, 948
   hand-off reporting in, 948
   home care in, 949
   implementation, 943
   inserting, 942–949, 942f, 944f, 945f, 946f, 947f
   interprofessional collaboration in, 942
   in older adults, 948
   patient education of, 948
   in pediatrics, 948
   planning, 943
   in populations with disabilities, 949
   removing, 942–949
Smallpox variola virus, 425–426t
Small-volume nebulizers, 649–657, 651f
   assessment, 650
   in children, 653
   delegation in, 649
   documentation in, 653
   equipment for, 649–652
   evaluation, 652
   hand-off reporting in, 653
   home care in, 653–657
   implementation, 651
   interprofessional collaboration for, 649
   in older adults, 653
   patient education in, 653–657
   planning, 650
   in populations with disabilities, 653
Smoking, 132, 134
Soapsuds enema (SSE), 1024t
Sodium-restricted diet, 926t
Soft diet, 926t
Soft extremity (ankle or wrist) restraint, 402, 402f
Soft fiber diet, 926t
Soft splints, 356t
Solutions (medication), 588t, 595
Source records, 58
Special beds, 362–380, 363–364t
   assessment, 374
   in children, 377
   delegation in, 374
   documentation in, 377
   equipment for, 374
   evaluation, 376
   flow diagram for ordering, 367f
   hand-off reporting in, 377
   home care and, 377
   implementation, 375
   interprofessional collaboration of, 374
   in older adults, 377
   patient education in, 377
   patient on, care for, 373–377
   planning, 375
   in populations with disabilities, 377
Specimen collection, 177–226
   arterial specimen for blood gas measurement, 220–225, 221f, 223f, 224f
   biohazard bag for, 272f
   blood glucose monitoring, 215–219, 215f, 217f, 218f
   blood specimens and culture by venipuncture (syringe and vacutainer method), 206–214, 209f, 210f, 211f, 212f, 213f
   evidence-based practice, 179
   nose specimens for culture, 192–196, 194f, 195f
   occult blood
      in gastric secretions (Gastroccult), 190–192, 191f
      in stool, 187–190, 187f, 189f
   person-centered care, 179
   practice standards, 178
   principles for practice, 179
   purpose, 178

Specimen collection (Continued)
   safety guidelines, 179
   sputum
      by expectoration, 199b
      by suction, 200–203, 202f
   throat specimens for culture, 192–196, 194f, 195f
   in transmission-based precautions, 272
   urine
      equipment for, 180–185
      in females, 182, 183f
      in males, 180f, 182, 182f
      midstream (clean-voided), 179–186, 180f, 182f, 183f
      screening for glucose, ketones, protein, blood, and pH, 179
      timed, 185–186b
      from urinary catheter, 179–186, 183f, 184f
   vaginal or urethral discharge specimens, 196–199
   wound drainage specimens, 203–206
Specimen hat, 180f
SPHM. see Safe patient handling and mobility
Sphygmomanometers, 1230
Spinal anesthesia, 1080t
Spiral turn, of bandage, 1188f, 1188t
Spiral-reverse turn, of bandage, 1188f, 1188t
Spirometer, use of, 1069f
Splint, 355
Splinting incisions, 1071f
Sponge bath, 525b
Standardized care plans, 60
Staples, removal of, 1122–1128, 1124f, 1125f
   in children, 1128
   delegation in, 1123
   documentation in, 1127
   equipment for, 1123–1127
   hand-off reporting in, 1127
   in older adults, 1128
   patient education in, 1127
   in pediatrics, 1128
START (Simple Triage and Rapid Treatment) triage system, 421–422, 421f
Stationary reservoir, 1240f
Status epilepticus, 411
Sterile field
   preparation of, 282–287, 284f, 285f, 286f
   solutions poured into receiving container on, 286, 286f
   sterile items added to, 286, 286f
Sterile gloving, 287–291, 289f, 290f
   assessment in, 288
   delegation in, 288
   documentation in, 291
   equipment for, 288–291
   hand-off reporting in, 291
   patient education for, 291
   planning, 289
Sterile gown, donning, 1102–1105, 1103f, 1104f
Sterile kit, 284, 284f, 285f
Sterile technique, 277–294
   cap, applying and removing, 279–282, 280f
   evidence-based practice, 278
   eyewear, applying and removing, 279–282, 280f
   gloving, 287–291, 289f, 290f
   mask, applying and removing, 279–282, 280f, 281f
   person-centered care, 278
   practice standards, 277
   principles for practice, 277, 278b
   purpose of, 277
   safety guidelines, 278
   sterile field. see Sterile field
Sterile urinary catheter, for urine specimen collection, 179–186, 183f, 184f
Sterile urine specimen, from urinary catheter, 180–185
Steri-Strips, 1126, 1126f
Sternal notch, 88f

Stethoscope, 114b
  acoustic, 86f
  for apical pulse assessment, 86
  for auscultation, 114–115, 114b
  Doppler ultrasonic, 102f
  use of, 1230
Stoma
  budded, 1041f
  measurement of, 1044f
  retracted, 1041f
Stool specimen, occult blood measurements in, 187–190, 187f, 189f
STOP-Bang questionnaire, 44
Stratum corneum, 1110
Stratum germinativum, 1110
Stratum granulosum, 1110
Stratum lucidum, 1110
Stratum spinosum, 1110
Stretch marks, 154
Stretcher, transferring patients to, 307, 308f, 309f, 310f
Subcutaneous injections, 677–685, 678f, 682f, 683f, 684f
  administration of
    heparin, 679–680, 679b
    insulin, 678–679, 679t
  assessment, 680
  in children, 685
  delegation in, 680
  documentation in, 685
  equipment for, 680–685
  evaluation, 684
  hand-off reporting in, 685
  home care in, 685
  implementation, 681
  interprofessional collaboration, 680
  in older adults, 685
  patient education in, 685
  planning, 681
  in populations with disabilities, 685
Subcutaneous tissue, 522
Subjective Global Assessment (SGA), 920b
Sublingual tablet, 616f
Suction, sputum collection by, 200–203, 202f
Sufentanil, 473
Suggesting, 20b
Supine position, 116t, 557–558t, 558f
Support surfaces, 362–380, 363–364t
  assessment, 370
  in children, 372–373
  delegation in, 369
  disabilities and, populations with, 373
  documentation in, 372
  evaluation, 376
  evidence-based practice of, 365
  hand-off reporting in, 372
  home care and, 373
  implementation, 375
  interprofessional collaboration of, 369
  nonpowered, 368
  in older adults, 373
  patient education in, 372
  person-centered care in, 364–365
  planning, 375
  practice standards of, 362
  pressure redistribution, 365–368b, 367f
  prevention of pressure injuries and, 365
  principles for, 362–363
  purpose of, 362
  safety guidelines for, 365–368
  supplemental standards of, 362
Suppository, 588t
  rectal, 655–657b, 656f
  vaginal, 653–655b, 653f, 654f, 655f
Suprapubic catheter, care for, 1013–1016, 1013f, 1015f
  assessment, 1013
  delegation in, 1013
  documentation in, 1016

Suprapubic catheter, care for (Continued)
  equipment for, 1013–1016
  evaluation, 1015
  hand-off reporting in, 1016
  home care, 1016
  implementation, 1014
  interprofessional collaboration in, 1013
  patient education, 1016
  planning, 1014
Surgery
  informed consent for, 1076t
  in older adults, 1074t
  patient preparation for, 1075–1079
  positive expiratory pressure device after, 1070f
Surgical hand antisepsis, 263, 1098–1101, 1099f, 1100f
  assessment, 1098
  delegation in, 1098
  documentation in, 1101
  equipment for, 1098
  evaluation, 1101
  hand-off reporting in, 1101
  implementation, 1099
  interprofessional collaboration, 1098
  planning, 1098
Surgical safety checklist, 1096, 1097f
Surgical site infections (SSIs), prevention of, 278
Suspension-based lotion, 627
Sustained release medication, 588t
Suture line, 1123
Sutures, removal of, 1122–1128, 1122f, 1125f
  in children, 1128
  continuous and blanket stitch, 1126, 1126f
  delegation in, 1123
  documentation in, 1127
  equipment for, 1123–1127
  hand-off reporting in, 1127
  interrupted, 1125f
  in older adults, 1128
  patient education in, 1127
  in pediatrics, 1128
Sweat glands, 522
Swing-through gait, 350
Swing-to gait, 351, 351f
Synchronized intermittent mandatory ventilation (SIMV), 742t
Syringe pumps, 699–705, 701f, 703f
  assessment, 699
  in children, 704
  delegation in, 699
  documentation in, 704
  equipment for, 699–704
  evaluation, 704
  hand-off reporting in, 704
  home care in, 705
  implementation, 700
  interprofessional collaboration, 699
  in older adults, 704–705
  patient education in, 704
  planning, 700
  in populations with disabilities, 705
Syringes, 662–663, 663f
  insulin, 663, 663f
  Luer-Lok, 662–663, 663f
  with magnifier, 1218f
  method, venipuncture, 209, 210f, 211f
  Non-Luer-Lok, 662–663, 663f
  tuberculin, 663, 663f
Syringes, for liquid medication, 614f
Syrup, 588t

T
Tablets, 588t
  buccal administration of, 616f
  crushing of, 614f
  orally disintegrating, 615
  sublingual, 616f

Tachycardia
  sinus, 145t, 790t, 822f
  ventricular, 790t, 822f
Tachypnea, 94b, 931–932
Tamper-evident syringe, 594f
Tap water, for irrigation, 570
Tap-water (hypotonic) enema, 1024t
Tears, 566–567b
Technological disasters, 418b
Teeth, 524, 524f
Telehealth, 1199
Telephone Interview for Cognitive Status (TICS), 1199
Telephone orders (TOs), 63, 63b
Temperature, body. see Body temperature
Temporal artery temperature, 73b, 80, 80f
Temporal artery thermometer, 74b, 74f
Temporal pulse, 82t
Tension pneumothorax, 800, 810t
Tertiary intention, wound healing, 1112
Test strip, 952f
Testes, palpation of, 161
Testicular self-examination, 157–158b
The Joint Commission (TJC)
  documentation guidelines, 52
  National Patient Safety Goals, 1075
  Patient and Family Education Standards, 1073b
  patient's rights, 42–43, 43b
Theme identification, 20b
Therapeutic communication, 17, 18, 20b, 22f
Therapeutic diet, 926t
Therapeutic effects, medication action, 589
Therapeutic foot boots, 316f
Thermometers
  chemical dot single-use, 74b, 74f
  electronic, 74b, 74f
  reusable, 74b
  temporal artery, 74b, 74f
  tympanic membrane, 74b, 74f
  types of, 74b
Thinking independently, 10–11, 11t
30-degree lateral side-lying position, 313, 1152f
  in bed, 318, 318f, 319f
Thoracentesis, 240–246, 241–242t
Thorax
  anterior, 138, 138f
  assessment of, 132–140, 132f
    in children, 139–140
    delegation in, 134
    documentation in, 139
    equipment for, 134
    evaluation in, 139
    hand-off reporting in, 139
    implementation in, 135
    interprofessional collaboration in, 134
    in older adults, 140
    patient education in, 139–140
    in pediatric patient, 139–140
    planning in, 135
  lateral, 137, 138f
  posterior, 136, 136f, 137f
Three-chamber water-seal system, 803–804
Three-point gait, 349, 351f
Throat specimens, for culture, 192–196, 195f
Thumb, range-of-motion in, exercise for, 332t, 333–336t
Ticks, 547–548t
Tidal volume (TV), 743t
Timed urine specimen, 185–186b
Time-out, 1096
Tincture, 588t
Tinea pedis, 551–552t, 551f
Toes, range-of-motion in
  assessment of, 167t
  exercise for, 332t, 333–336t
Topical medications, 623–628, 626f
  assessment, 624
  delegation in, 623
  documentation in, 628

Topical medications (Continued)
  equipment for, 623–628
  evaluation, 628
  hand-off reporting in, 628
  home care in, 628
  implementation, 625
  interprofessional collaboration for, 623
  in older adults, 628
  patient education in, 628
  planning, 624
  routes of, 609b
Touch, palpation and, 111
Tourniquet, 209f
Toxic effects, medication action, 591
Tracheal deviation, 800
Tracheobronchial tree, 137
Tracheostomy, 778–787, 778f, 779b, 779t, 782f,
    783f, 784f, 785f
  assessment, 780
  in children, 787
  evaluation, 786
  home care in, 787
  implementation, 781
  in older adults, 787
  patient education in, 786
  planning, 780
  in populations with disabilities, 787
Tracheostomy collar, 727, 729
Tracheostomy mask, 727, 727f, 729
Tracheostomy tubes, 742–743
  home care, 1243–1248, 1246f
Trade name, 587
TRALI. see Transfusion-related acute lung
    injury
Transdermal patch, 588t, 609
Transfer process, 45–47
  admitting process, 42–45
  assessment, 44–45
  evidence-based practice of, 41
  long-term care facilities, 47
  nurse role, 46
  person-centered care of, 41
  practice standards, 40
  principles for practice, 40–41
  purpose of, 40
  safety guidelines of, 41
  special considerations for, 45, 46–47
  supplemental standards, 40
Transferring patients
  assessment in, 299, 301f
  by assistive personnel, 298–299
  from bed to chair, 303, 305
  body mechanics during, 297b
  ceiling lift for, 306f
  in children, 311
  delegation in, 298–299
  disabilities and, populations with, 311
  documentation in, 311
  equipment for, 299–310, 299f
  gait belt for, 303, 304f
  hand-off reporting in, 311
  in home care, 311–312
  hydraulic lift for, 306f
  illustration for, 303f, 305f
  interprofessional collaboration of, 299
  lateral, from bed to stretcher, 307, 308f,
    309f, 310f
  in older adults, 311
  patient education in, 311
  rocking patient for, 305f
  slide board for, 307, 308f
  techniques for, 298–312
  to wheelchair, 311–312b, 312f
Transfusion-associated circulatory overload
    (TACO), 898–899t
Transfusion-associated graft-versus-host disease
    (TA-GVHD), 898–899t
Transfusion-related acute lung injury (TRALI),
    898–899t, 908

Transparent dressing, 1163–1164t
  application of, 1178–1181, 1180f
    in children, 1181
    delegation in, 1178
    documentation in, 1181
    equipment for, 1178–1181
    hand-off reporting in, 1181
    home care in, 1181
    interprofessional collaboration in, 1178
    in older adults, 1181
    patient education in, 1181
Transparent semipermeable membrane (TSM)
    dressings, 856, 857t
Transtracheal oxygen catheter, 1236
Traumatic pneumothorax, 800
Travel bath, 525b
Trendelenburg position, 557–558t, 557f
Trigeminal nerve, 168, 168f
Triple-lumen catheters, 987–998, 988f
Tripod position, 350f
Troche, 588t
Trochlear nerve, 168
Trough concentration, 589
T-tube, 727, 727f see also Briggs adapter
Tub bath, 525b, 536–538b, 537f
Tube feedings, 940 see also Enteral nutrition;
    Feeding tubes
Tuberculin syringe, 663, 663f
Tuberculosis, precautions, 267, 267b
Tumor, 124b
Tunneled catheter, for parenteral nutrition, 967f
Two-chamber dry suction water-seal system, 804
Two-person evacuation swing, 407f
Two-point gait, 350, 351f
Tympanic membrane temperature, 73b, 79, 79f
Tympanic membrane thermometer, 74b, 74f
Typhoidal tularemia, 425–426t

U
Ulcer, 124b see also Pressure injuries
Ulnar pulse, 82t, 148, 148f
Uncomplicated grief, 500–501
Unconscious or debilitated patient, mouth care
    for, 544–550
  assessment, 544
  delegation in, 544
  documentation in, 547
  equipment for, 544–546
  evaluation, 546
  hand-off reporting in, 547
  home care and, 547–550
  implementation, 545, 546f
  interprofessional collaboration of, 544
  in older adults, 547
  patient education in, 547
  in pediatrics, 547
  planning, 545
  in populations with disabilities, 547
Unit culture, in clinical decision making, 6
Unoccupied bed, making of, 561–562b
Upper extremities, range of motion in, assessment
    of, 167t
Upper gastrointestinal endoscopy, 254
Urethral discharge specimens, 196–199
Urethral meatus, cleaning, 1234
Urinalysis
  purpose of, 179
  routine, random urine specimen for, 179–180
Urinary catheter
  condom-type external, 1008
  indwelling
    care for, 998
    care of, 998–1004
    documentation in, 997
    in females, 991f
    hand-off reporting in, 997
    insertion of, 987–998, 987b, 988f, 989f, 992f,
      993f, 994f, 995f, 996f
    in males, 991f

Urinary catheter (Continued)
  in older adults, 997
    patient education, 997, 1008
    in pediatrics, 997
    removal of, 998–1004, 1000f
  latex, 1008
  single-use straight, 987, 988f
  size of, 987–988, 988f
  straight or indwelling, 987
  triple-lumen, 987–988, 988f
  urinary, insertion of, 987–998, 988f, 989f
  UTI and, 987
Urinary catheterization, 987
  drape for, 992f
  equipment for, 988–989, 989f
Urinary diversion
  catheterization, 1050–1052
  continent, 1039f
Urinary elimination, 983–1017
  bladder scan, 1003–1004b, 1003f, 1004f
  evidence-based practice for, 985
  person-centered care for, 985
  practice standards for, 984
  principles for practice, 984–985
  purpose of, 984
  safety guidelines for, 985–987
  urinals, 985b, 986f
Urinary incontinence, management of, 507
Urinary meatus, 993f, 994f
Urinary reservoir, 1038
Urinary tract infection (UTI), 987
Urine
  chemical properties of, 180
  culture and sensitivity of, 180
  specimen
    collection bag for, 185f
    collection containers, 180f
    equipment for, 180–185
    in females, 182, 183f
    for glucose, ketones, protein, blood, and
      pH, 179
    in males, 180f, 182, 182f
    midstream (clean-voided), 179–186, 180f,
      182f, 183f
    specimen hat, 180f
    timed, 185–186b
    from urinary catheter, 179–186, 183f, 184f
Urine "hat," 171f
Urine output, monitoring, 172f
Urostomy, 1039f
  pouching, 1046–1050, 1047f
Urticaria, 590t
Usual body weight (UBW), 921

V
Vacutainer method, 211f, 212f, 213, 213f
Vacutainer system, 210, 211f, 212f, 213f
VAD. see Vascular access devices
Vaginal discharge specimens, 196–199
Vaginal medications, 653–655b, 653f, 654f, 655f
Vaginal suppositories, 653–655b, 653f, 654f, 655f
Vagus nerve, 168
Vancomycin-resistant enterococcus (VRE), 267
VAP. see Ventilator-associated pneumonia
Vascular access devices (VAD), 843
  in blood transfusion, 902
  central. see Central vascular access devices
Vastus lateralis muscle, 686–687, 687f
Venipuncture, blood specimens and culture by,
    206–214, 209f, 210f, 211f, 212f, 213f
Venous insufficiency, 146t
Venous plexus foot pump, 1063f
Ventilator-associated events (VAEs), 744, 745b, 754
Ventilator-associated pneumonia (VAP), 742–743,
    744, 745b, 754
Ventricular fibrillation, 790t, 823f
Ventricular tachycardia, 790t, 822f
Ventrogluteal site, 686
Verbal orders (VOs), 63, 63b

Verbal reporting, 62–63
Vesicle, 124b
Veterans Health Administration (VHA), safe patient handling and mobility algorithm, 301f
Vials, 664–673, 665f, 667f, 668f, 669f
  assessment, 666
  delegation in, 665
  equipment for, 665–673
  evaluation, 670
  interprofessional collaboration, 665
  planning, 666
Video teleconferencing, 1199
Virtual care, 1199
Vital signs, 69–109
  blood pressure. see Blood pressure
  body temperature. see Body temperature
  evidence-based practice, 71
  measurement, 71b
  oxygen saturation, 105–107b, 107f
  person-centered care, 71
  practice standards, 70–71
  principles for practice, 71
  purpose of, 70
  respirations, 91–95, 91f, 94b
  safety guidelines in, 71–72
  supplemental standards, 71
  transmission-based precautions and, 271
Volume-control administration, 699
Volume-oriented incentive spirometer, 731, 731f

W

Walkers, use of, 345–355, 346f, 346t, 1200f
  assessment in, 347
  in children, 355
  delegation in, 347
  documentation in, 355
  equipment for, 347
  evaluation, 354
  hand-off reporting in, 355
  home care and, 355
  implementation, 348, 350f, 351f, 352f, 353f
  interprofessional collaboration of, 347
  in older adults, 355
  patient education in, 355
  planning in, 347
  in populations with disabilities, 355
Wandering, 1210
Water overlay, indications for, 363–364t
Weekly medication organizer, 1214f
Weight changes, nutrition status and, 922t
Wet suction water-seal systems, 803–804, 804t

Wheal, 124b
Wheelchair
  air-filled cushion for, 368f
  cushion for, 368f
  ROHO cushion for, 368f
  transferring patients to, 311–312b, 312f
Wheezes, 133, 133–134t
Whole blood, 900t
"Why" questions, 21
Workplace violence and safety, 35–38
  assessment, 35
  delegation in, 35
  documentation in, 38
  evaluation of, 37
  hand-off reporting in, 38
  implementation of, 36
  interprofessional collaboration of, 35–38
  planning, 36
World Health Organization, surgical safety checklist, 1096, 1097f
Wound
  assessment of, 1114–1116b, 1116f
  cleaning, 1170f
  color/tissue of, 1112t
  epithelialization of, 1111f
  full-thickness, 1113
  granulation tissue in, 1112f
  open, 1112f
  partial-thickness, 1113
Wound care, 1109–1140
  evidence-based practice in, 1113–1114
  negative-pressure wound therapy in, 1133–1138, 1133f, 1136f, 1137b
  person-centered care in, 1113
  practice standards in, 1110
  principles for practice in, 1110–1113, 1111b, 1111f, 1112f, 1113b
  purpose of, 1110
  removing sutures and staples in, 1122–1128, 1122f, 1124f, 1125f, 1126f
  safety guidelines for, 1114–1116, 1114f
  wound assessment in, 1114–1116b, 1116f
  wound drainage evacuation in, 1128–1132, 1128f, 1130f, 1131f
  wound irrigation in, 1117–1122, 1117f, 1119f
Wound drainage, 1128–1132, 1128f
  assessment, 1129–1132
  in children, 1132
  closed-drain system in, 1128
  delegation in, 1128
  documentation in, 1132

Wound drainage (Continued)
  equipment for, 1128
  evaluation, 1132
  hand-off reporting in, 1132
  Hemovac drain, 1130f
  home care in, 1132
  implementation, 1129
  Jackson-Pratt drain in, 1131f
  measurement of, 172f
  in older adults, 1132
  open-drain system in, 1128
  patient education in, 1132
  Penrose drain in, 1128, 1128f, 1169f
  planning, 1129
  types of, 1165b
Wound dressing, 1118t
Wound healing, 1111, 1112f, 1164
  factors that influence, 1113b
  phases of, 1111b
  by primary intention, 1111–1112
  by secondary intention, 1112
  by tertiary intention, 1112
Wound irrigation, 1117–1122, 1117f, 1117t, 1119f
  in children, 1122
  delegation in, 1117
  documentation in, 1122
  equipment for, 1117–1118
  hand-off reporting in, 1122
  home care in, 1122
  patient education in, 1122
  in pediatrics, 1122
  in populations with disabilities, 1122
Wound-cleaning considerations, 1117t
Wraparound belt, 396
Wrist, range-of-motion in
  assessment of, 167t
  exercise for, 332t, 333–336t

X

Xerostomia, 523–524

Y

Yankauer suction catheter, 755
Yersinia pestis, 425–426t
Y-tubing setup, in blood transfusion, 905, 905f

Z

Z-track method, in intramuscular injections, 686, 686f, 690

Index of Skills and Procedural Guidelines

Title (Skill number), page number

Abdominal Assessment (Skill 6.5), 151

Adapting the Home Setting for Clients With Cognitive Deficits (Skill 41.2), 1209

Administering an Enema (Skill 34.1), 1024

Administering Central Parenteral Nutrition (Skill 32.1), 970

Administering Ear Medications (Skill 21.5), 635

Administering Enteral Nutrition: Nasogastric, Nasointestinal, Gastrostomy, or Jejunostomy Tube (Skill 31.4), 955

Administering Intradermal Injections (Skill 22.2), 673

Administering Intramuscular Injections (Skill 22.4), 685

Administering Intravenous Medications by Piggyback and Syringe Pumps (Skill 22.6), 699

Administering Medications by Continuous Subcutaneous Infusion (Skill 22.7), 705

Administering Medications by Intravenous Push (Skill 22.5), 692

Administering Medications Through a Feeding Tube (Skill 21.2), 618

Administering Nasal Instillations (Skill 21.6), 638

Administering Ophthalmic Medications (Skill 21.4), 629

Administering Oral Medications (Skill 21.1), 610

Administering Oxygen Therapy to a Patient With an Artificial Airway (Skill 23.2), 727

Administering Peripheral Parenteral Nutrition With Lipid (Fat) Emulsion (Skill 32.2), 975

Administering Rectal Suppositories (PG 21.2), 655

Administering Subcutaneous Injections (Skill 22.3), 677

Administering Vaginal Medications (PG 21.1), 653

Adverse Event Reporting (PG 4.2), 64

Applying a Cardiac Monitor (Skill 25.2), 794

Applying a Dressing (Dry and Moist Dressings) (Skill 40.1), 1166

Applying a Hydrocolloid, Hydrogel, Foam, or Alginate Dressing (Skill 40.4), 1181

Applying a Pressure Bandage (Skill 40.2), 1175

Applying a Transparent Dressing (Skill 40.3), 1178

Applying an Abdominal Binder (PG 40.2), 1191

Applying an Incontinence Device (Skill 33.4), 1008

Applying an Oxygen-Delivery Device (Skill 23.1), 720

Applying and Removing Cap, Mask, and Protective Eyewear (Skill 10.1), 279

Applying Graduated Compression (Elastic) Stockings and Sequential Compression Device (PG 12.2), 337

Applying Physical Restraints (Skill 14.3), 398

Applying Rolled Gauze and Elastic Bandages (PG 40.1), 1187

Applying Topical Medications to the Skin (Skill 21.3), 623

Aspiration Precautions (Skill 30.3), 931

Assessing Apical Pulse (Skill 5.3), 86

Assessing Arterial Blood Pressure (Skill 5.5), 95

Assessing Radial Pulse (Skill 5.2), 82

Assessing Respirations (Skill 5.4), 91

Assisting an Adult Patient With Oral Nutrition (Skill 30.2), 925

Assisting With Ambulation (Without Assist Devices) (PG 12.3), 342

Assisting With Removal of Chest Tubes (Skill 26.2), 813

Assisting With Use of a Urinal (PG 33.1), 986

Assisting With Use of Canes, Walkers, and Crutches (Skill 12.2), 345

Autotransfusion of Chest Tube Drainage (Skill 26.3), 817

Bathing With Use of Chlorhexidine Chloride Gluconate (CHG) Disposable Washcloths, Tub, or Shower (PG 18.2), 536

Bladder Scan (PG 33.2), 1003

Blood Glucose Monitoring (Skill 7.9), 215

Cardiovascular Assessment (Skill 6.4), 140

Care and Removal of an Indwelling Catheter (Skill 33.2), 998

Care of a Gastrostomy or Jejunostomy Tube (PG 31.1), 962

Care of a Patient After a Natural Disaster (Skill 15.4), 438

Care of a Patient After Biological Exposure (Skill 15.1), 424

Care of a Patient After Chemical Exposure (Skill 15.2), 430

Care of a Patient After Radiation Exposure (Skill 15.3), 434

Care of a Patient on a Mechanical Ventilator (Skill 23.5), 742

Care of a Patient Receiving Noninvasive Positive Pressure Ventilation (Skill 23.4), 734

Care of a Patient Undergoing Bronchoscopy (Skill 8.4), 246

Care of a Patient Undergoing Endoscopy (Skill 8.5), 250

Care of a Patient With an Immobilization Device (Skill 12.3), 355

Care of Dentures (PG 18.3), 542

Care of Hearing Aids (Skill 19.3), 577

Care of Patients Undergoing Aspirations: Bone Marrow Aspiration/Biopsy, Lumbar Puncture, Paracentesis, and Thoracentesis (Skill 8.3), 240

Care of the Body After Death (Skill 17.3), 510

Care of the Patient on a Special Bed (Skill 13.2), 373

Care of the Patient on a Support Surface (Skill 13.1), 368

Caring for Patients Under Isolation Precautions (Skill 9.2), 267

Catheterizing a Urinary Diversion (Skill 35.3), 1050

Changing a Peripheral Intravenous Dressing (Skill 28.5), 874

Changing Infusion Tubing (Skill 28.4), 871

Changing Intravenous Solutions (Skill 28.3), 867

Closed (In-Line) Suction (PG 24.1), 769

Cold Application (Skill 16.8), 489

Collecting a Sputum Specimen by Expectoration (PG 7.2), 199

Collecting a Sputum Specimen by Suction (Skill 7.6), 200

Collecting a Timed Urine Specimen (PG 7.1), 185

Collecting Blood Specimens and Culture by Venipuncture (Syringe and Vacutaier Method) (Skill 7.8), 206

Collecting Nose and Throat Specimens for Culture (Skill 7.4), 192

Communicating With a Cognitively Impaired Patient (Skill 2.3), 31

Communicating With Colleagues (Skill 2.4), 33

Communicating With Patients Who Have Difficulty Coping (Skill 2.2), 26

Complete or Partial Bed Bath (Skill 18.1), 524

Contrast Media Studies: Arteriogram (Angiogram), Cardiac Catheterization, and Intravenous Pyelogram (Skill 8.2), 234

Designing a Restraint-Free Environment (Skill 14.2), 394

Discontinuing a Peripheral Intravenous Device (PG 28.1), 878

Donning a Sterile Gown and Closed Gloving (Skill 37.2), 1102

Ear Irrigation (Skill 19.2), 573

Epidural Analgesia (Skill 16.5), 472

Establishing the Nurse-Patient Relationship (Skill 2.1), 20

Eye Care for Comatose Patients (PG 19.1), 566

Eye Irrigation (Skill 19.1), 570

Fall Prevention in Health Care Settings (Skill 14.1), 384

Fire, Electrical, and Chemical Safety (PG 14.1), 405